Postgraduate Haematology

Postgraduate Haematology

EDITED BY

A Victor Hoffbrand MA, DM, FRCP, FRCPath, FRCP (Edin), DSc, FMedSci
Emeritus Professor of Haematology at University College London and Honorary Consultant Haematologist at the Royal Free Hospital, London, UK

Daniel Catovsky MD, DSc (Med), FRCPath, FRCP, FMedSci
Emeritus Professor of Haematology, Institute of Cancer Research, Sutton, Surrey, UK

Edward GD Tuddenham MD, FRCP, FRCPath, FMedSci
Professor of Haemophilia at University College London and Director of the Haemophilia Centre at Royal Free Hospital, London, UK

Anthony R Green PhD, FRCP, FRCPath, FMedSci
Professor of Haemato-oncology, Department of Haematology and Cambridge Institute for Medical Research, University of Cambridge; Honorary Consultant at Addenbrooke's Hospital, Cambridge, UK

Sixth edition

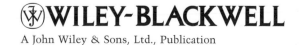

WILEY-BLACKWELL

A John Wiley & Sons, Ltd., Publication

This edition first published 2011 © 2005 by Blackwell Publishing Ltd

Blackwell Publishing was acquired by John Wiley & Sons in February 2007. Blackwell's publishing program has been merged with Wiley's global Scientific, Technical and Medical business to form Wiley-Blackwell.

Registered office: John Wiley & Sons Ltd, The Atrium, Southern Gate, Chichester, West Sussex, PO19 8SQ, UK

Editorial offices: 9600 Garsington Road, Oxford, OX4 2DQ, UK
The Atrium, Southern Gate, Chichester, West Sussex, PO19 8SQ, UK
111 River Street, Hoboken, NJ 07030–5774, USA

For details of our global editorial offices, for customer services and for information about how to apply for permission to reuse the copyright material in this book please see our website at www.wiley.com/wiley-blackwell

First published as *Tutorials in Postgraduate Haematology* © William Heinemann Ltd 1972
Reprinted 1975
Second edition 1981 published © Butterworth Ltd
Reprinted 1983, 1986
Third edition 1989 published © Butterworth Ltd
Reprinted 1992
Fourth edition 1999 published © Butterworth-Heinmann Ltd
Revised and reprinted 2001 by Arnold
Fifth edition 2005
Reprinted 2005

The right of the author to be identified as the author of this work has been asserted in accordance with the Copyright, Designs and Patents Act 1988.

Library of Congress Cataloging-in-Publication Data

Postgraduate haematology / edited by A. Victor Hoffbrand ... [et al.]. – 6th ed.
p. ; cm.
Includes bibliographical references and index.
ISBN 978-1-4051-9180-7
1. Blood–Diseases.   2. Hematology.   I. Hoffbrand, A. V.
[DNLM: 1. Blood.   2. Hematologic Diseases. WH 100 P857 2011]
RC633.P67 2011
616.1′5 dc22

2009046376

A catalogue record for this book is available from the British Library.

This book is published in the following electronic formats: ePDF 9781444323177; Wiley Online Library 9781444323160

Set in 9.5/12pt Minion by Toppan Best-set Premedia Limited
Printed and bound in Singapore by Fabulous Printers Pte Ltd

1   2011

Contents

Contents

www.wiley.com/go/hoffbrand/postgraduate

Companion website

This book has a companion website:

www.wiley.com/go/hoffbrand/postgraduate

with:

- Figures and tables from the book for downloading
- Interactive multiple-choice questions prepared by the authors

Contributors

Paul RJ Ames
Consultant Haematologist
Department of Haematology
Airedale General Hospital
Steeton
UK

Trevor Baglin
Consultant Haematologist
Department of Haematology
Cambridge University Hospitals NHS Trust
Addenbrookes Hospital
Cambridge
UK

Barbara J Bain
Department of Haematology
St Mary's Hospital
London
UK

John A Barbara
Emeritus Microbiology Consultant
NHS Blood and Transplant
Colindale
London
UK

Imelda Bates
Reader in Tropical Haematology
Liverpool School of Tropical Medicine
Liverpool
UK

Joan Bladé
Senior Consultant Haematologist
Servicio de Hematología
Hospital Clinic de Barcelona
Barcelona
Spain

Alan K Burnett
Department of Haematology
School of Medicine
Cardiff University
Cardiff
UK

Clara Camaschella
Professor of Medicine
Vita-Salut University;
Division of Genetics and Cell Biology
San Raffaele Scientific Institute
Milan
Italy

Dario Campana
Vice Chair for Laboratory Research
Departments of Oncology and Pathology
St Jude Children's Research Hospital
Memphis, TN
USA

Peter J Campbell
Cancer Genome Project
Wellcome Trust Sanger Institute
Cambridge
UK

Elias Campo
Clinical Director and Professor of Pathology
Center for Biomedical Diagnosis and Chief of
  Hematopathology Unit
Hospital Clinic
University of Barcelona
Barcelona
Spain

Daniel Catovsky
Emeritus Professor of Haematology
Institute of Cancer Research
Sutton
Surrey
UK

Ronjon Chakraverty
Royal Free and University College Medical School
London
UK

Timothy JT Chevassut
Senior Lecturer and Honorary Consultant in
  Haematology
Brighton and Sussex Medical School
Royal Sussex County Hospital
Brighton
UK

Peter W Collins
Senior Lecturer in Haematology
Department of Haematology
School of Medicine
Cardiff University
University Hospital of Wales
Cardiff
UK

Marcela Contreras
University College London and Blood Transfusion
  International
London
UK

Charles Craddock
Centre for Clinical Haematology
Leukaemia Unit
Queen Elizabeth Hospital
Birmingham
UK

Kate Cwynarski
Consultant Haematologist and Honorary Senior
  Lecturer
Department of Haematology
Royal Free Hospital
London
UK

Geoff Daniels
Consultant Clinical Scientist
Bristol Institute for Transfusion Sciences
NHS Blood and Transplant
Bristol
UK

Inderjeet S Dokal
Chair of Paediatrics and Child Health
Centre Lead
Barts and The London School of Medicine and
  Dentistry
Queen Mary University of London
Barts and The London Children's Hospital
London
UK

J Peter Donnelly
Department of Haematology
University Hospital Nijmegen
Nijmegen
The Netherlands

Mark T Drayson
Department of Immunology
University of Birmingham Medical School
Birmingham
UK

Elaine Dzierzak
Department of Cell Biology
Erasmus Stem Cell Institute
Erasmus Medical Centre
Rotterdam
The Netherlands

Ivy Ekem
Senior Lecturer and Head
Department of Haematology
University of Ghana Medical School
Accra
Ghana

Modupe O Elebute
Consultant Haematologist
King's College Hospital
London
UK

Simon DJ Gibbs
Clinical Academic Research Fellow (Haematology)
National Amyloidosis Centre
University College London Medical School;
Royal Free Hospital
London
UK

Nicola Gökbuget
Head of Study Center
Goethe University Hospital
Department of Medicine II
Hematology/Oncology
Frankfurt
Germany

John M Goldman
Department of Haematology
Imperial College School of Medicine
Hammersmith Hospital
London
UK

Anthony H Goldstone
Department of Haematology
University College London
London
UK

Keith Gomez
Senior Lecturer in Haematology
Haemophilia Centre and Thrombosis Unit
Royal Free and University College London
  Medical School
London
UK

Edward C Gordon-Smith
Department of Haematology
St George's Hospital Medical School
London
UK

Michael Greaves
Professor of Haematology
Head of School of Medicine and Dentistry
University of Aberdeen
Aberdeen
UK

Anthony R Green
Department of Haematology
University of Cambridge
Cambridge Institute for Medical Research
Cambridge
UK

Torsten Haferlach
MLL Munich Leukemia Laboratory GmbH
Munich
Germany

Paul Harrison
Clinical Scientist
Oxford Haemophilia and Thrombosis Centre
The Churchill Hospital
Headington
Oxford
UK

Philip N Hawkins
Clinical Director
National Amyloidosis Centre
University College London Medical School
Royal Free Hospital
London
UK

Chaim Hershko
Department of Medicine
Shaare Zedek Medical Centre;
Professor Emeritus
Hebrew U Hadassah Medical School
Jerusalem
Israel

Douglas R Higgs
Professor of Molecular Haematology
MRC Molecular Haematology Unit
Weatherall Institute of Molecular Medicine
John Radcliffe Hospital
Oxford
UK

Peter Hillmen
Department of Haematology
St James's University Hospital
Leeds
UK

Dieter Hoelzer
Professor of Internal Medicine
Onkologikum Frankfurt
Museum Embankment
Frankfurt
Germany

A Victor Hoffbrand
Emeritus Professor of Haematology
University College Medical School;
Honorary Consultant Haematologist
Royal Free Hospital
London
UK

Ronald Hoffman
Albert A and Vera List Professor of Medicine
Tisch Cancer Institute
Mount Sinai School of Medicine
New York, NY
USA

Derralynn A Hughes
Senior Lecturer in Haematology
Department of Academic Haematology
Royal Free and University College Medical School
London
UK

Beverley J Hunt
Thrombosis and Haemostasis
King's College;
Guy's and St Thomas' NHS Foundation Trust
London
UK

Michael A Laffan
Department of Haematology, Faculty of Medicine
Imperial College School of Medicine
Hammersmith Hospital
London
UK

Ashutosh Lal
Hematology/Oncology
Children's Hospital and Research Center at
    Oakland
Oakland, CA
USA

David Linch
Department of Haematology
UCL Medical School
London
UK

Ann-Margaret Little
Histocompatibility and Immunogenetics Service
Gartnavel General Hospital
Glasgow
UK

John H McVey
Weston Professor of Molecular Medicine
Molecular Medicine
Thrombosis Research Institute
London
UK

J Alejandro Madrigal
The Anthony Nolan Research Institute
Royal Free Hospital
London
UK

Pier M Mannucci
Professor and Chairman of Internal Medicine
A. Bianchi Bonomi Hemophilia and Thrombosis
    Center
IRCCS Cà Granada
Maggiore Hospital Foundation;
Department of Internal Medicine
University of Milan and Luigi Villa Foundation
Milan
Italy

Maurizio Margaglione
Associate Professor
Medical Genetics
Department of Biomedical Sciences
University of Foggia
Foggia
Italy

Judith CW Marsh
Department of Haematological Medicine
King's College Hospital
London
UK

Steven GE Marsh
The Anthony Nolan Research Institute
Royal Free Hospital
London
UK

John Mascarenhas
Assistant Professor of Medicine
Division of Hematology/Oncology
Tisch Cancer Institute
Mount Sinai School of Medicine
New York, NY
USA

Estella Matutes
Reader and Consultant Haematologist
Royal Marsden Hospital and Institute of Cancer
    Research
London
UK

Atul B Mehta
Consultant Haematologist
Department of Haematology
University College London School of Medicine
Royal Free Hospital
London
UK

Marzia Menegatti
A. Bianchi Bonomi Hemophilia and Thrombosis
    Center
IRCCS Cà Granada
Maggiore Hospital Foundation;
Department of Internal Medicine
University of Milan and Luigi Villa Foundation
Milan
Italy

Narla Mohandas
Vice President of Research
New York Blood Center
New York, NY
USA

Emili Montserrat
Director, Institute of Hematology and Oncology
Hospital Clinic
University of Barcelona
Barcelona
Spain

Paul AH Moss
Professor of Haematology and Head of School of
    Cancer Sciences
University of Birmingham
Birmingham
UK

Ghulam J Mufti
Head, Department of Haematological Medicine
King's College Hospital and Kings College London
London
UK

Tariq I Mughal
Guy's Hospital
London
UK

Adrian C Newland
Professor of Haematology
Department of Haematology
Queen Mary University of London
London
UK

Roberta Palla
A. Bianchi Bonomi Hemophilia and Thrombosis
    Center
IRCCS Cà Granada
Maggiore Hospital Foundation;
Department of Internal Medicine
University of Milan and Luigi Villa Foundation
Milan
Italy

K John Pasi
Centre for Haematology
Institute of Cell and Molecular Science
Barts and The London School of Medicine and
    Dentistry
London
UK

Flora Peyvandi
Associate Professor of Internal Medicine
A. Bianchi Bonomi Hemophilia and Thrombosis
    Center
IRCCS Cà Granada
Maggiore Hospital Foundation;
Department of Internal Medicine
University of Milan and Luigi Villa Foundation
Milan
Italy

Stefano A Pileri

Professor of Pathology
Department of Haematology and Oncological
  Sciences;
Director of the Haematopathology Unit
Bologna University School of Medicine
St Orsola Hospital
Bologna
Italy

Archibald G Prentice

Department of Haematology
Royal Free Hospital
London
UK

Drew Provan

Senior Lecturer in Haematology
Department of Haematology
Queen Mary University of London
London
UK

Ching-Hon Pui

Departments of Oncology and Pathology
St Jude Children's Research Hospital
Memphis, TN
USA

Farhad Ravandi

Department of Leukaemia
University of Texas MD Anderson Cancer Center
Houston, TX
USA

David Rees

Senior Lecturer
King's College Hospital;
Consultant Paediatric Haematologist
Department of Haematological Medicine
King's College London School of Medicine
London
UK

Irene AG Roberts

Professor of Paediatric Haematology
Centre for Haematology
Hammersmith Campus
Imperial College London
London
UK

Jesús San-Miguel

Professor and Chairman of Haematology
Department of Haematology
Hospital Universitario de Salamanca
Salamanca
Spain

Jonathan Sive

Department of Haematology
UCM Medical School
London
UK

Clare PF Taylor

Medical Director of SHOT
Medical Directorate
North London Blood Centre
London
UK

Jecko Thachil

Clinical Research Fellow in Haematology
School of Clinical Sciences
University of Liverpool
Liverpool
UK

Swee Lay Thein

Professor of Molecular Haematology
Department of Haematological Medicine
King's College Hospital;
Consultant Haematologist
Division of Gene and Cell Based Therapy
King's College London School of Medicine
London
UK

Cheng-Hock Toh

Professor of Haematology
School of Clinical Sciences
University of Liverpool
Liverpool
UK

Edward GD Tuddenham

Katharine Dormandy Chair of Haemophilia
Haemophilia Centre and Thrombosis Unit
Royal Free and University College London
  Medical School
London
UK

George Vassiliou

Wellcome Trust Sanger Institute
Wellcome Trust Genome Campus
Cambridge
UK

Adriano Venditti

Associate Professor
Department of Haematology
Policlinico Tor Vergata
Rome
Italy

Elliott P Vichinsky

Hematology/Oncology
Children's Hospital and Research Center at
  Oakland
Oakland, CA
USA

Stephen P Watson

BHF Chair in Cardiovascular Sceinces and
  Cellular Pharmacology
Division of Medical Sciences
Institute of Biomedical Research
Centre for Cardiovascular Sciences
University of Birmingham
Birmingham
UK

William G Wood

Professor in Haematology
Weatherall Institute of Molecular Medicine
John Radcliffe Hospital
Oxford
UK

Neal S Young

National Heart, Lung, and Blood Institute
National Institutes of Health
Bethesda, MD
USA

Alberto Zanella

Hematology 2 Unit
IRCCS Cà Granada
Maggiore Hospital Foundation
Milan
Italy

Preface to the sixth edition

Haematology continues to advance and change more rapidly than most areas of medicine. This sixth edition of *Postgraduate Haematology* includes much knowledge that has been gained in the five years since the previous edition. Professor Tony Green of the Department of Haematology, University of Cambridge has joined the editors of the last edition to help cover malignant diseases, where major changes have occurred in their classification (WHO, 2008) and in diagnostic procedures and treatment protocols. Haematological oncology now forms the major workload for many consultant haematologists. Nevertheless, benign conditions are a major source of work for the general haematologist and chapters concerning all these conditions have been extensively updated, often by new authors.

Despite increased understanding of the molecular basis of haematological diseases and advances in their investigation and management, we have kept the size of the book unchanged by omitting ten chapters from the fifth edition and incorporating their essential information into the remaining chapters.

As for previous editions, this book is aimed at providing haematologists in training and consultants with up-to-date knowledge of the aetiology of blood diseases combined with a practical guide to their investigation and treatment. The views expressed are those of the individual authors but relevant literature is listed at the end of each chapter to provide additional reference material.

Many of our authors are based outside the UK, particularly in Europe and the USA, and we hope this book will be used by haematologists practising in the UK, Europe and internationally. We are grateful to our publishers Wiley-Blackwell for their unstinting help during the publishing process and particularly to Rebecca Huxley and Jennifer Seward. We also thank Jane Fallows who, as previously, has with great expertise drawn all the scientific diagrams.

London and Cambridge, 2011
AVH, DC, EGDT, ARG

Preface to the first edition

In this book the authors combine an account of the physiological and biochemical basis of haematological processes with descriptions of the clinical and laboratory features and management of blood disorders. Within this framework, each author has dealt with the individual subjects as he or she thought appropriate. Because this book is intended to provide a foundation for the study of haematology and is not intended to be a reference book, it reflects, to some extent, the views of the individual authors rather than providing comprehensive detail and a full bibliography. For these the reader is referred to the selected reading given at the end of each chapter. It is hoped that the book will prove of particular value to students taking either the Primary or the Final Part of the examination for Membership of the Royal College of Pathologists and the Diplomas of Clinical Pathology. It should also prove useful to physicians wishing to gain special knowledge of haematology and to technicians taking the Advanced Diploma in Haematology of the Institute of Medical Laboratory Technology, or the Higher National Certificate in Medical Laboratory subjects.

We wish to acknowledge kind permission from the editors and publishers of the *British Journal of Haematology*, the *Journal of the Royal College of Physicians of London* and the *Quarterly Journal of Medicine* for permission to reproduce figures 4.1, 4.5, 4.10, 4.11, 4.12, 9.4 and 9.10, also the publishers of *Progress in Haematology* for figure 7.2, and many other publishers who, together with the authors, have been acknowledged in the text. We are particularly grateful to Professor J.V. Dacie for providing material which formed the basis of many of the original illustrations in Chapters 4–8. We are greatly indebted to Mrs T. Charalambos, Mrs J. Cope and Mrs D. Haysome for secretarial assistance and to Mrs P. Schilling and the Department of Medical Illustration for photomicrography, art work and general photography.

Finally, we are grateful for the invaluable help and forbearance we have received from Mr R. Emery and William Heinemann Medical Books.

London, 1972
AVH
SML

CHAPTER 1

Stem cells and haemopoiesis

1

Elaine Dzierzak

Erasmus Stem Cell Institute, Erasmus Medical Centre, Rotterdam, The Netherlands

Introduction

Haemopoietic stem cells (HSCs) are the foundation of the adult blood system and sustain the lifelong production of all blood lineages. These rare cells are generally defined by their ability to self-renew through a process of asymmetric cell division, the outcome of which is an identical HSC and a differentiating cell. Through a series of proliferation and differentiation events, mature blood cells are produced. In health, HSCs provide homeostatic maintenance of the system through their ability to generate the hundreds of millions of erythrocytes and leucocytes needed each day. In trauma and physiological stress, HSCs are triggered to replace the lost or damaged blood cells. The tight regulation of HSC self-renewal ensures the appropriate balance of blood cell production. Perturbation of this regulation and unchecked growth of HSCs and/or immature blood cells results in leukaemia. Over the last 50 years, bone marrow transplantation, and more recently cord blood transplantation, have underscored the medical value of stem cell regenerative therapy. However, insufficient numbers of HSCs are still a major constraint in clinical applications. As the pivotal cells in this essential tissue, HSCs are the focus of intense research to further our understanding of their normal behaviour and the basis of their dysfunction in haemopoietic disease and leukaemia, and to provide insights and new strategies into improved clinical transplantation therapies. This chapter provides current and historical information on the organization of the adult haemopoietic cell differentiation hierarchy, the ontogeny of HSCs, the stromal microenvironment supporting these cells,

and the molecular mechanisms involved in the regulation of HSCs.

Hierarchical organization and lineage relationships in the adult haemopoietic system

The haemopoietic system is the best-characterized cell lineage differentiation hierarchy and, as such, has set the paradigm for the growth and differentiation of tissue-specific stem cells (Table 1.1). HSCs are defined by their high proliferative potential, ability to self-renew and potential to give rise to all haemopoietic lineages. HSCs produce immature progenitors that gradually and progressively, through a series of proliferation and differentiation events, become restricted in lineage differentiation potential. Such restricted progenitors produce the terminally differentiated functional blood cells.

The lineage relationships of the variety of cells within the adult haemopoietic hierarchy (Figure 1.1) are based on results of *in vivo* transplantation assays in radiation chimeric mice and many *in vitro* differentiation assays that became available following the identification of haemopoietic growth factors. These assays facilitated measurement of the maturational progression of stem cells and progenitors, at or near the branch points of lineage commitment. Clonal analyses, in the form of colony-forming unit (CFU) assays, were developed to define the lineage differentiation potential of the stem cell or progenitor, and to quantitate the number/frequency of such cells in the population as a whole. In general, the rarer a progenitor is and the greater its lineage differentiation potential, the closer it is in the hierarchy to the HSC. *In vitro* clonogenic assays measure the most immature progenitor CFU-GEMM/Mix (granulocyte, erythroid, macrophage, megakaryocyte), bipotent progenitors

Postgraduate Haematology: 6th edition. Edited by A. Victor Hoffbrand, Daniel Catovsky, Edward G.D. Tuddenham, Anthony R. Green
© 2011 Blackwell Publishing Ltd.

Table 1.1

Transcription factors involved in haemopoietic and progenitor cell formation, survival and differentiation

Cell	Transcription factors
Stem cells from mesoderm	SCL/TAL-1; LMO2/RBTN-2
Generate and/or maintain stem cells	RUNX-1[a]/AML-1; TEL-1
Myelopoiesis	MLL; GATA2[a]
	PU.1; C/EBPα, C/EBPε
	GFI-1, EGR-1, NAB2
Erythroid/megakaryocyte/mast cells	GATA2
Erythropoiesis, megakaryopoeisis	GATA2; GATA1; FOG1
Lymphopoiesis	SCL; EKLF; p45NF-E2
	IKAROS1
B	E2A; EBF; PAX5
Plasma cell	BLIMP1
T	CSL; GATA3, T-BET, NFATc

Immunophenotype of haemopoietic stem cells

Positive	Negative
CD34	CD33
Thy1	CD38
AC133	Lineage markers
cKIT	HLA DR

[a]Based on mouse studies.

CFU-GM (granulocyte, macrophage) and restricted progenitors CFU-M (macrophage), CFU-G (granulocyte), CFU-E (erythroid) and BFU-E (burst forming unit-erythroid). While such *in vitro* clonogenic assays measure myeloid and erythroid potential, lymphoid potential is revealed only in fetal thymic organ cultures and stromal cell co-cultures in which the appropriate microenvironment and growth factors are present. Long-term culture assays (6–8 week duration), such as the cobblestone-area forming cell (CAFC) and the long-term culture-initiating cell (LTC-IC) assays, reveal the most immature of haemopoietic progenitors.

In vivo, the heterogeneity of the bone marrow population of immature progenitors and HSCs is reflected in the time periods at which different clones contribute to haemopoiesis. Short-term *in vivo* repopulating haemopoietic progenitor cells such as CFU-S (spleen) give rise to macroscopic erythromyeloid colonies on the spleen within 14 days of injection. Bona fide HSCs give rise to the long-term high-level engraftment of all haemopoietic lineages. Serial transplantations reveal the ability of the long-term repopulating HSCs to self-renew. The clonal nature of engraftment and the multilineage potential of HSCs has been demonstrated through radiation and retroviral marking of bone marrow cells. Moreover, such studies suggest that, at steady state, only a few HSC clones contribute to the haemopoietic system at any one time. Further analyses of bone marrow HSCs show that this compartment consists of a limited number of distinct HSC subsets, each with predictable behaviours as described by their repopulation kinetics in irradiated adult recipients. In general, the bone marrow haemopoietic cell compartment as measured by *in vitro* clonogenic assays and *in vivo* transplantation assays shows a progression along the adult differentiation hierarchy from HSCs to progenitors and fully functional blood cells with decreased multipotency and proliferative potential, and an increased cell turnover rate.

The use of flow cytometry to enrich for HSCs and the various progenitors in adult bone marrow has been instrumental in refining precursor–progeny relationships in the adult haemopoietic hierarchy. HSCs are characteristically small 'blast' cells, with a relatively low forward and side light scatter and low metabolic activity. Both mouse and human HSCs are negative for expression of mature haemopoietic lineage cell-surface markers, such as those found on B lymphoid cells (CD19, B220), T lymphoid cells (CD4, CD8, CD3), macrophages (CD15, Mac-1) and granulocytes (Gr-1). Positive selection for mouse HSCs relies on expression of Sca-1, c-kit, endoglin and CD150 markers and for human HSCs on expression of CD34, c-kit, IL-6R, Thy-1 and CD45RA markers. Similarly, cell types at lineage branch points have been identified, including the CMP (common myeloid progenitor), CLP (common lymphoid progenitor) and GMP (granulocyte macrophage progenitor). Recently, using the flt3 receptor tyrosine kinase surface marker along with many other well-studied markers, the LMPP (lymphoid primed multipotent progenitor) has been identified within the lineage negative, Sca-1 positive, c-kit positive (LSK) enriched fraction of HSCs. These cells have granulocyte/macrophage, B lymphoid and T lymphoid potential, but little or no megakaryocyte/erythroid potential. This suggests that the first lineage differentiation event is not a strict separation into common lymphoid and myeloid pathways. While these cell-surface marker changes and functional restriction events are represented by discrete cells in the working model of the haemopoietic hierarchy as depicted in textbooks and Figure 1.1, it is most likely that there is a continuum of cells between these landmarks. The currently identified progenitor cells in the hierarchy represent the cells present at stable and detectable frequencies and for which we currently have markers and functional assays. As more cell-surface markers are identified and sensitivity of detection is increased, more intermediate cell subsets are likely to be identified and it may be possible to determine, throughout the continuum, all the molecular events needed for the differentiation of the haemopoietic system and the transit times necessary for differentiation to the next subset.

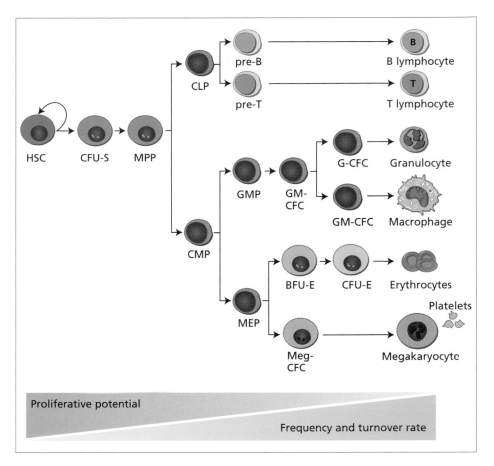

Figure 1.1 The adult haemopoietic hierarchy. Haemopoietic stem cells are at the foundation of the hierarchy. Through a series of progressive proliferation and differentiation steps the mature blood cell lineages are produced. Haemopoietic stem cells have the greatest proliferative and multilineage differentiation potential, while the mature blood cells are not proliferative and are lineage restricted. While large numbers of mature cells are found in the blood and turn over rapidly, the bone marrow contains long-lived quiescent haemopoietic stem cells at a very low frequency.

Sites of adult haemopoiesis

Bone marrow, spleen, thymus and lymph nodes are the haemopoietic sites in the adult, and each tissue plays a special role in supporting the growth and differentiation of particular haemopoietic cell lineages and subsets. Equally important is the blood itself, which is a mobile haemopoietic tissue, with mature blood cells travelling through the circulation to function in all parts of the body. Not only do the terminally differentiated cells, such as erythrocytes and lymphocytes, move by means of the circulation, but HSCs (at low frequency) also migrate through the circulation from the bone marrow to other haemopoietic tissues. HSCs are mostly concentrated in the bone marrow and are found in the endosteal and vascular niches (Figure 1.2). HSCs can be induced to circulate by administration of granulocyte colony-stimulating factor (G-CSF) and it is of great interest to determine whether these cells retain all the characteristics of stem cells. Recent improvements in confocal microscopy have allowed the visualization of the migration of circulating HSCs to the bone marrow endosteal niche by time-lapse imaging in the mouse.

The estimated frequency of HSCs is 1 per 10^4–10^5 mouse bone marrow cells and 1 per 20×10^6 human bone marrow cells.

HSCs are also found in the mouse spleen at approximately a 10-fold lower frequency and in the circulating blood at a 100-fold lower frequency. The capacity for HSCs to migrate and also be retained in the bone marrow is of relevance to clinical transplantation therapies. HSCs injected intravenously in such therapies must find their way to the bone marrow for survival and effective haemopoietic engraftment. For example, stromal-derived factor (SDF)-1 and its receptor CXCR4 (expressed on HSCs) are implicated in the movement of HSCs and the retention of HSCs in the bone marrow. Indeed, HSC mobilization can be induced through AMD3100, an antagonist of SDF-1, and by the administration of G-CSF. Mobilization strategies with G-CSF are used routinely to stimulate bone marrow HSCs to enter the circulation, allowing ease of collection in the blood rather than through bone marrow biopsy.

Development of HSCs

Waves of haemopoietic generation in embryonic development

Until the mid 1960s it was thought that blood cells were intrinsically generated in tissues such as the liver, spleen, bone marrow

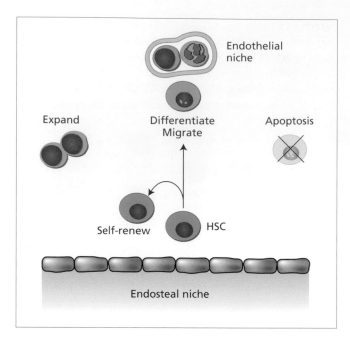

Figure 1.2 The bone marrow haemopoietic niches. Haemopoietic stem cells are found in the endosteal and endothelial niches of the bone marrow. These niches support the maintenance, self-renewal, expansion, differentiation, migration and survival of haemopoietic stem cells through local growth factor production, cell–cell interactions and more distance signals.

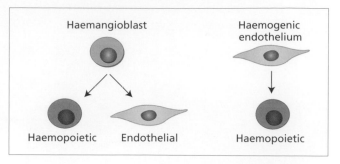

Figure 1.3 Precursors to haemopoietic cells in embryonic stages. The mesodermal precursor to haemopoietic and endothelial lineages at early stages of development is the haemangioblast. Later, haemogenic endothelial cells are the precursors to haemopoietic stem cells and progenitor cells. These cells appear to exist during a short window of developmental time.

and thymus. Survival studies in which cells from unirradiated tissues were injected into lethally irradiated mice showed that it was the bone marrow that contains the potent cells responsible for rescue from haemopoietic failure. Later, through clonal marking studies, it was demonstrated that bone marrow harbours HSCs during the adult stages of life. But where, when and how are HSCs generated during ontogeny? In the 1970s, examination of mouse embryo tissues suggested that adult haemopoietic cells are generated in the yolk sac, migrate and colonize initially the fetal liver and subsequently the bone marrow, where they reside throughout adult life. However, studies in non-mammalian vertebrate models (avian and amphibian) demonstrated that the aorta region in the body of the embryo generates the long-lived adult blood system, while the yolk sac (or equivalent tissue) produces the transient embryonic haemopoietic system. In agreement with these studies, the aorta–gonad–mesonephros (AGM) region of the mouse embryo was later found to generate the first adult HSCs.

The development of the mammalian adult haemopoietic system is complex and begins its development in the mouse embryo during mid-gestation. As a growing organism, the embryo itself needs rapid haemopoiesis to thrive before the adult system is generated. Thus, a simple transient haemopoietic system is generated during early development and rapidly produces primitive erythroid and myeloid cells. In the yolk sac

both haemopoietic and endothelial cells are simultaneously generated from a common mesodermal precursor cell, the haemangioblast (Figure 1.3). Thereafter, many haemopoietic progenitor and differentiated cell types are generated in both the yolk sac and the intraembryonic region of the dorsal aorta to create an intermediate haemopoietic system. It is likely that these cells also are derived from a haemangioblast-type precursor or from haemogenic endothelial cells, a specialized population of endothelial cells that have haemogenic potential. At both these early times in ontogeny, the mouse embryo contains no HSCs. Hence, in the absence of HSCs, the embryo generates a haemopoietic system that is short-lived and lacks the important qualitative characteristics (longevity and self-renewability) of the adult haemopoietic system. Independent and distinct waves of haemopoiesis supply the embryo and adult and do not arise from the same cohorts of mesodermal precursor cells (Figure 1.4).

The adult system has its foundation in a cohort of initiating HSCs. The first HSCs are *de novo* generated in the AGM region, only after embryonic haemopoietic cells are differentiated directly from mesodermal precursors. The first adult HSCs are autonomously generated in the mouse AGM at E10.5 and in the human AGM beginning at week 4 of gestation. Recently, the process of HSC generation has been visualized in real time in the mouse embryo (Boisset *et al.*, 2010). This remarkable observation demonstrating that HSCs are derived via a transdifferentiation event in which specialized endothelial cells lining the aorta bud into the lumen to form round cells with HSC fate, confirm the marking and static microscopic studies performed in avian embryos (Figure 1.5). The emerging mouse aortic HSCs are characterized by the loss of cell-surface markers for endothelium, such as Flk-1 and VE-cadherin, and the gain of expression of the haemopoietic markers c-kit, CD41 and CD45 and the HSC markers Sca1, c-kit and endoglin (Boisset *et al.*, 2010). Expression of HSC markers confirms that the emerging

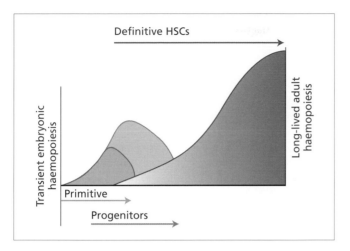

Figure 1.4 Waves of haemopoietic cell emergence during embryonic stages. The earliest haemopoietic cells are produced during the first wave of haemopoietic fate determination. The onset of this wave occurs in the yolk sac blood islands and produces transient primitive erythroid cells. This wave continues with the production of transient haemopoietic progenitors in the absence of bona fide haemopoietic stem cells. True long-lived definitive haemopoietic stem cells (adult repopulating stem cells) are generated in the second wave of haemopoietic cell emergence in the AGM region. In this wave, haemogenic endothelial cells bud into the aortic lumen as these cells take on haemopoietic stem cell fate.

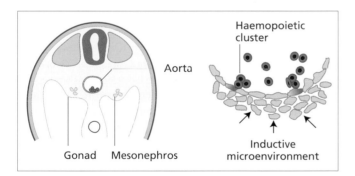

Figure 1.5 Schematic diagram of the aorta–gonad–mesonephros (AGM) region and haemopoietic cell clusters emerging from the dorsal aorta. The haemopoietic stem cell inductive microenvironment is localized in the ventral aspect of the aorta.

AGM cells are HSCs as functionally potent as bone marrow HSCs, since these sorted cells can form a complete long-term haemopoietic system in irradiated adult recipient mice.

Lineage tracing experiments in the mouse embryo have indicated that the adult haemopoietic system is generated during a short window of development, spanning E9–E11. Using Cre-lox recombination (temporally and cell lineage controlled) to mark VE-cadherin expressing endothelial cells in the mid-gestation embryo, it was found that almost all the blood cells in the circulation and haemopoietic tissues of the adult mice contained the recombination marker, unequivocally demonstrating that adult HSCs are the progeny of embryonic endothelial cells. Moreover, these cells require the Runx1 transcription factor as demonstrated by *Runx1* conditional deletion in this mouse model. Other lineage tracing experiments were also performed using Cre-lox technology so as to mark the earliest cells expressing the Runx1 and SCL transcription factors, both of which are known to be important for haemopoietic cell development. The progeny of marked SCL-expressing (endothelial and haemopoietic) cells and Runx1-expressing (definitive haemopoietic and haemogenic endothelial) cells also contributed to the bone marrow cells in the adult. Thus, the progeny of haemopoietic cells generated from haemogenic endothelium in the embryo contribute to a cohort of adult bone marrow HSCs that form the foundation of haemopoiesis throughout adult life.

Embryonic haemopoietic sites and haemopoietic migration

The AGM and yolk sac are not the only sites where haemopoietic cells are found in the early conceptus. The placenta is a highly haemopoietic tissue and has recently been shown to generate haemopoietic cells *de novo*. Much like the early-stage yolk sac, the mouse placenta can produce erythromyeloid progenitors. Embryos deficient for the *Ncx1* gene, lacking a heartbeat and circulation, have such progenitors in the yolk sac and placenta at early stages, suggesting that haemopoietic progenitors are generated in these tissues. Unfortunately, the embryos die before the onset of HSC generation at mid-gestation, precluding analysis of HSC production in the yolk sac and placenta. In normal embryos where the circulation is established between the embryo body and the extraembryonic tissues at E8.25, HSCs are detected in the placenta and yolk sac only beginning at E11, subsequent to the first HSC generation in the AGM at E10.5. Thus it is uncertain whether the placenta (or the yolk sac) can generate HSCs *de novo*. At present, there is no method by which cells can be uniquely marked in the specific developing tissues to examine this. Nonetheless, quantitative studies in which HSC numbers in each of these tissues was determined suggest that the AGM cannot generate all the HSCs that are eventually found in the fetal liver (a tissue that harbours haemopoietic cells but does not generate them) and later in the adult bone marrow (Figure 1.4). In particular, the placenta at mid-gestation contains an abundance of HSCs, suggesting that this highly vascularized tissue may generate HSCs from haemogenic endothelium and/or that the placenta is a highly supportive and expansive microenvironment for AGM-derived HSCs.

Like the mouse placenta, the developing human placenta contains HSCs. Already at week 6 in gestation HSCs can be detected, as analysed by *in vivo* xenotransplantation into immunodeficient mice. Also, haemopoietic progenitors are found at these early stages. Phenotypic characterization shows that HSCs and progenitors are in both the CD34-positive and CD34-negative fractions at week 6 of gestation and are exclusively in the CD34-positive fraction by week 19. These cells are in close association with the placental vasculature. Taken together, the development of the haemopoietic system in the human conceptus closely parallels that in the mouse conceptus. Interestingly, together with the umbilical cord blood harvested at birth, the placenta may provide additional haemopoietic progenitors and HSCs for preclinical studies and potential clinical therapies.

HSC quiescence, proliferation and ageing

Somatic stem cells undergo lifelong self-renewal and possess the potential to produce the differentiated cells of the tissue. HSCs are considered to be relatively dormant stem cells, dividing rather infrequently. They are enriched in the quiescent fraction of adult bone marrow and are resistant to antiproliferative drugs such as 5-fluorouracil. Recent studies using a label-retaining method for analysis of cycling versus non-cycling cells shows that dormant HSCs in homeostatic conditions cycle only once every 21 weeks. The adult mouse possesses approximately 600 of these dormant LSK $CD150^+CD48^-CD34^-$ HSCs. Interestingly, 38% of HSCs in G_0, considered to be the dormant HSCs, can be activated by injury, 5-fluorouracil or G-CSF. These cells can return to the dormant state after the re-establishment of homeostasis.

The maintenance of HSC dormancy is thought to be an important strategy for preventing stem cell exhaustion during adult life. It has been demonstrated by serial transplantation in the mouse that HSC self-renewal is limited to about six rounds of transplantation and that the ability of the transplanted stem cells to repopulate progressively decreases. Studies of chromosome shortening in human HSCs suggest that self-replication is limited to about 50 cell divisions. It has been suggested that accumulating DNA mutations and loss of telomere repeats affect HSC function. Recently, a set of experiments have demonstrated that HSCs are markedly reduced in number and/or function in ageing mice. Comparison of various inbred mouse strains has shown that the rate of haemopoietic cell cycling is inversely correlated with their mean lifespan. The decrease in HSC quantity or quality was due to cell-intrinsic genetic or epigenetic factors. Causative genes were identified by transcriptional profiling comparisons between the HSCs of the different strains. Of particular interest are chromatin modifiers involved in prevention of HSC exhaustion through maintenance of a stem cell-specific transcriptional programme. Changes in chromatin structure associated with high HSC turnover would result in stem cell senescence (which is thought to protect stem cells from malignant transformation by oncogenic events).

Haemopoietic supportive microenvironments

Adult bone marrow microenvironment

Most tissue-specific stem cells are maintained in a special microenvironment to support their long-term growth and self-renewal. To provide the continuous production of human blood over many decades, HSCs are also maintained in a specialized microenvironment, the haemopoietic supportive niches of the adult bone marrow (see Figure 1.2). The importance the bone marrow haemopoietic niche and the interactions between supportive cells and HSCs was first demonstrated in mice. In transplantation studies of anaemic mouse strains naturally deficient in the c-kit receptor tyrosine kinase (W mice) or kit-ligand (KL; Steel mice) it was revealed that bone marrow from W mutant mice could not repopulate the haemopoietic system of wild-type irradiated recipient mice, while bone marrow from Steel mutant mice could. In contrast, W mutant mice could be repopulated by wild-type donor bone marrow cells, whereas Steel recipients were defective for repopulation by wild-type donor cells. Thus, it was proposed that a receptor–ligand interaction was involved in the support of HSCs within the bone marrow microenvironment and it was subsequently shown that HSCs express c-kit and bone marrow stromal cells express KL. The development of *ex vivo* culture systems to study this complex microenvironment allowed further dissection of the cellular and molecular aspects of the bone marrow microenvironment. These studies were aided by the isolation of mesenchymal stromal cells.

Stromal cell lines have been derived from the adult mouse bone marrow and fetal liver tissues. These are generally of mesenchymal lineage as determined by cell-surface marker expression and their osteogenic and adipogenic potentials. Although widely heterogeneous in their ability to support haemopoiesis, some stromal lines (MS5 and AFT024, for example) have been shown to support the growth and/or maintenance of HSCs in co-cultures for long periods. Moreover, they have been instrumental in further characterization of these haemopoietic supportive niches. Comparative transcriptional profiling and database analysis of HSC supportive and non-supportive stromal cell lines has revealed a complex genetic programme involving a wide variety of known molecules and molecules whose function in haemopoiesis is unknown.

The *in vivo* bone marrow microenvironment is very complex, containing osteoblastic niches and vascular niches localized within the trabecular regions of the long bones. HSCs are maintained in close association with the so-called 'stromal cells' of the niches. Some of the key molecular regulators within the bone marrow niches include N-cadherin, CD150 and the SDF1/CXCR4, Notch, Wnt, Hedgehog, Tie2/angiopoietin, transforming growth factor (TGF), bone morphogenetic protein (BMP) and fibroblast growth factor (FGF) signalling pathway molecules. These regulators are implicated in a variety of cellular processes, such as HSC maintenance, differentiation, self-renewal and homing. Indeed, live tracking of haemopoietic progenitor/stem cells in the mouse model has shown the homing ability of these cells to bone marrow niches, and mouse models as well as *in vitro* culture systems are beginning to reveal the specific molecular mechanisms involved.

Microenvironments important for haemopoietic development in the conceptus

Prior to the necessity for an adult haemopoietic supportive microenvironment, the embryo contains several haemopoietic inductive microenvironments. The extraembryonic tissues, yolk sac and placenta, and the intraembryonic AGM generate haemopoietic progenitor cells, while the AGM region generates HSCs (Figure 1.6). Little is known about the differences between the microenvironments of these three tissues. However, the AGM microenvironment is the most well characterized due to the simplicity of its structure, with the aorta at the midline and the laterally located gonads and mesonephroi (see Figure 1.5). It is known that the avian AGM region contains different types of mesenchymal stem/progenitor cells and a population of aorta-associated stem cells called 'meso-angioblasts' contributes to cartilage, bone and muscle tissues and also to blood. In

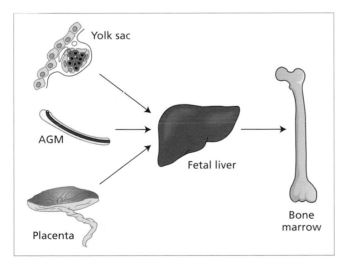

Figure 1.6 Haemopoietic sites during development. The first haemopoietic stem cells arise in the AGM region. Other haemopoietic cells and progenitors are generated in the yolk sac and placenta. It is as yet undetermined whether the yolk sac and placenta can generate haemopoietic stem cells. Haemopoietic cells generated in these three tissues migrate and colonize the fetal liver. Subsequently, the long-lived haemopoietic cells (primarily the haemopoietic stem cells) migrate and colonize the bone marrow, where they reside in the adult stages of life.

the mouse AGM region, cells more typical of mesenchymal stem/progenitor cells have been found. Interestingly, mapping and frequency analysis of mesenchymal progenitors in the mouse conceptus show that mesenchymal progenitors, with the potential to differentiate into cells of the osteogenic, adipogenic and/or chondrogenic lineages, reside in most of the sites harbouring haemopoietic cells, suggesting that both the HSC and mesenchymal stromal cell microenvironment develop in parallel in the AGM region.

Many stromal cell lines have been established from the AGM region, placenta and fetal liver. Stromal cell lines isolated from both the mid-gestation AGM and placenta can support immature haemopoietic progenitors. *In vivo* assays show that some of the AGM stromal clones are potent supporters of HSCs as compared with adult bone marrow and fetal liver cell lines. Indeed some of these lines can support the haemopoietic differentiation of embryonic stem (ES) cells. Although there is one report in the literature of an AGM stromal cell line with the capacity to induce HSC formation from early embryo cells, these results have not been reproduced. Phenotypic characterization of haemopoietic supportive AGM stromal lines places them in the vascular smooth muscle cell (VSMC) hierarchy, in between a mesenchymal stem cell and a VSMC. Thus, while AGM and other embryonic stromal cell lines can provide important signals for the maintenance of the first HSCs, the lack of firm evidence for HSC induction with such lines suggests that the AGM inductive microenvironment is likely to be complex with a variety of spatial and temporal cues emanating from several cell types.

Within the normal physiology of the embryo, the AGM lies between the ventral tissue that includes the endoderm-derived gut and the dorsal tissue including the notochord and the ectoderm-derived neural tube (see Figure 1.5). Mouse AGM explant culture experiments have shown that dorsal tissues/signals repress AGM HSC activity and ventral tissues/signals enhance HSC emergence. In both mouse and human AGM regions, cells expressing HSC markers are closely adherent to the vascular endothelium on the ventral aspect of the aorta. In the mouse, at precisely E10.5, single endothelial cells bud into the lumen as they take on HSC identity (see Figure 1.5). Importantly, HSC activity as determined by functional transplantation assays is localized exclusively to the ventral aspect of the mouse mid-gestation aorta. Thus there is a strong positive ventral positional influence on HSC generation in the AGM, and morphogens and local signals emanating from the ventral endodermal tissues may be responsible for establishing the HSC inductive microenvironment.

Haemopoietic transcription factors required for HSC generation such as Gata2 and Runx1 are expressed in cells of the ventral aortic clusters and endothelium. Deficiency of Gata2 and Runx1 in mice leads to mid-gestation embryonic lethality, with complete absence of adult haemopoiesis (although embryonic haemopoiesis occurs), thus demonstrating that these two pivotal transcription factors promote the HSC genetic programme. Zebrafish and frog embryos have been useful models for dissecting the cascade of upstream events that lead to HSC induction. Developmental growth factor signalling pathways, such as the BMP, Hedgehog and Notch pathways, converge to activate expression of the two transcription factors in aortic haemopoietic cells and promote the HSC programme. In both the mouse and human embryo, BMP4 is expressed in the mesenchyme underlying the ventral aspect of the aorta at the time of haemopoietic cluster formation. Culture experiments have demonstrated the positive influence of BMP4 exposure to mouse and human HSC-containing cell populations. However, it remains to be determined whether BMP4 acts directly on HSCs or stimulates the microenvironment to produce HSC effectors. Similarly, Hedgehog signalling regulates HSCs in the AGM region. However, while Hedgehog signalling acts ventrally in zebrafish embryos, in the mouse embryo Hedgehog-activated cells surround the aorta. This lack of ventral restriction suggests a more complex pattern of regulation of this signalling pathway in the mouse embryo. Other ventrally localized HSC regulators include the Notch signalling molecules, as well as Wnt3a and interleukin (IL)-1.

High-throughput chemical screens offer another means of identifying molecules involved in HSC growth, maintenance and expansion. Through such a screen in zebrafish embryos, prostaglandin E_2 (PGE$_2$) was recently identified as a regulator of HSC number. When tested in the murine transplantation model, *ex vivo* exposure of bone marrow cells to PGE$_2$ enhanced short-term repopulation by haemopoietic progenitors and increased the frequency of long-term repopulating bone marrow HSCs. It has been shown that PGE$_2$ modifies the Wnt signalling pathway, which in turn is thought to control HSC self-renewal and bone marrow repopulation. The zebrafish chemical screen also identified chemical blood flow modulators as regulators of HSC development. Nitric oxide synthetase inhibition or deficiency has also been shown to reduce transplantable murine bone marrow HSCs. Thus, these types of modulators hold promise for clinical treatments of bone marrow HSCs and the bone marrow haemopoietic niche. Together with more general physiological cues, such as the haemopoietic growth factors, KL, IL-3, Flt3 and thrombopoietin, these developmental regulators may be useful for expansion of HSC number and enhancement of HSC function for therapeutic purposes.

Haemopoietic regenerative and replacement therapies

Stem cell transplantation

For over 50 years, HSC transplantation has been the most successful and significant clinical cell regenerative therapy. Initially, whole bone marrow was the source of cells used in clinical transplantation, but through experience and much research new and/or improved sources of transplantable HSCs were found. These now include the CD34$^+$CD38$^-$ fraction of adult bone marrow, mobilized peripheral blood HSCs and the CD34$^+$CD38$^-$ fraction of umbilical cord blood. The cumulative data from the large number of patients worldwide receiving a bone marrow transplant provide valuable information on the success of autologous versus allogeneic transplantation, the number of human leucocyte antigen (HLA) differences that are tolerated by the recipient, the incidence of graft-versus-host disease (GVHD), and the unexpected and advantageous graft-versus-leukaemia effect.

Interestingly, umbilical cord blood (UCB) appears to offer an advantageous source of HSCs for several reasons: UCB HSCs are young, being harvested at the neonatal stage of development, thus circumventing concerns about the ageing of HSCs. UCB transplantation induces less frequent and less severe GVHD, since UCB contains many fewer activated T cells than adult bone marrow. Also, UCB HSCs are highly proliferative. However, only relatively small numbers of cells are harvested (approximately 10-fold lower than those in adult bone marrow) and this limits their use to paediatric patients, unless multiple UCB units are transplanted. Nonetheless, the large number of UCB units (400 000) in cord blood banks (>50) around the world (catalogued and recorded by EUROCORD and other coordinating efforts) offer greater availability and HLA donor-cell selection, especially for rare haplotypes.

New sources of HSCs for transplantation

The ability to expand HSCs *ex vivo* is a theoretically practical and attractive means to obtain an accessible and limitless source of HSCs for transplantation therapies. Unfortunately, despite many years of research using different culture systems and combinations of haemopoietic growth factors and proliferation stimulating agents, *ex vivo* expansion of HSCs has not been achieved. However, HSC developmental studies have begun to provide new insights into the processes directing the generation and growth of HSCs.

Haemogenic endothelial cells
As described in this chapter, the temporally and spatially limited production of HSCs in the embryonic aorta, examination of the specific microenvironment, and knowledge of the precursors to these stem cells has yielded insight into how HSCs may be induced and/or expanded without undergoing differentiation. If cells such as the haemogenic endothelial cells lining the ventral wall of the embryonic dorsal aorta are present in the adult vasculature, they could provide a novel source of inducible HSC precursors, particularly if they can be sustained and expanded to large numbers in culture. Alternatively, if haemogenic endothelial cells do not exist in the adult but it is possible to direct endothelium to be haemogenic, potential

therapeutic interventions could include the *in vivo* site-specific stimulation of HSC induction in the vasculature using the same developmental modulators and small molecules that affect the generation of HSCs in the embryonic aortic haemogenic endothelium. Some recent studies have suggested the presence of such cells in the human embryonic liver and fetal bone marrow.

Embryonic stem cells and induced pluripotent stem cells

Pluripotent ES cells have been used to generate differentiated cells in many tissue systems, including the haemopoietic system. Such haemopoietic-directed differentiation of human ES cells towards HSCs would be a potentially attractive alternative to conventional sources of HSCs. ES cells differentiated into embryoid bodies can be induced to differentiate into haemopoietic progenitors in cultures containing BMP4 and a cocktail of haemopoietic growth factors. These haemopoietic cells arise from haemangioblasts and/or primitive endothelial-like cells that express PECAM-1, FLK-1 (KDR) and VE-cadherin and are thought to represent the types of precursors, progenitors and differentiated cells found normally in the yolk sac. However, although ES cells can be induced to produce haemopoietic progenitors and differentiated cells of all haemopoietic lineages (and HoxB4 expression in mouse ES cells can promote granulocytic engraftment of adult irradiated mice), there are no convincing data showing the production of HSCs that are fully potent in adult transplantation scenarios. This could suggest that the relevant haemopoietic inductive environment such as the AGM region is missing. Bone marrow, fetal liver and AGM stromal cell lines have been used to promote human ES cell haemopoietic differentiation in co-cultures. An AGM stromal cell line appears to significantly enhance spontaneous haemopoietic differentiation in high-density human ES cell co-cultures and provide cells capable of primary and secondary haemopoietic engraftment into immunocompromised NOD/LtSz-*Scid IL2Rγ^{null}* recipients. Together, the induction of haemogenic endothelial cells from ES cells followed by haemopoietic induction with factors and/or cells of the AGM microenvironment may yield cells with the functions expected for definitive HSCs.

Recent reports of somatic cell reprogramming by means of induced pluripotency makes the human ES cell differentiation approach an exciting prospect for future cell-based therapies. The ability to produce patient-specific pluripotent cells (induced pluripotent stem or iPS cells) will eliminate all rejection issues that surround transplantation of HSCs from allogeneic donors. Indeed, a proof-of-principle study using gene-corrected mouse iPS cells from a thalassaemic mouse demonstrates the ability of such cells to form after transplantation normal functioning erythroid cells (Figure 1.7). Unfortunately, the presence of definitive adult HSCs was not demonstrated and hence future studies are needed to prove that HSCs can be generated *in vitro* from iPS/ES cells.

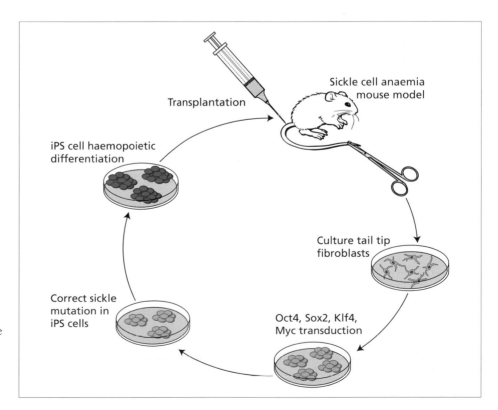

Figure 1.7 Experimental approach in which iPS cells were used to treat sickle cell anaemia in a mouse model. (From Hanna *et al.* 2007 with permission of the American Association for the Advancement of Science.)

Selected bibliography

Abramson S, Miller RG, Phillips RA (1977) The identification in adult bone marrow of pluripotent and restricted stem cells of the myeloid and lymphoid systems. *Journal of Experimental Medicine* **145**: 1567–79.

Adolfsson J, Mansson R, Buza-Vidas N *et al.* (2005) Identification of Flt3+ lympho-myeloid stem cells lacking erythro-megakaryocytic potential a revised road map for adult blood lineage commitment. *Cell* **121**: 295–306.

Arai F, Suda T (2007) Maintenance of quiescent haematopoietic stem cells in the osteoblastic niche. *Annals of the New York Academy of Sciences* **1106**: 41–53.

Blank U, Karlsson G, Karlsson S (2008) Signalling pathways governing stem-cell fate. *Blood* **111**: 492–503.

Boisset JC, Cappellen G, Andrieu C, Galjart N, Dzierzak E, Robin C (2010) *In vivo* imaging of hematopoietic stem cells emergence. *Nature* **464**: 116–20.

Breems DA, Blokland EA, Neben S *et al.* (1994) Frequency analysis of human primitive haematopoietic stem cell subsets using a cobblestone area forming cell assay. *Leukaemia* **8**: 1095–104.

Broudy VC (1997) Stem cell factor and hematopoiesis. *Blood* **90**: 1345–64.

Broxmeyer HE, Hangoc G, Cooper S *et al.* (2007) AMD3100 and CD26 modulate mobilization, engraftment, and survival of haematopoietic stem and progenitor cells mediated by the SDF-1/CXCL12-CXCR4 axis. *Annals of the New York Academy of Sciences* **1106**: 1–19.

Charbord P, Oostendorp R, Pang W *et al.* (2002) Comparative study of stromal cell lines derived from embryonic, fetal, and postnatal mouse blood-forming tissues. *Experimental Hematology* **30**: 1202–10.

Chen MJ, Yokomizo T, Zeigler BM *et al.* (2009) Runx1 is required for the endothelial to haematopoietic cell transition but not thereafter. *Nature* **457**: 887–91.

Cumano A, Dieterlen-Lievre F, Godin I (1996) Lymphoid potential, probed before circulation in mouse, is restricted to caudal intraembryonic splanchnopleura. *Cell* **86**: 907–16.

De Haan G, Gerrits A (2007) Epigenetic control of haematopoietic stem cell ageing the case of Ezh2. *Annals of the New York Academy of Sciences* **1106**: 233–9.

Durand C, Robin C, Bollerot K *et al.* (2007) Embryonic stromal clones reveal developmental regulators of definitive haematopoietic stem cells. *Proceedings of the National Academy of Sciences USA* **104**: 20838–43.

Dzierzak E, Speck NA (2008) Of lineage and legacy: the development of mammalian haematopoietic stem cells. *Nature Immunology* **9**: 129–36.

Gekas C, Dieterlen-Lievre F, Orkin SH *et al.* (2005) The placenta is a niche for haematopoietic stem cells. *Developmental Cell* **8**: 365–75.

Gluckman E, Rocha V (2009) Cord blood transplantation: state of the art. *Haematologica* **94**: 451–4.

Goessling W, North TE, Loewer S *et al.* (2009) Genetic interaction of PGE2 and Wnt signalling regulates developmental specification of stem cells and regeneration. *Cell* **136**: 1136–47.

Gothert JR, Gustin SE, Hall MA *et al.* (2005) *In vivo* fate tracing studies using the Scl stem cell enhancer: embryonic haematopoietic stem cells significantly contribute to adult hematopoiesis. *Blood* **105**: 2724–32.

Hackney JA, Charbord P, Brunk BP *et al.* (2002) A molecular profile of a haematopoietic stem cell niche. *Proceedings of the National Academy of Sciences USA* **99**: 13061–6.

Hanna J, Wernig M, Markoulaki S *et al.* (2007) Treatment of sickle cell anaemia mouse model with iPS cells generated from autologous skin. *Science* **318**: 1920–3.

Harrison DE, Astle CM (1982) Loss of stem cell repopulating ability upon transplantation. Effects of donor age, cell number, and transplantation procedure. *Journal of Experimental Medicine* **156**: 1767–79.

Jordan CT, Lemischka IR (1990) Clonal and systemic analysis of long-term hematopoiesis in the mouse. *Genes and Development* **4**: 220–32.

Kaufman DS. (2009) Toward clinical therapies using hematopoietic cells derived from human pluripotent stem cells. *Blood* **114**: 3513–23.

Kaufman DS, Hanson ET, Lewis RL *et al.* (2001) Haematopoietic colony-forming cells derived from human embryonic stem cells. *Proceedings of the National Academy of Sciences USA* **98**: 10716–21.

Kennedy M, D'Souza SL, Lynch-Kattman M *et al.* (2007) Development of the hemangioblast defines the onset of hematopoiesis in human ES cell differentiation cultures. *Blood* **109**: 2679–87.

Kumaravelu P, Hook L, Morrison AM *et al.* (2002) Quantitative developmental anatomy of definitive haematopoietic stem cells/long-term repopulating units (HSC/RUs): role of the aorta–gonad–mesonephros (AGM) region and the yolk sac in colonization of the mouse embryonic liver. *Development* **129**: 4891–9.

Ledran MH, Krassowska A, Armstrong L *et al.* (2008) Efficient haematopoietic differentiation of human embryonic stem cells on stromal cells derived from haematopoietic niches. *Cell Stem Cell* **3**: 85–98.

Lo Celso C, Fleming HE, Wu JW *et al.* (2009) Live-animal tracking of individual haematopoietic stem/progenitor cells in their niche. *Nature* **457**: 92–6.

Lux CT, Yoshimoto M, McGrath K *et al.* (2008) All primitive and definitive hematopoietic progenitor cells emerging before E10 in the mouse embryo are products of the yolk sac. *Blood* **111**: 3435–8.

Medvinsky A, Dzierzak E (1996) Definitive hematopoiesis is autonomously initiated by the AGM region. *Cell* **86**: 897–906.

Mendes SC, Robin C, Dzierzak E (2005) Mesenchymal progenitor cells localize within haematopoietic sites throughout ontogeny. *Development* **132**: 1127–36.

Metcalf D (1984) *The Hemopoietic Colony Stimulating Factors.* Elsevier Science Publishers, Amsterdam.

Minasi MG, Riminucci M, De Angelis L *et al.* (2002) The mesoangioblast: a multipotent, self-renewing cell that originates from the dorsal aorta and differentiates into most mesodermal tissues. *Development* **129**: 2773–83.

Moore KA, Ema H, Lemischka IR (1997) *In vitro* maintenance of highly purified, transplantable haematopoietic stem cells. *Blood* **89**: 4337–47.

Morrison SJ (ed.) (2002) *The Purification of Mouse Haematopoietic Stem Cells at Sequential Stages of Maturation.* Humana Press, Totowa, NJ.

North TE, Goessling W, Peeters M *et al.* (2009) Haematopoietic stem cell development is dependent on blood flow. *Cell* **137**: 736–48.

Oostendorp RA, Harvey KN, Kusadasi N *et al.* (2002) Stromal cell lines from mouse aorta–gonads–mesonephros subregions are potent supporters of haematopoietic stem cell activity. *Blood* **99**: 1183–9.

Orkin SH, Zon LI (2008) Hematopoiesis: an evolving paradigm for stem cell biology. *Cell* **132**: 631–44.

Ottersbach K, Dzierzak E (2005) The murine placenta contains haematopoietic stem cells within the vascular labyrinth region. *Developmental Cell* **8**: 377–87.

Ottersbach K, Smith A, Wood A *et al.* (2009) Ontogeny of haematopoiesis: recent advances and open questions. *British Journal of Haematology* **148**: 343–55.

Peeters M, Ottersbach K, Bollerot K *et al.* (2009) Ventral embryonic tissues and Hedgehog proteins induce early AGM haematopoietic stem cell development. *Development* **136**: 2613–21.

Rhodes KE, Gekas C, Wang Y *et al.* (2008) The emergence of haematopoietic stem cells is initiated in the placental vasculature in the absence of circulation. *Cell Stem Cell* **2**: 252–63.

Robin C, Bollerot K, Mendes S *et al.* (2009) Human placenta is a potent hematopoietic niche containing hematopoietic stem and progenitor cells throughout development. *Cell Stem Cell* **5**: 385–95.

Samokhvalov IM, Samokhvalova NI, Nishikawa S (2007) Cell tracing shows the contribution of the yolk sac to adult haematopoiesis. *Nature* **446**: 1056–61.

Spooncer E, Boettiger D, Dexter TM (1984) Continuous *in vitro* generation of multipotential stem cell clones from src-infected cultures. *Nature* **310**: 228–30.

Szilvassy SJ, Humphries RK, Lansdorp PM *et al.* (1990) Quantitative assay for totipotent reconstituting haematopoietic stem cells by a competitive repopulation strategy. *Proceedings of the National Academy of Sciences USA* **87**: 8736–40.

Taichman RS, Reilly MJ, Emerson SG (2000) The hematopoietic microenvironment: osteoblasts and the hematopoietic microenvironment. *Hematology (Amsterdam, Netherlands)* **4**: 421–6.

Takahashi K, Okita K, Nakagawa M, Yamanaka S (2007) Induction of pluripotent stem cells from fibroblast cultures. *Nature Protocols* **2**: 3081–9.

Taoudi S, Medvinsky A (2007) Functional identification of the haematopoietic stem cell niche in the ventral domain of the embryonic dorsal aorta. *Proceedings of the National Academy of Sciences USA* **104**: 9399–403.

Tavian M, Peault B (2005) Embryonic development of the human haematopoietic system. *International Journal of Developmental Biology* **49**: 243–50.

Tavian M, Zheng B, Oberlin E *et al.* (2005) The vascular wall as a source of stem cells. *Annals of the New York Academy of Sciences* **1044**: 41–50.

Till JE, McCulloch EA (1961) A direct measurement of the radiation sensitivity of normal mouse bone marrow cells. *Radiation Research* **14**: 213–22.

Trevisan M, Yan XQ, Iscove NN (1996) Cycle initiation and colony formation in culture by murine marrow cells with long-term reconstituting potential *in vivo*. *Blood* **88**: 4149–58.

Vaziri H, Dragowska W, Allsopp RC *et al.* (1994) Evidence for a mitotic clock in human haematopoietic stem cells: loss of telomeric DNA with age. *Proceedings of the National Academy of Sciences USA* **91**: 9857–60.

Wilkinson RN, Pouget C, Gering M *et al.* (2009) Hedgehog and Bmp polarize haematopoietic stem cell emergence in the zebrafish dorsal aorta. *Developmental Cell* **16**: 909–16.

Wilson A, Trumpp A (2006) Bone-marrow haematopoietic-stem-cell niches. *Nature Reviews Immunology* **6**: 93–106.

Wilson A, Laurenti E, Oser G *et al.* (2008) Haematopoietic stem cells reversibly switch from dormancy to self-renewal during homeostasis and repair. *Cell* **135**: 1118–29.

Xie Y, Yin T, Wiegraebe W *et al.* (2009) Detection of functional haematopoietic stem cell niche using real-time imaging. *Nature* **457**: 97–101.

Yokomizo T, Dzierzak E (2010) 3 dimensional cartography of hematopoietic clusters in the vasculature of whole mouse embryos. *Development*, in press.

Zambidis ET, Oberlin E, Tavian M *et al.* (2006) Blood-forming endothelium in human ontogeny: lessons from in utero development and embryonic stem cell culture. *Trends in Cardiovascular Medicine* **16**: 95–101.

Zeigler BM, Sugiyama D, Chen M *et al.* (2006) The allantois and chorion, when isolated before circulation or chorio-allantoic fusion, have haematopoietic potential. *Development* **133**: 4183–92.

Zhang Y, Li C, Jiang X *et al.* (2004) Human placenta-derived mesenchymal progenitor cells support culture expansion of long-term culture-initiating cells from cord blood CD34$^+$ cells. *Experimental Hematology* **32**: 657–64.

CHAPTER 2

Erythropoiesis

Douglas R Higgs and William G Wood

Weatherall Institute of Molecular Medicine, John Radcliffe Hospital, Oxford, UK

2

Introduction

The process of erythropoiesis includes all steps of haemopoiesis, starting with the initial specification of haemopoietic stem cells (HSCs) from mesoderm during embryogenesis. HSCs either undergo self-renewal or, through the process of lineage specification, differentiate and proliferate to form committed erythroid progenitors. Finally, they undergo terminal differentiation through a series of erythroblastic maturation stages to develop into red blood cells.

In a normal adult, the numbers of circulating red blood cells and their precursors remain more or less constant with a balance between the continuous loss of mature cells by senescence and new red cell production in the marrow. There also needs to be adequate reserves to cope rapidly with increased demand as a result of physiological or pathological circumstances. This balance is maintained by an oxygen-sensing system that is affected by the red cell mass and responds via the production of erythropoietin (Epo), which in turn controls red cell production by binding and signalling to committed erythroid progenitors. Many other cytokines, growth factors and hormones also influence erythroid proliferation, differentiation and maturation.

Over the past 20 years, key transcription factors controlling the internal programmes of erythroid progenitors have been identified and some insights into their roles in lineage specification and erythroid differentiation have been discovered. Understanding the basic biology of erythropoiesis provides a

Postgraduate Haematology: 6th edition. Edited by A. Victor Hoffbrand,
Daniel Catovsky, Edward G.D. Tuddenham, Anthony R. Green
© 2011 Blackwell Publishing Ltd.

logical basis for the diagnosis and treatment of the inherited and acquired anaemias that are so frequently encountered in clinical practice.

The origins of blood during development

Primitive haemopoiesis in humans (predominantly erythropoiesis) first appears in the blood islands of the extraembryonic yolk sac at around day 21 of gestation. About 1 week later (days 28–40), definitive HSCs emerge from the aorta–gonad–mesonephros (AGM) region, within the ventral wall of the dorsal aorta and are also found in the vitelline and umbilical arteries and the placenta. Both primitive (embryonic) and definitive (fetal/adult) HSCs arise in close association with endothelial cells. Several lines of evidence now suggest that haemopoietic and endothelial cells may emerge from a common progenitor, the haemangioblast, giving rise to both blood cells and blood vessels (see Chapter 1). At about 30–40 days, definitive haemopoiesis starts to occur in the fetal liver and definitive erythroid cells are released into the circulation at about 60 days. By 10–12 weeks, haemopoiesis starts to migrate to the bone marrow, where eventually erythropoiesis is established during the last 3 months of fetal life (Figure 2.1).

Primitive and definitive erythropoietic cells are distinguished by their cellular morphology, cell-surface markers, cytokine responsiveness, growth kinetics, transcription factor programmes and more general patterns of gene expression. In particular, the types of haemoglobin produced are quite distinct in embryonic (Hb Gower I $\zeta_2\varepsilon_2$, Gower II $\alpha_2\varepsilon_2$ and Hb Portland $\zeta_2\gamma_2$), fetal (HbF $\alpha_2\gamma_2$) and adult (HbA $\alpha_2\beta_2$ and HbA$_2$ $\alpha_2\delta_2$) erythroid cells. These specific patterns of globin expression have provided critical markers for identifying the developmental

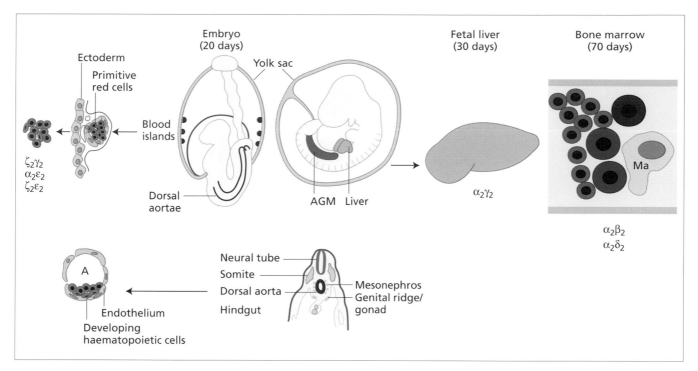

Figure 2.1 An outline of the origin and development of erythropoiesis during embryogenesis. Although both primitive (blood islands) and definitive (AGM, liver and bone marrow) haemopoiesis are derived from mesoderm, probably via a haemangioblast, the true origin of these early cells is not yet clear. The figure shows the formation of embryonic blood islands in the extraembryonic yolk sac and the formation of definitive haemopoiesis initially in the AGM region, with subsequent migration to the liver and bone marrow. 'A' denotes a magnified image of the early embryonic aortic region. Ma denotes a macrophage. The specific types of haemoglobin formed at each stage of erythropoiesis are indicated. The approximate times at which CD34+ cells first appear at each site are given in days of gestation. (Adapted from Dzierzak E, Medvinsky A, de Bruijn M (1998) Qualitative and quantitative aspects of haematopoietic cell development in the mammalian embryo. *Immunology Today* 19: 228–36 with permission.)

stages of erythropoiesis. Nevertheless, it is still not clear whether primitive and definitive haemopoiesis in mammals have entirely separate origins or if they are both derived from common stem cells that arise during early development. Accurately defining the embryological origins of these cells continues to be of considerable importance for understanding the normal mechanisms that establish and maintain HSCs and how these programmes are subverted in common haematological disorders.

Differentiation of HSCs to form erythroid progenitors

At all stages of development there is a continuous need to renew senescent blood cells that are ultimately lost from the peripheral blood days, weeks or months after undergoing terminal differentiation. For example, throughout adult life approximately 10^{11} senescent red cells must be replaced every day, and there are similar requirements for other mature blood cells (e.g. gran-

ulocytes). To prevent depletion of the haemopoietic cells requires a system that not only maintains a self-renewing stem cell pool, but also has the potential to differentiate into all types of highly specialized mature blood cells through a process referred to as lineage specification.

At present, the mechanisms underlying self-renewal and the early events committing multipotential HSCs to an increasingly restricted repertoire of lineage(s) are not fully understood. The probability of commitment to any particular lineage may be influenced by a complex interplay between the internal transcriptional programmes and epigenetic patterns (e.g. changes in nuclear position, replication timing, chromatin modification, DNA methylation) with external signals from the microenvironment (e.g. cytokines, growth factors and cell–cell interactions) acting via signal transduction pathways.

Microarray analyses of HSCs and their progeny consistently show a very wide range of gene expression in the earliest cell populations. Furthermore, many of the genes that are specific to individual lineages (e.g. erythroid, myeloid or lymphoid) are already transcribed, albeit at low levels, in HSCs. In other words, HSCs appear to show 'multilineage priming' and, as their progeny become committed to one pathway of differentiation, that lineage-specific gene expression programme becomes reinforced, whereas those of other lineages are suppressed.

In human adult bone marrow, approximately 1 per 10^4–10^6 nucleated cells are long-lived, multipotential HSCs that can be enriched on the basis of their cell-surface markers (e.g. CD33+ and CD34+ and lack of lineage-specific markers; see Figures 2.2 and 2.3), but such markers do not exclusively select stem cells

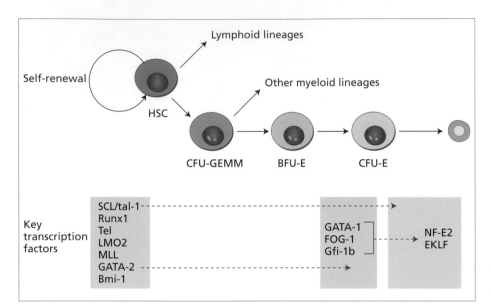

Figure 2.2 Summary of some steps in self-renewal, lineage specification and differentiation of haemopoietic stem cells to red cells. Some of the key transcription factors involved in this process are summarized beneath the diagram.

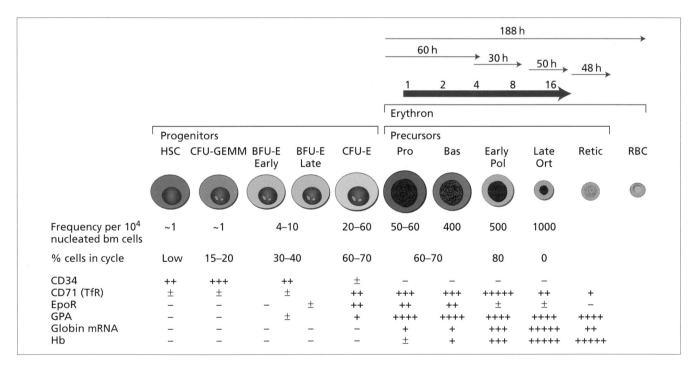

	Progenitors					Precursors					
	HSC	CFU-GEMM	BFU-E Early	BFU-E Late	CFU-E	Pro	Bas	Early Pol	Late Ort	Retic	RBC
Frequency per 10^4 nucleated bm cells	~1	~1	4–10		20–60	50–60	400	500	1000		
% cells in cycle	Low	15–20	30–40		60–70	60–70		80	0		
CD34	++	+++	++		±	–	–	–	–		
CD71 (TfR)	±	±	±		++	+++	+++	+++++	++	+	
EpoR	–	–	–	±	++	++	++	±	±	–	
GPA	–	–	±		+	++++	++++	++++	++++	++++	
Globin mRNA	–	–	–	–	–	+	+	+++	+++++	++	
Hb	–	–	–	–	–	±	+	+++	+++++	+++++	

Figure 2.3 The specification and terminal differentiation of erythroid cells from haemopoietic stem cells. At the top, the estimated times for maturation of terminally differentiating cells are shown. The precursors are as follows: pronormoblasts (Pro), basophilic erythroblasts (Bas), polychromatic erythroblasts (Pol), orthochromatic erythroblasts (Ort), reticulocytes (Retic), mature red blood cells (RBCs). The number of divisions from pronormoblasts to orthochromatic normoblasts (1–16) are also shown. Some examples of the expression patterns of key cell-surface markers are shown below.

(see Chapter 1). The only rigorous assay for bona fide HSCs is to measure their ability to contribute, throughout life, to all haemopoietic lineages *in vivo*. This has been amply demonstrated in mice, and the repeated, predictable success of human bone marrow transplantation clearly demonstrates the existence of such cells in humans.

The pathway of differentiation from HSCs to committed erythroid progenitors is still the topic of some debate. One model (proposed by Weissman) posits a common myeloid progenitor from which the granulocyte/monocyte, erythroid and megakaryocyte lineages develop. In a second model (Jacobsen) erythroid/megakaryocytic progenitors split before the separation of lymphoid and granulocyte/monocyte lineages. As stem cells differentiate, they form multipotential progenitor cells that have short-term repopulating ability but have lost long-term repopulating ability. Such cells can be assayed *in vitro* by their ability to form 'cobblestone' areas under stromal cells in long-term marrow cultures. Further differentiation progressively restricts the lineage potential of these cells as well as reducing their proliferative capacity, resulting in tripotential, bipotential and unipotential progenitors. These progenitor cells are functionally defined by their ability to produce clonal colonies in semisolid medium supplemented with a cocktail of haemopoietic cell growth factors permissive for the growth of all lineages.

Erythroid cells can be found in multilineage colonies (CFU-GEMM), which include granulocytes, macrophages and megakaryocytes, and in bipotential colonies with megakaryocytes (CFU-E/Mk). The earliest progenitors that are restricted to the erythroid lineage produce large colonies *in vitro*, consisting of several subunits, known as erythroid bursts (BFU-E, containing from several hundred up to 30 000 cells) after 12–14 days of growth. Their frequency in bone marrow is approximately 4–10 per 10^4 nucleated cells. Late erythroid progenitors form colonies (CFU-E) of 8–64 cells after about 7 days *in vitro* and constitute 20–60 per 10^4 bone marrow cells. CFU-Es defined in these culture systems most closely correspond *in vivo* to pronormoblasts (also known as proerythroblasts), the earliest morphologically recognizable erythroid precursor in the bone marrow. Once formed, these cells are destined to undergo terminal differentiation to form mature red cells, as discussed later.

Erythroid differentiation and maturation within the adult bone marrow *in vivo* is dependent on the microenvironment provided by the stromal cells (fibroblasts, fat cells, endothelial cells, macrophages and smooth muscle cells). There are also immunoregulatory cells (monocytes, macrophages and lymphocytes) that contribute to local cytokine production. Erythroblasts are not randomly distributed in the bone marrow but are organized into erythroblastic islands containing one or two central macrophages, surrounded by layers of erythroblasts at different stages of maturation (Figure 2.1).

A number of techniques have been described for the production of erythroblasts in liquid cultures. The great advantage of these techniques is that they allow the production of large numbers of erythroblasts from peripheral blood samples, enabling functional analyses of normal or abnormal erythropoiesis without the need for bone marrow sampling.

The transcription factor programme underlying erythropoiesis

As discussed above in the stochastic model of cell differentiation, many factors must be integrated for a cell to make the decision to undergo self-renewal or differentiation, become quiescent, proliferate or undergo apoptosis. Over the past few years, it has emerged that key transcription factors play a major role in regulating the formation, survival, proliferation and differentiation of multipotent stem cells as they undergo the transition to erythroid cells. These transcription factors may operate on their own or as members of multicomponent complexes involved in activation and/or repression. Many of the key transcription factors were originally identified because they are associated with chromosomal translocations found in leukaemia. This supports a model in which dysregulation of the normal transcriptional programme plays a causal role in haematological malignancies.

At present, the key transcription factors known to be involved in specifying HSCs as they develop during embryogenesis and in maintaining them throughout life include Runx1 (AML-1), SCL (tal-1), LMO2 (rhombotin), Tel (ETV6), MLL and GATA-2 (see Figure 2.2). In addition, the homeobox (Hox) genes and proteins that modify their expression (e.g. Bmi-1) have also been shown to play a role in haemopoiesis. Many of these factors (e.g. SCL, Runx1) appear to act quite differently in primitive as opposed to definitive haemopoiesis. Furthermore, not only is their importance in early definitive progenitors well established, but also many of these transcription factors play additional roles, later in differentiation, in specific haemopoietic lineages, including erythropoiesis.

Once progenitor cells have been committed to become erythroid cells, the most important transcription factors that enable them to proceed through terminal differentiation are GATA-1 and its cofactor FOG-1 (friend of GATA-1). GATA-1 was first identified by its ability to bind functionally important regulatory sequences in the globin genes. Since then, GATA-binding motifs have been found in the promoters and/or enhancers of virtually all erythroid-specific genes studied, including haem biosynthetic enzymes, red cell membrane proteins (including blood group antigens) and erythroid transcription factors such as erythroid Kruppel-like factor (EKLF) and GATA-1 itself. GATA-1 expression is restricted to erythroid, megakaryocytic, eosinophilic, mast cell and multipotential progenitors of the haemopoietic system. However, GATA-1 expression is highly upregulated in pronormoblasts and basophilic erythroblasts (see Figures 2.2 and 2.3).

Gene targeting studies in mice have shown that GATA-1 is essential for normal erythropoiesis. Mice that produce no GATA-1 die from severe anaemia. Although they produce adequate numbers of erythroid colonies (CFU-E), there is an arrest in erythroid maturation at the pronormoblast stage of differentiation. *In vitro* differentiated mouse embryonic stem cells lacking GATA-1 also fail to mature past the pronormoblast stage and undergo rapid apoptosis, indicating a role for GATA-1 in survival and maturation of erythroblasts.

GATA-1 may protect mature erythroblasts from apoptosis by directly or indirectly inducing expression of the anti-apoptotic protein Bcl-X_L. GATA-1 almost certainly regulates gene expression working as part of multiprotein complexes interacting, for example, with FOG-1, LMO2, SCL and a variety of ubiquitously expressed transcription factors. FOG-1 is a protein containing multiple zinc fingers, four of which interact with GATA-1. Like GATA-1, FOG-1 is expressed in erythroid and megakaryocytic cells and is coexpressed and directly interacts with GATA-1 during development. Genetically modified mice that express no FOG-1 also die in mid-gestation as a result of severe anaemia with arrest in erythroid maturation at the pronormoblast stage.

GATA-2 is a second member of the GATA family of proteins that is involved in haemopoiesis. Both GATA-1 and GATA-2 are particularly relevant for erythropoiesis. Both are expressed in multipotent progenitors, although GATA-2 appears to be more important than GATA-1 at this stage, when GATA-2 plays an important role in the expansion and maintenance of haemopoietic progenitors. During erythroid differentiation the level of GATA-2 declines as GATA-1 increases. In mouse embryos lacking GATA-2, erythrocytes are present, but in severely reduced numbers. There appears to be some overlap and redundancy between the roles of GATA-1 and GATA-2; in the absence of GATA-1 increased levels of GATA-2 may fulfil some, but not all, of the normal roles of GATA-1. Furthermore, there is evidence that the level of GATA-2 is regulated by the level of GATA-1. During normal erythroid development, it appears that GATA-2 may initiate the erythroid programme to be replaced later by GATA-1 during terminal erythroid maturation.

Expression of the two related zinc-finger DNA-binding proteins Gfi-1 and Gfi-1b is restricted to haemopoietic cells. Gfi-1b is expressed only in multipotent progenitors, megakaryocytes and erythroblasts, in which its pattern of expression mimics that of GATA-1. Gfi-1b-deficient mouse embryos die with a failure to produce mature red cells, although early precursors are formed normally. This is very similar to the phenotype observed in GATA-1-deficient embryos. However, from *in vitro* colony assays in which Gfi-1b is overexpressed, it appears that its effect is not on erythroid commitment, but rather it promotes the proliferation of erythroid progenitors as they undergo the transition from late BFU-Es to CFU-Es.

EKLF is a zinc finger-like protein of the Kruppel family, which binds the consensus sequence 5′-NCNCNCCCN-3′ and is mainly restricted to erythroid cells. These binding sites are found in the regulatory elements of several erythroid-specific genes, including the β-globin gene. Disruption of binding at this site gives rise to β thalassaemia. Mice in which EKLF is absent die from severe anaemia at the fetal liver stage caused in part by β thalassaemia, but also due to the failure to synthesize correctly other EKLF-regulated proteins (e.g. the red cell membrane protein Band3 and the α-globin stabilizing protein AHSP) required for red cell maturation. Therefore, EKLF may play a wider role than originally predicted in coordinating erythroid cell maturation and globin gene regulation.

Sequence motifs of the general class (T/C)GCTGA(G/C)TCA(T/C), called Maf recognition elements (MAREs), have been found in the enhancers of many erythroid-specific genes (e.g. globins, haem synthesis enzymes), and it was shown that they bind the transcription factor NF-E2. Purification of NF-E2 revealed that it consists of two subunits, p45NF-E2 and p18NF-E2 (now known as MafK). Both proteins contain basic zipper (B-ZIP) domains through which they form heterodimers and bind DNA. p45 is expressed mainly in erythroid cells, whereas p18 is widely expressed, although it is the predominant small Maf family member in erythroid cells. Furthermore, it is now known that both p45 and p18 are members of larger groups of proteins with overlapping functions. Other p45-like molecules include Nrf1, 2 and 3 and Bach1 and 2. All these proteins bind as obligate heterodimers with Maf proteins. It seems likely that binding to MARE elements is an important aspect of erythroid-specific activation, but it is not clear which proteins in this family bind the key sites or whether there is redundancy in the need for specific members of this family.

At present it is not fully understood how these transcription factors combine to commit cells to the erythroid lineage and terminal erythroid differentiation. However, this could involve the presence or absence of specific transcription factors, changes in the levels of the proteins and/or protein modification. One principle that seems to be emerging is that factors affiliated with different lineages such as GATA-1 (erythroid) and PU1 (lymphocytes and granulocytes) are both present in uncommitted progenitors, reflecting the potential to develop along alternative different pathways (so-called multilineage priming). It is now known that GATA-1 and PU1 interact and cross-antagonize each other. Therefore, as cells differentiate, reinforcement of the transcriptional programme of one lineage may actively suppress an alternative lineage.

Terminal maturation of committed erythroid cells

After the erythroid programme has been specified, the final phase of erythropoiesis involves the maturation of committed erythroid progenitors to fully differentiated red cells. The earliest recognizable erythroid precursor cell in the bone marrow is

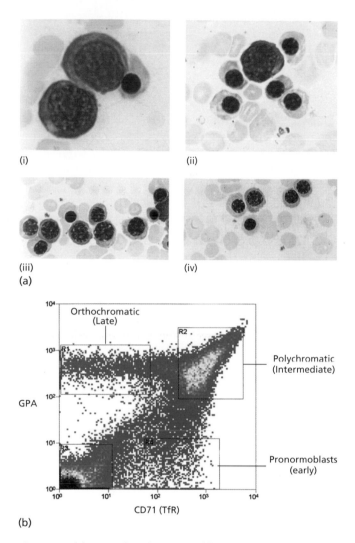

(a)

(b)

Figure 2.4 (a) Examples of pronormoblasts (i), basophilic and polychromatic erythroblasts (ii) and polychromatic and orthochromatic erythroblasts (iii and iv). All these different cell types can also be conveniently viewed at http://hsc.virginia.edu/medicine/clinical/pathology/educ/innes/text/nh/mature.html. (b) An example of early (pronormoblasts), intermediate (polychromatic erythroblasts) and late (orthochromatic erythroblasts) erythroid precursors separated on the basis of their cell-surface markers (CD71 and GPA).

the pronormoblast (Figure 2.4a, i) which, as discussed above, corresponds to the CFU-Es identified *in vitro*. The pronormoblast is a relatively large cell (12–20 μm) with a non-granular deep-blue cytoplasm and a large nucleus occupying about three-quarters of the cell that has a finely stippled chromatin pattern containing one or more prominent nucleoli.

The cytoplasm contains numerous ribosomes, several mitochondria, centrioles, a prominent Golgi apparatus and a few strands of rough endoplasmic reticulum. Division of these cells leads to smaller (10–16 μm) basophilic normoblasts (Figure 2.4a, ii). Again, the cytoplasm stains deep blue and the nucleus occupies a large proportion of the cell but has a coarser reticular chromatin pattern with a few small masses of condensed chromatin adjacent to the nuclear membrane. Further divisions form early polychromatic and late polychromatic normoblasts (10–12 μm), with increasing development of a pink cytoplasm and condensed (6 μm) nuclei (Figure 2.4a, iii). Late polychromatic/orthochromatic normoblasts (Figure 2.4a, iv) are non-dividing cells with deeply staining structureless nuclei.

As the cell proceeds through terminal differentiation, nucleoli disappear and the nucleus condenses further and is eventually extruded. Such nuclei are phagocytosed and degraded by the macrophages of the bone marrow. Ultrastructural studies have shown that nuclear extrusion usually occurs outside the sinusoids of the bone marrow, and that newly formed reticulocytes usually pass through pre-existing gaps in the walls of these sinusoids by diapedesis. Thus, the mature reticulocyte has no nucleus but has a few mitochondria and ribosomes and its cytoplasm stains predominantly pink because of the high concentration of haemoglobin. The cytoplasm still has a greyish tint due to the presence of ribosomes. When stained supravitally, the ribosomes precipitate into basophilic granules or a reticulum. Reticulocytes continue to synthesize haemoglobin for 24–48 hours after release from the bone marrow. On average, these cells are about 20% larger than mature red cells, which are circular, flat, biconcave discs with a mean diameter of 8.5 μm.

It has been estimated that, on average, four divisions occur within the morphologically recognizable proliferating precursor pool, so that each newly formed pronormoblast develops into 16 red cells (see Figure 2.3). As a small amount of cell death (ineffective erythropoiesis) normally occurs, the average amplification is slightly less than 16-fold. The majority (60–80%) of pronormoblasts, basophilic normoblasts and early polychromatic normoblasts are in cell cycle, mostly in S phase, with G_1 and G_2 stages lasting only a few hours. At any time, about 3% pronormoblasts, 5% basophilic erythroblasts and 6% polychromatic normoblasts are undergoing mitosis, which has been variously estimated to last for between 60 and 100 min. Erythroid cells eventually exit the cell cycle and, consistent with this, late polychromatic/orthochromatic erythroblasts are post-mitotic, non-dividing cells.

Changes in the cell-surface phenotype that accompany erythroid differentiation and maturation

The cell-surface phenotypes of erythroid progenitors and precursors are quite distinctive, reflecting the different signalling programmes of the cells as they differentiate. These markers are also of value in the analysis of erythroid progenitors and precursors as they can be used to identify and purify subpopulations of cells. CD34 is present on nearly all multipotent progenitors and committed BFU-Es but is lost on later erythroid progenitors (CFU-E) and all precursors.

A similar pattern of expression is shown for the receptor c-Kit. Epo receptor (see below) first appears in small numbers (20–50 copies per cell) on late BFU-Es, increases in CFU-Es and pronormoblasts (~1000 copies per cell) and subsequently declines and disappears in later erythroid precursors. CD71 (transferrin receptor, TfR) allows transferrin-bound iron to be taken into the cell and is present on early haemopoietic cells but is considerably upregulated on cells that are actively synthesizing haemoglobin, reaching a peak of 800 000 molecules per cell on polychromatic normoblasts. CD71 levels diminish in the late phase of terminal differentiation and the receptor is not detectable on mature erythrocytes. Glycophorin A (GPA) is a membrane sialoglycoprotein whose expression is highly upregulated as erythroid progenitors mature from pronormoblasts. Combinations of these cell-surface markers can be used to distinguish early, intermediate and late erythroid precursors (Figure 2.4b). Developing erythroid cells express cell-surface adhesion molecules that interact with the extracellular matrix; these include ICAM-1 (a member of the immunoglobulin superfamily) and integrin $\alpha_4\beta_1$ VLA4 (CD29/CD49d), which interacts with fibronectin. These adhesion molecules are most highly expressed in the early precursors and lost as maturation proceeds, freeing erythroid cells to exit the bone marrow.

Changes in gene expression in erythroid differentiation and maturation

As cells go through the final divisions of erythropoiesis and post-mitotic maturation there is progressive condensation of chromatin accompanied by complex changes in gene expression. When assessed by microarray analysis, many mRNAs are downregulated as multipotent progenitors enter terminal differentiation, reflecting the commitment of multipotent cells to a single specialized lineage. A subset of general mRNAs associated with proliferation, replication and cell cycle control show alterations as the growth characteristics of the cells change. mRNAs encoding proteins that characterize the red cell phenotype are, in general, upregulated. Examples include blood group antigens, red cell membrane proteins (e.g. spectrin, ankyrin, actin, protein 4.1), red cell glycolytic pathway enzymes, carbonic anhydrase and enzymes of the haem synthesis pathway such as δ-aminolaevulinic acid synthase (ALAS). A full catalogue of these changes in gene expression can be found at http://hembase.niddk.nih.gov.

The main purpose of erythropoiesis is to synthesize large amounts of haemoglobin (Figures 2.3–2.5). Globin mRNA sequences are first expressed in pronormoblasts and early basophilic erythroblasts. Globin chain synthesis parallels accumulation of globin mRNA, increasing at the polychromatic and orthochromatic stages. The amount of globin mRNA reaches 20 000 molecules per cell in late polychromatic and

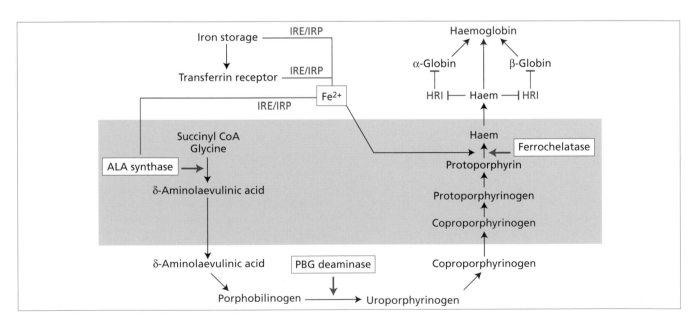

Figure 2.5 Coordination of globin synthesis, haem synthesis and iron regulation. Blue lines indicate some of the known regulatory feedback systems. The red shaded box indicates reactions occurring in the mitochondria. Rate-limiting controls of haem synthesis are shown in black boxes. ALA, δ-aminolaevulinic acid; PBG, porphobilinogen.

orthochromatic erythroblasts. During the later stages of erythroid cell maturation, the amount of RNA per cell and the rate of total protein synthesis declines, but the relative stability of globin mRNA ensures that globin becomes the predominant polypeptide made in late erythroblasts and reticulocytes.

The individual components of the haemoglobin synthetic pathway (iron, free porphyrins, haem and monomeric globin chains) are all extremely toxic to the cell, and consequently many positive and negative feedback loops have evolved and been incorporated into this process. The synthesis of globin must be very accurately matched with the synthesis of haem in which some steps occur in the cytoplasm and others in the mitochondria (Figure 2.5). mRNAs encoding many components of the haem biosynthetic pathway (e.g. ALAS and porphobilinogen deaminase) are coordinately upregulated in terminal erythroid differentiation and their genes contain similar *cis*-regulatory elements.

Continued translation of globin chains from mRNA only occurs in the presence of adequate haem. Reduced levels of haem rapidly trigger the formation of the haem-regulated inhibitor (HRI), a kinase that interacts with the translation initiating factor eIF-2α and prevents translation of α- and β-globin mRNA. The synthesis of haem itself is also regulated at many points and is particularly sensitive to the levels of available iron. Via a well-characterized pathway involving the iron-regulatory proteins (IRP1 and IRP2), binding to iron response elements (IREs) in the mRNA transcripts of ferritin, TfR and ALAS, the level of intracellular iron thus controls the translation of RNAs involved in iron storage, iron transport and haem synthesis (see Chapter 3). The discovery of hepcidin, which controls the uptake of iron from the gut, iron transport across the placenta and iron release from macrophages, adds another level of control to this complex system (see Chapter 3). Not surprisingly, diseases affecting the supply of iron (iron deficiency and the anaemia of chronic disease), the synthesis of haem (sideroblastic anaemia, lead poisoning, alcohol ingestion) or the synthesis of globin (thalassaemia) have interrelated effects on globin synthesis, haem synthesis and iron metabolism (Figure 2.5).

No mechanistic connection between haemoglobin synthesis and erythroid proliferation or differentiation has yet been established. However, it has been postulated that haemoglobin content and/or haemoglobin concentration *per se* may be a negative regulator of cell division. When haemoglobin synthesis is reduced or delayed, as in iron deficiency, the cells may undergo an extra division, yielding smaller hypochromic cells. Alternatively, when haemoglobin synthesis exceeds DNA synthesis, as in megaloblastic anaemias, the cells may skip a division and nuclear extrusion may occur early, resulting in macrocytosis. Although plausible, these hypotheses remain unproven.

The regulation of erythropoiesis by signalling pathways

The normal red cell lifespan is 120 days and therefore, to maintain equilibrium, approximately 1% of the circulating red cell pool must be replaced daily. For a total of about 3×10^{13} circulating erythrocytes and a lifespan of 120 days, the erythrocyte production rate needs to be maintained at approximately 10^{10}/hour in the steady state. Erythropoiesis accounts for about 20% of the nucleated cells in a normal bone marrow reflected in the myeloid/erythroid ratio (usually about 4:1). As committed erythroid cells become late BFU-E and CFU-E, they upregulate expression of the receptor for erythropoietin (EpoR). It is estimated that in the steady state, with low levels of circulating Epo, a high proportion of erythroid cells die through apoptosis. This provides a reserve that can be rescued by the increase in Epo levels that accompany anaemia. Signalling through EpoR not only prevents apoptosis but also stimulates proliferation. It is at the late progenitor/early precursor stages (CFU-E/pronormoblast) that there is considerable proliferative potential for expanding the overall level of erythropoiesis. Soon after reaching the CFU-E stage, erythroid cells enter the phase of terminal differentiation, after which there is only limited potential for further expansion. The two major components regulating erythropoiesis include sensing hypoxia and regulating the supply of erythroid precursors, mainly by controlling the numbers of erythroid progenitors via the Epo–EpoR signalling pathway.

Sensing hypoxia

Tissue hypoxia induces a variety of physiological responses in addition to activation of the Epo–EpoR pathway (see below). Parallel responses include the stimulation of new blood vessels by vascular endothelial growth factor (VEGF) and metabolic changes (e.g. in glycolytic pathway enzymes) that enable continued energy production despite inadequate oxygen availability. In addition, expression of TfR is upregulated. Over the past 20 years the mechanisms by which cells sense hypoxia and orchestrate their response have been discovered. It has been shown that the most important mediator of this cellular response is a transcription factor called HIF (hypoxia-inducible factor), which activates the genes that influence the adaptive responses to hypoxia including those encoding Epo, glycolytic pathway enzymes, TfR and VEGF (Figure 2.6).

HIF is a heterodimer constituting one of three α-subunits (HIF1-α, HIF2-α or HIF3-α) bound to the aryl hydrocarbon receptor nuclear translocator (ARNT), also known as HIF1-β. HIF1-α is a member of the basic helix–loop–helix (bHLH) family of transcription factors in which the HLH domains mediate subunit dimerization, whereas the basic domains bind

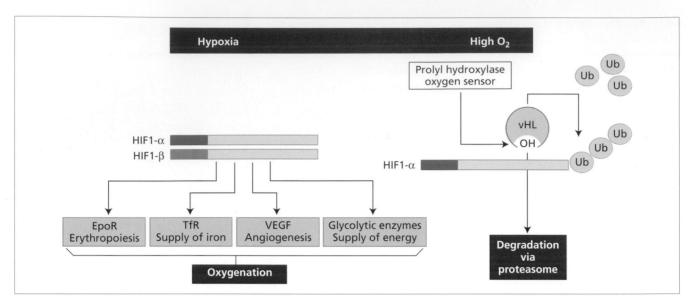

Figure 2.6 The oxygen-sensing system. Ub, ubiquitination; vHL, von Hippel–Lindau protein.

DNA. HIF binds to hypoxia-response elements (HREs, 5′-TACGTG-3′) located in the regulatory regions of hypoxia-inducible genes such as the gene encoding Epo (see below). Whereas changes in oxygen levels do not affect the levels of HIF1-β, which is expressed constitutively, hypoxia elevates the levels of HIF1-α subunits by increasing protein stability.

The oxygen sensor is a ferrous iron prolyl hydroxylase that requires molecular oxygen as a cosubstrate to hydroxylate specific proline residues in the α-subunits of HIF. Once hydroxylated, HIF1-α subunits become targets for ubiquitination by the widely expressed von Hippel–Lindau (vHL) protein and are thus targeted for proteosomal degradation. Under normal circumstances the α-subunits are undetectable but, when cells are exposed to hypoxic stimuli, the oxygen sensor can no longer hydroxylate the α-subunits of HIF. In this situation, α-subunits accumulate as they are no longer polyubiquitinated and degraded. This allows the α-subunits to heterodimerize with HIF1-β and activate the hypoxia-response genes. If the vHL protein is mutated (vHL syndrome), there is prolonged stimulation by HIF, leading to the development of polycythaemia (Epo stimulation) and vascular tumours (VEGF stimulation).

Erythropoietin and the erythropoietin receptor

The main initial site of Epo production is the fetal liver, with production largely switching to the kidney shortly after birth. Under normoxic conditions, little or no Epo mRNA is detectable in the kidneys but hypoxia results in its accumulation within 30 min in the peritubular interstitial cells and levels can increase 200-fold over baseline. Epo is a 166-amino-acid 34.4-kDa glycoprotein, found in serum at baseline levels of 1–30 mU/mL that can be elevated 1000-fold by severe anaemia. It contains about 40% carbohydrate, rich in sialic acid residues, and has a half-life of 7–8 hours in plasma, whereas non-glycosylated Epo is cleared rapidly from the circulation. There are no preformed stores of Epo and, normally, 90% of the hormone is produced in the kidney and 10% in the liver and elsewhere.

The Epo gene contains a hypoxia-response element at its 3′-end, and in the kidney and liver a cooperative interaction of HIF with HNF-4, including recruitment of the coactivator CBP/p300, leads to a significant increase in transcription and increased serum levels of the protein. The binding of Epo to EpoR results in signal transduction to the nucleus, and this constitutes the most important pathway for controlling definitive erythropoiesis. Careful clinical and haematological studies, together with the analysis of experimental animal models, have been important in establishing exactly which aspects of erythropoiesis are regulated by the Epo–EpoR system. Fetal livers of genetically modified mice in which Epo or EpoR has been deleted are devoid of late erythroid cells but contain normal numbers of BFU-E, demonstrating that this signalling system is not required for lineage specification but is essential for proliferation and differentiation of erythroid precursors into mature cells.

When tissue oxygenation is compromised owing to reduced ambient oxygen tension, blood loss, shortened red cell survival or any uncompensated need for increased oxygen delivery, the level of Epo rises, stimulating red cell production. The low numbers (20–50) of EpoRs on BFU-E explain the relative Epo non-responsiveness of these cells, and much higher levels (~1000) are found in CFU-E, pronormoblasts and basophilic erythroblasts. When circulating Epo increases, apoptosis of these erythroid progenitors decreases and CFU-Es rapidly respond by proliferating and differentiating. Therefore, the most important effect of Epo is to increase the number of progenitor cells that develop into viable pronormoblasts. It has also been suggested that Epo is able to speed up the rate of terminal differentiation by shortening the cell cycle and maturation times of erythroblasts, thereby explaining the macrocytosis that often accompanies 'stress' erythropoiesis; this remains to be confirmed.

The erythropoietin signalling system is relatively well understood. EpoR belongs to the cytokine receptor superfamily. Like other members of this family (growth hormone, prolactin and G-CSF), Epo was thought to induce dimerization of cell-surface receptors (EpoRs), triggering autophosphorylation and activation of the Janus family of protein tyrosine kinases (JAK2). More recent data suggest an alternative model in which unliganded EpoR dimers exist in a conformation that prevents activation of JAK2, but the receptor may undergo a ligand-induced conformational change that allows JAK2 to be activated. JAK2 and/or other kinases then phosphorylate specific tyrosine residues in EpoR, creating docking sites for the SH2 domains of several signal transduction proteins, which eventually results in the activation of at least three signal transduction pathways: STAT5, Ras/MAP kinase and phosphatidylinositol 3-kinase (PI3-K) (Figures 2.7 and 2.8).

Considerable interest has concentrated on the JAK2–STAT5 pathway. JAK2 is essential for erythropoiesis, and genetically modified mice in which JAK2 expression has been eliminated

die as embryos, with a phenotype similar to mice deficient in Epo or EpoR. However, the numbers of erythroid progenitors are more severely diminished, suggesting that JAK2 is required earlier in erythropoiesis than Epo–EpoR. JAK2 is rapidly phosphorylated in response to Epo stimulation. Dimerization or conformational changes of EpoR brings the associated JAK2 molecules into close proximity, enabling them to transphosphorylate and activate each other (Figures 2.7 and 2.8). STAT5 is phosphorylated and activated by EpoR. Phosphorylated STAT5 dissociates from the receptor, dimerizes and moves to the nucleus, where it activates gene expression and is thought to be important as an anti-apoptotic signal. Both fetal and adult mice defective in STAT5 have a defect in regulating survival of early erythroblasts, leading to a persistent anaemia.

Activation of the PI3-K and Ras-MAP kinase pathway (Figure 2.8) may be sufficient for normal erythroid differentiation, although they may not be essential as other pathways can compensate for loss of signalling through PI3-K. Therefore, in erythroid cells, activation of several, apparently redundant intracellular signalling pathways can support differentiation. Nevertheless, it is thought at present that these pathways may converge by activating a few important anti-apoptotic proteins, including Bcl-2, Bcl-X$_L$ and protein kinase B (also known as Akt) (Figure 2.8).

The full control of this system is complex and it should be noted that the EpoR pathway can also be activated by other mechanisms. For example, activation of c-Kit by its ligand, stem cell factor (SCF), causes tyrosine phosphorylation of EpoR and

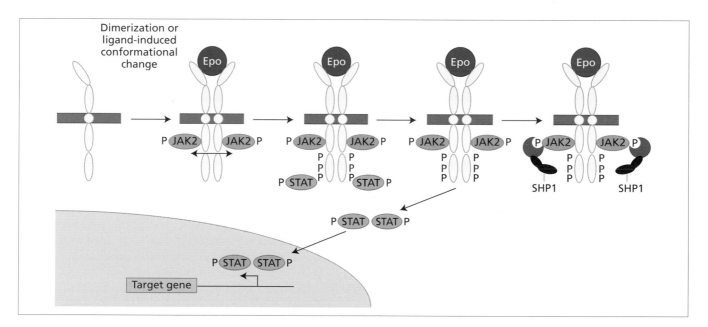

Figure 2.7 A summary of signalling via the erythropoietin (Epo) receptor as described in the text. P denotes regions of phosphorylation. The diagram shows Epo-induced dimerization or conformational change with transphosphorylation of JAK2, followed by phosphorylation of the Epo receptor. This is followed by binding and phosphorylation of STAT5. Binding of SHP1 (far right) to the Epo receptor activates its phosphatase activity, which can then dephosphorylate JAK2 and terminate signalling.

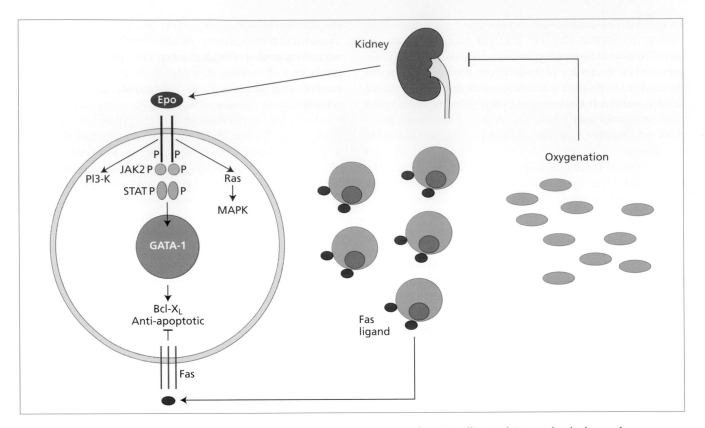

Figure 2.8 A summary of the apoptotic pathways (Epo and Fas) in erythroid progenitors. These cells (BFU-E and CFU-E) undergo apoptosis in the absence of Epo signalling or in the presence of Fas signalling. Bcl-X_L may be the key pathway through which these effects are mediated.

a functional interaction between the two receptors is essential for normal erythropoiesis.

Mechanisms for switching off the Epo–EpoR signalling pathway also exist. Specific phosphorylated tyrosines that occur on the Epo-stimulated dimerized EpoR provide docking sites for the SH2 domains of protein tyrosine phosphatases such as SHP1. Binding activates the phosphatase, which removes the activating phosphates from JAK2, terminating the positive signal from this pathway (Figure 2.7).

Other signalling pathways

Erythropoiesis is also influenced by pathways other than Epo–EpoR. Erythroid progenitors express receptors for SCF, insulin-like growth factor (IGF-1) and insulin. After Epo, the second most important signalling system for erythropoiesis involves SCF (Kit ligand) and its receptor (c-Kit). Activation by SCF induces tyrosine phosphorylation of its own receptor. SCF was originally identified by its ability to stimulate proliferation of multipotent haemopoietic progenitors, but it is also effective in supporting growth of committed progenitors, including erythroid progenitors, acting synergistically with Epo.

In addition to SCF and Epo, recent observations have shown that stimulation of the nuclear hormone receptors for dexamethasone (glucocorticoid receptor) and estrogen (estrogen receptor) produces sustained proliferation of erythroid progenitors. Furthermore, the nuclear hormone receptors for thyroid hormone (c-ErbA/thyroid hormone receptor), all-*trans* retinoic acid (retinoic acid receptor) and 9-*cis*- retinoic acid (RXR) were found to promote erythroid differentiation. Such observations are consistent with previous reports showing that patients with a wide range of endocrine disorders (hypothyroidism, hypopituitarism, Addison's disease and male hypogonadism) all have variable degrees of normochromic normocytic anaemia. It appears, therefore, that many hormones of the endocrine system can modify erythropoiesis.

Apoptosis during normal erythropoiesis

Programmed cell death (apoptosis) plays an important role in normal erythropoiesis (Figure 2.8), helping to regulate the accumulation of erythroid precursors to match the need for new mature red cells. Excess erythroid precursors are removed by apoptosis, and at least two pathways seem to be involved. First, it appears that late BFU-E, CFU-E and pronormoblasts may all require continuous signalling via EpoR, which is highly expressed on the surface of these cells, to prevent apoptosis. In the absence of Epo, these cells rapidly undergo programmed cell death in culture. It has been shown that, in part, this reflects a need for signals from EpoR, via the JAK2–STAT5 pathway, to induce or stabilize expression of the anti-apoptotic protein Bcl-X_L.

Apoptosis of erythroid precursors may also occur as a result of activation of the Fas receptor (FasR, known as CD95) that is present on both early and late erythroid precursors, although its activating ligand (FasL, known as CD95L) appears only on late erythroblasts. Binding of FasL to FasR activates proteolytic caspases that cleave intracellular proteins, possibly including the erythroid transcription factor GATA-1, with subsequent loss of Bcl-X_L. This regulation of erythropoiesis by negative feedback is thought to take place in the erythropoietic islands of the bone marrow, where the number of mature erythroblasts may control the expansion and differentiation of their less mature precursors.

As well as extracellular anti-apoptotic signals, erythroblasts also use internal programmes to ensure their own survival. The transcription factor GATA-1 is essential for maturation of erythroblasts; the absence of GATA-1 leads to apoptosis and a block in maturation. Some of the target genes regulated by GATA-1 are likely to be important for cell survival. Although many of the targets are unknown, it is clear that GATA-1 strongly induces expression of Bcl-X_L and may therefore cooperate with EpoR signalling. In this way, Epo signalling, Fas-mediated signalling and GATA-1 converge on Bcl-X_L, which represents a key target of the erythroid cell survival programme.

Erythropoiesis in clinical practice

Erythropoiesis is disturbed to a greater or lesser extent in almost all multisystem diseases and so the reader is referred to other chapters and references for specific examples. The aim of this chapter is to provide a framework for thinking about the process of erythropoiesis in clinical practice. The first stage involves the production of committed erythroid progenitors. The second involves controlling red cell production, which is mainly achieved via the oxygen sensor influencing the level of Epo, which in turn controls the numbers of late BFU-Es and CFU-Es, although many other hormones, cytokines and growth factors may modify the response. The third phase requires terminal erythroid differentiation to mature red cells containing large amounts of specific proteins such as haemoglobin. This phase makes significant demands on a variety of nutritional factors and cofactors, particularly iron, vitamin B_{12} and folate, but also manganese, cobalt, vitamin C, vitamin E, vitamin B_6 (pyridoxine), thiamine, riboflavin, pantothenic acid and amino acids. Absolute or relative deficiencies of these cofactors can negatively regulate erythropoiesis. The output from this process (red cell mass) is required to meet the demands for adequate tissue oxygenation, which itself has a major influence on the production of Epo, thus completing the regulatory loop (Figure 2.9).

Simple diagnostic tools are available to test the circuit in a logical manner (see also Chapter 6). First, one can evaluate the overall level of erythropoiesis by estimating the ratio of myeloid precursors to erythroid precursors in the marrow (normally about 4:1, but with a very broad normal range). Total erythropoiesis can be measured accurately using radioactive (^{59}Fe) ferrokinetic assays. The plasma iron turnover measures the total (i.e. effective and ineffective) amount of erythropoiesis, whereas the red cell iron utilization assay measures effective erythropoiesis. To a large extent, these two parameters can now be assessed much more easily by measuring the levels of soluble TfR and the reticulocyte count. Soluble TfR is a truncated form of the receptor that circulates in a complex with transferrin. The erythroblasts rather than the reticulocytes are the main source of soluble TfR and, when iron stores are adequate and available, measuring the level of soluble TfR (normal range 5.0 ± 1.0 mg/mL) is a good guide to the total level of erythropoiesis. Soluble TfR levels are increased when erythropoiesis is stimulated and

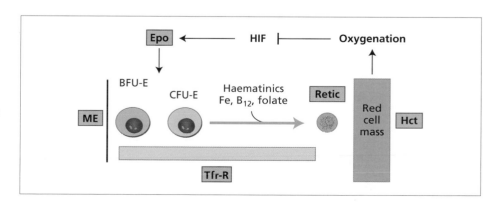

Figure 2.9 Summary of the regulation of erythropoiesis with the key points for assessment boxed in blue. ME denotes assessment of the myeloid/erythroid ratio in the bone marrow. Hct, haematocrit.

decreased when diminished. The interpretation of soluble TfR levels is complicated in iron deficiency as this condition independently raises the level of soluble TfR. The reticulocyte count (0.5–2.0% or 25–75 × 10^9/L) is raised in proportion to the degree of anaemia when erythropoiesis is effective (e.g. uncomplicated response to bleeding), but is relatively low when erythropoiesis is ineffective (e.g. β thalassaemia) or an abnormality prevents a normal response (e.g. nutritional deficiency).

The output of the system, the red cell mass, can be accurately measured by radioactive dilution techniques using ^{51}Cr, but can often be reliably estimated from the haematocrit or concentration of haemoglobin. Changes in red cell size, shape and haemoglobin content, often reflected in the red cell morphology, may provide important guides to specific abnormalities in red cell maturation (e.g. haemoglobinopathies, thalassaemia, nutritional deficiencies). If the red cell mass is appropriate to meet the demands for oxygenation, then Epo production will be suppressed and the serum level will be in the normal range (~25–50 mU/mL in cord blood and ~10–30 mU/mL in adults). If there is inadequate oxygenation, the level of Epo will generally be raised in proportion to the degree of anaemia (e.g. up to 3–10 U/mL after severe blood loss) unless there is some impediment to Epo production (e.g. chronic renal failure, anaemia of chronic diseases). For any given degree of anaemia the level of Epo in the blood may vary depending on the underlying conditions. For example, levels tend to be very high in aplastic anaemia and less than anticipated in thalassaemia. This may reflect the different numbers of precursors in the marrow that are able to bind available Epo molecules, thus altering the number of free Epo molecules that are measured.

These apparently straightforward assessments may be more difficult to interpret when there are multiple causes of abnormal erythropoiesis, and in particular when complicated by nutritional deficiencies, which should always be evaluated in parallel with these studies. In addition to the common nutritional anaemias, the vast number of specific diagnostic tests to determine the inherited or acquired disorders that may perturb each phase of erythropoiesis are described elsewhere in this book.

Proper oxygen delivery to the tissues requires sufficient circulating mature red cells, and any appropriate therapy should be aimed at correcting this. An important caveat is that excessive red cells may cause a sluggish circulation that can cause ischaemia, leading to serious complications (e.g. myocardial infarction and stroke). The simplified circuit presented here to describe the process of erythropoiesis (Figure 2.9) indicates three potential routes for therapeutic intervention. The first is to correct nutritional deficiencies, usually iron and less commonly folate or vitamin B$_{12}$. The discovery of the role of the iron-regulatory peptide hepcidin in the anaemias of chronic disorders suggests that some remaining common forms of anaemia related to this class (caused by inability to use stored iron) may be amenable to rational treatment in the not too distant future. A second frequently used approach is to correct anaemia, of any cause, with red cell transfusion, and the criteria for such treatment are set out in other sections of this book. The final approach is to increase erythropoiesis by administering recombinant human erythropoietin (rHuEpo). Following its considerable benefit to patients with the anaemia of chronic renal failure who are not capable of producing normal levels of Epo, rHuEpo has been assessed in a wide range of disorders (e.g. aplastic anaemia, red cell aplasia, thalassaemia intermedia, cancer of all types, haematological malignancy, myelodysplastic syndrome, rheumatoid arthritis, autologous blood donors, after stem cell transplantation and more). Modified forms of Epo, with a higher carbohydrate content and longer half-lives *in vivo*, have been developed and approved for clinical use, while small-molecule Epo mimetics with higher affinity for EpoR are under investigation. A review of the effectiveness of these therapeutic alternatives is beyond the scope of this chapter, but the considerable expense involved in treating patients, often over relatively long periods of time, with a hormone that does not always directly address the known pathophysiology of the anaemia requires careful consideration.

Finally, there are some conditions in which hormonal deficiency is known to contribute to anaemia (e.g. hypothyroidism, Addison's disease). In these cases appropriate correction of the hormonal deficiency logically helps correct the anaemia. Some rare forms of anaemia respond to a variety of therapies for unexplained reasons. For example, some cases of Diamond–Blackfan anaemia respond to corticosteroids, and some cases of congenital dyserythropoietic anaemia respond to interferon alfa, suggesting that there are still many unknown aspects to this clinically important and intellectually fascinating process of erythropoiesis.

Selected bibliography

Erythropoiesis in the context of general haemopoiesis

Cross MA, Enver T (1997) The lineage commitment of haemopoietic progenitor cells. *Current Opinion in Genetics and Development* **7**: 609–13.

Dzierzak E, Speck NA (2008) Of lineage and legacy: the development of mammalian haematopoietic stem cells. *Nature Immunology* **9**: 129–36.

Joshi C, Enver T (2003) Molecular complexities of stem cells. *Current Opinion in Hematology* **10**: 220–8.

Murre C (2007) Defining the pathways of early adult hematopoiesis. *Cell Stem Cell* **1**: 357–8.

Orkin SH, Zon LI (2008) Hematopoiesis: an evolving paradigm for stem cell biology. *Cell* **132**: 631–44.

Palis J (2008) Ontogeny of erythropoiesis. *Current Opinions in Haematology* **15**: 155–61.

Tavian M, Hallais M-F, Péault B (1999) Emergence of intraembryonic haematopoietic precursors in the pre-liver human embryo. *Development* **126**: 793–803.

Wickramasinghe SN (1975) Erythropoiesis. In: *Human Bone Marrow* (SN Wickramasinghe, ed.), pp. 162–232. Blackwell Scientific Publications, Oxford.

Regulation and differentiation of erythroid cells

Beguin Y (2003) Soluble transferrin receptor for the evaluation of erythropoiesis and iron status. *Clinica Chimica Acta* **329**: 9–22.

Bunn HF (2007) New agents that stimulate erythropoiesis. *Blood* **109**: 868–73.

De Maria R, Zeuner A, Eramo A *et al.* (1999) Negative regulation of erythropoiesis by caspase-mediated cleavage of GATA-1. *Nature* **401**: 489–93.

Panzenbock B, Bartunek P, Mapara MY *et al.* (1998) Growth and differentiation of human stem cell factor/erythropoietin-dependent erythroid progenitor cells *in vitro*. *Blood* **92**: 3658–68.

Schofield CJ, Ratcliffe PJ (2004) Oxygen sensing by HIF hydroxylases. *Nature Reviews. Molecular Cell Biology* **5**: 343–54.

Transcription factors controlling erythropoiesis

Bungert J, Engel JD (1996) The role of transcription factors in erythroid development. *Annals of Medicine* **28**: 47–55.

Cantor AB, Orkin SH (2002) Transcriptional regulation of erythropoiesis: an affair involving multiple partners. *Oncogene* **21**: 3368–76.

Gubin AN, Njoroge JM, Bouffard GG *et al.* (1999) Gene expression in proliferating human erythroid cells. *Genomics* **59**: 168–77.

Shivdasani RA, Orkin SH (1996) The transcriptional control of hematopoiesis. *Blood* **87**: 4025–39.

Sieweke MH, Graf T (1998) A transcriptional factor party during blood cell differentiation. *Current Opinion in Genetics and Development* **8**: 545–51.

Erythropoiesis in clinical practice

Beguin Y (2003) Soluble transferrin receptor for the evaluation of erythropoiesis and iron status. *Clinica Chimica Acta* **329**: 9–22.

Eschbach JW (2000) Current concepts of anaemia management in chronic renal failure: impact of NKF-DOQI. *Seminars in Nephrology* **20**: 320–9.

Muirhead N, Bargman JA, Burgess E *et al.* (1995) Evidence-based recommendations for the clinical use of recombinant human erythropoietin. *American Journal of Kidney Disease* **26**: S1–S24.

Samol J, Littlewood TJ (2003) The efficacy of rHuEPO in cancer-related anaemia. *British Journal of Haematology* **121**: 3–11.

Unger FE, Thompson AM, Blank MJ *et al.* (2010) Erythropoiesis-simulating agents – time for a reevaluation. *The New England Journal of Medicine* **362**: 189–192.

CHAPTER 3

Iron metabolism, iron deficiency and disorders of haem synthesis

3

A Victor Hoffbrand[1], Chaim Hershko[2] and Clara Camaschella[3]

[1]University College Medical School and Royal Free Hospital, London, UK
[2]Shaare Zedek Medical Center, Jerusalem, Israel
[3]Vita-Salute University, Milan, Italy

Introduction

Iron (atomic weight 55.85) is essential for many metabolic processes. It shares with other transition metals two properties of particular importance in biology: the ability to exist in more than one relatively stable oxidation state and the ability to form many complexes. Its ability to exist in both ferric and ferrous states underlies its role in critical enzyme reactions concerned with oxygen and electron transport and the cellular production of energy. As well as physiologically active iron compounds, many of which are haem proteins, there are also specialized proteins of iron transport and storage. The latter are necessary to enable iron to remain in solution at neutral pH, at which ferric iron is insoluble, and to limit the potential toxicity of this reactive metal. The insolubility of ferric iron also means that although the earth's crust contains approximately 4% iron and iron may be plentiful in the diet, much of this is unavailable. As

a result, the body is limited in the adjustments it can make to excessive loss of iron, which frequently occurs due to haemorrhage, and iron deficiency is the most common cause of anaemia throughout the world. The general need to conserve the metal is reflected in the absence of any physiological mechanism for excretion of iron, control of iron balance being at the level of iron absorption. This is important in the rarer but potentially fatal disorders of iron overload (see Chapter 4).

Distribution of body iron

The concentration of iron in the adult human body is normally about 50 mg/kg in males and 40 mg/kg in females. The largest component is circulating haemoglobin, with 450 mL (1 unit) of whole blood containing about 200 mg of iron (Figure 3.1). Much of the remainder is contained in the storage proteins ferritin and haemosiderin. These are found mainly in the reticuloendothelial cells of the liver, spleen and bone marrow (which gain iron from breaking down red cells), and in parenchymal liver cells (which normally gain most of their iron from the plasma iron-transporting protein transferrin).

Postgraduate Haematology: 6th edition. Edited by A. Victor Hoffbrand, Daniel Catovsky, Edward G.D. Tuddenham, Anthony R. Green
© 2011 Blackwell Publishing Ltd.

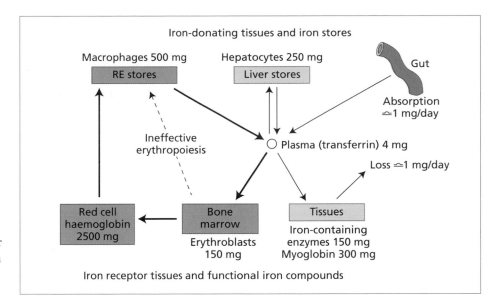

Figure 3.1 The major compartments of iron in a 70-kg man. Iron supply for erythropoiesis and release of iron from senescent red cells dominate internal iron exchange. RE, reticuloendothelial.

Proteins important in iron metabolism

Haemoglobin

Haemoglobin (molecular weight 64 500) contains four haem groups linked to four globin chains, and can bind four molecules of oxygen. Myoglobin (molecular weight 17 000) accounts for 4–5% of body iron and has a single haem group attached to its one polypeptide chain. It has a higher affinity for oxygen than haemoglobin and behaves as an oxygen reserve in muscles. The mitochondria contain a series of haem and non-haem iron proteins (including the cytochromes *a*, *b* and *c*, succinate dehydrogenase and cytochrome oxidase) that form an electron transport pathway responsible for the oxidation of intracellular substrates and the simultaneous production of adenosine triphosphate (ATP). Haem is an essential component of microsomal and mitochondrial cytochrome P450, which is concerned with hydroxylation reactions (including drug detoxification by the liver), and of cyclooxygenase, involved in prostaglandin synthesis. Other haem proteins include the enzymes catalase and lactoperoxidase, which are concerned with peroxide breakdown, and tryptophan pyrrolase, involved in the oxidation of tryptophan to formylkynurenine. There is a smaller group of iron sulphur proteins (e.g. xanthine oxidase, reduced nicotinamide adenine dinucleotide dehydrogenase and aconitase). Iron is also necessary for the function of ribonucleotide reductase, a key enzyme in DNA synthesis.

Ferritin and haemosiderin

Ferritin is the primary iron storage protein and provides a reserve of iron. It consists of an approximately spherical apo-protein shell (molecular weight 480 000) enclosing a core of ferric hydroxyphosphate (up to 4000 iron atoms). Human ferritin is made up from 24 subunits (molecular weight about 20 000) of two immunologically distinct types: H and L. There are multiple gene copies, which are mostly pseudogenes, on 12 different chromosomes. The coding loci are located at 11q12–q13 for the heavy chain and 19q13.3–q13.4 for the light chain. An intronless gene on chromosome 5 (q23.1) codes for mitochondrial ferritin, a novel H-type ferritin. The internal cavity of the ferritin molecule communicates with the exterior via six channels, through which ferrous iron may enter (to interact with a ferroxidase centre on the ferritin H subunit) or leave (after reduction, e.g. by dihydroflavins or ascorbic acid).

The way in which ferritin iron is mobilized is poorly understood, and a process in which the entire ferritin molecule is degraded within lysosomes prior to iron release has also been suggested. Variation in the proportion of H to L subunits explains the heterogeneity of ferritin from different tissues on isoelectric focusing: L-rich ferritins (from spleen and liver) are more basic than H-rich ferritins (from heart and red cells). The small amount of ferritin normally present in serum contains little iron and consists almost exclusively of L subunits. It is also heterogeneous, owing to glycosylation. This glycosylation and the direct relationship of serum concentration to storage iron in macrophages suggest that serum ferritin is secreted by macrophages in response to changing iron levels.

Haemosiderin, unlike ferritin, is a water-insoluble, crystalline, protein–iron complex that is visible by light microscopy when stained by the Prussian blue (Perls') reaction. It has an amorphous structure, with a higher iron/protein ratio than ferritin, and is probably formed by the partial digestion of ferritin aggregates by lysosomal enzymes. In normal subjects, the majority of storage iron is present as ferritin, and haemosiderin is predominantly found in macrophages rather than hepatocytes. In iron overload, the proportion present as haemosiderin increases considerably in both cell types.

Transferrin and transferrin receptors

Transferrin is a single-chain polypeptide (molecular weight 79 500) present in plasma (1.8–2.6 g/L) and extravascular fluid (Table 3.1). It has a plasma half-life of 8–11 days. The protein is synthesized predominantly by the liver, synthesis being inversely related to iron stores. Two atoms of ferric iron bind to each molecule. Although transferrin contains only about 4 mg of body iron at any time, it is vital to iron transport, with over 30 mg iron passing through this compartment each day (Figure 3.1). The binding sites (N-terminus and C-terminus) contain three tyrosine and two histidine residues and an arginine group. The uptake of iron from transferrin requires that the protein is attached to specific receptors on the cell surface. The transferrin receptor gene (*TFRC*) codes for TFR1, a transmembrane protein (identified as CD71), each molecule of two subunits binding one transferrin molecule. A second receptor, TFR2, also binds transferrin (Table 3.1). Through their binding with HFE, TFR1 and TFR2 are involved in regulating hepcidin synthesis (see Figure 3.2).

Lactoferrin is a glycoprotein (molecular weight 77 000) that is structurally related to transferrin. It is found in milk and other secretions and in neutrophils. It is thought to have a bacteriostatic action at secreting surfaces by depriving microorganisms of the iron needed for their growth.

Divalent metal transporter 1

Divalent metal transporter (DMT)1 is an electrogenic pump that requires proton cotransport in order to transfer Fe^{2+} across cell membranes. This occurs at the apical membrane and subapical endosomes of the duodenal enterocyte and the transferrin-cycle endosome, both of which have a low pH. The intestinal DMT is produced by different mRNA splicing from that which produces endosomal DMT1. DMT1 expression is upregulated in iron deficiency (see later) and may be involved in absorption of other divalent metal cations including Mn^{2+}, Co^{2+}, Zn^{2+}, Cu^{2+} and Pb^{2+}, although this is not established as a major function.

Ferroportin (SLC40A1)

This transmembrane domain protein is the basolateral transporter of iron, essential for iron release from macrophages, the intestinal absorptive enterocyte and placental syncytiotrophoblasts. It is also present in intracellular compartments. Caeruloplasmin is required for the cell surface localization of ferroportin, whose concentration is controlled by hepcidin, which triggers its tyrosine phosphorylation, internalization and degradation by ubiquitin in lysosomes.

Growth differentiation factor and twisted gastrulation protein

Growth differentiation factor (GDF)-15 is a member of the transforming growth factor (TGF)-β superfamily of proteins, which also includes the bone morphogenetic proteins (BMPs). GDF-15 exerts different functions according to the cell context, inhibiting hepcidin synthesis, macrophage activation, proliferation of immature haemopoietic progenitors and growth of tumour cell lines. It is strongly expressed during erythroblast maturation with lower levels in the other tissues. It is inducible by iron depletion and by hypoxia but is independent of hypoxia-inducible transcription factors (HIFs).

A second erythroid regulator of hepcidin expression, twisted gastrulation protein (TWSG1), has been identified. It is produced during the early stages of erythropoiesis and interferes with BMP-mediated hepcidin synthesis.

Other proteins

The roles in iron metabolism of hemojuvelin (HJV), BMP-6, SMADs, ferrioxidative and reduction enzymes, and caeruloplasmin are discussed under the headings of hepcidin regulation, iron absorption, iron uptake by erythroid cells and haem synthesis.

Hepcidin

Hepcidin has a central role in the regulation of iron metabolism and absorption (Figure 3.2). A product of the *HAMP* gene (Table 3.1), it is a small peptide (25 amino acids) with several isoforms and is released from a large prepropeptide of 84 amino acids. It is predominantly expressed in the liver. It regulates iron homeostasis by binding to cell-surface ferroportin, causing its tyrosine phosphorylation, internalization, ubiquitination and degradation in lysosomes. It therefore acts to inhibit iron absorption, iron release from macrophages and iron transport across the placenta. It is bound in plasma to α_2-macroglobulin and the major route of clearance is the kidney. Hepcidin can be measured in serum or urine by ELISA or mass spectrometry-based techniques. These have shown low or undetectable levels in iron deficiency and extremely high levels in inflammatory conditions, with inappropriately low levels in haemochromatosis and iron-loading anaemias.

Regulation of hepcidin expression

The regulation of hepcidin expression is transcriptional. Hepcidin expression is increased in response to raised serum iron, iron overload and inflammation, and is suppressed by

Table 3.1 Iron transport proteins, oxidoreductases, storage proteins and regulators.

Protein (gene)	Chromosome location	Tissue expression	Structure	Function	Regulation	Mutations and disease
Duodenal cytochrome b_1 (CYBRD1)	2q31	Enterocyte +	TMP, 6TMD	Ferric reductase	Fe (hepcidin)	–
DMT1 (SLC11A2)	12q13	Widespread	TMP, 568 aa	Fe uptake	Fe (3′-IRE)	Mk mouse, Belgrade rat Human microcytic anemia
Hemojuvelin (HFE2)	1q21.2	Liver, heart, muscle	Membrane-bound receptor or secreted protein	Regulator of hepcidin synthesis	?	Juvenile HC
Frataxin (FXN)	9q21.11	Heart, spinal cord, cerebellum	Mitochondrial protein, 210 aa	Mitochondrial iron donor		Friedreich ataxia
FLVCR (FLVCR1)	1q32.3	Erythroid	Major facilitator family	Receptor for feline leukaemia virus C; haem export		
Ferroportin 1 (SLC11A3)	2q32	Liver, spleen, enterocyte	TMP, 571 aa, 9TMD	Fe export	Fe (5′-IRE)	Human HC, autosomal dominant
Hepcidin (HAMP)	19q13.1	Plasma (liver)	20–25 aa	Regulator of iron homeostasis	Fe (HFE)	Juvenile HC (digenic HC)
Hephaestin (HEPH)	Xq11–q12	Enterocyte	TMP, 1TMD, copper protein with homology to caeruloplasmin	Fe^{2+} oxidase	–	Sla mouse
Haemochromatosis (HFE)	6p21.3	Widespread	HLA class I heavy chain	Regulates TFRC, iron uptake and hepcidin expression	?	Human HC, autosomal recessive
Mitoferrin (SLC25A37)	8p21.2	Erythroid	Mitochondrial inner membrane	Mitochondrial iron importer	?	
STEAP3	2q14.2	Erythroid, placenta (with TFR1)	Six-transmembrane epithelial antigen of the prostate-3	Ferric reductase (also reduces copper)	?	Erythropoietic protoporphyria
Transferrin receptor (TFR)	3q26.2-qter	Widespread: highest number in erythroblasts	TMP dimer of 90kDa polypeptide	Binds transferrin	Fe (3′-IRE)	(Lethal in knockout mouse)

Table 3.1 *Continued*

Protein (gene)	Chromosome location	Tissue expression	Structure	Function	Regulation	Mutations and disease
Transferrin receptor 2 (*TFR2*)	7q22	Liver, erythroid cells	60% similarity in extracellular domain to TFRC	Binds transferrin, iron homeostasis, regulator of hepcidin synthesis	No IRE	Human HC, autosomal recessive
Transferrin (*TF*)	3q21	Plasma, extravascular space	Single-chain polypeptide, glycoprotein	Iron transport	Iron stores	Atransferrinaemia
Ferritin heavy chain (*FTH1*)	11q13	Widespread, cytosolic	Subunit of ferritin	Iron storage (catalytic subunit for iron incorporation)	Fe (IRE)	Autosomal dominant Fe overload (very rare)
Ferritin light chain (*FTL*)	19q13.3–q13.4	Widespread, cytosolic	Subunit of ferritin	Iron storage	Fe (IRE)	Hyperferritinaemia and cataract syndrome Neuroferritinopathy*
IRP1 (*ACO1*)	9p21.1	Widespread	Cytoplasmic, 98 kDa with 4Fe–4S cluster	Regulation of synthesis of FTH, FTL, TFRC, DMT1, ferroportin 1, ALAS2	Cell iron	Not known
IRP2 (*IREB2*)	15	Widespread	Cytoplasmic, 105 kDa, no 4Fe–4S cluster	As IRP1	Cell iron	Not known
Matriptase-2 (*TMPRSS6*)	22q13.1	Mainly liver	Type II transmembrane protease from plasma membrane	Cleaves hemojuvelin	Unknown	Homozygous mutation leads to IRIDA

*In hyperferritinaemia/cataract syndrome, mutations affect the 5′-UTR IRE. In neuroferritinopathy, mutations affect *FTL* coding sequences. aa, amino acid; HC, haemochromatosis; IRIDA, iron refractory iron deficiency anaemia; IRE, iron response element; IRP, iron regulatory protein; TMD, transmembrane domain; TMP, transmembrane protein.

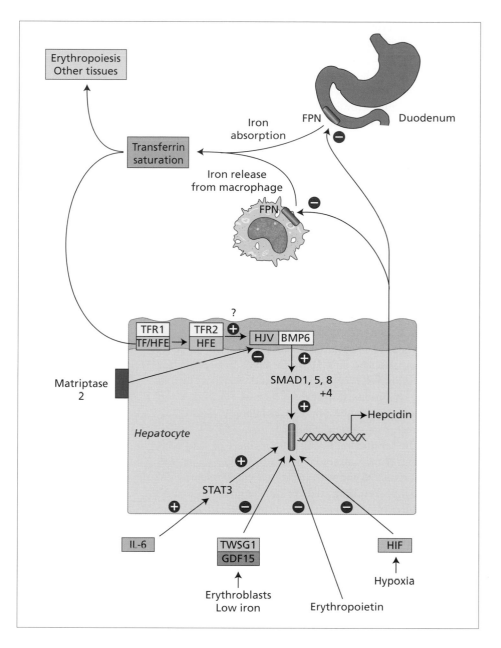

Figure 3.2 Stimulatory and inhibitory signals of hepcidin regulation. Hepcidin, as well as hemojuvelin (HJV), transferrin receptor 2 (TFR2) and HFE, are all produced in the hepatocyte. High plasma iron and inflammation stimulate hepcidin synthesis. This is mediated by SMADs and STAT3 respectively. Conversely, low plasma iron, increased rates of erythropoiesis (including ineffective erythropoiesis) and hypoxia inhibit hepcidin production. This is mediated by matriptase, growth differentiation factor (GDF)-15, twisted gastrulation protein (TWSG1) and HIF1-α respectively. Hepcidin binds ferroportin (FPN), causing its destruction and so inhibits iron absorption and iron release from macrophages into plasma and from intracellular compartments. BMP, bone morphogenetic protein.

iron deficiency, hypoxia and increased erythropoietic activity. Under basal conditions, expression depends on signalling through the BMP/SMAD pathway (Figure 3.2). HJV is a member of the repulsive guidance molecules (RGM) family that is highly expressed in liver, skeletal muscles and the heart. It is either associated with cell membranes through a glycosyl-phosphatidylinositol anchor or released as a soluble form. Membrane-bound HJV participates in the pathway regulating hepcidin expression as a BMP coreceptor, whereas soluble HJV antagonizes BMP-6. BMP-6 is the master hepcidin activator *in vivo*.

HFE and TFR2 are also involved in hepcidin expression (Figure 3.2). HFE is able to bind TFR1 and TFR2. During low or basal serum iron conditions, HFE and TFR1 exist as a complex at the plasma membrane, TFR1 serving to sequester HFE to silence its activity. Diferric serum transferrin (Fe^{2+}-TF) competes with HFE for binding to TFR1. Increased serum transferrin saturation therefore results in dissociation of HFE from TFR1. Acting as an iron sensor, HFE then binds to TFR2 and conveys the Fe^{2+}-TF status to the signal transduction effector complex. HJV binds to BMP, then phosphorylates SMADs to form an SMAD-1/-5/-8–SMAD-4 complex, which translocates to the nucleus and stimulates hepcidin production by activating its promoter. In keeping with this model, genetic mutations of HFE, TFR2, HJV and hepcidin all result in haemochromatosis with low serum hepcidin levels (see

Chapter 4). Iron levels also seem to control BMP-6 production but whether this is through liver iron or circulating transferrin is unclear.

A second type of transcriptional hepcidin regulation occurs in inflammation. Interleukin (IL)-6 and IL-1β induce transcription of the hepcidin gene by activating STAT3 (signal transducer and activator of transcription 3) and its binding to a regulatory element in the hepcidin promoter. It may converge on a final shared SMAD-4-dependent pathway.

The hepcidin response is remarkably rapid. In humans, iron ingestion results in a sharp increase in urinary hepcidin excretion within 12–24 hours of starting treatment. Likewise, infusion of recombinant IL-6 results in significant increase in urinary hepcidin and decreased serum iron and transferrin saturation within 2 hours of infusion. These observations imply that hepcidin expression is directly controlled by serum iron (probably by transferrin saturation) and IL-6 and not by long-term gradual accumulation of iron in tissues.

Response to anaemia and hypoxia

Hepcidin levels can be measured in patient serum or urine by ELISA or mass spectrometry. Hepcidin levels are reduced or undetectable in iron deficiency anaemia and extremely high in inflammatory conditions. Iron absorption is accelerated in iron deficiency, ineffective erythropoiesis and hypoxia (Figure 3.2). Erythroid precursors secrete GDF-15 and TWSG1, which inhibit hepcidin production by the liver. Serum concentrations of GDF-15 are grossly increased in thalassaemia major and other conditions associated with ineffective erythropoiesis and in iron deficiency, resulting in hepcidin suppression and so inability to turn off intestinal iron absorption. In addition, other studies indicate that the von Hippel–Lindau hypoxia inducible factors (HIFs), which stimulate erythropoietin synthesis, control iron homeostasis by the downregulation of hepcidin, repressing its promoter with the upregulation of ferroportin. Under normal conditions, HIFs play a useful role by mobilizing iron and supporting erythrocyte production in response to anaemia/hypoxia. However, the same mechanism may contribute to the harmful accumulation of iron in response to chronic anaemia associated with ineffective erythropoiesis in thalassaemia and other dyserythropoietic anaemias. In addition, soluble HJV *in vitro* and *in vivo* and erythropoietin itself in cell models are able to inhibit hepcidin transcription.

Matriptase-2 (TMPRSS6)

This is a type 2 member of the transmembrane serine protease family mainly expressed in the liver. Membrane-bound matriptase-2 regulates hepcidin expression by cleaving membrane-bound HJV, releasing soluble HJV fragments. The reduction in membrane-bound HJV and the presence of soluble HJV both result in reduced hepcidin transcription. The factors which regulate matriptase-2 expression need to be elucidated. Matriptase-2 activity overrides all known activating stimuli of hepcidin synthesis. Homozygous $TMPRSS6^{-/-}$ mutations in mice and humans result in marked upregulation of hepcidin and blockade of intestinal and macrophage iron transport into plasma, leading to a refractory hypochromic microcytic anaemia (see pp. 41, 51).

Intracellular iron homeostasis

Synthesis of several of the proteins involved in iron metabolism is regulated at the level of RNA translation by two cytoplasmic iron-dependent proteins, namely IRP1 and IRP2 (Table 3.1). These are capable of binding to mRNAs that contain a sequence forming a stem-and-loop structure called an *iron-responsive element* or IRE (Figure 3.3). IRP1 (molecular weight 98 000) contains an iron–sulphur (4Fe–4S) cluster and functions as a cytoplasmic aconitase with low affinity for the IRE when intracellular iron is abundant. When iron is scarce, however, the iron–sulphur cluster is no longer present and IRP1 binds to the IRE with high affinity. IRP2 (molecular weight 105 000) is expressed ubiquitously but is less abundant than IRP1. IRP2 has an extra section of 73 amino acids rich in proline, serine and cysteine that mediates IRP2 degradation in iron-replete cells. Activation of IRP2 requires accumulation of the protein as a result of new synthesis. Degradation takes place in the proteosome after addition of iron.

The 3′-untranslated region (3′-UTR) of TFR1 contains five IREs, whereas the 5′-UTR region of ferritin mRNA contains a single IRE. Binding of IRP when there are low levels of intracellular iron protects TFR1 mRNA from cytoplasmic degradation but inhibits translation of ferritin mRNA by interfering with the binding of initiation factors. In contrast, when intracellular iron is increased, the opposite effects occur. Thus, coordinated regulation of TFR1 and ferritin acts to maintain a constant intracellular iron content over the short term by balancing cellular iron uptake and storage.

Erythroid δ-aminolaevulinic acid synthase (ALAS2) mRNA also has an IRE in its 5′-UTR region, whereas 'housekeeping' ALAS1 mRNA does not. The IRP–IRE system is therefore involved in matching iron supply to haem synthesis, with repression of protoporphyrin synthesis in iron-deficient erythroblasts (see p. 38). Mitochondrial aconitase interconverts citrate and isocitrate and has a putative IRE at the 5′-UTR of its mRNA. DMT1 like TFR1 has a 3′-IRE and is upregulated in iron deficiency. Ferroportin 1 has a 5′-IRE (Table 3.1) but binding of IRP is weak compared with the TFR1, ferritin and DMT1 IREs. However, as occurs for DMT1, ferroportin 1 may be translated in a non-IRE isoform that escapes the IRP control in some tissues, for example in duodenal cells.

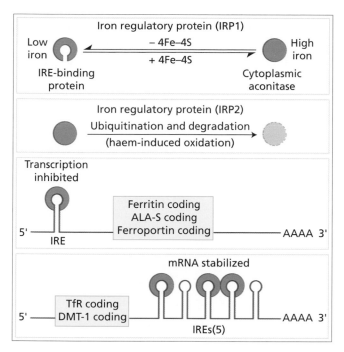

Figure 3.3 Coordinate regulation of expression of ferritin and transferrin receptor: the role of the iron response element (IRE)–iron regulatory protein (IRP) mechanism. When cellular iron levels are low, IRP binds to the IRE stem and loop structures of mRNA to inhibit translation of ferritin and ALA-S, but increases translation of transferrin receptors (TFR) and DMT1 by preventing degradation of the mRNA. When iron levels are high, the IRP functions as a cytoplasmic aconitase and no longer binds to the IREs. Ferritin synthesis can thus proceed, while TFR synthesis is reduced. IRP2 binds to IREs when iron levels are low, but is degraded after ubiquitination (initiated by haem-induced oxidation) when iron levels are high. The IRPs therefore provide two ways of sensing iron requirements either involving Fe–S proteins or haem proteins.

Normal iron balance

The amount of iron in the body at birth depends on the blood volume and haemoglobin concentration, the birth weight (which determines blood volume) being particularly important. Delay in clamping the cord leads to an increased red cell mass by placental transfusion. The level of maternal iron stores has little effect on fetal iron. The newborn contains about 80 mg/kg at full term. Neonatal iron reserves are utilized for growth, and from 6 months to 2 years virtually no iron stores are present. Thereafter, iron stores gradually accumulate during childhood to around 5 mg/kg. In men, there is a further increase between 15 and 30 years to about 10–12 mg/kg (total up to approximately 1 g), whereas iron stores remain lower in women (average

Table 3.2 Daily iron losses and requirements.

Group (age, years)	Daily loss (mg)		Requirement for growth (mg)	Total (mg)
	Urine, skin, faeces, etc.	Menses		
Children				
0.5–1	0.17	–	0.55	0.72
1–3	0.19	–	0.27	0.46
4–6	0.27	–	0.23	0.50
7–10	0.39	–	0.32	0.71
Males				
11–14	0.62		0.55	1.17
15–17	0.90	–	0.60	1.50
18+	1.05	–	–	1.05
Females				
11–14*	0.65	–	0.55	1.20
11–14	0.65	0.48[†]	0.55	1.68
15–17	0.79	0.48[†]	0.35	1.62
18+	0.87	0.48[†]	–	1.35
Post menopause	0.87	–	–	0.87
Lactating[‡]	1.15	–	–	1.15

*Non-menstruating.
[†]Median loss.
[‡]Average dietary requirement during pregnancy is 3–4 mg.
Source: WHO (2001).

300 mg) until the menopause. It would take 4 years or more for a man to deplete body iron stores and start developing iron deficiency anaemia solely due to lack of dietary intake or malabsorption.

Requirements are higher in menstruating women and during periods of rapid growth in infancy and adolescence (Table 3.2). Menstrual blood loss has a median value of 30 mL, but the 95th centile value is 118 mL per month (equivalent to 1.9 mg iron per day), which has been found to be significantly associated with iron deficiency. Requirements are highest of all in pregnancy.

Iron absorption

Iron absorption depends not only on the amount of iron in the diet but also, and more importantly, on the bioavailability of that iron, as well as the body's needs for iron. A normal Western diet provides approximately 15 mg of iron daily. Of that iron, digestion within the gut lumen releases about half in a soluble form, from which about 3 mg may be taken up by mucosal cells and only about 1 mg (or 5–10% of dietary iron) transferred to

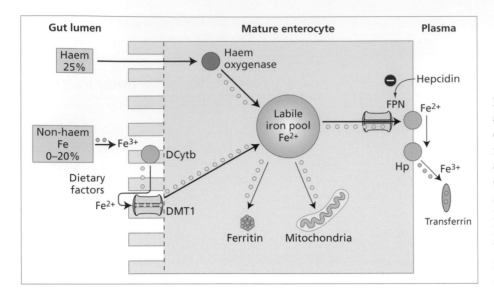

Figure 3.4 Molecular pathways of iron absorption. The area enclosed in the dotted box refers to the uptake of iron from the plasma in the developing enterocyte in the intestinal crypt. Otherwise, the diagram refers to iron absorption by the villous epithelial cell. DMT1, divalent metal transporter 1; FPN, ferroportin; Hp, hephaestin; TF, transferrin; TFR, transferrin receptor. For further details see text and Table 3.1.

the portal blood in a healthy man. Iron absorption can thus be influenced at several different stages.

Dietary and luminal factors

Much of dietary iron is non-haem iron derived from cereals (commonly fortified with additional iron in the UK), with a lesser component of haem iron from meat and fish. Even in iron deficiency, the maximum iron absorption from a mixed Western diet is no more than 3–4 mg daily. This figure is much less with the predominantly vegetarian, cereal-based diets of most of the world's population. Iron is better absorbed from animal than vegetable sources.

Iron is released from protein complexes by acid and proteolytic enzymes in the stomach and small intestine, and haem is liberated from haemoglobin and myoglobin. Iron is maximally absorbed from the duodenum and less well from the jejunum, probably because the increasingly alkaline environment leads to the formation of insoluble ferric hydroxide complexes. Acid pH, vitamin C and some low-molecular-weight chelates (e.g. sugars, amino acids) enhance absorption. Therapeutic ferrous iron salts are well absorbed on an empty stomach, but when taken with a meal absorption is reduced as a result of the same ligand-binding processes that affect dietary non-haem iron; phytates, tannates in tea and bran inhibit absorption.

Mucosal factors: molecular aspects of iron absorption and its regulation

A variety of mechanisms for the binding of non-haem iron to the mucosal membrane have been described. Specific, saturable and receptor-mediated mechanisms, and passive diffusion at higher doses, may occur.

The proposed process is illustrated in Figure 3.4. Non-haem iron is released from food as Fe^{3+} and reduced by duodenal cytochrome b_1 (DCytb) to Fe^{2+}. This is transported across the brush border membrane by DMT1, which is upregulated in iron deficiency. It is assumed that iron enters the labile pool and some may be incorporated into ferritin and lost when the cells are exfoliated. Iron destined for retention by the body is transported across the serosal membrane by ferroportin before uptake by transferrin as Fe^{3+}. The regulation of duodenal cell iron release by hepcidin through its action on ferroportin is rapid and occurs for all absorptive cells, including those at the tip of the villus. Hephaestin is a copper-containing ferroxidase expressed predominantly in villous cells of the small intestine that converts Fe^{2+} to Fe^{3+} in the basolateral transfer step of iron absorption.

Haem iron is initially bound by haem receptors at the brush border membrane and released intracellularly by haem oxygenase before entering the labile iron pool and following a common pathway with iron of non-haem origin.

Iron absorption is regulated both at the stage of mucosal uptake and at the stage of transfer to the blood. DMT1 levels increase when intracellular iron is low and ferroportin concentration is also high due to low plasma hepcidin levels. The amount of iron transported to the plasma through ferroportin is hepcidin-dependent.

Iron uptake by erythroid cells

About 85% of transferrin iron normally enters developing red cells for incorporation into haemoglobin. This tissue distribution of transferrin-bound iron reflects the expression of transferrin receptors, which are present in high concentration on cells with a high iron requirement. The latter includes any rapidly dividing cells but is normally dominated by the cells of the erythron. A soluble truncated form of the transferrin receptor derived from these cell surfaces is detectable in serum.

Transferrin receptors have the highest affinity for diferric transferrin. The transferrin–receptor complex is taken up by a process of receptor-mediated endocytosis (Figure 3.5). The iron is released at the low pH of the endosome, reduced from Fe^{3+} to Fe^{2+} by STEAP3, a ferrireductase, before the apotransferrin and receptor are recycled to the plasma and the cell membrane respectively. Iron release from the endosome is via DMT1 (Figure 3.5) and the iron is transported into mitochondria by mitoferrin or enters ferritin. Recently, direct endosome–mitochondrial iron transfer has also been suggested. A mitochondrial version of ferritin exists, coded by a gene on chromosome 5. Its physiological role is unknown but it is elevated in sideroblastic anaemias due to ALAS2 defects or myelodysplasia. Direct transfer of storage iron from macrophages to erythroblasts (rhopheocytosis) may also occur.

Some 80–90% of iron taken into developing erythroblasts is converted to haem within 1 hour. Any iron taken up in excess of the requirement for haem synthesis is incorporated in ferritin (Figure 3.5). The red cell ferritin content is therefore increased when haemoglobin synthesis is impaired, as in thalassaemia syndromes or sideroblastic anaemia. Excess iron may be seen in the cytoplasm of mature red cells as one or more siderotic granules. These are composed of haemosiderin and stain blue with Perls' reaction and purplish blue with Romanowsky stains,

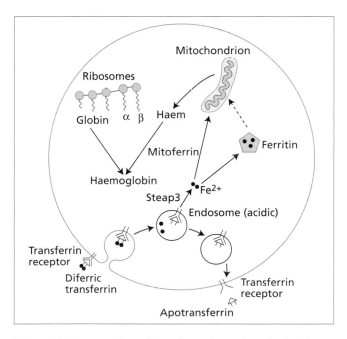

Figure 3.5 Incorporation of iron from plasma transferrin into haemoglobin in developing red cells. Uptake of transferrin iron is by receptor-mediated endocytosis.

when they are called Pappenheimer bodies. The spleen removes these granules by its pitting action.

Haem synthesis and mitochondrial iron metabolism

Haem consists of a protoporphyrin ring with an iron atom at its centre. Haem is synthesized from the precursors succinyl-CoA and glycine, which condense to form δ-aminolaevulinic acid (ALA) under the action of ALAS, with pyridoxal phosphate as a coenzyme (see Chapter 2; see also p. 39). Housekeeping ALAS (ALAS1) is coded by a gene on chromosome 3, but in erythroid cells erythroid-specific ALAS2 predominates and is encoded on the X chromosome. ALA can be utilized for the formation of both purines and haem. Four molecules of porphobilinogen condense under the influence of porphobilinogen deaminase and uroporphyrinogen cosynthase to form the tetrapyrrole ring compound uroporphyrinogen III. The latter is converted to protoporphyrin IX. Finally, iron in the ferrous form is incorporated under the influence of the enzyme ferrochelatase. Iron in haem has six coordinating valencies: four link the iron to nitrogen atoms in each pyrrole ring, whereas the remaining two link haem to histidine residues in the globin chain, the distal bond being unstable and easily replaced by oxygen to form oxyhaemoglobin.

The mitochondria play a major role in haem synthesis as they contain ALAS, coproporphyrinogen oxidase and ferrochelatase, the enzyme sequence from ALA to coproporphyrinogen being situated in the cytoplasm. Besides haem, mitochondria utilize iron in the synthesis of iron–sulphur clusters, prosthetic groups essential for the function of several mitochondrial (respiratory chain complexes, ferrochelatase) and cytosolic (aconitase) proteins. A connection exists between haem synthesis and sulphur cluster biogenesis, because the activity of the iron regulatory protein IRP1, which controls ALAS2, is iron–sulphur cluster-dependent and because ferrochelatase, the last enzyme in haem synthesis, has an iron–sulphur cluster.

The assembly of iron–sulphur clusters is a complex, incompletely understood process that requires multiple proteins. The best known is frataxin, a likely iron donor in this pathway. The gene encoding frataxin is mutated in Friedreich ataxia (see pp. 43, 44, 53). An enzyme active in the pathway, whose function is still unclear, is glutaredoxin-5, which has been found mutated in a rare recessive form of sideroblastic anaemia (see pp. 43, 44). ABCB7, a member of a family of transmembrane proteins characterized by the ABC domain that binds and hydrolyses ATP, transfers iron–sulphur clusters from mitochondria to the cytosol. Mutations of ABCB7 cause an X-linked form of sideroblastic anaemia with ataxia (see pp. 43, 44).

The mitochondria are also the site of the citric acid cycle, which supplies succinate. The mature red cell, which lacks mitochondria, is therefore unable to synthesize haem.

A number of porphyrins are formed by side reactions during the synthesis of protoporphyrin. In the porphyrias (see p. 41), many of these compounds accumulate in the major sites of haem synthesis, the liver and the red cells. A haem exporter, FLVCR (Table 3.1), is present in erythroid cells and rids the cell of any haem made in excess.

Intracellular transit iron and plasma non-transferrin-bound iron

It has been suggested but not proved that there is a transit pool of 'metabolically active' or 'labile' iron within cells, which receives iron from degraded haem or ferritin, exchanges with transferrin and is incorporated into newly synthesized iron-containing proteins. This iron is considered to be sensed by iron regulatory proteins and available for chelation. Within cells, low-molecular-weight chelates (e.g. with citrate) may be present. However, recent work questions the existence of these chelates and a model of iron transfer requiring direct protein–protein interaction that could involve interaction of organelles has been proposed. It is suggested that transferrin-containing endosomes may transfer iron directly to mitochondria. Within plasma in iron overload, non-transferrin-bound iron may also exist as oligomeric iron oxide, either free or bound to albumin, and is particularly toxic to various organisms (see Chapter 4).

Breakdown of haemoglobin

After phagocytosis by macrophages, haem from senescent red cells is broken down by haem oxygenase (HMOX1) to release iron (see Chapter 8). As ferrous iron, it can then either enter ferritin (where it is oxidized to ferric iron by the ferritin protein) or be released into plasma (via ferroportin 1), where its binding to transferrin (also as the ferric form) may be facilitated by a plasma ferrous oxidase (e.g. caeruloplasmin). The release of macrophage iron is controlled by hepcidin, with high levels, as in inflammation or iron overload, reducing iron release. Changes in the release of iron from macrophages are thought to account for the diurnal rhythm of serum iron concentration, which is highest in the morning and lowest in the evening. A diurnal increase in serum hepcidin at noon and 8 p.m. is observed in healthy volunteers.

Diagnostic methods for investigating iron metabolism

The large amount of iron present as haemoglobin means that the degree of any anaemia must always be considered in assessing iron status. Reduced amounts of haemoglobin accompany an overall reduction in body iron in iron deficiency anaemia or after acute blood loss. In other anaemias, including the anaemia of chronic disease and most haemolytic and megaloblastic anaemias, iron is redistributed from the red cells to macrophage iron stores, with a corresponding increase in marrow-stainable iron and serum ferritin. The various measurements of iron status are listed in Table 3.3 and described below. No single measurement is ideal for all clinical circumstances, as all are affected by confounding factors (Table 3.3) and changes may develop sequentially (as in progressive negative iron balance) or may affect particular body iron compartments. Reference ranges for haemoglobin and the various measures of iron status are given in Appendix 1. Table 3.4 summarizes the changes in measures of iron status accompanying various types of hypochromic anaemia. The assessment of *iron overload* is discussed in Chapter 4.

Storage iron

Serum ferritin
In healthy subjects, the serum ferritin concentration correlates with iron stores, as assessed by quantitative phlebotomy or tissue biopsy. Normal concentrations of serum ferritin range from about 15 to 300 μg/L, and are higher in men (median about 90 μg/L) than in premenopausal women (median 30 μg/L). In neonates, the concentration in cord blood (median approximately 100 μg/L) rises further over the first 2 months of life as fetal haemoglobin is broken down, and thereafter falls to low levels (median 20–30 μg/L) throughout childhood and adolescence.

Serum ferritin concentrations below 15 μg/L are virtually specific for storage iron depletion, but normal values do not exclude this and values above 300 μg/L do not necessarily, or even usually, indicate iron overload. This is because ferritin synthesis is influenced by factors other than iron (in particular, it behaves as an acute-phase reactant in many inflammatory diseases). For this reason, serum ferritin concentrations below 50 μg/L may be associated with a lack of storage iron in patients with the anaemia of chronic disease. A ferritin concentration above 100 μg/L suggests the presence of storage iron.

Bone marrow aspiration
Staining the bone marrow for iron gives an indication of reticuloendothelial iron stores as well as erythroblast iron (Figure 3.6a). In iron deficiency anaemia, reticuloendothelial iron and erythroblast iron are absent (Figure 3.6b).

Iron supply to the tissues

Serum iron and iron-binding capacity
The serum iron and, more particularly, the saturation of the total iron-binding capacity of transferrin (TIBC) give a measure of the iron supply to the tissues. A serum transferrin saturation

Table 3.3 Potential confounding factors in the interpretation of measures of iron status.

Measurement	Confounding factors
Iron stores	
Serum ferritin	Increased: as an acute-phase protein (e.g. in infection, inflammation or malignancy) and by release of tissue ferritins by damage, especially to iron-rich organs (e.g. with hepatic necrosis, chronic liver disease, splenic or bone marrow infarction in sickle cell disease) Decreased: by ascorbate deficiency
Tissue iron supply	
Serum iron and transferrin saturation	Labile measures: normal short-term fluctuations mean that a single value may not reflect iron supply over a longer period
Serum transferrin receptor	Directly related to extent of erythroid activity as well as being inversely related to iron supply to cells
Red cell protoporphyrin/red cell ferritin/% hypochromic red cells/ reticulocyte haemoglobin content	Stable measures: reduced iron supply at time of red cell formation leads to increases in protoporphyrin and reticulocyte haemoglobin content and hypochromic red cells, and reduced red cell ferritin. However, values may not reflect current iron supply. May be affected by other causes of impaired iron incorporation into haem (e.g. lead poisoning, sideroblastic anaemias)
Functional iron	
Haemoglobin concentration	Other causes for anaemia besides iron deficiency; a reciprocal relationship with iron stores should be expected in all anaemias except in iron deficiency anaemia
Red cell MCV, MCH	May be reduced in other disorders of haemoglobin synthesis (e.g. thalassaemia, sideroblastic anaemias) in addition to iron deficiency

MCH, mean corpuscular haemoglobin; MCV, mean corpuscular volume.

Table 3.4 Differential diagnosis of hypochromic anaemia.

	Iron deficiency	Chronic disease	Thalassaemia trait (α or β)	Sideroblastic anaemia	IRIDA
MCV/MCH	↓	↓ or N	↓	↓ (congenital) ↑N (acquired)	↓
Serum iron	↓	↓	N	↑	↓
TIBC	↑	↓ or N	N	N	
Transferrin saturation	↓	↓	N	↑	↓
Serum ferritin	↓	N or ↑	N	↑	N
Serum TFR	↑	N	N	N or ↑	↑
Serum hepcidin	↓	↑	N	↓	N or ↑
Bone marrow iron stores	↓	N or ↑	N	N or ↑	↑
Erythroblast iron	↓	↓	N	Ring forms	

IRIDA, iron refractory iron deficiency anaemia; MCH, mean corpuscular haemoglobin; MCV, mean corpuscular volume; N, normal; TFR, transferrin receptor; TIBC, total iron-binding capacity.

less than 15% is insufficient to support normal erythropoiesis. A rise in TIBC is characteristic of iron deficiency. A reduced serum iron concentration with a normal or reduced TIBC is a characteristic response to inflammation (see below).

Serum transferrin receptors

Plasma concentrations reflect both the number of erythroid precursors and iron supply to the bone marrow. In clinical practice, these two factors must be considered in interpreting

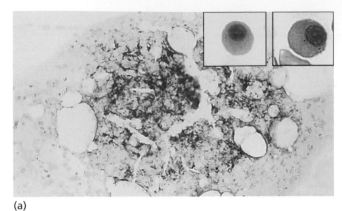

(a)

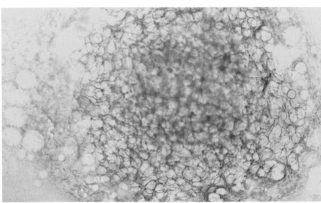

(b)

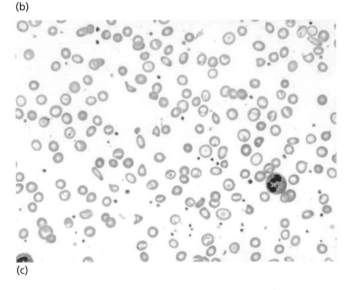

(c)

Figure 3.6 (a) Normal bone marrow showing plentiful iron in macrophages (Perls stain) with iron granules in erythroblasts (insets). (b) Iron deficiency: bone marrow showing absence of stainable iron (Perls stain). (c) Iron deficiency: peripheral blood film showing hypochromic microcytic red cells.

transferrin receptor levels. In the anaemia of chronic disease, the assay provides a valuable indicator of deficiency of body iron stores. Serum transferrin receptor levels only increase in this situation in the absence of storage iron.

Red cell protoporphyrin

When iron supply to the erythron is limited, iron incorporation into haem is restricted, leading to accumulation of the immediate precursor, protoporphyrin IX. This is lost only slowly from circulating red cells; concentrations greater than the normal upper limit of 80 μmol/mol haemoglobin therefore indicate that a reduction in iron supply has been present over the previous few weeks. Protoporphyrin levels may also increase in patients with sideroblastic anaemias and lead poisoning. Analysers that are portable and easy to operate are useful in large-scale field studies of iron deficiency anaemia as an initial screening test.

Percentage of hypochromic red cells

As iron supply to the erythron diminishes, the new red cells produced are increasingly hypochromic. Assessment of the haemoglobin content of individual red cells, which is possible using some automated cell counters, allows measurement of the percentage of hypochromic cells. Values rising to above 6% may help in the early identification of impaired iron supply in patients with chronic renal failure who are receiving treatment with recombinant erythropoietin, when associated inflammatory disease means that other measures of iron status can be misleading.

Reticulocyte haemoglobin content

Reticulocyte haemoglobin content (CHr) is useful in screening iron status, particularly in dialysis patients. A CHr cut-off value of 32 pg is appropriate for the assessment of iron-deficient erythropoiesis. Moreover, CHr may serve as a predictor of the response of anaemia to iron treatment. When response to treatment is favourable, an increase in CHr may be discerned within a few days of starting treatment before overall mean corpuscular haemoglobin (MCH) has changed.

Iron deficiency anaemia

Sequence of events

Depletion of iron stores

When the body is in a state of negative iron balance, the first event is depletion of body stores, which are mobilized for haemoglobin production. Iron absorption is increased when stores are reduced, before anaemia develops and even when the serum iron level is still normal, although the serum ferritin will have already fallen.

Iron-deficient erythropoiesis

With further iron depletion, manifested by a serum ferritin below 15 μg/L and fall in serum transferrin saturation to less than 15%, iron-deficient erythropoiesis develops with increasing concentrations of serum transferrin receptor and red cell protoporphyrin. At this stage, the haemoglobin, mean corpuscular volume (MCV) and MCH may still be within the reference range, although they may rise significantly when iron therapy is given.

Iron deficiency anaemia

If the negative balance continues, frank iron deficiency anaemia develops. The red cells become obviously microcytic and hypochromic (Figure 3.6c), and poikilocytosis becomes more marked. The MCV and MCH are reduced, and target cells may be present. The reticulocyte count is low for the degree of anaemia. The serum TIBC rises and the serum iron falls, so that the percentage saturation of TIBC is usually less than 10%.

The number of erythroblasts containing cytoplasmic iron (sideroblasts) is reduced at an early stage in the development of deficiency, and siderotic granules are entirely absent from these cells when iron deficiency anaemia is established. The erythroblasts have a ragged vacuolated cytoplasm and relatively pyknotic nuclei. The bone marrow macrophages show a total absence of iron, except where very rapid blood loss outstrips the ability to mobilize the storage iron. Platelets are frequently increased.

Tissue effects of iron deficiency

When iron deficiency is severe and chronic, widespread tissue changes may be present, including koilonychia (ridged nails, breaking easily), hair thinning, angular stomatitis (especially in those with badly fitting dentures), glossitis and pharyngeal webs (Paterson–Kelly syndrome). Partial villous atrophy, with minor degrees of malabsorption of xylose and fat, reversible by iron therapy, has been described in infants suffering from iron deficiency, but not in adults. Pica is sometimes present; in some who eat clay or chalk, this may be the cause rather than the result of iron deficiency.

Iron-dependent enzymes in the tissues are usually better preserved than other iron-containing compounds. In severe iron deficiency, however, these enzymes are not inviolate and their levels may fall. This may be partly responsible for the general tissue changes, with mitochondrial swelling in many different cells (including, in the experimental animal, hepatic and myocardial cells), poor lymphocyte transformation and diminished cell-mediated immunity, and impaired intracellular killing of bacteria by neutrophils.

A particular concern has been the finding that infants with iron deficiency anaemia may have impaired mental development and function, and that this deficit may not be completely restored by iron therapy. There is recent evidence that premature labour is more frequent in mothers with iron deficiency anaemia. It remains controversial whether impaired work performance seen in adults results from the anaemia or from depletion of mitochondrial iron-containing enzymes. It is also unclear to what extent some of the other tissue effects of iron deficiency can occur even in the absence of anaemia.

Table 3.5 Causes of iron deficiency.

Blood loss
Uterine: menorrhagia, post-menopausal bleeding, parturition
Gastrointestinal: oesophageal varices, hiatus hernia, *Helicobacter pylori*, peptic ulcer, aspirin ingestion, hookworm, hereditary telangiectasia, carcinoma of the stomach, caecum or colon, ulcerative colitis, angiodysplasia, Meckel diverticulum, diverticulosis, haemorrhoids, etc.
Renal tract: haematuria (e.g. renal or bladder lesion), haemoglobinuria (e.g. paroxysmal nocturnal haemoglobinuria)
Pulmonary tract: overt haemoptysis, idiopathic pulmonary haemosiderosis
Widespread bleeding disorders
Self-inflicted

Malabsorption
Gluten-induced enteropathy (child or adult), gastrectomy, atrophic gastritis, chronic inflammation, clay eating, etc.

Dietary
Especially vegetarian diet

Causes of iron deficiency (Table 3.5)

Diet

Defective intake of iron is rarely the sole or major cause of iron deficiency in adults in Western communities. The diet may contain insufficient or poorly available iron as a result of poverty, religious tenets or food faddism. Iron deficiency is more likely to develop in subjects taking a largely vegetarian diet – the majority of the world's population – who also have increased physiological demands for iron.

Increased physiological iron requirements

Iron deficiency is common in infancy, when demands for growth may be greater than dietary supplies. It is aggravated by prematurity, infections and delay in mixed feeding. It is also frequent in adolescence, in females and in pregnancy (Table 3.2). The fetus acquires about 280 mg of iron and a further 400–500 mg is required for the temporary expansion of maternal red cell mass. Another 200 mg of iron is lost with the placenta and with bleeding at delivery. Although iron absorption increases throughout pregnancy and increased requirements are partly offset by amenorrhoea, this may not be sufficient to meet the resultant net maternal outlay of over 600 mg iron.

Blood loss

Blood loss is the most common cause of iron deficiency in adults. A loss of more than about 6–8 mL of blood (3–4 mg iron) daily becomes of importance, as this equals the maximum amount of iron that can be absorbed from a normal diet. The loss is usually from the genital tract in women or from the gastrointestinal tract in either sex. The most common cause on a worldwide basis is infestation with hookworm, in which anaemia is related to the degree of infestation. In the UK, menorrhagia, haemorrhoids and peptic ulceration are common, as well as gastric bleeding because of salicylates or other non-steroidal anti-inflammatory drugs, hiatus hernia, colonic diverticulosis and bowel tumours (Table 3.5). Some unusual causes of blood loss deserve mention. Cow's milk intolerance in infants may lead to gastrointestinal haemorrhage. Self-induced haemorrhage may occur as an unusual form of Munchausen syndrome. Chronic intravascular haemolysis, such as that in paroxysmal nocturnal haemoglobinuria or mechanical haemolytic anaemia, may be a serious source of urinary iron loss.

Malabsorption

Malabsorption may be the primary cause of iron deficiency or it may prevent the body adjusting to iron deficiency from other causes. Dietary iron is poorly absorbed in gluten-induced enteropathy, in both children and adults. Gluten-induced enteropathy is encountered in about 5% of patients presenting with unexplained iron deficiency anaemia and, conversely, about 50% of patients with newly diagnosed coeliac disease have coexistent iron deficiency anaemia. Patients with this disease often show decreased or no response to oral therapy with inorganic iron.

Helicobacter pylori gastritis appears to be a common cause of iron deficiency, responding favourably to eradication with triple therapy. *Helicobacter pylori* gastritis inhibits gastric hydrochloric acid secretion, interfering with the solubilization and absorption of inorganic food iron but it is also possible that gastrointestinal blood loss plays a significant role in the causation of iron deficiency associated with *H. pylori* infection. Lastly, achlorhydria associated with autoimmune gastritis, an entity preceding and closely related to pernicious anaemia, is an important cause of iron malabsorption due to impaired food iron solubilization. It is encountered in about 20% of patients with unexplained or refractory iron deficiency anaemia, mostly women of fertile age in whom achlorhydria aggravates the consequences of menstrual blood loss.

Iron deficiency occurs in congestive heart failure due to malabsorption and iron loss and these patients may also have the features of the anaemia of chronic disorders. Intravenous iron benefits functional capacity and quality of life even in the absence of anaemia.

Management of iron deficiency

Management entails (i) identification and treatment of the underlying cause and (ii) correction of the deficiency by therapy with inorganic iron. Iron deficiency is commonly due to blood loss and, wherever possible, the site of this must be identified and the lesion treated.

Oral therapy

In most patients, body stores of iron can be restored by oral iron therapy. Iron is equally well absorbed from several simple ferrous iron salts, and as ferrous sulphate is the cheapest, this is the drug of first choice – 200 mg of ferrous sulphate contains 67 mg of iron. Where smaller doses are required, 300 mg of ferrous gluconate provides 36 mg of iron. It is usual to give 100–200 mg of elemental iron each day to adults and about 3 mg/kg per day as a liquid iron preparation to infants and children. The side-effects of oral iron, such as nausea, epigastric pain, diarrhoea and constipation, are related to the amount of available iron they contain. If iron causes gastrointestinal symptoms, these can usually be ameliorated by reducing the dose or taking the iron with food, but this also reduces the amount absorbed. Enteric-coated and sustained-release preparations should not be used, as much of the iron is carried past the duodenum to sites of poor absorption. Iron reduces absorption of tetracyclines (and vice versa) and of ciprofloxacin.

The minimum rate of response should be a 20 g/L rise in haemoglobin every 3 weeks, and the usual rate is 1.5–2.0 g/L daily. This will be slower when the dose tolerated is less than 100 mg/day, but this is seldom of clinical importance. It is usually necessary to give iron for 3–6 months to correct the deficit of iron in circulating haemoglobin and in stores (shown by a rise in serum ferritin to normal).

Failure to respond to oral iron is most commonly due to the patient not taking it, although there may be continued haemorrhage or malabsorption. In non-responding patients it is important to reassess the diagnosis to exclude other causes of microcytic anaemia such as iron-loading anaemias. For instance, many patients with thalassaemia trait, sideroblastic anaemia or other anaemias have been treated with iron before haemoglobin studies, bone marrow examination or other tests have revealed the correct diagnosis. A poor response may also be obtained if the patient has an infection, renal or hepatic failure, an underlying malignant disease or anaemia of inflammation due to high hepcidin levels (which inhibits absorption of therapeutic oral iron) and any other cause of anaemia in addition to iron deficiency.

Parenteral iron therapy

This is usually unnecessary, but it may be given if subjects genuinely cannot tolerate oral iron, particularly if gastrointestinal disease, such as inflammatory bowel disease, is present. It is also occasionally necessary in gluten-induced enteropathy and when it is essential to replete body stores rapidly (e.g. where severe iron deficiency anaemia is first diagnosed in late pregnancy) or when oral iron cannot keep pace with continuing haemorrhage (e.g. in patients with hereditary haemorrhagic telangiectasia). Patients with chronic renal failure who are being treated with recombinant erythropoietin are also likely to require parenteral iron therapy. In this situation, the demand for iron by the expanded erythron may outstrip the ability to mobilize iron from stores, leading to a 'functional' iron deficiency. Increased red cell loss at dialysis contributes to iron needs and oral iron therapy is usually inadequate to prevent an impaired response to erythropoietin. Serum ferritin in this setting is, as in other chronic inflammatory conditions, an unreliable indicator of iron deficiency. The use of transferrin iron saturation, percentage of hypochromic red cells or reticulocyte haemoglobin content for detection of functional iron deficiency is discussed on p. 38. A transferrin saturation of less than 20% indicates functional iron deficiency. Intravenous ferric carboxymaltose has been shown to benefit patients with congestive heart failure and iron deficiency with or without anaemia.

From all parenteral preparations, the iron complex is taken up by macrophages of the reticuloendothelial system, from which iron is released to circulating transferrin, which then transports it to the marrow. In the UK, three preparations are available. Iron dextran (CosmoFer) is given intravenously by slow injection or infusion or deep intramuscularly into the gluteal muscle. An iron–sucrose complex, Venofer, is given by slow intravenous infusion or injection. The deficit in body iron should be calculated from the degree of anaemia; it is usually 1–2 g. In patients receiving erythropoietin treatment in chronic renal failure, smaller intravenous doses of Venofer (25–150 mg/week) may be used, with regular monitoring of serum ferritin to avoid iron overload. Ferrinject is a macromolecular iron(III)-hydroxide carbohydrate complex (molecular weight approximately 150 000). It can be administered as an intravenous bolus (maximum single dose 200 mg) or slow infusion (maximum single dose 1000 mg). Newer intravenous preparations including ferumoxytol and ferrous gluconate (Ferrlecit) may become available.

Parenteral iron should not be used if there is a history of allergy as anaphylaxis occasionally occurs. For iron dextran, a test dose should therefore be given slowly, followed by close medical supervision of the rest of the infusion. Headache, flushing, nausea, skin rashes, urticaria, shivering, general aches and pains, dyspnoea and syncope are possible immediate adverse effects. Delayed reactions, including arthralgia, fever and lymphadenopathy, are well described and can persist for several days. An exacerbation of rheumatoid arthritis may also be precipitated.

Iron refractory iron deficiency anaemia

Homozygous or doubly heterozygous germline frameshift, splice junction or missense mutations of matriptase-2 (*TMPRSS6*) are a cause of iron refractory iron deficiency anaemia. The mutations may affect different conserved domains of the protein, including a trypsin-like serine protease domain. The patients show a microcytic hypochromic anaemia with normal or raised serum and urine hepcidin levels and low serum iron and percentage saturation of iron-binding capacity.

The patients absorb iron poorly and are refractory to oral iron therapy but are partially responsive to parenteral iron.

A microcytic hypochromic anaemia with liver iron overload has also been described in a few patients with homozygous or doubly heterozygous mutations of DMT1. Liver iron stores are increased but erythroid iron utilization is impaired and serum hepcidin levels are low for the degree of iron overload. These patients may respond to erythropoietin injections. The patients are susceptible to infections.

Deficiency of serum transferrin due to mutations of the transferrin gene causes a hypochromic microcytic anaemia with tissue iron overload caused by increased plasma non-transferrin-bound iron and low hepcidin levels. Treatment has been with infusions of fresh frozen plasma or apotransferrin. Deficiency of caeruloplasmin also causes a mild hypochromic microcytic anaemia with iron overload in the liver and progressive neurodegeneration. There is failure of ferroxidase activity, which impairs iron mobilization from stores.

Pathological alterations in haem synthesis

Porphyrias

These are a group of inherited or acquired diseases, each characterized by a partial defect in one of the enzymes of haem synthesis (see Chapter 2). Increased amounts of the intermediates of haem synthesis accumulate, the disorders being classified by whether the effects are predominantly in the liver or the erythron (Table 3.6). A full discussion of these disorders is beyond the scope of this chapter, but those with a particular haematological overlap are mentioned briefly.

Congenital erythropoietic porphyria

This is a very rare autosomal recessive disorder that is due to reduced uroporphyrinogen III synthase activity. Most patients are heteroallelic for mutations in the uroporphyrinogen III synthase gene. A single case with a germline mutation of the X-linked erythroid-specific transcription factor GATA binding protein (GATA-1) has been described. Large amounts of porphyrinogens accumulate, and their conversion by spontaneous oxidation to photoactive porphyrins leads to severe, and disfiguring, cutaneous photosensitivity and dermatitis, as well as a haemolytic anaemia with splenomegaly. Increased amounts of uroporphyrin and coproporphyrin, mainly type I, are found in bone marrow, red cells, plasma, urine and faeces. Ring sideroblasts have been found in the marrow in some cases but rarely in large numbers. The age of onset and clinical severity of the disease are highly variable, ranging from non-immune hydrops fetalis to a later onset in which there are only cutaneous lesions. Treatment, including avoidance of sunlight and splenectomy to improve red cell survival, is only partially effective. High-level

Table 3.6 Human porphyrias.

Form	Inheritance	Enzyme defect	Clinical features*
Hepatic			
Acute intermittent porphyria	Autosomal dominant	Porphobilinogen deaminase	A
Hereditary coproporphyria	Autosomal dominant	Coproporphyrinogen oxidase	A + P
Porphyria variegate	Autosomal dominant	Protoporphyrinogen oxidase	A + P
Porphyria cutanea tarda	Acquired or (rare) autosomal dominant	Uroporphyrinogen decarboxylase	P
Erythropoietic			
Congenital erythropoietic porphyria	Autosomal recessive	Uroporphyrinogen cosynthase	P
Erythropoietic protoporphyria	Autosomal dominant	Ferrochelatase	P

*Acute attacks (A) of the gastrointestinal and/or nervous system are related to the accumulation of porphyrin precursors (δ-aminolaevulinic acid and porphobilinogen). Photosensitive skin lesions (P) are seen when the level of the enzyme defect in the haem synthetic pathway leads to the accumulation of formed porphyrins.

blood transfusions to suppress erythropoiesis (combined with iron chelation therapy) have been used to reduce porphyrin production sufficiently to abolish the clinical symptoms. Allogeneic bone marrow transplantation has been successful.

Erythropoietic protoporphyria

This is the most common erythropoietic porphyria and is usually caused by an autosomal dominant inherited deficiency of ferrochelatase, which results in increased free (not Zn) protoporphyrin concentrations in bone marrow, red cells, plasma and bile. Bone marrow reticulocytes are the primary source of the excess protoporphyrin. This leaks from cells and is excreted in the bile and faeces. Molecular analysis of the ferrochelatase gene has revealed a variety of missense, nonsense and splicing mutations as well as deletions and insertions. The onset of the disease is usually in childhood.

Expression of the gene is variable, and photosensitivity and dermatitis range from mild or absent to moderate in degree. There is little haemolysis, but a mild hypochromic anaemia may occur, and accumulation of protoporphyrins can occasionally lead to severe liver disease. Treatment is by the avoidance of sunlight; β-carotene may also diminish photosensitivity. Iron deficiency should be avoided as this may increase the amount of free protoporphyrin.

Other groups of patients with a variant of erythropoietic protoporphyria have been discovered to have mutations of mitoferrin or gain-of-function mutation of ALAS2.

Porphyria cutanea tarda

This is the most common of the hepatic porphyrias and occurs worldwide. The incidence in the UK has been estimated at 2–5 per million. Type I or 'sporadic' porphyria cutanea tarda (PCT) accounts for 80% of cases of PCT. The underlying metabolic abnormality is decreased activity of uroporphyrinogen decarboxylase (UROD) in the liver. Type II disease is an autosomal dominant disorder caused by mutations in the *UROD* gene. Type III disease is a rare familial form and appears to result from unknown inherited defects that affect hepatic UROD activity. There is a marked increase in porphyrins in liver, plasma, urine and faeces. In the urine, uroporphyrin and heptacarboxylporphyrin predominate, with lesser amounts of coproporphyrin and pentacarboxylporphyrin and hexacarboxylporphyrin. The disease is characterized by photosensitivity and dermatitis. It is precipitated in middle or later life, more often in men than women, by factors such as liver disease, alcohol excess or estrogen therapy. A modest increase in liver iron is a common feature.

Either the homozygous or heterozygous presence of the C282Y and H63D mutations in the *HFE* gene may predispose to the development of PCT. Prevalence of the C282Y mutation is increased in both sporadic (type I) and familial (type II) PCT. In the UK, only homozygosity for C282Y (found in about 25% of patients) is significantly more common than in the general population (0.7%). In southern Europe, where C282Y is much less common, the H63D mutation is associated with PCT. Iron is known to inhibit UROD. Removal of the iron by repeated phlebotomy is standard treatment, usually leading to remission.

Lead poisoning

Chronic ingestion of lead in humans causes an anaemia that is usually normochromic or slightly hypochromic. Red cell lifespan is shortened and there is a mild rise in reticulocytes, but jaundice is rare. Basophilic stippling is a characteristic, though not universal, finding and it is thought to be due to precipitation of RNA, resulting from inhibition of the enzyme pyrimidine 5′-nucleotidase. Siderotic granules, and occasionally Cabot rings, are found in circulating red cells. The bone marrow shows increased sideroblasts, in some patients with ring sideroblasts. Red cell protoporphyrin and coproporphyrin are raised, as is urinary excretion of ALA, coproporphyrin III and uroporphyrin I.

The cause of the anaemia appears to be multifactorial. Haemolysis, probably due to the blocking of sulphydryl groups with consequent denaturation of structural proteins, and damage to mitochondria, with defective haemoglobin production due to inhibition of the enzymes of haem synthesis, are the major factors.

Sideroblastic anaemia

The sideroblastic anaemias comprise a group of refractory anaemias (Table 3.7) in which there are variable numbers of hypochromic cells in the peripheral blood, with an excess of iron in the bone marrow; at least 15% of the developing eryth-

roblasts in the primary forms of anaemia contain iron granules arranged in a ring around the nucleus (Figure 3.7). These ring sideroblasts (Table 3.8) (more than four perinuclear granules per cell and covering one-third or more of the nuclear circumference) are the diagnostic feature of the anaemia. Ring sideroblasts may comprise a small (<15%) population of the erythroblasts in a wide variety of clinical disorders.

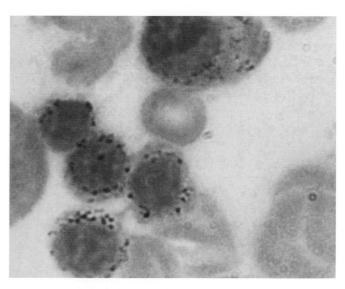

Figure 3.7 Sideroblastic anaemia. Erythroblasts showing perinuclear rings of iron (Perls stain).

Table 3.7 Sideroblastic anaemias.

Hereditary

X-linked
Erythroid-specific ALAS2 (Xp11.21) mutations
Associated with spinocerebellar ataxia: mitochondrial ATP-binding cassette (*ABCB7*) mutations

Autosomal
Thiamine responsive, THTR-1 (*SLC19A2*) mutations: DIDMOAD syndrome
Glutaredoxin-5 (*GLRX5*) mutations
Associated mitochondrial myopathy: pseudouridine synthase-1 mutations
SLC25 family transporter mutations

Mitochondrial
Pearson (marrow–pancreas) syndrome
Kearns–Sayre syndrome

Acquired

Primary
Refractory anaemia with ring sideroblasts

Secondary
Drugs: isoniazid, pyrazinamide, cycloserine, chloramphenicol, penicillamine
Mitochondrial toxicity: alcohol, lead poisoning
Copper deficiency systemic disease: carcinoma, rheumatoid arthritis

DIDMOAD, diabetes insipidus, diabetes mellitus, optic atrophy and deafness.

Table 3.8 Siderocytes and sideroblasts.

Siderocyte	Mature red cell containing one or more siderotic granules (Pappenheimer bodies)
Normal sideroblast	Nucleated red cell containing one or more siderotic granules, granules few, difficult to see, randomly distributed in the cytoplasm, reduced proportion of sideroblasts in iron deficiency and anaemia of chronic disorders
Abnormal sideroblasts	Cytoplasmic iron deposits (ferritin aggregates): increased granulation, granules larger and more numerous than normal, easily visible and randomly distributed, proportion of sideroblasts usually parallels the percentage saturation of transferrin (e.g. haemolytic anaemia, megaloblastic anaemia, iron overload, thalassaemia disorders) Mitochondrial iron deposits (non-ferritin iron): ring sideroblasts in inherited and acquired sideroblastic anaemias

Inherited sideroblastic anaemias

These are rare disorders manifesting mainly in males, usually in childhood or adolescence, but occasionally presenting late in life, when they need to be distinguished from the more common acquired form termed 'refractory anaemia with ring sideroblasts'.

X-linked

ALAS2 mutations

In most reported families, inheritance has followed an X-linked pattern. More than 25 different mutations of the gene for erythroid-specific ALAS2, located at Xp11.21, have been identified. All have been single-base substitutions. Most lead to changes in protein structure, causing instability or loss of function. They are found scattered over the seven exons (out of 11) encoding the C-terminal, catalytically active part of the protein. Mutations affecting the promoter have also been shown to cause disease. Function may be rescued to a variable degree by administration of pyridoxal phosphate (the essential cofactor for ALAS2), the best responses occurring when the mutation affects the pyridoxal phosphate-binding domain of the enzyme. The response is better if iron overload is reduced by phlebotomy or chelation.

Female carriers of X-linked sideroblastic anaemia may show partial haematological expression, usually with only mild or no anaemia, although rarely a severe dimorphic anaemia occurs. This may depend on variation in the severity of the defect, as well as the degree of lyonization of the affected X chromosome. Late onset in some patients suggests that the degree of lyonization may change with age. Iron loading may also aggravate the defect in haem synthesis in both males and females with sideroblastic anaemia.

Patients with X-linked sideroblastic anaemia show a hypochromic, often microcytic, anaemia. There may be a few circulating siderocytes, normoblasts and cells with punctate basophilia, but these features become pronounced only if the spleen has been removed. The bone marrow shows erythroid hyperplasia and the erythroblasts tend to be microcytic with a vacuolated cytoplasm. There are more than 15% ringed sideroblasts. The ineffective erythropoiesis is not usually accompanied by bone deformities, but some bossing of the skull and enlargement of the facial bones may result from the erythroid expansion. The spleen may be enlarged. Patients may present with severe iron overload even when the anaemia is relatively mild, but the rate of iron loading is accelerated if red cell transfusions are needed. Iron loading, however, aggravates the anaemia.

ABCB7 mutations

A rare form of X-linked sideroblastic anaemia is caused by abnormalities in the ATP-binding cassette transporter gene (ABCB7) at Xq13.3. This form is associated with early-onset, non-progressive cerebellar ataxia. A useful diagnostic distinction is the presence within the red cells of increased zinc pro-

toporphyrin, despite adequate iron stores, rather than the low/normal levels found in patients with abnormalities in ALAS2. The anaemia is mild to moderately severe. Three abnormalities of protein structure have been described, and these lie within 34 amino acids of one another at the C-terminal end of the transmembrane domain. The enzyme deficiency induces disruption in the maturation of cytosolic iron–sulphur clusters. The ataxia may be due to iron damage to mitochondria in neural cells.

Autosomal

Mitochondrial myopathy and sideroblastic anaemia

This results from a homozygous mutation in the nuclear-encoded gene for pseudouridine synthase. As in Pearson syndrome, there are defects of the mitochondrial electron transport chain affecting reduced access to ferrochelatase. It has been proposed that deficient pseudouridylation of mitochondrial tRNAs underlies this condition.

Abnormalities of a high-affinity transporter of thiamine

A gene (SLC19A2) encoding a putative thiamine transporter (THTR-1) that is widely and variably expressed has now been mapped to the long arm of chromosome 1 (1q23.3). Abnormalities in this gene are responsible for thiamine-responsive megaloblastic anaemia (Roger syndrome). This syndrome is inherited in an autosomal recessive manner and combines diabetes insipidus, diabetes mellitus, optic atrophy and deafness (DIDMOAD), which respond in varying degrees to pharmacological doses of thiamine (vitamin B_1). Ring sideroblasts in varying numbers are typically present and onset is usually in childhood, although some symptoms may be present in infancy. A direct link between the presence of the mutation and mitochondrial iron loading has yet to be demonstrated.

There are still a substantial number of cases of inherited sideroblastic anaemias in which the exact underlying genetic defect remains obscure. These cases may or may not show sex-linked inheritance and often show a macrocytic or dimorphic picture.

Mutations of glutaredoxin-5 (GLRX5)

This enzyme participates in iron–sulphur cluster formation. A single patient has been described with autosomal recessive hypochromic microcytic anaemia with ring sideroblasts with inherited mutations of the enzyme.

SLC25A38 mutations

This protein is a transporter that may be involved in glycine transfer to the mitochondria, an essential step in synthesis of ALA. Mutation in congenital sideroblastic anaemia is described.

Mitochondrial DNA mutations

Deletions of mitochondrial DNA, sometimes associated with duplications, are known to be the cause of the Pearson marrow–

pancreas syndrome, typically consisting of sideroblastic anaemia, pancreatic exocrine dysfunction and lactic acidosis. This is a severe disorder of early onset, presenting usually with failure to thrive, persistent diarrhoea and lactic acidosis. All haemopoietic cell lineages can be affected, and the anaemia is typically macrocytic with prominent vacuoles in cells of both myeloid and erythroid lineages.

Mitochondrial DNA has its own genetic code and encodes mitochondrial tRNA and ribosomal RNA as well as several mitochondrial proteins. In Pearson syndrome, deletions may encompass tRNA as well as mitochondrial genes and therefore have an effect on the function of all mitochondrion-encoded proteins, causing considerable loss of mitochondrial function. The presence of many different mitochondria within nucleated cells enable the coexistence of normal and abnormal species, the proportion of which is likely to vary within different tissues, a phenomenon known as *heteroplasmy*. The extent to which different tissues are affected depends to some extent on this proportion and detection often requires the study of different tissues. Inheritance is difficult to determine for the same reason and most cases are described as of 'sporadic' occurrence.

Acquired sideroblastic anaemias (see also Chapter 28)

Refractory anaemia with ring sideroblasts

This is a form of myelodysplasia and arises as a clonal disorder of haemopoiesis. The anaemia is often macrocytic with raised red cell protoporphyrin concentrations, in contrast to X-linked sideroblastic anaemia. Marked erythroid hyperplasia may be present, together with increased iron stores. In these patients, abnormalities in the white cell or platelet precursors are usually absent and the risk of transformation to acute myeloid leukaemia appears less than in other myelodysplastic disorders. Smaller numbers (<15%) of ring sideroblasts may be present in patients with any of the other myelodysplastic and myeloproliferative diseases. Recent data suggest that acquired defects of mitochondrial DNA may underlie iron transport abnormalities in refractory anaemia with ring sideroblasts.

Secondary sideroblastic anaemias

Sideroblastic anaemia associated with pyridoxine deficiency has been described, although not completely documented, in a few patients with gluten-induced enteropathy, in pregnancy, and with haemolytic anaemias, such as sickle cell disease and mechanical or autoimmune haemolytic anaemia. Sideroblastic anaemia may be found as a complication of antituberculous chemotherapy, particularly with isoniazid and cycloserine (pyridoxine antagonists). Sideroblastic anaemia occurs in alcoholism if there is associated malnutrition and folate deficiency. Suggested mechanisms include interference with haem formation and pyridoxine metabolism. The anaemia rapidly reverses with abstinence from alcohol, a normal diet and pyridoxine therapy. Chloramphenicol inhibits mitochondrial protein synthesis and in some patients causes ring sideroblast formation, presumably as a result of impaired haem formation in the mitochondria. Lead inhibits several enzymes involved in haem synthesis and may damage structural mitochondrial proteins. In some cases, ring sideroblasts are visible in the marrow. Ring sideroblasts may occur in erythropoietic porphyrias (see p. 41).

Treatment

Pyridoxine

Some patients with X-linked sideroblastic anaemia respond to pyridoxine, given initially in doses of 100–200 mg daily. The response is usually partial. Patients may require only small doses (less than 10 mg daily) to maintain a higher haemoglobin concentration.

Pyridoxine therapy is almost always ineffective in refractory anaemia with ring sideroblasts. However, some secondary sideroblastic anaemias may be completely reversed by pyridoxine therapy. This has been described in alcoholism, haemolytic anaemia and gluten-induced enteropathy, as well as in patients receiving antituberculous chemotherapy, in whom the drugs have been stopped and pyridoxine administered.

Other forms of treatment

Folic acid may benefit patients with secondary anaemia. For refractory patients, the anaemia may remain stable and, if the patient is transfusion independent, no treatment is needed. Patients requiring regular red cell transfusions require iron chelation therapy. Iron loading may aggravate the anaemia and, in some patients, improvement in the anaemia has followed iron removal by phlebotomy or iron chelation therapy. Splenectomy should usually be avoided, as it does not benefit the anaemia and leads to persistently high platelet counts postoperatively, with a high incidence of thromboembolism.

Selected bibliography

Anderson GJ, Frazer DM (2006) Iron metabolism meets signal transduction. *Nature Genetics* 38: 503–4.

Andrews NC (2008) Forging a field: the golden age of iron biology *Blood* 112: 219–30.

Andriopoulos B Jr (2009) BMP6 is a key endogenous regulator of hepcidin expression and iron metabolism. *Nature Genetics* 41: 482–7.

Anker SD, Colet JC, Filippatos G *et al.* (2009) Ferric carboxymaltose in patients with heart failure and iron deficiency. *New England Journal of Medicine* 361: 2436–48.

Babitt JL, Huang FW, Xia Y *et al.* (2007) Modulation of bone morphogenetic protein signalling *in vivo* regulates systemic iron balance. *Journal of Clinical Investigation* 117: 1933–9.

Barrett TG, Bundey S, Macleod AF (1995) Neurodegeneration and diabetes: UK nationwide study of Weifrom (DIDMOAD) syndrome. *Lancet* 346: 1458–63.

Beguin Y (2003) Soluble transferrin receptor for the evaluation of erythropoiesis and iron status. *Clinica Chimica Acta* **329**: 9–22.

Bottomley, S (2006) Congenital sideroblastic anemias. *Current Hematology Reports* **5**: 41–49

Camaschella, C (2008) Recent advances in the understanding of inherited sideroblastic anaemia. *British Journal of Haematology* **143**: 27–38.

Cazzola M (2002) Hereditary hyperferritinaemia/cataract syndrome. *Best Practice and Research. Clinical Haematology* **15**: 385–98.

De Domenico I, McVey Ward D, Kaplan J (2008) Regulation of iron acquisition and storage: consequences for iron-linked disorders. *Nature Reviews. Molecular Cell Biology* **9**: 72–81.

Drysdale J, Arosio P, Invernizzi R *et al.* (2002) Mitochondrial ferritin: a new player in iron metabolism. *Blood Cells, Molecules and Diseases* **29**: 376–83.

Du X, She E, Gelbart T (2008) The serine protease TMPRSS6 is required to sense iron deficiency. *Science* **320**: 1088–92.

Finberg KE, Heeney MM, Campagna DR *et al.* (2008) Mutations in TMPRSS6 cause iron-refractory iron deficiency anaemia (IRIDA). *Nature Genetics* **40**: 569–71.

Goswami T, Andrews NC (2006) Hereditary hemochromatosis protein, HFE, interaction with transferrin receptor 2 suggests a molecular mechanism for mammalian iron sensing. *Journal of Biological Chemistry* **281**: 28494–8.

Hershko C, Hoffbrand AV, Keret D (2005) Role of autoimmune gastritis, *Helicobacter pylori* and coeliac disease in refractory or unexplained iron deficiency anaemia. *Haematologica* **90**: 585–95.

Hoffbrand AV (ed.) (2009) Recent advances in the understanding of iron metabolism and iron-related diseases. *Acta Haematologica* **122**: 75–184, 12 articles covering all aspects of iron metabolism and related diseases.

Iolascon A, De Falco L, Beaumont C (2009) Molecular basis of inherited microcytic anaemia due to defects in iron acquisitions or haem synthesis. *Haematologica* **94**: 395–408.

Lakhal S, Talbot NP, Crosby A *et al.* (2009) Regulation of growth differentiation factor 15 expression by intracellular iron. *Blood* **113**: 1555–63.

Lebay V, Ras T, Baran D *et al.* (1999) Mutations in SCL19AZ cause thiamine-responsive megaloblastic anaemia associated with diabetes mellitus and deafness. *Nature Genetics* **22**: 300–4.

Locatelli F, Aljama P, Bárány P *et al.* (2004) Revised European best practice guidelines for the management of anaemia in patients with chronic renal failure. *Nephrology, Dialysis, Transplantation* **19** (Suppl. 2): 1–47.

Lozoff B, De Andraca I, Castillo M *et al.* (2003) Behavioural and developmental effects of preventing iron-deficiency anaemia in healthy full-term infants. *Pediatrics* **112**: 846–54.

Mehta A, Beck M, Eyskens F *et al.* (2010) Fabry disease: a review of current management strategies. *Quarterly Journal of Medicine*, epub ahead of print.

Meynard D, Kautz L, Darnaud V *et al.* (2009) Lack of the bone morphogenetic protein BMP6 induces massive iron overload. *Nature Genetics* **41**: 478–81.

Online Mendelian Inheritance in Man (OMIM) Available at www.ncbi.nlm.nih.gov/OMIM/. Knowledge base of human genes and genetic disorders.

Peyssonnaux C, Zinkernagel AS, Schuepbach RA *et al.* (2007) Regulation of iron homeostasis by the hypoxia-inducible transcription factors (HIFs). *Journal of Clinical Investigation* **117**: 1926–32.

Ramsay AJ, Hooper JD, Folgueras AR *et al.* (2009) Matriptase-2 (TMPRSS6): a proteolytic regulator of iron homeostasis. *Haematologica* **94**: 840–9.

Silvestri L, Pagani A, Nai A *et al.* (2008) The serine protease matriptase-2 (TMPRSS6) inhibits hepcidin activation by cleaving membrane hemojuvelin. *Cell Metabolism* **6**: 502–11.

Srai SK, Bomford A, McArdle HJ (2002) Iron transport across cell membranes: molecular understanding of duodenal and placental iron transport. *Best Practice and Research. Clinical Haematology* **15**: 243–59.

Tanno T, Bhanu NV, Oneal PA *et al.* (2007) High levels of GDF15 in thalassemia suppress expression of the iron regulatory protein hepcidin. *Nature Medicine* **13**: 1096–101.

WHO (2001) *Iron Deficiency Anaemia. Assessment, Prevention and Control. A Guide for Programme Managers*. World Health Organization, Geneva.

Wrighting DM, Andrews NC (2006) Interleukin-6 induces hepcidin expression through STAT3. *Blood* **108**: 3204–9.

Zhang AS, Enns CA (2009) Iron homeostasis: recently identified proteins provide insight into novel control mechanisms. *Journal of Biological Chemistry* **284**: 711–15.

Iron overload

4

Clara Camaschella[1] and A Victor Hoffbrand[2]

[1]Vita-Salute University, Milan, Italy
[2]Royal Free and University College Medical School, Royal Free Hospital, London, UK

Introduction

Excessive iron accumulation may eventually lead to tissue damage. Iron overload of the parenchymal cells of the liver commonly arises when there is excessive iron absorption, whereas iron administered parenterally (e.g. as multiple transfusions) is first taken up in senescent red cells by macrophages. However, there is no absolute distinction between the two sources of iron loading, as iron in macrophages is slowly released to transferrin, from which it can be taken up by parenchymal cells. Causes of iron overload are shown in Table 4.1. Severe iron overload, arbitrarily defined as an excess of more than 5 g, is confined to the genetic haemochromatoses, together with the iron-loading anaemias and sub-Saharan African dietary iron overload.

Genetic haemochromatosis

Classification

Genetic haemochromatosis is now classified according to the genetic defect causing iron overload (Table 4.2). The vast majority of cases are of type 1, involving the *HFE* gene (see Chapter 3). In populations of northern European origin, about 90% of patients with haemochromatosis are homozygous for the *HFE* Cys282Tyr mutation (C282Y). In southern Europe, homozygosity for C282Y is found in only about 60% of patients

Postgraduate Haematology: 6th edition. Edited by A. Victor Hoffbrand, Daniel Catovsky, Edward G.D. Tuddenham, Anthony R. Green
© 2011 Blackwell Publishing Ltd.

with haemochromatosis. Type 2, the severe juvenile haemochromatosis caused by mutations of the hemojuvelin or hepcidin genes, type 3, due to mutations of transferrin receptor 2, and type 4, due to mutations of ferroportin, are all very rare disorders reported mainly in European countries but also identified in some Asian patients with novel mutations. Types 1, 2 and 3 are autosomal recessive diseases and share common features due to hepcidin deficiency, including high transferrin saturation and hepatocyte iron accumulation. Type 4 haemochromatosis, inherited as a dominant condition, is a heterogeneous disease with variable clinical phenotype.

Type 1 haemochromatosis

This is one of the most common genetic conditions found in populations of northern European origin but it also occurs in African and Asian populations at very low gene frequency. In the UK, about one in eight people are carriers of the C282Y mutation of the *HFE* gene, and about 1 in 200 are homozygous for this mutation. Homozygosity is strongly associated with haemochromatosis, with about 90% of patients with genetic iron overload having this genotype. In homozygotes, there is a gradual accumulation of iron, leading to tissue damage, which may present as cirrhosis of the liver, diabetes, hypogonadism, cardiomyopathy, arthritis and a slate-grey skin pigmentation. Hepatocellular carcinoma develops in 25% of established cases with cirrhosis. Most patients present between the ages of 40 and 60 years, but the clinical penetrance is low (see p. 50). Full phenotypic expression of the disorder is dependent on other factors, including dietary iron intake, blood donations or blood loss and other genetic factors modifying the genotype. Menstrual losses and pregnancies account for a generally delayed onset in women.

Nature of the defect

A defect in the regulation of intestinal iron absorption leading to increased mucosal iron transfer to plasma is due to deficient hepcidin production. The responsible gene, *HFE*, is an atypical MHC class I-like gene that maps to the short arm of chromosome 6. The reported association with HLA-A3 and, to a lesser extent, B7 suggested a founder mutation in a chromosome carrying the A3, B7 haplotype. In over 80% of patients there is homozygosity for a G→A substitution at nucleotide 845 of the *HFE* gene that results in a cysteine to tyrosine substitution at

Table 4.1 Causes of iron overload.

Severe iron overload (>5 g excess)

Excess iron absorption

Hereditary haemochromatosis

Massive ineffective erythropoiesis (e.g. β-thalassaemia intermedia, sideroblastic anaemia, congenital dyserythropoietic anaemia)

Increased iron intake

Sub-Saharan dietary iron overload (in combination with a genetic determinant of increased absorption)

Excess parenteral iron therapy

Repeated red cell transfusions

Congenital anaemias (e.g. β-thalassaemia major, sickle cell anaemia, red cell aplasia)

Acquired refractory anaemias (e.g. myelodysplasia, aplastic anaemia)

Modest iron overload (<5 g excess)

Chronic liver disease (e.g. alcoholic cirrhosis)

Porphyria cutanea tarda

Rare genetic disorders of iron metabolism (e.g. atransferrinaemia, acaeruloplasminaemia, DMT1 mutations)

Focal iron overload*

Pulmonary haemorrhage, idiopathic pulmonary haemosiderosis

Chronic haemoglobinuria (e.g. paroxysmal nocturnal haemoglobinuria)

---

*May occur in association with general body iron deficiency.

amino acid 282 (C282Y). A second variant (187C→G) results in a histidine to aspartic acid substitution at amino acid 63 (His63Asp or H63D). This is carried by about 20% of the general population. In the UK, about 90% of patients presenting with haemochromatosis are homozygous for *HFE* C282Y, and another 4% are compound heterozygotes for the two mutations. That *HFE* was the haemochromatosis gene was confirmed by the demonstration that *HFE* knockout mice and mice homozygous for the C282Y mutation develop iron overload.

Hepcidin synthesis requires expression of *HFE* and in mice lacking *HFE* or expressing the C282Y protein hepcidin is low or at least inappropriate to the degree of iron overload (see Chapter 3). In addition, tissue-specific inactivation of HFE protein in hepatocytes but not in duodenal cells or macrophages leads to iron overload, indicating a specific function of HFE in the liver. Hepcidin is a negative regulator of iron absorption by binding ferroportin and causing its internalization and lysosomal degradation. Lack of hepcidin upregulates ferroportin expression in duodenal mucosa, thus increasing mucosal iron transfer to transferrin and leaving the duodenal cells iron deficient. Hepcidin also controls iron release from macrophages. Low hepcidin explains the findings in the early stages of haemochromatosis: increased iron absorption, a raised serum iron and a paucity of iron in macrophages. Most recent data suggest that all types of haemochromatosis (except Type 4; Table 4.2) are characterized by low hepcidin secretion, the defect being the most severe in juvenile haemochromatosis. The more recent model of the pathophysiology of the disease suggests that HFE competes with diferric transferrin for TFR1 binding and that when diferric transferrin binds TFR1, HFE is free to bind TFR2, thus forming a complex that results in hepcidin synthesis (see Chapter 3). Lack of HFE on the hepatic cell plasma membrane in the case of C282Y homozygosity will lead to decreased hepcidin synthesis.

HFE mutation frequencies worldwide

HFE genotypes have been reported from large population studies throughout the world. In a study of 100 000 multiethnic participants from primary care practices, the estimated prevalence of the C282Y homozygous genotype was higher in white

Table 4.2 Classification of genetic haemochromatosis.

Type	Gene	Inheritance and phenotype	Severity	Incidence
1	*HFE*	AR, parenchymal iron overload	Highly variable	Common
2 (juvenile)	Hemojuvelin (*HFE2*)	AR, parenchymal iron overload	Severe	Rare
	Hepcidin (*HAMP*)	AR, parenchymal iron overload	Severe	Rare
3	*TFR2*	AR, parenchymal iron overload	Variable	Rare
4	Ferroportin 1 (*SLC11A3*)	AD, RE iron or parenchymal iron	Variable	Rare

AD, autosomal dominant; AR, autosomal recessive; RE, reticuloendothelial.

For gene symbols see Table 3.1.

(1 in 227, 0.44%) than in black or Asian people, in whom it was extremely rare. The frequency is higher in northern Europe and lower in southern Italy and Greece. The H63D mutation is found throughout the world but is most common in Europe, where allele frequencies vary from 10 to 20%, with a mean of 15%. Other *HFE* gene mutations associated with iron accumulation have been described mostly in individual families.

HFE mutations and iron status

The haemochromatosis gene may have increased in frequency because of a selective advantage for heterozygotes, namely protection against iron deficiency anaemia. Homozygotes would be unlikely to suffer the effects of iron overload before reproducing. Transferrin saturation and serum ferritin are significantly higher in C282Y/C282Y subjects than in other genotypes. Increased levels of iron parameters are present in 75–100% of males and 40–60% of females in different studies. In population surveys slight but significantly higher values for serum iron and transferrin saturation have been found in heterozygotes for either C282Y or H63D compared with subjects lacking these mutations. The differences in ferritin levels are smaller and not significant. In compound heterozygotes, and those homozygous for H63D, there are larger increases in transferrin saturation and serum ferritin, although significant iron accumulation is rare. In heterozygotes for C282Y or H63D, haemoglobin levels are slightly higher than in subjects lacking these mutations, but it has not been clearly demonstrated that this leads to a lower prevalence of anaemia among women carrying either mutation.

HFE mutations and morbidity

Although advanced haemochromatosis is characterized by diabetes, arthritis and cirrhosis, there is no evidence that possession of *HFE* mutations is a risk factor for these conditions except through iron overload. The frequency of homozygosity or heterozygosity for C282Y or H63D mutations is not generally increased in patients with arthritis, diabetes and heart disease. Homozygosity for C282Y is more frequent in patients with cirrhosis and hepatoma than in the general population. Alcohol is a definite risk factor for the development of cirrhosis in patients homozygous for C282Y. The significance of other genetic modifiers remains uncertain.

Diagnosis: clinical

The variety of clinical presentations and their lack of specificity for haemochromatosis means that a high degree of clinical suspicion is needed. Fatigue, diabetes mellitus, signs and symptoms of gonadal failure and arthritis may be present for several years before the diagnosis is made. Arthritis particularly affects the second and third metacarpophalangeal joints (Figure 4.1), and destructive arthropathy of hip and knee joints occurs in 10% of patients. There is chondrocalcinosis with pyrophosphate deposition in the joints. Abdominal pain may result from

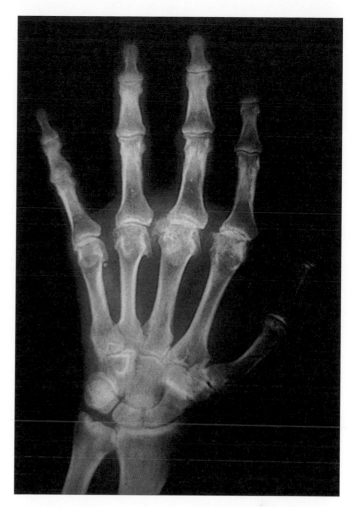

Figure 4.1 Radiograph of hand: patient with haemochromatosis showing loss of joint space and erosion of cartilage at the metacarpophalangeal joints.

hepatic enlargement or hepatocellular carcinoma. Grey skin pigmentation results from excess melanin deposition.

Diagnosis: iron status

Transferrin saturation and serum ferritin

In asymptomatic subjects, iron accumulation is indicated by a raised transferrin saturation (> 45%). Most men and about 50% of women who are homozygous for *HFE* C282Y will have a raised transferrin saturation. As iron accumulates, the serum ferritin concentration rises, and values in excess of 200 µg/L (women) and 300 µg/L (men) suggest iron overload. Serum ferritin concentrations largely reflect iron turnover in phagocytic cells and do not provide an early indication of iron accumulation in liver parenchymal cells. Thus, measurement of transferrin saturation is essential for early detection of iron loading. However, in patients with infection, inflammation or malignancy or in those undergoing surgery, transferrin saturation may be depressed and the serum ferritin concentration elevated. In most cases, *HFE* genotyping will confirm the diagnosis of haemochromatosis.

Liver biopsy

Since the advent of genetic testing, confirmation of iron overload by liver biopsy is not usually performed and is not necessary in the absence of liver damage. In patients homozygous for C282Y with evidence of liver disease and serum ferritin concentration above 1000 μg/L, liver biopsy is essential to assess tissue damage. In patients with an unexplained raised transferrin saturation and serum ferritin, who are not homozygous for C282Y, a liver biopsy may be required to confirm iron overload and to address the subsequent diagnostic process (Figure 4.2). The availability of non-invasive measurement of liver iron concentration has restricted the diagnostic use of liver biopsy.

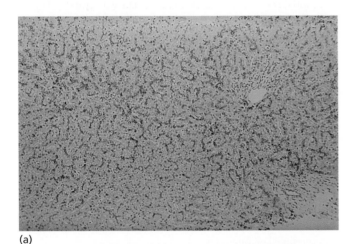

(a)

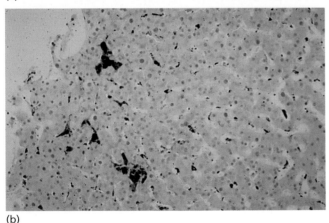

(b)

Figure 4.2 Liver histology (Perls stain). (a) Liver biopsy from a patient with type 1 haemochromatosis, showing staining predominantly in parenchymal cells. (b) Liver biopsy from a patient with type 4 haemochromatosis, showing iron staining predominantly in Kupffer cells.

Liver iron concentration can be measured on a dried fragment of liver biopsy. Values in excess of 80 μmol/g dry weight (4.5 mg/g dry weight) indicate iron overload. Since in haemochromatosis there is a progressive increase in liver iron concentration with age in some cases, it is useful to express the result as the 'hepatic iron index' (μmol iron/g dry weight divided by age in years).

Non-invasive methods

Techniques using magnetic resonance imaging (MRI) are being increasingly used as an indirect non-invasive measure of both liver and heart iron (see p. 55). They require special analytical skill. Although most experience is with secondary iron overload, MRI is also increasingly used in genetic haemochromatosis.

The superconducting quantum interface device (SQUID) biosusceptometry technique is sensitive, accurate and reproducible. It depends on the paramagnetic properties of haemosiderin and ferritin. Unlike MRI, it does not distinguish parenchymal from reticuloendothelial iron, but the result closely correlates with chemical estimation of liver iron, except when fibrosis is present. Machines are expensive to build and run and at present there are only four worldwide (none in the UK).

Mobilization of iron by phlebotomy to calculate iron stores

The amount of iron removed to reach iron depletion can be calculated (see Treatment) and provides a good estimate of total body iron. Since the advent of genetic testing, confirmation of iron overload by liver biopsy is not necessary in the absence of liver damage and quantitative phlebotomy provides the only practical way of confirming the presence of iron overload. The amount of iron removed at each venesection is calculated by weighing the blood bag before and after venesection (density of blood is 1.05 g/mL) and assuming that 450 mL of blood (haemoglobin concentration 13.5 g/dL) contains 200 mg of iron. Iron absorption should be allowed for at the rate of 3 mg daily (20 mg/week). With these assumptions, 25 weekly venesections will remove 4.5 g of iron. The amount of storage iron measured by the technique in normal adults has been shown to be about 750 mg in men and 250 mg in women.

Clinical penetrance

Before the discovery of the *HFE* gene, it was assumed that every family member who was homozygous for haemochromatosis would eventually accumulate sufficient iron to cause tissue damage. Recent studies, in which subjects homozygous for *HFE* C282Y have been compared with 'wild-type' subjects, have shown that the frequencies of lethargy, arthralgia and diabetes are the same. There is, however, a small but significant increase in the percentage of subjects with either raised serum transaminase activity or fibrosis/cirrhosis in the C282Y homozygous group in several studies. Population surveys have shown that less than 5% of subjects homozygous for C282Y ever receive a diagnosis of haemochromatosis. Despite much debate about ascertainment bias in family and population surveys, it is becoming clear that most men who are homozygous for C282Y will have a raised transferrin saturation before the age of 30 years; a proportion will have an elevated serum ferritin concentration, but only a minority will eventually develop fibrosis and cirrhosis of the liver. Studies in Australia and Norway found that 5% of homozygote males but no females showed cirrhosis. There is evidence that ferritin concentration above 1000 μg/L is a risk factor for liver fibrosis in different studies. These patients should undergo liver biopsy and complete cardiac and endocrinological evaluation. Only about 50% of homozygous women have a raised transferrin saturation, and progression through iron accumulation and tissue damage is usually, but not always, slower. In one population study in the USA, based on reported clinical complications, the clinical penetrance was estimated to be as low as 1%. In a more recent study, which evaluated for 12 years a cohort of C282Y homozygous patients of middle age (40–69 years) using strict criteria to define liver disease, this clinical complication was estimated to be present in about 30% of males and 1% of females. However, the iron accumulation rate of C282Y patients is not constant and may vary greatly from patient to patient. Many homozygotes followed for 10 years or more have shown no change in serum ferritin.

Family testing

Physicians should discuss with the patient the desirability of testing all first-degree relatives over the age of consent in order to identify those at risk. Transferrin saturation and serum ferritin concentration should be measured along with *HFE* genotyping. Genetic testing may identify other family members homozygous for *HFE* C282Y. If the serum ferritin concentration is normal and there is no evidence of liver disease, transferrin saturation and serum ferritin should be measured at yearly intervals and treatment instituted if necessary. Compound heterozygotes are at lesser risk of iron overload but should also be tested by measuring transferrin saturation and serum ferritin, perhaps at 3-yearly intervals. Iron status should be determined in heterozygotes and, if normal, reassessed after 5 years to ensure that no other iron-loading genes are present.

Associations with other conditions

The *HFE* C282Y mutation is relatively common; heterozygosity, and even homozygosity, may occur with other haematological conditions, including inherited sideroblastic anaemia. The occasional presence of iron overload in patients with haematological disorders such as congenital spherocytosis, in whom it is otherwise uncommon, may be due to a combined effect on iron absorption of increased erythropoiesis and coincidental inheritance of the heterozygous state for haemochromatosis.

Porphyria cutanea tarda, which may be associated with iron overload, an important trigger of disease manifestations, is discussed in Chapter 3.

Population screening

Widespread population screening by iron status or genetic testing is considered unwarranted as the level of risk for a C282Y homozygote developing iron overload appears to be low. Once the factors that convey a high risk of developing significant iron overload and tissue damage have been identified, it may be appropriate to reconsider this question but at present screening should be limited to at-risk populations.

Treatment

Removal of excess iron by regular phlebotomy greatly reduces the mortality from cardiac and hepatic failure, although hepatocellular carcinoma accounts for a substantial proportion of deaths in those with established disease. Early diagnosis is therefore a priority, as patients identified and treated before the onset of cirrhosis of the liver have a normal life expectancy.

Since no test is available to identify those patients who will progress to fibrosis and those who will not, the present recommendation is to phlebotomize all patients with evidence of iron overload. Phlebotomy should be at a rate of 450 mL of blood each week and should be performed until iron depletion is reached (serum ferritin <20 μg/L and transferrin saturation <16%). Haemoglobin levels should be measured weekly and the rate of venesection reduced if anaemia develops. Serum ferritin should be monitored monthly. The transferrin saturation should be measured weekly when the ferritin concentration drops below 50 μg/L.

Weekly phlebotomy will need to be continued for at least 6 months to remove total iron excess, which is usually greater than 5 g in established symptomatic disease but may be more than 20 g. When iron stores are exhausted, the frequency of phlebotomy should be reduced to two to four units each year, to continue indefinitely. The aim is to maintain a normal transferrin saturation (<50%) and a serum ferritin in the low-normal range (<50 μg/L). Fatigue and transaminase elevation usually reverse on venesection. In some patients, diabetes mellitus, hypogonadism and arthralgia improve, but cirrhosis and arthritis are not reversible. Early cardiac disease may respond to phlebotomy but severe cardiomyopathy does not and requires iron chelation.

Iron chelation with subcutaneous desferrioxamine (DFX) may be used in patients who do not tolerate phlebotomy or have concomitant anaemia. DFX given as a continuous intravenous infusion with or without an oral iron chelator (see below) may have a role in the short-term management of patients with life-threatening cardiac failure. Well-tolerated oral iron chelators are likely to become an option for treatment of selected patients in the future.

Type 2 (juvenile) haemochromatosis

Juvenile haemochromatosis is a rare autosomal recessive disease, with clinical symptoms related to iron overload appearing in the second and third decades of life. The disease is genetically heterogeneous since it can be due either to hemojuvelin mutations or, more rarely, to mutations in the hepcidin (*HAMP*) gene (see Chapter 3). More than 30 hemojuvelin mutations have been reported in European and Asian families with G320V being the most frequent. The age of onset has been as low as 5 years but the disease usually presents in teenagers or those in their early twenties. Hemojuvelin modulates hepcidin expression by acting as a coreceptor of bone morphogenetic proteins (see Chapter 3). Inactivation of hemojuvelin strongly decreases hepcidin production. This explains why the clinical phenotypes of *HAMP* or hemojuvelin (*HFE2*) mutations are indistinguishable. In both cases iron absorption is greater than in type 1 haemochromatosis and iron deposition occurs not only in the hepatocytes but also in cardiac myocytes, pancreas and pituitary; liver disease is present but symptoms related to cardiomyopathy, diabetes and hypogonadism are more prominent.

Digenic disease has been rarely described in patients with severe disease expression who are heterozygous for *HFE* C282Y and have a mutation in the *HAMP* (hepcidin) gene.

Type 3 haemochromatosis

Haemochromatosis type 3 is a rare autosomal recessive disease reported in those of European and Asian ancestry. It is phenotypically similar to type 1 haemochromatosis, although it may have an earlier age of onset. It is due to mutations in the gene for transferrin receptor 2 (*TFR2*) (see Table 4.2). TFR2 shows moderate homology to TFR1, may bind transferrin but is not iron regulated. Hepcidin levels are very low in type 3 haemochromatosis, disproportionate to the degree of iron overload (see Table 3.1). TFR2 binds HFE when transferrin saturation is high and this complex activates hepcidin (see Chapter 3). Thus mutations of either *HFE* or *TFR2* cause a similar disorder.

Type 4 haemochromatosis (ferroportin disease)

Haemochromatosis type 4 has peculiar genetic and clinical features compared with the other forms. First, it is inherited as an autosomal dominant trait. Second, all patients have increased serum ferritin levels, but some have a normal transferrin saturation. Third, at liver biopsy iron is usually increased in the reticuloendothelial cells, as well as in hepatocytes, features that suggest a different pathophysiology of the disease. Haemochromatosis type 4 is due to heterozygous missense mutations in the gene for the iron exporter ferroportin, located on chromosome 2q32. In the typical form (type 4a), so-called ferroportin disease, the phenotype differs from haemochromatosis and is similar to that found in the anaemia of chronic disease (see Figure 4.2b), with iron accumulation predominantly in the macrophages and normal or low transferrin saturation. These cases are due to loss-of-function ferroportins that are unable to target correctly to the cell surface and so export iron from macrophages. It seems that reticuloendothelial iron is less toxic than parenchymal iron. For this reason and because some of these patients develop mild anaemia, tolerance to phlebotomy should be carefully monitored and intensive regimens are not indicated. In the rare type 4b with mutations occurring in the binding site of ferroportin for hepcidin, mutant ferroportins reach the cell surface but are resistant to the effect of hepcidin, causing increased iron export to plasma, saturation of transferrin and iron deposition in hepatocytes similar to *HFE* haemochromatosis.

In people of African origin, the Gln248His mutation in ferroportin is a common variant that may be associated with a tendency to iron loading and mild anaemia.

Neonatal haemochromatosis

This is a condition that is recognized at birth but may occur *in utero*. It is characterized by heavy parenchymal iron deposition in several organs and irreversible liver failure. The only therapeutic option used to be liver transplantation. No mutations in the known haemochromatosis genes have been reported and a genetic cause has been more recently doubted in favour of an immunological pathogenesis, but heterogeneous causes cannot be ruled out. Neonatal haemochromatosis has been linked in some cases to the presence of a maternal factor, for example an antiribonuclear factor antibody. Infusions of gammaglobulin in pregnancy appear to reduce the severity of the condition and it has been proposed that the disease is due to an alloantibody (as rhesus incompatibility) but the target antigen is unknown.

Increased iron intake

African iron overload (Bantu siderosis) results from the combination of a dietary component (a traditional beer that contains iron) and an unknown susceptibility gene. Mutations in the *HFE* gene have been excluded but mutations of the ferroportin gene may play a role (see above). Iron deposition, as in type 4 haemochromatosis, occurs in both hepatocytes and reticuloendothelial cells. Serum ferritin is usually elevated, but transferrin saturation may be normal. The condition occurs in sub-Saharan Africa. It is a cause of hepatic fibrosis and cirrhosis, and associations with diabetes mellitus, peritonitis, scurvy and osteoporosis have been described. The iron overload is associated with a poor outcome of tuberculosis, an infection that is highly prevalent in sub-Saharan Africa.

Other causes of iron overload

Atransferrinaemia

This is a rare recessive genetic disorder associated with a severe hypochromic anaemia with, in some cases, excessive deposition of non-transferrin-bound iron (NTBI) in the parenchymal cells. In all cases tested, some iron-transferrin has been detected by iron-binding ability or immunologically defining a type of hypotransferrinaemia. Complete absence of transferrin would presumably lead to fetal death.

Iron and neurodegeneration

Acaeruloplasminaemia

This is also a rare recessive disorder in which there is a deficiency of ferroxidase activity as a consequence of mutations in the caeruloplasmin gene. Clinically, the condition presents in middle age, with progressive degeneration of the retina and basal ganglia and with diabetes mellitus. Iron accumulates in the liver, pancreas and brain with smaller amounts in the heart, kidneys, thyroid, spleen and retina. The serum iron is low and mild anaemia may be present. The total iron-binding capacity of transferrin (TIBC) is normal and ferritin is normal or raised. Unfortunately, no effective treatment is available to reduce neurodegeneration but deferiprone, which penetrates the blood–brain barrier, may be an option.

Hallervorden–Spatz syndrome

This is an autosomal recessive neurodegenerative disorder associated with iron accumulation in the brain. Clinical features include extrapyramidal dysfunction, onset in childhood and a relentlessly progressive course. Histological study reveals iron deposits in the basal ganglia. Hallervorden–Spatz syndrome is caused by a defect in a novel pantothenate kinase gene that causes accumulation of cysteine. Iron binding by cysteine may cause iron accumulation and oxidative stress, which is a likely explanation for the pathophysiology of the disease.

Neuroferritinopathy

A rare, dominantly inherited, late-onset basal ganglia disease that variably presents with extrapyramidal features similar to those of Huntington disease or parkinsonism also shows iron accumulation in the forebrain and cerebellum. The responsible gene (*FTL*) codes for ferritin light-chain polypeptide. An adenine insertion at position 460–461 was found that was predicted to alter carboxy-terminal residues of the gene product. Abnormal aggregates of ferritin and iron in the brain contrasted with low serum ferritin levels.

These diseases may serve as a model for complex neurodegenerative diseases such as Parkinson disease, Alzheimer disease and Huntington disease, in which accumulation of iron in the brain is also observed. Possession of the C282Y mutation of the *HFE* gene does not appear to be a risk factor for these conditions.

Friedreich ataxia

This is a neurodegenerative disease characterized by loss of sensory neurones in the spinal cord and dorsal root ganglia. There is mitochondrial iron overload and loss of activity of iron–sulphur cluster-containing enzymes. Patients frequently die from cardiomyopathy. The majority of cases of Friedreich ataxia result from the expansion of triple nucleotide repeats within an intron of the *FXN* gene, leading to reduced expression of frataxin mRNA and protein. Point mutations have also been identified in a small number of cases. Frataxin is found in the mitochondria where, in Friedreich ataxia, there is increased oxidative stress and decreased activity of iron–sulphur proteins. Oxidative damage following iron accumulation is thought to precipitate the neurone loss. This is confirmed by experiments in yeast that show that iron is redistributed to the mitochondria of Yfh (yeast frataxin homologue)-deficient yeast and that this iron accumulation precedes oxidative damage. Frataxin shows structural similarity to ferritin, suggesting that frataxin may regulate mitochondrial iron homeostasis by storing excess iron. A preliminary trial of deferiprone therapy has shown some improvement in neuropathy and gait in the youngest patients and larger-scale trials are now in progress.

Hereditary hyperferritinaemia–cataract syndrome

This syndrome is characterized by elevated serum ferritin levels, early-onset bilateral cataracts and normal or low serum iron and transferrin saturation. It is usually due to heterozygous point mutations in the L-ferritin iron-response element so that a monoclonal ferritin is synthesized due to impaired negative feedback of ferritin synthesis. There is no general tissue iron overload and serum transferrin saturation is normal, but ferritin accumulates in the lens causing cataracts. In a few cases, the mutation is in the coding regions of the gene.

Iron-loading anaemias

Removal of iron is essential in patients with transfusion-dependent anaemias, such as thalassaemia major, to prevent death from iron overload, usually caused by cardiac failure or arrhythmia. Red blood cell requirements are about 160 mL/kg annually in non-splenectomized and 120 mL/kg annually in splenectomized patients with thalassaemia major. The iron content of each transfusion is determined by volume (mL) × haematocrit × 1.16 mg. Intake of iron ranges from 0.32 to 0.64 mg/kg body weight daily. Patients with anaemias associated with increased iron absorption (e.g. thalassaemia intermedia), who are too anaemic to be venesected to remove iron, may also require iron chelation therapy, although the rate of iron loading is considerably lower at about 0.1 mg/kg daily. The iron-chelating drug widely available is desferrioxamine (DFX).

Table 4.3 Characteristics of desferrioxamine, deferiprone and deferasirox.

	Desferrioxamine	*Deferiprone*	*Deferasirox*
Structure	Hexadentate	Bidentate	Tridentate
Molecular weight	560	139	373
Iron–chelator complex	1:1	1:3	1:2
Plasma clearance ($t_{1/2}$)	20 min	53–166 min	1–16 hours
Absorption	Negligible	Peak 45 min	Peak 1–2.9 hours
Iron excretion	Urine + faecal	Urine	Faecal
Therapeutic daily dose	40 mg/kg	75–100 mg/kg	20–30 mg/kg
Route	Parenteral	Oral	Oral
Clinical experience	>40 years	>20 years	>8 years
Side-effects	Ototoxicity, retinal toxicity, growth defects, cartilage and bone abnormalities	Agranulocytosis, arthropathy, gastrointestinal disturbance, transient transaminitis, zinc deficiency	Skin rashes, gastrointestinal disturbance, rising serum creatinine

This is orally inactive and given by slow subcutaneous or intravenous infusion. Deferiprone, an orally active iron chelator first used clinically in 1987, is now licensed in 61 countries. A third drug, deferasirox, is orally active and was introduced into clinical practice in 2002 and is now widely prescribed (Table 4.3 and see Figure 4.5).

Iron chelation therapy is monitored by:
1 tests of body iron burden;
2 tests of function of the organs sensitive to iron overload (Table 4.4);
3 tests to detect potential side-effects of the particular chelating drug being used.

Tests (1) and (2) are discussed first. The results and side-effects with the individual iron-chelating drugs are then described.

Tests of body iron burden

Serum ferritin
Serum ferritin is useful in monitoring changes in body iron, although the absolute level is an imprecise measure of total body iron. There is a wide range of liver iron at any given serum ferritin level. This is partly because serum ferritin mainly reflects reticuloendothelial iron and partly because inflammation, (e.g. hepatitis C infection) raises the level, whereas vitamin C deficiency, frequent in iron overload, lowers it. The Thalassaemia International Federation (TIF) guidelines recommend maintaining the level below 1000 µg/L in thalassaemia major.

Liver iron
Liver iron may be measured chemically after liver biopsy, by MRI or, in a few specialized units, by SQUID (see p. 50). Chemical estimation is the gold standard but can be inaccurate

Table 4.4 Monitoring for iron-induced organ damage.

Cardiac function
ECG ± exercise
24-hour monitoring
Echocardiography, MUGA ± stress test
Doppler echography, MRI

Liver structure and function
Liver function tests
Liver histology

Bone
Osteoporosis: bone density (Dexa scan)

Endocrine system
Diabetes: urine glucose, HbA_{1c}, glucose tolerance test, IGF-1
Growth and sexual development: sitting and standing height, Tanner staging, radiography for bone age, testosterone, estradiol, LH, FSH, SHBG, pulsatile GnRH release, sperm tests
Thyroid: T_4, TSH
Parathyroid: calcium, phosphate, PTH

ECG, electrocardiogram; FSH, follicle-stimulating hormone; GnRH, gonadotrophin-releasing hormone; HbA_{1c}, glycated haemoglobin; IGF, insulin-like growth factor; LH, luteinizing hormone; MRI, magnetic resonance imaging; MUGA, multigated acquisition scan; PTH, parathyroid hormone; SHBG, sex hormone-binding globulin; TSH, thyroid-stimulating hormone.

if fibrosis is present. Levels greater than 15 mg/g dry weight have been associated in DFX-treated patients with a high risk of cardiac disease, liver fibrosis and cirrhosis. Levels between 7 and 15 mg/g dry weight are associated with liver damage only if

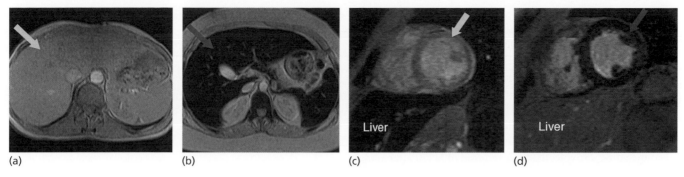

(a) (b) (c) (d)

Figure 4.3 Magnetic resonance imaging T2* technique. Tissue appearances of liver and spleen: (a) normal; (b) tissue iron overload; (c) severe liver iron overload with normal cardiac iron; (d) severe cardiac iron deposition with minimal liver iron deposition. (From Anderson *et al*. 2001 with permission.)

there is also hepatitis C infection and have been considered indicative of relative safety from cardiac disease but are associated with damage to the endocrine organs. Levels less than 7 mg/g dry weight are found in carriers of haemochromatosis and are considered safe.

MRI techniques are being increasingly used as indirect measures of liver and cardiac iron (Figure 4.3). They have the advantage of being non-invasive and are more widely available than SQUID (which is suitable for liver but not cardiac iron). MRI is also the only practical method of performing sequential studies of iron in the heart, pituitary or other endocrine organs. Different MRI techniques have been used. They all rely on a shortening of relaxation time and thus reduction in signal intensity with iron overload. Gradient-echo imaging with the calculation of the T2* has a short total imaging time, reducing movement artefacts. It is also extremely sensitive and reproducible. The spin-echo technique is less sensitive to iron and requires longer imaging time, making it less valuable for testing cardiac iron.

Cardiac iron

As cardiac failure or arrhythmia is the usual cause of death in transfusional iron overload, it is essential to monitor cardiac iron. Iron is deposited in myocytes and interstitial fibrosis develops. Direct measurement of cardiac iron by endomyocardial biopsy is inappropriate as the technique is highly invasive and inaccurate as iron localizes mainly in the ventricular myocardium and epicardium. T2* cardiovascular magnetic resonance offers a reproducible (around 5% coefficient of variation between different observers or between two studies of the same patient), sensitive, albeit indirect measure: the lower the T2* value, the greater the cardiac iron (Figure 4.3). The majority of patients with T2* greater than 20 ms have normal left ventricular function. A T2* below 20 ms correlates with the presence of cardiac dysfunction detected by echocardiography (left and right ventricles) or by 24-hour rhythm monitoring or the need for cardiac therapy (Figure 4.4). The great majority of patients

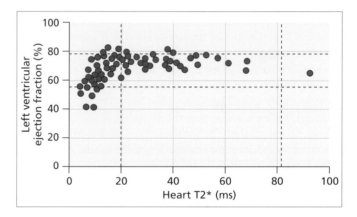

Figure 4.4 Relationships of myocardial T2* and left ventricular ejection fraction in patients with thalassaemia major and iron overload. (From Anderson *et al*. 2001 with permission.)

who develop cardiac failure have T2* less than 10 ms. Poor correlation has been found between myocardial iron and liver iron (MRI derived) or serum ferritin in patients receiving DFX, so serum ferritin and liver iron cannot be used as surrogate measures of cardiac iron.

Urine iron excretion

Iron excretion after a single infusion of a standard dose of DFX or oral dose of deferiprone is related to body iron. Urine iron is derived from the labile iron pool chelated mainly extracellularly with DFX and probably intracellularly with deferiprone. With DFX (but not deferiprone) urine iron excretion is increased by ascorbate and is proportionately higher if the haemoglobin is lower. The test is useful when commencing therapy with DFX or deferiprone, with which iron excretion is highly dose related, and for monitoring therapy, in some studies correlating closely with liver and cardiac iron. However, several estimations must be performed at any given dose in view of the variability found.

Non-transferrin-bound iron

This is present in plasma in patients with gross iron overload and 100% saturation of transferrin. It is highly toxic, promoting the formation of free radicals that cause peroxidation of membrane lipids. Part of the early improvement in liver and cardiac function with chelation therapy may be due to removal of this fraction, even before iron burden is substantially lowered. Its clearance by DFX is short-lived as it reappears in plasma within hours of stopping an infusion. Deferasirox, with its long clearance time, provides 24-hour removal of NTBI after a single oral dose. Deferiprone removes NTBI for about 6 hours after a single dose. NTBI is absent from plasma of well-chelated patients.

Tests of organ function

The tests that are usually needed are listed in Table 4.4. Heart function is best tested by measurement of left ventricular ejection fraction and by tests for rhythm disturbance. Liver function assessment requires routine liver function tests as well as liver biopsy to assess liver structure and liver iron burden (histologically and chemically). The endocrine system is also damaged by iron and appropriate tests are listed in Table 4.4. The anterior pituitary is particularly sensitive, with damage resulting in reduced growth and impaired sexual maturation. Direct damage to the ovaries or testes may also occur but is usually less important. Hypogonadic hypogonadism, defects of growth hormone secretion and in its receptor, and deficiency of insulin-like growth factor mainly account for growth failure; DFX may also cause this. Diabetes mellitus and pre-diabetes, due to iron deposition in the pancreatic islets, are frequent, especially in patients with genetic susceptibility. Hypothyroidism and hypoparathyroidism are also common in poorly chelated patients. Osteoporosis is well recognized in iron-overloaded thalassaemia patients; it is due to multiple factors and is detected by bone density studies.

Iron chelation therapy

Desferrioxamine

Pharmacokinetics

Desferrioxamine mesylate is licensed in all countries. It is not absorbed orally, and after parenteral injection is rapidly cleared from the plasma, being excreted in the urine, taken up by hepatocytes or metabolized in the tissues (Table 4.3). This accounts for the much greater mobilization of iron by continuous intravenous or slow subcutaneous infusions, which allow more prolonged exposure of the drug to the chelatable iron than with intramuscular injection.

DFX is a trihydroxamic acid (hexadendate) (Figure 4.5), one molecule binding covalently to all six oxygen sites on one ferric ion to form the red chelate, ferrioxamine. This is excreted in

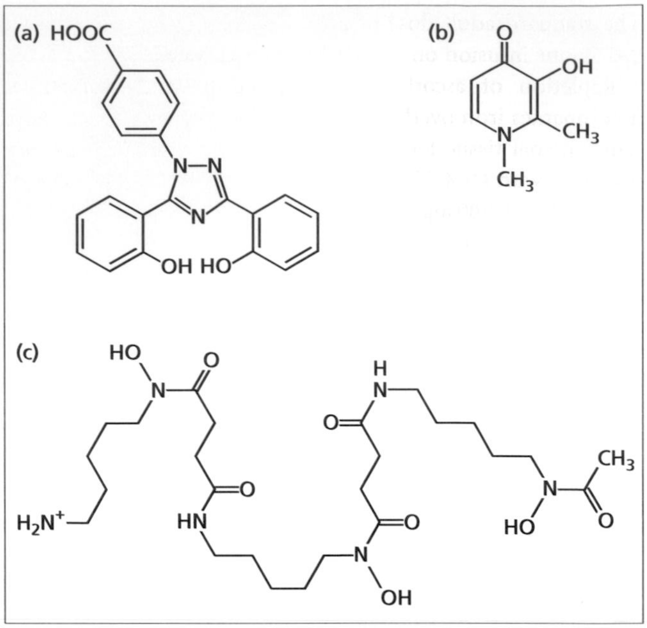

Figure 4.5 Chemical structures of three iron chelators: (a) deferasirox; (b) deferiprone; (c) desferrioxamine.

urine and bile. Faecal iron is derived from hepatocytes. Urine iron also derives, at least partly, from hepatocytes, although other body sources, especially iron released from macrophages, contribute. Urinary iron excretion tends to level off at higher doses, but this does not occur with bile excretion so bile iron may therefore predominate at high doses, and this is also the major route of excretion when total body iron has been reduced to relatively low levels. Increased erythropoiesis, as in haemolytic anaemias, is associated with an increase in urine iron excretion in relation to body iron stores.

Clinical studies

Most studies have involved thalassaemia major, but patients with other inherited anaemias (e.g. Diamond–Blackfan syndrome, Fanconi anaemia, sickle cell anaemia, sideroblastic anaemia) or acquired disorders, especially myelodysplasia, myelofibrosis, red cell aplasia or aplastic anaemia, may require iron chelation therapy. In these conditions, as well as in elderly patients with acquired, transfusion-dependent, refractory anaemias and otherwise good prognosis, deferasirox is widely used if iron overload is likely to cause significant morbidity or mortality. In children, tissue damage from iron may be present from very early life; regular iron chelation should begin in thalassaemia major after transfusion of about 12 units of blood or when serum ferritin exceeds 1000 µg/L. In young children, treatment with DFX should be started at 20 mg/kg to prevent tissue damage due to iron without causing toxicity due to excess DFX. A local anaesthetic cream (e.g. EMLA) reduces pain from the needle insertion. Oral chelation may be preferred to DFX.

The standard adult dose of DFX is 40 mg/kg s.c., given as an 8–12 hour infusion on at least 5 days each week.

Repletion of ascorbic acid deficiency, which sometimes accompanies iron overload, or ascorbate therapy even in those with normal tissue levels of ascorbate, increases urinary iron excretion with DFX. Vitamin C supplements should be given at a dose of 100–200 mg per day.

For those with iron-induced cardiomyopathy, continuous intravenous DFX may be given via an indwelling catheter (e.g. Hickman) or Port-a-Cath chamber. Removal of liver iron is more rapid than removal of cardiac iron with this intensive chelation regimen. Combined therapy with deferiprone may also be used. Studies with deferasirox are in progress.

Body iron stores can be restricted to 5–10 times normal in well-chelated, regularly transfused patients. There is improved cardiac function and survival in patients who comply with DFX therapy. Growth and pubertal development are improved in many, but not all, patients; diabetes and other endocrine abnormalities still occur frequently. Serum ferritin levels in well-chelated with DFX thalassaemia major patients usually plateau between 1500 and 2500 μg/L. Unfortunately, through lack of compliance with DFX, premature deaths usually from iron-induced cardiac damage may occur in a proportion of thalassaemia major patients. Combination therapy or orally active drugs alone should be used in these patients.

Side-effects

These include rare generalized sensitivity reactions, local soreness related to the site of injection (usually due to the needle being inserted too superficially) and exacerbation of some infections, notably of the urinary tract and precipitation of *Yersinia* enterocolitis. Auditory (high-tone sensorineural hearing loss) and visual neurotoxicity (night blindness, visual field loss, retinal pigmentation and changes on electrical tests) are relatively frequent. Growth and bone defects may also occur. The spine may be affected, with sitting height reduced; rickets-like bone lesions, genu valgum and metaphyseal changes are described, especially in children (Figure 4.6).

Auditory, visual and growth side-effects of DFX occur mainly if the body iron burden is low and doses of DFX high, particularly in children. A therapeutic index can be calculated as follows: mean daily dose (mg/kg)/current serum ferritin (μg/L). If this is below 0.025 at all times, these side-effects of DFX do not occur.

Deferiprone

Pharmacokinetics

Deferiprone (1,2-dimethyl-3-hydroxypyrid-4-one) is rapidly absorbed, appearing in plasma within 15 min of ingestion (see Table 4.3). The chelator–iron complex is excreted with the free drug and glucuronide derivative in urine. Its iron chelation site

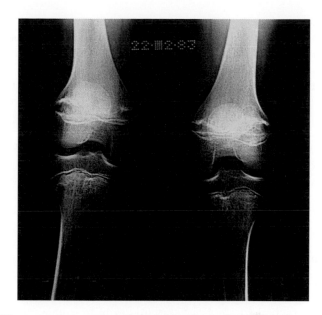

Figure 4.6 Bone and cartilage defects due to desferrioxamine.

is inactivated by glucuronidation, the speed of which varies from patient to patient. This explains much of the individual variation in response. It is available both as tablets (500 mg) and as a liquid formulation containing 100 mg/mL.

Deferiprone mobilizes iron from parenchymal and reticuloendothelial pools and from transferrin, ferritin and haemosiderin. The enhanced ability of deferiprone to cross cell membranes may underlie its superior ability compared with DFX to protect the heart from iron and also the 'shuttle' effect for iron when the two drugs are given simultaneously (see p. 59 and Figure 4.7). Deferiprone crosses the blood–brain barrier to treat neurological conditions with iron loading in the brain. Few balance studies have been performed. These suggest that, on average, deferiprone 75 mg/kg is about as effective as DFX 40 mg/kg. Wide individual variations occur, especially with deferiprone. Moreover, it is easier for patients to comply with deferiprone than DFX on all 7 days each week.

Clinical studies

The usual dose used has been 75–100 mg/kg daily. Serum ferritin levels tend to plateau around 2000–2500 μg/L. MRI studies suggest that liver iron may generally be higher in patients treated with deferiprone (75 mg/kg 7 days per week) compared with those treated with DFX (40 mg/kg 5 days per week). In the liver, DFX has the advantage of facilitated transport into cells by an active mechanism. Deferiprone, on the other hand, may have greater penetration of myocardial cells because of its lower molecular weight and because it is lipophilic. Retrospective and prospective studies have shown, on the basis of T2* MRI measurement of cardiac iron, echocardiography, clinical incidence of cardiac disease, need for cardiac therapy and survival, that

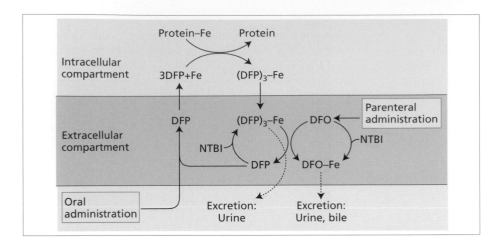

Figure 4.7 The concept of combination therapy: DFO, desferrioxamine; DFP, deferiprone; NTBI, non-transferrin-bound iron.

deferiprone 75 mg/kg is more effective than DFX at protecting the heart from iron-induced cardiomyopathy in routine clinical practice.

Side-effects

The most severe is agranulocytosis (neutrophils $< 0.5 \times 10^9$/L on two consecutive counts), with an estimated incidence of around 0.5–1.0% (0.2–0.3 episodes per 100 patient-years). It is most frequent in the first year of therapy. Lesser degrees of neutropenia ($0.5–1.5 \times 10^9$/L) are more frequent, around 3.5–8.5%, occurring more frequently in non-splenectomized patients. Agranulocytosis and neutropenia spontaneously recover when the drug is discontinued, usually within 4–28 days (median duration 9 days) but occasionally are more prolonged. Granulocyte colony-stimulating factor produces a faster recovery. The mechanism appears to be idiosyncratic, more common in females, with no definite evidence of an immune mechanism established. Patients should be monitored by blood counts every week for at least the first 8–12 weeks of therapy and every 2 weeks thereafter for 2 years. Agranulocytosis may be more frequent in patients with stem cell or progenitor cell defects, for example aplastic anaemia, Diamond–Blackfan syndrome or myelodysplasia. Deferasirox may be safer for these conditions.

Painful joints, especially the knees, occur in around 5–10% in most large series. The incidence has been highest in Indian patients. Some but not all studies show that this complication is most frequent in the most iron-loaded patients and with higher doses of deferiprone. It usually, but not invariably, resolves with withdrawal of the drug and it is often possible to reintroduce the drug, commencing with lower doses. About 2.0% of patients permanently discontinue therapy because of joint symptoms.

Gastrointestinal side-effects (e.g. nausea and abdominal pain) occur in about 30% of patients in the first year but decrease to 3% in subsequent years. In most the drug can be reintroduced long term, initially at a lower dose. The liquid preparation appears to produce fewer gastrointestinal symptoms. Zinc deficiency has been described in diabetic and pre-diabetic patients. Rarely, it can lead to clinical features, such as skin rashes and hair loss. It is easily treated by oral zinc therapy. Liver fibrosis was suggested as a complication of deferiprone therapy in one study, but larger studies show that liver fibrosis is not a consequence of deferiprone. Nevertheless, transient increases in liver enzymes have been associated with deferiprone therapy in about 7% of patients and about 1% of patients have been withdrawn from therapy because of a persistent rise in liver enzyme levels. There have been no reports of renal, cardiac or neurological side-effects. Embryo toxicity and teratogenicity have been reported in non-iron-loaded animals treated with deferiprone. Women of childbearing age should be counselled to avoid the drug or use contraception but a few uneventful pregnancies with healthy newborns have been reported.

Combination therapy

Urine iron excretion when DFX and deferiprone are given simultaneously is equivalent to the sum of the excretion when the drugs are given on separate days. There is evidence for a 'shuttle' effect in which deferiprone enters cells, chelates iron and then returns to plasma, where the iron is transferred to DFX for excretion in urine or bile (Figure 4.7). All studies of combination therapy, for example deferiprone on 7 days a week and DFX on 2 days, have shown a significant fall in serum ferritin and improvement in cardiac and liver iron over 6–18 months. It has been associated with improved survival and reversal of endocrinological complications including diabetes, hypothyroidism and hypogonadism. The combination has also proved successful in reversing severe myocardial siderosis. Alternating therapy has also been studied, for example 4 or 5 days of deferiprone and 2 or 3 days of DFX each week, with improved compliance and improved iron status in previously poorly compliant (with DFX) children or adults.

Deferasirox

Pharmacokinetics

Deferasirox, 4-[3,5-bis(2-hydroxyphenyl)-1,2,4-triazol-1-yl] benzoic acid (Figure 4.5), is a tridentate chelator forming a 2:1 chelator–iron complex and increases predominantly faecal iron excretion. After a single oral dose, only 6% of iron excretion occurs in the urine (see Table 4.3). It is highly selective for iron. Peak plasma concentration after a single oral dose occurs at about 2 hours, and the drug is still detectable in plasma in almost all patients at 24 hours, with a mean elimination half-life of between 11 and 19 hours after multiple-dose administration. The single daily dose ranges from 20 to 40 mg/kg.

Clinical studies

Deferasirox has been shown to be effective at eliminating NTBI in plasma and reducing serum ferritin and liver iron in heavily iron-loaded patients. The effect is dependent on dose and on transfusion requirements of the patient. The drug has been shown to be safe and effective in children as young as 2 years. The starting dose in children is 20 mg/kg daily with subsequent dose adjustments. In adults 30–40 mg/kg daily may be required according to iron stores. Trials lasting for up to 5 years on children and adults have not shown any progressive renal, hepatic or bone marrow dysfunction and there are no reports of deferasirox having negative impact on growth or sexual development.

Emerging data suggest that deferasirox is effective at removing cardiac iron and preventing cardiac siderosis in thalassaemia major. It has also been shown to maintain or reduce iron overload in transfusion-dependent patients with myelodysplasia, Diamond–Blackfan anaemia and aplastic anaemia and in iron-loaded sickle cell anaemia patients. Adverse effects in these groups appear similar to those with thalassaemia major. The use of deferasirox is also being explored in hereditary haemochromatosis, chronic hepatitis C infection, porphyria cutanea tarda and mucormycosis.

The most common adverse effects have been abdominal pain, nausea, diarrhoea, vomiting and skin rashes. These decrease in frequency annually. They usually respond to dose adjustments, taking the drug in the evening or adding products such as Lactaid to the diet. Non-progressive increases in serum creatinine (defined as a rise above the mean pretreatment measurement by more than 33% on two consecutive tests) occur in about one-third of patients. These increases are dose dependent and resolve spontaneously. Serum creatinine should be measured in duplicate before therapy and then monthly, with significantly increased levels managed by dose reduction or interruptions.

Thalassaemia intermedia

For these patients, and other severely anaemic patients who are not transfusion dependent or only need a few transfusions each year, iron loading occurs mainly through increased iron absorption. When anaemia is too severe for venesection, DFX has been used but oral iron chelation with deferasirox or deferiprone, more easily managed and with better patient compliance, has been shown effective in 'de-ironing' such patients, potentially reducing serum ferritin and liver iron to normal. A rise in haemoglobin level may occur. This may be due to removal of iron from the renal oxygen sensor, augmenting the effect of hypoxia and increasing erythropoietin secretion from the kidney. The rise in haemoglobin may also be a result of deferiprone directly removing iron from erythroblasts and mature red cells, reducing ineffective erythropoiesis and haemolysis. Improved haemopoiesis has also been described in myelodysplasia after chelation with DFX.

Acute iron poisoning

Acute oral iron poisoning produces a severe necrotizing gastritis and enteritis, followed by metabolic acidosis and, after a day or two, cardiovascular collapse and evidence of liver damage. DFX should be given both orally and parenterally. The instillation of 5 g into the stomach after a 1% sodium bicarbonate gastric lavage (to reduce further absorption) and an injection of 1–2 g i.m. may be tried. If a large number of tablets have been taken, an intravenous DFX infusion up to a maximum dose of 80 mg/kg in 24 hours should be used. Deferiprone and deferasirox have not yet been used in this setting.

Selected bibliography

Adams PC, Barton JC (2007) Haemochromatosis. *Lancet* **370**: 1855–60.

Anderson LJ, Holden S, Davis B et al. (2001) Cardiovascular T2-star (T2*) magnetic resonance for the early diagnosis of myocardial iron overload. *European Heart Journal* **22**: 2171–9.

Anderson LJ, Wonke B, Prescott E et al. (2002) Improved myocardial iron levels and ventricular function with oral deferiprone compared with subcutaneous desferrioxamine in thalassaemia. *Lancet* **360**: 516–20.

Angelucci E, Barosi G, Camaschella C et al. (2008) Italian Society of Haematology practice guidelines for the management of iron overload in thalassemia major and related disorders. *Haematologica* **93**: 741–52.

Beutler E, Felitti VJ, Koziol JA et al. (2002) Penetrance of 845G→A (C282Y) HFE hereditary haemochromatosis mutation in the USA. *Lancet* **359**: 211–18.

Boddaert N, Le Quan Sang KH, Rotig A et al. (2007) Selective iron chelation in Friedreich ataxia: biologic and clinical implications. *Blood* **110**: 401–8.

Camaschella C, Poggiali E (2009) Towards explaining 'unexplained hyperferritinemia'. *Haematologica* **94**: 307–9.

Camaschella C, Poggiali E (2009) Rare types of genetic hemochromatosis. *Acta Haematologica* **122**: 140–5.

Capellini MD, Cohen A, Piga A *et al.* (2006) A phase 3 study of deferasirox (ICL 670), a once-daily oral iron chelator, in patients with β-thalassemia. *Blood* **107**: 3455–62.

Cappellini MD, Porter JB, El-Beshlawy A *et al.* (2010) Tailoring iron chelation by iron intake and serum ferritin: prospective EPIC study of deferasirox in 1744 patients with transfusion-dependent anemias. *Haematologica*, in press.

Farmaki K, Tzoumari I, Pappa C *et al.* (2009) Normalisation of total body iron with very intensive combined therapy reverses cardiac and endocrine complications of thalassaemia major. *British Journal of Haematology* **148**: 466–75.

Galanello R, Piga A, Alberti D *et al.* (2003) Safety, tolerability and pharmokinetics of ICL 670, a new, orally active iron chelating agent in patients with transfusion-dependent iron overload due to beta-thalassemia. *Journal of Clinical Pharmacology* **43**: 565–72.

Gordeuk VR, Caleffi A, Corradini E (2003) Iron overload in Africans and African-Americans and a common mutation in the SCL40A1 (ferroportin 1) gene. *Blood Cells, Molecules and Diseases* **31**: 299–304.

Gurrin LC, Osbourne NJ, Constantine CC *et al* (2008) The natural history of serum iron in HFE C282Y homozygosity associated with hereditary hemochromatosis. *Gastroenterology* **135**: 1945–52.

Hoffbrand AV (ed.) (2009) Recent advances in the understanding of iron metabolism and iron-related diseases. *Acta Haematologica* **122**: 75–7. 12 articles covering all aspects of this topic.

Hoffbrand AV, Cohen A, Hershko C (2003) Role of deferiprone in chelation therapy for transfusional iron overload. *Blood* **102**: 17–24.

Ke Y, Qian ZM (2003) Iron misregulation in the brain: a primary cause of neurodegenerative disorders. *Lancet Neurology* **2**: 246–53.

Kirk P, Roughton M, Porter JB *et al.* (2009) Cardiac T2* magnetic resonance for prediction of cardiac complications in thalassemia major. *Circulation* **109**: 1961–8.

Lee PL, Beutler E (2009) Regulation of hepcidin and iron-overload disease. *Annual Review of Pathology* **4**: 489–515.

Lok CY, Merryweather-Clarke AT, Viprakasit V *et al.* (2009) Iron overload in the Asian community. *Blood* **114**: 20–5.

McLaren GD, McLaren CE, Adams PC *et al.* (2008) Clinical manifestations of hemochromatosis in HFFE homozygotes detected by screening. *Canadian Journal of Gastroenterology* **22**: 923–30.

Modell B, Khan M, Darlison M *et al.* (2008) Improved survival of thalassaemia major in the UK and relation to T2* cardiovascular magnetic resonance. *Journal of Cardiovascular Magnetic Resonance* **10**: 42.

Pennell DJ, Berdoukas V, Karagiorga M *et al.* (2006) Randomized controlled trial of deferiprone or deferoxamine in beta-thalassemia major patients with asymptomatic myocardial siderosis. *Blood* **107**: 3738–44.

Pennell DJ, Porter JB, Cappellini DM *et al.* (2010) Efficacy of deferasirox in reducing and preventing cardiac iron overload in beta-thalassemia. *Blood* **115**: 2364–71.

Pootrakul PS, Sirankapracha P, Sankote J *et al.* (2003) Clinical trial of deferiprone iron chelation therapy on β-thalassaemia/haemoglobin E patients in Thailand. *British Journal of Haematology* **122**: 305–10.

Porter JB, Galanello L, Saglio G *et al.* (2008) Relative response of patients with myelodysplastic syndromes and other transfusion-dependent anaemias to deferasirox (ICL670): a 1-yr prospective study. *European Journal of Haematology* **80**: 168–76.

Taher A, Cappellini MD, Vichinsky E *et al.* (2009) Efficacy and safety of deferasirox doses >30 mg/kg per day in patients with transfusion-dependent anaemia and iron overload. *British Journal of Haematology* **147**: 752–9.

Tanner MA, Galanello R, Dessi C *et al.* (2007) A randomized, placebo-controlled double blind trial of the effect of continued therapy with deferoxamine and deferiprone on myocardial iron in thalassemia major using cardiovascular magnetic resonance. *Circulation* **115**: 1876–84.

Tanner MA, Galanello R, Dessi C *et al.* (2008) Combination chelation therapy in thalassemia major for the treatment of severe myocardial siderosis with left ventricular dysfunction. *Journal of Cardiocasicular Magnetic Resonance* **10**: 12.

Voskaridou E, Plata E, Douskou M *et al.* (2010) Treatment with deferasirox (Exjade) effectively decreases iron burden in patients with thalassaemia intermedia: results of a pilot study. *British Journal of Haematology* **148**: 332–4.

Megaloblastic anaemia

5

A Victor Hoffbrand

University College Medical School, Royal Free Hospital, London, UK

Introduction

The megaloblastic anaemias are a group of disorders characterized by the presence of distinctive morphological appearances of the developing red cells in the bone marrow. The cause is usually deficiency of either cobalamin (vitamin B_{12}) or folate, but megaloblastic anaemia may arise because of inherited or acquired abnormalities affecting the metabolism of these vitamins or because of defects in DNA synthesis not related to cobalamin or folate (Table 5.1).

Underlying basic science

Biochemical basis of megaloblastic anaemia

The common feature of all megaloblastic anaemias is a defect in DNA synthesis that affects rapidly dividing cells in the bone marrow and other tissues. All conditions that give rise to megaloblastic changes share in common a disparity in the rate of synthesis or polymerization of the four immediate precursors

Postgraduate Haematology: 6th edition. Edited by A. Victor Hoffbrand,
Daniel Catovsky, Edward G.D. Tuddenham, Anthony R. Green
© 2011 Blackwell Publishing Ltd.

of DNA: the deoxyribonucleoside triphosphates (Figure 5.1). In deficiencies of either folate or cobalamin there is a failure to convert deoxyuridine monophosphate (dUMP) to deoxythymidine monophosphate (dTMP). The coenzyme 5,10-methylene tetrahydrofolate polyglutamate is needed for this reaction and the availability of this coenzyme is reduced in either cobalamin deficiency or folate deficiency (see below).

The reduced supply of deoxythymidine triphosphate (dTTP) in megaloblastic anaemia owing to folate or cobalamin deficiency slows elongation of newly originated replicating segments from multiple sites of origin. Thus small fragments accumulate, single-stranded areas become points of weakness where mechanical or enzymatic breakage may occur, and the failure to form bulk DNA impairs contraction of newly replicated lengths of DNA, leaving the chromosomes elongated, despirillated and with random breaks. Late-replicating DNA is particularly affected and some cells become arrested and die at this stage by apoptosis, which can be prevented *in vitro* by preformed thymidine. Surprisingly, measurements of dTTP concentration in megaloblasts have not shown a deficiency. This may be because the overall cell concentration masks a localized deficiency at the multienzyme complex directly concerned with DNA replication.

An alternative hypothesis for megaloblastic anaemia in cobalamin or folate deficiency is the misincorporation of uracil into DNA because of a build-up of deoxyuridine triphosphate

Table 5.1 Causes of megaloblastic anaemia.

Cobalamin deficiency or abnormalities of cobalamin metabolism
 (Table 5.4)
Folate deficiency or abnormalities of folate metabolism
 (Table 5.7)
Therapy with antifolate drugs (e.g. methotrexate)
Independent of either cobalamin or folate deficiency and
 refractory to cobalamin and folate therapy:
 Some cases of acute myeloid leukaemia, myelodysplasia*
 Therapy with drugs interfering with DNA synthesis (e.g.
  cytarabine, hydroxycarbamide, 6-mercaptopurine,
  azidothymidine)
 Orotic aciduria (responds to uridine)
 Lesch–Nyhan syndrome (? responds to adenine)

*Folate deficiency also occurs frequently in these diseases.

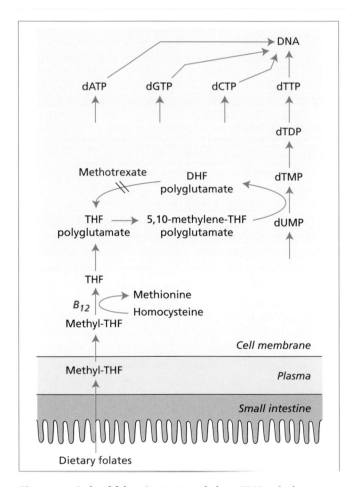

Figure 5.1 Role of folate (as 5,10-methylene-THF polyglutamate and methylcobalamin) in DNA synthesis. THF, tetrahydrofolate; MP, monophosphate; TP, triphosphate; d, deoxyribose; A, adenine; T, thymine; C, cytosine; G, guanine.

(dUTP) at the replication fork as a consequence of the block in conversion of dUMP to dTMP (Figure 5.1). There is a mechanism for recognition of this aberrant material for excision and repair, but with dTTP in short supply this may not be possible. Repeated cycles of futile excision and misrepair may occur, with disruption of the normal programme of DNA synthesis leading to apoptotic cell death. Data on this hypothesis are conflicting. It does not explain megaloblastic anaemia due to defects of DNA synthesis at sites other than thymidylate synthesis, for example with drugs such as hydroxycarbamide (hydroxyurea), cytarabine or 6-mercaptopurine, or with enzyme deficiencies such as orotic aciduria or thiamine-responsive megaloblastic anaemia (see below).

Cobalamin–folate relationship

Folate is required for many other reactions in mammalian tissues, including two in purine synthesis (Table 5.2), but impairment of these is far less important clinically.

 Only two reactions in the body are known to require cobalamin (Figure 5.2). Methylmalonyl-CoA isomerization, which requires deoxyadenosyl(ado)-cobalamin, is discussed later. The methylation of homocysteine to methionine requires both 5-methyltetrahydrofolate (methyl-THF) as methyl donor and methylcobalamin as coenzyme (Figure 5.3). This reaction, which is almost completely irreversible, is the first step in the pathway by which methyl-THF, which enters bone marrow and other cells from plasma, is converted into all the intracellular folate coenzymes (Figure 5.3). The coenzymes are all polyglutamated (the larger size aiding retention in the cell), but the enzyme folate polyglutamate synthase requires THF and not methyl-THF as substrate. In cobalamin deficiency, methyl-THF accumulates in the plasma, while intracellular folate concentrations fall due to failure of formation of intracellular folate polyglutamates because of 'THF starvation' or 'methylfolate trapping'.

 This theory explains the abnormalities of folate metabolism that occur in cobalamin deficiency (high serum folate, low cell folate, reduced thymidylate synthesis, positive purine precursor AICAR excretion; Table 5.2) and also why the anaemia that occurs in cobalamin deficiency will respond to folic acid in large doses. The explanation of why serum cobalamin falls in folate deficiency may also be related to impairment of the homocysteine–methionine reaction, with reduced formation of methylcobalamin, the main form of cobalamin in plasma, but other mechanisms may be responsible.

Clinical features

Many symptomless patients are detected through the finding of a raised mean corpuscular volume (MCV) on a routine blood

Table 5.2 Biochemical reactions of folate coenzymes.

Reaction	Coenzyme form of folate involved	Single-carbon unit transferred	Importance
Formate activation	THF	–CHO	Generation of 10-formyl-THF
Purine synthesis			
Formation of glycinamide ribonucleotide	5,10-Methenyl-THF	–CHO	Formation of purines needed for DNA, RNA synthesis, but reactions probably not rate limiting
Formylation of amino-imidazole-carboxamide-ribotide (AICAR)	10-Formyl-THF	–CHO	
Pyrimidine synthesis			
Methylation of deoxyuridine monophosphate (dUMP) to thymidine monophosphate (dTMP)	5,10-Methenyl-THF	–CH$_3$	Rate limiting in DNA synthesis Oxidizes THF to DHF Some breakdown of folate at the C-9–N-10 bond
Amino acid interconversion			
Serine–glycine interconversion	THF	=CH$_2$	Entry of single-carbon units into active pool
Homocysteine to methionine	5-Methyl-THF	–CH$_3$	Demethylation of 5-methyl-THF to THF; also requires cobalamin, flavine adenine dinucleotide, ATP and adenosylmethionine
Forminoglutamic acid to glutamic acid in histidine catabolism	THF	–HN–CH=	Basis of the Figlu test (now obsolete)

DHF, dihydrofolate; THF, tetrahydrofolate.

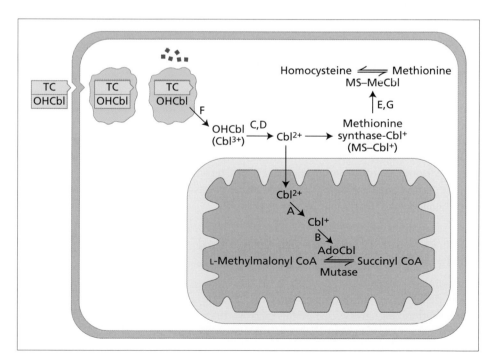

Figure 5.2 Intracellular cobalamin metabolism. Cbl^{1+}, Cbl^{2+} and Cbl^{3+} refer to the oxidation state of the central cobalt atom of cobalamin. A–G refer to the sites of blocks that have been identified by complementation analysis in infants with metabolic defects. AdoCbl, adenosylcobalamin; MeCbl, methylcobalamin; TC, transcobalamin. The mitochondrial, lysosomal and cytoplasmic compartments are indicated. (From Lilleyman JS, Hann IM, Blanchette VS (eds) (1999) *Paediatric Haematology*, 2nd edn. Churchill Livingstone, Edinburgh with permission.)

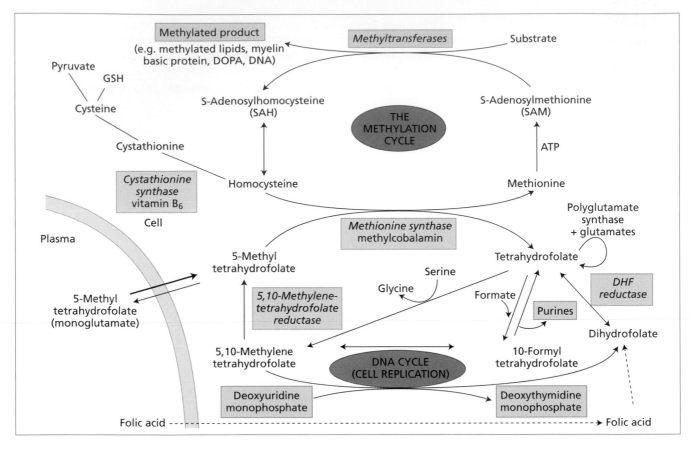

Figure 5.3 The role of folates in DNA synthesis and in formation of *S*-adenosylmethionine (SAM), which is involved in numerous methylation reactions. Enzymes are shown in yellow boxes. (Figure prepared in conjunction with Professor John Scott.)

count. The main clinical features in more severe cases are those of anaemia. Anorexia is usually marked and there may be weight loss, diarrhoea or constipation. Other particular features include glossitis, angular cheilosis, a mild fever in the more severely anaemic patients, jaundice (unconjugated) and reversible melanin skin hyperpigmentation, which may occur with either deficiency. Thrombocytopenia sometimes leads to bruising (and this may be aggravated by vitamin C deficiency in malnourished patients. The (anaemia and) low leucocyte count may predispose to infections, particularly of the respiratory or urinary tracts. Cobalamin deficiency has also been associated with impaired bactericidal function of phagocytes.

General tissue effects of cobalamin and folate deficiencies

Epithelial surfaces
These deficiencies, when severe, affect all rapidly growing (DNA-synthesizing) tissues. After the marrow, the next most affected tissues are the epithelial cell surfaces of the mouth, stomach, small intestine and respiratory, urinary and female genital tracts. The cells show macrocytosis, with increased

numbers of multinucleate and dying cells. The deficiencies may cause cervical smear abnormalities.

Complications of pregnancy
The gonads are also affected and infertility is common in both men and women with either deficiency if severe. Maternal folate deficiency has been implicated as a cause of prematurity and both folate and cobalamin deficiency have been implicated in recurrent fetal loss.

Neural tube defects
Folic acid supplements at the time of conception and in the first 12 weeks of pregnancy reduce by about 70% the incidence of neural tube defects (NTDs) – anencephaly, meningomyelocele, encephalocele and spina bifida – in the fetus. Most of this protective effect can be achieved by taking folic acid 0.4 mg daily. The incidence of cleft palate and harelip can also be reduced by prophylactic folic acid. There is no clear simple relationship between maternal folate status and these fetal abnormalities, although the lower the maternal folate, the greater the risk to the fetus. NTDs can also be caused by antifolate and antiepileptic drugs.

An underlying maternal folate metabolic abnormality has also been postulated. One abnormality has been identified: reduced activity of the enzyme 5,10-methylenetetrahydrofolate reductase (MTHFR) (Figure 5.3) caused by a common 677C→T polymorphism in the *MTHFR* gene. In one study, the prevalence of this polymorphism was found to be higher in the parents of NTD fetuses and in the fetuses themselves: homozygosity for the TT mutation was found in 13% compared with 5% in control subjects. The polymorphism codes for a thermolabile form of MTHFR. The homozygous state results in lower mean serum and red cell folate compared with control subjects, as well as significantly higher serum homocysteine levels. Tests for mutations in other enzymes possibly associated with NTDs, for example methionine synthase or serine–glycine hydroxymethylase, have been negative. Autoantibodies to folate receptors (see p. 77) had been suggested to cause NTDs but this has not been confirmed in a recent large study.

Cardiovascular disease

Children with severe homocystinuria (blood levels of 100 μmol/L or more) due to deficiency of one of three enzymes, methionine synthase, MTHFR or cystathionine synthase (Figure 5.3), suffer from vascular disease (e.g. ischaemic heart disease, cerebrovascular disease or pulmonary embolus) as teenagers or in young adulthood. Meta-analysis shows a significant association between lesser degrees of raised serum homocysteine (normal range 5–15 μmol/L) and of homozygosity for mutated *MTHFR* with ischaemic heart disease, stroke, deep vein thrombosis and pulmonary embolism. The odds ratios for a 5-μmol/L increase in serum homocysteine were 1.42 in 72 genetic (MTHFR) studies and 1.32 in 20 prospective studies of serum homocysteine, 1.60 for deep vein thrombosis with or without pulmonary embolism in genetic studies, and for stroke 1.65 in genetic studies and 1.59 in prospective studies. As the genetic and prospective studies do not share the same potential sources of error but both yield highly significant results, the authors considered the results strong evidence of a causal association between homocysteine and cardiovascular disease.

Heterozygosity for the C677T mutation has also been shown to be associated with an increase in the risk of thrombosis in subjects heterozygous for factor V Leiden. It remains possible that homocysteine levels may be high as a consequence of the vascular damage or may merely be a marker for some other underlying factor that is responsible for both the vascular damage and the raised homocysteine. Folate deficiency, for example, may be such a factor. Folate levels have been found in various studies to be lower in patients with myocardial infarct and carotid artery disease than control subjects. There are some reports of prevention of arterial disease recurrence or progression by prophylactic folic acid or cobalamin but the results are conflicting. Meta-analysis of data from large multicentre prospective trials of folic acid in prevention of coronary vascular disease do not show a positive effect. Meta-analysis does suggest that folic acid supplementation reduces the risk of stroke by 18% but even this is not certain, depending on which data are included in the analysis. Extremely high levels of homocysteine (>50 μmol/L) are toxic to endothelia. When homocysteine levels are only mildly (15–25 μmol/L) or moderately (25–50 μmol/L) elevated, then another mechanism needs to be invoked to explain vascular damage or increased risk of thrombosis. Several mechanisms have been proposed, including oxidant damage through the generation of peroxide produced during thiol oxidation to form disulphides and interaction of free reduced homocysteine with cysteine residues on coagulation factors, platelets, adhesion molecules or endothelial cells. Promotion of vascular wall inflammation through the generation of proinflammatory cytokines and interference with key methylation reactions are also possible mechanisms.

Malignancy

Prophylactic folic acid in pregnancy has been found in some but not all studies to reduce the subsequent incidence of acute lymphoblastic leukaemia (ALL) in childhood. A significant negative association has been found with the *MTHFR* 677C→T and 1298A→C polymorphisms and the incidence of both paediatric and adult ALL. There are various positive and negative associations between polymorphisms in other folate-dependent enzymes and the incidence of paediatric and adult ALL. Other tumours that have been associated with folate polymorphisms or status include follicular lymphoma, breast cancer and gastric cancer.

The C677T polymorphism is thought to lead to increased thymidine pools and 'better quality' of DNA synthesis by shunting one-carbon groups towards thymidine and purine synthesis. This may also explain its reported association with a lower risk for colorectal and gastric cancer. The incidence of colon cancer was also lower in subjects taking vitamin supplements containing folic acid and in those with higher folate intake compared with control subjects in the Nurses Health Study, and increased folate intake may mask the protective effect of the C677T and A1298C polymorphisms. There is no correlation between pre-diagnostic plasma folate and risk of death in patients with colorectal cancer. One study showed no overall difference in incidence of colonic adenoma in subjects taking folic acid or controls but a higher incidence of multiple (>3) adenomas in those taking folic acid. However, the statistics have been questioned and other studies have shown a lower incidence of colonic adenoma with higher folate intake. Folate deficiency is postulated to predispose to malignancy by reducing the ratio of *S*-adenosylmethionine (SAM) to *S*-adenosylhomocysteine (SAH), causing DNA hypomethylation and, by resulting in uracil misincorporation into DNA, possibly leading to double-strand breaks. Most recent data from large prospective trials suggest no significant effect of folic acid on the incidence or progress of any cancer.

Other tissues

Folate deficiency causes reduced regeneration of cirrhotic liver. Patients with gluten-induced enteropathy and those with sickle cell anaemia have also been reported to show stunted growth, which has been improved coincidentally with commencement of folic acid therapy, but it is not certain how much the growth improvement in these children was due to folic acid and how much to other, simultaneously administered vitamins. In the fragile X syndrome, sister chromatid exchange and DNA breaks are increased *in vitro* in a folate-deficient medium, apparently at the Xq28 site. No *in vivo* abnormality of folate metabolism can be detected.

Neurological manifestations

Cobalamin deficiency may cause bilateral peripheral neuropathy or degeneration (demyelination) of the posterior and pyramidal tracts of the spinal cord and, less frequently, optic atrophy or cerebral symptoms. The patient classically presents with paraesthesiae, muscle weakness or difficulty in walking and sometimes dementia, psychotic disturbances or visual impairment. Long-term nutritional cobalamin deficiency in infancy leads to poor brain development and impaired intellectual development. Folate deficiency may cause mental changes such as depression and slowness and has been suggested to cause organic nervous disease, but this is uncertain. Autoantibodies to the folate receptor involved in transport of folate into cerebrospinal fluid have been postulated to be associated with autism-associated neurological abnormalities. Methotrexate injected into the cerebrospinal fluid may cause brain or spinal cord damage. Neural tube defects in the fetus are discussed above.

The biochemical basis for cobalamin neuropathy remains obscure. Its occurrence in the absence of methylmalonic aciduria in transcobalamin deficiency, and in monkeys given nitrous oxide (N_2O), suggests that the neuropathy is related to the defect in conversion of homocysteine to methionine. Accumulation of SAH in the brain, resulting in inhibition of transmethylation reactions due to an altered SAM to SAH ratio, has been suggested. SAM is needed in methylation of biogenic amines (e.g. dopamine), as well as of proteins, phospholipids and neurotransmitters in the brain (see Figure 5.3). A reduced ratio of SAM to SAH is postulated to result in reduced methylation. However, measurements of methylation of arginine in myelin basic protein in fruit bats with cobalamin neuropathy, or in rats exposed to N_2O, showed no defect of methylation. Psychiatric disturbance is common in both folate and cobalamin deficiencies. Loss of cognitive function in the elderly has been associated with high plasma homocysteine and low vitamin B_{12} and folate levels. This, like the neuropathy, has been attributed to a failure of the synthesis of SAM.

Plasma homocysteine is a risk factor for dementia and Alzheimer disease, shown in a median follow-up period of 8 years in one study of 1092 subjects. Studies showing an association between lower serum levels of folate or cobalamin and higher homocysteine levels and Alzheimer disease, loss of cognitive function or brain volume loss have been reported. However, trials of supplementation with folic acid, vitamin B_{12} and vitamin B_6 have not shown a benefit in preventing progression of the dementia compared with a control group, or in improving cognitive function.

Haematological findings

Peripheral blood

Oval macrocytes, usually with considerable anisocytosis and poikilocytosis, are the main feature (Figure 5.4a). The MCV is usually more than 100 fL unless a cause of microcytosis (e.g. iron deficiency or thalassaemia trait) is present, when there is a raised red cell distribution width (RDW) and the film is dimorphic. In other cases, the MCV may be normal owing to excess fragmentation of red cells. Some of the neutrophils are hypersegmented (more than five nuclear lobes). Both macrocytosis and hypersegmented neutrophils may also occur in other situations (Table 5.3). Together, however, they strongly suggest megaloblastic haemopoiesis. There may be leucopenia due to a reduction in granulocytes and lymphocytes; the platelet count may be moderately reduced, rarely to less than $40 \times 10^9/L$. Occasionally, a leucoerythroblastic blood picture is seen. In the non-anaemic patient, the presence of a few macrocytes and

Table 5.3 Conditions in which macrocytosis or hypersegmented neutrophils may occur in the absence of megaloblastic anaemia.

Macrocytosis
Alcohol
Liver disease (especially alcoholic)
Reticulocytosis (haemolysis or haemorrhage)
Aplastic anaemia or red cell aplasia
Hypothyroidism
Myelodysplasia
Myeloma and macroglobulinaemia
Leucoerythroblastic anaemia
Myeloproliferative disease
Pregnancy
Newborn
Congenital dyserythropoietic anaemia (type II)
? Chronic respiratory failure

Hypersegmented neutrophils
Renal failure
Congenital (familial)
? Iron deficiency

Note: Falsely high MCV recorded when cold agglutinins, paraproteins or marked leucocytosis are present.

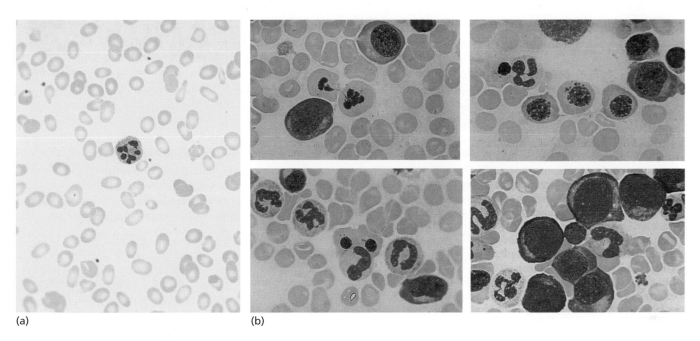

(a) (b)

Figure 5.4 Severe megaloblastic anaemia: (a) peripheral blood; (b) bone marrow.

hypersegmented neutrophils in the peripheral blood may be the only abnormalities.

Bone marrow

In the severely anaemic patient, the marrow is hypercellular with accumulation of primitive cells due to selective death of more mature forms. The most characteristic finding is dissociation between nuclear and cytoplasmic development in the erythroblasts, with the nucleus maintaining a primitive appearance despite maturation and haemoglobinization of the cytoplasm; fully haemoglobinized (orthochromatic) erythroblasts, which retain nuclei, may be seen. The nucleus of the megaloblast has an open, fine, lacy appearance; the cells are larger than normoblasts and an increased number of cells with eccentric lobulated nuclei or nuclear fragments may be present (Figure 5.4b). Mitoses and dying cells are more frequent than normal. Giant and abnormally shaped metamyelocytes and enlarged hyperpolyploid megakaryocytes are characteristic. Severe florid megaloblastic changes may be confused with acute erythroid leukaemia. Rarely, the marrow may be hypocellular or red cell precursors are lost almost completely from the marrow and a mistaken diagnosis of myeloid leukaemia may be made. Iron staining shows increase in both reticuloendothelial stores and in the developing megaloblasts.

In less anaemic patients, the changes in the marrow may be difficult to recognize. The terms 'intermediate', 'mild' and 'early' have been used. The changes may be mild and difficult to recognize, even in a severely anaemic patient, if the anaemia is largely due to other factors (e.g. iron deficiency, infection,

malignant disease, haemolysis) and the megaloblastosis is an incidental phenomenon. The term 'megaloblastoid' has several different connotations including the dysplastic changes seen in the myelodysplastic syndromes and is best avoided.

Chromosomes

Bone marrow cells, transformed lymphocytes and other proliferating cells in the body show a variety of changes including random breaks, reduced contraction, spreading of the centromere, and exaggeration of secondary chromosomal constrictions and overprominent satellites. Similar abnormalities may be produced by antimetabolite drugs (e.g. cytarabine, hydroxycarbamide and methotrexate) that interfere with either DNA replication or folate metabolism and which also cause megaloblastic appearances.

Ineffective haemopoiesis

There is accumulation of unconjugated bilirubin in plasma due to the death of nucleated red cells in the marrow (ineffective erythropoiesis). Other evidence for this includes raised urine urobilinogen, reduced haptoglobins and positive urine haemosiderin, raised serum lactate dehydrogenase to values between 1000 and 10 000 IU/dL, and raised serum iron, non-transferrin-bound iron and ferritin levels. Carbon monoxide production is also increased. Serum lysozyme may also be raised, suggesting ineffective granulopoiesis.

In rare patients, ineffective haemopoiesis is associated with features of disseminated intravascular coagulation, with raised serum fibrin degradation products. Thrombocytopenia, when it occurs, is usually caused by ineffective megakaryopoiesis. A weakly positive direct antiglobulin test due to complement can lead to a false diagnosis of autoimmune haemolytic anaemia.

Cobalamin

Cobalamin (vitamin B_{12}) exists in a number of different chemical forms. The molecule consists of two halves: a planar group and a nucleotide set at right angles to it (Figure 5.5). The planar group is a corrin ring and the nucleotide consists of a base, 5,6-dimethylbenzimidazole, and a phosphorylated sugar, ribose-5-phosphate. In nature, the vitamin is mainly in the 5′-deoxyadenosyl (ado) form. This is the main form in human tissues and is located in the mitochondria. It serves as the cofactor for methylmalonyl-CoA mutase. The other major natural cobalamin is methylcobalamin, the main form in human plasma and cell cytoplasm. It serves as the cofactor for methionine synthase. There are also minor amounts of hydroxocobalamin, the form to which methyl- and ado-cobalamin are rapidly converted by exposure to light, hydroxocobalamin having its cobalt atom in the fully oxidized Cbl^{3+} state, whereas the cobalt exists as reduced Cbl^{1+} in the methyl- and ado-cobalamin forms (see Figure 5.2). A glutathionyl cobalamin form has also been identified.

Dietary sources and requirements

Cobalamin is synthesized solely by microorganisms. Ruminants obtain cobalamin from the foregut but the only source for

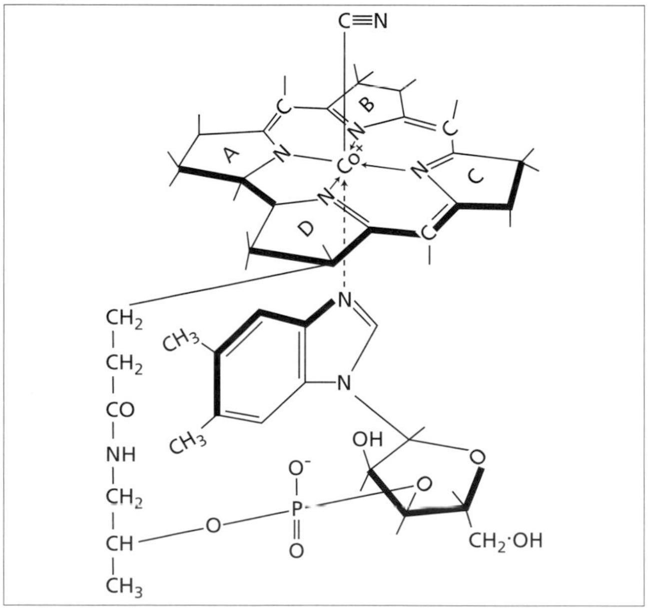

Figure 5.5 The structure of vitamin B_{12} (cyanocobalamin).

humans is food of animal origin. The highest amounts are found in liver and kidney (up to $100\,\mu g$ per $100\,g$), but it is also present in shellfish, organ and muscle meats, fish, chicken and dairy products (eggs, cheese and milk) in small amounts ($6\,\mu g/L$). Vegetables, fruits and all other foods of non-animal origin are free from cobalamin unless they are contaminated by bacteria. Cooking does not usually destroy cobalamin.

A normal Western diet contains 5–$30\,\mu g$ of cobalamin daily. Adult daily losses (mainly in the urine and faeces) are about 1–$2\,\mu g$ (about 0.1% of body stores) and because the body does not have the ability to degrade cobalamin, daily requirements are also about $1\,\mu g$. Body stores are of the order of 2–$3\,mg$ and are sufficient for 3–4 years if supplies are completely cut off.

Absorption

Two mechanisms exist for cobalamin absorption. One is passive, occurring equally through the duodenum and the ileum; it is rapid but extremely inefficient as less than 1% of an oral dose can be absorbed by this process. Passive absorption of cobalamin can also occur through other mucous membranes such as the sublingual and nasal mucosae. The other mechanism is active; it occurs through the ileum in humans and is efficient for small (a few micrograms) oral doses of cobalamin. This is the normal mechanism by which the body acquires cobalamin and is mediated by gastric intrinsic factor (IF).

Dietary cobalamin is released from protein complexes by enzymes in the stomach, duodenum and jejunum; it combines rapidly with a salivary glycoprotein (R binder) related to plasma transcobalamin I (TCI). These belong to the family of cobalamin-binding proteins known as haptocorrins (HCs), which differ only in glycosylation. They are products of a single gene (*TCN1*), and they occur in saliva, gastric juice, bile, milk and other body fluids. Subsequently, HC is digested by pancreatic trypsin and the cobalamin transferred to IF. Binding of cobalamin to IF is favoured by an alkaline pH; it binds one molecule for one molecule. All forms of cobalamin are absorbed by the same IF mechanism (Figure 5.6). Pseudo-cobalamin compounds, in which the 5,6-dimethylbenzimidazole nucleotide is replaced by other nucleotides that may attach to HC, do not attach to IF and therefore remain unabsorbed.

Intrinsic factor is a glycoprotein (molecular weight 45 000) encoded by a gene on chromosome 11q13. It is produced in gastric parietal cells in the fundus and body of the stomach. The IF–cobalamin complex, in contrast with free IF, is resistant to enzyme digestion, having a more closed structure. The IF–cobalamin complex passes to the ileum, where IF attaches to a specific receptor (cubilin, molecular weight 460 000) on the microvillus membrane of the brush border surface of the ileal absorptive cells. Cubilin (gene located on chromosome 10p12.1) is also present in yolk sac and renal proximal tubular epithelium. The attachment of the IF–cobalamin complex requires calcium ions and a pH around neutral. It is probably a physical

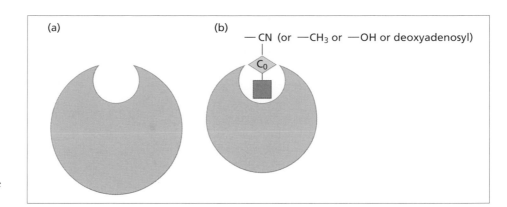

Figure 5.6 (a) Intrinsic factor; (b) intrinsic factor–cobalamin complex. Intrinsic factor has been estimated to have a molecular radius of 3.6 nm, vitamin B_{12} 0.8 nm and the complex 3.2 nm.

process, not requiring energy. Cubulin traffics by means of the protein amnionless (AMN, molecular weight 480 000). Cubulin and AMN are subunits of a novel complex in which AMN binds tightly to cubulin and directs sublocalization and endocytosis of cubulin with its ligand (IF–cobalamin complex). Defects in cubulin and AMN are implicated in autosomal recessive megaloblastic anaemia, characterized by intestinal malabsorption of cobalamin (see p. 73). A third protein, megalin (LRP2), has been suggested to play a role in stabilizing the cubulin–AMN complex.

Cobalamin then enters the ileal cell, but the exact fate of IF is unknown. IF does not enter the bloodstream as such, as after a delay of about 6 hours absorbed cobalamin appears in portal blood attached to transcobalamin (TCII), which is probably synthesized in the ileum, either by mucosal cells or by venous endothelial cells in the submucosa.

The ileum has a restricted capacity to absorb cobalamin because of limited receptor sites. Although 50% or more of a single dose of 1 μg of cobalamin may be absorbed, with doses above 2 μg the proportion absorbed falls rapidly. Moreover, after one dose of IF–cobalamin complex has been presented, the ileal cells become refractory to further doses for about 6 hours.

Enterohepatic circulation

Between 0.5 and 5.0 μg of cobalamin enter the bile each day. This binds to IF and a portion of biliary cobalamin is normally reabsorbed together with cobalamin derived from sloughed intestinal cells. Bile may enhance cobalamin absorption. Cobalamin deficiency develops more rapidly in individuals who malabsorb cobalamin than it does in vegans, who ingest no cobalamin but in whom reabsorption of biliary cobalamin is intact.

Transport

Two main cobalamin-binding proteins exist in human plasma; they both bind cobalamin one molecule for one molecule

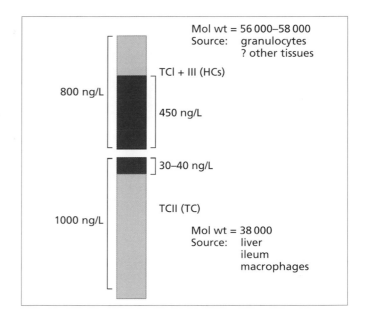

Figure 5.7 The serum cobalamin-binding proteins (TCs, transcobalamins). Dark blue rectangles indicate endogenous serum cobalamin; light blue rectangles indicate unsaturated cobalamin-binding protein; HCs, haptocorrins.

(Figure 5.7). One HC (also known as TCI) is a glycoprotein. TCIII was a name used to describe a minor isoprotein of TCI in plasma. These HCs are derived primarily from the specific granules in neutrophils and are normally about two-thirds saturated with cobalamin, which they bind tightly. They do not enhance cobalamin entry into tissues. Glycoprotein receptors on liver cells are concerned in the removal of HCs from plasma, and HC may have a role in the transport of cobalamin analogues to the liver for excretion in bile. The gene, *TCN1*, is located on chromosome 11q11–q12.3, has nine exons and codes a protein of 433 amino acids. Heterozygous, homozygous or compound heterozygous mutations in the gene may cause mild or severe reductions in serum vitamin B_{12} respectively with no known clinical consequences.

The other major cobalamin transport protein in plasma is transcobalamin (TC, also known as TCII). TC is a β-globulin (molecular weight 38 000) synthesized by liver, and by other tissues including macrophages, endothelial and possibly ileal cells. It normally carries only 20–60 ng of cobalamin per litre of plasma and readily gives up cobalamin to marrow, placenta and other tissues, which it enters by receptor-mediated endocytosis via clathrin-coated pits. TC is not reutilized. The gene is on chromosome 22q11–q13.1 and, as for IF and HC, there are nine exons. The three proteins are likely to have a common ancestral origin. TC has 20% amino acid homology and more than 50% nucleotide homology with human HC and with rat IF. The regions of homology of HC, TC and IF are involved in cobalamin binding. Five different inherited isoproteins of TC, separated by polyacrylamide gel electrophoresis, have been described; all are functionally active. TC occurs in cerebrospinal fluid and binds cobalamin (approximately 10 ng/L) there. Alterations may occur in TC and HC levels in a variety of disease states (Table 5.4). In general, an increase in HC causes an increase in serum cobalamin, whereas an increase in TC does not.

The TC receptor belongs to the low-density lipoprotein receptor family. It is composed of 282 amino acids and is heavily glycosylated; the gene is located at chromosome 19p15.2. It is more heavily expressed in dividing than quiescent cells, and is recycled to the cell surface. Megalin (LRP-2) is also involved in the endocytosis of TC–cobalamin.

Cobalamin analogues

Cobalamin analogues are corrinoids, which exist as cobamides (containing substitutions in the place of ribose, e.g. adenosyl) or as cobinamides (which have no nucleotide whatever). HC may carry analogues to the liver for excretion in the bile. It is unclear whether they are inert or inhibit cobalamin-dependent reactions. The proportion of analogues derived from diet, gut bacteria or endogenous breakdown of cobalamins is unknown. They are present in fetal blood and tissues.

Causes of cobalamin deficiency

Cobalamin deficiency is usually due to malabsorption. The only other cause is inadequate dietary intake. Cobalamin deficiency due to excess degradation occurs as a result of exposure to the anaesthetic gas N_2O. N_2O causes irreversible oxidation of the active Cbl^{1+} during catalytic shunting of labile methyl groups in the methionine synthase reaction (see Figure 5.2).

Inadequate dietary intake

Adults

Dietary cobalamin deficiency arises in vegans who omit meat, fish, eggs, cheese and other animal products from their diet. The largest group in the world consists of Hindus, and many millions of Indians are at risk of deficiency on a nutritional basis. However, not all vegans develop cobalamin deficiency of sufficient severity to cause anaemia or neuropathy, even though subnormal cobalamin levels have been found in up to 50% of randomly selected, young, adult Indian vegans. Dietary cobalamin deficiency may also arise rarely in non-vegetarian subjects who exist on grossly inadequate diets because of poverty or psychiatric disturbance. Explanations of why nutritional cobalamin deficiency may not progress to megaloblastic anaemia include the following.

1 The diet of most vegans is probably not totally lacking cobalamin. The serum cobalamin level may not be an accurate measure of their body stores.

2 The enterohepatic circulation of cobalamin is still intact in vegans and thus losses are less (about 1 μg daily) than in conditions of malabsorption (about 2 μg gdaily).

3 Daily losses of cobalamin are thought to be related to body stores; therefore, as the body stores become depleted, daily losses become smaller and the amount of cobalamin needed to maintain the status quo may also become smaller.

Table 5.4 Alterations in plasma cobalamin-binding proteins in disease.

Haptocorrin
Increased (usually with elevated serum cobalamin)
    Myeloproliferative diseases, especially chronic myeloid leukaemia, myelosclerosis, polycythaemia vera
    Hepatoma
    Increased granulocyte production (e.g. inflammatory bowel disease, liver abscess)
    Eosinophilia due to hypereosinophilic syndrome
Congenital absence
    Low total serum cobalamin
    No clear clinical abnormality

Transcobalamin (II)
Increased (sometimes with no elevation of serum cobalamin)
    Liver disease
    Gaucher disease
    Autoimmune disease
    Long-continued hydroxocobalamin therapy
Congenital absence
    Normal or decreased total serum cobalamin
    Megaloblastic anaemia or pancytopenia within a few weeks of birth
    Impaired cobalamin absorption, may be associated with defective cellular and humoral immunity

Table 5.5 Causes of cobalamin deficiency causing megaloblastic anaemia.

Nutritional
Vegans

Malabsorption
Pernicious anaemia

Gastric causes
Congenital intrinsic factor deficiency or functional abnormality
Total or partial gastrectomy

Intestinal causes
Intestinal stagnant loop syndrome: jejunal diverticulosis, ileocolic fistula, anatomical blind loop, intestinal stricture, etc.
Ileal resection and Crohn's disease
Selective malabsorption with proteinuria
Tropical sprue
Transcobalamin deficiency
Fish tapeworm

Table 5.6 Malabsorption of cobalamin may occur in the following conditions but is not usually sufficiently severe and prolonged to cause megaloblastic anaemia.

Gastric causes
Simple atrophic gastritis (food cobalamin malabsorption)
Zollinger–Ellison syndrome
Gastric bypass surgery
Use of proton pump inhibitors

Intestinal causes
Gluten-induced enteropathy
Severe pancreatitis
HIV infection
Radiotherapy
Graft-versus-host disease

Deficiency states
Cobalamin, folate, protein, ?riboflavin, ?nicotinic acid

Drug therapy
Colchicine, *p*-aminosalicylate, neomycin, slow-release potassium chloride, anticonvulsant drugs, metformin, phenformin, cytotoxic drugs

Alcohol

Infants

Cobalamin deficiency has been described in infants born to severely cobalamin-deficient mothers. These infants develop megaloblastic anaemia at about 3–6 months of age since they are born with low stores of cobalamin and are then fed breast milk of low cobalamin content. This occurs most commonly in Indian vegans, but a similar condition has also been described in unrecognized maternal pernicious anaemia and in strict practitioners of veganism living in Western countries whose offspring have shown growth retardation, impaired psychomotor development and other neurological sequelae.

Gastric causes of cobalamin malabsorption
(Tables 5.5 and 5.6)

Pernicious anaemia

Pernicious anaemia (PA) may be defined as a severe lack of IF due to gastric atrophy. It is a common disease in northern Europeans but occurs in all countries and ethnic groups. The overall incidence is about 120 per 100 000 population in the UK, but there is wide variation between one area and the next. The prevalence rate in Western countries may be as high as 2–3%. The ratio of incidence in men and women is approximately 1:1.6 and the peak age of onset is 60 years, with only 10% of patients presenting being less than 40 years of age. In some ethnic groups, notably black people and Latin Americans, the age of onset of PA is generally lower. The disease occurs more commonly than by chance in close relatives, in subjects with other organ-specific autoimmune diseases (see below), in those

with premature greying, blue eyes and vitiligo, and in persons of blood group A. An association with human leucocyte antigen (HLA)-3 has been reported in some but not all series and in those with endocrine disease, with HLA-B8, -B12 and -BW15. The life expectancy has been estimated as normal in women once regular treatment has begun. Men have a slightly subnormal life expectancy as a result of a higher incidence of carcinoma of the stomach than in control subjects.

Diagnosis

This is usually suspected from the clinical picture and the findings of megaloblastic anaemia due to cobalamin deficiency. A lack of IF has been demonstrated by cobalamin absorption studies but this test is no longer available in most countries. Tests for circulating gastric autoantibodies are also important. Direct measurements on gastric juice following pentagastrin stimulation are now rarely performed. Hydrochloric acid or pepsin production and IF output were previously measured. The serum gastrin level is usually raised in PA (>200 μg/L), the hormone coming from endocrine cells in the gastric fundus. Raised serum gastrin also occurs in simple atrophic gastritis. Serum pepsinogen I levels are low (< 30 μg/L) in over 90% of those affected and a low ratio of serum pepsinogen I to pepsinogen II correlates with the presence of chronic atrophic gastritis.

Gastric biopsy

This usually shows atrophy of all layers of the body and also fundal atrophy, with loss of glandular elements, an absence of parietal and chief cells and replacement by mucous cells, a mixed inflammatory cell infiltrate and perhaps intestinal metaplasia. The infiltrate of plasma cells and lymphocytes contains an excess of CD4 cells. The antral mucosa is usually well preserved. *Helicobacter pylori* infection is infrequent in PA, but it has been suggested that *H. pylori* gastritis may represent an early phase of atrophic gastritis, which is gradually replaced, in some individuals, by an immune process with disappearance of *H. pylori* infection.

Immune phenomena

In addition to the appearance of the gastric mucosa, there is a large body of evidence that suggests that immune mechanisms play an important role in the pathogenesis of PA. This aspect of the disease is discussed under four main headings.

Antibodies to gastric antigens

1 *IF antibodies.* Two types of IF antibody may be found in the sera of patients with PA, both being IgG. One, the 'blocking' or 'type I' antibody, prevents the combination of IF and cobalamin, whereas the other, the 'binding', 'type II' or 'precipitating' antibody, which attaches to IF whether joined to cobalamin or not, prevents attachment of IF to ileal mucosa. The blocking antibody occurs in the serum of about 55% of patients and the binding antibody in 35%. IF antibodies cross the placenta and cause temporary IF deficiency in the newborn infant. Patients with PA also show cell-mediated immunity to IF. An increased CD4/CD8 lymphocyte ratio in blood has been described in PA patients with IF antibodies. IF antibodies are rarely found in conditions other than PA. Type I antibody has been detected rarely in the sera of patients without PA but with thyrotoxicosis, myxoedema, Hashimoto disease or diabetes mellitus, and in relatives of PA patients. IF antibodies have also been detected in gastric juice in about 80% of patients with PA. These antibodies may reduce absorption of dietary cobalamin by combining with small amounts of remaining IF in the gastric juice. Achlorhydria favours the formation of this antigen–antibody complex.

2 *Parietal cell and gastrin receptor antibodies.* Parietal cell antibody is present in the sera of almost 90% of adult patients with PA, but it is frequently present in other subjects. Thus, it occurs in as many as 16% of randomly selected female subjects aged over 60 years and in a smaller proportion of younger control subjects; it is found more frequently than in control subjects in relatives of PA patients. These antibodies are also found more frequently in patients with simple atrophic gastritis, chronic active hepatitis and thyroid disorders and their relatives, as well as in Addison disease, rheumatoid arthritis and other conditions. The parietal cell antibody is directed against the α- and β-subunits of the gastric proton pump (H^+/K^+-ATPase). The sera of PA patients may also contain an autoantibody to the gastrin receptor, although this test is not used clinically.

Association with other 'autoimmune' diseases

There is a clinical association between PA and thyroid diseases, vitiligo, hypoparathyroidism and Addison disease. These diseases are often found in close relatives of patients with overt disease due to one of these conditions.

Response to steroid therapy

Steroid therapy improves the gastric lesion, at least temporarily, in a proportion of patients with PA. There may be regeneration of the mucosa with a return of secretion of acid and IF, and an improvement in cobalamin absorption. When steroid therapy is withdrawn, there is relapse within a few weeks. These findings suggest that an autoimmune process is continuously damaging the gastric mucosa in PA and preventing regeneration.

Hypogammaglobulinaemia

PA is found more often than by chance in patients with a deficiency of IgA or with complete hypogammaglobulinaemia. These subjects resemble others with PA, except that they often present relatively early (before the age of 40 years), they have a lower incidence of serum IF and parietal cell antibodies, and they may show intestinal malabsorption. They may also have a history of recurrent infections. The gastric lesion is similar to that in other causes, except that plasma cells are absent from the inflammatory cell infiltrate and the antrum is involved. Serum gastrin levels are normal.

Juvenile pernicious anaemia

This usually occurs in older children and resembles PA of adults. Gastric atrophy, achlorhydria and serum IF antibodies are all present, although parietal cell antibodies are usually absent. About half of these patients show an associated endocrinopathy such as autoimmune thyroiditis, Addison disease or hypoparathyroidism; in some, mucocutaneous candidiasis occurs.

Congenital intrinsic factor deficiency or functional abnormality

The affected child usually shows no demonstrable IF but has a normal gastric mucosa and normal secretion of acid. The inheritance is autosomal recessive. These patients usually present with megaloblastic anaemia in the first, second or third year of life when stores of cobalamin accumulated from the mother *in utero* are used up; a few have presented as late as the second decade. Parietal cell and IF antibodies are absent. Variants have been described in which the child is born with IF that can be detected immunologically but which is unstable or functionally inactive, being unable either to bind cobalamin or to facilitate its uptake by the ileum.

Gastrectomy

Following total gastrectomy, cobalamin deficiency is inevitable and prophylactic cobalamin therapy should be commenced immediately following the operation. After partial gastrectomy, 10–15% of patients also develop this deficiency. The exact incidence and time of onset are most influenced by the size of the resection and the pre-existing size of the cobalamin body store.

Simple atrophic gastritis (food cobalamin malabsorption)

The normal IF-mediated mechanism of cobalamin absorption requires adequate gastric output of acid and pepsin to ensure the release of food cobalamin. Failure of this mechanism is believed to be responsible for a condition more common in the elderly known as *food cobalamin malabsorption*, but there is no definitive proof of this. The syndrome has also been described in association with *H. pylori* infection, long-term use of histamine H_2-receptor antagonists and proton-pump inhibitors, chronic alcoholism, pancreatic exocrine failure, Sjögren syndrome and systemic sclerosis. The syndrome is associated with low serum cobalamin levels, with or without evidence of cobalamin deficiency, such as raised serum levels of methylmalonic acid and homocysteine. A minority of patients with food cobalamin malabsorption may go on to develop clinically significant cobalamin deficiency including polyneuropathy, confusion, dementia and subacute combined degeneration of the cord and anaemia, but the frequency of occurrence and reasons for this progression are not clear.

Intestinal causes of cobalamin malabsorption

Malabsorption of cobalamin occurs in a variety of intestinal lesions in which there is colonization of the upper small intestine by faecal organisms. This may occur in patients with jejunal diverticulosis, enteroanastomosis, intestinal stricture or fistula, or with an anatomical blood loop due to Crohn's disease, tuberculosis or an operative procedure. Bacterial overgrowth in the small intestine may also cause spurious elevation of serum methylmalonate (see below). Some bacteria produce copious quantities of propionate, the immediate precursor of methylmalonate. Removal of 1.2 m or more of terminal ileum causes malabsorption of cobalamin. In some patients, following ileal resection, particularly if the ileocaecal valve is incompetent, colonic bacteria may contribute further to the onset of cobalamin deficiency.

Nearly all patients with acute and subacute tropical sprue show malabsorption of cobalamin; this may persist as the principal abnormality in the chronic form of the disease, when the patient may present with megaloblastic anaemia or neuropathy due to cobalamin deficiency. Absorption of cobalamin usually improves after antibiotic therapy and, in the early stages, after folic acid therapy. Malabsorption of cobalamin occurs in about 30% of untreated patients with gluten-induced enteropathy and correlates with the degree of steatorrhoea. Cobalamin defi-

ciency is not usually severe in these patients and is probably never the cause of megaloblastic anaemia unless another lesion causing malabsorption of cobalamin (e.g. stagnant loop syndrome) is present. The absorption improves when these patients are treated with a gluten-free diet.

Selective malabsorption of cobalamin with proteinuria (also known as Imerslünd syndrome, Imerslünd–Grasbeck syndrome, congenital cobalamin malabsorption or autosomal recessive megaloblastic anaemia MGA1) is an autosomal recessive disease and is the most common cause of megaloblastic anaemia due to cobalamin deficiency in infancy in Western countries. More than 200 cases have been reported, with familial clusters in Finland, Norway, the Middle East and North Africa. The patients usually present with megaloblastic anaemia between the ages of 1 and 5 years, and secrete normal amounts of IF and gastric acid. In some cases, such as in Finland, impaired synthesis, processing or ligand binding of cubilin due to inherited mutations, for example 391C→T (named FM1) and a mutation at an intron causing a truncated protein (FM2), have been implicated. In others, for example in Norway, mutation of the gene for AMN has been reported. Other tests of intestinal absorption are normal. Over 90% of these patients show non-specific proteinuria but renal function is otherwise normal and renal biopsy has not shown any consistent renal defect. A few of these patients have shown aminoaciduria and congenital renal abnormalities, such as duplication of the renal pelvis.

The fish tapeworm (*Diphyllobothrium latum*) lives in the small intestine of humans and accumulates cobalamin from food, rendering this unavailable for absorption. People acquire the worm by eating raw or partly cooked fish. Infestation is common around the lakes of Scandinavia, Germany, Japan, North America and Russia. Megaloblastic anaemia or cobalamin neuropathy occurs only in those with a heavy infestation, with the worm high in the small intestine. Many carriers have no cobalamin deficiency.

In severe chronic pancreatitis, lack of trypsin is thought to be the reason why dietary cobalamin attached to gastric non-IF (R) binder is unavailable for absorption. It has also been proposed that in pancreatitis, the concentration of calcium ions in the ileum falls below the level needed to maintain normal cobalamin absorption.

Serum cobalamin levels tend to fall in patients with HIV infection and are subnormal in 10–35% of those with AIDS. Increased levels of apoTC, possibly derived from macrophages, are usual. Malabsorption of crystalline cobalamin not corrected by IF has been shown in some, but not all, patients with subnormal serum cobalamin levels. Cobalamin deficiency sufficiently severe to cause megaloblastic anaemia or neuropathy is rare.

Malabsorption of cobalamin has been reported in Zollinger–Ellison syndrome. It is thought that there is a failure to release cobalamin from R binding protein due to inactivation of pancreatic trypsin by high acidity, as well as interference with IF binding of cobalamin.

Both total body irradiation and local radiotherapy to the ileum (e.g. as a complication of radiotherapy for carcinoma of the cervix) may cause malabsorption of cobalamin. Graft-versus-host disease commonly affects the small intestine: malabsorption of cobalamin due to abnormal gut flora, as well as damage to ileal mucosa, is frequent.

Neomycin, colchicine, phenytoin, p-aminosalicylic acid, phenformin, metformin, slow-release potassium chloride and alcohol have all been reported to cause malabsoption of cobalamin; rarely, megaloblastic anaemia due to cobalamin deficiency has been reported with phenformin therapy. The use of histamine H_2-blockers for treatment of peptic ulcer disease causes a decrease in cobalamin absorption, and continued use may lead to lowering of the serum cobalamin level.

Both severe cobalamin and folate deficiencies affect the function of the small intestine; malabsorption of cobalamin due to ileal dysfunction may be found in patients with either deficiency. It may take several weeks of cobalamin therapy to correct the ileal absorptive defect in patients with PA. Deficiencies of protein, riboflavin and pyridoxine have also been reported to cause malabsorption of cobalamin.

Abnormalities of cobalamin metabolism

Congenital transcobalamin deficiency or abnormality

Infants with TC deficiency usually present with megaloblastic anaemia within a few weeks of birth. Serum cobalamin and folate levels are normal but the anaemia responds to massive (e.g. 1 mg three times weekly) injections of cobalamin, which cause free cobalamin to enter marrow cells by passive diffusion in the absence of functional TC. Some cases show neurological complications. In some cases, the protein is present in normal amounts but is unable to bind cobalamin or to attach to the cell surface and so is functionally inert. Genetic abnormalities so far found include mutations of an intra-exonic cryptic splice site, extensive or single nucleotide deletion, nonsense mutation and an RNA editing defect. These infants do not show methylmalonic aciduria, but malabsorption of cobalamin occurs in all cases and reduced immunoglobulins in some. Less severe cases present later in childhood. Failure to institute adequate cobalamin therapy or treatment with folic acid may lead to neurological damage.

Congenital methylmalonic acidaemia and aciduria

Infants with this abnormality are ill from birth, with vomiting, failure to thrive, severe metabolic acidosis, ketosis and mental retardation. Anaemia, if present, is normocytic and normoblastic. The condition may arise as a result of a functional defect in either the mitochondrial methylmalonyl-CoA mutase or its cofactor ado-cobalamin (see Figure 5.2). Mutations in methylmalonyl-CoA mutase are not responsive, or only poorly responsive, to treatment with cobalamin. Two disorders result in cobalamin-responsive methylmalonic acidaemia. In cobalamin (Cbl)A disease, there is failure of reduction of cobalamin III (Cbl^{3+}) or cobalamin II (Cbl^{2+}) to cobalamin I (Cbl^{1+}) in mitochondria; in CblB disease, there is a defect of an adenosyltransferase required for synthesis of ado-cobalamin (see Figure 5.2). A proportion of infants with CblA and CblB disease respond to cobalamin in large doses, whereas others are unresponsive. In those who do not respond to cobalamin, the enzyme methylmalonyl-CoA mutase is lacking (mut^0) or defective (mut^-). Some children have combined methylmalonic aciduria and homocystinuria due to defective formation of both cobalamin coenzymes. The defects are in the transfer of cobalamin from the endocytic compartment of lysosomes to the cytoplasm (CblF disease) or in the reduction of cobalamin 3^+ to cobalamin 2^+ after transfer to the cytoplasm (CblC and CblD diseases). Over 100 cases of CblC disease have been described. It usually presents in the first year of life with feeding difficulties, developmental delay, microcephaly, seizures, hypotonia and megaloblastic anaemia.

Some patients present with homocystinuria and megaloblastic anaemia, often with neurological defects but without methylmalonic aciduria. There is a selective deficiency of methylcobalamin. These conditions have been termed CblE and CblG disease (lack of association of methylcobalamin with methionine synthase).

Acquired abnormality of cobalamin metabolism: nitrous oxide inhalation

N_2O irreversibly oxidizes methylcobalamin from its active, fully reduced Cbl^{1+} state to an inactive Cbl^{2+} precursor. This has been shown to inactivate methylcobalamin and methionine synthase. This occurs in both humans and experimental animals and was of importance in the megaloblastic anaemia that occurred in patients undergoing prolonged N_2O anaesthesia (e.g. in intensive care units). A neuropathy resembling cobalamin neuropathy has been described in dentists and anaesthetists who are repeatedly exposed to N_2O and in monkeys exposed to the gas for many months. In patients with low cobalamin stores, megaloblastic anaemia or cobalamin neuropathy may be precipitated after shorter exposure to N_2O. Recovery from N_2O exposure requires regeneration of methionine synthase, as this protein is damaged by active oxygen derived from the N_2O–cobalamin reaction. Methylmalonic aciduria does not occur at first as ado-cobalamin is not inactivated by N_2O. Later, however, after generalized depletion of cobalamin, methylmalonate levels in serum, urine and cerebrospinal fluid rise.

Diagnosis of cobalamin deficiency

The diagnosis of cobalamin or folate deficiency has traditionally depended on the recognition of the relevant abnormalities in the peripheral blood and/or bone marrow and subsequent analysis of the blood levels of the vitamins. Other causes of macrocytosis and hypersegmented neutrophils are listed in Table 5.3. However, assays of serum methylmalonic acid and homocysteine (see below) have shown these to be raised in some subjects without haematological abnormalities, including a proportion with normal levels of serum cobalamin and folate in whom, nevertheless, the levels of the metabolites fall to normal with cobalamin and/or folate therapy. The significance of these biochemical changes remains controversial. They may imply functional cobalamin or folate deficiency, not reflected by subnormal levels of the vitamins or by disturbed haemopoiesis. If so, it would imply that the accepted normal serum and red cell levels of the vitamins reflect body stores which are sufficiently high to prevent haematological changes but which in some subjects may not be optimal for prevention of other complications of the deficiencies including vascular disease and NTDs in the fetus.

Measurement of serum cobalamin

Serum cobalamin is usually measured by one of a number of enzyme-linked immunosorbent assays. These are frequently automated. Normal serum cobalamin levels range from 160–200 ng/L to about 1000 ng/L (ng × 0.738 = pmol, so 200 ng/L = 148 pmol/L). In patients with megaloblastic anaemia due to cobalamin deficiency, the level is usually less than 100 ng/L. In general, the more severe the deficiency, the lower the serum cobalamin level. In patients with spinal cord damage due to the deficiency, levels are very low even in the absence of anaemia. Values of between 100 and 200 ng/L are regarded as borderline. They may occur, for instance, in pregnancy, in patients with megaloblastic anaemia due to folate deficiency, and in patients with heterozygous, homozygous or compound heterozygous mutations of the *TCN1* gene that codes for HC (TCI). The relative concentrations of HC and TC also influence the total serum cobalamin level. Raised serum cobalamin levels (if not due to recent therapy) are usually due to a rise in HC (Table 5.4), or to liver or renal disease with increased saturation of HC and TC.

Serum holotranscobalamin (holoTCII, holoTC)

Since TC is the plasma cobalamin transport protein that is responsible for cellular uptake and delivery of cobalamin, the notion was put forward that measurement of circulating cobalamin that was bound to TC (holoTC) would provide a more meaningful measure of cobalamin status than total serum cobalamin. However, measurement of holoTC is not available or used diagnostically except in research studies.

Serum methylmalonate and homocysteine levels

In patients with cobalamin deficiency sufficient to cause anaemia or neuropathy, the serum methylmalonate (MMA) and homocysteine levels are raised. Sensitive methods for measuring MMA and homocysteine in serum have been introduced and recommended for the early diagnosis of cobalamin defi-

ciency, even in the absence of haematological abnormalities or subnormal levels of serum cobalamin or folate. However, serum MMA fluctuates in patients with renal failure. Mildly elevated serum MMA and/or homocysteine levels occur in up to 30% of apparently healthy volunteers, with serum cobalamin levels up to 350 ng/L and normal serum folate levels; 15% of elderly subjects, even with cobalamin levels above 350 ng/L, have this pattern of raised metabolite levels. These findings bring into question the exact cut-off points for normal MMA and homocysteine levels. It is also unclear at present whether these mildly raised metabolite levels have clinical consequences and how many of the subjects will progress to clinically overt cobalamin deficiency. When cobalamin supplies to the cell are suboptimal, there may be preferential use of methylcobalamin for methionine synthesis compared with ado-cobalamin for MMA metabolism. Urinary MMA excretion may also be used to screen for cobalamin deficiency but this is also increased in aminoaciduria (e.g. Fanconi syndrome).

Homocysteine exists in plasma as single molecules, as two molecules linked together (homocystine) and as mixed homocysteine–cysteine disulphides. Serum homocysteine levels are raised in both early cobalamin and folate deficiency, but they may be raised in other conditions, for example chronic renal disease, alcoholism, smoking, pyridoxine deficiency, hypothyroidism, therapy with steroids, ciclosporin and other drugs. Levels are also higher in serum than in plasma, in men than in premenopausal women, in women taking hormone replacement therapy or oral contraceptive users and in elderly subjects and patients with several inborn errors of metabolism affecting enzymes in trans-sulphuration pathways of homocysteine metabolism. Thus, homocysteine levels are not widely used for diagnosis of cobalamin or folate deficiency. However, homocysteine levels are used in thrombophilia screening and in assessing for cardiovascular risk factors (see Chapter 46).

Tests for the cause of cobalamin deficiency

Studies of cobalamin absorption were used but because of the unavailability of radioactive cobalamin have become obsolete. The urinary excretion (Schilling) test is therefore only briefly described here. Serum tests for gastrin and antibodies to parietal cells and intrinsic factor aid in the diagnosis of PA. Upper GI endoscopy including gastric biopsy helps to confirm the diagnosis and exclude gastric neoplasms.

Cobalamin absorption

The urinary secretion (Schilling) test was carried out with an oral trace dose of crystalline radioactive cyanocobalamin with or without oral IF and a 'flushing' intramuscular dose of hydroxocobalamin or cyanocobalamin so that any labelled cobalamin absorbed would appear in a 24-hour urine. Radioactive cyanocobalamin is no longer available and the test is obsolete, as are similar tests of food absorption using radio-actively labelled cobalamin.

Folate

Dietary folate

Folic acid (pteroylglutamic acid) is a yellow, crystalline, water-soluble substance (molecular weight 441). It is the parent compound of a large family of folate compounds. Pteroylglutamic acid consists of three parts: pteridine, *p*-aminobenzoate and L-glutamic acid (Figure 5.8). It is only a minor component of normal food folates (probably less than 1%), which differ from it in three respects (Figure 5.8): (i) they are partly or completely reduced at positions 4, 5, 7 and 8 in the pteridine portion to dihydrofolate or THF derivatives; (ii) they usually contain a single carbon unit of varying degrees of reduction, such as a methyl group at N-5 or N-10; and (iii) 70–90% of natural folates contain a chain of three or more glutamate residues linked to each other by the unusual γ-peptide bond and are called pteroyl- or folate-polyglutamates. In human cells, four, five and six glutamate residues are usual.

Most foods contain some folate. The highest concentrations are found in liver and yeast (>200 μg per 100 g), spinach, other greens and nuts (>100 μg per 100 g). The total folate content of an average Western diet is about 250 μg daily, but the amount varies widely according to the type of food eaten and the method of cooking. Folate is easily destroyed by heating, particularly in large volumes of water; over 90% may be lost.

Body stores and requirements

Total body folate in the adult is about 10 mg, the liver containing the largest store. Daily adult requirements are about 100 μg. Up to 13 μg of folate is lost as such in the urine each day, but breakdown products of folate are also lost in urine. Losses of folate also occur in sweat and skin; faecal folate is largely derived from colonic bacteria. Stores are only sufficient for about 4 months in normal adults, so severe folate deficiency may develop rapidly.

Absorption

The principal site of folate absorption is the upper small intestine, and there is a steep fall-off in absorptive capacity in the lower jejunum and ileum. The absorption of all forms tested is rapid, a rise in blood level occurring within 15–20 min of ingestion.

The small intestine has a tremendous capacity to absorb folate monoglutamates: about 90% of a single dose is absorbed regardless of whether this is small (100 μg) or large (15 mg). A proton-coupled high-affinity folate transporter with a low pH optimum, termed PCFT/HCP1, is located at the apical brush border of the duodenal, and to a lesser extent jejunal mucosa and in other cells, including the blood–brain barrier. It accounts for the bulk of folate absorption including of folic acid itself, and loss of function in hereditary folate malabsorption is not compensated by other folate transporters expressed on intestinal cells.

The absorption of folate polyglutamates with higher numbers of glutamate residues is less. This may be due to the limited capacity of the small intestine to hydrolyse these compounds or to their limited transfer in the mucosal cell. On average, about 50% of food folates is absorbed.

Polyglutamate forms are hydrolysed by pteroylpolyglutamate hydrolase (PPH, also known as folylpoly-γ-glutamate carboxypeptidase) to the monoglutamate derivatives, either in the lumen of the intestine or within the mucosa; they do not enter portal blood intact. Monoglutamate or polyglutamate forms of dietary folate, which are already partly or completely reduced, are converted to 5-methyl-THF within the small intestinal mucosa before entering the portal plasma. The monoglutamates are actively transported across the enterocyte by a carrier-mediated mechanism. Pteroylglutamic acid at doses greater than 400 μg is absorbed largely unchanged and converted to natural folates in the liver. Lower doses are converted to 5-methyl-THF during absorption through the intestine.

Enterohepatic circulation

About 60–90 μg of folate enters the bile each day and is excreted into the small intestine. Loss of this folate, together with the folate of sloughed intestinal cells, accelerates the speed with which folate deficiency develops in malabsorption conditions.

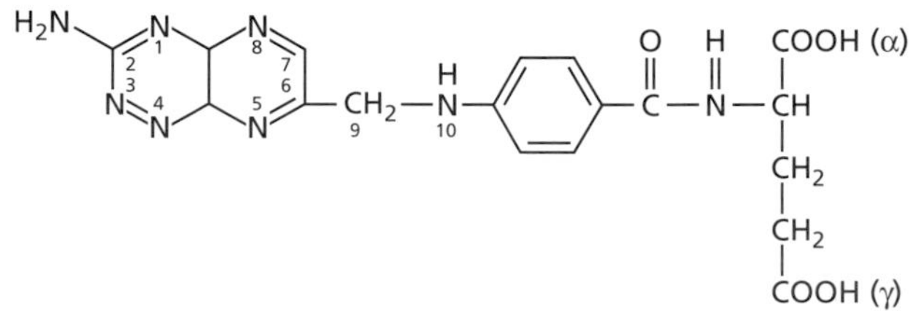

Figure 5.8 The structure of folic acid (pteroylglutamic acid).

Transport

Folate is transported in plasma, about one-third loosely bound to albumin and two-thirds unbound. In all body fluids (plasma, cerebrospinal fluid, milk, bile) folate is largely, if not entirely, 5-methyl-THF in the monoglutamate form. A carrier-mediated active process is involved in the entry of folate into cells, the rate of uptake being linked to the rate of folate polyglutamate synthesis in the cell, which in replicating cells is related to the rate of DNA synthesis. Reduced folates are more rapidly taken up than oxidized folates. In most cells, folates are retained with tight binding to folate-binding proteins, three of which are enzymes involved in methyl group metabolism (sarcosine dehydrogenase, dimethylglycine dehydrogenase and glycine N-methyltransferase), until the cell dies. Intact liver cells can release folate. Two types of folate-binding protein are involved in entry of methyl-THF into cells. The reduced folate carrier SLC19A1 is a facilitative transporter with a pH optimum of 7.4 and the characteristics of an anion exchanger. Two glycosyl-phosphatidylinositol (GPI)-linked folate receptors mediate cellular folate uptake by an endocytic mechanism, with internalization in a vesicle (caveola) which is then acidified, releasing folate into the vesicle lumen. Folate is then carried by the membrane folate transporter PCFT/HCPI into the cytoplasm; the caveola recycles to the cell surface, where its high-affinity receptors are reutilized. The GPI-linked transporters may be involved in transport of oxidized folates and folate breakdown products to the liver for excretion in bile.

Biochemical functions

Folates (as the intracellular polyglutamate derivatives) act as coenzymes in the transfer of single-carbon units from one compound to another (see Figure 5.3 and Table 5.2). Two of these reactions are involved in purine and one in pyrimidine synthesis necessary for DNA and RNA replication. Folate is coenzyme in another reaction, methionine synthesis, in which cobalamin is also involved and THF is regenerated. THF is the acceptor of single-carbon units newly entering the active pool via conversion of serine to glycine. Methionine, the other product of the methionine synthase reaction, is the precursor for SAM, the universal methyl donor involved in over 100 methyltransferase reactions.

During thymidylate synthesis, 5,10-methylene-THF is converted to dihydrofolate (Figure 5.3). The enzyme dihydrofolate reductase converts this to THF. The drugs methotrexate, pyrimethamine and, mainly in bacteria, trimethoprim inhibit dihydrofolate reductase, and this prevents formation of the active folate coenzymes from dihydrofolate. A small fraction of the folate coenzyme is not recycled during thymidylate synthesis but is degraded at the C-9–N-10 bond.

Table 5.7 Causes of folate deficiency.

Dietary
Particularly in old age, infancy, poverty, alcoholism, chronic invalids and the psychiatrically disturbed; may be associated with scurvy or kwashiorkor

Malabsorption
Major causes of deficiency
Tropical sprue, gluten-induced enteropathy in children and adults, and in association with dermatitis herpetiformis, specific malabsorption of folate, intestinal megaloblastosis caused by severe cobalamin or folate deficiency

Minor causes of deficiency
Extensive jejunal resection, Crohn's disease, partial gastrectomy, congestive heart failure, Whipple disease, scleroderma, amyloid, diabetic enteropathy, systemic bacterial infection, lymphoma, sulfasalazine

Excess utilization or loss
Physiological
Pregnancy and lactation, prematurity

Pathological
Haematological diseases: chronic haemolytic anaemias, sickle cell anaemia, thalassaemia major, myelofibrosis
Malignant diseases: carcinoma, lymphoma, leukaemia, myeloma
Inflammatory diseases: tuberculosis, Crohn's disease, psoriasis, exfoliative dermatitis, malaria
Metabolic disease: homocystinuria
Excess urinary loss: congestive heart failure, active liver disease
Haemodialysis, peritoneal dialysis

Antifolate drugs
Anticonvulsant drugs (phenytoin, primidone, barbiturates), sulfasalazine
Nitrofurantoin, tetracycline, anti-tuberculosis (less well documented)

Mixed causes
Liver diseases, alcoholism, intensive care units

Note: In severely folate-deficient patients with causes other than those listed under Dietary, poor dietary intake is often present.

Causes of folate deficiency (Table 5.7)

Nutritional

Dietary folate deficiency is common. Indeed, in most patients with folate deficiency a nutritional element is present. Certain individuals are particularly likely to have diets containing inadequate amounts of folate, including the old, edentulous, poor, alcoholic and psychiatrically disturbed, and patients after gastric operations. In relation to the size of the total body folate stores, which are in the order of 15–25 mg, the daily requirement of 100–200 mg is large. Consequently, with total cessation of intake or absorption, depletion of stores will occur in 3–6 months. In the USA and other countries where fortification of the diet with folic acid has been adopted to reduce the incidence of NTDs, the prevalence of folate deficiency has dropped dramatically and is now almost restricted to high-risk groups with increased folate needs. Nutritional folate deficiency occurs in kwashiorkor and scurvy, and in infants with repeated infections or who are fed solely on goats' milk, which has a low folate content (6 μg/L) compared with human or cows' milk (50 μg/L) as well as high concentrations of a high-affinity folate-binding protein.

Malabsorption

Malabsorption of dietary folate occurs in tropical sprue and in gluten-induced enteropathy in children and in adults, when it is associated with dermatitis herpetiformis. In the rare recessive congenital syndrome of selective malabsorption of folate, there is an associated defect of folate transport into the cerebrospinal fluid, and these patients show megaloblastic anaemia from the age of a few months, responding to physiological doses of folic acid given parenterally but not orally or large oral doses of 5-formyl-THF. These patients also show mental retardation, convulsions and other central nervous system abnormalities. Loss-of-function mutations, usually homozygous in the gene coding for the low pH transporter PCFT/HCPI, underlie the disease. Minor degrees of malabsorption may also occur following jejunal resection or partial gastrectomy, in Crohn's disease and in systemic infections but, in these conditions, if severe deficiency occurs, it is usually largely due to poor nutrition.

Malabsorption of folate has been described in patients receiving sulfasalazine, cholestyramine and triamterene. It has also been associated with anticonvulsant drug therapy, alcohol abuse and folate deficiency, but these relationships are less well established. In the intestinal stagnant loop syndrome, the predominant effect of the small intestinal bacteria is to cause a rise in serum, red cell and urinary folate by synthesizing folate, which is then absorbed.

Excess utilization or loss

Pregnancy

Folate requirements are increased by 200–300 μg to about 400 μg daily in a normal pregnancy, partly because of transfer of the vitamin to the fetus, but mainly because of increased folate catabolism due to cleavage of folate coenzymes in rapidly proliferating tissues at the C-9–N-10 bond. Megaloblastic anaemia due to this deficiency is now largely prevented by prophylactic folic acid therapy. It occurred in 0.5% of pregnancies in the UK and other Western countries, but the incidence is much higher in countries where the general nutritional status is poor. The deficiency is more common in pregnant women who also suffer from iron deficiency, probably because these patients have a poor diet. The usual presentation of the anaemia is similar to that of other megaloblastic anaemias, but occasionally, when there is an associated infection, acute arrest of haemopoiesis with pancytopenia may occur; this resembles aplastic anaemia, except that the marrow shows obvious megaloblastic changes.

A number of consequences of folate deficiency in pregnancy have been described, including antenatal and postpartum haemorrhages, prematurity and congenital malabsorption in the fetus. These have not been fully established, but several studies have shown that prophylactic folic acid therapy reduces the incidence of NTDs (see p. 64).

Prematurity

The newborn infant, whether full term or premature, has higher serum and red cell folate concentrations than the adult, but the newborn infant's demand for folate has been estimated to be up to 10 times that of adults on a weight basis and the neonatal folate level falls rapidly to the lowest values at about 6 weeks of age. The falls are steepest and liable to reach subnormal levels in premature babies, a number of whom develop megaloblastic anaemia responsive to folic acid at about 4–6 weeks of age. This occurs particularly in the smallest babies (<1500 g birth weight) and in those who have feeding difficulties or infections, or who have undergone multiple exchange transfusions. In these babies, prophylactic folic acid should be given.

Haematological disorders

Folate deficiency frequently occurs in chronic haemolytic anaemia, particularly in sickle cell disease, autoimmune haemolytic anaemia and congenital spherocytosis. In these and other conditions of increased cell turnover, folate deficiency arises because it is not completely reutilized after performing coenzyme functions, and it is partly lost as pteridines in the urine due to cleavage at the C-9–N-10 bond. Patients with primary myelofibrosis may develop folate deficiency at some stage of the illness. There is also a high incidence of mild folate deficiency in patients with leukaemia, lymphoma, myeloma or carcinoma, although it is unusual for this to progress to megaloblastic anaemia. Treatment with folic acid should be avoided (as it may 'feed' the tumour) unless severe megaloblastic anaemia due to folate deficiency is clinically important.

Inflammatory conditions

Chronic inflammatory diseases, such as tuberculosis, rheumatoid arthritis, Crohn's disease, psoriasis, exfoliative dermatitis, bacterial endocarditis and chronic bacterial infections, cause deficiency by reducing the appetite and by increasing the demand for folate. Systemic infections may also cause malabsorption of folate. Severe deficiency is virtually confined to those patients with the most active disease and the poorest diet. Fever *per se* has also been suggested to interfere with folate metabolism by inhibiting temperature-dependent folate enzymes. In patients with subclinical folate deficiency from causes other than infections, intercurrent infections often precipitate severe megaloblastic anaemia.

Homocystinuria

This is a rare metabolic defect in the conversion of homocysteine to cystathionine. Folate deficiency occurring in most of these patients may be due to excessive utilization because of compensatory increased conversion of homocysteine to methionine.

Long-term dialysis

As folate is only loosely bound to plasma proteins, it is easily removed from plasma by haemodialysis or peritoneal dialysis (in contrast, cobalamin is not removed from plasma by dialysis as it is firmly protein bound). The amount of body folate that can be removed in this way is relatively small. Nevertheless, in patients with anorexia, vomiting, infections and haemolysis, folate stores may become depleted and megaloblastic anaemia can supervene. Routine folate prophylaxis is now given.

Congestive heart failure, liver disease

Excess urinary folate losses of more than 100 µg per day may occur in some of these patients. The explanation appears to be release of folate from damaged liver cells.

Antifolate drugs

A large number of epileptics who are receiving long-term therapy with phenytoin (Dilantin) or primidone (Mysoline), with or without barbiturates, develop low serum and red cell folate levels. In some of these patients, megaloblastic anaemia supervenes. A number of mechanisms have been suggested: inhibition of folate absorption, inhibition of the action or synthesis of folate-dependent enzymes, displacement of folate from its plasma transport protein and induction of folate-utilizing enzymes. A dietary element is present in the patients with the severest deficiencies.

Alcohol may also be a folate antagonist, as patients who are drinking spirits may develop megaloblastic anaemia that will respond to normal quantities of dietary folate or to physiological doses of folic acid only if the alcohol is withdrawn. Chronic alcohol intake is associated with macrocytosis even when folate levels are normal. Inadequate folate intake is the major factor in the development of deficiency in spirit-drinking alcoholics. Beer is relatively folate-rich in some countries, depending on the technique used for brewing.

The drugs that inhibit dihydrofolate reductase include methotrexate, pyrimethamine and trimethoprim. Methotrexate has the most powerful action against the human enzyme, whereas trimethoprim is most active against the bacterial enzyme and is only likely to cause megaloblastic anaemia when used in conjunction with sulfamethoxazole in patients with pre-existing folate or cobalamin deficiency. The activity of pyrimethamine

is intermediate. The antidote to these drugs is folinic acid (5-formyl-THF).

Congenital abnormalities of folate metabolism

A number of infants have been described with congenital defects of folate enzymes (e.g. cyclohydrolase or methionine synthase). Some had megaloblastic anaemia.

Diagnosis of folate deficiency

Serum folate

This is measured by an enzyme-linked immunosorbent assay (ELISA). The serum folate level is low in all folate-deficient patients. In most laboratories, the normal range is from 2.0 µg/L (11 nmol/L) to about 15 µg/L. The serum folate is markedly affected by recent diet; inadequate intake for as little as 1 week may cause the level to become subnormal.

The serum folate level rises in severe cobalamin deficiency because of blockage in conversion of methyl-THF, the major circulating form, to THF; raised levels have also been reported in the intestinal stagnant loop syndrome, acute renal failure and active liver damage. (High levels are also obtained when the patient is receiving folic acid therapy, when the serum is contaminated with folate or folate-producing bacteria or, if a sample is haemolysed, because of the high concentration of folate in red cells.)

Red cell folate

The red cell folate assay is a valuable test of body folate stores. It is less affected by recent diet and traces of haemolysis than is the serum assay. In normal adults, concentrations range from 160 to 640 µg/L of packed red cells. Subnormal levels occur in patients with megaloblastic anaemia due to folate deficiency but also occur in nearly two-thirds of patients with megaloblastic anaemia due to cobalamin deficiency. If cobalamin deficiency is excluded, however, a low red cell folate can be used as an indication that severe folate deficiency is present and warrants full investigation and treatment. False normal results may occur if the folate-deficient patient has received a recent blood transfusion (as the folate content of the transfused red cells will be measured) or if the patient has a raised reticulocyte count (e.g. due to haemorrhage or haemolytic anaemia).

Serum homocysteine (see p. 75)

General management of megaloblastic anaemia

It is usually possible to establish which of the two deficiencies, folate or cobalamin, is the cause of the anaemia and to treat only with the appropriate vitamin. In patients who enter hospital severely ill, however, it may be necessary to treat with both vitamins in large doses once blood samples have been taken for cobalamin and folate assay and a bone marrow has been performed (if deemed necessary). Transfusion is usually unnecessary and inadvisable. If it is essential, packed red cells should be given slowly and one or two units will be ample. Exchange transfusion, as well as the usual treatment for heart failure, should be considered in patients with extreme anaemia and congestive heart failure. Platelet concentrates are of value in reducing spontaneous bleeding in the rare patients with severe thrombocytopenia. Potassium supplements have been recommended to obviate the danger of the hypokalaemia that has been recorded in some patients during the initial haematological response, but there is little evidence for this.

Treatment of cobalamin deficiency

It is usually necessary to treat patients who have developed cobalamin deficiency with lifelong regular cobalamin therapy. In the UK, the form used is hydroxocobalamin; in the USA cyanocobalamin is used. In a few instances, the underlying cause of cobalamin deficiency can be permanently corrected, for instance the fish tapeworm, tropical sprue or an intestinal stagnant loop that is amenable to surgery.

The indications for starting cobalamin therapy are a well-documented megaloblastic anaemia or neuropathy due to the deficiency. It is also necessary to treat any patients with haematological abnormalities due to cobalamin deficiency, even in the absence of anaemia (e.g. hypersegmented neutrophils or megaloblastic erythropoiesis). Patients with borderline serum cobalamin levels but no haematological or other abnormality should if practicable be followed, for example at yearly intervals, to ensure that the cobalamin deficiency does not progress. If malabsorption of cobalamin or rises in serum MMA levels have also been demonstrated, patients should also be given regular maintenance cobalamin therapy. Cobalamin should be given routinely to all patients who have had a total gastrectomy or ileal resection. Patients who have undergone gastric reduction for control of obesity or who are receiving long-term treatment with proton pump inhibitors should be screened and given cobalamin replacement as necessary.

Replenishment of body stores should be complete with six 1000-µg intramuscular injections of *hydroxocobalamin* given at 3–7 day intervals. More frequent doses are usually used in patients with cobalamin neuropathy, but there is no evidence that these produce a better response. For maintenance therapy, hydroxocobalamin 1000 µg i.m. once every 3 months is satisfactory. In the USA, hydroxocobalamin has not yet been approved and marketed for purposes of routine cobalamin replacement. Because of the poorer retention of cyanocobalamin maintenance treatment, protocols generally use higher and more frequent doses (1000 µg i.m. monthly).

Toxic reactions to cobalamin therapy are extremely rare and are usually due to contamination in its preparation rather than to cobalamin itself. Even when there is complete failure of the physiological IF-dependent mechanism, large daily oral doses (1000 µg) of cyanocobalamin can be used for replacement and maintenance of normal cobalamin status, for example in those who cannot have injections. If this approach is used, it is important to monitor compliance, particularly with elderly forgetful patients. Sublingual and nasal routes have also been proposed but no long-term follow-up data are available.

Treatment of folate deficiency

There is probably never any need to give folic acid parenterally, except in patients receiving parenteral nutrition who cannot swallow tablets. Oral doses of 5–15 mg folic acid daily are satisfactory, as sufficient folate is absorbed from these extremely large doses even in patients with severe malabsorption. The length of time therapy must be continued depends on the underlying disease. It is customary to continue therapy for about 4 months, when all folate-deficient red cells will have been eliminated and replaced by new folate-replete populations.

Before large doses of folic acid are given, cobalamin deficiency must be excluded and, if present, corrected, otherwise cobalamin neuropathy may develop, despite response of the anaemia of cobalamin deficiency to folate therapy. Studies suggest that there has been no increase in the proportion of subjects with low serum cobalamin levels and no anaemia since fortification of the diet in the USA.

Long-term folic acid therapy is required when the underlying cause of the deficiency cannot be corrected and the deficiency is likely to recur, for instance in chronic haemolytic anaemias such as thalassaemia major and sickle cell anaemia, and in primary myelofibrosis. It may also be necessary in gluten-induced enteropathy if this does not respond to a gluten-free diet. Where mild but chronic folate deficiency occurs, it is preferable to encourage any improvement in the diet after correcting the deficiency with a short course of folic acid. In any patient receiving long-term folic acid therapy, it is important to measure the serum cobalamin level at regular (e.g. once yearly) intervals to exclude the coincidental development of cobalamin deficiency.

Folinic acid (5-formyl-THF)

This is a stable form of fully reduced folate. It is given orally or parenterally to overcome the toxic effects of methotrexate or other dihydrofolate reductase inhibitors (as present in co-trimoxazole).

Prophylactic folic acid

In many countries, food is fortified with folic acid (in grain or flour) to reduce the incidence of NTDs. As yet there is no definite proof that folic acid prevents cardiovascular (other than stroke), neurological or psychiatric disease. There is some evidence it may reduce the risk of certain forms of cancer, but this remains controversial.

Pregnancy

Folic acid 400 µg daily should be given as a supplement throughout pregnancy. In women who have had a previous fetus with an NTD, 5 mg daily is recommended when pregnancy is contemplated and throughout the subsequent pregnancy. In women of childbearing age, a supplementary intake of folic acid 400 µg daily is recommended, so that this extra intake will be present from conception.

Prematurity

The incidence of folate deficiency is so high in the smallest premature babies during the first 6 weeks of life that folic acid (e.g. 1 mg daily) should be given routinely to babies weighing less than 1500 g at birth and to larger premature babies who require exchange transfusions or develop feeding difficulties, infections or vomiting and diarrhoea.

Haemolytic anaemia and dialysis

Prophylactic folic acid is usually also given to patients with chronic haemolytic anaemia or those who are undergoing long-term haemodialysis.

Megaloblastic anaemia not due to cobalamin or folate deficiency or altered metabolism

This may occur with many antimetabolic drugs (e.g. hydroxy-carbamide, cytarabine, 6-mercaptopurine) that inhibit DNA replication at a particular point in the supply of precursors or by inhibiting DNA polymerase. In the rare disease orotic aciduria, two consecutive enzymes in purine synthesis are defective. The condition responds to therapy with uridine, which bypasses the block. In thiamine-responsive megaloblastic anaemia, there is a genetic defect in the high-affinity thiamine transport (*SLC19A2*) gene. This causes defective RNA ribose synthesis through impaired activity of transketolase, a thiamine-dependent enzyme in the pentose cycle. This leads to reduced nucleic acid production and consequent induction of cell cycle arrest or apoptosis. It may be associated with diabetes mellitus and deafness and the presence of many ringed sideroblasts in the marrow (see p. 44). The biochemical explanation is unclear for megaloblastic changes in the marrow in patients with acute myeloid leukaemia, and other leukaemias and myelodysplasia in the absence of cobalamin or folate deficiency.

Other nutritional anaemias

Protein deficiency

Anaemia is usual in children and adults with severe protein deficiency (kwashiorkor). The anaemia, which may be partly masked by haemoconcentration, is usually normoblastic, but megaloblastic changes have been described in 10–60% of patients in different series. Hypoplasia, or even aplasia, of the marrow has also been reported. The mechanism by which protein deficiency causes anaemia is not completely understood. Lack of protein does not seem to reduce haemoglobin synthesis directly. Studies in experimental animals suggest that the major factor is diminution of erythropoietin secretion. This is probably due to a reduction in general tissue metabolism and therefore oxygen consumption, with a consequent reduced stimulus for erythropoietin secretion. In most patients, other factors contribute to the anaemia. These include infections, deficiencies of folate and iron, and also, possibly, deficiencies of vitamins C, E and B_{12} and other trace substances. Riboflavin deficiency may also contribute to the anaemia and become apparent only during the response to protein.

Scurvy

There is usually a moderate or severe normocytic, normochromic anaemia in scurvy because of external haemorrhage and haemorrhage into tissues, and from impaired erythropoiesis. In some patients, the anaemia is megaloblastic, which appears to be partly due to associated nutritional folate deficiency and partly due to impairment of folate metabolism caused by vitamin C deficiency. However, vitamin C is not established as playing a role in normal folate metabolism.

Other deficiencies

Deficiencies of nicotinic acid and panthothenic acid cause anaemia in experimental animals but have not been shown to do so in humans. However, riboflavin deficiency may cause anaemia in humans, resembling the anaemia of protein deficiency. Copper is essential for haemopoiesis and normal iron metabolism, and deficiency of copper causes an anaemia resembling that in iron deficiency in experimental animals. However, anaemia due to copper deficiency has never been documented in humans. Copper excess (as in Wilson disease) causes a haemolytic anaemia.

Selected bibliography

Boccia S, Hung R, Ricciardi G *et al.* (2008) Meta- and pooled analyses of the methylenetetrahydrofolate reductase C677T and

A1298C polymorphisms and gastric cancer risk: a huge-GSEC review. *American Journal of Epidemiology* **167**: 505–16.

Boros LG, Steinkamp MP, Fleming JC *et al.* (2003) Defective RNA ribose synthesis in fibroblasts from patients with thiamine-responsive megaloblastic anaemia (TRMA) *Blood* **102**: 3556–61.

Carmel R (2008) How I treat cobalamin (vitamin B12) deficiency. *Blood* **112**: 2214–21.

Carmel R, Parker J, Kelman Z (2009) Genomic mutations associated with mild and severe deficiencies of transcobalamin I (haptocorrin) that cause mildly or severely low serum cobalamin levels. *British Journal of Haematology* **147**: 386–91.

Christensen EI, Birn H (2002) Megalin and cubilin: multifunctional endocytic receptors. *Nature Reviews. Molecular Cell Biology* **3**: 256–66.

Dali-Youcef N, Andrès E (2009) An update on cobalamin deficiency in adults. *Quarterly Journal of Medicine* **102**: 17–28.

de Jonge R, Tissing WJ, Hooijberg JH *et al.* (2009) Polymorphisms in folate-related genes and risk of paediatric acute lymphoblastic leukaemia. *Blood* **113**: 2284–9.

Drake B, Colditz GA (2009) Assessing cancer prevention studies – a matter of time. *Journal of the American Medical Association* **302**: 2152–3.

Ebbing M, Bonaa KH, Nygard O *et al.* (2009) Cancer incidence and mortality after treatment with folic acid and vitamin B_{12}. *Journal of the American Medical Association* **302**: 2119–26.

Eichholzer M, Tonz O, Zimmerman R (2006) Folic acid: a public health challenge. *Lancet* **367**: 1352–61.

Fyfe JC, Madsen M, Hojrup P *et al.* (2004) The functional cobalamin (vitamin B_{12}) intrinsic factor receptor is a novel complex of cubulin and aminonless. *Blood* **103**: 1573–9.

He K, Anwar M, Rimm E *et al.* (2004) Folate, vitamin B_6 and B_{12} intakes in relation to risk of stroke among men. *Stroke* **35**: 169–74.

Koppen IJN, Hermans FJR, Caspers GJL (2009) Folate related gene polymorphisms and susceptibility to develop childhood acute lymphoblastic leukaemia. *British Journal of Haematology* **148**: 3–14.

Kozyraki R, Kristiansen M, Silahtraroglu A *et al.* (1998) The human intrinsic-factor–vitamin B_{12} receptor: molecular characterization and chromosomal mapping of the gene to 10p within the autosomal megaloblastic anaemia (MAI) region. *Blood* **91**: 3593–600.

Lasry I, Berman B, Straussberg R *et al.* (2008) A novel loss-of-function mutation in the proton-coupled folate transporter from a patient with hereditary folate malabsorption reveals that Arg 113 is crucial for function. *Blood* **112**: 2055–8.

Lewerin C (2008) Serum biomarkers for atrophic gastritis and antibodies against *Helicobacter pylori* in the elderly: implications for vitamin B12, folic acid and iron status and response to oral vitamin therapy. *Scandinavian Journal of Gastroenterology* **43**: 1502–8.

Matthew LH, Goldman ID (2003) Membrane transplant of folates. *Vitamins and Hormones* **66**: 403–56.

Miller JW, Ramos MI, Garrod MG *et al.* (2002) Transcobalamin II 775G→C polymorphism and indices of vitamin B12 status in healthy older adults. *Blood* **100**: 718–20.

Mills JL, VonKohirin I, Conley MR *et al.* (2003) Low vitamin B_{12} concentrations in patients without anaemia: the effect of folic acid fortification of grain. *American Journal of Clinical Nutrition* **77**: 1474–7.

Morris MS, Jacques PF, Resenberg IH, Selhub J (2007) Folate and vitamin B-12 status in relation to anaemia, macrocytosis, and cognitive impairment in older Americans in the age of folic acid fortification. *American Journal of Clinical Nutrition* **85**: 193–200.

Qiu A, Jansen M, Sakaris A *et al.* (2007) Identification of an intestinal folate transporter and the molecular basis for hereditary folate malabsorption. *Cell* **127**: 917–28.

Quadros EV (2009) Advances in the understanding of cobalamin assimilation and metabolism. *British Journal of Haematology* **148**: 195–204.

Quadros EV, Nakayama Y, Sequeira JM (2009) The protein and the gene encoding the receptor for the cellular uptake of transcobalamin-bound cobalamin. *Blood* **113**: 186–92.

Ramaekers VT, Blau N, Sequeira JM, Nassogne MC, Quadros EV (2007) Folate receptor autoimmunity and cerebral folate deficiency in low-functioning autism with neurological deficits. *Neuropediatrics* **38**: 276–81.

Savage DG, Lindebaum J (1995) Neurological complications of acquired cobalamin deficiency: clinical aspects. *Clinical Haematology* **8**: 657–78.

Seshadri S, Beiser A, Selhub J *et al.* (2002) Plasma homocysteine as a risk factor for dementia and Alzheimer's disease. *New England Journal of Medicine* **346**: 476–83.

Shaw GM, Lammer EJ, Wasserman CR *et al.* (1995) Risks of facial clefts in children born to women using multi-vitamins containing folic acid periconceptually. *Lancet* **346**: 393–6.

Tanner SM, Aminoff M, Wright FA *et al.* (2003) Amnionless, essential for mouse gastrulation, is mutated in recessive hereditary megaloblastic anaemia. *Nature Genetics* **33**: 426–9.

Wald DS, Low M, Morris JK (2002) Homocysteine and cardiovascular disease: evidence of causality from a meta-analysis. *British Medical Journal* **325**: 1202–6.

Wolpin BM, Wei EK, Ng K *et al.* (2008) Prediagnostic plasma folate and the risk of death in patients with colorectal cancer. *Journal of Clinical Oncology* **26**: 3222–8.

Haemoglobin and the inherited disorders of globin synthesis

6

Swee Lay Thein[1,2] and David Rees[1,2]

[1]Division of Gene and Cell Based Therapy, Kings College London School of Medicine, London, UK
[2]Department of Haematological Medicine, King's College Hospital, London, UK

Introduction

The inherited disorders of haemoglobin are the commonest single-gene disorders, with an estimated carrier rate of 7% among the world population. They occur at particularly high frequencies in populations of the tropical and subtropical belt, and consist mainly of the α and β thalassaemias, and the haemoglobin variants S, C and E. In many developing countries, as economic conditions improve and infant death rates from infection and malnutrition fall, the genetic disorders of haemoglobin start to place a major burden on the health services, a phenomenon that has already been observed in many parts of the world. As a result of migrations of populations, these conditions are being seen with increasing frequency in many countries in which they had not been recognized previously.

The structure, genetic control and synthesis of haemoglobin

Different haemoglobins are synthesised in the embryo, fetus and adult, each adapted to their particular oxygen requirements. They all have a tetrameric structure made up of two different pairs (one α-like and one β-like) of globin chains, each

Postgraduate Haematology: 6th edition. Edited by A. Victor Hoffbrand, Daniel Catovsky, Edward G.D. Tuddenham, Anthony R. Green
© 2011 Blackwell Publishing Ltd.

attached to one haem molecule, the moiety responsible for the reversible binding and transfer of oxygen (Figure 6.1).

The embryonic haemoglobins include Hb Portland ($\zeta_2\gamma_2$), Hb Gower 1 ($\zeta_2\varepsilon_2$), and Hb Gower 2 ($\alpha_2\varepsilon_2$). In the fetus, HbF ($\alpha_2\gamma_2$) predominates; in adults, HbA ($\alpha_2\beta_2$) comprises over 95% of the total haemoglobin, with a minor component of HbA_2 ($\alpha_2\delta_2$) in the red blood cells. There are two kinds of HbF composed of γ-chains that differ in their amino acid composition at position 136, where they have either glycine or alanine; those with glycine are called $^G\gamma$-chains and those with alanine $^A\gamma$-chains. The $^G\gamma$ and $^A\gamma$ chains are the products of separate globin gene loci ($^G\gamma$ and $^A\gamma$). These different types of haemoglobin are adapted to the changes in physiological requirements that occur during development. Fetal haemoglobin (HbF) exhibits a higher oxygen affinity than adult haemoglobins *in vivo*; the higher oxygen affinity of HbF relative to adult haemoglobin facilitates the transfer of oxygen across the placenta from the maternal to the fetal circulation.

The sigmoid shape of the oxygen dissociation curve, which reflects the allosteric properties of haemoglobin, ensures that oxygen is rapidly taken up at the high oxygen tensions found in the lungs and is released readily at the low tensions encountered in the tissues. It is quite different to myoglobin, a molecule that consists of a single globin chain with haem attached to it and which has a hyperbolic dissociation curve. The transition from a hyperbolic to a sigmoid curve reflects cooperativity between the four haem molecules. When one haem takes on oxygen, the affinity for oxygen of the remaining haems of the tetramer increases markedly. This is because haemoglobin can exist in

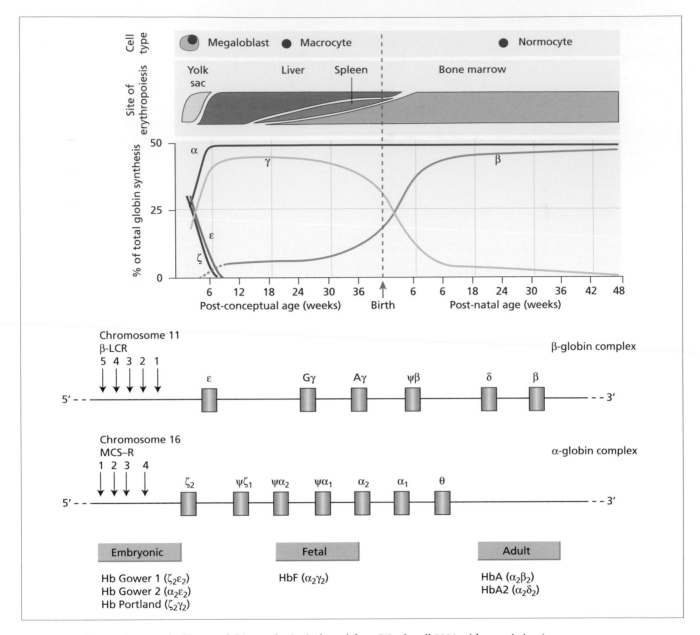

Figure 6.1 The genetic control of haemoglobin synthesis. (Adapted from Weatherall 2001 with permission.)

two configurations, deoxy(T) and oxy(R) (T and R stand for tight and relaxed states respectively). The T form has a lower affinity than the R form for ligands such as oxygen. At some point during the sequential addition of oxygen to the four haems, transition from the T to R configuration occurs and the oxygen affinity of the partially liganded molecule increases dramatically. The oxygen dissociation curve, which reflects these changes, can be modified in several ways. First, oxygen affinity is decreased with increasing CO_2 tensions – the Bohr effect. This facilitates oxygen loading to the tissues, where a drop in pH due to CO_2 influx lowers oxygen affinity. In contrast, in the lungs, efflux of CO_2 and an increase in intracellular pH increases

oxygen affinity and hence uptake. Oxygen affinity is also modified by the level of 2,3-diphosphoglycerate (2,3-DPG) in the red cell. Increasing concentrations shift the oxygen dissociation curve to the right (i.e. reduce oxygen affinity), whereas diminishing concentrations have the opposite effect.

Genetic control, regulation and synthesis

Human haemoglobin production is characterized by two 'switches'. The switch from embryonic to fetal haemoglobin production begins as early as week 5 of gestation and is completed by week 10 (Figure 6.1). Expression of β-globin starts as early as week 8 but synthesis remains low, increasing to approximately 10% at weeks 30–35 of gestation with a dramatic upregulation of β-globin synthesis just before birth, coinciding with a decrease in γ-globin expression that constitutes the fetal to adult haemoglobin switch. At birth, HbF ($\alpha_2\gamma_2$) comprises 60–80% of the total haemoglobin, falling to about 5% at 6 months of age and eventually reaching the adult level of 0.5–1.0% at 2 years. The relative synthesis of $^{G}\gamma$ and $^{A}\gamma$ chains also changes with the switch, from a $^{G}\gamma/^{A}\gamma$ ratio of 3:1 in fetal life to a ratio of 2:3 in adults. The switch from fetal to adult haemoglobin production is not total, production of variable levels of HbF persisting throughout adult life. These residual amounts are unevenly distributed; erythrocytes that contain measurable amounts of HbF are termed F cells.

Each of the α-like and β-like globin chains is encoded by genetically distinct loci, the α-like cluster on the tip of chromosome 16p and the β-like cluster on chromosome 11p15.5 (Figure 6.1). In both clusters, the genes are arranged along the chromosome in the order in which they are expressed during development: 5′-ε-$^{G}\gamma$-$^{A}\gamma$-ψβ-δ-β-3′ and 5′-ζ-ψζ-ψα2-ψα1-α2-α1-3′. The ψβ, ψζ and ψα genes are pseudogenes, that is they have sequences that resemble the β, ζ or α genes but contain inactivating mutations that prevent them from being expressed. They may be 'burnt out' remnants of genes that were functional at an earlier stage of evolution. Like most mammalian genes, the globin genes have one or more non-coding inserts, called intervening sequences or introns, interrupting the coding sequences or exons.

The β-like globin genes have similar structures, with three exons (coding regions) interrupted by two intervening sequences or introns of 122–130 and 850–900 bp, respectively. The β genomic sequence codes for 146 amino acids; intron 1 interrupts the sequence between codons 30 and 31, and intron 2 between codons 104 and 105. The α-globin genes code for 141 amino acids and contain similar but smaller introns between codons 30 and 31 and between codons 99 and 100. Within each α- and β-globin complex, in addition to the primary *cis* determinants of individual globin gene expression which are found in the immediate vicinity and within each gene, there are other local regulatory elements known as enhancers which are located at variable distances from the individual genes.

The local *cis*-acting sequences controlling globin gene expression include the promoter region, splicing donor and acceptors, and poly-A addition sites. The promoter, in the 5′ flanking region, includes blocks of nucleotide homology that are found in analogous positions in many species (Figure 6.2). The three positive *cis*-acting elements include the TATA box (position −28 to −31, i.e. between 28 and 31 bases upstream from the mRNA 'cap' site), a CCAAT box (position −72 to −76), and a CACCC motif which may be inverted or duplicated (position −80 to −140). These promoter elements are recognized by transcription factors and are involved in the initiation of transcription. It is interesting that while the CCAAT and TATA

elements are found in many eukaryotic promoters, the CACCC sequence is found predominantly in erythroid cell-specific promoters.

The 5′ untranslated region (UTR) occupies a region of about 50 nucleotides between the 5′ terminus or 'cap' site of globin mRNA and the initiation (ATG) codon. The cap appears to be important for maintaining the stability of the nuclear precursor mRNA. Within the 5′-UTR of the various globin genes there are conserved sequences that are important in the regulation of gene expression. The 3′-UTR constitutes the region between the termination codon and the poly-A tail. It consists of about 130 nucleotides with one conserved sequence, AATAAA, located 20 nucleotides upstream of the poly-A tail. The conserved hexanucleotide AATAAA acts as a signal for cleavage of the 3′ end of the primary transcript and addition of the poly-A tail, which confers stability on the processed mRNA and enhances translation. The importance of all these *cis* elements for normal globin gene expression has been validated by the discovery of thalassaemias caused by several mutations affecting these regions, as well as by deletion experiments.

Throughout development, the appropriate genes of the α- and β-globin gene clusters are coordinately expressed, maintaining a balance in the production of α- and β-like globins needed for the synthesis of normal haemoglobin. The regulation of globin gene expression is mediated at several levels; although most occurs at the transcriptional level, there is some fine-tuning during and after translation. Most DNA that is not involved in gene transcription is tightly packaged into a compact, chemically modified form that is inaccessible to transcription factors and polymerases and which is heavily methylated. Activity is associated with a change in the structure of the chromatin surrounding a gene, which can be identified by enhanced sensitivity to nucleases. Erythroid lineage-specific nuclease hypersensitivity sites are found at several locations in both the β-globin and α-globin gene clusters. A set of five DNase I hypersensitivity sites (designated HSs1–5), distributed 5–25 kb 5′ of the ε-globin gene, constitute the β locus control region (β LCR) (see Figure 6.1). This region was originally implicated in the control of the β-globin complex by the discovery of natural mutants that removed sequences upstream but left the globin genes intact and yet resulted in no output from the cluster. The human β LCR was the first LCR to be identified and was functionally defined as a DNA element that provides high levels of tissue-specific expression to a *cis*-linked gene in a copy number-dependent manner, and which is independent of host-genome integration site. The corresponding region in the α-globin cluster consists of four multispecies conserved sequence (MCS) regions lying 30–70 kb upstream of the α-globin genes called MCS-R1 to MCS-R4. Of these elements, only MCS-R2, which consists of a single DNase hypersensitive site, has been shown to be essential for α-globin expression. MCS-R2, which lies 40 kb upstream of the cluster, is also known as HS-40. The β LCR establishes a transcriptionally active

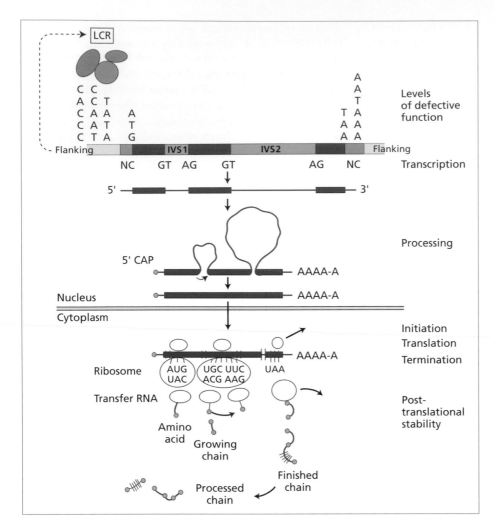

Figure 6.2 A prototype globin gene and the genetic control of globin chain synthesis. Levels of action of mutations are indicated on the right.

chromatin domain that encompasses the whole β-globin cluster and acts as a unique enhancer, whereas the α-globin MCS-R2 is most similar to HS2 of the β LCR and acts as an enhancer. In both clusters, expression of the respective genes is critically dependent on the presence of the upstream regulatory elements.

Several other enhancer sequences have also been identified in both globin gene clusters. All these regulatory regions bind a number of erythroid-specific transcription factors, notably GATA-1, NF-E2 and EKLF, as well as factors that are more ubiquitous in their tissue distribution such as Sp1. Tissue-specific expression may be explained by the presence of binding sites for the erythroid-specific transcription factors. The binding of haemopoietic-specific factors activates the LCR, which renders the entire β-globin gene cluster transcriptionally active. Transcription factors also bind to enhancer and local promoter sequences within each gene, which work in tandem to regulate the expression of the individual genes in the clusters. Some of the transcription factors are developmental stage specific and

may be involved in the (still poorly understood) differential expression of embryonic, fetal and adult globin genes.

The mechanisms by which developmental regulation is controlled are less clear. A dual mechanism has been proposed: autonomous gene silencing and gene competition for a direct interaction with the upstream LCR. It appears that the ε and ζ genes are switched on in embryonic cells and autonomously switched off in definitive cells (liver and bone marrow) in which they cannot be substantially reactivated. The second switch, from γ to β gene expression, is more complex and involves both autonomous silencing of the γ genes and competition between the γ and β genes for the β LCR. The transcriptional factor environment is critical in determining the balance between γ and β gene expression and is thought to be mediated by changes in the repertoire and/or abundance of various nuclear factors favouring particular promoter–LCR interactions. So far, the best-defined example of a developmental stage-specific regulatory factor is the erythroid Krüppel-like factor (EKLF) without which the β genes cannot be fully activated in the definitive cells. Not only is EKLF expression restricted mainly to erythroid cells but it is also a highly promoter-specific activator, binding with high affinity to the β-globin CACCC box. Its greater affinity for the β-globin than the γ-globin promoter accelerates the shutdown of γ in transgenic mice overexpressing EKLF, which suggests a role for EKLF in the γ-globin to β-globin switching process. However, EKLF is unlikely to be the only factor because (i) γ-globin silencing can also occur in the absence of a competing β-globin promoter and (ii) EKLF expression is equivalent at all developmental stages. The erythroid-specific transcription factors can be part of multiprotein complexes that also involve ubiquitous transcription factors such as Sp1.

Transcription and processing of mRNA

Genetic information in the DNA of the globin genes is transcribed into an RNA copy which is then translated into a specific globin chain (Figure 6.2). The TATA box acts as the initial DNA target for the progressive assembly of an initial transcription complex, which involves the interaction of transcription factors, TATA-binding protein and other proteins with the β LCR or α MCS, mediated by RNA polymerase II.

The primary transcript is a large mRNA precursor (pre-mRNA) that contains both introns and exons. While in the nucleus, it undergoes a number of modifications before it can be translated into protein (Figure 6.2). This includes the removal of introns by a complex series of reactions involving several different proteins that constitute the spliceosome, and splicing of the exons. Consensus sequences are universally found encompassing the 5′ (donor) and 3′ (acceptor) ends. Each intron invariantly starts with the dinucleotide GT (5′) and finishes with AG (3′). Mutations that alter the normal consensus sequences or mutations that create similar consensus sequences at new sites in globin genes cause aberrant splicing and constitute the molecular basis of many types of thalassaemia. Other modifications of the nascent mRNAs include the addition of a 'cap' structure at the 5′ end and the addition of a string of adenylic acid residues (poly-A) at the 3′ end. Proper cleavage of the primary RNA transcript and polyadenylation of the 3′ ends of mRNA is guided by a consensus hexanucleotide (AATAAA) sequence about 20 nucleotides upstream of the poly-A tail. The processed mRNA now moves into the cytoplasm to act as a template for globin chain production on defined organelles known as ribosomes.

Translation

Amino acids are transported to the mRNA template on carriers called transfer RNAs; there are specific transfer RNAs for each amino acid. The order of amino acids in a globin chain is determined by the order of nucleotides (reading frame); three bases (codon) code for a particular amino acid. The transfer RNAs also contain three bases, the anticodon, which are complementary to mRNA codons for particular amino acids. The transfer

RNAs carry amino acids to the template, where they find the right position by codon–anticodon base-pairing. The mRNA is translated from the 5′ to the 3′ end (left to right) starting with a specific initiation codon (AUG) and ending with a termination codon (UAA, UAG, UGA). When the ribosome reaches the termination codon, translation ceases, the completed globin chain is released, and the ribosomal subunits fall apart and are recycled. Individual globin chains combine with haem, which is synthesized through a separate pathway, and with themselves to form definitive haemoglobin molecules.

Terminations codons are also called nonsense codons because they do not usually encode any amino acid. Approximately 50% of the mutations causing β thalassaemia are caused by termination codons that are premature. Premature termination codons (PTCs) can result from different types of mutations. Single nucleotide substitutions can convert a sense codon to a nonsense codon and are often referred to as nonsense mutations. Frameshift mutations are insertions or deletions of a few bases that are not multiples of three that shift the reading frame, resulting in a nonsense codon that is premature (i.e. PTC). mRNAs with PTCs lead to production of encoded truncated proteins that are potentially harmful. They are kept in check by a cellular surveillance mechanism referred to as nonsense-mediated mRNA decay (NMD). NMD is usually triggered when translation stops prematurely at PTCs, resulting in termination of the mutant mRNA transcript and thus absence of abnormal protein. However, PTCs situated less than 50–55 nucleotides upstream of the 3′-most exon–exon junction or downstream of this junction generally fail to trigger NMD, and result in production of abnormal mRNA species. In the case of the β-globin gene, PTCs within the last exon (exon 3) and 3′ half of exon 2 result in the production of highly unstable β-globin variant chains and a dominantly inherited form of β thalassaemia, illustrating the importance of downregulating mRNAs that encode truncated proteins. However, there are exceptions to the 50–55 rule; PTCs within β-globin exon 1 and a PTC within exon 2 have been reported to fail to elicit NMD efficiently despite residing more than 55 nucleotides upstream of the exon 2–exon 3 junction.

The multistep process in the conversion of DNA into protein offers numerous opportunities for mishaps to occur that result in downregulation of gene expression, clearly illustrated by the different mutations causing thalassaemias and haemoglobinopathies (Figure 6.2).

Classification of the disorders of haemoglobin

Mutations in the globin genes can cause either a quantitative reduction in output from that gene or alter the amino acid sequence of the protein produced (Table 6.1). Quantitative

Table 6.1 The thalassaemias and related disorders.

β Thalassaemia
$β^0$
  Deletion
  Non-deletion
$β^+$
'Silent'
Normal HbA$_2$
Dominant

α Thalassaemia
$α^0$
$α^+$
  Deletion $(/−α)$
  Non-deletion $(/α^Tα)$

δβ Thalassaemia
$^Gγ^Aγ\ (δβ)^0$
$^Gγ\ (^Aγδβ)^0$
$(δβ)^+$

γ Thalassaemia

δ Thalassaemia

εγδβ Thalassaemia

Hereditary persistence of fetal haemoglobin
Deletion
Non-deletion
  $^Aγ$
  $^Gγ$

---

defects cause thalassaemia whereas qualitative changes, referred to as haemoglobin variants, cause a wide range of problems including sickle cell disease, unstable haemoglobins, decreased oxygen affinity, increased oxygen affinity and methaemoglobinaemia; however, the majority of qualitative mutations cause no significant change in haemoglobin properties or clinical problems. Some mutations combine both features, resulting in a haemoglobin variant which is made in reduced amounts; HbE (β26 Glu→Lys) is the most common example of this. The substitution at codon 26 (GAG→AAG) which causes HbE also causes alternative splicing of the β-globin mRNA, leading to a reduction in the normally spliced β message encoding the variant, and a thalassaemia phenotype. Other haemoglobin variants result in a thalassaemia phenotype caused by extreme instability and functional deficiency of the globin chain variant; for example, Hb Geneva, a dominantly inherited β thalassaemia. Other mutations in the globin gene complex might alter the switch from fetal to adult haemoglobin synthesis, and result in hereditary persistence of fetal haemoglobin (HPFH).

The thalassaemias and related disorders

The thalassaemias are the commonest single-gene disorders. Thalassaemia was first recognized by Cooley and Lee in 1925 as a form of severe anaemia associated with splenomegaly and bone changes in children. The term 'thalassaemia' is derived from the Greek θαλασσα (meaning 'the sea') since many of the early cases came from the Mediterranean region. However, it is now clear that the disorder is not just limited to the Mediterranean region but occurs throughout the world, prevalent in the tropical and subtropical regions including the Middle East, parts of Africa, Indian subcontinent and Southeast Asia. It appears that heterozygotes for thalassaemia are protected from the severe effects of malaria and natural selection has increased and maintained their gene frequencies in these malarious regions.

Definition and classification

The thalassaemias are classified into α, β, δβ, γδβ, δ, γ and εγδβ thalassaemias according to the type of globin chain(s) that is produced in reduced amounts (Table 6.1). The two major categories are the α and β thalassaemias while the rare forms include the γ, δ and εγδβ thalassaemias.

Functionally, some thalassaemia mutations cause a complete absence of globin chain synthesis, and these are called $α^0$ or $β^0$ thalassaemias; in others, the globin chain is produced at a reduced rate and these are designated $α^+$ or $β^+$ thalassaemias. The δβ thalassaemias are subdivided in the same way. HPFH syndromes refer to the group of disorders in which the switch from fetal to adult haemoglobin production is incomplete and fetal haemoglobin levels are variably increased in otherwise normal individuals. Because of their concomitant increased HbF levels, the δβ and γδβ thalassaemias are often considered with the HPFH syndromes.

Because thalassaemia occurs in populations in which structural haemoglobin variants are common, it is not unusual to inherit a thalassaemia gene from one parent and a gene for a structural haemoglobin variant from the other. Furthermore, both α and β thalassaemia occur commonly in some countries, and individuals may co-inherit genes for both types. These different interactions produce a clinically diverse family of genetic disorders that range in severity from death *in utero* to extremely mild, symptomless, hypochromic anaemias.

Most thalassaemias are inherited in a Mendelian recessive fashion. Heterozygotes are mostly symptomless, although usually they can be recognized by simple haematological analysis. More severely affected patients are either homozygotes for α or β thalassaemia or compound heterozygotes for different molecular forms of α or β thalassaemia or for one or other form of thalassaemia and a gene for a haemoglobin variant. Clinically, the thalassaemias are classified according to their severity into major, intermediate and minor forms. Thalassaemia major is a severe and transfusion-dependent disorder. Thalassaemia minor is the symptomless trait or carrier state. Thalassaemia intermedia is characterized by anaemia (with or without splenomegaly), though not of such severity as to require regular transfusion. In practice, thalassaemia intermedia encompasses a wide spectrum of clinical severities intermediate between the two extremes of thalassaemia major and trait.

The β thalassaemias

The β thalassaemias pose by far the most important public health problems because they are common and usually produce severe anaemia in their homozygous and compound heterozygous states.

Distribution

The β thalassaemias occur widely in a broad belt, ranging from the Mediterranean and parts of North and West Africa through the Middle East and Indian subcontinent to Southeast Asia. The disease is particularly common in Southeast Asia, where it occurs in a line starting in southern China and stretching down through Thailand and the Malay peninsula and Indonesia to some of the Pacific island populations. In this region, and in some of the Mediterranean island and mainland countries, gene frequencies range between 2 and 30%. It should be remembered that β thalassaemia is not confined entirely to these high-incidence regions and it occurs sporadically in every racial group.

Genetic basis of disease: molecular pathology

The β thalassaemias are considered to be autosomal recessive disorders since individuals who have inherited one abnormal β gene (carrier) are asymptomatic and the inheritance of two abnormal β globin genes is required to produce a clinically detectable phenotype. Molecular analysis of the β thalassaemia genes has demonstrated a striking heterogeneity. Although almost 300 β thalassaemia alleles (including deletions) have been characterized, population studies indicate that probably only 20 β thalassaemia alleles account for more than 80% of the β thalassaemia mutations in the whole world. This is because in each of the high-frequency areas, only a few (four to six) mutations are common, reflecting local selection due to malaria, with a varying number of rare ones. Each of these populations thus has its own unique group of mutations.

The vast majority (approximately 250) of β thalassaemia mutations are point mutations (i.e. single-base substitutions) and small insertions or deletions of one to two bases. These may involve any step in globin chain production: transcription, translation or post-translational stability of the globin gene product (Figure 6.2). Approximately half of these mutations completely inactivate the β gene with no β-globin production resulting in β^0 thalassaemia. Mutations that allow the production of some β-globin cause β^+ or β^{++} thalassaemia depending

on whether there is a marked or mild reduction in the output of β chains, respectively.

Transcription

The mutations that interfere with transcription include deletions and point mutations involving the globin gene promoter regions. With the exception of a deletion of about 600 bases at the 3′ end of the β-globin gene, which is restricted to certain Indian populations, major deletions are uncommon. A large number of point mutations involve the promoters or adjacent regions, most of which downregulate the β-globin gene to a variable degree and cause relatively mild forms of β thalassaemia.

A couple of β thalassaemia mutations in this class are 'silent': carriers do not have any evident haematological phenotypes, with red cell indices and HbA_2 levels within the normal range, the only abnormality being imbalanced globin chain synthesis. These β thalassaemia mutations have usually been 'discovered' in individuals with thalassaemia intermedia resulting from compound heterozygosity for one of those 'silent' mutations in combination with a typical β thalassaemia mutation. In this case, one parent has typical β thalassaemia trait and the other is apparently normal. Overall, the 'silent' β thalassaemia alleles are uncommon except for the -101 C→T mutation that has been observed fairly frequently in the Mediterranean region, where it interacts with a variety of more severe β thalassaemia mutations to produce milder forms of β thalassaemia intermedia.

Processing

A wide variety of mutations interfere with processing of the primary mRNA transcript. Those involving the invariant GT or AG sequences at intron–exon junctions prevent splicing altogether and cause β^0 thalassaemia. Mutations involving the consensus sequences adjacent to the GT or AG dinucleotides in the introns allows some normal splicing and causes β^+ thalassaemia. Several β thalassaemia mutations involve other parts of the introns; alternative splicing sites are produced leading to variable degrees of both normal and abnormal mRNA synthesis. An incorrectly spliced mRNA is not functional because it contains intron sequences, generating a frameshift and a PTC. Sequences that resemble the consensus sequences at intron–exon junctions are also present in exons. Mutations may activate these 'cryptic' sites, again leading to abnormal splicing.

Translation

About half of the β thalassaemia alleles completely inactivate the gene, mostly by generating PTCs, either by single-base substitution to a nonsense codon or through a frameshift mutation. As part of the surveillance mechanism that is active in quality control of the processed mRNA, mRNA harbouring a PTC is destroyed and not transported to the cytoplasm (a phenomenon called NMD) to prevent the accumulation of mutant mRNAs coding for truncated peptides. However, some in-phase PTCs that occur later in the β sequence, in the 3′ half of exon 2 and in exon 3, escape NMD and are associated with substantial amounts of mutant β mRNA, leading to synthesis of β-chain variants that are highly unstable and non-functional with a dominant negative effect (see next section). Other mutations of RNA translation involve the initiation (ATG) codon. Nine of these have been described; apart from an insertion of 45 bp, all are single base substitutions and again result in β^0 thalassaemia.

Mutations affecting post-translational stability

Instability of the β-globin gene product is the basis for the dominantly inherited β thalassaemias (Figure 6.3). As discussed earlier, in-phase PTCs within the 3′ half of exon 2 and in exon 3 cannot efficiently elicit NMD and hence abnormal mRNA containing the PTCs are transported to the cytoplasm and translated. However, these truncated variant β-chains are highly unstable, non-functional and not able to form viable tetramers. They precipitate in the erythroid precursors together with the redundant α chains, causing premature death of these cells, and accentuating the ineffective erythropoiesis. Severe anaemia and clinical disease results even in the heterozygous state. Highly unstable β-globin chains can also result from single-base substitutions or minor insertions/deletions that affect a critical amino acid of the β-globin peptide that is involved in α/β dimer formation or haem binding. In other cases, the minor insertions/deletions lead to shifts in the reading frame resulting in long unstable β-globin gene products that form prominent inclusion bodies in red cell precursors.

Deletions restricted to the β-globin gene

β Thalassaemia is rarely caused by deletions (Figure 6.4). Of these, only the 619-bp deletion at the 3′ end of the β gene is common, but even that is restricted to the Sind populations of India and Pakistan where it constitutes about 30% of the β thalassaemia alleles. The other deletions, although extremely rare, are of particular clinical interest because they are associated with an unusually high levels of HbA_2 and HbF in heterozygotes. The increase in HbF is adequate to compensate for the complete absence of HbA in homozygotes for these deletions. The mechanism underlying the elevated levels of HbA_2 and HbF appears to be related to removal of the 5′ promoter region of the β-globin gene, which removes competition for the upstream β LCR and limiting transcription factors, resulting in increased interaction of the LCR with the γ and δ genes in *cis*, thus enhancing their expression. This mechanism may also explain the unusually high HbA_2 levels that accompany the point mutations in the β promoter region.

Unusual causes of β thalassaemia

These are extremely rare and are mentioned here not just for the sake of completeness but also to illustrate the numerous molecular mechanisms that downregulate the β-globin gene. Transposable elements may occasionally disrupt human genes and result in their activation. The insertion of such an element, a retrotransposon of the LI family, into intron 2 of the β-globin gene has been reported to cause β^+ thalassaemia. Rarely, mutations in other genes distinct from the β-globin complex can downregulate β-globin expression. Such *trans*-acting mutations have been described affecting the XPD protein that is part of the general transcription factor TF11H, and the erythroid-specific GATA-1. Somatic deletion of the β-globin gene contributed to thalassaemia intermedia in three unrelated families of French and Italian origins. The affected individuals with thalassaemia intermedia were constitutionally heterozygous for β^0 thalassaemia but subsequent investigations revealed a somatic deletion of chromosome 11p15, including the β-globin gene

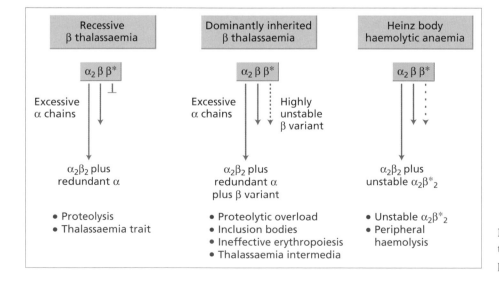

Figure 6.3 Heterozygous mutations in the β-globin gene and the different phenotypes.

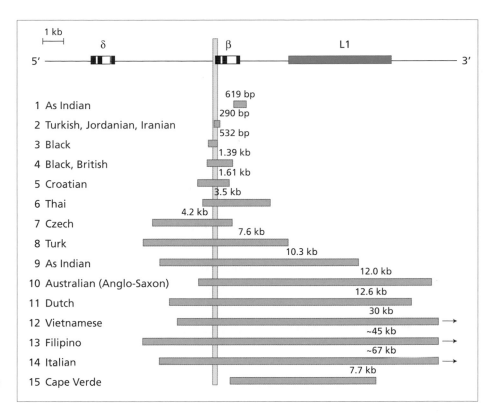

Figure 6.4 Deletions causing β thalassaemia. The vertical bar indicates the β-globin promoter region that is removed in common by these deletions, except for the 619 bp deletion. The horizontal arrows indicate that the 3′ end of the deletions have not been defined.

complex, in *trans* to the mutation in a subpopulation of erythroid cells. This results in a somatic mosaic: 10–20% of the cells were heterozygous with one normal copy of the β-globin gene, and the rest hemizygous (i.e. without any normal β-globin gene). In another case, thalassaemia major in a Chinese patient was caused by homozygosity for a paternal β thalassaemia allele due to uniparental isodisomy of chromosome 11p15.5 that encompassed the β-globin gene cluster.

Pathophysiology

The molecular defects in β thalassaemia result in absent or reduced β-chain production while α-chain synthesis is unaffected. The imbalance in globin chain production leads to an excess of α-chains. The free α-globin chains are highly unstable and precipitate in red cell precursors, forming intracellular inclusions that interfere with red cell maturation (Figure 6.5). Hence there is a variable degree of intramedullary destruction of erythroid precursors (i.e. ineffective erythropoiesis) that characterizes all β thalassaemias. Those red cells which mature and enter the circulation contain α-chain inclusions that interfere with their passage through the microcirculation, particularly in the spleen. However, the damage to red cell precursors and their progeny in β thalassaemia is not entirely mechanical. The degradation products of excess α-chains, particularly haem and iron, produce a wide range of deleterious effects on red cell membrane proteins and lipids, manifest by marked abnormalities of electrolyte homeostasis and membrane deformability.

The end result is an extremely rigid red cell with a shortened survival.

Thus, the anaemia of β thalassaemia results from a combination of ineffective erythropoiesis and haemolysis. It stimulates erythropoietin production, which causes expansion of the bone marrow and may lead to serious deformities of the skull and long bones. Because the spleen is being constantly bombarded with abnormal red cells, it hypertrophies. The resulting splenomegaly, together with bone marrow expansion, causes a major increase in plasma volume, which also contributes to the anaemia.

As mentioned previously, HbF production almost ceases after birth. However, some adult red cell precursors retain the ability to produce a variable number of γ-chains. Because the latter can combine with excess α-chains to form HbF, cells which make relatively more γ-chains in the bone marrow of β thalassaemics are partly protected against the deleterious effect of α-chain precipitation. These F cells come under selection in the marrow and peripheral blood and thus individuals with β thalassaemia have variable increases in HbF due to selective survival of these F cells. In some cases, there is also a genuine increase in HbF production as well as selection of F cells due to co-inheritance of a genetic determinant, or quantitative trait locus (QTL), for increased HbF production. Because δ-chain synthesis is unaffected, the disorder is characterized by a relative or absolute increase in HbA$_2$ ($\alpha_2\delta_2$) production.

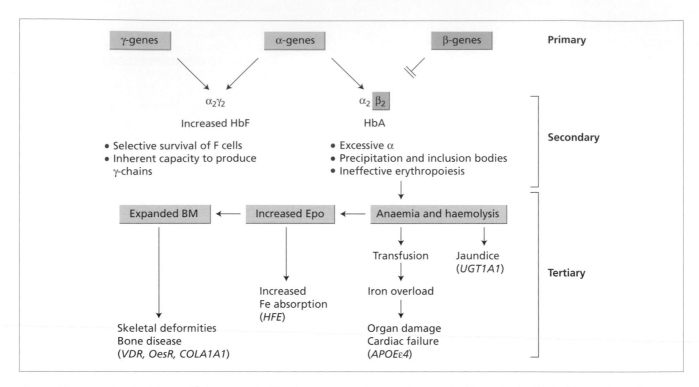

Figure 6.5 The pathophysiology of β thalassaemia. BM, bone marrow; Epo, erythropoietin. (From Thein 2004 with permission.)

It follows therefore that if the anaemia is corrected with blood transfusion, the erythropoietin drive is shut off, growth and development are normal, bone deformities do not occur and splenomegaly is less marked. On the other hand, each unit of blood contains 200–250 mg of iron, and with regular transfusion there is steady accumulation of iron in the liver, endocrine glands and myocardium. Thus, although well-transfused thalassaemic children grow and develop normally, they die of iron overload unless steps are taken to remove iron.

Genotype–phenotype relationships

The β thalassaemias show remarkable phenotypic variability, ranging from severe life-threatening anaemia to an extremely mild condition that may be identified only by chance. The molecular basis for this diversity is at least partly understood.

The genetic modifiers of the β thalassaemia phenotype can be divided into primary, secondary and tertiary (Figure 6.5). Primary modifiers are the different mutations that affect the β-globin gene. These have variable effects on β-globin gene expression that may affect the output of β-globin chains, ranging from zero to a very mild reduction. Secondary modifiers are those that reduce the degree of imbalance of globin chain synthesis. They include the co-inheritance of α thalassaemia and a variety of genetic modifiers of γ-chain production in adult life. Three major QTLs – $Xmn1$-$^{G}\gamma$ site, $HBS1L$-MYB intergenic poymorphisms ($HMIP$) on chromosome 6q, and $BCL11A$ gene on chromosome 2 – have recently been mapped, and it seems likely that many remain to be discovered.

While co-inheritance of α thalassaemia reduces chain imbalance and disease severity in individuals who have inherited two copies of β thalassaemia alleles, the increased output of α-globin through co-inheritance of extra α-globin genes in β thalassaemia heterozygotes increases chain imbalance, converting a typically asymptomatic state to that of thalassaemia intermedia. The outcome depends on the number of α-globin genes inherited as one or two copies of triplicated (/ααα) or quadruplicated (/αααα) α-globin complexes, and the type of β thalassaemia mutation (β^0 or β^+). More recently, another mechanism of inheriting extra α-globin genes involving segmental duplication of the whole α-globin gene cluster has also been described.

Tertiary modifiers are those that affect the complications of disease; the severity of bone disease, iron loading and jaundice may be affected by polymorphisms of genes involved in the metabolic pathways concerned with these complications. Bone mass, like HbF, is a quantitative trait under strong genetic control involving multiple QTLs, those implicated including estrogen receptor gene, vitamin D receptor (VDR) gene, collagen type α1 genes and transforming growth factor β1 ($TGFB1$) gene. Studies have shown that the levels of bilirubin and incidence of gallstones are related to a polymorphic variant (seven TA repeats) in the promoter of the uridine diphosphate glucuronosyltransferase 1A ($UGT1A1$) gene, also referred to as Gilbert syndrome. Iron loading in β thalassaemia results not just from blood transfusion but also from increased iron absorption. Variants in the HFE gene have a modulating effect on iron absorption, and as other genes in iron homeostasis become uncovered, it is likely that there will be genetic variants in these loci that influence the different degrees of iron loading in β thalassaemia. Similarly, it seems very likely that the propensity to infection is modified by polymorphisms involving the immune system and its regulation. Finally, it should be remembered that environmental factors, long neglected, may also play an important role in modifying the β thalassaemic phenotype.

Clinical findings in severe β thalassaemia

In many developed countries, neonatal screening programmes will first identify infants with more severe forms of β thalassaemia, before the development of any symptoms; in some cases, antenatal screening of the parents and possibly prenatal diagnosis will have identified the infant to be at high risk of β thalassaemia before birth. Mutations in the β-globin gene almost never cause clinical symptoms *in utero* or neonatally due to the predominance of γ-globin at this stage. In many countries, neonatal screening programmes do not exist and diagnosis in the child will depend on their symptomatic presentation. Severe β thalassaemia usually presents in the first year of life. Typically there is failure to thrive, with poor weight gain and growth with developmental delay. The parents may have noticed that the infant is pale and jaundiced, with a protruding abdomen. There may be a family history of severe anaemia, and typically the family will not be of northern European origin. Examination confirms the pallor and jaundice, with palpable hepatosplenomegaly. There may be evidence of marked erythroid hyperplasia, with signs of the typical 'thalassaemic facies' including expansion of the skull vault and maxillary bones. The symptoms and signs are not specific and differential diagnoses include gastrointestinal or hepatic disease, and malignancy.

Laboratory diagnosis of severe β thalassaemia

The full blood count shows a low haemoglobin, usually less than 5 g/dL. Mean corpuscular haemoglobin (MCH) and mean corpuscular volume (MCV) are low, with a very wide red cell distribution width. The nucleated cell count may be very high due to the presence of large numbers of nucleated red cells. A blood film shows marked anisopoikilocytosis, with basophilic stippling and small red cell fragments (Figure 6.6). The reticulocyte count is elevated but less than expected for the degree of anaemia, in keeping with the ineffective erythropoiesis. Renal function is normal, but liver function tests show elevation of bilirubin, aspartate aminotransferase and lactate dehydrogenase, with a normal alanine aminotransferase. Erythropoietin levels will be high, with soluble transferrin receptor levels up to 30 time greater than normal. White cell and platelet counts should be normal unless there is hypersplenism. A bone marrow aspirate is not essential to make the diagnosis, but if performed shows very marked erythroid hyperplasia, with dyserythropoiesis. Many of the erythroid precursors show inclusions after

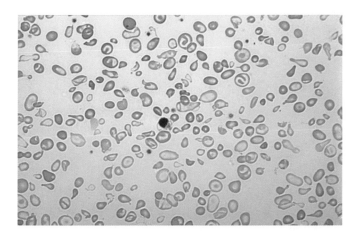

Figure 6.6 The peripheral blood appearances in β thalassaemia.

incubation with methyl violet; similar inclusions are found in the peripheral red cells after splenectomy. Immunoelectron microscopy confirms that the inclusions in β thalassaemia consist of precipitated α-globin chains.

Haemoglobin analysis is needed to confirm the diagnosis, typically using either electrophoretic or chromatographic techniques. This will usually show an increased amount of HbA$_2$, with the vast majority of the remainder consisting of HbF; small amounts of HbA may be present depending on the β-globin mutation, the age of the child and whether the child has been transfused. Absence of HbA confirms a diagnosis of β^0 thalassaemia, while presence of HbA (pre-transfusion sample) confirms β$^+$ thalassaemia. Testing of the parents should confirm the diagnosis, both typically being carriers of β thalassaemia, with HbA$_2$ levels greater than 3.5% and MCH below 27 pg. These findings are sufficient to make a diagnosis of severe β thalassaemia, although where DNA analysis is available it is often used to identify the mutations and confirm the diagnosis.

Management of severe β thalassaemia

Any child presenting in the first year of life with the features described above is likely to require regular red cell transfusions to grow and develop normally; this is referred to as thalassaemia major. If such children are not transfused regularly, as happened historically in all countries, and as happens currently in many poorer areas, progressive deterioration occurs. Growth and development continue to be severely impaired. The child often has muscle wasting due to increased metabolic demands, and in particular may become folate deficient. The spleen and liver become progressively enlarged; the spleen can become massive with hypersplenism and resulting cytopenias. There is marked erythroid hyperplasia with bony distortion and extramedullary haemopoiesis. Bones become enlarged, and this is most apparent in the face, with maxillary hyperplasia, dental malocclusion and development of a 'tower' skull. Extramedullary haemopoiesis is typically paraspinal and may

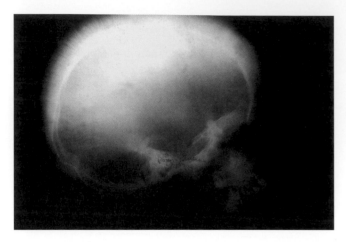

Figure 6.7 Radiograph of a skull of a thalassaemia major patient showing 'hair-on-end' appearance.

cause compression of spinal nerves with resulting symptoms; intracranial haemopoiesis may cause cranial neuropathies and symptoms of raised intracranial pressure. There is an increased tendency to infection, and without transfusion the child typically dies from either infection or high-output cardiac failure. Radoigraphy may show lacey trabecular patterns in long bones and a 'hair-on-end' appearance of the skull (Figure 6.7).

This picture is completely transformed by an appropriate transfusion regimen. Occasional blood transfusions may be necessary because of an acute exacerbation of anaemia, often related to infection. It is a bigger decision to institute a regular transfusion regimen, in that typically transfusions are then continued lifelong. Stopping transfusions in a child or adult who is adapted to a high haemoglobin level inevitably results in a prolonged period of symptomatic anaemia and ill health which may not be tolerated. Regular transfusions should be started if the child is failing to thrive, or if erythroid expansion is causing bony distortion or hypersplenism; abnormal facial appearances, if allowed to progress, may be irreversible without maxillofacial surgery.

Blood transfusions

The aim of regular transfusions is to correct anaemia and suppress the abnormal erythroid hyperplasia. Correcting anaemia improves oxygen delivery to the tissues and facilitates normal growth and development. Suppression of erythropoiesis stops bony distortion, limits excessive iron absorption and reduces extramedullary haemopoiesis. Measurement of soluble transferrin receptor levels, which are proportionate to the size of the erythron, suggest that suppression of erythropoiesis requires trough haemoglobin to be kept above 9.5 g/dL; in practice this means aiming for a pretransfusion haemoglobin of 9–10 g/dL. This can usually be achieved by regular red cell transfusions every 2–4 weeks, with a post-transfusion haemoglobin target of

13–15 g/dL. If venous access is difficult, as is often the case in young children, it is sometimes beneficial to insert a semi-permanent central venous access device, such as a Portacath or Hickman line. The majority of thalassaemia patients are treated with simple top-up transfusions as described. An alternative involves regular exchange transfusion in which blood is both venesected and transfused; this can be performed either manually or automatically using an apheresis machine. The main advantages are that transfusion can be less frequent, at intervals of up to 6 weeks, and iron loading is significantly less as blood is also removed. Disadvantages include increased expense and time, increased donor exposure with risk of infection and alloimmunization, and difficulties with venous access.

Ideally transfusions are with packed red cells. Leucodepleted blood reduces the risk of transfusion reactions and cytomegalovirus infection, and should be used where available. When the ethnicity of the blood donor population differs from that of the recipient thalassaemia population, as occurs in northern Europe, the USA and Australia, the transfused red cells should be matched for an extended range of blood groups to minimize the risk of alloimmunization; typically, full matching for all Rh and Kell groups, in addition to ABO, is of benefit. Before starting transfusions the patient should be vaccinated against hepatitis B, and ideally also hepatitis A.

Iron overload

Iron overload inevitably complicates regular blood transfusions and is the source of many serious complications. Each unit of transfused blood contains about 200–250 mg iron, compared with the 1 mg iron normally absorbed each day. Despite the increased iron, serum hepcidin remains inappropriately low, which further contributes to iron loading through increased intestinal iron absorption. Recent studies show that the low hepcidin is caused by an inhibitory effect of growth differentiation factor (GDF)-15 that is secreted by erythroid precursors and significantly increased in patients with thalassaemia major (see Chapter 4). Iron is initially stored in macrophages within the liver, and is chaperoned around the body bound to transferrin. As transferrin becomes saturated, labile, more toxic forms of iron appear in cells and plasma, referred to as non-transferrin-bound iron (NTBI). It is thought that NTBI is responsible for most of the iron toxicity, including iron loading into cardiac and endocrine tissues. Once in cells, the iron causes oxidative tissue damage, mostly through the generation of free radicals.

Iron overload and chelation is discussed in more detail in Chapter 4. Before iron chelation was available, most regularly transfused thalassaemics died in their late teens, mainly from cardiac iron deposition. Endocrine failure was also inevitable, with diabetes mellitus, hypothyroidism, hypoparathyroidism, hypogonadism and pituitary failure all occurring. With good iron chelation life expectancy is open-ended, and there is an established link between the efficacy of iron chelation and life expectancy.

The body has no mechanism for excreting iron and iron-chelating drugs are necessary to avoid toxic iron accumulation. Iron chelation is usually started after about 1 year of monthly blood transfusions. Ideally, children delay starting chelation until they are 3 years old, as drug toxicity is thought to be highest in the young; it is usually necessary to start chelation earlier in children who start transfusions in the first year of life, although in general low doses are used.

Currently, three drugs are used for iron chelation: desferrioxamine, deferiprone and deferasirox. Desferrioxamine has been in clinical use since the 1970s and is known to be safe and effective; side-effects seem only to occur when the drug is used in high doses or iron stores are low. Important side-effects include ocular and retinal toxicity, growth impairment and cartilaginous dysplasia. *Yersinia enterocolitica* infection is increased in iron overload, particularly if desferrioxamine is also in use. Regular use of desferrioxamine has been found to prolong survival in several observational studies. The main problem is that it has to be given by injection; the most commonly used regimen involves subcutaneous infusions given over 8 hours using a syringe driver or balloon-pump. To achieve negative iron balance in a regularly transfused person requires a dose of 40 mg/kg five times a week, and this is usually given overnight. The subcutaneous route is inevitably a cause of poor adherence to treatment regimens because of the pain and inconvenience. Historically, therefore, many patients have developed life-threatening iron overload despite the availability of desferrioxamine, with median age of death being 30–40 years. Deferiprone was developed in the UK about 30 years ago and was licensed in Europe in 1999. Initial trials demonstrated its efficacy, although subsequent studies suggested that there may be individual variation in response requiring higher dosage up to 100 μg/kg instead of 75 μg/kg. Arthropathy and agranulocytosis are potentially serious side-effects and it is currently recommended that people taking the drug have full blood counts every week. Despite concerns about its safety and efficacy, deferiprone seems to be particularly effective at removing cardiac iron, which is possibly linked to improved cardiac function and reduced cardiac mortality. It is increasingly used in combination with desferrioxamine. Deferasirox is a rationally designed oral iron chelator that has been approved in the USA and Europe since the mid-2000s. Large clinical trials have demonstrated its efficacy in thalassaemia. It effectively removes hepatic iron, with increasing evidence that it also removes cardiac iron to some extent.

It is important to monitor iron stores regularly in transfusion-dependent patients who are receiving iron chelation. Monitoring the volume of transfused blood allows the iron input to be calculated, which can guide what dose of iron chelator to use. Serum ferritin is proportional to the amount of stored iron in the liver and can be used to effectively monitor iron overload, particularly if serial measurements are used. Ferritin is artificially elevated by any inflammatory process, which can cause misleading results. Liver iron can be accurately assessed using liver biopsy, but this is invasive with a risk of complications. Increasingly, magnetic resonance imaging (MRI) is used to quantitate liver iron, with the R2 method being approved by both European and North American authorities. Cardiac MRI is also emerging as an important way of identifying those thalassaemics with significant cardiac iron, which allows chelation to be targeted to that organ, using either continuous intravenous desferrioxamine or one of the oral iron chelators. Iron monitoring and chelation is very expensive and not available to most patients in the world with thalassaemia major.

Monitoring and annual review of patients with thalassaemia major

The aim of regular transfusions is to allow the child to grow and develop normally, and for the quality and quantity of life to be as close to normal as possible. This requires the child to be closely monitored, and this is ideally done in a centre with expertise in the condition, often in the form of an annual review. Each year the volume of transfused blood (expressed as mL/kg) should be recorded; if the transfusion requirement is high, exceeding 200–250 mL/kg, this suggests the possibility of hypersplenism, and if the spleen is enlarged splenectomy may significantly reduce the rate of transfusion and iron loading. Splenectomy would not normally be considered before the age of 6 years, and there is emerging concern that it may increase the risk of pulmonary hypertension and other vascular complications in later life.

Growth should be carefully monitored in children, including annual measurement of sitting height to assess spinal growth; desferrioxamine toxicity has been specifically linked to impaired spinal growth. Blood tests should be performed each year to look for endocrinopathy, including fasting glucose, thyroid-stimulating hormone, parathyroid hormone, insulin-like growth factor 1 and sex hormone levels. Hepatic and renal function should be monitored regularly, together with hepatitis serology. Cardiac assessment should include an ECG, echocardiogram and increasingly MRI, which can assess both ejection fraction and iron loading; MRI is not tolerated by children under the age of 7 years without general anaesthesia or sedation, and is not usually justified at this age unless there is strong suspicion of cardiac or other problems. Osteopenia is more common in children and adults with thalassaemia major, and vitamin D levels should be measured, with bone densitometry from the age of about 10. There is evidence that osteopenia with falling bone density may benefit from treatment with bisphosphonates. All patients on iron chelation should also be monitored regularly for audiometric, ocular and retinal toxicity.

Dietary and psychological support are also often beneficial. In general, the organization and provision of all this care requires a multidisciplinary team, including paediatricians, haematologists, cardiologists, endocrinologists, nurse specialists and psychologists.

Bone marrow transplantation in severe thalassaemia

Bone marrow transplantation is generally seen as the treatment of choice if there is an HLA-identical sibling and it is clear that the child is transfusion dependent. The success of bone marrow transplantation is generally reduced as children get older, iron overload increases and iron-related organ damage increases. In optimal circumstances the transplant is successful in more than 90% of cases. The main complications are severe infection during the period of transplantation and either acute or chronic graft-versus-host disease. Significantly reduced fertility is also almost inevitable. Recent improvements in the outcome of medical treatment, related to oral iron chelation and better cardiac monitoring, have possibly shifted the balance away from transplantation. One limitation of transplantation is the availability of suitable donors; cord blood transplants are potentially important in this respect. In a small number of cases preimplantation genetic diagnosis has allowed the selection of HLA-matched embryos to produce siblings who can act as bone marrow donors. Efforts are also being made to develop mini- and micro-transplants, which may be less toxic, preserve fertility and potentially allow the use of alternative donors, such as haploidentical or matched unrelated donors.

Prognosis in severe thalassaemia

In theory, with adequate transfusion and effective chelation, survival in thalassaemia major should approach that of the normal population, although historically this has never been the case because of the difficulties patients encounter in adhering to subcutaneous chelation regimens. In Europe and North America, median survival has improved with each decade since the introduction of desferrioxamine in the 1970s. Most deaths are related to cardiac iron overload and improved survival is primarily related to earlier and more rational use of chelation. Recent studies suggest that death of cardiac origin has become much less common in the last 5–10 years, probably related to improved treatment of iron-related cardiomyopathy with intravenous desferrioxamine and combination therapy with both desferrioxamine and deferiprone. Earlier detection, using cardiac T2* MRI, and prevention of cardiac iron loading, with oral chelation, seem likely to improve prognosis further.

Heterozygous β thalassaemia

Carriers for β thalassaemia are usually symptom-free except in periods of stress such as pregnancy, when they may become more anaemic. Transfusion is sometimes necessary during pregnancy but no other treatment or follow-up is necessary.

Palpable splenomegaly is rare. Carriers may have mild anaemia; haemoglobin values are in the range 9–12 g/dL. The red cells show hypochromia and microcytosis with characteristically low values. The reticulocyte count is normal. The bone marrow shows moderate erythroid hyperplasia with corresponding increase in soluble transferrin receptor levels. The characteristic finding is an elevated HbA_2 level, usually greater than 3.5%. There is a slight elevation of HbF in the 1–3% range in about 50% of cases. Silent or near-silent carriers of β thalassaemia occur fairly rarely, in which the HbA_2 level is normal with only slight hypochromia; this is typically associated with mildly thalassaemic mutations in the promoter region of the gene. Failure to identify this state antenatally can result in significant and unexpected thalassaemia in the offspring, if the partner also carries β thalassaemia.

β Thalassaemia in association with haemoglobin variants

In many populations, because there is a high incidence of both β thalassaemia and various haemoglobin variants, it is quite common for an individual to inherit a β thalassaemia allele from one parent and a gene for a structural haemoglobin variant from the other. Although numerous interactions of this type have been described, only three are common: HbS/β thalassaemia, HbC/β thalassaemia and HbE/β thalassaemia.

HbS/β thalassaemia

HbS/β thalassaemia causes sickle cell disease, with the severity varying from very mild to severe. This interaction does not result in the thalassaemia phenotype. The principal determinant of the severity of sickle cell disease is the nature of the β thalassaemia mutation, and to what extent $β^A$ is reduced compared with normal. $HbS/β^0$ thalassaemia is broadly similar in severity to HbSS, with no HbA present and an average haemoglobin of 7–8 g/dL. It differs in that red cells are markedly hypochromic and contain excess α-globin chains. Clinically marked splenomegaly is more common than in HbSS, affecting up to 30% of adults. The severity of $HbS/β^+$ thalassaemia varies from severe to very mild, depending on how much HbA is produced. Some $β^+$ thalassaemia alleles produce less than 10% of the normal HbA output and result in a clinical picture identical to $HbS/β^0$ thalassaemia. At the other end of the spectrum, promoter mutations typically reduce HbA output by only 10% and result in a condition which is only marginally more symptomatic than sickle cell carriers. These mild forms of $HbS/β^+$ thalassaemia occur most often in populations of African origin, whereas the more severe forms are most often found in Mediterranean countries and India.

HbC/β thalassaemia

This is restricted to West Africans and some North African and southern Mediterranean populations. It is largely asymptomatic and characterized by a mild haemolytic anaemia associated with splenomegaly. The peripheral blood film shows numerous target cells and thalassaemic red cell changes with a moderately elevated reticulocyte count. Haemoglobin electrophoresis shows a preponderance of HbC. The diagnosis is confirmed by finding the HbC trait in one parent and the β thalassaemia trait in the other.

HbE/β thalassaemia

This the commonest severe form of thalassaemia in Southeast Asia and parts of the Indian subcontinent. The β^E allele is mildly thalassaemic due to the activation of a cryptic splice site, and when it is inherited together with β^0 thalassaemia, there is a marked deficiency of β-chain production. HbE is slightly unstable *in vitro*, although it is not clear that this has any clinical significance. The clinical and haematological changes are variable. There is nearly always anaemia and splenomegaly, with typical thalassaemic bone changes. Haemoglobin values are in the range 4–9 g/dL, with an average of 6–7 g/dL; in developed countries about half of the patients with this condition are regularly transfused. There are thalassaemic red cell changes and the bone marrow shows marked erythroid hyperplasia.

Although little is known about the natural history of this disorder, it is clear that in many parts of Southeast Asia and India it causes a very high mortality in early life. Clinically it is indistinguishable from other forms of β thalassaemia, although the link between genotype and phenotype is less predictable, with some patients having thalassaemia major and others growing and developing with few complications.

The diagnosis is confirmed by finding only HbE and HbF on haemoglobin electrophoresis and by demonstrating HbE trait in one parent and β thalassaemia trait in the other. In other cases of HbE/β^+ thalassaemia, variable quantities of HbA are present and the condition is milder.

Variant forms of β thalassaemia

Despite the vast heterogeneity of mutations, the increased levels of HbA$_2$ in β thalassaemia heterozygotes is remarkably uniform, in the range 3.5–5.5%, and rarely exceeds 6%. Unusually high HbA$_2$ levels in excess of 6.5% seem to characterize the subgroup caused by lesions (point mutations or small deletions) that affect the regulatory elements in the promoter region of the β-globin gene (see Figure 6.4). The unusually high HbA$_2$ levels are usually accompanied by higher than usual increases in HbF, resulting in a milder thalassaemia phenotype despite the absence of HbA$_2$ in some cases. Otherwise, the haematological picture is identical to the common forms of β thalassaemia. Some β thalassaemia heterozygotes have normal HbA$_2$ levels despite the typical hypochromic microcytosis. In most cases, this is due to the co-inheritance of δ thalassaemia. Other cases of normal HbA$_2$ β thalassaemia are extremely mild forms of β thalassaemia that is completely silent in heterozygotes and is only identified when it is co-inherited with a common form of β thalassaemia. Heterozygotes do not have any evident haematological phenotype, the only abnormality being a mild imbalance of globin chain synthesis.

β Thalassaemia occasionally follows a dominant pattern of inheritance, whereby it is symptomatic in heterozygotes (see Figure 6.3). The clinical picture is characterized by a moderate degree of anaemia and splenomegaly with marked thalassaemic changes of the red cells, and ineffective erythropoiesis with intracellular inclusion bodies. Although not usually transfusion dependent, such individuals develop iron overload from hyperabsorption due to ineffective erythropoiesis and may develop liver or endocrine damage. The common denominator of these dominantly inherited β thalassaemias is the synthesis of hyperunstable β-chain variants, caused by a spectrum of mutations; those resulting from PTCs are typically found in exon 3 of the β-globin gene. Unlike the recessive forms that are prevalent in malarious regions, dominantly inherited β thalassaemias are rare, occurring in dispersed geographical regions. Most of the dominant β thalassaemia alleles have been described in single families, many as *de novo* mutations. Dominantly inherited β thalassaemia should be suspected in any patient with a thalassaemia intermedia phenotype, even if both parents are haematologically normal, and the patient is from an ethnic background where β thalassaemia is rare. The diagnosis is confirmed by DNA sequence analysis of the β-globin genes.

δβ Thalassaemia and hereditary persistence of fetal haemoglobin

HPFH and δβ thalassaemia are much less common than β thalassaemia and manifest as a range of disorders characterized by decreased or absent HbA production and a variable compensatory increase in HbF synthesis. The distinction between them is subtle and originally made on what appeared to be clear-cut clinical and haematological grounds. However, as more cases became recognized and their underlying mutations delineated, it became evident that there is considerable overlap between the two groups of disorders.

The level of compensatory increase is higher in HPFH compared with δβ thalassaemias. HPFH heterozygotes have essentially normal red cell indices, normal HbA$_2$ levels and HbF levels of 10–35%, whereas heterozygotes for δβ thalassaemia have hypochromic microcytic erythrocytes and normal HbA$_2$ levels and the HbF increases are lower (5–15%). A distinguishing feature is the heterocellular distribution of HbF in δβ thalassaemia compared with a pancellular (or homogeneous) distribution in HPFH, although the intercellular distribution of HbF may be a reflection of the magnitude of increase and the sensitivity of the technique used to stain F cells. Clinically, HPFH homozygotes are asymptomatic with slightly reduced MCV and MCH, and compound heterozygotes with β thalassaemia have very mild disease. Compound heterozygotes of δβ thalassaemia with β thalassaemia, and δβ thalassaemia homozygotes have disease severity that ranges from mild anaemia to transfusion dependence.

Two types of mutations underlie this group of disorders: deletions that remove substantial regions of the β-globin cluster, including the β-globin gene (Figure 6.8), and point mutations in the promoters of either of the γ-globin genes ($^{G}\gamma$ or $^{A}\gamma$) (Figure 6.9). Six deletion forms of HPFH have been described in Africans, Mediterraneans, Indians and Southeast Asians, with deletions ranging from 13 to 86 kb in size. The commonest forms are Black HPFH-1 and HPFH-2, the latter also referred to as Ghanaian HPFH. Included within the HPFH conditions is Hb Kenya, a rare condition found largely in East Africa and

characterized by production of a hybrid $^{A}\gamma\beta$-globin chain and increased $^{G}\gamma$-chain (Figures 6.8 and 6.10). The first type of δβ thalassaemia to be described was Hb Lepore, which consists of hybrid δβ-globin chains produced by misaligned crossing-over between the δ and β globin genes (Figures 6.8 and 6.10). Heterozygotes for Hb Lepore have hypochromic microcytic red cells, normal HbA$_2$ and variably increased HbF. The more common forms of δβ thalassaemia result from different length deletions of the β-globin gene cluster (Figure 6.8). Deletions that leave both the γ-globin genes intact are called $^{G}\gamma^{A}\gamma$ $(\delta\beta)^{0}$ thalassaemias, and they all include parts or all of the δ and β globin genes. $^{G}\gamma(^{A}\gamma\delta\beta)^{0}$ thalassaemia deletions include part or all of the $^{A}\gamma$-globin gene and hence produce HbF containing

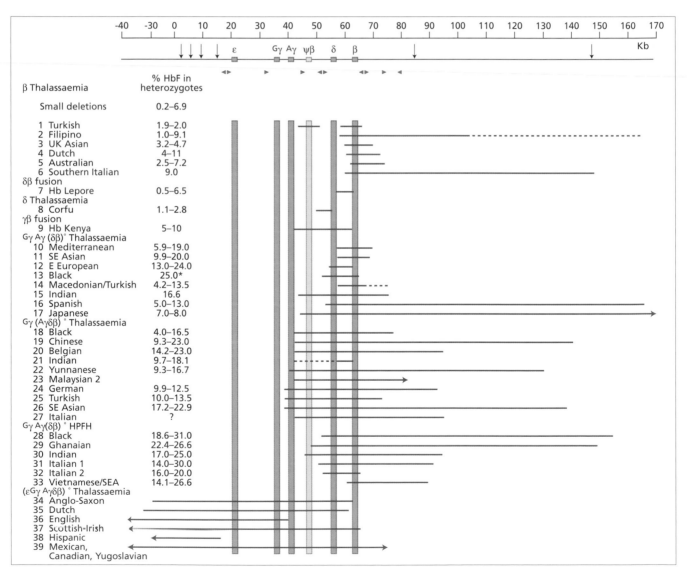

Figure 6.8 The deletions that underlie δβ thalassaemia and hereditary persistence of fetal haemoglobin. The upper arrows represent DNase I-hypersensitive sites. (From Weatherall & Clegg 2001 with permission.)

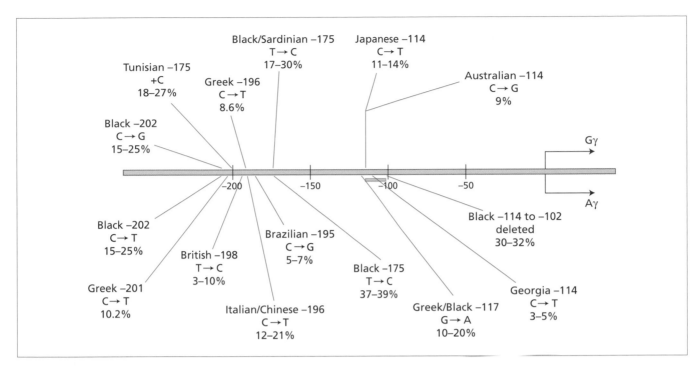

Figure 6.9 Non-deletion HPFH due to mutations in $^{G}\gamma$ and $^{A}\gamma$ promoter regions. (From Weatherall & Clegg 2001 with permission.)

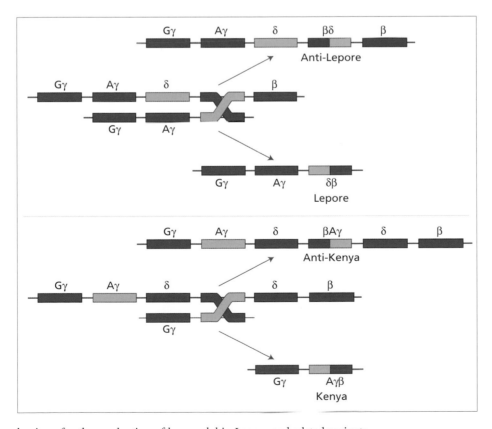

Figure 6.10 The mechanisms for the production of haemoglobin Lepore and related variants.

only $^{G}\gamma$-chains. A couple of the $(\delta\beta)^{0}$ thalassaemias include two deletions separated by an inverted region.

Non-deletion HPFH is caused by mutations within the promoters of either of the γ-globin genes, and lead to variably increased HbF with a preponderance of only one of the γ-chains (Figure 6.9). The mutations (single-base substitutions or minor deletions) are clustered in three regions of the promoters, around positions -114, -175 and -200. These regions contain binding sites for ubiquitous and erythroid-specific factors. Altered binding pattern of the transcription factors due to the point mutations are thought to be the cause of the elevated HbF levels, which vary from 5 to 35% in heterozygotes. Deletion and non-deletion HPFH and $\delta\beta$ thalassaemias are clearly inherited in a Mendelian pattern as alleles of the β-globin gene complex. Heterozygotes have significant elevations of HbF ranging from 10 to 40%.

Inherited increases in HbF have also been reported in families with β thalassaemia and sickle cell disease; these increases had a modulating effect on the severity of disease and the inheritance appeared to segregate independently of the β-globin gene cluster. Healthy members of the families may also have slight increases in HbF, and historically these individuals were said to have co-inherited heterocellular HPFH. Heterocellular HPFH was originally recognized in a group of Swiss army recruits; the HbF elevation was modest and unevenly distributed among the erythrocytes, the distinct HbF-carrying red blood cells being termed F cells. Hence Swiss HPFH was also referred to descriptively as heterocellular HPFH. It is now clear that HbF is a highly variable quantitative trait, and that heterocellular HPFH represents the upper tail of the natural continuous distribution that includes approximately 10% of the population with HbF levels between 0.8 and 5%. Unlike the Mendelian forms caused by major deletions or point mutations in the γ-globin promoters, the inheritance of heterocellular HPFH is complex with an overwhelming genetic contribution. The sequence variant (C→T) at position -158 of the $^{G}\gamma$-globin gene, also referred to as the $Xmn1$-$^{G}\gamma$ site (or rs74821440), was the first QTL to be implicated through family studies. Subsequent genetic association studies have confirmed $Xmn1$-$^{G}\gamma$ as one of the three major QTLs modulating HbF production in adults, the other two being the $HBS1L$-MYB intergenic region on chromosome 6q and $BCL11A$ on chromosome 2p. These three QTLs account for a relatively large proportion (20–50%) of the common variation in HbF levels, not only in healthy adults but also in patients from diverse ethnic groups with β thalassaemia and sickle cell disease. In African-American patients with sickle cell disease, the three loci contribute more than 20% to the HbF variation with a corresponding reduction in frequency of acute pain. Co-inheritance of the $Xmn1$-$^{G}\gamma$ site delays transfusion requirements in β thalassaemia. In Sardinia, β thalassaemia patients who have co-inherited certain $BCL11A$ variants have higher HbF levels and a milder disease.

$\varepsilon\gamma\delta\beta$ Thalassaemia

These are rare conditions and result from large deletions of the β-globin gene cluster that involve the β LCR. The deletions fall into two categories: group I removes all, or a greater part of, the complex including the β-globin gene and the β LCR, and group II removes extensive upstream regions including the β LCR but leaving the β-globin gene itself intact. There is no output from the globin genes of the affected cluster. Clearly, the homozygous state would not be compatible with survival. Heterozygotes have severe haemolytic disease of the newborn, with anaemia and hyperbilirubinaemia. The severity of anaemia and haemolysis is variable, even within a family, and in some cases blood transfusions are necessary during the neonatal period. If they survive the neonatal period, the infants grow and develop normally; in adult life they have the haematological picture of heterozygous β thalassaemia, with mild anaemia, hypochromic microcytic red cells and a haemoglobin pattern of normal HbA$_2$ β thalassaemia.

The α thalassaemias

Distribution

The α thalassaemias follow a similar distribution to the β thalassaemias, extending throughout sub-Saharan Africa, the Mediterranean region, the Middle East, the Indian subcontinent and Southeast Asia, in a line stretching from southern China through Thailand, the Malay peninsula and Indonesia, to the Pacific Island populations.

In some prevalent areas, carrier frequency for the mild form (α^{+}) reaches 80% or more. The more severe forms (α^{0} thalassaemias) reach their highest frequency in Southeast Asia, where carrier frequency can reach 10%.

Genetic basis of disease: molecular pathology

Normal individuals have four α-globin genes arranged as linked pairs, $\alpha2$ and $\alpha1$, at the tip of each chromosome 16, the normal α genotype being represented as $\alpha\alpha/\alpha\alpha$ (Figure 6.11). The α thalassaemias can be classified as α^{0} thalassaemia, in which no α-chains are produced from the linked pair, and α^{+} thalassaemia, in which production of α-chain from the affected chromosome is reduced.

The α^{0} thalassaemias are caused by deletion of both α-globin genes (Figure 6.12). The deletions vary in size and tend to be geographically isolated, with two particularly common ones in Southeast Asia $(/--^{SEA})$ and the Mediterranean region $(/--^{MED})$. Rarely, α^{0} thalassaemia can also arise from deletions of the upstream α-globin regulatory elements (MCS) in which the α-globin genes remain intact but completely inactivated. In other cases, more extensive deletions are associated with monosomy for a segment of the tip of chromosome 16p that result in the syndrome of α thalassaemia and mental retardation

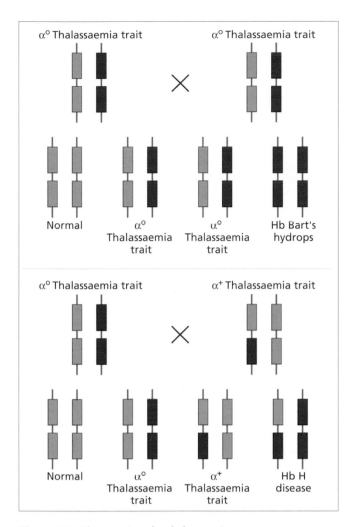

Figure 6.11 The genetics of α thalassaemia.

(ATR-16). The molecular basis of the α⁺ thalassaemias is more complicated; the commonest forms result from deletions that remove one of the linked pairs of α-globin genes, leaving the other intact (−α/αα). The linked α-globin genes are embedded in two highly homologous duplicated units of 4 kb within which are three homologous subsegments designated X, Y and Z (Figure 6.13), Misalignment and recombination between the Z segments, which are 3.7 kb apart, produces chromosomes with one α-globin gene (/−α³·⁷ or *rightward* deletion) and others with three α-globin genes (/ααα^anti-3.7). Similarly, crossover between the X boxes, which are 4.2 kb apart, produces the *leftward* deletion /−α⁴·² and the /ααα^anti-4.2 allele.

Less commonly, both the α-globin genes are intact and α⁺ thalassaemia results from a point mutation that partially or completely inactivates one of them (α^Tα/αα). In contrast to the β thalassaemias, non-deletional mutations are much less common causes of α thalassaemia but like those that cause β thalassaemia, the non-deletional α thalassaemia variants act at

different stages of gene regulation and expression. Almost 70 types of non-deletional α thalassaemia have been described; more than two-thirds of these are found on the dominant α2 gene, less than one-third on the α1 gene, and the others on an /−α chromosome (/−α^T). In general, the non-deletional α⁺ thalassaemia variants (/α^Tα) give rise to a more severe reduction in α-chain output than the single α gene deletion (/−α) due to the lack of compensatory increase in α output from the linked α1 gene as observed in deleted cases. One particularly common form of non-deletional α thalassaemia found in Southeast Asia is Hb Constant Spring (/α^CSα), which is due to a single-base substitution (TAA→CAA) in the α₂-globin termination codon. Instead of terminating at the stop codon, mRNA is read through the 3′-UTR until another in-phase termination codon is encountered 31 codons later. This results in an elongated α-globin chain of 172 residues, 31 amino acids from the natural arginine at codon 141. Of the six predicted α₂-chain termination variants, five have been described: Hb Constant Spring (α142 Gln), Hb Icaria (α142 Lys), Hb Koya Dora (α142 Ser), Hb Seal Rock (α142 Glu) and Hb Pakse (α142 Tyr). Hb Constant Spring is by far the most common of these variants, reaching frequencies of up to 4% in Thailand.

Non-deletional α thalassaemia can also arise from single-base substitutions causing structural α-globin variants that are highly unstable, for example Hb Quong Sze α125 Leu→Pro (/α^QSα).

Unusual causes of α thalassaemia

This includes a single case report of α⁰ thalassaemia arising from a deletion involving the α1 gene that also inactivated the intact linked α2 gene. Subsequent studies showed that the deletion results in juxtaposition of a downstream gene (*LUC7L*) next to the structurally normal upstream α2 gene. Transcription of antisense mRNA from *LUC7L* led to silencing of the linked α2 gene. Another novel form of non-deletional α thalassaemia results from a single nucleotide substitution in a non-genic region between the α-globin genes and their upstream regulatory elements. The single-base substitution leads to the creation of a new promoter-like element that interferes with normal activation of all the downstream α-like globin genes, resulting in α⁰ thalassaemia.

Pathophysiology

The pathophysiology of α thalassaemia is different to that of β thalassaemia. A deficiency of α-chains leads to the production of excess γ or β chains, which form Hb Bart's (γ₄) and HbH (β₄), respectively. These soluble tetramers do not precipitate extensively in the bone marrow and hence erythropoiesis is more effective than in β thalassaemia. However, HbH is unstable and precipitates in red cells as they age. The inclusion bodies cause red cell membrane damage and obstruction in the spleen leading to shortened red cell survival. Furthermore, both Hb

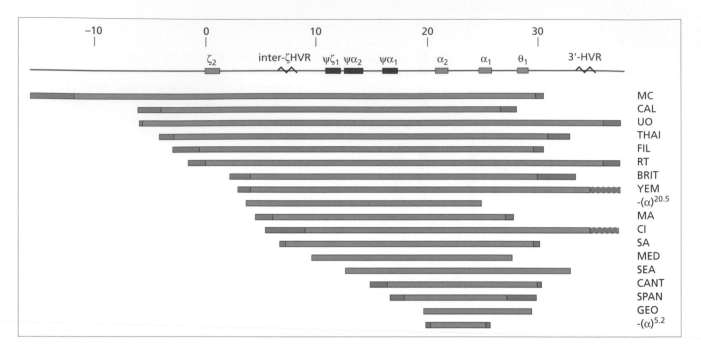

Figure 6.12 The α-globin gene cluster deletions that underlie α⁰ thalassaemia. (From Weatherall & Clegg 2001 with permission.)

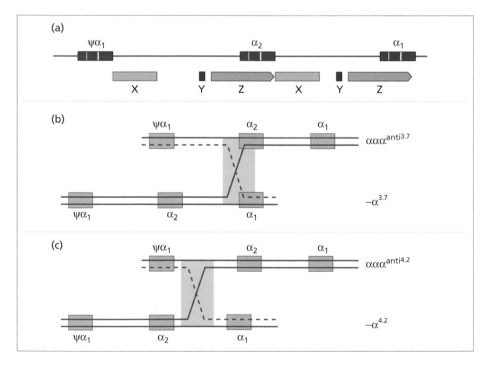

Figure 6.13 The molecular mechanisms that underlie the deletion forms of α thalassaemia: (a) normal cluster showing X, Y and Z homology boxes; (b) 3.7-kb deletion; (c) 4.2-kb deletion. (From Weatherall & Clegg 2001 with permission.)

Bart's and HbH have a very high oxygen affinity and their oxygen dissociation curves resemble myoglobin. Thus, the severe forms of α thalassaemia are due to defective haemoglobin production, the synthesis of homotetramers that are physiologically useless and a haemolytic component.

Genotype–phenotype relationship

Loss of one functioning α gene (αα/−α) is almost completely silent, with normal or only slightly hypochromic red cells. Loss of two α genes (− −/αα or −α/−α) produces a mild hypochromic microcytic anaemia, the α thalassaemia trait. Homozygotes for α^0 thalassaemia $(--/--)$ have a lethal condition with intrauterine haemolytic anaemia called Hb Bart's hydrops fetalis syndrome (see Figure 6.11). As Hb Bart's hydrops fetalis syndrome follows the homozygous inheritance of α^0 thalassaemia, this condition occurs only in populations in which α^0 thalassaemia is common, notably those of Southeast Asia and the Mediterranean islands. Deficiency of α-chains gives rise to an excess of γ-chains (in fetal life) or β-chains (in adult life), which form γ_4 tetramers (Hb Bart's) or β_4 tetramers (HbH). The presence of Hb Bart's or HbH is thus diagnostic of α thalassaemia. Due to their very high oxygen affinity, Hb Bart's and HbH are not functional haemoglobins; HbH is unstable and precipitates in older red cells forming H inclusions.

HbH disease lies between the two ends of the clinical spectrum, the asymptomatic α thalassaemia trait and Hb Bart's hydrops fetalis. As in β thalassaemia intermedia, HbH disease spans a wide range of clinical and haematological phenotypes, with equally heterogeneous genotypes, varying with the geographic distribution of the different α thalassaemia variants. HbH disease most commonly results from the interaction of α^0 and α^+ thalassaemia $(--/-\alpha)$ and thus, similar to Hb Bart's hydrops syndrome, is also restricted to populations where α^0 thalassaemia is common. Less often, it can result from the interaction of α^0 thalassaemia with non-deletional forms of α thalassaemia $(/\alpha^T\alpha)$ or from homozygous non-deletional α thalassaemia $(\alpha^T\alpha/\alpha^T\alpha)$. HbH disease in Southeast Asia commonly arises from homozygosity or compound heterozygosity for Hb Constant Spring $(\alpha^{CS}\alpha/\alpha^{CS}\alpha$ or $\alpha^{CS}\alpha/--)$.

As the non-deletional forms of α^+ thalassaemia tend to have a more severe phenotype than the deletional forms, in some cases the homozygous state $(\alpha^T\alpha/\alpha^T\alpha)$ may be associated with the phenotype of HbH disease. In a small number of cases, Hb Bart's hydrops syndrome can arise from the genotype $--/\alpha^T\alpha$.

Haemoglobin Bart's hydrops syndrome

This is a common cause of fetal loss throughout Southeast Asia and is also encountered in the eastern Mediterranean. There is no production of α-chains and hence neither fetal nor adult haemoglobin. The fetus is usually stillborn between 28 and 40 weeks or, if liveborn, takes a few gasping respirations and then expires within the first hour after birth. Affected neonates show the typical picture of hydrops fetalis, with gross pallor, generalized oedema and massive hepatosplenomegaly. There is an increased frequency of congenital abnormalities and a very large friable placenta. All these findings are due to severe intrauterine anaemia. The haemoglobin is in the range 6–8 g/dL and there are gross thalassaemic changes of the red cells, with many nucleated forms in the blood. The haemoglobin consists of approximately 80% Hb Bart's and 20% Hb Portland $(\zeta_2\gamma_2)$. It is believed that these infants survive to term because they continue to produce embryonic haemoglobin. Apart from fetal death, this syndrome is characterized by a high incidence of toxaemia of

pregnancy and obstetric complications due to the large placenta.

Haemoglobin H disease

This condition is characterized by a variable degree of anaemia and splenomegaly but it is unusual to find severe thalassaemic bone changes or growth retardation. Patients usually survive into adult life, although the course may be interspersed with severe episodes of haemolysis associated with infection or worsening of the anaemia due to progressive hypersplenism. In addition, oxidant drugs may increase the rate of precipitation of HbH and exacerbate the anaemia. Haemoglobin values range from 7 to 10 g/dL and the blood film shows typical thalassaemic changes. There is a moderate reticulocytosis and, on incubation of the red cells with brilliant cresyl blue, numerous inclusion bodies are generated by precipitation of HbH under the redox action of the dye. After splenectomy large preformed inclusions can be demonstrated on incubation of blood with methyl violet. Haemoglobin analysis reveals 5–40% HbH, together with HbA and a normal or reduced level of HbA_2.

α Thalassaemia traits

α^0 Thalassaemia trait is characterized by very mild hypochromic anaemia with red cell indices similar to those of β thalassaemia trait; the MCH is less than 25 pg and the HbA_2 level is normal. Occasional HbH bodies may be present in the red cell on supravital staining. There are no diagnostic tests with which to identify this condition with certainty except DNA analysis. Deletional α^+ thalassaemia carriers have near-normal haematological findings. The heterozygous states for the non-deletional forms of α^+ thalassaemia are sometimes associated with very mild hypochromic anaemia; the type associated with Hb Constant Spring can be identified by the presence of trace amounts of the variant on haemoglobin electrophoresis at an alkaline pH.

α^0 Thalassaemia carriers can be identified with more certainty in the neonatal period, when they have 5–10% Hb Bart's, which disappears over the first few months of life and is not replaced by HbH. Some α^+ thalassaemia carriers have slightly increased levels of Hb Bart's, in the 1–3% range, but its absence does not exclude the diagnosis.

Other forms of α thalassaemia

There are several other forms of α thalassaemia that are completely unrelated in their pathogenesis and distribution to the conditions described in the previous sections. They comprise the α thalassaemia mental retardation syndromes and the association of α thalassaemia with myelodysplasia.

α Thalassaemia with mental retardation syndromes

There are two forms of α thalassaemia associated with mental retardation, one encoded on chromosome 16 (ATR-16), the other on the X chromosome (ATR-X). ATR-16 results from large chromosomal rearrangements and extensive deletion of 1–2 Mb from the subtelomeric end of the short arm of chromosome 16. Affected children usually have a relatively mild degree of mental retardation and no dysmorphic features. On the other hand, ATR-X, which because of its mode of inheritance affects boys, is associated with widespread dysmorphic features and severe mental retardation. It results from many different mutations of the *ATRX* gene, which is located on the X chromosome. The ATRX protein has many features in common with DNA helicases, transcription factors that are involved in the modelling of chromatin and gene regulation. ATRX also appears to play an important role in the transcription of the α-globin genes and undoubtedly many other genes during early development. The *ATRX* gene has also been reported to be involved in a considerable number of X-linked mental retardation syndromes without an α thalassaemia phenotype.

α Thalassaemia associated with myelodysplasia

An α thalassaemic phenotype is also found in association with forms of myelodysplasia in elderly patients. The blood films of such patients show dimorphic features, with populations of red cells containing HbH inclusion bodies and a variable level of HbH in peripheral blood. Acquired mutations in the *ATRX* gene have been identified in the blood cells of patients with this syndrome. The relationship of the mutations in *ATRX* to the neoplastic phenotype remains to be determined.

Thalassaemia intermedia

Definition and molecular pathology

The term *thalassaemia intermedia* is used to describe patients with the clinical picture of thalassaemia which, although not transfusion dependent, is associated with a much more severe degree of anaemia than is found in carriers for α or β thalassaemia. Whether a patient is classified as having thalassaemia intermedia or thalassaemia major depends on a doctor deciding that the patient would benefit from regular blood transfusions; this decision is based not only on the clinical factors mentioned in the section on thalassaemia major, but also on non-clinical factors such as the availability of blood transfusions, the experience of the clinician and the wishes of the patient. Many different genotypes may underlie thalassemia intermedia, as mentioned earlier, with HbE/β thalassaemia perhaps being the commonest (Table 6.2). HbH disease is sometimes considered as a type of thalassaemia intermedia, but its pathophysiology is quite different to that caused by β thalassaemia.

Clinical and haematological changes

At one end of the spectrum are individuals who, except for mild anaemia, are symptom-free. At the other, there are patients who have haemoglobin values of 5–7 g/dL and who develop marked splenomegaly, osteopenia and skeletal deformities due to expansion of bone marrow; the severity may change with

Table 6.2 Molecular basis of β thalassaemias intermedia.

Homozygous or compound heterozygous state for β thalassaemia
Inheritance of mild β thalassaemia alleles (homozygous or compound heterozygotes)
Compound heterozygosity for a mild and a more severe allele
Co-inheritance of α thalassaemia
Increased HbF response
    β-Globin gene promoter mutations (deletional or non-deletional)
    Co-inheritance of HbF quantitative trait loci
        Linked: *Xmn*1-$^G\gamma$ polymorphism
        Unlinked: *BCL11A* gene (chromosome 2p), *HBS1L-MYB* intergenic polymorphisms (chromosome 6q)

Heterozygous state for β thalassaemia
Co-inheritance of extra α-globin genes as triplicated (/ααα) or quadruplicated (/αααα) globin complexes or segmental duplication of entire α-globin cluster
Dominantly inherited β thalassaemia (hyperunstable β-globin chain variants)

Compound heterozygosity for β thalassaemia and β-chain variants
HbE/β thalassaemia

Compound heterozygosity for β thalassaemia and HPFH or δβ thalassaemia

Homozygosity for δβ thalassaemia

increasing age, due to iron loading because of increased intestinal absorption and decreased tolerance of anaemia because of reduced cardiovascular fitness. A wide range of other problems are particularly associated with thalassaemia intermedia, including pulmonary hypertension, hypercoagulability, pseudoxanthoma elasticum and other connective tissue disorders, hypersplenism, leg ulceration, folate deficiency, extramedullary haemopoietic tumour masses in the chest and skull, gallstones and a marked proneness to infection. Because of the heterogeneity of these disorders, management is highly dependent on the course that evolves in an individual patient; all patients should be followed up very carefully from early childhood. The haemoglobin constitution of the intermediate forms of β thalassaemia depends on the contributing genotypes, and in many cases is similar to that found in the major forms.

Treatment

Intermittent blood transfusions are often necessary due to falls in haemoglobin caused by fever and infection, particularly with parvovirus B19, which causes reticulocytopenia. It can be difficult to decide who would benefit from more regular blood transfusions and when to start them. In countries with a ready supply of safe blood, there is an increasing tendency to start regular transfusions even in children, maintaining the haemoglobin at greater than 8 g/dL in order to avoid the emerging complications of skeletal deformities, pulmonary hypertension and osteopenia. There is also some evidence that this improves the quality of life, particularly with emerging options for oral iron chelation. This is not possible in much of the world and management consists of reserving transfusion for severe symptomatic anaemia.

Pharmacological treatment to increase HbF and total haemoglobin levels is potentially applicable to thalassaemia intermedia, in that relatively small increases in haemoglobin levels with a corresponding reduction in ineffective erythropoiesis could help a patient thrive who would otherwise require regular transfusions. Hydroxycarbamide (hydroxyurea) is the most widely used drug in this context, and while some patients undoubtedly benefit, in general results are disappointing. Butyrate and other short-chain fatty acids also promote HbF synthesis and have been used with limited clinical success in thalassaemia intermedia. A number of newer drugs are being developed which may boost HbF to a greater extent, most notably the new generation of short-chain fatty acid derivatives and immunomodulatory drugs such as pomalidomide and lenalidomide.

Screening for thalassaemias

Pre-conception, antenatal and neonatal screening programmes are important in the clinical care and public health management of haemoglobinopathies. Thalassaemia is prevalent in many developing and poorer countries, where either treatment is not available or the cost of regular blood transfusions and chelation is a major drain on limited medical resources. In other countries, including parts of Europe, Australia and North America, it is important to identify the antenatal risk of having a baby with thalassaemia to provide informed parental choice. Apart from bone marrow transplantation, there is no definitive treatment, and many countries in which the disease is common are putting a major effort into programmes for its prevention.

Premarital and pre-conception screening

Ideally, individuals know their thalassaemia status before they decide to have children, and potentially use this information to choose a suitable partner. Some areas therefore concentrate on screening teenagers at school. Other countries insist that a couple are screened for thalassaemia status before they can get married; this latter approach has been successful in Cyprus, where social pressures have reduced the number of at-risk marriages.

Antenatal screening, prenatal diagnosis and preimplantation genetic diagnosis

Many screening programmes concentrate on identifying pregnant women who are thalassaemia carriers in the first trimester of pregnancy. This is done by varying combinations of blood tests and identifying women at high risk of carrying thalassaemia based on their ethnic origin; this latter approach is particularly effective in areas with a low prevalence of thalassaemia in the native population, such as northern Europe. If a woman is found to be a carrier, screening is then offered to her partner, and if both are carriers, they are counselled about the risk of the fetus inheriting a severe form of thalassaemia and offered prenatal diagnosis (PND).

PND of the thalassaemias was first carried out by fetal blood sampling, typically for β thalassaemia, between 18 and 20 weeks' gestation. At about 20 weeks in the normal fetus, β-globin synthesis constitutes about 10% of the total haemoglobin, giving a β/γ ratio of 0.1. A fetus heterozygous for β thalassaemia has a β/γ ratio of about 0.05, while one with β thalassaemia major produces either none or traces of β-globin with a β/γ ratio of less than 0.025. Fetal blood sampling has now been replaced by fetal DNA analysis. DNA analysis was applied to PND of the haemoglobinopathies in the late 1970s and early 1980s. Fetal DNA is obtained at 11–12 weeks' gestation by chorionic villus sampling or amniocentesis. Initially, detection of the mutations was indirect, relying on linkage analysis of restriction fragment length polymorphisms (RFLPs) and Southern blot hybridization, which required relatively large amounts of DNA and the whole procedure took 7–10 days. The development of polymerase chain reaction (PCR) for specific amplification of DNA has revolutionized the molecular diagnostic field, and mutations can now be detected directly using PCR-based techniques in 1 day, enabling PND to be carried out rapidly within 3 days.

Couples can then make an informed choice as to whether to terminate the pregnancy if the fetus is affected. Some couples find PND helpful in preparing for the birth of a potentially ill child, even though they would not contemplate termination. The main complication of invasive PND is the increased risk of miscarriage of about 1%. This has led to research to develop non-invasive methods of PND based on maternal blood sampling. Maternal blood contains small numbers of fetal cells and also cell-free fetal DNA, both of which could potentially be used to diagnose fetal thalassaemia. The low concentration of fetal material relative to maternal has made this technically very difficult, although advances in methods of DNA analysis seem likely to make this feasible in the near future.

Some couples want to avoid having a fetus without thalassaemia but find PND and selective termination unacceptable. Preimplantation genetic diagnosis involves the use of *in vitro* fertilization techniques to generate 5–15 embryos; at the eight-cell stage, one embryonic cell can be removed and tested for thalassaemia alleles; it is then possible to only implant embryos without thalassaemia. While appealing, it is currently a difficult, stressful and expensive procedure, with only 10–20% of couples taking home a baby. Again, advances in reproductive biology and DNA technology seem likely to make this more applicable in the future.

Neonatal screening

It is possible to detect the majority of babies with severe thalassaemia by neonatal testing, either as cord blood or more commonly from the neonatal blood spot, which is taken up on a piece of blotting paper and also screened for other conditions such as phenylketonuria. If haemoglobin analysis shows HbF only, with no HbA or other haemoglobin variants, it is likely that the baby has inherited a severe form of β thalassaemia and may be transfusion dependent; less severe possibilities include thalassaemia intermedia and homozygosity for HPFH. Babies identified in this way can then be followed up closely rather than waiting until they present following a period of prolonged illness. Parents can also be tested and given advice concerning the risk to future pregnancies.

Structural haemoglobin variants related to thalassaemia (Table 6.3)

The unstable haemoglobin disorders

The unstable haemoglobin disorders are a rare group of inherited haemolytic anaemias that result from structural changes in the haemoglobin molecule, which cause its intracellular precipi-

Table 6.3 Diseases due to structural haemoglobin variants.

Sickle syndromes causing haemolysis and vaso-occlusion
HbSS
Compound heterozygosity for HbS with other β haemoglobin variants (HbS/C, HbS/D Punjab, HbS/O Arab)
Compound heterozygosity for HbS with β thalassaemia (HbS/β thalassaemia)

Haemolytic anaemia
Unstable haemolytic variants

Congenital polycythaemia
High-oxygen-affinity haemoglobin variants

Congenital cyanosis
Low-oxygen-affinity haemoglobin variants
M haemoglobins

Hypochromic microcytic anaemia (thalassaemia phenotype)
Variants with inefficient synthesis due to alternative splicing, e.g. HbE
Lepore haemoglobins
Unstable chain termination variants, e.g. Hb Constant Spring

Drug-induced haemolysis
e.g. Hb Zurich

---

tation with the formation of Heinz bodies. Their true incidence is not known and there have been several well-documented instances in which patients with one of these variants have had no affected relatives, suggesting that they have arisen by a new mutation.

Molecular pathology and pathogenesis

Most of the unstable haemoglobins result from single amino acid substitutions or small deletions. For example, substitutions in or around the haem pocket can disrupt its anatomy and allow in water, with subsequent oxidative damage to haem, leading to precipitation of haemoglobin. Some substitutions, such as those involving proline residues, cause a marked disturbance of the secondary structure of globin chains. A few variants result from deletions of either single amino acids or several residues. For example, in Hb Gun Hill, five amino acids are missing, including the haem-binding site. As the unstable haemoglobins precipitate in the red cells or their precursors, they produce intracellular inclusions (Heinz bodies) which, together with oxidant damage to their membranes, make the cells more rigid and hence cause their premature destruction in the microcirculation.

Clinical features

All these conditions are characterized by a haemolytic anaemia and splenomegaly. Like all chronic haemolytic anaemias, there is an increased incidence of pigment gallstones with their associated complications; the risk is particularly high if there is co-inheritance of Gilbert syndrome (polymorphic variant in the promoter of the *UGT1A1* gene). The condition may become worse during periods of infection and, in the more severe forms, such episodes are associated with life-threatening anaemia that requires blood transfusion. Some oxidant drugs may increase the rate of haemolysis, and parvovirus B19 infection may cause temporary reticulocytopenia. Apart from icterus and splenomegaly, there are no characteristic physical findings.

Laboratory diagnosis

The peripheral blood film shows typical features of haemolysis but the red cell morphology may be normal. Occasionally, there is mild hypochromia and microcytosis. Heinz bodies are present in the peripheral blood after splenectomy. The most characteristic feature of the unstable haemoglobins is their heat instability. If a dilute haemoglobin solution is heated at 50°C for 15 min, the unstable haemoglobins precipitate as a dense cloud. A similar effect can be induced by isopropanol at lower temperatures. Some of these variants can be seen on haemoglobin electrophoresis but others, because they result from a neutral amino acid substitution, produce no electrophoretic changes and can be demonstrated only by the heat precipitation test. DNA analysis can provide definitive diagnosis, typically by sequencing of the α or β globin genes.

Treatment

Splenectomy seems to be beneficial in some cases, although experience is inevitably limited. Intermittent blood transfusions may be necessary. If haemolysis is very severe, the patient may benefit from regular blood transfusions and bone marrow transplantation should be considered.

High-oxygen-affinity haemoglobin variants

Some haemoglobin variants cause increased oxygen affinity, which results in varying degrees of polycythaemia.

Molecular pathology

Some high-oxygen-affinity haemoglobin variants result from single amino acid substitutions at critical parts of the haemoglobin molecule that are involved in the configurational changes which underlie haem–haem interaction and the production of a sigmoid oxygen dissociation curve at the junctions between the α and β subunits. Others involve the amino acids concerned with the binding of 2,3-DPG to haemoglobin. Reduced 2,3-DPG binding moves the oxygen dissociation curve to the left, reducing the P_{50} and causing the haemoglobin to hold on to oxygen more avidly than normal. This causes functional anaemia, with tissue hypoxia, which in turn causes an increased output of erythropoietin and an elevated red cell mass.

Clinical features

Most affected persons are completely healthy and are identified only when a routine haematological examination shows an unusually high haemoglobin level or packed cell volume. There is no splenomegaly and, apart from a raised red cell mass, there are no associated haematological findings. Although it might be expected that a high-oxygen-affinity haemoglobin would cause defective oxygenation of the fetus, none of the reported families has a history of such problems.

Diagnosis

The condition should be suspected in any patient with a pure red cell polycythaemia associated with a left-shifted oxygen dissociation curve. The diagnosis can be confirmed by haemoglobin analysis using chromatography, mass spectrometry or DNA analysis.

Treatment

In asymptomatic persons, no treatment is necessary. The difficulty arises if there is associated vascular disease, particularly coronary or cerebral artery insufficiency. As these patients require a high haemoglobin level for oxygen transport, venesection should be carried out with great caution. Venesection is undertaken because of increased risk of vascular complications, and typically the aim is to keep the haematocrit below 0.55, although there is little evidence to support this.

Low-oxygen-affinity haemoglobin variants

More than 50 haemoglobin variants with reduced oxygen affinity have been identified, often associated with other abnormal properties such as instability. The first to be described, Hb Kansas (β102 Asn→Thr), was found in a mother and son with unexplained cyanosis. The subjects were asymptomatic and had normal haemoglobin levels without any evidence of haemolysis. Like many of the high-affinity variants, the amino acid substitution in this variant was at the interface between the α and β globin chains. For reasons that are not clear, some substitutions in this region give rise to variants with a relatively low oxygen affinity. This condition should be thought of in any patient with unexplained congenital cyanosis.

Congenital methaemoglobinaemia due to haemoglobin variants

Several α and β globin variants associated with methaemoglobinaemia have been discovered. These disorders, unlike the genetic methaemoglobinaemias due to enzyme defects, follow a dominant pattern of inheritance. The patients are blue in colour, and may have mild polycythaemia as methaemoglobin does not carry oxygen. Diagnosis is based on measuring methaemoglobin levels, and analysis of haemoglobin and DNA.

Acknowledgement

Parts of the present chapter are based on the corresponding previous edition chapter, and for this we acknowledge the contribution of Professor Sir David Weatherall. We also thank Claire Steward for help on the preparation of the chapter.

Selected bibliography

Anderson LJ, Holden S, Davis B et al. (2001) Cardiovascular T2-star (T2*) magnetic resonance for the early diagnosis of myocardial iron overload. European Heart Journal 22: 2171–9.

Angelucci E, Barosi G, Camaschella C et al. (2008) Italian Society of Haematology practice guidelines for the management of iron overload in thalassemia major and related disorders. Haematologica 93: 741–52.

Borgna-Pignatti C (2007) Modern treatment of thalassaemia intermedia. British Journal of Haematology 138: 291–304.

Borgna-Pignatti C, Rugolotto S, De Stefano P et al. (2004) Survival and complications in patients with thalassemia major treated with transfusion and deferoxamine. Haematologica 89: 1187–93.

Borgna-Pignatti C, Cappellini MD, De Stefano P et al. (2006) Cardiac morbidity and mortality in deferoxamine- or deferiprone-treated patients with thalassemia major. Blood 107: 3733–7.

Cappellini M-D, Cohen A, Eleftheriou A, Piga A, Porter J, Taher A (eds) (2008) Guidelines for the Clinical Management of

Thalassaemia. Thalassaemia International Federation, Nicosia, Cyprus.

Chakalova L, Carter D, Debrand E *et al.* (2005) Developmental regulation of the beta-globin gene locus. *Progress in Molecular and Subcellular Biology* **38**: 183–206.

Chang JG, Tsai WC, Chong IW, Chang CS, Lin CC, Liu TC (2008) Beta-thalassemia major evolution from beta-thalassemia minor is associated with paternal uniparental isodisomy of chromosome 11p15. *Haematologica* **93**: 913–16.

Cohen AR, Glimm E, Porter JB (2008) Effect of transfusional iron intake on response to chelation therapy in beta-thalassemia major. *Blood* **111**: 583–7.

De Gobbi M, Viprakasit V, Hughes JR *et al.* (2006) A regulatory SNP causes a human genetic disease by creating a new transcriptional promoter. *Science* **312**: 1215–17.

Galanello R, Perseu L, Perra C *et al.* (2004) Somatic deletion of the normal beta-globin gene leading to thalassaemia intermedia in heterozygous beta-thalassaemic patients. *British Journal of Haematology* **127**: 604–6.

Harteveld CL, Refaldi C, Cassinerio E, Cappellini MD, Giordano PC (2008) Segmental duplications involving the alpha-globin gene cluster are causing beta-thalassaemia intermedia phenotypes in beta-thalassaemia heterozygous patients. *Blood Cells, Molecules and Diseases* **40**: 312–16.

Hershko C (2006) Oral iron chelators: new opportunities and new dilemmas. *Haematologica* **91**: 1307–12.

Higgs DR, Weatherall DJ (2009) The alpha thalassaemias. *Cellular and Molecular Life Sciences* **66**: 1154–62.

Higgs DR, Wood WG (2008) Long-range regulation of alpha globin gene expression during erythropoiesis. *Current Opinion in Hematology* **15**: 176–83.

Hoffbrand AV (ed.) (2009) Recent advances in understanding of iron metabolism and iron related diseases. *Acta Haematologica* **122** (2–3) Special Issue.

Lettre G, Sankaran VG, Bezerra MA *et al.* (2008) DNA polymorphisms at the BCL11A, HBS1L-MYB, and beta-globin loci associate with fetal haemoglobin levels and pain crises in sickle cell disease. *Proceedings of the National Academy of Sciences USA* **105**: 11869–74.

Maquat LE (2002) Nonsense-mediated mRNA decay. *Current Biology* **12**: R196–R197.

Menzel S, Garner C, Gut I *et al.* (2007) A QTL influencing F cell production maps to a gene encoding a zinc-finger protein on chromosome 2p15. *Nature Genetics* **39**: 1197–9.

National Health Service Sickle Cell and Thalassaemia Screening Programme. Available at http://sct.screening.nhs.uk/

Palstra RJ, de Laat W, Grosveld F (2008) Beta-globin regulation and long–range interactions. *Advances in Genetics* **61**: 107–42.

Pennell DJ, Berdoukas V, Karagiorga M *et al.* (2006) Randomized controlled trial of deferiprone or deferoxamine in beta-thalassemia major patients with asymptomatic myocardial siderosis. *Blood* **107**: 3738–44.

Percy MJ, Lappin TR (2008) Recessive congenital methaemoglobinaemia: cytochrome b(5) reductase deficiency. *British Journal of Haematology* **141**: 298–308.

Pinto FO, Roberts I (2008) Cord blood stem cell transplantation for haemoglobinopathies. *British Journal of Haematology* **141**: 309–24.

Premawardhena A, Fisher CA, Olivieri NF *et al.* (2005) A novel molecular basis for beta thalassemia intermedia poses new questions about its pathophysiology. *Blood* **106**: 3251–5.

Quek L, Thein SL (2007) Molecular therapies in beta-thalassaemia. *British Journal of Haematology* **136**: 353–65.

Rund D, Rachmilewitz E (2005) Beta-thalassemia. *New England Journal of Medicine* **353**: 1135–46.

Sankaran VG, Menne TF, Xu J *et al.* (2008) Human fetal haemoglobin expression is regulated by the developmental stage-specific repressor BCL11A. *Science* **322**: 1839–42.

Sankaran VG, Xu J, Orkin SH (2010) Advances in the understanding of haemoglobin switching. *British Journal of Haematology* **149**: 181–94.

Steinberg MH, Forget BG, Higgs DR, Weatherall DJ (eds) (2009) *Disorders of Haemoglobin*. Cambridge University Press, New York, USA.

Taher A, Isma'eel H, Cappellini MD (2006) Thalassemia intermedia: revisited. *Blood Cells, Molecules and Diseases* **37**: 12–20.

Tanno T, Bhanu NV, Oneal PA *et al.* (2007) High levels of GDF15 in thalassemia suppress expression of the iron regulatory protein hepcidin. *Nature Medicine* **13**: 1096–101.

Thein SL (2004) Genetic insights into the clinical diversity of beta thalassaemia. *British Journal of Haematology* **124**: 264–74.

Thein SL (2005) Genetic modifiers of beta-thalassemia. *Haematologica* **90**: 649–60.

Thein SL (2008) Genetic modifiers of the beta-haemoglobinopathies. *British Journal of Haematology* **141**: 357–66.

Thein SL, Menzel S (2009) Discovering the genetics underlying foetal haemoglobin production in adults. *British Journal of Haematology* **145**: 455–67.

Thein SL, Menzel S, Peng X *et al.* (2007) Intergenic variants of HBS1L-MYB are responsible for a major quantitative trait locus on chromosome 6q23 influencing fetal haemoglobin levels in adults. *Proceedings of the National Academy of Sciences USA* **104**: 11346–51.

Tufarelli C, Stanley JA, Garrick D *et al.* (2003) Transcription of antisense RNA leading to gene silencing and methylation as a novel cause of human genetic disease. *Nature Genetics* **34**: 157–65.

Uda M, Galanello R, Sanna S *et al.* (2008) Genome-wide association study shows BCL11A associated with persistent fetal haemoglobin and amelioration of the phenotype of beta-thalassemia. *Proceedings of the National Academy of Sciences USA* **105**: 1620–5.

UK Thalassaemia Society (2008) *Standards for the Clinical Care of Children and Adults with Thalassaemia in the UK*. The UK Thalassaemia Society, London.

Vichinsky E (2008) Clinical application of deferasirox: practical patient management. *American Journal of Hematology* **83**: 398–402.

Weatherall DJ (2001) Phenotype–genotype relationships in monogenic disease: lessons from the thalassaemias. *Nature Reviews. Genetics* **2**: 245–55.

Weatherall DJ, Clegg JB (2001) Inherited haemoglobin disorders: an increasing global health problem. *Bulletin of the World Health Organization* **79**: 704–12.

Weatherall DJ, Clegg JB (2001) *The Thalassaemia Syndromes*. Blackwell Science, Oxford.

CHAPTER 7

Sickle cell disease

Ashutosh Lal and Elliott P Vichinsky

Children's Hospital and Research Center, Oakland, California, USA

Introduction

Sickle cell disease (SCD) is an inherited chronic haemolytic anaemia whose clinical manifestations arise from the tendency of the haemoglobin (HbS or sickle haemoglobin) to polymerize and deform red blood cells into the characteristic sickle shape. This property is due to a single nucleotide change in the β-globin gene leading to substitution of valine for glutamic acid at position 6 of the β-globin chain ($\beta^{6glu \to val}$ or β^s). The homozygous state (HbSS or sickle cell anaemia) is the most common form of sickle cell disease, but interaction of HbS with thalassaemia and certain variant haemoglobins also leads to sickling. The term 'sickle cell disease' is used to denote all entities associated with sickling of haemoglobin within red cells (Table 7.1).

Geographic distribution of sickle mutation

Several distinct β-globin gene haplotypes are associated with the sickle mutation, and their distribution provides evidence for

Postgraduate Haematology: 6th edition. Edited by A. Victor Hoffbrand, Daniel Catovsky, Edward G.D. Tuddenham, Anthony R. Green
© 2011 Blackwell Publishing Ltd.

origin of the mutation in several locations within Africa (the Senegal, Benin and Bantu haplotypes) and Asia (the Arab–Indian haplotype). The sickle trait bestows survival benefit in areas endemic for falciparum malaria, and the distribution of SCD historically paralleled this disease. The sickle haemoglobin-containing red cells inhibit proliferation of *Plasmodium falciparum*, and are more likely to become deformed and removed from the circulation. In recent times, the dissemination of the sickle mutation in different areas of the world took place from the movement of populations via trade routes and the slave trade (Table 7.2). The prevalence of SCD varies tremendously among ethnic and tribal groups within a geographic area. The disease is observed occasionally among the white population: 10% of patients with HbSS identified by the California newborn screening programme are not of African descent.

Pathophysiology

Molecular basis of sickling

Deoxygenation of HbS leads to a conformational change that exposes a hydrophobic patch on the surface of the β^s-globin chain at the site of β^6 valine (Figure 7.1). Binding of this site to a complementary hydrophobic site on a β-subunit of another haemoglobin tetramer triggers the formation of large polymers. The polymers consist of staggered haemoglobin tetramers that

Table 7.1 The sickling syndromes.

Genotype	Mean haemoglobin (g/dL)	MCV	Haemoglobin electrophoresis (%)				
			S	A	F	A_2	Other
SS	8.1	N	80–95	–	2–20	N	–
SS $-\alpha/\alpha\alpha$, SS $-\alpha/-\alpha$	8.6, 9.2	↓, ↓	80–90, 80–90	–, –	2–20, 2–20	3.3–3.8, 3.3–3.8	–, –
SC	11.0	↓	40–50	–	1–4		C: 40–50
S/β^0 thalassaemia	8.8	↓	75–90	–	2–20	4–6	–
S/β^+ thalassaemia	11.5	↓	50–85	5–30	2–20	4–6	–
SD Punjab	8.2	N	40	–	2.5–5	2–3	D Punjab: 50
SO Arab	8.1	N	45	–	4–7		O Arab: 45
S Lepore	11.0	↓	75	–	3.5–40	2	Lepore: 10
SE	13.0	↓	60	–	4		E: 30–35
S/HPFH	13.7	N or ↓	60–70	–	25–35	1.5–2.5	–
AS*	N	N	30–45	50–65	2–5	N	–

*Sickle cell trait is asymptomatic.

MCV, mean corpuscular volume.

Table 7.2 Areas of high prevalence of sickle mutation.

Geographic region	Heterozygote rate (%)
Africa	
Northern	1–2
Western	10–30
Central	7–37
Southern	0–5
Mediterranean	
Northern Greece	1–27
Southern Italy	
Americas	
United States: African ancestry	8
Caribbean: African ancestry	10
Brazil: non-white	7
Asia	
Saudi Arabia: south-west	5
Saudi Arabia: eastern province	25
India: central India – tribal population	20–30

aggregate into 21-nm diameter helical fibres, with one inner and six peripheral double strands. The polymerization proceeds after a delay, the length of which is extremely sensitive to the intracellular deoxy-HbS concentration. Even a small increase in deoxy-HbS concentration, such as might occur with cellular dehydration, profoundly shortens the delay time and augments sickling. The process of polymerization is highly cooperative and its kinetics are best explained by the double nucleation model. The haemoglobin tetramers first aggregate into a nucleus, which rapidly expands into a fibre (homogeneous nucleation). The newly formed fibre provides nuclei on its surface for aggregation of haemoglobin tetramers to form several more fibres (heterogeneous nucleation).

The polymerization of HbS in the circulating red cells is influenced by the oxygenation status, the intracellular haemoglobin concentration and the presence of non-sickle haemoglobins. Acidosis and elevated level of 2,3-diphosphoglycerate (2,3-DPG) promote polymer formation by reducing the oxygen affinity of haemoglobin. The presence of HbA within the red cells, as in sickle trait, inhibits polymerization by diluting HbS. The inhibitory effect of HbF on polymerization of HbS is more profound owing to the greater amino acid disparity between the β^s- and γ-globin chains.

Effect on erythrocytes

Red cells acquire the sickle or elongated shape upon deoxygenation as a result of intracellular polymerization of HbS, a phenomenon that is reversible on reoxygenation. Even in the normally shaped red cells, however, the presence of HbS polymer reduces deformability, with consequent increase in blood viscosity. Repeated or prolonged sickling progressively damages the red cell membrane, which is a phenomenon of primary importance in the pathophysiology of SCD. Membrane damage causes movement of potassium ions and water out of the cell by the Gardos pathway and potassium–chloride cotransport, leading to dehydration of red cells. The intracellular haemoglobin concentration rises (producing dense cells), which shortens the delay time to sickle polymer formation. A second key consequence of membrane damage is alteration of the chemistry of the red cell membrane. Perturbation of lipid organization causes negatively charged phosphatidylserine to

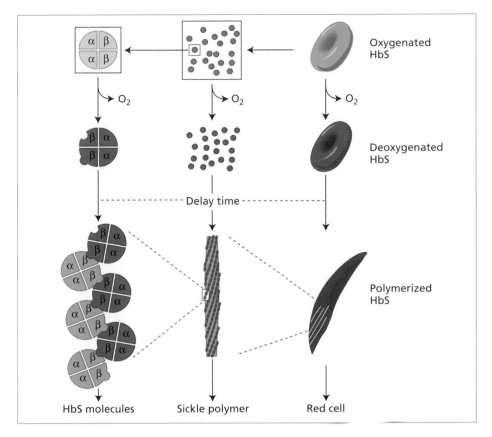

Figure 7.1 Induction of red cell sickling. As red cells traverse the microcirculation, oxygen is released from oxy-HbS (red circles), generating deoxy-HbS (purple circles). Conformational change exposes a hydrophobic patch at the site of the β^6-valine replacement, shown as a projection (left column), which can bind to a complementary hydrophobic site on a subunit of another haemoglobin tetramer, shown as an indentation. Only one of the two β^6-valine sites in each HbS tetramer makes this contact. The middle column shows the assembly of deoxy-HbS into a helical 14-strand fibre, shown as a twisted rope-like structure. The delay time is inversely proportional to the intracellular haemoglobin concentration raised to the 15th power. As deoxy-HbS polymerizes and fibres align, the red cell is distorted into an elongated banana or 'sickle' shape (right column). (From Bunn 1997 with permission.)

appear on the red cell surface instead of its normal location in the inner monolayer. In addition, the red cells become abnormally adherent to the vascular endothelium through vascular cell adhesion molecule (VCAM)-1, thrombospondin and fibronectin.

and is promoted by leucocytosis, platelet activation and inflammatory cytokines. Genetic influences independent of the sickle mutation probably modulate the tendency for vaso-occlusion in individuals and account for some phenotypic variation seen in this disease.

Vaso-occlusion

Several processes contribute to development of vaso-occlusion in SCD. Slowing of blood flow arises from abnormal regulation of vascular tone as a result of diminished nitric oxide (NO)-induced vasodilatation. This is aggravated by increase in blood viscosity, resulting from less deformable red cells, a phenomenon called abnormal rheology. Vaso-occlusion is initiated by adhesion of young deformable red cells to the vascular endothelium, and is followed by trapping of rigid irreversibly sickled cells (Figure 7.2). Adhesion occurs in the post-capillary venules

Haemolysis

SCD is characterized by chronic intravascular and extravascular haemolysis. Sickling-induced membrane fragmentation and complement-mediated lysis cause intravascular destruction of red cells. Membrane damage also leads to extravascular haemolysis through entrapment of poorly deformable cells or uptake by macrophages. The red cell survival measured by ^{51}Cr assay is 4–25 days, with dense cells surviving for a considerably shorter time than red cells containing some HbF (F cells). Patients have greatly expanded bone marrow space, but the serum erythro-

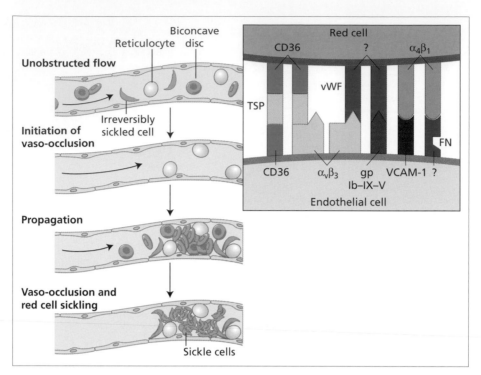

Figure 7.2 Endothelial red cell adhesion and vaso-occlusion in sickle cell disease. Adhesive sickle reticulocytes initiate vaso-occlusion by becoming attached to the endothelium of vessel walls. Thereafter, poorly deformable red cells begin to accumulate behind the site of adhesion, ultimately resulting in an occluded vascular segment containing many sickled red cells. The inset shows the site of red cell attachment to an endothelial cell and several adhesion mechanisms that could participate in the vaso-occlusive process. On the red cell, the relevant adhesion receptors include CD36, which binds thrombospondin (TSP), and integrin $\alpha_4\beta_1$, which binds both fibronectin (FN) and vascular cell adhesion molecule (VCAM)-1. On the endothelial cell, the receptors include CD36; integrin $\alpha_v\beta_3$; the complex of glycoproteins Ib, IX and V (gp Ib–IX–V), which binds von Willebrand factor (VWF); and VCAM-1. Adhesive interactions between the red cell and endothelial cells may be direct ($\alpha_4\beta_1$ to VCAM-1) or mediated by a plasma factor (CD36 to TSP to $\alpha_v\beta_3$). The list of molecules identified as involved in mediating adhesion continues to increase and redundancy in the system is likely. Question marks indicate unidentified receptors. (From Hebbel RP (2000) Blockade of adhesion of sickle cells to endothelium by monoclonal antibodies. *New England Journal of Medicine* **342**: 1910–12 with permission.)

poietin level is lower than expected for the extent of anaemia because of the decreased oxygen affinity of HbS. Individuals with concomitant deletion of one or two α-globin genes, or the Senegal or Arab–Indian haplotypes, have higher baseline haemoglobin levels. The significance of chronic intravascular haemolysis in SCD extends beyond anaemia, since the release of free haemoglobin causes depletion of NO in the plasma. This is linked to endothelial dysfunction and the development of several complications including pulmonary hypertension.

Clinical manifestations

Clinical symptoms vary tremendously between patients with SCD for several reasons. The disease is more severe in patients with HbSS or HbS/β⁰ thalassaemia than in those with HbS/β⁺ thalassaemia or HbSC disease. The Arab–Indian haplotype produces a less severe disease than the African haplotypes. The co-inheritance of one or two α-gene deletions also modifies the clinical picture. The high HbF level observed in hereditary persistence of fetal haemoglobin (HPFH) is associated with very mild disease. However, for poorly recognized reasons, the disease severity varies enormously even within the subgroup of patients with HbSS.

In countries with inadequate healthcare, SCD is associated with high mortality in the first 3 years of life as a result of sepsis and splenic sequestration. In the developed world, the typical patient with SCD has moderately severe anaemia, leads a relatively normal life interrupted by 'crises' as a result of vaso-occlusion, and has a life expectancy of over 45 years.

Anaemia

The underlying β-globin genotype primarily determines the baseline haemoglobin value in SCD, but exacerbation of anaemia can occur for numerous reasons. Patients with more severe anaemia at baseline have a greater probability of developing stroke and renal dysfunction. On the other hand, a higher haemoglobin level is associated with a higher incidence of painful episodes, avascular necrosis and acute chest syndrome. Infants with SCD have lower than normal haemoglobin levels after the neonatal period, and the decline continues until it reaches a nadir between 12 and 15 months of age. Boys are slightly more anaemic than girls in the first decade, whereas adult men have higher haemoglobin values than women. Gradual exacerbation of anaemia is observed in both sexes beginning in the fifth decade.

A gradual decrease in haemoglobin level from the baseline value may indicate an underlying folate or iron deficiency. In older patients, however, inadequate erythropoietin production due to chronic renal insufficiency is the most important aetiology of worsening anaemia. Many such patients will become transfusion dependent, although recombinant human erythropoietin therapy can improve the anaemia.

Acute exacerbations of anaemia are observed with aplastic crises and splenic sequestration. The transient arrest of erythropoiesis and the resultant reticulocytopenia in aplastic crisis is most often due to parvovirus B19 infection. Severe anaemia is the consequence of the shortened lifespan of red cells and the course is similar to other chronic haemolytic anaemias. Aplastic crisis is typically preceded by fever and upper respiratory or gastrointestinal symptoms, and several family members may fall ill over a period of days. The reticulocytopenia begins 5 days after exposure, lasts for 7–10 days and is followed by recovery with reticulocytosis and normoblasts in peripheral blood. Blood transfusion is often required in the short term. Parvovirus B19 infection is followed by development of lifelong protective immunity.

Splenic sequestration is a serious complication in young children whose spleen has not yet undergone fibrosis due to recurrent vaso-occlusion. The peak incidence of first episode of sequestration is between 6 and 12 months of age and it affects 30% of all patients. Approximately 15% of patients die during the acute episode and the condition recurs in half of the survivors. Episodes may be triggered by a viral illness and the rapid acute enlargement of the spleen traps a significant proportion of the blood volume. Clinically, the child presents with acutely worsening anaemia (> 2 g/dL fall in haemoglobin), reticulocytosis, enlarging spleen and hypovolaemic shock. Prompt restoration of the blood volume and correction of anaemia is required. Splenectomy is recommended following a sequestration crisis due to the risk of recurrences. Chronic transfusion therapy or partial splenectomy is sometimes used in infants with life-threatening anaemic episodes. Parent education to detect splenic enlargement and seek early medical attention significantly reduces the risk of death from sequestration crisis.

Acute painful episode

Acute episode of pain due to vaso-occlusion is the most frequent symptom for which patients with SCD seek medical attention. More frequent painful episodes are observed in patients with HbSS, low HbF level, α thalassaemia and higher baseline haemoglobin levels. Painful episodes are more common in young adults and tend to diminish in older patients. One-third of the patients with SCD rarely experience pain, whereas a small subgroup of patients suffer from recurrent episodes. When patients maintain a pain diary, painful events are noted on up to half of the days but are not severe enough to require visit to a physician. Painful episodes vary in intensity and generally last for a few days. The majority of the episodes have no identifiable cause, although some attacks are precipitated by cold, dehydration, infection, stress or menses.

In young children, the initial pain episode typically presents as dactylitis or hand–foot syndrome, with swelling over the dorsal surface of hands and feet. It arises from bone infarction affecting the small bones and the swelling subsides over 1–2 weeks. The radiographs show thinning of cortex and destructive changes of the affected small bones several weeks after onset. In older children and adults, the common sites of pain are the back, chest, extremities and abdomen. Chest pain is of special significance as it can precede development of acute chest syndrome. Frequent incapacitating painful episodes that are inadequately managed have adverse psychosocial consequences and stress the physician–patient relationship.

Growth and development

Children with SCD are born with normal weight but fall behind other children by the end of the first year. The weight deficit persists through adulthood and imparts a thin habitus to the typical patient, although obesity is seen in some cases. The rate of growth is lower than normal in SCD patients, and the pubertal growth spurt is delayed by 1–2 years, but the final adult height is normal. Delays also occur in skeletal maturation and onset of puberty, and female patients achieve menarche 1–2 years later than their peers.

Infections

Early loss of splenic function from recurrent vaso-occlusion and the inability to make specific IgG antibodies to polysaccharide antigens increases the risk of fulminant sepsis. Pneumococcal infection is a serious problem in SCD, particularly in children under 3 years (Figure 7.3). Meningitis can accompany pneumococcal sepsis, and the overall mortality rate is 20–50%. Patients who have had previous pneumococcal sepsis are at increased risk for recurrent episodes and must remain on lifelong penicillin prophylaxis. *Haemophilus influenzae* type B is the next most common organism and affects older children. There is considerable variation in the relative incidence of bacterial organisms causing sepsis in young children with SCD in various regions of the world. In Africa, *Salmonella* spp., *Klebsiella* spp., *Escherichia coli* and *Staphylococcus* spp. are more commonly isolated from the blood of febrile children than *Streptococcus pneumoniae*. Pneumococcal infections are particularly infrequent in the eastern province of Saudi Arabia and Nigeria. Furthermore, the incidence of pneumococcal and *H. influenzae* sepsis has declined as a result of penicillin prophylaxis and vaccination of infants. The risk of death during septic episodes has decreased considerably owing to empirical use of antibiotics to treat fever in SCD.

Of the other infections, pneumonia is particularly common in SCD and can be difficult to differentiate from non-infective causes of acute chest syndrome. The most frequent organisms responsible for pneumonia are *Mycoplasma pneumoniae*, *Chlamydia pneumoniae*, *S. pneumoniae* and *H. influenzae*. Lung infections can also arise due to respiratory viruses. In adults, bacteraemia and urinary tract infections due to *E. coli* and other Gram-negative organisms are more frequent. Patients with SCD are susceptible to osteomyelitis caused by bone infarction resulting from vaso-occlusion. The infection is typically due to *Salmonella* spp. or *Staphylococcus aureus*.

Neurological complications

Neurological complications are an important cause of morbidity in SCD. Transient ischaemic attacks or stroke due to cerebral infarction or haemorrhage occur in 25% of patients with SCD (Figure 7.4a). The risk of stroke is increased with lower baseline haemoglobin, low HbF level, high leucocyte count or high systolic blood pressure. Vascular damage results from elevated cerebral blood flow velocities and interaction of rigid or adherent sickle cells with the vessel wall. Angiography demonstrates stenosis or occlusion of vessels in the circle of Willis and internal carotid arteries, sometimes with aneurysm formation or development of moya moya disease (Figure 7.4b). Increased blood flow velocity due to stenosis can be detected by transcranial Doppler ultrasonography in asymptomatic patients, and flow rates in excess of 200 cm/s correlate with a high risk of stroke.

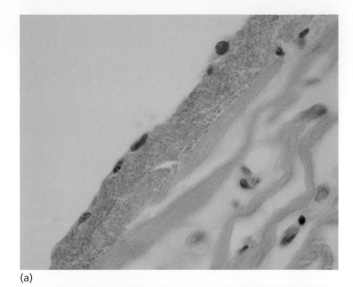
(a)

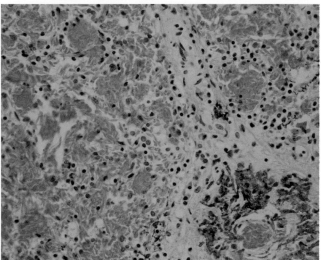
(b)

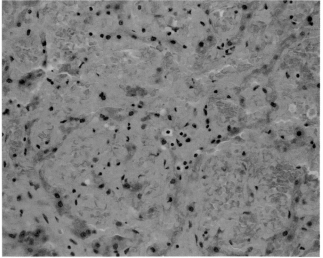
(c)

Figure 7.3 Overwhelming pneumococcal sepsis in a 7-year-old child. (a) Numerous bacteria in the blood adjacent to the right ventricular wall. Massive sequestration of the spleen (b) and the liver (c).

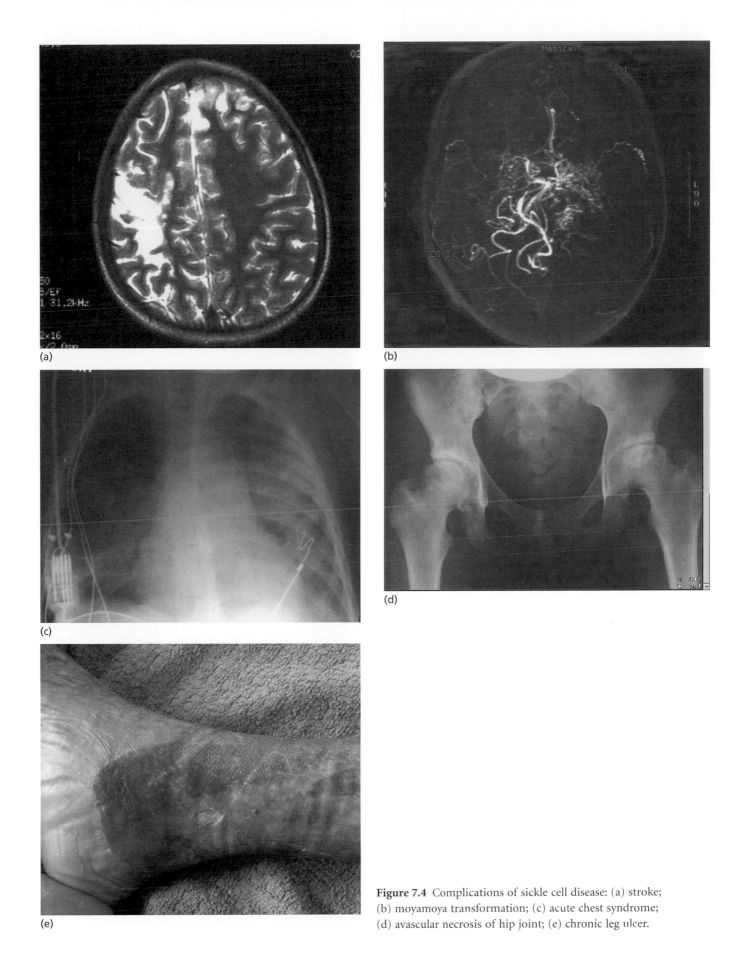

Figure 7.4 Complications of sickle cell disease: (a) stroke; (b) moyamoya transformation; (c) acute chest syndrome; (d) avascular necrosis of hip joint; (e) chronic leg ulcer.

Stroke due to infarction is more frequent in younger children and those over 30 years of age, whereas haemorrhage is more common between 20 and 30 years. Stroke is rare in infants, increases to 1 in 100 patients per year between 2 and 9 years, and then diminishes to half that incidence in older patients. The incidence of stroke is 5–10 times greater in HbSS compared with HbSC, HbS/β^+ thalassaemia or HbS/β^0 thalassaemia. Focal seizures or transient ischaemic attacks are common presenting symptoms of stroke, followed by hemiparesis, coma and speech or visual disturbances. The site of bleeding in haemorrhagic stroke is frequently subarachnoid, and these patients present with severe headache, vomiting and coma. Death can occur during the acute event, particularly with haemorrhagic stroke. Patients with neurological symptoms should be evaluated by computed tomography (CT) or magnetic resonance imaging (MRI) to distinguish thrombosis from haemorrhage. Immediate exchange transfusion to lower HbS level to less than 30% is required. Patients with haemorrhage may require surgical intervention to ligate accessible aneurysms. Surgical vascular bypass procedure with extracranial arteries (encephalodural synangiosis) should be considered in children with moyamoya disease.

As stroke recurs in two-thirds of the survivors within 3 years, all such patients should be maintained on regular transfusions to lower HbS level for several years. Development of first stroke in children at risk, who are identified by elevated cerebral Doppler blood flow velocity, can be prevented effectively through regular transfusions. As an alternative to transfusions, hydroxycarbamide (hydroxyurea) treatment can also reduce the high cerebral blood flow velocity, and its use for primary or secondary prevention of stroke is being explored. Even in the absence of overt stroke, silent cerebral infarcts are commonly observed on MRI in SCD and are linked to progressive neuropsychiatric and neurological damage, and poor school performance. Early detection and treatment is important in preventing further neurocognitive impairment.

Pulmonary complications

Acute and chronic pulmonary complications are the leading cause of death in older patients. The acute chest syndrome is characterized by hypoxia, tachypnoea, fever, chest pain and pulmonary infiltrate on chest radiography (Figure 7.4c). Acute chest syndrome often follows a painful event, particularly in adults (Table 7.3). The pathogenesis of acute chest syndrome involves vaso-occlusion, infection or embolization of bone marrow fat. Infections due to *Mycoplasma*, *Chlamydia*, *Legionella*, pneumococcus, *H. influenzae* and viruses are more likely in children. Fat-laden pulmonary macrophages in the airways due to fat embolization from the bone marrow are present in half of the cases. Hypoxia due to acute chest syndrome can result in widespread sickling and vaso-occlusion, with risk of multiorgan failure. Patients should receive supplemental oxygen, incentive spirometry and antibiotic therapy

Table 7.3 Presenting symptoms of acute chest syndrome.

Symptom	Children (%)	Adults (%)
Fever	86	70
Shortness of breath	31	58
Chest pain	27	55
Extremity pain	22	58
Rib pain	14	30

Adults are more likely than children to have pain preceding the onset of pulmonary symptoms.

directed towards the common organisms. One commonly used regimen consists of cefuroxime and erythromycin, although antibiotics should be guided by local experience. Most patients have a bronchoreactive component and should receive bronchodilator therapy. Patients require close monitoring for persistent hypoxia or worsening lung consolidation for which blood transfusion should be provided. Partial exchange transfusion and mechanical ventilation is sometimes needed in rapidly progressive cases. NO and steroids may be beneficial in life-threatening cases.

Chronic pulmonary problems seen in SCD are restrictive and obstructive lung disease, hypoxaemia and pulmonary hypertension. Chronic complications are more frequent in patients with a history of acute chest syndrome. Echocardiography can detect elevated pulmonary artery systolic pressure (>35 mmHg), which is observed in 20% of patients. Pulmonary hypertension is more frequent among patients with high rates of chronic haemolysis, reflected by marked elevation in plasma lactate dehydrogenase (LDH). The diagnosis of pulmonary hypertension is associated with a 10-fold increase in relative risk of dying compared with patients who have normal pulmonary artery systolic pressure, although most deaths are not from cardiac failure. Hydroxycarbamide therapy should be strongly considered in SCD patients with pulmonary hypertension. Severely affected patients have been treated with regular transfusions, vasodilators, anticoagulation and oxygen inhalation.

Hepatobiliary complications

The liver can be affected by intrahepatic trapping of sickle cells, transfusion-acquired infection and transfusional haemosiderosis. Episodes of cholestasis due to intrahepatic sickling can lead to liver failure in rare instances. Pigmented gallstones are seen in two-thirds of patients, particularly those with HbSS, and can occur in young children. Patients with abdominal symptoms attributable to gallstones should undergo cholecystectomy, although the management of asymptomatic gallstones is less clear. Laparoscopic cholecystectomy can be safely performed, but associated common duct bile stones first require endoscopic retrograde cholangiopancreatography.

Pregnancy

The steady-state haemoglobin level falls in SCD during pregnancy, similar to the decline in haemoglobin observed in normal pregnant women. Folate deficiency can exacerbate the anaemia and supplements should be provided throughout pregnancy. Painful episodes become more common in the last trimester. The incidence of pre-eclampsia is higher than normal in SCD patients and there is a slight increase in maternal mortality. Risk to the fetus from abortion, stillbirth, low birth weight and neonatal death is also increased. Prophylactic transfusions during pregnancy or the type of delivery do not alter the outcome for mother or newborn. It is safe to use oral contraceptives for birth control in SCD.

Renal complications

The hypoxic, acidotic and hypertonic renal medulla favours vaso-occlusion, leading to destruction of the vasa recta and hyposthenuria in the first year of life. It presents clinically as enuresis or nocturia, and patients are susceptible to dehydration in hot weather. Haematuria as a result of papillary necrosis usually originates from the left kidney. Management is generally by bed rest and hydration, although sometimes blood transfusion and ε-aminocaproic acid are required. The prevalence of essential hypertension in SCD is lower than in the general population, although elevated systolic blood pressure is a risk factor for stroke. Proteinuria due to glomerular injury precedes development of nephrotic syndrome and eventual chronic renal insufficiency in one-quarter of adults. The progression to renal failure can be delayed by angiotensin-converting enzyme inhibitors. Careful control of blood pressure, avoidance of non-steroidal anti-inflammatory drugs (NSAIDs) and aggressive treatment of urinary tract infection and anaemia are important objectives for patients with chronic renal insufficiency. Patients with end-stage renal disease are treated with dialysis and renal transplantation. Some renal complications, such as hyposthenuria and haematuria, are also observed in individuals with sickle trait, as is the rare renal medullary carcinoma.

Priapism

Priapism occurs in two-thirds of males with SCD, with a peak incidence in the second and third decades. It is caused by vaso-occlusion leading to obstruction of venous drainage from the penis. It typically affects the corpora cavernosa alone, resulting in a hard penis with a soft glans. Episodes can be brief (stuttering) or prolonged, when they last for longer than 3 hours. Recurrent priapism leads to fibrosis and eventual impotence. Young boys require explanation of symptoms and the need to seek early help for priapism. At the onset of priapism, patients should drink extra fluids and attempt to urinate. An oral dose of pseudoephedrine or terbutaline can be given. Persistent priapism requires intravenous hydration and opioid analgesia. If priapism persists for more than 2–3 hours, aspiration and irrigation of the corpora with dilute phenylephrine or etilefrine solution should be performed. A simple intracavernosal injection with these agents tried early may induce detumescence and avoid the need for aspiration and irrigation.

Ocular complications

Vaso-occlusion of retinal and other vascular beds in the eye can lead to grave complications. Patients with SCD can develop abnormal (comma-shaped) conjunctival vessels, iris atrophy, retinal pigmentary changes and retinal haemorrhages. However, much more serious is neovascularization causing proliferative retinopathy, appearing as a 'sea fan', with its potential for vitreous haemorrhage and retinal detachment. Such patients are treated with laser photocoagulation or vitrectomy. The incidence of proliferative changes is substantially higher in HbSC and HbS/β^+ thalassaemia patients than in HbSS. All patients with SCD should have annual ophthalmological evaluation, beginning in the second decade.

Sudden change in vision in a patient with SCD is an ocular emergency. Central retinal artery occlusion requires immediate treatment with hyperoxygenation and reduction of intraocular pressure, but the prognosis for vision is poor. Hyphaema, which can arise after minor trauma, leads to glaucoma due to sickling of blood in the anterior chamber. The elevated intraocular pressure causes ischaemic optic atrophy and retinal artery occlusion. Individuals with sickle trait are also vulnerable to this complication. Urgent surgical attention is required to wash out blood from the anterior chamber.

Bone complications

The chronic haemolytic process results in expansion of the medullary space, although the resultant bony changes are less pronounced than in thalassaemia. Bone infarction due to vaso-occlusion produces tenderness, warmth and swelling, which can be difficult to distinguish from osteomyelitis. In such cases, cultures from blood and direct aspiration are negative and radiography later shows patchy sclerosis and cortical thickening. Collapse of vertebral end plates due to infarction produces the codfish appearance. Patients are managed with analgesia and hydration until resolution of symptoms.

Avascular necrosis of the femoral head is a serious complication that is difficult to treat and leads to chronic disability and pain (Figure 7.4d). Patients with coexisting α thalassaemia have a higher incidence of osteonecrosis at a younger age. The condition also affects the humeral head but with less functional consequences. The outcome is better in young patients with immature capital epiphysis, who should be treated with analgesics and avoidance of weight-bearing for 3–6 months. In older adolescents and adults the condition is more likely to progress to degenerative arthritis with conservative management. Aggressive physical therapy or combination of early core decompression followed by physical therapy can postpone the need for additional surgical intervention. Hip arthroplasty may be required for patients with severe symptoms.

Leg ulcers

Chronic leg ulcers are frequent in adult patients with SCD, particularly affecting males with the HbSS genotype (Figure 7.4e). Ulcers arise near the medial or lateral malleolus and may be single or multiple. Occlusion of skin microvasculature from sickle red cells predisposes to ulcers, which are made worse by trauma, infection or warm climate. Ulcers are always colonized with pathogenic bacteria (*Pseudomonas aeruginosa*, *S. aureus* and *Streptococcus* spp.) and acute infection can occur. The ulcers are painful and resistant to healing, and although bed rest and elevation of the leg are efficacious, they may not be practical owing to the chronic nature of the problem. Treatment requires débridement, elastic dressings, zinc sulphate and, in some cases, red cell transfusions and skin grafting.

Variant sickle cell syndromes

Sickle cell trait

Sickle cell trait (HbAS) is a benign condition that has no haematological manifestations and is associated with normal growth and life expectancy. The ratio of HbA to HbS is 60:40, owing to the greater affinity of α-globin chains for β^A-globin chains. Sickle cell trait affects 8–10% of African-Americans and up to 25–30% of the population in West Africa. Sickle trait reduces the risk of severe falciparum malaria, but not the prevalence of parasitaemia. There appears to be no effect on infections with other forms of malaria. Impaired urine-concentrating ability and haematuria can occur, and an increased incidence of urinary tract infection is observed in pregnant women with sickle cell trait. Splenic infarction is possible at very high altitudes, and varies in severity from mild discomfort to occasional splenic rupture. A slight risk of sudden death during exercise has been reported predominantly in two settings. Army recruits with sickle cell trait have a 25-fold higher rate of unexplained death, with greatest risk during basic training or at high altitude. The second risk group is young athletes engaged in intensive exercise that leads to dehydration, hyperthermia and acidosis. Sickling and vaso-occlusion under these extreme circumstances cause rhabdomyolysis, acute renal failure and cardiac arrhythmias. These individuals are advised to gradually increase exercise intensity, avoid dehydration, and to stop physical activity with the onset of muscle cramp or fatigue. Treatment of sudden collapse consists of rapid intravenous hydration and oxygen supplementation. Genetic counselling should be provided to individuals with sickle cell trait.

HbSC disease

HbC is found among individuals of African descent and the compound heterozygote state HbSC accounts for 25–50% of patients with SCD. The vaso-occlusive complications seen in patients with HbSC resemble those seen in patients with HbSS but are less severe. Splenomegaly and the risk of sequestration can persist into adult life. Of particular note is the higher incidence of proliferative retinopathy in HbSC beginning in the second decade. The haemoglobin level (10–12 g/dL) is higher than in HbSS, and the red cells are relatively microcytic with a higher mean corpuscular haemoglobin concentration (MCHC). Peripheral blood smear reveals frequent target cells, intraerythrocytic crystals and rare sickle cells. The pathogenesis of sickling in HbSC involves membrane damage with resultant water and cation loss and increase in intraerythrocytic concentration of HbS. Equal amounts of HbS and HbC are present in the red cells and the solubility test for sickle haemoglobin is positive. The electrophoretic appearance of HbSC, HbSE and HbSO Arab at pH 8.4 is similar, but a distinction can be made based on ethnicity and by performing isoelectric focusing or agar gel electrophoresis at pH 6.5.

Sickle cell/β thalassaemia

Sickle cell/β thalassaemia compound heterozygotes account for less than 10% of patients with sickle syndromes. The majority of these patients have the β^+ phenotype, with the proportion of HbA ranging from 3 to 25%. The clinical phenotype is mild and disease severity correlates with the amount of HbA present. The clinical manifestations of the less frequent HbS/β^0 genotype are similar in severity to those of HbSS. The red cells are microcytic and hypochromic, and variable numbers of target cells and sickle cells are observed. Reticulocytosis (10–20%) is present and the level of HbA_2 is elevated.

Sickle cell anaemia with coexistent α thalassaemia

Co-inheritance of α thalassaemia ($-\alpha/\alpha\alpha$ or $-\alpha/-\alpha$) with SCD is common, and such patients have less severe anaemia and demonstrate hypochromia and microcytosis. In general, the clinical severity is similar to that seen in HbSS patients with a normal complement of α-globin genes.

Sickle cell/HPFH

Approximately 1 in 100 patients with HbSS has an elevated HbF level due to deletional or non-deletional mutations that maintain γ-globin gene expression after birth. Such individuals have

20–30% HbF and less than 2.5% HbA_2. The haemoglobin level is normal with microcytosis, and target cells are observed in the peripheral smear. The clinical course is benign, and vaso-occlusive complications are rare because of the inhibition of sickling by elevated HbF.

Other sickling syndromes

Sickle cell/Hb Lepore disease

Co-inheritance of Hb Lepore with sickle cell mutation produces a clinical picture similar to that of HbS/β thalassaemia but with a low HbA_2 level.

Sickle cell/HbD disease

Of all the D or G haemoglobins, HbD Punjab (D Los Angeles) alone interacts with HbS to produce moderately severe haemolytic anaemia in compound heterozygotes. Target cells and irreversibly sickled cells (ISCs) are observed in the peripheral smear, and the clinical manifestations resemble mild sickle cell anaemia.

Sickle cell/HbO Arab disease

HbO Arab resembles HbC on alkaline electrophoresis and produces a moderately severe haemolytic anaemia in association with HbS. The disease is more severe than HbSC, and numerous sickled erythrocytes are observed on the peripheral smear.

Sickle cell/HbE disease

HbSE disease causes mild haemolysis and no remarkable abnormality of red blood cell morphology. HbE comprises only 30% of the total haemoglobin because of the thalassaemic nature of the mutation. Patients are generally asymptomatic, although occasionally significant vaso-occlusive complications and anaemia have been observed.

Diagnosis

Peripheral blood findings

The peripheral blood picture depends on the type of sickle cell syndrome. The haemoglobin level is normal in the newborn period, but anaemia develops and sickle or cigar-shaped ISCs can be observed in the peripheral blood by 3–4 months of age as HbF declines. In HbSS disease, the red cells are normocytic and normochromic, with polychromasia, many ISCs and fewer target cells (Figure 7.5a). The average reticulocyte count is 10% (4–20%) and normoblasts may be observed. Red cells are microcytic in the presence of coexisting α thalassaemia or iron deficiency. In HbS/β thalassaemia, ISCs, target cells and hypochromic microcytic red cells are prominent. The red cell morphology in HbSC disease is characterized by predominant target cells and rare ISCs. The occasional Howell–Jolly body, indicative of loss of splenic function in SCD, may be observed.

The white cell count is elevated ($12–20 \times 10^9$/L) as a result of an increase in mature neutrophils. The platelet count is also elevated to $300–500 \times 10^9$/L as a result of decreased splenic function.

Other laboratory tests

The measurement of clotting factors in SCD indicates mild ongoing activation of the coagulation system, even in the steady state. The erythrocyte sedimentation rate is consistently low. Serum levels of unconjugated bilirubin and LDH are elevated, and haptoglobin is decreased.

Haemoglobin electrophoresis

HbS can be identified by cellulose acetate electrophoresis at pH 8.4 (Table 7.1 and Figure 7.5b). HbD and HbG have the same electrophoretic mobility with this method, but can be distinguished using citrate agar electrophoresis at pH 6.2 or thin-layer isoelectric focusing. Distinction cannot be made between HbSS and HbS/$β^0$ thalassaemia on electrophoresis. The diagnosis of HbS/$β^0$ thalassaemia is suggested by microcytosis and elevated HbA_2, and confirmed by finding β thalassaemia trait in one of the parents. HbA and HbS are observed upon electrophoresis in both sickle cell trait and HbS/$β^+$ thalassaemia; however, the HbA fraction is greater than 50% in the former, but ranges from 5 to 30% in the latter. The level of HbF is variably elevated, with higher levels observed in patients with the Arab–Indian and Senegal haplotypes.

Other tests to detect sickle haemoglobin

Sickling of red cells can be induced by sealing a drop of blood under a coverslip to exclude oxygen or by adding 2% sodium metabisulphite. The solubility test for HbS utilizes a reducing agent such as sodium dithionite, which is added to the haemolysate. Deoxy-HbS is insoluble and renders the solution turbid (Figure 7.5c). Both these tests are unable to distinguish sickle cell trait from sickle cell anaemia and cannot be used for primary diagnosis. They are useful aids in the identification of an abnormal electrophoretic band as HbS and for identifying sickle cell trait in units of red cells prior to transfusion. High performance liquid chromatography (HPLC) can be used instead of electrophoresis to identify and quantitate HBS and other haemoglobins.

Newborn screening

Universal newborn screening is recommended for identifying SCD in the neonatal period. The efficacy of penicillin prophylaxis in preventing death from early sepsis in SCD provided the rationale for development of screening programmes. Blood samples obtained by heel prick are spotted onto filter paper and

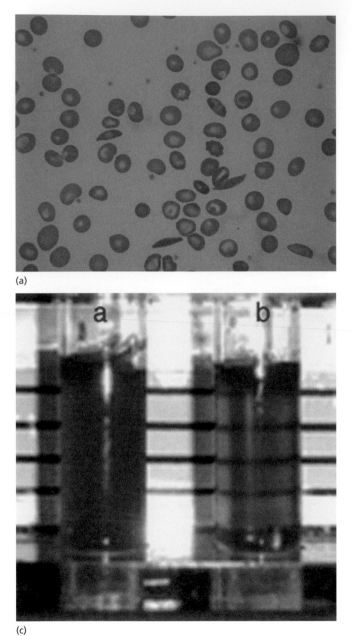

(a)

(c)

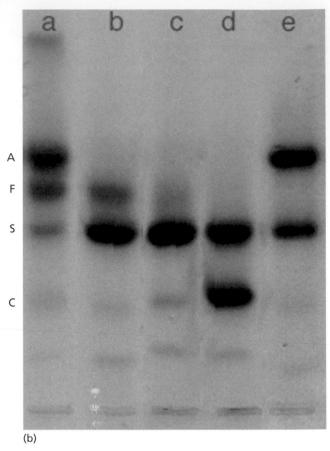

(b)

Figure 7.5 (a) Peripheral blood smear from an individual with sickle cell anaemia. (b) Haemoglobin electrophoresis showing standard (lane a), HbSS (lanes b and c), HbSC (lane d) and sickle trait (lane e). (c) Sickle solubility assay is positive (tube a) in all three conditions.

tested by electrophoresis or chromatography. Neonates with HbSS disease and HbS/β^0 thalassaemia have an FS pattern (the order of haemoglobins indicates their relative abundance in the sample). In sickle cell trait, the haemoglobin pattern is FAS, whereas newborns with HbS/β^+ thalassaemia have an FSA pattern. Finally, the presence of the FSC pattern suggests HbSC disease. Family studies help to make the definitive diagnosis and, when both parents are unavailable, DNA-based testing is useful.

Prenatal diagnosis

Prenatal diagnosis is available through direct detection of the GAG→GTG mutation responsible for SCD in fetal cells. Genetic counselling is difficult owing to the marked variability in clinical manifestations within the same genotype, and the lack of ability at present to predict individual phenotype. Preimplantation diagnosis and selection of healthy embryos may offer a solution to this ethical problem.

Therapy

This section discusses general issues in the management of sickle cell disease. The treatment of specific complications is addressed in the section Clinical manifestations.

Routine healthcare

The majority of children with SCD can be managed by paediatricians or community physicians in coordination with a haematologist. Adults with SCD should also continue to have routine office visits. Patients who suffer from more severe complications or who need therapy to modify the course of SCD require specialized care at experienced centres.

The level of healthcare available to patients with SCD varies tremendously in different countries. Where resources are limited, the primary focus should be on penicillin prophylaxis, vaccination, education and analgesia for painful episodes. Where comprehensive care is available, both medical and psychosocial needs should receive attention (Figure 7.6). Sickle cell centres should have specialists in several fields who are available to address complications that may affect different organs.

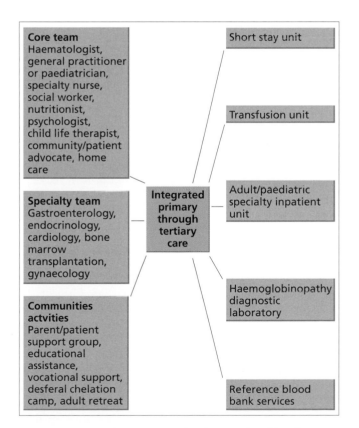

Figure 7.6 Comprehensive care of patients with sickle cell disease.

In cases when diagnosis is made on newborn screening, the infant should be seen within 1–2 months to instruct parents about infections and splenic enlargement. Routine immunization should include pneumococcal, *H. influenzae*, hepatitis B and influenza vaccines. All children receive prophylactic penicillin (phenoxymethylpenicillin orally twice daily or benzathine benzylpenicillin by intramuscular injection once per month), which may be stopped after the age of 5 years in the absence of any episode of pneumococcal sepsis or splenectomy. Folic acid supplementation (1 mg daily) is recommended. Evaluation of cerebral blood flow by transcranial Doppler should be performed on all children after 2 years to identify those at risk for stroke. Annual retinal examination is begun at 10 years. Sexually active women should have routine pelvic examinations and receive instructions about birth control.

Infections

Fever in children with SCD requires urgent attention in the office or emergency room. A complete blood count, blood and urine cultures and chest radiographs should be obtained, and lumbar puncture should be performed if meningitis is suspected. Very young children with fever or older children who appear septic should be hospitalized for intravenous antibiotics. The choice of antibiotics depends on causative agents prevalent locally and the pattern of resistance. In the USA, cefuroxime or ceftriaxone are preferred, whereas high-dose penicillin is used in several other countries. Many patients older than 2 years who do not look septic or seriously ill can be managed at home after receiving ceftriaxone in the emergency department. Antibiotics should continue for 1 week when bacteraemia is documented. In the presence of pneumonia, a macrolide should be added to cover *Mycoplasma* or *Chlamydia*. Antibiotics for osteomyelitis should provide coverage for *Salmonella* and *S. aureus* and are given for a period of 4–6 weeks.

Transfusion therapy

Blood transfusion in SCD is used to treat severe anaemia or to reduce the amount of circulating sickle haemoglobin. Only sickle-negative blood, which can be identified by negative sickle solubility test, is used for transfusions. The blood should also be leucodepleted, and matched for common minor E, C and Kell antigens. A simple transfusion is used to treat severe anaemia that is often associated with aplastic crisis and splenic sequestration. Older patients with renal failure may also need transfusions for declining haemoglobin level.

Dilution of circulating sickle haemoglobin can be accomplished by simple transfusion if the baseline haemoglobin level is low. Exchange transfusion or erythrocytapheresis is required to prevent hyperviscosity from the significant rise in haemoglobin when the patient has high baseline haemoglobin or when a greater reduction in HbS is desired. The final haemoglobin level should not exceed 12 g/dL after simple or exchange transfusion. Conditions in which a reduction in the proportion of HbS is required include stroke, progressive acute chest syndrome, persistent priapism or preparation for general anaesthesia. Longer-term reduction in HbS through regular transfusions is advocated to prevent recurrence of stroke and sequestration, and in selected patients with leg ulcers or chronic pain. Routine blood transfusion is not needed for pain episodes, infections, minor surgery or uncomplicated pregnancy.

It is possible to eliminate most complications of SCD with the use of chronic transfusions to suppress endogenous sickle haemoglobin production. However, alloimmunization, iron overload and transmission of viruses are significant risks that limit the use of transfusions to the management of severe complications. In addition, because of the limited availability and decreased safety of blood, criteria for transfusion are more stringent in less developed countries. The high incidence of alloimmunization from minor blood group incompatibility (Rh, Kell, Duffy and Kidd) between donors and recipients can be avoided by use of phenotypically matched units. Patients on long-term transfusions develop iron overload, which requires chelation with desferrioxamine or deferasirox. The prevalence of iron-induced organ damage appears to be lower in SCD compared with thalassaemia despite similar amounts of iron burden. Liver biopsies or MRI are usually necessary to measure iron burden because the serum ferritin is unreliable. Because iron accumulation can be reduced or prevented by erythrocytapheresis, this technique is now preferred when venous access is available.

Pain management

Prompt management of pain is essential, given its frequent occurrence and potential adverse psychological consequences. Patients with recurrent pain are best managed in a familiar ambulatory setting rather than the emergency ward. The patient should be evaluated for potential infectious, traumatic or surgical causes of pain. Pain assessment tools are available for young patients and are also helpful in older patients to follow the response to therapy. Adequate hydration should be provided, along with analgesia using narcotics and NSAIDs. Several narcotic agents are available for oral and parenteral use and the choice of medicine depends on local experience as well as the patient's preference. The use of incentive spirometry reduces the potential for developing hypoxia and acute chest syndrome secondary to hypoventilation. Under-treatment of pain can be avoided by using patient-controlled analgesia, which has the added benefit of reducing apparent drug-seeking behaviour. Narcotic addiction is no more frequent in sickle cell patients than in others requiring analgesia. NSAIDs improve pain control with or without narcotics. Providing psychosocial support and reassurance, and allaying anxiety are important

goals. Chronic pain is rare in SCD and may require long-acting narcotics for management.

Hydroxycarbamide

Hydroxycarbamide is a tremendously important drug in the management of patients with SCD who have severe clinical manifestations. Hydroxycarbamide inhibits ribonucleotide reductase, leading to S-phase arrest of replicating cells, and is used in SCD because of its ability to stimulate production of HbF. Hydroxycarbamide increases HbF as a result of stress erythropoiesis induced by its myelosuppressive effect. Patients show variable response in the degree of rise in HbF, and some experience no change from the baseline value. Other biological effects of hydroxycarbamide play an equally significant role in the beneficial clinical effects observed during therapy. Erythrocytes of patients on hydroxycarbamide have increased water content and deformability and decreased adherence to vascular endothelium. There is elevation of the haemoglobin level, mean corpuscular volume (MCV), HbF and F cells, whereas total white cell and neutrophil count, reticulocyte count and the number of dense sickle cells decrease. Patients on hydroxycarbamide experience 50% reduction in the incidence of acute painful episodes and acute chest syndrome. Transfusion needs, frequency of hospital admissions and the risk of death are also decreased. Hydroxycarbamide does not improve leg ulcers, while the effect on priapism is unclear. Hydroxycarbamide may reduce risk of stroke, and its role in children with elevated cerebral blood flow velocities and previous stroke is under intense study.

The efficacy of hydroxycarbamide therapy is now well established in adults and there is growing evidence to support its use in children. Prospective trials are underway to evaluate safety and efficacy in infants, and to specifically examine if end-organ damage to spleen, brain and kidney can be reduced. In young patients with severe disease, stem cell transplantation should also be considered as an alternative to chronic transfusions or long-term hydroxycarbamide therapy. The overall benefit of hydroxycarbamide to the patient is closely related to compliance, for which monitoring in the clinic and psychological support should be provided. Patients should be made aware that 3–6 months may elapse before clinical benefits are realized. Hydroxycarbamide is offered to patients (adults and children over 6 years) with frequent pain episodes or acute chest syndrome. It is started at a dose of 20 mg/kg per day and increased by 5 mg/kg every 2–3 months until the absolute neutrophil count is close to 2.5×10^9/L. Compliance with prescribed dose should be ascertained before each dose escalation, up to the maximum dose of 35 mg/kg or 2000 mg/day. Patients require frequent monitoring of blood counts, as well as renal and hepatic function. Myelosuppression is the most commonly encountered side-effect and temporary cessation of therapy and dose reduction is required for neutropenia, thrombocytopenia, reticulocytopenia or fall in haemoglobin. Dose modification is necessary for patients with renal failure. Skin pigmentation affecting the nails, palms and soles is commonly observed. There may be a temporary decline in sperm production among men while on hydroxycarbamide treatment. Despite concerns about the leukaemogenic and teratogenic effects of hydroxycarbamide, no convincing increase has been reported in SCD so far. Men and women should practise contraception while taking hydroxycarbamide, and women who become pregnant should stop the drug. No decrease in growth rate is observed in children over 5 years using hydroxycarbamide, while the growth effects of the drug in younger children are under evaluation. Overall, the risks associated with hydroxycarbamide therapy appear to be low and are certainly tolerable compared with the perils of untreated SCD in the severely affected patient.

New therapeutic modalities

A better appreciation of the pathophysiology of SCD will make it possible to exploit new therapeutic mechanisms (Table 7.4). Agents under development include membrane-active chemicals that improve hydration of sickle cells by blocking Gardos channels and potassium–chloride cotransport, or inhibit red cell adherence to endothelium. Decreased availability of NO has an important role in vaso-occlusion in SCD, and agents that correct NO deficiency may have significant therapeutic benefit. Newer agents to induce HbF synthesis that are being studied include orally effective butyrate compounds and decitabine, an analogue of 5-azacytidine. Decitabine can improve HbF level in patients who do not respond to hydroxycarbamide.

Haemopoietic stem cell transplantation

Allogeneic haemopoietic stem cell transplantation (HSCT) from a matched sibling donor cures 85% of children with SCD less than 16 years of age. Both bone marrow and umbilical cord blood from related donors are suitable sources for the stem cells. Studies are underway to evaluate the use of unrelated donors or reduced intensity conditioning regimens. However, 5% of patients die of complications related to HSCT and another 10% experience graft rejection with the return of SCD (Figure 7.7). Additional long-term risks after HSCT are infertility and second malignancy. Selection of candidates for HSCT is complex owing to the uncertain long-term course of the disease. HSCT should be considered in children (age < 16 years) with SCD (any genotype) who have a human leucocyte antigen (HLA)-identical related donor and evidence of target organ damage involving the brain, lungs, kidneys or eyes. Children who are placed on long-term blood transfusions for any indication should also be evaluated for HSCT. Although it is clear that high-risk patients benefit from this treatment, the role of HSCT in asymptomatic children is not defined. Severe organ dysfunc-

Table 7.4 Advances in the management of sickle cell disease.

Category	Intervention
Newborn screening	Counselling
	Comprehensive care
Infection	Prophylactic penicillin
	Immunization
Brain injury prevention	Screening with TCD, MRI
	Neurocognitive testing
	Chronic transfusions
Transfusion safety and iron overload prevention	Phenotypically matched red cells
	Erythrocytapheresis
	Iron chelation
Lung injury prevention	Incentive spirometry
	Antibiotics (including macrolides)
	Transfusion
	Echocardiographic screening for PHT
	Prevention with hydroxycarbamide
Surgery/anaesthesia	Preoperative transfusion
Avascular necrosis of the hip	Physical therapy
	Hip joint replacement
Priapism	Adrenergic agonist
	Antiandrogen therapy
Pain	Prevention with hydroxycarbamide
	Patient-controlled analgesic devices
	Non-steroidal anti-inflammatory drugs
Renal	ACE inhibitors for proteinuria
	Improved renal transplantation
Gallbladder disease	Laparoscopic cholecystectomy
Severe disease	Allogeneic bone marrow transplantation
	Chronic transfusions
	Hydroxycarbamide

ACE, angiotensin-converting enzyme; MRI, magnetic resonance imaging; PHT, pulmonary hypertension; TCD, transcranial Doppler.

tion increases the risks from the procedure, and hence discussion for HSCT should be started early when eligible indications are identified.

Gene therapy

Correction of SCD by gene therapy requires efficient insertion of a gene into repopulating haemopoietic cells and regulated expression in erythropoietic lineages. An anti-sickling haemoglobin, constituting 20–30% of the total haemoglobin, would be enough to produce clinical response. Mouse models of sickle cell disease have considerably helped in the effort to develop

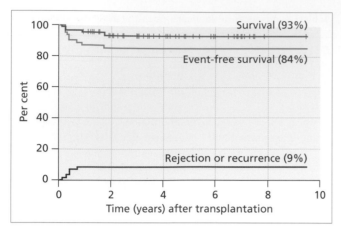

Figure 7.7 Outcome after transplantation for 59 children with advanced symptomatic sickle cell disease. Kaplan–Meier estimates for survival and event-free survival following marrow transplantation are shown. An event is defined as death, graft rejection or recurrence of sickle cell disease. A cumulative incidence curve for graft rejection and return of sickle cell disease is also depicted. (From Walters MC, Patience M, Leisenring W *et al.* (2001) Stable mixed hematopoietic chimerism after bone marrow transplantation for sickle cell anemia. *Biology of Blood and Marrow Transplantation* 7: 665–73 with permission.)

gene therapy, and correction of the sickling phenotype has been demonstrated in such animals.

Psychosocial issues

Recurrent pain and the unpredictable course of the illness place SCD patients at higher risk of depression and poor family relationships. Despite this, with integrated medical care and social support most patients with SCD are well adjusted. Addiction to narcotics is an uncommon phenomenon and is the result of social influences rather than analgesic therapy. Attention to psychological well-being as well as educational and vocational support are important components of the care provided to SCD patients.

Selected bibliography

Adams RJ (2007) Big strokes in small persons. *Archives of Neurology* **64**: 1567–74.

Adeyoju AB, Olujohungbe AB, Morris J *et al.* (2002) Priapism in sickle-cell disease: incidence, risk factors and complications. An international multicentre study. *BJU International* **90**: 898–902.

Anie KA (2005) Psychological complications in sickle cell disease. *British Journal of Haematology* **129**: 723–9.

Bhatia M, Walters MC (2008) Haematopoietic cell transplantation for thalassemia and sickle cell disease: past, present and future. *Bone Marrow Transplantation* **41**: 109–17.

Brawley OW, Cornelius LJ, Edwards LR *et al.* (2008) National Institutes of Health Consensus Development Conference statement: hydroxyurea treatment for sickle cell disease. *Annals of Internal Medicine* **148**: 932–8.

Bulas D (2005) Screening children for sickle cell vasculopathy: guidelines for transcranial Doppler evaluation. *Pediatric Radiology* **35**: 235–41.

Bunn HF (1997) Pathogenesis and treatment of sickle cell disease. *New England Journal of Medicine* **337**: 762–9.

Charache S, Terrin ML, Moore RD *et al.* (1995) Effect of hydroxyurea on the frequency of painful crises in sickle cell anaemia. Investigators of the Multicenter Study of Hydroxyurea in Sickle Cell Anaemia. *New England Journal of Medicine* **332**: 1317–22.

Geller AK, O'Connor MK (2008) The sickle cell crisis: a dilemma in pain relief. *Mayo Clinic Proceedings* **83**: 320–3.

Gladwin MT, Vichinsky E (2008) Pulmonary complications of sickle cell disease. *New England Journal of Medicine* **359**: 2254–65.

Hankins J, Aygun B (2009) Pharmacotherapy in sickle cell disease: state of the art and future prospects. *British Journal of Haematology* **145**: 296–308.

Hebbel RP (2008) Adhesion of sickle red cells to endothelium: myths and future directions. *Transfusion Clinique et Biologique* **15**: 14–18.

Hsieh MM, Kang EM, Fitzhugh CD *et al.* (2009) Allogenic hematopoietic stem-cell transplantation for sickle cell disease. *The New England Journal of Medicine* **361**: 2309–17.

Josephson CD, Su LL, Hillyer KL *et al.* (2007) Transfusion in the patient with sickle cell disease: a critical review of the literature and transfusion guidelines. *Transfusion Medicine Reviews* **21**: 118–33.

Madani G, Papadopoulou AM, Holloway B *et al.* (2007) The radiological manifestations of sickle cell disease. *Clinical Radiology* **62**: 528–38.

Neumayr LD, Aguilar C, Earles AN *et al.* (2006) Physical therapy alone compared with core decompression and physical therapy for femoral head osteonecrosis in sickle cell disease. Results of a multicenter study at a mean of three years after treatment. *Journal of Bone and Joint Surgery. American Volume* **88**: 2573–82.

Ohene-Frempong K, Weiner SJ, Sleeper LA *et al.* (1998) Cerebrovascular accidents in sickle cell disease: rates and risk factors. *Blood* **91**: 288–94.

Pham PT, Pham PC, Wilkinson AH *et al.* (2000) Renal abnormalities in sickle cell disease. *Kidney International* **57**: 1–8.

Quinn CT, Lee NJ, Shull EP *et al.* (2008) Prediction of adverse outcomes in children with sickle cell anaemia: a study of the Dallas Newborn Cohort. *Blood* **111**: 544–8.

Rogers ZR (2005) Priapism in sickle cell disease. *Hematology/ Oncology Clinics of North America* **19**: 917–28, viii.

Section on Hematology/Oncology Committee on Genetics, American Academy of Pediatrics (2002) Health supervision for children with sickle cell disease. *Pediatrics* **109**: 526–35.

Serjeant GR, Serjeant BE, Mohan JS *et al.* (2005) Leg ulceration in sickle cell disease: medieval medicine in a modern world. *Hematology/Oncology Clinics of North America* **19**: 943–56, viii–ix.

Smith WR, Penberthy LT, Bovbjerg VE *et al.* (2008) Daily assessment of pain in adults with sickle cell disease. *Annals of Internal Medicine* **148**: 94–101.

Strouse JJ, Lanzkron S, Beach MC *et al.* (2008) Hydroxyurea for sickle cell disease: a systematic review for efficacy and toxicity in children. *Pediatrics* **122**: 1332–42.

Thein SL (2008) Genetic modifiers of the beta-haemoglobinopathies. *British Journal of Haematology* **141**: 357–66.

Trompeter S, Roberts I (2009) Haemoglobin F modulation in childhood sickle cell disease. *British Journal of Haematology* **144**: 308–16.

Tsaras G, Owusu-Ansah A, Boateng FO *et al.* (2009) Complications associated with sickle cell trait: a brief narrative review. *American Journal of Medicine* **122**: 507–12.

Tshilolo L, Kafando E, Sawadogo M *et al.* (2008) Neonatal screening and clinical care programmes for sickle cell disorders in sub-Saharan Africa: lessons from pilot studies. *Public Health* **122**: 933–41.

Vichinsky EP, Neumayr LD, Earles AN *et al.* (2000) Causes and outcomes of the acute chest syndrome in sickle cell disease. National Acute Chest Syndrome Study Group. *New England Journal of Medicine* **342**: 1855–65.

Voskaridou E, Dimitrios C, Antonios B *et al.* (2010) The effect of prolonged administration of hydroxyurea on morbidity and mortality in adult patients with sickle cell syndromes: results of a 17 year, single-centre trial (LaSHS). *Blood* **115**: 2354–63.

CHAPTER 8

Hereditary disorders of the red cell membrane

Edward C Gordon-Smith[1] and Narla Mohandas[2]

[1]St George's Hospital Medical School, London, UK
[2]New York Blood Center, New York, USA

Introduction

This chapter and the next deal with genetically determined disorders of the red cell, other than those of haemoglobin, which cause its premature destruction. In this chapter, genetic changes that affect the structure and function of the red cell membrane are described. Chapter 9 describes the inherited defects in red cell metabolism that shorten red cell survival.

Whereas the primary genetic changes underlying these disorders are quite heterogeneous, many of the manifestations are similar, as they result mainly from the increased rate of red cell destruction and from the consequent hyperactivity of the erythroid component of the bone marrow. Therefore, the description of individual conditions will be prefaced with a brief consideration of the pathophysiology of haemolysis.

Haemolysis

Definitions

Haemolysis indicates that the destruction of red cells is accelerated. Normally, in adults, the bone marrow output is well below its maximal capacity. Red cell production can be increased about sixfold in the adult by increasing the cellularity of existing haemopoietic marrow, as well as by expansion of haemopoietic

marrow into the long bones. In the newborn, and during infancy, marrow expansion depends on expanding the medullary cavity of bones, leading to thinning of cortical bone. These bony changes are most extreme in the β thalassaemia syndromes, but some skeletal changes, usually some bossing of the frontal bones, may be seen in more extreme hereditary haemolytic anaemias of other causes.

Increased red cell destruction is often completely matched by increased production, resulting in compensated haemolysis. When the rate of haemolysis exceeds the maximum erythropoietic capacity of the bone marrow, or when the latter is limited (e.g. because of inadequate supply of iron or folate or by ineffective erythropoiesis), the result is haemolytic anaemia. As in any haemolytic disorder, with or without anaemia, the consequences of haemolysis are always present, and as the same underlying pathogenetic process may cause at different times, even in the same patient, either a compensated haemolytic disorder or haemolytic anaemia, the two terms are often used, somewhat loosely, as though they are interchangeable.

General features of haemolysis

The clinical and laboratory aspects of haemolysis depend on the consequences of increased red cell destruction and production as well as the main process by which destruction takes place. Increased red cell destruction leads to an increase in unconjugated bilirubin from increased haemoglobin turnover. Unconjugated bilirubin does not appear in the urine, although there will be an increase in urinary urobilinogen. The bilirubin level is usually not more than two to three times normal because the normal liver is able to increase excretion to compensate for

Postgraduate Haematology: 6th edition. Edited by A. Victor Hoffbrand, Daniel Catovsky, Edward G.D. Tuddenham, Anthony R. Green
© 2011 Blackwell Publishing Ltd.

at least some of the increased production. Jaundice is usually mild in hereditary haemolytic anaemias although there are important exceptions.

In the neonate, particularly premature infants, liver function is not fully developed and more severe jaundice requiring urgent therapeutic intervention may occur. A rare but potentially confusing problem is the co-inheritance of Gilbert syndrome, which comprises a group of congenital liver enzyme deficiencies that impair bilirubin conjugation. On its own, Gilbert syndrome does not produce clinical jaundice except when there is inadequate calorie intake, but in conjunction with haemolytic anaemia the hyperbilirubinaemia may be considerable. The increased bilirubin of haemolysis does increase the risk of gallstones and cholecystitis, which in turn may lead to an increase in serum bilirubin.

In the degradation of haemoglobin, the molecule is broken down to two $\alpha\beta$ subunits, which are bound to haptoglobin, the complex being rapidly internalized in the hepatocyte after binding to the haptoglobin complex receptor. In the presence of haemolysis, serum haptoglobin levels are greatly reduced or absent. However, haptoglobin is an acute-phase protein and levels will increase in the presence of inflammation. Haemopexin is another haem-binding protein produced by the liver, which is decreased in haemolysis. Chronic haemolytic anaemia may increase the iron content of the body through increased iron absorption as a result of anaemia coupled to the retention of the haem iron following binding to haptoglobin and haemopexin. In rare cases of inherited haemolytic anaemia, this iron overload may be sufficient to produce clinically important effects, particularly if there is co-inheritance of a haemochromatosis gene. In most haemolytic anaemias, owing to membrane defects, the destruction of red cells takes place extravascularly in the reticuloendothelial system and the iron is retained as described. When destruction is intravascular, free haemoglobin will be released into the plasma, producing haemoglobinaemia and methaemalbuminaemia, and will pass through the glomerulus to produce haemoglobinuria and haemosiderinuria. Iron deficiency is thus more likely than overload in intravascular haemolysis.

Increased red cell production leads to expansion of the red cell precursor compartment of the bone marrow as described above. There are also changes in the structure of the marrow as a consequence of the chronic anaemia, which allows the early release of reticulocytes and, in more marked cases of haemolytic anaemia, nucleated red cells and even myelocytes. In the peripheral blood, the polychromasia and macrocytosis of reticulocytosis are the result of this increased throughput and release. The increased cell production requires an increased supply of folate which, at least theoretically, can produce folate deficiency unless supplements are given. It is usual to give folic acid (400 μg daily or 5 mg once weekly) to people with chronic haemolytic anaemia. The main features of haemolytic anaemia are summarized in Table 8.1.

Table 8.1 Main features of haemolytic anaemia.

Increased red cell destruction
Unconjugated hyperbilirubinaemia
    Mild jaundice
    Increased risk of gallstones
Increased urinary and faecal urobilinogen
Decreased serum haptoglobin and haemopexin
Extravascular changes
    Increased iron stores
    Splenomegaly
Intravascular changes
    Haemoglobinaemia and haemoglobinuria
    Haemosiderinuria
    Methaemalbuminaemia
    Decreased iron stores

Increased red cell production
Marrow expansion: bone changes
Increased erythropoiesis: ↓ myeloid/erythroid ratio
Reticulocytosis: polychromasia
Increased folate requirements: macrocytosis

Classification

Because of the unique structural and functional specialization of the mature red cell, the impact on it of a wide range of exogenous or endogenous changes is relatively uniform: the cell will be destroyed prematurely. According to the site of the primary change, haemolytic disorders have been traditionally classified as being due either to intracorpuscular or to extracorpuscular causes. According to the nature of the primary change, haemolytic disorders have also been classified as inherited or acquired. These two classifications correlate almost completely with each other, in that extracorpuscular causes are usually acquired, whereas intracorpuscular causes are usually inherited. One notable exception is paroxysmal nocturnal haemoglobinuria, a disease in which an intracorpuscular defect is acquired as a result of a somatic mutation (see Chapter 11).

Although in every cell all molecules and organelles are naturally interdependent, it is convenient to consider the red cell as a conveyance for a large amount of haemoglobin contained in a plasma membrane, the stability of which is maintained by an appropriate metabolic machinery. Unfavourable genetic changes in any of these components may cause haemolysis. Accordingly, inherited haemolytic disorders can be classified into three major groups: (i) genetic disorders of haemoglobin (see Chapter 6); (ii) abnormal membrane (including the cytoskeleton); and (iii) abnormal metabolism (enzymopathies) (see Chapter 9).

Red cell metabolism

The details of red cell metabolism are considered in Chapter 9. Suffice to say in this chapter that the red cell membrane requires a supply of both ATP and reducing power to maintain its proper integrity. The way in which energy is supplied to the membrane is intimately related to its structure. The main pathway for metabolizing ATP in the membrane is via Na^+/K^+-ATPase. The enzyme glyceraldehyde-3-phosphate dehydrogenase (Ga3PD) is closely associated with the inner layer of the membrane. It catalyses the conversion of glyceraldehyde-3-phosphate (Ga3P) to 1,3-diphosphoglycerate (1,3-DPG), with the production of NADH. ATP is produced in the next step of the glycolytic pathway, the conversion of 1,3-DPG to phosphoglycerate, which occurs in intimate contact with the membrane.

The red cell membrane

The red cell membrane, like all other cell membranes, consists of a lipid bilayer that is stabilized and given specific properties by the proteins, glycolipids and other specialized molecules and structures with which it is associated.

The lipid bilayer consists of approximately equal molar quantities of phospholipids and cholesterol molecules. The charged phosphatidyl groups of the phospholipids are hydrophilic and form the outer and inner surfaces of the bilayer. The interior of the membrane is formed by hydrophobic bonding of the acyl chains and cholesterol, which form the internal parts of the two leaflets (Figure 8.1). The arrangement is energy efficient but the two leaflets are not symmetrical. The outer leaflet consists mainly of phosphatidylcholine and sphingomyelin, the inner leaflet of phosphatidylethanolamine and phosphatidylserine (Figure 8.2). Maintenance of the asymmetry and the proper function of the membrane requires energy. In mature red cells this is provided by ATP from the glycolytic pathway and reducing power mainly in the form of glutathione.

The normal biconcave shape and function of the red cell membrane are determined by the membrane proteins and their interactions with the lipid bilayer and with each other. There are two main sorts of protein–membrane associations. The integral proteins have strong hydrophobic domains that associate with the hydrophobic part of the bilayer. Many of these integral proteins span the membrane and provide channels between the plasma and cytosolic compartments. The cytostolic inner domains of these proteins interact with each other and with the second main group, the proteins of the cytoskeleton. The integral proteins that provide the links between the plasma surface and the cytoskeleton have conveniently been referred to as 'vertical connections', whereas the proteins of the cytoskeleton that comprise the inner network of the cell membrane are characterized as 'horizontal connections'. Genetic abnormalities that produce spherocytes mainly have mutations affecting the vertical connections. Mutations of the horizontal system usually produce elliptocytosis or more bizarre-shaped changes. The main proteins are listed in Table 8.2, and their arrangement is shown schematically in Figure 8.3.

In addition to the compartments mentioned so far, there are numerous surface proteins that provide the main interface with the plasma, including the blood group systems and other receptors. Many of these molecules are heavily glycosylated, as are

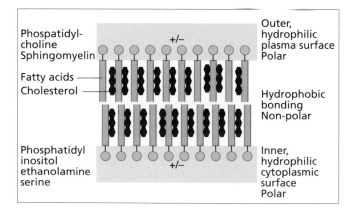

Figure 8.1 Arrangement of membrane lipids. The acyl chains of the diacyl phosphatidylglycerides are hydrophobic non-polar domains and they form hydrophobic bonds with the acyl groups of the opposite layer. Cholesterol is present in roughly equimolar amounts and determines the fluidity of the membrane.

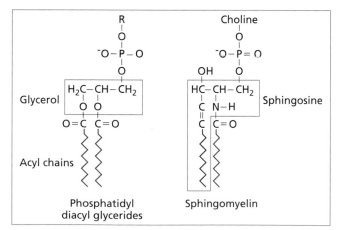

Figure 8.2 Main lipids of the red cell membrane. The outer, plasma, layer contains mostly neutral lipids, sphingomyelin and phosphatidylcholine (lecithin). The inner, cytoplasmic, layer contains mostly acidic groups, phosphatidylserine, phosphatidylethanolamine and phosphatidylinositol. R may be choline, serine, ethanolamine or inositol.

Table 8.2 Proteins of the red cell membrane.

Band*	Protein	Gene location	Function	Associated haemolytic anaemias
1	α-Spectrin	SPTA1, 1q21	Cytoskeleton network	HE, HS
2	β-Spectrin	SPTB, 14q24.1–q24.2	Cytoskeleton network	HPP HE, HS
2.1	Ankyrin	ANK1, 8p21.1–11.2	Vertical contact	HS
2.9	Adducin	ADD1 (α-chain), 4p16.3; ADD2 (β-chain), 2p13.3	Promotes spectrin binding to actin, binds Ca^{2+}/ calmodulin	(HS, HE in mice)
3	Band 3. Solute carrier family 4 (anion exchanger) member 1	SLC4A1, 17q12–q21	Anion exchange channel, Ii blood groups, binds glycolytic enzymes	HS, SAO, HAC
4.1	Protein 4.1	EPB41, 1p33–p32	Stabilizes spectrin–actin contact	HE
4.2	Protein 4.2 (pallidin)	EPB42 (PLDN), 15q15–q21	Spectrin–ankyrin complex	HS (Japan)
5	β-Actin	ACTB, 7p15–p12	Spectrin network junction	?
6	Ga3PD	GAPDH, 12p13.31	Links ATP production to membrane	?
PAS-1†	Glycophorin A	GYPA, 4q28–q31	MN blood groups	?
PAS-2	Glycophorin C	GYPC, 2q14–q21	Gerbich blood groups	HE
PAS-3	Glycophorin B	GYPB, 4q28–q31	Ss blood groups	?

*Band numbers refer to the position on SDS-PAGE electrophoresis.
†Periodic acid–Schiff stain: bands seen only on PAS-stained gels.
HAC, hereditary acanthocytosis; HE, hereditary elliptocytosis; HS, hereditary spherocytosis; HPP, hereditary pyropoikilocytosis; SAO, Southeast Asian ovalocytosis; Ga3PD, gyceraldehyde-3-phosphate dehydrogenase.

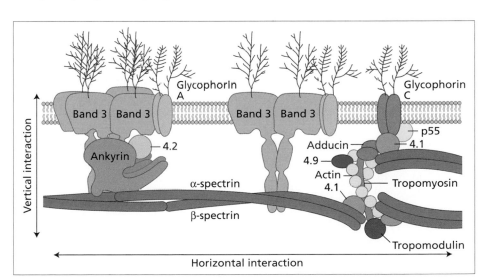

Figure 8.3 Arrangement of membrane proteins.

the integral proteins the glycophorins. Sialic acid, which comprises the main side-chain of the glycophorins, contributes the most to the negative surface change of the erythrocyte. Many of these surface proteins are linked to the membrane by the glycosylphosphatidylinositol (GPI) anchor, which provides the hydrophobic domain required for association with the inner hydrophobic part of the membrane. Somatic mutations in the gene for phosphatidylinositol glycan A (PIGA) leads to a failure to produce the anchor and to paroxysmal nocturnal haemoglobinuria (discussed in Chapter 11).

The integral proteins and vertical interaction

The two major integral proteins that span the lipid bilayer are band 3 (the anion channel protein) and the glycophorins A, B and C. Band 3 and associated molecules, 4.2 (pallidin) and ankyrin (2.1), form one major vertical interactive pathway with binding to the β-chain of the spectrin tetramer through ankyrin. Glycophorin C and protein 4.1 also provide a vertical interaction but the association with spectrin is through a link with actin, which is a key part of the horizontal network.

The band 3–4.2–ankyrin–spectrin complex is a central part of the organization of the lipid bilayer and loss of part of this complex leads to loss of lipid from the outer leaflet of the bilayer, reducing the surface area to volume ratio of the red cell and leading to the characteristic spherocytes of hereditary spherocytosis.

The main protein of the cytoskeleton is spectrin. Spectrin consists of two subunits, α and β, which associate side by side to produce a heterodimer. The dimers associate head to head to form tetramers about 200 nm long. The tail end of the dimer makes contact with a short actin filament composed of 14 monomers, and the interaction between spectrin and actin is stabilized by protein 4.1. Binding of spectrin dimers to actin filaments produces the more or less hexagonal network of spectrin tetramers on the inner surface of the membrane associated with the lipid bilayer. Spectrin–actin–4.1 interactions provide much of the flexibility of the red cell membrane. Deficiencies of spectrin that affect these horizontal interactions tend to induce a loss of flexibility in the membrane and elliptocytosis.

The clinical phenotypes of hereditary membrane disorders

Mutations in the genes that control the proteins of the membrane and their interaction mainly produce changes in the shape of red cells, which is characteristic in any individual. Many of the conditions are inherited as autosomal dominant disorders, homozygosity for major defects mainly being lethal. Severe, bizarre or unexpected red cell morphology is often produced by double heterozygosity or inheritance of more than one defect of the membrane proteins. The mutations affecting the red cell membrane are many and heterogeneous, but the effect on the phenotype can be classified in five main categories: (i) hereditary spherocytosis; (ii) hereditary elliptocytosis and hereditary pyropoikilocytosis; (iii) Southeast Asian ovalocytosis; (iv) hereditary acanthocytosis; and (v) hereditary stomatocytosis.

Hereditary spherocytosis

As the name implies, hereditary spherocytosis (HS) is a genetically determined haemolytic anaemia characterized by the

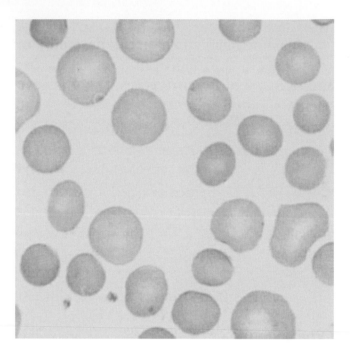

Figure 8.4 Hereditary spherocytosis, peripheral blood. Small spherocytic red cells lack area of central pallor. Large polychromatic red cells (reticulocytes) result in normal MCV, although MCHC may be increased.

spherical shape of the affected red cells. The spherical shape produces a characteristic appearance in the stained blood film of round cells with smaller than normal diameter, which lack the area of central pallor of the normal biconcave discs (Figure 8.4). The old name, 'familial acholuric jaundice', emphasizes the presence of jaundice in the absence of bile in the urine, distinguishing this jaundice from that caused by hepatobiliary problems. The disorder is generally inherited as a dominant condition with a wide spectrum of severity. The usual clinical picture is of mild to moderate haemolytic anaemia but varies from severe neonatal haemolysis with kernicterus (rare) to clinically silent and asymptomatic (usual) haemolysis. Autosomal recessive inheritance occurs in a few mutations, often producing severe haemolysis.

In white populations, HS is one of the most common haemolytic anaemias due to membrane defects, with a prevalence of clinically apparent disease of 200–300 per million population. The occurrence of clinically silent cases probably means that the overall prevalence is slightly higher.

Clinical features

The commonest forms of HS present as mild anaemia and jaundice, with a modestly enlarged spleen. However, the genetic heterogeneity of HS (see below) is reflected in the clinical presentation. As the main site of increased red cell destruction in HS is the spleen, it is not surprising that the size of the spleen tends to reflect the severity of the haemolysis, although splenomegaly is rarely marked, enlargement below the umbilicus being very uncommon. When HS presents in adolescence or adult life, it needs to be distinguished from other causes of microspherocytosis, particularly warm autoimmune haemolytic anaemia.

HS may present at birth. The functions of the spleen become mature only after birth, so severe anaemia *in utero* is rare. Erythropoiesis is highly active before birth but enters a phase of reduced activity in the neonatal period. Severe anaemia, developing over 5–30 days post delivery and requiring transfusion, may result from this double physiological development of reduced production and increased destruction, but the anaemia may greatly reduce during the first year of life as compensatory erythropoiesis develops. Decisions about splenectomy do not need to be taken during this time.

Molecular pathology

About 60% of HS cases result from a defect in the ankyrin–spectrin complex, with the genes for the α and β subunits of the spectrin dimer (*SPTA1*, *SPTB*) or for ankyrin (*ANK1*) being implicated in different genetic types (Table 8.2). A further 25% involve deficiency in band 3, the anion channel. In the remainder of the dominantly inherited HS families there is a deficiency of protein 4.2 or no abnormality has yet been identified. Deficiency of protein 4.2 is particularly common in Japanese families with HS (Table 8.2). These defects involving spectrin–ankyrin–band 3 interactions affect the vertical interactions described by Jiri Palek and colleagues.

It will be appreciated that the genetic defect that produces the dominant form of HS affects only one of a pair of genes. The presence of one abnormal protein influences the protein–protein interactions of these complexes, leading to partial deficiency of several proteins, even if they are not genetically disturbed. This is particularly true of spectrin. Complete loss of complex function is probably not viable, so homozygous children are not found. Double heterozygosity or inheritance of separate membrane defects does occur and is associated with usually severe haemolytic anaemia. Other recessive forms of HS are also seen in which the inheritance of one defective gene involving the spectrin subunit produces no clinical effect, whereas homozygosity produces a severe defect and haemolysis.

Laboratory diagnosis

The typical findings of extravascular haemolysis are present in HS (see Table 8.1). The diagnosis is usually made on the basis of morphology of the blood, backed up where possible with a family history. The mean corpuscular haemoglobin concentration (MCHC) is often increased above 35 g/dL in HS, but the presence of macrocytic reticulocytes usually results in a low normal mean corpuscular volume (MCV) rather than true microcytosis. These changes result not only from the reduction

of the surface area to volume ratio but also from the slight dehydration of HS cells. A number of variants of the typical HS features have been described, usually the more severe forms that may have denser and less perfectly round cells in the peripheral blood. In infancy, the morphology may be more difficult to interpret. The effect of immature splenic function and the macrocytosis and anisocytosis of infancy combine with the HS phenotype to produce red cell appearances not typical of the developing HS. Family studies may assist in the diagnosis.

Osmotic fragility test

The osmotic fragility test measures the sensitivity of red cells to lysis *in vitro* to swelling caused by incubation in increasingly hypotonic saline solutions. Red cells are able to swell with increasing volume until the pressure disrupts the unstretchable membrane and lysis occurs. In normal red cells with the biconcave disc shape, 50% lysis occurs when the saline solution reaches about 0.5% sodium chloride. The more rigid HS cells have less ability to swell and so lyse at higher concentrations, producing a right-shifted osmotic fragility curve. One of two patterns may be seen in HS: a generally right-shifted curve, which is the more common finding, and one where there appears to be a 'tail' of lysis-sensitive cells. Incubation of blood for 24 hours at 37°C accentuates the fragility (Figure 8.5).

The acidified glycerol lysis test (AGLT) uses glycerol to slow the entry of water into the cells *in vitro*. The time taken for lysis to occur is a function of the osmotic resistance of the cells. HS cells lyse more rapidly than normal cells. The test is easier to perform than the osmotic fragility test.

Autohaemolysis test

The autohaemolysis test examined the ability of red cells to withstand metabolic deprivation by incubation *in vitro* for 24 hours with and without the addition of glucose. It is a crude insensitive test which has generally been abandoned.

Identification of protein abnormalities or gene defects

Methods that identify the defective gene or its product are the most specific for membrane defects but are beyond the scope of most routine haematology laboratories. The original identification of membrane proteins using sodium dodecyl sulphate-solubilized polyacrylamide gel (SDS-PAGE) electrophoresis has led to the classification according to the banding system indicated in Table 8.2. The identification of specific genetic abnormalities may be important in compound haemolytic syndromes but requires specialist laboratories.

One screening test for HS makes use of the binding of eosin-labelled maleimide, in the form of eosin-5-maleimide, to lysine 430 in band 3 and cysteine molecules in surface proteins, particularly rhesus blood groups. In about 25% of HS patients there is a deficiency of band 3 and a loss of surface proteins caused by the instability of the lipid bilayer. HS red cells bind eosin-5-maleimide less than normal cells, by about 25–30%.

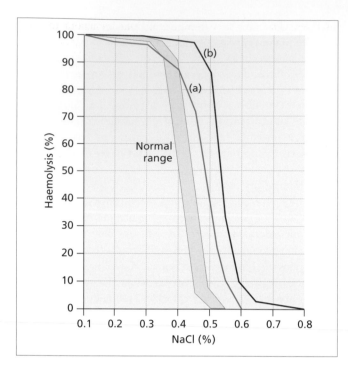

Figure 8.5 Osmotic fragility test in hereditary spherocytosis. Osmotic fragility is increased in the microspherocytes (right shift), but there is also a small population of resistant cells due to increased reticulocytes (a). After splenectomy, the microspherocytes remain but the proportion of reticulocytes is reduced to normal values and the resistant cells are not seen (b).

Even when the main defect is not in band 3, there may be sufficient loss of eosin-5-maleimide binding to indicate HS. The screening test has to be used in conjunction with morphology because Southeast Asian ovalocytosis, congenital dyserythropoietic anaemia type II and cryohydrocytosis also give reduced fluorescence.

Clinical course and complications

In most kindred, the course of the disorder is similar in affected members although, as with most inherited defects, there is some variable penetrance and it is not rare to find a very mildly affected parent with more severely affected offspring.

As with all congenital haemolytic anaemias, the anaemia may be aggravated by environmental factors. This may be consequent on an increase in the red cell destruction or a decrease in production. Increased jaundice may occur during viral infections or bacterial sepsis, the anaemia also being aggravated by a decrease in production consequent on the effects of the acute-phase response or the inhibition of erythropoiesis by interferon (IFN)-γ.

Primary infection with parvovirus 19 produces a specific and marked inhibition of erythropoiesis, often characterized as an aplastic crisis. In patients with shortened red cell survival, severe

anaemia may be produced by the inhibition, which lasts for some 4–7 days. In normal individuals with a red cell lifespan of 120 days, such an inhibition produces no clinical effect. The anaemia associated with parvovirus infection in HS may require urgent transfusion. The diagnosis is made by finding absent parvovirus antibodies with subsequent appearance of IgM antibodies. The presence of IgG antibodies at the time of the anaemia excludes the diagnosis.

Acute anaemia due to splenic sequestration is a relatively uncommon complication of HS in childhood. The pathogenesis is probably increased splenic size and activity leading to increased trapping of HS cells within the spleen. This complication may also require urgent transfusion.

Malnutrition may increase anaemia because of folate deficiency but also from increased jaundice through the effect of low-calorie input on unconjugated bilirubin levels in the blood.

The anaemia of pregnancy may aggravate a haemolytic anaemia and hence bring the condition to the attention of clinicians and patients. Classical HS is not a risk to mother or child in pregnancy.

Gallstones are an expected complication in HS as in other chronic haemolytic anaemias. Silent gallstones require no intervention. Recurrent cholecystitis or biliary colic may require cholecystectomy accompanied by splenectomy (see below). Leg ulcers are a rare but well-recognized complication of HS, as with other chronic haemolytic anaemias. Extramedullary haemopoietic masses, usually paravertebral, occur rarely in more severe HS.

Management

Patients with well-compensated haemolysis and no transfusion requirements need no treatment other than reassurance and folic acid supplements (e.g. 400 μg daily or 5 mg weekly). For people with a well-balanced and adequate diet, folic acid supplements are probably unnecessary, but custom dictates the practice should be continued. Radiolucent gallstones, if detected by chance on ultrasound, are common and need no treatment unless complications arise. Gallstones without recurrent inflammation are not a risk factor for carcinoma of the gallbladder. Recurrent cholecystitis or obstruction would be an indication for cholecystectomy, which would also be an indication for splenectomy.

Splenectomy

For the great majority of patients with autosomal dominant forms of HS, and most patients with *de novo* disease, splenectomy restores the lifespan of the red cells to normal and hence cures the haemolysis and hyperbilirubinaemia. In HS, the spleen is responsible for the removal of the older red cells that have lost the most surface through lipid loss from the outer layer. This removal of damaged but functional cells shortens the lifespan and causes jaundice and reticulocytosis. However, splenectomy carries short- and long-term risks that must be weighed against the benefits in any individual patient. After splenectomy, the blood film continues to show spherocytosis together with changes of a splenectomy film. The osmotic fragility remains increased.

Risks of splenectomy (see also Chapter 20)
The immediate risks associated with splenectomy include those of any abdominal operation together with an increased risk of thrombosis, associated with a marked rise in platelet count that occurs promptly after splenectomy. In HS, in which the erythropoietic drive returns to normal following splenectomy, the platelet count also returns to normal and the risk diminishes. In conditions where haemolysis persists, the platelet count remains elevated, sometimes markedly, and the increased risk of thrombosis continues. The long-term cardiovascular risks are discussed by Schilling (2008, 2009).

The major hazard of splenectomy is the long-term susceptibility to severe infection, so-called overwhelming postsplenectomy infection (OPSI) (see also Chapter 20). The spleen plays an important role in filtering and phagocytosing bacteria, and removing parasitized red cells from the blood. The spleen is the major source for mounting the rapid, specific IgM response to organisms that enter through the gut. The main organisms of this class are the encapsulated organisms, *Streptococcus pneumoniae*, *Haemophilus influenzae* type B and *Neisseria meningitidis*. Pneumococcal infection is responsible for about 70% of OPSI and has a 60% mortality. Lack of a spleen greatly increases the virulence of the infection, with progression from the first feeling of fever and non-specific flu-like symptoms to irreversible endotoxic shock occurring in a matter of hours. Patients may present with purpura, evidence of disseminated intravascular coagulation, multiorgan failure, hypotension and peripheral limb ischaemia. Diarrhoea and vomiting are common prodromes. It is this speed of progression that makes the prophylaxis of this fortunately uncommon complication so important. Prophylaxis depends on education and awareness for the patient, specific measures to reduce the risk from particular organisms and the provision of information concerning the splenectomy for healthcare workers (Table 8.3). There is no direct evidence that phenoxymethylpenicillin (e.g. 250 mg twice daily) reduces the risk of OPSI in splenectomized patients but good evidence that it does so in homozygous sickle cell patients who have functionally inactive spleens. It is on this evidence that such antibiotic prophylaxis (or erythromycin 250 mg b.d. for those sensitive to penicillin) is recommended (see also Chapter 7). The actual incidence of OPSI is difficult to calculate. The overall risk has been stated as 0.04 per 100 patient-years for patients without added immunosuppression, but considerably higher for those immunocompromised by malignancy or chemotherapy. The risk is greatest in the first 2 years after splenectomy but continues lifelong. Children under the age of 5 years are particularly susceptible and splenectomy should be avoided in this group if at all possible.

Table 8.3 Guidelines for prevention and management of infection in the splenectomized patient.

All patients receive polyvalent pneumococcal immunization, preferably 2 weeks prior to splenectomy, with a booster dose every 5–10 years

Any unimmunized patient should receive *Haemophilus influenzae* type B vaccine

Meningococcal immunization (types A and C) are not routinely recommended but should be given to travellers to countries where meningitis is possible, and during outbreaks in the UK

Influenza immunization may be beneficial and should be given

Lifelong prophylactic antibiotics (oral phenoxymethylpenicillin or an alternative)

Awareness of risks of malaria and scrupulous prophylaxis if at risk

Animal, particularly dog and tick, bites may be dangerous

Leaflet card for patients to alert health professionals to risk of OPSI

Patients developing infection despite measures should receive systemic antibiotics and be admitted urgently to hospital

Source: After Working Party of the British Committee for Standards in Haematology Clinical Haematology Work Force (1996).

Indications for splenectomy
Patients with marked haemolysis producing symptoms or requiring transfusion should be splenectomized, although preferably not before the age of 5 years (later if possible). Recurrent aplastic crises are also an indication. Attacks of cholecystitis or biliary colic warrant cholecystectomy and splenectomy, but symptomless gallstones are not a necessary indication.

Hereditary elliptocytosis and hereditary pyropoikilocytosis

Deficiency of spectrin tetramers, the horizontal links of the cytoskeleton, produces a wide spectrum of disease from fully compensated haemolysis with mildly elliptocytic red cells to severe and life-threatening anaemia with grossly distorted cells. When the morphological characteristic is a relatively uniform elliptical shape, the condition is referred to as hereditary elliptocytosis (HE). Haemolytic anaemia associated with the more distorted forms, which are also heat labile, is called hereditary pyropoikilocytosis (HPP). Recent evidence implies that HPP is a severe form of HE. Within a family, HE and HPP may both be present, the more severely affected individuals having both a total spectrin deficiency as well as a relative deficiency of spectrin tetramers. This may be caused by co-inheritance of a low-expression allele for α-spectrin, compound heterozygosity for two HE alleles or HE homozygosity. A number of families have been described in which mutations involving the initiation codon of the protein 4.1 gene result in failure to produce the protein. In heterozygotes with this variant, elliptocytosis occurs without haemolysis; in homozygotes, there is a severe haemolysis with extensive cell fragmentation.

Clinical features

As mentioned above, the HE/HPP group of haemolytic anaemias has a heterogeneous clinical presentation and molecular basis. Heterogeneity is amplified by the not uncommon co-inheritance of a mutated gene in *trans* (see below) with the HE gene, usually resulting in a more marked decrease in spectrin tetramer assembly.

Mild common hereditary elliptocytosis

Frequently, HE is discovered by chance from a blood film (Figure 8.6) or the presence of marginally raised bilirubin. Some affected people have no evidence of shortened red cell survival, whereas others have a well-compensated haemolytic anaemia. No treatment is required, although the blood film of partners should be examined if there is consanguinity, making homozygosity in offspring possible. For patients with mild haemolysis, anaemia may increase during infections, in pregnancy, with folate deficiency or with other conditions likely to enhance anaemia.

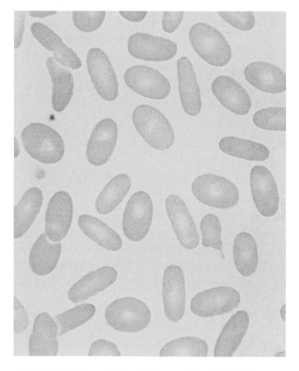

Figure 8.6 Hereditary elliptocytosis, peripheral blood. Characteristic elliptocytes of mild common hereditary elliptocytosis.

Silent carriers: low-expression genes

Mutations that produce low expression of α-spectrin may lead to no haematological abnormality because of the normal overexpression of α-spectrin in red cells compared with β-spectrin. However, when these defects are inherited in *trans*, on the other allele from an HE gene, HPP may result. Several mutations have been described, particularly commonly in codon 28, which produces low-expression genes. A common polymorphism, intron $45C \rightarrow T$, is spectrin α^{LELY} (LELY denoting 'low-expression allele Lyon').

Hereditary elliptocytosis and poikilocytosis in the neonate

In the neonate, the manifestations of HE may be a more marked poikilocytosis resembling HPP, with more fragmented red cells. These red cells are susceptible to fragmentation above 46°C, whereas normal cells only fragment above 50°C. The morphological changes and haemolysis gradually decrease over the first year until the typical picture of mild HE remains. Treatment of neonatal pyropoikilocytosis is required only if the anaemia is such as to warrant transfusion.

Spherocytic hereditary elliptocytosis

In rare white families with HE, haemolysis with modest splenomegaly is found with a blood film that has a low proportion of abnormally shaped cells, ranging from spherocytes to elliptocytes. Splenectomy is not usually indicated.

Hereditary pyropoikilocytosis

The characteristics of HPP are densely contracted and fragmented cells (Figure 8.7), moderate to severe haemolysis and heterogeneity of manifestations within a family. In general, patients with HPP have spectrin deficiency in addition to the abnormalities of spectrin–spectrin contacts that produce the heterotetramer deficiency of HE. One parent of an HE propositus may have normal haematology but carry a mutation in *trans*, which leads to spectrin deficiency. The affected cells show thermal lability and fragmentation at lower temperatures than normal. HPP is more common in black people.

Hereditary elliptocytosis in Africa

In some parts of West Africa, a high incidence of HE has been found (up to 1.6% of the population). Interestingly, there is considerable molecular heterogeneity for the basis of the condition in this area. *In vitro*, *Plasmodium falciparum* is less able to parasitize HE cells that have mutations in α-spectrin, glycophorin C or protein 4.1. Invasion is reduced in red cells from homozygous patients, and intracellular multiplication reduced, particularly in homozygous 4.1$^{(-/-)}$ red cells. It seems possible that the varieties of HE offer some protection against the clinical manifestations of falciparum malaria.

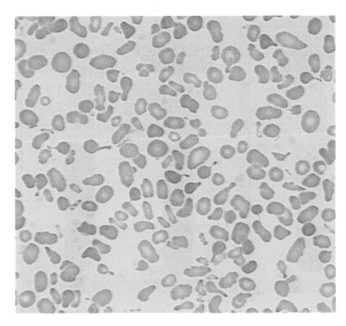

Figure 8.7 Hereditary pyropoikilocytosis, peripheral blood. Marked anisocytosis and poikilocytosis from a child with homozygous hereditary elliptocytosis.

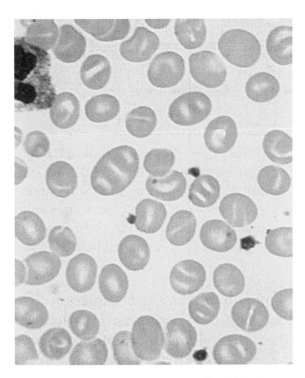

Figure 8.8 Hereditary stomatocytosis, peripheral blood.

Laboratory investigation

The standard approach to the diagnosis of HE/HPP is the identification of haemolysis, coupled to a careful examination of the blood film of the patient and as many first-degree relatives as possible. Examples of blood films are shown in Figures 8.6 and 8.7. Other acquired causes of elliptocytic or fragmented red cells need to be excluded, including iron, folate or vitamin B$_{12}$ deficiency, and the microangiopathic haemolytic anaemias. Congenital dyserythropoietic anaemia and thalassaemia intermedia also need to be excluded.

As with the investigation of HS, SDS-PAGE may reveal protein abnormalities, although more specific identification requires a sophisticated approach beyond the abilities of most haematology laboratories.

Treatment

Patients with chronic haemolysis should be given folate supplements. Splenectomy is indicated for severe haemolytic anaemia in patients with HPP or homozygous HE. Response in HPP may not be complete, but the anaemia is usually markedly alleviated. There may be a theoretical risk of increased thrombotic tendency due to remaining high platelet count, but the risk is small. The precautions against OPSI are the same as for HS.

Hereditary stomatocytosis and related disorders

Stomatocytes are so called from the mouth-like slit or 'stoma' that appears on blood films (Figure 8.8). The appearance seems to be produced by folding of cells during preparation. Stomatocytes are leaky to cations. There are other variations with Na$^+$ or K$^+$ leaks that are clinically similar to stomatocytosis without the obvious morphological changes. All these conditions are inherited in autosomal dominant fashion, and mostly produce moderate haemolytic anaemia (haemoglobin 10 g/dL or above) and macrocytosis. There are two main variants: overhydrated hereditary stomatocytosis, in which MCHC is low, and dehydrated hereditary stomatocytosis, with an increased MCHC.

The blood film may show stomatocytosis but more commonly the film is unremarkable, apart from macrocytosis and polychromasia. The group is rare, estimates suggesting that 1 in 10000 to 1 in 100000 of the population are affected. However, associated features make the conditions important beyond their rarity (Table 8.4). Pseudohyperkalaemia may occur because K$^+$ leaks rapidly from the red cells at room temperature. In some individuals, there is no evidence of haemolysis, only macrocytosis and pseudohyperkalaemia. Unless the cause of the apparent hyperkalaemia is diagnosed, unnecessary, and even dangerous, investigation and treatment may be undertaken. In some families, the K$^+$ leak is greatly increased *in vitro* by cold (cryohydrocytosis). In dehydrated hereditary stomatocytosis, there may be marked perinatal ascites that resolves spontaneously over the first year of life, but which again can lead to extensive unnecessary investigation. The third problem with hereditary stomatocytosis, both overhydrated and dehydrated varieties, is that splenectomy is followed by very marked

Table 8.4 Features of hereditary stomatocytosis and related disorders.

Characteristic	Expression	Group affected
Haemolytic anaemia	Mild to moderate	All variants
	Absent	Hereditary pseudohyperkalaemia
Morphology	Macrocytosis	All variants
	Stomatocytosis	Variable
MCHC	Decreased	Overhydrated HSt (hydrocytosis)
	Increased	Dehydrated HSt (hereditary xerocytosis, desiccocytosis)
Serum [K⁺]	Raised *in vitro*	Pseudohyperkalaemia Dehydrated HSt Cryohydrocytosis
Thrombotic tendency	Post splenectomy	All variants
Fluid balance	Perinatal oedema	Dehydrated HSt

HSt, hereditary stomatocytosis; MCHC, mean corpuscular haemoglobin concentration.

thrombotic tendencies such that splenectomy should not be performed.

Laboratory investigations

Tests for haemolysis and examination of the blood film of the patient and close relatives are the first steps in diagnosis. The finding of a raised serum potassium, together with macrocytosis, especially with some evidence of haemolysis, indicates the pseudohyperkalaemia of dehydrated hereditary stomatocytosis.

Definitive studies involve the measurement of intracellular $[Na^+]$ or $[K^+]$ and their flux through the membrane at different temperatures. Four subgroups have been defined according to the intracellular sodium concentration (normal 5–10 mmol/L). Patients with the pseudohyperkalaemia of dehydrated hereditary stomatocytosis may have normal or slightly high sodium concentrations (12–18 mmol/L); in families with cryohydrocytosis (temperature-sensitive leak) the sodium concentration is 20–50 mmol/L, and in overhydrated hereditary stomatocytosis the sodium concentration is 60 mmol/L or more.

Treatment

There is rarely a need for measures to raise the haemoglobin and splenectomy should be avoided because of the risk of thrombosis, including hepatic and portal vein thrombosis. If splenectomy is necessary, lifelong anticoagulation should be introduced.

Rh$_{null}$ syndrome

The Rh system forms a large complex traversing the lipid bilayer several times, containing extracellular thiol groups. In the Rh$_{null}$ phenotype, the complex is absent. The condition is very rare and is inherited as a recessive disorder. Patients have mild to moderate haemolytic anaemia that may respond to splenectomy, and the blood film shows occasional stomatocytes. The Rh complex involves two genes, one encoding the D polypeptide, the other the Cc and Ee polypeptides, depending on post-translational splicing. Mutation of one or other of the genes encoding these proteins is the molecular basis underlying the Rh$_{null}$ phenotype.

Southeast Asian ovalocytosis

A dominantly inherited ovalocytosis is found in parts of Southeast Asia, where falciparum malaria is common, particularly in Papua New Guinea, Borneo and the Philippines. The red cell morphology is ovalocytic rather than elliptocytic. Stoma-like slits may be present and transverse banding in the red cells is seen (Figure 8.9). Most individuals have no haemolysis but, in a few, mild anaemia may be present. Cells have increased rigidity, unlike HE in which rigidity is decreased. The molecular defect is a deletion of nine amino acids at the transmembrane cytosol junction of band 3, a defect that possibly limits the mobility of band 3 within the membrane. Homozygosity is not found and is presumably lethal *in utero*.

Abnormalities of membrane lipids

Acanthocytosis

Acanthocytes, or spur cells, show prominent, somewhat regular projections on the surface, best demonstrated by scanning electron microscopy. They are formed when the outer lipid layer of the membrane acquires additional lipid. Acanthocytosis is an acquired characteristic of severe liver disease, usually end stage, and the result of interaction of altered plasma lipids.

Abetalipoproteinaemia

Abetalipoproteinaemia is a rare inherited defect with absent β-apolipoprotein, which results in low serum cholesterol but increased sphingomyelin, which enters the cell membrane and produces the acanthocytes. The main clinical features are retinitis pigmentosa, fat malabsorption and hepatic encephalopathy.

McLeod phenotype

In the McLeod phenotype, acanthocytosis occurs (Figure 8.10), together with decreased expression of the Kell antigen. The defective gene is on the X chromosome (Xp21), close to genes

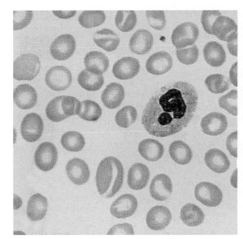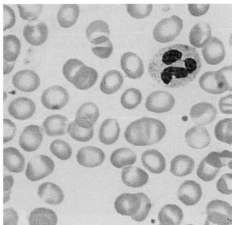

Figure 8.9 Southeast Asian ovalocytosis, peripheral blood films. Mild ovalocytosis and some stomatocytosis. Some cells have apparent transverse ridge.

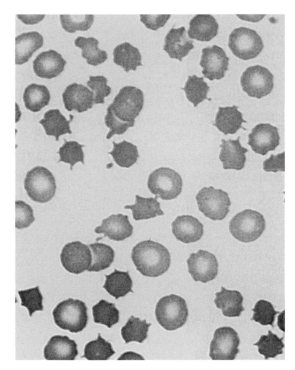

Figure 8.10 McLeod syndrome, peripheral blood. Note the marked acanthocytosis.

for Duchenne muscular dystrophy and retinitis pigmentosa, conditions with which the phenotype has been linked. The gene codes for the Kx protein that carries the Kell blood group protein. There may be mild anaemia.

Selected bibliography

Reviews

Chu X, Thompson D, Yee LJ, Sung LA (2000) Genomic organization of mouse and human erythrocyte tropomodulin genes encoding the pointed end capping protein for the actin filaments. *Gene* **256**: 271–81.

Davies KA, Lux SE (1989) Hereditary disorders of the red cell membrane skeleton. *Trends in Genetics* **5**: 222–7.

Delaunay J (2002) Molecular basis of red cell membrane disorders. *Acta Haematologica* **108**: 210–18.

Delaunay J, Dhermy D (1993) Mutations involving the spectrin heterodimer contact site: clinical expression and alterations in specific function. *Seminars in Hematology* **30**: 21–33.

Elgsaeter A, Stokke BT, Mikkelsen A, Branton D (1986) The molecular basis of erythrocyte shape. *Science* **234**: 1217–23.

Gilligan DM, Bennett V (1993) The junctional complex of the membrane skeleton. *Seminars in Hematology* **30**: 74–83.

McKusick VA (1973) Phenotypic diversity of genetic disease resulting from allelic series. *American Journal of Human Genetics* **25**: 446–56.

Mohandas N, Gallagher PG (2008) Red cells: past, present and future. *Blood* **112**: 3939–48.

Palek J, Jarolin P (1993) Clinical expression and laboratory detection of red blood cell membrane protein mutations. *Seminars in Hematology* **30**: 249–83.

Pawloski JR, Hess DT, Stamler JS (2001) Export by red blood cells of nitric oxide bioactivity. *Nature* **409**: 622–6.

Tanner MJA (1993) Molecular and cellular biology of the erythrocyte anion exchanger (AE1) *Seminars in Hematology* **30**: 34–57.

Tse WT, Lux SE (1999) Red cell membrane disorders. *British Journal of Haematology* **104**: 2–13.

Hereditary spherocytosis

Agre P, Asimos A, Casella JF, McMillan C (1986) Inheritance pattern and clinical response to splenectomy as a reflection of erythrocyte spectrin deficiency in hereditary spherocytosis. *New England Journal of Medicine* **315**: 1579–83.

Barry M, Scheuer PJ, Sherlock S, Ross CF, Williams R (1968) Hereditary spherocytosis with secondary haemochromatosis. *Lancet* **ii**: 481–5.

Bolton-Maggs PH, Stevens RF, Dodd NJ, Lamont G, Tittensor P, King MJ; General Haematology Task Force of the British Committee for Standards in Haematology (2004) Guidelines for the diagnosis and management of hereditary spherocytosis. *British Journal of Haematology* **126**: 455–74.

Bruce LJ, Ghosh S, King MJ *et al.* (2002) Absence of CD47 in protein 4.2-deficient hereditary spherocytosis in man: an interaction between the Rh complex and band 3 complex. *Blood* **100**: 1878–85.

Delhommeau F, Cynober T, Schischmanoff PO *et al.* (2000) Natural history of hereditary spherocytosis during the first year of life. *Blood* **95**: 393–7.

Dhermy D, Galand C, Bournier O *et al.* (1997) Heterogenous band 3 deficiency in hereditary spherocytosis related to different band 3 gene defects. *British Journal of Haematology* **98**: 32–40.

Eber SW, Gonzalez JM, Lux ML *et al.* (1996) Ankyrin-1 mutations are a major cause of dominant and recessive hereditary spherocytosis. *Nature Genetics* **13**: 214–18.

Gallagher PG, Forget BG (1998) Hematologically important mutations: spectrin and ankyrin variants in hereditary spherocytosis. *Blood Cells, Molecules and Diseases* **24**: 539–43.

Gallagher PG, Ferreira JDS, Costa FF *et al.* (2000) A recurrent frameshift mutation of the ankyrin gene associated with severe hereditary spherocytosis. *British Journal of Haematology* **111**: 1190–3.

Hanspal M, Yoon S-H, Yu H *et al.* (1991) Molecular basis of spectrin and ankyrin deficiencies in severe hereditary spherocytosis: evidence implicating a primary defect of ankyrin. *Blood* **77**: 165–73.

Ideguchi H, Nishimura J, Nawata H *et al.* (1990) Genetic defect of erythrocyte band 4.2 protein associated with hereditary spherocytosis. *British Journal of Haematology* **74**: 347–53.

Iwamoto S, Kajii E, Omi T *et al.* (1993) Point mutation in the band 4.2 gene associated with autosomal recessively inherited erythrocyte band 4.2 deficiency. *European Journal of Haematology* **50**: 286–91.

Jacob HS, Jandl JH (1964) Increased cell membrane permeability in the pathogenesis of hereditary spherocytosis. *Journal of Clinical Investigation* **43**: 1704–20.

King MJ, Behrens J, Rogers C *et al.* (2000) Rapid flow cytometric test for the diagnosis of membrane cytoskeleton-associated haemolytic anaemia. *British Journal of Haematology* **111**: 924–33.

Korsgren C, Lawler J, Lambert S *et al.* (1990) Complete amino acid sequence and homologies of human erythrocyte membrane protein band 4.2. *Proceedings of the National Academy of Sciences USA* **87**: 613–17.

Lefrere JJ, Courouce A-M, Girot R *et al.* (1986) Six cases of hereditary spherocytosis revealed by human parvovirus infection. *British Journal of Haematology* **62**: 653–8.

Miraglia del Giudice E, Perrotta S, Pinto L *et al.* (1992) Hereditary spherocytosis characterized by increased spectrin/band 3 ratio. *British Journal of Haematology* **80**: 133–6.

Miraglia del Giudice E, Francese M, Nobili B *et al.* (1998) High frequency of de novo mutations in ankyrin gene (ANK1) in children with hereditary spherocytosis. *Journal of Pediatrics* **132**: 117–20.

Miraglia del Giudice E, Perrotta S, Nobili B *et al.* (1999) Coinheritance of Gilbert syndrome increases risk for developing gallstones in patients with hereditary spherocytosis. *Blood* **94**: 2259–62.

Miraglia del Giudice E, Nobili B, Francese M *et al.* (2001) Clinical and molecular evaluation of non-dominant hereditary spherocytosis. *British Journal of Haematology* **112**: 42–7.

Okamoto N, Wada Y, Nakamura Y *et al.* (1995) Hereditary spherocytic anaemia with deletion of the short arm of chromosome 8. *American Journal of Medical Genetics* **58**: 225–9.

Perrotta S, Gallagher PG, Mohandas N (2008) Hereditary spherocytosis. *Lancet* **372**: 1411–26.

Reinhart WH, Wyss EJ, Arnold D *et al.* (1994) Hereditary spherocytosis associated with protein band 3 defect in a Swiss kindred. *British Journal of Haematology* **86**: 147–55.

Rybicki AC, Heath R, Wolf JL *et al.* (1988) Deficiency of protein 4.2 in erythrocytes from a patient with a Coombs negative haemolytic anaemia: evidence for a role of protein 4.2 in stabilizing ankyrin on the membrane. *Journal of Clinical Investigation* **81**: 893–901.

Splenectomy

Anon (1985) Splenectomy: a long term risk of infection [Editorial]. *Lancet* **ii**: 928–9.

Anon (1998) The place of pneumococcal vaccination [Editorial]. *Drug and Therapeutics Bulletin* **36**: 73–6.

Bader-Meunier B, Gauthier F, Archambaud F *et al.* (2001) Long term evaluation of the beneficial effect of subtotal splenectomy for management of hereditary spherocytosis. *Blood* **97**: 399–403.

Crary SE, Buchanan GR (2009) Vascular complications after splenectomy for hematologic disorders. *Blood* **114**: 2861–8.

McMullin M, Johnston G (1993) Long term management of patients after splenectomy [Editorial]. *British Medical Journal* **307**: 1371–2.

Schilling RF (2009) Risks and benefits of splenectomy versus no splenectomy for hereditary spherocytosis – a personal view. *British Journal of Haematology* **145**: 728–32.

Schilling RF, Gangnon RE, Travers MI (2008) Delayed adverse vascular events after splenectomy in hereditary spherocytosis. *Journal of Thrombosis and Haemostasis* **6**: 1289–95.

Working Party of the British Committee for Standards in Haematology Clinical Haematology Work Force (1996) Guidelines for the prevention and treatment of infection in patients with an absent or dysfunctional spleen. *British Medical Journal* **312**: 430–4.

Hereditary elliptocytosis

Gallagher PG, Forget BG (1996) Hematologically important mutations: spectrin variants in hereditary elliptocytosis and hereditary pyropoikilocytosis. *Blood Cells, Molecules and Diseases* **22**: 254–8.

Glele-Kakai C, Garbarz M, Lecomte MC *et al.* (1996) Epidemiological studies of spectrin mutations related to hereditary elliptocytosis and spectrin polymorphisms in Benin. *British Journal of Haematology* **95**: 57–66.

Marchesi SL, Letsinger JT, Speicher DW *et al.* (1987) Mutant forms of spectrin alpha-subunits in hereditary elliptocytosis. *Journal of Clinical Investigation* **80**: 191–8.

Randon J, Boulanger L, Marechal J *et al.* (1994) A variant of spectrin low-expression allele alpha-LELY carrying a hereditary elliptocytosis mutation in codon 28. *British Journal of Haematology* **88**: 534–40.

Hereditary pyropoikilocytosis

Agre P, Orringer EP, Chui DHK *et al.* (1981) A molecular defect in two families with haemolytic poikilocytic anaemia: reduction of high affinity membrane binding sites for ankyrin. *Journal of Clinical Investigation* **68**: 1566–76.

Gallagher PG, Petruzzi MJ, Weed SA *et al.* (1997) Mutation of a highly conserved residue of beta-1 spectrin associated with fatal and near-fatal neonatal haemolytic anaemia. *Journal of Clinical Investigation* **99**: 267–77.

Goel VK, Li X, Chen H *et al.* (2003) Band 3 is a host receptor binding merozoite surface protein 1 during the *Plasmodium falciparum* invasion of erythrocytes. *Proceedings of the National Academy of Sciences USA* **100**: 5164–9.

Liu S-C, Palek J, Prchal J *et al.* (1981) Altered spectrin dimer–dimer association and instability of erythrocyte membrane skeletons in hereditary pyropoikilocytosis. *Journal of Clinical Investigation* **68**: 597–605.

Hereditary stomatocytosis, pseudohyperkalaemia

Delaunay J, Stewart G, Iolascon A (1999) Hereditary dehydrated and overhydrated stomatocytosis: recent advances. *Current Opinion in Hematology* **6**: 110–14.

Grootenboer S, Schischmanoff PO, Cynober T *et al.* (1998) A genetic syndrome associating dehydrated hereditary stomatocytosis, pseudohyperkalaemia and perinatal oedema. *British Journal of Haematology* **103**: 383–6.

Grootenboer S, Schischmanoff PO, Laurendeau I *et al.* (2000) Pleiotropic syndrome of dehydrated hereditary stomatocytosis, pseudohyperkalemia, and perinatal oedema maps to 16q23–q24. *Blood* **96**: 2599–605.

Stewart GW, Turner EJ (1999) The hereditary stomatocytoses and allied disorders: congenital disorders of erythrocyte membrane permeability to Na and K. *Baillière's Best Practice and Research. Clinical Haematology* **12**: 707–27.

Stewart GW, Corrall RJ, Fyffe JA *et al.* (1979) Familial pseudohyperkalaemia. A new syndrome. *Lancet* **ii**: 175–7.

Stewart GW, Amess JA, Eber SW *et al.* (1996) Thrombo-embolic disease after splenectomy for hereditary stomatocytosis. *British Journal of Haematology* **96**: 303–10.

Southeast Asian ovalocytosis and malaria

Goel VK, Li X, Chen H *et al.* (2003) Band 3 is a host receptor binding merozoite surface protein 1 during the *Plasmodium falciparum* invasion of erythrocytes. *Proceedings of the National Academy of Sciences USA* **100**: 5164–9.

Hadley T, Saul A, Lamont G *et al.* (1983) Resistance of Melanesian elliptocytes (ovalocytes) to invasion by *Plasmodium knowlesii* and *Plasmodium falciparum* malaria parasites *in vitro*. *Journal of Clinical Investigation* **71**: 780–2.

Liu S-C, Zhai S, Palek J *et al.* (1990) Molecular defect of the band 3 protein in South-East Asian ovalocytosis. *New England Journal of Medicine* **323**: 1530–8.

CHAPTER 9

Disorders of red cell metabolism

9

Alberto Zanella[1] and Edward C Gordon-Smith[2]

[1]Fondazione IRCCS Ca'Granada, Ospedale Maggiore Policlinico, Milan, Italy
[2]St George's Hospital Medical School, London, UK

Introduction

The main function of the red cell is to carry haemoglobin around the circulation in high concentration and in a functional state so that gas exchange may occur efficiently in the lungs and in the tissue capillaries. Oxygen is thus taken up in the lungs in exchange for carbon dioxide and delivered to the tissues at physiological pH and gas pressure. The structure and function of haemoglobin is discussed in Chapter 6. In order to fulfil its function, the red cell needs a supply of energy in the form of ATP and a source of reducing power.

A mature red cell contains no DNA or RNA and hence is incapable of protein synthesis, and the mitochondria which are present in reticulocytes have been lost during maturation, so that the only source of energy as ATP is derived from anaerobic glycolysis and the linked reducing system of the hexose monophosphate shunt (pentose phosphate pathway) and the glutathione cycle. ATP is required to maintain the membrane is its deformable state, with asymmetric lipid layers, and to regulate ion and water exchange. Reducing power is required to reduce methaemoglobin to its functional state of deoxyhaemoglobin and to counteract the strong oxidative stresses which a cell carrying molecular oxygen around the circulation is likely to encounter. The main process that reduces methaemoglobin utilizes reduced nicotinamide adenine dinucleotide (NADH), produced from nicotinamide adenine dinucleotide (NAD$^+$) by the glycolytic pathway. Reduction and detoxification of free oxygen radicals and hydrogen peroxide produced during reactions to infection is provided by reduced nicotinamide adenine dinucleotide phosphate (NADPH) generated by the first steps of the pentose phosphate pathway, catalysed by glucose-6-phosphate dehydrogenase (G6PD) and the linked enzyme 6-phosphogluconate dehydrogenase. NADPH drives the glutathione cycle, glutathione (GSH) being the major reducing agent within the red cell.

The lack of protein synthesis in the mature red cell means that none of the enzymes in the metabolic pathways can be replaced during the red cell lifespan. Over the 120 days of normal red cell survival, enzyme activities decline at variable but predictable rates. This decline probably contributes to the ageing process of the red cell. Many of the mutations that affect red cell metabolism and provoke haemolytic anaemia cause instability and premature inactivation of the enzyme; other mutations directly affect catalytic activity.

The glycolytic pathway (Embden–Meyerhof pathway)

Glycolysis (or, more correctly, glucolysis) is the process by which glucose is converted to pyruvate through a number of steps, with a net gain of two moles of ATP generated for each mole of glucose metabolized by the pathway. Glucose is derived from the plasma by facilitated transfer through the membrane. Pyruvate and lactic acid are in equilibrium determined by the redox potential of the cell (NAD$^+$/NADH) and can diffuse out of the cell. The internal milieu of the cell, with its high K$^+$ concentration and presence of other cations such as magnesium necessary for efficient glycolysis, is maintained through the activity of various ion and cation channels in the membrane, with energy linked by appropriate ATPases. The glycolytic

Postgraduate Haematology: 6th edition. Edited by A. Victor Hoffbrand, Daniel Catovsky, Edward G.D. Tuddenham, Anthony R. Green
© 2011 Blackwell Publishing Ltd.

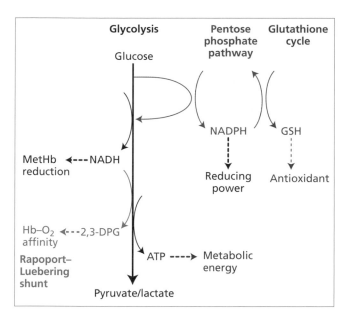

Figure 9.1 Principal pathways of energy production in the mature red cell. The glycolytic pathway provides energy in the form of ATP. Under normal conditions, methaemoglobin (MetHb) is reduced by the coupled reaction with NADH$^+$. The Rapoport–Luebering shunt provides 2,3-diphosphoglycerate (2,3-DPG) for control of haemoglobin oxygen affinity. Reducing power is produced by the pentose phosphate pathway and is linked to redox reactions through the glutathione cycle.

pathway also provides the redox reaction to convert methaemoglobin to deoxyhaemoglobin by utilizing NADH in a reaction catalysed by methaemoglobin-NADH reductase (cytochrome b_3). The various products and functions of glucose metabolism are shown schematically in Figure 9.1 and in more detail in Figure 9.2.

The Rapoport–Luebering shunt

One of the essential roles of metabolism in the red cell is to provide sufficient 2,3-diphosphoglycerate (2,3-DPG) to regulate the oxygen affinity of haemoglobin. 2,3-DPG is produced from 1,3-DPG under the influence of the enzyme diphosphoglycerate mutase in linked reactions that form the Rapoport–Luebering shunt (Figure 9.2). 2,3-DPG is broken down to 3-phosphoglycerate by a phosphatase and thus re-enters the glycolytic pathway. It should be noted that when metabolism takes place via the Rapoport–Luebering shunt, there is bypass of the stage of ATP production. The shunt thus not only provides the 2,3-DPG for interaction with the haemoglobin tetramer but also acts as an energy control mechanism for glycolysis.

Disorders of the glycolytic pathway

Mutations of most of the enzymes in the glycolytic pathway have been described in association with congenital non-spherocytic haemolytic anaemia (CNSHA). However, deficiency of pyruvate kinase is far and away the most common enzyme to be affected. The haemolysis is the result of a failure to produce sufficient ATP.

Pyruvate kinase

Pyruvate kinase (PK) catalyses the final steps of the glycolytic pathway with the conversion of phosphoenolpyruvate to pyruvate, with the concomitant phosphorylation of ADP to ATP, leading to overall net gain of ATP from this pathway. There are four types of PK in different tissues derived from two separate genes. The *PKM2* gene, on chromosome 15, produces PKM1 and PKM2 through differences in post-transcriptional splicing. PKM1 is present in skeletal muscles, PKM2 in leucocytes, kidneys, adipose tissue and lungs. The *PKLR* gene, on chromosome 1, gives rise to PKL in the liver and PKR in red cells. The isoenzymes are transcribed differently through the influence of tissue-specific promoters. The active enzymes are homotetramers. PKM2, PKR and PKL all demonstrate marked allosteric reactions with several ligands. PKM1, on the other hand, has no allosteric interactions.

The main ligands involved in the allosteric control of PKR in the erythrocyte are shown in Figure 9.3. PK is one of the dominant controlling steps in glucose metabolism (together with hexokinase), exerting its effect through major feedback loops, especially by its requirement for activation by fructose-1,6-diphosphate.

Pyruvate kinase deficiency

PK deficiency leads to chronic non-spherocytic haemolytic anaemia with extravascular haemolysis.

Molecular biology

PK deficiency is the commonest of the enzymopathies of the glycolytic pathway, at least 300 times more common than any other. Best estimates based on gene frequency in the white population suggest a prevalence of about 50 per million. About 200 different mutations have been described in PK deficiency, the majority involving point mutations or deletions in the transcribed gene but a few involving the promoter region. Haemolytic anaemia due to PK deficiency is an autosomal recessive disorder. Many individuals are compound heterozygotes. Not surprisingly, there is enormous genetic heterogeneity between affected individuals, reflected in the multiplicity of quantitative and kinetic defects detected (Figure 9.3). Because PKR is a homotetramer composed of four chains derived from the products of the two alleles, enzyme kinetic variations are many and genotype–phenotype correlates are difficult to predict. First attempts to delineate the genotype–phenotype

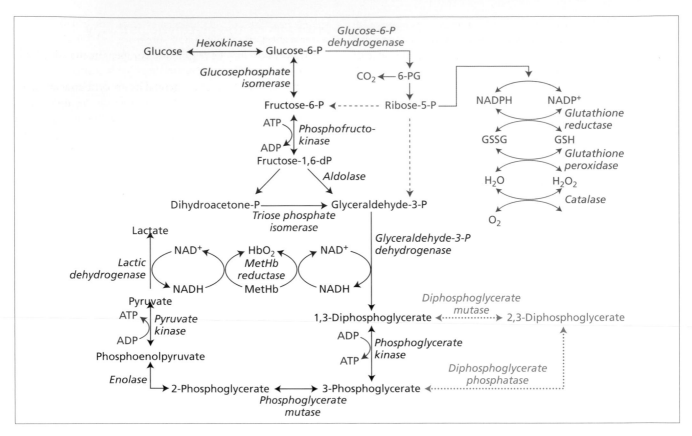

Figure 9.2 The glycolytic pathway and its interactions with the pentose phosphate pathway and the Rapoport–Luebering shunt.

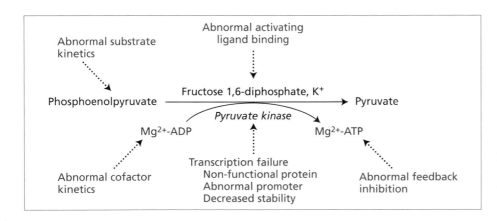

Figure 9.3 The reactions of pyruvate kinase showing the main ligands that influence activity and the sites affected by various mutations encountered in PK deficiency.

association were mainly based on analysis of the enzyme's three-dimensional structure and observation of the few homozygous patients. More recently, comparison of recombinant mutants of human red cell PK with wild-type enzymes has revealed the effect of amino acid replacements on the molecular properties of the enzyme. However, the clinical manifestations of red cell enzyme defects are not merely dependent on the molecular properties of the mutant protein but rather reflect the complex interactions of additional factors,

including genetic background, concomitant functional polymorphisms of other enzymes, post-translational or epigenetic modifications, ineffective erythropoiesis and differences in splenic function.

PK catalyses the ultimate step in the glycolytic pathway. Deficient activity leads to accumulation of substrates further up the pathway, including 2,3-DPG. The increased concentration of 2,3-DPG in PK-deficient red cells shifts the oxygen dissociation curve to the right, indicating low oxygen affinity.

Patients with PK deficiency tolerate apparent anaemia well because the lower haemoglobin content will deliver the same amount of oxygen to the tissues as normal haemoglobin, at least under normal conditions, though oxygen reserve would be limited.

Reticulocytes have alternative means of producing energy in the form of ATP via the oxidative respiratory pathway of the remaining mitochondria. They can also synthesize enzyme in those defects where lack of stability is the major cause of enzyme deficiency in the mature cell. Reticulocytes thus have a metabolic advantage over mature red cells in PK deficiency.

Clinical features

The genetic heterogeneity is reflected by the wide variation in the phenotype. The presenting features may vary from severe neonatal jaundice and anaemia (Figure 9.4), rarely even presenting with hydrops fetalis, severe chronic non-spherocytic haemolytic anaemia requiring repeated transfusions, moderate haemolysis with exacerbation during infections or pregnancy, to symptomless compensated haemolysis with only a minor apparent anaemia. The majority of reported cases have pre-sented in childhood. PK deficiency does not usually have an adverse effect on the outcome of pregnancy, although occasionally transfusion may be required to compensate the added dilutional anaemia (Figure 9.5).

Jaundice, as with other congenital haemolytic anaemias, may be exacerbated by co-inheritance of other genes, for example Gilbert syndrome. The haemolysis is nearly always extravascular, though rare examples with some intravascular haemolysis have been detected. Gallstones are common in PK deficiency and may lead to bouts of choelcystitis and biliary colic (Figure 9.6). Jaundice may also be increased by administration of drugs that affect bile excretion. As with other cases of congenital haemolytic anaemia with extravascular haemolysis, excess iron accumulation may occasionally develop even in the absence of transfusion or co-inheritance of a haemochromatosis gene.

The spleen is usually palpable in cases where there is significant haemolysis, though in milder cases it may only be evident by ultrasound or other imaging techniques.

PK deficiency is not associated with abnormalities of other tissues, since the deficient enzyme is unique to the red cells, but occasionally individuals are seen with associated

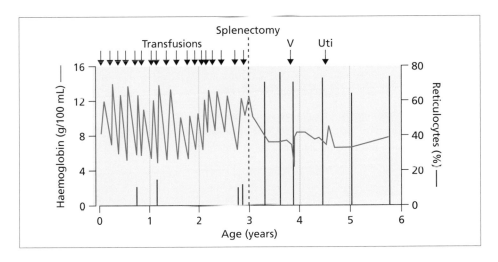

Figure 9.4 Effect of splenectomy in a child with severe CNSHA due to pyruvate kinase deficiency. Splenectomy was delayed until the child was 3 years old. Note the marked reticulocytosis post splenectomy (V, viral infection; Uti, urinary tract infection). The child grew normally despite haemoglobin of around 8 g/dL (see text).

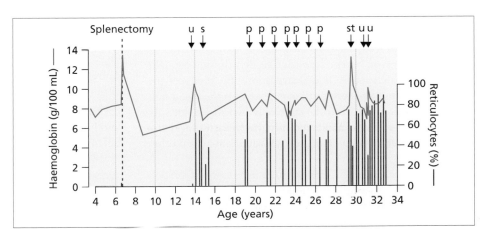

Figure 9.5 Multiple successful pregnancies in a splenectomized patient with pyruvate kinase deficiency. Transfusion was required during pregnancy (p) and before surgery (st, sterilization) and during infection (u, urinary tract infection; s, sepsis).

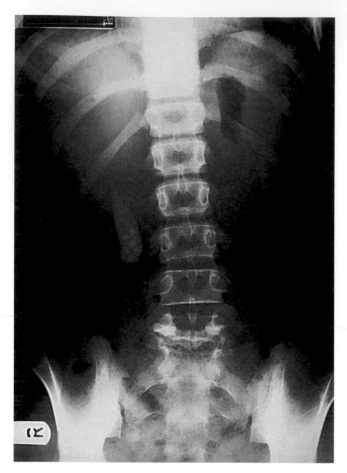

Figure 9.6 Plain radiograph of a patient with pyruvate kinase deficiency showing a calcified gallbladder with mixed calcified pigment stones as a result of repeated attacks of inflammatory cholecystitis.

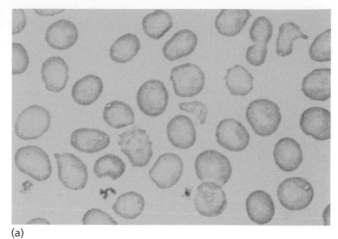

(a)

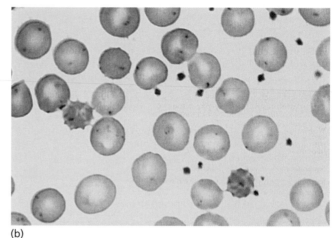

(b)

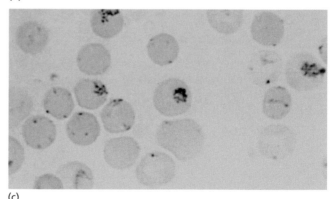

(c)

Figure 9.7 Pyruvate kinase deficiency, peripheral blood. (a) Red cell anisocytosis and poikilocytosis before splenectomy. (b) After splenectomy showing acanthocytes or 'prickle' cells. (c) Gross reticulocytosis after splenectomy (supravital new methylene blue stain).

abnormalities due to deletions within chromosome 1 close to the *PKLR* gene.

Laboratory diagnosis

The blood count reveals a normochromic anaemia with reticulocytosis, sometimes producing a slight macrocytosis. An increased mean corpuscular haemoglobin concentration is occasionally seen in severe cases due to dehydration brought about by ATP deficiency. This dehydration also produces the characteristic spur cells or acanthocytes seen on the blood film (Figure 9.7a,b). Apart from the spur cells (which are not specific) and the very large reticulocytosis post splenectomy (Figure 9.7c), there is nothing to distinguish PK deficiency from other causes of CNSHA.

The autohaemolysis test, involving the incubation of defibrinated red cells with and without glucose for 48 hours at 37°C, has traditionally been used for screening tests. The haemolysis in the unfortified aliquot is uncorrected by the addition of glucose (type II). The test is not specific and has mainly been abandoned in favour of the enzyme assay.

The definitive diagnosis depends on the analysis of enzyme activity and kinetics, although the finding of an elevated 2,3-

DPG level (two to three times normal) may be a useful pointer. Characterization of the enzyme requires measurement of maximal activation under optimal conditions (V_{max}), kinetic studies to determine the substrate(s) concentration at which the enzyme shows 50% V_{max} (K_m), thermal stability, pH optimum and electrophoretic mobility. Meaningful enzyme levels can only be achieved after total removal of leucocytes, which have up to 300 times the PK activity of red cells. The effect of reticulocytes also has to be taken into account. International guidelines for investigation of PK deficiency have been published. Typically, homozygotes have about 25% of normal V_{max} activity, allowing for the age of the red cells, and heterozygotes 50–60% but the range is great and there is much overlap in V_{max} between the groups, emphasizing the need for kinetic and other studies (Figure 9.8).

Management

The mainstay of management of patients who have sufficiently severe haemolysis to warrant treatment is splenectomy. Assessment of the need for splenectomy should take into account the symptoms of the patient not the haemoglobin level. The low haemoglobin (even as low as 7.0 g/dL) may be well tolerated because of the right-shifted oxygen dissociation curve. Indications for splenectomy include severe neonatal haemolysis and chronic transfusion requirements. The dangers of splenectomy, particularly the risk of overwhelming sepsis, have been discussed in Chapter 8. Splenectomy raises the effective haemoglobin so that transfusion is not required but does not prevent hyperbilirubinaemia so biliary complications may still arise after splenectomy. Following splenectomy for PK deficiency, there is a huge elevation in the reticulocyte count, which may reach 80% or more of the peripheral blood cells (see Figure 9.4).

Although pregnancy may exacerbate this anaemia, there is no indication that PK deficiency itself has an adverse effect on the pregnancy or outcome, so long as the anaemia is managed as necessary (see Figure 9.5). As with all chronic haemolytic anaemias, folic acid 5 mg per week or 400 μg daily is a sensible supplement.

Other defects of the enzymes of the glycolytic system

Compared with PK deficiency, the other defects of the glycolytic pathway are very rare. The main features of these disorders are summarized in Table 9.1.

Hexokinase

Hexokinase (HK1) catalyses the phosphorylation of glucose to glucose-6-phosphate (G6P), the first step in the glycolytic pathway. The enzyme in the red cell differs from that in nucleated cells, which have oxidative respiration, by lacking a porin-binding domain that links the enzyme to the mitochondrial membrane. The red cell enzyme is derived from alternative splicing of the gene product. The enzyme provides a major rate-limiting step in glycolysis and has extensive allosteric interactions: it is highly pH sensitive and its activity is regulated by its products, G6P, P_i, 2,3-DPG and disulphide compounds. The enzyme activity decays predictably with age of the normal red cell, and may be used as a comparator for other enzyme activities where absolute levels may be difficult to interpret because of the age distribution of the red cells.

Hexokinase deficiency

Hexokinase deficiency has been recorded in only 17 families, but even within this small number there is evidence of molecular and phenotypic heterogeneity. Complete hexokinase deficiency is probably lethal. Most patients have moderately reduced activity for the age of the red cell, and in the majority of cases it is the stability of the enzyme that is affected by the mutation. Combined heterozygosity for complete gene deletion and a nonsense mutation affecting activity has been recorded as a typical example of compound genetic inheritance. In most recorded cases, the activity of the enzyme is reduced to 10–20% of normal. As with other glycolytic enzyme deficiencies, there is variable non-spherocytic haemolytic anaemia, in this case mostly relatively mild. Obligate heterozygotes have reduced levels of the enzyme, but assaying the activity in patients with

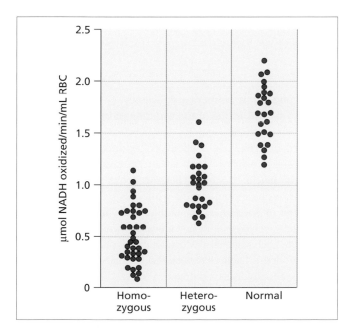

Figure 9.8 Pyruvate kinase activity (V_{max}) measured in patients, obligate heterozygotes and normal control subjects. Note the wide overlap of values between the two groups, indicating the importance of kinetic studies as well as the effect of reticulocytosis.

Table 9.1 Main features of glycolytic enzyme deficiencies.

Enzyme	Gene (chromosome, inheritance)	Haematology	Other systems affected	Comment
Hexokinase	HK1, 10q22 AR	CNSHA High O_2 affinity	None directly*	Very rare, occasional AD
Glucose phosphate isomerise	GPI, 19q13.1 AR	CNSHA	None directly*	Most common after PK deficiency
Phosphofructokinase	PFKL (L subunit), 21q22.3 PFKM (M subunit), 12q13.11 Complex	Erythrocytosis Minimal haemolysis	Dominated by myopathy	Tarui disease, subunit genes
Fructose diphosphate aldolase A	ALDOA, 16p11.2 AR	CNSHA Intermittent HA	Dysmorphism, myopathy	Very rare (three families)
Triose phosphate isomerase	TPI1, 12p13 AR	CNSHA Infections	Neuromuscular, cardiac	Neuromuscular defects dominate, sudden death, splenectomy not helpful
Phosphoglycerate kinase	PGK1, Xq13.3 X-linked	CNSHA	CNS, myopathy, rhabdomyolysis	Rare (28 families), variable systems involved
Diphosphoglycerate mutase	BPGM, 7q31–q34 AR	Erythrocytosis	None	Very rare, low 2,3-DPG
Glyceraldehyde-3-phosphate dehydrogenase	GAPDH, 12p13.31 AD	None	None	Membrane protein band 6, gene syntenic with TPI
Pyruvate kinase	PKLR, 1q22 AR rarely AD	CNSHA	None	Commonest CNSHA

*Neurological signs may be secondary to hypoxia or ischaemia.
AD, autosomal dominant; AR, autosomal recessive; CNSHA, congenital non-spherocytic haemolytic anaemia; HA, haemolytic anaemia.

haemolytic anaemia due to hexokinase deficiency may be difficult to interpret because of the higher activity in reticulocytes and in young cells. Typically, reduced hexokinase activity is associated with a fall in the concentration of 2,3-DPG within the cells. Patients have less exercise tolerance for a given level of haemoglobin than would be expected because of the left shift in the oxygen dissociation curve.

Glucose phosphate isomerase

Glucose phosphate isomerase (GPI) catalyses the second step of the Embden–Meyerhof pathway, the interconversion of G6P to fructose-6-phosphate (F6P). The enzyme is also known as phosphohexose isomerase, phosphoglucose isomerase, autocrine motility factor and neuroleukin. The names 'autocrine motility factor' and 'neuroleukin' indicate that the protein has other actions in other cells. The interconversion of the hexose phosphates is driven towards F6P by the rapid metabolism of that product along the metabolic pathway so that the concentration of F6P in the red cell is low and drives the reaction towards its formation.

Glucose phosphate isomerase deficiency

Deficiency of GPI is one of the commonest causes of CNSHA after G6PD deficiency and PK deficiency. About 50 families have been described; it is about as common as pyrimidine 5′-nucleotidase deficiency (see later). The mutations that give rise to GPI deficiency are very heterogeneous. About 30 different mutations have been identified but only seven of them have been found in more than one family; 17 of the 27 cases were compound heterozygotes. The clinical picture perhaps reflects this genetic heterogeneity. Most reported cases present with mild to moderate haemolytic anaemia, but in one Indian family stillbirths and hydrops occurred in several sibs before early delivery and exchange transfusion for hydrops allowed survival. The mutations described mainly affect the stability of GPI, which is perhaps why there are no associated anomalies found in nucleated cells. In T lymphocytes, GPI acts as neuroleukin, a lymphokine that induces the formation of antibody-secreting cells. It is also present in neutrophils, but there is no increase in infections in deficient subjects. In some severely deficient patients, neurological retardation has been thought to be related to hypoxia or ischaemia *in utero* rather than to direct metabolic effects.

Phosphofructokinase

Phosphofructokinase (PFK) catalyses a reaction in which F6P is phosphorylated to fructose-1,6-diphosphate, ATP being the donor of the phosphate group. Under normal physiological conditions this may be the major rate-limiting step in glycolysis in the red cell. PFK is a tetramer, which in the red cell is a heterotetramer composed of M or L subunits. Two separate genes code for the two subunits. PFK is a homotetramer of M subunits (M4) in muscle and of L subunits (L4) in liver. In the red cell, there may be five isoenzymes composed of different numbers of L and M subunits. A third subunit is found in platelets.

Phosphofructokinase deficiency

Deficiency of the M subunit leads to glycogen storage disease type 7 (Tarui disease). It is characterized by muscle cramps and myoglobinuria on exertion. Shortened red cell viability may be a minor component of this disease. Evidence of haemolysis may be accompanied by mild erythrocytosis as a result of decreased production of 2,3-DPG. To date, 15 PFK-deficient *PFKM* alleles from more than 30 families have been characterized.

Fructose diphosphate aldolase A

Fructose-1,6-diphosphate aldolase A (ALDOA) catalyses the conversion of fructose-1,6-diphosphate to Ga3P and dihydroxyacetone phosphate (DHAP). There are three aldolases in human tissues, A, B and C, of which only A is expressed in the red cell. ALDOA is produced in the developing embryo and also forms the bulk of the enzyme in muscle, where it may be as much as 5% of the total cellular protein. In the red cell, the reaction catalysed by the enzyme is virtually irreversible.

Fructose diphosphate aldolase A deficiency

The condition is extremely rare, with only three families having been definitely identified as having ALDOA deficiency. Two families have been described in which the propositus presented with CNSHA, mental retardation and dysmorphic features similar in the two families. In at least one family, the mutation produced an unstable enzyme. In a third patient, symptoms were mainly of myopathy with weakness and premature fatigue. Anaemia and jaundice were intermittent, and rhabdomyolysis occurred. There was severe deficiency of both muscle and red cell enzyme activity.

Triose phosphate isomerase

Triose phosphate isomerase (TPI) catalyses the interconversion of DHAP and Ga3P. In the glycolytic pathway of the red cell, all DHAP is converted to Ga3P, which is then metabolized down the glycolytic pathway, providing the ultimate two molecules of ATP for each molecule of glucose metabolized by that pathway. The enzyme is a homodimer present in all tissues. In tissues other than the red blood cell, DHAP is an important precursor for the biosynthesis of ether glycerolipids (plasmalogens).

Triose phosphate isomerase deficiency

TPI deficiency produces a severe syndrome present from birth, consisting of CNSHA, a progressive neurological disorder with spasticity and central nervous system (CNS) degeneration. Cardiac failure and sudden death due to arrhythmias are also features. Death occurs usually about 5 years of age. There is, as usual, some variation and haemolysis without neurological degeneration, and the opposite, have been described. Splenectomy does not appear to be effective in modifying the haemolysis and does not influence the neurological complications. The diagnosis is made based on clinical suspicion together with the appropriate enzyme assay. A number of point mutations have been identified that lead to the syndrome, but by far the most predominant is Glu104Asp, a mutation linked by common haplotypes suggesting descent from a common ancestor.

Phosphoglycerate kinase

Phosphoglycerate kinase (PGK) catalyses the reversible conversion of 1,3-DPG to 3-phosphoglycerate, generating one molecule of ATP for each molecule of 1,3-DPG metabolized by this pathway. It should be noted that two molecules of 1,3-DPG are produced for each molecule of glucose metabolized by this pathway. PGKA, the active enzyme in the red blood cell, is the product of a gene (*PGK1*) on the X chromosome. The enzyme is monomeric and is expressed in all tissues (a testis has an additional *PGK2* gene coded on an autosome).

Phosphoglycerate kinase deficiency

A total of 28 families with PGK deficiency have been reported, and sequencing data are available for 17 families. Overall, 17 different mutations in the *PGK1* gene, mostly missense, have been described in association with PGK deficiency. Of the 28 families, CNSHA occurred in 17, CNS disorders in 13 and myopathy with or without rhabdomyolysis in 13. All three systems were involved in only one of the families. Anaemia when present is usually well tolerated because of the increased concentration of 2,3-DPG produced by the increased flow of 1,3-DPG to 2,3-DPG via the Rappaport–Leubering shunt in the presence of the mutated PGK deficiency. Splenectomy has been effective in some cases of severe anaemia, but less so in others.

Defence against oxidative stress: the production of reducing power

As with all cells, but perhaps more urgently, red blood cell needs to be protected against the effects of free radicals, hydrogen peroxide and other highly oxidative material in order to maintain membrane integrity and functional activity. In addition, haemoglobin has to be maintained in its functional state, and the steady production of methaemoglobin reversed to deoxyhaemoglobin, which is able to combine reversibly with oxygen. The major generator of reducing power within the red cell

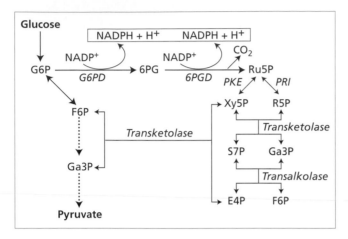

Figure 9.9 The pentose phosphate pathway. Substrates: G6P, glucose-6-phosphate; 6PG, 6-phosphogluconate; Ru5P, ribulose-5-phosphate; R5P, ribose-5-phosphate; Ga3P, glyceraldehyde-3-phosphate; F6P, fructose-6-phosphate; Xy5P, xylose-5-phosphate; S7P, septulose-7-phosphate; E4P, erythrose-4-phosphate. Enzymes: G6PD, glucose-6-phosphate dehydrogenase; 6PGD, 6-phosphogluconate dehydrogenase; PKE, phosphoketoepimerase; PRI, phosphoribose isomerase.

is the pentose phosphate pathway (hexose monophosphate shunt), which generates reducing power in the form of NADPH from $NADP^+$ coupled to the oxidation of G6P to 6-phosphogluconate (6PG) and the subsequent oxidation of that compound to ribose-5-phosphate, the two reactions catalysed by G6PD and 6-phosphogluconate dehydrogenase (Figure 9.9).

GSH is important for protecting cells from oxidative damage by these free radicals, protecting against the effects of infection, maintaining protein sulphydryl goups in the reduced state and maintaining membrane transport. A constant supply of GSH is provided by the glutathione cycle linked to the pentose phosphate pathway through the action of glutathione reductase (Figure 9.10).

Oxidative stress that exceeds the reducing power of the red cell leads to intravascular haemolysis following denaturion of haemoglobin and precipitation as Heinz bodies and peroxidation of the red cell membrane. Methaemoglobinaemia may occur. The clinical features that emerge – acute intravascular haemolysis, Heinz body haemolytic anaemia or methaemoglobinaemia – depend on the nature of the oxidative stress and the size of the imbalance between the stress and the redox potential.

Pentose phosphate pathway (hexose monophosphate shunt)

The reactions of the pentose phosphate pathway are shown schematically in Figure 9.2 and in more detail in Figure 9.9. In most cells the pentose phophate pathway is an essential pathway

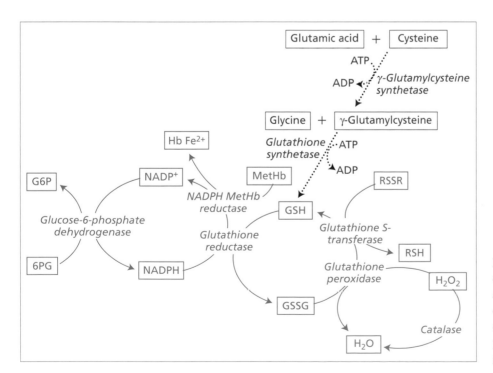

Figure 9.10 The glutathione (GSH) cycle and synthetic pathways. GSH is synthesized in two linked steps. Redox control is exercised by the glutathione cycle linked to the NADPH of the pentose phosphate pathway by glutathione reductase.

for the production of ribose and its incorporation into RNA. In the red cell its only function is the production of reducing power in the form of NADPH. The first step of the pathway, catalysed by G6PD, utilizes G6P as substrate. G6P is also a substrate for the glycolytic pathway. Under normal circumstances, about 10% of glucose is metabolized by the pentose phosphate pathway, the activity of that pathway being determined by the availability of NAD^+ and feedback inhibition by ATP. Under conditions of oxidative stress, the flux through the pentose phosphate pathway can be greatly increased. The products of the pathway re-enter the glycolytic pathway through F6P or Ga3P.

From the point of view of haematological disorders, G6PD deficiency is far and away the most important step in the pathway. However, other enzymes of the pathway can be important in acquired disorders, some steps being inhibited by drugs, including estrogen/progesterone contraceptive pills.

Glucose-6-phosphate dehydrogenase

G6PD catalyses the first step of the pentose phosphate pathway and is the enzyme controlling flux through the pathway. The activity is controlled by the availability of $NADP^+$. Conversion of G6P to 6PG is accompanied by the reduction of $NADP^+$ to NADPH and the second step in the pathway, the oxidation of 6PG to ribose-5-phosphate, produces a second molecule of NADPH.

The gene for G6PD is located on the X chromosome at Xq28. The gene has 13 exons and 12 introns. The gene is transcribed as a monomer of 514 amino acids that assemble to produce an equilibrium of dimers and tetramers (Figure 9.11). Each monomer has an $NADP^+$-binding domain and a large domain with the active site between the two. The gene is a household gene, active in all cells, with an essential role in the production of RNA in nucleated cells. Not surprisingly, the gene is highly conserved in evolutionary history. Complete inactivity of the enzyme in nucleated cells would not be compatible with life. The clinical consequences of G6PD deficiency are virtually confined to the red blood cell, with occasional evidence of leucocyte malfunction in some variants. The majority of mutations affect the stability of the transcribed enzyme so that there is a rapid decline in activity in the mature enucleate red cell as it ages.

In the red cell, G6PD determines the reduction of $NADP^+$ to NADPH (Figure 9.9); $NADP^+$ availability is determined by the activity of the glutathione cycle, which is linked to the pentose phosphate pathway through the activity of the enzyme glutathione reductase (Figure 9.10). The availability of $NADP^+$ is the major rate-limiting step for the pentose phosphate pathway.

Glucose-6-phosphate dehydrogenase deficiency

G6PD deficiency is the commonest genetically determined enzyme deficiency in the world, with an estimated 400 million people being affected. At least 127 different variants associated with deficient enzyme activity have been described, as well as a number of polymorphisms that do not affect enzyme activity. The G6PD variants have been classified into five groups according to their activity relative to the wild-type G6PD type B (Table 9.2). In Africa, the variant G6PD type A^- is the predominant polymorphism, with equivalent activity to G6PD type B.

Epidemiology

G6PD deficiency is widely disseminated throughout Africa, the Mediterranean basin, the Middle East, Southeast Asia and indigenous populations of the Indian subcontinent. G6PD-A^- (with two mutations in the *G6PD* gene; see Figure 9.12) is common in Africa, the Mediterranean variant is comon in southern Italy, Sardinia and other places around the Mediterranean basin, and G6PD-Canton is common in southern China. These variants are only the most common among

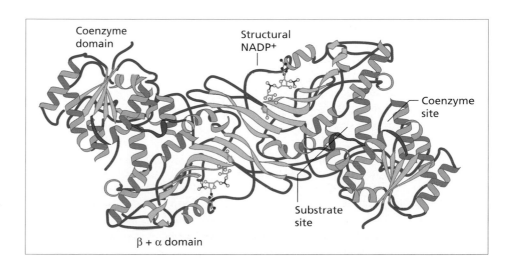

Figure 9.11 Structure of glucose-6-phosphate dehydrogenase in dimer form showing active sites for glucose-6-phosphate and $NADP^+$. Mutations that affect interactions of the monomers lead to CNSHA.

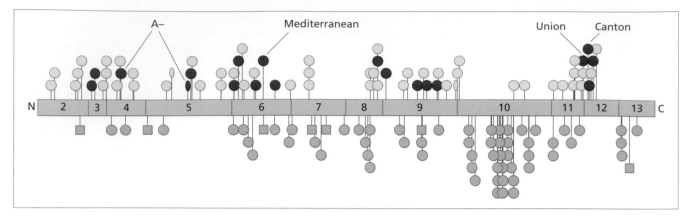

Figure 9.12 Map of glucose-6-phosphate dehydrogenase (*G6PD*) gene showing mutation sites. Numbered boxes refer to the location of *G6PD* exons. Yellow circles, class I and II variants; yellow ellipses, class IV variants; red circles, polymorphic variants; green circles and squares, class I variants caused by amino acid substitutions and small in-frame deletions, respectively. (Courtesy of Tom Vulliamy, Hammersmith Campus, Imperial College, London.)

Table 9.2 World Health Organization classification of G6PD deficiency (1989).

Class	Enzyme activity (% normal)	Examples	Clinical effects
I	Severe (usually <20)	Santiago de Cuba (Gly447Arg)	CNSHA, acute exacerbations
II	<10	Mediterranean (Ser188Phe)	Favism, acute intravascular haemolysis (drug induced), neonatal jaundice
		Canton (Arg459Leu)	
		Orissa (Ala44Gly)	
III	Moderate (>10, <60)	A⁻ (Val68Met, Asn126Asp)	Acute intravascular haemolysis (drug induced), neonatal jaundice
IV	100	B (wild type)	None
		A (Asn126Asp)	None

CNSHA, congenital non-spherocytic haemolytic anaemia.

many different mutations in these areas and throughout the rest of the affected world (Figure 9.13). This distribution of the deficiency equates with areas where *Plasmodium falciparum* malaria is common, and this is thought to be the evolutionary drive that has produced such widespread polymorphisms (Figure 9.13). It has subsequently been confirmed that G6PD deficiency does indeed protect against lethal falciparum malaria, particularly in childhood, and this protection, especially in hyperendemic areas, more than outweighs the haematological problems associated with deficiency.

Clinical features
There are four main syndromes associated with G6PD deficiency. In all four, haemolysis is aggravated or promoted by exposure to oxidative stress through infection or ingestion of oxidative foods or drugs, but the clinical presentations differ. Age always modifies the clinical effects, not always as might be expected. The four syndromes are neonatal jaundice, favism,

chronic non-spherocytic haemolytic anaemia and drug-induced haemolytic anaemia. The neonatal jaundice syndrome has been described in class I, II and III variants, favism in mainly, though not exclusively, class II, CNSHA in class I, and the drug-induced haemolytic anaemias mainly class III. While G6PD deficiency is most common in males, the prevalence of the gene in many parts of the world (Figure 9.13) means that female homozygotes are not uncommon and heterozygous females are often susceptible to oxidative stress because of the effects of X-inactivation and marked lyonization in leaving a significant population of deficient red cells.

Neonatal jaundice and G6PD deficiency in infancy
Neonatal jaundice is a severe manifestation of G6PD deficiency and is a major source of potential morbidity from kernicterus. Most common variants have been associated with the syndrome, including the A⁻ and Mediterranean variants. In parts of the world where the mutations are common, the deficiency

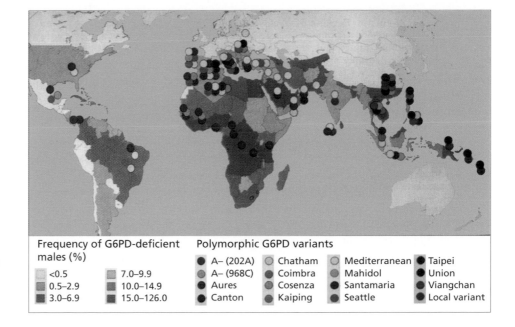

Figure 9.13 Global distribution of *G6PD* gene variants causing G6PD deficiency. Shaded areas indicate the prevalence of G6PD deficiency. The coloured dots depict the distribution of 16 of the most common variants. (From Luzzatto & Notaro 2001 with permission.)

Frequency of G6PD-deficient males (%)	Polymorphic G6PD variants			
<0.5	● A− (202A)	○ Chatham	○ Mediterranean	● Taipei
0.5–2.9	● A− (968C)	● Coimbra	● Mahidol	● Union
3.0–6.9	● Aures	● Cosenza	● Santamaria	● Viangchan
7.0–9.9	● Canton	○ Kaiping	● Seattle	● Local variant
10.0–14.9				
15.0–126.0				

Table 9.3 Association between G6PD deficiency and jaundice in male newborns.*

Groups of newborns	N	G6PD deficiency (%)
Normal	500	22.5
Mild jaundice (bilirubin 150–200 μmol/L)	38	45
Severe jaundice (bilirubin > 230 μmol/L)	70	60
Admitted with kernicterus	20	78

*Data collected in Ibadan, Nigeria.

Table 9.4 Characteristic features of haemolytic attack in G6PD deficiency.

Phase	Clinical	Laboratory
Acute	Abrupt onset	
	Malaise, prostration	
	Pallor	Anaemia, Heinz bodies, reticulocytosis, G6PD deficient
	(Abdominal pain)	
	Fever	Leucocytosis
	Dark urine	Haemoglobinuria, haptoglobin absent
	Haemoglobinaemia	
	Methaemalbuminaemia	
	Jaundice	Hyperbilirubinaemia
	(Renal failure)	↑ Urea, ↑ creatinine
Recovery	Gradual but rapid cessation of haemolysis	Reticulocytes peak days 5–8
	Urine clears in few days	G6PD increases but rarely to normal range
	Jaundice clears in 1–2 weeks	

is the most prevalent cause of neonatal jaundice (Table 9.3). The jaundice probably starts *in utero* in the perinatal period, but the clinical problem only becomes apparent about the second or third day after birth. Between 10 and 50% of deficient infants are affected. Phototherapy or exchange transfusion may be required to prevent neurological sequelae. Anaemia is not a feature, and it is thought that this is a manifestation of liver enzyme deficiency coupled perhaps to the physiological underdevelopment of neonatal liver function or the co-inheritance of the UDP-glucuronyltransferase 1 deficiency of Gilbert syndrome.

Acute haemolytic crises may occur in G6PD-deficient infants, usually through exposure to oxidative stress, including nitrites or nitrates in water or the ingestion of fava beans by the mother, but in some cases of severe acute haemolysis, even fatal, no cause has been obvious.

Favism

Favism is the term given to the G6PD syndrome where acute intravascular haemolysis may be precipitated by exposure to the broad bean *Vicia fava*, usually about 24 hours after the meal (Table 9.4). Fresh, dried or frozen beans or even exposure to pollen may precipitate the crisis. The offending agent is divicine, or its aglycone isouramil, which can produce free oxygen radicals on autoxidation. Divicine is not present in peas or beans of other types, which may be eaten without effect. The amount of haemolysis is dose-related, which may explain the marked variation in susceptibility not only between children and adults but also in the same individual at different times. There is variation in divicine content between different cultivars; some fungi can break down the compound and the amount may vary in different seasonal environments. In children acute haemolysis, sometimes life-threatening, is common but renal failure is uncommon, although there may be systemic symptoms of fever and loin pain. Renal failure occurs more often in adults, possibly because of co-morbidity. Favism is usual in class II variants, for example Mediterranean and Canton, but may occur in others, including the African A- variant. Acute haemolysis after eating fava beans has also been described in glutathione reductase deficiency. Although fava beans give the syndrome its name, some other compounds with which affected individuals may come in contact can cause acute haemolysis, including topical henna and some of the pulses used to make local sweetmeats.

Between attacks of favism or exposure to oxidizing substances, the blood count is normal with no evidence of haemolysis. The co-occurrence of infection, which promotes the formation of hydrogen peroxide following the oxygen burst in neutrophils and macrophages, with ingestion of oxidizing substances, even mild ones such as chloramphenicol, may promote haemolysis even though the drug on its own does not.

Chronic non-spherocytic haemolytic anaemia

Sporadic cases in virtually all populations of CNSHA are found with underlying G6PD deficiency. Many of the mutations that cause CNSHA occur on exon 10 and affect the formation of dimers or tetramers (see Figures 9.11 and 9.12). The haemolysis is extravascular, although additional oxidative stress may provoke an acute intravascular episode.

Drug-induced acute haemolysis

The introduction of primaquine and its derivative pamaquine as antimalarials to replace quinine during the Pacific phase of the Second World War and the later Korean War revealed that a proportion of men exposed, particularly in the black population, suffered from severe acute intravascular haemolysis. Intensive studies by Carson and others from the University of Chicago, working at the Statesville Penitentiary Malaria Project, finally identified the problem as G6PD deficiency and identified that young red cells and reticulocytes had sufficient activity to withstand the oxidative stress so that haemolysis lessened as the reticulocyte level rose. It became apparent that many other drugs could also produce haemolysis, but mostly fava beans did not. The common African A⁻ variant is the main example of class III mutations producing this type of haemolysis.

The haemolysis is dose-related and may be self-limiting. Although it is important to recognize which drugs are likely to produce haemolysis (Table 9.5), it is also important to realize that the disease for which the drugs may be needed, for example falciparum malaria, may be fatal and thus the haemolysis is a lesser problem.

Laboratory diagnosis

Acute intravascular haemolysis raises the suspicion of G6PD deficiency. The blood film shows red cells with contracted haemoglobin in 'ghost' membranes (Figure 9.14). Haemoglobinuria may be gross, producing almost black urine without red cells in the centrifuge deposit.

Several screening tests have been devised to identify G6PD deficiency in red blood cells. The most widely used tests have been the brilliant cresyl blue decolorization test, the methaemoglobin reduction test and an ultraviolet spot test. These tests can reliably distinguish between deficient and non-deficient individuals, but are not reliably quantitative. Hemizygous deficient males and homozygous deficient females will be identified, the threshold being a G6PD activity of about 30% of normal.

If a screening test indicates deficiency or is doubtful, the ideal follow-up test for definitive diagnosis is quantitation of G6PD activity by spectrophotometric assay. Standardized methods have been published. There are two clinical situations in which quantitation is especially important. First, during a haemolytic attack, the oldest red cells (with the least G6PD activity) are destroyed selectively and therefore the surviving red cells have a relatively higher (but still deficient) G6PD activity. This increases further as the reticulocyte response sets in over the following days. During this time, a screening test might yield a

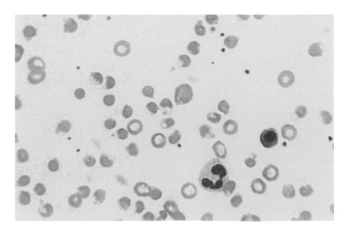

Figure 9.14 Glucose-6-phosphate dehydrogenase deficiency. Peripheral blood film following acute oxidant drug-induced haemolysis shows an erythroblast and damaged red cells, including 'blister' and 'bite' cells.

Table 9.5 Drugs to be avoided in G6PD deficiency.*

Antimalarials
Primaquine (can be given at reduced dosage, 15 mg daily or
   45 mg twice weekly under survelliance)
Pamaquine

Sulphonamides and sulphones
Sulfanilamide
Sulfapyridine
Sulfadimidine
Sulfacetamide (Albucid)
Sulfasalazine (Salazopyrin)
Dapsone[†]
Sulfoxone[†]
Glucosulfone sodium (Promin)
Septrin

Other antibacterial compounds
Nitrofurans: nitrofurantoin, furazolidone, nitrofurazone,
   nalidixic acid

Analgesics
Acetylsalicylic acid (aspirin): moderate doses can be used
Acetophenetidin (phenacetin): paracetamol is a safe alternative

Anthelminthics
β-Naphthol
Stibophan
Niridazole

Miscellaneous
Vitamin K analogues (1 mg menadoxime can be given to babies)
Naphthalene (mothballs)[†]
Probenecid
Dimercaprol (BAL)
Methylene blue
Toluidine blue

*This list is compiled on the basis of data available for patients
with the A⁻ variant of G6PD deficiency. It can be generally
assumed to be applicable to patients from Africa and of African
descent. For patients with the Mediterranean type of G6PD
deficiency, with an unknown variant, or with CNSHA, the
following should also be added: acetanilide, chloramphenicol,
chloroquine (may be used under surveillance when required for
prophylaxis or treatment of malaria), mepacrine, *p*-aminosalicylic
acid and thiazosulfone. Many other drugs may produce
haemolysis in particular individuals.
[†]These drugs may cause haemolysis in normal individuals if taken
in large doses.

false-normal result and, rarely, even a quantitative test might
do so. In such cases, the best counsel is to repeat the test a
couple of weeks later. Alternatively, the oldest remaining cells
can be isolated by differential centrifugation and they can be
shown to have low G6PD activity. The diagnosis of heterozygous females can be especially difficult; in extreme cases, it
can only be done by family studies. However, from the practical
point of view, it must be borne in mind that the probability of
clinically significant haemolysis in a heterozygote roughly correlates with the proportion of G6PD-deficient red cells in her
blood. Therefore, if a normal level of G6PD activity is found in
a heterozygote, she is unlikely to be at risk of G6PD-related
haemolysis. In regions where G6PD has a high prevalence and
the main variants are known, DNA analysis is the most effective
way of identifying heterozygotes.

Management

Management is mostly dictated by the symptoms and signs in
the patient, although education in the avoidance of oxidizing
substances is important (Table 9.5). In many populations the
condition is well known and the need for avoidance recognized.
Neonatal jaundice may need urgent therapy to prevent neurological damage (Table 9.3). Extreme hyperbilirubinaemia can
be prevented by administration of Sn-mesoporphyrin if the
diagnosis is known at birth. Acute intravascular haemolysis may
require transfusion but the anaemia is often self-limiting (Table
9.4). High fluid intake should be encouraged to prevent renal
damage. CNSHA may be severe enough to warrant active treatment and splenectomy may be helpful.

Glutathione

GSH is the major intracellular thiol in aerobic cells, and is
equally important in the red blood cell. It is thought to have a
number of critical functions: protecting cells against oxidative
damage, participation in detoxification of foreign compounds,
maintenance of protein sulphydryl groups in a reduced state,
and possibly transport of amino acids. In the red cell, its main
function is as an antioxidant. GSH is synthesized from glutamate, cysteine and glycine by the link reactions of two enzymes,
γ-glutamylcysteine synthetase and glutathione synthetase (see
Figure 9.10). GSH exerts its function in preserving thiol groups
and reducing hydrogen peroxide and free oxygen radicals
through reactions catalysed by the enzymes glutathione-*S*-
transferase and glutathione peroxidase, respectively. Oxidized
glutathione (GSSG) is reduced to GSH by the action of glutathione reductase, the hydrogen donor being NADPH (see Figure
9.10). Failure to maintain the GSH level as a result of deficiency
in the synthetic pathways or deficiency in the recycling process
leads to chronic haemolytic anaemia and increased susceptibility to oxidative stress.

Table 9.6 Enzymopathies of the glutathione cycle and synthetic pathways.

Enzyme	Gene	Haematology	Other systems	Comments
Glutathione synthetase	GSS, 20q11.2 AR	CNSHA, Heinz bodies, oxidative HA	Neurological, metabolic acidosis	5-Oxoprolinaemia/uria, RBC deficiency, may have no neurological disease, nine families
γ-Glutamylcysteine synthetase	GCLC, 6p12 GCLM, 1p21 AR	CNSHA, oxidative HA, basophilic stippling	Neurological	Variable neurological features, five families
Glutathione reductase	GSR, 8p21.1 AR	Favism	None	Most reports due to FAD deficiency, one family
Glutathione peroxidase	GPX1, 3p21.3 AR	HDN, acute intravascular haemolytic anaemia	None	Self-limited neonatal jaundice, one Japanese family

AR, autosomal recessive; CNSHA, congenital non-spherocytic haemolytic anaemia; FAD, flavin adenine dinucleotide; HDN, haemolytic disease of the newborn.

Glutathione deficiency

Complete loss of GSH synthesis is probably lethal. Severe deficiency leads to 5-oxoprolinuria, metabolic acidosis and mental retardation. A milder deficiency limited to red cells is associated with haemolytic anaemia aggravated by oxidative stress. Low levels of GSH caused by γ-glutamylcysteine synthetase or glutathione synthetase deficiency, with CNSHA, have been described. Haemolytic anaemia due to deficiency of glutathione reductase and glutathione peroxidase has also been reported (Table 9.6).

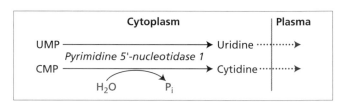

Figure 9.15 Pyrimidine nucleotide catabolism in the reticulocyte. Pyrimidine 5′-nucleotidase converts the nucleotides to monophosphates, which diffuse out of the cell.

Nucleotide metabolism

Adenosine nucleotides – ATP (85–90%), ADP (10–12%) and AMP (1–3%) – comprise the main nucleotide pool in the mature red cell. The cell has no mechanism for making nucleotides once the RNA of the reticulocytes has been degraded. The cell does have an effective salvage mechanism for maintenance of the adenine pool, with the enzymes adenosine deaminase (ADA) and adenylate kinase involved in regulation. Deficiency of the enzymes in the salvage pathway does not lead to haemolysis. ADA deficiency is associated with severe combined immunodeficiency and excess activity is found in Diamond–Blackfan anaemia. During maturation of reticulocytes the RNA is broken down to pyrimidine and purine nucleotides, which are dephosphorylated to nucleosides that can diffuse out of the cell. The purine nucleotides enter the salvage pathway. Deficiency of pyrimidine 5′-nucleotidase leads to accumulation of pyrimidine nucleotides that interferes with the adenine nucleotide pool, producing haemolysis.

Pyrimidine 5′-nucleotidase

Pyrimidine 5′-nucleotidase (P5N), also called pyrimidine 5′-monophosphate hydrolase, catalyses the dephosphorylation of the pyrimidine 5′-monophosphates uridine monophosphate (UMP) and cytidine monophosphate (CMP) to corresponding nucleosides (Figure 9.15). In red blood cells, there are two isoforms of P5N, type 1 (P5N1), which has a high affinity for UMP and CMP, and type 2 (P5N2), which hydrolyses deoxypyrimidine nucleotide monophosphates. It is deficiency of P5N1 that leads to haemolytic anaemia. The gene (NT5C3, also named P5′N1) is located on chromosome 7p14.3. The gene consists of 10 exons with alternative splicing at exon 2, which gives rise to isoforms with 286 and 297 amino acids. The P5N1 enzyme corresponds to the 286-amino-acid isoform. The enzyme is strongly inhibited by lead.

Pyrimidine 5′-nucleotidase deficiency
P5N1 deficiency is not uncommon: more than 60 patients have been reported worldwide, with presumably large numbers

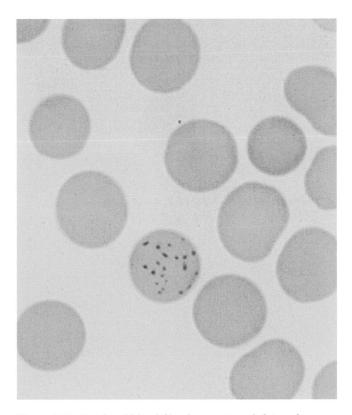

Figure 9.16 Peripheral blood film from patient deficient for pyrimidine 5′-nucleotidase showing basophilic stippling (a similar appearance is seen in chronic lead poisoning).

undetected. The prevalence of P5N1 deficiency is unknown. It is probably the third most common enzyme deficiency causing haemolytic anaemia, perhaps equal to GPI deficiency. Nearly all reported cases have shown homozygosity for the mutation, and the mutation has been specific for individual families. However, there is a suggestion that certain mutations (del G576 and ins GG743) might be more prevalent in southern Italy or southern Mediterranean regions. One compound heterozygote was found in this region.

Deficiency of P5N1 is associated with a recessively inherited haemolytic anaemia characterized by marked basophilic stippling in the red cells (Figure 9.16) and accumulation of high concentrations of pyrimidine nucleotides. The haemolysis is usually mild to moderate, although more severe cases have been reported. Splenectomy is usually of little value, though benefit has been reported in some cases. The appearance of the blood film is similar to that seen in lead poisoning, and the mechanism of the anaemia in lead poisoning certainly involves the inhibition of P5N.

Selected bibliography

General and reviews

Dacie JV (1999) *The Haemolytic Anaemias*, 3rd edn, Vol. 1. Churchill Livingstone, London.

Durand PM, Coetzer TL (2008) Hereditary red cell disorders and malaria resistance. *Haematologica* **93**: 961–3.

Roper D, Layton M, Lewis SM (2001) Investigation of the hereditary haemolytic anaemias: membrane and enzyme abnormalities. In: *Dacie and Lewis Practical Haematology* (SM Lewis, BJ Bain, I Bates, eds), 9th edn, pp. 167–98. Churchill Livingstone, London.

Steiner LA, Gallagher PG (2007) Erythrocyte disorders in the perinatal period. *Seminars in Perinatology* **31**: 254–61.

van Wijk R, van Solinge WW (2005) The energy-less red blood cell is lost: erythrocyte enzyme abnormalities of glycolysis. *Blood* **106**: 4034–42.

Zanella A (2000) Inherited disorders of red cell metabolism. *Baillières Best Practice andt Research. Clinical Haematology* **13**: 1–148.

Enzyme deficiencies of the Embden–Meyerhof pathway

Pyruvate kinase deficiency

Beutler E, Gelbart T (2000) PK deficiency prevalence and the limitations of a population-based survey [Letter]. *Blood* **96**: 4005–6.

Hipkins R, Thompson J, Naidoo P, Bishay E, Djearaman M, Pratt G (2009) Paravertebral extramedullary haemopoiesis associated with pyruvate kinase deficiency. *British Journal of Haematology* **147**: 275.

Marshall SR, Saunders PWG, Hamilton PJ *et al.* (2000) The dangers of iron overload in pyruvate kinase deficiency. *British Journal of Haematology* **120**: 1090–1.

Wax JR, Pinette MG, Cartin A, Blackstone J (2007) Pyruvate kinase deficiency complicating pregnancy. *Obstetrics and Gynecology* **109**: 553–5.

Zanella A, Bianchi P (2000) Red cell pyruvate kinase deficiency: from genetics to clinical manifestations. *Baillières Best Practice and Research. Clinical Haematology* **13**: 57–81.

Zanella A, Bianchi P, Fermo E (2007) Pyruvate kinase deficiency. *Haematologica* **92**: 721–3.

Zanella A, Fermo E, Bianchi P, Chiarelli LR, Valentini G (2007) Pyruvate kinase deficiency: the genotype–phenotype association. *Blood Reviews* **21**: 217–31.

Other enzymes of the Embden–Meyerhof pathway

Beutler E (2007) PGK deficiency. *British Journal of Haematology* **136**: 3–11.

Corrons JL, Alvarez R, Pujades A *et al.* (2001) Hereditary nonspherocytic haemolytic anaemia due to red blood cell glutathione synthetase deficiency in four unrelated patients from Spain: clinical and molecular studies. *British Journal of Haematology* **112**: 475–82.

Fujii H, Miwa S (2000) Other erythrocyte enzyme deficiencies associated with non-haematological symptoms: phosphoglycerate kinase and phosphofructokinase deficiency. *Baillières Best Practice and Research. Clinical Haematology* **13**: 141–8.

Kanno H (2000) Hexokinase: gene structure and mutations. *Baillières Best Practice and Research. Clinical Haematology* **13**: 83–8.

Kreuder J, Borkhardt A, Repp R *et al.* (1996) Brief report: inherited metabolic myopathy and hemolysis due to a mutation in aldolase A. *New England Journal of Medicine* **334**: 1101–4.

McCann SR, Finkel B, Cadman S *et al.* (1976) Study of a kindred with hereditary spherocytosis and glyceraldehyde-3-phosphate dehydrogenase deficiency. *Blood* **47**: 171–81.

Morimoto A, Ueda I, Hirashima Y *et al.* (2003) A novel missense mutation (1060G→C) in the phosphoglycerate kinase gene in a Japanese boy with chronic haemolytic anaemia, developmental delay and rhabdomyolysis. *British Journal of Haematology* **122**: 1009–13.

Murakmi K, Kanno H, Tancabelic J *et al.* (2002) Gene expression and biological significance of hexokinase in erythroid cells. *Acta Haematologica* **108**: 204–9.

Nakajima H, Raben N, Hamaguchi T, Yamasaki T (2002) Phosphofructokinase deficiency: past, present and future. *Current Molecular Medicine* **2**: 197–212.

Orosz F, Oláh J, Ovádi J (2006) Triosephosphate isomerase deficiency: facts and doubts. *IUBMB Life* **58**: 703–15.

Valentin C, Pissard S, Martin J *et al.* (2000) Triose phosphate isomerase deficiency in three French families: two novel null alleles, a frameshift mutation (TPI Alfortville), and an alteration in the initiation codon (TPI Paris). *Blood* **96**: 1130–5.

Yao DC, Tolan DR, Murray MF *et al.* (2004) Haemolytic anaemia and severe rhabdomyolysis caused by compound heterozygous mutations of the gene for erythrocyte/muscle isozyme of aldolase, ALDOA(Arg303X/Cys338Tyr). *Blood* **103**: 2401–3.

Glucose-6-phosphate dehydrogenase deficiency

Reviews

Cappellini MD, Fiorelli G (2008) Glucose-6-phosphate dehydrogenase deficiency. *Lancet* **371**: 64–74.

Kwok CJ, Martin ACR, Au SWN *et al.* (2002) G6PDdb, an integrated database of glucose-6-phosphate dehydrogenase (G6PD) mutations. *Human Mutation* **19**: 217–24.

Mason PJ, Bautista JM, Gilsanz F (2007) G6PD deficiency: the genotype–phenotype association. *Blood Reviews* **21**: 267–83.

Glucose-6-phosphate dehydrogenase deficiency, evolution and malaria

Beutler E, Duparc S (2007) G6PD Deficiency Working Group. Glucose-6-phosphate dehydrogenase deficiency and antimalarial drug development. *American Journal of Tropical Medicine and Hygiene* **77**: 779–89.

Luzzatto L, Notaro R (2001) Malaria. Protecting against bad air. *Science* **293**: 442–3.

Notaro R, Afolayan A, Luzzatto L (2000) Human mutations in glucose 6-phosphate dehydrogenase reflect evolutionary history. *FASEB Journal* **14**: 485–94.

Tishkoff SA, Varkonyi R, Cahinhinan N *et al.* (2001) Haplotype diversity and linkage disequilibrium at human G6PD: recent origin of alleles that confer malarial resistance. *Science* **293**: 455–62.

Glucose-6-phosphate dehydrogenase deficiency in newborn

Kappas A, Drummond GS, Valaes TA (2001) Single dose of Sn-mesoporphyrin prevents development of severe hyperbilirubinemia in glucose-6-phosphate dehydrogenase-deficient newborns. *Pediatrics* **108**: 25–30.

Watchko JF (2009) Identification of neonates at risk for hazardous hyperbilirubinemia: emerging clinical insights. *Pediatric Clinics of North America* **56**: 671–87.

Molecular pathology

Beutler E, Westwood B, Prchal JT *et al.* (1992) New glucose-6-phosphate dehydrogenase mutations from various ethnic groups. *Blood* **80**: 255–6.

Vulliamy TJ, D'Urso M, Battistuzzi G *et al.* (1988) Diverse point mutations in the human glucose-6-phosphate dehydrogenase gene cause enzyme deficiency and mild or severe haemolytic anaemia. *Proceedings of the National Academy of Sciences USA* **85**: 5171–5.

Vulliamy T, Beutler E, Luzzatto L (1993) Variants of glucose-6-phosphate dehydrogenase are due to missense mutations spread throughout the coding region of the gene. *Human Mutation* **2**: 159–67.

Susceptibility to infection

Costa E, Vasconcelos J, Santos E *et al.* (2002) Neutrophil dysfunction in a case of glucose-6-phosphate dehydrogenase deficiency. *Journal of Pediatric Hematology/Oncology* **24**: 164–5.

Mallouh AA, Abu-Osba YK (1987) Bacterial infections in children with glucose-6-phosphate dehydrogenase deficiency. *Journal of Pediatrics* **111**: 850–2.

van Bruggen R, Bautista JM, Petropoulou T *et al.* (2002) Deletion of leucine 61 in glucose-6-phosphate dehydrogenase leads to chronic nonspherocytic anaemia, granulocyte dysfunction, and increased susceptibility to infections. *Blood* **100**: 1026–30.

Assays

Beutler E (1984) *Red Cell Metabolism. A Manual of Biochemical Methods*, 2nd edn. Grune and Stratton, Orlando, FL.

Beutler E, Blume KG, Kaplan JC *et al.* (1979) International Committee for Standardization in Haematology: recommended screening test for glucose-6-phosphate dehydrogenase (G-6-PD) deficiency. *British Journal of Haematology* **43**: 465–7.

Roper D, Layton M, Lewis SM (2001) Investigation of the hereditary haemolytic anaemias: membrane and enzyme abnormalities. In: *Dacie and Lewis Practical Haematology* (SM Lewis, BJ Bain, I Bates, eds), 9th edn, pp. 167–198. Churchill Livingstone, London.

WHO Working Group (1989) Glucose-6-phosphate dehydrogenase deficiency. *Bulletin of the World Health Organization* **67**: 601–11.

Clinical

Kamerbeek NM, van Zwieten R, de Boer M *et al.* (2007) Molecular basis of glutathione reductase deficiency in human blood cells. *Blood* **109**: 3560–6.

Ronquist G, Theodorsson E (2007) Inherited, non-spherocytic haemolysis due to deficiency of glucose-6-phosphate dehydrogenase. *Scandinavian Journal of Clinical and Laboratory Investigation* **67**: 105–11.

Pyrimidine 5′-nucleotidase deficiency

Chiarelli LR, Fermo E, Zanella A, Valentini G (2006) Hereditary erythrocyte pyrimidine 5′-nucleotidase deficiency: a biochemical, genetic and clinical overview. *Hematology* **11**: 67–72.

Rees DC, Duley JA, Marinaki AM (2003) Pyrimidine 5′-nucelotidase deficiency. *British Journal of Haematology* **120**: 375–83.

Vives-Corrons JL (2000) Chronic non-spherocytic anaemia due to congenital pyrimidine 5′-nucleotidase deficiency: 25 years later. *Baillières Best Practice and Research. Clinical Haematology* **13**: 103–18.

Zanella A, Bianchi P, Fermo E, Valentini G (2006) Hereditary pyrimidine 5′-nucleotidase deficiency: from genetics to clinical manifestations. *British Journal of Haematology* **133**: 113–23.

CHAPTER 10

Acquired haemolytic anaemias

10

Edward C Gordon-Smith[1] and Modupe O Elebute[2]

[1]St George's Hospital Medical School, London, UK
[2]King's College Hospital, London, UK

Introduction

Acquired haemolytic anaemias are usually divided into two main categories depending on the mechanism by which the premature destruction of red blood cells is produced. In the immune haemolytic anaemias, antibodies are the main agents of destruction. The non-immune acquired haemolytic anaemias include diverse causes and mechanisms of haemolysis. In most anaemias, there is some shortening of red cell survival, but in the haemolytic anaemias this shortening of red cell lifespan is the major cause of the anaemia and produces the classical features of haemolysis.

Immune haemolytic anaemias

Antibody-mediated haemolysis is an important cause of acquired haemolytic anaemia. Antibodies may be autoantibodies produced by the patient's own immune system and directed against epitopes of his/her own red cell antigens or they may be alloantibodies. Alloantibodies may be produced by the patient and directed against antigens not present on that person's own red cells, but either introduced as foreign red cell antigens by blood transfusion or secondarily acquired by the patient's red cells, as in drug-induced haemolysis. Alloantibodies directed against the patient's red cell antigens might also be introduced from outside the patient, most notably from the mother in haemolytic disease of the newborn. A simple classification of immune haemolytic anaemias is given in Table 10.1. Typically, the immune haemolytic anaemias are distinguished from the

Postgraduate Haematology: 6th edition. Edited by A. Victor Hoffbrand, Daniel Catovsky, Edward G.D. Tuddenham, Anthony R. Green
© 2011 Blackwell Publishing Ltd.

non-immune by detecting antibody on the surface of red cells by the direct antiglobulin test (DAT), also known as the Coombs test.

Autoimmune haemolytic anaemia

Autoimmune haemolytic anaemia (AIHA) is characterized by a positive Coombs test or DAT, which detects antibody, with or without complement, on the red blood cell surface. AIHA is classified into warm and cold types, depending on whether the antibody reacts more strongly with red blood cells at 37°C or at 4°C and whether IgG (warm) or IgM (cold) autoantibody predominates. Haemolysis is mainly extravascular in AIHA, although complement-mediated intravascular haemolysis may sometimes occur in either type. Red blood cells coated with IgG only are preferentially destroyed in the spleen, but if they are also coated with complement or with complement alone, their main site of destruction is the liver. The site and severity of red cell destruction depend on structural and functional characteristics of the antibody and efficiency of the mechanism of destruction. The degree of anaemia depends on the rate and acuteness of the destruction and the capacity of the bone marrow to compensate.

AIHA may occur without any underlying cause (as primary or idiopathic conditions) or may be associated with other systemic autoimmune disease (such as systemic lupus erythematosus and rheumatoid arthritis), malignancy (lymphoma, thymoma and chronic lymphocytic leukaemia) or drug exposure. In many cases, the pathogenesis involves a disturbance of the immune system in which T-lymphocyte control of autoreactive B lymphocyte clones is reduced.

Antibody characteristics

Antibody characteristics that influence the site and intensity of red cell destruction in AIHA can be evaluated using the DAT.

Table 10.1 Classification of immune haemolytic anaemias.

Antigen type	Antibody	Diseases	Associations
Autoimmune	Warm antibody	Primary	Idiopathic
		Secondary	Autoimmune diseases (SLE, etc.)
			Lymphoproliferative disorders
			Infections (EBV)
			Ovarian cysts
			Some cancers
			Drugs
	Cold antibody	Cold haemagglutinin disease	
		Cold antibody syndromes	Infections, lymphoproliferative disorders
	Donath–Landsteiner	Paroxysmal cold haemoglobinuria	Post viral, syphilis
Alloimmune	Induced by red cell antigens	Haemolytic transfusion reactions	
		Haemolytic disease of the newborn	
		Post-stem cell allografts	
	Drug dependent	Antibody/macrophage mediated	
		Antibody/complement mediated	
		Membrane modification	

EBV, Epstein–Barr virus; SLE, systemic lupus erythematosus.

The thermal range of antibody binding also characterizes the antibody.

Immunoglobulin class

Monospecific antihuman globulin reagents for the DAT are routinely available for the detection of IgG, IgM and IgA and for complement components C3c and C3d. Multispecific reagents are also available, as are reagents specific for IgG subclasses, but the latter are difficult to standardize.

Warm-acting antibodies

Warm-acting antibodies are most active *in vitro* at 37°C. The antibodies are polyclonal, and IgG antibodies predominate. Where the specificity of the antibody can be determined, it is most commonly in the rhesus blood group complex. The most frequent patterns detected by the DAT on the red cell surface are as follows: IgG alone; IgG and complement; and complement alone. Antibodies may be detected in the serum at 37°C by the indirect antiglobulin test in about 50–60% of patients; this will rise to more than 90% when the red cell membrane of the reagent cells is modified with papain or another proteolytic enzyme. Antibody may also be eluted from the red cell membrane in a majority of cases and the specificity determined. A subtype of warm AIHA has been defined in which both warm- and cold-type antibodies are found. Both tend to be lytic, and this 'mixed type' AIHA tends to produce a more severe haemolysis with an intravascular component. It is most commonly associated with systemic lupus erythematosus (SLE) or lymphoproliferative disease.

Cold-acting antibodies

Cold-acting antibodies are predominantly IgM and are most actively bound to antigen in the cold (4°C). Cold antibodies act as both agglutinins and lysins *in vitro*; the two functions may have different thermal ranges. The clinical significance of the antibody depends purely on the thermal range: how the antibody binds to red cells at or near 37°C, not the titre in the cold. IgM antibodies active against I (auto)antigen at 4°C are a normal finding but produce no clinical disturbance if not active above 31°C. The IgM antibodies have specificity mainly for the I antigen, although i specificity may be found in Epstein–Barr virus (EBV)-associated antibodies and some cases of lymphoproliferative disease. Rarely, anti-P activity is found. *In vitro*, the IgM antibodies elute off the red cell membrane, usually leaving bound complement to be detected by anti-C3d in the DAT. In cold haemagglutinin disease (CHAD) and most cases associated with lymphoproliferative disease, the cold antibodies are monoclonal (IgM κ). Those associated with viral infections are polyclonal.

The antibodies in a subtype of cold AIHA, paroxysmal cold haemoglobinuria (PCH), are IgG in type and bind to antigen below 20°C. When the temperature is raised to 37°C in the presence of complement, lysis occurs. This biphasic reaction is the basis of the Donath–Landsteiner reaction.

Complement activation

Autoantibodies against red cell antigens may activate complement on the red cell membrane. Antibody binding to two adjacent sites on the red cell membrane is required to activate the C1 complement component by the classical pathway. IgM molecules are pentameric and a single molecule can bind adjacent sites. IgG molecules will activate complement if they form a 'doublet': IgG1, IgG2 and IgG3 can activate complement, whereas IgG4 and IgA do not. In AIHA, complement activation usually stops at the C3 stage, where C3b is bound to the membrane and further proteolysed to form the inactive component C3d, which is detected by the appropriate DAT. Complement beyond the C3 stage may lead to the formation of the membrane attack complex and intravascular haemolysis. AIHA due to IgG2 alone is very rare, and that due to IgG4 or IgA alone is uncommon. It is interesting that in the rare case of IgA AIHA, complement does become activated on the cell surface. In general, when there is more than one class or subclass of antibody on the cell surface, the haemolysis is more intense and may be intravascular.

Specificity of red cell autoantibodies

Warm-type autoimmune haemolytic anaemia

In most cases, the antibody detected in the patient's serum is pan-reacting with all cells in a routine group O panel. Some 10–15% of antibodies show specificity for rhesus antigens, particularly anti-e, anti-D or anti-c. A greater proportion show specificity by reacting with all cells except –/– Rh^{null} cells. Other rare specificities against high-frequency antigens include anti-En^a, anti-Wr^b or anti-U. Usually, autoantibodies show reactivity against a number of antigens and are not as specific as alloantibodies.

Cold-type autoimmune haemolytic anaemia

In cold agglutinin syndrome, anti-i specificity is usually seen. Occasionally, there is specificity for anti-I, and even more rarely for anti-Pr, anti-P, anti-M or anti-N, and even cold-reacting anti-A or anti-B. In PCH, the specificity is anti-P.

Effector mechanisms for immune red cell destruction in vivo

Two main effector mechanisms exist *in vivo*: (i) cell-mediated, predominantly extravascular, immune destruction and (ii) complement-mediated intravascular haemolysis.

Cell-mediated immune red cell destruction

Human macrophages and monocytes have cell-surface receptors for the Fc portion of IgG and for antigenic determinants present on activated C3. Cellular immune destruction is mediated through these receptors. Neutrophils and lymphocytes also have these receptors, but macrophages of the reticuloendothelial system within the spleen, liver and bone marrow are the main site of destruction *in vivo*.

Fc receptor mechanism

Macrophages have Fc receptors for IgG1 and IgG3 molecules, but not for IgG2, IgG4, IgM or IgA. Only IgG-coated red cells are destroyed in this way, but this is clinically important in warm AIHA as 70–75% of autoantibodies are IgG. Phagocytosis and antibody-dependent cell-mediated cytotoxicity are the major Fc receptor-dependent modes of antibody-coated cell destruction.

The role of the spleen

The splenic vasculature is adapted to make the spleen an efficient filter for such particles as effete red cells, bacteria and immune complexes. As blood passes through the central arteries towards the red pulp, the branches of these arteries have a plasma-skimming effect that raises the haematocrit of the blood as it passes towards the splenic cords. There, red cells come into close contact with the splenic macrophages. The low plasma content and the relative lack of free plasma IgG molecules allow red cell-bound IgG to interact preferentially with the macrophage Fc receptors, leading to phagocytosis of the coated red cells. When phagocytosis is partial, so that only portions of the cell membrane are removed, the remaining circulating red cell becomes spherocytic, although the somewhat rigid spherocytes may themselves be trapped in the splenic sinusoids and destroyed. The spleen is thus most commonly the major site of red cell destruction when IgG alone is the main Fc-binding protein on the red cell surface (see Chapter 20).

The role of the liver

Kupffer cells are macrophages that are present in the liver sinusoids and which express Fc receptors on their surface. Blood flow through the sinusoids is rapid compared with the spleen and there is no plasma-skimming effect. IgG-coated red cells are not preferentially destroyed in this situation, where there is competition for Fc receptors from circulating IgG. Here, red cell destruction is more dependent on cells being coated with C3.

C3 receptor mechanisms

Two types of C3 receptor have been identified on macrophages, CR1 and CR3. CR1 is specific for an antigenic site in the C3c region of activated C3b that is not exposed on native C3. The breakdown product of C3b (iC3b) is also a major ligand for CR1 and is the only ligand for CR3. Immune adherence of C3b-coated red cells to macrophages occurs mainly through CR1, whereas CR3 binding triggers phagocytosis. The largest concentration of C3b-binding macrophages is found in the liver sinusoids so that the liver becomes the major site for trapping and phagocytosing C3b-coated red cells. There is no competition for complement receptor sites from non-activated C3 in the plasma. If the spleen is very large, this too becomes an important site of cell destruction.

In cold AIHA, IgM agglutinins bind most avidly to red cells in the peripheral circulation, where the temperature may be as low as 10–20°C. Complement activation occurs and leads to C3b and iC3d expression on the red cell membrane. Macrophage destruction of red cells is the main mechanism of haemolysis in IgM cold antibody-coated cells and also occurs in warm AIHA as a result of complement-fixing IgG and IgM antibodies.

Complement-mediated intravascular haemolysis

Intravascular complement-mediated haemolysis is a minor mechanism for red cell destruction in most patients with AIHA. In a small proportion of patients, such a mechanism may predominate and produce severe intravascular haemolysis. Complement-induced intravascular haemolysis in warm AIHA is most likely to occur when more than one class or subclass of immunoglobulin is present on the red cell surface. Intravascular haemolysis has been reported with IgA-coated red cells, although the mechanism is obscure, as IgA does not itself fix complement.

In cold AIHA syndromes, intravascular haemolysis may be precipitated by exposure to cold. In such cases, lytic as well as agglutinating antibodies with a high thermal range may be demonstrated *in vitro*. This pattern is not uncommon in cold AIHA associated with *Mycoplasma pneumoniae*. Acute intravascular haemolysis is the usual presentation in PCH, where the antibody is IgG in type.

Other factors influencing red cell destruction and production

Bone marrow function

The ability of the marrow to increase erythropoiesis may be impaired. Autoantibodies may be produced, which act against reticulocytes and erythroblasts, as well as mature red cells. Red cell production may also be reduced by folate deficiency secondary to the increased demand. Lymphoproliferative diseases may impair production through infiltration of the marrow.

Reticuloendothelial function

The severity of cellular immune red cell destruction depends largely on macrophage function. Reticuloendothelial function may be reduced in SLE by the clearance of immune complexes, a process known as reticuloendothelial blockade. In methyldopa-induced AIHA, the drug has been shown to reduce reticuloendothelial clearance of IgG-coated red cells, which might explain why many patients with a strongly positive DAT due to methyldopa have little or no haemolysis.

Hypocomplementaemia

Partial protection from complement-mediated lysis may occur in patients with chronic CHAD, in which continuous complement activation may lead to relative complement deficiency. Hypocomplementaemia is common in SLE and may also be caused by chronic activation of the complement pathway. In addition, there is a strong association between SLE and the occurrence of null alleles for the C2 and C4 genes, which causes a genetically determined complement deficiency.

Warm-type autoimmune haemolytic anaemias

Clinical features

Warm-type AIHA affects all age groups and accounts for up to 70% of AIHA cases. Haemolysis is caused by high-affinity IgG antibodies produced by reactive polyclonal B cells. An underlying or associated disorder can be identified in 50–70% of cases. Presentation is variable and depends on the speed with which anaemia develops, the capacity of the bone marrow to compensate and the effects of any associated disease. Most commonly, the onset is insidious, with the gradual awareness of symptoms of anaemia or the observation of pallor or icterus by friends or relatives. Occasionally, the onset is acute, with rapidly developing anaemia and, in older patients, the risk of heart failure. Rarely, severe cases can occur with fulminating haemolysis, resulting in life-threatening anaemia. Mild jaundice is present. A moderate increase in unconjugated serum bilirubin and excess urinary urobilinogen occurs as a result of extravascular haemolysis. Intravascular haemolysis occurs occasionally, leading to dark urine caused by haemoglobinuria and haemosiderinuria. More marked icterus (bilirubin >90 μmol/L) suggests coexisting liver disease or biliary tract obstruction due to pigment gallstones or biliary sludge. Mild splenomegaly is common, rarely more than 2–3 cm below the costal margin at presentation. Marked splenomegaly suggests the possibility of a lymphoproliferative disease. Reticulocytosis is present, and the peripheral blood film is characterized by polychromasia, spherocytes (Figure 10.1), circulating nucleated red cells and, in some cases, red cell agglutination. Rarely, there may be reticu-

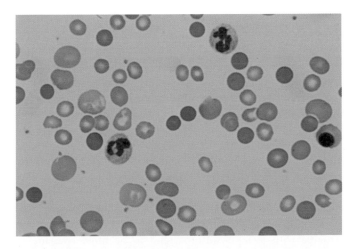

Figure 10.1 Warm autoimmune haemolytic anaemia. Blood film showing spherocytosis, polychromasia and nucleated red blood cell (×40).

locytopenia associated with a positive DAT. There is an increase in lactate dehydrogenase (LDH) due to lysis of red cells, but other liver function tests are normal unless there is associated liver or biliary tract disease. The DAT is positive, most commonly as a result of the presence of red cells coated with IgG alone (mainly IgG1 and IgG3 subclasses) or IgG and complement (the latter pattern commonly seen in SLE). Autoantibody in the serum may show specificity within the rhesus system (e.g. auto-anti-e), but in most cases is pan-reactive with all red blood cells. The autoantibody reacts at 37°C. In very rare cases the amount of antibody remaining on the red cell surface is insufficient to be detected by the conventional DAT.

Idiopathic warm AIHA

In approximately 30% of patients with a DAT-positive haemolytic anaemia, no associated disorder is found. Idiopathic AIHA may occur at any age. There is a peak incidence during infancy and early childhood and a second rise during the third decade, with the majority of cases occurring after the fifth decade. There is a preponderance of female patients in both idiopathic and secondary AIHA. A careful drug history should always be taken to exclude drug-induced AIHA, and chemical exposure at work or in the domestic environment must be assessed. In girls, AIHA may precede clinical or immunological evidence of SLE, so that negative serology for SLE does not exclude the disease at a later date. As mentioned above, the presentation may vary from the gradual onset of anaemia to an acute haemolytic process. Systemic symptoms are rare other than those of anaemia. Pallor, jaundice and mild splenomegaly (usually to between one and a half to five times its normal size) are present. Enlargement of the spleen to the umbilicus or below is not a feature of idiopathic AIHA and suggests a secondary cause.

Evans syndrome

This is defined as the combination of AIHA and immune thrombocytopenia (ITP) in the absence of any underlying disease. The occurrence of thrombocytopenia may coincide with the haemolysis or may arise as separate episodes. The platelet and red cell antibodies are distinct and do not cross-react. Rarely, episodes of immune neutropenia or pancytopenia have also been described in association with a positive DAT.

The diagnosis is important because there appears to be a higher incidence of underlying illness such as immunodeficiency or autoimmune lymphoproliferative disease in children and SLE or T-cell lymphoma in adults. Typically, the disease runs a chronic course characterized by relapses and remissions. Management is as for warm AIHA or ITP (see Chapter 49) but patients with Evans syndrome tend to be more resistant to initial therapy with prednisolone. Options for second-line therapy include immunosuppressive drugs such as vincristine, danazol, ciclosporin and mycophenolate mofetil as single agents or in combination regimens. Splenectomy is usually considered but responses are inferior to those seen in uncomplicated ITP. More recently, the anti-CD20 antibody rituximab has produced remission of both cytopenias in a high proportion of children and adults with steroid-refractory Evans syndrome. Stem cell transplantation offers the only hope for long-term cure for severe refractory patients but carries a significant risk of transplant-related morbidity and mortality.

Warm AIHA in infancy and childhood

AIHA of unknown cause occurs in infancy and in young children. In infancy, the onset is often acute and anaemia may be profound and difficult to control. The majority of cases in children are transient. It is interesting that in this group the sex difference is reversed, with more boys being affected. In childhood, the haemolytic episode is frequently precipitated by infection. IgG antibodies may be transferred from a mother with AIHA across the placenta to produce haemolysis in the newborn.

Warm AIHA associated with other autoimmune diseases

AIHA is often associated with SLE, especially in young women. Autoantibodies are usually IgG, and both IgG and C3d are found on the red cell surface. Occasionally, the DAT may be positive because of immune complexes adsorbed onto the red cell surface. The spleen is important for clearing such coated cells and splenectomy should be avoided if possible. Otherwise, treatment is as for idiopathic AIHA (see below). This condition is also described with other autoimmune or presumed autoimmune diseases, notably rheumatoid arthritis, Sjögren syndrome and ulcerative colitis; AIHA is also part of the spectrum of autoimmune diseases associated with agammaglobulinaemia.

Warm AIHA in lymphoproliferative diseases

The most common association is with B-cell chronic lymphocytic leukaemia (CLL), low-grade B-cell non-Hodgkin lymphoma or Hodgkin disease. The AIHA may precede the diagnosis of lymphoma, sometimes by months or years. On other occasions, the presentations may be simultaneous or the AIHA may be delayed. The antibodies are polyclonal and have no distinct pattern of antibody type or specificity. The formation of antibodies in this group is thought to be due to immune dysregulation rather than direct production by the malignant clone. Both fludarabine and alemtuzumab, used in the treatment of CLL, are associated with an increased incidence of often somewhat refractory autoimmune cytopenias, probably the result of their powerful effect on the immune system.

Warm AIHA due to drugs

Haemolytic anaemia caused by antibodies directed against self antigens has been described with a number of drugs. Mefenamic acid, levodopa and procainamide have been reported to provoke this condition. The mechanism by which AIHA is produced by exposure to drugs is not known. Alteration to the red cell membrane or modulation of the immune response by the drug have both been suggested. Treatment of patients with CLL with fludarabine and other purine analogues may provoke a very severe and life-threatening acute AIHA and, less commonly, other autoimmune cytopenias. The mechanism may be related to a decrease in autoregulatory T cells caused by treatment with fludarabine.

Warm AIHA and carcinoma

AIHA has been recorded with a number of malignancies, but it is not clear that there is a true association. It may be associated with ovarian cysts, with the cyst fluid containing the agglutinin. It has been suggested that there is also an association with ovarian carcinoma.

Warm AIHA and viral infections

In children, but rarely in adults, AIHA may follow a viral infection. Haemolysis is usually brisk but self-limiting. It is possible that the virus alters the red cell membrane, which provokes 'auto' antibodies against the altered antigens, or that antiviral antibodies cross-react with membrane antigens. A third possibility is that immune complexes form between the virus and specific antibodies and are secondarily adsorbed onto the red cell surface, leading to immune destruction.

Treatment
Corticosteroids

First-line treatment of warm AIHA is with corticosteroids. The initial dose should be prednisolone 1–2 mg/kg body weight daily. The dose may be given once daily if tolerated and should be continued for 10–14 days, according to response. In patients who respond, the dose should then be reduced steadily, down to half the starting dose over the next 2 weeks and more gradually thereafter. In practice, the reduction in dose is tailored to individual patients and their response. It is important not to stop the steroids too quickly and allow relapse. About 70–80% of patients improve their haemoglobin initially but only 15–20% maintain this response long term. For patients who do not respond or who require unacceptably high doses of prednisolone (>20 mg/day) to maintain a reasonable haemoglobin, other measures should be tried as they are at risk of serious steroid side-effects such as avascular necrosis, osteoporosis, infections and diabetes mellitus. A proton pump inhibitor or histamine H_2 antagonist should be given at the same time as the steroids to reduce the risk of gastric erosions. Folic acid supplements should be given to patients with chronic haemolysis.

Cytotoxic immunosuppressive drugs

These agents are used for patients who are refractory to steroids or those who relapse following steroid withdrawal. On its own,

azathioprine is largely ineffective and is used for its steroid-sparing action at a dose of 1.5–2.0 mg/kg daily. Cyclophosphamide 1.5–2.0 mg/kg daily or ciclosporin, starting at 5 mg/kg daily in two divided doses to achieve trough plasma levels of 100–200 mg/L, can also be used. There has been recent interest in the use of mycophenolate mofetil as an alternative immunosuppressive agent for severe refractory AIHA. Response to these drugs is not usually seen for 4–6 weeks and they should be continued for at least 3 months before being deemed ineffective. The mechanism of action of these agents is relatively non-selective, resulting in significant systemic toxicity including bone marrow suppression, renal toxicity and the potential long-term risk of malignancy. It should be emphasized that there are no controlled trials to prove the worth of cytotoxic drugs in AIHA but there are small case reports of success with each agent.

Intravenous immunoglobulin

Intravenous immunoglobulin has been used in AIHA, particularly when IgG is the main component on the red cell surface. The dose used is the same as for ITP, 0.4 mg/kg daily for 5 days. AIHA responds less frequently to intravenous immunoglobulin than does ITP. Side-effects include headache, fever-chill reactions and a small but present risk of viral transmission.

Splenectomy

The spleen is the primary site of clearance of antibody-coated red cells and splenectomy is considered if there is no response to corticosteroids after 3 months' trial. Patients with predominantly IgG on the red cell surface respond best, and those with complement often respond poorly. Splenectomy may be performed laparoscopically; of selected patients, about 30% achieve a complete remission and do not require steroids, 30% have a significantly reduced steroid requirement and the remainder show no or only transient response. There is no certain way to determine who will respond to splenectomy. There is an increased risk of overwhelming sepsis after splenectomy and all patients should receive pneumococcal, meningococcal and *Haemophilus influenzae* B vaccination at least 2 weeks before the procedure, and prophylactic penicillin indefinitely. The complications of splenectomy are dealt with in more detail in Chapter 8. Because of the emergence of monoclonal antibody therapy as an effective alternative treatment for AIHA, there is a trend towards delaying splenectomy as an option for more resistant/refractory cases.

Monoclonal antibody therapy

Recently, rituximab, a chimeric murine–human monoclonal antibody that binds to the CD20 antigen on B cells and immature plasma cells and largely used in the treatment of CD20-positive B-cell non-Hodgkin lymphoma, has been shown to be effective in idiopathic and secondary warm AIHA as well as in cold agglutinin disease. The standard dose and treatment schedule used in follicular lymphoma (375 mg/m^2 i.v. weekly for 4 weeks) is used for autoimmune cytopenias, although more recent studies in ITP suggest that lower doses may be as effective. Response has been shown in patients who are steroid-refractory and who have received multiple treatment modalities, and some patients who relapse after rituximab have been found to respond to retreatment. Overall response rates of 45–75% have been reported, with durable responses of up to 3 years in patients of all ages. Side-effects are minimal and mainly infusion related, such as fever, chills and hypotension. There are concerns about the long-term effects of the profound B-cell depletion that occurs immediately following rituximab therapy. However, naive and memory B cells can be detected by 4–6 months after therapy and the incidence of viral infections remains low in treated patients. In contrast, the results with alemtuzumab (Campath 1H), the anti-CD52 antibody, have been disappointing in AIHA and ITP.

Blood transfusion

Blood transfusion must be given if the clinical situation demands it, if the haemoglobin continues to fall or heart failure develops, despite the impossibility of achieving a satisfactory cross-match in the presence of a positive DAT. The least incompatible grouped blood should be used and transfused slowly. Some authors recommend the use of blood lacking antigens to which the autoantibodies react, but others point out that specificity is rarely absolute and that there is a risk of provoking an alloantibody response.

Prognosis

The prognosis in warm AIHA depends on a number of variables, including age, associated diseases and severity of haemolysis. In all patients, AIHA should be considered a serious and potentially life-threatening disease. Estimates of mortality of idiopathic AIHA in adults vary from 10% at 5 years to 40% at 7 years. The higher figures are mainly in patients aged over 50 years. Most deaths occur in the first 2 years after diagnosis and are related to associated disease. In children, mortality is much lower, probably about 5%, with the majority of patients recovering completely. AIHA may carry considerable morbidity, often from prolonged high-dose steroid therapy.

Cold-type autoimmune haemolytic anaemias

The clinical features of the cold haemagglutinin syndromes vary with the pathogenesis of the disorder. Serological tests are useful in identifying the cause and in determining treatment. The serological characteristics of the antibodies found in these syndromes are shown in Table 10.2.

Clinical features

Idiopathic cold haemagglutinin disease

Primary CHAD, a relatively uncommon disorder accounting for only 15% of AIHA, is mainly seen in older people and runs a chronic course. Although the condition is mostly benign, the clinical features may be very distressing and disabling. Purplish skin discoloration, maximal over the extremities (acrocyanosis), may be present in cold weather. Acrocyanosis is due to stasis in the peripheral circulation secondary to red cell agglutination. On warming the skin, the colour returns to normal or there is transient erythema. This sequence distinguishes acrocyanosis from Raynaud syndrome. Haemolysis resulting in anaemia is usually present and the patient may be mildly icteric. Occasionally, haemolysis dominates the clinical picture, depending on the ability of the antibody to activate complement on the red cell surface. The cold agglutinins are monoclonal IgM κ, with heavy chain variable regions encoded by the IGHV4–34 gene segment but serum electrophoresis may not reveal a monoclonal band because the concentration of the protein is too low. CHAD may be thought of as a premalignant B-cell disorder, which only presents clinically because of the specificity of the antibody for red cell surface antigens. This is highlighted by the fact that although, traditionally, CHAD has been defined by the absence of an underlying disorder, recent studies using sensitive flow cytometric and immunohistochemical assessments have demonstrated a monoclonal CD20-positive κ-positive B-lymphocyte population in the bone

Table 10.2 Serological characteristics of cold-acting antibodies in the cold agglutinin syndromes.

Disorder	Specificity		
	Anti-I	Anti-i	Anti-P, -Pr
Idiopathic (CHAD)	Monoclonal IgM κ		Monoclonal (rare)
Secondary to			
Lymphoproliferative disease	Monoclonal IgM κ/λ (IgG)	Monoclonal (rare)	
Mycoplasma pneumoniae	Polyclonal		
Infectious mononucleosis	Polyclonal	Polyclonal	
Paroxysmal cold haemoglobinuria	Donath–Landsteier (biphasic)		Polyclonal (anti-P)

CHAD, cold haemagglutinin disease; mono.

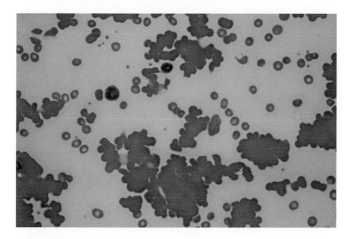

Figure 10.2 Cold haemagglutinin disease. Blood film showing gross haemagglutination (×20).

marrow of 90% of patients and lymphoplasmacytic lymphoma is a frequent finding.

In the laboratory, spontaneous agglutination of red cells is frequently observed, both macroscopically and on the peripheral blood film if made at room temperature (Figure 10.2). Automated blood cell counters detect the agglutinates and record erroneously high mean corpuscular volume and low haemoglobin values, unless the sample is tested at 37°C. The DAT shows only C3d on the red cell surface; IgM cold agglutinins are not detected because they elute from the cell surface *in vitro*. They are usually anti-I, although anti-Pr, anti-P and other rarer specificities have been described.

Cold agglutinin syndromes and lymphoproliferative disorders

Occasionally, the cold agglutinin syndrome accompanies or precedes a B-cell lymphoma or CLL. In these cases, the antibody is monoclonal and is a product of the malignant clone. The serological specificity is either anti-I or anti-i. Haemolysis is often more troublesome than symptoms of agglutination. The prognosis is usually that of the underlying lymphoproliferative disease.

Cold agglutinin syndromes and infections

Haemolysis due to cold agglutinins may follow infections, almost always due to *M. pneumoniae*, or infectious mononucleosis. Rare cases following *Listeria* or *Toxoplasma* infections have been reported. The antibodies are mostly polyclonal IgM in type but occasional IgG cold antibodies are found. The antibodies develop in response to the infecting organism and cross-react with the red cell antigens. Haemolysis appears 2–3 weeks after the infection and is usually mild and self-limiting. Occasionally, very severe and even fatal acute intravascular haemolysis develops after *M. pneumoniae* infection. Blood transfusion through a blood warmer may be urgently required.

Treatment
General

Management of cold haemagglutinin syndromes is difficult. All patients should avoid exposure to cold, and electrically heated gloves and socks are available for use in winter. Wintering in a warm climate is a pleasant alternative. Folic acid supplements should be given to patients with chronic haemolysis.

Alkylating agents

Chlorambucil may be effective in reducing antibody production when there is an underlying B-cell neoplasm such as in CLL. Intermittent regimens such as 10 mg/day for 14 days every 4 weeks or continuous treatment of 2–4 mg/day are both effective. Long-term treatment carries the risk of bone marrow suppression and the development of myelodysplasia and acute myeloid leukaemia. Alkylating agents including chlorambucil, purine analogues such as cladribine and interferon alfa are usually ineffective in idiopathic CHAD.

Corticosteroids

Corticosteroids are rarely of use. They should be used only in exceptional circumstances when the antibodies are present in low titres and have a high thermal range. Their use should be avoided in other cases.

Splenectomy

Removal of the spleen is rarely of any use. The cells are coated with C3b and destruction occurs mainly in the liver.

Blood transfusion

Blood transfusions should be given with due regard to the difficulty in cross-matching in the presence of cold haemagglutinins. Blood should be given through an in-line blood warmer. The patient should be nursed in a warm environment, preferably at 37°C. Special precautions are needed for surgical procedures to keep the patient warm.

Plasma exchange

The titre of cold agglutinin may be lowered temporarily by plasma exchange. The procedure may be useful in the control of severe symptoms but has no effect on the underlying disease.

Monoclonal antibody therapy

The anti-CD20 monoclonal antibody rituximab has been shown to be an effective therapeutic option for both idiopathic CHAD and cold agglutinin syndromes with associated B-lymphoproliferative disorders. Response rates of up to 50% have been reported in Phase II studies but with relatively short response duration of only 11 months.

Paroxysmal cold haemoglobinuria

This rare syndrome usually occurs in children following acute viral infections. The original cases were described by Donath,

Landsteiner and Ehrlich in congenital and tertiary syphilis but such cases are no longer encountered. A history of cold exposure is not always present and presentation is with sudden intravascular haemolysis resulting in pallor, dark urine (haemoglobinuria), abdominal pain and sometimes collapse. The cold antibody is a biphasic polyclonal IgG antibody (Donath–Landsteiner antibody) that reacts with red cells below 20°C in the peripheral circulation, causing lysis by complement activation as the red cells are warmed to 37°C in the central vessels. The antibody has specificity for the P antigen.

Treatment depends on keeping the patient warm, preferably at an ambient temperature of 37°C. Haemolysis is usually self-limiting but blood transfusion is often required. The rare pp cells are not usually available and transfusion of ABO- and rhesus-compatible P-positive blood should be given through a blood warmer.

Alloimmune haemolytic anaemia

Drug-induced immune haemolytic anaemia

Antibody-induced haemolytic anaemia caused by drugs is rare but in some cases may be acute, severe and even life-threatening. Four main mechanisms have been proposed for antibody-dependent drug-induced haemolytic anaemias: drug adsorption, immune complex and membrane modification mechanisms that lead to antibodies reacting with novel epitopes, and true autoantibody-induced haemolytic anaemia (see above). The same drug at different doses or repeated usage may activate different mechanisms and there are recent suggestions that membrane modification may underlie most of the mechanisms. The diagnosis of drug-induced immune haemolytic anaemia should be made in three stages: (i) diagnosis of a DAT-positive haemolytic anaemia; (ii) careful drug history; and (iii) serological demonstration of drug-specific antibody, which interacts with red cells.

Pathogenesis
Drug adsorption mechanism: IgG antibodies and extravascular haemolysis

Penicillin is the prototype drug, although cephalosporins and other penicillin derivatives have also been implicated. Drugs in this group readily form hapten–carrier complexes with plasma proteins, which enhance drug-specific antibody production. It has been estimated that 90% of individuals receiving penicillin produce clinically insignificant IgM anti-penicillin antibodies. When high-dose intravenous penicillin is administered, the drug is adsorbed onto the red cell surface, where it becomes non-specifically attached to red cell surface proteins. A minority of patients on high-dose intravenous penicillin therapy (>1 million units daily) develop high-titre IgG anti-penicillin antibodies that attach to the drug bound to the red cell surface and cause predominantly extravascular haemolysis. The clinical picture is usually of mild to moderate haemolysis but if unrec-

ognized, so that large doses of the drug are continued in the presence of increasing antibody levels, complement fixation and acute intravascular haemolysis may occur. The DAT becomes positive after some weeks of treatment and is due to IgG only on the red cell surface. When the drug is stopped, the DAT rapidly becomes negative and haemolysis stops. Antibody in the patient's serum or eluate from the red cells will react with normal red cells only in the presence of the drug. The clinical and serological features are shown in Table 10.3.

Immune complex mechanism: complement-activated acute intravascular haemolysis

Several drugs have been reported to cause immune haemolytic anaemia by this mechanism. Those most frequently reported are rifampicin, phenacetin, quinine, quinidine, hydrochlorothiazide and chlorpropamide and, more recently, intravenous cephalosporins and diclofenac (see below). Hapten–carrier complexes are formed between these drugs and plasma proteins, leading to the production of drug-specific antibodies. Once drug antibodies are present, reintroduction of the drug causes immune complexes to form, which are adsorbed onto the red cell membrane and complement is activated.

Classically, haemolysis occurs on the second or subsequent exposure to the drug and may develop within minutes or hours of drug ingestion. Severe intravascular haemolysis may occur with fever, rigors or nausea and, in extreme cases, acute renal failure. Several groups have reported fatal immune haemolysis with the third-generation cephalosporin ceftriaxone, and cefotaxime and ceftazidime have also been reported to cause immune haemolytic anaemia. Second-generation cephalosporins have also been implicated, although there are fewer reports with them than with third-generation antibiotics. Diclofenac can also cause an immune haemolytic anaemia with intravascular haemolysis, and this is thought to be mediated by both immune complex and drug adsorption mechanisms.

Membrane modification mechanism

Cephalosporin, in addition to the drug adsorption mechanism, can cause a positive DAT by modifying red cell membrane components. Cisplatin and carboplatin have also been reported to cause immune haemolytic anaemia by this mechanism. As a result, a variety of plasma proteins, including immunoglobulin and complement, may attach via a non-immune mechanism to the red cell membrane. This may result in the finding of a positive DAT but rarely causes immune haemolytic anaemia.

Ribavirin in combination with interferon alfa or peginterferon alfa is the treatment for chronic hepatitis C infection. The main dose limiting toxicity is haemolytic anaemia. Ribavirin enters cells and is phosphorylated to ribavirin triphosphate. In nucleated cells the triphosphate is hydrolysed back to ribavirin, which leaves the cells as the serum level declines. Red cells lack the hydrolysing enzymes: the triphosphate accumulates and alters the deformability of the membrane and extravascular

Table 10.3 Drug-induced immune haemolytic anaemias: clinical and serological features.

	Drug adsorption mechanism	Immune complex mechanism	Autoimmune mechanism	Membrane modification mechanism
Examples	Penicillin	IV third-generation cephalosporins	Methyldopa	Cephalosporins
	Cephalosporins	Quinidine	Procainamide	Cisplatin
		Diclofenac	Mefenamic acid	Carboplatin
			Fludarabine*	
			Cladribine*	
Dose/duration	Large therapeutic doses/prolonged	Very low dose on second or subsequent exposure/short	Therapeutic About 6 weeks	Therapeutic
Haemolysis	Extravascular	Intravascular	Extravascular	Rare
	Subacute	Acute	Mild/subacute	
DAT	IgG ± C'3	C'3 only	IgG only	IgG
Serum reaction	To drug-treated cells	Only in presence of drug or metabolite	To normal cells	To drug-treated cells
Eluate reaction	To drug-treated cells	Non-reactive	To normal cells	To drug-treated cells

*May change T-cell regulation.

haemolysis occurs. With ribavirin monotherapy the haemolysis may be compensated by increased marrow activity but the marrow suppression caused by interferon alfa inhibits the response and severe anaemia may result. Occasionally, autoantibodies have been detected, presumably generated to antigens in the altered membrane. Haemolytic anaemia may require dose reduction (<800 mg/day) or erythropoietin in 10–30% of patients.

Autoimmune mechanism

Methyldopa was the paradigmatic drug in drug-induced AIHA. Ther was a delay of some 6 weeks before the DAT became strongly positive due to IgG on the red cell surface. Haemolysis was absent or trivial, although this is not true with some other drugs that produce haemolysis by this route, notably mefenamic acid (Ponstan). The antibodies usually show no Rh specificity when tested against Rh_{null} cells. It should be noted that some drugs may produce haemolysis by both the immune complex and autoimmune mechanisms, depending on the circumstances.

Serological diagnosis of drug-induced haemolytic anaemia
Drug adsorption and membrane modification mechanisms

The DAT is usually positive with IgG1, or IgG and C3 on the red cell surface. The red cell eluate and serum do not react against normal or enzyme-modified red cells. Warm-reacting drug-specific antibody in the eluate and serum is only detected after preincubation of the test red cells with the appropriate drug.

Immune complex mechanism

The DAT is usually positive but may be negative if performed immediately after a brisk episode of haemolysis. The red cell eluate is not reactive even in the presence of the drug. The drug-specific antibody is best detected by preincubating the patient's serum with the drug in solution to allow immune complexes to form. The preincubated serum is then tested against normal and enzyme-modified groups of cells in the presence of fresh complement. In some cases the antibodies may be specific for metabolites rather than for the parent drug. Drug metabolite antibodies may be detected by preincubating drug metabolite obtained from the serum or urine of a volunteer (who has taken the drug) with the patient's serum. A simplified summary of the serological investigation of a patient with suspected drug-induced immune haemolysis is shown in Table 10.3.

Alloimmune haemolytic anaemia with anti-D

Intravenous anti-D immunoglobulin (WinRho) is licensed for the treatment of ITP in unsplenectomized RhD-positive patients. Some intravenous anti-D immunoglobulin preparations have been licensed for treatment of ITP in unsplenectomized RhD-positive patients. Higher doses than those used in prevention of haemolytic disease of the newborn are indicated by the manufacturers. The mechanism of action is thought to be inhibition of platelet destruction by the spleen due to phagocytosis of coated red cells. In some patients, severe acute intravascular haemolysis may occur 1–24 hours after treatment. The onset is with loin pain, fever, prostration and dark red or black urine. Oliguria and disseminated intravascular coagulation (DIC) may ensue with renal failure. A number of deaths have been reported. The reaction is similar to that seen in acute intravascular haemolytic reaction in mismatched transfusion reactions (see Chapter 16), but so far no culpable antibodies other than anti-D have been detected in different batches of the anti-D preparations tested. The reaction does not happen at the doses used with any of the preparations given to prevent rhesus sensitization in pregnancy.

Non-immune acquired haemolytic anaemias

Haemolysis and haemolytic anaemia may be the consequence of a wide variety of acquired conditions that do not lend themselves to a precise and logical classification. Classification tends to be based on causes rather than mechanisms, although there are some common pathogenetic mechanisms that lead to red cell destruction. The main groups of agents causing haemolysis are infections, vascular disorders (mechanical disorders) and chemical and physical agents, and disorders affecting the red cell membrane. A classification is shown in Table 10.4.

Infections causing haemolytic anaemia

A variety of infections may produce haemolysis through several different pathways. Haemolysis may be a consequence of direct invasion of the red cell by a microorganism or may arise from alterations in the microcirculation, leading to mechanical haemolysis. The intracellular organisms tend to produce the more severe haemolysis.

Malaria

Some degree of haemolysis is seen in all types of malarial infection, but the most severe abnormalities are found in *Plasmodium falciparum* infection. *Plasmodium falciparum* infection is one of the most common causes of anaemia in the world. Many factors may contribute to the anaemia, including marrow suppression, dyserythropoiesis, folate deficiency, hypersplenism and red cell sequestration, as well as haemolysis. The condition has two main components: extravascular destruction of parasitized cells in the reticuloendothelial system, particularly the spleen, and intravascular lysis when the sporozoites break out of the red cells in the circulation. In most patients, the systemic symptoms of malaria dominate the clinical picture but, occasionally, acute intravascular haemolysis is the presenting emergency problem. Haemolysis in malaria is often associated with a positive DAT.

Blackwater fever

Acute intravascular haemolysis leading to the passing of black or dark-red urine is an uncommon but well-described and feared complication of falciparum malaria. The syndrome usually occurs after a few days of typical malaria fever. The appearance of black urine is usually accompanied by further

Table 10.4 Non-immune acquired haemolytic anaemias.

Cause	Examples	Mechanisms
Infections	Falciparum malaria	Intracellular organisms
	Babesiosis	
	Bartonella	
	Meningococcal sepsis	Endotoxin-induced DIC
	Pneumococcal sepsis	
	Gram-negative sepsis	
	Atypical mycobacterial infections	Haemophagocytic syndromes
	HIV	
	Viruses	
	Clostridium perfringens	Enzyme toxins
	Snake, spider bites	
Chemical and physical agents	Drugs	Oxidative damage
	Industrial/domestic substances	
	Burns	Heat
	Drowning	Osmotic lysis (fresh water), dehydration of red cells (salt water)
	Lead poisoning	
	Copper (Wilson disease)	Enzyme inhibition
Fragmentation (mechanical)	Cardiac haemolysis	Lysis on prosthetic surfaces
	Perivalvular leak	
	Microangiopathic haemolytic anaemia	Vasculitis, endothelial cell swelling, fibrin shear
	March haemoglobinuria	
Acquired membrane disorders	Liver disease	Lipid/cholesterol changes
	Paroxysmal nocturnal haemoglobinuria	Somatic mutation

DIC, disseminated intravascular coagulation.

fever and often back pain in the renal angle. Oliguric renal failure may ensue, particularly if the patient becomes hypotensive and hypovolaemic from dehydration. Pulmonary and cerebral symptoms may develop. The condition was first described in white people, most of whom had been treated with quinine, and the importance of this association was stressed. However, the condition is seen in all populations in endemic areas and certainly does not seem to be confined to non-immune individuals. In indigenous populations, glucose-6-phosphate dehydrogenase (G6PD) deficiency may play a part in the pathogenesis as well as quinine exposure. The spread of chloroquine-resistant malaria in the Far East has led to increased use of quinine and an increase in the incidence of blackwater fever.

The degree of parasitaemia is very variable. In about half of the cases the parasite count may be high, whereas in others the count may be low, perhaps because of the intense intravascular haemolysis. The red cell count may fall to 1×10^{12}/L within 24 hours of the start of the haemoglobinuria. There is usually a rise in fibrin degradation products in the serum, but this rise is not often marked and is compatible with a degree of renal failure. Intravascular coagulation does not seem to play a major role in pathogenesis.

Immediate treatment is directed towards correction of the fluid and electrolyte loss, counteracting the anaemia and eradication of the parasite. Renal dialysis may be required and may have to be continued for 1 month or more before renal function returns. Subsequent attacks of falciparum malaria are likely to produce further episodes of blackwater fever in susceptible individuals, so scrupulous prophylaxis should be followed.

Babesiosis

Infection with the intracellular protozoan *Babesia* is uncommon and symptomatic disease is mostly confined to splenectomized patients, at least in the European variety. *Babesia* is a tick-borne organism, the tick in Europe being *Ixodes ricinus*, associated with cattle, and in North America, *Ixodes dammini*, carried by rodents and deer. It may be transmitted by blood transfusion.

In splenectomized patients, the disease has an acute onset and is often fatal. There is a 1–3 day period of malaise, sometimes with vomiting and diarrhoea, followed by high fever, rigors, jaundice, acute intravascular haemolysis, haemoglobinuria, renal failure and death. In North America, unsplenectomized patients may experience a milder self-limiting disease, although intravascular haemolysis does occur. The diagnosis is made from the peripheral blood film, where the parasites, looking very similar to *P. falciparum*, are seen in the red cells. There may be a history of tick bite or of exposure to potential vectors. Treatment is difficult. Clindamycin and quinine are the standard therapy for severe infection; exchange transfusion and renal support may be required in severely affected patients.

Bartonella (Oroya fever)

Infection with *Bartonella bacilliformis* is an arthropod-transmitted infection found only in the western Andes of Peru and neighbouring countries. The diagnosis is made from the peripheral blood film. The organism is an intracellular Gram-negative rod during the acute attack, becoming coccoid in

recovery. In non-immune individuals, there may be splenomegaly and haemolytic anaemia, partly intravascular, partly through erythrophagocytosis. The organism is rapidly killed by chloramphenicol, tetracyclines, penicillin and aminoglycosides.

Clostridium perfringens

Clostridium perfringens septicaemia causes an intense intravascular haemolysis with prominent microspherocytosis and ghost cells in the peripheral blood film. The spherocytosis is the result of membrane destruction by lipases and proteases produced by the organism. Although the organism is sensitive to a variety of antibiotics, the appearance of intravascular haemolysis is usually a harbinger of death because of the toxaemia.

Toxoplasmosis

Infection with *Toxoplasma gondii* acquired *in utero* may produce haemolysis and a syndrome similar to haemolytic disease of the newborn. In adults, toxoplasmosis is not associated with haemolysis, except perhaps in the immunocompromised host.

Bacterial infections

Intravascular coagulation produced by bacterial infection may be accompanied by some degree of intravascular haemolysis with fragmentation of red cells. Septicaemia from meningococcal or pneumococcal infection may show evidence of haemolysis, but such features are not clinically significant compared with the other effects of the septicaemia.

Haemorrhagic fevers

Haemorrhagic fevers may be accompanied by haemolysis. Dengue fever is widespread in many parts of the world and may cause intravascular haemolysis. Other haemorrhagic fevers, for example yellow fever and West African haemorrhagic fevers, may also produce haemolysis.

Haemophagocytic syndrome

The haemophagocytic syndrome (HPS) is characterized by proliferation of macrophages in the bone marrow, spleen, liver and lymph nodes, with inappropriate phagocytosis of erythroid precursors, granulocytes and platelets. In some variations, the skin may be involved. It may occur in severe systemic infections, such as cytomegalovirus, fungal infection and tuberculosis. Clinically, the patient presents with persistent fever, pancytopenia, jaundice and evidence of liver dysfunction, often with a coagulopathy. The manifestations may be acute or subacute, with the patient exhibiting severe malaise, weight loss and rapidly developing pancytopenia. The jaundice is partly the result of the destruction of red cells and their precursors in the marrow, spleen or liver, usually associated with a marked rise in LDH. There is an acute-phase response, with greatly elevated serum ferritin levels (>20 000 μg/L) and increases in interferon (IFN)-γ and tumour necrosis factor (TNF)-α with variable changes in other cytokines. The syndrome is associated with abnormal T-cell activation, which triggers the macrophage response and which may be the consequence of a T-cell lymphoma or may be unmasked by a variety of infections. The two main subdivisions of the syndrome are infection-associated HPS and malignant HPS. Clinically, the distinction may be very difficult because in the lymphomas the proliferation may be trivial, the syndrome being derived from the release of cytokines, and because in malignant HPS superadded infection is common. Likewise, in infection-associated HPS it may be impossible to identify the underlying infection. In children, infection-associated HPS seems to be more common, whereas in adults the majority of cases are associated with lymphoma.

Fragmentation haemolysis: mechanical haemolytic anaemias

The relationship between the vascular endothelium, the cellular elements of the blood and the mechanisms of haemostasis and fibrinolysis is clearly intricate and complex. The integrity of the red blood cell may be destroyed by contact with abnormal endothelial surfaces, although not all abnormalities of vessels cause haemolysis. It may be that some adherence between the red cell and the abnormal vessel wall is necessary for fragmentation of the red cell to occur, and that this usually happens in the context of abnormal flow as well as an altered endothelium. The situations in which fragmentation haemolysis may occur are the presence of prosthetic material and altered flow following cardiovascular surgery, the trapping or adherence of red cells in arteriovenous malformations, and the destruction of red cells in pathologically altered small blood vessels (microangiopathic haemolytic anaemia).

The characteristic features of fragmentation haemolysis are the appearance of the blood film (Figure 10.3) and the presence of intravascular haemolysis. Depending on the underlying vascular pathology, there may be a reduction in the platelet count and evidence of DIC. The rate of red cell destruction also varies

according to the pathogenesis, so the signs of intravascular haemolysis vary from absence of haptoglobin, elevated LDH and minimal haemosiderinuria to acute intravascular destruction with haemoglobinaemia and haemoglobinuria. The major causes of fragmentation haemolysis are shown in Table 10.5.

Cardiac haemolytic anaemia

This syndrome was so called because it mainly occurred after cardiac surgery in which prosthetic valves, patches or grafts were inserted. Haemolysis usually becomes significant only when there is turbulent flow that brings the circulating red cells into intimate contact with the prosthetic material. There are certain situations in which the haemolysis may be of considerable clinical importance.

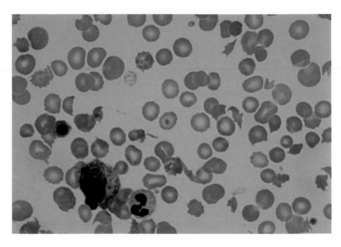

Figure 10.3 Microangiopathic haemolytic anaemia. Blood film from a patient with carcinoma and bone marrow metastases. Note fragmentation of red cells, leucoerythroblastic changes with nucleated red cell and metamyelocyte and low platelets suggesting possible disseminated intravascular coagulation (×40).

Vascular origin	Pathogenesis	Platelets
Cardiac haemolysis	Prosthetic heart valves	Normal
	Patches, grafts	
	Paraprosthetic or perivalvular leaks	
Arteriovenous malformations	Kasabach–Merritt syndrome	Very low
	Malignant haemangioendotheliomas	
Microangiopathic	TTP/HUS	Low
	Malignant disease	Normal/low
	Vasculitis	Normal/low
	Pre-eclampsia, HELLP	Low
	Renal vascular disorders	Normal/low
	Disseminated intravascular coagulation	Low

Table 10.5 Classification of mechanical anaemias caused by fragmentation haemolysis.

HELLP, haemolysis with elevated liver function tests and low platelets; HUS, haemolytic–uraemic syndrome; TTP, thrombotic thrombocytopenic purpura.

Periprosthetic or perivalvular leaks

If after insertion of a prosthesis or repair of a heart valve a leak occurs around the valve or through a suture track, there may be severe intravascular haemolysis without evidence of haemodynamic distress. A difficulty may be that fragmentation of red cells is not always prominent, although spherocytes may be present. However, once autoimmune haemolysis is ruled out, the diagnosis can scarcely be anything other than cardiac haemolysis in a patient who has had cardiac surgery. The haemolysis can be cured only by further surgery.

Ambulatory haemolysis

A patient who has undergone valve replacement may show only slight evidence of haemolysis while in hospital but experience significant anaemia after discharge. This is thought to occur because the higher cardiac output associated with the greater exercise as an outpatient produces more turbulence and hence greater opportunity for red cell fragmentation. A similar mechanism is thought to operate if the patient becomes iron deficient as a result of chronic intravascular haemolysis. Iron replacement and advice about the level of exercise may prevent or delay the need for further surgery.

Cardiopulmonary post-perfusion syndrome

Acute intravascular haemolysis may occur in patients who have undergone cardiopulmonary bypass surgery. The haemolysis may be accompanied by neutropenia and pulmonary distress. The syndrome does not strictly belong in this section as the haemolysis seems to be caused by complement activation and binding of the membrane attack complex to the red cell surface. The blood film shows ghost red cells rather than fragmentation. The condition is self-limiting and the patient requires only supportive care.

Arteriovenous malformation

Fragmentation of red cells may be seen in Kasabach–Merritt syndrome, in which platelets are trapped in the vascular network of giant arteriovenous malformations, sometimes with evidence of a consumption coagulopathy. The bleeding disorder is of greater significance than the haemolysis in these patients. A similar picture, usually with clear evidence of a consumptive coagulopathy with evidence of DIC, may be seen in malignant haemangio-endothelioma, in which the tumour tends to invade and grow along veins.

Microangiopathic haemolytic anaemias

Microangiopathic haemolytic anaemia (MAHA) is a condition in which intravascular haemolysis with fragmentation of red cells is caused by their destruction in an abnormal microcirculation. Proof of microangiopathy may be lacking in those not subjected to a post-mortem, and MAHA should be considered a clinical syndrome. The three main pathological lesions that give rise to MAHA are deposition of fibrin strands, often associ

Table 10.6 Causes of microangiopathic haemolytic anaemia.

Disease	Microangiopathy
Haemolytic–uraemic syndrome	Endothelial cell swelling, microthrombi in renal vessels
Thrombotic thrombocytopenic purpura	Platelet plugs, microaneurysms, small-vessel thrombi
Renal cortical necrosis	Necrotizing arteritis
Acute glomerular nephritis	
Malignant hypertension	
Pre-eclampsia	Fibrinoid necrosis
HELLP	
Polyarteritis nodosa	Vasculitis
Wegener granulomatosis	
Systemic lupus erythematosus	
Homograft rejection	Microthrombi in transplanted organ
Mitomycin C	Uncertain
Ciclosporin	Renal vessel anomalies
Carcinomatosis	Abnormal tumour vessels, intravascular coagulation (disseminated or localized)
Primary pulmonary hypertension	Abnormal vasculature
Cavernous haemangioma (Kasabach–Merritt)	Local vascular changes, thrombosis

HELLP, haemolysis with elevated liver function tests and low platelets.

ated with DIC; platelet adherence and aggregation; and vasculitis. The vessel abnormalities may be generalized or confined to particular sites or organs. In most cases, the haemolysis is of less consequence than the underlying cause of the microangiopathy, but the fragmentation of red cells may be important in pointing to the diagnosis. Some of the disorders producing MAHA are given in Table 10.6. Only well-defined clinical syndromes are described in detail here.

Microangiopathic haemolytic anaemia and malignant disease

Fragmentation of red cells with chronic intravascular haemolysis may occur in malignant disease. Clinically significant anaemia may occur, especially when there is invasion of the tumour into a large blood vessel (as in haemangiopericytoma), but more commonly the haemolysis is trivial or well compensated. The fragmentation may simply be noted on the blood film. A blood film that shows evidence of MAHA together with leucoerythroblastic changes is virtually diagnostic of malignant disease with secondary deposits in the bone marrow (Figure

10.3). Mucin-secreting tumours are most likely to produce MAHA.

In acute leukaemia, particularly but not exclusively promyelocytic (M3), there may be intense intravascular coagulation that may be accompanied by MAHA. The coagulation changes dominate the clinical picture.

Microangiopathic haemolytic anaemia and infection

Infections, particularly septicaemia, may provoke intravascular coagulation and MAHA. Generally, the coagulation changes and septic shock overshadow the mild fragmentation but, occasionally, infections produce a chronic state of partially compensated intravascular haemolysis and marked red cell fragmentation. Haemolytic–uraemic syndrome may be precipitated by infection, particularly *Escherichia coli* 0157. Haemolytic–uraemic syndrome is discussed in Chapter 44.

Thrombotic thrombocytopenic purpura

Thrombotic thrombocytopenic purpura is an acute syndrome characterized by fever, neurological signs, haemolytic anaemia with fragmented red cells and thrombocytopenia. The diagnosis is made on the basis of the clinical presentation and evidence for haemolytic anaemia with fragmented red cells and thrombocytopenia. Bilirubin is elevated, as is serum LDH, indicating intravascular haemolysis. LDH is a useful marker for measuring the activity of the microangiopathic process, as is the persistence of red cell fragments in the blood film. It may take up to 1 week for all fragments to be removed from the circulation after the haemolytic process stops. The destruction of red cells occurs at the site of intravascular occlusions; at post-mortem, platelet and fibrin plugs are found in capillaries (Figure 10.4). The condition, including the pathophysiology, is discussed in detail in Chapter 44.

March haemoglobinuria

Haemoglobinuria following running has been documented for about 100 years. Its origin is mechanical, with destruction of red cells occurring in the feet. It can be cured by wearing soft shoes or running on soft ground. The disorder may arise in joggers and is benign except that it may lead to extensive invasive investigations unless recognized. The blood film does not show any red cell fragmentation or consistent abnormality. Occasionally, haemoglobinuria after running is accompanied by nausea, abdominal cramps and aching legs, and enthusiastic athletes with this condition may exhibit mild splenomegaly and jaundice.

Chemical and physical agents

Oxidative haemolysis

Oxidative substances may cause haemolysis in people with normal red cell metabolism and normal HbA if the oxidative stimulus is large enough. The major causes of oxidative haemo-

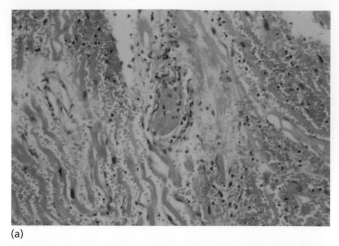

(a)

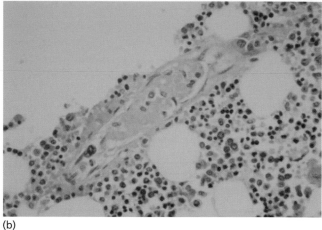

(b)

Figure 10.4 Thrombotic thrombocytopenic purpura. Microthrombi in capillaries: (a) section from the myocardium; (b) thrombus in a bone marrow capillary (haemotoxylin and eosin, ×100). (Courtesy of Dr Margaret Burke.)

lysis in normal subjects are shown in Table 10.7. The clinical features of this condition are dependent on the main sites of oxidative attack, whether on the membrane of the red cell (intravascular haemolysis), the globin chains (Heinz body formation) or the haem group (methaemoglobin accumulation).

Chronic intravascular haemolysis with Heinz bodies

Dapsone and sulfasalazine (Salazopyrin) will cause oxidative intravascular haemolysis in normal subjects if taken in sufficiently high dosage. Red cells show the 'bite' abnormality of the chemically damaged cell (Figure 10.5). Heinz bodies may be absent or scanty in patients with an intact spleen. Dapsone may be used in the treatment of G6PD-deficient subjects with leprosy and in the treatment of dermatitis herpetiformis, in which functional hyposplenism occurs; Heinz bodies appear in the latter case, acute intravascular haemolysis in the former. Haemosiderinuria may be detected in patients taking these

Table 10.7 Substances causing oxidative haemolysis and/or methaemoglobinaemia in normal people.

Substance	Use	Remarks
Dapsone	Leprosy, dermatitis herpetiformis	Chronic haemolysis; slow acetylators more susceptible
Maloprim	Antimalarial	Methaemoglobinaemia in NADH methaemoglobin reductase-depleted subjects
Sulfasalazine	Ulcerative colitis	Chronic intravascular haemolysis
Phenazopyridine	Analgesic in urinary tract infections	Methaemoglobinaemia
Menadiol	Water-soluble vitamin K analogue	Haemolysis/kernicterus in infants
Nitrites	Fertilizer; present in well water, some vegetable juices	Methaemoglobinaemia in infants
Nitrates	Amyl nitrate, butyryl nitrite; abused recreationally	Methaemoglobinaemia/haemolysis
Chlorate	Weed killer	Acute i.v. haemolysis; renal failure; >30 g fatal
Arsine	Gas produced in smelting and other industrial processes	Acute i.v. haemolysis; renal failure

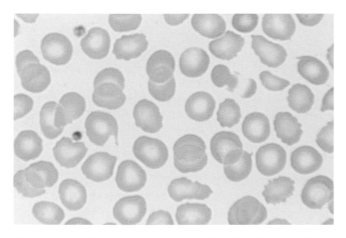

Figure 10.5 Oxidative haemolysis caused by drug (phenacetin). Note red cells with contracted haemoglobin.

drugs, and there may be polychromasia and macrocytosis. Haemolysis is usually well compensated and there is no need to stop the treatment unless the anaemia is severe. A dose reduction may sometimes be needed. Methaemoglobinaemia is uncommon unless the patient is partially deficient in NADH methaemoglobin reductase. The gene for this abnormality may not be very uncommon, and it may account for some people becoming cyanosed after taking dapsone-containing antimalarial preparations.

Methaemoglobinaemia with or without haemolysis

Nitrites in water or vegetable juices may cause methaemoglobinaemia in infants who have a physiological impairment of the reducing systems. Well-water that comes from land with an excess of nitrites and which is used to reconstitute artificial feeds has produced cyanosis in infants. Cases have also been described following the enthusiastic feeding of juice from carrots grown on organically fertilized land and of spinach juice (spinach has a high concentration of nitrogen-fixing bacteria on its leaves). Nitrate drugs, for example amyl nitrate, also produce methaemoglobinaemia and have proved fatal when taken in sufficiently high dosage for 'recreational' purposes. Water-soluble analogues of vitamin K (menadiol sodium diphosphate) cause haemolysis with or without methaemoglobinaemia in infants and *in utero* if given to the mother during the third trimester. Fat-soluble vitamin K preparations must be used if required in these situations. Methaemoglobinaemia due to oxidative drugs rarely causes problems with oxygen delivery but severe cases (>40% methaemoglobin) may be treated with intravenous methylene blue 1–2 mg/kg. Ascorbic acid by mouth may also be used. These measures are ineffective in G6PD-deficient patients and when very strong oxidant substances are implicated. In these circumstances, methylene blue should be avoided because it acts as an oxidant and makes the condition worse.

Acute intravascular haemolysis, methaemoglobinaemia and renal failure

These conditions occur following exposure to strong oxidizing substances found mainly in industrial or horticultural settings, for example sodium chlorate is a popular weedkiller and arsine is a gas produced in various industrial situations, including dross removal in smelting procedures and drain clearances where arsenic is a contaminant. Acute intravascular haemolysis and haemoglobinuria develop 1–24 hours after exposure depending on the dose. The serum becomes brown, often very dark, so that blood cells cannot be seen in anticoagulated preparations, due to the presence of methaemalbumin, methaemoglobin and free haemoglobin. Vomiting, abdominal pain and oliguric renal failure usually develop over about 24 hours. The blood film shows microspherocytosis, ghost cells and bizarre forms. Plasma exchange and renal dialysis are the mainstays of treatment, methylene blue being ineffective. Poisoning with arsine is usually reversible with these measures. Chlorate poisoning is more difficult, 30 g being a generally fatal dose. It is mostly ingested deliberately in suicide attempts.

Thermal injury

Normal red cells when heated *in vitro* show no changes when heated to 46°C for 1 hour but show temperature- and duration-dependent changes above 47–50°C. Some hereditary membrane defects produce red cells that have increased thermal fragility (see Chapter 8).

Haemolysis following burns

Severe burns may be accompanied by intravascular haemolysis with haemoglobinuria. The intravascular haemolysis is related to the extent and severity of the burns. The gross haemoglobinuria occurs over the first 24 hours after the burns and ceases thereafter. The blood film shows spherocytosis and schistocytes, the morphological abnormalities reflecting the thermal damage and the amount of lysis. Prolonged anaemia after burning is related to inflammation, occult blood loss and infection rather than haemolysis.

Lead poisoning

Haemolysis is an important contributor to the anaemia associated with excessive lead exposure. Lead is a potent inhibitor of pyrimidine 5′-nucleotidase 1 (P5N1). This is the prime mechanism of lead-induced haemolysis, producing the same gross basophilic stippling of the red cells as seen in the inherited deficiency of the enzyme (see Chapter 9). P5N1 activity is a good surrogate marker for lead exposure.

Acquired disorders of the red cell membrane

The most common acquired disorder is paroxysmal nocturnal haemoglobinuria, caused by somatic mutation of the phosphatidylinositol glycan A (*PIGA*) gene on the X chromosome, which leads to failure to produce the glycosylphosphatidylinositol (GPI) anchor needed to transport and attach many proteins to the red cell membrane. Intravascular haemolysis occurs through the unchecked action of activated complement. Paroxysmal nocturnal haemoglobinuria is described in detail in Chapter 11.

The mature red cell does not have the capacity to repair its membrane. The lipids of the membrane are in equilibrium with the lipids of the plasma and changes in the ratio of free cholesterol to phospholipids in plasma may affect red cell shape and, in some instances, lead to haemolysis. This is most commonly seen in liver disease, but other inherited lipid disorders may affect the red cell secondarily.

Liver disease

Some degree of shortening of red cell survival occurs in most cases of acute hepatitis, cirrhosis and Gilbert disease, but anaemia is not present and there is only a slight rise in reticulocytes, which may not be detectable. Biliary obstruction is associated with the appearance of target cells and fulminant hepatitis with acanthocytosis, both consequent on changes in the plasma lipid composition.

Zieve syndrome is an uncommon disorder seen mainly in alcoholics. It comprises intravascular haemolysis and acute abdominal pain. These patients usually have cirrhosis and jaundice. The cause is unknown but is probably related to lipid changes in the blood. Spherocytes are seen in the peripheral blood.

Wilson disease may present as acute intravascular haemolysis. This is probably not a membrane disorder but is consequent on the high levels of copper ions in the blood. The haemolysis may antedate the development of hepatic or neurological features, but Kayser–Fleischer rings are usually present. The blood film may show spherocytosis. The diagnosis is made once the condition is suspected. Apart from caeruloplasmin deficiency, patients have a specific aminoaciduria.

Hereditary acanthocytosis (abetalipoproteinaemia)

This rare inherited deficiency of low-density lipoproteins is characterized by retinitis pigmentosa, steatorrhoea, ataxia and mental retardation. The haemolysis that occurs is of minor importance to such patients, but the blood film may indicate the diagnosis, with the red cells showing marked acanthocytosis.

Vitamin E deficiency

Deficiency of vitamin E may occur in infants who are fed a diet rich in polyunsaturated fatty acids. There is haemolysis with contracted cells and a thrombocytosis. Oedema may be present. Vitamin E is an antioxidant, and oxidative damage to the red cell membrane is thought to be the cause of the haemolysis.

Selected bibliography

General

Dacie JV (1992) *The Autoimmune Haemolytic Anaemias. The Haemolytic Anaemias*, 3rd edn, Vol. **3**. Churchill Livingstone, Edinburgh.

Dacie JV (1995) *Secondary or Symptomatic Haemolytic Anaemias. The Haemolytic Anaemias*, 3rd edn, Vol. **4**. Churchill Livingstone, Edinburgh.

Petz LD, Garraty G (2004) *Acquired Immune Haemolytic Anemias*, 2nd edn. Churchill Livingstone, Philadelphia.

Autoimmune haemolytic anaemias

Warm type

D'Arena G, Califano C, Annunziata M *et al.* (2007) Rituximab for warm-type idiopathic haemolytic anaemia: a retrospective study of 11 adult patients. *European Journal of Haematology* **79**: 53–8.

Garvey B (2008) Rituximab in the treatment of autoimmune haematological disorders. *British Journal of Haematology* **141**: 149–69.

Jeffries LC (1994) Transfusion therapy in autoimmune haemolytic anaemia. *Hematology/Oncology Clinics of North America* **8**: 1087–104.

Norton A, Roberts I (2006) Management of Evans syndrome. *British Journal of Haematology* **132**: 125–37.

Passweg JR, Rabusin M, Musso M *et al.* (2004) Haematopoietic stem cell transplantation for refractory autoimmune cytopenias. *British Journal of Haematology* **125**: 749–55.

Provan D, Butler T, Evangelita ML *et al.* (2007) Activity and safety profile of low-dose rituximab for the treatment of autoimmune cytopenias in adults. *Haematologica* **92**: 1695–8.

Cold type

Berentsen S, Klaus B, Geir ET (2007) Primary chronic cold agglutinin disease: an update on pathogenesis, clinical features and therapy. *Haematology* **12**: 361–70.

Drug induced

Gaines AR (2005) Disseminated intravascular coagulation associated with acute hemoglobinemia or hemoglobinuria following Rh(0)(D) immune globulin intravenous administration for immune thrombocytopenic purpura. *Blood* **106**: 1532–7.

Gaines AR, Lee-Stroka H, Byrne K *et al.* (2009) Investigation of whether the acute hemolysis associated with Rho(D) immune globulin intravenous (human) administration for treatment of immune thrombocytopenic purpura is consistent with the acute hemolytic transfusion reaction model. *Transfusion* **49**: 1050–8.

Marani TM, Trich MB, Armstrong PM (1996) Carboplatin induced immune haemolytic anaemia. *Transfusion* **36**: 1016–18.

Myint H, Copplestone JA, Orchard J *et al.* (1995) Fludarabine-related autoimmune haemolytic anaemia in patients with chronic lymphocytic leukaemia. *British Journal of Haematology* **91**: 341–4.

Salama A (2009) Drug-induced immune haemolytic anaemia. *Expert Opinion on Drug Safety* **8**: 73–9.

Salama A, Kroll H, Wittmann G *et al.* (1996) Diclofenac-induced immune haemolytic anaemia: simultaneous occurrence of red blood cell autoantibodies and drug dependent antibodies. *British Journal of Haematology* **95**: 640–4.

Shiffman ML (2004) Side effects of medical therapy for hepatitis C. *Annals of Hepatology* **3**: 5–10.

Shiffman ML (2009) What future for ribavirin? *Liver International* **29** (Suppl. 1): 68–73.

Wright MS (1999) Drug induced haemolytic anemias: increasing complications to therapeutic interventions. *Clinical Laboratory Science* **12**: 115–18.

Non-immune haemolytic anaemias

Infections

Bruneel F, Gachot B, Wolff M, Regnier B, Danis M, Vachon F (2001) Resurgence of blackwater fever in long-term European expatriates in Africa: report of 21 cases and review. *Clinical Infectious Diseases* **32**: 1133–40.

Daly JJ, Haeusler MN, Hogan CJ, Wood EM (2006) Massive intravascular haemolysis with T-activation and disseminated intravascular coagulation due to clostridial sepsis. *British Journal of Haematology* **134**: 553.

Ekvall H (2003) Malaria and anaemia. *Current Opinion in Hematology* **10**: 108–14.

McArthur HL, Dalal BI, Kollmannsberger C (2006) Intravascular hemolysis as a complication of *Clostridium perfringens* sepsis. *Journal of Clinical Oncology* **24**: 2387–8.

Vannier E, Gewurz BE, Krause PJ (2008) Human babesiosis. *Infectious Disease Clinics of North America* **22**: 469–88.

Mechanical haemolytic anaemias

Davidson RJL (1969) March or exertional haemoglobinuria. *Seminars in Hematology* **6**: 150.

Hall GW (2001) Kasabach–Merritt syndrome: pathogenesis and management. *British Journal of Haematology* **112**: 851–62.

Cardiac haemolysis

Maraj R, Jacobs LE, Ioli A, Kotler MN (1998) Evaluation of hemolysis in patients with prosthetic heart valves. *Clinical Cardiology* **21**: 387–92.

Shapira Y, Vaturi M, Sagie A (2009) Hemolysis associated with prosthetic heart valves. A review. *Cardiology in Review* **17**: 121–4.

Thrombotic thrombocytopenic purpura

Aqui NA, Stein SH, Konkle BA *et al.* (2003) Role of splenectomy in patients with refractory or relapsed thrombotic thrombocytopenic purpura. *Journal of Clinical Apheresis* **18**: 51–4.

Fontana S, Kremer Hovinga JA, Studt J-D *et al.* (2004) Plasma therapy in thrombotic thrombocytopenic purpura: review of the literature and the Bern experience in a subgroup of patients with severe acquired ADAMTS-13 deficiency. *Seminars in Hematology* **41**: 48–59.

Kremer Hovinga JA, Meyer S (2008) Current management of thrombotic thrombocytopenic purpura. *Current Opinion in Hematology* **15**: 445–50.

Levy GC, Nichols WC, Lian EC *et al.* (2001) Mutations in a member of the ADAMTS gene family cause thrombotic thrombocytopenic purpura. *Nature* **413**: 488–94.

Pisoni R, Ruggementi P, Remuzzi G (2001) Drug induced thrombotic microangiopathy. Incidence, prevention and management *Drug Safety* **24**: 491–501.

Sadler JE (2009) Von Willebrand factor, ADAMTS13, and thrombotic thrombocytopenic purpura. *Blood* **112**: 11–18.

Yarranton H, Machin SJ (2003) An update on the pathogenesis and management of acquired thrombotic thrombocytopenic purpura. *Current Opinion in Neurology* **16**: 367–73.

Chemical and physical agents

Kim Y, Yoo CI, Lee CR *et al.* (2002) Evaluation of activity of erythrocyte pyrimidine 5′-nucleotidase (P5N) in lead exposed workers: with focus on the effect on hemoglobin. *Industrial Health* **40**: 23–7.

CHAPTER 11

Paroxysmal nocturnal haemoglobinuria   11

Peter Hillmen

St James's University Hospital, Leeds, UK

Introduction

Paroxysmal nocturnal haemoglobinuria (PNH) has fascinated haematologists since its first definitive description in 1882 by Paul Strübbing. PNH is unique as an acquired haemolytic disorder in which the defect is intrinsic to the red cell. Patients have a propensity to develop thromboses that are frequently life-threatening. PNH is also associated with bone marrow failure and indeed may provide a unique insight into the pathophysiology of a variety of bone marrow failure syndromes.

Recently, the development of the terminal complement inhibitor eculizumab has revolutionized the treatment of PNH but in turn has revealed further insights into the pathophysiology of the disease and into normal physiology. The treatment of PNH with eculizumab is not without problems in that a minority of patients have suboptimal responses and require modifications to maximize the benefits of therapy.

Pathophysiology

Glycosylphosphatidylinositol defect

PNH results from the expansion of an abnormal haemopoietic clone that arises following an acquired mutation in a gene critical for the biosynthesis of glycosylphosphatidylinositol (GPI) structures. These GPI anchors are highly conserved

throughout evolution from yeast to humans, having an identical core structure. GPI anchors are glycolipid structures through which a large number of cell surface antigens are attached to the cell membrane. All patients with PNH have the same biosynthetic defect in one of the early steps of the pathway, namely the transfer of *N*-acetylglucosamine from UDP-*N*-acetylglucosamine to phosphatidylinositol. In 1993, Miyata and colleagues reported the cloning of the phosphatidylinositol glycan complementation class A (*PIGA*) gene, which is part of the enzyme complex involved in this step of the pathway and which has subsequently been shown to be mutated in all cases of acquired PNH reported to date.

Mutations of the *PIGA* gene are different between patients as they are acquired somatic mutations not inherited. It appears that the mutation rate of *PIGA* is similar to that of other genes and in fact populations of PNH-like GPI-deficient cells can be observed at extremely low levels (1–10 per million cells) in most normal individuals, indicating that occasional haemopoietic stem cells by chance acquire *PIGA* mutations. Since the *PIGA* gene is located on the X chromosome (Xp22.1), each somatic cell, male or female, only has a single active copy and therefore a somatic mutation of this active gene leads to deficiency of GPI biosynthesis. GPI-deficient clones only expand if there is an additional factor that encourages their selection. The mechanism of this selective growth advantage of PNH clones is of key importance in understanding the pathophysiology of PNH. This could involve a second genetic event intrinsic to the PNH clone, as described in two separate cases where a chromosomal translocation of the *HMGA2* gene has been reported. However, *HMGA2* abnormalities have not been discovered in the analysis of a large number of cases of PNH. A much more likely explanation is indicated by the association between PNH and other bone marrow failure syndromes.

Postgraduate Haematology: 6th edition. Edited by A. Victor Hoffbrand,
Daniel Catovsky, Edward G.D. Tuddenham, Anthony R. Green
© 2011 Blackwell Publishing Ltd.

Association with bone marrow failure

PNH clones frequently occur at very low levels in normal individuals but very rarely expand to become routinely detectable let alone replace virtually all haemopoiesis, as is frequently observed in haemolytic PNH. In addition, PNH clones are detectable in up to 50% of patients with aplastic anaemia and in a smaller proportion of patients with myelodysplastic syndrome. This suggests that such bone marrow failure syndromes are permissive for the expansion of PNH clones. There is overwhelming evidence that aplastic anaemia is an autoimmune disorder in which there is an aberrant immune attack, probably by CD8 cytotoxic T cells directed against the haemopoietic stem cell. It would therefore appear likely that PNH stem cells, presumably due to GPI deficiency, evade this immune attack. This implies that the immune attack in bone marrow failure syndrome is, at least in part, directed through a GPI-linked structure. Understanding PNH may well provide an insight into the mechanism of a variety of bone marrow failure syndromes and provide a unique therapeutic target for these conditions.

Epidemiology

If PNH is defined as the presence of a PNH clone identified during the investigation of bone marrow failure, haemolysis or thrombosis, then the incidence of PNH in a series from the UK was found to be 1.3 newly diagnosed patients per million per year and the prevalence 15.9 patients per million population. However, of these patients, 57% have less than 10% PNH neutrophils, indicating that they are unlikely to have clinically significant haemolysis and only one-third reported macroscopic haemoglobinuria. Thus in the region of 5 patients per million population have haemolytic PNH, and of these only a proportion will be severely affected with symptoms requiring transfusion.

Clinical features

Clinical triad

The clinical picture in PNH depends on the balance between three components: intravascular haemolysis, bone marrow failure and thrombotic complications.

Haemolysis

PNH, the disorder with perhaps the most intense chronic intravascular haemolysis, is characterized by episodes of haemoglobinuria, during which the patient's urine is often black and which, for unknown reasons, is worse in the morning. This episodic haemoglobinuria is frequently associated with disabling symptoms including profound lethargy out of keeping with the patient's anaemia, abdominal pain sometimes requiring opiates, dysphagia that can be temporarily absolute, and erectile dysfunction. The degree of haemolysis is associated with the size of the PNH clone and particularly the proportion of PNH type III (completely deficient) red cells. Macroscopic haemoglobinuria is rarely seen unless there are at least 10% type III red cells. However, patients with apparently identical PNH clones can have a wide range of disease severity, from very occasional attacks of haemoglobinuria without anaemia to severe recurrent or even continuous haemoglobinuria and transfusion dependence, suggesting that other important factors influence the severity of the symptoms. It is possible that this variation is due to the severity of underlying bone marrow failure, to an inherent variation in complement activity or to some other unidentified factor.

Many of the symptoms and complications of PNH result directly from intravascular haemolysis. The presence of extracellular haemoglobin is deleterious as is suggested by the elaborate mechanisms to remove even the smallest quantity. Free plasma haemoglobin is immediately bound to haptoglobin and removed, explaining why haptoglobin is depleted in every patient. Free haemoglobin binds to and removes other gases such as nitric oxide (NO). This depletion of NO in PNH results in smooth muscle dysfunction, vasoconstriction and pulmonary and systemic hypertension. This leads to dysphagia, abdominal discomfort, possibly due to intestinal spasm, erectile dysfunction, severe lethargy, pulmonary hypertension and possibly thrombosis, all classic symptoms of PNH. This syndrome of NO consumption has only become clear since the development of eculizumab (see below), which stops intravascular haemolysis in almost all patients and abrogates the clinical features of PNH.

Bone marrow failure

The degree of anaemia and other cytopenias is a composite of the activity of intravascular haemolysis and the degree of persisting bone marrow failure. The platelet count in many patients is a suitable surrogate for marrow function but in some patients, for example those with previous intra-abdominal thrombosis and subsequent hypersplenism, there may be other causes for a low platelet count. The presence of a PNH clone in patients with bone marrow failure probably indicates that there is a significant immune component to the marrow failure and may suggest that immune suppression is a reasonable therapeutic option. The degree of bone marrow failure will also impact on the efficacy of eculizumab as this will only treat the component due to complement activity, such as intravascular haemolysis and thrombosis.

Thrombosis

The precise cause of thrombosis in PNH is not entirely clear and is probably multifactorial. The activation of PNH platelets

Table 11.1 Sites of thrombotic events in haemolytic PNH.

Venous thrombosis	
Deep vein thrombosis	41 (33.1%)
Lower extremity	23 (18.5%)
Other	18 (14.5%)
Mesenteric/splenic vein thrombosis	23 (18.5%)
Hepatic/portal vein thrombosis	21 (16.9%)
Pulmonary embolus	8 (6.5%)
Cerebral/internal jugular thrombosis	7 (5.6%)
Superficial vein thrombosis	5 (4.0%)
Arterial thrombosis	
Cerebrovascular accident/TIA	17 (13.7%)
Myocardial infarction/unstable angina	2 (1.6%)
Total	124 (100%)

Source: This research was originally published in *Blood*. Hillmen P, Muus P, Duhrsen U *et al.* Effect of the complement inhibitor eculizumab on thromboembolism in patients with paroxysmal nocturnal hemoglobinuria. *Blood* 2007;110:4123–8. © American Society of Hematology.

by complement is at least part of the cause. Also, intravascular haemolysis and NO consumption may lead to endothelial damage and thrombosis. Recent data indicate that the thrombotic tendency in PNH is in arterial as well as venous sites, with several patients reported as having cerebrovascular accidents and myocardial infarctions at an early age. Thrombosis occurs in 40–50% of patients with haemolytic PNH, with a predilection for certain veins such as the hepatic veins (Budd–Chiari syndrome), other intra-abdominal veins or the cerebral veins (Table 11.1). Approximately 10% of patients present with a thrombosis as their initial clinical manifestation of PNH. After the first thrombosis, patients have a 7.8-fold increased risk of dying compared with those patients who have not had a thrombosis. A classical clinical scenario is that of downward spiralling thrombotic events: after a first thrombosis, patients continue to experience further apparently discrete thromboses despite what would be considered adequate anticoagulation with warfarin and/or heparin until they eventually succumb. Eculizumab has a marked effect on thrombosis in PNH and can interrupt this spiral of thrombosis.

Other clinical sequelae

Consequences of haemolysis

Even before the development of targeted therapy for PNH, patients usually survived for prolonged periods, with a median survival in the region of 20 years. A minority of patients experienced spontaneous remissions and therefore the majority of patients had decades of life in which they experienced a con-

tinuous high level of intravascular haemolysis. This leads to several complications of the disease.

Renal disease

All patients with haemolytic PNH develop heavy renal tubular iron loading due to the continuous filtration of haemoglobin. This is evident on both magnetic resonance imaging (MRI) and post-mortem studies. The majority of patients will eventually develop chronic renal disease, with a minority progressing to established chronic renal failure requiring dialysis. In addition, during times of very intense intravascular haemolysis and haemoglobinuria, patients can rarely develop acute renal failure, which is potentially fully reversible even though it may require dialysis. Some patients may develop repeated episodes of acute renal dysfunction. The use of nephrotoxic therapies, such as ciclosporin, adds to the renal insult, as do rare complications such as renal vein thrombosis.

Cholelithiasis

Patients with PNH have both intravascular and extravascular haemolysis, which increases the risk of developing gallstones. In patients who develop abdominal pain, a common symptom in PNH, and particularly if there is any additional change in liver function tests, then the presence of gallstones should be considered.

Leukaemic transformation

There have been a number of case reports of myelodysplastic syndrome and acute myeloid leukaemia (AML) in patients with PNH. These have led to the suspicion that PNH may be pre-leukaemic. However, this is almost certainly not the case for two principal reasons. Firstly, in patients with PNH who develop AML, GPI-linked antigens on myeloid blasts have been reported to be deficient in some but normal in others, indicating that the leukaemia can develop in either the residual normal or the GPI-deficient haemopoietic cells. Secondly, less than 5% of PNH patients in the larger series develop AML. This is similar to the incidence of AML in aplastic anaemia and since it seems the majority, if not all, patients with PNH have an underlying aplasia, then the rate of AML is no higher than would be expected if GPI deficiency has no impact on leukaemogenesis. Therefore it is aplastic anaemia that predisposes to both AML and PNH, and the development of PNH does not increase the development of AML.

Spontaneous remission

PNH often develops in young adults between 20 and 40 years old. Historically, most patients with PNH have either died as a direct or indirect result of their disease or have suffered from the disease for the remainder of their life. In a series of 80 haemolytic PNH patients reported in 1995, initially diagnosed between 1940 and 1970, median survival was 10 years and 12 of the 35 patients surviving at least 10 years experienced spontaneous remission. Analysis of GPI-linked antigens on blood

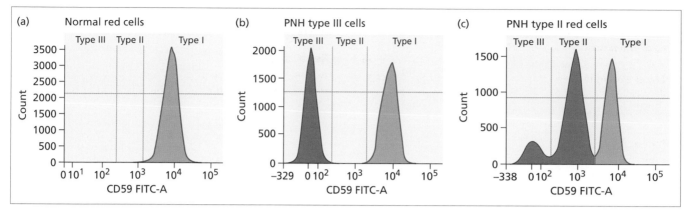

Figure 11.1 Identification of PNH red cells by flow cytometry. (a) GPI anchor protein (e.g. CD59) expression on normal red cells (type I). (b) A total of 46% of red cells are completely GPI anchor-deficient (type III). (c) A mixture of all three types of red cells are shown: type III, 10%; type II (partial GPI anchor expression), 54%; normal type I cells, 36%. (Figure courtesy of S.J. Richards.)

cells up to 20 years after spontaneous clinical remission demonstrated that the myeloid series was entirely normal with no residual PNH cells, whereas there was a small PNH clone in the lymphoid compartment (presumably these are long-lived memory cells). Early reports suggest that a proportion of patients treated with eculizumab have a progressive decrease in the size of their PNH clone, perhaps suggesting that remission may occur.

Nitric oxide consumption

Intravascular haemolysis leads to the release of cell-free haemoglobin into the plasma. There is now a growing body of evidence in other haemolytic disorders, such as sickle cell anaemia, that many of the symptoms and complications are due to the deleterious effects of free haemoglobin. Free haemoglobin absorbs NO, which is a key mediator in homeostasis and smooth muscle function. Since PNH has extremely high and chronic levels of intravascular haemolysis, it is perhaps not surprising that many of the symptoms of the disease – severe lethargy out of keeping with the level of haemoglobin, dysphagia, abdominal pain, erectile dysfunction, pulmonary hypertension – are most probably due to intravascular haemolysis and NO consumption.

deficiency) nor do they provide information about the proportion of PNH leucocytes. The proportion of PNH neutrophils and monocytes probably gives a more accurate assessment of the true size of the PNH clone as they are not influenced by the intensity of intravascular haemolysis or by transfusions. The modern diagnosis of PNH depends on the flow cytometric analysis of at least two cell lineages (e.g. neutrophils and red cells), with a transmembrane marker to positively identify the cell type and at least two separate GPI-linked antigens to clearly separate PNH cells from their normal counterparts (Figures 11.1 and 11.2). In most patients there is a population of red cells with complete deficiency of GPI-linked molecules (PNH type III cells, the most complement-sensitive cells) and in some an additional population with partial GPI deficiency (PNH type II cells, intermediate complement sensitivity). Type II and III are usually not evident in the neutrophils. The size of the PNH clone correlates with the risk of complications, such as thrombosis, and the severity of haemolysis. In addition, the evolution of the clone – either its expansion, leading to more haemolytic disease, or its reduction, ultimately leading to spontaneous remission – can be tracked. Flow cytometry has superseded the complement sensitivity tests in the diagnosis of PNH.

Investigation

The diagnosis of PNH was historically made by demonstrating the sensitivity of red cells to lysis by activated complement. The method used to activate complement varied, for example by acidification in the Ham test or by low ionic solutions in the sucrose lysis test. However, these tests only give an indirect assessment of the proportion of PNH red cells and do not assess the type of PNH red cells (complete versus partial GPI

Treatment

Supportive care

Conventional management in PNH has been supportive. The severity of haemolysis varies greatly between patients, in part dependent on the size of the PNH clone and the degree of underlying bone marrow failure. However, even patients with no evidence of clinically apparent marrow failure and large

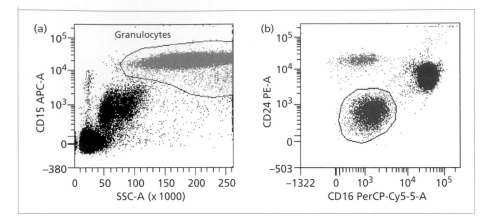

Figure 11.2 Identification of PNH granulocytes by multicolour flow cytometry. (a) Granulocytes identified based on CD15 expression and side scatter. (b) Analysis of CD16 and CD24 (both GPI-linked proteins) reveals a small population of PNH granulocytes (10%) that are deficient in both proteins. (Figure courtesy of S.J. Richards.)

PNH clones can have highly variable levels of haemolysis: some patients experience recurrent, even continuous, haemoglobinuria and are transfusion dependent, whereas others experience haemoglobinuria only rarely, or not at all, do not require any transfusions and have a well-compensated haemolytic anaemia. Patients with a significant degree of haemolysis should receive folic acid supplementation. The constant haemosiderinuria means that patients, even those who require regular transfusions, have a tendency to become iron deficient. This iron deficiency can result in failure of the marrow to compensate for the increased red cell destruction and therefore increasing anaemia. Iron supplementation has been reported to precipitate episodes of intravascular haemolysis but usually patients tolerate oral iron supplements well and should be treated where iron deficiency is present.

Patients should be transfused according to their symptoms. In most patients the severity of haemoglobinuria lessens immediately after a transfusion but then increases, with a progressive fall in haemoglobin level until the patient requires a further transfusion. Incidental infections lead to an increase in haemolysis, presumably due to activation of the complement system, and frequent sudden drops in the level of haemoglobin. These episodes are often associated with severe symptoms of abdominal pain, dysphagia and debilitating lethargy.

Corticosteroids have been widely used in the treatment of haemolysis in PNH. At high doses steroids do appear to have an effect of reducing the activity of complement and some patients report an improvement in symptoms. However, high doses are required to have a clinically useful effect and as the haemolysis in PNH is chronic, the required dose is too high. Steroids are therefore not generally recommended in PNH as the long-term side-effects outweigh the potential benefits.

Thrombosis

The major cause of morbidity and mortality in PNH is thrombosis, which usually affects the venous system, particularly the intra-abdominal and cerebral vessels, but also appears to result in arterial thrombosis (Table 11.1). The chance of developing a thrombosis depends on the size of the PNH clone and the severity of haemolysis, two variables that are closely related; half of patients with over 50% PNH neutrophils will develop a thrombosis at some point in their disease course. In most series, approximately one-third of patients will eventually die as a result of thrombosis. In a series reported by Hall and colleagues, 39 patients with PNH who had not previously experienced a thrombosis were treated with warfarin to maintain an International Normalized Ratio (INR) of 2.0–3.0. None of these 39 patients developed a thrombosis compared with a 36.5% chance of thrombosis at 10 years for the 56 patients with large PNH clones who elected not to have warfarin prophylaxis. However, two patients on warfarin experienced intracranial haemorrhage and one of these died as a result. Therefore it appears that primary prophylaxis with warfarin is effective in preventing thrombosis but carries a significant risk in this patient group. Aspirin does not appear to be protective against thrombosis and has no effect on the symptoms of PNH such as abdominal pain (Peter Hillmen, unpublished observation). It seems very likely that primary prophylaxis with warfarin is unnecessary for patients receiving the anti-complement monoclonal antibody eculizumab, as this agent significantly reduces the risk of thrombosis in PNH (see below).

The treatment of established thrombosis is similar to the management of thrombosis in patients without PNH. However, in view of the risk of recurrent thrombosis, patients should remain on lifelong anticoagulation after their first episode of thrombosis. Hepatic vein thrombosis (Budd–Chiari syndrome) is one of the more common thromboses seen in PNH and there have been reports of the successful lysis of such thromboses using tissue plasminogen activator; this should be considered even in patients who present with a relatively long history suggesting that their thrombosis occurred days or even weeks before.

Allogeneic bone marrow transplantation

The only curative strategy for PNH is allogeneic stem cell transplantation but this carries a considerable risk of mortality. From the reported series and in view of the fact that a proportion of patients will eventually experience a spontaneous remission of PNH and with the advent of potentially effective novel therapies such as eculizumab, transplantation should only be considered in selected cases, such as those with a syngeneic donor or with associated bone marrow failure. In these patients the indications for transplantation are similar to those for aplastic anaemia.

Complement blockade

The development of eculizumab (Soliris), a humanized monoclonal antibody that blocks the activation of terminal complement, has dramatically altered the management and almost certainly the prognosis in PNH. The complement cascade can be activated by the classical pathway (antibody dependent), the alternative pathway (directly through microbial membranes) or the lecithin pathway, which all converge at the fifth component of complement (C5). C5 is cleaved and releases C5a (a potent anaphylatoxin) and C5b, to which C6, C7, C8 and numerous C9 molecules bind to form a pore (the membrane attack complex) that punches holes in the membrane of the target. Eculizumab binds to C5 and stops it being cleaved and, as long as trough plasma levels remain above 35 mg/L, prevents any activation of terminal complement. Individuals with inherited terminal complement deficiency are either asymptomatic or present with recurrent *Neisseria meningitidis* (meningococcus) infections and this highlights the main concern with eculizumab. The clinical features of PNH are due largely to the absence of CD59 from haemopoietic cells and therefore the uncontrolled activity of terminal complement on PNH cells, making eculizumab an ideal candidate for the targeted therapy of PNH. In the initial study, 11 patients with transfusion-dependent haemolytic PNH were treated with eculizumab using a schedule designed to maintain trough levels to ensure that complement was completely blocked. The responses were dramatic, with an immediate resolution of the symptoms of intravascular haemolysis. This study was followed by a randomized placebo-controlled Phase III trial (TRIUMPH) and a non-randomized trial (SHEPHERD). In total, 195 patients were included in these three trials, which led to the licensing of eculizumab in the USA and Europe in 2007. The results of these trials are summarized below.

Efficacy of eculizumab

Intravascular haemolysis

Eculizumab has a profound and immediate effect on intravascular haemolysis in PNH. The lactate dehydrogenase (LDH) concentration, which is typically as much as 10–20 times normal in PNH, falls immediately in all patients treated with eculizumab to normal or just above normal. Other markers of haemolysis, such as aspartate aminotransferase, fall to normal and in some patients the haptoglobins become detectable, at least temporarily. In general this results in increasing haemoglobin level which, depending on the degree of coexistent bone marrow failure as well as the extent of extravascular haemolysis (see below), will reach a plateau usually between 9 and 12 g/dL. The most dramatic effect of eculizumab is on the symptoms, with resolution of the abdominal pain and dysphagia and improvement in the severe lethargy and the other features of haemolysis. In the vast majority of patients transfusion requirements improve, with over half of patients becoming transfusion independent. The dramatic improvement in PNH-related symptoms is due to a marked reduction in NO consumption during therapy as a result of the improvement in intravascular haemolysis and thereby the reduction in free haemoglobin. This probably explains many of these benefits of the drug and provides insights into the pathophysiology of the symptoms of PNH. There is a dramatic and clinically significant improvement in the quality of life of patients as measured by validated questionnaires. There is now evidence that the adverse consequences of intravascular haemolysis, such as renal damage and pulmonary hypertension, are ameliorated by eculizumab.

Thrombosis

Eculizumab also protects patients from thrombosis. Compared with thrombosis before patients commencing eculizumab (effectively using patients as their own controls), the thrombotic rate reduces by fivefold to tenfold. In patients who have had a previous thrombosis and who are on anticoagulation, there is still a high recurrent thrombosis rate prior to starting eculizumab. However, since eculizumab became available, such recurrent thromboses are extremely uncommon. Patients who commence eculizumab during a 'spiral' of thrombotic events stop having further thromboses, indicating that eculizumab specifically targets the mechanism of thrombosis in PNH and that this is a more effective strategy than conventional anticoagulation alone. There is now increasing confidence that the catastrophic thrombotic complications of PNH can be much more successfully managed with a combination of eculizumab and anticoagulation. This observation will have an impact on the decision to use warfarin prophylaxis: in cases where there are concerns over the safety or requirement for warfarin prophylaxis, such as those with low platelets or with borderline PNH clone sizes, it is clearly safer to withhold anticoagulation as long as the use of eculizumab is an option for the patient should a thrombosis occur.

Renal dysfunction

In the 195 patients entering the eculizumab trials, renal dysfunction or damage was observed in 65% of patients before they were treated with eculizumab. In this series, 27% of patients had developed major clinical kidney disease within 10 years from their initial diagnosis of PNH and 21% of patients developed late-stage chronic kidney disease (stage 3 or 4 as defined by the Kidney Disease Outcomes Quality Initiative) or kidney failure (stage 5). The early analysis of patients treated with eculizumab suggests that many of the patients with early renal dysfunction (stages 1 and 2) will improve, and the deterioration in renal function in patients with advanced renal dysfunction (stages 3–5) is frequently stabilized. Thus eculizumab appears to have a beneficial effect on renal function in PNH and this is presumably due to the marked reduction in intravascular haemolysis and therefore in haemoglobinaemia and haemoglobinuria.

Extravascular haemolysis with eculizumab

Despite the impressive impact on intravascular haemolysis, most patients remain somewhat anaemic, maintaining their haemoglobin between 9 and 12 g/dL. Virtually all have a persisting reticulocytosis and many continue to have a raised bilirubin. These features are suggestive of ongoing extravascular haemolysis, which has previously been unreported in PNH. On further investigation it transpires that approximately two-thirds of PNH patients on eculizumab develop a positive direct antiglobulin test to complement only. Flow cytometry demonstrates that the PNH red cells are coated by early complement components (C3b and C3d), possibly because PNH red cells, as well as being deficient in the principal controller of terminal complement, namely CD59, do not express the inhibitor of C3 convertase decay-accelerating factor (DAF). It appears that preventing terminal complement activation leads to a build-up of the early complement components, which accumulate on PNH red cells due to their deficiency of DAF. If intense, this extravascular haemolysis results in a poor increase in haemoglobin and a minority of patients continuing to require transfusions. If the transfusions are due to poor marrow reserves and a lack of compensation, particularly in patients with evidence of renal dysfunction, then treatment with erythropoietin can lead to a clinically meaningful increase in haemoglobin. If this fails, then it does not appear that steroids have a major role. When patients become generally unwell, particularly with coexistent infections, there can be an increase in the level of extravascular haemolysis and/or a decrease in marrow compensation, leading to a fall in the level of haemoglobin. When patients recover from infection, they usually goes back to their steady state.

Eculizumab administration and dosing

Eculizumab is given as a 30-min intravenous infusion. The aim is to rapidly block complement and to maintain complement blockade continuously. The standard dosage schedule for eculizumab comprises a loading dose of 600 mg every week for 4 weeks, followed by 900 mg the next week and then 900 mg every 2 weeks indefinitely. In the majority of patients this is adequate to maintain trough levels of eculizumab above 35 mg/L and

therefore to block complement completely. In approximately 5% of patients this dose is inadequate and patients break through complement blockade. Patients appear well with no signs of haemolysis until immediately before a dose of eculizumab but then develop dark urine often with abdominal pain, sometimes with dysphagia, and a sudden deterioration in the laboratory measures of haemolysis, such as LDH and bilirubin, and a fall in the level of haemoglobin. In this situation the maintenance dose of eculizumab is too low and an increase, either by reducing the interval or more conveniently by increasing the dose (from 900 mg every 2 weeks to 1200 mg every 2 weeks is usually effective), will raise trough levels of eculizumab above 35 mg/L and re-establish continuous control of haemolysis (Figures 11.3 and 11.4).

Infectious risk with eculizumab

Eculizumab is generally very well tolerated with few infusion-related reactions. However, as noted above, blocking terminal complement activity would be expected to increase the risk of infection with *Nesseria meningitidis* (meningococcus). All patients commencing eculizumab should be vaccinated with a wide-spectrum meningococcal vaccine (ACWY Vax). Unfortunately, the current vaccines do not cover serotype B, which is common in the UK. Although the risk of meningococcal infection is a concern, the observed risk is less than 0.5 cases of meningococcal infection per 100 patient-years on eculizumab. However, when these infections occur they can be life-threatening and it is vitally important to impress on patients that they should seek medical help if they suffer any symptoms suggestive of infection, and these are usually of septicaemia rather than meningitis. The role of antibiotic prophylaxis with penicillin is currently being explored. There is no convincing evidence as yet of an increased risk to any other organism except for *N. meningitidis*.

Pregnancy in PNH

It is difficult to estimate the true risk of pregnancy in PNH but there is undoubtedly an increased risk of maternal morbidity and mortality. The reported maternal mortality, mainly from thrombosis, is between 12 and 21%, although this is likely an overestimate due to biased reporting. In addition, an increased fetal loss rate has been reported, although again this is difficult to substantiate and is probably due to maternal factors. There have now been a number of successful pregnancies in women receiving eculizumab either later in pregnancy or throughout the pregnancy from conception to delivery. The reports to date are positive with little or no eculizumab crossing the placenta into the fetus. It does appear that the metabolism of eculizumab may be altered in pregnancy and women seem more likely to break through complement blockade and may need higher doses in the latter part of pregnancy.

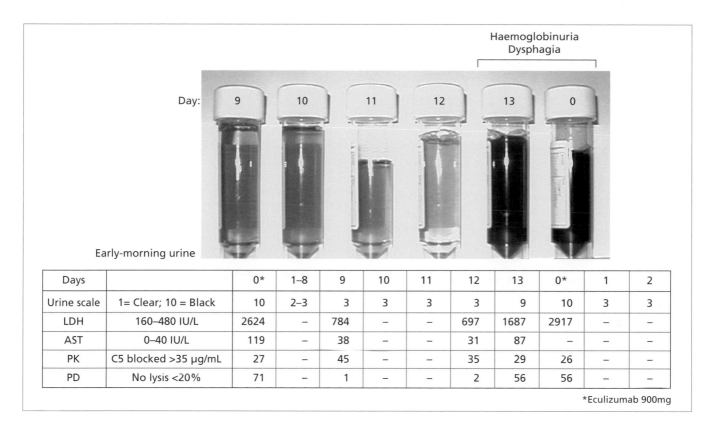

Days		0*	1–8	9	10	11	12	13	0*	1	2
Urine scale	1= Clear; 10 = Black	10	2–3	3	3	3	3	9	10	3	3
LDH	160–480 IU/L	2624	–	784	–	–	697	1687	2917	–	–
AST	0–40 IU/L	119	–	38	–	–	31	87	–	–	–
PK	C5 blocked >35 µg/mL	27	–	45	–	–	35	29	26	–	–
PD	No lysis <20%	71	–	1	–	–	2	56	56	–	–

*Eculizumab 900mg

Figure 11.3 Breakthrough from complement blockade by eculizumab due to inadequate dose level. The urine is clear with lactate dehydrogenase (LDH) just above normal and no haemolytic activity in the patient's serum at day 12 after a 900-mg dose of eculizumab. On day 13, the patient suddenly begins to haemolyse as the level of eculizumab falls below 35 mg/L (the level at which complement is blocked). Immediately after the next dose (day 0), the haemolysis stops. Urine scale: patient assesses urine colour first thing in the morning (red or black urine at 6+). AST, aspartate aminotransferase; PK, pharmacokinetics (serum level of eculizumab); PD, pharmacodynamics (haemolytic potential of the patient's serum *in vitro*).

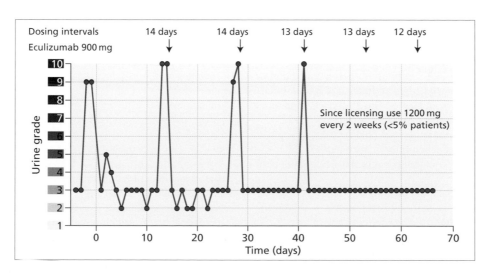

Figure 11.4 Urine colour with increasing eculizumab dose. Patient records early-morning urine colour according to scale on *y*-axis. He is breaking through from complement blockade for 2 days when receiving 900mg eculizumab every 14 days. When the frequency of eculizumab 900mg is increased to every 12 days, his breakthroughs cease. He is now maintained on 1200mg eculizumab every 14 days.

Prognosis

A series of 80 patients with haemolytic PNH diagnosed between 1940 and 1970 were reported in 1995 to reveal a median survival of approximately 10 years from initial diagnosis of PNH. In this series, spontaneous remissions of PNH were reported in 12 of the 34 patients who survived over 10 years from diagnosis. A more recent series of 465 patients reported from France, including patients with small PNH clones as well as haemolytic PNH, reported a median survival of 22 years. The major causes of death in haemolytic PNH are thrombotic and since these are virtually abolished by eculizumab therapy, it is anticipated that treatment will have a major impact on survival in PNH.

Future challenges and developments

The development of targeted therapy for PNH promises to alter the natural history of the disease. Recently, a global PNH registry has been established to document the changes in the natural history of the disease as well as to record any unexpected complications of the newer therapeutic interventions. The current therapy of PNH controls rather than cures the disease. It is hoped that with more detailed understanding of the pathophysiology of PNH a curative strategy may be developed.

Selected bibliography

Araten D, Nafa K, Pakdeesuwan K, Luzzatto L (1999) Clonal populations of haematopoietic cells with paroxysmal nocturnal hemoglobinuria genotype and phenotype are present in normal individuals. *Proceedings of the National Academy of Sciences USA* **96**: 5209–14.

Armstrong C, Schubert J, Ueda E *et al.* (1992) Affected paroxysmal nocturnal hemoglobinuria T lymphocytes harbour a common defect in assembly of *N*-acetyl-D-glucosamine inositol phospholipid corresponding to that in class A Thy-1- murine lymphoma mutants. *Journal of Biological Chemistry* **267**: 25347–51.

Brodsky RA, Young NS, Antonioli E *et al.* (2008) Multicenter phase 3 study of the complement inhibitor eculizumab for the treatment of patients with paroxysmal nocturnal hemoglobinuria. *Blood* **111**: 1840–7.

De Latour RP, Mary JY, Salanoubat C *et al.* (2008) Paroxysmal nocturnal hemoglobinuria: natural history of disease subcategories. *Blood* **112**: 3099–106.

de Planque MM, Bacigalupo A, Würsch A *et al.* (1989) Long-term follow-up of severe aplastic anaemia patients treated with antithymocyte globulin. Severe Aplastic Anaemia Working Party of the European Cooperative Group for Bone Marrow Transplantation (EBMT). *British Journal of Haematology* **73**: 121–6.

Hall C, Richards SJ, Hillmen P (2003) Primary prophylaxis with warfarin prevents thrombosis in paroxysmal nocturnal hemoglobinuria (PNH). *Blood* **102**: 3587–91.

Hill A, Hillmen P, Richards SJ *et al.* (2005) Sustained response and long-term safety of eculizumab in paroxysmal nocturnal hemoglobinuria. *Blood* **106**: 2559–65.

Hill A, Wang X, Sapsford RJ *et al.* (2005) Nitric oxide consumption and pulmonary hypertension in patients with paroxysmal nocturnal hemoglobinuria. *Blood* **106**: Abstract 1046.

Hill A, Platts PJ, Smith A *et al.* (2006) The incidence and prevalence of paroxysmal nocturnal hemoglobinuria (PNH) and survival of patients in Yorkshire. *Blood* **108**: Abstract 985.

Hill A, Rother RP, Arnold L *et al.* (2010) Eculizumab prevents intravascular hemolysis in patients with paroxysmal nocturnal hemoglobinuria and unmasks low-level extravascular hemolysis occurring through C3 opsonization. *Haematologica* **95**: 567–73.

Hill A, Rother RP, Wang X *et al.* (2010) Effect of eculizumab on haemolysis-associated nitric oxide depletion, dyspnoea, and measures of pulmonary hypertension in patients with paroxysmal nocturnal haemoglobinuria. *British Journal of Haematology* **149**: 414–25.

Hillmen P, Bessler M, Mason PJ *et al.* (1993) Specific defect in *N*-acetylglucosamine incorporation in the GPI anchor synthetic pathway in cloned cell lines from patients with paroxysmal nocturnal hemoglobinuria. *Proceedings of the National Academy of Sciences USA* **90**: 5272–6.

Hillmen P, Lewis SM, Bessler M *et al.* (1995) Natural history of paroxysmal nocturnal hemoglobinuria. *New England Journal of Medicine* **333**: 1253–8.

Hillmen P, Hall C, Marsh JC *et al.* (2004) Effect of eculizumab on hemolysis and transfusion requirements in patients with paroxysmal nocturnal hemoglobinuria. *New England Journal of Medicine* **350**: 552–9.

Hillmen P, Young NS, Schubert J *et al.* (2006) The complement inhibitor eculizumab in paroxysmal nocturnal hemoglobinuria. *New England Journal of Medicine* **355**: 1233–43.

Hillmen P, Elebute MO, Kelly R *et al.* (2007) High incidence of progression to chronic renal insufficiency in patients with paroxysmal nocturnal hemoglobinuria (PNH). *American Journal of Hematology*.

Hillmen P, Muus P, Duhrsen U *et al.* (2007) Effect of the complement inhibitor eculizumab on thromboembolism in patients with paroxysmal nocturnal hemoglobinuria. *Blood* **110**: 4123–8.

Inoue N, Izui-Sarumaru T, Murakami Y *et al.* (2006) Molecular basis of clonal expansion of hematopoiesis in 2 patients with paroxysmal nocturnal hemoglobinuria. *Blood* **108**: 4232–6.

Kelly R, Arnold L, Richard SJ *et al.* (2008) Modification of the standard eculizumab dose to successfully manage intravascular hemolysis breakthrough in patients with paroxysmal nocturnal hemoglobinuria. *Blood* **112**: Abstract 3441.

Kelly R, Arnold L, Richards SJ *et al.* (2010) The management of pregnancy in paroxysmal nocturnal haemoglobunuria on long term eculizumab. *British Journal of Haematology* **149**: 446–50.

Kelly RJ, Tooze RM, Doody GM *et al.* (2007) The investigation of *HMGA2* dysregulation and promoter mutations in *PIG-M* in the molecular pathogenesis of paroxysmal nocturnal haemoglobinuria (PNH). *Blood* **110**: Abstract 3671.

McMullin MF, Hillmen P, Jackson J *et al.* (1993) Tissue plasminogen activator for hepatic vein thrombosis in paroxysmal nocturnal haemoglobinuria. *Journal of Internal Medicine* **235**: 85–9.

Miyata T, Takeda J, Iida Y *et al.* (1993) The cloning of PIG-A, a component in the early step of GPI-anchor biosynthesis. *Science* **259**: 1318–20.

Miyata T, Yamada N, Iida Y *et al.* (1994) Abnormalities of PIG-A transcripts in granulocytes from patients with paroxysmal nocturnal hemoglobinuria. *New England Journal of Medicine* **330**: 249–55.

Moyo VM, Mukhina GL, Garrett ES, Brodsky RA (2004) Natural history of paroxysmal nocturnal haemoglobinuria using modern diagnostic assays. *British Journal of Haematology* **126**: 133–8.

Nishimura J, Kanakura Y, Ware RE *et al.* (2004) Clinical course and flow cytometric analysis of paroxysmal nocturnal hemoglobinuria in the United States and Japan. *Medicine (Baltimore)* **83**: 193–207.

Parker CJ (2002) Historical aspects of paroxysmal nocturnal haemoglobinuria: defining the disease. *British Journal of Haematology* **117**: 3–22.

Parker CJ, Omine M, Richards S *et al.* (2005) Diagnosis and management of paroxysmal nocturnal hemoglobinuria. *Blood* **106**: 3699–709.

Ray JG, Burrows RF, Ginsberg JS *et al.* (2000) Paroxysmal nocturnal hemoglobinuria and the risk of venous thrombosis: review and recommendations for management of the pregnant and non-pregnant patient. *Haemostasis* **30**: 103–17.

Richards SJ, Hill A, Hillmen P (2007) Recent advances in the diagnosis, monitoring and management of patients with paroxysmal

nocturnal hemoglobinuria. *Cytometry. Part B, Clinical Cytometry* **72**: 291–8.

Rimola J, Martin J, Puig J *et al.* (2004) The kidney in paroxysmal nocturnal haemoglobinuria: MRI findings. *British Journal of Radiology* **77**: 953–6.

Risitano AM, Notaro R, Marando L *et al.* (2009) Complement fraction 3 binding on erythrocytes as additional mechanism of disease in paroxysmal nocturnal hemoglobinuria patients treated by eculizumab. *Blood* **113**: 4094–100.

Rother RP, Bell L, Hillmen P, Gladwin MT (2005) The clinical sequelae of intravascular hemolysis and extracellular plasma haemoglobin: a novel mechanism of human disease. *Journal of the American Medical Association* **293**: 1653–62.

Rother RP, Rollins SA, Mojcik CF *et al.* (2007) Discovery and development of the complement inhibitor eculizumab for the treatment of paroxysmal nocturnal hemoglobinuria. *Nature Biotechnology* **25**: 1256–64.

Saso R, Marsh J, Cevreska L *et al.* (1999) Bone marrow transplants for paroxysmal nocturnal haemoglobinuria. *British Journal of Haematology* **104**: 392–6.

Socié G, Hillmen P, Muus P *et al.* (2007) Sustained improvements in transfusion requirements, fatigue and thrombosis with eculizumab treatment in paroxysmal nocturnal hemoglobinuria. *Blood* **110**: Abstract 3672.

Takahashi M, Takeda J, Hirose S *et al.* (1993) Deficient biosynthesis of *N*-acetylglucosaminyl-phosphatidylinositol, the first intermediate of glycosyl phosphatidylinositol anchor biosynthesis, in cell lines established from patients with paroxysmal nocturnal hemoglobinuria. *Journal of Experimental Medicine* **177**: 517–21.

Takeda J, Miyata T, Kawagoe K *et al.* (1993) Deficiency of the GPI anchor caused by a somatic mutation of the PIG-A gene in paroxysmal nocturnal hemoglobinuria. *Cell* **73**: 703–11.

CHAPTER 12

Inherited aplastic anaemia/bone marrow failure syndromes

Inderjeet S Dokal

Barts and The London School of Medicine and Dentistry, Queen Mary University of London, Barts and The London Children's Hospital, London, UK

Introduction

A number of inherited (constitutional/genetic) disorders are characterized by aplastic anaemia (AA)/bone marrow failure, usually in association with one or more somatic abnormalities (Table 12.1). The features of some of these are summarized in Table 12.2. The precise incidence/prevalence of these remains unclear but, collectively, they represent approximately 10–20% of patients presenting with AA and constitute a significant clinical burden, as many are associated with premature mortality. The bone marrow failure may present at birth or at a variable time thereafter, including in adulthood in some cases. The bone marrow failure may involve all lineages or a single lineage; in some cases it may initially be associated with a single cytopenia and then progress to pancytopenia. Scientifically, they constitute an important group of diseases as recent advances in understanding the genetics of some of these are not only beginning to unravel their pathophysiology but are also providing important insights into normal haemopoiesis.

The two syndromes that are frequently associated with generalized bone marrow failure/AA are Fanconi anaemia (FA) and dyskeratosis congenita (DC). These two syndromes are now also two of the best characterized and are discussed in some detail in this chapter (followed by sections on Shwachman–Diamond syndrome, Diamond–Blackfan anaemia, congenital

dyserythropoietic anaemia, congenital neutropenia, thrombocytopenia with absent radii and congenital amegakaryocytic thrombocytopenia) to demonstrate their clinical and genetic heterogeneity, management and possible impact on our understanding of the pathophysiology of the more common 'idiopathic aplastic anaemia'. Indeed, patients with both FA and DC can sometimes present with AA alone as their initial manifestation and can thus pose a diagnostic/management challenge.

Fanconi anaemia

Clinical features

Since the first description by Guido Fanconi in 1927, FA has become to be recognized as an autosomal recessive disorder (X-linked in a rare subset) in which there is progressive bone marrow failure and an increased predisposition to malignancy, especially acute myeloid leukaemia (AML). Most, but not all, affected individuals also have one or more somatic abnormalities, including skin (café-au-lait spots), skeletal (absent thumbs, radial hypoplasia, scoliosis), genitourinary (underdeveloped gonads, horseshoe kidneys), gastrointestinal, cardiac and neurological anomalies (Table 12.3). Some of these somatic abnormalities are shown in Figure 12.1. The course of the disease and the pattern of somatic abnormalities show considerable variation, with approximately one-third of patients having no physical abnormalities. This makes diagnosis based on clinical criteria alone difficult and unreliable.

Postgraduate Haematology: 6th edition. Edited by A. Victor Hoffbrand, Daniel Catovsky, Edward G.D. Tuddenham, Anthony R. Green
© 2011 Blackwell Publishing Ltd.

Table 12.1 The inherited bone marrow failure syndromes.

Pancytopenia (usually associated with a global haemopoietic defect)
Fanconi anaemia
Dyskeratosis congenita
Shwachman–Diamond syndrome
Reticular dysgenesis
Pearson syndrome
Familial aplastic anaemia (autosomal and X-linked forms)
Myelodysplasia
Non-haematological syndromes (Down, Dubowitz syndromes)

Single cytopenia (usually)
Anaemia
  Diamond–Blackfan anaemia
  Congenital dyserythropoietic anaemia
Neutropenia
  Severe congenital neutropenia including Kostmann syndrome
Thrombocytopenia
  Congenital amegakaryocytic thrombocytopenia
  Amegakaryocytic thrombocytopenia with absent radii

Table 12.3 Somatic abnormalities in FA.

Abnormality	Percentage of patients
Skeletal (radial ray, hip, vertebral, scoliosis, rib)	71
Skin pigmentation (café-au-lait, hyper- and hypo-pigmentation)	64
Short stature	63
Eyes (microphthalmia)	38
Renal and urinary tract	34
Male genital	20
Mental retardation	16
Gastrointestinal (e.g. anorectal, duodenal atresia)	14
Heart	13
Hearing	11
Central nervous system (e.g. hydrocephalus, septum pellucidum)	8
No abnormalities	30

Source: modified from Auerbach *et al.* (2001) with permission.

Table 12.2 Characteristics of the bone marrow failure syndromes.

	FA	DC	SDS	DBA	CDA	TAR	SCN	IAA
Inheritance pattern	AR, XLR	XLR, AR, AD	AR	AD	AR, AD	AR	AD, AR	?
Somatic abnormalities	Yes	Yes	Yes	Yes	Rare	Yes	Rare	?None
Bone marrow failure	AA (> 90%)	AA (~ 80%)	AA (20%)	RCA	Eryth	Megs	Neutropenia	Yes (100%)
Short telomeres	Yes	Yes	Yes	?	?	?	?	Yes
Malignancy	Yes	Yes	Yes	Yes	?No	?No	Yes	Yes
Chromosome instability	Yes	Yes	Yes	?	?	?	?	Yes
Genes identified	13	6	1	7	1	No	3	*

*Heterozygous mutations in TERC and TERT are risk factors for some cases of AA.
AA, aplastic anaemia; AD, autosomal dominant; AR, autosomal recessive; CDA, congenital dyserythropoietic anaemia; DBA, Diamond–Blackfan anaemia; DC, dyskeratosis congenita; FA, Fanconi anaemia; IAA, idiopathic aplastic anaemia; Eryth, ineffective erythropoiesis; Megs, low megakaryocytes; RCA, red cell aplasia; SCN, severe congenital neutropenia; SDS, Shwachman–Diamond syndrome; TAR, thrombocytopenia with absent radii; XLR, X-linked recessive.

The cumulative incidence of bone marrow failure by the age of 40 years is estimated to be around 90%. At birth the blood count is usually normal. Pancytopenia develops insidiously and presents in most cases between the ages of 5 and 10 years (median age 7 years). However, in some cases the pancytopenia develops in adolescence or even in adult life. The haemoglobin and platelet count are usually first to fall; the granulocytes are usually well preserved in the early stages. As the pancytopenia develops, the bone marrow becomes progressively hypocellular. There is often a marked increase in macrophage activity with evidence of haemophagocytosis. Bone marrow failure leading to fatal haemorrhage or infection is the main cause of death in FA patients. In an analysis from the International Fanconi Anaemia Registry (IFAR), the median survival time was 24 years; this is changing with improvements in clinical care.

FA is associated with an increased risk of leukaemia and other malignancies. The leukaemias are usually of the acute myeloid type, particularly FAB types M4 (myelomonocytic) and M5 (monocytic). In some cases, leukaemia may be the initial event leading to the diagnosis of FA. The cumulative incidence of haematological malignancy by the age of 40 years is 33%. Besides these haematological malignancies, there is a significant risk of hepatic tumours and squamous cell carcinoma, including squamous cell carcinomas of the vulva, oesophagus, head

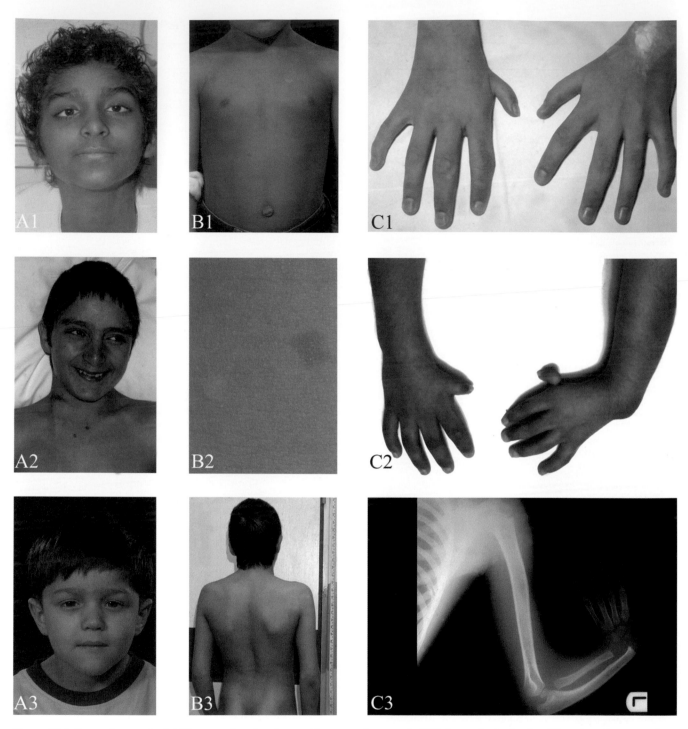

Figure 12.1 Fanconi anaemia. (a) Photographs of patients with FA (A1–A3) with small mouth and chin ('Fanconi facies'). (b) Abnormalities of pigmentation (hyper- and hypo-pigmentation) on the abdomen (B1) with a close-up (B2) of a café-au-lait spot and a hypopigmented patch. The bottom photograph (B3) shows the back of an FA patient demonstrating lumbar scoliosis. (c) Hands/forearms of FA children showing hypoplastic thumbs (C1), rudimentary ('dangling') thumbs (C2) and a radiograph (C3) showing rudimentary thumb (skeletal) development.

and neck. The cumulative incidence of solid tumours is calculated to be 28% by the age of 40 years. The impression is that malignancies occur mainly in patients with late-onset bone marrow failure and longer survival, with a median age of 13 years for leukaemia and 25 years for solid tumours. Recent analysis from the German FA registry largely concurs with these earlier observations. Furthermore, long-term follow-up in FA patients who have been treated by haemopoietic stem cell transplantation (HSCT) is showing a higher incidence of non-haematological malignancies in patients with FA than patients with other types of bone marrow failure who underwent HSCT, again emphasizing the predisposition to malignancy.

Cell and molecular biology

Over the last three decades many advances have been made in our understanding of the pathophysiology of FA. FA cells characteristically display a high frequency of spontaneous chromosomal breakage and hypersensitivity to DNA cross-linking agents such as diepoxybutane (DEB) and mitomycin C (MMC). This genomic instability (Figure 12.2) led to the development of a diagnostic test (i.e. increased chromosomal breakage in FA cells compared with normal controls after exposure to DEB/MMC) over two decades ago and this remains a useful FA screening test today. This 'FA cell phenotype' has also facilitated many advances in our understanding of FA, including elucidation of the complex genetics of this disease, with 13 subtypes/complementation groups currently characterized. The genes responsible for these subtypes have all been identified and are designated *FANCA, FANCB, FANCC, FANCD1, FANCD2,*

FANCE, FANCF, FANCG, FANCI, FANCJ, FANCL, FANCM and *FANCN* (Table 12.4).

Studies from several research groups around the world have demonstrated that the proteins encoded by the FA genes participate in a complicated network important in DNA repair. Specifically, eight of the FA proteins (FANCA, FANCB, FANCC, FANCE, FANCF, FANCG, FANCL and FANCM) interact with each other and form a nuclear complex called the FA core complex (Figure 12.3). The FA core complex is required for activation of the FANCD2 protein to a monoubiquitinated isoform (FANCD2-Ub). In normal (non-FA) cells, FANCD2 is monoubiquitinated in response to DNA damage and is targeted to chromatin containing the DNA damage (e.g. DNA cross-link). FANCD2-Ub then interacts with DNA repair proteins (including BRCA2 and RAD51) leading to repair of the DNA damage. In cells from FA-A, FA-B, FA-C, FA-E, FA-F, FA-G, FA-L or FA-M patients, FANCD2 monoubiquitination is not observed. It has been recently observed that FANCI (the protein mutated in the FA-I subtype) is a paralogue of FANCD2. FANCI associates with FANCD2 as the FANCI–FANCD2 (I–D2) complex. Like FANCD2, FANCI is also monoubiquitinated. FA-D1 patients have biallelic mutations in BRCA2. These observations have linked the FA proteins (FANCA, FANCB, FANCC, FANCD2, FANCE, FANCF, FANCG, FANCI, FANCL and FANCM) with BRCA1 and BRCA2 (FANCD1) in a DNA damage response pathway called the FA–BRCA pathway. The BRCA2 protein is important in the repair of DNA damage by homologous recombination. Cells lacking BRCA2 inaccurately repair damaged DNA and are hypersensitive to DNA cross-linking agents. It has also been established that FANCJ is BRIP1

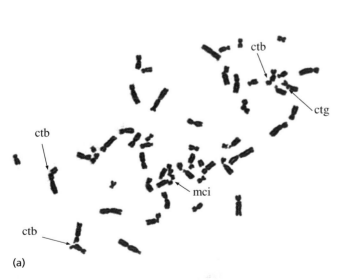

(a)

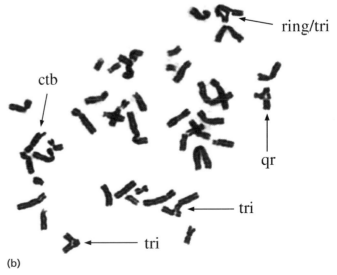

(b)

Figure 12.2 (a, b) Chromosomal abnormalities seen in FA lymphocytes following incubation with diepoxybutane. ctb, chromatid break; ctg, chromatid gap; mci, multiple chromatid

interchanges (complex rearrangement); tri, triradial; qr, quadriradial. (Courtesy of Nicola Foot, Cytogenetics Section, Hammersmith Hospital.)

Table 12.4 FA complementation groups/genetic subtypes.

Complementation group/gene	Approximate percentage of FA patients	Chromosome location	Protein (amino acids)	Exons
A (*FANCA*)	65	16q24.3	1455	43
B (*FANCB*)*	< 1	Xp22.2	859	10
C (*FANCC*)	12	9q22.3	558	14
D1 (*FANCD1*)†	< 1	13q12.3	3418	27
D2 (*FANCD2*)	< 1	3p25.3	1451	44
E (*FANCE*)	4	6p21.3	536	10
F (*FANCF*)	4	11p15	374	1
G (*FANCG*)	12	9p13	622	14
I (*FANCI*)	< 1	15q26.1	1328	35
J (*FANCJ/BRIP1*)‡	< 5	17q23.2	1249	20
L (*FANCL*)	< 1	2p16.1	375	14
M (*FANCM*)	< 1	14q21.3	2048	23
N (*FANCN/PALB2*)§	< 1	16p12.1	1186	13

FANCB is on the X chromosome.
†*FANCD1* is *BRCA2*.
‡FANCJ is BRIP1 (BRCA1 interacting protein).
§FANCN is PALB2 (partner and localizer of BRCA2).

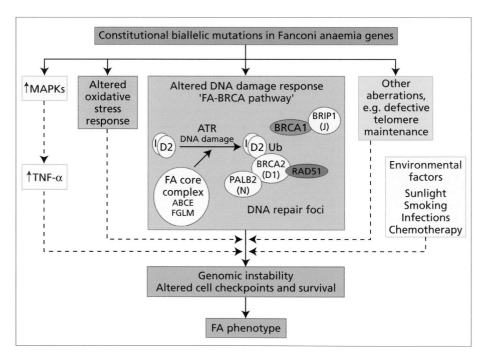

Figure 12.3 Schematic representation of the FA–BRCA pathway and related networks. The diagram shows that the constitutional mutations in FA cells lead to aberration of the FA–BRCA pathway, abnormal handling of oxidative stress, aberrant activation of mitogen-activated protein kinases (MAPKs), defective telomere maintenance as well as possibly other biological aberrations. The net impact of these is increased genomic instability and altered cell survival/checkpoints. The diagram also highlights the potential role of environmental factors such as smoking and sunlight in adding to the effect of the FA mutations. Within the FA–BRCA pathway, the proteins shown in yellow are those mutated in different FA patients. The FA core complex consists of eight FA proteins (A, B, C, E, F, G, L and M) and this, together with ATR (ataxia telangiectasia and RAD3-related protein), is essential for activation (ubiquitination) of the I–D2 complex after DNA damage. Activated I–D2-Ub translocates to DNA repair foci where it associates with other DNA damage response proteins including BRCA2 and RAD51 and participates in DNA repair. TNF, tumour necrosis factor; Ub, ubiquitination.

(partner of BRCA1) and that FANCN is PALB2 (partner of BRCA2). These findings further strengthen the connection between the FA and BRCA proteins and DNA repair.

The FA–BRCA pathway is activated in response to DNA damage (e.g. replication fork arrest) and involves ATR (ataxia telangiectasia and RAD3-related protein) (Figure 12.3). The pathway is inactivated by the de-ubiquitinating enzyme USP1. ATR appears to directly regulate the FA pathway as it is required for the monoubiquitination of FANCD2 and FANCI. ATR is mutated in a subset of patients with Seckel syndrome, a disease exhibiting some clinical similarity to FA. ATR and ATM (ataxia telangiectasia mutated) are known to phosphorylate FANCD2 and FANCI. Interestingly, ATR-Seckel cells also exhibit defects in FANCD2 monoubiquitination. Furthermore, Nijmegen breakage syndrome (NBS) cells (mutated in *NBN*) show defects in FANCD2 monoubiquitination. This suggests that as well as clinical overlap between patients with FA, NBS and Seckel syndrome, there is also overlap in the biological defects observed in cells from these patients. This highlights the complexity of physical interactions between the different molecules involved in this matrix of pathways. Equally it is clear that FA cells also display other abnormalities in addition to DNA repair (Figure 12.3). This includes hypersensitivity to oxygen, accelerated telomere shortening, abnormal cell cycle kinetics, and overactivation of the mitogen-activated protein kinase (MAPK) pathways leading to overproduction of tumour necrosis factor (TNF)-α. These observations suggest that our understanding of the molecular events responsible for all the FA pathology is currently incomplete.

It is noteworthy that the phenotypes associated with biallelic *BRCA2* (FA-D1) and *PALB2* (FA-N) mutations are markedly similar to each other but different from the other FA genes. Specifically, FA-D1 and FA-N are associated with high risks of solid childhood malignancies (e.g. Wilms tumour and medulloblastoma) which are not usually seen in the other FA subtypes. Furthermore, heterozygous mutations in *BRCA2* (FA-D1), *PALB2* (FA-N) and *BRIP1* (FA-J) confer an elevated risk of breast cancer yet this is not the case for the other FA genes. These differences highlight that the relationship between the FA proteins and their interactions with other molecules is complex at both the clinical and molecular levels.

In vitro gene transfer studies have demonstrated that introduction of the appropriate wild-type FA gene into FA human lymphoid and haemopoietic cells markedly enhances their growth and normalizes their response to MMC; in lymphoid lines, cell kinetics (G_2 phase) and chromosomal breakage are normalized. Thus the transfer of the wild-type FA genes corrects the extreme sensitivity to DNA cross-linking agents, the hallmark of the FA cell phenotype. These studies provide the rationale for haemopoietic gene therapy (discussed below).

Murine mouse models of FA have shown that haemopoietic progenitors are hypersensitive to TNF-α and interferon (IFN)-γ. This differential hypersensitivity to IFN-γ is thought to be mediated by *fas*-induced apoptosis and may turn out to be an important mechanism in the development of progressive bone marrow failure in FA. It is noteworthy that patients with idiopathic AA usually have raised IFN-γ levels, thus providing a possible link in the pathophysiology of bone marrow failure in both idiopathic and FA-associated AA. The presence of short telomeres in cells from patients with both FA and idiopathic AA can also be expected to be important in the pathophysiology of bone marrow failure in both diseases. This feature is discussed further in relation to DC.

Treatment

The major cause of premature mortality in FA patients is the development of bone marrow failure. Until the advent of HSCT, treatment consisted largely of supportive care and attempts to stabilize and improve haemopoietic function by administrating androgens (oxymetholone) and corticosteroids (prednisolone). Oxymetholone treatment can produce useful trilineage haematological responses in 50–70% of patients but many will become refractory after a variable time. Oxymetholone is associated with side-effects, including liver dysfunction and increased risk of hepatic tumours. It is a very good holding treatment until more definitive treatment can be planned using HSCT, which has now become the treatment of choice. From the *in vitro* and *in vivo* studies it has become clear that cells from FA patients are hypersensitive to agents such as cyclophosphamide and high-dose irradiation compared with non-FA patients. Therefore, HSCT conditioning regimens have been modified by reducing the dose of cyclophosphamide and radiation. Initially, using low-dose cyclophosphamide (20 mg/kg) and 4.5–6 Gy of thoracoabdominal irradiation, the actuarial survival for patients transplanted using HLA identical sibling donors was found to be around 70% at 2 years. The results using unrelated donors were less good, with 2 year survival between 20 and 40%. More recently, the use of fludarabine is being explored in conditioning protocols. Additionally, long-term follow-up of patients who have survived after HSCT shows a much higher incidence of malignancies, particularly of the head and neck, usually 8–10 years after the transplant. This partly relates to the inherent predisposition of FA patients to malignancy (which can perhaps now be explained given the link to defects in DNA repair) and partly to factors such as the use of radiotherapy in the conditioning. Transplant groups are therefore exploring low-dose cyclophosphamide (20–40 mg/kg) HSCT protocols that avoid the use of radiotherapy. Preliminary results using fludarabine (120–150 mg/m^2) in association with low-dose cyclophosphamide are very encouraging for both sibling and unrelated HSCT. Longer follow-up is necessary to determine if such protocols will be associated with a lower risk of malignancy.

In addition to HSCT, alternative treatment strategies are being explored. The identification of the FA genes, combined with the *in vitro* gene transfer data which show that FA haemopoietic stem cells rescued by gene therapy should have a selective growth advantage within the hypoplastic bone marrow environment, has resulted in clinical studies of retroviral-mediated gene therapy for FA patients. The pilot study on FA-C patients was associated with no serious side-effects but efficacy was limited. Further studies on this approach are being undertaken but none have yet shown significant efficacy in the clinic.

The identification of FA *mosaic* patients strengthens the case for future trials of gene therapy. In such cases, the DEB/MMC test may be negative or only demonstrate chromosomal instability in a subgroup of cells. Somatic mosaicism is due to reversion of a pathogenic allele to 'wild' type in a single haemopoietic (somatic) cell. The mechanism of how this occurs can vary, but in each case it generates one 'normal' FA allele and the resulting cell effectively becomes a 'heterozygous cell', which would be expected to have a growth/survival advantage in the background of FA cells. These mosaic patients can have an improvement in their haematological profile, suggesting that a single pluripotent stem cell may be sufficient to restore adequate haemopoiesis. FA patients with somatic mosaicism can thus be regarded as having undergone natural haemopoietic gene therapy.

Over the last 20 years there has been significant progress in treating the bone marrow failure associated with FA. For the future the major challenge will relate to the treatment of malignancies and in the management of patients with atypical presentations.

Dyskeratosis congenita

Clinical features

Classical DC is an inherited disease characterized by the mucocutaneous triad of abnormal skin pigmentation, nail dystrophy and mucosal leucoplakia (Figure 12.4). Since its first description by Jacobi in 1906 and Zinsser in 1910, a variety of non-cutaneous (dental, gastrointestinal, genitourinary, neurological, ophthalmic, pulmonary and skeletal) abnormalities have also been reported (Table 12.5). Bone marrow failure is the principal cause of early mortality, with an additional predisposition to malignancy (haematological and non-haematological) and fatal pulmonary complications. X-linked recessive, autosomal dominant and autosomal recessive forms of the disease are recognized. It is therefore now acknowledged that DC is a very heterogeneous disorder, both clinically and genetically.

Clinical manifestations in DC often appear during childhood. The skin pigmentation and nail changes typically appear first, usually by the age of 10 years. Bone marrow failure usually develops below the age of 20 years; 80–90% of patients will have developed bone marrow abnormalities by the age of 30 years. In some cases, the bone marrow abnormalities may appear before the mucocutaneous manifestations and the patients may be categorized as having 'idiopathic aplastic anaemia'. The main causes of death are bone marrow failure/immunodeficiency

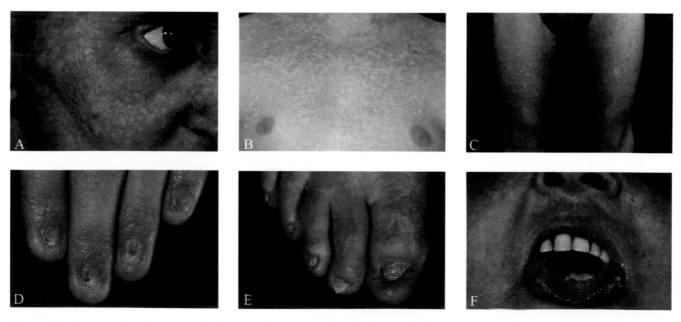

Figure 12.4 Photographs of patients with dyskeratosis congenita showing abnormal skin pigmentation (A, B, C), nail dystrophy (D, E) and leucoplakia of tongue (F).

Table 12.5 Somatic abnormalities in dyskeratosis congenita.

Abnormality	Percentage of patients
Abnormal skin pigmentation	89
Nail dystrophy	88
Bone marrow failure	85.5
Leucoplakia	78
Epiphora	30.5
Learning difficulties/developmental delay/mental retardation	25.4
Pulmonary disease	20.3
Short stature	19.5
Extensive dental caries/loss	16.9
Oesophageal stricture	16.9
Premature hair loss/greying/sparse eyelashes	16.1
Hyperhidrosis	15.3
Malignancy	9.8
Intrauterine growth retardation	7.6
Liver disease/peptic ulceration/enteropathy	7.3
Ataxia/cerebellar hypoplasia	6.8
Hypogonadism/undescended testes	5.9
Microcephaly	5.9
Urethral stricture/phimosis	5.1
Osteoporosis/aseptic necrosis/scoliosis	5.1
Deafness	0.8

(about 60–70%), pulmonary complications (about 10–15%) and malignancy (about 10%).

Cell and molecular biology

DC has many features in common with FA, in which cells display hypersensitivity to clastogenic agents such as MMC. Although the occasional DC patient may show some evidence of chromosome breakage, in general there is no significant difference in chromosomal breakage between DC and normal lymphocytes with or without the use of bleomycin, DEB, MMC and γ-irradiation. This observation enables DC patients to be distinguished from FA.

Primary DC skin fibroblasts are abnormal in both morphology and growth rate. Furthermore, they show unbalanced chromosomal rearrangements (dicentrics, tricentrics, translocations, end-to-end fusions) in the absence of any clastogenic agents. In addition, peripheral blood and bone marrow metaphases from some patients show unbalanced chromosomal rearrangements in the absence of any clastogenic agents. These studies provide evidence for a defect that predisposes DC cells to developing chromosomal rearrangements. DC, like FA, may thus be regarded as a chromosome/genomic instability disorder but with a predisposition principally to chromosomal rearrangements rather than the gaps and breaks seen in FA.

Haemopoietic progenitor studies have shown reduced numbers of all progenitors compared with control subjects and there is usually a downwards decline with time. The degree to which the progenitors are reduced can vary from patient to patient and they can be reduced even when the peripheral blood count is normal. The demonstration of abnormalities of growth and chromosomal rearrangements in fibroblasts suggests that the bone marrow failure is likely to be a consequence of abnormalities in both haemopoietic stem cells and stromal cells.

X-chromosome inactivation patterns (XCIPs) have been studied in peripheral blood cells of women from X-linked DC families by investigating a methylation-sensitive restriction enzyme site in the polymorphic human androgen receptor locus (*HUMARA*) at Xq11.2–q12. All carriers of X-linked DC showed complete skewing in XCIP. The presence of the extremely skewed pattern of X-inactivation in peripheral blood cells suggests that cells expressing the defective gene have a growth/survival disadvantage over those expressing the normal allele. Furthermore, a skewed XCIP provides important information about carrier status for use in the counselling of families at risk of DC. In addition, XCIP allow us to distinguish an inherited mutation from a *de novo* event in sporadic male DC cases, as well as autosomal from X-linked forms of the disease.

The majority of DC patients recruited to the Dyskeratosis Congenita Registry in London are male. This observation suggests that the X-linked recessive form of DC represents a major subset of cases. Initially, through linkage analysis in one large family with only affected males, it was possible to map the gene for the X-linked form to Xq28. The availability of polymorphic genetic markers from the Xq28 and additional X-linked families facilitated positional cloning of the gene (*DKC1*) that is mutated in X-linked DC. Identification of the *DKC1* gene in 1998 made available a genetic test that can be used to confirm diagnosis in suspected cases and provide antenatal diagnosis in X-linked families. It also led to the demonstration that another rare syndrome, Hoyeraal–Hreidarsson (HH) syndrome, is due to mutations in the *DKC1* gene. HH syndrome is a severe multisystem disorder characterized by severe growth failure, abnormalities of brain development (particularly cerebellar hypoplasia), aplastic anaemia and immunodeficiency (T+ B− NK− severe combined immunodeficiency). The recognition that HH syndrome is a severe variant of DC has further highlighted the considerable variability of the DC phenotype.

In addition to providing an accurate diagnostic test, this genetic advance has provided insights into the pathogenesis of DC. The *DKC1* gene is expressed in all tissues of the body, indicating that it has a vital housekeeping function in the human cell. This correlates well with the multisystem phenotype of DC. The *DKC1* gene and its encoded protein, dyskerin, are highly conserved throughout evolution. Dyskerin is a nucleolar protein associated with the H/ACA class of small nucleolar RNAs (snoRNAs) and is involved in pseudo-uridylation of specific residues of ribosomal RNA (rRNA). This step is essential for ribosome biogenesis and therefore initially suggested that DC arises largely because of defective ribosome production.

Subsequent studies have shown that dyskerin also associates with the RNA component of telomerase (TERC), which also contains an H/ACA consensus sequence. Telomerase is an enzyme complex that is important in maintaining chromosomal telomere length after cell division. The precise composition of the telomerase complex is unknown, but two essential components, the RNA component (TERC) and the catalytic reverse transcriptase (TERT), have been well characterized. Telomerase activity can be reconstituted *in vitro* using just

TERC and TERT. In patients with X-linked DC, it was initially demonstrated that the level of TERC was reduced and that telomere lengths were much shorter than in age-matched normal controls. Subsequently, it was found that telomeres are also shorter in cells from patients with autosomal forms of DC. This therefore suggested that DC might principally be a disease of defective telomere maintenance rather than of ribosome biogenesis. Further clarification came from linkage analysis in one large DC family, which showed that the gene for autosomal dominant DC is on chromosome 3q, in the same area where the gene for TERC had been previously mapped. This led to *TERC* mutation analysis in this and other DC families and the demonstration that autosomal dominant DC is due to mutations in the *TERC* gene.

As the *DKC1*-encoded protein dyskerin and TERC are both components of the telomerase complex (Figure 12.5), it now appears that DC arises principally from an abnormality in tel-

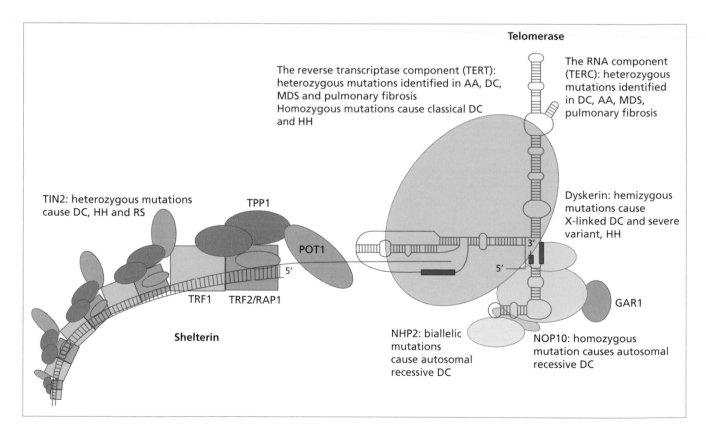

Figure 12.5 A schematic representation of the telomerase complex (dyskerin, GAR1, NHP2, NOP10, TERC and TERT), the shelterin complex and their association with different categories of dyskeratosis congenita and related diseases. The telomerase complex is an RNA–protein complex since TERC is a 451-base RNA molecule that is never translated. The other molecules (dyskerin, GAR1, NHP2, NOP10 and TERT) are proteins. Recent studies suggest that the minimal active telomerase enzyme is composed of two molecules each of TERT, TERC and dyskerin. Dyskerin, GAR1, NHP2 and NOP10 are believed to be important for the stability of the telomerase complex. The shelterin complex is made up of six proteins (TIN2, POT1, TPP1, TRF1, TRF2 and RAP1) and is important in protecting the telomere. Mutations in components of the telomerase complex or the shelterin complex, as occurs in different subtypes of DC, result in telomere shortening. AA, aplastic anaemia; DC, dyskeratosis congenita; HH, Hoyeraal–Hreidarsson syndrome; MDS, myelodysplastic syndrome; RS, Revesz syndrome.

Table 12.6 Genetic subtypes of dyskeratosis congenita (DC).

DC subtype	Approximate percentage of DC patients	Chromosome location	RNA/protein product	Exons
X-linked recessive	30	Xq28	Dyskerin	15
Autosomal dominant	< 5	3q26.2	TERC	1
	< 5	5p15.33	TERT	16
	10	14q12	TIN2	6
Autosomal recessive	< 1	15q14–q15	NOP10	2
	< 1	5p15.33	TERT	16
	< 1	5q35.3	NHP2	4
Uncharacterized*	40–50	?	?	?

*These are likely to represent more than one genetic locus and include the genetically heterogeneous autosomal recessive DC.

omerase activity. Affected tissues are those that need constant renewal, consistent with a basic deficiency in stem cell activity due to defective telomerase activity. The demonstration of *DKC1* and *TERC* mutations in DC families provides an accurate diagnostic test, including antenatal diagnosis, in a significant subset of cases (Table 12.6). For DC patients, this now also provides the basis for designing new treatments. For the wider community it provided the first direct genetic link between a human disease characterized by features of premature ageing (premature grey hair/hair loss, early dental loss, abnormalities of skin pigmentation, nail dystrophy, bone marrow failure, increased predisposition to malignancy) and short telomeres. Therefore, unravelling the biology of this rare disease has had important implications not only for patients with DC but also for the more common disorders, such as ageing, cancer and AA, that are also associated with abnormal telomeres.

Recently, heterozygous *TERC* mutations have been observed in a subset of patients with AA and myelodysplastic syndrome (MDS) but who lacked classical features of DC. Furthermore, AA patients associated with *TERC* mutations had significantly shorter telomeres than age-matched controls. These data indicate that, in a subset of patients with AA and MDS, the disorder is associated with a genetic defect in the telomere maintenance pathway. They also highlight the diverse manifestations of DC: its severe variant form (HH syndrome), its classical form and its 'cryptic' form (AA or MDS). The similarities between DC and AA are given in Table 12.2.

These findings also suggest that treatments aimed at restoration of telomere length might be useful in this group of patients. Heterozygous mutations in *TERT* have also recently been found in some patients with bone marrow failure and autosomal dominant DC. These findings further support the model that DC is principally a disorder of telomere maintenance. Additionally, telomerase dysfunction (heterozygous mutations in *TERT* or *TERC*) has also been identified as the likely cause of a subset of familial idiopathic pulmonary fibrosis, a disease in which fibrotic tissue forms in the lungs, eventually leading to respiratory failure. More recently, a subset of DC patients have been found to have heterozygous mutations in a component of the shelterin complex TIN2. Patients with *TIN2* mutations also have very short telomeres, providing further evidence that DC is principally a disorder of defective telomere maintenance.

Recently, the genetic basis of some cases of autosomal recessive DC has been elucidated. In one large family with autosomal recessive DC, the disease has been found to be due to homozygous mutations in the telomerase-associated protein NOP10. Patients with homozygous *NOP10* mutations, like patients with *DKC1* and *TERC* mutations, were also found to have very short telomeres, further highlighting that DC is principally a disease of defective telomere maintenance. In some autosomal recessive families it has been found that the disease is due to biallelic mutations in *TERT*, suggesting that a pure but severe deficiency in telomerase can produce a phenotype of classical autosomal recessive DC and its severe variant, HH syndrome. Very recently, in two autosomal recessive families biallelic mutations have been found in the telomerase component NHP2 and these patients also had very short telomeres.

Treatment

Transient successful responses to granulocyte/macrophage colony-stimulating factor (GM-CSF), granulocyte colony-stimulating factor (G-CSF) and erythropoietin have been reported. As in FA, the anabolic steroid oxymetholone (0.5–2.0 mg/kg daily) can produce an improvement in haemopoietic function in many (> 50%) patients for a variable period of time. The use of oxymetholone and growth factors may be synergistic in some patients. However, the main treatment for severe bone marrow failure is allogeneic HSCT, and there is some experience using both sibling and alternative stem cell donors. Unfortunately, because of early and late fatal pulmonary/

vascular complications after HSCT, the results of conventional transplants have been less successful than in FA. The presence of pulmonary disease in a significant proportion of DC patients perhaps now explains the high incidence of fatal pulmonary complications in the setting of HSCT. It also highlights the need to avoid therapies (such as busulfan and radiotherapy) associated with pulmonary toxicity. As bone marrow failure is the main cause of premature death in DC patients and HSCT is the only curative option for bone marrow failure at present, HSCT should continue to be performed on carefully selected patients. Perhaps the best candidates for HSCT are patients with no preexisting pulmonary disease and who have sibling donors. HSCT using fludarabine-based protocols that avoid radiotherapy and busulfan appears to be giving encouraging preliminary results.

DC is theoretically a good candidate for haemopoietic gene therapy. In any given patient, DC is a single-gene disorder and the cells that need to be targeted (haemopoietic stem cells) are accessible. Furthermore, there is evidence from fibroblast culture studies and from skewed XCIPs in X-linked DC carriers that cells transfected with the normal gene would have a growth/survival advantage compared with uncorrected cells. Such an advantage would also be predicted from the role of the DC genes in telomere maintenance. It remains to be seen whether treatments aimed at restoration of telomere length will prove to be of clinical benefit in DC and related disorders.

Shwachman–Diamond syndrome

Clinical features

Shwachman and Bodian and their colleagues first reported this disease independently in 1964. Shwachman–Diamond syndrome (SDS) is now recognized as an autosomal recessive disorder characterized by exocrine pancreatic insufficiency (100%), bone marrow dysfunction (100%) and other somatic abnormalities (particularly involving the skeletal system). Signs of pancreatic insufficiency (malabsorption, failure to thrive) are apparent early in infancy (note that pancreatic function can improve in a subset of patients with SDS by 5 years of age). Other common somatic abnormalities include short stature (~ 70%), protuberant abdomen and an ichthyotic skin rash (~ 60%). Metaphyseal dysostosis is seen on radiographs in about 75% of patients. Other abnormalities include hepatome-

galy, rib/thoracic cage abnormalities, hypertelorism, syndactyly, cleft palate, dental dysplasia, ptosis and skin pigmentation.

The spectrum of haematological abnormalities includes neutropenia (~ 60%), other cytopenias (~ 20% have pancytopenia), myelodysplasia and leukaemic transformation (~ 25%). The age at which leukaemia develops varies widely, from 1 to 43 years. AML is the commonest category and there is an unexplained preponderance of cases of leukaemia in males (male to female ratio approximately 3 : 1).

Exocrine pancreatic insufficiency and haematological abnormalities are also seen in Pearson syndrome (PS), and this is therefore an important differential diagnosis. In PS, the anaemia is usually more prominent than neutropenia and the marrow usually shows ringed sideroblasts along with vacuolation of myeloid and erythroid precursors. In addition, acidosis, abnormalities of liver function and mitochondrial DNA rearrangements are seen in PS. PS has a worse prognosis than SDS, with many patients dying before the age of 5 years from liver or marrow failure. Other differential diagnoses to be excluded are cartilage hair syndrome and cystic fibrosis.

Cell and molecular biology

The SDS gene (*SBDS*) on 7q11.22 was identified in 2003. The majority (> 90%) of SDS patients have been found to have mutations in this gene (Table 12.7). Its precise function is unknown but, based on the function of its homologues, it is predicted to have an important role in RNA metabolism and/or ribosome biogenesis. Recent data from yeast studies provide compelling evidence that the SBDS protein has an important role in the maturation of the 60S ribosomal subunit (Figure 12.6). Several abnormalities in SDS cells have been observed, including haemopoietic stem and stromal defects, increased rates of apoptosis and short telomeres. It will be interesting to see how mutations in the *SBDS* gene lead to all these cell defects, the increased frequency of isochromosome 7q and the clinical abnormalities characteristic of SDS. More immediately, this advance provides a genetic test that will facilitate diagnosis in difficult cases. It will also enable researchers to determine the role of the *SBDS* gene in AA, MDS and leukaemia in general. In this regard it has recently been shown that the SBDS protein can act to stabilize the mitotic spindle, preventing genomic instability, and that cells from SDS patients exhibit an increased incidence of abnormal mitoses.

Table 12.7 Genetic subtypes of Shwachman–Diamond syndrome (SDS).

SDS subtype	Approximate percentage of SDS patients	Chromosome location	Protein product	Exons
Autosomal recessive	> 90	7q11.22	SBDS	5
Uncharacterized	< 10	?	?	?

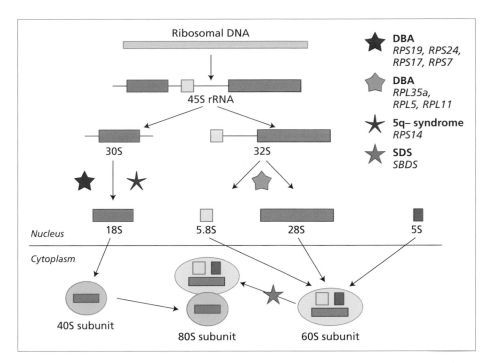

Figure 12.6 Schematic diagram showing scheme of ribosomal (r) RNA processing in human cells and the points at which this is possibly disrupted in the different bone marrow failure syndromes. The rRNAs are transcribed by RNA polymerase I as a single precursor transcript (45S rRNA). The 45S rRNA is then processed to 18S, 5.8S and 28S rRNAs. The 18S is a component of the 40S ribosomal subunit. The 5.8S and 28S together with 5S (synthesized independently) are components of the 60S ribosomal subunit. The 40S and 60S subunits are assembled to form the 80S ribosomes. The processing steps affected in Diamond–Blackfan anaemia (due to heterozygous mutations in *RPS19, RPS17, RPS24, RPS7, RPL35a, RPL5* and *RPL11*), 5q– syndrome (haploinsufficiency of *RPS14*) and Shwachman–Diamond syndrome (biallelic mutations in *SBDS*) are indicated by the different coloured stars. DBA, Diamond–Blackfan anaemia; SDS, Shwachman–Diamond syndrome.

Treatment

The malabsorption in SDS responds to treatment with oral pancreatic enzymes. For those with neutropenia, G-CSF may produce an improvement in the neutrophil count. Some patients with anaemia and/or thrombocytopenia may achieve haematological responses with oxymetholone treatment. As in other cases of bone marrow failure, supportive treatment with red cell and platelet transfusions and antibiotics is very important. The main cause of death is infection or bleeding.

Recent analysis of SDS patients has showed that the incidence of myelodysplasia and transformation to AML (about 15–25%) is higher than reported previously. The development of leukaemia, often with features of myelodysplasia, usually has a poor prognosis. SDS patients with leukaemia treated with conventional courses of chemotherapy usually fail to regenerate normal haemopoiesis. As this is a constitutional disorder all somatic cells, including haemopoietic stem cells, are abnormal. In addition, the haemopoietic stem cells may have accumulated secondary abnormalities as suggested by complex karyotypes (especially involving chromosome 7) often observed in the bone marrow from such patients. Therefore, for those who develop leukaemia, the only approach likely to be successful is allogeneic HSCT, perhaps in the future using low-intensity conditioning regimens that include fludarabine. The similarities between SDS and the other common inherited bone marrow failure syndromes emphasize that SDS should be regarded as a disorder with high propensity to develop both AA and leukaemic transformation, particularly AML with erythroid differentiation (AML-M6). As these complications may not develop until adult life, it is important to continue close haematological follow-up throughout life. It is noteworthy that non-haematological malignancies have not been observed in SDS patients.

Diamond–Blackfan anaemia

Clinical features

Red cell aplasia was first reported in 1936 by Josephs. In 1938, Diamond reported on four children with hypoplastic anaemia

197

and this has now come to be recognized as Diamond–Blackfan anaemia (DBA) or congenital pure red cell aplasia. DBA usually presents in early infancy, with features of anaemia such as pallor or failure to thrive. The hallmark of classical DBA is a selective decrease in erythroid precursors and normochromic macrocytic anaemia associated with a variable number of somatic abnormalities such as craniofacial, thumb, cardiac and urogenital malformations. Hitherto the diagnostic criteria for DBA have comprised (i) normochromic, usually macrocytic, but occasionally normocytic anaemia developing in early childhood; (ii) reticulocytopenia; (iii) normocellular bone marrow with selective deficiency of erythroid precursors (erythroblasts < 5%); (iv) normal or slightly decreased leucocyte counts; and (v) normal or often increased platelet counts. More recently, elevated erythrocyte deaminase activity, macrocytosis and elevated fetal haemoglobin have been added to the list of supportive features of DBA. It has also been recognized that in a subset of cases the presentation may be in adulthood.

There is considerable heterogeneity in the associated somatic abnormalities, pattern of inheritance and response to therapy. Analysis of 420 cases recruited to the DBA Registry of North America (DBAR) has confirmed previous findings as well as highlighting new features. The annual incidence of DBA is about 5 per million live births. The median age at presentation was 8 weeks and 93% of patients presented in the first year of life. In total, 79% were initially responsive to steroids, 17% were non-responsive and 4% were never treated with steroids; 31% of patients were receiving transfusions at analysis. The actuarial survival rates at older than 40 years were 100% for those in sustained remission, 87% for steroid-maintained patients and 57% for transfusion-dependent patients. Of the 36 deaths reported to the DBAR, 25 were treatment related: five from infections, five from complications of iron overload, one related to vascular access and 14 from transplant-related complications.

In the DBAR, 8.8% of families had more than one affected individual. Most of the familial cases displayed an autosomal dominant pattern of inheritance. Somatic anomalies, excluding short stature, were found in 47% of patients. Of these, 50% were craniofacial (high-arched palate, cleft lip, hypertelorism and flat nasal bridge), 38% were upper limb and hand (flat thenar eminence, triphalangeal thumb), 39% genitourinary and 30% cardiac. Height was below the third centile for age in about 30%.

MDS and AML have been reported in a few patients with DBA, suggesting an increased predisposition to haematological malignancies. There are also cases that have evolved into AA; neutropenia and thrombocytopenia are relatively common after the first decade. Giri and colleagues reported on moderate to severe bone marrow hypocellularity in 21 of 28 (75%) patients with steroid-refractory DBA; marrow hypoplasia correlated with the development of neutropenia (9 of 21, 43%) and/or thrombocytopenia (6 of 21, 29%). Furthermore, using

in vitro long-term culture-initiating cell assay, they provided evidence for a trilineage haemopoietic defect in patients with refractory DBA. Thus, although DBA has been regarded classically as a pure red cell aplasia, a more global haemopoietic defect is likely to be present, and this may be seen more frequently in the future as patients are surviving longer due to improved medical care.

Cell and molecular biology

The classical haematological profile in DBA patients consists of normochromic macrocytic anaemia, reticulocytopenia and a normocellular marrow with selective deficiency of red cell precursors. A number of different defects of *in vitro* erythroid progenitor proliferation, differentiation and cytokine responsiveness have been reported but have not clarified the mechanism of *in vivo* erythroid failure. For many years, based on the typical selective deficiency in red cell precursors, many researchers believed that DBA was due to an intrinsic problem with erythroid proliferation/differentiation. On the other hand, the observation of a wide range of somatic abnormalities in a significant proportion of patients and case reports of thrombocytopenia, neutropenia and AA, together with the recent evidence for a trilineage haemopoietic defect, suggest that the primary problem in DBA is not confined to the erythroid lineage.

The establishment of DBA registries, advances in genetics and the identification of a female with a balanced X;19 translocation has facilitated a change in research strategy in DBA. Genetic mapping studies localized a gene responsible for DBA to a 1-Mb region on 19q13 on the basis of (i) the identification of a *de novo* balanced reciprocal X;19 translocation breakpoint in a girl with DBA; (ii) linkage analysis in multiplex DBA families; and (iii) *de novo* microdeletions associated with the disease. Cloning of the chromosome 19q13 breakpoint demonstrated that this breakpoint interrupts the gene encoding ribosomal protein S19 (*RPS19*). The subsequent finding of *RPS19* mutations in about 25% of DBA patients led to the first genetic characterization of DBA and has paved the way for subsequent studies. Interestingly, mutations in the *RPS19* gene were also found in some apparently unaffected individuals from DBA families presenting only with an isolated elevation of erythrocyte adenosine deaminase activity. The lack of a genotype–phenotype correlation implies that other factors modulate the phenotypic expression of the primary genetic defect in families with *RPS19* mutations.

Over the last 10 years, heterozygous mutations in other genes encoding ribosomal proteins of the small (RPS214, RPS17, RPS7) and large (RPL5, RPL11 and RPL35a) ribosomal subunits have also been reported (Table 12.8); collectively the genetic basis of approximately 50% of DBA patients can now be substantiated at the genetic level. It has also been demonstrated that mutations in these genes are associated with diverse defects in the maturation of rRNAs in the large or the small ribosomal

Table 12.8 Genetic subtypes of Diamond–Blackfan anaemia (DBA).

DBA subtype	Approximate percentage of DBA patients	Chromosome location	Protein product	Exons
Autosomal dominant	25	19q13.2	RPS19	6
	2	10q22–23	RPS24	7
	< 1	15q25.2	RPS17	5
	7	1p22.1	RPL5	8
	5	1p36.1–p35	RPL11	6
	3	3q29–qter	RPL35a	5
	< 1	2p25	RPS7	7
Uncharacterized*	~ 50	?	?	?

*These are likely to represent more than one genetic locus.

subunit production pathway (see Figure 12.6). These studies therefore suggest that the primary defect in DBA is defective ribosome biogenesis, which then leads to other biological defects including increased apoptosis and alterations in molecules such as c-Myc and p53. It will now be important to establish how precisely mutations in these ribosomal protein genes lead to altered cell growth (and anaemia), developmental anomalies and increased susceptibility to cancer. Review of clinical and genetic data has shown that patients with mutations in the *RPL5* gene tend to have multiple physical abnormalities, including craniofacial, thumb and heart anomalies, whereas isolated thumb malformations are predominantly seen in patients with heterozygous *RPL11* mutations. Some genotype–phenotype correlations are therefore beginning to emerge.

In summary, it is noteworthy that the recent advances in the genetics of DBA have demonstrated that (i) DBA is caused by mutations in genes important in the biogenesis of the small (*RPS19, RPS24, RPS17* and *RPS7*) and large (*RPL11, RPL5* and *RPL35a*) ribosomal units; (ii) the *SBDS* gene mutated in SDS (see above) is required for the maturation of the large ribosomal unit; and (iii) the 5q– syndrome (a recognized subtype of acquired myelodysplasia) is associated with haploinsufficiency of the gene encoding the ribosomal protein RPS14. These advances have thus provided a very interesting connection between DBA, SDS, MDS and defective ribosome biogenesis (see Figure 12.6). They also highlight the importance of studies on rare syndromes, as often they can provide significant insights into the pathology of more common diseases.

Treatment

The first line of treatment for DBA remains corticosteroids. Once a maximal haemoglobin response has been achieved, the dose of prednisolone should be tapered slowly until the patient is on the lowest dose possible on an alternate-day regimen. The dose required to achieve this can vary considerably from patient to patient. For those patients who fail to respond or become refractory to steroids, blood transfusion is the mainstay of treatment. As in thalassaemia, the major complication from transfusions is iron overload, and chelation of iron with desferrioxamine should therefore be commenced as soon as patients have increased iron stores. The promising results with the new oral iron chelator deferasirox are likely to have a positive impact in the management of this group of DBA patients. Splenectomy may be indicated in the event of an increased transfusion requirement secondary to hypersplenism. For patients who are transfusion dependent and who have a compatible sibling donor, HSCT may be appropriate and is potentially curative.

Congenital dyserythropoietic anaemia

Congenital dyserythropoietic anaemia (CDA) comprises a heterogeneous group of inherited disorders of erythropoiesis characterized by anaemia, increased ineffective erythropoiesis and frequently morphological evidence of dyserythropoiesis. The first description of this group of disorders was in 1966 by Crookston and colleagues. In 1968 Wendt and Heimpel classified CDA into three types (I, II and III) (Table 12.9). Over the years many additional subtypes (IV, V, VI and VII) have been added to the list, often based on case report studies. Much of the work of establishing diagnostic features and criteria for classification of CDA has been done by Wickramsinghe and colleagues. With the emerging genetics it will be interesting to see how this classification will evolve.

CDA type I

Over 150 cases have been published. The majority of patients present with splenomegaly and mild to moderate anaemia. In some cases non-haematological features (e.g. skeletal abnormalities, abnormal skin pigmentation) have been observed. In

Table 12.9 Characteristics of common subtypes of congenital dyserythropoietic anaemia.

Feature	Type I	Type II	Type III
Inheritance	AR	AR	AD, AR
Erythrocytes	Macrocytic	Normocytic	Macrocytic
Erythroblasts			
Light microscopy	Megaloblastic, internuclear chromatin bridges	Normoblastic, binuclearity	Megaloblastic, up to 12 nuclei/cell
Electron microscopy	'Swiss-cheese' appearance	Peripheral double membranes	Non-specific
Serology			
Ham test	Negative	Usually positive	Negative
Anti-i-agglutinability	Normal/strong	Strong	Normal/strong
SDS-PAGE	Normal	Band 3 thinner and migrates faster than normal	Band 3 migrates faster than normal
Gene location	15q15.2	20q11.2	15q21–q25
Genes identified*	CDAN1	?	?

*It is not known how many genes are mutated in each CDA subtype.
Source: modified from Wickramasinghe & Wood (2005) with permission.

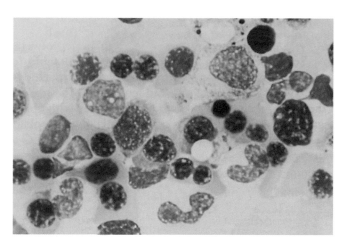

Figure 12.7 Congenital dyserythropoietic anaemia type I. Bone marrow aspirate showing internuclear bridging in normoblasts.

a review by Wickramasinghe and colleagues, the steady-state haemoglobin varied between 6.6 and 11.6 g/dL and approximately 70% had macrocytosis. Ineffective erythropoiesis was evidenced by morphological abnormalities in the peripheral blood (anisocytosis) and in the marrow (megaloblastic erythroid precursors, internuclear chromatin bridging, binuclearity affecting 3–7% of erythroblasts; Figure 12.7), as well as by increased markers of haemolysis (elevated lactate dehydrogenase and bilirubin). The defining ultrastructural feature is a spongy ('Swiss cheese') appearance of the heterochromatin in the majority of erythroblasts on electron microscopy.

Recognized to be an autosomal recessive disorder, the gene responsible for CDA type 1 (CDAN1) was identified in 2002 and is located on chromosome 15q15.2. Subsequent studies have shown that not all patients previously classified as CDA type 1 have mutations in this gene, suggesting that there is genetic heterogeneity within this subtype. The precise function of this gene (and its encoded protein, codanin-1) remains unkown.

CDA type II

This is the most common subtype of CDA (over 300 reported cases) and was initially described as hereditary erythroblastic multinuclearity with a positive acidied serum lysis test (HEMPAS) in 1969. It is inherited as an autosomal recessive trait and has been described in several ethnic groups. The anaemia is variable (haemoglobin 8–11 g/dL). It is important to recognize that about 10% of cases require regular transfusions and that some cases present with anaemia at birth. The clinical presentations include a variable degree of jaundice, hepatomegaly and splenomegaly and cirrhosis. Mental retardation has been reported in some cases.

Peripheral blood morphology shows moderate to marked red cell anisocytosis. Bone marrow features include normoblastic erythroid hyperplasia with usually more than 10% binucleate erythroblasts (Figure 12.8). At the electron microscope level, the erythroid cells have a characteristic peripheral arrangement of the endoplasmic reticulum giving the appearance of a 'double membrane' (Figure 12.9). Red cells from patients with CDA type II are haemolysed by some acidified sera but not by the patient's own serum. The primary defect in CDA type II remains unknown. There is some evidence to suggest that CDA type II is associated with defects in the synthesis of complex N-linked oligosaccharides. The gene for CDA type II has been mapped to chromosome 20q11.2.

CDA type III

This subtype is rare, with three large families having been described as well as some sporadic cases. In one of the largest (Swedish) families investigated the disease was characterized by giant multinucleated erythroblasts in the marrow (Figure 12.10). There appears to be an increased prevalence of lymphoproliferative disorders in CDA type III. The disease in the Swedish family appears to be autosomal dominant and the gene has been mapped to chromsome 15q21–q25.

Treatment

Those with mild anaemia require no major intervention. Folate supplementation should be given to prevent folate deficiency. If regular transfusions are necessary, early attention to iron chelation is essential. Splenectomy may be of benefit in some patients (CDA type II) and there are rare case reports of successful HSCT. In CDA type I there are also case reports of improvement in the haemoglobin after treatment with interferon alfa. The mechanism of this therapeutic benefit remains unclear.

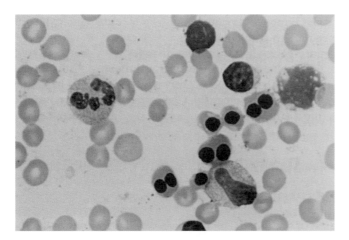

Figure 12.8 Congenital dyserythropoietic anaemia type II (HEMPAS). Bone marrow aspirate showing typical multinuclearity.

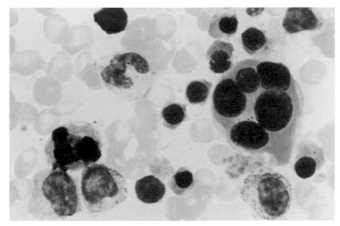

Figure 12.10 Congenital dyserythropoietic anaemia type III. Giant multinucleated erythroblast from the marrow.

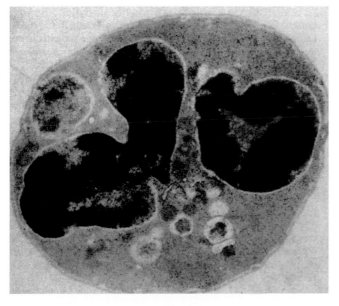

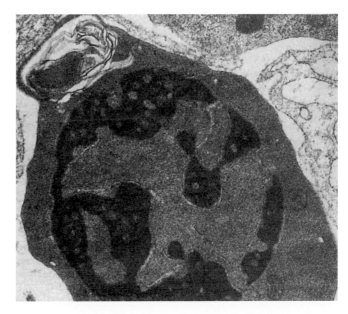

Figure 12.9 Congenital dyserythropoietic anaemia type II. Electron micrographs of erythroblast showing peripheral arrangement of endoplasmic reticulum with 'double membrane' appearance.

Congenital and cyclical neutropenias

Congenital neutropenia is a heterogeneous disorder (Table 12.10). It includes Kostmann syndrome, which was first described in 1954. Although the original description by Kostmann was of an autosomal recessive disorder, other congenital neutropenia subtypes (both sporadic and autosomal dominant) have subsequently been included in this category. The neutropenia is usually recognized at birth and the neutrophil count is often below 0.2×10^9/L. The haemoglobin and platelet count are usually normal and the bone marrow shows maturation arrest of myelopoiesis at the level of the promyelocyte/myelocyte (with abundant promyelocytes but with selective reduction in myelocytes, metamyelocytes and neutrophils).

The neutropenias are associated with severe infections and early death. No patient has developed AA but myeloid leukaemias ($\sim 25\%$ by 25 years) can occur. The availability of G-CSF has revolutionized the outcome of these children. However, somatic mutations in the gene that encodes the G-CSF receptor have been documented during the evolution to leukaemia in patients receiving G-CSF. The precise contribution of G-CSF therapy to the development of G-CSF receptor mutations remains unclear. For patients who become refractory to G-CSF or who develop leukaemia, HSCT may be appropriate and curative.

Cyclical neutropenia is characterized by a neutrophil count that usually reaches a nadir with a 21-day periodicity. Around the nadir, patients may develop fever and mouth ulcers. In cyclical neutropenia, the pattern of inheritance is usually autosomal dominant. Linkage analysis in affected families resulted in the localization of the disease gene to 19p13.3. Subsequent studies identified mutations in the gene (*ELA2*) encoding neutrophil elastase. An extraordinary twist to the story was the identification of *ELA2* mutations in many patients with congenital neutropenia as well. In cyclical neutropenia, the mutations are usually clustered around the active site of the molecule, whereas the opposite face of the molecule tends to be mutated in congenital neutropenia. Neutrophil elastase is a serine protease that is synthesized predominantly at the promyelocytic stage and can be expected to be important in neutrophil development. Recent studies suggest that *ELA2* mutations lead to accumulation of the non-functional protein, which in turn triggers an unfolded protein response leading to maturational arrest. The precise mechanism leading to maturation arrest of promyelocytes remains unclear. The original family described by Kostmann had autosomal recessive severe congenital neutropenia, and has recently been shown to be associated with biallelic mutations in the *HAX1* gene, predicted to lead to defects in cell death. Biallelic mutations in *HAX1* account for approximately 10% of congenital neutropenia. The HAX1 protein is a critical regulator of the mitochondrial membrane potential and cellular viability. While there are data which suggest that HAX1 is important in controlling apoptosis, it is unclear why premature death of neutrophils is consistently associated with HAX1 deficiency. Mutations in other genes (*GFI1*, *WASP*) are also known to be rarely associated with severe congenital neutropenia, demonstrating genetic heterogeneity.

Thrombocytopenia with absent radii

Thrombocytopenia with absent radii (TAR) is an autosomal recessive disorder characterized by hypomegakaryocytic thrombocytopenia and bilateral radial aplasia. Babies with TAR often have haemorrhagic manifestations at birth, when the diagnosis is usually made because of the characteristic physical appearance combined with thrombocytopenia. Additional skeletal abnormalities (absent ulnae, absent humeri, clinodactyly) and other somatic abnormalities (microcephaly, hypertelorism, strabismus, heart defects) may be seen in some patients.

The platelet count is usually below 50×10^9/L. The leucocyte count can be normal or raised, sometimes up to 100×10^9/L ('leukaemoid reaction'). Bone marrow cellularity is normal and myeloid and erythroid lineages are normal or increased. Megakaryocytes are absent or decreased. Most patients bleed in infancy and then improve after the first year. The mainstay of management is prophylactic and therapeutic use of platelet

Table 12.10 Genetic subtypes of neutropenia.

Subtype	Approximate percentage of patients	Chromosome location	Gene/protein product	Exons
Autosomal dominant	50–60	19p13.3	*ELA2*/neutrophil elastase	5
Autosomal recessive	10–15	1q21.3	*HAX1*	7
Autosomal dominant	< 1	1p22	*GFI1*	
Uncharacterized*	30–40	?	?	?

*This is likely to be a heterogeneous group. Furthermore, some patients initially presenting as isolated neutropenia may turn out to be cryptic presentations of other syndromes, such as Wiskott–Aldrich and Shwachman–Diamond syndromes.

Table 12.11 Genetic subtypes of congenital amegakaryocytic thrombocytopenia (CAMT).

CAMT subtype	Approximate percentage of CAMT patients	Chromosome location	Gene/protein product	Exons
Autosomal recessive	?	1p34	MPL	12
Uncharacterized	?	?	?	?

Table 12.12 Laboratory tests useful in the investigation of patients with bone marrow failure.

Test	Diagnostic value
Peripheral blood	
Fetal haemoglobin	High level suggestive of generalized bone marrow failure
DEB/MMC chromosomal breakage	Increased in FA
Mutation analysis of specific genes	
FANCA–FANCN	Mutated in FA
DKC1, TERC, TERT, NOP10, NHP2, TINF2	Mutated in DC
SBDS	Mutated in SDS
RPS19, RPS24, RPS17, RPL5, RPL11, RPL35a, RPS7	Mutated in DBA
CDAN1	Mutated in CDA type I
ELA2, HAX1, GFI1	Mutated in congenital and cyclic neutropenia
MPL	Mutated in CAMT
Mitochondrial DNA analysis	Deletions seen in PS
X-chromosome inactivation patterns	Skewed in carriers of X-linked DC
Ham test (CD59 analysis)	Abnormal in paroxysmal nocturnal haemoglobinuria
Telomere length	Short in AA, very short in DC
Constitutional karyotype	Abnormality suggestive of constitutional AA
Other investigations	
To identify somatic abnormalities	
Skeletal survey	Presence of somatic abnormalities in association with AA is suggestive of constitutional/inherited AA
Ultrasound of abdomen	
Pulmonary function tests	
Echocardiogram	
Exocrine pancreatic function	Abnormal in SDS and PS
Neutrophil chemotaxis	Abnormal in SDS
Fibroblast cultures	Abnormalities seen in DC

AA, aplastic anaemia; CAMT, congenital amegakaryocytic thrombocytopenia; CDA, congenital dyserythropoietic anaemia; DBA, Diamond–Blackfan anaemia; DC, dyskeratosis congenita; DEB/MMC, diepoxybutane/mitomycin C; FA, Fanconi anaemia; PS, Pearson syndrome; SDS, Shwachman–Diamond syndrome.

transfusions. Patients with TAR have a very good prognosis after infancy. There have been no reports of AA or leukaemia.

The pathophysiology of TAR is unknown. Thrombopoietin levels are usually elevated and thrombopoietin receptor expression on the surface of TAR platelets is normal. Therefore, defec-tive megakaryocytopoiesis/thrombocytopoiesis does not appear to be caused by a defect in thrombopoietin production. There is some evidence that it may be due to a lack of response to thrombopoietin in the signal transduction pathway of the thrombopoietin receptor (c-mpl).

Congenital amegakaryocytic thrombocytopenia

Congenital amegakaryocytic thrombocytopenia (CAMT) is a rare disorder that usually presents in infancy and is characterized by isolated thrombocytopenia and reduction/absence of megakaryocytes in the bone marrow, usually with no somatic abnormalities. It is genetically heterogeneous with autosomal recessive and X-linked subtypes. Approximately 50% of patients will develop AA, usually by the age of 5 years. For patients with severe thrombocytopenia or AA, the treatment of choice is HSCT if a compatible donor is available.

In a subgroup of patients with CAMT, mutations in the gene encoding the thrombopoietin receptor (*MPL*) have been identified (Table 12.11). As patients with *MPL* mutations can also have abnormalities in the leucocyte count and haemoglobin level and central nervous system (CNS) abnormalities (e.g. cerebral and cerebellar hypoplasia), this study highlights the important role of the thrombopoietin receptor in haemopoiesis in general and in CNS development. It also substantiates the genetic heterogeneity of CAMT.

Conclusion

Since the identification of the first FA gene (*FANCC*) in 1992, there have been significant advances in our understanding of FA, DC and other bone marrow failure syndromes. This is already facilitating diagnosis, as highlighted in Table 12.12. It can be anticipated that further studies of the pathophysiology of these disorders is likely to lead to a better understanding of normal haemopoiesis and how this becomes defective in many patients presenting with the more common forms of AA and MDS. Indeed, recent studies have already established a link between DC and AA and, in turn, to defective telomere maintenance. Equally, a link between DBA, SDS and MDS and, in turn, defective ribosome biogenesis has been recognized. These advances also suggest that new treatment strategies, based on correction of the primary defect in each syndrome, may now emerge.

Acknowledgements

I would like to thank all my research colleagues past (Stuart Knight, Anna Marrone, David Stevens and Philip Mason) and present (Richard Beswick, Upal Hossain, Michael Kirwan, Amanda Walne and Tom Vulliamy) and all the patients and clinicians on whom research in our laboratory depends. The research work is supported by funding from the Wellcome Trust and the Medical Research Council UK.

Selected bibliography

All inherited bone marrow failure syndromes
Alter BP, Young NS (1998) The bone marrow failure syndromes. In: *Haematology of Infancy and Childhood* (DG Nathan, HS Orkin, eds), pp. 237–335. WB Saunders, Philadelphia.

Fanconi anaemia
Auerbach AD, Buchwald M, Joenje H (2001) Fanconi anaemia. In: *The Metabolic and Molecular Basis of Inherited Disease* (CR Scriver, AL Beaudet, WS Sly, D Valle, eds), 8th edn, pp. 753–68. McGraw-Hill, New York.

de la Fuente J, Reiss S, McCloy M *et al.* (2003) Non-TBI stem cell transplantation protocol for Fanconi anaemia using HLA-compatible sibling and unrelated donors. *Bone Marrow Transplantation* **32**: 653–6.

D'Andrea AD (2010) Susceptibility pathways in Fanconi's anemia and breast cancer. *The New England Journal of Medicine* **362**: 1909–10.

Guardiola P, Socie G, Pasquini R *et al.* (1998) Allogeneic stem cell transplantation for Fanconi anaemia. *Bone Marrow Transplantation* **21** (Suppl. 2): 24–7.

Guardiola P, Pasquini R, Dokal I *et al.* (2000) Outcome of 69 allogeneic stem transplantations for Fanconi anaemia using HLA-matched unrelated donors: a study on behalf of the European Group for Blood and Marrow Transplantation. *Blood* **95**: 422–9.

Howlett NG, Taniguchi T, Olson S *et al.* (2002) Biallelic inactivation of BRCA2 in Fanconi anaemia. *Science* **297**: 606–9.

Joenje H, Patel KJ (2001) The emerging genetic and molecular basis of Fanconi anaemia. *Nature Reviews. Genetics* **2**: 446–57.

Liu JM, Kim S, Read EJ *et al.* (1999) Engraftment of haematopoietic progenitor cells transduced with the Fanconi anaemia group C gene (*FANCC*). *Human Gene Therapy* **10**: 2337–46.

Reid S, Schindler D, Hanenberg H *et al.* (2007) Biallelic mutations in PALB2 cause Fanconi anaemia subtype FA-N and predispose to childhood cancer. *Nature Genetics* **39**: 142–3.

Smogorzewska A, Matsuoka S, Vinciguerra P *et al.* (2007) Identification of the FANCI protein, a monoubiquitinated FANCD2 paralogue required for DNA repair. *Cell* **129**: 289–301.

Taniguchi T, Garcia-Higuera I, Xu B *et al.* (2002) Convergence of the Fanconi anaemia and ataxia telangiectasia signalling pathways. *Cell* **109**: 459–72.

Wagner JE, Eapen M, MacMillan ML *et al.* (2007) Unrelated donor bone marrow transplantation for the treatment of Fanconi anaemia. *Blood* **109**: 2256–62.

Waisfisz Q, Morgan NV, Savino M *et al.* (1999) Spontaneous functional correction of homozygous Fanconi anaemia alleles reveals novel mechanistic basis for reverse mosaicism. *Nature Genetics* **22**: 379–83.

Wang W (2007) Emergence of a DNA-damage response network consisting of Fanconi anaemia and BRCA proteins. *Nature Reviews. Genetics* **6**: 735–48.

Dyskeratosis congenita
Armanios MY, Chen JJ, Cogan JD *et al.* (2007) Telomerase mutations in families with idiopathic pulmonary fibrosis. *New England Journal of Medicine* **356**: 1317–26.

Dokal I (2000) Dyskeratosis congenita in all its forms. *British Journal of Haematology* 110: 768–79.

Heiss NS, Knight SW, Vulliamy TJ *et al.* (1998) X-linked dyskeratosis congenita is caused by mutations in a highly conserved gene with putative nucleolar functions. *Nature Genetics* 19: 32–8.

Knight SW, Heiss NS, Vulliamy TJ *et al.* (1999) Unexplained aplastic anaemia, immunodeficiency, and cerebellar hypoplasia (Hoyeraal–Hreidarsson syndrome) due to mutations in the dyskeratosis congenita gene, DKC1. *British Journal of Haematology* 107: 335–9.

Marrone A, Walne A, Tamary H *et al.* (2007) Telomerase reverse transcriptase homozygous mutations in autosomal recessive dyskeratosis congenita and Hoyeraal–Hreidarsson syndrome. *Blood* 110: 4198–205.

Mitchell JR, Wood E, Collins K (1999) A telomerase component is defective in the human disease dyskeratosis congenita. *Nature* 402: 551–5.

Savage SA, Giri N, Baerlocher GM, Orr N, Lansdorp PM, Alter BP (2008) TINF2, a component of the shelterin telomere protection complex, is mutated in dyskeratosis congenita. *American Journal of Human Genetics* 82: 501–9.

Vulliamy T, Marrone A, Goldman F *et al.* (2001) The RNA component of telomerase is mutated in autosomal dominant dyskeratosis congenita. *Nature* 413: 432–5.

Vulliamy T, Marrone A, Dokal I *et al.* (2002) Association between aplastic anaemia and mutations in telomerase RNA. *Lancet* 359: 2168–70.

Vulliamy T, Beswick R, Kirwan M *et al.* (2008) Mutations in the telomerase component NHP2 cause the premature ageing syndrome dyskeratosis congenita. *Proceedings of the National Academy of Sciences USA* 105: 8073–8.

Walne AJ, Vulliamy T, Marrone A *et al.* (2007) Genetic heterogeneity in autosomal recessive dyskeratosis congenita with one subtype due to mutations in the telomerase-associated protein NOP10. *Human Molecular Genetics* 16: 1619–29.

Yamaguchi H, Calado RT, Ly H *et al.* (2005) Mutations in TERT, the gene for reverse transcriptase, in aplastic anaemia. *New England Journal of Medicine* 352: 1413–24.

Shwachman–Diamond syndrome

Boocock GRB, Morrison JA, Popovic M *et al.* (2003) Mutations in *SBDS* are associated with Shwachman–Diamond syndrome. *Nature Genetics* 33: 97–101.

Dror Y, Freedman MH (2002) Shwachman–Diamond syndrome. *British Journal of Haematology* 118: 701–13.

Menne TF, Goyenechea B, Sanchez-Puig N *et al.* (2007) The Shwachman–Bodian–Diamond syndrome protein mediates

translational activation of ribosomes in yeast. *Nature Genetics* 39: 486–96.

Diamond–Blackfan anaemia

Dianzani I, Loreni F (2008) Diamond–Blackfan anaemia: a ribosomal puzzle. *Haematologica* 93: 1601–4.

Draptchinskaia N, Gustavsson P, Andersson B *et al.* (1999) The gene encoding ribosomal protein S19 is mutated in Diamond–Blackfan anaemia. *Nature Genetics* 21: 169–75.

Gazda HT, Sheen MR, Vlachos A *et al.* (2008) Ribosomal protein L5 and L11 mutations are associated with cleft palate and abnormal thumbs in Diamond–Blackfan anaemia patients. *American Journal of Human Genetics* 83: 769–80.

Lipton JM, Astidaaftos E, Zyskind I *et al.* (2006). Improving clinical care and elucidating the pathophysiology of Diamond Blackfan anaemia: an update from the Diamond Blackfan Anaemia Registry. *Pediatric Blood and Cancer* 46: 558–64.

Congenital dyserythropoietic anaemia

Dgany O, Avidan N, Delaunay J *et al.* (2002 Congenital dyserythropoietic anaemia type I is caused by mutations in codanin-1. *American Journal of Human Genetics* 71: 1467–74.

Wickramasinghe SN, Wood WG (2005) Advances in the understanding of congenital dyserythropoietic anaemia. *British Journal of Haematology* 131: 431–46.

Congenital and cyclical neutropenia

Dale DC, Person RE, Bolyard A *et al.* (2000) Mutations in the gene encoding neutrophil elastase in congenital and cyclic neutropenia. *Blood* 96: 2317–22.

Klein C, Grudzien M, Appaswamy G *et al.* (2006) HAX1 deficiency causes autosomal recessive severe congenital neutropenia (Kostmann disease). *Nature Genetics* 39: 86–92.

Person RE, Li FQ, Duan Z *et al.* (2003) Mutations in proto-oncogene GFI1 cause human neutropenia and target ELA2. *Nature Genetics* 34: 308–12.

Zeidler C, Germeshausen M, Klein C *et al.* (2008) Clinical implications of ELA2, HAX1 and GCSF-receptor mutations in severe congenital neutropenia. *British Journal of Haematology* 44: 459–67.

Congenital amegakaryocytic thrombocytopenia

Ihara K, Ishii E, Eguchi M *et al.* (1999) Identification of mutations in the c-mpl gene in congenital amegakaryocytic thrombocytopenia. *Proceedings of the National Academy of Sciences USA* 96: 3132–6.

CHAPTER 13

Acquired aplastic anaemia

Judith CW Marsh[1] and Neal S Young[2]

[1]King's College Hospital, London, UK
[2]National Heart, Lung and Blood Institute, National Institutes of Health, Bethesda, Maryland, USA

Characterization and definition

Aplastic anaemia (AA) is defined by pancytopenia with a hypocellular bone marrow in the absence of an abnormal infiltrate and with no increase in reticulin. The term 'aplastic anaemia' encompasses different entities, but here we discuss acquired idiosyncratic AA, most often idiopathic though sometimes a drug or chemical or a virus infection is implicated. 'Inevitable' AA/myelosuppression occurs after treatment with cytotoxic drugs or radiation; it is dose dependent and recovery is usually predictable, and is discussed no further here.

AA is a bone marrow failure disorder and shows considerable overlap with clonal disorders of bone marrow failure, including myelodysplastic syndrome (MDS), acute myeloid leukaemia (AML), paroxysmal nocturnal haemoglobinuria (PNH) and T-large granular lymphocyte leukaemia/lymphoproliferative disorder (T-LGL), and a tendency itself to later evolve to MOS/AML (Figure 13.1). The inherited forms of AA, such as Fanconi anaemia (FA), dyskeratosis congenita (DC) and Shwachmann–Diamond syndrome (SDS), are rarer than acquired AA and are discussed in detail in Chapter 12. However, the importance of excluding an inherited form of AA and the increasing proportion of adults with apparent acquired AA with related genetic lesions is highlighted in this chapter.

In AA there must be at least two of the following: (i) haemoglobin below 10 g/dL; (ii) platelet count below 50×10^9/L; and (iii) neutrophil count below 1.5×10^9/L. The severity of the disease is graded into very severe, severe and non-severe AA, according to the blood count parameters and bone marrow findings as summarized in Table 13.1. However, it is important to remember that routine use of the more accurate automated counting of reticulocytes overestimates the reticulocyte count used in the historical Camitta criteria for defining disease severity. The assessment of disease severity is important in treatment decisions but has less prognostic significance today in terms of correlation with response to antithymocyte globulin (ATG) (see section Predictors of response to ATG). Patients with bilineage or trilineage cytopenias that are less severe than this are not classified as AA. However, they should have their blood counts monitored to determine whether they will develop AA later.

Epidemiology

Incidence

Because AA is a rare disease, only large national and international prospective studies, with appropriate diagnostic criteria, will provide meaningful data on the aetiology of this condition. Studies indicate an incidence of AA in the West of 2 per million per year. There is a twofold to threefold higher incidence rate in Asia. In a large prospective study from Thailand, an incidence of 3.9 per million was reported from the metropolitan area of Bangkok compared with 5 per million in the northeast region of Khonkaen. An incidence of 7.4 per million was reported from a prospective study from China, although this may represent an

Postgraduate Haematology: 6th edition. Edited by A. Victor Hoffbrand, Daniel Catovsky, Edward G.D. Tuddenham, Anthony R. Green
© 2011 Blackwell Publishing Ltd.

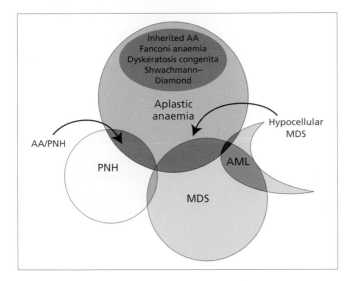

Figure 13.1 The overlap of acquired and inherited aplastic anaemia (AA) with the clonal disorders of myelodysplastic syndrome (MDS), acute myeloid leukaemia (AML) and paroxysmal nocturnal haemoglobinuria (PNH).

Table 13.1 Definition of disease severity of aplastic anaemia (AA).

Severe AA

Bone marrow cellularity < 25%, or 25–50% with < 30% residual haemopoietic cells

Two out of three of the following:

  Neutrophils < 0.5×10^9/L

  Platelets < 20×10^9/L

  Reticulocytes < 20×10^9/L

Very severe AA

As for severe AA but neutrophils < 0.2×10^9/L

Non-severe AA

Patients not fulfilling the criteria for severe or very severe AA

The definition of severe AA is based on the so-called Camitta criteria (Camitta *et al.* 1975). The reticulocyte count threshold was based on manual reticulocyte counts, but today automated reticulocyte counts are routinely estimated and these correlate poorly with manual counts. These criteria are still useful for management planning but are not predictive of response to immunosuppressive therapy.

overestimate as a bone marrow trephine was not required for the diagnosis of AA. There is a biphasic age distribution, with peaks at 10–25 years and over 60 years; it is possible that some cases diagnosed in older patients represent hypocellular MDS rather than AA. There is no significant difference in incidence between males and females.

Aetiology

The reasons for the differences in incidence are not known but may include environmental and genetic factors. The relative importance of genetic factors was examined in a hospital-based study of children with AA in Canada. A higher incidence was reported among Asian children who had emigrated to Canada, and an association with human leucocyte antigen (HLA) type demonstrated.

Post-hepatitic AA accounts for around 5–10% of cases; invariably such cases are negative for the known hepatitic viruses. AA may follow liver transplantation for severe hepatitis (also non-A, non-B, non-C hepatitis). Post-hepatitic AA is usually severe but responds well to immunosuppressive therapy, and similar oligoclonal expansion of activated cytotoxic T cells is observed as in idiopathic AA, suggesting a common pathogenesis for the hepatitis and bone marrow failure. However, the same therapeutic algorithm should be used for all cases of AA, with first-line allogeneic haemopoietic stem cell transplantation (HSCT) if the patient is young and has an HLA-matched sibling donor. Rarely, AA may be a sequela of infectious mononucleosis.

AA occurs in association with other systemic autoimmune disorders, especially eosinophilic fasciitis but also systemic lupus erythematosus (SLE), Sjögren syndrome and coeliac disease. There have been anecdotal reports of SLE-associated AA responsive to high-dose cyclophosphamide or ATG. SLE can also produce pancytopenia with a cellular bone marrow or it may occasionally be associated with myelofibrosis. A positive family history of rheumatoid arthritis occurs more frequently in patients with AA. AA may be associated with thymoma. Fatal AA is almost invariably the outcome of transfusion-associated graft-versus-host disease (GVHD); it is well documented clinically and can be reproduced *in vivo* in a mouse model (see next section on pathogenesis).

AA can rarely occur in pregnancy, although this may be due to chance and other possible causes should always be sought. A retrospective review from Leiden over a 24-year period of the frequency of pregnancy in 35 women of childbearing age and with a new diagnosis of AA found a similar frequency of pregnancy to that in the general population. However, due to the rarity of AA, this may not exclude a possible association in a larger number of patients. The disease may remit spontaneously after termination, whether spontaneous or therapeutic, and after delivery, but not in all cases. There is a risk of relapse in pregnancy in patients who have previously responded to immunosuppressive therapy. In contrast, after successful allogeneic HSCT, pregnancy does not trigger relapse.

In rural areas of Thailand, the use of non-bottled water, agricultural pesticides, non-medical needle exposures and exposure of farmers to ducks and geese are significant environmental risk factors for developing AA. There is good evidence for an association between benzene exposure and AA, but for other solvents, such as hair dyes and glycol ethers, the data are not strong. Occupational exposure to pesticides such as organophosphates, lindane, DDT, paraquat and carbamates has also been implicated. A wide variety of chemicals including cutting oils and lubricating agents were identified in a large British case–control study. However, confounding factors may complicate this picture, for example exposure to an infectious agent in the environment in individuals exposed to a pesticide. For these reasons, blacklists of implicated drugs and chemicals need to be interpreted cautiously in assigning causation in an individual case, including for legal purposes.

Many drugs and chemicals have been implicated in the aetiology of AA, but for only a few is there strong evidence for an association, and even then it is usually impossible to prove causality (Table 13.2). In most studies, drug exposure accounts for around 5–10% of cases of acquired AA, although in a recent epidemiological study from Spain AA was associated with drug exposure in 20.8% of cases. Confounding factors include exposure to viruses and systemic diseases such as rheumatoid arthritis, which may themselves contribute to an increased risk of AA. For these reasons, the proportion of cases attributed to drugs

Table 13.2 Drugs and occupational and environmental exposures reported to be associated with aplastic anaemia.

Drugs
Antibiotics: chloramphenicol, sulphonamides, co-trimoxazole, linezolid
Anti-inflammatory agents: phenylbutazone, indomethacin, diclofenac, naproxen, piroxicam, gold, penicillamine
Anticonvulsants: phenytoin, carbamazepine
Antithyroid agents: carbimazole, thiouracil
Antidepressants: dothiepin, phenothiazines
Antidiabetic agents: chlorpropamide, tolbutamide
Antimalarial agents: chloroquine
Others: mebendazole, thiazides, allopurinol, ticlopidine

Occupational and environmental exposures
Benzene: evidence base includes large industrial studies, case–control study from Thailand
Pesticides (organochlorines such as lindane; organophosphates; pentachlorophenol): evidence base includes literature review of case reports and UK case–control study
Cutting oils and lubricating agents: evidence base includes UK case–control study
Recreational drugs (e.g. methylenedioxymethamphetamine, Ecstasy): evidence base includes case reports

Source: Marsh JCW, Gordon-Smith EC (2009) Aplastic anaemia and other causes of bone marrow failure. In: *Oxford Textbook of Medicine* (DA Warrel, eds). Oxford University Press, Oxford, with permission.

may be declining in the literature as investigators become more sceptical of assigning aetiology based on putative association. Nevertheless, a careful drug history, including occupational exposures, should be obtained. Drug exposure in the year preceding presentation should be detailed. Earlier exposures should be recorded but are not likely to be relevant unless the particular drug or drug group has been readministered during the presumed critical period. If the patient is taking several drugs that may have been implicated in AA, even if the evidence is based on case reports alone, then all the putative drugs should be discontinued and the patient should not be rechallenged with the drugs after recovery of the blood count.

Since the 1950s chloramphenicol has been reported to be strongly associated with AA. It is likely that the risk has been overestimated, and more recent epidemiological studies, including the study from Thailand where chloramphenicol is still used, have failed to demonstrate an association. Drugs commonly associated with AA are listed in Table 13.2. European case–control epidemiological studies have reported relative risks for sulphonamides, gold, pencillamine, non-steroidal anti-inflammatory drugs, anticonvulsants, allopurinol, ticlopidine and sulphonylureas; a similarly designed study from Thailand incriminated sulphonamides, thiazide diuretics and mebendazole. More recently, the antibiotic linezolid has been implicated in bone marrow suppression but this has not been evaluated in population-based studies.

Pathogenesis and its clinical relevance

The haemopoietic defect in AA

AA is characterized by both a quantitative and qualitative defect in the haemopoietic stem cell compartment. The primitive long-term culture-initiating cells and more mature haemopoietic progenitors in the bone marrow (colony-forming cells) of all cell lineages are reduced or absent. The long-term bone marrow culture (LTBMC) system was modified using crossover experiments, in which AA CD34$^+$ cells were inoculated onto irradiated preformed LTBMC stromas; this demonstrated a lack of generation of CFU-GM over time, consistent with impaired marrow repopulating ability of AA bone marrow CD34$^+$ cells. There is a reduction in the percentage of CD34$^+$ bone marrow cells, and the CD34$^+$ cells are more apoptotic than normal CD34$^+$ cells. About 10–15% of patients with AA have shortened telomeres, as measured in blood leucocytes. This was initially presumed to reflect 'stressed' haemopoiesis, but subsequently mutations in the telomerase gene complex have been demonstrated in such patients with apparent acquired AA.

The bone marrow stromal cell microenvironment functions normally in most patients, as assessed by crossover LTBMC in which normal bone marrow CD34$^+$ cells are inoculated onto irradiated AA stromal layers. Such an *in vitro* system does not examine individual cellular components of the stromal cell microenvironment and thus defects in particular cells cannot be excluded. The frequencies of fibroblast colonies (CFU-F) are normal in AA, and mesenchymal stem cells showed normal phenotype as defined by CD34$^-$CD45$^-$CD44$^+$CD29$^+$CD90$^+$CD105$^+$CD106$^+$. The differentiation capacity of AA mesenchymal stem cells has not yet been formally evaluated. Cultured AA mesenchymal stem cells support *in vitro* haemopoiesis after addition of normal bone marow mononuclear cells.

AA is not due to a deficiency of any known haemopoietic growth factor (HGF). Long-term marrow culture studies have shown normal mRNA expression and/or secretion of granulocyte/macrophage colony-stimulating factor, granulocyte colony-stimulating factor (G-CSF), interleukin (IL)-6, stem cell factor and thrombopoietin from stromal cells. Serum levels of most HGFs, including the above and recombinant human erythropoietin, are markedly elevated. These observations explain the lack of striking effects of HGFs in most AA patients.

The immune-mediated nature of acquired AA

In acquired AA, it is proposed that an inciting event, such as a virus or drug, provokes an aberrant immune response, triggering oligoclonal expansion of cytotoxic T cells that destroy haemopoietic stem cells (Figure 13.2). Bone marrow transplantation (BMT) or immunosuppressive therapy leads to complete or partial response by eradicating or suppressing pathogenic T-cell clones (Figure 13.2a, middle panel). Relapse occurs with recurrence of the immune response, and the immunologically stressed and depleted stem-cell compartment also allows selection of abnormal haemopoietic clones that manifest as MDS and occasionally AML.

There is strong evidence that AA has an autoimmune nature in many patients based on the following observations.
1 Haematological recovery after immunosuppressive therapy with ATG and ciclosporin (CSA) occurs in the majority of patients.
2 There are activated autoreactive oligoclonal CD8$^+$ T cells present in blood and bone marrow that release interferon (IFN)-γ and tumour necrosis factor (TNF)-α, cytokines that inhibit haemopoiesis.
3 Intracellular IFN-γ levels in T cells correlate with response to immunosuppressive therapy.
4 Increased Fas expression on bone marrow CD34$^+$ cells indicates increased apoptosis.
5 T-cell repertoire analysis shows oligoclonal expansion of CD8$^+$ T cells in AA, MDS and PNH.
6 Transcription factor T-bet is upregulated and binds to the IFN-γ promoter, resulting in increased expression of IFN-γ.
7 CD4$^+$CD25$^+$FOXP3$^+$ regulatory T cells are reduced in AA patients.

Gene expression profiling in AA CD34$^+$ cells has shown that more than half the upregulated genes are related to the immune response, including genes for cytokines and cytokine receptors, signal transduction genes, as well as other immune response genes. Many apoptosis and cell death genes are upregulated and some anti-apoptotic genes downregulated.

It is unclear why T cells are activated in AA. HLA-DR2 and its split HLA-DR15 and DRB1*1501 and 1502 alleles are over-represented in AA, as a class I HLA-B*4002 and HLA-A*0206, indicating a possible role for antigen recognition. There is correlation between ATG response and DRB1*1501, but most of these HLA data come from studies of Japanese patients. Studies of cytokine gene polymorphisms that may reflect a heightened immune response in AA are limited; polymorphisms in the TNF-α promoter, IL-6 and IFN-γ genes have been reported, but a systematic assessment of all potentially relevant cytokine genes has not been reported.

The specific cytotoxic T-cell targets on haemopoietic stem and progenitor cells in AA have not been identified. Potential candidates, identified by screening antibodies in patients' serum against a peptide library using leukaemia cell lines, include kinectin, DRS-1 (diazepam-binding inhibitor-related protein-1), PMS1 (postmeiotic segregation increased 1), moesin and hnRNPK (heterogeneous nuclear ribonucleoprotein K). However, the relevance of these findings is unclear, and they may represent epiphenomena rather than primary targets of cytotoxic T-cell attack.

Alternatively, a defect in the glycosylphosphatidylinositol (GPI) anchor may be the trigger for the immune response against normal progenitor cells through aberrant expression of intracellular GPI-protein(s) while at the same time providing a protective mechanism for GPI-defective cells. The expansion of PNH clones in a subset of patients with AA and hypoplastic MDS is also a well-established finding but the mechanism(s) that leads to this expansion is poorly understood. PNH cells may show a selective clonal advantage because (i) GPI-negative haemopoietic stem cells are spared from autoimmune attack because the absent GPI anchor is the target of the immune attack; (ii) GPI-negative cells acquire a second mutation that confers a survival advantage; or (iii) *PIGA* mutation confers an intrinsic resistance to apoptosis. *PIGA* mutations are present in the blood of most healthy individuals but do not result in disease. They may also appear following treatment with the monoclonal antibody alemtuzumab, which recognizes the GPI-linked antigen CD52. ATG contains high levels of antibodies to the GPI-deficient proteins CD52 and CD48 and low levels of antibodies to CD16, which may contribute to the emergence of PNH clones after treatment of AA.

Mouse models

There is currently no ideal animal model of AA. An early mouse model was produced by high-dose chronic administration of

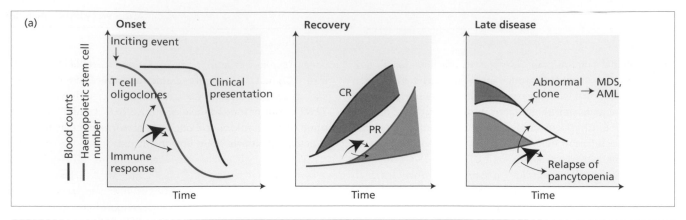

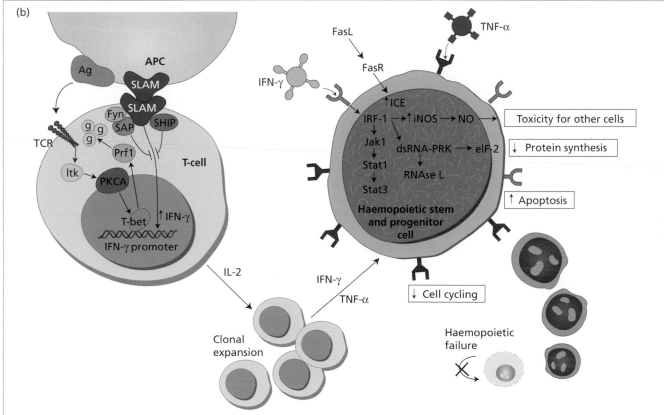

Figure 13.2 (a) Pathophysiology of acquired aplastic anaemia (AA). In acquired AA, it is proposed that an inciting event, such as a virus or drug, provokes an aberrant immune response, triggering oligoclonal expansion of cytotoxic T cells that destroy haemopoietic stem cells (left-hand panel, Onset). Bone marrow transplantation or immunosuppressive therapy leads to complete response (CR) or partial response (PR) by eradicating or suppressing pathogenic T-cell clones (middle panel, Recovery). Relapse occurs with recurrence of the immune response, and the immunologically stressed and depleted stem-cell compartment also allows selection of abnormal haemopoietic clones that manifest as myelodysplastic syndrome (MDS) and occasionally as acute myeloid leukaemia (AML) (right-hand panel, Late disease). (b) Immune destruction of haemopoiesis. Antigens are presented to T lymphocytes by antigen-presenting cells (APCs), which trigger T cells to activate and proliferate. T-bet, a transcription factor, binds to the interferon (IFN)-γ promoter region and induces gene expression. SAP binds to Fyn and modulates SLAM activity on IFN-γ expression, diminishing gene transcription. Patients with AA show constitutive T-bet expression and low SAP levels. IFN-γ and tumour necrosis factor (TNF)-α upregulate cellular receptors on other T cells and also the Fas receptor. Increased production of interleukin (IL)-2 leads to polyclonal expansion of T cells. Activation of Fas receptor by the Fas ligand leads to apoptosis of target cells. Some effects of IFN-γ are mediated through interferon regulatory factor (IRF)-1, which inhibits the transcription of cellular genes and entry into the cell cycle. IFN-γ is a potent inducer of many cellular genes, including inducible nitric oxide synthase (NOS), and production of the toxic gas nitric oxide (NO) may further diffuse toxic effects. These events ultimately lead to reduced cell cycling and cell death by apoptosis. Ag, antigen; TCR, T-cell receptor. (This research originally published in *Blood*. Young NS, Calado RT, Scheinberg P. Current concepts in the pathophysiology and treatment of aplastic anaemia. *Blood* 2006;108:2509–19. © American Society of Haematology.)

the cytotoxic drug busulfan. After a year, mice developed pancytopenia, aplasia and very low CFU-S frequency. This model is used for studying chemotherapy-induced myelosuppression and is consequently not a model of immune-mediated AA.

Workers at the National Institutes of Health (NIH) have infused parent lymph node cells into F₁ hybrid mice to induce a model based on transfusion-induced GVHD. Allogeneic lymphocytes present in the infused cells attacked and destroyed host cells in a graft-versus-host response, resulting in pancytopenia, hypocellular bone marrow, increased serum IFN-γ levels, a 35-fold increase in bone marrow CD4⁺ cells, a 400-fold increase in bone marrow CD8⁺ cells, and increased bone marrow CD95 expression. However, the nature of the effector cells was unclear and mice did not show a response to CSA. Using a similar model, but without sublethal irradiation, the same group also demonstrated oligoclonal T-cell expansion, recovery of blood counts and improved survival after administration of ATG or CSA, and improved survival after anti-IFN-γ or anti-TNF-α. This model involves transplanting cells that differ in major and minor histocompatibility antigens. Mismatch for minor histocompatibility antigens in the setting of HLA-identical sibling BMT is responsible for severe immune responses against host cells. Chen has recently shown that a single mismatch for the H60 minor histocompatibility antigen results in generation of H60-specific cytotoxic T lymphocytes that can trigger AA in this mouse model, which is prevented by administration of CSA or CD4⁺CD25⁺ T cells. Mice were engineered with a germline deletion of T-bet (T-bet⁻/⁻). Whereas T-bet⁺/⁺ lymph node cells induced severe aplasia, infusion of T-bet⁻/⁻ cells into sublethally irradiated F₁ hybrids did not result in severe aplasia, CD4⁺ and CD8⁺ cells were diminished, bone marrow IFN-γ was reduced but IL-4 and IL-7 were increased, indicating that the reduced Th1 response due to T-bet deficiency was partially compensated by increased Th2 and Th17 responses.

Genetic predisposition to AA

Inherited forms of AA have long been regarded as very rare causes of acquired AA, these including FA, DC and SDS (see Chapter 12). More recent awareness of these syndromes, with characterization of the genetic mutations in these and other bone marrow failure syndromes and the finding of very short telomeres in some patients with AA, indicate (i) a more common occurrence than previously realized, (ii) a shared defect in ribosomal biogenesis for SDS and Diamond–Blackfan anaemia (DBA), and (iii) a shared pathophysiology in DC and AA based on accelerated telomere attrition.

DC is due to mutations in the telomerase gene complex, a protein–RNA molecular machine for telomere repair, and also in the shelterin family, proteins that directly bind to and protect telomeres (Figure 13.3). The clinical features and gene mutations are discussed in further detail in Chapter 12. The DC

genes are involved in telomere maintenance, and all DC patients invariably have very short telomeres. About 10% of patients with apparent acquired AA have inherited mutations in TERC, TERT or one of the two shelterin genes, TERF1 and TERF2, with none or very mild mucocutaneous abnormalities. Families of affected individuals often show an increase in pulmonary fibrosis and cirrhosis.

SDS is an autosomal recessive inherited form of bone marrow failure, and another example of disordered ribosomal biogenesis and RNA processing. SDS usually occurs in childhood with neutropenia, but can present in adult life. The molecular and clinical features of SDS are discussed in Chapter 12.

In addition to mutations in the DC genes, other factors such as 'stressed' haemopoiesis as a result of reduced stem cell numbers in AA, and environmental factors such as smoking, contribute to the shortened telomeres. Telomeres are assumed to be short in all organs, but they are only measured in blood leucocytes (the tissue for which there are sufficient age-matched controls). The consequences of telomere shortening include genomic instability resulting in increased risk of malignant transformation (MDS, AML), bone marrow failure, and defects in repair and regeneration (pulmonary fibrosis, cirrhosis). The clinical consequences of missing an inherited form of AA include likely mortality after allogeneic HSCT using standard conditioning regimens and failure to screen potential family bone marrow donors for inherited bone marrow failure.

That not all patients with acquired AA respond to immunosuppressive therapy could be explained in pathogenetic terms by (i) complete stem cell depletion due to a severe autoimmune attack, (ii) insufficient degree of clinical immunosuppressive therapy, or (iii) a non-immune basis for the bone marrow failure, of which one mechanism may be a genetic predisposition resulting in genomic instability. The presence of shortened telomeres in AA does not preclude initial response to immunosuppressive therapy, but there are insufficient data in patients with TERC or TERT mutations on response to immunosuppressive therapy (see also section Predictors of response to ATG).

Clinical features

Patients with AA most commonly present with symptoms of anaemia and skin or mucosal haemorrhage (ecchymoses or petechiae), including buccal haemorrhages, or visual disturbance due to retinal haemorrhage. Infection, particularly sore throat or failure of minor infections to clear, may be a presenting feature but is less common. There is no lymphadenopathy or hepatosplenomegaly in the absence of infection. An important careful history and clinical examination help to exclude an inherited form of AA, especially in children and young adults. This also applies to older patients as it has more recently been

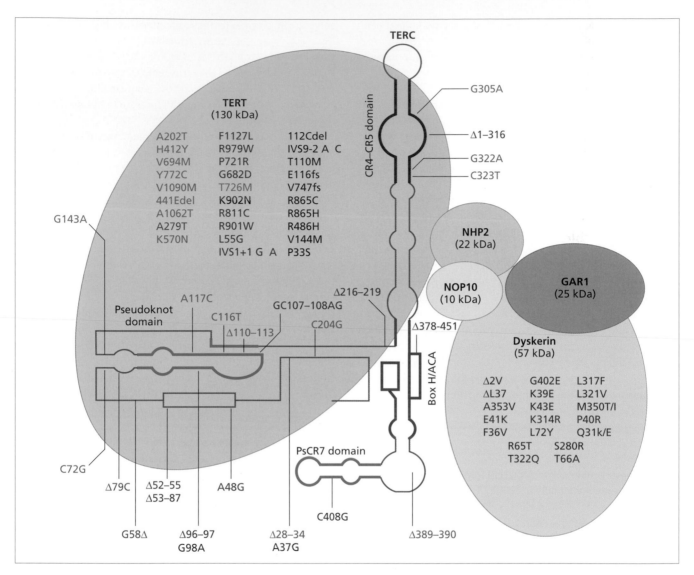

Figure 13.3 The components of the telomerase gene complex: TERT (reverse transcriptase), TERC (RNA template for TERT) and the nucleolar protein dyskerin, which forms a protein complex with the other proteins NHP2, NOP10, GAR1, that associates with TERC. Shown in red are the mutations found in dyskeratosis congenita, in green the mutations found in patients with AA, and in black mutations the mutations found in 'idiopathic' pulmonary fibrosis. The mutations shown in blue represent polymorphisms. (This research originally published in *Blood*. Calado RT, Young NS. Telomere maintenance and human bone marrow failure. *Blood* 2008;111:4446–55. © American Society of Hematology.)

realized that typical features of inherited bone marrow failure syndromes may be absent and/or other features may be present in older patients. The findings of short stature, abnormal thumbs and forearms, café-au-lait spots and skeletal anomalies would raise the possibility of an inherited form of AA, specifically FA, although FA can present in adults without physical anomalies. Patients with FA most commonly present between the ages of 3 and 14 years but can occasionally present later in their thirties or forties and very rarely early fifties. The findings of leucoplakia, nail dystrophy and pigmentation of the skin are characteristic of DC, with a median age at presentation of 7 years (range 6 months to 26 years). Some affected patients may have none of these clinical features and the diagnosis is made later after failure to respond to immunosuppressive therapy. For patients with AA and an inherited *TERC*/*TERT* mutation, the family history is very important as the pedigree may reveal pulmonary fibrosis, cirrhosis, osteoporosis or avascular necrosis of bone. A previous history of malabsorption or neutropenia may underlie a diagnosis of SDS in children or young adults, especially as the malabsorption often resolves in later life. A preceding history of jaundice, usually 2–3 months, may indicate a post-hepatitic AA.

Diagnostic investigations and differential diagnosis

To diagnose AA with certainty, it is important to consider other possible causes of pancytopenia with a hypocellular bone marrow and to exclude an inherited form of AA, as this will have important implications for treatment options, the choice of conditioning regimen for BMT, genetic screening and counselling of family members and the choice of donor for HSCT. All patients should be screened by cytogenetics and for a PNH clone.

The full blood count shows pancytopenia, although usually the lymphocyte count is preserved. In most cases the haemoglobin level and neutrophil and platelet counts are all uniformly depressed, but in the early stages isolated cytopenia, particularly thrombocytopenia, may occur. Such patients may be misdiagnosed as having immune thrombocytopenic purpura. There is anaemia with reticulocytopenia, and macrocytosis is common. The blood film should be examined to exclude the presence of dysplastic neutrophils and abnormal platelets, blasts and other abnormal cells such as hairy cells. In AA, anisopoikilocytosis is common and neutrophils may show toxic granulation. Platelets are reduced in number and are mostly of small size.

Both a bone marrow aspirate and trephine biopsy are required. Fragments should be readily obtained from the aspirate. A 'dry tap' should raise the suspicion of a diagnosis other than AA, such as primary myeloid metaplasia or myelofibrosis secondary to a malignancy. The bone marrow is hypocellular with prominent fat and variable amounts of residual haemopoietic cells. Erythropoiesis is reduced or absent; dyserythropoiesis is very common and often marked, and on its own does not indicate MDS. Megakaryocytes and granulocytic cells are reduced or absent; dysplastic megakaryocytes and granulocytic cells are not seen in AA. Lymphocytes, macrophages, plasma cells and mast cells appear prominent. In the early stages of the disease, one may also see prominent haemophagocytosis by macrophages, as well as background eosinophilic staining representing interstitial oedema. The trephine is needed to assess overall cellularity, the morphology of residual haemopoietic cells and to exclude an abnormal infiltrate. The trephine is hypocellular throughout but is sometimes patchy, with hypocellular and cellular areas. A 'hotspot' in a patchy area may explain why sometimes the aspirate is normocellular. Reticulin is not increased and abnormal cells are not present. Increased blasts are not seen in AA.

Liver function tests should be performed to detect antecedent hepatitis, but in post-hepatitic AA the serology is invariably negative for all the known hepatitis viruses. The onset of AA occurs 2–3 months after an acute episode of hepatitis and is more common in young males. Blood should be examined for hepatitis A antibody, hepatitis B surface antigen, hepatitis C antibody and Epstein–Barr virus (EBV). Cytomegalovirus (CMV) and other viral serology should be assessed if HSCT is being considered. HIV is not a recognized cause of AA but can cause isolated cytopenias. Appropriate investigations to exclude alternative aetiologies of cytopenias (vitamin B_{12}, red cell folate and HIV) should be performed, although bone marrow aplasia secondary to vitamin deficiency is exceedingly rare. Blood should be sent for antinuclear antibody to exclude SLE as another rare cause of AA.

The presence of a PNH clone is diagnosed by performing flow cytometry. Analysis of GPI-anchored proteins, such as CD55, CD59 and CD66b, is a sensitive and quantitative test for PNH that enables the detection of small PNH clones, which occur in up to 50% of patients with AA. Small clones are most easily identified in the neutrophil and monocyte lineages in AA and will be detected by flow cytometry and not by the Ham test. A recent blood transfusion does not prevent the diagnosis of a PNH clone, as flow cytometry will detect a GPI-deficient population of neutrophils and monocytes; a population of GPI-deficient red cells can be demonstrated in the presence of the transfused red cells. The clinical significance of a small PNH clone in AA as detected by flow cytometry remains uncertain. Such clones can remain stable, diminish in size, disappear or increase. A large PNH clone may be seen with clinical or laboratory evidence of haemolysis.

Cytogenetic analysis of the bone marrow should be attempted, although this may be difficult in a very hypocellular bone marrow and often insufficient metaphases are obtained. In this situation, fluorescence in situ hybridization analysis of chromosomes 5 and 7 can be attempted. The relevance of an abnormal cytogenetic clone in patients with no morphological features of MDS or AML remains controversial. Abnormal cytogenetic clones may be present in up to 12% of patients with otherwise typical AA at diagnosis. Common cytogenetic abnormalities include trisomy 6, trisomy 8, trisomy 15 and monosomy 7/del 7q. Monosomy 7 is associated with a high risk of MDS and poor response to immunosuppressive therapy. In contrast, trisomy 8 is associated with a good response to ATG and excellent survival. Abnormal cytogenetic clones may also arise during the course of the disease. If there is a lymphocytosis or prominent large granular lymphocytes on the blood film, immunophenotyping and analysis of T-cell receptor gene rearrangement should be performed to detect a clonal T-cell disorder such as T-LGL.

The diagnosis of FA is made by culturing peripheral blood lymphocytes for spontaneous and diepoxybutane (DEB)- or mitomycin C (MMC)-induced chromosomal breakages. This test should be performed in younger patients and is mandatory before stem cell transplantation. Rarely, FA has been diagnosed in the fifth decade of life. DC may be excluded by identifying a known mutation but there are probably other mutations yet to be identified. Along with measuring telomere lengths, this is not currently available as a routine clinical service in the UK, and at present remains a research investigation. Rarely, the chromosomal breakage test performed on peripheral blood may be falsely negative in patients with FA who have haemopoietic mosaicism due to genetic reversion in one allele. In this situation, skin fibroblast cultures will demonstrate hypersensitivity to DEB or MMC.

Chest radiography is useful at presentation to exclude infection and for comparison with subsequent films. Radiographs of the radii are not routinely indicated but may be helpful in inherited AA, especially FA. An abdominal ultrasound may be performed if an enlarged spleen and/or enlarged lymph nodes and a malignant haematological disorder are suspected. Abnormal anatomically displaced kidneys or a single kidney are features of FA.

Differential diagnosis

The following disorders may sometimes present with pancytopenia and a hypocellular bone marrow.
• Hypocellular MDS/AML, featuring dysplastic megakaryocytes and dysplastic granulocytic cells, increased reticulin fibrosis, blasts, ALIPs (abnormal localization of abnormal precursors), the presence of any ringed sideroblasts and an increase in CD34$^+$ cells.
• Aleukaemic leukaemia describes cases of hypocellular acute lymphoblastic leukaemia, or less often hypocellular AML, in children. It presents initially with pancytopenia and a hypocellular bone marrow but later evolves to overt leukaemia.
• Hairy cell leukaemia classically presents with pancytopenia, monocytopenia, an interstitial infiltrate of hairy cells and increased bone marrow reticulin. Splenomegaly is common.
• Lymphomas, either Hodgkin disease or non-Hodgkin lymphoma, and myelofibrosis. Myelofibrosis is usually accompanied by splenomegaly.
• Mycobacterial infections, especially atypical infection. Other bone marrow abnormalities include granulomas, fibrosis, marrow necrosis, haemophagocytosis and demonstrable acid alcohol-fast bacilli.
• Anorexia nervosa or prolonged starvation. The bone marrow may show hypocellularity and gelatinous transformation (serous degeneration/atrophy) with loss of fat cells as well as haemopoietic cells, and increased ground substance.

Management

Supportive care

Transfusions
Support with red cell and platelet transfusions is essential for patients with AA to maintain a safe blood count. Current practice in both the UK and USA is to give prophylactic platelets when the platelet count is below 10×10^9/L (or $< 20 \times 10^9$/L in the presence of fever, sepsis or bleeding). A trial to evaluate the use of prophylactic platelets in thrombocytopenic patients is currently ongoing in the UK (TRAP, Trial to Reduce Alloimmunization to Platelets). Predicting bleeding is difficult in an individual patient. Fatal haemorrhage, usually cerebral, is more common in patients who have less than 10×10^9/L platelets, extensive retinal haemorrhages, buccal haemorrhages or rapidly spreading purpura.

A common problem in multitransfused patients with AA, compared with leukaemia patients, is that they may develop alloimmunization to leucocytes present in red cell and platelet transfusions by generating HLA or non-HLA (minor histocompatibility) antibodies. In AA, rates of alloimmunization obtained prior to universal leucodepletion are around 30–50%. Leucodepletion, which has been universally applied to cellular blood components in the UK since November 1999, has probably reduced the incidence of alloimmunization. Alloimmunization can result in platelet refractoriness, as well as an increased risk of graft rejection after allogeneic BMT. Patients who become refractory to platelet transfusions should be screened for HLA antibodies, once other causes of platelet refractoriness have been excluded. If a patient does become sensitized to random donor platelets, HLA-matched platelets should be used. Current matching strategies in the UK and USA are based on counting the number of HLA-A and -B mismatches between patient and donor. This procedure requires the availability of a large HLA-typed donor panel and even then sometimes no suitable matches can be found. Novel approaches, including the use of HLA epitope-matched platelets, merit further evaluation.

Red cell and platelet transfusions should be given to maintain a safe haemoglobin level and platelet count and not be withheld for fear of sensitizing the patient. Directed blood and platelet donations from family members are not permitted within the National Blood Service, and not looked on favourably in the USA either; the recipient may become sensitized to minor histocompatibility antigens from the potential bone marrow donor, resulting in a high risk of graft rejection. In exceptional circumstances, a family donor may provide the most compatible platelets if a patient has developed multispecific HLA antibodies and requires platelets urgently.

If a patient is a candidate for early or later BMT, it is recommended that the patient is transfused with CMV-negative blood products until the patient's CMV status is known. CMV-negative blood products should then be continued only if both the patient and donor are CMV negative.

It is currently unclear whether red cell and platelet transfusions should be routinely irradiated in all AA patients who are potential HSCT candidates and in all patients undergoing treatment with ATG. The rationale for considering the use of irradiated blood products is twofold. Firstly, animal data demonstrate that irradiation of all red cell and platelet transfusions before HSCT further reduces the risk of sensitization to minor histocompatibility antigens (and hence reduced risk of graft rejection after allogeneic HSCT). Leucodepletion of blood products is likely to have reduced alloimmunization in AA patients. Secondly, irradiated blood products would abolish the potential risk of transfusion-associated GVHD associated with ATG therapy. Transfusion-associated GVHD has very rarely been reported after ATG. Rabbit ATG is more immunosuppressive than is horse ATG. Rabbit ATG also results in a more prolonged period of lymphopenia and has a longer half-life and higher-affinity IgG subtype to human lymphocytes than does horse ATG. For these reasons, even though there is no evidence base, the British Committee for Standards in Haematology now recommends empirically the use of irradiated blood components for all AA patients receiving ATG.

The use of granulocyte transfusions is being re-evaluated as supportive therapy in patients with life threatening neutropenia. Adverse events, such as febrile reactions, HLA alloimmunization and transfusion-related acute lung injury, are well-recognized complications following granulocyte transfusions. Irradiated granulocyte transfusions are used at specialized centres to support patients with fungal/mould disease or bacterial sepsis who are severely neutropenic and not adequately responding to maximal antibiotics, when the possible benefits outweigh the hazards.

Iron chelation therapy

Many AA patients require multiple red cell transfusions leading to transfusion haemosiderosis. Iron overload impacts adversely on outcome after allogeneic BMT. Iron chelation therapy should commence when the serum ferritin is above 1000 µg/L, although the evidence base for this is lacking. It may be difficult to deliver subcutaneous desferrioxamine to AA patients on account of local haemorrhage and infection from subcutaneous injections. If not tolerated, intravenous desferrioxamine through a central line may be considered. Alternative oral agents include deferiprone and deferasirox (Exjade). Because of a high incidence of agranulocytosis with deferiprone, it is not used routinely in patients with AA. In the USA, deferasirox is now widely prescribed in the marrow failure syndromes. There were initial concerns about cytopenias in patients treated with deferasirox, so its safety in AA patients was unclear. Results of a recent prospective study of deferasirox in 166 iron-over-loaded AA patients showed that after 1 year there was a median fall in serum ferritin of 946 µg/L from a baseline median of 3254 µg/L. There were no cases of myelosuppression due to deferasirox.

Infections

Patients with AA are at risk of bacterial and fungal infections, depending in part on the degree of neutropenia. Very severe neutropenia (neutrophils $< 0.2 \times 10^9$/L) carries a high risk of systemic bacterial and fungal infections. At neutrophil counts between 0.2 and 0.5×10^9/L, the risk of infection is less but acquired infection cannot be readily counteracted. If there is severe neutropenia, non-absorbable antibiotics are sometimes administered to reduce the potential pathogenic load from the gastrointestinal tract. An alternative option is an oral quinolone, although neither is standard practice in the USA. Oral hygiene is important. Entry sites for venous access are potential sources of systemic infection. Patients with AA are at high risk of fungal infection, including *Aspergillus*. Fluconazole provides no protection against *Aspergillus* species, for which the drugs of choice are itraconazole, which has clinically significant but manageable or avoidable interactions with other drugs, and posaconazole, which has not yet been shown to be superior in efficacy to itraconazole.

Fever should be treated with broad-spectrum antibiotics without waiting for laboratory isolation of organisms, and with early introduction of systemic antifungal therapy if fever fails to respond to antibiotics. Chest radiography should be part of the investigation of new or persistent fever, along with computed tomography of the chest. G-CSF is usually ineffective in severe AA due to a marked reduction or absence of myeloid progenitor cells, although it is reasonable to consider giving a short course to assess for a temporary increase in the neutrophil count.

General comments relating to the management of AA

Because AA is a rare disease, the haematologist responsible for the patient should contact a centre/specialist with expertise in AA soon after presentation to discuss a management plan for the patient. Patients should be offered the opportunity to be reviewed in a specialist centre. Whenever possible, patients should be enrolled into prospective national or international trials.

Prior to administration of specific treatment for the disease, the patient should be stabilized clinically in terms of controlling bleeding and treating infection. The presence of infection is an adverse factor for outcome after HSCT, although it may sometimes be necessary to proceed with HSCT in the presence of active infection, particularly fungal infection. In this setting, transplantation may offer the best chance of early neutrophil recovery, and delaying the transplant may risk progression of the fungal infection.

Indications for treatment of AA

The two main treatment options for AA are allogeneic HSCT or immunosuppressive therapy with ATG and CSA, based on disease severity, age of the patient, availability of a matched sibling donor, and patient choice. Young patients with a low neutrophil count have a significant advantage if treated with first-line HSCT. Older patients with a higher neutrophil count do better if given immunosuppressive therapy as first-line therapy. For patients with severe AA who are under 40 years of age, the first-line treatment is matched sibling donor HSCT. For all other patients who require treatment, namely those with non-severe AA or those older than 40 years, immunosuppressive therapy is the first option. An exception to this is children with non-severe AA who are transfusion dependent, where first-line treatment is matched sibling donor HSCT. Unrelated donor HSCT is indicated after failure to respond to one course of immunosuppressive therapy, for those patients who lack a matched sibling donor, and who are under 50 years of age, or older if of good performance status.

The currently recommended regimen for immunosuppressive therapy comprises the combination of ATG and CSA. There is no role for HGFs as specific therapy for AA. Corticosteroids should not be given to treat AA as they are ineffective and encourage fungal and bacterial infections. Figure 13.4 illustrates current treatment algorithms for severe and non-severe AA.

Immunosuppressive therapy

Antithymocyte globulin: properties, mechanism of action and administration

ATG is a polyclonal IgG antibody preparation produced by immunizing horses or rabbits with human thymocytes obtained at the time of cardiac surgery in children. It binds to T cells, B cells, monocyte/macrophages, dendritic cells and endothelial cells, and also reacts with molecules involved in the immune response, cell migration and adhesion and signal transduction. Its mechanism of action in AA is not entirely clear. Furthermore, the mode of action of rabbit and horse ATG preparations may differ. Possible mechanisms include the following:

1 T-cell depletion by complement-mediated lysis;
2 destruction of activated cytotoxic T lymphocytes by Fas-mediated apoptosis and antibody-dependent cellular cytotoxicity;
3 reduced apoptosis and Fas expression on AA CD34$^+$ bone marrow cells;

4 direct stimulation of normal and AA CD34$^+$ bone marrow cells and a mitogenic effect in the absence of complement resulting in release of HGFs;
5 direct stimulation of T-regulatory cells has been demonstrated when normal bone marrow mononuclear cells are incubated with rabbit ATG.

In the UK, most of Europe and many other countries, the standard preparation of ATG has until recently been horse ATG (Lymphoglobuline, Genzyme). In the USA, horse ATG (Atgam) is still widely used. The rabbit preparation (Thymoglobuline, Genzyme) was usually reserved for second or subsequent courses. From June 2007, horse ATG was withdrawn due to manufacturing difficulties in maintaining quality control.

ATG is a powerful immunosuppressive drug and its use in severely neutropenic patients requires very careful monitoring, the prophylaxis and treatment of fevers and infections, as well as adequate (and sometimes intensive) platelet transfusion support. Rabbit ATG is given for 5 days as a daily intravenous infusion over 12–18 hours through a central venous catheter. The daily dose of rabbit ATG is 1.5 vials per 10 kg body weight (1 vial of rabbit ATG contains 25 mg protein, so the daily dose is 3.75 mg/kg). A test dose must be given beforehand and if a severe systemic reaction or anaphylaxis occurs, further doses of that preparation of ATG must not be given. Instead of giving a separate test dose, some centres give the first 100 mL of the first infusion very slowly over 1 hour. Allergists maintain that this is inadequate to prevent anaphylaxis as the amounts delivered are relatively large. In the USA, a skin test for horse ATG sensitivity is routinely given but by custom not for rabbit ATG in the absence of published data. Horse ATG (Atgam) dosage is 40 mg/kg daily for 4 days.

Immediate side-effects are allergic and occur commonly, including fever, rigors, rash, hypertension or hypotension and fluid retention. Each daily dose should be preceded by intravenous methylprednisolone and chlorpheniramine. In the USA, patients are pretreated with diphenhydramine and pethidine if fever and chills have occurred. Platelet transfusions should be given to maintain a safe platelet count (ideally $> 30 \times 10^9$/L; in the USA, a threshold of $> 20 \times 10^9$/L is used). Prior to starting ATG, patients should be assessed to ensure adequate platelet increments with random donor platelets. Poor platelet increments should be investigated beforehand. Patients are often in isolation with reverse barrier nursing, but this is not standard practice in the USA. Fevers are treated with broad-spectrum antibiotics. Intravenous methylprednisolone (or oral prednisolone) and paracetamol are given at least 30 min before each daily dose of rabbit ATG 1–2 mg/kg, with reduction of the prednisolone dose by half every 5 days. Prednisolone is given to help prevent serum sickness. Serum sickness typically occurs between 7 and 14 days from the start of ATG treatment. The common symptoms of serum sickness include arthralgia, myalgia, rash,

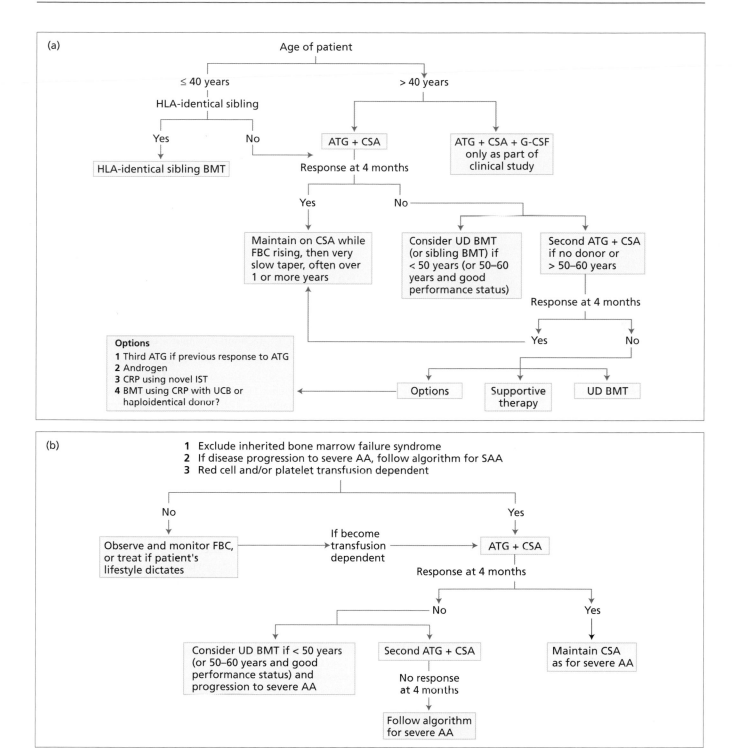

Figure 13.4 Algorithms for treatment of (a) severe acquired aplastic anaemia and (b) non-severe aplastic anaemia. AA, aplastic anaemia; ATG, antithymocyte globulin; BMT, bone marrow transplantation; CSA, ciclosporin; FBC, full blood count; IST, immunosuppressive therapy; UD, unrelated donor; HLA id sib BMT, HLA-identical sibling BMT; CRP, clinical research protocol; UCB, umbilical cord blood. (Modified from Marsh *et al.* (2009) *British Journal of Haematology* **147**: 43–70, with permission of Wiley Publishers.)

fever, mild proteinuria and platelet consumption often necessitating increased platelet transfusion support.

Evolution of ATG-based immunosuppression

ATG was first used in the treatment of AA by George Mathé, who observed autologous recovery after haploidentical BMT with ATG. Subsequent work confirmed that the responses seen were due to ATG and not the haploidentical bone marrow. During the late 1970s and early 1980s, ATG was given with high-dose methylprednisolone, on the (incorrect) assumption that high-dose methylprednisolone contributed to response. The addition of androgens (in most cases oxymetholone) to ATG and high-dose methylprednisolone during the early to mid 1980s failed to significantly improve response rates or survival after ATG. ATG in combination with CSA during the mid/late1980s resulted in a significant improvement in response rates and survival. For non-severe AA, the combined use of ATG and CSA resulted in 75% response compared with 45% for CSA alone. For severe AA, significantly better responses were seen with the combination of ATG and CSA compared with ATG alone.

The rationale for using daily G-CSF (administered for 3 months) with ATG and CSA was to help reduce infection and to improve response. There were concerns about an increase in later clonal disorders with G-CSF, particularly from studies in Japan; transformation could only be fully appreciated with follow-up of at least 10 years. Two prospective randomized studies comparing ATG, CSA and G-CSF with ATG and CSA alone demonstrated no difference in response and survival between the two groups. A further prospective study from Europe is awaiting analysis. A large retrospective study from the European Group for Blood and Marrow Transplantation (EBMT) of patients treated with ATG and CSA, of whom 43% also received G-CSF, reported an incidence of MDS/AML of 10.9% with G-CSF and 5.8% without G-CSF. *In vitro* studies have shown that incubation of AA CD34$^+$ bone marrow cells with G-CSF selected cells in which there was upregulation of the class IV mRNA isoform of G-CSFR, which is defective in cellular differentiation signalling. Incubation of bone marrow cells from AA patients with monosomy 7 with high doses of G-CSF increased the proportion of monosomy 7 cells. These studies showed that high doses of G-CSF did not induce monosomy 7 in AA but caused expansion of pre-existing monosomy 7 cells. Because of the above observations, and the continued need for longer follow-up in these studies, the routine use of G-CSF with ATG and CSA is not currently recommended.

There is a good rationale for considering the use of additional immunosuppressive drugs with ATG and CSA, as some non-responders may not have received adequate immunosuppression. Two separate studies from NIH evaluated the addition of mycophenolate mofetil (MMF) and sirolimus to ATG and CSA. There was no improvement in response or reduction in relapse using MMF in combination with ATG and CSA compared to therapy without MMF. The second study examined the addition of sirolimus in a prospective randomized study. Sirolimus was chosen because it has a different pathway of action to CSA, and in solid transplantation it is synergistic with CSA. Sirolimus blocks mTOR (mammalian target of rapamycin), a serine/threonine kinase, and so may target those autoreactive T cells that escape inhibition through calcium-independent or CSA-resistant pathways. However, no significant difference in response was demonstrated to ATG and CSA with or without sirolimus (37% at 3 months and 51% at 6 months in the arm with sirolimus; 57% at 3 months and 62% at 6 months without sirolimus).

Survival after ATG

Data from EBMT and large single centres confirm that over the last three decades overall survival after ATG therapy has improved steadily, with 5-year survival of 70–80% reported (Figure 13.5). The reasons for improved survival have been difficult to assess formally, but likely factors include (i) improved supportive care for prevention and treatment of infections, especially superior antifungals and better availability and quality of blood products, (ii) the use of CSA with ATG and (iii) successful second-line therapies including another round of ATG, unrelated donor BMT (UDBMT) in younger patients and allogeneic HSCT in older adults. A summary of large studies reporting outcomes after immunosuppressive therapy with ATG and CSA is shown in Table 13.3.

Predictors of response to ATG

Although disease severity does not impact on overall survival, patients with non-severe AA are more likely to respond than

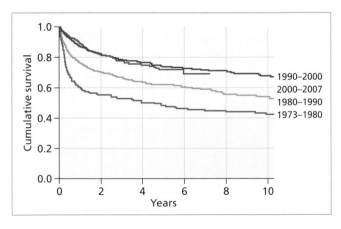

Figure 13.5 Survival of patients with severe aplastic anaemia: overall survival of 2400 patients reported to the EBMT database according to year of treatment with ATG with or without ciclosporin. (From Passweg JR, Tichelli A (2009) Immunosuppressive treatment for aplastic anaemia: are we hitting the ceiling? *Haematologica* **94**: 310–12 with permission.)

Table 13.3 Immunosuppressive therapy using ATG and CSA.

Study	N	Median age (years)	Response (%)	Relapse (%)	Clonal evolution (%)	Survival (%)
1	84	32	66	19	8	59 at 11 years
2	100	16	77	12	11	85 at 5 years
3	122	35	61	35	11	55 at 7 years
4	119	9	68	22	6	89 at 3 years
5	104	30	62	37	9	80 at 4 years

Only studies with more than 20 enrolled patients are shown. Responses to immunosuppressive therapy are usually partial; blood counts may not normalize but patients become transfusion independent and recovery of neutrophil count is sufficient to prevent infection. Study 4 included androgens with or without G-CSF; study 5 included mycophenolate mofetil.
Key to studies: 1, Frickhofen *et al.* (2003); 2, Bacigalupo A, Bruno B, Saracco P *et al.* (2000); 3, Rosenfeld *et al.* (2003); 4, Kojima *et al.* (2000); 5, Scheinberg *et al.* (2006).
Source: modified from table originally published in *Blood*. Young NS, Calado RT, Scheinberg P. Current concepts in the pathophysiology and treatment of aplastic anaemia. *Blood* 2006;108:2509–19. © American Society of Hematology.

are patients with severe or very severe AA. However, the classical Camitta criteria (see Table 13.1) were not designed to predict response to ATG. Furthermore, automated reticulocyte counting tends to overestimate at low levels and correlates poorly with manual counts.

In a recent multivariate analysis from NIH of response at 6 months, only younger age, absolute reticulocyte count (ARC) and absolute lymphocyte count (ALC) correlate with response to ATG. The lack of association with the absolute neutrophil count reflected a high number of early deaths in patients with very severe neutropenia. For patients with ARC 25×10^9/L or more and ALC 1.0×10^9/L or more, the response was 83% compared with 41% for those with lower counts. The better prognostic group also showed significantly better survival.

Several studies have examined whether the presence of a PNH clone is associated with response to ATG, with conflicting results. This may reflect differences in sensitivity of the test used to detect a PNH clone. Those using very sensitive tests to detect GPI-deficient clones of less than 0.003 cells show a strong correlation with response.

HLA type may also correlate with response to immunosuppressive therapy. A Japanese study showed that HLA-DRB1*1501 associated with response to CSA. Although HLA-DR15 or DRB1*1501 predicts response to ATG in white patients with MDS, no association was seen in AA patients. More recently, the same Japanese group demonstrated that of the 30 different DRB1 alleles, only DRB1*1501 and DRB1*1502 occurred more frequently in AA than in controls, and that response to ATG and CSA was only associated with DRB1*1501 in the presence of a PNH clone. Thus specific HLA haplotypes correlate with response to immunosuppressive therapy in Japanese patients, but similar studies in white Europeans are lacking.

Recent studies from NIH indicate that shortened telomere length does not preclude initial response to immunosuppressive therapy, but predicts relapse after ATG and is a risk factor for later cytogenetic abnormalities and evolution to MDS and AML. Thus telomere length at diagnosis may reflect depleted stem cell reserve so that prolonged stem cell division is not possible, resulting in later relapse; later clonal evolution reflects genomic instability of the critically shortened telomeres. In patients with *TERC* or *TERT* gene mutations, there are insufficient data on their response to immunosuppressive therapy.

Repeat courses of ATG

A second course of rabbit ATG may be administered if there is relapse after the first course or no response to the first course by 3–4 months. The response rate following a second course of horse ATG for relapse was 61%, and 64% in patients who did not respond to the first course. When rabbit ATG is given for the second course following an initial course of horse ATG, the response rate was only 30% for non-responders and 65% for relapsing patients. A recent study from Japan has examined prospectively the outcome of 52 children who failed one course of horse ATG, and who went on to receive either a second course of horse ATG or an unrelated donor HSCT. The response to a second course of ATG was only 11%, with a 5-year failure-free survival of only 9.5%; three children had anaphylaxis to the second course of ATG. Another study has assessed the value of giving three courses of ATG. Among those patients who showed no response to the first or second courses, there were no sustained responses, but for those who had relapsed after two previous courses, all responded to a third. Those patients treated with more than two courses of ATG had received various combinations of horse and rabbit ATG. Following the withdrawal of horse ATG (Lymphoglobuline), there are currently no data on using rabbit ATG more than twice in the same patient. For patients receiving more than one course of ATG, the risk of anaphylaxis may be higher. Serum sickness is still unpredictable though it may occur earlier following a second course of the same animal preparation of ATG.

Late complications after ATG

Relapse occurs in up to 30–35% of patients when CSA is withdrawn at 6 months. A more prolonged course of CSA with a later slow tapering of the drug reduces the relapse risk to around 13–16%. About one-third of patients are CSA dependent and require a small dose long term. CSA can be continued for at least 12 months after a maximal response before starting to taper the drug, followed by a very slow taper, for example by 25 mg every 3 months.

Patients treated with ATG are also at risk of developing clonal disorders, such as PNH, MDS and AML. A survey in 1993 from EBMT reported a 10-year incidence of developing MDS of 10%; the corresponding 10-year incidence for AML was 5%. Long-term follow-up of the prospective German national study of 84 patients treated with either the combination of ATG and CSA or ATG alone, between 1986 and 1989, reported overall survival of 58% and 54%, respectively, at 11 years. The actuarial probability of developing haemolytic PNH at 11 years was 10%, MDS or AML 8% and a solid tumour 11%. Risk factors for developing MDS/AML include repeated courses of ATG, older age, and high doses, prolonged duration of G-CSF with ATG and CSA, and shortened telomeres. Long-term follow-up from a large NIH cohort showed a 55% 7-year overall survival, 35% relapse at 5 years, and 10% risk of PNH and 15% risk of clonal evolution excluding PNH at 10 years.

ATG treatment in older patients and children

For older patients, the response rate and survival rate are lower compared with younger patients, with a higher risk of bacterial and fungal infections, bleeding and serious cardiac events after ATG. Although there is no upper age limit for ATG treatment, consideration for treatment should be preceded by medical assessment to exclude significant comorbidities and bone marrow examination to exclude hypocellular MDS. For older patients who are not candidates for ATG, CSA may be considered, but there is increased risk of renal toxicity and hypertension.

Excellent response to ATG is seen in children. Current response rates are around 75%, with 90% long-term survival. Hence, for children with severe AA who lack an HLA-identical sibling donor, first-line therapy should be ATG with CSA. If there is no response to a single course of immunosuppressive therapy, unrelated donor HSCT should be explored.

Other immunosuppressive drugs used in AA

Cyclophosphamide

High-dose cyclophosphamide (HDC) administered at 200 mg/kg has been used to treat AA in the absence of stem cell support, following the observation that complete autologous haematological recovery occurs in a small number of patients undergoing allogeneic sibling BMT using HDC. Although durable responses were seen, the predictable and markedly prolonged cytopenias exposed patients to a high risk of fatal fungal infections and a significant increase in use of blood and platelet transfusions, days of intravenous antibiotics and amphotericin, and inpatient days in hospital. In addition, HDC treatment did not eliminate the risk of clonal events. Consequently, the use of HDC in the treatment of AA has not been met with much enthusiasm.

Alemtuzumab

The anti-CD52 monoclonal antibody alemtuzumab (Campath-1H) is effective in other autoimmune disorders such as multiple sclerosis, autoimmune cytopenias and the vasculitides. It is currently being evaluated in the treatment of AA. It produces profound lymphocyte depletion by antibody-dependent cell-mediated cytotoxicity and complement-mediated lysis. A small prospective study combined with a retrospective review of cases reported to EBMT on the use of a single course of alemtuzumab (100 mg over 5 days) and CSA in AA showed response in 9 of 18 patients, although relapses were common. At the NIH, preliminary data from ongoing studies (but with a larger number of patients) suggest that alemutuzumab (100 mg over 10 days) is effective for patients refractory to horse ATG or who have relapsed.

Haemopoietic stem cell transplantation

Outcomes following allogeneic HSCT for acquired AA, whether from a matched sibling donor or a matched unrelated donor, have steadily improved over time. Matched sibling donor transplantation for severe AA results in a 75–90% chance of long-term cure in young patients, but is less successful in older patients (Figure 13.6). More recently, significant improvements have been observed for matched unrelated donor HSCT for AA patients failing immunosuppressive therapy, with 60–80% survival and the best results seen in younger patients. Major difficulties remain for older patients in general and for patients who have failed immunosuppressive therapy and who have no suitable bone marrow donor. For these patients, new transplantation approaches are needed.

Pretransplant assessment of the patient

A reassessment bone marrow examination with cytogenetics and flow cytometry for GPI-deficient cells should be performed to exclude a malignant, premalignant or PNH clone, along with a careful re-evaluation to ensure that a constitutional form of aplasia has been excluded, since this would influence the choice of transplant conditioning regimen. Patients with FA need a much reduced intensity conditioning regimen compared with that used for acquired AA. A repeat HLA antibody screen should be performed to exclude HLA alloimmunization.

Pretransplant comorbidities impact adversely on non-relapse mortality after HSCT, including iron overload. Iron status is

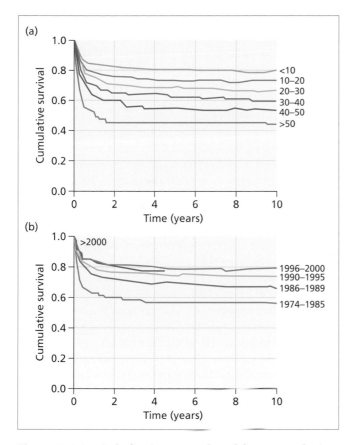

Figure 13.6 Survival of patients transplanted for severe aplastic anaemia according to (a) year of transplant and (b) patient age. (Data obtained from EBMT database, JR Passweg, 2007.)

especially relevant to patients with AA who have often been multiply transfused prior to HSCT. Efforts should be made to reduce the serum ferritin before transplantation, although there is no clear guidance on the target level to achieve. The issues relating to pre-existing comorbidities are of importance in older patients with AA, because their transplant-related mortality is higher than in younger patients.

HLA-matched sibling donor transplantation

Conditioning regimens

The standard conditioning regimen for younger patients is HDC 200 mg/kg, which results in survival of at least 80% in younger patients (< 30 years). HDC is relatively free of long-term side-effects, and fertility is usually preserved. The dose needs to be carefully calculated because it is close to a cardiotoxic dose. The commonly used transplant regimens for AA patients are non-myeloablative. Older patients may need modified conditioning, as discussed later.

ATG is widely used with HDC to reduce graft rejection, although a prospective randomized study from the Centre for International Blood and Marrow Transplant Research (CIBMTR) registry failed to show a significant difference in graft rejection, GVHD or survival when HDC alone was compared with HDC and ATG. Standard GVHD prophylaxis is with CSA and methotrexate. Alemtuzumab has also been used with CSA; one small single-centre study confirmed a significant reduction in GVHD compared with ATG-based conditioning regimens in AA. Because AA patients are at risk of late graft failure, CSA is usually continued for 12 months after HSCT.

Dose and source of haemopoietic stem cells

It is important to give at least 3×10^8 nucleated marrow cells/kg because at lower doses the risk of graft rejection increases significantly higher. Infusion of less than 2×10^6 CD34$^+$ cells/kg is associated with delay in neutrophil engraftment and increased risk of graft failure and bacterial infections.

There is thus a good theoretical rationale for considering using G-CSF mobilized peripheral blood stem cells in HSCT for AA as a means of obtaining a high stem-cell dose and early engraftment, although a retrospective study showed more chronic GVHD in younger patients after peripheral blood stem cell transplantation in younger patients, worse survival and graft rejection the same, compared with BMT. At present, routine use of peripheral blood stem cell transplantation for AA is not recommended, although data from the EBMT Registry show that its use in AA continues to increase.

Graft rejection

Historical data indicate that AA patients have a higher rate of graft rejection compared with patients transplanted for haematological malignancies, although this has not been re-evaluated in the light of now routine practice of giving only leucodepleted blood products. Graft rejection occurred in 5–15% of matched sibling donor and 10–30% of matched unrelated donor HSCT. Early (or primary) graft rejection results in either no evidence of engraftment following the transplantation, with persistent pancytopenia, or early engraftment with neutrophils and monocytes but followed by pancytopenia. Late (or secondary) graft rejection occurs after a period of established engraftment.

Factors associated with graft rejection in AA include:
1 Multiple blood transfusions, in most series classified as more than 50 transfusions prior to HSCT, can result in alloimmunization to HLA and minor histocompatibility antigens present on donor cells but lacking in recipients.
2 Pretransplant and post-transplant immunsuppression affect graft rejection, namely the use of CSA or irradiation.
3 A low dose of donor haemopoietic stem cells.
4 T-cell depletion of donor marrow.
5 Sex-mismatched HSCT when male donors used for female recipients.
6 Progressive mixed chimerism.

Chimerism

Using polymerase chain reaction for short tandem repeats on unfractionated bone marrow or peripheral blood mononuclear cells, the Dublin group in collaboration with EBMT reported mixed chimerism in 25% of HSCTs for AA. Full donor chimerism occurs in 75%. Patients with mixed chimerism may have either stable or progressive mixed chimerism. All the cases of graft failure occurred in the progressive mixed chimerism group, of whom 50% rejected their grafts. Patients with stable mixed chimerism had excellent survival and no chronic GVHD, suggesting a state of tolerance may be achieved. Regular monitoring of chimerism is especially important at the time of CSA withdrawal. Increasing recipient chimerism would indicate the need for continued CSA.

Treatment of graft rejection

If graft rejection occurs, a second HSCT may be indicated. If there is residual host haemopoiesis, reconditioning of the recipient is necessary. Graft rejection associated with inadequate donor haemopoiesis may benefit from 'booster' donor stem cells without the need for further immunosuppression. Late graft failure may respond to reintroduction of therapeutic doses of CSA if the rejection occurred after discontinuation or withdrawal of CSA. Outcome after second HSCT depends on performance status and timing of the second transplant, with better outcome if the patient is transplanted more than 3 months after the first HSCT. There have been anecdotal reports of using donor lymphocyte infusion in cases of late graft failure, but there have been no formal clinical trials to fully evaluate its effectiveness and safety. The major concern with this approach is the induction of chronic GVHD. Complete autologous recovery may occur after graft rejection, and is defined as normalization of the blood count with restoration of host haemopoiesis; it results in excellent long-term survival.

Adverse factors for outcome

The effect of age on matched sibling donor HSCT is an important factor determining outcome. An EBMT study showed actuarial survival of patients aged 16 years or less, 17–40 years and over 40 years to be 77%, 68% and 54%, respectively. Other adverse prognostic factors are prior failed immunosuppressive therapy, long interval between diagnosis and HSCT, heavy transfusion burden and active infection before HSCT. For patients transplanted for haematological malignancies, iron overload is an adverse factor for outcome.

The outcome of patients above 40 years of age undergoing HSCT with conventional intensity protocols is significantly inferior compared with younger patients. A recent CIBMTR study has compared outcomes in patients over 40 years of age. Older patients showed worse survival, more GVHD and slower platelet recovery. Factors impacting on survival in older patients included poor performance status, multiple blood transfusions and more than 6 months from diagnosis to transplant. Because

of worse outcomes in older patients transplanted for AA, new approaches are needed. There are encouraging preliminary results using minimal-intensity conditioning with fludarabine, low-dose cyclophosphamide and ATG, with improved survival.

Graft-versus-host disease

GVHD (especially chronic) is one of the most serious complications, as it adversely impacts on performance status, quality of life and survival after marrow transplantation, especially in a disease like AA where there is no advantage in having a graft-versus-disease effect. It is seen mainly in patients with complete donor chimerism. Using ATG-based conditioning regimens, the incidence of acute GVHD is 12–30% and of chronic GVHD 30–40%. Chronic GVHD remains one of the most important challenges in HSCT for AA.

The risk factors for chronic GVHD include (i) history of prior acute GVHD, (ii) infusion of unirradiated donor buffy coat cells (this manoeuvre was used previously to overcome the problem of graft rejection but abandoned because of the high incidence of chronic GVHD), (iii) older patient age, (iv) the use of peripheral blood stem cells and (v) the use of ATG compared with alemtuzumab-based conditioning regimens.

Long-term complications of HSCT

Infertility

Fertility is usually well preserved when irradiation is not used in the conditioning regimen, and the chances of pregnancy or fathering a child are much higher in patients who receive a marrow transplant for AA than for haematological malignancies. Pregnancies in patients transplanted for AA usually have a successful outcome. Fludarabine-based conditioning regimens in AA use much lower doses of cyclophosphamide and may therefore have a theoretical advantage over conventional intensity protocols in preserving fertility, but data are lacking.

Secondary malignancies

There is an increased frequency of solid tumour malignancies after marrow transplantation for AA, but the risk is lower than in patients transplanted for haematological malignancies when irradiation is avoided. A combined study from Seattle and Paris of 700 patients, of whom 79 had FA, reported an estimated risk of developing a secondary tumour at 20 years for AA patients (excluding FA) of 14% and a median time for developing a second tumour of 9 years. Significant risk factors were treatment of chronic GVHD with azathioprine, irradiation and age.

Risk factors for EBV post-transplant lymphoproliferative disease after allogeneic HSCT for acute and chronic leukaemia and AA include unrelated donor HSCT, mismatched related donor transplantation, T-cell depletion of donor marrow, use of ATG, older age (> 50 years) and patients receiving second transplants. For AA patients, immunosuppressive therapy with ATG prior to HSCT is also a risk factor. The use of alemtuzumab in the conditioning regimen instead of ATG is associated with a lower risk as it depeletes not only T cells but also B cells (including EBV-infected B cells).

Unrelated donor HSCT for AA

Indications and timing

Unrelated donor HSCT is considered for young adults and children with severe or very severe AA who have failed one course of ATG and CSA. In older patients a second course of ATG may be preferred before proceeding to matched unrelated donor BMT. They should ideally have a fully matched (at DNA level for both class I and II antigens) donor and be under 50 years old, although patients aged 50–60 years may be considered if they have a good performance status.

Improvements in outcome after unrelated donor HSCT for AA

Up until the late 1990s, the outcome after unrelated donor HSCT for severe AA was dismal, with only 30–40% long-term survival. Subsequently, the EBMT identified a significant improvement in 5-year survival, from 32% for patients transplanted before 1998 to 57% after 1998. Improved outcome may be due to better donor matching with high-resolution DNA typing and better supportive care. Because of improved outcomes, unrelated donor HSCT is now considered earlier, after one failed course of immunosuppressive therapy as compared with the previous practice of deferring unrelated donor HSCT until patients had failed at least two courses of immunosuppressive therapy. Earlier HSCT is likely to be more successful as there would be less chance of allosensitization from multiple transfusions, reduced iron overload and less risk of exposure to infections.

Two approaches have been used to improve outcome after unrelated donor HSCT, involving modification of the condition regimen using (i) irradiation-based conditioning and (ii) non-irradiation, fludarabine-based conditioning. Deeg and colleagues used a de-escalating dose of total body irradiation (TBI), from 6 Gy to 2 Gy, in combination with cyclophosphamide 200 mg/kg and ATG. Graft rejection was low (5%) and 7-year survival was 61% for matched unrelated donor HSCT. The risk of GVHD was high, 69% for grade II–IV acute GVHD and 52% for chronic GVHD. The optimal dose of TBI was 2 Gy: survival in patients under 20 years of age using this regimen was 80%. The Japan Marrow Donor Programme has reported 154 patients exposed to varying doses of TBI/limited field irradiation and cyclophosphamide 120–200 mg/kg, with or without ATG; survival at 5 years was 56% and graft failure 11%.

The European approach has been to use a radiation-free regimen, at least in younger patients. The initial regimen comprises fludarabine 30 mg/m^2 daily for 4 days, cyclophosphamide 300 mg/m^2 daily for 4 days and ATG 15 mg/kg. Survival is 73% at 2 years, and graft rejection 18%. For children (< 14 years) survival is excellent at 84% with only 5% graft rejection, but for older patients survival is 61% and rejection 32%. Acute GVHD occurs in 11% and chronic GVHD in 27%. For older patients, EBMT now recommend the addition of 2-Gy TBI and a reduction in ATG to 7.5 mg in order to reduce the risk of EBV post-transplant lymphoproliferative disorder. With this modification, graft rejection is 12% in older patients.

The exact degree of mismatch that can be tolerated is not clear. The Japanese study identified mismatching for HLA-A or HLA-B as important, but not HLA-DR. The importance of HLA matching was examined further in a French national study. 10/10 allelic matching for HLA-A, -B, -C, -DRB1 and -DQB1 was associated with better survival and less graft rejection and GVHD, but this was not the case for HLA-A, -B, -DRB1 and -DQB1 matched grafts, suggesting that mismatching for HLA-C could be particularly important. The current viewpoint is that (i) better outcomes follow high-resolution matching that approximates a matched sibling donor and (ii) the use of more aggressive conditioning regimens for mismatched UDBMT will likely increase the rate of late complications.

Alternative forms of HSCT

Umbilical cord blood transplantation

Experience in acquired AA is still limited. Recent studies show encouraging results, although graft rejection is the major issue. In a study of nine adult patients from China who received cyclophosphamide 60 mg/kg and ATG with CSA and methotrexate, seven survived, six with stable mixed chimerism and normal or near-normal blood counts, and one with complete donor chimerism. The incidence of GVHD was low. The Japan Cord Blood Network reported 31 patients undergoing single umbilical cord blood transplantation, with a median age of 27.9 years (range 0.8–72.7). Most patients received fludarabine, TBI and melphalan, with or without ATG. Sustained engraftment was seen in only 17 patients. Median time to absolute neutrophil count above 0.5×10^9/L was 19 days (range 12–35) and median time to platelet count above 50×10^9/L was 59 days (range 39–145). Cumulative incidence of greater than grade II acute GVHD was 17%, and 19.7% for chronic GVHD. Survival at 2 years was 41%, but 20% for patients aged over 40 years. Favourable outcome factors were conditioning with fludarabine, cyclophosphamide and TBI, and the absence of ATG. A study of nine children from Texas, using most often fludarabine, cyclophosphamide, TBI and ATG, reported graft rejection in three patients, two of whom received a second umbilical cord blood transplantation using alemtuzumab. Actuarial survival was 78% at 3 years, there were three cases of extensive chronic GVHD, a high incidence of bacterial and viral infections, and three cases of EBV post-transplant lymphoproliferative disorder.

Haploidentical HSCT

There are only anecdotal reports during the last 5 years, mostly in children, using very immunosuppressive conditioning and CD34$^+$-selected stem cells. These data show that some selected patients might benefit from this approach, but there are no large studies at present to evaluate its role further in AA.

Selected bibliography

Bacigalupo A (2007) Aplastic anaemia: pathogenesis and treatment. *Hematology. American Society of Hematology Education Program*, 23–8.

Bacigalupo A, Brand R, Oneto R *et al.* (2000) Treatment of acquired severe aplastic anaemia: bone marrow transplantation compared with immunosuppressive therapy. The European Group for Blood and Marrow Transplantation experience. *Seminars in Hematology* 37: 69–80.

Bacigalupo A, Bruno B, Saracco P *et al.* (2000) Antilymphocyte globulin, cyclosporine, prednisolone, and granulocyte colony-stimulating factor for severe aplastic anemia: an update of the GITMO/EBMT study on 100 patients. *Blood* 95: 1931–4.

Bacigalupo A, Locatelli F, Lanino E *et al.* (2005) Fludarabine, cyclophosphamide and ATG for alternative donor transplants in acquired severe aplastic anaemia: a report of the EBMT SAA Working Party. *Bone Marrow Transplantation* 41: 45–50.

Bacigalupo A, Locatelli F, Lanino E *et al.* (2009) Fludarabine, cyclophosphamide with or without low dose TBI for alternative donor transplants in acquired aplastic anemia (SAA): a report from the EBMT-SAA Working Party. *Biology of Blood and Marrow Transplantation* 15: 5.

Bennett JM, Orazi A (2009) Diagnostic criteria to distinguish hypocellular acute myeloid leukaemia from hypocellular myelodysplastic syndromes and aplastic anaemia: recommendations for a standardized approach. *Haematologica* 94: 264–8.

Buyck HC, Ball S, Junagade P, Marsh J, Chakrabarti S (2009) Prior immunosuppressive therapy with antithymocyte globulin increases the risk of EBV-related lymphoproliferative disorder following allo-SCT for acquired aplastic anaemia. *Bone Marrow Transplantation* 43: 813–16.

Calado RT, Young NS (2008) Telomere maintenance and human bone marrow failure. *Blood* 111: 4446–55.

Calado RT, Graf SA, Wilkerson KL *et al.* (2007) Mutations in the SBDS gene in acquired aplastic anaemia. *Blood* 110: 1141–6.

Camitta BM, Rappeport JM, Parkman R, Nathan DG (1975) Selection of patients for bone marrow transplantation in severe aplastic anaemia. *Blood* 45: 355–63.

Champlin RE, Perez WS, Passweg J *et al.* (2007) Bone marrow transplantation for severe aplastic anaemia: a randomized controlled study of conditioning regimens. *Blood* 109: 4582–5.

Cooper JN, Calado R, Wu C *et al.* (2008) Telomere length of peripheral blood leucocytes predicts relapse and clonal evolution after immunosuppressive therapy in severe aplastic anaemia [Abstract]. *Blood* 112, 442.

Deeg HJ, O'Donnell M, Tolar J *et al.* (2006) Optimization of conditioning for marrow transplantation from unrelated donors for patients with aplastic anaemia after failure of immunosuppressive therapy. *Blood* 108: 1485–91.

Feng X, Kajigaya S, Solomou EE *et al.* (2008) Rabbit ATG but not horse ATG promotes expansion of functional CD4$^+$CD25^{high}FOXP3$^+$ regulatory T cells *in vitro*. *Blood* 111: 3675–83.

Frickhofen N, Heimpel H, Kaltwasser JP *et al.* (2003) Antithymocyte globulin with or without cyclosporin A: 11-year follow-up of a randomized trial comparing treatments of aplastic anaemia. *Blood* 101: 1236–42.

Gupta V, Ball S, Yi Q *et al.* (2004) Favourable effect on acute and chronic graft-versus-host disease with cyclophosphamide and *in vivo* anti-CD52 monoclonal antibodies for marrow transplantation from HLA-identical sibling donors for acquired aplastic anaemia. *Biology of Blood and Marrow Transplantation* 7, 867–76.

Gupta V, Brooker C, Tooze J *et al.* (2006) Clinical relevance of cytogenetic abnormalities at diagnosis of acquired aplastic anaemia in adults. *British Journal of Haematology* 134: 95–9.

Islam MS, Anoop P, Datta-Nemdharry P *et al.* (2009) Implications of CD34$^+$ cell dose on clinical and haematological outcome after allo-HSCT for acquired aplastic anaemia. *Bone Marrow Transplantation*. doi: 10.1038/bmt.2009.267.

Issaragrisil S, Kaufman D, Anderson T and the Aplastic Anaemia Study Group (2006) The epidemiology of aplastic anaemia in Thailand. *Blood* 107: 1299–307.

Kao SY, Xu W, Brandwein JM *et al.* (2008) Outcomes of older patients (≥ 60 years) with acquired aplastic anaemia treated with immunosuppressive therapy. *British Journal of Haematology* 143: 738–43.

Kojima S, Hibi S, Kosaka Y *et al.* (2000) Immunosuppressive therapy using antithymocyte globulin, cyclosporine, and danazol with or without human granulocyte colony-stimulating factor in children with acquired aplastic anemia. *Blood* 96: 2049–54.

Kojima S, Matsuyama T, Kato S *et al.* (2002) Outcome of 154 patients with severe aplastic anaemia who received transplants from unrelated donors: the Japan Marrow Donor Program. *Blood* 100: 799–803.

Kosaka Y, Yagasaki H, Sano K *et al.* (2008) Prospective multicenter trial comparing repeated immunosuppressive therapy with stem-cell transplantation from an alternative donor as second-line treatment for children with severe and very severe aplastic anaemia. *Blood* 111: 1054–9.

Landgren O, Gilbert OS, Rizzo JD *et al.* (2009) Risk factors for lymphoproliferative disorders after allogeneic haematopoietic cell transplantation. *Blood* 113: 4992–5001.

Locasciulli A, Oneto R, Bacigalupo A *et al.* (2007) Outcome of patients with acquired aplastic anaemia given first line bone marrow transplantation or immunosuppression treatment in the last decade: a report from the European Group for Blood and Marrow Transplantation (EBMT). *Haematologica* 91: 11–18.

McCann S, Passweg J, Bacigalupo A *et al.* (2007) The influence of cyclosporin alone, or cyclosporin and methotrexate, on the incidence of mixed haematopoietic chimaerism following allogeneic sibling bone marrow transplantation for severe aplastic anaemia. *Bone Marrow Transplantation* 39: 109–14.

Mao P, Zhu Z, Wang H *et al.* (2005) Sustained and stable haematopoietic donor-recipient mixed chimerism after unrelated cord blood transplantation for adult patients with severe aplastic anaemia. *European Journal of Haematology* **75**: 430–5.

Marsh JCW, Testa NG (2000) Stem cell defect in aplastic anaemia. In: *Aplastic Anaemia. Pathophysiology and Treatment* (H Schrezenmeier, A Bacigalupo, eds), pp. 3–20. Cambridge University Press, Cambridge.

Marsh JC, Ball SE, Darbyshire P *et al.* (2003) Guidelines for the diagnosis and management of acquired aplastic anaemia. *British Journal of Haematology* **123**: 782–801. (The 2008 revised guidelines are available at www.bschguidelines.org.uk)

Marsh JCW, Ganser A, Stadler M (2007) Haematopoietic growth factors in the treatment of acquired bone marrow failure states. *Seminars in Hematology* **44**: 138–47.

Marsh JCW, Ball SE, Cavenagh J *et al.* (2009) Guidelines for the diagnosis and management of aplastic anemia. *British Journal of Haematology* **147**: 43–70.

Maury S, Balère-Appert M-L, Chir Z *et al.* (2007) Unrelated stem cell transplantation for severe acquired aplastic anaemia: improved outcome in the era of high-resolution HLA matching between donor and recipient. *Haematologica* **92**: 589–96.

Montané E, Ibáñez L, Vidal X *et al.* (2008) Epidemiology of aplastic anaemia: a prospective multicenter study. *Haematologica* **93**: 518–23.

Myers KC, Davies SM (2009) Haemopoietic stem cell transplantation for bone marrow failure syndromes in children. *Biology of Blood and Marrow Transplantation* **15**: 279–92.

Risitano A, Maciejewski J, Green S *et al.* (2004) In-vivo dominant immune responses in aplastic anaemia: molecular tracking of putatively pathogenetic T-cell clones by TCR b-CDR3 sequencing. *Lancet* **364**: 355–64.

Rosenfeld S, Follmann D, Nunez O, Young NS (2003) Antithymocyte globulin and cyclosporine for severe aplastic anaemia: association between hematologic response and long-term outcome. *Journal of the American Medical Association* **289**: 1130–5.

Saracco P, Quarello P, Iori AP *et al.* (2008) Cyclosporin A response and dependence in children with acquired aplastic anaemia: a multicentre retrospective study with long-term observation follow-up. *British Journal of Haematology* **140**: 197–205.

Scheinberg P, Nunez O, Wu C, Young NS (2006) Treatment of severe aplastic anaemia with combined immunosuppression: anti-thymocyte globulin, ciclosporin and mycophenolate mofetil. *British Journal of Haematology* **133**: 606–11.

Scheinberg P, Wu CO, Nunez O, Young NS (2008) Long-term outcome of pediatric patients with severe aplastic anemia treated with antithymocyte globulin and cyclosporine. *Journal of Pediatrics* **153**: 814–19.

Scheinberg P, Wu CO, Nunez O, Young NS (2009) Predicting response to immunosuppressive therapy and survival in severe aplastic anaemia. *British Journal of Haematology* **144**: 206–16.

Scheinberg P, Wu CO, Nunez O *et al.* (2009) Treatment of severe aplastic anaemia with a combination of horse antithymocyte globulin and cyclosporine, with or without sirolimus: a prospective randomized study. *Haematologica* **94**: 348–54.

Schrezenmeier H, Passweg JR, Marsh JCW *et al.* (2007) Worse outcome and more chronic GVHD with peripheral blood progenitor cells than bone marrow in HLA-matched sibling donor transplants for young patients with severe acquired aplastic anaemia. *Blood* **110**: 1397–400.

Siegal D, Xu W, Sutherland R *et al.* (2008) Graft-versus-host disease following marrow transplantation for aplastic anemia: different impact of two GVHD prevention strategies. *Bone Marrow Transplantation* **42**: 51–6.

Sloand EM, Yong ASM, Ramkissoon S *et al.* (2006) Granulocyte colony-stimulating factor preferentially stimulates proliferation of monosomy 7 cells bearing the isoform IV receptor. *Proceedings of the National Academy of Sciences USA* **103**: 14483–8.

Socie G, Henry-Amar M, Bacigalupo A *et al.* (1993) Malignant tumours occurring after treatment of aplastic anaemia. *New England Journal of Medicine* **329**: 1152–7.

Socie G, Rosenfeld S, Frickhofen N *et al.* (2000) Late clonal diseases of treated aplastic anaemia. *Seminars in Hematology* **37**: 91–100.

Socie G, Mary J-Y, Schrezenmeier H *et al.* (2007) Granulocyte colony stimulating factor for severe aplastic anaemia: a survey by the European Group for Blood and Marrow Transplantation. *Blood* **109**: 2794–6.

Solomou EE, Rezvani K, Mielke S *et al.* (2007) Deficient CD4$^+$ CD25$^+$ FOXP3$^+$ T regulatory cells in acquired aplastic anaemia. *Blood* **110**: 1603–6.

Sugimori C, Chuhjo T, Feng X *et al.* (2005) Minor populations of CD55$^-$CD59$^-$ blood cells predict response to immunosuppressive therapy and prognosis in patients with aplastic anaemia. *Blood* **107**: 1308–14.

Teramura M, Kimura A, Iwasse S *et al.* (2007) Treatment of severe aplastic anaemia with antithymocyte globulin and cyclosporine A with or without G-CSF in adults: a multicentre randomized study in Japan. *Blood* **110**: 1756–61.

Tisdale JF, Dunn DE, Geller N *et al.* (2000) High dose cyclophosphamide in severe aplastic anaemia: a randomized trial. *Lancet* **356**: 1554–7.

Viollier R, Socie G, Tichelli A *et al.* (2007) Recent improvement in outcome of unrelated donor transplantation for aplastic anemia. *Bone Marrow Transplantation* **41**: 45–50.

Walne AJ, Dokal I (2009) Advances in the understanding of dyskeratosis congenita. *British Journal of Haematology* **145**: 164–72.

Yamaguchi H, Calado R, Ly H *et al.* (2005) Mutations in TERT, the gene for telomerase reverse transcriptase, in aplastic anaemia. *New England Journal of Medicine* **352**: 1413–24.

Yoshimi A, Kojima S, Taniguchi S *et al.* (2008) Unrelated cord blood transplantation for severe aplastic anemia. *Biology of Blood and Marrow Transplantation* **14**: 1057–63.

Young NS, Calado RT, Scheinberg P (2006) Current concepts in the pathophysiology and treatment of aplastic anaemia. *Blood* **108**: 2509–19.

Red cell immunohaematology: introduction

14

Marcela Contreras[1] and Geoff Daniels[2]

[1]University College London and Blood Transfusion International, London, UK
[2]Bristol Institute for Transfusion Sciences, Bristol, UK

Introduction

The primary purpose of transfusion medicine is to provide 'safe' blood when the clinician requires it. However, blood groups and immunohaematological problems of blood transfusion and transplantation are extremely interesting in their own right and their solutions have much to offer to haematology in general.

Blood group serology or immunohaematology includes the study of antigenic molecules present on the various cellular and soluble components of whole blood, together with study of the antibodies and lectins that recognize them and their interactions. However, in practice the term 'blood group serology' is generally restricted to red cell surface antigens and their interactions with specific antibodies. In this narrower sense, the complexities of human leucocyte antigen (HLA), granulocyte, platelet and plasma protein determinants do not normally fall within the blood group serologist's realm, even though all are likewise genetically polymorphic and play a role in blood transfusion.

The narrower definition of blood group serology encompasses (i) determination of the phenotype of red cells using antibodies and reagents of known specificity; (ii) the search for and identification of antibodies using red cells of known phenotype; and (iii) compatibility testing of patients' sera against cell samples from donor units. At present, more than 2 million units of red cells are transfused to patients each year in the UK alone.

The aim of this chapter is to provide an introduction to blood group serology and to include aspects of immunology, biochemistry and molecular genetics that contribute to our understanding of blood group antigens, antibodies and antigen–antibody reactions.

The red cell membrane and chemistry of blood group antigens

The red cell membrane is composed of about 40% (w/w) lipids and up to 10% carbohydrates, the remainder being proteins. The exact arrangement of its components is still unresolved, but a rough model is shown in Figure 14.1.

The lipids of the red cell membrane can be subdivided into 60% (w/w) phospholipids, 30% (w/w) neutral lipids (mainly cholesterol) and 10% (w/w) glycolipids. The phospholipids and glycolipids play a role in the structure of the membrane and are important in the maintenance of red cell shape. These lipids have a molecular arrangement reminiscent of a tuning fork,

Postgraduate Haematology: 6th edition. Edited by A. Victor Hoffbrand, Daniel Catovsky, Edward G.D. Tuddenham, Anthony R. Green
© 2011 Blackwell Publishing Ltd.

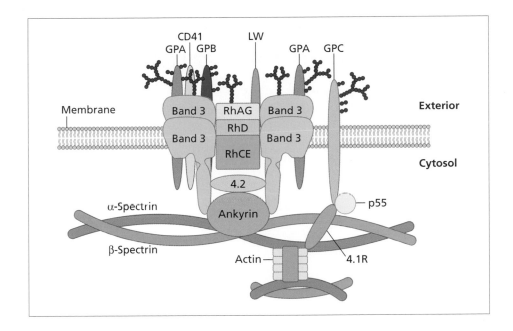

Figure 14.1 Diagrammatic representation of some integral red cell membrane proteins, including the band 3/Rh macrocomplex and components of the membrane cytoskeleton.

with the hydrophobic fatty acids forming the 'prongs' and the polar group the 'handle'. They are arranged in a bilayer with the 'prongs' pointing inwards and the hydrophilic 'handle' pointing out towards the plasma or towards the cytoplasmic surface of the membrane. Cholesterol is inserted between the other lipids. This arrangement allows the interior of the membrane to be in a semi-fluid state and the whole membrane to be very flexible. The lipid bilayer does not allow the passive transfer of ions. The carbohydrates are attached to the lipids and proteins, and occur only on the external surface of the membrane. They are composed of chains of monosaccharides, the majority of which are hexoses.

About 60–80% of the proteins of the membrane are released only after drastic treatment with detergents. These are the integral proteins that penetrate the lipid bilayer and, in some cases, are bound to the membrane skeleton or cytoskeleton. Cell surface proteins are not necessarily discrete units within the cell membrane. They may congregate together in lipid rafts or might be part of complexes of proteins in which the components contribute to the function of the whole. There are four types of integral proteins in the red cell membrane (Figure 14.1). Type 1 glycoproteins, typified by the glycophorins, cross the membrane once, with the amino-terminal domain on the outside and the carboxy-terminal domain in the cytosol. The Kell glycoprotein is a type 2 structure. It also crosses the membrane once, but has the carboxy-terminal domain on the outside and the amino-terminal domain in the cytosol. Type 3 glycoproteins are polytopic: they cross the membrane several times giving rise to a series of extracellular loops, one of which is usually glycosylated. These N-glycans express ABO, H and Ii blood group activity. In most of these type 3 proteins both terminal domains are cytosolic (e.g. Rh proteins, band 3, Kidd

glycoprotein), but the Duffy glycoprotein has an extracellular amino-terminal domain. Type 5 membrane glycoproteins, which include the Dombrock and Cromer glycoproteins, reside in membrane microdomains rich in cholesterol known as lipid rafts and are attached to the lipid bilayer by a glycolipid, the glycosylphosphatidylinositol (GPI) anchor.

On the inside of the lipid bilayer is a network of glycoproteins that comprise the membrane skeleton, often called the cytoskeleton, which is responsible for maintenance of the shape and integrity of the red cell as it squeezes through the tiniest capillaries. The main components of the membrane skeleton are the α and β subunits of spectrin, which form long flexible rods, plus actin, ankyrin, proteins 4.1R and 4.2, and several other glycoproteins. Band 3, the anion exchanger and Diego blood group antigen, has an extended N-terminal domain attached to the membrane skeleton through ankyrin and proteins 4.2 and 4.1R. Glycophorin (GP)C and GPD, the Gerbich glycoproteins, have C-terminal domains attached to the membrane skeleton through protein 4.1R and p55. In addition there is evidence that several other integral membrane proteins interact with components of the membrane skeleton. Absence or reduced levels of these integral membrane proteins that interact with the membrane skeleton often result in some degree of abnormal red cell morphology.

Blood group antigens have been found in the polypeptide and carbohydrate moieties of membrane glycoproteins and in the carbohydrate moieties of glycolipids (Table 14.1). Most blood groups represent amino acid sequence changes in glycoproteins, although the Rh antigens are non-glycosylated proteins containing two or three molecules of palmitic acid. ABH and Ii antigens are found predominantly on the carbohydrate moieties of the major red cell glycoproteins band 3 (anion

Table 14.1 Blood group active proteins.

Protein	Blood group	Molecular mass (kDa)*	Copies per cell (×10³)	Function
Band 3 (CD233)[†]	Diego, ABH[‡], I	100	1000	Anion transport; cytoskeletal attachment
UT-B1	Kidd, ABH[‡]	46–60	14	Urea transport
Aquaporin 1	Colton, ABH[‡]	40–60	200	Water channel
Aquaporin 3	GIL	45		Glycerol and water channel
GLUT-1	ABH[‡]	55	500	Glucose transport
RhD and RhCcEe proteins (CD240D and CE)[†]	Rh	30–34	100–200	Unknown
RhAG (CD241)[†]	RHAG, ABH[‡]	35–100	100–200	Involved in NH_3^+ or CO_2 transport?
Xk	Kx	37		Neurotransmitter transport?
Duffy glycoprotein (CD234)	Duffy	40–50	6–12	Chemokine receptor
Lutheran glycoprotein (CD239)	Lutheran	78 and 85	2–4	Adhesion (to laminin)
ICAM-4 (CD242)[†]	LW	37–47	3–5	Adhesion
CD44	Indian	80	6–10	Adhesion (to hyaluronan)
Xg and CD99 glycoproteins	Xg	23–28 and 32	1–10	Adhesion?
ERMAP	Scianna	60–68		Adhesion?
EMMPRIN (CD147)	Ok	35–68		Signal transduction?
CD108	JMH	76	1–3	Adhesion?
Kell glycoprotein (CD238)	Kell	93	4–8	Endopeptidase
Acetylcholinesterase	Yt	72	7–10	Acetylcholinesterase
Dombrock glycoprotein	Dombrock	47–57		ADP-ribosyltransferase
DAF (CD55)	Cromer	70	6–14	Complement regulation
CR1 (CD35)	Knops	190	0.2–1	Complement regulation
Glycophorin A (CD235A)[†]	MN	43	1000	Sialic acid carrier
Glycophorin B (CD235B)[†]	Ss	25	250	Sialic acid carrier
Glycophorins C and D (CD236)	Gerbich	40 and 30	143 and 82	Sialic acid carrier; cytoskeletal attachment

*Apparent molecular weight determined by electrophoresis.
[†]Part of the band 3/Rh protein macrocomplex.
[‡]Carbohydrate antigens.

exchanger) and on the glucose transporter, although they are also present on some other minor glycoproteins and on the carbohydrate portions of membrane glycolipids. P, P1 and P^K antigens are expressed on the carbohydrate of glycolipids. The M and N antigens arise from interactions between the carbohydrate and polypeptide in the glycoprotein GPA. In addition to the antigens on integral membrane components, the Lewis and Chido/Rogers antigens are not of erythroid origin and are adsorbed from the plasma. Structural details of selected antigens are given in Chapter 15.

Antigens

Originally, an antigen was defined as the part of a molecule that is bound by a specific antibody. More recently, it has become customary to define an antigen as a substance that can stimulate an immune response (immunogenicity). Immune responses can be either positive or negative. Positive responses lead to the production of antibodies (humoral immunity) and/or proliferation of immunocompetent cells (cellular immunity) that can bind and eliminate their stimulatory antigen. In negative responses, the cells that mediate humoral and cellular immune responses are rendered non-responsive. This state is described as acquired immunological tolerance and is important in preventing autoimmune disease, as well as in establishing the 'take' or acceptance of transplanted syngeneic and allogeneic tissues.

The hallmark of the adaptive immune response is its specificity: specific immunocompetent cells and/or antibodies are produced, which can distinguish molecules that differ only by two or three atoms (e.g. trinitrophenol versus dinitrophenol).

As described later, even the difference between the A and B antigens is minimal. However, antibodies can often react with antigens similar, but not identical, to the stimulatory antigen (cross-reactivity). As far as is known, specific immune responses to human red cells are mediated by antibodies only; *specific cell-mediated immunity to red cell alloantigens or autoantigens has not been described.*

The parts of an antigen that bind antibodies or cellular receptors are called epitopes, and those parts of the antibodies that bind to them are called paratopes. Most antigens that occur naturally are of high molecular weight, and each antigenic molecule may have several different or several identical epitopes. As antibodies are specific for the individual epitopes and not for the antigen as a whole, antisera will usually be a collection of antibodies specific for different regions of the antigen in question, arising from different clones of immunocompetent cells (polyclonal antibodies); such antibodies can sometimes be distinguished serologically by anti-idiotype reagents (see below).

The biological significance of blood group antigens

The functions of many red cell membrane protein structures bearing blood group antigenic determinants are known, or can be deduced from their structure (Table 14.1). Some are membrane transporters, facilitating the transport of biologically important molecules through the lipid bilayer: band 3 membrane glycoprotein, the Diego antigen, provides an anion exchange channel for HCO_3^- and Cl^- ions; the Kidd glycoprotein is a urea transporter; the Colton glycoprotein is aquaporin 1, a water channel; and the GIL antigen is aquaporin 3, a glycerol transporter. The Rh proteins and the Rh-associated glycoprotein (RhAG) together with band 3 and other proteins form a protein macrocomplex. RhAG probably functions as a channel for rapid CO_2 transfer in and out of the cell. CO_2 in the red cell is converted to bicarbonate ions by carbonic anhydrase II and then transported rapidly out of the cell to the plasma by band 3, where it is carried rapidly to the lungs.

The Lutheran, LW and Indian (CD44) glycoproteins are adhesion molecules, possibly serving their functions during erythropoiesis. The Duffy glycoprotein is a chemokine receptor and might function as a 'sink' or scavenger for unwanted chemokines. The Cromer and Knops antigens are markers for decay accelerating factor and complement receptor 1, respectively, which protect the cells from destruction by autologous complement. Some blood group glycoproteins have enzyme activity: the Yt antigen is acetylcholinesterase and the Kell antigen is an endopeptidase with the ability to cleave a biologically inactive peptide to produce the vasoconstrictor endothelin-3. The C-terminal domains of the Gerbich antigens, GPC and GPD, and the N-terminal domain of the Diego glycoprotein, band 3, are attached to components of the cytoskeleton and function to anchor the membrane to it skeleton. The carbohydrate moieties of the membrane glycoproteins and glycolipids, especially those of the most abundant glycoproteins, band 3 and GPA, constitute the glycocalyx, an extracellular coat that protects the cell from mechanical damage and microbial attack.

The difference between red cell antigens that represent the products of alleles (e.g. A and B, K and k, Fy^a and Fy^b) is small, often being just one monosaccharide or one amino acid. The biological importance of these differences is unknown and there is little evidence to suggest that one antigen confers any significant advantage over another. Most blood group systems have a null phenotype in which the whole blood group protein is absent from the red cells or any other cells. These usually result from homozygosity for gene deletions or inactivating mutations within the genes. In most cases, individuals with these null phenotypes are apparently healthy, suggesting that whatever the precise function of the missing structure may be, some other structure must be able to substitute in its absence. However, there are exceptions; 15% of whites lack the D protein of the Rh system with no ill effect, but those rare Rh_{null} individuals who lack D and CcEe Rh proteins, as well as RhAG, have chronic haemolysis, which may be compensated by increased red cell production, but may require splenectomy for stabilization. Absence of the Xk protein causes weakness of expression of all Kell system antigens, as a result of linkage between the two proteins in the membrane, but is also associated with acanthocytosis and neurological and muscular disorders. Very rare patients lacking the RAPH glycoprotein, CD151, have disruption of basement membranes causing hereditary nephritis, epidermolysis bullosa and neurosensory deafness. A patient lacking the Diego antigen, the anion transporter, only survived with extreme medical intervention, and no person with the Yt_{null} phenotype and thus absence of neurotransmitter acetylcholinesterase has been found. On the other hand, people with the rare Bombay phenotype lack ABH antigens from all cells and tissues, with no apparent ill effect or red cell abnormality.

Some blood group antigens are exploited by pathological microorganisms as receptors for attaching and entering cells. Consequently, in some cases absence of antigens can be beneficial. The Duffy glycoprotein, expressing Fy^a or Fy^b, is used by *Plasmodium vivax* to penetrate red cells. The Fy(a−b−) phenotype is common in Africans and confers resistance to *P. vivax* malaria. Fy(a−b−) in Africans results from homozygosity for a mutation in an erythroid-specific transcription factor binding site, leading to absence of the Duffy glycoprotein from red cells but expression in other tissues. *Plasmodium falciparum* malaria appears to have played a part in the establishment of the ABO polymorphism. The geographic distribution of group O is consistent with selection pressure by *P. falciparum* in favour of group O individuals in malaria endemic regions and there is evidence that blood group O protects against severe *P. falciparum* malaria through reduced rosetting.

Table 14.2 Effector functions of the immunoglobulin isotypes.*

	IgG1	IgG2	IgG3	IgG4	IgA1	IgA2	Secretory IgA	IgM	IgE
Complement fixation: classical pathway[†]	+	(+)	++	–	–	–	–	++++	–
Complement fixation: alternative pathway	–	–	–	–	+[‡]	++	–	–	–[‡]
Placental transfer/lymphocyte binding	++	+	+	+	–	–	–	–	–
Monocyte/macrophage Fc receptor binding	++	–	+++	–	–	–	–	–	?[§]
Mast cell binding	–	–	–	(?)	–	–	–	–	+++
Binding to *Staphylococcus aureus* protein A	+	+	–	+	–	–	–	–	–

*No biological function has been ascribed to IgD, but it might be intimately involved in maturation of B cells into competent effector cells and/or memory cells.

[†]IgG molecules fix complement only up to C3.

[‡]Aggregated molecules can activate the alternative pathway.

[§]Human IgE has been reported to bind to macrophages.

Antibodies

Antibodies are immunoglobulins produced by the B lymphocytes of the adaptive immune system in response to an antigen for which they exhibit specific binding. Depending on the origin of the antigenic stimulus, antibodies can be termed (i) alloantibodies, when produced by an individual against epitopes present in another individual of the same species; (ii) autoantibodies, when reactive with determinants present on the individual's own antigens; and (iii) xenoantibodies (or heteroantibodies), when produced against antigenic determinants present on the cells of another species. The first two are the antibodies encountered routinely in the blood bank; xenoantibodies can be used as antiglobulin sera or typing reagents when raised in animals against human antigens and are often present in reagents as monoclonal antibodies.

There are five classes of immunoglobulins: IgM, IgG, IgA, IgD and IgE. Antibodies with specificity for blood group antigens are found only in the IgG, IgM and, rarely, IgA classes. IgA antibodies play a minor role in blood group serology as they only appear as alloantibodies together with IgM and/or IgG. Some of the biochemical and biophysical differences between IgG, IgM and IgA are listed in Table 14.2.

Biochemistry and genetics of immunoglobulins

Figure 14.2 shows a diagram of the basic immunoglobulin molecule. This consists of four polypeptide chains arranged as two light (L) chains and two identical heavy (H) chains. The light and heavy chains are held together by disulphide (S–S) bonds. IgG and serum IgA molecules are mainly monomers of this basic immunoglobulin structure; secretory IgA is mainly dimeric. IgM molecules are pentamers, with the basic immu-

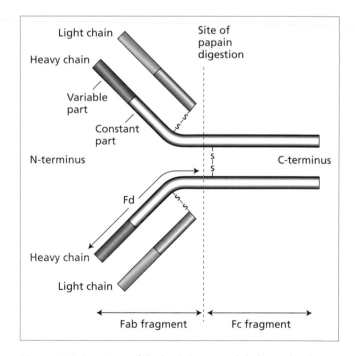

Figure 14.2 Structure of the basic immunoglobulin molecule.

noglobulin molecules held together by S–S bonds and a joining (J) chain (Figure 14.3).

There are two distinct types of light chain, kappa (κ) and lambda (λ). These are common to all immunoglobulins. Either of these chains may combine with any heavy chain, but in any one immunoglobulin molecule both light chains are of the same type and are identical; κ chains occur in about 65% and λ chains in about 35% of the normal immunoglobulins in each class. Each class has an immunologically distinct heavy chain: γ for IgG, μ for IgM, α for IgA, δ for IgD and ε for IgE (Figure 14.3).

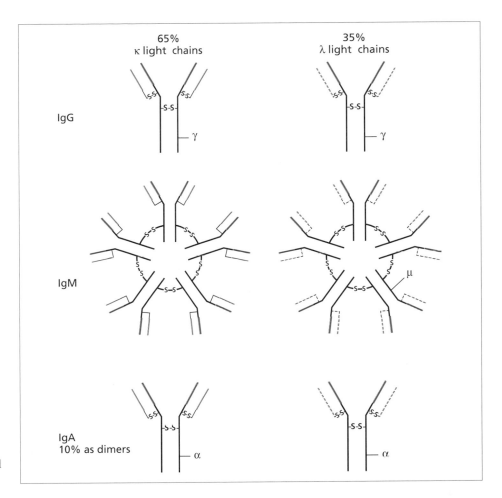

Figure 14.3 Structure of IgG, IgM and IgA molecules.

There are four subclasses of human IgG (IgG1, IgG2, IgG3 and IgG4, with γ1, γ2, γ3 and γ4 heavy chains), and two IgA subclasses (IgA1 and IgA2, with α1 and α2 heavy chains).

Analyses of various light chains from different sources show that the amino acid sequence differs in half of the chain (variable region), whereas in the other half the sequence remains remarkably constant (constant region) between light chains of the appropriate κ or λ groups. Similarly, in the corresponding heavy chain, there is a variable region and a constant region when different chains are analysed.

Papain can split the basic immunoglobulin molecule into three fragments at a site near the S–S bonds that hold the heavy chains together (Figure 14.2). One fragment contains the C-termini of the heavy chains and is called the Fc fragment. The other two are called Fab fragments, each of which consists of the N-terminus of the heavy chain (Fd portion) and the whole of the light chain, and contains the antigen-binding site of the molecule.

Repetition of amino acid sequences within the heavy chain constant regions indicates that there are either three (for IgG and IgA) or four (for IgM, IgD and IgE) constant region domains for H chains. These are designated C_H1, C_H2, C_H3 and C_H4. In contrast, there is only one constant region domain for light chains and only one variable region domain for heavy and light chains. The segment between C_H1 and C_H2 is called the *hinge region*. This area imparts flexibility to the immunoglobulin molecule so that antigen-binding sites can span varying distances.

The vast majority of the differences between antibodies of various specificities occurs in three or four short amino acid sequences in the L- and H-chain variable regions. These hypervariable sequences contact the antigen on binding and provide the basis of antibody specificity. The remaining sequences within the variable region are known as the framework determinants. These are believed to provide the general skeleton of the antigen-recognizing region, within which variations in and between hypervariable sequences generate specificity for the different epitopes bound by different antibodies.

Amino acid sequences within framework and hypervariable segments can sometimes be recognized by specific antisera, usually from another species, raised by deliberate immunization with a particular antibody. The sequences recognized are referred to as idiotopes, and the sera that define them are called anti-idiotypes. The idiotype of the particular immunoglobulin molecule represents the sum of all the idiotopes of all its framework and hypervariable sequences.

The binding of anti-idiotype sera that recognize idiotopes within hypervariable sequences of the immunizing immunoglobulin can be inhibited by the specific hapten recognized by that immunizing antibody. This is because contact between the hapten and the hypervariable sequences blocks access of the idiotype-specific antibody. In contrast, binding of anti-idiotypes to framework determinants of the immunizing antibody is usually not blocked by binding of the hapten recognized by that antibody.

The great diversity in the repertoire of antibodies generated by the immune system in response to the immense variety of antigens that it encounters is a direct reflection of the immune system's ability to generate variations within the three hypervariable sequences. This ability is partly genetic in origin and arises from the random selection and joining of several separate genetic elements that produce a single intact variable region gene coding for the final variable region amino acid sequence.

The variable region genes comprise (i) genes coding for a large number of V-region sequences, with approximately 150 κ-chain, 125 λ-chain and 500 or so H-chain variable region genes; each of these genes is arranged in three exons, the random joining of which provides the variations that generate the first and second hypervariable sequences; (ii) in H chains only, approximately 10–20 D (diversity) genes; and (iii) in both H and L chains, five or six J (joining) genes.

The random joining of numerous choices, in a variety of combinations of V–J genes in L chains and V–D–J genes in H chains, during ontogeny of the immune response, generates the third hypervariable sequence and provides an additional somatic contribution for increasing the repertoire of the immune system. Following V–J/V–D–J joining, which is achieved by splicing together of certain DNA sequences and deletion of others during B-cell maturation, a further increase in antibody diversity is achieved by mutation in the spliced V gene DNA of mature B cells, during their proliferation in an ongoing immune response.

Biological and physical properties of immunoglobulins

Immunoglobulins are essentially multifunctional; not only do they bind antigen, but they also perform various other functions depending on the class. Most of these additional functions reside in the Fc fragment and are listed in Table 14.2. The most important include the following.
1 Complement fixation (IgM > IgG3 > IgG1 > IgG2); IgA does not bind complement in the classical pathway.
2 Binding to Fc receptors of mononuclear phagocytic cells, particularly monocytes and macrophages (IgG3 >> IgG1). After IgG-coated cells bind to Fc receptors on mononuclear phago-

cytic cells, they are destroyed by phagocytosis or cytotoxicity (see Chapter 16).
3 Transplacental passage: there is preferential active transport of IgG1 relative to the other IgG subclasses.

Some functions can be ascribed to particular domains, for example C_H2 or C_H2/C_H3 for complement (C1q) binding and control of catabolic rate; the hinge region for binding to the Fc receptors of macrophages and monocytes; C_H2 and C_H3 for binding to staphylococcal protein A (IgG3 does not bind) and to the Fc receptors on placental syncytial trophoblasts and lymphocytes.

For blood group-specific antibodies, these class-dependent biological functions contribute to their clinical significance. In the majority of cases, antigen–antibody binding does not cause red cell destruction per se; immune-mediated red cell destruction is usually a consequence of these secondary effector functions.

As only IgG passes the placental barrier, only IgG blood group antibodies can cause haemolytic disease of the fetus and newborn (HDFN) and only IgG1 and IgG3 will mediate significant immune red cell destruction. The IgG level in cord blood will be much the same as the level in the mother. Passively transferred maternal IgG gradually disappears from the infant after birth and is almost gone by 3 months of age. The serum of newborn infants contains a small amount of IgM of fetal origin and almost no IgA; the production of IgA and IgG starts at about 1–2 months of age.

There are many ways of separating IgG and IgM molecules by physical methods (e.g. gel filtration and affinity chromatography). In routine serology, IgG is easily distinguishable from IgM by treating sera with mild reducing agents such as 2-mercaptoethanol or dithiothreitol at low concentrations. These agents split the S–S bonds of the J chains, which link the IgM subunits, thereby rendering them non-agglutinating; IgA is either slightly affected or not affected by such reducing agents.

Blood group antibodies

Several terms have been used in the past and are still sometimes used to describe different types of blood group antibodies, including 'naturally occurring' and 'immune' antibodies, 'cold' and 'warm' antibodies, and 'complete' (or 'saline') and 'incomplete' antibodies. They are described below and an attempt is made to correlate these terms with the class of immunoglobulin involved.

Naturally occurring and immune antibodies

Antibodies are naturally occurring when they are produced without any obvious immunizing stimulus, such as during pregnancy, transfusion or injection of blood. These antibodies are not present at birth and, in the case of anti-A and anti-B, start to appear in the serum at about 3–6 months of age. ABO antibodies are probably produced in response to antigens of bacteria, viruses and other substances that are inhaled or ingested; many Gram-negative organisms have antigens that are structurally similar to the A and B antigens. Despite this probable antigenic stimulus, the term 'naturally occurring' is retained for these 'non-red cell-induced' antibodies. 'Immune' blood group antibodies are only produced after pregnancy or following transfusion or injection of blood or blood group substances.

Cold and warm antibodies

Cold antibodies give higher agglutination titres at low temperatures (0–4°C) and many of them will not agglutinate red cells at 37°C. Most naturally occurring antibodies are cold reacting. Some, such as naturally occurring anti-A,B, have a wide thermal range and will still react at 37°C, at which temperature they will activate complement and lyse red cells, but the titre will be much higher at 0–4°C. Cold antibodies that fail to react above 30°C are of no clinical significance and can be ignored for blood transfusion purposes.

The thermal optimum of warm antibodies is 37°C and this implies that higher titres are obtained at this temperature. Immune antibodies are warm reacting. Any red cell antibody reacting above 30°C should be considered potentially capable of destroying red cells *in vivo*.

IgM and IgG antibodies

IgM or 'complete' antibodies agglutinate red cells when they are suspended in saline. They are often called saline or directly agglutinating antibodies in laboratory parlance. Conversely, 'incomplete' IgG antibodies will not agglutinate saline-suspended red cells. However, lack of agglutination does not mean that the antibodies have not bound to their antigen, and it can be shown that they have reacted by using antiglobulin reagents, which facilitate agglutination of antibody-coated cells (see below). Most naturally occurring antibodies are cold reacting, complete and IgM. Immune antibodies are always warm reacting; most are partly IgG, but some may be IgM. Exceptionally, and when very potent, IgG complete antibodies are found.

Monoclonal antibodies

Animal sera have generally been a poor source of blood grouping reagents. Deliberate immunization of laboratory animals to produce blood group-specific xenoantibodies has had limited success as only a few polyclonal specificities have been made in rabbits, goats and chickens. The most useful reagents have been anti-A, -B, -M, -N, -P₁, -Leᵃ, -Leᵇ and -LW.

The advent of monoclonal antibody technologies has increased the repertoire of blood grouping reagents. By fusing the spleen cells of immunized mice or rats with drug-sensitive myeloma cells and selecting for drug-resistant hybrids, it has been possible to establish permanently growing cloned cell lines in tissue culture that secrete antibodies of desired specificities. Several murine hybrids secreting human blood group-specific monoclonal antibodies have now been established, many of which were raised using immunogens other than intact red cells (e.g. anti-A, -B, -Leᵃ, -Leᵇ, -M and -N). Unfortunately, rodents have proved remarkably resistant to efforts to produce antibodies to the human D antigen.

Attempts to produce human monoclonal antibodies by the cell fusion approach have been of limited success owing to the lack of suitable human myelomas. Nevertheless, human monoclonal antibodies specific for D, other Rh antigens, Jkᵃ and Jkᵇ, and several other antigens, have been obtained by alternative approaches involving transformation of isolated peripheral blood lymphocytes from immunized individuals with Epstein–Barr virus or by fusion of human lymphocytes with mouse myelomas to form heteromyelomas. Monoclonal antibodies of murine and human origin have widely replaced polyclonal blood grouping reagents in everyday ABO and D grouping.

The future of antibody reagent production may lie in recombinant DNA technology, but a useful blood grouping reagent is still to be produced by these methods.

Lectins

Lectins are sugar-binding proteins, mostly extracted from plants and lower vertebrate animals. They are useful tools for routine and experimental blood group serology. They combine with simple sugars (e.g. fucose, galactose, N-acetylgalactosamine) present on the glycolipids and glycoproteins of cell membranes and body fluids. Most lectins agglutinate red cells irrespective of target cell phenotype; hence only a handful are used with any regularity in blood group serology. The three most commonly used blood group-specific lectins are extracts from *Dolichos biflorus*, *Vicia graminea* and *Ulex europaeus*, which have anti-A₁, anti-N and anti-H specificities, respectively. Several other lectins have proven valuable in investigating red cell polyagglutinability (see Chapter 15). In addition to blood grouping, lectins are also used for determining ABH secretor status and for partially purifying and identifying blood group-active membrane glycoproteins.

Complement

Complement consists of a series of proteins, mainly enzymes present in fresh plasma as inactive precursors, which react sequentially with each other to form products that are important in the immune destruction of cells, including bacteria. In complement activation there are two stages of relevance. The first stage is the generation of the active form of the third component, C3b, which leads to the coating, or opsonization, of the cell with a large amount of protein. There are two pathways by which active C3b may be generated: the classical and alternative pathways (Figure 14.4). The second stage is the lytic stage: activation of the proteins of the membrane attack complex, comprising components C5 through C9, leads to the destruction of red cells in the circulation.

In general terms, the complement cascade is analogous to the clotting sequence. Activation of one component or group of components leads to the generation of enzyme activity for activation of the next components. To lead to haemolysis, however, the activated components in the plasma must bind to the red cell membrane (except C1, which binds only to a specific binding site on the antibody), which they do with varying degrees of efficiency. Moreover, some activated components, for example C1, C4 and C3, have specific inactivators in the plasma as well as (for C3b and C4b) in the red cell membrane itself; even though these components bind to the red cell membrane, their active life may be very short (half-life 2–25 min). As a consequence, and as happens with several IgG blood group antibodies such as anti-Jk^a and -Fy^a, the whole sequence is not completed and there is no intravascular haemolysis. In these cases, early components can be detected on the red cell surface with suitable antiglobulin reagents.

Complement components in the classical pathway are designated C1 to C9 in their native form. Apart from C4, which is activated before C2 and C3, the components are activated sequentially according to their numerical order. Complement components in the alternative pathway include factor B, factor D and properdin. During activation of the 'classical' components, small-molecular-weight fragments (C4a, C3a, C5a) are released, which have important chemotactic and anaphylactic activity. Release of C3a and C5a, as well as vasoactive amines and cytokines, leads to most of the signs and symptoms observed in severe haemolytic transfusion reactions and also in febrile non-haemolytic transfusion reactions caused by white cell antibodies.

The opsonization phase of the complement sequence (Figure 14.4)

The classical pathway

The classical pathway can be activated by many factors, including antigen–antibody complexes, enzymes (trypsin, plasmin, lysosomal enzymes), endotoxins and low-ionic-strength media. Only one molecule of IgM on a cell membrane is necessary to activate the complement system, although at least two of the five IgM subunits must attach to the cell membrane, in close proximity, for activation to occur. At least two IgG molecules must combine with antigen sites very close together on the cell membrane to bring about complement activation.

The first component of complement is a complex of three protein molecules, C1q, C1r and C1s. After complement-fixing antibodies have bound to their red cell antigens (EA is often used to denote the resulting erythrocyte–antibody complex), C1 binding sites are exposed on the Fc fragments. If two such sites

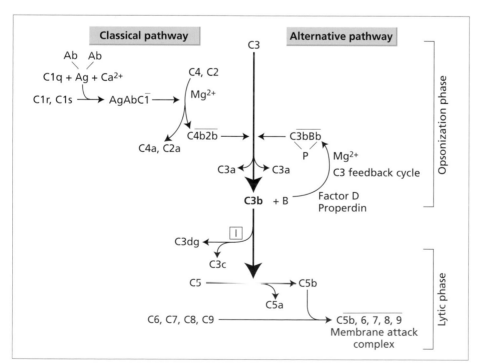

Figure 14.4 The complement cascade. Component C3b plays a central role in the classical and alternative pathways.

are sufficiently close together (approximately 25–40 nm), the C1 complex is fixed through its C1q subunits. C1q is a complex molecule with six immunoglobulin-binding sites. Binding of C1q activates C1r, which in turn cleaves the third molecule, C1s, yielding the active enzyme form of the C1 complex, which is held together by calcium. In the presence of EDTA or other chelating agents, the complex falls apart and the whole process of complement fixation will not occur.

C1s can now activate sequentially C4 and C2 in the presence of magnesium, generating a second enzyme, C4b2b, called C3 convertase.

The cell-bound C4b2b can optimally activate several thousand C3 molecules by splitting them into C3a and C3b. As C3 is present in large amounts (100–150 mg/dL) in the serum, the fixation of C3b can considerably increase the globulin coating of the red cells. While C3b is still intact, opsonized red cells will adhere to monocytes and macrophages through their C3b receptors and may then be phagocytosed. C3b has a short half-life and there is no free C3b in plasma. Hence, C3b coating of IgG-sensitized cells neutralizes the inhibitory effect of free plasma IgG on immune adherence to macrophage Fc receptors and amplifies erythrophagocytosis and antibody-mediated cytotoxicity 100-fold. Thus, C3b-coated IgG-sensitized cells are destroyed mainly in the liver, where there are numerous phagocytic cells with receptors able to bind cells coated with IgG and C3b. On the other hand, cells coated with non-complement-fixing IgG antibodies can only be destroyed in the spleen where there is haemoconcentration and less competition of IgG-coated cells for Fc receptors with fresh IgG in plasma. The active phase of C3 is transient because C3b is rapidly degraded by an enzyme (C3b inactivator, C3bINA or factor I) and its accelerator (βIH or factor H) so that only C3dg remains on the red cell surface. C3dg is an end product of the complement sequence and, by occupying the C3 sites, can prevent further binding of C3b and therefore haemolysis of the red cell. C3dg, unlike C3b, is not capable of adhering to receptors on macrophages and monocytes, so that cells coated with C3dg may return to the circulation and will be resistant to further lysis. This explains the existence of a population of C3dg-coated cells refractory to lysis in chronic cold haemagglutinin disease. C3dg-coated cells can be detected by anti-complement in the antiglobulin test.

C4b2b3b will 'trigger' the fixation of C5, C6, C7, C8 and C9, leading to the formation of the membrane attack complex on normal red cells and bringing about their lysis.

The alternative pathway
The alternative pathway does not necessarily involve antibody and represents non-specific 'innate' immunity. The proteins of the alternative pathway form a feedback loop for the conversion of C3 to C3b; the latter is both a product and reactant of this loop.

The alternative pathway can be activated by aggregated IgA, zymosan, bacterial cells or lipopolysaccharides. Initiation of the alternative pathway is a two-step process: (i) binding of C3b to an activator and (ii) interaction of bound C3b with neighbouring surface structures. Initially, spontaneously generated fluid-phase C3b interacts with factor B to form a complex. Factor B is activated through cleavage by the protease factor D, releasing a fragment Ba into the plasma and yielding a transient alternative C3 convertase, C3bBb. The latter can be stabilized by properdin, which is essential for preventing the dissociation of C3bBb by factor H.

The alternative C3 convertase splits serum C3 into C3a and C3b. C3b attaches to the cell surface and can then combine with more factor B and D, thereby restarting the feedback loop. The amount of C3b deposited by the alternative pathway is low owing to the small amount of convertase generated and to the inefficient deposition of C3b from plasma. This contrasts with the vast numbers of C3b molecules generated by the classical pathway. The two sources of C3b are indistinguishable; both act on C5 to start the lytic phase.

The classical and alternative pathways cannot be separated from each other *in vivo*. The alternative pathway amplifies the classical pathway because, when C3b is generated, factors B and D may be activated and complexed with it to generate further C3b.

The lytic phase of the complement sequence (Figure 14.4)
The lytic phase starts with the activation of C5 by C3b, yielding membrane-bound C5b and fluid-phase C5a. This step is followed by non-enzymatic interaction of C5b with C6, C7, C8 and C9. These molecules adhere to each other to form the membrane attack complex and insert themselves into the lipid bilayer of the red cell membrane. C8 catalysed by C9 produces protein-lined cylinders in the red cell membrane that are about 10 nm in diameter. They form pores through which ions and water can enter. The osmotic pressure exerted by haemoglobin draws water into the cell until it swells and bursts.

Optimum temperature and pH for complement lysis
Many of the active complement components are enzymes and as such are very sensitive to changes in pH and temperature. The optimum pH for haemolysis to occur is 6.8 and the optimum temperature is 32–37°C. At temperatures below 15°C, the red cell cannot be haemolysed by complement and it is assumed that the last stages of complement fixation do not occur. However, the early stages of complement fixation can occur at 15°C and the components can be detected on the red cell surface with anti-complement reagents.

Ability of the antibody to bind complement
Why some antibody molecules bind complement easily and others do not is not fully understood, but several factors seem to be important.

1 The immunoglobulin class and subclass of the antibody, as discussed later.

2 At least two C1q-binding sites properly aligned and close together are necessary for complement fixation. One molecule of IgM antibody carries several C1q-binding sites, whereas one molecule of IgG carries only one and will therefore need another molecule of IgG alongside it (IgG doublet) in order to fix C1q. Therefore, for IgG antibodies to cause lysis by complement, there must be many more molecules available. It has been shown that only one molecule of IgM anti-sheep red cell antibody is needed to lyse a sheep red cell, but at least 700–1000 molecules of IgG antibody are needed to ensure that two IgG molecules are aligned in order to start the whole complement cascade.

3 If the antigen site density is low or moderate, it may be difficult for two IgG molecules to be properly aligned regardless of quantity of antibody available. This may partly explain the poor performance of IgG antibody molecules in complement fixation compared with IgM.

4 Flexibility at the hinge region is important; the wider the angle at this junction, the greater the ability of the IgG antibody to fix complement.

In red cell destruction caused by complement-fixing lytic antibodies, the number of red cells that can be rapidly destroyed is limited only by the amount of antibody and complement available. In ABO-incompatible transfusions, there may be no surviving A or B red cells in the circulation within 1 hour of transfusion. If antibodies are partially able to fix complement up to C3b (most anti-Jk^a, -K and -Fy^a), red cell destruction will be extravascular and will proceed more slowly.

Clinical significance of red cell antibodies

The clinical significance of different red cell antibodies depends partly on their destructive capacity and partly on their frequency. For example, anti-PP_1P^K (anti-Tj^a) is a very potent haemolysin, but it is of minimal importance in blood transfusion practice owing to its rarity. Conversely, ABO and D antibodies are by far the most significant, owing to their prevalence and destructive capacity.

Several factors influence immune red cell destruction *in vivo*.

1 *Plasma concentration and avidity of the antibody.*

2 *Thermal amplitude of the antibody.*

3 *Immunoglobulin class and subclass.* The complement-fixing ability of most warm-reacting IgM antibodies makes them clinically significant. Of the IgG subclasses, IgG1 and IgG3 have clinical importance because of the ability of some to fix complement up to C3b and their capacity to bind to the Fc receptors of mononuclear phagocytic cells, the effector cells of extravascular immune red cell destruction.

4 *Antibody specificity.* Several warm-reacting antibodies are incapable of causing *in vivo* red cell destruction (e.g. anti-Ch, -Rg, -Cs^a, -Kn^a, -Xg^a and most examples of anti-Yt^a).

5 *Antigen density on the red cell membrane.* The likelihood and degree of sensitization of a red cell with antibody and complement increases with the number of antigen sites on the surface.

6 *Volume of incompatible red cells transfused.* A small volume of incompatible red cells will be destroyed more rapidly than a large volume from the same donor. Larger volumes of cells may exhaust the circulating antibody available and saturate the mononuclear phagocytic system.

7 *Presence of antigen in donor plasma.* Lewis antigens (Le^a and Le^b) and the Chido and Rogers antigens are primarily in plasma and are only secondarily adsorbed onto red cells. The free antigen in plasma can react with the antibody and inhibit its binding to red cells. Also, the amount of Lewis antigen on red cells depends on the ABO group. Hence, cross-match-compatible blood, of the same ABO group, unscreened for Lewis phenotype is transfused to patients with Lewis antibodies. Furthermore, when Lewis-positive blood is transfused to patients with antibodies, the cells lose their Lewis antigens and become Le(a−b−). For this reason, Lewis antibodies are unable to cause delayed haemolytic transfusion reactions.

8 *Activity of cells of the mononuclear phagocyte system.* The ability of macrophages to remove sensitized red cells varies between individuals. Splenectomy and drugs such as corticosteroids will decrease the clearance of IgG-sensitized cells.

9 *Sensitivity of red cells to complement.* Because of the absence of cell-bound complement regulators, patients with paroxysmal nocturnal haemoglobinuria have red cells that are highly sensitive to lysis by complement activation.

10 *Extent of complement activation.* Some antibodies regularly bind complement and others do so rarely or not at all. Of the complement-binding antibodies, IgM (e.g. anti-A, -B, -PP_1P^K) will activate the complement cascade through to C9, resulting in intravascular destruction, but IgG antibodies, such as anti-Fy^a, -Jk^a and -K, the cascade is interrupted at the C3 stage. Red cells coated with IgG and C3b will be destroyed extravascularly in the liver. As a rule, Rh antibodies do not fix complement.

Blood group antigen–antibody reactions

In blood group serology, the interaction between the antigen sites on the cells and the corresponding antibody is normally detected by observing agglutination of the cells concerned. Agglutination is the result of the cross-linking of individual red cells by antibody molecules and can be thought of as occurring in two stages. The first stage is the fundamental reaction, i.e. the combination of the antibody molecules with their specific antigen sites. The second stage is the actual linkage of the individual antibody-coated red cells.

First stage of agglutination: combination of antibody with antigen

The combination of antigen with antibody cannot be observed directly; it arises from the fit of the antigen into a structurally complementary site within the antibody molecule. The resulting complex is then stabilized by various short-range forces between the chemical groups of the antigen-binding site in the antibody and the antigenic determinant itself. These weak short-range forces include ionic attraction, hydrogen bonding, van der Waals forces and hydrophobic interactions. Individually, these forces are weak; however, when in close apposition, the simultaneous formation of a large number of bonds stabilizes antigen binding. The greater the interface between antigen and antibody, the stronger the binding forces generated and the greater the affinity of the antibody for its specific antigen.

The association of antigen (Ag) with antibody (Ab) is reversible and obeys the law of mass action, so that at equilibrium:

$$(Ag) + (Ab) \underset{k_2}{\overset{k_1}{\rightleftharpoons}} (AgAb)$$

where k_1 and k_2 are rate constants of association and dissociation respectively. Hence, at equilibrium:

$$K = k_1/k_2 = \frac{(AgAb)}{(Ag)(Ab)}$$

where K is the equilibrium constant for the reaction and reflects the strength of association between antigen and antibody. The greater the value of K, the greater the amount of antigen–antibody complex formed.

Factors affecting the first stage of agglutination

Factors that affect the equilibrium constant include pH, ionic strength and temperature.

pH

Most antibodies are not affected by changes in pH within the range 5.5–8.5. Below pH 4 and above pH 9, antigen–antibody complexes are largely dissociated and the antibody can be recovered in the supernatant. This is the basis of some techniques for eluting antibodies from red cells.

Ionic strength of the medium

In saline of normal ionic strength, the ionized groups of both antigen and antibody are partially neutralized by oppositely charged ions in the medium. By lowering the ionic strength while maintaining tonicity, the ions become exposed and theoretically there should be an increase in attraction. Decreasing

the ionic strength increases the rate of association (k_1) of antigen with antibody but has little effect on their rate of dissociation (k_2). Low-ionic-strength saline (LISS) solutions have been used routinely in some blood banks to increase the speed and sensitivity of pretransfusion tests. Regrettably, LISS can lead to failure to detect some clinically important antibodies, in particular anti-K.

LISS solutions are also used to coat red cells with complement components via the alternative pathway. For this reason, the use of LISS under uncontrolled conditions can lead to unwanted positive direct and indirect antiglobulin tests.

Temperature of the reaction

The effect of temperature on antigen–antibody reactions includes (i) an alteration in the equilibrium constant and (ii) an alteration of the rate of encounter. With warm antibodies, the equilibrium constant is not changed by variations in temperature, but decreasing the temperature from 37°C to 4°C slows the rate of reaction 20-fold. With cold antibodies, there is an increase in the equilibrium constant with decreasing temperature and, even though the encounter rate is reduced, stronger reactions and higher titres are found at lower temperatures.

Second, or 'visual', stage of agglutination

Factors that affect the second stage of agglutination

These include the degree of contact of the antibody-coated red cells with each other, the span of the antibody molecules, the electrical charge of the red cells, the location and density of the antigen sites on the red cells, and the capacity of the antibody to bind complement after reacting with the antigen.

Degree of contact of antibody-coated cells

This contact can be achieved by allowing the cells to settle by gravity, although full settling does not occur in a saline serum medium until 1–2 hours have elapsed. Settling can be accelerated by centrifugation, but as red cell drifts mimicking agglutination may be formed, it is best to centrifuge at quite low speeds for not more than 1 min.

Electrical charge of the red cells

Red cells suspended in 9 g/L of NaCl are negatively charged; because of this charge and the repulsive force that it generates, there is always a gap between individual red cells. The minimum distance of approach of unsensitized cells is approximately 18 nm between their membranes. This is considerably greater than the maximum distance between the two arms of an IgG molecule (12 nm). IgM molecules, with a greater distance (~ 30 nm) between the antigen-combining sites, are able to bridge this gap and thus cause agglutination of appropriate cells suspended in saline. For this reason IgM antibodies are called 'complete'. Conversely, cells coated with IgG (e.g. anti-D) approach each other to within 6 nm between the Fc ends of the coating IgG. Agglutination of IgG-coated cells can then be brought about by various agents that bring them closer together or by molecules that cross-link coating IgG, such as proteases or neuraminidase, or antiglobulin reagents.

Span of the antibody molecule

The span of an IgG molecule can be increased by mild reduction and alkylation, which opens up the hinge region by cleaving S–S bonds. Antibodies treated in this way can be used as direct agglutinins.

Location and density of antigen sites

IgG anti-A, -B, -M and -N may agglutinate the appropriate red cells in saline. This could be due to the comparatively high number of the corresponding antigen sites (see Chapter 15 and Table 14.1). For those antigens that protrude from the cell surface (e.g. ABO, MN, I, i), agglutination by the corresponding antibodies will occur more readily than for antigens embedded in the membrane (e.g. Rh).

The number of antigen sites is, for some blood group systems, a reflection of the genotype; *MM* cells will carry twice the number of M antigens as *MN* cells and will be more readily agglutinated by the appropriate antibody (dosage effect). In other systems (e.g. ABO), zygosity dosage is not apparent.

Capacity of the antibody to bind complement

If an antibody binds complement, there might be no agglutination. The simplest explanation of this absence of agglutination is that the added presence of complement molecules, close to the antibody, prevents the antibody molecules from linking up individual cells. This lack of agglutination can be dangerous. In grouping or compatibility tests, for instance, anti-A,B in a patient's fresh serum may cause partial lysis of the red cells and no agglutination of the unlysed cells. If this lysis is not noticed, the test may be read as negative and grossly incompatible blood might be regarded as compatible.

Use of enzyme-treated red cells

Several proteases (papain from papaya, trypsin from calf spleen, bromelin from pineapple, ficin from figs) are used to treat red cells and potentiate agglutination. Whether enzyme treatment of the red cells enhances agglutination by an antibody depends on the nature of the appropriate antigen. Agglutination by Rh, Lewis, P₁, Kidd, I and i antibodies is enhanced regardless of whether the antibodies are IgM or IgG. Agglutination by most examples of anti-K is not enhanced with enzyme-treated cells. Several protein antigens are destroyed by protease treatment of intact red cells. These include M, N, S, Fy^a, Fy^b, Xg^a, In^a, In^b, Yt^a, Ch, Rg, Pr and Tn (see Chapter 15).

Detection of red cell antigen–antibody reactions

Principles of agglutination techniques

There are various ways of detecting antigen–antibody reactions *in vitro*. In manual methods, tubes, microplates or gels can be used. The most widely used methods employ the following techniques.

Direct agglutination

Most IgM antibodies will directly agglutinate the appropriate red cells suspended in saline. This method is used routinely for ABO and RhD grouping using monoclonal antibodies.

Indirect agglutination

Apart from ABO, antibodies against most blood group antigens are IgG and generally will not produce direct agglutination of red cells. Such antibodies can be detected with the aid of agents that enhance agglutination, for example proteases, albumin and other colloids, and aggregating agents such as polybrene.

Antiglobulin or Coombs test

The antiglobulin test is used to detect IgG antibodies that do not cause direct agglutination of red cells carrying the corresponding antigen when suspended in saline. The technique can be used to test directly, with an antiglobulin reagent, for the presence of antibodies or complement components that are bound to the red cells *in vivo*, as in autoimmune haemolytic anaemias or haemolytic transfusion reactions; this is the so-called direct antiglobulin test (DAT). Alternatively, the test can be used before transfusion to detect IgG antibodies in a patient's serum by adding the appropriate screening test red cells and then, after incubation and thorough washing of the cells, adding an antiglobulin reagent that will agglutinate cells coated *in vitro* with antibody or complement components; this is the so-called indirect antiglobulin test (IAT).

IATs are also used with many reagent antibodies for determining blood group phenotypes. If an IAT is undertaken with red cells suspended in normal-ionic-strength saline (NISS) solution, maximum antibody uptake, and hence maximum sensitivity, is achieved within a 60–90 min incubation period. The incubation phase for IATs can be reduced to 10–15 min by using LISS solutions. LISS IATs may be performed by either suspending the test red cells in LISS before adding the patient's serum or by adding LISS to the red cell–serum mixture. LISS IAT is less sensitive than NISS IAT for the detection of some examples of anti-K if the incubation time is reduced below 15 min. A further disadvantage of LISS IAT is that, if used in the cold, clinically insignificant antibodies such as anti-P₁ and anti-Le^a may be detected more readily because of their increased uptake under low ionic strength conditions. In view of the many

LISS preparations available, it is important that the manufacturer's instructions are followed strictly.

When the DAT and IAT are performed in tubes or microplates, it is essential that the red cells are washed three or four times with a large volume of saline before adding the antiglobulin reagent, as any free IgG or complement will neutralize the anti-IgG or anti-complement reagent and lead to false-negative reactions. This test was previously mainly carried out in tubes, but the use of microplates and microcolumns containing a matrix of either a gel or glass beads is becoming increasingly popular. With columns, the wash phase, as described below, has been eliminated.

Anti-human globulin (AHG) serum was originally made by injecting animals, usually rabbits, sheep or goats, with human serum. Of particular relevance to the antiglobulin test are antibodies against IgG and complement, which should always be present in polyspecific AHG reagents. The anti-IgG component is essential for pretransfusion antibody screening and crossmatching, as the vast majority of clinically significant antibodies, apart from anti-A and -B, are IgG. The anti-complement component is needed for the detection of occasional examples of weak complement-binding antibodies (e.g. some anti-Jk^a) and for the detection of *in vivo* complement coating of red cells (i.e. in the DAT). Antiglobulin reagents are now generally produced from monoclonal antibodies to C3d and polyclonal antibodies to IgG, made in animals.

The basic composition of a polyspecific reagent is a blend of anti-IgG and anti-C3d. Anti-C4d should be avoided and antibodies against IgA and IgM are not necessarily always present in polyspecific reagents. Pure anti-IgG, anti-IgA and anti-IgM serum can be made in animals by injecting the appropriate purified immunoglobulin and removing any antibody against L chains by absorption.

Most IgM blood group antibodies can be detected readily by direct agglutination. On those occasions when it is desirable to detect subagglutinating amounts of IgM active at 37°C, the lack of anti-IgM in polyspecific reagents can be offset by the ability of most IgM antibodies to fix complement in the presence of fresh serum. Moreover, as only a few molecules of IgM are needed to start the complement sequence and lead to the binding of many hundreds of molecules of C3, the agglutination of complement-coated cells by anti-complement sera can be a very sensitive method of detecting IgM antibodies. Complement-fixing IgG antibodies will also be detected with anti-complement sera but, in most cases, they can be detected effectively by anti-IgG. However, there are exceptional examples of complement-fixing IgG red cell alloantibodies (e.g. anti-Jk^a) that are not detectable with anti-IgG, and anti-complement is essential for their identification.

Polyspecific antiglobulin reagents composed of anti-IgG and anti-C3d are perfectly suitable for pretransfusion testing, including the cross-match. For those rare cases of autoimmune haemolytic anaemia in which the test with polyspecific AHG is negative, it is necessary to test with anti-IgA and anti-IgM, which are now available ready for use in gel microcolumns. Polyclonal and monoclonal reagents against the four human IgG subclasses are commercially available and are generally used in research for characterizing clinically significant red cell alloantibodies.

Standardization of AHG reagents

All antiglobulin reagents available at present, monospecific or polyspecific, are standardized by the producer and issued prediluted for immediate use or within the gel or bead matrix of a microcolumn.

When new batches of an AHG reagent or IAT microcolumns are acquired by a laboratory, they should be subjected to a minimum *verification* with several IgG antibodies of different specificities to ensure that all are detectable. Laboratories should confirm that, on each day of use, the AHG reagent is reacting according to the manufacturer's specifications, with control red cells coated weakly with IgG. The control IgG-coated cells are the same cells as those used to check the validity of negative antiglobulin tests when a washing step is part of the process; the weakly coated cells are added to each tube that has given a negative result, followed by repeat centrifugation and reading. Agglutination of these cells confirms that the AHG reagent in the tube had not been neutralized by residual unbound IgG that was not removed during washing of the original test cells.

Agents that enhance agglutination

Various agents may be added to serological mixtures to enhance the agglutinability of red cells. These include albumin and LISS, as described above, as well as polybrene and polyethylene glycol.

Inhibition of agglutination

Expected agglutination reactions with known antigens and antibodies can be neutralized by soluble antigens of the appropriate specificity. For example, the saliva of group A secretors inhibits the agglutination of group A cells by anti-A. Hydatid cyst fluid with P$_1$P^K activity can be used to confirm the presence of anti-P$_1$ in sera. Soluble antigens produced by recombinant DNA technology will become useful in reference laboratories as aids to sorting out complex serological problems.

Haemolysis

Red cell lysis indicates a positive antigen–antibody reaction mediated by IgM complement-fixing antibodies. A pink or red coloured supernatant after settling or centrifugation of red cell–antibody mixtures is an indication of red cell lysis.

Adsorption and elution tests

Specific antibodies can be removed from serum by adsorption on red cells carrying the corresponding antigen. Bound antibodies can be subsequently recovered from the washed

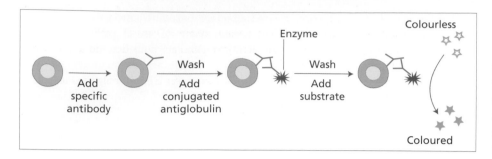

Figure 14.5 Enzyme-linked immunosorbent assay (ELISA) for cell-bound antibodies. Enzyme substrate is represented by open and closed stars, for colourless and coloured derivatives respectively.

sensitized red cells by elution with heat treatment, freeze-thawing, low pH or chloroquine treatment.

Specialized serological methods

Flow cytometry and enzyme-linked immunosorbent assays (ELISAs) are used for the estimation of the number of antigen sites on red cells and when more sensitive antiglobulin techniques are required. The essence of these approaches is the use of a labelled antiglobulin: in flow cytometry, fluorescent anti-IgG is used (or antibodies can be directly coupled with a fluorescent dye); in the case of ELISA, enzymes are attached covalently (i.e. conjugated) to the antiglobulin.

The execution of these assays requires antibody-coated cells or particles to be incubated with the labelled antiglobulin reagent. After incubation, excess unbound antiglobulin is washed away and bound labelled antiglobulin is then measured. For flow cytometry, a cytofluorimeter is used to measure fluorescence of each cell. For ELISA, the bound enzyme conjugate is detected through the enzyme's ability to modify, and usually effect a colour change, in its substrate (Figure 14.5). The colour intensity of the modified substrate can then be measured with a spectrophotometer.

Microcolumn tests (gel and beads)

The principle of microcolumn tests is the separation of agglutinated from non-agglutinated red cells by centrifugation through a miniature filtration column. For blood grouping, red cells are layered on microcolumns impregnated with blood grouping sera; for antibody screening and identification, phenotyped panel red cells are mixed with patients' sera within the incubation chamber of the microcolumn. After centrifugation, agglutinated red cells are retained towards the top of the microcolumn because the agglutinates are trapped by the column matrix, whereas unagglutinated red cells form a button at the bottom of the column (Figure 14.6).

Positive and negative results are discriminated by the appearance of cells trapped within the matrix or at the bottom of the microcolumn respectively. Antiglobulin tests can be accomplished by centrifuging the preincubated mixture of red cells and patient's serum through a column impregnated with

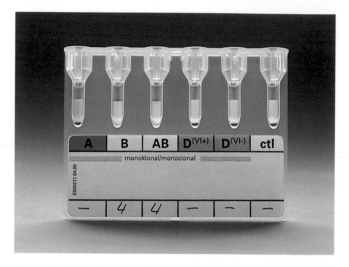

Figure 14.6 Results of a gel microcolumn test. The subject is group B D-negative. Red cells remaining at the top of the gel represent a positive result; red cells collected at the bottom of the tube represent a negative result.

anti-IgG or polyspecific AHG. Any red cells coated with IgG will be agglutinated by the free anti-IgG in the matrix of the column, giving a positive result. No washing of sensitized cells is required as IgG in the serum does not penetrate the column and so does not neutralize the anti-IgG in the column. The advantages of microcolumn techniques are the ease of reading and reproducibility, and the fact that the tests can be stored for later examination, checking, photocopying or photographing. In the Diamed ID system, Sephadex gels are used. The Ortho Biovue system uses glass beads rather than gels. Both systems can be automated and the agglutination results evaluated by image analysis.

Microplate techniques

Semi-automated blood grouping and antibody screening can be performed in microtitre plates, which can also be used for extended phenotyping of red cells, antibody identification and large-scale screening for rare red cells and antibodies. A single microplate is equivalent to 96 short test tubes and the same basic principles of discrete analysis of agglutination apply. The advantages of these techniques include enhanced sensitivity, speed of performance, reduced reagent requirements, simplicity and reduced requirements for laboratory space and expensive equipment. Several commercial microplate-based blood grouping systems are now available that incorporate the use of bar codes to identify samples, automated liquid handling of samples and reagents, and plate readers linked to computers for easy and accurate record-keeping.

Solid-phase systems, involving microplates containing red cells adhered to the surface of the plastic, help to reduce the variability between tests that is inherent in liquid-phase systems when undertaken by different operators, and easily lend themselves to automated reading of results. Blood grouping (e.g. for ABO and D groups) by solid phase can be accomplished by the use of U-shaped microplate wells coated with the relevant antibody (e.g. anti-A, -B, -D); suspensions of patients' or donors' red cells are added to the wells and then centrifuged. Positive results appear as a carpet of cells coated over the bottom of the well. Negative results appear as a tight pinhead of unattached cells in the centre of the well.

Antibody screening and identification by a solid-phase technique can be achieved with microplates coated with a panel of phenotyped red cell ghosts. The wells are incubated with patient serum and LISS, washed and then anti-IgG is added. Anti-IgG will bind to those wells where the patient's IgG red cell antibody has bound to the relevant red cell ghost; bound anti-IgG is then easily detected by adding indicator red cells coated with IgG (e.g. D-positive cells coated with anti-D), followed by brief centrifugation, as described above.

Automated techniques

Fully automated blood grouping and antibody screening, using microcolumn techniques or microplates, are carried out in transfusion centres, where large numbers of donor samples are tested daily, and increasingly in hospital transfusion laboratories. In automated systems such as the Olympus PK, test samples are mixed with typing sera or screening cells in individual wells of a special microplate that are constructed to have a terraced surface at the bottom of the well. After incubation and settling of the red cells in the reaction mixtures, agglutination patterns are distinguished either on the basis of light transmission or by image analysis with the aid of a computer-controlled CCD camera.

Other automated systems are available for use with microcolumns, for example ID-GelStation (Diamed) and AutoVue systems (Ortho). These are fully automated walk-away systems using bar codes to identify samples, reagents and test cards. Each has a pipetting (liquid handling) station, incubator, centrifuge and reader linked to a computer to maintain the identity of the sample being tested throughout the entire testing process. Similar walk-away systems are available for use with solid-phase

microplate systems, for example Tango (Biotest), Galileo (Immucor). The Qwalys system (Diagast) applies magnetized red cells for antigen typing and antibody detection, in order to avoid centrifugation.

A continuous-flow autoanalyser is commonly used for quantification of anti-D or anti-c, especially in antenatal patients and immunized volunteers, as well as in plasma pools used for the manufacture of anti-D immunoglobulin. Manual titration is simple, but provides only a fairly crude semi-quantitative estimate of the concentration of anti-D.

Quantitative haemagglutination methods using continuous-flow automated analysers and appropriate anti-D or anti-c international standards are sensitive (e.g. as low as 0.02 IU/mL for anti-D), relatively simple, objective, rapid, of acceptable reproducibility, and amenable to routine use and standardization. The method involves the agglutination of D-positive red cells by the anti-D to be quantified, in the presence of an agglutination enhancer, while being pumped through a series of coils at set temperatures to allow the desired incubation of the segments of reactants. The agglutinates are sedimented and removed, whereas the remaining unagglutinated red cells are haemolysed by a detergent. The absorbance of the haemolysate is proportional to the amount of haemoglobin and is thus inversely proportional to the number of agglutinated cells removed. This reflects the antibody concentration, which can be calculated (in IU/mL) using the values obtained from the standard, run in parallel.

Flow cytometry can also be used for antibody quantitation, but is probably less reliable than the autoanalyser technology described above.

Blood grouping reagents

To avoid potential fatalities resulting from errors in ABO and D grouping, it is essential that the chosen ABO and RhD typing reagents have suitable potency and comply with the European Directive on in vitro diagnostic devices and the associated Common Technical Specifications and carry the 'CE' mark to show they are in conformance.

Blood grouping reagents prepared from polyclonal antisera should be free of unwanted antibodies and should have been exhaustively tested with an extensive panel of cells to exclude common and rare specificities before they are issued for routine use. Unwanted contaminating antibodies are generally not a problem with monoclonal reagents as they have to be extensively tested before being placed on the market. IgM monoclonal reagents are generally used for ABO, Rh and K typing.

Strict adherence to the manufacturer's instructions for each reagent is essential. Standard operating procedures should include completing the worksheet prior to testing, labelling all tubes, microplates or gels, recording results immediately after reading, repeating discrepancies and using adequate controls. Any other equipment used in an investigation (centrifuge, incubator) must be calibrated and in range at the time that the test is undertaken.

ABO grouping has an in-built control in the reverse grouping (serum check; see Chapter 15). Controls for D typing must always be used in order to prevent a D-negative patient being mistyped as D-positive. At least two potent anti-D reagents should be used in Rh typing and these reagents must be selected to detect or not detect variants of D, as appropriate (see Chapter 15).

Antibody screening and identification

With plenty of anticipation prior to transfusion, patients' sera should be screened against unpooled group O cells from selected individuals known to carry the following antigens between them: D, C, E, c, e, M, N, S, s, P_1, Le^a, Le^b, K, k, Fy^a, Fy^b, Jk^a and Jk^b. Ideally, one cell sample should be R_1R_1 (DCe/DCe) and the other R_2R_2 (DcE/DcE), so that the Rh antigens are all in double dose. A minimum homozygous expression (i.e. double dose) of Fy^a and Jk^a should be present on one of the red cell samples. It is generally possible to meet these requirements with two cells but if more antigens are required with homozygous expression, it might be necessary to use three cells. Zygosity can be checked by molecular genetic methods.

The techniques employed for antibody screening of patient's sera need only include a well-controlled sensitive IAT, commonly using microcolumn techniques. If the antibody screening is positive, antibody identification with a second sensitive technique (e.g. enzyme-treated cells or the polyethylene glycol or manual polybrene test), in addition to the IAT, should be used against a panel of fully phenotyped red cells. Saline tests are not essential for antibody screening or identification and all incubations should be performed at 37°C; antibodies reacting at lower temperatures are of no clinical importance.

It is recommended that an autologous control be used by incubating the patient's serum with the patient's cells, by the methods used for antibody identification. All tests must follow a written standard operating procedure. Immunohaematologists should not forget that the main aim of blood group serology is to provide hazard-free transfusions.

Molecular techniques for blood grouping

Almost all the genes for human blood groups have now been cloned and the molecular bases for all the clinically important blood group polymorphisms have been determined. Consequently, it is now possible to predict blood group phenotypes from DNA with a high degree of accuracy. This is usually performed when a blood group phenotype is required but a suitable red cell sample is not available. The most important application is the determination of fetal blood groups. When a pregnant woman has a blood group antibody with the potential to cause HDFN (see Chapter 16), it is beneficial to be able to determine whether her fetus has the corresponding antigen and consequently whether it is at risk from HDFN. Such tests usually involve RhD typing, but may also involve typing for Rhc and K antigens, and rarely other blood group antigens. The usual source of fetal DNA used to be amniocytes, obtained by amniocentesis, an invasive procedure with a small risk of spontaneous abortion and a 20% risk of transplacental haemorrhage, which could boost the mother's antibody. Non-invasive testing for D and other antigens is now used routinely in some countries, in which fetal blood group phenotype is predicted from the small quantity of free fetal DNA present in the maternal plasma. Such testing will also be useful for unsensitized RhD-negative pregnant women in order to genotype the fetus they are carrying and thus avoid giving antenatal Rh immunoglobulin prophylaxis when the fetus is shown to be D negative.

Another use of molecular methods for blood grouping is for transfusion-dependent patients, where serological methods are not possible because of the presence of transfused red cells that are always present in the patient's blood. If genotypes can be determined for all clinically important blood group polymorphisms in transfusion-dependent patients, then matched blood can be provided to prevent the patient from making multiple antibodies to blood group antigens. Tests are carried out on DNA that is isolated from whole blood from the transfused patient. Another application is blood grouping of patients with autoimmune haemolytic anaemia, whose red cells are coated with immunoglobulin, making serological typing difficult.

Several types of tests are commonly used in blood group genotyping.

1 Amplification of a portion of a blood group gene to determine whether it is present. This only applies to *RHD* of the Rh system. Presence of the amplified product can be detected by gel electrophoresis, although monitoring of the amplification by the use of a fluorescent probe in a 'real-time' system is the usual method for detecting fetal *RHD* in maternal plasma.

2 Amplification of a portion of a gene followed by detection of the polymorphism with restriction endonucleases (see Chapter 15). Kits for blood group testing by this technology are available commercially.

3 Selective amplification of a specific allele by the use of an allele-specific primer (see Chapter 15).

4 Amplification of a portion of a gene followed by direct sequence of the amplified product.

5 Allelic discrimination by polymerase chain reaction (PCR) incorporating allele-specific fluorescently labelled probes, in which relative quantities of a pair of alleles are measured.

6 Application of some sort of microarray technology in which numerous polymorphisms can be tested from a relatively small quantity of DNA.

It is unlikely that molecular genetics will be used for routine ABO and Rh typing of donors and patients, at least in the near future. However, there may be other roles for molecular blood grouping in the future. One such function could be genotyping large numbers of blood donors for multiple blood groups in order to establish a database of donors typed for all clinically significant blood groups. This would be valuable for the treatment of transfusion-dependent patients, as it would facilitate the provision of compatible blood for those patients who have made blood group antibodies and matched blood for those who have not. To perform such testing, high-throughput methods will be required. High-throughput techniques for detecting DNA polymorphisms are available, and some are being developed for blood group testing.

Selected bibliography

General

Klein HG, Anstee DJ (2005) *Mollison's Blood Transfusion in Clinical Medicine*, 11th edn. Blackwell Publishing, Oxford.

Roback JD, Combs MR, Grossman BJ, Hillyer CD (2008) *AABB Technical Manual*, 16th edn. American Association of Blood Banks, Bethesda, MD.

Immunology

Abbas AK, Lichtman AH, Pober IS (2000) *Cellular and Molecular Immunology*, 4th edn. Saunders, Philadelphia.

Delves P, Martin S, Burton D, Roitt IM (2006) *Roitt's Essential Immunology*, 11th edn. Wiley Blackwell, Oxford.

Janeway CA, Travers P, Walport M *et al.* (2001) *Immunobiology*, 5th edn. Garland Publishing, New York.

Red cell membrane

Bruce LJ, Beckmann R, Ribeiro ML *et al.* (2003) A band 3-based macrocomplex of integral and peripheral proteins in the RBC membrane. *Blood* **101**: 4180–8.

Daniels G (2002) *Human Blood Groups*, 2nd edn. Blackwell Science, Oxford.

Daniels G (2007) Functions of red cell surface proteins. *Vox Sanguinis* **93**: 331–40.

Mohandas N, Gallagher PG (2008) Red cell membrane: past, present, and future. *Blood* **112**: 3939–48.

Yawata Y (2003) *Cell Membrane: The Red Cell as a Model*. Wiley-VCH, Weinheim.

Antigen–antibody reactions

Bell CA (1982) *Seminar on Antigen–Antibody Reactions Revisited*. American Association of Blood Banks, Arlington, VA.

International Forum (1995) What is the best technique for the detection of red cell alloantibodies? *Vox Sanguinis* **69**: 292–300.

Knight RC, de Silva M (1996) New technologies for red cell serology. *Blood Reviews* **10**: 101–10.

Siegel DL (2007) Phage display-based molecular methods in immunohematology. *Transfusion* **47** (1 Suppl.): 89S–94S.

Sinor LT (1990) Advances in solid phase red cell adherence methods and transfusion serology. *Transfusion Medicine Reviews* **6**: 26–31.

Clinical significance of blood group antibodies

International Forum (2004) Red cell transfusions and blood groups. *Vox Sanguinis* **87**: 210–22.

Poole J, Daniels G (2007) Blood group antibodies and their significance in transfusion medicine. *Transfusion Medicine Reviews* **21**: 58–71.

Blood grouping methods

Avent ND (2007) Large scale blood group genotyping. *Transfusion Clinique et Biologique* **14**: 10–15.

Chapman JF, Elliott C, Knowles SM, Milkins CE, Poole GD. Working Party of the British Committee for Standards in Haematology Blood Transfusion Task Force (2004) Guidelines for compatibility procedures in blood transfusion laboratories. *Transfusion Medicine* **14**: 59–73.

Daniels G, Finning K, Martin P, Massey E (2009) Non-invasive prenatal diagnosis of fetal blood group phenotypes: current practice and future prospects. *Prenatal Diagnosis* **29**: 101–7.

Hillyer C, Shaz BH, Winkler AM, Reid M (2008) Integrating molecular technologies for red blood cell typing and compatibility testing into blood centres and transfusion services. *Transfusion Medicine Reviews* **22**: 117–32.

Judd J, Johnson ST, Storry JR (2008) *Judd's Methods in Immunohematology*, 3rd edn. American Association of Blood Banks, Bethesda, MD.

National Blood Service (2005) *Guidelines for the Blood Transfusion Services in the United Kingdom*, 7th edn. The Stationery Office, London (available at http://www.tsoshop.co.uk/bookstore.asp).

CHAPTER 15

Antigens in human blood

15

Marcela Contreras[1] and Geoff Daniels[2]

[1]University College London and Blood Transfusion International, London, UK
[2]Bristol Institute for Transfusion Sciences, Bristol, UK

Introduction

The main topic of this chapter is red cell antigens and their antibodies. However, in human blood there are many other antigenic structures that stimulate the production of antibodies in recipients of blood transfusions. Leucocyte antibodies are an important cause of febrile transfusion reactions in patients who have had previous transfusions or pregnancies. Lymphocytotoxic antibodies and, rarely, platelet antibodies may be a cause of failure of the platelet count to rise after platelet transfusions. Thus, a description of granulocyte and platelet antigens and antibodies is also included. The human leucocyte antigen (HLA) system is covered in Chapter 37. Antibodies against proteins present in plasma may lead to urticarial or anaphylactic transfusion reactions; these are considered briefly.

The International Society of Blood Transfusion recognizes 308 red cell surface antigens, 270 of which belong to one of 30 blood group systems (Table 15.1). Each system represents either a single gene locus or two or three very closely linked loci of homologous genes. Each system is genetically discrete from all the others. In addition, there are 38 antigens that have not been included in systems. Most blood groups are inherited as Mendelian characters, although environmental factors may occasionally affect blood group expression. The 35 genes representing the 30 systems have been located on a specific chromosome (Table 15.1). All are autosomal except *XG* and *XK*, which are on the X chromosome, and *CD99*, which is located on both the X and Y chromosomes. All the genes have been cloned.

Blood group antigens may be integral proteins or glycoproteins of the red cell membrane, or they may be membrane glycolipids. In proteins and glycoproteins, blood group polymorphisms and variants may represent differences in the amino acid sequence (e.g. Rh and Kell antigens). In glycoproteins and glycolipids, the blood group activity may reside in the carbohydrate moiety and polymorphism is associated with differences in the oligosaccharide sequence (e.g. ABO). In some glycoproteins, blood group polymorphism may be caused by amino acid substitutions, but antigen expression is also dependent on glycosylation of the polypeptide.

The ABO system

The clinical importance of a blood group system in blood transfusion lies in the frequency of its antibodies and in the possibility that such antibodies will destroy incompatible cells *in vivo*.

Postgraduate Haematology: 6th edition. Edited by A. Victor Hoffbrand, Daniel Catovsky, Edward G.D. Tuddenham, Anthony R. Green
© 2011 Blackwell Publishing Ltd.

Table 15.1 Human blood group systems.

No.	Name	Symbol	No. of antigens	Gene name(s)	Chromosome	CD number
001	ABO	ABO	4	ABO	9	
002	MNS	MNS	46	GYPA, GYPB, GYPE	4	CD235a/b
003	P	P1	1	P1	22	
004	Rh	RH	50	RHD, RHCE	1	CD240D/CE
005	Lutheran	LU	19	BCAM	19	CD239
006	Kell	KEL	31	KEL	7	CD238
007	Lewis	LE	6	FUT3	19	
008	Duffy	FY	6	DARC	1	CD234
009	Kidd	JK	3	SLC14A1	18	
010	Diego	DI	21	SLC4A1	17	CD233
011	Yt	YT	2	ACHE	7	
012	Xg	XG	2	XG, CD99	X/Y	CD99
013	Scianna	SC	7	ERMAP	1	
014	Dombrock	DO	6	ART4	12	CD297
015	Colton	CO	3	AQP1	7	
016	Landsteiner–Wiener	LW	3	ICAM4	19	CD242
017	Chido–Rodgers	CH/RG	9	C4A, C4B	6	
018	H	H	1	FUT1	19	
019	Kx	XK	1	XK	X	
020	Gerbich	GE	8	GYPC	2	CD236
021	Cromer	CROM	15	CD55	1	CD55
022	Knops	KN	9	CR1	1	CD35
023	Indian	IN	4	CD44	11	CD44
024	Ok	OK	1	BSG	19	CD147
025	Raph	RAPH	1	CD151	11	CD151
026	John Milton Hagen	JMH	5	SEMA7A	15	CD108
027	I	I	1	GCNT2	6	
028	Globoside	GLOB	1	B3GALT3	3	
029	Gill	GIL	1	AQP3	9	
030	RHAG	RHAG	3	RHAG	6	CD241

ABO was the first system to be recognized and remains the most important in transfusion and transplantation (histo-blood group system). Almost everybody over the age of about 6 months has clinically significant anti-A and/or anti-B in their serum if they lack the corresponding antigens on their red cells. Thus, if we consider the incidence of ABO blood groups in the UK (Table 15.2), transfusions given without regard to ABO would result in a major incompatibility (patient has the antibody and the antigen is on the transfused red cells) about once in every three cases.

Antigens of the ABO system

The vast majority of human bloods can be grouped into six main ABO phenotypes (Table 15.3), although several other rare weak variants can be distinguished serologically. The incidence of ABO groups varies very markedly in different parts of the

Table 15.2 Incidence of ABO groups in southern England.

Phenotype	Frequency (%)	
O	44.9	
A$_1$	30.8	} 41.1
A$_2$	10.3	
B	10.1	
A$_1$B	2.7	} 3.9
A$_2$B	1.2	

world and in different races. Even in the UK, there is some variation between north and south, and in some cities the frequencies will reflect racial differences. In such areas, the blood groups of the patient population do not reflect those of the predominantly white blood donors.

Table 15.3 ABO grouping.

Agglutination of test cells with				Agglutination by test serum of			ABO group of test sample	Possible genotype
Anti-A	Anti-A$_1$	Anti-B	Anti-A,B*	A cells	B cells	O cells		
−	−	−	−	+	+	−	O	O/O
+	+	−	+†	−	+	−†	A$_1$	A^1/A^1, A^1/O, A^1/A^2
+	−	−	+	−/+‡	+	−	A$_2$	A^2/A^2, A^2/O
−	−	+	+	+	−	−	B	B/B, B/O
+	+	+	+	−	−	−†	A$_1$B	A^1/B
+	−	+	+	−/+‡	−	−	A$_2$B	A^2/B

*Anti-A,B (group O serum) is not generally used in routine laboratories.
†Some group A$_1$ and A$_1$B individuals may have weak anti-H in their plasma.
‡Serum from a proportion of A$_2$ (1–8%) and A$_2$B (22–35%) individuals contain anti-A$_1$.

A$_1$ and A$_2$ subgroups

The distinction between the A$_1$ and A$_2$ subgroups is usually made by using anti-A$_1$, which will agglutinate A$_1$, but not A$_2$, red cells. Anti-A$_1$ can be obtained in several ways: (i) it can be made by absorbing anti-A (from group B people) with A$_2$ red cells; (ii) it is found in the serum of some A$_2$ and A$_2$B persons (Table 15.3); (iii) it can be made from a saline extract of the seeds of the hyacinth bean *Dolichos biflorus*; and (iv) mouse monoclonal anti-A$_1$. Anti-A$_1$ is not used routinely as it is not necessary to distinguish group A$_1$ from group A$_2$ blood for most transfusion recipients. There is no specific antibody for A$_2$ red cells; if anti-A is absorbed with A$_1$ cells, all the antibody is removed. Group B serum can therefore be thought of as containing two antibodies: anti-A, which agglutinates both A$_1$ and A$_2$ red cells, and anti-A$_1$, which agglutinates only A$_1$ red cells. The anti-A component of group O serum also has both antibodies.

The presence of the A^2 allele in the presence of A^1 cannot be determined by serology. Among people who are genotypically A/O or A/B, approximately three possess the A^1 gene for every one who possesses A^2 (Table 15.2).

The difference between the A$_1$ and A$_2$ subgroups is partly quantitative: the red cells of A$_1$ and A$_1$B subjects have more A antigen sites than A$_2$ and A$_2$B subjects, respectively. For practical purposes, A$_2$ can be regarded as a weaker form of A. Table 15.4 shows quantitative differences in the number of A antigen sites on A$_1$ and A$_2$ red cells. When both the A and B antigens are present, there are less sites for each than when either is present alone. The practical importance of this lies in the fact that the A antigen of A$_2$B red cells may give an extremely weak reaction with anti-A, which could be missed in routine grouping tests if reagents of inadequate potency are used. Moreover, if the same person's serum contains anti-A$_1$ and is tested in the reverse grouping only with A$_1$ and not A$_2$ red cells, they will be grouped as B. For this reason, potent anti-A reagents reacting with A$_2$B cells must be used in routine blood grouping.

Table 15.4 Numbers of A and B antigen sites on red cells of various ABO groups.

Blood group of red cell	Approximate no. of A antigen sites	Approximate no. of B antigen sites
A$_1$ adult	1 000 000	−
A$_1$ cord	300 000	−
A$_1$B adult	500 000	−
A$_1$B cord	220 000	−
A$_2$ adult	250 000	−
A$_2$ cord	140 000	−
A$_2$B adult	120 000	400 000
B adult	−	700 000

There is also a qualitative difference between A$_1$ and A$_2$, but this must be very subtle because A$_2$ red cells can absorb all the anti-A from group B serum if the absorption is carried out at 0–4°C for sufficient time. The chemical basis is unresolved, but A-active oligosaccharide structures called type 3A and type 4A (see p. 249) might represent A$_1$: they are of relatively low abundance on A$_1$ cells, but may be absent from A$_2$ red cells.

H antigen

Group O cells have no antigens of the ABO system (Table 15.3) but do possess H antigen, the precursor upon which the products of the *ABO* genes act. The H gene (called *FUT1*) segregates independently from *ABO* and is on a different chromosome: *ABO* on chromosome 9, *FUT1* on chromosome 19. The H antigen is present to some extent on almost all red cells, regardless of the ABO group, but the amount of H antigen varies with the ABO group as follows: O > A$_2$ > A$_2$B > B > A$_1$ > A$_1$B.

Individuals with the rare Bombay phenotype are homozygous for inactive *FUT1* alleles (*h/h*). Their red cells are not agglutinated by anti-A or anti-B, regardless of *ABO* genotype, but are not group O as they are also not agglutinated by anti-H. The serum of Bombay subjects contains potent anti-H, anti-A and/ or anti-B that will only allow them to be transfused with the scarce Bombay blood. Parents and offspring of Bombay individuals, who are heterozygous for the inactive *FUT1* allele (*H/h*), have H and red cells of normal ABO phenotype.

Development of the A, B and H antigens
The A and B antigens can be detected on the red cells of very young fetuses, but their reactions are weaker than those of adults. Table 15.4 shows that there are fewer A and B antigen sites on cord than on adult red cells. Similarly, the H antigen is less well developed at birth than in adult life. After birth, the expression of the A, B and H antigens increases until about 3 years of age, and thereafter, in health, remains stable throughout life.

Distribution of the A, B and H antigens
ABH antigens are often referred to as histo-blood group antigens because they are widely distributed in the body. They are therefore very important in transplantation. They are present on white cells, platelets and epidermal and other tissue cells. They are also present in the plasma, whether individuals are secretors or non-secretors of A, B or H, and in the saliva and other secretions of ABH secretors (see later).

Rare ABO variants
Rare ABO variants are usually disclosed because an expected ABO antibody is missing. A sample typed as group O that has anti-B but no anti-A will usually prove to be a weak A variant. The presence of weak A or B antigens can be demonstrated either by using potent antisera or by adsorption and elution. Rare ABO variants can arise as follows.

1 *Rare ABO genes.* These include A₃, Ax, Aend, Am and Ael variants. All are extremely rare and are usually recognized by their variable reactions with anti-A and/or anti-A,B sera. Similarly, subgroups of B have been described; all are very rare.

2 *Genes segregating independently of* ABO. These rare variants are the H-deficiency or Bombay phenotypes described on p. 250.

3 *Environmental effects.* Weakening of the A antigen can occur in various types of leukaemia (usually acute myeloid). The A antigen may revert to almost normal in remission. Similar weakening of B, H and I has been described. B-like antigens may be acquired by group A individuals who are suffering from bowel infections, usually associated with carcinoma or strictures of the large bowel. Red cells with an acquired B antigen are agglutinated by some anti-B, including some monoclonal anti-B, but not by the patient's own anti-B. Bacterial deacetylases convert *N*-acetylgalactosamine, the immunodominant sugar of the A antigen, into galactosamine, a structure similar to galactose, the immunodominant sugar of the B antigen (see p. 248). In some cases, acquired B may also be associated with polyagglutination (see p. 261).

Antibodies of the ABO system

Anti-A, anti-B and anti-A,B
Sera taken from people over the age of about 6 months that do not contain the expected A and B antibodies (Table 15.3) are very rare. They should always be investigated thoroughly; often, some interesting explanation will be found, for example a rare subgroup of A, a blood group chimera or congenital absence of IgM.

It is likely that ABO antibodies arise in response to A- and B-like antigens present on bacterial, viral or animal molecules. Titres of ABO antibodies vary considerably with age, reaching a peak in young adults and then declining in old age. Titres vary depending on the techniques used: normal adult sera can have anti-A titres, by direct agglutination in saline medium, in the range 16–1024 and anti-B titres in the range 4–256, but most have saline titres below 100. The anti-A and anti-B titres of group O subjects are much higher than in group B or A subjects.

Naturally occurring anti-A and anti-B have a wide thermal range. Although they are active at 37°C, they react better at lower temperatures. The antibodies always have some IgM component and, in group A and B persons, they are almost entirely IgM. Antibodies from group O individuals, even before immunization, usually have some IgG anti-A,B, an antibody that cross-reacts with both A and B structures.

Following immunization with red cells or blood group substances, the thermal characteristics of the antibodies change, but group A and B subjects continue to produce antibodies that are mainly IgM. Most group O persons, however, will produce IgG as readily as IgM anti-A,B. Consequently, mothers of children with ABO haemolytic disease of the fetus and newborn (HDFN) are almost always group O. Immune anti-A,B are mainly IgG2, which does not cause HDFN because there are no Fc receptors for IgG2 on the cells of the mononuclear phagocyte system. When the maternal serum contains potent IgG1 and/or IgG3 ABO antibodies, HDFN may occur, although this is usually mild compared with Rh HDFN. Some IgA anti-A or anti-B is produced following immunization with A or B substances. Some differences in the serological properties of immune and naturally occurring anti-A and anti-B are shown in Table 15.5, which also indicates ways of detecting IgG anti-A or anti-B in the presence of IgM anti-A or anti-B, which has relevance to ABO HDFN, as discussed in Chapter 17.

Dangerous 'universal' donors
Good practice in pretransfusion testing requires compatibility testing, which consists of incubating the patient's serum with donor red cells. Group O red cells can be given to A, B or AB recipients and group O donors were formerly, and inappropriately, called 'universal donors'. Group O donors have anti-A, anti-B and anti-A,B in their plasma, which will react with the recipient's A or B cells. Normally, if group A, B or AB recipients

Table 15.5 Some properties of immune and naturally occurring anti-A and anti-B.

	Naturally occurring IgM	Immune IgM	IgG
Complement binding (at 37°C)	++/+++	+++	++
Agglutination of appropriate cells	+++	+++	+++
Cross the placenta	–	–	+++
Detection enhanced by anti-IgG	–	–	+++
Inhibited by soluble A or B substances (e.g. saliva)	+++	+++	–*
2-ME or DTT sensitive	+++	+++	–

*IgG ABO antibodies are usually inhibited only by large amounts of specific substance.

2-ME, 2-mercaptoethanol; DTT, dithiothreitol.

are transfused with a relatively small number of group O units of whole blood, the anti-A or anti-B that is transfused will be diluted out and neutralized by the plasma of the adult recipient, especially if plasma-reduced blood, or red cells in additive solution are used. However, if the transfused units of red cells contain potent immune haemolytic antibodies, this neutralization and dilution effect could be insufficient and the antibodies may cause marked destruction of the A or B red cells of the recipient, leading to a severe acute haemolytic transfusion reaction (HTR). For this reason, the practice of transfusing group O whole blood, or even plasma-reduced red cells, to non-O recipients should be strongly discouraged.

There is usually a shortage of group O blood, and not infrequently a surplus of group A blood. In the vast majority of cases, including emergencies, there is enough time to perform a rapid ABO group on the patient's cells, which will allow the transfusion of group-specific blood. If there is no time to do an ABO group before transfusion, red cells in optimal additive solution, devoid of plasma, should be given until the patient's blood group is known. The practice of transfusing group O platelets to non-O patients should be discouraged as the dose of adult platelets will contain at least 300 mL of plasma, unless part of it has been replaced by platelet-additive solution. Group O fresh-frozen plasma and cryoprecipitate should only be given to group O recipients. This matter is discussed again in Chapter 17.

Anti-A$_1$

Anti-A$_1$, reactive at room temperature (18–22°C), can be found in the serum of 1–8% of group A$_2$ and 22–35% of group A$_2$B

persons. Most of these antibodies are more of a nuisance in compatibility tests than of clinical importance because they often do not agglutinate A$_1$ red cells at 30°C and above, and so are unable to cause increased *in vivo* red cell destruction. Very rarely, anti-A$_1$ able to agglutinate A$_1$ red cells at 37°C may lead to significant destruction of A$_1$ red cells *in vivo*. The appropriate group A$_2$ or A$_2$B red cells should be cross-matched in these rare instances.

Anti-H

Several forms of anti-H exist.

1 Clinically significant 'true' anti-H occurs in the serum of the very rare persons with Bombay phenotype. When it does occur, it is active at 37°C and only Bombay phenotype blood may be transfused.

2 Anti-H and anti-HI, commonly found in the serum of group A$_1$, B and A$_1$B persons, react much more strongly with adult than with cord red cells. Anti-H is inhibited by secretor saliva; anti-HI is not. Although these antibodies agglutinate O red cells at 20°C, they do not usually agglutinate them at temperatures above 30°C. Very occasionally, anti-H/anti-HI may cause rapid destruction of at least some of the transfused O red cells *in vivo*. However, these antibodies will not interfere with the survival of transfused cells if ABO identical units, i.e. A$_1$, B or A$_1$B donor units, are chosen for A$_1$, B or A$_1$B recipients respectively.

ABH secretor status

About 80% of the UK population are ABH secretors as they have H antigen, plus A or B according to their ABO genotype, in a water-soluble form in their body secretions. The remaining 20% are non-secretors and have no secreted ABH antigens, regardless of ABO genotype.

Biochemistry and biosynthesis of ABH antigens

ABH antigens

A, B and H antigens on red cells are predominantly glycoproteins, the majority being on the N-glycans of the anion exchanger (band 3) and the glucose transporter. ABH antigens on red cells are also expressed on glycosphingolipids, which include paraglobosides (Table 15.6). Soluble ABH antigens are glycoproteins. Differences in the terminal sugars of the glycoproteins and glycolipids determine the specificity of these antigens: L-fucose (Fuc) for H; L-fucose plus N-acetyl-D-galactosamine (GalNAc) for A; and L-fucose plus D-galactose (Gal) for B.

Two major types of carbohydrate chain endings serve as acceptors for the fucosyltransferases that synthesize H antigen: type 1 and type 2 chains have Gal joined to N-acetylglucosamine (GlcNAc) through $1\rightarrow3$ and $1\rightarrow4$ linkages, respectively. A- and B-transferases synthesize the transfer of GalNAc and Gal, respectively, from their donor substrates UDP-GalNAc and

Table 15.6 Some glycolipids of the red cell surface expressing H, A, B, P_1, P^K, P and LKE activity.

Structure	Antigen	Name
Paragloboside series		
Galβ1→4GlcNAcβ1→3Galβ1→4Glc-Cer	–	Paragloboside
Fucα1→2Galβ1→4GlcNAcβ1→3Galβ1→4Glc-Cer	Type 2H	
Fucα1→2Galβ1→4GlcNAcβ1→3Galβ1→4Glc-Cer 3 ↑ 1 GalNAc	Type 2A	
Fucα1→2Galβ1→4GlcNAcβ1→3Galβ1→4Glc-Cer 3 ↑ 1 Gal	Type 2B	
Galα1→4Galβ1→4GlcNAcβ1→3Galβ1→4Glc-Cer	P_1	
Globoside series		
Galβ1→4Glc-Cer	–	Lactosylceramide, Gb2
Galα1→4Galβ1→4Glc-Cer	P^K	Globotriosylceramide, Gb3
GalNAcβ1→3Galα1→4Galβ1→4Glc-Cer	P	Globoside, Gb4
NeuAcα2→3Galβ1→3GalNAcβ1→3Galα1→4Galβ1→4Glc-Cer	LKE	Sialosylgalactosylgloboside
Fucα1→2Galβ1→3GalNAcβ1→3Galα1→4Galβ1→4Glc-Cer	Type 4H	Globo-H

Cer, ceramide; Fuc, fucose; Gal, galactose; GalNAc, *N*-acetylgalactosamine; Glc, glucose; GlcNAc, *N*-acetylglucosamine.

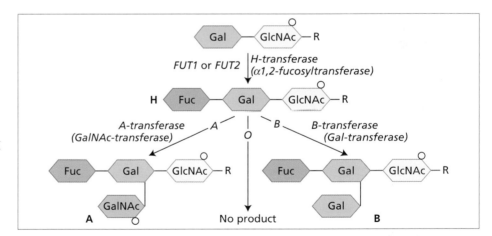

Figure 15.1 Biosynthetic pathway of H antigen from its precursor, and of A and B antigens from H. H remains unconverted in the absence of *A* or *B* gene products. R, remainder of molecule.

UDP-Gal to the terminal galactosyl residue of type 1 H and type 2 H, creating A and B epitopes and masking H specificity (Figure 15.1).

Secretory glycoproteins possess both type 1 and type 2 linkages, whereas red cells synthesize type 2 chains only. Plasma glycolipids, passively adsorbed onto the red cells, have only type 1 chains; these also carry Lewis antigens (see p. 250). Other chains, called type 3 and 4, are also present in low numbers on red cells, but probably only on glycolipids.

ABO genes

The *ABO* gene is located on the long arm of chromosome 9, comprises seven exons and encodes proteins with a structure characteristic of glycosyltransferases. Products of the *A* and *B* alleles differ by four amino acids encoded by exon 7, two of which determine whether the enzyme product has GalNAc-transferase (A) or Gal-transferase (B) activity.

The majority of *O* alleles (called *O¹*) resemble *A*, but have a single-base deletion in exon 6, which creates a shift in the reading frame and scrambles the amino acid sequence after the first quarter of the transferase polypeptide; introduction of a premature stop codon truncates any putative polypeptide. About 3% of O alleles (called O^2) have a single-nucleotide polymorphism (SNP) that changes one of the vital amino acids in the catalytic site, inactivating the enzyme.

The A^2 allele has a single-base deletion immediately before the usual termination codon, creating a reading frameshift and abolition of this stop codon. This creates an A-transferase with an extraneous 21 amino acids on its C-terminus, which accounts for its reduced efficiency as a GalNAc-transferase.

Gene sequences for many variants of A, B and O alleles have been determined and in most cases there is heterogeneity, with more than one mutation accounting for similar phenotypes.

H genes

At least two genes, *FUT1* and *FUT2*, are responsible for production of H antigen. Both encode α1,2-fucosyltransferases that catalyse the transfer of fucose to the terminal galactose residue of the H precursor chain (Figure 15.1). *FUT1* is active in mesodermally derived tissues, including haemopoietic tissues, and is responsible for H expression on red cells. Homozygosity for inactivating mutations in *FUT1* gives rise to Bombay and related phenotypes. *FUT2* is responsible for the expression of H antigen in endodermally derived tissues, including those responsible for secretions, and hence is the gene responsible for ABH secretion. Secretors are homozygous or heterozygous for an active allele (*Se*) at *FUT2*; non-secretors are homozygous for an inactive allele (*se*) usually containing a nonsense mutation.

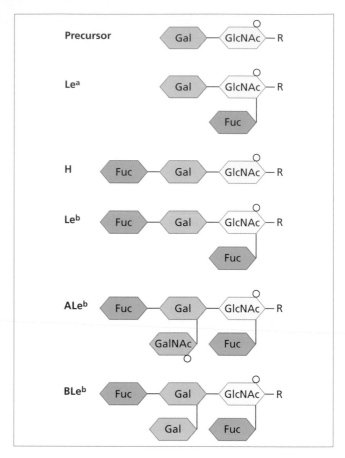

Figure 15.2 Diagrammatic representation of H and Lewis antigens. Le^a requires the action of the Lewis α1,4-fucosyltransferase, H the action of the H α1,2-fucosyltransferase, Le^b the action of both Lewis and H fucosyltransferases, and ALe^b and BLe^b the action of Lewis and H fucosyltransferases and the A or B glycosyltransferases.

The Lewis system

Antigens of the Lewis system and their biosynthesis

The Lewis system differs from all other blood group systems in that it is primarily a system of soluble antigens present in secretions and in plasma. The Lewis antigens on red cells are adsorbed passively from the plasma, and a constant presence of plasma is needed to maintain Lewis antigen on the red cells. There are two basic Lewis antigens: Le^a and Le^b. Expression of either requires the presence of an active Lewis gene, but Lewis phenotypes are also governed by the gene controlling H secretion (*FUT2*). Lewis antigens in saliva and plasma are glycoproteins and glycolipids, respectively.

The Lewis gene, *FUT3*, encodes an α1,4-fucosyltransferase that catalyses the addition of L-fucose in 1→4 linkage to the subterminal GlcNAc of type 1 chains (Figure 15.2). If the type 1 core structure has been unmodified, Le^a antigen is produced. If the secretor α1,2-fucosyltransferase has already modified the type 1 chains to produce type 1H, the action of the Le-transferase

leads to the formation of Le^b. In a white population, 75% have active Lewis and secretor genes and hence Le(a−b+) red cells; 20% have an active Lewis gene but are H non-secretors and have Le(a+b−) red cells; and 5% are homozygous for Lewis genes with inactivating mutations and are Le(a−b−) (Table 15.7). In Oriental populations there is a low incidence of non-secretors, but a high incidence of a weak secretor allele of *FUT2*. Competition between the Lewis and weak-secretor transferases leads to the Le(a+b+) red cell phenotype.

Adsorption of the Lewis substances by red cells

Le(a+b−) and Le(a−b+) red cells incubated in Le(a−b−) plasma lose their Lewis antigens into the plasma. Similarly, if Le(a+b−) or Le(a−b+) red cells are transfused into an Le(a−b−) person, the transfused cells will gradually lose their Lewis antigens and will group as Le(a−b−) within 1 week of transfusion. So, if the patient has clinically significant anti-Le^a or anti-Le^b, the red cells

Table 15.7 The Lewis system and secretion of ABH.

Genotype		Antigens in saliva			Plasma/red cells*	
FUT2 *(secretor)*	FUT3 *(Lewis)*	*Le*^{a}	*Le*^{b}	ABH	*Le*^{a}	*Le*^{b}
Se/Se, Se/Se^w or *Se/se*	*Le/Le* or *Le/le*	+	++	++	w/−	++
Se/Se, Se/Se^w or *Se/se*	*le/le*	−	−	++	−	−
Se^w/*Se*^{w} or *Se*^{w}/*se*	*Le/Le* or *Le/le*	++	++	++	++	++
Se^w/*Se*^{w} or *Se*^{w}/*se*	*le/le*	−	−	++	−	−
se/se	*Le/Le* or *Le/le*	+++	−	−	++	−
se/se	*le/le*	−	−	−	−	−

*Le^a and Le^b on red cells are passively adsorbed from plasma.
Le, active allele at *FUT3* locus; *le*, inactive allele; *Se*, active allele at *FUT2* locus; *Se*^{w}, weakly active allele; *se*, inactive allele; w, weak.

that were not destroyed in the first few days will not be haemolysed once they become Le(a−b−).

Development of Lewis antigens on red cells

The Lewis antigens are poorly developed at birth and red cells from cord blood are usually Le(a−b−). Thereafter, Le^a develops first, followed by Le^b if the relevant Lewis and secretor genes are present. The cells of children between the ages of 6 months to 4 years often type as Le(a+b+) if they are destined to become Le(a−b+). The definitive adult Lewis phenotype may not be reached until the age of 4–5 years.

Antibodies of the Lewis system

Lewis antibodies are generally made only by individuals with the Le(a−b−) red cell phenotype. Anti-Le^a occurs fairly frequently. The incidence of Le(a−b−) is much higher in people of African and Southeast Asian origin than in whites and Lewis antibodies detectable at 22°C or above may be found in up to 10% of random serum samples from black people.

Anti-Le^b commonly accompanies anti-Le^a. Pure anti-Le^b is uncommon and is made by people who are non-secretors and whose red cells are Le(a−b−). Very rarely, anti-Le^b can be made by Le(a+b−) individuals.

Serological characteristics of Lewis antibodies

Lewis antibodies are predominantly IgM, even after deliberate stimulation. They usually agglutinate the appropriate cells at 20°C. All Lewis antibodies that react at 37°C will bind complement and may lyse antigen-positive cells. Usually, Lewis antibodies do not agglutinate red cells in saline at 37°C, but can be detected with anti-complement in an indirect antiglobulin test (IAT).

Clinical significance of Lewis antibodies

Some patients may have Lewis antibodies reacting at 37°C. Anti-Le^a is usually more haemolytic than anti-Le^b, and there are some anti-Le^{a+b} that can be very potent, leading to increased intravascular red cell destruction in the initial stages of transfusion. However, all Lewis antibodies lead to two-component survival curves of transfused incompatible red cells, i.e. the first cells are destroyed at an accelerated rate and the remainder, which have been stripped of their adsorbed Lewis antigens, will have a normal survival.

For patients with Lewis antibodies reacting at 37°C, it is recommended that ABO-identical red cells, compatible in an IAT cross-match at 37°C, should be transfused. It is important to choose ABO-identical cells as group A, B and AB cells carry less Lewis antigens than group O cells routinely used in antibody screening. This is because the A- and B-transferases compete with the Lewis transferase for the same precursor substrate. The provision of pretyped Le(a−b−) blood for patients with Lewis antibodies is not necessary, as it is always easy to find cross-match-compatible red cells at 37°C.

Lewis antibodies do not cause HDFN as they are almost always IgM and newborn infants have Le(a−b−) red cells.

P blood groups

P$_1$ was discovered by Landsteiner and Levine, who used suitably adsorbed sera of rabbits injected with human red cells. About 75% of subjects tested were positive for P$_1$, which is inherited as a Mendelian dominant character. P$_1$ frequency varies in different populations and the P$_1$-negative phenotype is called P$_2$. P$_1$ is weakly expressed at birth and its strength varies considerably in adults. For this reason, identification of anti-P$_1$ can be difficult, as panel cells will have varying expression of the antigen.

Anti-P$_1$ is a naturally occurring antibody commonly found in the serum of P$_2$ individuals. Unlike anti-A and anti-B, anti-P$_1$ rarely causes transfusion reactions because it is usually a cold-reacting IgM antibody, often not reactive above 30°C.

P_1 is a structure in the paragloboside series of glycolipids. The *P1* gene is an α1,4-galactosyltransferase that adds galactose to the P_1 precursor, paragloboside (see Table 15.6). A precursor of paragloboside is lactosylceramide, which is converted to the P^K antigen by α1,4-galactosyltransferase-1. In most people, almost all P^K is further converted to P antigen (globoside) by β1,3-*N*-acetylgalactosaminyltransferase-1. The very rare 'p' phenotype results from deficiency of α1,4-galactosyltransferase-1 and leads not only to absence of P^K and P, but also P_1 because α1,4-galactosyltransferase-1 is also the enzyme responsible for P_1 synthesis. Deficiency of β1,3-*N*-acetylgalactosaminyltransferase-1 causes the P^K phenotype, in which the red cells express P^K antigen strongly, but no P (globoside). P^K red cells may be P_1 or P_2.

Anti-PP_1P^K and anti-P invariably occur in the sera of the very rare individuals with p and P^K phenotypes, respectively. Anti-PP_1P^K react with all red cells except those of the p phenotype; anti-P react with all red cells except those of the P^K and p phenotypes. They are usually strong IgM antibodies, often lytic at 37°C, and can cause severe transfusion reactions if incompatible red cells are transfused. Occasionally, IgG anti-P or anti-PP_1P^K are found and have been associated with spontaneous early abortion.

The biphasic Donath–Landsteiner autoantibody is found in the sera of patients suffering from paroxysmal cold haemoglobinuria. It is always IgG and usually has anti-P specificity.

I and i antigens

The antigens I and i are not controlled by alleles: i is the biosynthetic precursor of I. I and i antigens are carbohydrates and are on the interior structures of the complex oligosaccharides that carry ABO, H and Lewis antigens. The i antigen represents linear structures that are converted to I-active branched structures by the product of the I gene (*GCNT2*), a β1,6-*N*-acetylglucosaminyltransferase. This enzyme is not active in neonates. Consequently, red cells of most adults are agglutinated strongly by anti-I and only weakly by anti-i, whereas red cells from cord blood give the opposite result. The agglutinability of an infant's red cells with anti-I increases, and with anti-i decreases, with maturity; at about 18 months of age the red cells give the reactions of adult cells. Adults who are homozygous for rare inactivating mutations in *GCNT2* have the adult i phenotype; their red cells react weakly with anti-I and strongly with anti-i, and their serum contains anti-I.

In haematological disorders such as thalassaemia, megaloblastic anaemia, sideroblastic anaemia, hereditary spherocytosis, paroxysmal nocturnal haemoglobinuria and some aplastic and dyserythropoietic anaemias, agglutinability by anti-i is increased without a reciprocal decrease in the agglutinability by anti-I.

Anti-I

Autoanti-I that agglutinates the patient's own and other adult ABO-compatible red cells at 20°C, but not at 30°C, occurs in a variety of disorders and after blood transfusions. These patients' red cells give a negative direct antiglobulin test (DAT). A transient increase in strength, titre and thermal range of anti-I regularly occurs after infections with *Mycoplasma pneumoniae* and occasionally leads to acute haemolysis; red cells of such patients give a positive DAT, as do those of patients suffering from chronic cold haemagglutinin disease (CHAD). In CHAD, the autoantibody is nearly always monoclonal and usually has anti-I specificity. All anti-I in CHAD are IgM and complement binding.

Anti-i

Autoanti-i is found transitorily in many patients suffering from infectious mononucleosis. Very occasionally, the titre and thermal range of this antibody may lead to acute haemolysis, particularly if the patient's red cells are more agglutinable than normal with anti-i. Red cells of these patients give a positive DAT. Autoanti-i may occasionally be the antibody specificity in chronic CHAD. Such patients often have an underlying lymphoma.

The Rh system

The Rh blood group system, the fourth to be discovered, is the second most important in blood transfusion. This is not because Rh antibodies are usually present when the Rh antigen is absent, but because anti-RhD is formed readily when RhD-positive blood is transfused to an RhD-negative person. Moreover, as these immune antibodies are normally IgG, they are able to cross the placenta and cause HDFN. The Rh system now contains a total of 50 antigens, but D (RH1), because of its high immunogenicity, is by far the most important because of its ability to cause severe HDFN and HTRs.

Rh antigens

The D antigen (RH1)

In 1939, Levine and Stetson described a patient who had an antibody that agglutinated the red cells of 85% of ABO-compatible donors. She had delivered a stillborn infant and then suffered a severe reaction to transfusion of her husband's blood. In 1940, Landsteiner and Wiener found that guinea pigs and rabbits injected with rhesus monkey red cells made an antibody that not only agglutinated rhesus monkey red cells, but also the red cells of 85% of people of European origin. The human and animal antibodies were originally thought to be the same and the human antibody was called anti-Rhesus.

Table 15.8 Eight Rh haplotypes and their frequencies in English, Nigerian and Hong Kong Chinese populations.

Haplotype			Frequencies (%)		
CDE	Rh-Hr	Numerical	English	Nigerian	Chinese
DCe	R^1	RH 1,2,−3,−4,5	42	6	73
dce	r	RH −1,−2,−3,4,5	39	20	2
DcE	R^2	RH 1,−2,3,4,−5	14	12	19
Dce	R^0	RH 1,−2,−3,4,5	3	59	3
dcE	r″	RH −1,−2,3,4,−5	1	Very rare	Very rare
dCe	r′	RH −1,2,−3,−4,5	1	3	2
DCE	R^z	RH 1,2,3,−4,−5	Rare	Very rare	Rare
dCE	r^y	RH −1,2,3,−4,−5	Very rare	Very rare	Rare

Results of testing with anti-D, -C, -c, -E and -e red cells from 2000 English donors, 274 Yoruba of Nigeria and 4648 Cantonese from Hong Kong.

Many years later, it was realized that the human antibody (now called anti-D of the Rh system) does not identify the same antigen as the rabbit and guinea pig rhesus antibody, the error arising out of a phenotypic association between the antigens. As it was now too late to change the name of the whole system, Levine suggested that the antigen defined by the original rhesus antibody should be called LW in honour of Landsteiner and Wiener. The blood group system originally identified by the human antibody is now called the Rh system.

For clinical purposes, individuals can be classified as Rh-positive (have the D antigen) and Rh-negative (lack the D antigen).

The expansion to include C, E, c and e (RH2–RH5)

By the end of 1943, four antisera detecting genetically related antigens were available to Fisher and Race, who noticed that two of them appeared to give antithetical results. They proposed that the antigens recognized by these two antisera were allelic and called them C and c. They gave further letters, D (the original Rh antigen) and E, to the antigens recognized by the other two antisera and postulated that each had an alternative, which they called d and e. Anti-e was found in 1945. Anti-d has never been found as no d antigen exists. Fisher and Race proposed that the Rh antigens were controlled by three closely linked genes, giving rise to eight gene complexes or haplotypes: CDe, cDE, cDe, CDE, cde, Cde, cdE and CdE. At about the same time, Wiener proposed that there was only one Rh gene, controlling a number of blood factors, equivalent to C, c, D, E and e.

Molecular genetics has shown that there are two Rh genes, one encoding D, the other encoding the Cc and Ee antigens. As the Cc and Ee polymorphisms are determined by separate regions of a single gene, the CDE terminology of Fisher and Race is still suitable for understanding Rh at most levels (although the Wiener terminology is often used as a shorthand; Table 15.8). The approximate frequencies of the Rh gene complexes in three populations are shown in Table 15.8. In a white

Table 15.9 The most common Rh genotypes in the UK population.

Genotype		Frequency (%)
DCe/dce	R^1r	31
DCe/DCe	R^1R^1	16
dce/dce	rr	15
DCe/DcE	R^1R^2	13
DcE/dce	R^2r	13
DcE/DcE	R^2R^2	3

population, the first three complexes form 94% of the total and combinations of these three will give the most common genotypes (Table 15.9). Genotype frequencies vary considerably in different parts of the world. For instance, dce/dce varies from about 35% in Basques to 0.3% in Japanese and Chinese.

Probable Rh genotype

When a person's Rh phenotype is known, the probable genotype can be discerned and its likelihood calculated from known genotype frequencies within the same population (Table 15.10). When probable genotype determinations are carried out, it is very important that the ethnic origin of the person is known; figures for one population will not apply to people of other populations. For example, in white populations, dce is 15 times more common than Dce, whereas in African populations Dce has a slightly higher frequency than dce. Consequently, the phenotype D+ C+ c+ E− e+ represents a probable genotype of DCe/dce in a white person, but of DCe/Dce in a black person.

Levels of D antigen expression are affected by the presence of other Rh antigens on the red cells. Table 15.10 shows the

Table 15.10 Determining probable Rh genotype in the UK population and the number of D antigen sites on red cells of those phenotypes.

Reactions with anti-					Common genotypes	Genotype incidence (%) for each phenotype		No. of D antigen sites
D	C	c	E	e		Unselected persons	Fathers of infants with anti-D HDN	
+	+	+	−	+	DCe/dce*	94	79	9900–14600
					DCe/Dce	6	21	
+	+	−	−	+	DCe/DCe*	96	99	14500–19300
					DCe/dCe	4	1	
+	−	+	+	+	DcE/dce*	94	79	14000–16000
					DcE/Dce	6	21	
+	−	+	+	−	DcE/DcE*	86	96	15800–33000
					DcE/dcE	14	4	
+	+	+	+	+	DCe/DcE*	90	97	23000–31000
					DcE/dce	⎫	⎫	
					DcE/dCe	⎬ 10	⎬ 3	
					DCe/dcE	⎭	⎭	
					DCE/Dce			
−	−	+	−	+	dce/dce	100	0	0

*Probable genotype.

number of D antigen sites on red cells of different phenotypes as estimated by the use of ^{125}I-labelled anti-IgG to quantify bound IgG anti-D. The *DcE* haplotype produces high levels of D expression and, for reasons still to be explained, *C* causes depression of D antigen produced by the Rh haplotype on the opposite chromosome.

Molecular genetics of Rh

Rh genes and proteins

Rh antigens are encoded by two closely linked genes with 92% sequence homology. *RHD* encodes the D antigen and *RHCE* the Cc and Ee antigens. Each consists of 10 exons and, unusually for homologous genes, the two genes are in opposite orientation on the chromosome (Figure 15.3). Each gene encodes a 416-amino-acid polypeptide of 30–32 kDa that is palmitoylated but not glycosylated. The polypeptides encoded by *RHD* and *RHCE* differ by 31–35 amino acids, depending on the *RHCE* genotype.

There is substantial evidence that the Rh polypeptides traverse the lipid bilayer 12 times, with both termini in the cytoplasm and six extracellular loops that provide the putative sites for antigenic activity (Figure 15.3). Rh antigen activity is very dependent on the conformation of the proteins within the membrane and may involve interactions between two or more of the extracellular loops. Removal of the proteins from the membrane generally ablates all antigenic activity.

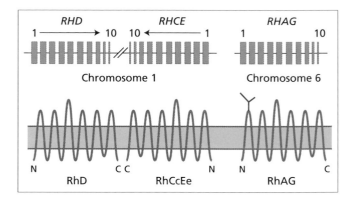

Figure 15.3 Rh and related genes and the polypeptides they encode, showing the 10 exons of *RHD* and *RHCE* in reverse orientation on chromosome 1 and of *RHAG* on chromosome 6, and the RhD and RhCcEe polypeptides and RhAG glycoprotein crossing the membrane 12 times.

D, C/c and E/e polymorphisms

In white people, the D-negative phenotype almost always results from homozygosity for a complete deletion of the *RHD* gene. Consequently, D-negative represents the absence of the whole RhD protein from the membrane. Anti-D can detect epitopes on any of the external loops of the RhD protein. D-positive people may be homozygous or hemizygous for the presence of *RHD*. However, most D-negative black Africans have an inactive *RHD*, called the *RHD* pseudogene (*RHD*ψ), that contains a 37-bp duplication in exon 4 and a translation stop codon in exon 6.

The Cc polymorphism is associated with three or four amino acid substitutions encoded by exons 1 and 2 of *RHCE*, although the definitive change is Ser103 for C and Pro103 for c in the second extracellular loop of the RhCcEe protein. E and e are associated with Pro226 and Ala226, respectively, in the fourth extracellular loop.

The Band 3/Rh molecular macrocomplex

The two Rh proteins are closely associated in the red cell membrane with a glycoprotein, the Rh-associated glycoprotein (RhAG). RhAG is homologous to the Rh proteins and has a similar conformation in the membrane, spanning the membrane 12 times, but is glycosylated on the first extracellular loop (Figure 15.3). Unlike *RHD* and *RHCE*, which are on chromosome 1, the gene encoding RhAG is on chromosome 6. The complex of Rh proteins and RhAG is part of a membrane macrocomplex or metabolon, with band 3 (the anion exchanger and Diego blood group antigen) at its core and also containing the LW glycoprotein (ICAM-4), CD47 and glycophorin (GP)A and GPB. This macrocomplex is attached to the membrane skeleton (see Chapter 14), primarily through ankyrin and protein 4.2.

The function of the Rh/RhAG complex is unknown, although evidence exists that RhAG might function as a gas channel for CO_2 and possibly O_2. The Rh proteins are only present on erythroid cells, but RhAG and non-erythroid related proteins (RhBG, RhCG) are more widely distributed and homologues are found throughout the animal and plant kingdoms where they often function as ammonium transporters.

Variants of D

Most D-negative individuals lack the whole RhD protein from their red cells and, when immunized by D-positive red cells, can make antibodies to an array of epitopes on the external loops of the RhD protein. About 30 D epitopes have been defined using monoclonal antibodies. There are numerous variants of D, which have, for convenience, been divided into two types, weak D (formerly D^u) and partial D, though in reality the boundaries have been blurred and the situation is more complex than that. Numerous variants of e are known, generally found only in people of African origin.

Weak D

By definition, weak D red cells express all epitopes of D at a low level and individuals with weak D phenotype cannot make anti-D. Red cells that have the weak D phenotype should, for most transfusion purposes, be regarded as D-positive. Weak D red cells have fewer D sites per cell than normal D-positive red cells. In a white population, the gene for weak D is commonly accom-

panied by *RHCE* encoding either a C or E antigen (D^weak^Ce or D^weak^cE); D^weak^ce is rare. Weak D is more common in Africans and is usually produced by D^weak^ce. It is important that anti-D typing reagents should detect most weak D phenotypes, especially in blood donors, although very weak forms of D will be typed as D-negative. The weakest form of weak D, named DEL, can only be detected serologically by absorption and elution tests.

In the UK, the recommended method for D typing of patients requires direct agglutination tests, in duplicate, with potent IgM monoclonal anti-D reagents. An antiglobulin test is not required. This means that very weak D red cells will by typed as D-negative. This is not considered important, as the patient will be harmlessly transfused with D-negative red cells. Donors are not typed any longer for D by an antiglobulin test, as this is not necessary because it is unlikely that transfusion of very weak D red cells to a D-negative patient will result in immunization of the patient.

Partial D

Partial D antigens have some or many of the D epitopes missing; those that are present may be expressed normally or weakly. If immunized with normal D-positive red cells, individuals with partial D can make antibody to the D epitopes they lack. This antibody will not react with the subject's own cells, or with partial D red cells of the same type, but will behave as anti-D when tested with red cells of common Rh phenotypes. Over 40 different types of partial D have been recognized and the classification of these D variants can only be made by serological methods in a few specialized reference laboratories.

The most important partial D antigen, from a transfusion perspective, is called DVI ('D six'). It is not the most common, but lacks most of the D epitopes and is the most commonly encountered partial D associated with the production of anti-D. In the UK it is recommended that anti-D reagents for typing patients should not detect DVI. Consequently, DVI patients will be transfused with D-negative red cells and DVI pregnant women will be given anti-D prophylaxis. Ideally, one of the anti-D reagents used for typing donor red cells should detect DVI. Consequently, DVI individuals should be considered D-negative patients but D-positive donors.

Molecular basis of D variants

Partial D antigens result either from missense mutations in *RHD*, encoding single amino acid changes, or from *RHD* in which a segment has been replaced by the equivalent segment of an *RHCE* gene. For example, the most common form of DVI is produced by an *RHD–CE–D* hybrid gene in which exons 4–6 have the nucleotide sequence of *RHCE*, and external loops 3 and 4 of the encoded hybrid protein have the amino acid sequence of an RhCe protein. Hence, a protein is produced with a sequence similar enough to *RHD* to be stable in the membrane, but different enough to lack many epitopes of D. A variety of names have been used to denote the different types of partial D, for example DIII1, DVI, DFR, DAR, DBT. These can mostly be distinguished by sophisticated serological techniques.

Weak D results from missense mutations in *RHD* that encode amino acid changes that are predicted to be in the cytoplasmic or membrane-spanning domains of the D protein, but not in any of the loops exposed to the exterior of the cells. Based on molecular genotyping, at least 60 different types of weak D have been identified, and these have been numbered. They cannot be distinguished serologically. The three most common weak D types are weak D type 1 (70%, Val270Gly), type 2 (18%, Gly385Ala) and type 3 (5%, Ser3Cys).

Unfortunately, some D variants, for example weak D type 4.2 and weak D type 15, have been given weak D numbers based on their molecular background, but have subsequently been found in a number of cases to be associated with anti-D production and so are really partial D. Clearly a new terminology is needed and care must be taken in making transfusion decisions based on the terminology derived from molecular testing.

Other Rh antigens

Table 15.11 lists the antigens of the Rh system recognized by the International Society of Blood Transfusion. A few of these are described below.

C^w and C^x antigens (RH8 and RH9)

C^w and C^x occur in about 2% and 0.2% of white people, respectively, although substantially higher frequencies are found in Finns. They appear to have an allelic relationship, although C^w and C^x represent Gln41Arg and Ala36Thr substitutions in an RhCcEe protein, respectively. Anti-C^w and anti-C^x have caused HDFN but on the rare occasions on which this has occurred, it has usually been mild.

G antigen (RH12)

With only rare exceptions, G is expressed when either D or C, or both, are present. Anti-G recognizes a determinant common to the products of *RHD* and the *C* allele of *RHCE*. Anti-G usually occurs with anti-D (see p. 257).

Table 15.11 Antigens of the Rh system.

Number	Alternative names	Frequency*	Number	Alternative names	Frequency*
RH1	D	Polymorphic	RH32	R^N	Low
RH2	C	Polymorphic	RH33	Har	Low
RH3	E	Polymorphic	RH34	Hr^B	High
RH4	c	Polymorphic	RH35	R^N-like	Low
RH5	e	Polymorphic	RH36	Be^a	Low
RH6	ce, f	Polymorphic	RH37	Evans	Low
RH7	Ce	Polymorphic	RH39	C-like	Polymorphic
RH8	C^w	Polymorphic	RH40	Tar	Low
RH9	C^x	Low	RH41	Ce-like	Polymorphic
RH10	V	Polymorphic†	RH42	Cce^s	Polymorphic†
RH11	E^w	Low	RH43	Crawford	Low
RH12	G	Polymorphic	RH44	Nou	High
RH17	Hr$_o$	High	RH45	Riv	Low
RH18	Hr	High	RH46	Sec	High
RH19	hr^s	Polymorphic	RH47	Dav	High
RH20	VS	Polymorphic†	RH48	JAL	Low
RH21	C^G	Polymorphic	RH49	STEM	Low
RH22	CE	Low	RH50	FPTT	Low
RH23	D^w	Low	RH51	MAR	High
RH26	c-like	Polymorphic	RH52	BARC	Low
RH27	cE	Polymorphic	RH53	JAHK	Low
RH28	hr^H	Polymorphic†	RH54	DAK	Low
RH29	Total Rh	High	RH55	LOCR	Low
RH30	Go^a	Low	RH56	CENR	Low
RH31	hr^B	Polymorphic	RH57	CEST	High

*Polymorphic indicates > 1%, < 99% in at least one major population.
†Only polymorphic in black people, low in other populations.

VS and V antigens (RH20 and RH10)

VS and V have frequencies of about 40% and 10%, respectively, in Africans, but are rare in other ethnic groups. Both are associated with an *RHCE* mutation encoding Leu245Val, but only VS is expressed when a Gly336Cys mutation is also present. Neither anti-VS nor anti-V have caused HDFN or an HTR.

Compound antigens

Antibodies to the compound antigens, anti-ce (-f, -RH6), anti-Ce (-RH7), anti-cE (-RH27) and anti-CE (-RH22), define pairs of CcEe antigens present only when they are encoded by the same *RHCE* gene. For example, anti-Ce and anti-cE will react with D+ C+ c+ E+ e+ cells of *DCe/DcE* genotype, but not *DCE/dce*, whereas the reverse applies to anti-ce and anti-CE.

Rh$_{null}$, Rh$_{mod}$ and D−−

Rh$_{null}$ and Rh$_{mod}$

Rh$_{null}$ red cells lack all antigens of the Rh system and people with this rare phenotype can make an antibody, anti-RH29, that reacts with all red cells except those of the Rh$_{null}$ phenotype. They also lack RhAG, LW, and Fy5 of the Duffy system, and have weakened expression of CD47 and of S, s and U antigens on GPB. Rh$_{null}$ subjects have a chronic haemolytic stomatocytic anaemia, which is usually compensated but may require splenectomy.

There are two modes of inheritance of the Rh$_{null}$ phenotype.
1 Homozygosity for a deletion of *RHD* (characteristic of most D-negatives) plus homozygosity for an inactivating mutation in *RHCE*. Consequently, neither Rh protein is produced. Both parents are heterozygous for the mutations and possess only half of the usual quantity of Rh antigens. This is the rarer of the two types.
2 Homozygosity for inactivating mutations (frameshift, splice site, missense) in *RHAG*, the gene encoding RhAG. In the absence of RhAG, no Rh antigens are expressed, despite the presence of normal Rh genes. Consequently, individuals with this type of Rh$_{null}$ inherit normal Rh genes from their parents and pass them on to their offspring. These parents and offspring are heterozygous for the *RHAG* mutation and have apparently normal Rh antigens, although there may be some weakening of expression. The parents of both types of Rh$_{null}$ individuals are usually consanguineous.

Rh$_{mod}$ arises from partial inactivation of *RHAG*, caused by mutations encoding single amino acid substitutions. This results in weakened expression of all Rh antigens. Rh$_{mod}$ individuals cannot make anti-RH29.

D−− and related phenotypes

Homozygosity for a rearranged *RHCE* gene, together with an active *RHD*, results in a series of phenotypes, called D−−, D··, Dc− and DC^w−, in which no E or e antigens and, in the case of D−− and D··, no C or c is produced. These phenotypes are very rare and have enhanced expression of D. If transfused, individuals with these phenotypes produce anti-Hr$_o$ (-RH17), an antibody that reacts with all red cells except for Rh$_{null}$ cells and cells with D−− and related phenotypes.

Antibodies of the Rh system

Naturally occurring antibodies

Generally, Rh antibodies are only produced following immunization with red cells. However, anti-E is often naturally occurring; about half may occur without a history of pregnancy or transfusion. Rarely, naturally occurring anti-D and anti-C^w are found. All such naturally occurring Rh antibodies react optimally with enzyme-treated cells.

Immune antibodies

The clinical importance of the Rh system lies in the readiness with which anti-D arises in D-negative subjects after stimulation with D-positive red cells by pregnancy or transfusion. Prophylaxis against D immunization with anti-D immunoglobulin has led to a significant decrease in the incidence of anti-D, but it still remains the most common immune antibody of clinical relevance detected in a routine blood transfusion laboratory. D is considerably more immunogenic than the other Rh antigens, which have the following order of immunogenicity: c > E > e > C.

About 20–30% of anti-D sera also appear to contain anti-C. Usually, this anti-C is not a separable antibody and is probably more correctly called anti-G (see p. 256). About 1–2% of anti-D sera also contain anti-E. Anti-C (and anti-G) in the absence of anti-D is very uncommon.

The incidence of other Rh antibodies is much lower, but together they are more common than anti-K (Kell), which is the most immunogenic antigen after D. In routine screening, pure anti-E is the most common, followed by anti-c, although anti-c is a more common cause of HDFN, which can be severe. This is probably because about half of the examples of anti-E are weak, naturally occurring antibodies. Anti-e, like anti-C, is very rare.

The vast majority of Rh antibodies are IgG and do not fix complement. Anti-D may occasionally be partly IgA. IgM anti-D is very rare.

D immunization

The realization that D-negative women without anti-D who had just delivered a D-positive child could be protected from forming anti-D by the injection of IgG anti-D soon after delivery has been a powerful stimulus for experimental work on D-negative volunteers. About 90% of D-negative people will make anti-D after the transfusion of a large volume of D-positive cells, and 70% will respond to repeated small volumes.

It has been shown that 20 μg (100 IU) of anti-D immunoglobulin given intramuscularly will give complete protection from 1 mL of concentrated D-positive red cells (approximately 2 mL of blood). This figure is the basis for the standard dose of 100 μg (500 IU) anti-D immunoglobulin given post partum in the UK, as it will cover the vast majority of cases of transplacental haemorrhage (TPH). A dose of 3.2–4.0 mg of anti-D immunoglobulin given intravenously will protect a D-negative recipient against the consequences of inadvertently transfusing a unit of D-positive whole blood (c. 200 mL of red cells). If D-positive platelets need to be given to D-negative girls and women of childbearing age, they should be protected with a dose of intravenous anti-D immunoglobulin.

The mechanism of protection by anti-D immunoglobulin is not really known. Two explanations have been suggested. The first is that the passively administered antibody leads to phagocytosis of antibody-coated red cells and their rapid destruction by mononuclear phagocytic cells in the spleen before they can combine with receptors of immunologically competent cells. The second is a central mechanism by which the Fc fragment of the antibody combined to antigen might give a suppressive or inactivating signal to the immunocompetent cells. It has been calculated that the amount of passive antibody needed to protect the recipient from antibody formation is less than that needed to cover all the D antigen sites on the injected Rh-positive cells.

Prior to the advent of Rh immunoprophylaxis, the first ABO-compatible, D-positive baby resulted in the primary immunization of about 17% of D-negative women. In about half of these women, the antibodies appeared within 6 months of delivery; in the other half, the antibodies became detectable by the end of the second pregnancy.

Source of anti-D for immunoprophylaxis

Anti-D is usually obtained from immunized D-negative volunteer men and from women unable to bear children from the USA. Those with low levels of anti-D are deliberately restimulated with D-positive red cells. Plasma from these donors is harvested by apheresis and sent to a fractionation plant for processing. It is unlikely that the use of human monoclonal anti-D for prophylaxis will become a reality in the near future, since clinical trials have been fraught with difficulty.

Detection of fetal red cells in the maternal circulation

Fetal red cells can be detected in a sample of maternal blood by the acid elution method of Kleihauer, which depends on the fact that fetal haemoglobin is more resistant to elution in an acid medium than adult haemoglobin. Thus, fetal haemoglobin is retained in the cell and the fetal red cell stains darkly with the counterstain, whereas adult haemoglobin elutes and the mother's red cells appear as ghosts. Fetal D-positive cells can also be quantified in the maternal circulation by flow cytometry after fluorescent staining with anti-D, with as few as 0.05% of fetal cells being detected.

Fetal red cells can frequently be detected in the mother's circulation, particularly during the last trimester of pregnancy and after delivery. In about 85% of blood samples taken soon after delivery, the proportion of fetal cells to adult cells is less than 1 in 20 000 (equivalent to a TPH of less than 0.5 mL). In two to three samples per 1000 deliveries, the TPH will be of the order of 10 mL of whole blood (5 mL of red cells) or more. Such women, if D-negative and delivering a D-positive infant, will not be protected by the standard UK anti-D immunoglobulin dose of 100 μg and additional protection should be given. All laboratories should standardize the conditions of the acid elution technique (or any other quantitative technique) in order to estimate the absolute amount of fetal red cells present in the maternal circulation.

Immunization by abortion, miscarriage and obstetric intervention

Abortion and miscarriage can induce the immunization of D-negative women; the incidence is greater if the abortion is therapeutic and if it occurs in the second trimester rather than in the first. Amniocentesis, chorionic villus sampling, fetal blood sampling and other obstetric manoeuvres can also lead to immunization of D-negative women carrying a D-positive fetus.

Prediction of fetal Rh genotype by molecular methods

Knowledge of the molecular basis for D-negative phenotypes has made it possible to devise tests for predicting fetal D type from fetal DNA. This is valuable in determining whether the fetus of a woman with anti-D is at risk from HDFN. Most methods involve polymerase chain reaction (PCR)-based tests that detect the presence or absence of *RHD*, but it is also important to test for more than one region of *RHD*, so that hybrid genes responsible for partial D antigens do not give a false result, and to test for the *RHD* pseudogene (*RHDψ*), so that this does not give rise to a false-positive result.

Although fetal DNA can be obtained by amniocentesis, this procedure is associated with a significant risk of fetal loss and fetomaternal haemorrhage. An alternative source of fetal DNA for determining fetal D type in D-negative pregnant women is the small quantities of free fetal DNA present in maternal plasma. This non-invasive form of fetal D typing is now provided for pregnant women with significant levels of anti-D as a reference service in the UK and some other parts of Europe.

It is a common practice to offer all D-negative pregnant women one or two doses of anti-D immunoglobulin at around 28–30 weeks' and 34 weeks' gestation to prevent antenatal immunization. However, in a predominantly white population about 40% of these women will have a D-negative fetus and receive the treatment unnecessarily. Several successful trials have been carried out on high-throughput methods for determining fetal D type from DNA in maternal plasma, and it is likely that fetal D testing of all D-negative pregnant women will be available in some countries within the next few years. The testing will make it possible to discern which women are in need of routine antenatal prophylaxis because they are carrying a D-positive fetus.

The MNS system

MNS was discovered by Landsteiner and his colleagues in 1927 and the MNS genes were the first blood group genes to be cloned, in 1986 and 1987. The MNS system now contains 46 antigens.

Antigens of the MNS system

M and N are inherited as codominant Mendelian traits, giving rise to three common genotypes *M/M*, *M/N* and *N/N*. The *Ss* locus, which is closely linked to *MN*, also consists of two codominant alleles, at least in Europeans and Asians, producing S or s antigens. In northern Europeans, haplotype frequencies are as follows: *MS*, 25%; *Ms*, 28%; *NS*, 8%; *Ns*, 39%. The system also contains many variants. About 2% of black West Africans and 1.5% of African-Americans are S– s– and most of these lack the U antigen that is present when either S or s is expressed.

The MN antigens are carried on GPA, which is encoded by the *GYPA* gene on chromosome 4. M and N differ by amino acids at positions 1 and 5 of the external N-terminus of GPA. There are about 1 million molecules of GPA per cell, yet their absence in the rare En(a–) phenotype does not affect red cell function or survival. The negative charge of the red cells is mainly due to the ionized COOH groups of sialic acid (neuraminic acid), which is mostly carried on the oligosaccharides of GPA and can be removed with neuraminidase. En(a–) cells therefore have a reduced negative charge and behave serologically as if they have been treated with neuraminidase. GPB carries the S and s determinants, which represent an amino acid substitution at position 29. GPB is encoded by *GYPB*, which is closely linked and homologous to *GYPA*. S– s– U– red cells lack GPB. The sequence of the N-terminal amino acids of GPB is identical to that of N-specific GPA and accounts for the weak 'N' reactivity of *M/M* cells, provided they are S+ or s+. The numerous MNS variants mostly result from amino acid substitutions in GPA and GPB and from the formation of hybrid GPA–GPB molecules, formed by intergenic recombination between *GYPA* and *GYPB*. GPA and GPB are exploited as receptors by the malaria parasite *Plasmodium falciparum*.

Antibodies of the MNS system

Anti-M is uncommon and reacts with about 80% of random samples. It is usually naturally occurring, but can be immune and, very rarely, causes HDFN.

Anti-N is also rare and reacts with about 70% of random samples. It is nearly always a cold-reactive IgM antibody. Because of the 'N' activity of GPB at low temperatures, anti-N reacts with, and can be completely absorbed by, *M/M* cells, except those of the M+ N– S– s– phenotype. Useful anti-N lectin can be prepared from the seeds of *Vicia graminea*.

Anti-S, the rarer anti-s and anti-U are usually immune, IgG and can cause HDFN. They have also been implicated in HTRs. Anti-U only occurs in S– s– black people and reacts with all cells that have the S or s antigens and up to 50% of cells that are S– s–. Finding compatible blood for a patient with anti-U can prove difficult.

The Lutheran blood group system

Lutheran is a complex system comprising four pairs of allelic antigens: Lu^a and Lu^b, Au^a and Au^b, Lu6 and Lu9, Lu8 and Lu14. These represent single amino acid substitutions in the Lutheran glycoproteins. There are another 11 antigens of very high frequency in this system. The incidence of Lu^a/Lu^b phenotypes in the UK population is as follows: Lu(a+b–), 0.1%; Lu(a+b+), 7.5%; Lu(a–b+), 92.4%. The extremely rare Lu$_{null}$ phenotype, in which no Lutheran antigens are expressed, results from homozygosity for an inactive Lutheran gene; anti-Lu3 may be produced. Individuals heterozygous for a dominant suppressor gene, *In(Lu)*, have very low levels of Lutheran antigens and reduced levels of some other blood group antigens, including P$_1$ and In^b. *In(Lu)* represents mutations in the erythroid transcription factor gene *EKLF*.

Lutheran antibodies are uncommon and are not generally considered clinically significant, although anti-Lu^b may have caused mild delayed HTRs. Lu^a may be omitted from antibody screening cells.

The Lutheran glycoproteins bind the extracellular matrix glycoprotein laminin and might function as adhesion molecules with a role in erythropoiesis.

The Kell blood group system

The Kell system consists of one triplet and four pairs of allelic antigens – K and k; Kp^a, Kp^b and Kp^c; Js^a and Js^b; K11 and K17; K14 and K24 – all of which represent amino acid substitutions in the Kell glycoprotein, plus 15 high-frequency and five low-frequency antigens.

In European whites, the incidence of the K/k phenotypes, the most important clinically, is as follows: K+ k–, 0.2%; K+ k+, 8.7%; K– k+, 91.1%. K is rare in populations other than those of white people. Js^a is present in about 20% of black people, but is extremely rare in other ethnic groups. The very rare null phenotype of the Kell system, in which no Kell system antigens are expressed, is called K_o, and results from homozygosity for a variety of inactivating mutations in the *KEL* gene.

The Kell antigens are located on a glycoprotein of 93 kDa, which crosses the cell membrane once and has a large glycosylated C-terminal extracellular domain, maintained in a folded conformation by multiple disulphide bonds. Reduction of these bonds by 2-aminoethylisothiouronium bromide (AET) results in loss of expression of all Kell system antigens. The Kell glycoprotein has sequence and structural homology with a family of neutral endopeptidases that processes biologically important peptides. The Kell glycoprotein cleaves the biologically inactive peptide big endothelin-3 to produce endothelin-3, an active vasoconstrictor. Whether Kell performs this function *in vivo* is not known.

The Kell glycoprotein is linked by a single disulphide bond to the Xk protein, which is produced by an X-linked gene, *XK*. Absence of Xk protein, resulting from hemizygosity in males of a deletion of *XK* or *XK* inactivating mutations, gives rise to the McLeod phenotype, in which there is no expression of Kx antigen and weak expression of all Kell system antigens. This rare phenotype is also associated with McLeod syndrome, a neuroacanthocytosis that is usually characterized by late-onset muscular, neurological and, occasionally, psychiatric disorders, and abnormally shaped red cells. In some cases, an X chromosome deletion is large enough to encompass *XK* and *CYBB*, a gene for a subunit of flavocytochrome b_{558}, which leads to McLeod syndrome and chronic granulomatous disease (CGD). If boys with McLeod syndrome and CGD are transfused, they are liable to make anti-Kx, which can cause severe HTRs and makes compatible blood very difficult to find.

Anti-K is an important antibody in white populations; it is nearly always immune, IgG and complement-binding. It causes severe HTRs and HDFN. K antigen stimulates the formation of anti-K in about 10% of K-negative people who are given one unit of K-positive blood. About 0.1% of all cases of HDFN are caused by anti-K; most of the mothers will have had previous blood transfusions. HDFN caused by anti-K differs from Rh HDFN in that anti-K appears to cause fetal anaemia by suppression of erythropoiesis, rather than immune destruction of mature fetal erythrocytes. Kell antigen is expressed by erythroid cells at a very early stage of erythropoiesis and anti-K probably facilitates immune destruction of early erythroid progenitors, before they become haemoglobinized. Anti-K is best detected by the IAT; anti-K does not always agglutinate red cells treated with enzymes or suspended in low-ionic-strength solution.

Anti-k is a very rare antibody, which reacts with 99.8% of random blood samples. It is always immune and has been incriminated in HDFN. Most other Kell system antibodies are rare and best detected by the IAT.

The Duffy blood group system

Fy^a and Fy^b antigens represent a single amino acid substitution in the extracellular N-terminal domain of the Duffy glycoprotein. Their incidence in the UK is as follows: Fy(a+b−), 20%; Fy(a+b+), 46%; Fy(a−b+), 34%. About 70% of African-Americans and close to 100% of West Africans are Fy(a−b−). They are homozygous for an Fy^b allele containing a mutation in a binding site for the erythroid-specific GATA-1 transcription factor, which means that Duffy glycoprotein is not expressed in red cells, although it is present in other tissues. The Duffy glycoprotein is the receptor essential for penetration of *Plasmodium vivax* merozoites into erythroid cells and the Fy(a−b−) phenotype confers resistance to *P. vivax* malaria. An identical GATA mutation is found in an Fy^a allele in Papua New Guinea and in Brazil.

The Duffy glycoprotein (also called Duffy-antigen chemokine receptor, DARC) is a red cell receptor for a variety of chemokines, including interleukin 8. It might function as a 'sink' or scavenger for the removal of unwanted chemokines.

Anti-Fy^a is not infrequent and is found in previously transfused patients who have usually already made other antibodies. It is IgG, often complement-fixing and can cause HTRs, but seldom HDFN. It is best detected by IAT and does not react with red cells treated with the proteases papain and ficin. Anti-Fy^b is very rare and is always immune.

The Kidd blood group system

Kidd has two alleles, Jk^a and Jk^b, which represent a single amino acid change in the Kidd glycoprotein. Phenotype frequencies in the UK population are as follows: Jk(a+b−), 25%; Jk(a+b+), 50%; Jk(a−b+), 25%. A Kidd null phenotype, Jk(a−b−), results from homozygosity for inactivating mutations in the Kidd gene, *SLC14A1*. It is very rare in most populations, but reaches an incidence of greater than 1% in Polynesians. The Kidd glycoprotein is a urea transporter in red cells and in renal endothelial cells.

Anti-Jk^a is uncommon and anti-Jk^b is very rare, but they may both cause severe transfusion reactions and, to a lesser extent, HDFN. Kidd antibodies have often been implicated in delayed HTRs; they are IgG and predominantly complement-fixing up to C3b, but may be difficult to detect because they tend to disappear and then reappear promptly in an anamnestic response. The antiglobulin test is the best method for detection; reactions will be enhanced if the cells have been protease-treated or if fresh serum is added as a source of complement. Patients who have made Kidd antibodies should always be given an antibody card.

The Diego blood group system

Diego is a large system of 21 antigens: two pairs of allelic antigens – Di^a and Di^b, Wr^a and Wr^b – plus 17 antigens of very low frequency. All represent single amino acid substitutions in band 3, the red cell anion exchanger. The original Diego antigen, Di^a, is very rare in white and black people, but relatively common in Mongoloid people, with frequencies varying between 1% in Japanese and 50% in some native South Americans. Anti-Di^a and anti-Di^b are immune and rare, but can cause HDFN. Wr^a has a frequency of about 0.1%. Its high-frequency antithetical antigen, Wr^b, is dependent on an interaction between GPA and band 3 for its expression. Naturally occurring anti-Wr^a is present in approximately 1% of blood donors. Anti-Wr^a is often found in the serum of patients who have made other antibodies or who are suffering from autoimmune haemolytic anaemia. Very rarely, anti-Wr^a causes HDFN.

The Dombrock blood group system

Do^a and Do^b antigens represent a single amino acid substitution on the Dombrock glycoprotein, a member of the ADP-ribosyltransferase family, which also expresses the high-incidence antigens Gy^a, Hy, Jo^a and DOYA. Approximately 67% of northern Europeans are Do(a+) and 82% Do(b+). Gy(a−) red cells are Do(a−b−) Hy− Jo(a−). Dombrock antibodies are extremely rare, immune and are best detected by IAT; they have been implicated in severe acute and delayed HTRs. Anti-Do^a and anti-Do^b reagents are rare and unreliable, so Dombrock typing is best achieved by molecular methods.

The Colton blood group system

Co^a and Co^b represent a single amino acid substitution in the water channel aquaporin-1. Colton phenotype frequencies in white people are as follows: Co(a+b−), 90.5%; Co(a+b+), 9.0%; Co(a−b+), 0.5%. The extremely rare Colton null phenotype, Co(a−b−), results from homozygosity for inactivating mutations in the Colton gene, AQP1. Colton antibodies are very uncommon. Anti-Co^a has caused severe HDFN, and has been implicated in acute and delayed HTRs.

Some other blood group systems

Yt^a and Yt^b of the Yt system represent a single amino acid change in red cell membrane acetylcholinesterase. Yt^a and Yt^b have frequencies of about 99.8% and 8% respectively. Anti-Yt^a

and anti-Yt^b are exceptional and most are of no clinical significance.

The Scianna system consists of seven antigens, including the allelic antigens Sc1 and Sc2 of high and low frequency, respectively. They are located on the adhesion protein ERMAP. Scianna antibodies are very rare and little is known of their clinical significance.

The Xg system comprises two antigens, Xg^a and CD99, encoded by separate but homologous genes on the X chromosome; CD99 is also expressed on the Y chromosome. The corresponding antibodies are rare and of no clinical significance.

The eight antigens of the Gerbich system, three of high frequency and five of low frequency, are located on GPC and GPD, which are encoded by a single gene, GYPC. The 15 antigens of the Cromer system and nine antigens of the Knops system are carried on the complement regulatory glycoproteins decay accelerating factor (CD55) and complement receptor 1 (CD35), respectively. Antibodies of these three systems are not generally considered clinically significant, although antibodies of the Knops system are relatively common and may obscure identification of other, clinically important antibodies in the same serum. Once identified, Knops antibodies can be ignored from a clinical point of view.

Antigens with high or low frequency

There are many other antigens, of either very high or very low incidence, that have not been assigned to blood group systems. Anti-Vel, -Lan, -At^a, -AnWj and -MAM are examples of antibodies to high-frequency antigens that have caused HDFN and/or HTRs. For those rare individuals who have formed antibodies to high-frequency antigens, the provision of compatible blood can be a problem; it is often necessary to approach the national or international panels of rare donors for compatible units.

Antibodies to low-frequency antigens are usually naturally occurring; they may occasionally give rise to unexpected incompatible cross-matches. Some antibodies to low-frequency antigens have caused HDFN.

Polyagglutinable red cells

Erythrocyte polyagglutination is the agglutination of red cells irrespective of blood group by many sera from normal adults. Polyagglutinable red cells are not agglutinated by the patient's own serum. The abnormality is a property of the red cells, not of the sera, in contrast to panagglutination, which is the agglutination of most red cells by one serum.

There are two main categories of polyagglutination, acquired and inherited. The acquired forms can be subdivided into

Table 15.12 Some characteristics of T, Tk, Tn and Cad polyagglutinable red cells.

	T	Tk	Tn	Cad
MN antigens	↓	Normal	↓	Normal
ABH antigens	Normal	↓	Normal	Normal
Most normal sera	+	+	+	+
Glycine soja lectin	+	−	+	+
Arachis hypogaea lectin	++	+	−	−
Bandeiraea simplicifolia lectin	−	+	−	−
Salvia sclarea lectin	−	−	+	−
Dolichos biflorus lectin (other than group A₁)	−	−	+	+
Polybrene* solution	−	+	+mf	+

*Polybrene is a positively charged polymer that agglutinates cells with a negative charge and fails to aggregate sialic acid-deficient cells.
↓, reduced reactivity of MN or ABH antigens; mf, mixed field.

Table 15.13 Structure of T, Tn and Tk antigens.

O-linked oligosaccharide of GPA and GPB

NeuNAcα2→3Galβ1→3GalNAc–Ser/Thr	Normal
$\quad\quad\quad\quad\quad\quad$ 6	
$\quad\quad\quad\quad\quad\quad$ ↑	
$\quad\quad\quad\quad\quad\quad$ 2	
$\quad\quad\quad\quad\quad\quad$ NeuNAc	T
Galβ1→3GalNAc–Ser/Thr	Tn
GalNAc–Ser/Thr	

A-, B- or H-active chains modified by endo-β-galactosidase

GlcNAcβ1→3Galβ1→4GlcNAc–R	Tk

Gal, galactose; GalNAc, *N*-acetylgalactosamine; GlcNAc, *N*-acetylglucosamine; NeuNAc, *N*-acetylneuraminic acid (sialic acid); R, remainder of molecule; Ser/Thr, serine or threonine.

(i) microbial polyagglutination, which results either from the passive coating of red cells with bacteria or their products or from the action of microbial enzymes on red cell surface oligosaccharides (T, Tk, acquired B); and (ii) non-microbial polyagglutination, which is caused by somatic mutation (Tn). There are four types of inherited polyagglutination: Cad (strong expression of Sdᵃ), congenital dyserythropoietic anaemia type II (CDAII or HEMPAS), NOR and Hyde Park. Lectins are required for the identification of the different types of polyagglutination (Table 15.12).

T activation

T activation occurs transiently in some patients with an obvious microbial infection, especially *Vibrio cholerae*, *Clostridium perfringens*, *Streptococcus pneumoniae*, various other streptococci and the influenza virus. These microbes produce sialidases, which remove sialic acid (*N*-acetylneuraminic acid) from the oligosaccharides of membrane sialoglycoproteins (Table 15.13) to expose the hidden T antigen (galactose linked to *N*-acetylgalactosamine), with an accompanying loss of negative surface charge.

Most adult sera contain naturally occurring, cold-reacting, complement-fixing, IgM anti-T. Most cases of T activation and other forms of polyagglutination were detected by the discrepancy in results of cell and serum ABO grouping, but with the introduction of monoclonal antibody reagents polyagglutination is found much less often.

T polyagglutination may be associated with (i) haemolytic anaemia, (ii) HTRs (especially in children) caused by anti-T in transfused plasma, although this is still questionable, (iii) haemolytic–uraemic syndrome and (iv) neonatal necrotizing enterocolitis.

Peanut (*Arachis hypogaea*) lectin is the most effective tool for identification of T-activated cells (Table 15.12).

Tk activation

Tk activation, like T activation, is transient and associated with infection. Endo-β-galactosidases produced by *Bacteroides fragilis*, various clostridia or *Candida albicans* remove β-galactose from ABH polysaccharide chains, exposing *N*-acetylglucosamine (see Tables 15.7 and 15.13), with the consequent depression of ABH expression, without affecting the quantity of sialic acid on the red cell. Tk cells are specifically agglutinated by BSII lectin, an extract from *Bandeiraea simplicifolia* (see Table 15.12). These cells are also agglutinated by peanut lectin, probably owing to the exposure of galactose, the next sugar in the chain.

Tn activation

Tn activation, unlike T and Tk, is a persistent abnormality caused by an abnormal clone of stem cells arising by somatic mutation. Tn is often associated with other haematological abnormalities, such as chronic haemolytic anaemia, leucopenia or thrombocytopenia, but may be present in healthy individuals. Somatic mutation in a gene encoding a molecular chaperone leads to a deficiency of T-synthase, the galactosyltransferase that elongates the O-linked oligosaccharides on GPA. Consequently, many of the O-glycans consist of only *N*-acetylgalactosamine, the immunodominant sugar of Tn (see Table 15.13). This loss results in a depression of M and N antigens, a loss of sialic acid and a negative charge similar to that found in T activation. Only some of the red cells are agglutinated by the anti-Tn present in all normal adult sera, giving a mixed field appearance in agglutination tests. Platelets also show two populations. *Salvia sclarea* lectin specifically agglutinates Tn-activated cells, and the exposed *N*-acetylgalactosamine molecules can be detected with *D. biflorus* lectin (but only in people who are not group A$_1$).

White cell and platelet antigens and antibodies

HLA and transfusion

The HLA system is covered in Chapter 37. Leucocyte-reactive antibodies have in the past been reported, albeit transiently, in up to 96% of massively transfused patients. Complement-fixing lymphocytotoxic antibodies have been found in as many as 50% of patients receiving multiple transfusions of platelet concentrates over a 4-week period. This frequency is lower in immunosuppressed patients. In contrast, some patients never become HLA immunized, despite repeated transfusions, and are considered to be non-responders to HLA. Pregnancy can lead to HLA antibodies in approximately 15%, 25% and 35% of women after a first, second or third pregnancy, respectively. Such antibodies are generally of class I specificity, with anti-HLA-B being approximately twice as prevalent as anti-HLA-A.

HLA antibodies stimulated by pregnancy or transfusion are usually IgG and complement-fixing; naturally occurring IgM antibodies produced without a known stimulus, usually HLA-B8 specific, can be found in about 1% of individuals. The clinical importance of HLA antibodies relates to their ability to mediate graft rejection. In pregnant women, IgG antibodies may cross the placenta but are not considered to be a cause of neonatal leucopenia or thrombocytopenia. HLA antibodies are the usual cause of immunological refractoriness to random donor platelet transfusions, but not all patients with HLA antibodies are refractory to platelet transfusions, because platelets carry HLA

class I antigens, and a small proportion of immunologically refractory patients have no detectable lymphocytotoxic antibodies. Currently, the most sensitive and specific technique for detecting and identifying cytotoxic and non-cytotoxic HLA antibodies is Luminex. In this technique the relevant recombinant or purified proteins (antigens) are bound to coloured polystyrene beads of uniform size. These beads are then incubated with the patient's serum. The reaction is visualized using a phycoerythrin-conjugated anti-human IgG; following washing, the beads are run on a LabScan 100 flow-based machine to detect the reactions against the different beads. Two laser beams are used: one laser discriminates between different coloured beads and the other quantifies the fluorescent reporter molecule. The management of patients who become immunologically refractory to platelet transfusions is described in Chapter 16.

Residual HLA antigens, often referred to as Bg antigens, are also present on red cells of some individuals and HLA antibodies have been implicated in rare cases of delayed and acute HTRs.

Neutrophil-specific antigens and antibodies

Neutrophils carry not only HLA class I antigens but also neutrophil-specific antigens, now termed the HNA system (Table 15.14). Antibodies showing specificity to the following antigens are clinically important.
1 Alloimmune neonatal neutropenia (HNA-1a, HNA-1b, HNA-1c, HNA-2, HNA-3a, HNA-4a).
2 Febrile transfusion reactions (HNA-1a, HNA-1b, HNA-2, and other unidentified antigens on FcγRIIIb and CD18).
3 Transfusion-related acute lung injury, caused by the passive transfer of mainly HLA antibodies, but also HNA antibodies in donor plasma (HNA-1a, HNA-1b, HNA-2, HNA-3a, NB2).
4 Autoimmune neutropenia, in adults or in infancy.
The antigens of the HNA-1 system are expressed on FcγRIIIb; those of HNA-4 and HNA-5 on the integrins $\alpha_M\beta_2$ (MAC-1) and $\alpha_L\beta_2$ (LFA-1), respectively. In addition, neutrophils express polymorphic antigens that also occur on endothelial cells (EM

Table 15.14 Neutrophil antigens.

System	Antigen	Previous names	Frequency (%)*	Glycoprotein	Amino acid change
HNA-1	HNA-1a	NA1	61.2	FcγRIIIb	Arg36, Asp65, Asp82, Val106
	HNA-1b	NA2, NC1	89.6		Ser36, Ser65, Asp82, Ile106
	HNA-1c	SH	< 0.01		Asp78
HNA-2	HNA-2a	NB1	90.8	58–64 kDa glycoprotein	
HNA-3	HNA-3a	5b		SLC44A2, CTL2	Arg154
HNA-4	HNA-4a	Mart^a		CD11b, Mac-1, CR3, $\alpha_M\beta_2$ integrin	Arg61
HNA-5	HNA-5a	Ond^a		CD11a, LFA-1, $\alpha_L\beta_2$ integrin	Arg766

*In white people.

antigens), monocytes (HMA antigens), monocytes plus lymphocytes (HNA-4, HNA-5), and granulocytes and lymphocytes (SL).

Working with granulocytes is cumbersome and typing, as well as antibody screening, should be left to specialized laboratories. The techniques most widely used to detect neutrophil antigens and antibodies are the granulocyte agglutination test (GAT), the granulocyte immunofluorescence test (GIFT) and the monoclonal antibody immobilization of granulocyte antigens (MAIGA) assay. GAT and GIFT will detect HLA antibodies, including non-complement fixing ones that are not detectable by the lymphocytotoxicity test (LCT). Genotyping is also used for determining phenotype, but is not applicable to HNA-2, because the HNA-2 null phenotype results from a transcription defect.

The discrimination of granulocyte-specific antibodies from granulocyte-reactive antibodies such as anti-HLA, which also react with other leucocyte subsets, requires access to large panels of HLA-typed granulocytes and lymphocytes and the application of tests that detect non-complement-fixing lymphocyte-binding antibodies (e.g. GIFT and MAIGA). More recently, the Luminex technique (see above) LABScreen[R] has been described, using recombinant antigens for HNA-1a, HNA-1b, HNA-1c and HNA-2a and purified HNA antigens for HNA-4a and HNA-5a.

Neutrophil antibodies can be found in as many as 3% of pregnant women, especially if their serum is tested against their partner's neutrophils. However, neonatal alloimmune neutropenia is very rare and, as expected, associated with the presence of potent IgG antibodies. Neutrophil autoantibodies are usually IgG, although some cold-reacting IgM antibodies have also been reported; some may be cytotoxic. Soluble IgG-containing immune complexes, rather than granulocyte-binding (auto) antibodies, may cause the neutropenia associated with Felty syndrome. Autoimmune neutropenia may also be caused by antibodies that prevent neutrophil precursor maturation rather than by destroying mature neutrophils, and some drug-dependent antibodies may also act by binding to neutrophil precursors.

Platelet-specific antigens and antibodies

Platelets carry ABH, Lewis, Ii and P antigens, as well as HLA class I antigens and the platelet-specific human platelet antigens (HPA). The HLA class I antigens are predominantly HLA-A and HLA-B; HLA-C is only weakly expressed on platelets. In some individuals, HLA-A and HLA-B are barely detectable, or undetectable, on the platelet surface. HLA antibodies are the single most important cause of immunological refractoriness to random donor platelet transfusions, although platelet-specific antibodies occur in 3–9% of cases, usually in association with HLA antibodies. HPA antibodies are also responsible for post-transfusion purpura (PTP) and neonatal alloimmune thrombocytopenia (NAIT) and, very occasionally, febrile transfusion reactions.

Over 20 antigens have been described as platelet-specific (Table 15.15). These include the antigens of the various HPA systems, most of which are composed of a high-incidence 'a' allele (e.g. *HPA-1a*) and a low-incidence 'b' allele (*HPA-1b*). However, some of the HPA antigens are not truly platelet specific; the HPA-1 antigens are also found on endothelial cells, which might contribute to the severity of NAIT and PTP caused by anti-HPA-1a. The HPA-5 antigens have been described on activated T cells and probably also on endothelial cells, on the VLA-2 (very late antigen-2) membrane protein. The genetic basis of the HPA alleles is known for all HPA systems. Almost all represent SNPs encoding amino acid substitutions at different positions on platelet glycoproteins (Table 15.15).

The platelet antibody specificity that most frequently causes PTP is anti-HPA-1a, found in 85% of cases; anti-HPA-1b has been reported in 5% and anti-HPA-3a in 7% of cases in Europe. Similarly, anti-HPA-1a is the most common cause of NAIT, having been reported in 80% of HPA-1a-negative mothers at the time of birth of an affected infant. Anti-HPA-5b has been found in 15% of NAIT cases, as have occasional examples of anti-HPA-1b and anti-HPA-3a, in HPA-1a-positive mothers in Europe.

Serological methods for platelet typing and antibody detection

Typing for platelet antigens by serology is difficult: sera with appropriate specificity are rare, usually contaminated by HLA antibodies, and generally lack the adequate potency required for reliable typing. Serology is now often replaced by PCR-based DNA typing methods.

Serological techniques for platelet antibody detection in patients' sera include the platelet suspension immunofluorescence test (PIFT), a solid-phase technology and an antigen-capture ELISA technique known by the acronym MAIPA (monoclonal antibody immobilization of platelet antigens). In the PIFT, HPA-typed platelets are incubated with the patient's serum, washed, and any bound immunoglobulin detected with a fluorescent anti-immunoglobulin conjugate is visualized by ultraviolet microscopy or flow cytometry. In the solid-phase method, platelets are anchored onto the bottom of U-well microtitre plates by a polyclonal rabbit/anti-human platelet serum. Following incubation with the patient's serum, platelet-bound IgG is subsequently detected using anti-human IgG-coated indicator red cells. In the MAIPA assay, donor platelets are incubated successively with the patient's serum and a mouse monoclonal antibody that recognizes a specific platelet membrane glycoprotein complex (e.g. anti-GPIIb/IIIa, anti-GPIa/IIa or anti-GPIb/IX), and are then solubilized in a mild detergent such as Triton X-100. Immune complexes in the resulting supernatant are captured into the wells of an ELISA plate coated with goat-anti-mouse IgG. Any human antibody present in a

Table 15.15 Platelet antigens.

System	Antigen	Previous names	Frequency (%)*	Glycoprotein	Amino acid change
HPA-1	HPA-1a	Zwᵃ, Pl^A1	97.6	GPIIIa	Leu33
	HPA-1b	Zwᵇ, Pl^A2	26.8		Pro33
HPA-2	HPA-2a	Koᵇ	99.4	GPIbα	Thr145
	HPA-2b	Koᵃ, Sibᵃ	14.3		Met145
HPA-3	HPA-3a	Bakᵃ, Lekᵃ	87.7	GPIIb	Iso843
	HPA-3b	Bakᵇ	64.1		Ser843
HPA-4	HPA-4a	Yukᵇ, Penᵃ	> 99.9	GPIIIa	Arg143
	HPA-4b	Yukᵃ, Penᵇ	< 0.2†		Gln143
HPA-5	HPA-5a	Brᵇ, Zavᵇ	99.0	GPIa	Glu505
	HPA-5b	Brᵃ, Zavᵃ, Hcᵃ	20.0		Lys505
HPA-6	HPA-6(b)	Caᵃ, Tuᵃ	< 0.01	GPIIIa	Arg489
					Gln489
HPA-7	HPA-7(b)	Mo	0.01	GPIIIa	Pro407
					Ala407
HPA-8	HPA-8(b)	Srᵃ	< 0.01	GPIIIa	Arg636
					Cys636
HPA-9	HPA-9(b)	Maxᵃ	< 0.01	GPIIb	Val837
					Met837
HPA-10w	HPA-10w(b)	Laᵃ	< 0.01	GPIIIa	Arg62
					Gln62
HPA-11w	HPA-11w(b)	Groᵃ	< 0.01	GPIIIa	Arg633
					His633
HPA-12w	HPA-12w(b)	Iyᵃ	< 0.01	GPIbβ	Gly15
					Glu15
HPA-13w	HPA13w(b)	Sitᵃ	< 0.01	GPIa	Thr799
					Met799
HPA-14w	HPA-14w(b)	Oeᵃ	< 1	GPIIIa	Lys611 deleted
HPA-15	HPA-15a	Govᵇ	80	CD109	Tyr703
	HPA-15b	Govᵃ	60		Ser703
HPA-16w	HPA 16w(b)	Duvᵃ	< 1	GPIIIa	Ile140
					Thr140

*In white people.
†In Japan.

captured monoclonal antibody–platelet glycoprotein trimolecular complex is detected with an anti-human immunoglobulin ELISA conjugate. Other techniques that have been used for platelet serology, although much less frequently, include platelet agglutination, the platelet radioactive antiglobulin test, ELISA, ⁵¹Cr release, monocyte chemiluminescence and complement fixation.

A new Luminex-based aproach, similar to one described for HLA antibodies, is currently being developed for the detection of HPA antibodies.

Molecular methods for platelet typing

Two alternative strategies for PCR typing have been widely used. In the first (PCR-RFLP), the relevant HPA genes are amplified with appropriate primers and the alleles encoded subsequently discriminated with allele-specific restriction enzymes. The length of the DNA fragments produced on cleavage by the enzymes are analysed by gel electrophoresis. In PCR-SSP, allele sequence-specific primers are used to amplify individual alleles and the PCR product is visualized after electrophoresis through agarose and staining with ethidium bromide. In these PCR-based typing methods, DNA extracted from lymphocytes is used because platelets, being anucleate, lack DNA. Amplification of genomic DNA by PCR-SSP can be used to type donors and patients, even when the latter are thrombocytopenic. Alternatively, platelet mRNA can be converted to cDNA with reverse transcriptase before PCR amplification by a 5′-nuclease (Taqman) assay.

Platelet provision and matching for immunologically refractory patients

The major cause of immunological refractoriness to platelet transfusion is the presence of HLA-A and/or HLA-B antibodies in multitransfused patients. Quite often, such antibodies are found to react with the lymphocytes from the majority (and sometimes all) of the donors included in the panel. Platelet-specific antibodies may occur in 3–9% or less of refractory patients. Implicated specificities have included anti-HPA-1a and anti-HPA-1b, as well as anti-HPA-3a, anti-HPA-2b and anti-HPA-15b, and in this setting platelet-specific antibodies are usually accompanied by HLA antibodies.

Management of immunological refractoriness can often be accomplished by transfusion of platelets obtained by apheresis from HLA-typed donors that match the HLA type of the immunologically refractory patient. The best matched platelets are theoretically from 'A-matched' donors which do not express HLA-A or HLA-B antigens that are not present on the recipient's lymphocytes. Some degree of mismatching of donor-recipient phenotypes may be permissible. 'HLA-B-matched' platelets, which differ by one or more antigens (B1 to B4 matches) within a serologically cross-reactive group of HLA-A or HLA-B antigens, can often provide satisfactory increments in platelet counts, for example by transfusing platelets from an HLA-A1-A11-B8-B27 donor to an A1-A11-B8-B7 patient (B7 and B27 are cross-reactive). Donors with apparently 'homozygous' HLA phenotypes (e.g. A1-X-B8-X) can often provide 'A-matched' platelets for a variety of recipients (e.g. A1-A2-B8-B44) who have an HLA haplotype in common with the homozygous donor. All matched donor platelets must be gamma-irradiated before transfusion to prevent potentially fatal transfusion-associated graft-versus-host disease.

The provision of HLA-matched platelets is an extremely expensive service, so it is strongly recommended that their use is properly justified by taking post-transfusion platelet counts 1 or 24 hours after transfusion. In immunological refractoriness to platelet transfusions, the provision of HLA-matched platelets may not be sufficient per se for obtaining satisfactory post-transfusion platelet increments; it could be that a previously unrecognized HLA specificity, detectable by cross-matching the donor's lymphocytes by LCT, might be present, or that platelet-specific antibodies might be involved. If a patient does not show good increments when transfused with HLA-matched platelets that gave negative LCT cross-matches, then cross-matching the donor's platelets by a method such as the solid-phase technique could prove valuable in selecting compatible donors.

If HLA-matched or cross-match (by LCT or solid phase) compatible platelets still do not provoke satisfactory increments and the presence of platelet-specific antibodies has been excluded, then it is recommended to revert to the transfusion of platelets from random donors. Larger than normal doses of platelet concentrates may be needed.

Plasma protein antigens and antibodies

Many components of human plasma can be antigenic when whole blood or plasma is transfused. Problems associated with such antibodies represent one of the less well investigated areas in blood transfusion. Urticarial reactions following the transfusion of blood or plasma components are not infrequent, although the culprit proteins are only rarely disclosed and are most likely to consist of haptens present in donor plasma derived from food ingested recently (e.g. chocolate, prawns, drugs). Quite often the antibodies causing the reactions are IgE, present in atopic recipients. Antibodies to factor VIII are not known to cause transfusion reactions, although they will cause inhibition of the activity of transfused factor VIII. Antibodies to IgA can lead to serious anaphylactic reactions. Antibodies to IgG determinants may cause problems in blood grouping, but their role in transfusion reactions is debatable.

Selected bibliography

General

Klein HG, Anstee DJ (2005) *Mollison's Blood Transfusion in Clinical Medicine*, 11th edn. Blackwell Publishing, Oxford.

Red cell antigens

Avent ND, Reid ME (2000) The Rh blood group system: a review. *Blood* **95**: 375–87.

Chester MA, Olsson ML (2001) The ABO blood group gene: a locus of considerable genetic diversity. *Transfusion Medicine Reviews* **15**: 177–200.

Daniels G (2002) *Human Blood Groups*, 2nd edn. Blackwell Science, Oxford.

Daniels G (2005) The molecular genetics of blood group polymorphism. *Transplant Immunology* **14**: 143–53.

Daniels G, Bromilow I (2006) *Essential Guide to Blood Groups*. Blackwell Publishing, Oxford.

Daniels GL, Fletcher A, Garratty G *et al.* (2004) Blood group terminology 2004. From the ISBT Committee on Terminology for Red Cell Surface Antigens. *Vox Sanguinis* **87**: 304–16.

Hadley TJ, Peiper SC (1997) From malaria to chemokine receptor: the emerging physiologic role of the Duffy blood group antigen. *Blood* **89**: 3077–91.

Henry S, Samuelsson B (2000) ABO polymorphisms and their putative biological relationships with disease. In: *Human Blood Cells. Consequences of Genetic Polymorphism and Variations* (M-J King, ed.), pp. 1–103. Imperial College Press, London.

Kumpel BM (2007) Efficacy of Rh D monoclonal antibodies in clinical trials as replacement therapy for prophylactic anti-D immunoglobulin: more questions than answers. *Vox Sanguinis* **93**: 99–111.

Poole J, Daniels G (2007) Blood group antibodies and their significance in transfusion medicine. *Transfusion Medicine Reviews* **21**: 58–71.

Wagner FF, Flegel WA (2000) *RHD* gene deletion occurred in the Rhesus box. *Blood* **95**: 3662–8.

Watkins WM (2001) The ABO blood group system: historical background. *Transfusion Medicine* **11**: 243–65.

Yamamoto PI, Clausen H, White T *et al.* (1990) Molecular genetic basis of the histo-blood group ABO system. *Nature* **345**: 229–33.

Yu L-C, Twu Y-C, Chou M-L *et al.* (2003) The molecular genetics of the human *I* locus and molecular background explaining the partial association of the adult I phenotype with congenital cataracts. *Blood* **101**: 2081–8.

White cell and platelet antigens

Blanchette VS, Johnson J, Rand M (2000) The management of alloimmune neonatal thrombocytopenia. *Baillière's Best Practice and Research: Clinical Haematology* **13**: 365–90.

Bux J (2008) Human neutrophil alloantigens. *Vox Sanguinis* **94**: 277–85.

Chapman CE, Strainsby D, Jones H *et al.* on behalf of the Serious Hazards of Transfusion Steering Group (2009) Ten years of haemovigilance reports of the transfusion-related acute lung injury in the UK, and the impact of preferential use of male donor plasma. *Transfusion* **49**: 440–52.

Hod E, Schwartz J (2008) Platelet transfusion refractoriness. *British Journal of Haematology* **142**: 348–60.

International Forum (2003) Detection of platelet-reactive antibodies in patients who are refractory to platelet transfusions, and the selection of compatible donors. *Vox Sanguinis* **84**: 73–88.

Lemnrau AG, Cardoso S, Creary L *et al.* (2009) HPA typing of neonatal alloimmune thrombocytopenia (NAIT) patients using whole genome amplified DNA and a 5′-nuclease assay. *Transfusion* **49**: 953–8.

Lucas GF, Metcalfe P (2000) Platelet and granulocyte polymorphisms. *Transfusion Medicine* **10**: 157–74.

Metcalfe P, Watkins NA, Ouwehand WH *et al.* (2003) Nomenclature of human platelet antigens. *Vox Sanguinis* **85**: 240–5.

Murphy MF, Navarrete C, Massey E (2009) Donor screening as a TRALI risk reduction strategy. *Transfusion* **49**: 1779–82.

Webert KE, Blajchman MA (2003) Transfusion related acute lung injury. *Transfusion Medicine Reviews* **17**: 252–62.

CHAPTER 16

Clinical blood transfusion

16

Marcela Contreras[1], Clare PF Taylor[2] and John A Barbara[1]

[1]University College London and Blood Transfusion International, London, UK
[2]National Blood Service, North London Centre, London, UK

Introduction

This chapter describes pretransfusion testing of the recipient's blood, complications and adverse effects of blood transfusion, appropriate use of components and, finally, a description of the features of haemolytic disease of the newborn. The first section deals with aspects of blood donation and collection, and the preparation and storage of blood components.

The blood donor (Tables 16.1 and 16.2)

Blood donation shall in all circumstances be voluntary. Financial profit must never be a motive for the donor or for those collecting the donation.

These statements sum up the attitude of the World Health Organization (WHO) and the International Society of Blood Transfusion towards the principle of blood donation. However, in a number of countries worldwide, whole blood donation and apheresis plasma donation are remunerated. There are data showing that the microbiological safety of donations from paid donors is inferior, and stringent post-donation testing and viral inactivation, when possible, are required to enhance blood safety.

In general, blood donors should be healthy adults between the ages of 17–18 and 65–70 years. These age limits vary slightly worldwide, but a lower limit is set to take account of the high iron requirements of adolescence. An upper limit is necessary because with age there is an increase in medical conditions that might make blood donation more hazardous and which increase the probability that coincidental accidents may be attributed to the act of giving blood. Pregnant and lactating women are not accepted as donors of allogeneic blood, again because of high iron requirements.

Because donors should be fit healthy individuals, no donations should be accepted from those who have ever suffered from cancer, diabetes, or heart or kidney disease. Those with severe allergic disorders should not give blood because recipients may develop temporary hypersensitivity reactions due to passively transfused antibodies.

Minor red cell abnormalities

Donors with minor red cell abnormalities, such as thalassaemia trait, sickle cell trait and hereditary spherocytosis, are perfectly acceptable, providing that the haemoglobin (Hb) screening test excludes anaemia. Red cells containing HbS have limited sur-

Postgraduate Haematology: 6th edition. Edited by A. Victor Hoffbrand, Daniel Catovsky, Edward G.D. Tuddenham, Anthony R. Green
© 2011 Blackwell Publishing Ltd.

Table 16.1 Measures to protect the donor.

Age 17–70 years (60 at first donation)
Weight above 50 kg (7 st 12 lb)
Haemoglobin > 13 g/dL for men, 12 g/dL for women
Minimum donation interval of 12 weeks (16 weeks advised) and
    three donations per year maximum
Pregnant and lactating women excluded because of high iron
    requirements
Exclusion of those with:
    Known cardiovascular disease, including hypertension
    Significant respiratory disorders
    Epilepsy and other CNS disorders
    Gastrointestinal disorders with impaired absorption
    Insulin-dependent diabetes
    Chronic renal disease
    Ongoing medical investigation or clinical trials
Exclusion of any donor returning to occupations such as driving
    bus, plane or train, heavy machine or crane operator,
    mining, scaffolding, etc. because delayed faint would be
    hazardous

Table 16.2 Conditions in the donor that lead to deferral.

All potential donors provided with information, so those at risk
    of HIV through lifestyle will refrain from donation (sexual
    practices, piercing, tattooing)
Donors with history of hepatitis deferred until 12 months after
    recovery
Exclusion of all potential donors who have themselves received a
    blood component transfusion since 1980 (due to risk of third
    party vCJD transmission)
Exclusion of those who have received pituitary-derived hormones
    or cadaveric dura mater or corneal grafts, and those with
    family history of CJD
Exclusion of those whose travel history places them at risk of
    malaria, Chagas disease (unless antibody test available) and
    SARS
Permanent exclusion of any donor who has had filariasis,
    bilharzia, yaws or Q fever
Exclusion for varying time periods following vaccinations
Exclusion after known exposure to infectious illnesses such as
    varicella
Exclusion of anyone with a malignant condition except fully
    excised BCC of skin
Exclusion of those with diseases of unknown origin, e.g. Crohn's
    disease
Donor deferral for most drugs based on the underlying illness,
    e.g. cardiovascular, diabetes, malignancy, anaemia
Exclusion of those taking teratogenic drugs or those that
    accumulate in the tissues

BCC, basal cell carcinoma; SARS, severe acute respiratory
syndrome; vCJD, variant Creutzfeldt–Jakob disease.

vival under conditions of reduced oxygen tension and so should not be transfused to newborn infants and patients with hypoxia or sickle cell disease. Red cells with HbS obstruct leucodepletion filters and it is therefore advisable, in the UK, to defer such people from blood donation. Blood from donors with glucose-6-phosphate dehydrogenase deficiency survives normally, unless the recipient is given oxidant drugs.

Volume of blood taken

Modern blood collection packs are designed to hold 450 ± 45 mL of blood, mixed with 63 mL of citrate-phosphate-dextrose-adenine (CPD-A) anticoagulant. The ratio of anticoagulant to blood must be maintained at the optimal level, and donations of less than 405 mL or more than 495 mL of blood should not be issued for clinical use. Healthy donors can generally withstand the loss of 450 mL of blood without any ill effect, but vasovagal reactions become more common in those who weigh less than 50.0 kg, as the standard donation represents a greater proportion of their total blood volume. The allowable donation frequency is generally 16 weeks in the UK, with a minimum of 12 weeks. In some countries, such as China and Japan, 'underweight', otherwise healthy, donors may donate smaller volumes (250 mL) of blood into specially designed packs containing the appropriate volume of anticoagulant. In several countries, including the UK, double doses of red cells are collected by apheresis from suitable large donors; such units are very useful for decreasing donor exposure in multitransfused patients such as those with β-thalassaemia major.

Haemoglobin estimation

A test to exclude anaemia is performed before donation. A convenient and widely used method depends on the specific gravity of a drop of blood, obtained by means of a fingerprick. An estimate of the haemoglobin value can be made, depending on whether the drop of capillary blood sinks in a copper sulphate solution of known specific gravity. According to the EU Blood Directive, the haemoglobin standard for male donors is 13.4 g/dL and for female donors is 12.4 g/dL, although lower limits have been introduced in some countries. The copper sulphate method tends to underestimate the haemoglobin value and may lead to unnecessary rejection of donors. On the other hand, the specific gravity of whole blood does not depend solely on the haemoglobin content of red cells and a pathological rise in plasma protein level or total white cell count (e.g. myeloma, chronic myeloid leukaemia) can lead to an anaemic donor passing the haemoglobin test. An alternative rapid simple colorimetric test using filter paper has been tried by WHO and is used in some countries. Many transfusion services use portable haemoglobinometers on donors who fail the copper sulphate test, or as an alternative screening test. A relatively inexpensive portable haemoglobinometer can significantly reduce the number of unnecessary rejections.

Donation intervals

A donation of 450 mL of blood contains approximately 200 mg of iron, which is lost to the body. Studies have shown depletion of iron stores in those who give three or four blood donations per year, but overt iron deficiency anaemia is uncommon except in female donors of childbearing age. In general, donors are given the opportunity to donate two or three times per year in the UK (minimum interval 16 weeks), but some donors are able to donate more frequently without any significant iron depletion. When it is standard practice to take donations at shorter intervals, appropriate monitoring and/or iron supplements are recommended.

Hazards of blood donation

The most common hazard of blood donation is fainting, reported in 2–5% of all donors, but being especially common in young people and in those donating for the first time, particularly if they are nervous or apprehensive. A sympathetic approach by blood collection staff, provision of a drink prior to donation, enforcement of an adequate rest period, and constant vigilance to detect warning signs of an impending vasovagal attack can help avert this problem. Once a faint occurs, the standard treatment of rest in a horizontal position and elevation of the legs is usually sufficient. Delayed faints occurring after a donor has left the clinic are potentially hazardous and a contraindication to further donation. For this reason, those donors who are drivers, machine operators, scaffolders and so on should not return to work on the day of donation. Infection of the venepuncture site should be avoided by meticulous attention to skin cleansing and aseptic techniques.

All blood collection packs are manufactured as integral sets; each needle is sterile, to be used only once. No pack should be reused (even on the same donor) if the initial venepuncture attempt fails. Bruising of the arm may occur, particularly when venous access has been difficult; firm pressure over the site for 2–3 min and an explanation to the donor are usually sufficient. In the very rare event of arterial puncture, elevation of the limb and firm pressure over the site for 10–15 min should be combined with prolonged rest if a whole donation has been taken, as the rate of blood donation under such circumstances is usually very rapid. Very occasionally, attempted venepuncture may result in trauma to the nerves in the arm, resulting in pain, paraesthesiae and numbness. Such symptoms generally resolve in a few days, but very rarely may take several months of recovery. Even rarer complications are aneurysms and arteriovenous fistulae, following arterial punctures.

Hazards of allogeneic blood transfusion

A number of diseases have the potential to be transmitted by transfusion of blood or its components. Donor selection criteria and subsequent testing of all donations are designed to prevent such transmission (Table 16.3).

The viruses that pose the greatest potential risk for transmission by transfusion are those that have long incubation periods (often causing subclinical infection), and especially those that may be carried by asymptomatic individuals for many years, or even lifelong. Alternatively, some viruses that are transfusion transmissible exhibit cell-associated latency. If the virus is latent in white blood cells, recrudescence of that virus, stimulated by allogeneic transfusion, can cause infection of the recipient.

More rarely, a few viruses causing acute infection can be transmitted in the short presymptomatic viraemic phase if this coincides with the time of blood donation. Such agents pose a risk only if recipients have not been previously infected and donors have become infected during an epidemic period (e.g. parvovirus B19) or after visiting endemic countries (e.g. hepatitis A). Theoretically, respiratory infections such as influenza and severe acute respiratory syndrome (SARS) may also pose a potential risk.

Bacteria, especially skin contaminants and blood-borne parasites, are also potentially transmissible by blood transfusion. The key transfusion-transmissible agents are summarized in Table 16.4.

Table 16.3 Measures to protect the recipient.

Measure	UK currently
Donor selection	Yes
Donor deferral/exclusion	Yes
Stringent arm cleansing	Yes
Diversion of the first 20–30 mL of blood collected	Yes
Microbiological testing of donations	Yes
Immunohaematological testing of donations	Yes
Leucodepletion of cellular blood components	Yes
Post-collection viral inactivation of FFP (e.g. MB or SD treatment)	For at-risk patients
Safest possible sources of donors for plasma-based products	For at-risk patients
Monitoring and testing for bacterial contamination	Under evaluation
Pathogen inactivation of cellular components (e.g. psoralens)	No
Prion filtration	No

MB, methylene blue; SD, solvent-detergent.

Table 16.4 Transfusion-transmissible agents.

Agents		Characteristics related to transfusion
Viruses		
Hepatotropic	HAV	Very rarely transfusion transmitted during incubation; no carrier state; faecal–oral transmission
	HEV	As above but person-to-person spread is rare
	HBV	2–6 month incubation period; carrier state; readily transmissible by blood
	HCV	Majority of cases asymptomatic; carrier state; readily transmissible by blood
Retroviruses	HIV-1 and HIV-2	Carrier state and latent in WBCs; readily transmissible by blood
	HTLV-I and HTLV-II	Latent in WBCs
Herpesviruses	CMV	50% of UK adults have been infected; latent in WBCs
	EBV	Most UK adults have been infected (therefore already exposed pre transfusion); latent in WBCs
Others	Parvovirus B19	Generally mild or asymptomatic, posing no transfusion risk except for non-immune aplastic anaemia patients and fetuses
		Approximately two-thirds of UK adults have been infected
		Seasonal variation (and epidemic years) in incidence rate
	West Nile virus	Recently exhibiting epidemic rates of transmission in summer months in North America
	Dengue virus	Transfusion transmission has been reported in Asia
Bacteria		
Endogenous	*Treponema pallidum*	Inactivated by storage at 4°C
		No transfusion transmissions reported in the past 15 years
	Yersinia enterocolitica	Very occasional transmissions, usually contaminated red cells transfused late in the storage period
Exogenous	For example *Staphylococcus epidermidis, Micrococcus, Sarcina*	Mainly skin commensals or contaminants
		Most common cause of platelet contamination
Parasites		
	Malaria	Only five verified transfusion cases reported in UK in 25 years (all *Plasmodium falciparum*)
	Chagas disease	No transmission of *Trypanosoma cruzi* by transfusion has been reported in UK; many cases in Latin America
Prions		
	Abnormal PrP	Transfusion risk from vCJD. Only five possible cases of transmission in 12 years (three with disease)

WBCs, white blood cells.

Hepatitis viruses

Donors with a history of hepatitis are deferred for 12 months. The hepatitis viruses can be transmitted in cellular and plasma components, as well as plasma products.

When serum from an individual with hepatitis B virus (HBV) is ultracentrifuged and examined with the electron microscope, three types of particle may be seen. The large (42-nm diameter) Dane particle is the actual virus with its central nucleocapsid core, which has its own antigenic constituent HBc. The core contains partially double-stranded DNA and DNA polymerase, and is surrounded by a lipoprotein coat carrying the hepatitis B surface antigen (HBsAg). The other two types of particles are 18–22 nm rods and spheres and represent overproduction of surface antigen material. HBsAg can be detected for a few months only in cases of acute HBV infection, or for years in chronic carriers. The HBe antigen is in soluble form and is present in the incubation period, during acute infection and during the first years of the carrier phase. HBeAg is a marker of high infectivity. Dane particles are very rare in the plasma of low-infectivity carriers. When HBc disappears, anti-HBc appears, persisting for a long time, in the presence or absence of HBsAg. All donations are tested for the presence of HBsAg by sensitive enzyme-linked immunosorbent assays (ELISAs) that can detect at least 0.2 IU/mL of HBsAg.

Hepatitis C virus (HCV) is recognized as the cause of the majority of cases of what was previously known as non-A non-B (NANB) hepatitis. Although electron microscopic visualization of HCV has not been verified, its genome has been cloned and ELISAs have been developed in which cloned and/or synthetic peptides can react with antibody to HCV. Combined antigen plus antibody detection tests are also available.

Individuals with a history of jaundice may be accepted as donors, provided that they have been shown to be negative for markers of HBV and HCV. Clinical jaundice may be due to causes other than HBV and HCV, including non-viral causes; also, the majority of donors who are positive for HBsAg have no such history, so there is no sense in rejecting all people who give a history of clinical jaundice. In the UK, the incidence of HBsAg in first-time blood donors is approximately 1 in 2000 and in established donors (i.e. new infections) less than 1 in 100 000. HBsAg-positive subjects are permanently excluded from donation, and should be under specialist follow-up, as they have an increased risk of developing chronic liver disease and hepatocellular carcinoma.

Although the transmission of HBV by blood and blood components has been virtually eliminated, HBsAg testing will not exclude all donors capable of transmitting HBV, as the sensitivity of presently available serological techniques may allow as many as 10^4–10^6 HBV genome copies per mililitre of plasma to remain undetected. The introduction of screening for anti-HBc and/or HBV DNA would reduce the very low risk of transmission of HBV yet further. Although reports of clinically apparent post-transfusion hepatitis are very rare in the UK, HBV DNA testing (as part of a 'triplex' assay that also detects HIV and HCV RNA) has been introduced in the UK in line with several other countries.

In the USA, before screening for anti-HCV was introduced, about 10% of transfusions caused significant increases in transaminase activity in recipients, the so-called NANB hepatitis. There were also occasional cases of symptomatic hepatitis. Acute HCV infection is usually mild, but a proportion of patients do develop chronic liver disease, with a risk of hepatocellular carcinoma. Confirmed rates of HCV positivity in the UK are 1 in 2000 for new donors and less than 1 in 100 000 for repeat donors. Methods of heat inactivation and solvent-detergent treatment of factors VIII and IX prevent transmission of HCV. Haemophiliacs who have received effectively inactivated factor VIII have proved negative for anti-HCV, in contrast with those who received untreated concentrate.

Hepatitis A virus is rarely transmitted by transfusion. Any donor who has been in close contact with a case (e.g. household contact) or developed hepatitis A is deferred for 12 months.

Hepatitis E virus is similarly rarely transmitted by transfusion. Like hepatitis A virus, hepatitis E has a short incubation period and no carrier state. Unlike hepatitis A it is rarely transmitted from person to person.

The so-called 'hepatitis G' virus (more correctly classified as GB virus-C) is not hepatotropic. Although transmissible by transfusion, it is asymptomatic and has not been associated with any pathology.

Human immunodeficiency virus (HIV-I and HIV-2)

The classical descriptions and the vast majority of the literature on AIDS refer to HIV-1; a second retrovirus capable of causing AIDS, HIV-2, mainly occurs in West Africa.

Human immunodeficiency virus (HIV) can be transmitted in both cellular and plasma components (platelets, white cells, single donor plasma, fresh-frozen plasma and cryoprecipitate). Most of the patients infected by the transfusion of blood components were transfused before the introduction of screening of blood donations for HIV antibodies. Moreover, the majority of recipients of blood products who were infected in the past were transfused before 1985 with unheated non-pasteurized pooled plasma products, mainly factor VIII and factor IX concentrates. Thus, HIV infection became an important sequel to transfusion of factor VIII concentrates to haemophiliacs in the early 1980s, before the introduction of heat treatment and other viral inactivation methods. HIV is more heat labile than HBV, especially when in solution. Prolonged heat treatment and other viral inactivation methods of plasma products are effective means of protecting haemophiliacs from infection.

Albumin solutions are pasteurized, and carry no risk of HIV transmission. Similarly, intramuscular immunoglobulin preparations are rendered safe from HIV infectivity by their manufacturing processes.

Certain behaviour patterns place individuals at greater risk of HIV infection. Accordingly, male homosexuals and bisexuals, intravenous drug users and prostitutes are permanently deferred from blood donation. The sexual partners of such individuals and of haemophiliacs treated with blood products are also excluded. In addition, large areas of sub-Saharan Africa and Southeast Asia have a high incidence of HIV seropositivity in the general population. Inhabitants of these areas and their partners are also considered to be at greater risk of HIV infection than heterosexual non-drug users in other areas of the world. Donor education and encouragement of those whose behaviour may have exposed them to HIV to exclude themselves from blood donation are highly cost-effective methods for the prevention of transmission of HIV infection by blood transfusion. Systems for donor selection and deferral should continue to be in place, even in the presence of sensitive assays for the detection of infectious donors.

In most HIV-infected subjects, antibody develops within 3–4 weeks and coexists with the virus thereafter. Hence, HIV seropositivity is an indicator of infectivity. The tests that lend themselves most readily to the rapid mass screening required in blood transfusion are all ELISA or chemiluminescence based. As many of the commercially available kits have some false-positive reactions, mainly due to cross-reactivity, confirmatory tests using alternative methodologies are carried out before a positive result is reported.

Routine screening, combined with the well-established donor education and self-deferral schemes, have reduced even further the already small risk of the transfusion of a contaminated donation. There have been only four documented cases of HIV transmission by transfusion in the UK since screening began in 1985. The small residual number of HIV transmissions through screened blood will arise through donations given in the 'window period' of infectivity, i.e. soon after the donor has been infected but before anti-HIV has become detectable (as in the four UK documented cases referred to), or potentially through system errors. With current combined antigen–antibody screening techniques, the window period has been estimated to be less than 2 weeks on average. With the recently introduced nucleic acid test (NAT) for HIV RNA, the window period has decreased to approximately 7 days. The prevalence of HIV antibodies in repeat UK blood donors is less than 1 in 100 000, and is 1 in 25 000 in new donors; there is no doubt that energetic donor education has contributed to this very low rate by excluding high-risk individuals. In areas of low HIV incidence, the number of extra donors detected by NAT screening will be extremely small. In the UK, combined antigen–antibody serological testing has proved extremely effective, although NAT for HIV has been introduced as part of a triplex assay for HCV, HIV and HBV (see above).

In England and Wales in 2008, it was estimated that the residual risk of HIV infection by transfusion, per donation, was approximately 1 in 5.4 million. Although small, the risk of HIV transmission by transfusion is greater in the USA (approximately 1 per million donations) than in the UK.

Human T-cell leukaemia viruses

Human T-cell leukaemia viruses (HTLV-I and HTLV-II) are related retroviruses. The importance of HTLV-II is not clear; it appears to be associated with intravenous drug use in the Western world and has no known association with any clinical condition. However, HTLV-I is endemic in the Caribbean, parts of Africa and in Japan, where 3–6% of the population are seropositive. The virus is transmitted from mother to child through breast-feeding. Infection with HTLV-I is associated with at least two distinct clinical conditions; it can occasionally lead to adult T-cell leukaemia, with an incubation period of approximately 20 years, and, on even rarer occasions, to tropical spastic paraparesis (also known as HTLV I-associated myelopathy), with a shorter incubation period. Only about 1% of patients who are seropositive develop T-cell leukaemia. Both

HTLV-I and HTLV-II are cell associated and not transmitted in plasma. In highly endemic areas, transmission of HTLV-I by transfusion was relatively common before mandatory screening was introduced. Both tropical spastic paraparesis and adult T-cell leukaemia have been associated with transfusion-transmitted HTLV-I.

In areas of low prevalence of HTLV-I and HTLV-II infection, the cost benefit of mandatory screening of blood donations has been a matter for debate. Routine serological screening is by ELISA, but confirmation of positive results can still cause difficulties because other retroviruses may cross-react. In certain cases, it may also be difficult to differentiate between HTLV-I and HTLV-II in the laboratory. The prevalence of anti-HTLV in previously untested UK blood donors is roughly 1 in 50 000. Screening using a sensitive ELISA for anti-HTLV-I/II on pooled plasma samples became mandatory in 2002. In the UK the residual risk of transmission of HTLV by transfusion is estimated to be approximately 1 in 24 million donations (figures for UK residual risk 2006–2008 courtesy of Lisa Brant).

Cytomegalovirus

Although most cases of post-transfusion cytomegalovirus (CMV) infection are subclinical, the syndrome of post-transfusion infectious mononucleosis-like illness is well recognized, especially after the transfusion of large amounts of blood. The infection is characterized by fever, splenomegaly and atypical lymphoid cells in the peripheral blood, with a negative Paul Bunnell test. The usually benign course of CMV infection in recipients and the high prevalence of CMV antibodies in the general population have meant that there has been no necessity to screen all donors for evidence of past infection. However, immunosuppressed individuals are at great risk from potentially fatal pneumonitis or disseminated CMV infection, and these recipients require special measures to prevent CMV transmission.

The groups at particular risk include premature babies weighing less than 1500 g, bone marrow and other organ transplant recipients, and pregnant women (the fetus is at risk). In such cases, if the patient (and the organ/cell donor) or the mother (in the case of neonates) lacks evidence of past CMV infection, then anti-CMV-free blood and blood components should be provided. This may cause logistical problems, especially with platelet supplies, as the prevalence of anti-CMV in the UK adult population is 50–60%. Although only a small number of antibody-positive donors may be capable of transmitting the infection, there is no test for infectivity. Thus, all antibody-positive donors should be considered as having the potential to transmit CMV. As CMV is cell associated, effective leucodepletion should provide similar levels of safety as serological testing. This has not been demonstrated by prospective parallel studies, although observational studies are supportive.

Syphilis

According to WHO data, the global incidence of syphilis has increased in recent years. Each donation is tested by a serological test for syphilis. Although *Treponema pallidum* does not survive well at 4°C and red cell preparations are likely to be non-infective after 4 days' refrigeration, passive transmission of the antibody to a recipient could cause diagnostic confusion. The organism is more likely to be transmitted in platelet concentrates, due to their room temperature storage and short shelf-life. Any donation from an individual giving a positive result is discarded, and subjects with positive tests are permanently debarred from donation, even after effective therapy. In the past, syphilis testing was believed valuable as a surrogate marker for lifestyles known to be associated with high risk of HIV infection. Sensitive HIV assays have reduced this usefulness.

Malaria

Malarial parasites remain viable in blood stored at 4°C and are readily transmissible by blood transfusion. In some endemic areas, all recipients are treated with antimalarial drugs. In non-endemic areas, there is a real risk of failure to recognize post-transfusion malaria owing to the rarity and unexpectedness of the infection. This fact, combined with increasing travel to tropical areas, necessitates the careful vetting of blood donors by direct questioning and, in some centres, by tests for malarial antibodies. In the UK, donors with a history of possible malaria exposure (provided it was more than 6 months previously and they are free of symptoms) can be accepted if they are negative by ELISA for malarial antibodies.

Other infections

There are no other protozoal or microbiological diseases (for which tests are available) that pose a significant problem in the context of blood transfusion in the UK. However, diseases such as Chagas disease cause significant problems for the blood transfusion services in Latin America, and potential exposure of UK donors necessitates stringent donor selection criteria and specific serological testing of those individuals to exclude the possibility of infection.

Babesia microti, the agent of Nantucket fever, still poses a risk in certain areas of the USA. There are very few reports of possible transmission of *Leishmania donovani*, all outside Europe. Subjects giving a history of brucellosis are not accepted as donors in the UK due to the risk of transmission of this agent.

Other viral risks of transfusion

Acute infections, although associated with short phases of viraemia, can pose transmission risk by transfusion especially if their incidence is high. This has been amply demonstrated by West Nile virus (WNV) in North America. WNV is an arthropod-borne infection of birds, with humans and horses as incidental hosts. The annual outbreaks in recent years in the USA and Canada have resulted in several transmissions by transfusion, with severe morbidity and mortality in immunosuppressed and elderly patients. This has necessitated the introduction of NAT screening of donors in these countries and the temporary exclusion, in non-endemic countries such as the UK, of donors who have visited North America. A similar situation pertains with two other arboviruses, dengue virus (which has caused two reported instances of transfusion transmission to date) and Chikungunya fever virus in French departments.

Hepatitis A and hepatitis E viruses, both acute infections with short periods of viraemia and no carrier state, have also occasionally been transmitted by transfusion. The possible risk from respiratory viruses with transient viraemia such as SARS and influenza viruses is being monitored internationally. No transmissions by transfusion have been reported.

Bacteria

Although rare in absolute terms (approximately three to four cases are reported and confirmed per year in the UK), bacterial transmissions by transfusion constitute two-thirds of all reported microbial transmissions by this route in the UK and often prove fatal. The vast majority of such cases are due to contaminated platelet preparations that are more than 3 days old, because bacteria (mostly skin commensals) proliferate easily at room temperature. This risk is now far greater than that posed by viruses because of the introduction of viral screening of blood donations by sensitive ELISAs and NAT. UK blood services have introduced enhanced methods of donor arm cleansing, and 'diversion' of the first 20 mL of the donation to reduce the risk from skin contaminants. Routine bacterial screening of platelet preparations is in place in Scotland and Wales. In England, a proportion of platelet concentrates undergo bacterial screening during long weekends, in order to extend the shelf-life from 5 to 7 days. The UK Serious Hazards of Transfusion (SHOT) 2008 report cites four (platelet) units transmitting bacteria. These resulted in one fatality directly caused by the transfusion, one fatality in which the transfusion was implicated and one case of major morbidity. Three other 'possible' bacterial transmission complications were noted.

Prions

Variant Creutzfeldt–Jakob disease (vCJD), the human form of bovine spongiform encephalopathy (BSE), is considered a potential threat to blood safety. This risk remains mainly applicable to the UK, where nearly 170 cases of vCJD had been reported by 2009. Therefore, plasma for fractionation (and fresh-frozen plasma for infants and children not exposed to the risk of BSE in food) is obtained from the USA. Appropriate donor exclusions and the introduction of leucodepletion of all blood components are other precautionary interventions. It has been shown experimentally that BSE acquired in sheep, by eating contaminated beef, can be transmitted by blood transfusion to other sheep. As it is not known how many people could be infected with vCJD and because of the reports of at least three possible transfusion-associated cases of vCJD transmission, recipients of blood and blood products have been excluded as blood donors in the UK. In addition, vCJD prion has been detected in spleen and/or lymph nodes in two recipients of blood and blood products from donors diagnosed with vCJD subsequent to donation. Both recipients died of unrelated causes, with no clinical manifestations of vCJD. Interestingly, one was a haemophilia patient. The implicated blood donations were all made prior to the introduction of leucodepletion. As yet no screening tests are available for testing blood donations, although several companies are claiming to have made progress. In addition, two companies have reported success with a special filter to remove abnormal prions from red cell units; these claims are under investigation.

Laboratory tests on blood donations
(Table 16.5)

Samples for laboratory testing are taken at the time of donation in order to avoid later entry into the sterile blood pack. The routine tests are automated if large numbers of donor samples are tested daily, as is the case in blood centres in the UK.

All blood donors in the UK are tested at each donation for syphilis, HBsAg, anti-HIV-1 and anti-HIV-2 and HIV antigen, anti-HCV, HCV and HIV RNA, HBV DNA, and anti-HTLV. ABO and RhD grouping are determined routinely on each occasion. Typing for other Rh antigens (C, E, c and e) and K is now routinely performed on all blood donations in the UK. Phenotyping for antigens other than ABO, Rh and K is only performed on a restricted number of units in order to match blood for special cases, such as alloimmunized patients and

Table 16.5 Microbial testing in England and North Wales.

HIV	ELISA (combined HIV-1 antigen plus anti-HIV-1 and anti-HIV-2); NAT for RNA
HBV	HBsAg ELISA; NAT for DNA
HCV	Anti-HCV ELISA plus NAT for RNA
HTLV	Anti-HTLV ELISA (on pools of samples)
CMV	Anti-CMV for immunosuppressed recipients only
Malaria	Antibody screening of potentially exposed donors
Chagas disease	Antibody screening of potentially exposed donors
Bacteria	All donations are tested for antibody to syphilis; the option to test platelet preparations by culture methods is under review

sickle cell disease patients. Ideally, girls and women of child-bearing age should be matched for c and K, as anti-c and anti-K are, after anti-D, the major causes of severe haemolytic disease of the newborn (HDN) in the UK.

All donations are also screened for the presence of atypical red cell alloantibodies by testing against group O red cells that are selected to bear the most common blood group antigens, ideally in double dose. The incidence of clinically significant red cell alloantibodies in blood donors is very low (0.3%) compared with the incidence in potential recipients (1–2%). Donations with potent clinically significant alloantibodies are not issued to hospitals. Group O blood for emergency or 'flying squad' use, which in exceptional circumstances may be given to ungrouped recipients, should be given as red cells in additive solution such as saline-adenine-glucose-mannitol (SAGM) in order to avoid problems that might be caused by high-titre anti-A,B in donor plasma. As soon as the patient's group is known, group-specific blood should be given. If group O platelets have to be given to non-O recipients, donors with high-titre anti-A,B should be excluded as the providers of the plasma used to suspend the platelets; alternatively, platelet-additive solutions can be used to replace most of the plasma.

Some donations are screened for CMV antibodies for patients in need of CMV-negative blood. Units from donors at risk are screened for malaria antibodies, Chagas disease antibodies and for HbS (sickle trait).

Residual microbial risk of allogeneic blood transfusion

The residual risks of microbial transmission are now so low in the UK that the prospective studies to determine them would be too large to be practical. Risk is therefore calculated from the length of the window period (prior to laboratory detectability of the infection) and the rate of new infections (incidence) for specific viruses. The calculated residual risks per donation in England and Wales for HIV, HBV and HCV are approximately 1 in 5.4 million, 1 in 0.9 million and 1 in 72 million respectively (figures for UK residual risk 2006–2008 courtesy of Lisa Brant). These calculations are consistent with 'haemovigilance' reports in the UK SHOT scheme. Indeed, acute microbial transmissions in 2008 constituted less than 1% of all reported hazards, with 'incorrect blood component transfused' being the major reported risk. The low microbial risk is a result of a series of incremental safety interventions becoming ever more complex and costly. Bacterial transmissions continue to pose the major microbial risk of blood transfusion.

In this context, reduction in pathogen-inactivation techniques is likely to prove cost-*ineffective*, unless a safe single treatment becomes available for blood prior to component separation, existing safety interventions can be reduced or discontinued, or 'emerging' microbial risks are considered to pose a sufficient threat. In any case, if pathogen-inactivation techniques such as photochemical inactivation are introduced, we need to ensure that the blood component is not affected in its immunogenicity or efficacy, and that the benefits of their introduction outweigh the risks.

In the UK, because of the risk of vCJD, fresh-frozen plasma (FFP) for paediatric use is imported from the USA. It has recently been recommended that all FFP for use in the UK should be imported. However, because the residual risk of viral transmission by transfusion is greater in the USA than in the UK, all imported plasma is subjected to pathogen inactivation with methylene blue.

Storage of blood

When blood is stored in a liquid state there is a progressive loss of viability of the red cells, and of red cell ATP, and depletion of 2,3-diphosphoglycerate (2,3-DPG). The purpose of modern anticoagulants used for the collection of blood, and additive solutions used to store red cells and platelets, is to reduce these changes to a minimum.

Anticoagulants

The vast majority of whole blood donations are collected into CPD (citrate-phosphate-dextrose) anticoagulant. The addition of 'rejuvenating' agents or purine nucleosides such as adenine to standard anticoagulant solutions (e.g. CPD-AI) has been shown to improve significantly the viability of red cells by restoring their ATP or 2,3-DPG content. However, for some clinical indications, such as neonatal or intrauterine transfusion, there have been theoretical concerns regarding toxicity of additives such as adenine and mannitol. In the UK, the majority of blood for neonatal or intrauterine transfusion is now prepared from CPD whole blood. Heparinized blood for neonatal cardiac surgery and exchange transfusion has been replaced by CPD or CPD-AI blood, less than 5 days old, with no untoward effects. Platelet preparations from apheresis are usually collected into acid-citrate-dextrose. CPD is used to collect both double-dose red cells and plasma from apheresis donors.

Optimal additive solutions (e.g. SAGM)

Optimal additive plasma replacement solutions have been developed to improve the viability of plasma-depleted red cells on storage, by maintaining both ATP and 2,3-DPG levels. SAGM (as well as ADSOL and Nutricel) medium provides good red cell storage conditions and is now the most usual preservative solution for red cells in the UK. The majority of red cells for transfusion are stored in additive solutions rather than autologous plasma. There are few clinical indications for red cells stored in plasma and but include red cells for neonatal exchange transfusion and those for intrauterine transfusion. Red cells in SAGM are now usually used for top-up and large-

volume transfusions to neonates (e.g. cardiac surgery). Currently in the UK, platelets are normally stored in CPD-plasma either from one of the four pooled donations, in the case of 'buffy coat' platelets (see below), or as part of the apheresis collection. Alternatively they can be resuspended in 70% platelet additive solution and 30% plasma, especially for patients in whom exposure to plasma is contraindicated or when the potency of anti-A,B in group O platelets needs to be reduced for non-O recipients. For patients with severe allergic reactions to plasma proteins, platelets can be suspended in 100% additive solution, but this limits the shelf-life to 24 hours due to the lack of plasma to maintain platelet function.

Blood components

Preparation and storage of blood components

There are no specific clinical indications for the transfusion of whole blood, and the vast majority of blood that is transfused is therefore separated into its component parts. This is achieved by the collection and separation of whole blood donations, or by collection of specific components from donors by apheresis. A multiple 'bottom and top' blood collection pack is used (Figure 16.1) if the donation will be used to make platelets; otherwise, a simpler 'top and top' system is used to make red cells and plasma. The blood donation is taken into the main pack, which contains standard CPD anticoagulant. In the bottom and top system, after centrifugation, whole blood is separated into plasma at the top, a buffy coat in the middle and red cells at the bottom (Figure 16.1). Fresh plasma is expressed from the top and red cells from the bottom of the pack, leaving the buffy coat in the original pack. The red cells are transferred to a pack containing an optimal additive solution to preserve red cell function during storage. The resulting red cells have a shelf-life of 35–42 days (35 days in the UK).

The plasma is then kept to resuspend the platelets, or frozen either for clinical use as FFP or it can be subjected to a fractionation process for the manufacture of intravenous immunoglobulin, albumin, anti-D, specific antiviral immunoglobulins and coagulation factors. However, at present it is not permitted to use UK plasma for fractionation because of concerns over the possible transmission of vCJD by blood products.

The buffy coat layer contains most of the platelets, over 80% of the white cells and 5–10% of the red cells. This is pooled with three other buffy coats and more than 200 mL of plasma from one of the donations, preferably from a male donor, using a sterile connecting device (Figure 16.2). The pool undergoes a second gentle centrifugation step and the supernatant is used to produce a platelet preparation. The residue from the buffy coat pool, containing mainly white cells and red cells, is then discarded.

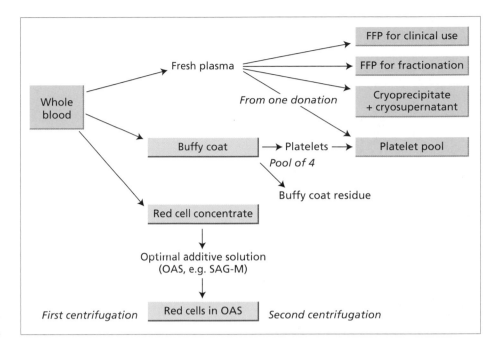

Figure 16.1 Diagrammatic representation of the preparation of components from whole blood by the 'top and bottom' or 'buffy coat' method. Items in boxes represent final components. FFP, fresh-frozen plasma.

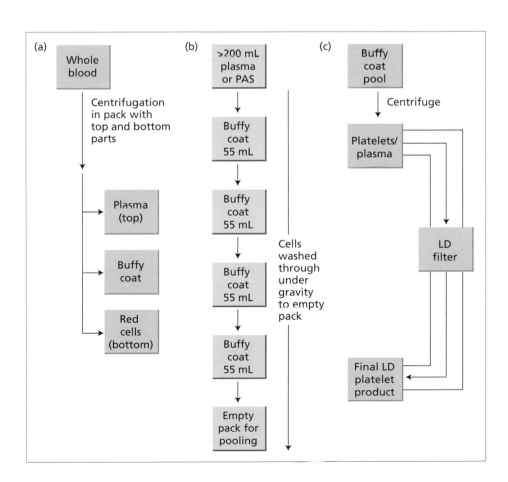

Figure 16.2 Preparation of leucodepleted pooled, buffy coat-derived platelet preparations. PAS, platelet additive solution; LD, leucodepletion.

The systems that enable the separation of buffy coats in a semi-automated manner are called blood separators, examples of which include Optipress and Compomat (Figure 16.2). Cellular components (red cells and platelets) and plasma may, at this stage, be individually filtered to leucodeplete to a level below 5×10^6 white cells per unit. The alternative is to use leucodepletion filters at the initial stage on whole blood, before separation of components. These two alternative methods are necessary because most whole blood filters also remove a significant number of platelets, making production of platelet concentrates from filtered whole blood impossible. In the UK, leucodepletion of all blood components has been mandatory since 1999, as a measure which might decrease the risk of vCJD transmission by transfusion. Added benefits of leucodepletion include a significant decrease in the incidence of febrile non-haemolytic transfusion reactions, in the risk of human leucocyte antigen (HLA) alloimmunization and in the risk of transmission of intracellular viruses such as CMV and HTLV.

Platelet preparations

Unlike red cells, platelets must be stored at 20–22°C, since storage at 4°C results in poor survival of platelets following transfusion. Platelets have a shelf-life of 5 days, and are stored in permeable bags that allow the diffusion of oxygen into the pack, which, with constant gentle agitation, maintains aerobic metabolism and reduces the rate of fall of pH. The shelf-life of platelet preparations can be extended to 7 days provided that systems are in place to monitor bacterial contamination or to inactivate pathogens in platelet concentrates (e.g. photochemical inactivation with psoralens).

Platelet pools provide an adequate adult dose of platelets and contain, on average, 3×10^{11} platelets, usually from four donations suspended in the plasma from one donation, preferably from a male donor, in order to avoid the risk of transfusion of donor white cell antibodies that might cause transfusion-related acute lung injury (TRALI) (Figure 16.2).

In the USA, platelets are prepared from individual donations by a method which leaves the platelet-rich plasma as a supernatant. Each platelet concentrate contains a minimum of 5.5×10^{10} platelets, suspended in 50 mL of plasma. An adult dose of platelets prepared in this way contains significantly more leucocytes than the platelet concentrates prepared by 'top and bottom' systems and which are considered to be leucocyte poor, even before leucodepletion.

The equivalent of two or even three adult doses of platelets (minimum 2.4×10^{11} each) may be obtained from one donor, with adequate platelet counts, by an apheresis procedure lasting approximately 90 min. At present, in the UK, approximately 80% of platelets are produced by this method. These preparations reduce donor exposure and are invaluable for the treatment of immunologically refractory thrombocytopenic patients requiring HLA-matched platelets. However, they are expensive

to produce and demanding on both staff and donors. A large HLA-typed donor panel is available in England to provide HLA-matched platelets for immunologically refractory patients. Most apheresis platelet donors are also human platelet antigen (HPA) typed in order to provide HPA-1a-negative platelets for newborns affected with neonatal alloimmune thrombocytopenia and also for some of the HPA-1a-negative patients who have become immunologically refractory to platelet transfusions.

Frozen platelets can be preserved in dimethyl sulphoxide (DMSO) or glycerol. The platelet recovery is significantly lower than with fresh preparations, but the post-transfusion survival is normal. Frozen platelets are very seldom used and are not available in the UK, due to the remaining concerns about their safety and loss of efficacy.

Systems to kill pathogens that may be present in platelet preparations are now available, but none are yet in routine use in the UK or the USA.

Granulocyte concentrates

With the increase in intensive chemotherapy regimens, demand for granulocytes has risen in order to prevent or treat fungal or other serious infections in severely neutropenic patients.

Granulocytes are extremely labile; they must be separated from whole blood immediately after collection and transfused within hours of preparation. Granulocytes prepared from routine blood donations (buffy coats) are heavily contaminated with red cells and platelets. Buffy coats from at least 10 donors are required to produce a therapeutic dose for an adult (at least 1×10^{10} granulocytes). Ten buffy coats also contain the equivalent of two units of red cells and 2.5 pools of platelets. Venesection of the recipient may therefore be required if daily buffy coats are indicated. A new pooled granulocyte component produced from whole blood donations that has reduced volume and red cell contamination is under clinical assessment in the UK. However, due to the heavy red cell contamination of available buffy coats, they should be ABO and RhD compatible with the recipient and cross-matched against the recipient's serum. Granulocyte concentrates prepared by apheresis are the only satisfactory means of achieving a therapeutic dose for an adult neutropenic patient. Sedimenting agents (gelatin, hydroxyethyl starch) must be added to the blood or given to the donor in order to obtain an adequate yield, unless the donor has chronic granulocytic leukaemia.

A directed donation from a suitable relative may sometimes be possible. Consent may then be obtained for the donors to have their counts boosted using steroids and granulocyte colony-stimulating factor (G-CSF), resulting in an excellent yield of granulocytes. In the UK, it is not permitted for non-directed volunteer donors to receive this medication. Average yields from unstimulated apheresis collections are 0.7×10^{10}; with the use of G-CSF and steroids, this can be increased to $5–10 \times 10^{10}$.

All granulocyte concentrates should be cross-matched against the recipient's serum by lymphocytotoxicity, as white cell antibodies may cause severe transfusion reactions, with respiratory distress.

Fresh-frozen plasma

This plasma has been separated from whole blood (Figure 16.1) or obtained by apheresis, and frozen within 24 hours to a temperature that will maintain the activity of the labile factors V and VIII. FFP contains all coagulation factors and should be stored at −30°C or below for up to 24 months or even longer. When needed, the plasma is thawed rapidly at 37°C and then transfused without delay. A dose of 15 mL/kg is appropriate to correct abnormal coagulation in acquired coagulopathies when no concentrate is available. The main use of FFP is for multiple acquired coagulation factor deficiency, but it is also used to treat inherited single coagulation factor deficiencies if the appropriate factor concentrates are not available. Evidence is gathering in favour of the early and more liberal use of FFP, together with red cells and platelets, in the massive haemorrhage of trauma (see below).

Single units of FFP can be treated with photosensitizing chemicals such as methylene blue (MB), riboflavin or amotosalen and exposed to visible or ultraviolet light to inactivate pathogens that may be present in the plasma. If required, the residual chemicals can be removed before the plasma is rapidly frozen to −30°C. Alternatively, FFP can be pooled with around 1500 other units and treated with solvent-detergent (SD) in order to inactivate pathogens. All methods of viral inactivation reduce the levels of labile clotting factors in FFP. The current recommendation from the UK Department of Health is that the treatment of choice for children is MB-FFP and that SD-FFP should be used for plasma exchanges in the treatment of thrombotic thrombocytopenic purpura (TTP). Both types of FFP are produced from plasma collected outside the UK in order to reduce the risk of vCJD.

In recent years in the UK, every effort is made to prepare FFP only from male donors in order to minimize the risk of passive transfer of donor white cell antibodies that can give rise to TRALI.

Cryoprecipitate

Cryoprecipitate is prepared from FFP that is allowed to thaw slowly (classically at 4°C overnight). After removal of the supernatant, factor VIII:C, von Willebrand factor (VWF), fibrinogen, fibronectin and factor XIII are left as a precipitate, which is then refrozen in approximately 30 mL of plasma and stored at −30°C or below for up to 24 months. Each unit should contain a minimum of 70 IU of factor VIII:C and 140 mg of fibrinogen. Cryoprecipitate is now used mainly as a source of fibrinogen in cases of disseminated intravascular coagulation (DIC), hepatic failure and hypofibrinogenaemia. A standard adult dose of cryoprecipitate is 10 units, which are thawed at 37°C in about 10 min and should be used immediately. Pools of 5 single units are available in the UK. Fibrinogen concentrate, a safer low-volume alternative to cryoprecipitate, is now available in the UK.

Cryoprecipitate-poor plasma (cryosupernatant)

This term is used for the remaining plasma after the removal of cryoprecipitate. It is stored frozen at −30°C or below for up to 24 months. The only specific indication for cryosupernatant is for plasma exchange in TTP. This is an immune-mediated condition in which there is an autoantibody directed against a VWF-cleaving metalloproteinase. The resulting accumulation of high-molecular-weight VWF multimers contributes to the pathophysiology of the condition, with thrombosis in the microvasculature. Although cryosupernatant has reduced levels of high-molecular-weight multimers compared with FFP, there is no evidence that plasma exchange for TTP with cryosupernatant is any more effective. FFP or cryosupernatant are therefore alternatives to the current product of choice (SD-FFP); however, they are derived from UK donors, who might have been exposed to vCJD.

Storage changes of blood components

Loss of red cell and platelet viability are the most important practical considerations. Progressive loss of viability varies according to the combination of anticoagulant used, how blood is stored prior to component separation, what storage medium the components are stored in, and the pack systems used. The time limit for storage of blood or its component parts is set taking all these into consideration. After transfusion of stored red cells or platelets, a proportion is removed from the circulation within the first 24 hours. The remainder appear to survive normally. There are various changes in the *in vitro* characteristics of red cells during storage (the so-called storage lesion), including depletion of metabolic substrates such as ATP and 2,3-DPG, leakage of potassium and changes in red cell morphology. Some of these changes can be partially reversed *ex vivo* by incubation with purine nucleosides, or following transfusion *in vivo*. ATP seems to be an important determinant of red cell viability, although not the only one. 2,3-DPG is almost completely depleted in red cells after 14–21 days storage. Red cell 2,3-DPG is restored to normal by approximately 24–48 hours after transfusion. The clinical significance of the low 2,3-DPG level of stored red cells is only likely to be an important consideration in recipients with severe anaemia or coronary artery insufficiency.

During storage of red cells, potassium gradually leaks out through the cell membrane once active transport has been halted by the cooling of blood to 4°C. There is rapid restoration of electrolyte levels after transfusion. The pH of blood decreases with storage, but most recipients can handle the acid load during transfusion without ill effect.

Likewise there are a number of changes in platelet function that occur during platelet storage, including increased platelet activation and decreased responsiveness to agonists such as ADP. For both red cells and platelets, the relationship between these changes *in vitro* and the function of the cells following transfusion is complex, and it is notoriously difficult to predict post-transfusion viability from the results of laboratory testing.

As the storage time of either red cells or platelets increases, the viability decreases. Acceptable limits for the recovery of red cells and platelets following transfusion are as follows: greater than 75% of red cells 24 hours following transfusion, and greater than 66% of platelets (compared with that of fresh platelets).

Frozen red cells

Red cells can be stored for a prolonged period (up to 30 years) without damage if glycerol is added before freezing. Thawed red cells must be washed free of glycerol before transfusion. This method of storage is expensive and time-consuming but is invaluable as a means of storing red cells with rare phenotypes. National banks for frozen rare cells have been established for this purpose. Freezing, thawing and washing is also an efficient way of removing plasma, platelets and leucocytes from red cells.

The recipient

Preoperative assessment (Table 16.6)

The need to correct anaemia with haematinics preoperatively and avoid unnecessary transfusions, in addition to the growing pressure on hospital beds and increasing use of day surgery, suggest that a preoperative assessment should be performed before admission. This allows for efficient use of hospital resources and limits the number of cancelled operations. The key aims are to assess a patient's fitness to undergo surgery and anaesthesia (including haemoglobin optimization), anticipate complications, arrange for supportive therapy to be available perioperatively and to liaise with the appropriate specialists regarding non-surgical management. This assessment needs to take place at a presurgical clinic at least 1 month before the planned date of surgery. After the clinic, it is imperative that the results are evaluated so that the necessary action, such as the treatment of ferropenic anaemia, can be taken for each patient.

Only a small proportion (1–2%) of potential recipients will have red cell alloantibodies other than anti-D; however, a sample taken at the pre-assessment clinic for pretransfusion antibody screening will allow blood bank staff to identify those samples that need detailed investigation, well in advance of the planned transfusion, so that antigen-negative blood can be available as required.

Table 16.6 Preoperative assessment.

Take a full history and examination, including previous surgical episodes and bleeding history, transfusion and obstetric history

Arrange full blood count (FBC), group and antibody screen, routine chemistry, coagulation screen (if indicated) and tube for haematinics assessment (ferritin level for iron stores, vitamin B_{12} and folic acid), which can be put on hold pending FBC results

Make cell salvage available if there is a likelihood of significant blood loss requiring transfusion and a 'clean' surgical procedure

Consider using recombinant erythropoietin (600 IU/kg weekly for 4 weeks preoperatively) and/or intravenous iron preparations in order to optimize haemoglobin even when within normal range

Prescribe iron and folic acid supplement if any suspicion of iron deficiency

Establish whether patient is taking regular aspirin, clopidogrel, non-steroidal anti-inflammatory drugs or warfarin and, whenever possible, make necessary arrangements to stop this drug 7 days preoperatively

Laboratory tests

Pretransfusion group and screen

The ABO and RhD groups of all potential recipients should be determined before transfusion. No other blood groups are routinely tested or matched when selecting blood for transfusion. The need for blood is rarely so urgent that there is insufficient time to perform the ABO and RhD groups before transfusion, as rapid testing need take only 5–10 min. The patient's serum should also be screened for the presence of atypical red cell antibodies using a sensitive indirect antiglobulin test (IAT), with two or three individual (not pooled) group O red cells selected to express, between them, all the common red cell antigens, ideally in double dose. If a positive result is obtained, further investigation using a red cell panel of 8–10 cells is required to identify the antibody.

For patients who have preformed antibodies, because they are already good responders, an antibody screen using a panel of cells that are negative for the pertinent antigen(s) should be used (i.e. panel of rr cells in the case of preformed anti-D). Only 1–2% of patients have clinically significant red cell alloantibodies other than anti-D. About 75% of these antibodies have Rh and/or K specificity. Therefore, patients with haematological diseases (e.g. sickle cell anaemia, β-thalassaemia) who are likely to need repeated transfusion over many years should ideally be phenotyped for the major red cells antigens; if this is not possible, at least RhD, C, c, E, e and K typing should be performed.

Blood that is compatible with the patient's Rh and K type should be transfused, as this reduces the probability that they will produce alloantibodies. It is not difficult to implement this policy in England, as all red cell units are typed for all Rh antigens and for K. Because, after RhD, the K and Rhc antigens are the most immunogenic and the antibodies that can lead to severe HDN, ideally girls and women of childbearing age should be transfused with K-negative red cells, although K typing is not necessary as only 9% will be positive. On the other hand, girls and women of childbearing age should be typed for the Rhc antigen and those found to be negative should be given c-negative blood.

Red cells for transfusion are selected to be of the same ABO and RhD group as the recipient. If clinically significant red cell alloantibodies are present in the recipient, units of blood lacking the relevant antigens are selected for compatibility testing, even if the maximum (or standard) surgical blood ordering schedule (SBOS, see below) only requires group and screen for that surgical procedure.

Compatibility testing (cross-match)

The donor red cells are routinely tested against the recipient serum or plasma in order to detect any potential incompatibilities, i.e. identify any antibodies in the recipient that are reactive with antigens on the red cells of the selected donor. This test will provide a means of checking the ABO compatibility of donor and recipient. If the antibody screen is negative, then the cross-match should be as simple as possible, for example an immediate spin or IAT at 37°C. This will detect ABO incompatibilities resulting from clerical or technical errors such as sample switching or erroneous group in the bag, as well as the presence of antibodies missed in the screening. The antiglobulin test can be performed in low-ionic-strength saline (LISS) solution in tubes or using gel (column) techniques (see Chapter 14) that decrease the incubation time and increase the sensitivity for the detection of most antibodies. Tests should be carried out at 37°C, not at room temperature, otherwise clinically insignificant cold antibodies will be detected, especially when LISS is used. This may cause confusion and inconvenience to the recipient (e.g. cancellation of planned surgery). Any clinically significant antibody will react at 37°C (see Chapter 14), and the techniques chosen should take this into account.

A group and screen policy used in combination with a maximum (or standard) surgical blood ordering schedule (MSBOS, SBOS) can reduce the number of compatibility tests performed and avoid the reservation of red cell units unlikely to be transfused.. Each hospital should agree its own SBOS among the blood bank, surgeons and anesthetists, through the hospital transfusion committee. The SBOS is based on a retrospective comparison of the number of units of blood cross-matched and the number actually transfused for each elective surgical procedure. Procedures that are likely to require blood have a ratio of cross-matched to transfused blood below 2.5:1. All patients awaiting surgery have blood samples taken for grouping and antibody screening. As long as no atypical alloantibodies are detected, cross-matching is reserved for those in whom the need for blood is fairly certain. Operations for which blood is not usually required (such as hysterectomy and cholecystectomy) are not covered by cross-matched blood. If blood is unexpectedly needed, an abbreviated cross-match (using an immediate spin technique to ensure ABO compatibility) may be used safely, with minimal risk to the recipient. If atypical antibodies are detected, antigen-negative blood should be cross-matched before surgery if there is any minimal likelihood of blood being required, regardless of the SBOS.

Electronic cross-match

An increasing number of hospitals with suitable blood bank computing systems now use a so-called electronic cross-match or 'electronic issue'. A patient has group and screen performed on two separate occasions. If both screen results on the laboratory's computer system are negative and if no blood has been transfused during this period, ABO and Rh compatible blood is issued directly via the computer with no further wet testing being performed. This makes it possible to reduce the number of operations for which blood is issued in advance even further, as the electronic cross-match is very quick. It also saves laboratory time, which can then be dedicated to more complex problems.

Antenatal testing

All women should have blood samples taken at antenatal booking for blood grouping and antibody screening. If no clinically significant antibody is detected, further samples should be tested at 28 weeks' gestation (see p. 294) before routine antenatal prophylaxis is given to RhD-negative women. Much of the emergency compatibility testing for possible Caesarean sections can be avoided by performing another antibody screen and group at admission, using either an abbreviated or electronic cross-match, should blood be required.

Repeated transfusions

Patients who require repeat transfusion after an interval of more than 72 hours must have a new sample screened before the next transfusion to detect any clinically significant antibody that may have been stimulated in an anamnestic response by the recent transfusion. Severe haemolytic transfusion reactions (HTRs) still occur due to failure to observe this simple rule; many could be avoided. In the case of an HTR, in addition to the antibody screen, a direct antiglobulin test (DAT) should be performed on the red cells of the new sample to detect, in mixed field agglutination, any alloantibodies attached to donor red cells but not free in the serum.

Massive transfusion

If the total blood volume has been replaced within less than 24 hours, compatibility testing becomes academic. In such patients, inter-donor incompatibility is a possible problem, but all donor sera should have been screened at the transfusion centre for the presence of potent atypical antibodies. When a pretransfusion alloantibody screen on the recipient has not detected any atypical antibodies and blood has been cross-matched without a problem, then continued compatibility testing may be omitted. If a pretransfusion screen reveals the presence of an atypical antibody, the blood selected should be negative for the relevant antigen. Once transfusion has commenced, the antibody will be 'diluted out' and compatibility testing may no longer be reliable, unless the original serum sample is used for all testing. In practice, once 10 units have been transfused there is no need to continue to cross-match red cells for further transfusions, or to select antigen-negative red cells, if these are scarce. If unimmunized RhD-negative men or postmenopausal women are likely to need massive transfusion, RhD-positive red cells should be transfused from the start.

Transfusion in autoimmune haemolytic anaemia

Ideally, patients with this condition should not be transfused. However, if transfusion is imperative, special serological techniques such as elution and absorption should be used to exclude the presence of alloantibodies, which may be masked by autoantibodies. Blood should then be selected that is compatible with the alloantibody, if present, even though transfused red cells will be destroyed by the autoantibody at the same rate as the patient's own blood. Whenever possible, red cells should also be Rh and K compatible to reduce the possibility of further alloimmunization. Blood that does not express the antigen to which the autoantibody is directed should be issued only when the autoantibody has restricted specificity and mimics an alloantibody such as anti-e. However, if the patient is a female of childbearing age and is RhD-negative, with an autoantibody mimicking anti-e, then R_2R_2 (*cDE/cDE*) cells should not be given because of the high risk of RhD immunization.

Neonatal 'top-up' transfusion

Premature infants are among the most widely transfused patients, with 'top-up' transfusions being very frequent. Only the first pretransfusion sample needs to be tested, with no further sample testing until 4 months of age, as infants are not capable of making clinically significant antibodies in the first months of life. Ideally, the unit of red cells used for the first transfusion should be aliquoted into several (six to eight) satellite (or 'paedi') packs and used for the same infant until expiry in order to decrease exposure to multiple donors. Measures should be in place in all neonatal units and their supporting laboratories to minimize the quantities of blood required for testing, by use of microsampling techniques and near-patient testing. Anaemia in this group is largely due to 'bleeding into the laboratory'. Erythropoietin has been extensively studied as an alternative to transfusion in the anaemia of prematurity but it does not consistently reduce the need for transfusion in this patient group.

Complications of blood transfusion

The frequency of the complications of blood transfusion will vary inversely with the care exercised in preparation for, and especially in supervision of, the transfusion.

Although the majority of side-effects are mild, the overall incidence of complications is estimated at 2–5%. Immediate fatalities, although difficult to quantify accurately, are of the order of 1 in 100 000 to 1 in 500 000 patients transfused; 50% of these are caused by ABO incompatibilities, mainly due to failure to correctly identify the donor or recipient at the time of sampling or at the time of transfusion. The wrong pack of blood, i.e. one intended for a different recipient, is reported to be given in 1 in 6000 to 1 in 30 000 transfusions. This is likely to be an underestimate due to underdetection and non-reporting of incidents. It follows that transfusions of blood and blood components should only be prescribed when there is a definite and appropriate clinical indication, when there are no feasible alternatives and when the benefits of transfusion are judged by the prescribing clinician to outweigh its short- and longer-term risks.

The complications of blood transfusion can be conveniently divided into acute and delayed, immunological and non-immunological categories (Table 16.7).

Immunological complications

Sensitization to red cell antigens
As only the ABO and RhD antigens are routinely matched in blood transfusion, there is a constant possibility of sensitization to other red cell antigens, although all red cell antigens are significantly less immunogenic than D. Alloimmunization is more likely in multitransfused patients. The consequences may be negligible but can lead to difficulty with compatibility testing, HDN and HTRs.

Haemolytic transfusion reactions
This is premature destruction of transfused red cells reacting with antibodies in the recipient. Naturally occurring antibodies, such as ABO antibodies, are IgM and, if warm-reacting, can destroy red cells *in vivo* by complement fixation. Red cell alloantibodies are usually IgG and form in response to exposure, through previous transfusions or pregnancies. HTRs may occur

Table 16.7 Hazards of transfusion.

Immediate (hours)

Non-immune complications
Bacterial: acute sepsis or endotoxic shock
Hypothermia
Hypocalcaemia ($\downarrow Ca^{2+}$) in infants

Immune complications
Febrile non-haemolytic transfusion reactions
Acute haemolytic transfusion reactions: intravascular (IgM),
    extravascular (IgG)
Allergic reactions (urticarial)
Anaphylactic reactions (anti-IgA)
Transfusion-related acute lung injury
Transfusion-associated circulatory overload

Delayed (days to years)

Non-immune complications
HIV, HCV, HBV, CMV
Others: parvovirus B19, HAV, HEV, WNV, dengue, malaria,
    Chagas disease, brucellosis, syphilis, vCJD

Immune complications
Delayed haemolytic transfusion reactions (due to anamnestic
    immune responses with red cell alloantibodies)
Post-transfusion purpura
Transfusion-associated graft-versus-host disease (immune
    modulation)

CMV, cytomegalovirus; HAV, hepatitis A virus; HEV, hepatitis E
virus; WNV, West Nile virus.

immediately after the transfusion or may be delayed for anything up to 2–3 weeks.

Immediate or acute haemolytic transfusion reactions

These may be intravascular or extravascular.

Immediate intravascular red cell destruction is the most dangerous type of HTR; it is associated with activation of the full complement cascade by IgM antibodies and is practically always due to ABO-incompatible blood transfusions (haemolytic anti-A,B, anti-A or anti-B present mainly in the recipient or, rarely, in the donor plasma). Most of these ABO-incompatible transfusions are due to errors, and occur with an approximate frequency of 1 in 100 000 patients transfused. The mortality rate in such ABO-incompatible cases is 5–10%. In a further 10–15% of cases there is major morbidity.

In the 20–25% of recipients of ABO-incompatible blood with serious reactions, the symptoms are usually dramatic and severe; most are due to the anaphylatoxins C3a and C5a that are liberated during complement activation, releasing vasoactive amines and hydrolases from mast cells and granulocytes (see Chapter 14). The cytokines interleukin (IL)-1, IL-8 and tumour necrosis factor (TNF) also play an important role, causing inflammation, smooth muscle contraction, platelet aggregation, increased capillary permeability, and hypotension. Typically, within less than 1 hour of the start of the transfusion, when the reaction is symptomatic, the patient complains of heat or pain in the cannulated vein, throbbing in the head, flushing of the face, chest tightness, nausea and lumbar pain. These symptoms are usually accompanied by tachycardia and hypotension. In severe cases, there is profound hypotension, leading to shock and renal failure. Rigors and pyrexia usually follow. Intravascular destruction of red cells brings about liberation of thromboplastin-like substances that activate coagulation and lead to DIC. The bleeding diathesis and increased destruction of red cells (which may eventually involve the recipient's cells) further exacerbates the problem. Intravascular destruction of red cells liberates haemoglobin into the circulation. Once haptoglobins are saturated, haemoglobin will also appear in the urine. If haemoglobinuria is very severe, haemosiderinuria may be seen. Renal complications consist of acute renal failure with oliguria and anuria, possibly the result of hypotension and/or the action of activated complement. The initial symptoms may of course be modified or abolished in anaesthetized or heavily sedated patients, in whom evidence of DIC, hypotension or the presence of haemoglobinuria may be the first signs.

Immediate intravascular destruction of recipient red cells should be avoidable. In practice, the main cause is error, when the incorrect blood component is transfused. The most severe reactions occur in major incompatibility, when a group O recipient with high-titre anti-A,B is transfused with group A, B or AB red cells. Less severe intravascular haemolysis occurs when group A red cells are transfused to a group B recipient, or vice versa, because group B and A subjects have less potent ABO antibodies than those of group O. More rarely, intravascular red cell destruction may occur when group O plasma is transfused by mistake to A, B or AB recipients. For this reason, group O red cells, even in additive solution, should not routinely be used for non-O recipients; furthermore, this practice leads to unnecessary shortages of group O blood. If unavoidable, the group O blood must first be screened for the presence of high-titre haemolysins or be devoid of plasma. In the UK, screening for high-titre ABO antibodies is routinely carried out at the blood centre and marked on the bag. ABO-compatible cryoprecipitate, FFP and platelet transfusions should be selected for all recipients, especially for children because of their smaller blood volume. Group A, B or AB plasma components are safe for group O recipients.

Occasionally, there is a laboratory error when tubes are transposed or there are transcription errors or misrecording of results, or there is insufficient time to complete an antibody screen or compatibility test. In the UK haemovigilance (SHOT) system, approximately 30% of cases of incorrect blood component transfusion reported in the last 12 years have been primarily due to clerical or technical errors that originated in the

Postgraduate Haematology

hospital laboratory. Obviously, not all the errors led to ABO-incompatible transfusions; in fact 10% of errors led to ABO incompatibilities. The remainder of reports (70%) relate to clerical or administrative errors in the ward, collection of the blood from the blood bank, failure to confirm the identity of the patient when taking samples, mislabelling of the sample of blood or failure to perform proper checks before removing the units from the refrigerator or transfusing the blood. The potentially serious consequences of failures resulting in ABO-incompatible transfusions emphasize the need for set protocols with meticulous checking at all stages. If an identification mistake has been made, it is important to check, as a matter of urgency, that the units intended for the patient under investigation have not also been misdirected to another recipient.

Haemoglobinaemia and haemoglobinuria may also be seen in severe extravascular HTRs (see below) and, occasionally, after the transfusion of lysed red cells. This may occur in the following circumstances: inappropriate warming and overheating of blood; exposure to extreme cold due to faulty storage conditions; lysis due to mechanical problems during administration; or due to the injection of 5% dextrose with the transfused red cells. Severe fulminant toxic symptoms leading to death, similar to those of intravascular HTRs, can be seen after the transfusion of bacterially infected blood, especially if it contains endotoxin-producing organisms (e.g. *Staphylococcus* and *Yersinia* species). Haemoglobinaemia and haemoglobinuria may also follow transfusion of blood to a patient with severe autoimmune haemolytic anaemia, due to an increase in the number of red cells in the circulation which will be subject to immune lysis.

Extravascular red cell destruction is mediated by IgG antibodies (Table 16.8). Mononuclear phagocytic cells have receptors for the Fc fragment of IgG1 and IgG3; the binding of IgG-coated cells to these receptors is inhibited by free IgG in plasma. There are no receptors for IgM on macrophages. Red cells sensitized with IgG1 and/or IgG3 antibodies may or may not activate complement up to C3b only. If they do not, they are removed extravascularly (by phagocytosis or cytotoxicity) by mononuclear phagocytic cells, predominantly in the red pulp of the spleen, where the plasma is largely excluded and the IgG on the red cells can compete with free IgG in the plasma. However, cells coated with IgG antibodies, which activate complement up to C3b, adhere to the C3b receptor on macrophages and monocytes. The presence of C3b on red cells greatly enhances the extravascular destruction of IgG-coated cells. This is because the binding to C3b receptors is not inhibited as there is no native C3b in plasma and consequently IgG/C3b-coated cells are destroyed by phagocytosis or cytotoxicity, predominantly in the liver, where there are abundant macrophages (Kupffer cells) and a generous blood flow. As C3b is rapidly inactivated and converted into C3dg by the action of factors H and I and proteases, a proportion of the cells re-enter the circulation, coated with C3dg, and are resistant to further lysis (Figure 16.3). Red

Table 16.8 Antibodies associated with haemolytic transfusion reactions.

Blood group system	Antibodies implicated in intravascular haemolysis	Antibodies implicated in extravascular haemolysis
ABO	A, B	
Hh	H (Bombay)	
Rh		All
Kell		K, k, Kp^a, Kp^b, Js^a, Js^b
Kidd		Jk^a, Jk^b, Jk^3
Duffy		Fy^a, Fy^b, Fy^3
MNS		M, S, s, U (some)
Lutheran		Lu^b (some)
Lewis	Le^a, Le^b, Le^{a+b}	
Cartwright		Yt^a (some)
Vel	Vel	Vel (some)
Colton		Co^a, Co^b
Dombrock		Do^a, Do^b

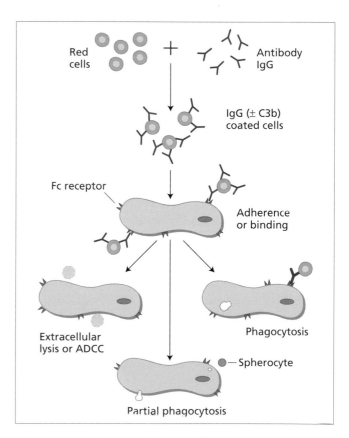

Figure 16.3 Mechanisms of extravascular destruction of red cells coated with IgG1 or IgG3 (± C3b). ADCC, antibody-dependent cell-mediated cytotoxicity.

cells coated with potent IgG antibodies, especially if they are C3b-binding, are destroyed mainly by cytotoxicity. Red cells coated with less potent antibodies are mostly destroyed by phagocytosis. Very rarely, red cell alloantibodies too weak to be detectable by routine pretransfusion testing may destroy donor red blood cells carrying the corresponding antigen.

The features of an immediate HTR vary according to a number of factors: whether the red cells are destroyed within the circulation or in the mononuclear phagocytic system; the strength, class and subclass of the antibody; the nature of the antigen; the number of incompatible red cells transfused; and the clinical state of the patient. When antibodies are present in the circulation in low titres and a large volume of incompatible blood is given, all circulating antibody will bind to the incompatible red cells, coating them weakly, without destroying them. There will then be no antibody detectable in the serum for a number of days until secondary antibody production is stimulated by the immune challenge. On the other hand, in the presence of an overloaded or poorly functioning mononuclear phagocytic system, large volumes of IgG-sensitized incompatible red cells can be present in the circulation with minimal or no premature removal, so the haemoglobin level may be stable with little evidence of haemolysis. The DAT will be positive, but as there is no free antibody, elution techniques will be necessary for antibody identification.

Immediate extravascular destruction of red cells may be accompanied by hyperbilirubinaemia, occasionally haemoglobinaemia due to antibody-dependent cytotoxicity (in severe cases), fever and failure to achieve the expected rise in haemoglobin level. The signs and symptoms are less severe and dramatic than in intravascular haemolysis and usually appear more than 1 hour after the start of transfusion (Table 16.8). There may be no signs or symptoms at all. Renal failure is very rare,

even when the antibody binds the earlier components of the complement cascade. Symptoms are attributed in large degree to liberation of cytokines from mononuclear phagocytic cells after binding to IgG-coated red cells and to liberation of C3a when complement is bound up to C3b. The mortality is extremely low, but in an already sick patient the added complication of destruction of transfused red cells may contribute to death.

The management of immediate HTRs should be to terminate the transfusion immediately the patient develops the appropriate signs or symptoms. The identity of the patient and the units transfused should be checked against the appropriate documentation. Blood samples must be taken for investigation (Table 16.9). The circulating blood volume should be restored and blood pressure and urinary flow maintained using fluid challenges and furosemide (frusemide) infusion. Monitoring on a high-dependency unit may be required. The renal team should be involved early if urine output is poor (< 1 mL/kg per hour) and haemofiltration may be necessary. Appropriate blood component therapy will be required if there is DIC.

All packs of transfused units should be returned to the blood bank. Pretransfusion samples should be tested in parallel. If no identification mistake is discovered immediately, a sample should be sent for bacteriological testing and all urine passed during the first 24 hours should be measured and examined for haemoglobin. Subsequent management depends upon awareness of the possible complications and prompt therapy if these occur. If the patient develops only a rise in temperature, unaccompanied by other symptoms, red cell incompatibility is unlikely and the transfusion should be slowed, under strict monitoring, but need not be stopped.

New technologies to prevent patient identification errors are being evaluated in a number of countries. These generally

Table 16.9 Investigation of suspected acute haemolytic transfusion reaction.

Blood test	Rationale/findings
Full blood count	Baseline parameters, red cell agglutinates on film
Plasma/urinary Hb, haptoglobin, bilirubin	Evidence of intravascular or extravascular haemolysis
Blood group of patient and units transfused	Compare with retested pretransfusion sample, to detect ABO error
	Unexpected ABO antibodies may arise from transfusion of incompatible plasma. Rechecking labels is often sufficient
DAT	Positive in majority. Compare with retested pretransfusion sample. May be negative if all incompatible cells destroyed
Compatibility testing	Repeat antibody screen and compatibility testing on pre- and post-transfusion samples. Elution of antibody from post-transfusion cells may aid antibody identification or confirm specificities in plasma in cases of non-ABO incompatibility
Urea, electrolytes and creatinine	Baseline renal function
Coagulation screen	Detection and monitoring of DIC
Blood cultures of patient and units	In event of possible septic reaction caused by bacterial contamination of unit

involve bar-coded patient identification details on the patient's wristband and the use, both on the wards and in the laboratory, of a hand-held bar-code reader with all data collated by the transfusion computer system. These systems are likely to be developed in tandem with similar arrangements for pharmacy and drug prescriptions, as well as ordering of blood tests and other investigations for patients.

Delayed haemolytic transfusion reactions

Such reactions are neither predictable nor preventable. They are always caused by IgG antibodies. In the majority of cases, an individual has been previously sensitized to one (or more) red cell antigen(s) by previous transfusion or pregnancy. Antibody is not detectable in routine pretransfusion testing, but the transfusion of blood containing the antigens to which the recipient has been sensitized previously provokes a brisk anamnestic response that is characteristic of the secondary immune response. Within days, the antibody level rises and the transfused cells are removed from the circulation. The effects of the secondary immunization are usually seen about 5–10 days after the transfusion, when the recipient may already have left hospital.

Most of these reactions are asymptomatic, but when manifest the clinical features include the triad of fever, hyperbilirubinaemia and anaemia. The degree of reduction in haemoglobin level will of course depend on the number of incompatible units transfused.

The possibility of delayed HTRs underlines the importance of always taking fresh serum samples for antibody screening, DAT and compatibility testing if a transfusion has been given more than 72 hours previously. Awareness of this complication may avoid unnecessary investigations to exclude infection when fever develops a few days after a transfusion. Most importantly, it will detect any alloantibody that will have been boosted by the transfusion, thus enabling the provision of compatible blood.

Reactions due to white cell and platelet antibodies

Non-haemolytic febrile transfusion reactions

Febrile reactions are most frequently due to the transfusion of blood components containing white cells to patients sensitized to white cell antigens and, more rarely, to platelet antigens. Together with urticaria, these are the most common types of immunological reactions to blood transfusion. Antibodies are directed usually against HLA antigens, or sometimes against granulocyte and platelet-specific antigens; they are stimulated by previous transfusions or pregnancies. Cytokines released from white cells during storage may also be pyrogenic. Characteristically, the onset of the reaction is delayed until 30–90 min after the start of the transfusion (depending on the strength of antibody and the speed of transfusion). A rise in temperature may be the sole symptom, but the recipient may suffer chills, headache or rigors. There is no associated hypotension, lumbar pain or chest discomfort. These reactions are usually only troublesome rather than dangerous, except in very sick patients or when caused by very potent lymphocytotoxic HLA antibodies.

The management of a simple mild febrile transfusion reaction is to slow the rate of transfusion and treat the patient with an antipyretic such as paracetamol. Antihistamines are of no benefit. It is usually not necessary to discontinue the transfusion: more blood is probably wasted by premature termination of a unit due to a simple febrile reaction than for any other reason.

When a patient requiring repeated transfusions has a history of simple febrile reactions, the rate of transfusion should be kept slow and antipyretics should be prescribed prophylactically. If severe symptoms persist, tests for HLA antibodies (lymphocytotoxicity) should be carried out. If these are negative, platelet antibodies should be sought. In the UK, the incidence of febrile transfusion reactions has decreased significantly since the introduction, first, of buffy-coat removal (leucoreduction) and, since 1999, of universal leucodepletion of blood components. Modern pre-storage leucodepletion filters are highly efficient and can remove more than 98% of the white cells; the specification is that 99% of leucodepleted components should have less than 5×10^6 leucocytes. Red cells and platelets should be filtered as soon as possible after collection in the transfusion centre. In countries where there is no universal leucodepletion policy, there is no need to administer white cell-depleted blood prophylactically, except in cases where prevention of sensitization to HLA and leucocyte/platelet antigens is essential (i.e. possible future consideration for bone marrow transplantation, especially in patients with aplastic anaemia). In such countries, the provision of buffy coat-poor red cell and platelets will prevent most non-haemolytic febrile transfusion reactions.

Transfusion-related acute lung injury

TRALI consists of non-cardiogenic pulmonary oedema with bilateral pulmonary infiltrates on chest radiography, accompanied by chills, fever, cough and dyspnoea with low oxygen saturation and low or normal central venous pressure. The clinical picture, depending on the severity, will be the same as acute lung injury or acute respiratory distress syndrome (ARDS) due to other causes, and a differential diagnosis is essential. Symptoms develop very rapidly, usually within 1–2 hours, or up to 6 hours after infusion of a plasma-containing component.

Management is essentially supportive, requiring care in a high-dependency unit, and careful attention to fluid balance. The reaction is due in most cases to passive transfer of leucoagglutinins (mostly anti-HLA class I or class II or granulocyte antibodies, i.e. anti-HNA) in donor plasma, leading to endothelial and epithelial injury, alveolar damage and inflammatory changes, mediated by cytokines and other inflammatory mediators. The donors are usually multiparous women. Once identified as the source of a reaction, such donors should be removed from the panel, even though it is known that their plasma does not always lead to TRALI in recipients with the pertinent antigens. The incidence is unclear but may be in the region of 1 in 5000 transfusions. There appears to be a significant mortality rate from this condition, but not as high as from other causes of ARDS.

In the UK, the incidence of TRALI has been declining in recent years since the introduction of the policy to produce FFP and use plasma to suspend platelet pools mainly from male donors.

Post-transfusion purpura

Post-transfusion purpura is a rare complication of blood transfusion, characterized by sudden onset of severe thrombocytopenia 7–10 days after the transfusion of platelet-containing blood components, usually red cells. The patient always has a history of previous blood transfusions or pregnancies (thus it is far more common in women). The most frequent cause is the presence in the recipient of an antibody (anti-HPA-1a) against the platelet-specific antigen HPA-1a (PI^{A1}); next in frequency is anti-HPA-5b. It appears that the antigen–antibody reaction between the recipient's antibody and the donor platelets causes both transfused and autologous platelets to be prematurely destroyed, either by the formation of immune complexes (in a manner similar to the 'innocent bystander' mechanism) or by cross-reaction of the causative antibody with the patient's own platelets. The disease is self-limiting, but in severe cases or if bleeding occurs, prompt therapy with intravenous immunoglobulin or plasma exchange is indicated. Platelet transfusion is not recommended, as this may exacerbate the disease process.

Transfusion-associated graft-versus-host disease

Transfusion-associated graft-versus-host disease is a very rare but usually fatal complication of blood transfusion, caused by the engraftment and clonal expansion of HLA-compatible donor lymphocytes in the recipient. It is characterized by fever, skin rash, diarrhoea, hepatitis and pancytopenia. The diagnosis is made by detecting donor-derived cells or DNA in the peripheral blood or affected tissues of the patient. The first SHOT (haemovigilance) reports included 13 cases of transfusion-associated graft-versus-host disease, all fatal, in patients for whom gamma-irradiated blood components were not indicated at the time. In recent years there have been no reprts of this condition.

Reactions due to plasma protein antibodies

Mild urticarial reactions without other symptoms are not uncommon during blood transfusion; they occur with an approximate incidence of 1% and are mediated by IgE antibodies, usually against plasma proteins or other allergens present in donor plasma. Mild urticarial reactions may be treated effectively with antihistamines, and do not always recur. There is no necessity to avoid transfusion of standard 'bank blood' unless symptoms are recurrent and severe. On the other hand, anaphylactic reactions accompanied by dyspnoea, wheezing, collapse and shock are rare and potentially fatal. Such severe reactions are associated with the presence of anti-IgA in an IgA-deficient recipient. These antibodies react with IgA in the transfused plasma and complement is activated, with the consequent liberation of anaphylatoxins C3a and C5a, leukotrienes and cytokines. Milder anaphylactoid reactions may be associated with anti-IgA of limited specificity.

If an anaphylactic reaction occurs, the recipient should be treated promptly with adrenaline and tested for the presence of plasma protein antibodies. If anti-IgA is detected, plasma from IgA-deficient donors should be used in future, as well as well-washed red cells and platelets. Occasionally, washed cells may be indicated for patients with serious urticarial or severe hypersensitivity reactions due to non-IgA antibodies.

Non-immunological complications

Disease transmission
See p. 270.

Reactions due to bacterial pyrogens and bacteria

The presence of bacteria in transfused blood may lead either to febrile reactions in the recipient (due to pyrogens) or to the far more serious manifestations of septic or endotoxic shock. Bacterial-transmitted infections are considerably more frequent than serious acute manifestations of virus-transmitted infections in countries such as the UK (see p. 274).

Bacterial pyrogens are rarely the cause of reactions with present-day methods of manufacture and the sterilization of fluids and disposable equipment. Infection of stored blood is also rare, but has a very high mortality in recipients. Skin contaminants are sometimes present in freshly donated blood but many (e.g. staphylococci) do not survive storage at 4°C. However, they will grow profusely in platelet concentrates stored at 22°C. A number of Gram-negative, psychrophilic, endotoxin-producing contaminants found in dirt, soil and faeces (pseudomonads, coliforms) may very rarely enter a unit and grow readily under the storage conditions of blood (and even more rapidly at room temperature).

Healthy individuals who are bacteraemic at the time of donation may also act as a source of infection. The majority of such cases relate to transmission of *Yersinia enterocolitica*, which grows well in red cell components due to its dependence on citrate and iron.

Transfusion of heavily contaminated blood will usually lead to sudden dramatic symptoms, with collapse, high fever, shock and DIC with haemorrhagic phenomena. These symptoms resemble, and may be more severe than, those of ABO incompatibility. Prompt recognition of the cause and administration of broad-spectrum intravenous antibiotics, in conjunction with the treatment of shock, are vital. The diagnosis should be confirmed by direct microscopic examination of the blood, and blood cultures from both the recipient and the blood bag.

Prevention of this potentially disastrous complication of blood transfusion rests on stringent observation of procedures for aseptic technique during arm cleansing prior to blood collection and for the manufacture of anticoagulant solutions and packs. Diversion of the first 20–30 mL of blood into a satellite pouch further reduces the contamination of units of blood with skin bacteria. Packs should never be opened for sampling, and the unit should be transfused within 24 hours if any open method of preparation has been used (e.g. washed red cells, frozen–thawed blood). Blood should always be kept in accurately controlled refrigerators (with alarms), maintained strictly at 2–6°C, and a unit of blood should never be removed and taken to the ward or theatre until it is required. The practice of ordering multiple units of blood for the same patient and leaving unused units at room temperature (or in uncontrolled ward refrigerators) until needed must not be tolerated. Handling and storage errors are increasingly reported to SHOT and comprised 13% of all reports in 2008. Bacteria may cause haemolysis or clotting of blood and all units should be inspected for these before transfusion. Platelets should be inspected for discoloration, foaming and absence of swirling.

Baseline observations and regular monitoring of patients undergoing transfusion, with repeat observations at 15–30 min after commencement, are essential so that reactions are detected and acted upon at the earliest opportunity.

Transfusion-associated circulatory overload

All patients, except those who are actively bleeding or fluid depleted, will experience a temporary rise in blood volume and venous pressure after the transfusion of blood and/or plasma. In young people with normal cardiovascular function, this will not cause any embarrassment, providing the total volume given and the transfusion rate are not excessive. In contrast, pregnant women, patients with severe anaemia, and the elderly with compromised cardiovascular function will not tolerate the increase in plasma volume, and acute pulmonary oedema may develop. In view of this possibility, concentrated red cells should be given to these patients slowly over 4 hours. Patients with severe chronic anaemia and cardiac failure may require partial exchange transfusion. In less severe cases, diuretics (oral or intravenous furosemide) should be given at the start of the transfusion and only one or two units of concentrated red cells should be transfused in any 24-hour period. Faster correction of anaemia is rarely required in a non-bleeding patient. The patient should be observed carefully for early signs of cardiac failure (raised jugular venous pressure, crepitations at the lung bases, and symptoms of pulmonary oedema, cough and breath-lessness). For this reason alone, transfusions should be given during the day, when staff are able to monitor the patient closely. Overnight transfusions should be avoided for the patient's safety and comfort. If circulatory overload occurs, transfusion should be discontinued, the patient propped upright and intravenous diuretics given. Emergency venesection for fluid overload should not be necessary if all precautions have been taken.

Thrombophlebitis

Thrombophlebitis is a complication of indwelling venous cannulae, and not specifically related to blood transfusion.

Air embolism

This is now practically unknown, as blood and blood components are administered from plastic bags.

Transfusion haemosiderosis

Haemosiderosis is a very real complication of repeated blood transfusions, and is being seen more commonly as long-term blood transfusion therapy improves the survival of patients suffering from some chronic anaemias. It is most commonly seen in thalassaemic individuals, who commence transfusions in early childhood. Each unit of blood contains approximately 200 mg of iron, whereas the daily excretion rate is about 1 mg, and the body has no way of excreting the excess. Unless a patient is actively bleeding, and therefore losing iron, iron accumulation is inevitable. Significant iron overload is generally present after approximately 50 units of blood have been transfused to an average-sized adult. It is routine practice to give thalassaemic patients the parenteral iron-chelating agent desferrioxamine or the oral iron chelator deferiprone when available, or a combination of both or deferasirox orally. This does not completely overcome the iron load administered with blood, but has substantially delayed the onset of problems due to haemosiderosis (see Chapters 4 and 6).

Patients who are transfusion dependent should receive blood which is less than 1 week old, which may help to increase the transfusion interval and therefore reduce the overall number of units required. Transfusion of neocytes, or young red cells, looked promising as a means of decreasing the frequency of transfusions and of reducing the iron load. However, this practice is expensive and time-consuming and the trial results were not as favourable as expected.

Complications of massive transfusion

Massive transfusion is usually defined as the replacement of the total blood volume within a 24-hour period. Although a number of different problems may result from changes that occur in stored blood, it should not be forgotten that any patient who needs a massive blood transfusion is by definition already seriously ill. Too much attention may be paid to the theoretical problems caused by metabolic changes in stored blood and not enough to the underlying clinical condition. The coagulopathy problems derived from massive transfusion are different in trauma from those in elective surgery.

Although the transfusion problems encountered in cardiac surgery were in the past similar to those of massive transfusion, the volume of blood transfused to such patients is now insufficient to merit the routine administration of fresh blood or FFP. When postoperative bleeding occurs, this is usually due to platelet dysfunction and/or reduced numbers. Platelet transfusion is then indicated. Whenever possible, antiplatelet and antithrombotic drugs should be suspended 5–7 days prior to elective surgery.

Replacement of the total blood volume will inevitably lead to some dilution of platelets. Blood effectively has no functional platelets after 48 hours of storage and once 8–10 units of blood have been given to an adult, thrombocytopenia will usually be seen. Regular monitoring of the platelet count in these situations is essential, preferably employing reliable point-of-care testing techniques for rapidly available results; platelet administration may then be judged on the clinical condition and the platelet count. As a guide, platelet transfusion is indicated if the platelet count falls below $80 \times 10^9/L$ in the face of continued bleeding or surgical intervention. Red cell transfusion contributes to normal haemostasis by helping with the margination of platelets and responsiveness of activated platelets, so it is recommended to aim for haemoglobin levels around 10 g/dL if possible.

Coagulation factors will also be diluted as stored blood is administered. Whole blood that has been stored for less than 14 days has adequate levels of most coagulation factors for haemostasis (whole blood is not available in the UK). Factors V and VIII are the most labile but, in conditions of patient 'stress', factor VIII is released from endothelial cells; deficiency of factor VIII sufficient to cause bleeding does not usually occur in these circumstances. If stored blood more than 14 days old is given, or if plasma reduced blood or red cells in optimal additive solution have been used, replacement of coagulation factors may become necessary. Treatment should be monitored by coagulation studies and DIC screen; FFP and cryoprecipitate, as a source of fibrinogen, should be prescribed on the basis of results from the laboratory or point-of-care testing, such as the thromboelastograph. DIC associated with massive transfusion is most usually due to the underlying condition, such as trauma and/or prolonged shock, and not due to transfused blood per se.

Recent evidence, especially from military practice, has suggested that in cases of major trauma with massive haemorrhage, aggressive early platelet and FFP transfusion reduces overall component usage and improves outcome, especially in patients with High Injury Severity Score. Although further good-quality data are still required, some practitioners in this area favour the issue of a 'shock pack' from the blood bank in these circumstances, so that platelets and FFP as well as red cells are available for immediate transfusion. Fibrinogen concentrate, pro-thrombin complex concentrate and recombinant FVIIa are increasingly used to aid the control of massive haemorrhage. Well-designed randomized controlled studies are difficult in this area, but case series show encouraging results.

Metabolic changes in stored blood include low pH, hypocalcaemia and hyperkalaemia. The reduced oxygen-carrying capacity of stored blood becomes significant only after 21 days' storage (for CPD-AI blood) and is due to low 2,3-DPG levels (see Chapter 20, p. 376). Although excess citrate in transfused blood could cause toxicity theoretically, its metabolism in the liver is usually rapid. In practice, the only situations when citrate toxicity is a real problem is with extremely rapid transfusion (1 unit every 5 min), or in infants, especially if premature, having exchange transfusion with blood stored in citrate for longer than 5 days. Hypocalcaemia and hyperkalaemia are usually transient and rapidly corrected once the transfused blood is circulating. Acidosis is not generally significant, as citrate metabolism leads to an alkalosis. However, if a patient is severely shocked and under-transfused, acidosis may be a clinical problem. All these changes due to stored blood are exacerbated by hypothermia. Cardiac irregularities, in particular ventricular fibrillation, may result from transfusion of large quantities of cold blood. The optimal functioning of coagulation factors and of platelets is also temperature dependent and effectiveness is reduced by hypothermia. Thus, the use of a blood warmer and keeping the patient warm may be the most important measures to prevent the complications of massive transfusion. Unfortunately, this inevitably reduces the speed at which blood can be transfused, which may be a serious disadvantage when rapid transfusion is needed. When replacement therapy has failed, recombinant activated factor VII (rFVIIa) has been reported as successful in treating the coagulopathy of massive transfusion. However, more evidence is needed. The utilization of prothrombin complex concentrates in this setting also requires evaluation. Tranexamic acid is also being tried in a controlled trial.

The most important consideration in massive blood transfusion is to replace blood loss quickly and adequately with maintenance of normal tissue perfusion, and to prevent development of coagulopathy or thrombocytopenia by aggressive early replacement. Too little blood too late has far more serious consequences than massive blood transfusion itself.

Haemovigilance and SHOT

The interest in transfusion-transmitted infections (TTIs) has meant that transfusion medicine has developed significantly in the last two to three decades and great emphasis has been put on quality, audit and good manufacturing practice. However, there were no surveillance systems in place to assess the incidence and prevalence of transfusion risks. France instituted the first system of national haemovigilance in 1994. Haemovigilance is defined by the International Haemovigilance Network as 'a set of surveillance procedures organized from the collection of blood and its components to the follow-up of its recipients, with the purpose of collecting and evaluating information on the undesirable and unexpected effects resulting from the therapeutic use of labile blood components and of preventing their occurrence or recurrence'.

The UK's professionally led haemovigilance system, SHOT, was introduced in 1996 (Figure 16.4). SHOT receives reports of adverse incidents surrounding the transfusion of single or small pool blood components supplied by the UK National Blood Services (red cells, platelets, FFP including MB and SD treated, cryoprecipitate and cryodepleted plasma). The vast majority of incidents reported are from hospitals, with at least 50% arising from clinical areas. SHOT does not comprehensively cover complications of fractionated plasma products but does report on incidents related to anti-D immunoglobulin administration. In the past, reporting to SHOT has been voluntary. In recent years a number of quality, inspection and accreditation bodies within the UK have made reporting to SHOT a requirement. These include Clinical Pathology Accreditation UK, the National Patient Safety Agency and the Department of Health (via HSC 30/2007).

There is now a statutory requirement to report serious adverse reactions and serious adverse events arising in blood establishments or hospital blood banks to the European Commission under Directive 2005/61. In the UK, reporting to both SHOT and the regulatory authority, the Medicines and Healthcare Products Regulatory Agency, is completed online via a shared portal called SABRE (Serious Adverse Blood Reactions and Events). Hospitals report incidents to SHOT in the following categories.

1 Error-related incidents
   (a) Incorrect blood component transfused, regardless of harm to recipients.
   (b) Handling and storage errors.
   (c) Inappropriate and unnecessary transfusion.
2 Physiological reactions
   (a) Acute transfusion reaction within 24 hours.
   (b) Delayed transfusion reaction beyond 24 hours.
   (c) Transfusion-associated graft-versus-host disease.
   (d) TRALI.
   (e) Transfusion-associated circulatory overload.
   (f) Transfusion-associated dyspnoea.
   (g) Post-transfusion purpura.
3 Transfusion-transmitted infection
   (a) Bacterial contamination.
   (b) Post-transfusion viral infection.
   (c) Other post-transfusion infection (e.g. malaria, vCJD).
4 'Near-miss' events (this has been introduced more recently).
5 Anti-D-related events.

Since 1996, SHOT has collected data on serious transfusion complications in the UK and has used these to make firm recommendations for improvements in transfusion safety. The four UK Blood Services currently issue approximately 3 million blood components each year. Since 1996 there has been a year-on-year increase in the number of reports, with over 400 eligible hospitals registered on the scheme. Participation in the scheme continues to increase, and a greater number of hospitals are

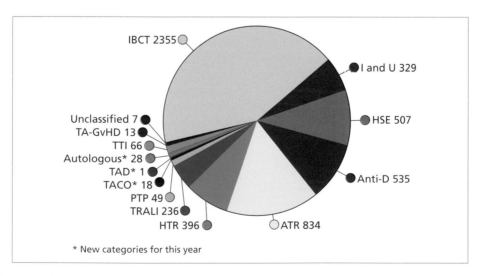

Figure 16.4 Cumulative numbers of cases reviewed 1996–2008. ATR, acute transfusion reaction; HSE, handling and storage errors; HTR, haemolytic transfusion reaction; I&U, inappropriate and unnecessary transfusion; IBCT, incorrect blood component transfused; PTP, post-transfusion purpura; TACO, transfusion-associated circulatory overload; TAD, transfusion-associated dyspnoea; TA-GvHD, transfusion-associated graft-versus-host disease; TRALI, transfusion-related acute lung injury; TTI, transfusion-transmitted infection.

sending in more than one report. There has been a consistent increase in reporting every year, with most recently an 85% increase between 2007 and 2008, affecting all categories except transfusion-transmitted infection.

Of 5374 fully analysed reports between 1996 and 2008, 2355 (44%) were 'wrong blood' incidents (excluding handling and storage errors and inappropriate and unnecessary transfusion, which were previously included in the category 'Incorrect blood component transfused'; see Figure 16.4). Of these, 233 were ABO-incompatible red cell transfusions. Immune complications constituted 28% of reports, with 236 cases of possible TRALI.

Over the 12 years of reporting, the trends observed by SHOT have borne the hallmarks of an effective vigilance system. The number of incidents reported overall has risen, while the frequency of the most serious events has fallen (Figure 16.5). There has been a decrease in the number of ABO-incompatible transfusions and a reduction in the number of cases of TRALI. These trends follow changes in national policies on training and competency for staff involved in blood transfusion, and a switch to male-only FFP, both instigated as a result of SHOT data. Overall mortality directly attributable to transfusion has decreased (Figure 16.6). TTI constituted just 1.2% of reports. There were 64 confirmed TTIs, of which the majority (38 cases)

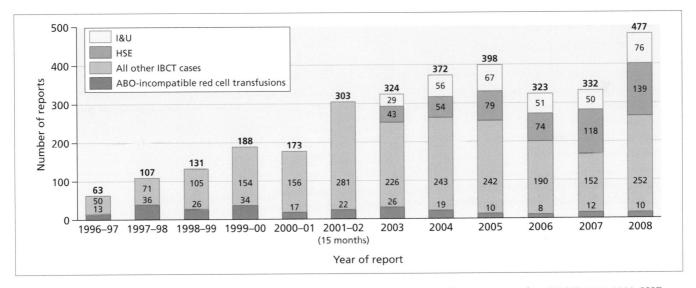

Figure 16.5 Incorrect blood component transfused (IBCT) and ABO-incompatible red cell cases reported to SHOT 1996–2008. HSE, handling and storage errors; I&U, inappropriate and unnecessary transfusion.

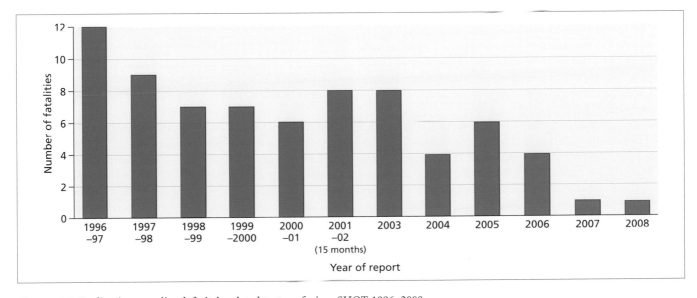

Figure 16.6 Decline in mortality definitely related to transfusion, SHOT 1996–2008.

were of bacterial contamination, 32 from platelets and six from red cells. In 2008 there were four incidents involving bacterially contaminated platelets affecting six patients, two of whom died.

The SHOT data demonstrate that in high-resource countries, virological safety of the blood supply is advanced. Efforts should now be concentrated on preventing bacterial contamination and in other areas of transfusion medicine, such as the encouragement of appropriate use of blood, safe administration of blood components, and accurate patient and sample identification.

Appropriate use of blood and alternatives to allogeneic blood transfusion

In view of the inherent risks of blood transfusion and difficulties with donor recruitment due to escalating stringent donor selection criteria, blood components should only be transfused when the benefits outweigh the risks.

There are several reasons for aiming to reduce unnecessary allogeneic blood transfusion:

1 safety of the patient, by avoiding errors, as well as microbiological and immunological risks;
2 shortages of blood and increasing difficulties in the recruitment of blood donors;
3 cost containment;
4 high anxiety levels in patients that are disproportionate to the real residual infectious risk of transfusion.

There are several alternatives to allogeneic blood transfusion, and these can be classified as operational, biological and pharmacological.

Operational alternatives

• Treatment of preoperative anaemia with haematinics, if appropriate, in a timely way through pre-assessment clinics for elective surgery. Optimization of preoperative haemoglobin using haematinics (including intravenous iron) and erythropoietin.
• Autologous transfusion. Cell salvage is most cost-effective if applied to patients undergoing surgical procedures with a high risk of requirement for blood transfusion. Preoperative autologous deposit is becoming less favoured as evidence of efficacy is patchy and contradictory. European regulation (Directive 2002/98, UK Blood Safety and Quality Regulations 2005) mandates that this process can only be carried out at a blood establishment. The value of preoperative haemodilution needs further assessment.
• Re-evaluation of transfusion triggers and algorithms for estimation of acceptable blood loss in surgery. Adherence to guidelines.

• Alternative fluid replacement, i.e. replace use of FFP or albumin with crystalloids or colloids when appropriate.
• Anaesthetic methods to reduce blood loss (e.g. hypotension, patient warming).
• Enhancement of surgical haemostasis and new surgical technologies (e.g. harmonic scalpels, laser, water jets).
• Non-invasive surgery (e.g. angioplasty, laparoscopic surgery).
• Stopping aspirin, non-steroidal anti-inflammatory drugs, clopidogrel and anticoagulants preoperatively.
• Postoperative haematinics.
• Point-of-care testing in theatre.
• Miniaturizing blood sampling in intensive care units for premature babies and adults.
• Stem cell transplantation for transfusion-dependent patients (e.g. thalassaemia).

Biological alternatives

• Recombinant erythropoietin.
• G-CSF.
• Recombinant clotting factors.
• Recombinant activated factor VII (rFVIIa).
• Fibrin glue in surgery.
• In the future: haemoglobin solutions and platelet substitutes?

Pharmacological alternatives

• Tranexamic acid infusion intraoperatively or postoperatively.
• DDAVP preoperatively in mild haemophiliacs.
• Intravenous iron, with or without recombinant erythropoietin preoperatively, especially in patients intolerant or unresponsive to oral iron.
• In the future: oxygen carriers such as fluorocarbons?

Haemolytic disease of the fetus and newborn

Haemolytic disease of the fetus and newborn is a condition in which the lifespan of the fetal/neonatal red cells is shortened due to maternal alloantibodies against red cell antigens inherited from the father. Maternal IgG can cross the placenta, and thus IgG1 and IgG3 red cell alloantibodies can gain access to the fetus. If the fetal red cells contain the corresponding antigen, then binding of antibody to red cells will occur. When the antibody is of clinical significance (e.g. anti-D, -c, -E, -K, -Jk^a), and of sufficient potency, the coated cells will be prematurely removed by the fetal mononuclear phagocytic system. The effects on the fetus/newborn infant may vary according to the characteristics of the maternal alloantibody.

The antibodies giving rise to HDN most commonly belong to the Rh or ABO blood group systems. The morbidity of Rh HDN is explained by the great immunogenicity of the D antigen; HDN due to anti-c is also important and its incidence comes second among the cases of severe HDN, closely followed by the non-Rh antibody, anti-K. (The disease caused by anti-K is more properly called *alloimmune anaemia of the fetus and newborn* as it is due to direct inhibition of erythropoiesis by the antibody and haemolysis is not a feature.) Antibodies against antigens in almost all the blood group systems (e.g. Duffy, Kidd), and against the so-called 'public' and 'private' antigens, have also been occasionally responsible for HDN. However, IgM cannot cross the placenta and Lewis and P_1 antibodies, which occur frequently during pregnancy, are usually IgM and do not lead to HDN. Furthermore, the Lewis antigens are not red cell antigens per se and are not fully developed at birth.

All women who have had previous pregnancies or blood transfusions may become immunized against 'foreign' red cell antigens. However, red cell antibodies may be found in those with no such history, either because the antibodies are 'naturally occurring' or because a spontaneous abortion early in a previous pregnancy was unrecognized as such. Blood samples from all pregnant women must be tested early for the presence of atypical red cell antibodies (usually at 12–16 weeks, during the booking visit), and again at 28 weeks' gestation, even if no antibody was found at booking.

When anti-D, anti-c or anti-K are detected at booking, the strength of the antibody and the rate of rise (if any) in titre, or level in micrograms, during pregnancy must be carefully monitored by regular monthly blood sampling during the second trimester and fortnightly thereafter. If the level of any other clinically significant antibody is moderately high or high at 28 weeks, it should be monitored fortnightly until term. If the level of anti-D is greater than 10 IU/mL (2 μg/mL) or anti-c greater than 20 IU/mL, or if other antibodies have an IAT titre of 32 or greater, the fetus should be monitored by ultrasound/Doppler for evidence of anaemia and cardiac decompensation. At these levels, in the case of anti-D, anti-c or anti-K, referral to a fetomaternal unit is advised. It should be noted that, in the case of potent anti-K, severe anaemia may occur relatively early during gestation.

Fetal and neonatal anaemia due to anti-D and anti-K tends to be more severe than that due to any other alloantibody. The next important, in terms of severity, is that due to anti-c. Anti-A,B is a common cause of HDN in group O mothers delivering group A or B infants (1 in 150 births), but the disease is usually mild; death *in utero* is unknown though exchange transfusion after birth may occasionally be required.

There are many significant differences between HDN due to ABO and Rh incompatibilities. The low incidence of infants requiring treatment for ABO HDN contrasts with the situation in Rh HDN. Furthermore, ABO HDN is found as frequently in the first pregnancy as in later pregnancies; subsequent infants may not be affected. In Rh HDN, a first pregnancy is usually unaffected (unless there has been prior immunization by abortion or transfusion), and subsequent Rh-incompatible infants are affected to an equal degree or more severely. The majority of neonates affected with Rh HDN require some form of therapy.

Clinical features

In its least severe form, HDN manifests itself as mild haemolytic anaemia. The infant's red cells, coated with maternal IgG alloantibody, are removed prematurely from the circulation, causing slight jaundice (maximum on the second to third days of life) and mild anaemia during the second week of life. More severely affected infants show severe hyperbilirubinaemia in the neonatal period, a condition that was called *icterus gravis neonatorum*. Prompt treatment with exchange transfusion is necessary to prevent bilirubin impregnation of the basal ganglia and neurological damage, a condition known as *kernicterus*. This condition may be fatal, or lead to serious neurological deficit, with deafness, mental retardation, choreoathetosis and spasticity.

In the most severely affected cases, profound anaemia develops *in utero*, and intrauterine death may occur at any time from the 18th week of gestation. Affected fetuses are pale and oedematous, with marked ascites. The placenta is bulky, swollen and friable. This condition is known as *hydrops fetalis*, and had a high mortality rate until ultrasound-guided intravascular transfusions and improved intensive care facilities for very premature babies were introduced. The pathophysiology of hydrops is not fully understood, but extravascular haemolysis with fetal anaemia seems to play a major role by stimulating extramedullary erythropoiesis in the liver, with distortion of the hepatic circulation, leading to portal hypertension and impaired albumin production. Hypoalbuminaemia leads to ascites, oedema and pleural/pericardial effusions. In addition, the severe anaemia leads to cardiac failure and tissue hypoxia, which damages the endothelium, leading to fluid extravasation into the extravascular space.

The blood film of a fetus affected by HDN shows polychromasia and increased numbers of nucleated red cells (Figure 16.7). In most cases (except a few due to ABO antibodies), the DAT (Coombs test) on the infant's cells is positive owing to IgG coating.

Rh haemolytic disease of the newborn

Until the early 1970s (when Rh immunoprophylaxis was introduced), 0.5–0.75% of all births gave rise to infants affected by Rh HDN. Anti-D accounted for over 90% of all cases. Although anti-D HDN has decreased significantly as a cause, it remains the most important. Of all infants affected by Rh HDN, 10–20% died *in utero* or in the early neonatal period before effective

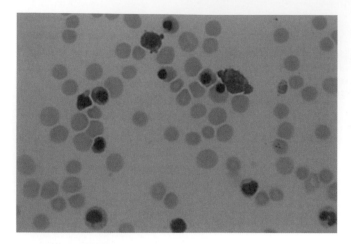

Figure 16.7 Blood film of a fetus affected by HDN showing polychromasia and increased numbers of normoblasts.

therapy was possible. The disease due to anti-D is more severe than that due to most other alloantibodies (e.g. anti-c, -E) except for some cases of anti-K. Early detection of maternal alloantibodies, regular fetal monitoring and assessment of rises in antibody titres are prerequisites to a successful outcome.

Antenatal assessment of maternal blood

Rarely, anti-D may develop in a first pregnancy in a woman who has had no previous transfusions. However, it is not common for the antibody to reach high levels, and it is not usually detectable before 28 weeks; most of such cases become apparent after delivery. Conversely, in women who have had previous pregnancies or transfusions with Rh-positive red cells, anti-D may be detected early in pregnancy; regular monitoring of the level is necessary in order to plan the best type and timing of intervention. At present, the most objective means of quantifying anti-D levels routinely is with an automated analyser or, rarely, by flow cytometry and not by manual titration. More important than the anti-D levels in determining the severity of HDN is the obstetric assessment of the fetus.

The ABO, Rh groups and antibody screen should be performed in all pregnant women at booking (usually around 16 weeks' gestation). All women should have the testing repeated once more at about 28 weeks to confirm the Rh group and to detect the presence of atypical antibodies. If clinically significant antibodies are detected, more frequent testing will be required (see below). If the mother is RhD negative with no anti-D by 28 weeks, routine antenatal prophylaxis should be given (see below). Following delivery, all RhD-negative women who are unsensitized for RhD should be given prophylactic anti-RhD immunoglobulin if the infant is RhD positive (Figure 16.8).

The level of anti-D in the serum correlates approximately with the clinical severity of the HDN, but this is also affected by factors such as IgG subclass, rate of rise of antibody, past history and presence of maternal blocking antibodies. As a rough guide, levels below 4.0 IU/mL (0.8 μg/mL) require no action, whereas a level above 4 and up to 10 IU/mL (2.0 μg/mL) indicates moderate risk; 10–20 IU/mL indicates high risk of HDN and levels greater than 20 IU/mL indicate a high risk of hydrops. Anti-D, anti-c and anti-K should be monitored monthly to 28 weeks and 2-weekly thereafter. Other red cell antibodies reacting by IAT should be retested at 28 weeks, titrated and the maternal serum should be tested for the presence of Kell alloantibodies. If the anti-D level is above 10 IU/mL, anti-c above 20 IU/mL or for other antibodies the IAT titre is above 32, the fetus should be monitored by the fetal medicine specialist for evidence of anaemia. The strength and trend in titre of other maternal alloantibodies should be reported to the obstetrician, for fetal monitoring as appropriate.

Antenatal assessment of disease severity and treatment of haemolytic disease

The severity of the haemolytic process may be assessed by fetal medicine specialists using clinical and ultrasound monitoring, including Doppler flow velocity. The systolic velocity of the fetal middle cerebral artery is a reliable indicator of fetal anaemia (Figure 16.9). Measurement of bile pigments in the amniotic fluid by spectrophotometry from week 28 onwards is less commonly used now in the UK. The absorbance of normal amniotic fluid over the range of wavelengths 400–600 nm forms a smooth curve when plotted on semi-logarithmic graph paper. When there is an excess of bilirubin, the curve shows a greatly increased absorbance, with a peak at about 450 nm. The increase in density at this wavelength over the normal absorbance is the measurement of severity.

If the non-invasive parameters of severity indicate a severely affected infant, the fetal medicine specialist can perform ultrasound-guided fetal blood sampling from 18–20 weeks onwards. The fetal haemoglobin deficit is measured (Figure 16.10) and, if necessary, an intravascular transfusion with fresh (< 5 days old) group O, RhD-negative, CMV-negative, irradiated blood of the desired packed cell volume (PCV) can be administered. Such transfusions will be performed subsequently throughout pregnancy, with a frequency determined by the severity of the disease. Fetal blood sampling and amniocentesis carry a risk of immunizing a previously unsensitized RhD-negative woman carrying an RhD-positive fetus, due to leakage of fetal blood into the maternal circulation. Similarly, pre-existing low antibody levels may be 'boosted' by a new stimulus. Immunization to, or boosting of, other clinically significant red cell alloantibodies is not a rare occurrence. Although the risks of fetal blood sampling are small in experienced hands, there are possible adverse effects on the fetus (e.g. bleeding through puncture of fetal vessels).

Intraperitoneal transfusion involves injection of antigen-negative donor red cells into the peritoneal cavity of the fetus (now rarely used). Blood with the same specification as for intravascular transfusions is used from 24 weeks of gestation. If

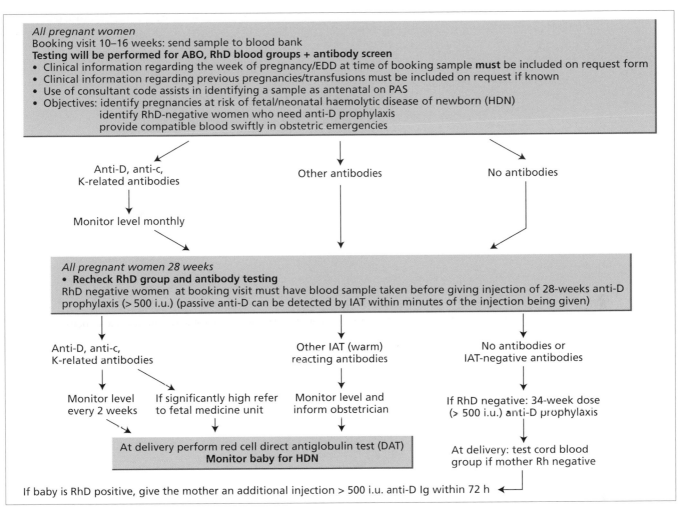

Figure 16.8 Blood group and antibody testing in pregnancy. (From British Committee for Standards in Haematology (1996) *Guidelines for Blood Grouping and Antibody Testing During Pregnancy*, with permission).

ascites is already present, absorption of the red cells into the fetal circulation is slow and intravascular transfusion will continue to be the treatment of choice.

It is possible to determine the Rh genotype of the fetus from amniotic cells through DNA typing, thus avoiding further manipulations when the fetus is RhD negative. Fetal RhD genotyping is now possible by DNA extraction from maternal plasma from 16–18 weeks' gestation; this non-invasive technique is replacing amniocyte typing (see Chapter 15). If the partner is available, he too may be tested for the presence of the relevant antigen.

Premature delivery

Modern neonatal intensive care has dramatically increased survival rates of very premature infants born at 24–30 weeks' gestation. Nevertheless, morbidity is high and premature delivery is now, due to the success of intrauterine transfusions, rarely performed. It is sometimes considered at 36 weeks for fetuses suf-

fering from haemolytic disease due to antibodies other than anti-D, anti-c or anti-K. When the previous obstetric history is poor, the mother starts with a high level of anti-D and the partner is homozygous for D, or the fetus is known to be D positive, intravenous immunoglobulin is given to carry the pregnancy to 20 weeks, when intrauterine transfusions can be started. In several countries, intravenous immunoglobulin is the mainstay of therapy throughout pregnancy.

Assessment of severity in the newborn

Cord blood samples should be taken at delivery. The DAT may be positive but is not a useful indication of severity or need for therapy. The best simple criterion of severity is the cord haemoglobin level; this is much more useful than a sample taken a few hours after birth, when rapid haemodynamic changes are occurring. The normal range of cord haemoglobin levels is 13.6–19.6 g/dL. Most infants with levels in this range do not require therapy; more than 50% of affected babies have a level

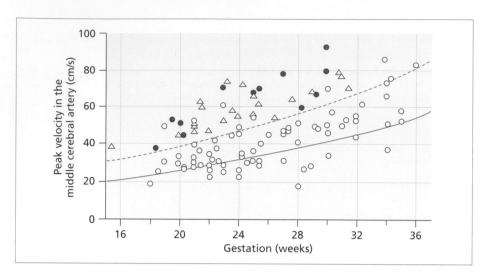

Figure 16.9 Middle cerebral artery Doppler. Peak velocity of systolic blood flow in the middle cerebral artery in 111 fetuses at risk for anaemia due to maternal red cell alloimmunization. Open circles indicate fetuses with either no anaemia or mild anaemia (≥ 0.65 multiples of the median Hb concentration). Triangles indicate fetuses with moderate or severe anaemia (< 0.65 multiples of the median Hb concentration). Solid circles indicate the fetuses with hydrops. Solid curve indicates the median peak systolic velocity in the middle cerebral artery and the dotted curve indicates 1.5 multiples of the median. (Courtesy of Professor Charles Rodeck.)

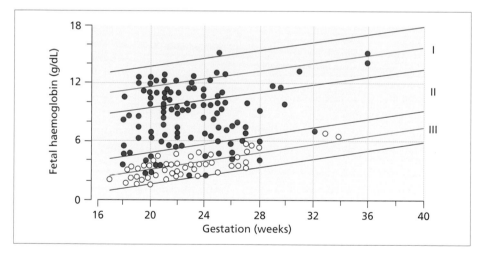

Figure 16.10 Fetal haemoglobin (Hb) concentration of 48 hydropic (open circles) and 106 non-hydropic (closed circles) fetuses from red cell isoimmunized pregnancies at time of first blood sampling. Values are plotted on the reference range of fetal Hb for gestation. The individual 95% confidence intervals of the normal Hb for gestation define zone I and the individual 95% confidence intervals of the Hb for gestation of the hydropic fetuses define zone III. Zone II indicates moderate anaemia. (Courtesy of Professor Charles Rodeck.)

in the normal range. Where the cord haemoglobin is below 12 g/dL, exchange transfusion will be necessary. It may also be indicated for a rising bilirubin level after birth, depending on the rate of rise and the maturity of the infant. Phototherapy may be given to reduce the rise in bilirubin levels but it is not a substitute for transfusion. Less severely affected infants may require small-volume transfusions of red cells at 2–3 weeks of age. In both these instances, careful follow up arrangements must be made as haemolysis may continue, causing further rises in bilirubin or need for additional top-up transfusion.

The infant's RhD group should be determined on the cord blood sample of all infants born to D-negative mothers with no preformed anti-D in order to give anti-D immunoglobulin prophylaxis if they type as D-positive. A DAT is only performed on cord bloods of mothers who have made anti-D; the cord bloods of women given antenatal Rh prophylaxis should not undergo DAT as it may be positive due to the passive anti-D given. If intrauterine transfusions have been given, the ABO and Rh groups may be those of the donor, and the DAT may be negative. A DAT should be performed on the cord blood of all women who have IAT-reactive antibodies. If the DAT is positive, the cord haemoglobin should be checked and the clinical state, haemoglobin and bilirubin of the infant monitored for signs of HDN for 1 month.

Exchange transfusion

Exchange transfusion is effective therapy for HDN, removing from the infant's circulation sensitized red cells and plasma containing both maternal antibody and bilirubin. It also treats the anaemia.

An exchange transfusion of one blood volume will replace approximately 75% of the infant's red cells. It is usual to exchange relatively large volumes of blood (e.g. 160 mL/kg) slowly, via an umbilical vein catheter. The donor blood should be ABO compatible with mother and infant, and lack the antigen against which the maternal antibody is directed. A compatibility test should be performed against maternal serum. Blood in CPD-AI of less than 5 days old with a PCV of 0.5–0.6 is suitable for exchange transfusions, regardless of the ABO group of the infant. If group O blood is used in all exchange transfusions, it should be devoid of high-titre ABO antibodies. CMV antibody-negative donations should be used for infants less than 1200 g in weight. If possible, the blood should be irradiated, but there should be no delay to the exchange on account of this. Irradiated blood must be given to infants who have been transfused *in utero*, because they are at greater risk of transfusion-associated graft-versus-host disease.

ABO haemolytic disease of the newborn

In 20% of births, the mother is ABO incompatible with her fetus. In A and B subjects, the anti-B and anti-A are predominantly IgM and do not enter the fetus. ABO HDN is usually restricted to group O mothers possessing IgG anti-A,B, in addition to IgM antibodies. In 15% of all pregnancies of white mothers, a group O mother carries a group A or B fetus, but the overall incidence of ABO HDN requiring treatment is extremely low. In absolute terms, however, exchange transfusion may be required in up to 1 in 3000 infants.

The lack of severity of ABO HDN can be accounted for by the widespread occurrence of A and B antigens, not only on red cells but also in plasma and on other cells, which will partially neutralize maternally derived ABO antibodies. Furthermore, the A and B antigens are not fully developed in the infant and the number of ABO sites is much smaller than in adults (see

Chapter 15, p. 247). Thus, only small amounts of the maternal antibody bind to infant red cells, and clinical sequelae are usually mild.

Serological findings

The mother is usually blood group O; IgG anti-A,B, anti-A and anti-B can be demonstrated in her plasma after inactivating or inhibiting the IgM component with a reducing agent (2-mercaptoethanol or dithiothreitol, ZZAP). When infants are affected and require therapy, the maternal IgG anti-A or anti-B is almost always present in a titre greater than 64.

The infant will be group A or B and the DAT may be positive, only weakly positive or negative. In most cases, spontaneous agglutination will be observed if a drop of whole blood from the cord is rocked gently on a tile, especially if the cells are suspended in ABO-compatible plasma. Testing eluates from the red cells by IAT will reveal anti-A or anti-B specificity. Examination of the infant's blood film may show spontaneous agglutination of red cells, spherocytosis (not seen with Rh HDN), reticulocytosis, polychromasia and increased numbers of nucleated red cells.

Treatment

Severe anaemia is uncommon. Hyperbilirubinaemia is more often a problem and often subsides with phototherapy, but may occasionally be serious enough to warrant exchange transfusion to prevent brain damage. Group O donor blood with low-titre anti-A,B should be used.

Haemolytic disease of the newborn due to other antibodies

After anti-D, the antibodies encountered most commonly as a cause of HDN are anti-c and anti-K (the former usually due to previous pregnancy and the latter to previous maternal blood transfusions). The disease is generally less severe than that caused by anti-D, but may sometimes be serious enough to warrant early delivery and/or exchange transfusion, and occasionally requires treatment of the fetus. Anti-K of high titre may cause severe fetal anaemia, because the K antigen is present in early red cell precursors. Assessment and treatment of the fetus and infant should be along the same lines as for anti-D. Blood that lacks the appropriate antigen should be given if intrauterine or exchange transfusion is required.

Although uncommon, practically all other red cell alloantibodies have been implicated in HDN, requiring no therapy, small-volume transfusion or, very rarely, exchange transfusions.

Prevention of haemolytic disease of the newborn

The major success in HDN in the last 15 years is because of the decrease in cases due to anti-D, so that other antibodies now account for a higher proportion of cases. This reduction has been achieved by the routine administration of a minimum dose of 500 IU (100 μg) anti-RhD immunoglobulin to all RhD-negative mothers within 72 hours following delivery of a RhD-positive infant. Extra doses of 50–75 IU (20–25 μg) per additional millilitre of red cells may be required for the small number of women (< 1%) who have a transplacental bleed greater than that covered by the standard dose (which covers 4 mL of packed cells). Anti-RhD immunoglobulin is also indicated after spontaneous or therapeutic abortion or threatened miscarriage and all procedures that might lead to a fetomaternal bleed (amniocentesis, external version, abdominal injury, chorionic villus sampling); the dose is 250 IU (50 μg) up to 20 weeks' gestation and 500 IU thereafter. It is critical that a Kleihauer acid elution test for detection and quantification of fetal red cells is performed on a maternal blood sample taken shortly after (within 1 hour of) delivery and after each sensitizing event after 20 weeks. If the test shows more than 4 mL of fetal cells, flow cytometry should be used to check the volume and give additional doses of anti-D as required. In several countries, and parts of the UK, the standard dose of anti-D immunoglobulin is 1250–1500 IU (250–300 μg). Where routine antenatal anti-D prophylaxis (see below) is being used, some lesser sensitizing events will be adequately covered. However, a Kleihauer test must still be performed.

Despite prophylaxis, new cases of sensitization to the D antigen still occur. Some may be due to an early unrecognized abortion and some to clerical and administrative errors (e.g. incorrect grouping of mother or child, or errors in the recording of groups). Failure of protection after delivery may result from omission of anti-D immunoglobulin (e.g. early discharge), an insufficient dose, or where primary immunization has already occurred during the pregnancy, now the most common cause of failure of conventional postnatal prophylaxis. Approximately 0.8–1.5% of Rh-negative women carrying a Rh-positive fetus become immunized during pregnancy.

To further reduce Rh immunization significantly, anti-RhD immunoglobulin should be given routinely during pregnancy to all RhD-negative women. A minimum of 500 IU (100 μg) should be administered intramuscularly at 28 and 34 weeks, with some centres administering up to 1250 IU. A single dose of 1500 IU (300 μg) at 28 weeks has also been recommended, although there are insufficient data regarding efficacy and the risk to mother and fetus if this single dose is missed is much more significant. Data from Canada suggest that a second dose of 300 μg may be needed for many women at 34 weeks, despite the larger dose at 28 weeks. The UK national policy is to offer routine antenatal prophylaxis to all pregnant RhD-negative women, as it significantly reduces the incidence of RhD sensitization in pregnant women. It is expected to offer D typing of the fetus from DNA extracted from maternal plasma before 28 weeks' gestation (see Chapter 15). This will avoid giving unnecessary routine antenatal Rh prophylaxis to women carrying RhD-negative fetuses.

The next most common causes of HDN requiring therapy are anti-c and anti-K. Any reduction in the cases due to anti-K could only be achieved by prevention of sensitization through transfusion of all women of childbearing potential with K-negative blood.

Neonatal alloimmune thrombocytopenia

This is a condition in which the platelets of the fetus and newborn are destroyed by maternal platelet-specific alloantibodies against platelet antigens inherited from the father. It is analogous to HDN, but for platelets. Although more than 15 human platelet antigen (HPA) systems have been described, most cases are due to anti-HPA-1a in alloimmunized HPA-1b mothers. The difference with neonatal alloimmune thrombocytopenia is that the offspring of the first pregnancy can be affected and that the potency of the platelet antibodies is often not correlated with the severity of the fetal or neonatal thrombocytopenia. The most serious complication is intracranial haemorrhage, which may lead to death or severe neurological sequelae. Treatment consists of intravenous immunoglobulin and/or transfusion of HPA-1a-negative platelets, available from stock throughout the National Blood Service.

Selected bibliography

Barbara JAJ, Regan FAM, Contreras MC (eds) (2008) *Transfusion Microbiology*. Cambridge University Press, Cambridge.

Beauregard P, Blajchman MA (1994) Haemolytic and pseudohaemolytic transfusion reactions: an overview of the haemolytic transfusion reactions and the clinical conditions that mimic them. *Transfusion Medicine Reviews* 7: 184–9.

Blood Safety and Quality Regulations (2005) Statutory Instrument 2005 No. 50. Available at www.opsi.gov.uk/si/si2005/20050050.htm

British Committee for Standards in Haematology Blood Transfusion Task Force (1996) Guidelines for pretransfusion compatibility procedures in blood transfusion laboratories. *Transfusion Medicine* 6: 273–83.

British Committee for Standards in Haematology Blood Transfusion Task Force (1998) Guidelines for the clinical use of blood cell separators. *Clinical and Laboratory Haematology* 20: 265–78.

British Committee for Standards in Haematology Blood Transfusion Task Force (1999) Guidelines for the estimation of fetomaternal haemorrhage. *Transfusion Medicine* 9: 87–92.

British Committee for Standards in Haematology Blood Transfusion Task Force (1999) Addendum for guidelines for blood grouping and red cell antibody testing during pregnancy. *Transfusion Medicine* 9: 99.

British Committee for Standards in Haematology Blood Transfusion Task Force (1999) Guidelines for the administration of blood and blood components and the management of transfused patients. *Transfusion Medicine* **9**: 227–38.

British Committee for Standards in Haematology Blood Transfusion Task Force (2000) Guidelines for blood bank computing. *Transfusion Medicine* **10**: 307–14.

British Committee for Standards in Haematology Blood Transfusion Task Force (2004) Guidelines for the use of fresh frozen plasma, cryoprecipitate and cryosupernatant. *British Journal of Haematology* **126**: 11–28.

British Committee for Standards in Haematology (2009) *Guidelines for Blood Transfusion*. Available at http://www.bcshguidelines.com/

Brown P (2001) Creutzfeldt–Jakob disease: blood infectivity and screening tests. *Seminars in Hematology* **38**: 2–6.

Chapman C, Stainsby D, Jones H *et al.* (2009) Ten years of hemovigilance reports of transfusion-related acute lung injury in the United Kingdom and the impact of preferential use of male donor plasma. *Transfusion* **49**: 440–52.

Commission Directive 2005/61/EC of 30 September 2005 implementing Directive 2002/98/EC of the European Parliament and of the Council as regards traceability requirements and notification of serious adverse reactions and events. Official Journal of the European Union.

Commission Directive 2005/62/EC of 30 September 2005 implementing Directive 2002/98/EC of the European Parliament and of the Council as regards Community standards and specifications relating to a quality system for blood establishments. Official Journal of the European Union.

Contreras M (ed.) (2009) *ABC of Transfusion*, 4th edn. Wiley-Blackwell/BMJ Books, Oxford/London.

Directive 2002/98/EC of the European Parliament and of the Council of 27 January 2003 setting standards of quality and safety for the collection, testing, processing, storage and distribution of human blood and blood components and amending Directive 2001/83/EC. Official Journal of the European Union.

Engelfriet C, Reesink H (1999) Haemovigilance systems. *Vox Sanguinis* **77**: 110–20.

Hunter N, Foster J, Chong A *et al.* (2002) Transmission of prion diseases by blood transfusion. *Journal of General Virology* **83**: 2897–905.

Lee D, Contreras M, Robson SC *et al.* (1999) Recommendations for the use of anti-D immunoglobulin for Rh prophylaxis. *Transfusion Medicine* **9**: 93–7.

Llewelyn CA, Hewitt PE, Knight RS *et al.* (2004) Possible transmission of variant Creutzfeldt–Jakob disease by blood transfusion. *Lancet* **363**: 411–12.

Malone DL, Hess JR, Fingerhut A (2006) Massive transfusion practices around the globe and a suggestion for a common massive transfusion protocol. *Journal of Trauma* **60** (6 Suppl.): S91–S96.

Mangano DT, Tudor JC, Dietzel C (2006) The risk associated with aprotinin in cardiac surgery. *New England Journal of Medicine* **354**: 353–65.

Mollison PL, Engelfriet CP, Contreras M (1997) *Blood Transfusion in Clinical Medicine*, 10th edn. Blackwell Scientific Publications, Oxford.

National Institute for Clinical Excellence (2008) Routine antenatal anti-D prophylaxis for women who are RhD-negative. TA156, August 2009. Available at www.nice.org.uk.

Slichter SJ, Kaufman RM, Assmann SF *et al.* (2010) Dose of prophylactic platelet transfusions and prevention of hemorrhag. *The New England Journal of Medicine* **362**: 600–13.

Stainsby D, Jones H, Asher D *et al.* (2006) Serious hazards of transfusion: a decade of hemovigilance in the UK. *Transfusion Medicine Reviews* **20**: 273–82.

Strauss RG (1994) Neonatal transfusion. In: *Scientific Basis of Transfusion Medicine* (KC Anderson, PM Ness, eds), pp. 421–42. Saunders, Philadelphia.

Taylor C, Cohen H, Mould D *et al.* (2009) on behalf of the Serious Hazards of Transfusion (SHOT) Steering Group. *The SHOT Annual Report 2009*. Available at www.shotuk.org.

Teixeira PG, Inaba K, Shulman I *et al.* (2009) Impact of plasma transfusion in massively transfused trauma patients. *Journal of Trauma* **66**: 693–7.

TRAP Study Group (1997) Leucocyte reduction and UV-B irradiation of platelets to prevent allo-immunization and refractoriness to platelet transfusion. *New England Journal of Medicine* **337**: 1861–9.

Turner M (2003) vCJD screening and its implications for transfusion: strategies for the future? *Blood Coagulation and Fibrinolysis* **14**: 565–8.

UK Blood Transfusion Services (2002) *Guidelines for the Blood Transfusion Services in the United Kingdom*, 6th edn. The Stationery Office, London. Available at http://www.transfusion-guidelines.org.uk.

van der Poel CL, Seifried E, Schaasberg WP (2002) Paying for blood donations: still a risk? *Vox Sanguinis* **83**: 285–93.

World Health Organization (2009) *Screening Blood Donations for Transfusion-transmissible Infections*. World Health Organization, Geneva.

CHAPTER 17

Phagocytes

John Mascarenhas[1], Farhad Ravandi[2] and Ronald Hoffman[1]

[1]Tisch Cancer Institute, Mount Sinai School of Medicine, New York, New York, USA
[2]University of Texas MD Anderson Cancer Center, Houston, Texas, USA

Introduction

White blood cells have fundamental roles in defence against invading microorganisms and the recognition and destruction of neoplastic cells as well as their role in acute inflammatory reactions. Furthermore, through their phagocytic function, white blood cells are influential in clearing senescent and apoptotic cells, hence allowing tissue repair and remodelling. Production of various cytokines by white blood cells influences the functions of other cells and affects processes such as cellular and humoral immunity, and allergic phenomena. The phagocytic actions of white blood cells can cause damage to the host tissue, leading to inflammation. This occurs either as a by-product of their microbial killing actions or as a direct attack on the host in autoimmune disorders.

Normal haemopoiesis, including generation of appropriate white blood cell number and constellation, is dependent upon intricately regulated signalling cascades that are mediated by cytokines and their receptors. Orderly function of these pathways leads to the generation of the normal constellation of haemopoietic cells, and their abnormal activation results in impaired apoptosis, uncontrolled proliferation and neoplastic transformation. Cytokines function in a redundant and pleiotropic manner; different cytokines can exert similar effects on the same cell type and any particular cytokine can have several differing biological functions. This complexity of function is a result of shared receptor subunits as well as overlapping downstream pathways, culminating in transcription of similar genes. Increased understanding of the role of cytokines and other

growth factors in the control of normal haemopoiesis has led to better delineation of the pathogenetic events that affect the function and number of these cells.

In this chapter, we consider the normal production and function of white blood cells involved in phagocytosis and describe various disorders causing their altered number and activity.

Mechanisms of phagocyte function

Locomotion

Phagocytes are an important part of the innate host defence system, performing their function either as resident cells in tissues (e.g. macrophages) or as circulating defenders (e.g. neutrophils, eosinophils and monocytes). Phagocytosis of invading microorganisms by both types of defenders involves the synthesis of highly toxic derivatives of molecular oxygen by the respiratory burst NADPH oxidases and the delivery of stored antimicrobial proteases into the vacuoles containing microbes.

Circulating phagocytes such as neutrophils respond to spatial gradients of chemotaxins and move by alternating the extrusion and retraction of broad frontal lamellipodia that determine the direction of movement. As a result, the body of the cell elongates along the axis defined by the lamellar protrusion. As little as a 2% change in the concentration of the chemoattractant can be recognized by neutrophils. The signals generated by such gradients activate the cytoplasm of the cell leading to propulsive and retractive events. The movement of neutrophils is achieved by the contraction of an actin filamentous network in the cortical gel at the leading front. This dynamic network provides strength for the forming protrusions and serves as an anchor for adhesion molecules. ATP provides the energy for the movement of the cell.

Postgraduate Haematology: 6th edition. Edited by A. Victor Hoffbrand, Daniel Catovsky, Edward G.D. Tuddenham, Anthony R. Green
© 2011 Blackwell Publishing Ltd.

Phagocytic cells possess a number of cell–cell adhesion receptors and ligands, which mediate their recruitment, migration and interaction with other immune cells (Table 17.1). These include members of the integrins, the immunoglobulin superfamily and the selectins. Migration of macrophages involves their adhesion to endothelial surfaces and their extravasation to the extravascular space. This process is mediated by cytokine-regulated expression of intercellular adhesion molecules (ICAMs) on the surface of both phagocytes and endothelial cell. ICAMs share similar structure to the immunoglobulin family and other immunoglobulin-like adhesion molecules such as vascular cell adhesion molecule (VCAM)-1, and serve as ligands for the β_2 integrins. The distribution and regulation of the three members of the ICAM family is different. ICAM-1 is expressed at a low level on endothelial cells; its expression is enhanced by the inflammatory cytokines such as interleukin (IL)-1, interferon (IFN)-α and IFN-γ. ICAM-2 is constitutively expressed on endothelial cells, with no response to the inflammatory cytokines. ICAM-3 is expressed by neutrophils, monocytes and lymphocytes. Another member of the endothelial immunoglobulin superfamily, PECAM-1 (CD31), serves an important role in transmigration of neutrophils into mucosal or other body tissues.

The β_2 integrin family consists of three leucocyte restricted integrins, LFA-1 (CD11a/CD18), CR3 (MAC-1, CD11b/CD18) and p150/95 (CD11c/CD18). They share a common β-subunit, CD18, and three unique α-subunits, CD11a, CD11b and CD11c. LFA-1 and ICAM-1 are both present on monocytes and mediate their attachment to endothelial cells and to lymphocytes bearing the corresponding receptor/ligand, thereby facilitating antigen presentation. Leucocyte adhesion deficiency type I, described later in the chapter, is caused by the genetic deficiency of all three CD18 integrins, and neutrophils in this condition bind poorly to IL-1-stimulated endothelial cells and do not undergo transendothelial migration.

Selectins are expressed on all leucocytes (L-selectins) as well as post-capillary endothelial surfaces (E-selectins) and in platelet α-granules and endothelial cell Weibel–Palade bodies (P-selectins). Neutrophils, eosinophils, monocytes and macrophages constitutively express L-selectin. E- and P-selectins recognize oligosaccharide ligands on macrophages. Selectins are implicated in the early interactions of phagocytes and endothelium. The interaction of E- and P-selectins on cytokine-activated endothelial cells, and L-selectins on macrophages with their appropriate ligands, targets phagocytic cells to the endothelium at sites of vascular injury and initiates the rolling movement of leucocytes along the vessel wall. The ligands for selectins have a similar structure, containing carbohydrate groups typically as terminal structures of glycoproteins and glycolipids. A major selectin ligand, a sialylated and fucosylated tetrasaccharide related to the sialylated Lewis X blood group, is heavily expressed on quiescent neutrophils and monocytes.

Paracellular diapedesis is the purposeful coordinated movement of leucocytes though the endothelial lining towards sites of inflammation. Neutrophil chemotaxis requires a series of sequential steps resulting in the recruitment of these cells at tissue sites away from the vessel lumen. Selectin-mediated leucocyte tethering and rolling across endothelial surfaces is followed by integrin-mediated firm adhesion and leucocyte polarization at endothelial cell junctions. CD157, a glycosylphosphatidylinositol (GPI)-anchored surface protein, is crucial to this process of locomotion and is expressed on the surface of neutrophils and vascular interendothelial junctions. As would be expected, neutrophils from patients with paroxysmal nocturnal haemoglobinuria, in which there is loss of GPI-linked proteins, demonstrate defective chemotaxis with impaired transendothelial migration.

Phagocyte receptors

Phagocytes express a number of surface receptors that are able to recognize microbial surfaces as well as altered tissue components and apoptotic bodies (Table 17.2). Furthermore, nonspecific components of the innate immune response, such as the components of the complement cascade, can tag and thereby identify invading microorganisms, thus allowing their opsonization via another family of receptors, leading to the uptake of complement-coated microorganisms. This complement fixation can occur either via the classical pathway, which is activated by the prior binding of immune IgG or IgM to the organism or particle, or by antibody-independent activation of the alternative pathway. Similarly, other molecules such as matrix proteins (i.e. fibronectin and vitronectin) can act as opsonins allowing recognition and uptake by the phagocytic cells. Interestingly, in order to evade phagocytes, pathogenic bacteria such as *Streptococcus pneumoniae*, *Haemophilus influenzae* and *Neisseria meningitidis* have developed strategies such as production of polysaccharide capsules, which provide a shield against complement binding and activation, and recognition by scavenger receptors.

Two types of complement receptors, CR1 (CD35) and CR3 (CD11b/CD18), have been described. CR1 is a glycosylated protein of 160–250 kDa and can be identified as CD35. CR1 is present on all phagocytes as well as some T lymphocytes. CR1 mediates phagocytosis of particles opsonized by C3b and regulates complement activation. CR3 is a member of the β_2 integrin family and is designated CD11b/CD18. It is composed of two polypeptide chains, an α-subunit of 185 kDa and a β-subunit of 95 kDa. CR3 is expressed on all phagocytes as well as natural killer cells and some $\gamma\delta$ T cells. Monocytes and macrophages express high levels of CR3; neutrophils have lower-level expression that can increase rapidly through release from intracellular stores. CR3 can bind particles opsonized with C3bi as well as determinants on unopsonized microbes. The avidity of CR3 is enhanced by an amphipathic anion lipid called integrin-

Table 17.1 Phagocytic cell adhesion molecules.

Adhesion molecule	CD number	Cellular distribution	Ligand	Function
Integrin family				
Very late-acting antigens				
$\alpha_1\beta_1$ (VLA-1)	CD49a/29	Mo, EC	Collagen I, IV, laminin	Cell adherence to ECM
$\alpha_2\beta_1$ (VLA-2)	CD49b/29	Mo, EC, platelets	Collagen I, IV, laminin	
$\alpha_3\beta_1$ (VLA-3)	CD49c/29	Mo	Collagen I, laminin, fibronectin	Cell adherence to ECM
$\alpha_4\beta_1$ (VLA-4)	CD49d/29	Mo, eos, bas	Fibronectin, VCAM-1	Cell adherence to ECM and cell–cell adhesion matrix
$\alpha_5\beta_1$ (VLA-5)	CD49e/29	Mo, neut, EC	Fibronectin	Cell adherence to ECM
$\alpha_6\beta_1$ (VLA-6)	CD49f/29	Mo	Laminin	Cell adherence to ECM
Leucocyte integrins (LFA-1 family)				
$\alpha_D\beta_2$	–/18	Ma	?	
$\alpha_L\beta_2$ (LFA-1)	CD11a/18	Mo, Ma, granulocytes	ICAM-1, ICAM-2, ICAM-3	Cell–cell adhesion and cell–matrix adhesion
$\alpha_M\beta_2$ (CR3, Mac-1)	CD11b/18	Mo, Ma, granulocytes	ICAM-1, C3bi, fibronectin, factor X, microbial antigens	Endothelium adherence/ extravasation
$\alpha_X\beta_2$ (p150,95)	CD11c/18	Mo, Ma, granulocytes	C3bi, fibronectin	Adhesion during inflammatory response
Cytoadhesins				
$\alpha_V\beta_3$ (vitronectin receptor)	CD51/61	Mo, EC	Vitronectin, fibronectin, collagen, thrombospondin, vWF	Cell adherence to ECM
$\alpha_R\beta_3$ (leucocyte response integrin)		Mo, granulocytes	Vitronectin, fibronectin, collagen, thrombospondin, vWF	Cell adherence to ECM
$\alpha_V\beta_5$	CD51/–	Mo	Vitronectin, fibronectin	Cell adherence to ECM
$\alpha_V\beta_7$	CD51/–	Ma	?	
Immunoglobulin superfamily				
ICAM-1	CD54	Mo, EC	$\alpha_L\beta_2, \alpha_M\beta_2$	Cell–cell adhesion
ICAM-2	CD102	Mo, EC	$\alpha_L\beta_2$	Cell–cell adhesion
ICAM-3	CD50	Mo, granulocytes	$\alpha_L\beta_2$	Cell–cell adhesion
VCAM-1	CD106	Ma, EC, dendritic cells	$\alpha_4\beta_1$	Recruitment
PECAM-1	CD31	Mo, EC, platelets	CD31, $\alpha_V\beta_3$	Transmigration
HCAM	CD44	Ubiquitous	Collagen I, IV, fibronectin	Extravasation
Selectin family				
L-selectin	CD62L	Mo, granulocytes	Carbohydrate determinants on EC	Migration, rolling on vessel wall
E-selectin	CD62E	Neutrophil, EC	Mo, neut, eos	Migration, rolling on vessel wall
P-selectin	CD62P	EC, platelets	Mo, neut, eos	Adhesion to activated platelets and EC

Bas, basophil; CD, cluster of differentiation; EC, endothelial cell; eos, eosinophil; ICAM, intercellular adhesion molecule; Mo, monocyte; Ma, macrophage; neut, neutrophil.

Table 17.2 Opsonic receptors mediating phagocytosis.

Receptor	Marker	Opsonic ligand	Binding affinity (K_a)	Cell type	Function
FcγRI	CD64	IgG1	High (50 nmol/L)	Monocytes, macrophages, neutrophils (after IFN-γ exposure)	Phagocytosis, respiratory burst
FcγRII	CD32	IgG1 = IgG3 ≥ IgG4 = IgG2	Low (1 μmol/L)	Neutrophils, monocytes, macrophages	Phagocytosis, respiratory burst
FcγRIII		IgG1 = IgG3	Low (110 nmol/L)	Neutrophils, monocytes, macrophages	IIIB: phagocytosis (requires CR1 or FcγRII)
IIIA	CD16a, 1 allotype NA1		Low (470 nmol/L)		
IIIB	CD16b, two allotypes NA1 and NA2				
FcαR	CD89 My43 IgM	IgA1, IgA2, secretory IgA1 and IgA2		Neutrophils, monocytes, macrophages, T and B cell subsets, NK cells, erythrocytes	Phagocytosis, respiratory burst, bacterial killing
CR1	CD35, four alleles	C3b and C4b dimers	High (0.5 nmol/L)	All phagocytes, some T lymphocytes	Phagocytosis
CR3	CD11b/CD18 Mac1	C3bi	High (0.5 nmol/L)	All phagocytes, NK cells, γδ T cells	Phagocytosis, respiratory burst

CR, complement receptor; NK, natural killer.

modulating factor (IMF-1) as well as by bacterial peptide fragments, C5a, leukotriene (LT)B₄, and cytokines such as tumour necrosis factor (TNF), granulocyte colony-stimulating factor (G-CSF) and granulocyte/macrophage colony-stimulating factor (GM-CSF). However, IFN-γ transiently decreases the binding capacity of both CR1 and CR3. Simultaneous cross-linking between two different receptor types also increases binding by CR3. For example, macrophages adhered to collagen ingest complement-coated particles less efficiently than macrophages adhered to fibronectin, which cross-links other integrin receptors. CR3 also plays a critical role in adherence-dependent potentiation of the respiratory burst and secretory responses of neutrophils.

Phagocytes also express a number of receptors for the Fc portion of immunoglobulin molecules IgA, IgE and IgG. They mediate opsonization of particles and microorganisms, enhancing their phagocytic uptake. The antigen-binding site (Fab) of IgG binds to bacteria exposing the Fc-binding site, which is in turn recognized by one of three classes of receptor, FcγRI, FcγRII or FcγRIII. FcγRIII is constitutively expressed by neutrophils, with 100 000–300 000 copies per cell, and is identified as CD16. Two isoforms, A and B, exist, which differ only with respect to their transmembrane and cytoplasmic domains. FcγRIIIB lacks both of these domains and is anchored by a GPI protein and is therefore absent in patients with paroxysmal

nocturnal haemoglobinuria. FcγRIIIB can trigger granule release but no associated respiratory burst. However, FcγRIIIB and CR3, together with FcγRII, act synergistically to activate the respiratory burst. FcγRII (identified as CD32) is a constitutive low-affinity receptor with low expression (1000–4000 copies per cell) requiring dimeric IgG for binding. Cross-linking FcγRII stimulates oxygen radical production. FcγRI, identified as CD64, is not expressed on quiescent neutrophils but its expression is highly increased after exposure to IFN-γ and a number of inflammatory mediators. It binds IgG1 and IgG2 with high affinity and promotes phagocytosis of bacteria opsonized by them. Polymeric IgA antibody can also function as an opsonin and is recognized by a specific IgA receptor (FcαR), which is widely distributed on the circulating haemopoietic cells but is more highly expressed in phagocytes found in secretions of the gut and the lung.

A number of miscellaneous receptors involved in phagocytosis have been described. The mannosyl/fucosyl receptors, otherwise known as the macrophage mannose receptors (MMR), are lectin-like molecules that bind mannose and fucose residues on the surfaces of yeast, bacteria and parasites. These receptors are present only on the surface of macrophages and their expression is increased by IFN-γ. Their activation mediates endocytosis, phagocytosis and cytotoxicity by reactive oxygen intermediates. The receptors described to date are composed of eight and ten contiguous C-type lectin domains. In addition to recognizing the haemoglobin–haptoglobin complex, the macrophage scavenger receptor CD163 has also been shown to bind Gram-positive and Gram-negative bacteria and elicit an inflammatory cytokine response as part of the innate immune response. CD14 is the receptor for complexes of lipopolysaccharide (LPS)-binding protein with LPS, which coat Gram-negative bacteria and enhance phagocytosis. CD14 is constitutively expressed on monocytes and macrophages but its expression is modulated by cytokines. TNF, IL-1 and IL-6 increase its expression, whereas IFN-γ and IL-4 decrease it. CD14 expression can also be induced on neutrophils by various cytokines. CD14 is also a GPI-linked protein and is shed by monocytes.

Several receptors have also been implicated in the recognition and phagocytosis of apoptotic cells. Defective clearance of apoptotic cells is believed to promote inflammatory responses leading to the development of autoimmunity and efficient removal of apoptotic cells maintains peripheral immunological tolerance. Epithelial cells, fibroblasts, mesangial cells and both professional and non-professional phagocytes contribute to the effective identification and removal of apoptotic bodies before their intracellular contents are released. Different subsets of dendritic cells and macrophages likely play distinct roles in the clearance of cells at different stages of apoptosis. IL-10-producing anti-inflammatory macrophages are the professional phagocytes involved in the recognition and clearance of early apoptotic cells. Morphological changes in the apoptotic cells, such as formation of characteristic membrane protuberances (blebs), lead to the exposure of phosphatidylserine and changes on surface sugars, which are recognized by phagocytic receptors. These include integrins of the $\alpha_v\beta_3$ or $\alpha_v\beta_5$ classes and the lipid scavenger receptors of both A and B classes. The membrane of apoptotic cells binds increased amounts of thrombospondin, a macrophage secretory product that is recognized by both CD36 (thrombospondin receptor) and integrin $\alpha_v\beta_3$ (vitronectin receptor). Similarly, phagocytic lectin receptors bind carbohydrate determinants exposed on the surface of apoptotic cells. A specific receptor for phosphatidylserine has also been described, which acts alone or in association with CD36 to recognize the exposed phosphatidylserine. CD14 has also been reported to be involved in tethering of apoptotic lymphocytes via interaction with ICAMs. Apoptotic cell-associated molecular patterns (ACAMPs) are highly conserved molecular changes expressed in cells undergoing apoptosis that are recognized by innate immune system receptors such as CD14, CD91, C1q, C3bi, collectins and pentraxins. ACAMPs can be visualized as a topological change in grouping of molecules in the apoptotic cell plasma membrane that form a pattern that is then recognized by phagocytic cells.

Neutrophils also recognize chemoattractant signals through receptors expressed on their cell surface. N-formyl-methionyl tripeptide receptors such as f-Met-Leu-Phe (FMLP) are similar to naturally occurring bacteria-derived factors. Each demonstrates time-dependent saturable binding kinetics and a high-affinity dissociation constant (K_D) for the specific chemoattractant. Approximately 50 000 FMLP receptors per cell with a K_D of 20 nmol/L have been demonstrated on human neutrophils. Thrombospondin also has chemotactic activity and binds neutrophils via specific receptors linked to G_{i2} proteins, a subpopulation of which is also associated with the FMLP receptors. Neutrophils also have a specific receptor for the chemotactic cleavage product of C5a, with receptor expression of approximately 50 000–100 000 per cell and a binding affinity of 2 nmol/L.

Chemokines are a family of proinflammatory cytokines with potent chemotactic activity. They are small proteins (8–10 kDa, characterized by a pattern of conserved cysteine residues. CXC chemokines such as IL-8 are specific to neutrophils and are distinguished by having their first two cysteine residues separated by an amino acid. CC chemokines, including macrophage inflammatory protein (MIP)-1α, have the first two cysteine residues adjacent, are inactive for neutrophils, but attract monocytes, basophils, eosinophils and T lymphocytes. Monocyte migration is also directed by monocyte chemotactic proteins. Eosinophil migration is directed by MIP-1α and RANTES (regulation on activation normal T-cell expressed and secreted protein), in addition to the CC chemokine eotaxin. Phagocytic cells in general have high expression of the receptors for these chemokines, enabling them to recognize and respond to the appropriate chemoattractants.

Phagocytic signalling

The complex process of phagocytosis is regulated by events related to the activation of various receptors such as the FcγRs. Such receptor activation results in initiation of downstream signalling events through immunoreceptor tyrosine-based activation motifs (ITAMs). As a result of cross-linking of these receptors under appropriate conditions, downstream effector functions are activated, resulting in phagocytosis, stimulation of the respiratory burst, degranulation of bactericidal proteins and activation of transcription factors, in turn leading to enhanced expression of genes encoding cytokines and other inducible proteins.

Members of the Src family of tyrosine kinases (e.g. Lyn, Fgr and Hk) associate with FcγRs and are probably responsible for their tyrosine phosphorylation. The tyrosine-phosphorylated ITAMs then serve as binding sites for downstream kinases such as Syk, which propagate signals important for phagocytosis. Downmodulation of Syk in monocytes using antisense oligonucleotides results in decreased ability of these cells to ingest IgG-coated particles. Furthermore, macrophages that lack Syk demonstrate a profound reduction in FcγR-mediated tyrosine phosphorylation of p85 subunit of phosphatidylinositol 3-kinase (PI3K), SHIP, Shc and other important signalling proteins.

Phosphorylation and activation of members of the Rho/Rac family of GTPases as well as the ARF6 family are probably involved in cytoskeletal remodelling necessary to trigger phagocytosis. For example, inhibition of Rac1 or Cdc42 in murine macrophage models leads to impaired focal actin assembly beneath bound IgG-coated particles and blocks subsequent ingestion without affecting particle binding. Cdc42 and Rac1 appear to control different steps in the phagocytic process, namely pseudopod formation for the former and phagosome closure for the latter. The role of phospholipase Cγ and protein kinase C (PKC) isoforms in actin assembly and the role of PI3K pathways in membrane remodelling during phagocytosis are under investigation. Treatment of macrophages with PI3K inhibitors such as wortmannin and LY 294002 results in the failure of pseudopods to extend around particles.

Degranulation and secretion

Degranulation and secretion are processes whereby the contents of phagocytic storage granules are released into the phagocytic vacuoles (degranulation) or into the extracellular space (secretion). Degranulation and secretion can be triggered by invading microorganisms, immune complexes, cytokines, chemotactic factors, and adhesion to tissue surfaces and activation of ICAMs. The processes of degranulation and secretion begin with the onset of phagocytosis. A number of morphological changes occur within the granules and they translocate and fuse their membranes with those of the phagocytic vacuoles formed by the invagination of the plasma membrane.

Cytoskeletal proteins are essential for this process, facilitating granule transfer to plasma membrane or phagolysosomes. The exact cause of membrane fusion is unknown but the process is likely to involve the activation of several phospholipases, leading to altered lipid composition of granule–phagosome or granule–plasma membrane contact points. Actin polymers act like a barrier between plasma membrane and granules, and in order for membrane fusion to occur the granules have to negotiate the physical barrier of such cytoskeletal elements in the cell periphery. Furthermore, the repulsive negative charge on the surface of both membranes, related to the negatively charged phospholipids phosphatidylserine and phosphatidylethanolamine, is a further barrier that needs to be overcome. A number of soluble molecules capable of provoking the release of granule content into the extracellular space have been described. These include many chemotactic factors such as C5a, FMLP, platelet-activating factor (PAF) and LTB_4, as well as phorbol myristate acetate and several non-chemotactic interleukins, cytokines and growth factors such as TNF-α, IL-1, IL-4, IL-6 and GM-CSF. Importantly, phagocytes are capable of

rapidly replenishing cellular stores of proteins and forming new granules, thus allowing repeated degranulation and secretion.

Regulation of granule release is mediated by a number of factors such as calcium, guanine nucleotides and G-proteins, which regulate changes in the cytoskeleton, resulting in actin polymerization and clearing of the cytoskeleton along the plasma membrane fusion site. These proteins include members of the annexin family, the calcium-binding protein calmodulin, PKC and phospholipases.

Phagocytic killing: the respiratory burst

Activation of phagocytes is associated with a rapid and dramatic increase in oxygen consumption described as the respiratory burst. This process is non-mitochondrial and is mediated by the activation of a latent enzyme system referred to as NADPH oxidase, which transfers a single electron to molecular oxygen (O_2) to form the superoxide anion (O_2^-). The superoxide anion then dismutates to hydrogen peroxide (H_2O_2), a process occurring either spontaneously or through the catalytic function of superoxide dismutase. H_2O_2 then reacts with superoxide anion, forming the highly reactive hydroxyl radical ($OH^{\bullet}$), which is highly microbicidal. This and other reactive oxidative products not only contribute to microbial killing but also activate metalloproteinases such as elastase and collagenase, leading to the surrounding tissue injury that often accompanies phagocyte activation.

The NADPH oxidase is a multicomponent enzyme, with several subunits located in various regions of the quiescent phagocytes (Figure 17.1). These subunits, called phox (phagocyte oxidase) proteins, are identified by their molecular weight (e.g. p40 phox). In the quiescent neutrophil, p47 phox protein resides in the cytosol, along with p67 phox complexed with p40 phox. Activation of NADPH oxidase results from PKC-mediated phosphorylation of p47 phox and the subsequent binding of the p47 phox phosphoprotein and the p67 phox–p40 phox complex to the membrane flavocytochrome b_{558} located primarily in the specific granules, gelatinase granules and secretory vesicles of neutrophils. The cytochrome b_{558} is the terminal component of the superoxide-generating system allowing the efficient transfer of electrons from the cytoplasmic NADPH to the surface of phagolysosome or the extracellular surface, where oxygen is reduced to the superoxide anion. Other GTP-binding proteins such as Rap1A and Rac2 associate with the above molecules and regulate phagocyte activation and oxidase activity through their preferred substrate GTP (Figure 17.1).

Phagocytic killing: nitric oxide

Generation of reactive nitrogen intermediates through nitric oxide synthase (NOS) is another mechanism for phagocytic

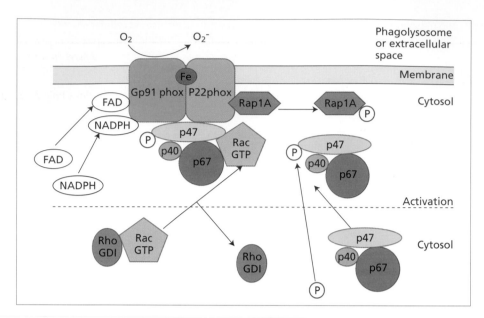

Figure 17.1 Components of the NADPH oxidase system. The components include a 47-kDa cytosolic protein (p47), a 67-kDa cytosolic protein (p67), a 40-kDa cytosolic protein (p40), cytosolic G-proteins (Rac and Rap1), and a membrane-bound cytochrome (b_{558}). The cytochrome consists of haem-containing p22-phox and gp91-phox. The gp91 subunit is an FAD-dependent flavoprotein shuttling electrons to molecular oxygen, forming O_2^-. The p47 component can be phosphorylated to various extents. In activated cells, the p40, p47 and p67 proteins translocate to the membrane to form an activation complex with cytochrome b_{558}. Similarly, the Rac and Rap1 proteins also translocate. The activated oxidase passes electrons from NADPH via FAD to oxygen, thereby generating superoxide.

killing of microbes. Nitric oxide (NO) is the highly reactive free radical product of the oxidation of L-arginine in phagocytes during inflammation. Three distinct isoforms of NOS have been described in blood cells. Two are found in endothelial and neuronal cells and the third, inducible NOS, is induced by cytokines, such as IFN-γ, in a number of cell types. Cofactors required for the activity of NOS include flavine adenine dinucleotide (FAD), flavine mononucleotide (FMN), NADPH and tetrahydrobiopterin. The calcium-binding protein calmodulin is tightly bound to the macrophage NOS. The activity of NOS is also regulated by kinases and phosphatases and its production is influenced by other cytokines such as IL-4, IL-10, IL-8 and transforming growth factor (TGF)-β.

NO has an important role in the antimicrobial activity of both neutrophils and mononuclear phagocytes. In contrast to NADPH oxidase, which is active at the plasma and phagolysosome membrane, NOS is located in the cytoplasm and mediates defence against facultative intracellular pathogens, as well as other prokaryotic and eukaryotic pathogens. Its inhibitory effects are due to nitrosylation of proteins and interaction with transition metals at the active sites of enzymes. Furthermore, NO scavenges superoxide to form peroxynitrite (OONO⁻), which can disrupt protein phosphorylation.

Phagocytic killing: antimicrobial proteins

Phagocytic cells such as neutrophils can kill microorganisms using proteins present in various granules. The importance of such non-oxidative killing is evident in chronic granulomatous disease neutrophils that are still capable of killing many potent microorganisms. Furthermore, this process is important for defence against organisms such as *Escherichia coli* and *Salmonella typhimurium*, which do not produce their own source of oxidants and are killed under anaerobic conditions. The contents of each phagocytic cell type are specific. Neutrophil antimicrobial proteins include defensins, serpocidins (including cathepsin G and azurocidin) and bacterial permeability-increasing protein (BPI). The antimicrobial proteins within neutrophils are summarized in Table 17.3.

These microbicidal proteins exert their killing effect through enzymatic means such as proteolysis or by non-catalytic mechanisms, and their combinations potentiate bactericidal activity. Cathepsin G is a serine protease that exerts its bactericidal action by binding to penicillin-binding proteins of bacteria and interfering with the synthesis of peptidoglycans. Azurocidin is another serine protease effective against a number of bacteria and fungi. Defensins constitute as much as 50% of neutrophil

Table 17.3 Neutrophil microbicidal proteins.

Protein	Characteristics	Target organisms	Effects on target
Non-enzymatic proteins			
BPI	Highly cationic, neutralizes LPS, most potent cidal protein, not released from granule	Gram-negative bacteria	Binds lipid A region of LPS, increases bacterial membrane permeability, activates bacterial degradative enzymes
Defensins	Comprise 30–50% of azurophil granule protein	Gram-positive > Gram-negative bacteria, fungi, viruses, mammalian cells	Increases membrane permeability
Lactoferrin	Cationic, stimulates hydroxyl radical formation	Gram-positive and Gram-negative bacteria, fungi	Oxidative damage
Catalytic proteins and analogues			
Proteinase 3	Serine proteinase	*Escherichia coli, Streptococcus faecalis, Candida albicans*	Growth inhibition
Cathepsin G	Serine proteinase	Gram-positive and Gram-negative bacteria, fungi	Inhibition of peptidoglycan synthesis
Azurocidin	Serine proteinase	Gram-negative bacteria	Non-catalytic mechanisms
Lysozyme	Cationic	Gram-negative bacteria, few Gram-positive bacteria	Potentiation of complement and H_2O_2 killing, cleavage of cell wall peptidoglycans
Elastase	No direct cidal activity		Co-active with lysozyme, potentiation of MPO–halide–H_2O_2 system

BPI, bacterial permeability-inducing factor; LPS, lipopolysaccharide; MPO, myeloperoxidase.

granule protein content and exert their cidal activity by inserting into hydrophobic channels, forming voltage-dependent ion channels in the lipid bilayer. BPI kills Gram-negative bacteria by binding to their LPS capsule and altering their bacterial membrane permeability to extracellular solutes. A mutant strain of *S. typhimurium* that is resistant to BPI has also been found to be resistant to neutrophil bactericidal activity under strict anaerobic conditions, demonstrating the importance of BPI in non-oxidative killing by neutrophils. Other neutrophil granule proteins include lactoferrin, which kills some Gram-negative bacteria by generating free radicals from iron bound to it, and lysozyme, which is involved in the digestion of killed bacteria in phagolysosomes of neutrophils. These antimicrobial proteins can also enhance the effects of other cidal mechanisms such as complement lysis and oxidative killing. Combinations of these proteins can also enhance their killing action, as seen with the combination of neutrophil lysozyme and elastase against Gram-negative bacteria. Some of the microbicidal proteins of the phagocytes have other effects at lower concentrations, such as stimulation of mast cell degranulation, release of proinflammatory molecules and monocytic chemotaxis, as well as regulation of phagocytosis and granulopoiesis.

Production, structure and dysfunction of phagocytes

White blood cells are produced from pluripotent haemopoietic stem cells located within the bone marrow. Development of white blood cells along different lineages is governed by external stimuli including cytokines, matrix proteins and other cellular products within the marrow environment. The combination of specific cytokines and growth factors influence the maturation of white blood cell progeny along specific lineages. Although there is significant overlap between these growth factors, certain cytokines have been found to be associated with specific maturation pathways. Some of these cytokines are now manufactured commercially and are in clinical use to influence the speed of recovery of white blood cells following administration of chemotherapy.

Neutrophils (Figure 17.2a)

Development and function
Neutrophils are the predominant white blood cells involved in phagocytic killing of bacteria and certain fungi. They are also

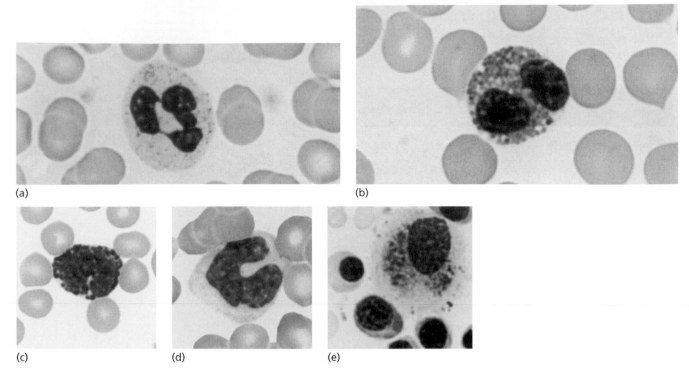

Figure 17.2 Morphology of phagocyte cell types: (a) neutrophil; (b) eosinophil; (c) basophil; (d) monocyte; (e) macrophage.

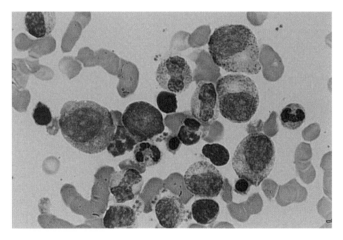

Figure 17.3 Stages of neutrophil maturation, showing a myeloblast, a promyelocyte, several myelocytes and metamyelocytes, a band cell and a segmented neutrophil.

referred to as polymorphonuclear or segmented leucocytes, owing to their characteristic lobulated nucleus (their nucleus is segmented into two to five lobes, connected by thin chromatin strands). They are at the end stage of maturation (Figures 17.3 and 17.4) and generally uniform in size (13 μm in diameter), with pink cytoplasm and fine azurophilic granules. The production of neutrophils involves the action of a variety of growth factors, including G-CSF, GM-CSF, IL-3 and macrophage

colony-stimulating factor. In addition to G-CSF-induced neutrophil production, G-CSF has also been implicated in leucocyte trafficking into tissues involved with active inflammation, such as inflamed joints in a collagen-induced arthritis murine model. Other factors such as IL-11, stem cell factor (SCF) and FLT-3 ligand enhance clonal neutrophil expansion *in vitro*. GM-CSF induces neutrophil, eosinophil and macrophage colony expansion *in vitro*, but there is no evidence that it induces neutrophil differentiation in the absence of G-CSF.

Granulopoiesis is the process of terminal differentiation from a pluripotent haemopoietic stem cell via a multipotent common myeloid progenitor and bipotent granulocyte–macrophage progenitor stage to a committed mature neutrophil. Granulocyte differentiation depends on the coordinated expression of certain transcription factors, including Pu.1, CCAAT enhancer-binding protein (C/EBPα), C/EBPε and GFI1. Microarray technologies utilized for the analysis of human bone marrow populations highly enriched for promyelocytes, myelocytes, metamyelocytes and neutrophils have been successful in defining the transcriptional programme of terminal granulocytic differentiation. Chemokine and cytokine receptors and ligand pairs are upregulated in the transition from myelocyte to neutrophil and involve the constitutive activation of NF-κB.

Neutrophils contain four types of granules that can be identified by marker enzymes or proteins (Table 17.4). The lysozyme-like azurophil granules, otherwise known as primary granules, are present in promyelocytes and all further stages of neutrophil

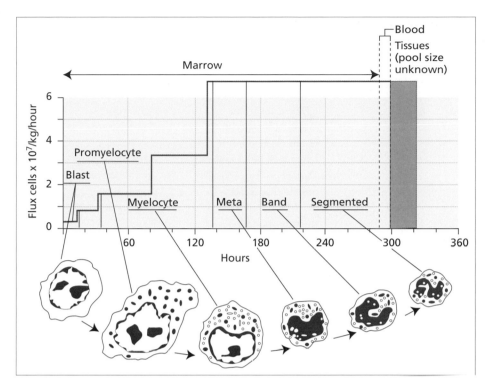

Figure 17.4 Neutrophil lifespan and stages of maturation. Of every 100 nucleated cells in the bone marrow, 2% are myeloblasts, 5% promyelocytes, 12% myelocytes, 22% metamyelocytes and bands, and 20% mature neutrophils (i.e. about 60% developing neutrophils). The times indicated for the various compartments were obtained by isotopic labelling techniques. The ordinate shows the flux, and the abscissa the time, in each compartment. The stepwise increase in cell numbers through the dividing compartments represents serial divisions. Note that no mitoses occur after the myelocyte stage. (From Bainton DF (1992) Developmental Biology of Neutrophils and Eosinophils. In: *Inflammation: Basic Principles and Clinical Correlates*, 2nd edn (JI Gallin, IM Goldstein, R Snyderman), pp. 303–324. Raven Press, New York, and Cronkite EP, Vincent PC (1969) Granulocytopoiesis. *Ser Haematology* **4:** 3–43, with permisssion).

differentiation and contain microbicidal proteins and acid hydrolases (e.g. myeloperoxidase, defensins, lysozyme) involved in oxidative and non-oxidative killing of bacteria and fungi. These granules release their contents exclusively into phagocytic granules, with little discharge outside the cell except for release from disintegrating neutrophils. Specific or secondary granules are smaller than azurophil granules and contain other distinct hydrolases, as well as chemotactic, opsonic and adhesion protein receptors. They release their contents into both phagocytic vesicles and the extracellular medium. Haptoglobin has been identified in specific granules of mature neutrophils and has been shown to be synthesized during the myelocyte–metamyelocyte stage of granulocytic differentiation. The release of haptoglobin from specific granules after neutrophil activation in sites of inflammation would act to reduce local tissue injury and bacterial growth. Other granules, collectively known as tertiary granules, include secretory vesicles, which contain alkaline phosphatase, and gelatinase granules rich in gelatinase. Degranulation of neutrophils begins with the onset of phagocytosis and involves their translocation and fusion with phagocytic vacuoles created by invagination of the plasma membrane.

Degranulation may also occur by reverse endocytosis as a result of the action of complement, aggregated immunoglobulin or certain cytokines. Although the release of granule contents is important for phagocytosis and bacterial killing, extracellular release can also lead to tissue injury and inflammation.

Neutrophil clearance of infectious organisms is critical to the immune response and neutrophil function is impaired in the septic state. Peroxisome proliferator-activated receptor (PPAR)-γ, a ligand-activated nuclear transcription factor, has been shown to be constitutively expressed on isolated human neutrophils and upregulated in the presence of inflammatory cytokines. Inhibition of PPAR-γ activation has been shown to restore *in vitro* neutrophil chemotaxis.

Neutrophils exist in one of three states: quiescent, activated or primed. They circulate in the blood in the quiescent state and react weakly to stimuli, thus limiting potential damage to vascular walls. Priming of neutrophils is a process that does not immediately stimulate an effector response but allows an exaggerated response upon later stimulation. Therefore, this is a mechanism whereby phagocytes are selectively activated on recruitment to sites of infection and inflammation. Three main

Table 17.4 Neutrophil granules and their contents.

Granule	Azurophilic (primary)	Specific (secondary)	Gelatinase (tertiary)	Secretory vesicles
Marker enzyme	Myeloperoxidase	Lactoferrin	Gelatinase	Alkaline phosphatase
Membrane	CD63, granulophysin, CD68, V-type H$^+$-ATPase	CD15, CD66, CD67, CD11b/CD18, cytochrome b, fMLP-R, fibronectin-R, G-protein α-subunit, laminin-R, NB-1 antigen, 19-kDa protein, 155-kDa protein, Rap-1, Rap-2, SCAMP, thrombospondin-R, TNF-R, urokinase-type plasminogen activator-R, VAMP-2, vitronectin	CD11b/CD18, cytochrome b, diacylglycerol-deacylating enzyme, fMLP-R, SCAMP, urokinase-type plasminogen activator-R, VAMP-2, V-type H$^+$-ATPase	CD10, CD13, CD45, CD14, CD16, CD35 (CR1), CD11b/CD18, alkaline phosphatase, fMLP-R, SCAMP, urokinase-type plasminogen activator-R, V-type H$^+$-ATPase, VAMP-2, C1q-receptor, decay activating factor
Matrix, microbicidal	Myeloperoxidase, nitric oxide synthase, lysozyme, BPI protein, defensins, serpocidins, elastase, cathepsins, proteinase 3, azurocidin (CAP 37)	Lactoferrin, lysozyme	Lysozyme	
Matrix, hydrolases	Acid β-glycerophosphatase, α-mannosidase, β-glucuronidase, β-glycerophosphatase, N-acetyl-β-glucosaminidase, sialidase	Gelatinase, collagenase, histaminase, heparanase, NGAL, sialidase	Gelatinase, acetyltransferase	
Matrix, other	Acid-mucopolysaccharide, heparin-binding protein	β$_2$-Microglobulin, urokinase-type plasminogen activator, vitamin B$_{12}$-binding protein	β$_2$-Microglobulin,	Plasma proteins (including tetranectin)

fMLP, f-Met-Leu-Phe; R, receptor; SCAMP, secretory carrier membrane protein; VAMP, vesicle-associated membrane protein.

types of agonists are responsible for priming neutrophils, including chemotactic inflammatory mediators, serum immunoglobulin and complement opsonins, and inflammatory cytokines and growth factors. On neutrophil activation, a significant increase in oxygen consumption, termed respiratory burst, occurs that leads to the production of reactive oxygen species responsible for microbial killing.

Neutrophils are the most numerous leucocytes, comprising 65% of circulating phagocytes, with a normal range in the peripheral blood of $1.5–7.7 \times 10^9$/L. The term 'granulocyte' is often used synonymously with neutrophil despite the fact that neutrophils, eosinophils and basophils can all be classified as granulocytes. Neutrophils are made in the bone marrow at a rate of 10^{12} per day, and once released into the circulation have a half-life of 6–8 hours. The largest proportion of neutrophils

are present within the marrow (reserve pool), with circulating and tissue pools comprising smaller fractions (Figure 17.4). The circulating pool itself consists of a marginated pool of cells that are loosely adherent to the vascular endothelium and a freely circulating pool with the compartments in a constant state of dynamic equilibrium. Several factors including corticosteroids, exercise and infection can lead to an increase in the free circulating pool. Corticosteroids promote the release of neutrophils from the reserve pool into the circulation and prevent migration from the blood into the tissue pool. On the other hand, endotoxin and some complement components (C5a) result in increased margination and reduction in the circulatory pool (Figure 17.4). The variations in neutrophil morphology are shown in Figure 17.5. These include (i) Barr body, a drumstick appendage to the neutrophils in females; (ii) Pelger–Huët

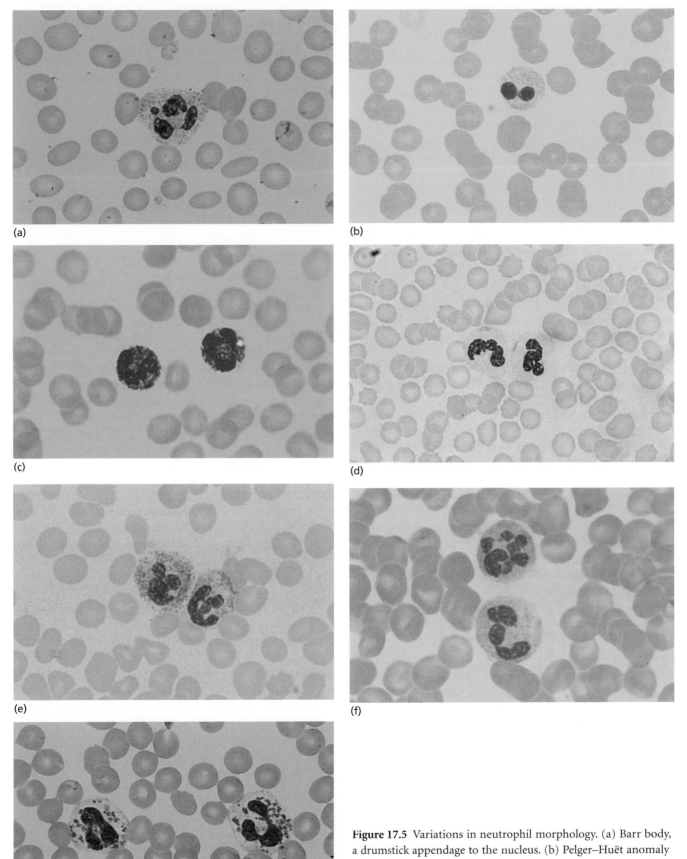

Figure 17.5 Variations in neutrophil morphology. (a) Barr body, a drumstick appendage to the nucleus. (b) Pelger–Huët anomaly with a bilobed nucleus. (c) Alder–Reilly anomaly with prominent purple granules (also in monocytes and lymphocytes). (d) May–Hegglin anomaly with Döhle bodies in the cytoplasm. (e) Toxic granulation. (f) Neutrophil with nuclear hypersegmentation and a normal neutrophil. (g) Chédiak–Higashi syndrome with giant granules.

anomaly, with bilobed nuclei; (iii) Alder–Reilly anomaly; (iv) May–Hegglin anomaly; (v) toxic granulation; (vi) hypersegmented neutrophils; and (vii) Chédiak–Higashi syndrome.

The May–Hegglin anomaly is a rare autosomal dominant condition characterized by thrombocytopenia and giant platelet forms. This disorder is due to a gene encoding a non-muscle myosin heavy chain II (*MYH9*) and results in neutrophils containing basophilic inclusions resembling Döhle bodies. Treatment is usually not needed except in severe cases when platelet transfusions are necessary due to severe thrombocytopenia.

Neutrophils undergo apoptosis within 24 hours of leaving the bone marrow through either intrinsic or extrinsic mechanisms. G-CSF plays an integral role in both the recruitment of neutrophils from the bone marrow and the inhibition of mature neutrophil apoptosis. Calpains are calcium-dependent cysteine proteases that activate pro-apoptotic factors such as Bax, and inhibit anti-apoptotic factors such as X-linked inhibitor of apoptosis (XIAP). G-CSF slows the influx of extracellular calcium and thus downregulates calpain activity, resulting in inhibition of caspase-3, the executioner of apoptosis. Neutrophil apoptosis is characterized by pyknocytosis and the loss of expression of L-selectin and CD16, and the increased expression of CD11b/CD18. Loss of functions including attachement, phagocytosis, degranulation and respiratory burst activity leave the apoptotic neutrophil without purpose and marked for clearance after an inflammatory response has been mounted. Certain drugs, cytokines and mediators of inflammation can delay/inhibit apoptosis in neutrophils, including glucocorticoids, G-CSF, GM-CSF, IL-3, IL-6, IL-15, endotoxin, TNF-α and IFN-γ.

Disorders of neutrophil function and number

Neutrophilia

Leucocytosis, or increased white blood cell count, may be due to either a primary (congenital or acquired) marrow disorder or secondary to a disease process, toxin or drug (Table 17.5). Neutrophil counts are high in neonates and decrease to normal adult levels with ageing. Secondary leucocytosis not associated with leukaemia but with a very high white cell count ($> 50 \times 10^9$/L) is often referred to as a 'leukaemoid reaction' and can be associated with the presence of Döhle bodies and toxic granulation within the cytoplasm (Figure 17.5), as well as with a 'left shift' (with the presence in blood of myelocytes, metamyelocytes and band forms) and an elevated leucocyte alkaline phosphatase score (compared with a low score in chronic myeloid leukaemia). In contrast with acute leukaemia, there is orderly maturation and proliferation of all normal myeloid elements in the bone marrow. Leukaemoid reactions have been described in patients with osteomyelitis, empyema, septicaemia, tuberculosis, Hodgkin disease, juvenile rheumatoid arthritis and dermatitis herpetiformis.

Table 17.5 Causes of neutrophilia.

Primary
Hereditary
Chronic idiopathic
Familial myeloproliferative disease
Leukaemoid reaction associated with congenital anomalies
Leucocyte adhesion deficiency (LAD) types I and II
Familial cold urticaria and leucocytosis

Secondary
Infection
Stress
Chronic inflammation
Drugs (steroids, lithium, tetracycline)
Non-haematological neoplasms
Asplenia and hyposplenism

Neoplastic
Chronic myeloid leukaemia
Other myeloproliferative disorders (myelofibrosis, polycythaemia vera, essential thrombocythaemia)

Leucocyte adhesion deficiency (LAD) is a congenital disorder that presents with persistent leucocytosis, delayed separation of the umbilical cord, recurrent infections, impaired wound healing and defects of neutrophil activation. The condition is caused by defects in adhesion of neutrophils to blood vessel walls. As a result, phagocytes do not migrate from the bloodstream to sites of infection. Two types of LAD have been described. In LAD type I, mutations of the gene encoding the β-subunit of the β₂ integrins (CD11b and CD18) have been detected. The molecular basis for the rare LAD type II is defective glycosylation of ligands on leucocytes recognized by the selectin family of adhesion molecules. The clinical features in the two types are similar, and because of the defect in neutrophil migration, abscesses and other sites of infection are devoid of pus despite the striking neutrophilia. Treatment involves the use of prophylactic antibiotics and aggressive therapy of periodontal disease. Stem cell transplantation can be considered in patients with severe disease. The LAD-I variant syndrome is a condition characterized by non-pussing bacterial and fungal infections, poor wound healing, mucosal bleeding and the potential for life-threatening intracranial bleeds that are seen early in life, with bone marrow transplantation as the only curative modality.

Hereditary neutrophilia has been described in a single family of four, with leucocyte counts chronically in the range 20–70×10^9/L as well as splenomegaly, widened diploë of the skull and a high leucocyte alkaline phosphatase but without serious medical problems. Neutrophil function and adhesion to vessel walls in these patients are normal and the condition appears to have an autosomal dominant inheritance.

Chronic idiopathic neutrophilia is an association of a chronically elevated neutrophil count (in the range $11–40 \times 10^9/L$) in healthy individuals without any associated clinical problems. In one series, several individuals were followed for up to 20 years without developing any disease.

Leukaemoid reactions have been described with congenital disorders such as amegakaryocytic thrombocytopenia, tetralogy of Fallot, dextrocardia with absent radii and in patients with Down syndrome. The neutrophilia in Down syndrome is transient but may be exaggerated in response to stress. The transient myeloproliferative disorder, or 'transient leukaemia', can be seen in up to 10% of children born with Down syndrome and is characterized by clonal proliferation of myeloid blasts that is asymptomatic and self-limiting in most cases. High white cell count, the presence of ascites, preterm delivery, bleeding diathesis and failure of spontaneous remission were all found to be positively correlated with the occurrence of early death in multivariable anlaysis. Approximately 20% of neonates with Down syndrome will develop an aggressive form of acute myeloid leukaemia (mostly FAB M7-like) requiring intensive chemotherapy. A syndrome of growth retardation, hepatosplenomegaly and leucocytosis has been described as a familial myeloproliferative disease, with some affected individuals dying in early life and others remaining stable or even improving with time. These patients had low leucocyte alkaline phosphatase scores and no detectable cytogenetic abnormalites. Others have reported families with several generations of affected individuals with a variety of myeloproliferative disorders but without cytogenetic abnormalities.

Familial cold urticaria and leucocytosis is a syndrome of fever, urticaria, rash and muscle and skin tenderness on exposure to cold that appears to be dominantly inherited. The onset of the disease is in infancy, with urticaria, rash and leucocytosis generally occurring several hours after cold exposure. The skin rash is histologically characterized by intense infiltration by neutrophils.

Non-malignant causes of neutrophilia include acute infections, with elevated counts in most bacterial infections. In response to overwhelming infection, marrow depletion of leucocytes can occur, resulting in neutropenia rather than neutrophilia. Neutrophilia in response to chronic inflammatory processes is usually more modest in degree and can be accompanied by monocytosis. Modest elevations of neutrophil counts are commonly seen in various forms of 'stress' such as exercise, adrenaline injection, myocardial infarction, in the postoperative period, in post-ictal states and with emotional distress. This is probably due to the migration of neutrophils from the marginated pool to the circulatory pool. Mild neutrophilia has also been reported with unipolar depression. A number of drugs and drug reactions are commonly associated with increased neutrophil counts. Steroids stimulate the release of neutrophils

from the bone marrow and diminish their egress from the circulation resulting in chronic neutrophilia. This can be distinguished from neutrophilia due to infection by the distinct lack of band forms in the former. The β-agonists produce an acute neutrophilia by releasing neutrophils from the marginated pool. Other drugs known to produce neutrophil leucocytosis include lithium, which increases the production of CSF and potentiates its effects on myeloid colony formation, and tetracycline, which has been associated with counts as high as $80 \times 10^9/L$. Growth factors such as G-CSF, GM-CSF and Neulasta (a pegylated form of G-CSF that has a prolonged half-life in circulation) are commercially available and are used commonly to reduce the duration of neutropenia associated with chemotherapy and to mobilize stem cells for transplantation. Their use in healthy individuals for the latter purpose is associated with significant neutrophilia and a left shift.

Neutropenia

Neutropenia can be due to impaired production by the bone marrow, shift from the circulating pool to marginated pool, increased peripheral destruction, or a combination of these (Table 17.6). It has been defined as an absolute neutrophil count (ANC) of more than two standard deviations below a normal mean value. There is variation of neutrophil counts among different ethnic groups, with black people generally having slightly lower counts (lower limit of normal $1.2 \times 10^9/L$) compared with white people (lower limit of normal $1.5 \times 10^9/L$). The lower count in black populations has been attributed to a relative decrease in the size of the marrow storage pool. In patients whose neutropenia is related to decreased production, the propensity to develop infections is directly related to the degree and duration of neutropenia.

On the other hand, in patients whose neutropenia is due to peripheral destruction or margination of neutrophils, there is no direct correlation between the degree of neutropenia and the propensity for infections. Neutropenia due to marrow failure states or associated with chemotherapy can predispose patients to severe life-threatening infections, although this is more likely in patients with neutrophil counts below $0.5 \times 10^9/L$. Common organisms encountered in this setting are *Staphylococcus aureus*, *Pseudomonas aeruginosa*, *E. coli* and *Klebsiella* species. On the other hand, patients with some congenital or immune forms of neutropenia can tolerate low counts for prolonged periods without any apparent increase in the incidence of infections. Moderate asymptomatic neutropenia associated with specific ethnic groups such as African-Americans and Yemenite Jews is associated with a dominant inheritance pattern and requires no specific intervention.

Several well-defined inherited syndromes associated with neutropenia have been described and are worth mentioning. *Severe congenital neutropenia* (SCN) is a multigene heterogeneous group of disorders characterized by severe neutropenia at birth (ANC $< 0.5 \times 10^9/L$) and maturation arrest at the

Table 17.6 Causes of neutropenia.

Decreased production

Inherited
Reticular dysgenesis
Dyskeratosis congenita
Schwachman–Diamond–Oski syndrome
Cyclic neutropenia
Kostmann syndrome
Hyper-IgM syndrome
Chronic idiopathic neutropenia

Acquired
Aplastic anaemia
Bone marrow infiltration (leukaemia, lymphoma, tumours,
    tuberculosis, etc.)
Severe infection
Drug induced (cytotoxic chemotherapy, radiation,
    chloramphenicol, penicillins, cephalosporins, phenothiazine,
    phenylbutazone, gold, antithyroid drugs, quinidine,
    anticonvulsants, alcohol)
Myelodysplastic syndrome
Vitamin B_{12} or folate deficiency
Pure white cell aplasia
T-γ lymphocytosis and neutropenia
Neutropenia associated with metabolic disorders
Acute leukaemia

Increased peripheral destruction
Hypersplenism
Immune mediated
Drug induced
Associated with collagen vascular disease (Felty syndrome,
    systemic lupus erythematosus)
Complement mediated (haemodialysis, cardiopulmonary bypass)

Altered distribution
Drugs
Stress

---

developmental stage of the promyelocyte/myelocyte. Kostmann syndrome is an autosomal recessive form involving mutations of the *HAX1* gene encoding a mitochondrial-associated protein with structural similarity to other anti-apoptotic BCL-2 family members. Autosomal dominant and sporadic cases are more closely linked to gene mutations of *ELA2*, which codes for neutrophil elastase 2. It is still unclear as to the exact pathogenetic mechanism by which the *ELA2* mutation leads to neutrophil apoptosis but may involve structural rather than functional properties of the mutated protein. Less common mutations in genes encoding p14, G6PC3, GFI1, CSF3R, TAZ and WASP have all been documented in SCN. SCN is usually diagnosed in infancy in the setting of recurrent severe infections. Monocytosis,

eosinophilia and hypergammaglobulinaemia are often present. Myelopoiesis is blocked and the increased number of promyelocytes found in the bone marrow are characterized by atypical nuclei and cytoplasmic vacuolization. SCN associated with *HAX1* and *ELA2* has an increased risk of leukaemic transformation that is not observed in cases of SCN linked to the other gene mutations. Importantly, the risk of developing infection is independent of the underlying genetic defect and can be correlated to the ANC nadir. First-line treatment of infections in such patients is antibiotics with G-CSF. G-CSF is the cornerstone of therapy in reducing the infectious risk. Stem cell transplantation offers the potential of cure for those who do not respond to antibiotics and G-CSF. Transformation to myelodysplastic syndrome (MDS)/acute myeloid leukaemia (AML) in SCN is also independent of genetic defect and is approximately 21% at 10 years. The Severe Chronic Neutropenia International Registry has identified a group of patients with SCN who were less responsive to G-CSF in achieving and maintaining an adequate ANC; these patients have a cumulative incidence of developing MDS/AML or dying of sepsis at 10 years of 40% and 14%, respectively. These patients should be considered for haemopoietic stem cell transplantation earlier in life. The acquisition of *CSF3R* point mutations has also been shown to increase the risk of transformation to MDS/AML irrespective of the underlying genetic defect, and detection of monosomy 7 in the bone marrow of MDS/AML-associated SCN may indicate the occult presence of a G-CSF-sensitive leukaemic clone.

Cyclic neutropenia is a rare autosomal dominant disorder with variable expression that is characterized by repetitive episodes of fever, pharyngitis, stomatitis and other bacterial infections attributable to recurrent severe neutropenia occurring every 15–35 days. The nadir neutrophil count, usually between zero and 200×10^9/L, lasts 3–7 days and is frequently associated with monocytosis. Cycling of red cell and platelet production is also observed in some cases. The bone marrow is characterized by transient arrest at the promyelocyte stage before each cycle. Both childhood and adult onset have been reported. Recent studies have shown that autosomal dominant and sporadic cases of this disease are due to a mutation in *ELA2*, the gene for neutrophil elastase (a chymotryptic serine protease of neutrophil and monocyte granules), located on chromosome 19p13.3. This enzyme is synthesized in neutrophil precursors early in the process of primary granule formation. The present hypothesis suggests that the mutant neutrophil elastase functions aberrantly within the cells to accelerate apoptosis of the precursors, resulting in oscillatory production. The cyclic nature of this disorder provides evidence of a regulatory mechanism gone awry, likely due to a defective feedback circuit in which neutrophils inhibit cell proliferation thereby regulating progenitor cell proliferation. Recently, the process has been shown to involve interactions between PFAAP5, a protein mediating transcriptional repressor GFI1, and neutrophil elastase. This disorder is effectively treated with G-CSF, and no transformation to AML or MDS has been observed in these patients, with or without G-CSF therapy.

Schwachman–Diamond–Oski syndrome is an autosomal recessive disorder characterized by exocrine pancreas insufficiency, metaphyseal dysostosis and bone marrow dysfunction (see Chapter 12). Recurrent severe bacterial infections and susceptibility to leukaemia are the major causes of morbidity and mortality, although many affected individuals have relatively few problems with infections. Neutrophil count is commonly less than 500×10^9/L and many patients are also anaemic and thrombocytopenic. Bone marrow is usually hypoplastic and a number of neutrophil functional disorders such as chemotactic defects may be present. A variety of physical anomalies including short stature, strabismus, syndactyly, cleft palate and microcephaly may exist. The propensity to develop leukaemia and aplastic anaemia suggests that a stem cell defect may be present. Treatment involves the use of G-CSF in patients with recurrent infections, and the use of pancreatic enzyme supplements for the gastrointestinal insufficiency and steatorrhoea. Some anaemic patients respond to steroids.

Reticular dysgenesis is associated with neutropenia, lymphoid hypoplasia, and thymic hypoplasia with normal erythropoiesis and megakaryopoiesis. Patients have a hypoplastic marrow and low levels of IgM and IgG and die from overwhelming infections usually in early infancy. Dyskeratosis congenita is a rare disease characterized by abnormal skin pigmentation, nail dystrophy and mucosal leucoplakia. More than 80% of the affected individuals develop bone marrow failure, which is the major cause of death. The disorder is caused by defective telomere maintenance in stem cells. The major X-linked form of the disease is due to mutations in the *DKC1* gene located at Xq28 and coding for dyskerin, a nucleolar protein (see Chapter 12). Dyskerin is part of small nucleolar ribonucleoprotein particles involved in processing ribosomal RNA. It is also found in the telomerase complex, pointing to a possible link between these two processes. An autosomal dominant form is due to mutations in the RNA component of telomerase. Patients with this form of the disease are more severely affected in the later generations carrying the mutations, possibly due to the inheritance of shortened telomeres, and may be considered to have aplastic anaemia.

Neutropenia has been seen with immunological abnormalities such as hyper-IgM syndrome and X-linked agammaglobulinaemia. Hyper-IgM syndrome is an X-linked disorder characterized by lymphoid hyperplasia, low concentrations of IgG and IgA but high concentration of IgM, and severe neutropenia. A genetic defect in the T-cell CD40 ligand has been implicated as the cause of the disease. CD40 ligand is a 39-kDa protein expressed on the surface of activated CD4$^+$ T cells that delivers contact-dependent signals to CD40-expressing cells: B cells, monocytes, dendritic cells, epithelial cells, endothelial cells and fibroblasts. The loss of interaction between CD40 and its ligand results in impairment of T-cell function, of B-cell differentiation and of monocyte function. Patients commonly die of overwhelming infections by the age of 5 years unless treated with intravenous immunoglobulin and long-term G-CSF.

Chronic benign neutropenia, chronic idiopathic neutropenia and *autoimmune neutropenia* are very similar in laboratory findings and differ only with regard to age of onset and association with other immune disorders. Chronic benign neutropenia commonly presents in older children or young adults. Patients are usually asymptomatic and have neutrophil counts in the range $0.2–0.5 \times 10^9$/L. Bone marrow examination is commonly normocellular or occasionally moderately hypocellular. They usually have a peripheral monocytosis and often a benign course, although occasional cases progressing to acute leukaemia have been reported. Anti-neutrophil antibodies, detected in some patients, are not commonly present but antibodies to the progenitor cells or other precursors may be the inciting factor in these patients. As these patients generally have a benign course, treatment to increase neutrophil counts should be reserved for those who have recurrent infections. Corticosteroids, splenectomy, cytotoxic agents and G-CSF have all been used successfully in this setting. Chronic benign neutropenia of infancy and childhood is probably a related disease, with the majority of patients presenting during the first year of life. There is no familial predisposition and anti-neutrophil antibodies are commonly detected. Furthermore, the neutropenia responds to immunosuppressive therapy, suggesting an immune mechanism. There is a compensatory increase in neutrophil precursors in the marrow. Some patients have a measurable defect of neutrophil mobility, otherwise described as 'lazy leucocyte syndrome'.

Infants of hypertensive mothers also commonly have moderate to severe neutropenia lasting for several days. This is probably related to bone marrow suppression. Moderate to severe neutropenia can also occur in newborn infants as a result of the transfer of maternal IgG anti-neutrophil antibodies in a manner similar to rhesus haemolytic disease of the newborn. This isoimmune neutropenia develops antenatally and is due to maternal production of antibodies against antigens on fetal neutrophils.

Pure white cell aplasia is a rare condition associated with recurrent pyogenic infections and with thymoma in 70% of the affected patients. There is almost complete absence of myeloid precursors without any abnormality of erythroid or megakaryocytic precursors in the marrow. In the majority of patients, the marrow inhibitory activity is in the IgG and IgM fractions of serum but, in some, the inhibition is due to the lymphocytes. The immunoglobulin is directed against progenitor cells or myeloid precursors. The disorder has been associated with therapy with ibuprofen, certain natural remedies and chlorpropamide. If associated with thymoma, surgical removal of the thymus gland can partially correct the neutropenia. Other treatment options include corticosteroids, ciclosporin, cyclophosphamide and intravenous immunoglobulin.

Humoral and cellular immune responses are responsible for the development of neutropenia in a number of settings. Autoimmune neutropenia due to circulating antibody can occur as an isolated condition or in association with other autoimmune disorders such as autoimmune thrombocytopenic purpura and autoimmune haemolytic anaemia. The antibodies may be directed at the mature neutrophils or morphologically identifiable myeloid precursors.

Inhibition of granulopoiesis by suppressor or cytotoxic T lymphocytes can occur in patients with collagen vascular disorders as well as in patients with T-γ lymphocytosis. Patients with T-γ lymphocytosis commonly present with recurrent infections at a median age of 55 years. There is clonal proliferation of either $CD3^+/CD56^+$ T cells or $CD3^-/CD56^+$ natural killer (NK) cells. NK cells do not express CD5 and T-cell receptor (TCR) proteins, and their TCR locus is not rearranged, whereas $CD3^+$ large granular lymphocytes have rearranged TCR genes and are thought to represent *in vivo* activated cytotoxic T cells. The characteristic findings include peripheral blood lymphocytosis with most lymphocytes being large granular lymphocytes. Patients may also have lymphadenopathy and hepatosplenomegaly; the bone marrow is commonly normocellular with increased lymphocytes and arrested myelopoiesis at the myelocyte stage. The $CD3^+$ subset of the disease most commonly has an indolent course, although most patients need treatment for recurrent episodes of life-threatening infections. G-CSF therapy is used in managing acute infections and methotrexate, prednisolone, cyclophosphamide or ciclosporin can be effective in improving neutrophil counts for sustained periods. In contrast, the $CD3^-/CD56^+$ NK-cell disorders are clinically aggressive, occurring in younger patients and presenting with fever, massive hepatosplenomegaly, jaundice and marrow infiltration with the abnormal clone. They typically have a rapidly progressive course unresponsive to combination chemotherapy.

Neutropenia is also associated with collagen vascular diseases such as systemic lupus erythematosus (SLE) and with rheumatoid arthritis. IgG or IgM antibodies may be directed against mature neutrophils or their precursors. Recent advances have allowed better understanding regarding the mechanism of neutropenia and improved options for treatment. Target antigens for anti-neutrophil antibodies have been identified for both Felty syndrome and SLE. In Felty syndrome, severe neutropenia is associated with rheumatoid arthritis, splenomegaly and leg ulcers. Therapy for neutropenia with methotrexate and ciclosporin has been attempted with variable success. The efficacy of both GM-CSF and G-CSF in reversing neutropenia and decreasing the risk of infections in Felty syndrome and SLE has been well documented. Of concern, however, have been flares of symptoms or development of leucocytoclastic vasculitis in some patients following the use of these cytokines. Recent results suggest that G-CSF should be administered at the lowest dose effective at elevating the neutrophil count above 1.0×10^9/L.

Neutrophil counts between 0.1 and 0.45×10^9/L are seen in WHIM syndrome, a rare disorder characterized by warts, hypogammaglobulinaemia, infections and myelokathexis. The bone marrow is usually hypercellular with normal-appearing early myeloid forms and abnormal metamyelocytes, bands and mature neutrophils with diploid and tetraploid nuclei. Autosomal dominant inheritance of a CXC-chemokine receptor (CXCR)4 mutation is associated with WHIM syndrome and leads to impaired receptor downregulation. Leucocyte CXCR4 engagement by stem cell-derived factor (SDF)-1 as presented by bone marrow stromal cells is an important signal promoting the retention of leucocytes within the bone marrow microenvironment niche. The overexpression of CXCR4 by leucocytes in WHIM leads to impaired egress of mature neutrophils from the bone marrow and resultant neutropenia. Decreased expression of BCL-X in myeloid precursors is also a feature of WHIM and is associated with an increased rate of apoptosis. G-CSF can be used to improve the neutropenia in WHIM syndrome.

Drug-induced neutropenia is probably the commonest cause of isolated neutropenia. A thorough evaluation of the medication history of a patient with neutropenia is important for excluding drugs as the inciting factor. Usually the mechanisms involve suppression of bone marrow activity or are immunological in nature. The neutropenia commonly develops 1–2 weeks after initiation of the drug and resolves soon after discontinuation of the offending agent. Agents most commonly associated with this side-effect include antibiotics (e.g. penicillins, cephalosporins, chloramphenicol), anticonvulsants (e.g. carbamazepine, phenytoin), anti-inflammatory agents (e.g. gold, phenylbutazone), antithyroid drugs (e.g. carbimazole, methylthiouracil), hypoglycaemic agents (e.g. chlorpropamide), diuretics (e.g. hydrochlorothiazide, bumetanide) and phenothiazine. The use of cytotoxic agents in cancer therapy is frequently associated with the development of neutropenia.

Neutropenia can also be a factor in aplastic anaemia. Other miscellaneous causes of neutropenia include the following.
• Viral infections: HIV, varicella, measles, rubella, infectious mononucleosis, influenza, hepatitis A and B, parvovirus and cytomegalovirus.
• Overwhelming bacterial infections (by exhausting the neutrophil reserve pool).
• Metabolic diseases: orotic aciduria, methylmalonic aciduria, glycogen storage disease type Ib.
• Nutritional deficiencies: vitamin B_{12}, folate (which causes hypersegmented nuclei; see Figure 17.5f) or copper.
• Hypersplenism.

Disorders of neutrophil function
A number of congenital and acquired conditions with abnormal neutrophil morphology (see Figure 17.2a) and/or function have been recognized (Table 17.7). Some of these are associated with abnormal neutrophil numbers and have been discussed earlier.

Table 17.7 Disorders of neutrophil morphology and/or function.

Functional defect	Congenital	Acquired
Minimal	Hereditary neutrophil hypersegmentation (AD)	Megaloblastic hypersegmentation
	Pelger–Huët anomaly (AD)	Mucopolysaccharidoses
	Alder–Reilly anomaly (AR)	
	May–Hegglin anomaly (AD)	
	Myeloperoxidase deficiency (AR)	
Adherence/migration	Leucocyte adhesion deficiency (AR)	Renal failure
	Neutrophil-specific granule deficiency (AR)	Diabetes
	Schwachman syndrome (?AR)	Neonates
	Hyper-IgE syndrome	Malnutrition
	Job syndrome (AR)	Leukaemia
	Familial Mediterranean fever (AR)	
Phagocytic killing	Chronic granulomatous disease	Malnutrition
	Papillon–Lefevre syndrome (AR)	Vitamin E deficiency
		Severe iron deficiency
		Neonates
		Diabetes
		Viral infections
		Sickle cell disease

AD, autosomal dominant; AR, autosomal recessive.

Chédiak–Higashi syndrome

Chédiak–Higashi syndrome is a rare autosomal recessive disorder characterized by oculocutaneous albinism, recurrent and severe bacterial infections, giant blue-grey granules in the cytoplasm of white blood cells (see Figure 17.5g), a mild bleeding diathesis, progressive peripheral neuropathy and cranial nerve abnormalities. Morbidity results from patients succumbing to frequent bacterial infections or to an 'accelerated phase', a progressive lymphoproliferative syndrome. Patients eventually succumb to a profound pancytopenia. Neutrophils contain a highly heterogeneous population of giant granules probably derived from coalescence of azurophil and secondary granules. The giant granules are seen more commonly in the bone marrow than peripheral blood, as many of the abnormal myeloid precursors are destroyed before release, leading to moderate neutropenia.

Chédiak–Higashi syndrome neutrophils also have a deficiency of antimicrobial proteins as well as disordered degranulation and chemotaxis. Dysfunction of other elements of the immune system, such as cytotoxic T lymphocytes and NK cells, contribute to the propensity for infection and the development of the accelerated phase of the disease. Mutations in the lysosomal trafficking regulator gene, *LYST*, located on chromosome 1q42.1–q42.2, have been implicated as the cause of this disease. At present, treatment for the disorder is allogeneic stem cell transplantation, which alleviates the immune problems and the accelerated phase but does not inhibit the development of neurological disorders that frequently become increasingly worse with age.

Chronic granulomatous disease

Chronic granulomatous disease (CGD) is an inherited disease characterized by severe and recurrent purulent bacterial and fungal infections, including pneumonia, lymphadenitis, hepatic abscesses and osteomyelitis. The majority of patients present in the first year of life with infections with catalase-positive organisms. Phagocytic cells of CGD patients have a defect in the phagosomal and plasma membrane-associated NADPH oxidase, resulting in impaired superoxide formation necessary for efficient bacterial and fungal killing. In addition, a failure to switch off the inflammatory response leads to the formation of granulomas, the distinctive hallmark of the disorder. All the subtypes of X-linked CGD are caused by mutations in the gene for the gp91-phox subunit of cytochrome *b* (*CYBB*) located at Xp21.1. There is significant heterogeneity in the mutations in the gene, with most being family specific. This accounts for the clinical heterogeneity seen in X-linked CGD. Other mutations in recessively inherited forms of the disease have also been described.

The incidence of CGD is 1 in 200000 to 1 in 250000 live births and the diagnosis is suggested by failure of neutrophils to reduce nitroblue tetrazolium (NBT slide test). The diagnosis can be further established by directly measuring respiratory burst activity as oxygen consumption, oxygen production or

H_2O_2 production. Severe deficiency of glucose-6-phosphate dehydrogenase (G6PD) in neutrophils, as seen in a rare X-linked disorder, can result in a greatly attenuated respiratory burst and a condition resembling CGD. Therapy involves prevention and early treatment of infections, aggressive parenteral antibiotic therapy for established infections, and use of prophylactic trimethoprim–sulfamethoxazole. In a prospective multicentre trial of CGD patients, recombinant human IFN-γ has been shown to augment host defence and reduce the incidence of life-threatening infections via unknown mechanisms other than reversing the respiratory burst defect; its efficacy in reducing serious bacterial and fungal infections has been confirmed in a prospective multicentre study in CGD. Haemopoietic stem cell transplantation, if performed at the first signs of a severe course of the disease, is a valid therapeutic option for children with CGD. Newer approaches using reduced conditioning stem cell transplantation are still being investigated; more recently, Phase I clinical trials with retrovirally transduced autologous peripheral blood CD34$^+$ stem cells may make gene therapy for CGD a possibility in the future.

Myeloperoxidase deficiency

Myeloperoxidase (MPO) deficiency is the most common inherited disorder of phagocytes and is inherited in an autosomal recessive manner. The gene encoding MPO is located at 17q21.3–q23 near the breakpoint of the translocation in acute promyelocytic leukaemia. Despite the key role of MPO in the microbicidal function of neutrophils, persons with MPO deficiency lack any clinical symptoms and therapy is not required, except for a higher incidence of fungal infections when aggressive antifungal therapy is indicated.

Neutrophil specific granule deficiency

Specific granule deficiency is a rare congenital disorder characterized by recurrent bacterial and fungal infections of skin and lungs. The inheritance is autosomal recessive and although the precise molecular defect has not been elucidated, recent data implicate functional loss of the myeloid transcription factor CCAAT/enhancer-binding protein, C/EBPε, as important in the development of specific granule deficiency. The neutrophils of these patients display atypical bilobed nuclei, lack expression of at least one primary and all secondary and tertiary granule proteins, and possess defects in chemotaxis, disaggregation, receptor upregulation and bactericidal activity. Similar neutrophil granule deficiencies have been described in some patients with leukaemia.

Papillon–Lefevre syndrome

This is a rare autosomal recessive disorder characterized by palmoplantar keratoderma and early-onset peridontitis. Pyogenic liver abscesses are an increasingly common complication. Consanguinity is common and the disease is commonly manifested in the first 6 months of life, with early progressive loss of both primary and secondary dentition. A phagocytic defect in microbicidal activity and degradation of ingested material is thought to be present. This is attributed to loss-of-function mutations of the *CTSC* gene located on chromosome 11q14.2, which encodes the protease cathepsin C.

Eosinophils (Figure 17.2b)

Development and function

Eosinophils, which account for 5–10% of leucocytes (0.2×10^9/L), are similar to neutrophils morphologically except for the presence of a bilobed nucleus and numerous bright-orange cytoplasmic granules. There are three distinct granule populations: the round, uniformly electron-dense primary granules present mainly in the eosinophilic promyelocyte/myelocyte stages; secondary or specific granules; and the less well characterized small granules (Table 17.8).

Primary granules contain eosinophil peroxidase and Charcot–Leyden crystal protein. The eosinophil peroxidase is distinct from neutrophil MPO and can mediate damage to microorganisms and tissues and bronchoconstriction in asthma. Charcot–Leyden crystal protein is found in tissues and fluids in association with eosinophil inflammatory reactions and may have a role in respiratory disease.

The large specific granules contain the eosinophil's cytotoxic and proinflammatory proteins and account for more than 95% of granules in the mature eosinophils, conferring the characteristic appearance of the cell. Eosinophil granules contain a number of enzymes similar to those found in the lysosomes of the neutrophil, but lack lysozyme. Different cationic polypeptides are the major constituents of eosinophil granules and include major basic protein (MBP), eosinophil cationic proteins (ECP) and eosinophil-derived neurotoxin (EDN). MBP is toxic to cells, including parasites and mammalian epithelial cells, and evokes release of mediators from basophils and mast cells. Eosinophils have a significant cytotoxic and proinflammatory function and play an important part in the pathogenesis of a number of allergic, parasitic and malignant disease processes.

Eosinophils are derived from bone marrow stem cell-derived myeloid progenitors in response to a number of T cell-derived cytokines and growth factors including IL-3, GM-CSF and IL-5. Mast cells, macrophages, NK cells, endothelial cells and stromal cells also produce these cytokines. IL-5 is the most lineage-specific factor and plays an important role in regulation of terminal differentiation and post-mitotic activation of eosinophils. Therefore, IL-5 is a late-acting cytokine that is both necessary and sufficient for eosinophil development *in vivo*, a finding that has been confirmed by IL-5 transgenic and IL-5 knockout mice.

In normal individuals, eosinophils exist transiently in the circulation and localize specifically to certain tissues and organs

Table 17.8 Contents of eosinophil granules.

Granule	Protein content	Comment
Primary granule (Charcot–Leyden granule)	Charcot–Leyden crystal (CLC) protein	Weak lysophospholipase, carbohydrate-crystal protein-containing binding properties
Specific granule (secondary granule)	Eosinophil peroxidase	
	Major basic protein (MBP)	Toxic to parasites
	Eosinophil cationic protein (ECP)	Ribonuclease, bactericidal, toxic to parasites
	Eosinophil-derived neurotoxin (EDN)	Ribonuclease, toxic to parasites
	Eosinophil peroxidase (EPO)	Antibacterial
	Lysophospholipase	
	Acid phosphatase	
	Arylsulphatase B	
	Phospholipase A_2 (secretory)	Antibacterial
	BPI protein	LPS binding, antibacterial
	NAMLAA	Antibacterial
	FAD	
	Catalase	
	Urokinase	
	CD63	Tetraspanin
	Proteoglycan	
	α_1 Antitrypsin	
Small-type granule	Arylsulphatase B	Lysosomal hydrolase
Secretory vesicle	Cytochrome b_{558}	NADPH oxidase component
	CR3	β_2 integrin

BPI, bactericidal permeability-increasing protein; FAD, flavin adenine dinucleotide; LPS, lipopolysaccharide; NAMLAA, N-acetylmuramyl-L-alanine amidase.

exposed to the external environment. Eosinophils are recruited in response to early- and late-phase components of immediate hypersensitivity reactions as well as other immunologically mediated reactions. Their activation and recruitment involves the interaction of several adhesion pathways and chemotactic agents including the complement fragment C5a, PAF, IL-3, IL-5, GM-CSF, IL-2, RANTES, eotaxins and the CD8$^+$ T cell-derived lymphocyte chemoattractant factor (LCF).

The specificity and intensity of the microbicidal function of eosinophils differ from those of other leucocytes; their bactericidal activity is less efficient than that of neutrophils, but not because of any deficiency of specific enzymes. In fact, eosinophil peroxidase is more bactericidal than MPO. However, the major protective role of eosinophils in host defence is the destruction of metazoan parasites. Eosinophils readily degranulate in response to stimulation by antigens, cytokines and complexed or secretory IgA, IgE and IgG. Proteins released from eosinophils result in histamine release from basophils and mast cells, and amplify the inflammatory response. These proteins are also powerful toxins towards host cells, leading to tissue injury. A further role of eosinophils is tissue repair and remodelling through regulation of the deposition of extracellular matrix proteins.

Disorders of eosinophils

Eosinophilia

Eosinophilia is considered as an absolute eosinophil count of 0.5×10^9/L or more. Blood and tissue eosinophilia can be seen in a number of parasitic, neoplastic, collagen vascular and allergic diseases (Table 17.9). Because of the varied causes of eosinophilia, diagnostic evaluation should include complete physical examination and history, routine chemistries, serum IgE, vitamin B_{12} levels, HIV serology, stool ova and parasites, electrocardiogram, echocardiogram, pulmonary function tests, chest and abdominal computed tomography, and bone marrow biopsy and aspirate.

In these disorders, a variety of abnormal stimuli lead to the increased production and tissue localization of eosinophils. When no underlying cause can be identified, the hypereosinophilic syndrome (HES) may be present. Several reactive pulmonary and cutaneous eosinophilic syndromes (e.g. Churg–Strauss syndrome, Loeffler syndrome and eosinophilic lymphofolliculosis or Kimura disease) as well as an eosinophilia–myalgia syndrome have also been described. Eosinophilia–myalgia syndrome is related to metabolites and contaminants in preparation of the drug L-tryptophan and presents with peripheral

Table 17.9 Causes of eosinophilia.

Infections
Parasitic: helminthic (filariasis, strongyloidiasis, hydatid disease,
  onchocerciasis, etc.), visceral larva migrans
Non-parasitic: coccidiomycosis, recovery from acute infections,
  cat scratch disease, *Cryptococcus*

Allergic disease
Atopic diseases
Drug hypersensitivity
Bronchopulmonary aspergillosis

Pulmonary
Allergic bronchopulmonary aspergillosis
Eosinophilic pneumonia
Transient pulmonary infiltrates (Loeffler syndrome)
Prolonged pulmonary infiltrates with eosinophilia
Tropical pulmonary eosinophilia
Allergic granulomatosis (Churg–Strauss syndrome)

Cutaneous
Eosinophilic lymphofolliculosis (Kimura disease)
Bullous pemphigoid
Granulomatous dermatitis with eosinophilia (Wells disease)
Eosinophilic fasciitis (Shulman syndrome)
Atopic dermatitis
Urticaria and angioedema

Connective tissue disorder
Vasculitis
Serum sickness
Eosinophilic fasciitis

Immunological disorders
Wiskott–Aldrich syndrome
Selective IgA deficiency
Graft-versus-host disease

Neoplastic conditions
Eosinophilic leukaemia
Lymphoma (Hodgkin, T cell)
Chronic myeloid leukaemia
Acute myeloid leukaemia, M4Eo
Some solid tumours

Miscellaneous
Eosinophilic myalgia syndrome
Toxic oil syndrome
Idiopathic hypereosinophilic syndrome

blood eosinophilia, fatigue and severe myalgia. It responds slowly to cessation of L-tryptophan therapy in a number of the patients.

HES is characterized by sustained eosinophilia of 30–70% of total leucocyte count ($> 1.5 \times 10^9$/L) for longer than 6 months, absence of other underlying causes of eosinophilia and evidence of organ dysfunction due to eosinophilic tissue infiltration. Presenting features include anorexia, weight loss, fever, sweating, thromboembolic episodes, heart failure, splenomegaly, and skin and central nervous system (CNS) disease. Peripheral blood eosinophils have a variety of cellular abnormalities, and bone marrow eosinophils are increased (30–60%) but myeloblasts are usually not. It has been difficult to assess the clonality of HES. Cases that are clonally derived, as demonstrated by clonal karyotypic abnormalities and the performance of restriction polymorphism analysis in females, are now reclassified by WHO (2008) as chronic eosinophilic leukaemia.

This clinically variable disorder has various subtypes, including the myeloproliferative variant (10–50%) (these are now classified as chronic eosinophilic leukaemia; see aso Chapters 27 and 36), lymphoproliferative variant (5–50%), familial form, episodic form and benign form. Patients with the myeloproliferative variant of HES are typified by male predominance, end-organ damage, elevated serum tryptase, splenomegaly, anaemia, thrombocytopenia and bone marrow myeloproliferation with reticulin fibrosis. This variant was historically recognized as unresponsive to steroid therapy, with a mortality greater than 50%, most commonly due to cardiac dysfunction from endomyocardial fibrosis. The myeloproliferative variant is usually caused by an interstitial deletion on chromosome 4q12, resulting in a *FIP1L1–PDGFRA* fusion gene. The protein product of this fusion gene is a tyrosine kinase with enhanced activity and particular sensitivity to low-dose imatinib therapy, leading to durable complete haematological and cytogenetic remission. Even rarer cases with often different haematological features are due to rearrangement of *PDGFRB* or *FGFR1* (see Chapter 36). In a prospective multicentre study of primary HES, all 27 patients with the *FIP1L1–PDGFRA* fusion gene achieved complete haematological and molecular remission at doses of imatinib between 100 and 400 mg daily. This response was durable with a median follow-up of 25 months, and re-emergence of the fusion gene was detectable by reverse transcriptase polymerase chain reaction in only three patients who stopped imatinib for several months. In HES patients negative for the *FIP1L1–PDGFRA* fusion gene, 14% achieved a complete haematological remission with imatinib therapy that was short-lived.

The lymphoproliferative variant of HES is a distinct clinical syndrome characterized by hypereosinophilia occurring in response to IL-5 stimulation by a clonal CD3⁻CD4⁺CD8⁻ activated T-cell population. Patients with this variant are more likely to have skin, gastrointestinal and pulmonary involvement and less likely to have endomyocardial fibrosis and myelofibrosis. Unique to this group of patients is the increased incidence of progression to lymphoma. The other variants of HES are rare and include a form with cyclic episodes of eosinophilia and angio-oedema (also referred to as Gleich syndrome) and a rare familial form with predominant autosomal dominant transmission and gene involvement at 5q31–33.

The goal of treatment in HES is to limit organ damage by controlling the eosinophil count and, except for treatment of *FIP1L1–PDGFRA* associated HES with tyrosine kinase inhibitors, steroids remain first-line therapy. In patients who are refractory or intolerant to the side-effects of steroids, cytotoxic agents such as hydroxycarbamide (hydroxyurea), vincristine and cytarabine have been used, as well as immunomodulatory therapy with interferon alfa, ciclosporin and intravenous immunoglobulins.

Basophils and mast cells (Figure 17.2c)

Development and function

The functions of basophils and mast cells are similar but not identical. They express the receptor that binds with high affinity the Fc portion of IgE antibody (FcεIR) on their surface and they have large metachromatic (purple-black) granules rich in histamine, serotonin and leukotrienes. Basophils have a bilobed nucleus, in contrast to mast cells, which have a unilobed nucleus. More recent studies have demonstrated that despite their significant similarities, basophils and mast cells are terminally differentiated progeny of distinct bone marrow progenitors. Basophils develop from haemopoietic stem cells and mature in the bone marrow and circulate in the blood, whereas mast cells mature in the tissues. They both play significant roles in the development of a number of allergic and inflammatory disorders as well as host defence mechanisms against parasites.

Mechanisms mediating the maturation of basophils and mast cells differ. Mast cells are derived from CD34$^+$, c-Kit-positive progenitors and leave the marrow before their terminal maturation and hone to vascularized peripheral tissues where they mature. A complex array of cytokines, elaborated by T cells, macrophages and stromal cells, regulates the production of basophils and mast cells. The major growth and differentiation factor for basophils is IL-3, whereas the growth and development of mast cells requires the presence of SCF.

Basophils are the least abundant leucocytes, accounting for less than 0.5% of bone marrow and peripheral blood leucocytes. Basophils arise from a common basophil–eosinophil progenitor cell, mature in the marrow over a period of 2–7 days and after release in the circulation last for up to 2 weeks. They are the key mediators of immediate hypersensitivity reactions such as asthma, urticaria and anaphylaxis. In addition, they have been implicated in the delayed cutaneous hypersensitivity reaction. Basophils are stimulated by a number of mediators, such as IgE, IL-3, C5a, GM-CSF, insect venoms and morphine, to release the contents of their granules such as histamine. Synergistic induction of both proinflammatory and immunoregulatory cytokines by IL-33-expressing resident tissue cells, IL-3-expressing mast cells, Th2 lymphocytes, and IgE receptor activation by allergen exposure may provide the mechanism by which basophils are activated without the required involvement of the adaptive immune system.

The interaction between IgE and basophil/mast cell FcεIR and antigen bridging results in basophil degranulation and initiation of their effects of granule contents. The granules of basophils and mast cells contain sulphated glycosaminoglycans responsible for their intense staining, as well as histamine, LTD$_4$, PAF, eosinophil chemotactic factor and kallikrein responsible for type I immediate hypersensitivity reactions and chronic inflammation (Table 17.10). Histamine is derived from histidine by decarboxylation and is stored as a complex with heparin or chondroitin sulphate proteoglycans. The primary protease of mast cells, tryptase, is mainly released during the early phase of allergic response and is a marker of mast cell activation in chronic inflammatory diseases. Other neutral proteases such as carboxypeptidase B, chymase and sulphatases are also released and degrade extracellular matrix proteins. Basophil and mast cell activation also leads to the elaboration of cytokines such as GM-CSF, TNF-α, IFN-γ, IL-3, IL-4 and IL-5, which serve to amplify the inflammatory response; TNF-α and GM-CSF recruit and prime neutrophils, IL-5 activates eosinophils and IL-4 enhances cell adhesion molecule expression on endothelial cells, recruits eosinophils into tissues and induces helper T cells to mediate IgE production by B cells.

Disorders of basophils and mast cells

High basophil numbers are commonly seen in patients with myeloproliferative disorders, in particular chronic myeloid leukaemia (CML). Basophil number can be strikingly elevated in patients with CML, accounting for over 20% of circulating leucocytes in the more advanced stages of the disease. They are a part of the neoplastic clone expressing the Philadelphia chromosome or the *BCR–ABL* fusion gene. In other myeloproliferative disorders such as primary myelofibrosis and polycythaemia vera, elevation of basophil numbers is usually more modest. Cases of AML with high levels of immature basophils have also been reported. Rarely, basophils may constitute over 80% of circulating leucocytes, a condition sometimes referred to as basophilic leukaemia. These patients may exhibit clinical features related to the release of histamine and other basophil granular contents, and their treatment can be difficult owing to the possibility of massive release of these mediators secondary to cellular lysis. Other causes of basophilia include ulcerative colitis, myxoedema, recovery from acute illness and drug allergies, although these conditions are usually associated only with modest elevations of circulatory basophils.

As discussed earlier, SCF or c-Kit ligand is an important factor in mast cell development. Therefore, it is plausible that conditions leading to its excessive production and mutation of

Table 17.10 Basophil and mast cell granules, and their contents.

Component	Function	Main physiological role	Other properties	Cell specificity
Protein				
Histamine	Binds to H_1, H_2, H_3 receptors	Hypersensitivity reactions and inflammation		Basophils, mast cells
Proteoglycan				
Heparin	Package of basic proteins into granules		Binds and stabilizes proteases	Connective tissue mast cells
Chondroitin sulphates	Package of basic proteins into granules		Binds and stabilizes proteases	Basophils
Enzymes				
Chymase	Inactivates bradykinin	Affects microcirculation		Connective tissue mast cells
	Activates angiotensin 1	Modulates microcirculation		
	Activates precursor IL-1β	Modulates skin inflammation		
Tryptase	Cleaves C3 to C3a and C3b	Proinflammatory, stimulates neutrophil chemotaxis and adherence	Tetrameric when bound to heparin, monomer inactive, restricted substrate specificity, raised levels in mast cell disorders	Mast cells
	Activates metalloproteinase 3, inactivates fibrinogen, degrades calcitonin gene-related peptide	Regulates collagenase, attenuates fibrin deposition		
Cathepsin G-like protease				Connective tissue mast cell
Carboxypeptidase	Inactivates bradykinin	Affects microcirculation		Connective tissue mast cell
Other				
Charcot–Leyden crystal protein	Lysophospholipase	Phospholipid metabolism	Neutralizes pulmonary surfactant	Basophil
Major basic protein		Disrupts membranes		Basophil
Sulphatase				
Exoglycosidase				

c-*kit*, leading to its constitutive activation, can cause mastocytosis. An increased number of tissue mast cells can be seen in a number of disorders, including atopy, parasitic diseases, Hodgkin disease and other lymphoproliferative disorders, some neoplasms and rheumatoid arthritis. The zebrafish has also been validated as an efficient *in vivo* system for studying mast cell development and has led to the identification of key transcription factors necessary for development and may serve as a potential model of human mast cell diseases.

Several conditions, ranging from isolated cutaneous mastocytomas to mast cell leukaemia, are associated with mast cell proliferation. Solitary mastocytomas generally regress spontaneously. The more common cutaneous mastocytosis or urti-

caria pigmentosa typically presents with multiple, small, round, reddish-brown maculopapular lesions that, when subjected to minimal trauma, lead to intense pruritus. In some patients, this disease progresses to the systemic variety, with involvement of bone marrow, spleen, liver and the gastrointestinal tract. Systemic mastocytosis can also occur without prior or concurrent cutaneous disease, and in association with haematological disorders, including leukaemias and lymphomas. Organ dysfunction may be secondary to the release of biochemical mediators by mast cells, such as peptic ulcer disease secondary to histamine release. Mast cell leukaemia, a rare condition, presents with circulating mast cells of abnormal morphology (accounting for up to 95% of circulating nucleated cells), peptic ulcer disease, constitutional symptoms, anaemia and hepatosplenomegaly. It should be distinguished from AML, which can develop in association with systemic mastocytosis.

Management of patients within all categories of mastocytosis includes careful counselling of patients and care providers, avoidance of factors triggering acute mediator release, treatment of acute and chronic mast cell mediator release, an attempt to treat organ infiltration by mast cells, and treatment of any associated haematological disorder. The agents and modalities commonly used in treating patients with mastocytosis include antihistamines, histamine H_2-receptor blockers, adrenaline, steroids, cromolyn sodium, proton pump inhibitors, psoralen with ultraviolet light (PUVA), chemotherapy, radiation, interferon alfa, ciclosporin, 2-chlorodeoxyadenosine and splenectomy. With increased availability of small-molecular-weight inhibitors of intracellular signalling pathways, targeting of the constitutively active mutated c-*kit* has attracted more attention. Two classes of constitutive activating c-*kit* mutations have been reported. The more frequent occurs in the catalytic pocket coding region, with substitutions at codon 816, and the other in the intracellular juxtamembrane coding region. Therefore, kinase inhibitors that block mutated c-*kit* activity might be used as therapeutic agents in systemic mastocytosis. Imatinib mesylate inhibits both wild-type and juxtamembrane mutant c-Kit kinase activity, but has no effect on the activity of the D816V mutant, commonly seen in patients with mastocytosis. Therefore, imatinib mesylate does not appear to be an effective therapy for this disease. However, activity of imatinib has been reported in a subset of mastocytosis patients with associated eosinophilia who express the *FIP1L1–PDGFRA* fusion gene.

Monocytes and macrophages (Figure 17.2d,e)

The mononuclear phagocyte system has been defined as a family of cells comprising bone marrow progenitors, blood monocytes and tissue macrophages. Monocytes develop from a pluripotent haemopoietic stem cell in the bone marrow termed CFU-GEMM (colony-forming unit – granulocyte, erythrocyte, monocyte, megakaryocyte) and the more committed CFU-GM. This progenitor cell can commit to both the neutrophil and monocytic pathways. Cytokines and growth factors, such as monocyte colony-stimulating factor, GM-CSF and IL-3, allow commitment along monocytic pathways. Monocyte colony-stimulating factor, also known as colony-stimulating factor (CSF)-1, is the most important factor in the development of monocytes and macrophages, and is necessary but not sufficient for their activation. Macrophage colony-stimulating factor is the primary macrophage growth factor detected in peripheral blood and has been shown in mouse models to be essential for macrophage differentiation, unlike GM-CSF. Macrophages stimulated by macrophage colony-stimulating factor can also clear apoptotic cells by macropinocytosis in the same fashion as dendritic cells.

Following their release into the circulation, monocytes rapidly partition between the marginating and circulating pools. The circulating monocytes have a highly convoluted surface and a lobulated nucleus. They can be further characterized by non-specific esterase and contain a single type of nucleus with staining characteristics of lysosomes. After migration into tissues, they become larger and acquire the characteristics of tissue macrophages. Monocytes contain lysosomal hydrolases and the intracellular enzymes elastase and cathepsin. After transformation into tissue macrophages they produce predominantly metalloproteases and metalloprotease inhibitors, lose expression of hydrolases, and express macrophage-specific genes and products such as inducible NOS and IFN-γ. Tissue macrophages are long-lived and self-sustaining cells.

Kupffer cells, phagocytic cells residing within the lumen of hepatic sinusoids, represent up to 90% of fixed tissue macrophages and are the first phagocytes to encounter bacteria originating from the colon. Recent advances in the understanding of Kupffer cells suggest that two subsets exist: a sessile radioresistant hepatic-derived population that does not participate in inflammatory reactions and a radiosensitive population that is replaced by bone marrow-derived precursor cells and is recruited to sites of inflammation by CD8$^+$ T cells. These two subsets can be distinguished by flow cytometry and immunohistochemical techniques. Phagocytosis by Kupffer cells may not be the principal mechanism of organism removal from the bloodstream but likely involves a complex interaction with neutrophils recruited to the liver within 2 hours of infection. Kupffer cells are also implicated in the removal of neutrophils after the clearance of an organism, downmodulating the inflammatory response and abrogating the tissue destruction sometimes seen in overwhelming sepsis.

Macrophage activation is the acquisition of competence to perform specific and complex functions as a result of exposure to a constellation of cytokines and other factors in their environment, rather than achievement of a universal activated state. Physiological factors from the host such as cytokines and growth factors as well as environmental factors from microorganisms constitute this constellation and their combined effect is synergistic. Macrophage activating factor, identified as IFN-γ, as well as IL-2, IL-4, macrophage colony-stimulating factor and GM-CSF are either directly or indirectly, through IFN-γ, responsible for macrophage activation. They stimulate monocyte/macrophage proliferation, increase adhesion receptor expression and stimulate the production of proteolytic agents responsible for pathogen clearance. The hypothalamic–pituitary–adrenal axis and autonomic nervous system communicate with the inflammatory system via catecholamine-induced activation of macrophage NF-κB and subsequent release of macrophage-derived proinflammatory cytokines.

Although production of IFN-γ by Th1 cells results in a cytocidal macrophage state, IL-4 and IL-13 produced by the Th2 population of T lymphocytes stimulate the antigen-presenting cell state. These cytokines then enhance macrophage stimulation of T cells by inducing class II MHC antigen and costimulatory molecule expression. Activated macrophages, in turn, produce cytokines that stimulate both types of helper T cells.

Several cytokines, including IL-4, IL-10, IL-13 and TGF-β, can inhibit different aspects of macrophage function. Furthermore, prostaglandin (PG)E$_2$, elaborated by macrophages, as well as corticosteroids can suppress various actions of macrophages. These provide a feedback mechanism for control of the immune response.

Recently, a subset of activated macrophages has been shown to express a folate receptor that can bind and internalize folate-linked drugs and dyes, which opens the possibility for folate-linked radioimaging techniques of joints as well as selective drug delivery to sites of active inflammation.

Disorders of monocyte/macrophages

Monocytosis and monocytopenia

Chronic inflammatory conditions, both infectious and immune in nature, are associated with monocytosis (Table 17.11). These include tuberculosis, bacterial endocarditis, syphilis, collagen vascular disease, sarcoidosis and ulcerative colitis. Monocytosis is also commonly seen in a number of haematological malignancies such as AML, Hodgkin disease, non-Hodgkin lymphomas and histiocytosis. Decreased number of circulating monocytes has been reported with endotoxaemia, corticosteroid administration and hairy cell leukaemia.

Histiocytic disorders

As described above, bone marrow monocytes enter the circulation and transform into tissue-specific macrophages under the influence of the local environment, thus becoming cells of the mononuclear phagocytic system. Dendritic cells also have their origin in the bone marrow and share common progenitors with macrophages. Progenitors of dendritic cells are released from the bone marrow and enter tissues in which they differentiate into functional antigen-presenting dendritic cells. The ordinary tissue macrophages have IgG Fc receptors, whereas the tissue-based dendritic cells comprising the dendritic cell system lack phagocytic capacity or Fc receptors and are predominantly antigen-presenting cells. The dendritic Langerhans cells are found in virtually all tissues except the brain and are the major immunological cellular components of the skin and mucosa. Their racquet-shaped ultrastructural inclusions (Birbeck bodies) distinguish them from other tissue cells. They interact with and process antigen, then migrate to lymphoid organs where, through interaction with T cells, they generate cellular and humoral immune responses. This ability of dendritic cells to interact with T cells and other inflammatory cells contributes to the often varied clinical manifestations of the histiocytic disorders.

Table 17.11 Causes of monocytosis.

Inflammatory conditions
Infections
Tuberculosis
Bacterial endocarditis
Fever of unknown origin
Syphilis

Other
Systemic lupus erythematosus
Rheumatoid arthritis
Temporal arteritis
Polyarteritis
Ulcerative colitis
Sarcoidosis
Myositis

Malignant disorders
Acute myeloid leukaemia
Hodgkin disease
Non-Hodgkin lymphomas
Histiocytoses
Carcinomas
Myelodysplastic syndrome

Miscellaneous
Cyclic neutropenia
Chronic idiopathic neutropenia
Kostmann syndrome
Post splenectomy

The histiocytic disorders comprise various haematological disorders, with cells of the mononuclear phagocytic system or the dendritic cell system involved in their pathogenesis. In general, diseases associated with proliferation of histiocytes can be grouped into two different categories: inflammatory disorders and neoplastic (clonal) disorders (Table 17.12). In the more recent classifications by the World Health Organization Committee on Histiocytic/Reticulum Cell Proliferations, other disorders in which histiocytes are implicated, such as storage diseases (Gaucher and Niemann–Pick), have been excluded. Abnormal immune responses mediated by cytokines has been proposed to be the inciting factor for the two more common disorders: Langerhans cell histiocytosis and haemophagocytic lymphohistiocytosis. However, it is unclear whether the histiocytes themselves or other immune cells are the defective cell population.

Langerhans cell histiocytosis

The offending cells in the disorders previously referred to as histiocytosis X (including eosinophilic granuloma, Letterer–

Table 17.12 Histiocytic disorders.

Disorders of varied biological behaviour
Related to dendritic cells
Langerhans cell histiocytosis
Juvenile xanthogranuloma and related disorders
Solitary dendritic cell histiocytoma

Related to macrophages
Haemophagocytic syndromes
   Primary: familial haemophagocytic histiocytosis
   Secondary: infectious, tumour associated, drug associated (e.g.
     phenytoin)
Rosai–Dorfman disease (sinus histiocytosis with massive
   lymphadenopathy)
Solitary macrophage histiocytoma

Clonal disorders
Related to monocytes
Leukaemia: FAB M4 and M5, acute myelomonocytic leukaemia,
   chronic myelomonocytic leukaemia, extramedullary monocytic
   tumours

Related to dendritic cells
Histiocytic sarcoma (malignant histiocytosis): localized or
   disseminated

Related to macrophages
Histiocytic sarcoma (malignant histiocytosis): localized or
   disseminated

Siwe disease and Hand–Schüller–Christian disease) have the characteristics of epidermal Langerhans cells. These disorders, now collectively referred to as Langerhans cell histiocytosis (LCH), have variable clinical features depending on the organs infiltrated by the responsible Langerhans and accompanying cells. The true prevalence of these disorders is seven cases per million. The majority of cases occur in children under 15 years of age, but they can occur at any age.

The aetiology of these disorders is far from clear, but a number of clues from their biology and epidemiology are emerging. Associations with malignancies and an inherited predisposition based on studies in identical twins have been suggested. No seasonal variations or geographic or racial clustering has been reported, disputing the possibility of an infectious aetiology. Flow cytometric and chromosomal analysis of cells from LCH infiltrates as well as methods to assess clonality based on restriction fragment length polymorphisms have suggested the possibility of a clonal nature, although no consistent chromosomal alterations have been reported so far.

It is now clear that LCH is characterized by clonal proliferation of CD1a-positive cells. The Langerhans cells from the lesions of patients demonstrate several phenotypic changes that distinguish them from their normal counterparts. Differences in staining by the lectin peanut agglutinin, expression of placental alkaline phosphatase, expression of the IFN-γ receptor, and expression of costimulatory receptors such as CD86 and CD80 allow one to distinguish between LCH lesional cells and their normal counterparts. There is extensive expression of GM-CSF, IL-1, IL-3, IL-4, IL-8, TNF and leukemia inhibitory factor (LIF) in the lesions of LCH, suggestive of activation of T lymphocytes as well as recruitment of macrophages, eosinophils and granulocytes. The accumulation of IL-1 and PGE_2 may explain the association of these lesions with bone loss. Such increases in immunostimulatory and tissue-damaging cytokines occur at local sites, usually without high systemic levels.

The diagnosis of LCH is based on a biopsy of the involved organs, with the key diagnostic feature being the presence of pathological Langerhans cells, which can be identified by demonstration of either CD1a surface antigen or the presence of Birbeck granules on electron microscopy. Mitoses are usually not present and when found have no prognostic significance. Early lesions are generally cellular and locally destructive, with abundance of essentially normal Langerhans cells. As the lesions mature, there are fewer Langerhans cells with occasional necrosis.

The lesions of LCH occur in skin, bone, lymph nodes, liver, spleen, bone marrow, lungs, the CNS and the gastrointestinal tract. Clinical features are varied and depend on the organs involved. It may involve single organs or involve multiple systems, and assessment of organ function is important as it can have prognostic significance. Initial investigations should include a full blood count, assessment of renal and hepatic function, a skeletal survey and a technetium bone scan; these latter studies are complementary, with the latter being more sensitive for early lesions. Other investigations include chest radiography and possibly magnetic resonance imaging (MRI) of the brain to rule out CNS involvement. Additional testing for diabetes insipidus and other organ involvement should be carried out as indicated.

Langerhans cells play an integral role in antigen recognition and presentation in immune responses throughout many tissues. Pulmonary Langerhans cell histiocytosis (PLCH) is a non-neoplastic collection of reactive Langerhans cells that causes interstitial lung disease in adult smokers. PLCH is uncommon and comprises 5% of all interstitial lung disease, predominantly afflicting middle-aged men and women smokers. PLCH typically presents with dyspnoea, non-productive cough and constitutional symptoms and radiographic features of reticulonodular changes with cyst formation. Diagnosis is made with open lung biopsy and, depending on the stage of the lesion, histopathology can range from an abundance of Langerhans cells, lymphocytes, eosinophils, plasma cells in a background of mild to dense fibrosis. Langerhans cells in PLCH are phenotypically similar to lymphostimulatory dendritic cells within the lymphoid organs and can be identified by positive immunostaining for CD1a, langerin, E-cadherin and S-100, as well as the presence of Birbeck granules. The treatment of PLCH is smoking cessation and although no randomized studies exist, reports can be found in the literature supporting the use of corticosteroids and chemotherapy for progressive disease. Prognosis is variable and cases of spontaneous regression even without intervention have been documented.

Solitary or multifocal eosinophilic granuloma occurs mainly in older children and young adults and accounts for the majority of cases of LCH. Hand–Schüller–Christian disease occurs in younger children (2–5 years) and often presents with exophthalmos due to a tumour mass in the orbital cavity. Letterer–Siwe disease is the rarest and often most severe form of LCH, typically presenting with a scaly, seborrhoeic, eczematoid and, occasionally, purpuric or ulcerative rash in infants younger than 2 years. Bone involvement in LCH can lead to a tender swelling (as a result of infiltration of adjacent tissues) and inability to bear weight. Radiographically, lesions appear as 'punched-out' holes sometimes with sclerotic edges. Other clinical manifestations include rashes, which may be maculopapular, nodular or vesicular; ear discharge; lymphadenopathy; diabetes insipidus, due to involvement of the hypothalamus and the pituitary; respiratory symptoms, with radiographic changes such as micronodular infiltrates due to lung involvement; hepatomegaly with laboratory evidence of liver dysfunction; splenomegaly; CNS disease, with ataxia, dysarthria and cranial nerve palsies; and, rarely, gut involvement with diarrhoea, malabsorption and protein-losing enteropathy.

The prognosis of patients with LCH depends on age of onset, number of involved organs and degree of dysfunction. In general, infants with multiorgan disease have the worst prognosis. There is also growing realization that multiple recurrences of the disease can occur indefinitely, and those patients with multisystem involvement can have long-term sequelae of their disease and/or its treatment. These include neurocognitive and psychosocial problems, neurological complications with a neurodegenerative pattern of CNS involvement, orthopaedic problems, hearing loss, and hypothalamic–pituitary axis deficiencies leading to stunted growth and other endocrine problems.

Spontaneous resolution in a significant proportion of patients with LCH can occur and patients with limited disease usually do not require systemic therapy. In contrast, patients with multifocal disease generally benefit from systemic therapy. Treatment options have included low-dose radiation for symptomatic single lesions, local injection of steroids, topical steroids, PUVA, non-steroidal anti-inflammatory drugs, high-dose systemic steroids, and systemic combination chemotherapy regimens with agents such as prednisolone, vinblastine, vincristine, etoposide and 6-mercaptopurine. Other treatments that have been tested in patients with disease progression while on

therapy include ciclosporin, antithymocyte globulin, 2-chlorodeoxyadenosine, thalidomide, TNF inhibitors, anti-CD1a antibodies and haemopoietic stem cell transplantation.

Haemophagocytic lymphohistiocytosis

These disorders include genetic (familial and immunodeficiency-related syndromes) and acquired forms. Familial forms affecting neonates and infants occur in 1 in 50 000 live births. Males and females are equally affected and over two-thirds of cases occur in siblings. The familial form is an autosomal recessive disease without a well-defined genetic defect. Recently, several defects in genes with important immune functions have been reported in patients with familial haemophagocytic lymphohistiocytosis (HLH) and include mutations in the genes for perforin (*PRF1*), Munc13-4 (*UNC13D*) and syntaxin 11 (*STX11*). The acquired form is associated with Chédiak–Higashi syndrome, Griscelli syndrome and X-linked lymphoproliferative syndrome.

It is hypothesized that the disease is caused by impaired lymphocyte-mediated cytotoxicity and defective triggering of apoptosis. Perforin, normally secreted by cytotoxic T cells and NK cells, can form cell death-inducing pores through which toxic granzymes may enter the target cell and trigger apoptosis. Mutations of the perforin gene have been reported in several patients with familial HLH and result in defective lymphocyte cytotoxic activity. The manifestations of the disease are thought to be mediated by hypersecretion of proinflammatory cytokines such as IFN-γ, TNF-α, IL-6, IL-10 and macrophage colony-stimulating factor (M-CSF). Such excess of proinflammatory cytokines results in tissue infiltration by lymphocytes and macrophages, leading to haemophagocytosis and the characteristic laboratory abnormalities including cytopenias, coagulopathies and hypertriglyceridaemia.

Both familial and acquired forms of HLH are commonly precipitated by viral (particularly Epstein–Barr virus and other herpesviruses), bacterial, fungal and protozoan infections, occurring frequently in an immunocompromised host. Other factors that have been associated with acquired HLH include malignancies (particularly lymphoproliferative disorders), drugs (such as phenytoin) and rarely with inborn errors of metabolism (lysinuric protein intolerance and multiple sulphatase deficiency). It is important to distinguish patients with the secondary form of the disease from individuals with familial HLH and a precipitant viral infection.

Symptoms of HLH commonly include high fever, anorexia, malaise, irritability and vomiting. Hepatosplenomegaly, lymphadenopathy and neurological signs such as cranial nerve palsies and seizures are also common. Laboratory features include pancytopenia, hypertriglyceridaemia, hypofibrinogenaemia, cerebrospinal fluid pleocytosis, coagulopathy, transaminitis and hyperbilirubinaemia. The marrow is often hyperplastic with increased numbers of haemophagocytic histiocytes. Histopathological features of the lymph nodes or other

Table 17.13 Diagnostic criteria for haemophagocytic lymphohistiocytosis.

Familial disease/known genetic defect

Clinical and laboratory criteria (5/8 criteria)
Fever
Splenomegaly
Cytopenia in two or more cell lines
    Haemoglobin < 9 g/dL (below 4 weeks < 12 g/dL)
    Platelets < 100×10^9/L
    Neutrophils < 1×10^9/L
Hypertriglyceridaemia and/or hypofibrinogenaemia
    Fasting triglycerides ≥ 3 mmol/L
    Fibrinogen < 1.5 g/L
Ferritin ≥ 500 µg/L
sCD 25 ≥ 2400 U/mL
Decreased or absent NK cell activity
Haemophagocytosis in bone marrow, CSF or lymph nodes

Supportive evidence includes cerebral symptoms with moderate pleocytosis and/or elevated protein, elevated transaminases and bilirubin, lactate dehydrogenase > 1000 U/L.
sCD 25, soluble interleukin-2 receptor.

involved tissue are often diagnostic, showing infiltration by lymphocytes and histiocytes and characteristic prominent erythrophagocytosis and haemophagocytosis, features required for diagnosis. During the acute phase of the illness, the plasma concentrations of inflammatory cytokines and the α-chain of the soluble IL-2 receptor as well as impaired NK cell activity are abnormal. Revised criteria from the Histiocyte Society for the diagnosis of HLH are shown in Table 17.13.

Treatment of familial HLH has included the use of corticosteroids (dexamethasone is preferred over prednisolone due to its ability to cross the blood–brain barrier), immunoglobulin infusions, ciclosporin and etoposide. Although early responses are observed, disease recurrence within months is common. Adequate control of CNS disease is important and intrathecal therapy using methotrexate with or without corticosteroids is merited in patients with recurrent CNS disease. Patients are at risk of developing opportunistic infections due to their underlying immune dysfunction and the effects of therapy. If a treatable infectious agent is identified, appropriate antimicrobial therapy should always be employed, regardless of whether the patient has genetic or acquired HLH. Haemopoietic stem cell transplantation from a matched sibling or unrelated donor remains the definitive treatment modality in patients with genetic forms of HLH.

Sinus histiocytosis with massive lymphadenopathy or Rosai–Dorfman syndrome is characterized as a benign, frequently chronic, painless lymphadenopathy involving the cervical nodes and less commonly other nodal areas and has no known aetiology. Other features may include fever, weight loss and extranodal disease in skin, soft tissues, orbits, upper respiratory mucosa, bone and other organs. Although the disease commonly occurs in the first two decades of life, all ages can be affected. Diagnostic evaluation of involved lymph nodes reveals infiltration by histiocytes and multinucleated giant cells associated with erythrophagocytosis. The proliferating histiocytes are morphologically distinguished from the Langerhans cells of LCH by the absence of Birbeck granules on electron microscopy as well as their surface phenotype. Nodal disease is often self-limited and regresses without intervention. However, bulky extranodal disease can cause symptoms and even organ impairment. Therapy depends on the extent of involvement and ranges from observation to surgical debulking and/or radiation. Chemotherapy plays no role in treatment.

Erdheim–Chester disease is a rare non-Langerhans cell histiocytosis that occurs in adults and may be of clonal origin. Bony pain with symmetric osteosclerosis of the metaphyses and diaphyses of long bones is characteristic of the disease. Extraosseous lesions can be found in approximately 50% of cases and can involve lung, heart, skin, kidney, CNS, muscle, breast and sinonasal mucosa. Because of the very rare nature of this disease, only anecdotal reports of treatment with steroids, interferon, chemotherapy, radiation and stem cell transplantation with variable rates of success are found in the literature. Prognosis is dependent on the extent of extraosseous disease and many patients die within a few years due to progressive pulmonary and retroperitoneal involvement.

Although monocytic leukaemias are included in the classification of histiocytic disorders, their discussion is beyond the scope of this chapter and are dealt with elsewhere.

Selected bibliography

Haemopoietic cell development
Metcalf D (1993) Haematopoietic regulators: redundancy or subtlety? *Blood* **82**: 3515–23.
Ogawa M (1993) Differentiation and proliferation of haematopoietic stem cells. *Blood* **81**: 2844–53.

Mechanisms of phagocyte function
Booth JW, Trimble WS, Grinstein S (2001) Membrane dynamics in phagocytosis. *Seminars in Immunology* **13**: 357–64.
Borregaard N, Cowland JB (1997) Granules of human neutrophilic polymorphonuclear leucocyte. *Blood* **89**: 3503–21.
Castellano F, Chavrier P, Caron E (2001) Actin dynamics during phagocytosis. *Seminars in Immunology* **13**: 347–55.
Clutterbuck EJ, Sanderson CJ (1990) Regulation of human eosinophil precursor production by cytokines: a comparison of recombinant human interleukin-1 (rhIL-1), rhIL-3 rhIL-5 rhIL-6 and rh granulocyte-macrophage colony-stimulating factor. *Blood* **75**: 1774–9.

Cox D, Greenberg S (2001) Phagocytic signalling strategies: Fc(gamma)receptor-mediated phagocytosis as a model system. *Seminars in Immunology* **13**: 339–45.

Dancey JT, Deubelbeiss KA, Harker LA *et al.* (1976) Neutrophil kinetics in man. *Journal of Clinical Investigation* **58**: 705–15.

Denburg JA (1992) Basophil and mast cell lineages *in vitro* and *in vivo*. *Blood* **79**: 846–60.

Duffield JS (2003) The inflammatory macrophage: a story of Jekyll and Hyde. *Clinical Science* **104**: 27–38.

Egesten A, Calafat J, Janssen H *et al.* (2001) Granules of human eosinophilic leucocytes and their mobilization. *Clinical and Experimental Allergy* **31**: 1173–88.

Fadok VA, Chimini G (2001) The phagocytosis of apoptotic cells. *Seminars in Immunology* **13**: 365–72.

Falcone FH, Haas H, Gibbs BF (2000) The human basophil: a new appreciation of its role in immune responses. *Blood* **96**: 4028–38.

Feger F, Varadaradjalou S, Gao Z *et al.* (2002) The role of mast cells in host defence and their subversion by bacterial pathogens. *Trends in Immunology* **23**: 151–8.

Garcia-Garcia E, Rosales C (2002) Signal transduction during Fc receptor-mediated phagocytosis. *Journal of Leucocyte Biology* **72**: 1092–108.

Gordon S (1995) The macrophage. *Bioessays* **17**: 977–86.

Gregory CD, Devitt A (2004) The macrophage and the apoptotic cell: an innate immune interaction viewed simplistically? *Immunology* **113**: 1–14.

Malech HL, Gallin JI (1987) Current concepts: immunology. Neutrophils in human diseases. *New England Journal of Medicine* **317**: 687–94.

Mansour MK, Levitz SM (2002) Interactions of fungi with phagocytes. *Current Opinion in Microbiology* **5**: 359–65.

Prussin C, Metcalfe DD (2003) IgE, mast cells, basophils, and eosinophils. *Journal of Allergy and Clinical Immunology* **111**: S486–S494.

Sanderson CJ (1992) Interleukin-5 eosinophils, and disease. *Blood* **79**: 3101–9.

Sansonetti P (2001) Phagocytosis of bacterial pathogens: implications in the host response. *Seminars in Immunology* **13**: 381–90.

Theilgaard-Monch K, Jacobsen LC, Nielsen MJ *et al.* (2006) Haptoglobin is synthesized during granulocyte differentiation, stored in specific granules, and released by neutrophils in response to activation. *Blood* **108**: 353–61.

Watts C, Amigorena S (2001) Phagocytosis and antigen presentation. *Seminars in Immunology* **13**: 373–9.

Xu W, Roos A, Schlagwein N, Woltman AM, Daha MR, van Kooten C (2006) IL-10-producing macrophages preferentially clear early apoptotic cells. *Blood* **107**: 4930–7.

Production, structure and dysfunction of phagocytes

Allen TC (2008) Pulmonary Langerhans cell histiocytosis and other pulmonary histiocytic diseases: a review. *Archives of Pathology and Laboratory Medicine* **132**: 1171–81.

Arceci RJ, Longley J, Emanuel PD (2002) Atypical cellular disorders. *Hematology. American Society of Hematology Education Program*, 297–314.

Baccarani M, Cilloni D, Rondoni M *et al.* (2007) The efficacy of imatinib mesylate in patients with FIP1L1–PDGFRalpha-positive hypereosinophilic syndrome. Results of a multicenter prospective study. *Haematologica* **92**: 1173–9.

Bernini JC (1996) Diagnosis and management of chronic neutropenia during childhood. *Pediatric Clinics of North America* **43**: 773–92.

Cham B, Bonilla MA, Winkelstein J (2002) Neutropenia associated with primary immunodeficiency syndromes. *Seminars in Hematology* **39**: 107–12.

Dinauer MC (2005) Chronic granulomatous disease and other disorders of phagocyte function. *Hematology. American Society of Hematology Education Program*, 89–95.

Etzioni A, Doerschuk CM, Harlan JM (1999) Of man and mouse: leucocyte and endothelial adhesion molecule deficiencies. *Blood* **94**: 3281–8.

Freedman MH, Alter BP (2002) Risk of myelodysplastic syndrome and acute myeloid leukaemia in congenital neutropenias. *Seminars in Hematology* **39**: 128–33.

Fuleihan RL (1998) The X-linked hyperimmunoglobulin M syndrome. *Seminars in Hematology* **35**: 321–31.

Germeshausen M, Welte K, Ballmaier M (2009) *In vivo* expansion of cells expressing acquired CSF3R mutations in patients with severe congenital neutropenia. *Blood* **113**: 668–70.

Herring WB, Smith LG, Walker RI *et al.* (1974) Hereditary neutrophilia. *American Journal of Medicine* **56**: 729–34.

Heyworth PG, Curnutte JT, Rae J *et al.* (2001) Hematologically important mutations: X-linked chronic granulomatous disease (second update). *Blood Cells, Molecules and Diseases* **27**: 16–26.

Janka G, Zur Stadt U (2005) Familial and acquired hemophagocytic lymphohistiocytosis. *Hematology. American Society of Hematology Education Program*, 82–8.

Klion AD (2005) Recent advances in the diagnosis and treatment of hypereosinophilic syndromes. *Hematology. American Society of Hematology Education Program*, 209–14.

Klusmann JH, Creutzig U, Zimmermann M *et al.* (2008) Treatment and prognostic impact of transient leukaemia in neonates with Down syndrome. *Blood* **111**: 2991–8.

Kyono W, Coates TD (2002) A practical approach to neutrophil disorders. *Pediatric Clinics of North America* **49**: 929–71, viii.

Lakshman R, Finn A (2001) Neutrophil disorders and their management. *Journal of Clinical Pathology* **54**: 7–19.

Lekstrom-Himes JA, Gallin JI (2000) Immunodeficiency diseases caused by defects in phagocytes. *New England Journal of Medicine* **343**: 1703–14.

Mason PJ (2003) Stem cells, telomerase and dyskeratosis congenita. *Bioessays* **25**: 126–33.

Putsep K, Carlsson G, Boman HG *et al.* (2002) Deficiency of antibacterial peptides in patients with morbus Kostmann: an observation study. *Lancet* **360**: 1144–9.

Roos D, Law SK (2001) Hematologically important mutations: leucocyte adhesion deficiency. *Blood Cells, Molecules and Diseases* **27**: 1000–4.

Rosenberg PS, Alter BP, Bolyard AA *et al.* (2006) The incidence of leukaemia and mortality from sepsis in patients with severe congenital neutropenia receiving long-term G-CSF therapy. *Blood* **107**: 4628–35.

Rothenberg ME (1998) Eosinophilia. *New England Journal of Medicine* **338**: 1592–600.

Salipante SJ, Rojas ME, Korkmaz B *et al.* (2009) Contributions to neutropenia from PFAAP5 (N4BP2L2), a novel protein mediating transcriptional repressor cooperation between Gfi1 and neutrophil elastase. *Molecular and Cellular Biology* **29**: 4394–405.

Shastri KA, Logue GL (1993) Autoimmune neutropenia. *Blood* **81**: 1984–95.

Starkebaum G (2002) Chronic neutropenia associated with autoimmune disease. *Seminars in Hematology* **39**: 121–7.

Ward DM, Shiflett SL, Kaplan J (2002) Chediak–Higashi syndrome: a clinical and molecular view of a rare lysosomal storage disorder. *Current Molecular Medicine* **2**: 469–77.

Ward HN, Reinhard EH (1971) Chronic idiopathic leukocytosis. *Annals of Internal Medicine* **75**: 193–8.

Welte K, Zeidler C (2009) Severe congenital neutropenia. *Hematology/Oncology Clinics of North America* **23**: 307–20.

CHAPTER 18

Lysosomal storage disorders

Atul B Mehta[1] and Derralynn A Hughes[2]

[1]Royal Free Hospital, London, UK
[2]Royal Free and University College Medical School, London, UK

18

Lysosomes

Lysosomes are membrane-bound intracellular organelles that represent the major degradative compartment of mammalian cells. They are morphologically heterogeneous and are distinguished from other organelles by the presence of a range of catalytic enzymes and lysosome-associated membrane proteins (LAMPs). More than 50 lysosomal hydrolases, active at acidic pH, catalyse the degradation of macromolecules (lipids, proteins, nucleic acids, glycosaminoglycans and oligosaccharides). These include breakdown products of blood cell membranes, gangliosides from neurones, and glycosaminoglycans derived from connective tissue and extracellular matrix. Substantial flows of substrate of intracellular origin are also generated as a product of intermediary metabolism and turnover of macromolecules. Substrate is delivered to the lysosome by the processes of endocytosis, pinocytosis, phagocytosis or autophagocytosis, or is imported from the cytoplasm using a system of biological chaperones.

The lysosomal membrane and its LAMPs protect cytoplasmic components from the acid hydrolases. LAMPs are transmembrane proteins with highly glycosylated intralysosomal domains, among the most densely N-glycosylated proteins so far reported. The lysosomal membrane is also involved in fusion with other organelles, in maintenance of an acidic intralysosomal pH and in the efflux of amino acids and monosaccharides and oligosaccharides produced by the lysosomal hydrolases.

Soluble lysosomal enzymes are synthesized on the rough endoplasmic reticulum and acquire N-linked oligosaccharide side-chains in the Golgi apparatus. Here, asparagine-linked high-mannose residues are phosphorylated at position 6. This modification is specific for lysosomal enzymes and is essential for the routing of the enzymes to the lysosomal compartment via mannose 6-phosphate receptors (Figure 18.1). The small proportion of newly synthesized enzyme that does not bind to the intracellular receptor is secreted into the interstitial fluid, where it may bind mannose 6-phosphate receptor located on the plasma membrane. This enzyme is then recovered by receptor-mediated endocytosis and transported to the lysosome. Trafficking signals for lysosomal membrane glycoproteins probably reside in the cytosolic tails of the proteins and differ from those of lysosomal enzymes. This knowledge of the sorting mechanism for lysosomal enzymes has allowed the development of enzyme replacement therapy of lysosomal storage disorders.

Pathophysiology of lysosomal storage disorders

In most lysosomal storage disorders, an inherited deficiency of a specific lysosomal enzyme results in the accumulation of undegraded substrates within the lysosome. In others, accumulation of storage product results from deficiency or malfunction of activator proteins or transport proteins. Individual mutations of the relevant genes give rise to variable levels of residual enzyme activity. The resulting diseases are grouped according to the major stored substance, for example the mucopolysaccharidoses, sphingolipidoses and glycoproteinoses. Storage product within the lysosomes causes disruption of cellular organization and disturbance of normal membrane functions including signal transduction and ion transport. Different lysosomal storage diseases have the characteristic organ distribution patterns of the stored metabolites. For example, in mucopolysaccharidosis (MPS) type III (Sanfilippo disease)

Postgraduate Haematology: 6th edition. Edited by A. Victor Hoffbrand, Daniel Catovsky, Edward G.D. Tuddenham, Anthony R. Green
© 2011 Blackwell Publishing Ltd.

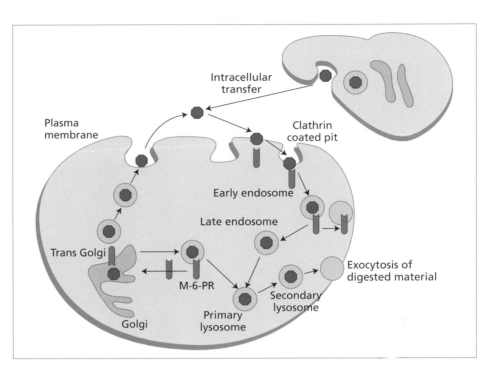

Figure 18.1 Routes of lysosomal enzyme cycling. Extracellular enzyme binds to the plasma membrane via mannose 6-phosphate receptors and is internalized by a clathrin-coated vesicle into an early endosome. As the early endosome acidifies to become a late endosome, the enzyme dissociates from the mannose 6-phosphate receptor, which recycles to the plasma membrane. The late endosome fuses with a primary lysosome derived from the Golgi apparatus to form a secondary lysosome, which may remain in the cell as a residual body or fuse with the plasma membrane in the process of exocytosis of digested products.

there is accumulation of heparan sulphate, an essential component of the neuronal membrane. This results in mental retardation. In contrast, in MPS type IV (Morquio disease) accumulation of keratan sulphate results in severe skeletal deformities. However, even within a discrete storage disorder there are often wide-ranging clinical manifestations and considerable interindividual heterogeneity. Furthermore, genotype–phenotype relationships are generally unclear and even siblings with the same mutation can have widely disparate clinical manifestations.

Although knowledge of the genetics and biochemistry of the disorders has recently improved, little is known of the pathological processes that actually result in end-organ damage. These processes do not simply relate to the burden of storage product but extend to involve a complex host reaction to abnormal cells. This may result in cytokine secretion, cellular proliferation, disturbed calcium homeostasis, exaggerated inflammation and perturbed control of apoptosis. In Gaucher disease, where storage cells are macrophages that play an essential role in host physiology and pathogenesis of inflammatory and immunological responses, a wide variety of enzymes, cytokines and coagulation factors are perturbed (Table 18.1). Interleukin (IL)-1, IL-6, IL-10 and tumour necrosis factor (TNF) have been implicated in the pathogenesis of Gaucher disease. Elevated serum levels of IL-6, which is produced by macrophages, endothelial cells, fibroblasts and T cells, have been found to correlate with an index of severity in patients with Gaucher disease, and may be instrumental in the pathogenesis of B-cell dysregulation and bone disease. IL-10, which in general inhibits the synthesis of other inflammatory cytokines,

is also elevated and may represent an abnormal state of immune activation.

Prevalence

Recent studies suggest that the true prevalence of lysosomal storage disorders may be higher than previously thought. This is because patients with minimal symptoms, such as homozygotes for the Gaucher N370S mutation, may not come to medical attention and also because of misdiagnosis of multisystem disorders such as Fabry disease. Studies in Europe, the USA and Australia suggest that although the diseases are individually rare, their combined overall birth prevalence is 1 in 5000–8000. In a study performed in the Netherlands, lipidoses were the most frequent as a group followed by mucopolysaccharidoses. Mucolipidoses and oligosaccharidoses were very rare. Metachromatic leucodystrophy, Krabbe disease and Gaucher disease were the most frequent individual disorders (Table 18.2). Attenuated forms of some lysosomal storage disorders (e.g. Fabry disease) may be much commoner and may underlie diverse late clinical manifestations in adults, including stroke, renal failure and left ventricular hypertrophy (see below).

Diagnosis

In the absence of an informative family history, diagnosis of lysosomal storage disorders requires a high degree of clinical

Table 18.1 Enzyme and cytokine disturbance in type I Gaucher disease.

	Elevated	Reduced
Plasma	Glucosylceramide	Total plasma cholesterol
	Apolipoprotein E	Low-density lipoprotein
	Transcobalamin II	High-density lipoprotein
	Ferritin	Apolipoprotein A-1
	β-Hexosaminidase	Apolipoprotein B
	α-Mannosidase	Factor XI
	β-Glucuronidase	Factors V and VIII (normalize post splenectomy)
	Angiotensin-converting enzyme	Factors II, VII, X, XII
	Lysozyme	
	Tartrate-resistant acid phosphatase	
	Chitotriosidase	
	Thrombin–antithrombin	
	Plasmin–antiplasmin	
	D-Dimer	
	Immunoglobulins	
	Paraprotein	
	IL-1	
	IL-6	
	IL-8	
	IL-10	
	TNF-α	
	M-CSF	
	Soluble CD14	
	CCL18/PARC	
Tissue	Glucosylceramide	
	β-Hexosaminidase	
	β-Glucuronidase	
	Galactocerebrosidase	
	Tartrate-resistant acid phosphatase	
	Non-specific esterase	
Hepatic	Alkaline phosphatase	
	Transaminases	

suspicion. Storage product may be identified within biopsy specimens, plasma or urine. These may have been requested incidentally, for example the finding of Gaucher disease in the bone marrow biopsy of a thrombocytopenic patient or Fabry disease in a renal biopsy, or may be a specific directed examination such as a skin biopsy in a patient with the characteristic rash of Fabry disease. Levels of lysosomal enzymes may be measured in plasma or leucocytes using commercially available synthetic or naturally occurring labelled substrates. Once a can-

didate enzyme is identified, analysis of the corresponding gene may identify a specific mutation and facilitate rapid screening of other family members. As effective treatment becomes available for a larger number of disorders, it is increasingly important that patients should be diagnosed as early as possible as presymptomatic individuals may be candidates for early intervention.

Therapy

Effective treatment of lysosomal storage disorders self-evidently involves reduction of the stored compound and prevention of its reaccumulation. This has been achieved by elevation of enzyme activity by stem cell transplantation, infusion of the missing enzyme (enzyme replacement therapy or ERT) or stabilization of protein folding variants by pharmacological chaperones. Conversely, reduction of the substrate can also be achieved by limiting its synthesis through inhibition of anabolic enzymes, so-called substrate reduction therapy (SRT).

Many patients with Gaucher disease, metachromatic leucodystrophy, Krabbe disease and MPS type I have undergone stem cell transplantation. Donation of stem cells has largely been from HLA-identical siblings but as the highest level of enzyme activity will be supplied by donor cells from non-carriers, cord blood from unrelated donors has recently been used with good results.

ERT is now available or under investigation for several lysosomal storage disorders (Table 18.2). A range of production platforms has been developed recently. Recombinant human enzyme can be produced in Chinese hamster ovary cells or plant (e.g. carrot) cells. Gene activation technologies have been applied to cultured human fibroblasts. The resulting translated proteins are chemically modified, purified and prepared for infusion. The effectiveness of ERT depends on the accessibility of the site of the pathology to exogenous enzyme and the ability of affected cells to internalize the enzyme. ERT is effective in reducing the non-neuronopathic manifestations of a number of disorders, including Gaucher disease type I, Fabry disease, Pompe disease and MPS types I, II, III and VI. However, infused enzymes do not cross the blood–brain barrier and ERT does not prevent the onset and progression of neurological symptoms. Intrathecal administration is under investigation but is likely to be of limited success. Furthermore, ERT for systemic therapy has to be given by intravenous infusion. Antibodies readily develop to infused enzyme and this certainly attenuates effectiveness in some diseases (e.g. Pompe disease) but data are lacking in other conditions (e.g. Gaucher disease, Fabry disease).

Recently, other treatment strategies have been developed. One approach, SRT, is to decrease the rate of synthesis of the stored component so that it is approximately equal to the rate of degradation. Analogues of small molecules are used to inhibit the activity of synthetic enzymes. Thus, glucose and ceramide

Table 18.2 Lysosomal storage disorders: biochemistry, prevalence and therapy.

Category	Disease	Alternative name	Enzyme deficiency	Stored material	Chromosome	Birth prevalence per 100000	Therapy
Mucopolysaccharidosis	MPS I	Hurler Scheie, Hurler/Scheie	Iduronidase	Dermatan sulphate Heparan sulphate	4p16.3	1.14	ERT SCT
	MPS II	Hunter	Iduronate-2-sulphatase	Dermatan sulphate Heparan sulphate	Xq27–28	0.74	ERT SCT
	MPS III	Sanfilippo				(1.89)	
		IIIA	Heparan-N-sulphatase	Heparan sulphate	17q25.3	0.88	SCT
		IIIB	N-Acetyl-glucosaminidase	Heparan sulphate	17q21.1	0.47	
		IIIC	Acetyl-CoA glucosamine N-acetyltransferase	Heparan sulphate	Uncertain	0.07	
		IIID	N-Acetyl-glucosamine-6-sulphatase	Heparan sulphate	12q14	0.09	
	MPS IV	Morquio				0.59	ERT under development
		IVA	Galactose-6-sulphatase	Keratan sulphate	16q24	(0.22)	
		IVB	β-Galactosidase	Keratan sulphate	3p21–pter	(0.14)	
	MPS VI	Maroteaux–Lamy	Galactosamine-4-sulphatase	Dermatan sulphate	5q13–q14	0.43	ERT
	MPS VII	Sly	β-Glucuronidase	Dermatan sulphate Heparan sulphate	7q21.1–q22	0.05	SCT ERT Preclinical
	MPS IX		Hyaluronidase	Hyaluronic acid	3p21.3		
Mucolipidoses	ML I	Sialidosis I	Neuraminidase	Sialic acid	10pter-q23	0.02	
	ML II	I cell	UDP-N-acetylglucosamine transferase	Many		(0.16)	SCT
	ML III	Pseudo-Hurler				(0.08)	
		IIIA	As ML II	Many	16p		
		IIIC	Transferase-D-subunit	Many			
	ML IV		Neuraminidase	Mucolipin	19p13.2–13.3		

Table 18.2 *Continued*

Category	Disease	Alternative name	Enzyme deficiency	Stored material	Chromosome	Birth prevalence per 100000	Therapy
Sphingolipidoses	GM1 gangliosidosis		β-Galactosidase	GM1-ganglioside, Keratan sulphate, Oligosaccharide, Glycolipids	3p21–3pter	0.5	SCT
	GM2 gangliosidosis	Tay–Sachs	β-Hexosaminidase A	GM2-ganglioside, Keratan sulphate, Oligosaccharide, Glycolipids	15q23–24	0.26	SCT SCT
		Sandhoff	β-Hexosaminidase A and B	GM2-ganglioside, Oligosaccharide	5q13		
	GM2 gangliosidosis		GM2 activator	GM2-ganglioside, Glycolipids	5q32–33		
	Globoid cell leucodystrophy	Krabbe	Galactocerebrosidase	Galactosylceramides	14q31	0.71	SCT
	Metachromatic leucodystrophy		Arylsulphatase A	Sulphatides	22q13–3	1.09	SCT
	Metachromatic leucodystrophy		Saposin B activator	Sulphatides, GM2-ganglioside, Glycolipids	10q21		
	Fabry disease		α-Galactosidase A	Globotriacylceramide	Xq22	0.85	ERT, EET (Phase III)
	Gaucher disease		Glucocerebrosidase	Glucosylceramide	1q21	1.75	ERT, SRT, SCT
	Gaucher disease		Saposin C activator	Glucosylceramide	10q21		
	Farber disease		Ceramidase	Ceramide	8q22–21.2		SCT
	Niemann–Pick disease A and B		Sphingomyelinase	Sphingomyelin	22q13.1–13.2	0.4	ERT, Preclinical
Oligosaccharidoses	α-Mannosidosis		α-Mannosidase	α-Mannosides	19p13.2–q12	0.09	SCT
	β-Mannosidosis		β-Mannosidase	β-Mannosides	4p	0.13	
	Fucosidosis		Fucosidase	Fucosides, glycolipids	1p24	0.05	SCT
	Aspartylglucosaminuria		Aspartylglucosaminidase	Aspartylglucosamine	4q32–33	0.05	
	Schindler disease		α-N-acetylgalactosaminidase	N-Acetylgalactosamine glycolipids	22q13.1–13.2		

Disease category	Disease	Phenotype/variant	Protein	Substrate	Gene locus	Incidence	Therapy
Glycogen	Pompe disease		α-Glucosidase	Glycogen	17q23	0.68	ERT
Lipid	Niemann–Pick disease C		Unknown	Cholesterol Sphingolipids	NPC1, 18q11–q12 NPC2, 14q24.3	0.47	SCT
	Wolman disease and cholesterol ester storage disease		Acid lipase	Cholesterol ester	10q23.2–23.3	0.19	SRT
Monosaccharide amino acids and monomers	ISSD	Infantile sialic acid storage disease	Sialic acid transporter	Sialic acid glucuronic	6q14–q15	0.19	SCT
	Salla disease		As ISSD	As ISSSD	As ISSD		ERT
	Cystine		Cystine transporter	Cystine	17p13	0.52	Preclinical
	Cobalamin F disease		Cobalamin transporter	Cobalamin	Unknown		
	Danon disease		LAMP-2	Cytoplasmic debris and glycogen	Xq24		
Peptides	Pycnodysostosis		Cathepsin K	Bone proteins	1q21		
S-acylated proteins, ceroid lipofuscinosis	CLN	Batten disease					
	CLN 1	Infantile	Palmitoyl protein thioesterase	Saposins	11p32		
	CLN 2	Late infantile	Pepstatin-insensitive carboxypeptidase	Subunit C mitochondrial ATP synthase	11p15.5		
	CLN 3	Juvenile	Membrane protein	As CLN 2	16p21		
	CLN 4	Adult, Kuf disease	Unknown	As CLN 2	Unknown		
	CLN 5	Late infantile, Finnish variant	Membrane protein	As CLN 2	13q22		
	CLN 6	Late infantile variant	Unknown	As CLN2	15q21–q23		
	CLN 7	Late infantile variant	Unknown	Unknown	Unknown		
	CLN 8	Progressive epilepsy with mental retardation	Membrane protein	As CLN 2	8p23		
Multiple enzyme deficiencies	Multiple sulphatase deficiency		Multiple sulphatase enzymes	Sulphatides, glycolipids, glycosaminoglycans	Unknown	0.07	
	Galactosialidosis		Neuraminidase and β-galactosidase protective protein	Oligosaccharides, sialic acid	20q13.3	(0.04)	

EET, enzyme enhancement therapy; ERT, enzyme replacement therapy; SCT, stem cell transplantation; SRT, substrate reduction therapy.

analogues can be used separately to reduce the activity of the enzyme glucosylceramide synthetase. This approach is only feasible in individuals with later-onset forms of the diseases who harbour mutations associated with detectable levels of residual enzyme activity. The small molecules used in SRT can be given orally, are easily absorbed and have a wide tissue distribution. Furthermore, SRT may have therapeutic utility in crossing the blood–brain barrier.

Some mutations lead to reduced levels of residual enzyme activity by causing misfolding of peptide chains or abnormal intracellular transport. The oral administration of small molecules (pharmacological chaperones) that can rescue misfolded or unstable enzymes is currently under active investigation for several lysosomal storage disorders. Such chaperones are designed to bind specifically to mutant peptides, aid their passage through the endoplasmic reticulum, rescue them from proteosomal degradation and guide them to the lysosome. They would dissociate from the enzyme within the acidic lysosomal environment. Combinations of ERT and chaperone therapy are also being evaluated in clinical trials.

Agents that bind to ribosomes (e.g. derivatives of gentamicin) and which modify the processing of RNA transcripts to allow 'read-through' of premature stop codon mutations are another class of mutation-specific therapy currently being evaluated in lysosomal storage disorders. Finally, gene therapy is under investigation in animal models of lysosomal storage disorders and has been reported as an adjunct to ERT in Gaucher disease.

Prognosis

The clinical course of infants diagnosed with a lysosomal storage disorder usually follows a predictable path of loss of learned skills and neurological deterioration until death results from infection and progressive organ damage. When onset is later, in adolescents and adults, the clinical course is more varied and the prognosis depends on the major organ systems affected. However, patient heterogeneity is such that it is not possible to predict which patients are most likely to experience significant morbidity or early mortality.

Clinical manifestations

The key clinical features of the major lysosomal storage disorders are presented in Table 18.3. In view of recent advances in therapy, Gaucher disease, Fabry disease and Pompe disease are presented in greater detail below.

Gaucher disease

Gaucher disease is due to deficiency of the enzyme β-glucocerebrosidase, a lysosomal enzyme that hydrolyses glucosylceramide to glucose and ceramide (Figure 18.2). It is an autosomal recessive condition arising as a result of mutation within the *GBA* gene. Affected individuals have a mutant enzyme with reduced activity, resulting in accumulation of the substrate (glucosylceramide) in lysosomes of reticuloendothelial cells. It is one of the commonest lysosomal storage disorders, with an estimated incidence of 1 in 60 000 to 1 in 80 000 individuals.

Clinical features

Clinical manifestations are due to cellular and tissue damage consequent upon accumulation of sphingolipid-laden macrophages in reticuloendothelial organs. Three main clinical phenotypes are observed (Table 18.4), determined in large part by the residual activity of the mutant enzyme. All three types are progressive disorders. Residual enzyme activity in type II is so low that abnormal cells accumulate in the central nervous system (CNS). This is the acute neuronopathic form of the disease, which presents with neurological complications in early infancy and usually leads to death before the age of 2 years. Type III disease is the subacute neuronopathic form that leads to a slowly progressive neurodegenerative disorder. Type I is the commonest form of Gaucher disease and typically does not cause neurological disease. It is particularly common among subjects of Ashkenazi Jewish origin; within this community, as many as 1 in 15–20 subjects are carriers, and approximately 1 in 800–1000 subjects are homozygous. Type I Gaucher disease is a heterogeneous disorder that may present in childhood or in late adult life (> 60 years old). It is likely that many undiagnosed subjects are asymptomatic. Symptomatic individuals have hepatosplenomegaly, skeletal disease and bone marrow infiltration, leading to pancytopenia. Rarer manifestations of type I Gaucher disease include pulmonary disease, skin involvement and peripheral neuropathy. Patients with type I Gaucher disease have an increased incidence of malignancy generally and an increased incidence of haematological malignancies, especially B-lymphocyte disorders (myeloma, monoclonal gammopathy of undetermined significance) and myelodysplasia. There is an increased incidence of Parkinson disease among affected individuals and carriers.

Laboratory features

Affected individuals have mutations within the *GBA* gene; more than 300 different mutations have been described. The commonest mutation causing type I disease is a single base-pair substitution in codon 370 (N370S), which accounts for approximately 70% of mutant alleles in affected Ashkenazi Jewish subjects. A base-pair substitution in codon 444 (L444P) is the commonest mutation underlying neuronopathic Gaucher disease. Diagnosis is confirmed by enzymatic assay of β-glucocerebrosidase activity in leucocytes, fibroblasts and urine. However, enzymatic assay does not always identify heterozygote subjects and measured enzyme activity correlates poorly with clinical severity.

Table 18.3 Lysosomal storage disorders: clinical features.

Category	Disease	Clinical features
Mucopolysaccharidoses	MPS I	Hurler disease: developmental delay, ENT infections, coarse facial features, macrocephaly, thick skin, corneal clouding, hepatosplenomegaly, bony deformity including large skull, pelvic dysplasia, deformed vertebrae and shortened tubular bones (dysostosis multiplex)
		Scheie disease: mild skeletal abnormalities, stiff joints, corneal opacities, carpel tunnel syndrome, cardiac valvular abnormalities and respiratory infections
	MPS II	Like MPS I but without corneal clouding
	MPS III	Loss of acquired skills, aggression, hyperactivity, coarse hair, hirsutism, seizures, may become tetraspastic
	MPS IV	Disproportionate dwarfism, joint contractures, kyphoscoliosis, corneal clouding
	MPS VI	Like Hurler disease but without neurological involvement
	MPS VII	Skeletal disease, hepatosplenomegaly, lethal hydrops, normal
Mucolipidoses	ML I	Early psychomotor retardation, hypotonia, truncal ataxia, upper motor neurone signs, corneal clouding
	ML II	Like Hurler disease, mild corneal clouding and hepatosplenomegaly, prominent gum hypertrophy, severe dysostosis multiplex
	MLIII	Progressive arthropathy, bone lesions, low intelligence, cardiac valvular lesions, corneal clouding
	ML IV	Like ML I
Sphingolipidoses	GM1 gangliosidosis	Infantile: coarse features, seizures, progression to decerebrate rigidity and spastic quadriplegia by 2 years
		Juvenile: psychomotor and neurological degeneration over 2–10 years
		Adult: progressive cerebellar impairment, spasticity and intellectual impairment
	GM2 gangliosidosis	Tay–Sachs disease: motor weakness, psychomotor retardation, blindness, lapsing into vegetative state with decerebrate rigidity
		Sandhoff disease: like rapidly evolving Tay–Sachs disease
	Globoid cell leucodystrophy	Developmental delay and progressive neurological degeneration aged 3–9 months
	Metachromatic leucodystrophy	Flaccid paresis, lack of coordination and hyporeflexia, psychomotor retrogression, juvenile and adult forms have later onset, intellectual deterioration
	Fabry disease	Left ventricular hypertrophy, renal impairment, angiokeratoma and acroparaesthesia
	Gaucher disease	Type 1: hepatosplenomegaly, skeletal disease and pancytopenia
		Type 2: death from neurological complications by 2 years
		Type 3: slowly progressive neurodegenerative disorder
	Farber disease	Hoarse cry, painful arthropathy, pulmonary infiltration, cherry-red spot, mental handicap, thickened heart valves
	Niemann–Pick disease	A: Hepatosplenomegaly, lymphadenopathy, neurological regression, epileptic seizures, macular cherry-red spot
		B: Hepatosplenomegaly and pulmonary infiltration
		C: Psychomotor delay and regression
Oligosaccharidoses	α-Mannosidosis	Mild skeletal deformity, coarse facial features and moderate to marked mental retardation
	β-Mannosidosis	Hearing loss and swallowing difficulties
	Fucosidosis	Neurological degeneration, neurological impairment, seizures, angiokeratoma and mild skeletal dysplasia
	Aspartylglucosaminuria	Progressive psychomotor retardation, coarse facial features and mild skeletal dysplasia
	Schindler disease	Progressive psychomotor retardation, blindness and seizures
Glycogen	Pompe disease	Cardiomegaly, hepatosplenomegaly, muscular weakness and macroglossia

Table 18.3 *Continued*

Category	Disease	Clinical features
Lipid	Wolman disease	Failure to thrive, malabsorption, adrenal gland enlargement and calcification, fatal by 1 year
	Cholesterol ester storage disease	Hypercholesterolaemia and premature atherosclerosis
Monosaccharide amino acids and monomers	ISSD	Visceral involvement, skeletal dysplasia, psychomotor retardation and early death
	Salla disease	Mental retardation, ataxia and near-normal lifespan
	Cystinosis	Polyuria, thirst, failure to thrive, renal tubular acidosis, rickets, photophobia and hypothyroidism
	Cobalamin F disease	Stomatitis, glossitis, convulsions and developmental delay
	Danon disease	Cardiomyopathy, myopathy, variable mental retardation
Peptides	Pycnodysostosis	Short stature, osteosclerosis, short fingers, open fontanelle, hypodontia
Ceroid lipofuscinosis	CLN	Mental impairment, seizures, loss of vision and motor skills
Multiple enzyme deficiencies	Multiple sulphatase deficiency	Resembles a combination of metachromatic leucodystrophy and Hurler disease
	Galactosialidosis	Hypotonia, coarse features with facial oedema, retinal cherry-red spot

Table 18.4 Clinical manifestations of Gaucher disease.

Manifestation	Type I	Type II	Type III
Onset	1 year	< 1 year	2–20 years
Hepatosplenomegaly	++	+/−	+
Bone disease	++	−	+/−
Cardiac valve disease	−	−	+
CNS disease	−	+++	+/−
Oculomotor apraxia	−	+	+/−
Corneal opacities	−	+/−	+/−
Age at death	60–90 years	< 5 years	< 30 years

Splenic enlargement and marrow infiltration frequently lead to anaemia, thrombocytopenia and leucopenia.

Changes in serum immunoglobulins are frequent. Polyclonal hypergammaglobulinaemia is found in more than one-third of patients, and monoclonal gammopathy of undetermined significance is seen in up to 20%. Liver function tests are often abnormal, reflecting infiltration of the liver by Gaucher cells leading to necrosis, fibrosis and, occasionally, even frank cirrhosis. There is an increased incidence of gallstones. The serum cholesterol level is typically lowered. Gaucher disease is associated with a bleeding diathesis, attributable to abnormal platelet function and thrombocytopenia. Factor XI deficiency is commonly observed and is largely due to co-inheritance of other genetic abnormalities that are also common among Ashkenazi Jews.

The abnormal lipid-laden macrophages are readily detected on tissue biopsy (e.g. bone marrow aspirate; Figure 18.3), although biopsy is no longer considered necessary to make the diagnosis. The serum levels of ferritin, angiotensin-converting enzyme (ACE) and acid phosphatase are typically elevated. The enzyme chitotriosidase is derived from macrophages and is typically grossly elevated in untreated Gaucher disease, and declines progressively with treatment. Levels may be as high as 30 000 U/L (normal range < 150 U/L); values below 1000 U/L generally indicate stable disease and with prolonged (> 7 years) ERT, values may even come down into the normal range (Figure 18.4). However, up to 6% of the population are deficient in this enzyme because of a 24-bp duplication in the chitotriosidase gene. These individuals cannot be monitored by measurement of plasma chitotriosidase activity. A new surrogate marker, pulmonary activation-regulated cytokine (PARC, CCL18), is also elevated in plasma of patients with Gaucher disease and is useful for monitoring those patients with chitotriosidase deficiency. PARC is a member of the CC chemokine family and its overexpression may be relevant to some of the pathophysiological features of Gaucher disease such as abnormalities in neutrophil chemotaxis.

Treatment

All patients with Gaucher disease should be evaluated by experienced physicians. Gaucher disease is the first lysosomal storage disorder to be treated by ERT, and a number of different ERT preparations are now available for the treatment of type I Gaucher disease. Indications for ERT include significant pancytopenia (e.g. Hb < 10 g/dL, platelets < 100×10^9/L), skeletal

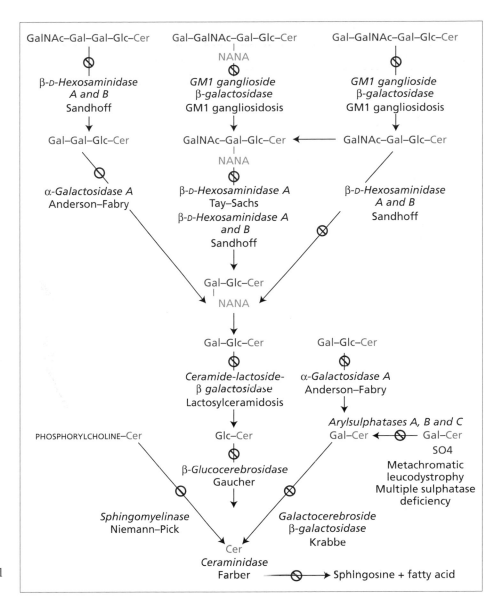

Figure 18.2 Biochemistry of lysosomal storage disorders.

disease and significant hepatosplenomegaly. High-dose ERT (> 100 U/kg every 2 weeks) has been evaluated in type II Gaucher disease but recombinant enzyme does not cross the blood–brain barrier and although hepatosplenomegaly improves, ERT has no discernible impact on CNS disease.

However, ERT has recently (2003) been licensed for patients with type III Gaucher disease, who typically have milder CNS abnormalities (e.g. ophthalmoplegia) in association with advanced systemic changes. SRT has been evaluated in combination with ERT in type III Gaucher disease but again no significant benefits on CNS manifestations have hitherto been demonstrated. ERT is administered by intravenous infusion (typically in the patient's home) every 1–2 weeks. The dose of therapy is titrated against the severity of clinical and laboratory changes. Type I patients with extensive bony disease and

hepatosplenomegaly require in excess of 30 U/kg every 2 weeks (> 60 U/kg for type III), and these high doses should be continued for 2–3 years or more. Patients are monitored regularly with blood tests (the chitotriosidase assay is particularly helpful) and an annual skeletal magnetic resonance scan. Some patients with advanced type I and III disease may benefit from more frequent infusions (e.g. weekly) for the first year or more. The dose of ERT is gradually lowered as the disease burden declines. Patients with less advanced disease may require lower doses, and some patients may only require monthly infusions. ERT is well tolerated and has been available for over 10 years. A small proportion of patients (< 10%) develop antibodies, but these are not usually neutralizing and do not affect treatment efficacy. Infusion reactions are rare and easily managed.

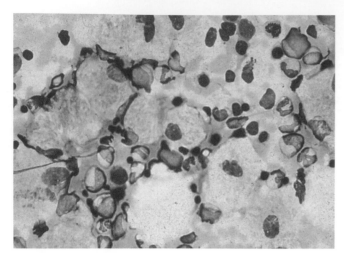

Figure 18.3 Gaucher cells in the bone marrow.

An oral form of therapy (miglustat, Zavesca) has recently been developed and is licensed for mild to moderate type I disease. It is a form of SRT (see above). It is a small molecule that reduces the amount of substrate (glucosylceramide) being produced within lysosomes, such that patients with reduced residual enzyme activity will benefit. It is being evaluated at present in other lysosomal storage disorders (e.g. Niemann–Pick type C) as its administration leads to reduction of a range of substrates in addition to glucosylceramide.

Supportive therapy is frequently required. The skeletal disease in Gaucher disease (Figure 18.5) is painful and patients may require analgesia. Prior to the use of ERT, patients frequently developed acute 'bone crisis' – episodic severe pain, typically in the limbs and often precipitated by dehydration. Bisphosphonate therapy is under evaluation for its potential to reduce pain and rate of progression of skeletal disease. Blood component therapy may be required for pancytopenic patients.

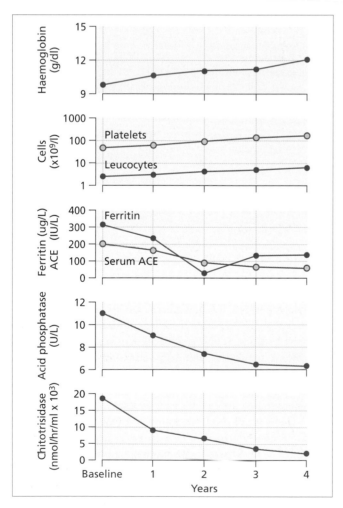

Figure 18.4 Clinical course in Gaucher disease treated with enzyme replacement therapy.

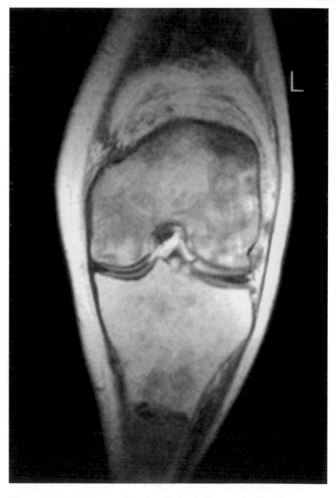

Figure 18.5 MRI scan showing skeletal changes in Gaucher disease.

Splenectomy should be avoided if possible as splenectomized subjects are more likely to develop tissue infiltration in other organs (e.g. liver, lungs, skeleton). Allogeneic stem cell transplantation is curative and has a definite role in carefully selected children with neuronopathic Gaucher disease.

Fabry disease

Fabry disease (or Anderson–Fabry disease) is an X-linked lysosomal storage disorder due to mutation within the gene for α-galactosidase A (GLA) (see Figure 18.2). The resulting inability to catabolize glycosphingolipids leads to progressive accumulation of the substrate globotriasylceramide in a range of tissues. In contrast to Gaucher disease, the lipid accumulation in Fabry disease affects a range of cells (e.g. endothelial cells, epithelial cells, myocytes) within a broad range of tissues and organs, particularly the kidneys (leading to renal failure), heart (causing ventricular hypertrophy and conduction disturbances) and vasculature of the CNS. It is one of the commonest lysosomal storage disorders, with an incidence of approximately 1 in 100 000. It is pan-ethnic. Milder variants of Fabry disease may be much commoner and may present as left ventricular hypertrophy, stroke/transient ischaemic attack and renal failure. Although it is X-linked, Fabry disease typically causes manifestations in females, though these occur later and are usually less severe than in males.

Diagnosis

Diagnosis is by assay of α-galactosidase A activity in leucocytes and detection of molecular abnormalities within the GLA gene. More than 200 different mutations have been described, and most lead to complete loss of enzyme activity. Tissue diagnosis is by renal, skin or cardiac biopsy.

Clinical features

Clinical features are legion. Although females are heterozygous, they are usually symptomatic and may be as severely affected as males. A skin rash (angiokeratoma) and pain in limbs (acroparaesthesia) are early symptoms (under 10 years old). In late childhood, reduced sweating, abdominal symptoms and lymphoedema are characteristic. Renal failure, cardiac failure, stroke, epilepsy and CNS/sensory organ involvement are later features. Life expectancy is 40–50 years for men and 50–65 years for most women.

Treatment

ERT for Fabry disease has been available since 2001. Two formulations are available: a recombinant galactosidase that is translated in Chinese hamster ovary cells and mannose-terminated (agalsidase beta, Genzyme Corporation, MA, USA); and an enzyme of identical amino acid sequence that is translated in a human fibroblast cell line wherein post-translational modification is performed within the human cell itself (Shire, MA, USA). The infused enzyme in Fabry disease must be taken up by lysosomes within cells in diverse organs and tissues, so targeting is of crucial importance. Beneficial clinical effects of ERT have been observed in renal and cardiac function, pain, hearing loss and gastrointestinal symptoms.

Pompe disease

Pompe disease (glycogen storage disease type II) is caused by deficiency of acid α-glucosidase. It is characterized clinically by an early infantile subtype associated with cardiomyopathy, hypotonia and reduced survival, and a later-onset form with features consistent with a limb girdle muscle disease phenotype and survival into adulthood. On blood film examination lymphocytes show glycogen vacuolation, which is positive on PAS staining. The prevalence of Pompe disease has been estimated to be 1 in 146 000, although it is higher in certain populations such as African-Americans (1 in 40 000) and Chinese (1 in 50 000). In untreated patients with the late-onset form of Pompe disease, muscle strength and pulmonary function deteriorate over time.

Alglucosidase alfa (Myozyme) is a recombinant formulation of human acid α-glucosidase generated from the transduction of Chinese hamster ovary cells. In infantile-onset patients, enzyme therapy has been shown to significantly extend overall and ventilator-free survival compared with data on historical controls. Trials involving the Chinese hamster ovary-derived enzyme in late-onset patients are in progress.

Niemann–Pick disease

Niemann–Pick disease is divided into subtypes A and B resulting from sphingomyelinase deficiency and subtype C resulting from defects in cellular cholesterol trafficking. Patients with type A exhibit neurodegenerative disease resulting in death in infancy, those with type B have lung but not neurological involvement, and those with type C show slowly progressive neurological disturbance. Hepatosplenomegaly may be found in all three types. Over 100 sphingomyelinase mutations causing Niemann–Pick disease type A or B have been described and DNA-based carrier screening has been implemented in the Ashkenazi Jewish community. Murine knockout mouse models have also been constructed and used to investigate disease pathogenesis and treatment. Based on these studies in the mouse model, a clinical trial of ERT has been initiated in adult patients with non-neurological sphingomyelinase-deficient Niemann–Pick disease. The use of inhibitors of glycolipid synthesis including miglustat appears promising in the therapy of Niemann–Pick disease type C. A recent 24-month randomized trial of miglustat in 29 patients with Niemann–Pick disease type C has recently been published and demonstrated improvement in, or stability of, several clinical markers including swallowing capacity and hearing acuity.

Selected bibliography

Beck M (2007) New therapeutic options for lysosomal storage disorders: enzyme replacement, small molecules and gene therapy. *Human Genetics* **121**: 1–22.

Berger J, Lecourt S, Vanneaux V *et al.* (2010) Glucocerebrosidase deficiency dramatically impairs human bone marrow haematopoiesis in an *in vitro* model of Gaucher disease. *British Journal of Haematology* **150**: 93–101.

Brady R (2006) Enzyme replacement therapy for lysosomal diseases. *Annual Review of Medicine* **57**: 283–96.

Grabowski GA (2008) Treatment perspectives for the lysosomal storage diseases. *Expert Opinion on Emerging Drugs* **13**: 197–211.

Grabowski GA (2008) Phenotype, diagnosis, and treatment of Gauchers disease. *Lancet* **372**: 1264–71.

Hughes D, Cappellini MD, Berger M *et al.* (2007) Recommendations for the management of the haematological and onco-haematological aspects of Gaucher disease. *British Journal of Haematology* **138**: 676–86.

Mehta A, Beck M, Eyskens F *et al.* (2010) Fabry disease: a review of current management strategies. *Quarterly Journal of Medicine* epub ahead of print.

Van der Ploeg AT, Reuser AJJ (2008) Pompe's disease. *Lancet* **372**: 1342–53.

Velloddi A (2004) Lysosomal storage disorders. *British Journal of Haematology* **128**: 413–31.

Zarate AY, Hopkin RJ (2008) Fabry disease. *Lancet* **372**: 1427–35.

Zimran A, Altarescu G, Phillips M *et al.* (2010) Phase ½ and extension study of velaglucerase alfa replacement therapy in adults with type 1 Gaucher disease: 48 month experience. *Blood* **115**: 4651–56.

Normal lymphocytes and non-neoplastic lymphocyte disorders

19

Paul AH Moss[1] and Mark T Drayson[2]

[1]University of Birmingham, Birmingham, UK
[2]University of Birmingham Medical School, Birmingham, UK

Introduction

The immune system has evolved to provide protection against infection and is believed to play an important role in the control of malignant disease. The immune response is often considered to comprise two functional components, known as the *innate* and *adaptive* arms of the immune response, but in reality these have a broad overlap. The innate immune system is responsible for the initial response to infection and inflammation and is mediated by cells such as macrophages, neutrophils and dendritic cells as well as lymphoid subsets such as natural killer (NK) cells, γδ T cells and B1 B cells. The adaptive or specific immune system is mediated by antigen-specific lymphocytes that are selected and expanded following recognition of antigen on antigen-presenting cells.

The anatomy of the immune system

The cells of the immune system are of haemopoietic origin and derive ultimately from the haemopoietic stem cell in the bone

marrow. The myeloid and lymphoid lineages diverge during differentiation, with separation of a common myeloid progenitor and a common lymphoid progenitor. There are three broad classes of lymphocyte – B cells, T cells and NK cells – and these have different developmental pathways.

T cells are generated in the thymus following the migration of prothymocytes from bone marrow to thymus followed by selection of thymocyte precursors. Over 95% of thymocytes die in the thymus, but the minority population emerges from the thymus as single-positive CD4⁺ or CD8⁺ T cells and enters the lymphoid system as naive precursors that can survive for many years. The antigen receptor on T cells, the T-cell receptor (TCR), exists only as a cell-surface molecule and is not secreted. T cells have extremely diverse functions including (i) providing signals that help induce T cells and B cells to proliferate and differentiate, (ii) specifically deleting virally infected cells or foreign cells, (iii) activating macrophages to enhance cellular cytotoxicity, and (iv) regulation of established immune responses.

Most *B cells* are generated from within the bone marrow, the 'B' in their name referring to an obscure avian structure called the bursa of Fabricius in which the B cells of birds develop. Naive mature B cells enter the lymphoid circulation but, if triggered by antigen in the periphery, a proportion of cells will return to the bone marrow as long-lived plasma cells that secrete immunoglobulin. B lymphocytes are the precursors of

Postgraduate Haematology: 6th edition. Edited by A. Victor Hoffbrand, Daniel Catovsky, Edward G.D. Tuddenham, Anthony R. Green
© 2011 Blackwell Publishing Ltd.

antibody-producing cells. Each B cell produces and expresses on its surface immunoglobulin with a distinct specificity for antigen. The specificity of the immunoglobulin is determined by the way the immunoglobulin variable-region genes are rearranged during B lymphopoiesis. B cells that bind antigen through their surface immunoglobulin have to obtain accessory signals if they are to proliferate and differentiate into antibody-secreting cells. These can be provided by helper T cells, which recognize antigen that has been taken up and presented by the B cell.

NK cells similarly appear to develop from within the environment of the bone marrow. They are able to kill cells that fail to express major histocompatibility complex (MHC) class I molecules on their surface or that express molecules associated with cellular stress.

The bone marrow and thymus are therefore the sites of lymphocyte development and are known as the *primary lymphoid organs*. However, immune responses are initiated when lymphocytes encounter antigen and this occurs primarily in *secondary lymphoid tissues* such as lymph nodes and the spleen.

Lymphocytes circulate around the body tissues via the blood and lymphatic vasculature. Lymphatic vessels drain extravascular spaces and lymph nodes are collections of lymphoid tissue in lymphatic vessels, which are organized to optimize encounters between lymphocytes and antigen. Afferent lymph drains into the lymph nodes, bringing circulating lymphocytes and populations of antigen-loaded dendritic cells from regional tissue. Efferent lymph returns lymphocytes to the bloodstream, where naive cells continue this circulatory pattern in a continuing quest for antigenic encounter. Antigen-experienced lymphocytes migrate to a variety of tissues in order to mediate their effector functions. The pattern of homing is largely determined by the chemokine receptor profile on the lymphocyte (see below).

Nature of the antigen-specific receptors on T and B cells

Antigen recognition by lymphocytes

Each B or T lymphocyte expresses approximately 20 000–100 000 antigen-specific receptors on their surface and all the receptors on a single T cell or B cell are identical. However, although the antigen receptors on a single cell are identical, they are different from the receptors on other B or T lymphocytes. During lymphoid development, a repertoire of billions of B and T cells is generated and all have slightly different antigen receptors on their surface. At the initiation of an immune response, only a few of these cells are able to recognize the antigen and these are then expanded during their differentiation into effector cells. This is the basis of the *clonal selection* theory of immunology. The mechanisms that generate this great diversity of antigen

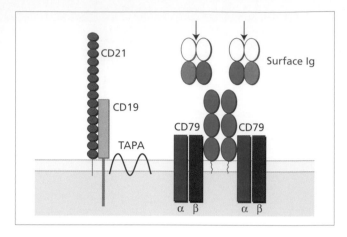

Figure 19.1 The structure of the antigen-specific receptor of B cells (BCR). Antibody (immunoglobulin) molecules on the surface of B cells provide their antigen-specific receptors. The green structures are the heavy (H) chains and the orange the light (L) chains. The antigen-combining (variable) regions are shown as open circles; the locations of the antigen-combining sites are indicated by arrows. The binding of antigen by B cells through their surface immunoglobulin can lead to antigen being internalized and can result, indirectly, in proliferation by the B cell and its differentiation to become an antibody-secreting cell or a memory cell. Signals delivered to the B cell when the surface immunoglobulin binds antigen are delivered through the α and β CD79 transmembrane signalling molecules and other surface immunoglobulin-associated molecules, including the complex of CD21 and CD19 with TAPA. CD21 binds the complement component C3d, which is derived from C3, and attaches to bacterial and other cell membranes; when CD21 and the surface immunoglobulin are cross-linked, the stimulus for B-cell activation is considerably more than that delivered through surface immunoglobulin alone. All B-cell surface immunoglobulin, such as plasma IgG and IgA, has two heavy and two light chains per molecule; IgA secreted from the body is a dimer and most IgM found in body fluids a pentamer of this basic four-chain structure.

receptors on lymphocytes are described in the next section. Figure 19.1 shows the structure of surface immunoglobulin on B cells.

T cells recognize peptides presented in association with MHC molecules. In humans, the MHC molecules are also known as human leucocyte antigens (HLAs) and there are two classes of MHC molecule. MHC class I molecules (Figure 19.2) are expressed by all nucleated cells except germ cells. They are not expressed by erythrocytes but are found on the surface of erythroblasts. The peptides recognized by T cells in association with class I MHC molecules are, in most circumstances, derived from proteins produced from within the cell. This places MHC class I molecules in an excellent position to present peptides

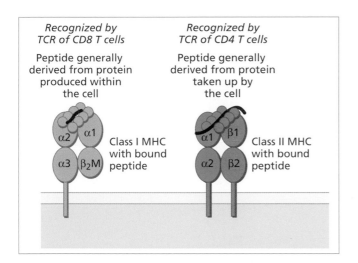

Recognized by TCR of CD8 T cells

Recognized by TCR of CD4 T cells

Peptide generally derived from protein produced within the cell

Peptide generally derived from protein taken up by the cell

α2 α1
α3 β2M

Class I MHC with bound peptide

α1 β1
α2 β2

Class II MHC with bound peptide

Figure 19.2 T cells recognize peptides held in MHC molecules. A class I MHC molecule is depicted on the left and a class II MHC molecule on the right. Some of the protein produced within each cell is broken down to peptides, which are presented on the cell surface in the peptide-binding groove of MHC molecules, usually class I (Figure 19.3). Extracellular molecules are taken up by antigen-presenting cells, broken down within the cell and presented on the cell surface in the peptide-binding groove of MHC molecules, usually class II (Figure 19.3). There are three isotypes of class II molecules, known as DP, DQ and DR, and three main class I isotypes, A, B and C. All of these are encoded within the MHC gene complex at 6p21.3. The genes encoding the peptide-binding grooves of each of these isotypes show extraordinary variability within the human population, so-called 'allelic polymorphism' (see Figure 19.5). The range of peptides that can be held by different MHC molecules varies. Consequently, this polymorphism is reflected in differences between individuals in the ability to recognize specific peptides. Any one T-cell receptor (TCR) will only recognize a particular peptide within a particular groove structure. β_2-Microglobulin is a non-polymorphic immunoglobulin-like domain that is non-covalently associated with HLA class I MHC molecules; it stabilizes peptide binding and is essential for the expression of class I on the cell surface.

derived from viral proteins following intracellular viral infection (Figure 19.3). It is now clear that antigen-presenting cells are also able to take up proteins from outside the cell and process them such that peptides gain access to the MHC class I presentation. This process is called *cross-presentation* and may be particularly important in generating CD8$^+$ T-cell responses to tumour-associated proteins.

MHC class I antigen presentation starts with the intracellular breakdown of proteins by a multimolecular proteolytic complex known as a *proteasome*. These peptides are actively transported by TAP (transporter associated with antigen processing) proteins into the endoplasmic reticulum, where empty MHC class

I molecules are being assembled. The nascent MHC molecules are able to 'fold' around the peptides, which make non-covalent interactions with the peptide-binding groove at the top of the molecule. This complex is then stabilized by the association of β_2-microglobulin before being transported to the cell surface. In this way, the cells are continuously advertising the peptide composition of the proteins that they are producing.

The selection of T cells during their development in the thymus involves the processes of negative selection and positive selection. T cells that have high affinity for self peptides held in the groove of a self MHC molecule are deleted by apoptosis in a process known as negative selection. T cells with lower affinity for self peptide–MHC complexes are positively selected and survive to become peripheral T cells. T cells that recognize peptide presented by MHC class I molecules express a molecule, CD8, that binds to the α3 domain of the MHC class I molecule (Figure 19.2). When any cell in the body presents immunogenic peptides, these may be recognized by a cytotoxic CD8 T lymphocyte that can then kill the target cell. This is most likely to occur as the result of virus infection when virus-encoded proteins are produced; it may also occur following the acquisition of a genetic mutation within a cell.

The other class of MHC molecule, MHC class II (Figure 19.2), is less widely expressed. The only cells that constitutively express large amounts of this class of MHC molecule are specialized antigen-presenting cells collectively known as dendritic cells, B lymphocytes and thymic epithelial cells. Dendritic cells are derived from haemopoietic stem cells and codevelop with monocytes; they can be derived from blood mononuclear preparations by culture with granulocyte/macrophage colony-stimulating factor (GM-CSF) and interleukin (IL)-4. They migrate to many tissues, particularly epithelia, where they remain until activated by local tissue injury. On activation, they take up fluid and particles from their surrounding environment (Figure 19.3). The pinocytotic activity in these cells can be induced by IL-1 and tumour necrosis factor (TNF) released at sites of injury. The pinocytotic vesicles fuse with an antigen-presenting endosomal compartment; proteolytic enzymes within this compartment are activated and proteins are broken down to peptides by the action of lysosomal enzymes. Class II molecules with peptide-binding grooves sealed by invariant chain (CD74) are inserted into the endosome wall. The invariant chain is digested and this allows peptides within the compartment to associate with MHC class II molecules. The MHC class II–peptide complex is then taken to the cell surface.

The scrutiny of antigen-presenting cells by T cells starts when dendritic cells have moved from peripheral tissues to the T cell-rich areas of adjacent secondary lymphoid organs. In this site they are known as interdigitating dendritic cells (IDCs), which express increased amounts of MHC class II and constitutively express other molecules associated with T-cell activation such as CD40, CD80 (B7.1) and CD86 (B7.2). In the T zones of secondary lymphoid organs, CD4$^+$, and to a lesser extent CD8$^+$,

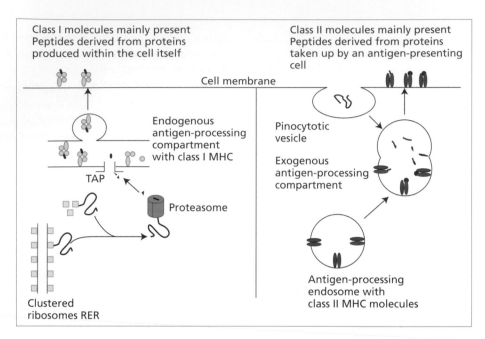

Figure 19.3 Antigen processing and presentation in association with MHC molecules. *Left*: Antigen presentation of proteins produced within cells is mainly the property of class I MHC molecules. A proportion of proteins (black ribbons) produced within a cell on ribosomes (yellow) are broken down to peptides (black fragments) within a cytoplasmic molecular complex known as a proteasome. The resulting peptides are actively transported by TAP proteins (blue) through the wall of specialized endoplasmic reticulum (ER) that has MHC class I molecules in its wall. The peptides and β_2-microglobulin associate with class I molecules and are then expressed on the cell surface (detailed in Figure 19.2). *Right*: Antigen presentation in association with class II MHC molecules involves pinocytosis of

antigen (black ribbon) and fusion with an antigen-processing endosome, which has class II MHC molecules (magenta and blue) inserted in its wall. The antigen-presenting grooves of the class II MHC molecules are kept empty by the association with invariant chain (CD74). Fusion of the pinosome with the endosome heralds the activation of proteolytic enzymes; the invariant chain and the ingested proteins are broken down to peptides. The resulting peptides (black fragments) are assembled into the antigen-presenting groove of class II MHC molecules that are held in the endosomal wall. The HLA class II molecules with bound peptides are then carried to the cell surface (detailed in Figure 19.2).

recirculating T cells are constantly migrating to the surface of IDCs, which they appear to scrutinize for the presence of an MHC–peptide complex to which they can bind with their TCR. In this way, the T cells continually screen for the presence of peptides derived from both extracellular and intracellular antigens (see section Immune responses).

The TCR (Figure 19.4) has certain similarities to immunoglobulin in that it is composed of two non-identical polypeptide chains that have constant and variable regions. In addition, as described in the next section, the genes that encode for TCR and immunoglobulin are remarkably similar. The TCR has only one antigen-binding site per molecule, as opposed to the two antigen-binding sites of immunoglobulin. There are two types of TCR, the most common being a heterodimer comprising an α-chain and a β-chain. The minority population of γδ TCRs is less well characterized, but they appear to recognize antigen in a different way from αβ TCR. A number of different molecules are associated with the two TCR polypeptide chains in order to

generate the TCR complex. This transmembrane signalling complex of molecules is collectively known as CD3 (detailed in Figure 19.4) and is linked to second messenger signalling molecules, whose expression varies between different T-cell subsets and at different stages of T-cell differentiation. CD4 or CD8 molecules are closely associated with the CD3 complex and determine the class of MHC molecule to which the TCR can bind.

Polymorphism of MHC molecules

There is extensive polymorphism of MHC class I and class II molecules (Figure 19.5). These were first recognized as targets for allograft rejection and the allelic forms of the MHC molecules differ in the fine structure of their MHC-binding grooves. This is reflected in differences in the range of peptides that different MHC alleles can present to T cells. Crossover during meiosis is relatively rare; consequently the alleles on each chromosome 6 are usually inherited en bloc and are named the MHC haplotype of that chromosome. It follows that approximately one in four siblings share the same MHC haplotype on both chromosomes. For the purposes of stem cell transplantation, the patient and donor must usually be fully matched for HLA alleles and thus only 25% of siblings are appropriate for donation.

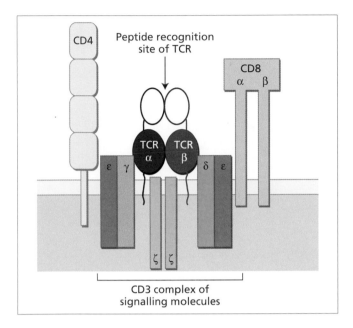

Figure 19.4 The αβ T cell receptor (TCR) complex. The αβ TCR is composed of two polypeptide chains, each with a variable (open ovoid) and constant (closed ovoid) domain. Peptide plus MHC is recognized by the combined variable regions. The TCR is surrounded by the CD3 complex of transmembrane signalling molecules. This is composed of four types of polypeptide chain, γ, δ, ε and ζ, that are present as three pairs: ε with δ, ε with γ and a pair of ζ-chains or ζ plus η (a splice variant of ζ with a longer intracellular tail). Most monoclonal antibodies against CD3 are directed against antigenic determinants on CD3ε. Most peripheral T cells express CD4 or CD8 with their TCR. In the thymus, the TCR is first expressed on thymocytes that express both CD4 and CD8, allowing the possibility for selection on the basis of either class II or class I-recognizing properties (see section on T-cell development).

Certain MHC alleles are associated with relative protection against specific infections. Conversely, some alleles, or combinations of alleles, are associated with a greater chance of developing autoimmunity. Many diseases, including diabetes mellitus, Graves disease and ankylosing spondylitis, are distinctly more common in individuals with a particular MHC allele or MHC haplotype. It seems logical that in evolution most alleles have been retained because they have certain advantages without too many disadvantages. The advantages of an allele might relate to a particular infection that is prevalent in one part of the world but almost unknown in another; for example, the HLA-B53 allele has a high prevalence in West Africa and is associated with relative protection from a potentially lethal form of malaria.

Generation of antigen-specific receptors on T and B lymphocytes

There are six pairs of genes that encode antigen-specific receptors: three for immunoglobulin (κ and λ light chains, and heavy chains) and three for TCRs (β, γ and a combined α and δ locus; see Table 19.1). These genes show marked similarities, indicating that the gene complexes evolved from a common precursor gene. The genetic organization of the variable-region genes and the way in which they are rearranged can generate a huge diversity of antigen recognition structures for subsequent display on the surface of mature B and T lymphocytes. For T cells, this is the only way in which diversity of V region structure is achieved. In B cells, there is an additional mechanism that increases the variable-region gene repertoire. This is called *somatic hypermutation*, which is activated during B-cell maturation in germinal centres and which introduces mutations into the rearranged immunoglobulin variable-region genes.

Both the immunoglobulin and TCR variable-region genes have to undergo a process of *gene rearrangement* from their germline configuration before they can encode an antigen recognition structure. As an example, the immunoglobulin heavy chain gene is located at 14q32.3 and the germline organization of the part of the gene that encodes for the variable region of IgH is shown at the top of Figure 19.6. The variable-region component of the immunoglobulin heavy chain gene is divided into three types of *gene segment*: V segments, D segments and J

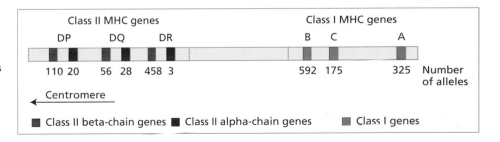

Figure 19.5 MHC polymorphism. This is a simplified diagram of the main genes that encode MHC class I and MHC class II molecules and their exceptional polymorphism.

Table 19.1 The variable region genes of human T-cell and B-cell antigen receptors.

Gene complex	Chromosomal location	Gene segments	
		Type	Approximate number
Immunoglobulin heavy chain	14q32.3	V_H	51
		D_H	~27
		J_H	6
		C_H	10
Immunoglobulin κ light chain	2p12	V_κ	40
		J_κ	5
		C_κ	1
Immunoglobulin λ light chain	22q11	V_λ	~29
		J_λ	4
		C_λ	4
TCR α-chain	14q11.2 (contains TCR δ locus)	V_α	~70
		J_α	61
		C_α	1
TCR δ-chain	14q11.2 (between Vα and Jα of TCR α)	V_δ	~4
		D_δ	3
		J_δ	3
		C_δ	1
TCR β-chain	7q32.5	V_β	52
		D_β	2
		J_β	13
		C_β	2
TCR γ-chain	7p15	V_γ	12
		J_γ	5
		C_γ	2

C, constant regions; D, diversity segments; J, joining segments; V, variable sements.

Where the number of functional gene segments is uncertain, this is denoted by '~'. There are many non-functional gene segments (pseudogenes); these are disregarded in this table. Because TCR α and δ genes are encoded in the same gene complex on chromosome 14, successful rearrangement of the TCR α genes inevitably results in looping out of the δ genes so that α and δ genes cannot be coexpressed.

segments. A large number of individual V gene segments are encoded within the genome. The V gene segments are longer than J or D segments and encode much of the framework of the variable-region domain, together with the first and second hypervariable regions (known as the complementarity-determining regions, CDR1 and CDR2). The CDR1 and CDR2 regions encode two of the three parts of the variable region that determine the antigenic specificity of the heavy-chain V region.

There are fewer D and J gene segments. The third hypervariable region (CDR3) is encoded at the site of joining of one of the functional D segments with any one of the functional J segments and includes the downstream end of one of the V segments. Heavy-chain rearrangement involves two looping-out manoeuvres (Figure 19.6). In the first of these, one of the J segments becomes spliced to one of the D segments and the intervening sequences are deleted. Next, one of the two rearranged D–J pairs becomes linked to one of the V segments and again the intervening sequences are deleted. The association of segments appears to occur at random and the theoretical number of different variable region genes that might be generated in this way is the product of the number of functional V, D and J segments, i.e. about 8262. In practice, D to J and V to D–J joining is not exact and additional random nucleotides may be added at the point where the gene segments join. This results in very much greater diversity, which is seen only in CDR3 and which includes both the D to J and V to D–J junctions.

The diversity of CDR1 and CDR2 is therefore much less than that of CDR3. Junctional diversity in CDR3 is sufficiently great to allow the conclusion that B cells with the same CDR3 sequence are almost certainly derived from the same clone and this fact is used widely to identify the origin and relationship of malignant B cells.

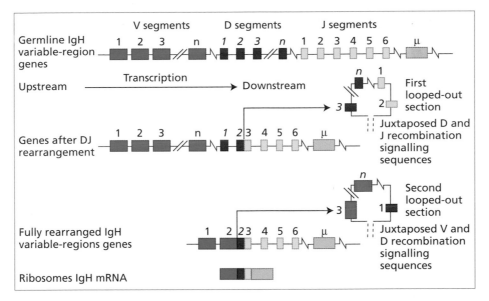

Figure 19.6 Immunoglobulin heavy-chain variable-region genes and their rearrangement. The germline structure of the variable-region gene complex is shown in the top line. The genes are present in this form in haemopoietic stem cells. The approximate number (n) of V_H, D_H and J_H segments are given in Table 19.1. The constant-region genes are downstream of the V-region genes. The first of these, μ, encodes the IgM heavy chain constant-region domain. This is followed in sequence by δ, $\gamma3$, $\gamma1$, a non-functional pseudo-ε gene, $\alpha1$, $\gamma2$, $\gamma4$, ε and $\alpha2$. The boxes represent exons and lines introns. During rearrangement, first one of the J segments becomes aligned with one of the D segments and the intervening sequences are deleted; DJ rearrangement is always attempted on both chromosomes 14. The aligned DJ pair on one chromosome 14 then becomes linked to one of the V segments on that chromosome, and again intervening sequences are deleted. If this V to DJ rearrangement is able to encode a variable region, then there is no V to DJ rearrangement on the other chromosome; if it has been unsuccessful (e.g. the rearrangement is out of frame) the cell goes on to attempt to rearrange a V segment to the DJ on the other chromosome. The D to J and V to DJ alignment is made possible by the presence of recombinase signalling sequences that flank (i) the upstream end of each J segment and the downstream end of each D segment and (ii) the upstream end of each D segment and the downstream end of each V segment. Additional diversity at the junctions between the rearranged V, D and J segments results in part from imprecise splicing and partially through the insertion of additional non-encoded (N) basepairs at the D to J and V to DJ junctions through the action of terminal deoxynucleotidyltransferase.

B lymphopoiesis

B-cell production starts in the fetal liver at the end of the first trimester of pregnancy and normally ceases at this site later in pregnancy. Subsequently, B cells are also produced in the bone marrow and production in this tissue continues throughout life such that approximately 2% of adult marrow mononuclear cells are B-cell progenitors.

The events that occur as cells differentiate towards B cells are summarized in Figure 19.7. The associated phenotypic changes are set out in Table 19.2. The earliest signs associated with differentiation of haemopoietic cells towards the B lineage are the expression of CD19, CD24 and MHC class II molecules on the cell surface and CD22 inside the cell. These changes are followed by the expression of molecules such as the recombinase-activating genes *RAG1* and *RAG2*, which are involved in immunoglobulin gene rearrangement.

Almost always, heavy-chain gene rearrangement precedes light-chain gene arrangement. The first rearrangements to occur are in the joining of one of the J segments to one D segment, with the looping out of the intervening sequences (see previous section for details). The rearrangement or attempted rearrangement of D to J is completed on both chromosomes 14 before an attempt is made to rearrange the D–J to a V segment on one of the chromosomes. If this is successful, the rearranged V–D–J sequence will be transcribed together with the genes encoding the μ constant region. After translation of this transcript, the cell has cytoplasmic μ heavy chain and is known as a *pre-B cell*. During all the preceding stages of B lymphopoiesis, cells showing differentiation towards B cells are known as *pro-B cells*.

When intact μ heavy chain is expressed, an essential further step has to take place if the B cell is to proceed to light-chain rearrangement. The μ chain is expressed on the cell surface at low level with a 'surrogate' light chain that is composed of two

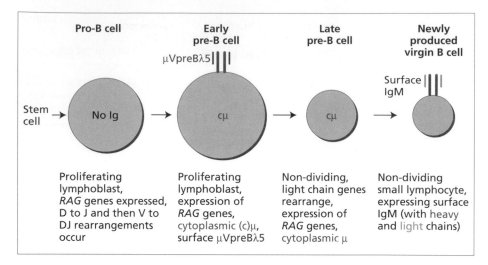

Figure 19.7 Outline of the main stages of B lymphopoiesis. The central process in B-cell formation is the rearrangement of immunoglobulin variable-region genes. For rearrangement of V-region genes to occur in either T or B cells, the recombinase-activating genes *RAG1* and *RAG2* have to be expressed. Absence of these genes totally blocks further differentiation towards B or T cells. After a successful heavy-chain VDJ has been made, a B cell must express the heavy chain with the surrogate light chain composed of V_{preB} and λ5 if further differentiation is to occur. Cells that fail to make either a productive heavy- or light-chain rearrangement destroy themselves by apoptosis.

Table 19.2 Phenotypic changes during B-cell lymphopoiesis.

	Surface CD34	Cytoplasmic CD22 with surface CD19 and CD24	Nuclear TdT	Surface CD10	Surface CD20	Cytoplasmic μ	Surface IgM
Pro-B cell	+	+	+	−	−	−	−
Early pre-B cell	+	+	+	+	−	−	−
Late pre-B cell	−	+	−	+	+	+	−
Virgin B cell	−	+	−	−	+	+	+

TdT, terminal deoxynucleotidyltransferase.

peptides, V_{preB} and λ5. If this surface expression does occur, the pre-B cell receives a signal for further differentiation to proceed, exits cell cycle and starts light-chain gene rearrangement. On the other hand, if the first attempt to rearrange V to D–J is not successful and no μ V_{preB}–λ5 complex is expressed at the surface, an attempt is made to rearrange a V segment to D–J on the other chromosome 14. If this also fails and the cell is still unable to express μ V_{preB}–λ5 at its surface, it will die by apoptosis. When the second heavy-chain rearrangement is successful, the cell proceeds, as above, towards light-chain gene rearrangement. The first expression of IgM on a B-cell surface marks the transition from pre-B cell to a newly produced virgin B cell.

Extensive analysis of variable-region genes in pre-B cells of mice has failed to identify cells with two functional VDJ rearrangements. One functional VDJ rearrangement can only be seen with a non-functional VDJ rearrangement or a D–J rearrangement. This *allelic exclusion* of antigen receptor genes means that only one functional antigen-binding protein is expressed on the surface of the cell.

The enzyme terminal deoxynucleotidyltransferase (TdT) is expressed during variable-region gene rearrangement and introduces non-encoded (N) sequences at the junctions of V to D–J and D to J. The enzyme is expressed both in pro-B cells in the marrow and in cortical thymocytes during TCR gene rearrangement. The expression of TdT is much greater in the bone marrow than in the fetal liver and, as a result, junctional diversity is less marked in the first B cells that are produced. These are mainly B1 cells, which are described later. The enzyme TdT is not expressed in late pre-B cells at the time of light-chain gene rearrangement and N sequences are not a feature of light chain

V–J junctions. Normally, B cells will express only light chains encoded by one of their four light-chain gene complexes, i.e. they express either a κ-chain or a λ-chain. The ratio of κ-expressing B cells to λ-expressing B cells is closely regulated and in humans is close to 60:40. Major deviation from this ratio has been observed only in B-cell neoplasia, when there is massive expansion of a neoplastic clone of B cells. Disturbance of the κ/λ B-cell ratio to more than 10:1 or less than 0.1:1 can therefore be taken as a reliable indicator of the presence of a neoplastic clone.

Intact heavy chains can be exported to the surface of a B cell only if they are complexed with light chain or surrogate light chain. This does not apply to free light chains, which are able to pass out of B cells and plasma cells. Physiological light chain production is always greater than that required to complex all the available heavy chain, and measurement of serum free light chain is now a useful tool in the management of paraproteinaemia. The heavy chains that are secreted in heavy chain disease are able to leave the cell only because they are truncated heavy chains.

T-cell production and selection in the thymus

Although the earliest progenitors of T cells are produced in the bone marrow, the development and selection of most mature immunologically competent T cells occurs in the thymus. The thymus is an encapsulated gland that is organized into lobules by capsular septa. Within each lobule, there is a complex meshwork of epithelial and other cells that are responsible for regulating the development of prothymocytes into mature T cells. The subcapsular region of the thymus is divided into the more peripheral cortex and the deeper medulla.

CD8 and CD4 thymocytes are selected on the basis of their potential to recognize peptides held in association with either MHC class I or MHC class II molecules respectively. Immature αβ TCR thymocytes are subject to two selection processes: *positive selection*, which allows cells that have the potential to recognize foreign peptide in association with self MHC to mature into functional T cells, and *negative selection*, which removes T cells that recognize self peptides in association with a self MHC molecule. During the development from prothymocytes to mature lymphocytes, T cells pass from the outer cortex, through the inner cortex and on through the medulla before emerging as immunocompetent T cells in the peripheral circulation. T cells whose TCR molecules fail to engage with MHC–peptide complexes within the thymus die by neglect, whereas those whose TCR can interact with these complexes are subject to positive and negative selection (see below). It has been estimated that 95% of all thymocytes die within the thymus either as a result of failure to rearrange their TCR genes in an express-

ible form or as a consequence of elimination during the T-cell selection process.

Thymic epithelial cells in the cortex are critical in the positive selection of thymocytes that have moderate affinity for MHC–peptide complexes. The boundary of the cortex and medulla is populated by macrophages (often called sentinel macrophages) that phagocytose cells undergoing apoptosis. The medulla contains bone marrow-derived dendritic cells that express MHC class I and II antigens. It is here that the process of negative selection is mediated, in which T cells with high affinity for self MHC–peptide complexes are deleted. Structures known as Hassall corpuscles, which are whorled aggregates of epithelial cells, can also be seen in the medulla though their function is uncertain.

TCR gene rearrangements and phenotypic changes

Bone marrow-derived T-cell progenitors (prothymocytes) seed the subcapsular region of the thymic lobule (Figure 19.8). At this stage of ontogeny the cells have not started to rearrange their TCR genes, do not express the mature T-cell markers CD3, CD4 or CD8, and may not be irreversibly committed to the T-cell lineage. They may be identified by expression of CD7 and CD34. Interaction with the thymic stroma is accompanied by proliferation and expression of CD2, soon followed by cytoplasmic expression of CD3 genes. By this stage, the cell is committed to the T-cell lineage and TCR gene rearrangement is underway.

The configuration of the TCR and its genes is discussed in the section on antigen-specific receptors on T and B cells and is summarized in Figure 19.4 and Table 19.1. During early fetal development, the first cells to leave the thymus as mature T cells have successfully rearranged their γ and δ genes and express the γδ form of the TCR. Many γδ T cells do not express CD8 or CD4, suggesting they may not be interacting with antigen in association with MHC class I or class II molecules. During later stages of human fetal development and throughout the rest of life, 85–98% of T cells that leave the thymus have undergone successful α and β gene rearrangement and express the αβ TCR.

Rearrangement of the gene encoding the TCR β-chain occurs first with D to J rearrangements followed by V to D–J rearrangements. Successful rearrangement leads to low-level expression of the β-chain at the cell surface in a complex with CD3 and a surrogate α-chain analogous to V_{preB}–λ5 in B-cell development. It is at this stage that the cell starts to express low levels of both CD4 and CD8; further β-chain gene rearrangement is halted and α-chain gene rearrangement starts (Figure 19.8). TCR α-chain gene rearrangement may involve sequential rearrangements of V–J pairs, which enables the cell to express different TCR α-chains until a successful TCR αβ heterodimer is generated.

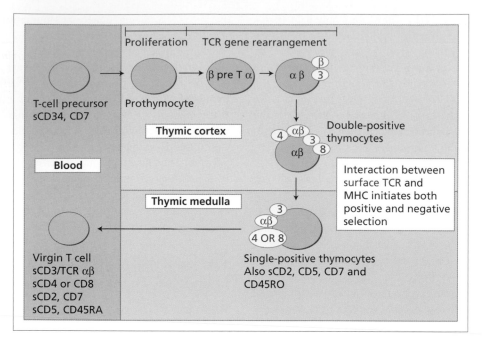

Figure 19.8 T-cell maturation in the thymus. Molecules within cells (red) or on a cell's surface (blue) are depicted without the prefix CD. T-cell progenitors enter the thymus from the marrow or other primary lymphoid site to become a prothymocyte. At this stage their T-cell receptor (TCR) genes are in germline configuration. The proliferative potential and lack of commitment of prothymocytes is reflected in the ability of a single prothymocyte to populate an entire thymic lobe and generate a full T-cell repertoire. Prothymocytes proliferate in the outer cortex. Towards the end of the proliferative phase, TCR rearrangement starts: first, β-chain genes are rearranged, then these are expressed with a surrogate α-chain (pre-T α–); after this, α-chain genes rearrange. As with B cells, these rearrangements require *RAG1* and *RAG2* genes to be expressed, and junctional diversity is increased by the addition of N sequences using terminal deoxynucleotidyltransferase. Selection occurs at the double-positive stage when the full TCR complex is expressed with CD3 and both CD4 and CD8. These cells are selected on their ability to recognize self peptide presented by a self MHC molecule at low avidity. Those cells recognizing peptide with class I go on to become single-positive CD8 expressors; those recognizing peptide with class II continue to express CD4 without CD8. Cells recognizing self peptide at high avidity and cells failing to recognize a self MHC molecule are deleted.

The B-cell repertoire

B cells constitute around 10–20% of the peripheral lymphoid pool and two broad lineages have been recognized, *B1 cells* and *conventional (or B2) cells*. B1 cells are the predominant B-cell subtype in fetal life and during the first year after birth, and are capable of antigen-independent self-renewal in the periphery. The antigen-binding specificity of the antibodies produced by these cells tends to have broad reactivity including autoreactivity. The function of B1 cells and the background IgM antibody they produce is still far from clear. It has been suggested that they may play a regulatory role in selection of the B-cell repertoire and they are highly conserved during evolution. B1 B cells often express CD5 and share many features in common with the malignant cells of B-cell chronic lymphocytic leukaemia.

The majority of B cells are conventional (B2) B cells and are produced in the marrow after the first year of life. Three stages of conventional B-cell differentiation can be identified: newly produced virgin B cells, recirculating B cells and marginal zone B cells (Table 19.3). Most recirculating B cells are virgin cells, whereas the B cells of the marginal zones do not recirculate and are a mixture of virgin and memory cells.

Naive B cells are small non-dividing virgin B lymphocytes that classically are positive for surface IgM and IgD. They are in a constant state of migration between the follicles of secondary lymphoid organs. On their way to the follicles, they migrate through the T cell-rich zones that contain antigen-presenting cells and have an average lifespan of 4 weeks or more.

Marginal zone cells, like recirculating B cells, respond to T cell-dependent antigens and to bacterial cell wall lipopolysaccharides (thymus-independent type 1, or TI-1, antigens).

Table 19.3 Differences between the three main types of human B cell found in adults.

	Marrow IgM⁺, IgD⁻	*Recirculating*	*Marginal zone*
Diameter		~ 8 μm	~ 10 μm
Chromatin	Condensed	Condensed	Open
Cytoplasm volume/basophilia	Scanty/little	Scanty/little	Moderate/moderate
Proliferating	No	No	No
Lifespan	About 3 days	4 weeks or more	3 weeks or more
Antigen-independent movement	Migrate from marrow to secondary lymphoid tissue	Migrate between the secondary lymphoid tissues	Remain in the marginal zones
Surface immunoglobulin	IgM	IgM and IgD	IgM or IgG or IgA
Memory or virgin	All virgin	Almost all virgin	Variable mixture of virgin and memory
Immunoglobulin V-region mutations	None	Not present	Present in memory cells
Molecules expressed on the cell surface			
CD19, CD20, CD37, CD40 and class II MHC	Positive	Positive	Positive
CD21, CD39	Negative	Positive	Positive
CD5	Negative	Some positive	Negative
CD23	Negative	Positive	Negative
CD25	Negative	Negative	Positive
CD38	Negative	Negative	Negative
Capacity to respond to different classes of antigen			
Bacterial cell wall lipopolysaccharide	+	+	+
Bacterial capsular polysaccharide	–	–	+
Protein-based antigens	+	+	+

IgM⁺, IgD⁻ cells of the marrow are representative of newly produced virgin B cells.

Unlike recirculating B cells, they will also respond to bacterial capsular polysaccharides. Capsular polysaccharides are thymus-independent type 2 (TI-2) antigens. These antigens do not evoke antibody responses until several months after birth, and levels of antibody produced in response to these antigens do not reach adult levels until 5 years of age.

The T-cell repertoire

The majority (around 95%) of peripheral T cells express αβ TCR. When these αβ T cells leave the thymus, most express either CD4 or CD8 on their surface and are restricted to the recognition of peptides in the context of MHC class II or class I molecules respectively. A minority of T cells express a γδ TCR and exhibit antigenic specificity for non-peptide molecules.

CD4⁺ and CD8⁺ T cells and their functions

CD4⁺ T cells can have one or more of a variety of functions. Their major role is in the provision of signals that induce proliferation or differentiation of T or B cells, generally known as *T-cell help*. They can also activate macrophages and may mediate HLA class II-restricted cytotoxic activity. Increasing attention is being given to their regulatory role in T-cell immune responses and this is mediated through a FoxP3-positive subset.

CD8⁺ T cells have a predominant role in the recognition of virally infected cells and recognize antigen in association with HLA class I. Antigen recognition is followed by lysis of the target cell or secretion of cytokines or interferon (IFN)-γ. There are two main killing mechanisms which both induce apoptosis in the target cell. Firstly, enzymes known as *granzymes* and pore-forming molecules termed *perforins* are transferred from the T cell to the target cell. Granzymes and perforins are present in granules that stain crimson and are easily seen against the featureless pale cytoplasm of cytotoxic T cells and NK cells in Jenner–Giemsa preparations. These features have given rise to the term 'large granular lymphocyte'. The second cytotoxic mechanism involves the expression of the Fas ligand (FasL) by the effector cell. The resulting engagement of Fas on the target cell induces the target to undergo apoptosis. Fas is a member of the TNF receptor family and FasL is an analogue of TNF-α and TNF-β.

Once the peripheral T-cell pool is established, it can maintain itself without further input from the thymus. Even neonatal thymectomy in humans during cardiac surgery does not cause clinically noticeable immunodeficiency. This indicates that T-cell clones can be very long-lived and this certainly applies to CD45RA^{high} virgin T cells. Unlike the peripheral pool of recirculating B cells, which cannot replenish itself when depleted, small numbers of transferred recirculating T cells will proliferate to fill a depleted peripheral T-cell pool in a process known as *homeostatic proliferation*. Some experiments suggest that memory T-cell clones persist only if there is periodic restimulation by antigen, but other experiments indicate that in some instances this is not required.

Natural killer cells

NK cells are cytotoxic lymphocytes that lack expression of a TCR and have a range of functional activities in the immune system. They express a range of inhibitory and activating receptors and it is the balance of signals received through these molecules that determines whether the target cell will be recognized. Inhibitory signals include (i) killer inhibitory receptors (KIRs) that bind to HLA-C or HLA-B alleles on the surface of the target cell and (ii) CD94–NKG2 heterodimers that bind to HLA-E. Activating receptors include (i) activating forms of KIR molecules, whose ligands are uncertain at present; (ii) NKG2D, which binds to proteins such as MICA and ULBP expressed on cells under physiological stress; and (iii) the immunoglobulin receptor (FcR) CD16.

HLA class I expression is often downregulated on the surface of cells following viral infection and is also a common feature of malignant cells. This provides some protection from recognition by CD8$^+$ T cells but renders the cell susceptible to lysis by NK cells (Figure 19.9). Thus, CD8$^+$ T cells and NK cells can be viewed as having complementary recognition systems based on the level of HLA class I on the target cell. The ability of NK cells to recognize ligands such as MIC-A, which are expressed on the surface of damaged or stressed cells, demonstrates that NK cells may also have the ability to target cells at the site of inflammation, irrespective of HLA class I expression level.

The lytic mechanisms of NK cells seem to be the same as those used by cytotoxic T cells. NK cells proliferate in the presence of IL-2 and their activity can be augmented by exposure

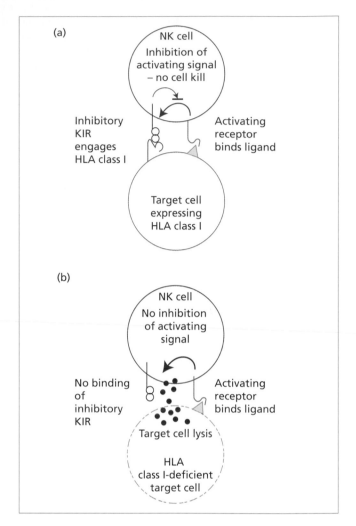

Figure 19.9 Mechanism by which NK cells kill target cells that fail to express HLA class I. NK cells express two classes of receptors which either activate (b) or inhibit (a) NK cell killing. Activating receptors can bind to a range of ligands on the target cell whose expression is often constitutive. In contrast, the major forms of inhibitory receptor bind to HLA class I molecules. If HLA class I expression is downregulated on the target cell, no inhibitory signal is delivered to the NK cells and the target cell is killed.

to IFN-γ. They characteristically express a range of receptors such as CD56 (NCAM) and CD57 but these are also expressed on a subset of T cells.

Natural killer T cells

Natural killer T (NKT) cells represent a small (< 1%) population of peripheral blood T cells and appear to be positioned somewhere between conventional T cells and NK cells in that they express a TCR but also a range of receptors typically associated with NK cells. Moreover, the TCR is invariant, with the same $V\beta11V\alpha24$ heterodimer being expressed on all cells. NKT cells recognize lipid antigens presented on the surface of CD1d molecules, CD1d being a protein with homology to MHC class I. It appears that NKT cells are activated very early in an immune response, although their functional significance is uncertain.

The immune response

In this section we consider how an immune response is developed within the secondary lymphoid tissue. The general structure of a lymph node is shown in Figure 19.10 to provide an anatomical context for immune physiology.

Lymph nodes have an afferent lymphatic supply that is fed by lymph draining the extravascular tissue spaces and this provides the main source of antigen for the node. Dendritic cells activated by local disturbance take up and process antigen, and then pass through afferent lymph into lymph nodes (Figure 19.11). The afferent lymph passes into the subcapsular sinus, which forms a lake of lymph that covers the cortical surface of the node. From the subcapsular sinus, lymph passes through intranodal lymph sinuses that surround and separate the cone-like segments that make up the solid tissue of the node. The intranodal lymphatics, as they pass the follicles and T zone, are difficult to see as they are crossed by fibrous cords. Attached to these and the walls of the tissue cones are macrophages and other poorly defined cells. Increased numbers of these cells in the intranodal lymph sinuses and similar cells in the subcapsular sinus are described by histopathologists as *sinus histiocytosis*. The intranodal lymph sinuses passing the medullary cords

contain fewer fixed cells and are easier to identify. In the medulla, the intranodal lymph sinuses feed into the efferent lymphatic vessel that returns the lymph to the venous blood supply; in the case of the gut and lower half of the body, via the thoracic duct to the left subclavian vein.

The solid tissue of the node is composed of variable numbers of roughly cone-like segments (Figure 19.10). The base of each cone abuts onto the subcapsular lymph sinus in the cortex of the node and the apex is in the medulla. These cones fit together, but are separated by the intranodal lymphatic sinuses, to form the roughly kidney-shaped structure of lymph nodes. The cones have three main zones: the follicles in the cortex, the T zones and the medullary cords. The medullary cords form a convoluted apex to the cone. The contents and functions of each of these zones are described in detail in subsequent sections. The blood supply to the node enters and leaves the node through the medulla, and the specialized small blood vessels termed *high endothelial venules* through which recirculating B and T cells and newly produced virgin B cells enter the node are located in the T zones. Virgin B and T cells, and some memory cells, enter the T zone by passing across the high endothelial venules. Here they encounter IDCs (Figure 19.11), which present peptides on MHC molecules and initiate immune responses. The series of stages leading to T cell-dependent B-cell activation in the T zones is shown in Figure 19.11. If a T cell is able to recognize a peptide–MHC complex, it is activated through TCR signalling. Costimulation is provided by interaction between molecules such as CD80 and CD86 expressed on IDCs and CD28, which is constitutively expressed by T cells. The effect of this interaction is to bring about changes in the T cell that are collectively called *T-cell priming* (Figure 19.12).

Cytokines are produced by the T cell following this interaction and the nature of the cytokines produced in different situations is considered later. Short-term proliferation of the T and B cells is also induced, and most B cells migrate to local sites of antibody production. In the spleen this is the red pulp, and in lymph nodes the medullary cords. The lifespan of most of these plasma cells is 3 days. The extent of immunoglobulin class switching will depend on the conditions of dendritic cell activation and T-cell priming. In primary antibody responses, the plasma cells generated by B-cell activation in T zones do not have somatic mutations in their immunoglobulin V-region genes. On the other hand, in secondary responses, marginal-zone memory B cells that have somatic mutations in their V-region genes can be induced to migrate to T zones on contact with antigen and give rise to short-lived plasma cells.

The other pathway of migration of T and B cells activated in T zones is to the follicles. Both antigen-specific B blasts and T blasts migrate to the follicles at an early stage in T-zone responses and give rise to *germinal centres*. Germinal centres are present in the first 3 weeks following an immune response and build around B blasts that migrate to follicles and undergo massive clonal expansion such that the spaces in the follicular dendritic

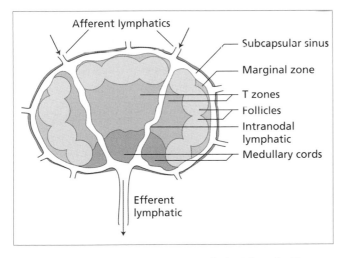

Figure 19.10 The main compartments of a lymph node. Note that the size of the marginal zone is variable; although it is often obvious in mesenteric lymph nodes, it may not be obvious in small nodes such as the popliteal nodes, particularly if these have not been sites of recent immune responses.

Labels in figure:
Afferent lymphatics
Subcapsular sinus
Marginal zone
T zones
Follicles
Intranodal lymphatic
Medullary cords
Efferent lymphatic

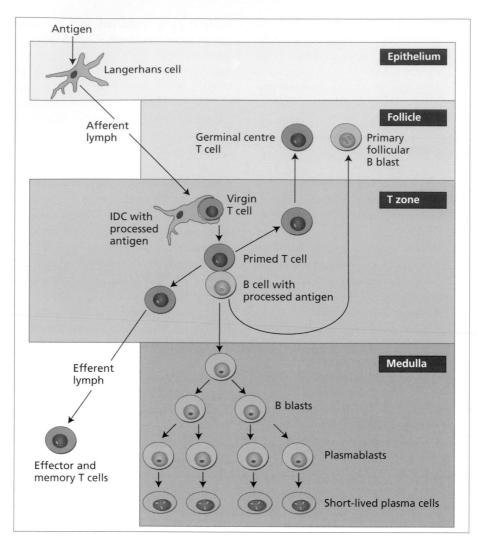

Figure 19.11 T-cell priming and T-cell-dependent B-cell activation in a lymph node. Local disturbance induces dendritic cells in the tissues to take up material from their surroundings. Ingested proteins are processed to peptides inside the cell (see Figure 19.3). Dendritic cells that have taken up antigen migrate through afferent lymphatics to draining lymph nodes or through the blood to the spleen. By the time they reach a T zone, they have differentiated into interdigitating cells (IDCs), which are specialized at presenting antigenic peptides, held in MHC molecules, to recirculating T cells. Virgin T cells migrating through the T zones move over the surface of the interdigitating cells and are activated if they meet antigen they recognize. As the result of this priming process, they move to the outer T zone and become targets for B cells that have taken up and processed antigen. The primed as opposed to virgin T cells are able to deliver costimulatory signals via CD40 and B7.1 and B7.2 to B cells that specifically engage their TCR. B cells activated in this way migrate to extrafollicular foci of B-cell proliferation – the medullary cords in lymph nodes – where they generate short-lived plasma cells. Other B cells migrate to follicles where they may form germinal centres. T cells, after a brief period of proliferation in the T zone, either leave the node as effector cells/recirculating memory T cells or migrate to follicles, where they proliferate further and participate in the selection of B cells that have mutated the immunoglobulin variable-region genes in germinal centres (see Figure 19.14). The consequences of this cognate T cell–B cell interaction are described in more detail in the text.

cell (FDC) network become filled with blasts. At this stage, changes occur whereby the classical germinal centre structures of dark and light zones develop. The dark zone is formed by the blasts moving to the edge of the FDC network next to the T zone. These blasts, now termed *centroblasts*, activate the somatic hypermutation mechanism that acts on their rearranged immunoglobulin V-region genes. Centroblasts continually give rise to *centrocytes*, non-dividing cells that migrate into the FDC

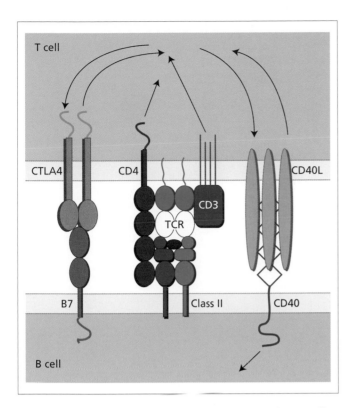

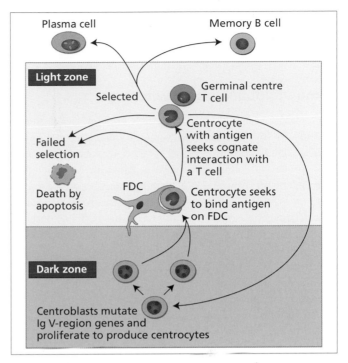

Figure 19.12 Surface molecules involved in T-dependent B-cell activation in T zones. B cells take up antigen that they bind specifically through their surface immunoglobulin. This is internalized, broken down to peptides and the peptides are presented on the B-cell surface, held in the peptide-binding grooves of MHC class II molecules (see Figure 19.3). Cross-linking of surface immunoglobulin by antigen induces the endocytosis of the antigen–antibody complex and signals upregulation of CD40 expression and *de novo* B7.1 and B7.2 expression. If this B cell interacts with a primed T cell that recognizes the peptide complex with class II MHC molecules, there will be costimulation through the molecule CD28, which is constitutively expressed by CD4 T cells, and this can result in further signalling through costimulatory molecules that are transiently expressed on the T-cell surface; CD40 ligand exemplifies these transiently expressed signalling molecules. These interactions can lead to B- and T-cell proliferation and differentiation and may also induce cytokine secretion by the cells. Cytokine receptor expression by the B cell and the T cell is initiated or upregulated. The arrows indicate that TCR engagement induces CD40 ligand expression and that engagement of these molecules by their counterstructures on the B cell delivers further signals to the T cell. CD40 ligation induces immunoglobulin class switching in the B cell and migration as indicated in Figure 19.11.

Figure 19.13 Selection of cells that have undergone immunoglobulin V-region gene hypermutation in germinal centres. The hypermutation mechanism is active in centroblasts, which are the rapidly dividing cells of the dark zone that give rise to centrocytes. Centrocytes die by apoptosis unless they (i) pick up and process antigen held on follicular dendritic cells (FDCs) and (ii) find a T cell in the germinal centre that recognizes the peptides from this antigen presented on centrocytes in association with self class II. The T cell-dependent selection mechanism makes it unlikely that centrocytes with mutated immunoglobulin V-region genes that encode self-reactive antibody will be selected. Most B cells that are selected leave the germinal centre to (i) migrate to distant sites of antibody production, the gut or bone marrow, where they differentiate to become plasma cells and (ii) differentiate into memory B cells. Some selected cells remain within the germinal centre and return to the dark zone as centroblasts.

network that forms the light zone of the germinal centre. Centrocytes either leave the light zone within 12 hours or die *in situ*. They can leave the light zone only if they receive antigen-specific selection signals (Figure 19.13).

Centrocytes pick up antigen from FDCs in order to process peptides for T-cell recognition. This requirement for the B cells to receive T-cell help in the germinal centre protects against potential autoimmune responses as those B cells that have developed reactivity against autoantigens are unlikely to receive selection signals from germinal centre T cells. Centrocytes that survive selection within germinal centres leave the light zone as either plasmablasts or memory B cells. The plasmablasts migrate to bone marrow or the lamina propria of the gut and differentiate into plasma cells.

Immunoglobulin class switching

Most plasma cells and memory B cells undergo *switch recombination* in which rearranged V-region genes become linked to heavy chain constant region genes downstream from IgD. This process is similar to immunoglobulin variable gene rearrangement, with the DNA forming loops between complementary switch region genes that lie upstream of each set of heavy chain gene exons. The order of the heavy chain constant-region genes that encode the different heavy chain isotypes is located downstream from the variable-region genes: μ, δ, $\gamma3$, $\gamma1$, a non-functional pseudo-ε gene, $\alpha1$, $\gamma2$, $\gamma4$, ε and $\alpha2$. Thus, switching to $\gamma2$ involves looping out μ, δ, $\gamma3$, $\gamma1$, pseudo-ε and $\alpha1$. Switch recombination within B cells is driven by cytokines produced following recognition by antigen-specific T cells, and variation in the distribution of immunoglobulin isotypes underlies disorders such as allergy in which there is excess IgE production.

Differentiation of primed T cells into effector cells

Following recognition of antigen, most CD8$^+$ T cells differentiate into cytotoxic effector cells. Differentiation of primed CD4$^+$ cells is directed into one of four major pathways (Figure 19.14) and it appears that factors such as the nature of the antigen, associated inflammatory stimuli and the affinity of T-cell engagement can influence the subtype of CD4 T cell that is produced. CD4$^+$ T cells stimulated in the presence of IL-12, which is produced by macrophages, and dendritic cells are more likely to differentiate into Th1 cells. IFN-γ secreted by NK cells or Th1 cells themselves has a similar effect, which is partly attributable to inhibition of differentiation towards Th2 cells. In contrast, IL-4 produced by either NKT cells or Th2 cells promotes production of Th2 cells and inhibits Th1 cell formation.

Th1 cells produce cytokines that are associated with macrophage activation, granuloma formation and delayed hypersensitivity. These cytokines are principally IL-2, IFN-γ and TNF-β. Macrophages work in concert with Th1 cells to provide a major mechanism by which mycobacteria and other pathogens are destroyed. Inflammatory CD4$^+$ T cells enhance this activity through the action of cytokines following recognition of peptides presented by MHC class II molecules on macrophages. Some Th1 cells have cytolytic potential and can kill infected macrophages through granzyme/perforin or Fas ligand.

Th2 cells produce cytokines associated with antibody production, particularly IL-4, IL-10 and, in some instances, IL-6,

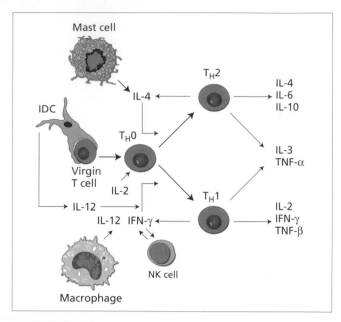

Figure 19.14 Maturation pathways of CD4$^+$ T helper cells. CD4$^+$ T cells that have been activated by antigen acquire the capacity to produce cytokines. The cytokines that they produce depends on the environment in which they are activated. Two major subsets of effector Th cell are recognized, Th1 and Th2 cells. The cytokines produced by Th1 cells tend to promote further Th1 cell formation and inhibit Th2 cell formation, and IL-4 produced by Th2 cells promotes further differentiation towards Th2 cells. Th1-promoting cytokines are also produced by activated macrophages, dendritic cells and NK cells, whereas mast cells produce IL-4. Th17 cells are an additional effector subset that is induced through the activity of IL-23 and produce large amounts of IL-17 and IL-22. T regulatory cells can be induced through the activity of transforming growth factor (TGF)-β and play an important role in the control of autoimmune responses. IDC, interdigitating dendritic cell.

although the last of these is mainly produced by macrophages and osteoclasts.

Th17 cells produce large amounts of the cytokine IL-17 and are associated with inflammatory disorders. They may play an important role in the control of fungal disease and could represent an important target for future immunotherapeutic interventions.

The balance between Th1 and Th2 cells can be an important determinant of immunopathology. Tuberculoid leprosy exemplifies apparent dominance of a Th1 response, while atopic disease seems to reflect an imbalance towards Th2. Nevertheless, manipulation of these cytokine networks provides a potential means of modifying established immune responses to avoid the complications associated with overactivity of either Th1 or Th2 cells.

Regulatory CD4⁺ T cells

Immunological tolerance is mediated by a number of mechanisms, including deletion of self-reactive B and T cells in the bone marrow and thymus respectively. In addition, it is now clear that a specialized population of T lymphocytes can actively suppress immune responses. These cells have been termed regulatory T (Treg) cells and their dominant phenotype is that of expression of the transcription factor FoxP3 in association with CD4. In addition, these cells usually express high levels of CD25, the IL-2 receptor α-chain, as well as low levels of CD127, a component of the IL-7 receptor. Treg cells are involved in maintenance of peripheral T-cell tolerance to self antigens and protection against autoimmunity. They constitute approximately 1–5% of peripheral blood CD4 lymphocytes and may be derived either from a discrete thymic lineage (natural Treg cells) or following the differentiation of CD4⁺CD25⁻ T cells in the presence of cytokines such as transforming growth factor (TGF)-β (induced Treg cells). The role of Treg cells in a range of human diseases is being explored at present and typically they are deficient, in either number or function, in autoimmune disorders while relative overactivity may be apparent in malignant disease. Immunotherapeutic strategies that involve cellular therapy with Treg cells, or which utilize reagents such as anti-CTLA-4 antibody to suppress their function, are now in clinical trial.

Cytokines and their classification

Cytokines are soluble proteins produced by leucocytes and other cells that influence the behaviour of cells that carry cytokine receptors. Many are secreted, but others, such as TNF-α, are cell membrane proteins that are active when bound to the cell that produced them but which also have activity as a soluble protein. The potency of cytokines *in vivo* has been exemplified clearly by the dramatic effects of recombinant granulocyte colony-stimulating factor (G-CSF) in inducing accelerated recovery of neutrophil counts after the administration of myelotoxic therapy and the effect of interferon alfa in the management of haematological malignancies. It seems likely that many cytokines act only at very short range and some appear to be more potent as membrane-bound forms than as released proteins. The families of cytokines are summarized in Table 19.4 and a fuller description of the known cytokines that act on cells of the immune system is given in Table 19.5.

Chemokines and their classification

Chemokines are a class of cytokines with chemoattractant properties and are all related in sequence. There are two groups, the CC chemokines, which have two adjacent cysteine residues in

Table 19.4 The cytokine and cytokine receptor families.

Cytokine family	Members of family	Type of receptor
β-Trefoil	IL-1α, IL-1β	Immunoglobulin family
Haematopoietins	IL-2, IL-3, IL-4, IL-5, IL-6, IL-7, IL-9, IL-13, IL-15, GM-CSF	Class I cytokine receptor
	IL-10, interferons	Class II cytokine receptor
Tumour necrosis factor	TNF-α, TNF-β	Nerve growth factor receptor family
Cysteine knot	NGF	Nerve growth factor receptor family
	TGF-β	Serine threonine kinase
Chemokines	IL-8, MIP-1α, MIP-1β, I-309, MCP-1, MCP-2, MCP-3, γIP-10	Rhodopsin family

their sequence, and the CXC chemokines, in which these two cysteine residues are separated by another amino acid. Chemokine receptors are integral membrane proteins linked to G-proteins and have seven membrane-spanning domains. They are classified according to the type of chemokine that they bind, i.e. CCR1–9 and CXCR1–5. Cells that express chemokine receptors are attracted towards an increasing concentration of chemokine molecules, and these interactions are critical to many functions of the innate and adaptive immune response (Table 19.6). Some chemokines are expressed in a constitutive fashion, whereas others are released in response to inflammation.

Interpretation of blood lymphocyte counts

Blood provides the most accessible view of the lymphoid system but it must be remembered that peripheral blood contains only around 2% of total body lymphocytes. The cells present in the blood are in transit and many are recirculating T and B lymphocytes that will pass rapidly into secondary lymphoid organs in less than 30 min.

The numbers of different lymphocyte subsets normally found in the blood in different age groups is given in Table 19.7. These numbers are derived from studies in which whole blood was labelled by fluorescent dye/monoclonal antibody conjugates, followed by red cell lysis and flow cytometry. When this method is used to measure the proportion of lymphocytes that belong to different subsets, much of the interlaboratory variation that

Table 19.5 The main cytokines that have been described as having activity on cells of the immune system.

Cytokine	Molecular family (molecular mass)	Cytokine produced by	Family and size of receptors	Receptors expressed by	Immunological actions
IL-1α	β-Trefoil (17.5 kDa)	Macrophage, epithelia	Immunoglobulin superfamily: type I (CD121a, 80 kDa), type I (CD121b, 60–68 kDa)	Very broad, including T, B and NK cells	Activates T, macrophage, is pyrogenic
IL-1β	β-Trefoil (17.3 kDa)	Macrophage, epithelia	As IL-1α	As IL-1α	Activates T, macrophage, is pyrogenic
IL-2 (TCGF)	Haematopoietin (15–20 kDa)	Th0 and Th1	CKR class I: α (CD25, 55 kDa) + β (CD122, 70–75 kDa) + γ_c (64 kDa)	Activated T, some B, NK, macrophage	Induces T growth and differentiation; also induces growth and differentiation of some B
IL-3 (multi-CSF)	Haematopoietin (14–30 kDa)	T, thymic epithelium	CKR class I: α (CD123, 70 kDa) + β_c (KH97, 120 kDa)	Haemopoietic, B, macrophage	Apart from effect on haemopoiesis, induces growth and differentiation of some B
IL-4	Haematopoietin (15–19 kDa)	Th2, mast, marrow stroma	CKR class I: α (CD124, 140 kDa) + γ_c	Activated B and some T, others	B growth, switch to IgG4 and IgE
IL-5	Haematopoietin (45 kDa)	T, mast, eosinophil	CKR class I: α (CD125, 60 kDa) + β_c	Eosinophil and basophil	Eosinophil growth and differentiation; growth and differentiation of mouse but not human B
IL-6	Haematopoietin (26 kDa)	T, macrophage, some B, osteoclast, others	CKR class I: CD126 (gp80) + CD130 (gp130)	Activated B, plasma, T, macrophage, others	Inflammatory; cytokine induces acute-phase reaction, plasmacytoma growth factor; influences T and B activity
IL-7	Haematopoietin (20–25 kDa)	Bone marrow and thymic stroma	CKR class I: CD127 (68 kDa) + γ_c	T and B progenitors, mature T	Pre-B and thymocyte growth, some action on mature T

IL-8	Chemokine (7 kDa)	Lymphocyte, macrophage, granulocyte, endothelia, others	Rhodopsin family: CDw128 (40 kDa)	Neutrophil, basophil, some lymphocyte	Chemoattractant neutrophil and basophil, inflammatory and angiogenic
IL-9	Haematopoietin (35 kDa)	Th2	CKR class I: IL-9R (64 kDa), may associate with γc	Th, macrophage	Growth T, erythroblast, mast and megakaryoblastic leukaemia lines
IL-10	Haematopoietin (35–40 kDa)	Th0, Th2, mφ	CKR class II (90–110 kDa)	B, T	Suppresses macrophage activation by Th1 and NK, with TGF-β induces B switch to IgA
IL-11	Haematopoietin? (23 kDa)	Fibroblasts	Unassigned: IL-11R (151 kDa)	Plasmacytoma, haemopoietic	Plasmacytoma, megakaryocyte and macrophage precursor growth factor
IL-12	Unassigned (35 + 40 kDa)	B, macrophage	CKR class I? IL-12R (180 kDa)	T, NK	Differentiation Th0 to Th1, promotes NK cytotoxic activity, induces IFN-γ secretion
IL-13	Haematopoietin (132 kDa)	T	CKR class I (IL-13R may share components with IL-4R)	?	Growth and differentiation of B; like IL-4, suppresses production of IL-1β, IL-6, TNF-α by activated macrophage
IL-14	Unassigned (60 kDa)	T, some B	Unassigned: IL-14R	B	B growth factor, inhibits immunoglobulin synthesis
IL-15	Probably haematopoietin (14 kDa)	Epithelial, macrophage	CKR class I: includes IL-2R β and γc but not CD25	?	Actions like IL-2
GM-CSF	Haematopoietin (22 kDa)	T cells, macrophage	CKR class I: α (CDw116) +βc	GM series, Langerhans, others	GM precursor growth and differentiation, some plasmablasts

Table 19.5 *Continued*

Cytokine	Molecular family (molecular mass)	Cytokine produced by	Family and size of receptors	Receptors expressed by	Immunological actions
IFN-γ	Haematopoietin (40–70 kDa)	T, NK	CKR class II: CDw119	Leucocyte, others	Macrophage and NK activation, expression MHC class I raised
IFN-α	Haematopoietin, many isoforms (16–21 kDa)	Leucocytes	CKR class II: complex includes CD118	Most cells	Growth, differentiation of some B, expression MHC class I raised
NGF	Cysteine knot (26 kDa)	Nervous system, prostate	NGFR (70–75 kDa)	Neurones, B, macrophage	Apart from role in nervous system, growth and differentiation B
TNF-α	TNF family (52 kDa)	Activated mφ, NK, T, B, fibroblast	NGF family: type I CD120a (gp55); type II CD120b (gp75)	Type I most cells, not resting T or red, type II haemopoietic	Induces apoptosis of some transformed cells synergizing with IFN-γ, inflammation, lymphocyte growth synergy with IL-6
TNF-β (lymphotoxin)	TNF family (soluble, 25 kDa)	Activated T and B	NGF family: as TNF-αRs		Induces apoptosis of some cells, inflammation, fibroblast growth factor
TGF-β	Cysteine knot (25 kDa × 2), there are three isoforms	Platelet, T, macrophage, others	Serine/threonine kinase: type I and II high affinity and type III low affinity (53, 65 and 250–350 kDa) act in concert	Most	Inhibits cell growth, involved in wound repair and bone remodelling

This list is not comprehensive and some of the information about the function of these molecules is based on studies *in vitro* that will not necessarily be found to be relevant to activity *in vivo*.

β_c and γ_c, common receptors shared by more than one of the class I cytokine receptor family; CKR, cytokine receptor family; CSF, colony-stimulating factor; 'growth', used to mean proliferation of cells; GM, granulocyte macrophage, IFN, interferon; IL, interleukin; NGF, nerve growth factor; R, receptor; TCGF, thymus cell growth factor; TGF, transforming growth factor; Th, helper T cell; TNF, tumour necrosis factor.
The word 'cell' has been omitted, e.g. T for T cell.

Table 19.6 The major chemokines within the CXC and CC subgroups.

Chemokine	Production	Receptors	Cells that are attracted	Effects
CXC subgroup				
IL-8	Monocytes	CXCR1	Neutrophils	Inflammation
	Macrophages	CXCR2	T cells	Angiogenesis
	Fibroblasts			
β-TG	Platelets	CXCR2	Neutrophils	Inflammation
GROα,β,γ	Monocytes	CXCR2	Neutrophils	Inflammation
	Endothelium		T cells	Angiogenesis
			Fibroblasts	
IP-10	Endothelium	CXCR3	T cells	Promotes Th1 immunity
	Monocytes		NK cells	Immunostimulation
	T cells		Monocytes	
	Fibroblasts			
SDF-1	Stromal cells	CXCR4	Stem cells	Stem cell homing
			Lymphocytes	Haemopoiesis
CC subgroup				
MIP-1α	Monocytes	CCR1, 3, 5	Monocytes	Th1 immunity
	T cells		NK and T cells	
	Fibroblasts		Dendritic cells	
MIP-1β	Monocytes	CCR1, 3, 5	Monocytes	Th immunity
	Macrophages		NK and T cells	
	Neutrophils		Dendritic cells	
	Endothelium			
MCP-1	Monocytes	CCR2B	Monocytes	Th2 immunity
	Macrophages		NK and T cells	
	Fibroblasts		Dendritic cells	
	Keratinocytes			
RANTES	T cells	CCR1, 3, 5	Monocytes	Inflammation
	Endothelium		NK and T cells	T-cell activation
	Platelets		Dendritic cells	
Eotaxin	Endothelium	CCR3	Eosinophils	Allergy
	Monocytes		Monocytes	
	Epithelium		T cells	

is observed in calculating absolute numbers of subsets can be attributed to the method of measuring the total white cell count and the percentage of lymphocytes. A wide range of results is to be expected between different individuals. The most consistent variation is seen in childhood, but from adolescence onwards age-related changes are small and there is also little difference in relation to ethnicity or gender.

Alteration of the lymphocyte count can result from an absolute change in the number of cells or alteration in the distribution of lymphocytes within tissues. Redistribution of lymphocytes accounts for much of the variation in lymphocyte subset numbers found in serial measurements within a healthy individual. Some of these changes in lymphocyte number follow a diurnal pattern, with peak levels at night and nadir in the

morning; accordingly, time of sampling should be taken into account.

Increased number of effector cells in the blood usually reflects an active immune response. Analysis of the phenotype of these effector cells provides some information on the type of immune response, especially in differentiating between cytotoxic and inflammatory CD4$^+$ T cells. Particularly in viral infections, this response may be of sufficient magnitude to cause a lymphocytosis. Some non-malignant causes of lymphocytosis are given in Table 19.8.

Redistribution of lymphocytes is probably the cause of the lymphocytosis seen in *Bordetella pertussis* infection. Although lymphocytosis is uncommon in bacterial infections, in children over the age of 6 months the second and third weeks of infection

Table 19.7 Normal ranges for lymphocyte subsets in the blood.*

Percentile	0–2 months		2–3 months		4–8 months		1–2 years		2–5 years		5–12 years		Adults	
	5	95	5	95	5	95	5	95	5	95	5	95	5	95
Total lymphocytes	3.2	8.5	2.9	8.8	3.6	8.8	2.2	8.3	2.4	5.8	1.8	5.8	1.0	3.4
CD3$^+$ (all αβ and γδ T cells)			2.1	6.5	2.3	6.5	1.5	5.4	1.6	4.2	0.9	2.6	0.6	2.5
CD4$^+$ (class II MHC-restricted αβ T cells)	1.2	5.3	1.4	5.6	1.4	5.7	1.0	3.6	0.9	2.9	0.5	1.4	0.35	1.5
CD8$^+$ (class I MHC-restricted αβ T cells, some γδ T cells and NK cells)			0.7	2.5	0.7	2.5	0.6	2.2	0.6	1.9	0.4	1.2	0.23	1.1
CD4/CD8 ratio	1.1	4.5	1.1	4.4	1.1	4.2	1.0	3.0	0.9	2.7			0.66	3.5
CD3$^-$CD57$^+$ or CD56$^+$ NK cells					0.3	0.7			0.2	0.6			0.2	0.7
CD19$^+$ or sκ$^+$ or sλ$^+$ total B cells					0.5	1.5			0.5	1.3			0.04	0.7

There is considerable variation in the normal ranges reported from different studies and this table is only intended to be illustrative.
*All values (except CD4/CD8 ratio) are ×10^9/L.

Table 19.8 Non-malignant causes of lymphocytosis.

Viral infections
Infectious lymphocytosis, infectious mononucleosis, cytomegalovirus infection; occasionally rubella, hepatitis, adenoviruses, varicella, HIV, human herpesvirus 6, mumps, chickenpox, dengue

Bacterial infections
Pertussis; occasionally healing tuberculosis, brucellosis, secondary and congenital syphilis, cat scratch fever, typhoid fever, diphtheria

Protozoal infections
Toxoplasmosis; occasionally malaria

Other conditions
Serum sickness, allergic drug reactions, splenectomy, dermatitis herpetiformis, metastatic melanoma, hyperthyroidism, congenital adrenal hyperplasia

with pertussis are usually associated with a lymphocytosis in excess of 10×10^9/L (in some cases $> 50 \times 10^9$/L). The lymphocytosis consists of small lymphocytes and is believed to be caused by a protein toxin from *B. pertussis* that prevents migration of lymphocytes across endothelium into tissue.

Acute infectious lymphocytosis is a benign disease, usually of children. In most cases there are no symptoms, but in some there is fever and in a small proportion gastrointestinal symp-

toms. Increase in the size of secondary lymphoid organs, anaemia and thrombocytopenia are rare. There is an increased number of small lymphocytes, persisting for 3–7 weeks, with an average peak level of $30–40 \times 10^9$/L. This is usually associated with an eosinophilia (average 2×10^9/L), but the aetiology of the condition is unknown.

Lymphopenia some lymphopenias predominantly reflect redistribution rather than a depletion of total body lymphocyte numbers. A dramatic short-term lymphopenia is induced by corticosteroids. This causes the retention of lymphocytes in secondary lymphoid organs but these are released again after about 2 days and the blood lymphocyte count returns to near-normal levels. Endogenous secretion of corticosteroids during acute illnesses may be partly responsible for the lymphopenias often seen in conditions such as heart failure or pneumonia. In many other conditions, lymphopenia reflects an increased rate of death of lymphocytes and/or a reduction in their rate of formation. Some of the causes of secondary lymphopenia are listed in Table 19.9. A normal absolute lymphocyte count can belie an underlying deficit of one or more lymphocyte subsets. This is often seen in HIV infection, when a severe deficit of CD4$^+$ T cells may be disguised by expansion of CD8$^+$ T cells.

Infectious mononucleosis

Infectious mononucleosis (IM) is caused by Epstein–Barr virus (EBV), which infects B lymphocytes. EBV enters B cells via CD21, a surface receptor for the C3d component of comple-

Table 19.9 Causes of secondary lymphopenia.

Infections
Influenza; occasionally other viral infections, colorado tick fever, miliary tuberculosis, pneumonia, septicaemia, malaria, HIV

Loss of lymphocytes
Intestinal lymphangiectasia, Whipple disease, severe right-sided heart failure, rarely inflammatory bowel disease, lymphatic fistula

Therapeutic procedures
Radiotherapy, anti-lymphocyte globulin, corticosteroids, cytotoxic drugs, purine analogues

Neoplastic conditions
Metastatic carcinoma, advanced Hodgkin disease

Nutritional/metabolic
B_{12} or folate deficiency, zinc deficiency, uraemia

Other conditions
Systemic lupus erythematosus and other collagen vascular diseases, myasthenia gravis, aplastic anaemia, graft-versus-host disease, pancreatic necrosis, sarcoidosis, idiopathic

ment. After the acute infection has been resolved, lifelong subclinical infection is maintained, with a low frequency of infected B cells and detectable virus in the saliva – a main vehicle for contagion.

EBV infection of children usually results in immunity without development of the typical clinical manifestations of IM. This immunity can be detected serologically and is associated with lifelong protection. Usually only after the age of 10 years is infection by EBV associated with the clinical manifestations of IM. In developing countries, the rate of seroconversion before the age of 10 years can be so high that clinically evident IM is rare. IM has its highest prevalence in young adults and a study of medical students showed that the syndrome was seen in 25% of individuals who underwent seroconversion. It is uncommon after the age of 30 years and rare after the age of 40 years. The determinants of clinical symptoms are unknown but may relate to host immunogenotype, viral load or viral polymorphisms.

Clinical features

The symptoms of IM usually develop abruptly, with fatigue, malaise and fever after an incubation period of up to 7 weeks. These symptoms last for about 3 weeks. Sore throat occurs in over 80% of cases and is usually accompanied by anorexia and nausea. The sore throat develops in the first week and subsides in the second week, rarely generating severe symptoms or massive tonsillar/pharyngeal oedema. Sharply defined red spots at the junction of the soft and hard palates are of diagnostic

value. Positive throat swabs for β-haemolytic streptococci are frequently found. Bilateral non-inflammatory cervical lymphadenopathy is almost invariable, and inguinal and axillary lymphadenopathy is usual. The spleen is palpable in more than half of cases, although only occasionally does it extend to the iliac crest. These secondary lymphoid organs increase in size in the first week and subside slowly after the second week. Slight hepatomegaly and jaundice occurs in about 10% of cases. Fever is present in most cases but of no characteristic type and may be transient. A few patients develop a fine macular rash, but rashes are more usually found as temporary reactions to penicillin and especially ampicillin.

Blood picture

In most patients, IM is associated with a leucocytosis; this peaks in the second and third weeks and usually persists for 1–2 months (the first week is occasionally associated with a leucopenia). In two-thirds of patients, the leucocytosis ranges from 10 to 20×10^9/L but in some cases may substantially exceed these levels. The leucocytosis is attributable to an absolute increase in numbers of both normal small lymphocytes and of activated T cells (atypical lymphocytes). Most of the activated cells are $CD8^+$ T cells but they also include $CD4^+$ T cells and $CD3^-$ NK cells. Most of these activated lymphocytes are cytotoxic for virus-infected cells and target viral peptides presented on MHC class I molecules. Although infection of B cells by EBV stimulates their proliferation, this appears to be controlled by the T-cell response such that the proportion of blood mononuclear cells that is EBV infected rarely exceeds 0.1%.

A peripheral neutrophilia may be seen early in the disease, but a neutropenia is equally common and eosinophilia is not unusual. Thrombocytopenia may occur and is occasionally severe. Anaemia is rare and then usually associated with anti-i antibodies. EBV infection may trigger a haemophagocytic syndrome in rare cases.

Serological changes

Three categories of antibody are produced as a result of EBV infection: virus specific, heterophile and autoimmune. The first virus-specific antibodies to appear are directed against the EBV capsid antigen (VCA). IgM anti-VCA antibodies probably develop during the incubation period and peak in the second week of the illness followed by a rapid decline. IgG anti-VCA antibodies peak in the second to third weeks and persist for life. Most patients also have a transient response to EBV early antigen (EA), which peaks in weeks 2–3. Antibodies to EBV nuclear antigen (EBNA) do not develop until some weeks into the illness but are present lifelong in all patients by 6 months. Serological diagnosis of acute IM is most accurately made by the presence of IgM anti-VCA and anti-EA antibodies and the absence of anti-EBNA antibodies.

Paul and Bunnell demonstrated that patients with IM have serum agglutinins directed against sheep erythrocytes (heterophile antibodies) and that a serum titre in excess of 1 : 112 is highly suggestive of IM. Similar agglutinins are found in low titre in healthy individuals (directed against Forssman antigen) and in some leukaemias and lymphomas as well as serum sickness. However, in these conditions the heterophile antibody can be absorbed onto guinea pig red cells. Formalin-treated horse erythrocytes appear to be agglutinated exclusively by heterophile antibodies of IM, and this forms the basis of the *Monospot test*. Heterophile antibodies provide the routine serological test for IM but are commonly negative, particularly in children and in patients over the age of 25 years. EBV-specific serodiagnostic tests should be applied in cases with strong clinical suspicion but negative heterophile antibodies. Total serum immunoglobulin levels increase around 4 weeks following onset of symptoms, and raised levels may persist for many months. The greatest proportional increase is in IgM, but IgG may also be raised. The specificity of most of these immunoglobulins is unknown but a variety of autoantibodies may be found, including cold-reactive anti-i antibodies, Donath–Landsteiner cold haemolysins and, occasionally, antibodies against smooth muscle, thyroid, stomach, rheumatoid factors and antinuclear antibodies.

Differential diagnosis and treatment

The diagnosis and course of IM are usually uncomplicated. Signs of significant respiratory, cardiovascular, intestinal, urinary or joint disease make consideration of other diseases mandatory; some of these other diseases are listed in Table 19.8. Perhaps the commonest problem is when the patient is heterophile antibody negative. In this situation, other viral infections, particularly cytomegalovirus (CMV), should be considered, with assay for CMV-specific IgM. Primary EBV infection is rare in older patients and there may not be conspicuous lymphadenopathy. Occasionally, the blood picture may raise the suspicion of a leukaemia, in which case immunophenotyping of the blood mononuclear cells may be appropriate. Persistent lymphadenopathy beyond a few weeks suggests the need for diagnostic biopsy, particularly if heterophile antibodies are negative, but the possibility of a false-positive Monospot test should also be considered. Virus-specific serology may be helpful in both these situations.

There is no specific therapy for IM. In patients with severe fever or lymphadenopathy, corticosteroids produce prompt lysis of fever and reduction of lymph node hyperplasia. Steroids may be indicated in management of associated haemolytic anaemia, thrombocytopenia, progressive neurological complications and incipient airway obstruction. Patients should be advised of the small risk of splenic rupture from minor abdominal trauma and contact sports should be avoided for several months.

X-linked lymphoproliferative syndrome (Duncan syndrome) is a rare inherited X-linked condition in which there is specific immunodeficiency against EBV. These individuals may die as a result of primary infection or the subsequent development of an EBV-driven B-cell lymphoma. Patients receiving immunosuppressive therapy for allografts and who are carriers of EBV can develop proliferations of B lymphocytes that carry the EBV genome. These cases of *post-transplant lymphoproliferative disease* are heterogeneous, and B-cell proliferations vary from a polyclonal diffuse B-cell hyperplasia to monoclonal B-cell lymphomas. There is evidence for a causal role of EBV in the development of Burkitt lymphoma, in association with both HIV infection and in the form endemic in African children. In less than 20% of sporadic cases of Burkitt lymphoma, EBV-associated DNA can be demonstrated in the lymphoma cells.

Secondary associations of infectious mononucleosis

In the 1950s it was reported that there was an increased incidence of Hodgkin lymphoma in individuals with a history of IM. Although the epidemiological challenges of confirming this association are profound, several very large studies have revealed

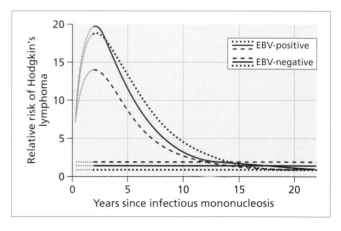

Figure 19.15 Relative risk of Epstein–Barr virus (EBV)-positive and EBV-negative Hodgkin lymphoma after infectious mononucleosis. Solid lines represent the relative risks of EBV-positive (blue) and EBV-negative (red) Hodgkin lymphoma, given that EBV status was determined in an unbiased way and that the missing data on viral status in 11 tumours were uninformative with respect to their true EBV status. Short dashed lines represent the relative risks of EBV-positive and EBV-negative Hodgkin lymphoma given that all tumours whose EBV status was unknown were EBV-positive. Long dashed lines represent the relative risks given that all tumours whose EBV status was unknown were EBV-negative. The analyses were restricted to the period 2 years or more after infectious mononucleosis. (From Hjalgrim *et al.* 2003 with permission.)

a definite association. Hjalgrim and colleagues studied 38 555 people with a confirmed diagnosis of IM and identified 29 cases of Hodgkin lymphoma, of which 16 had evidence of EBV. The study revealed a 4.1-fold increased risk of EBV-associated Hodgkin lymphoma in patients with a history of IM, with a median incubation time of just over 4 years to development of lymphoma (Figure 19.15).

IM is also associated with an increased risk of multiple sclerosis later in life. Thacker and colleagues have estimated this relative risk at 2.3 and this is likely to reflect the growing appreciation that EBV infection is associated with the pathogenesis of multiple sclerosis, although the mechanisms involved are unclear.

It is not yet clear whether individuals who suffer from IM carry a genetic predisposition to a variety of immunopathological disorders or if these secondary events are a direct consequence of the IM syndrome. However, these observations do offer important clues as to the pathogenesis of these important disorders.

Selected bibliography

General reading

Janeway CA, Travers P, Walport M et al. (2004) Immunobiology: The Immune System in Health and Disease, 6th edn. Current Biology, London.

Korn T, Bettelli E, Oukka M, Kuchroo VK (2009) IL-17 and Th17 cells. Annual Review of Immunology 27: 485–517.

Leucocyte molecules

Barclay AN, Birkland ML, Brown M (1998) The Leucocyte Antigen Facts Book. Academic Press, London.

Mason D (ed.) (2001) Leucocyte Typing VII. Oxford University Press, Oxford.

Infectious mononucleosis

Hjalgrim H, Askling J, Rostgaard K et al. (2003) Characteristics of Hodgkin's lymphoma after infectious mononucleosis. New England Journal of Medicine 349: 1324–1332.

Thacker EL, Mirzaei F, Ascherio A (2006) Infectious mononucleosis and risk for multiple sclerosis: a meta-analysis. Annals of Neurology 59: 499–503.

Clinical aspects of immunology

Chappel H, Haeny M (1994) Essentials of Clinical Immunology, 4th edn. Blackwell Scientific Publications, Oxford.

The spleen

20

Paul AH Moss

University of Birmingham, Birmingham, UK

The spleen has several important and diverse roles in homeostasis. Its normal functions are affected in a number of primary blood diseases as well as in other clinical disorders when its dysfunction can give rise to haematological abnormalities. These haematological effects are usually a minor phenomenon but in some cases may come to dominate the clinical presentation.

Evolution of the spleen

The spleen evolved around 500 million years ago with the appearance of the adaptive immune system between the origin of vertebrates and the development of the jawed vertebrates. It has undergone more functional and structural diversification than the thymus and this may reflect its varied physiological roles. The spleen shares a capsule of fibromuscular tissue in all animals and this extends inwards as a reticular network. The red pulp is present in all species but there have been marked changes in the anatomy of the white pulp and this is likely to reflect increasing sophistication of cellular immunity.

The spleen is derived from a condensation of mesenchymal cells that arise in the mesentery close to the pancreatic rudiment. The mesenchymal cells differentiate into reticulum cells, pluripotent stem cells and colony-forming units. Together with the liver, the spleen has a transient role in haemopoiesis from the third month, continuing until birth. From about 20 weeks the bone marrow becomes a site of haemopoiesis and this

Postgraduate Haematology: 6th edition. Edited by A. Victor Hoffbrand, Daniel Catovsky, Edward G.D. Tuddenham, Anthony R. Green
© 2011 Blackwell Publishing Ltd.

increases rapidly during the last trimester of pregnancy, whereas haemopoietic activity in the spleen disappears (Figure 20.1). There is no evidence for a specific inhibitor of haemopoiesis and the spleen remains a potential site for blood production in the adult, particularly for the maintenance of erythropoiesis. This occurs during pathological states and the development of such extramedullary haemopoiesis after birth is described below.

Structure and function

The major functions of the spleen are (i) filtration and 'quality control' of red cells within the circulation; (ii) capture and destruction of blood-borne pathogens; and (iii) generation of adaptive immune responses. In order to achieve these aims the spleen has evolved a unique anatomical structure that is based on the filtering of blood through two main systems. These constitute a white pulp, which is concerned mainly with immunological function, and a red pulp, which regulates the selection of red cells for re-entry into the circulation. A major feature is the presence of both 'open' and 'closed' circulatory systems and these are described in detail in the subsequent sections.

The spleen lies in the left hypochondrium with its long axis beneath the proximal half of the tenth rib. Its convex surface rests under the diaphragm whereas the visceral surface is in contact with the stomach and left kidney, with the tail of the pancreas reaching the hilum at the medial side. The normal spleen weighs about 150–250 g but there is considerable variation between normal individuals and at various ages in the same individual. At puberty it weighs about 200–300 g but after the age of 65 years this decreases to 100–150 g or less. In the adult

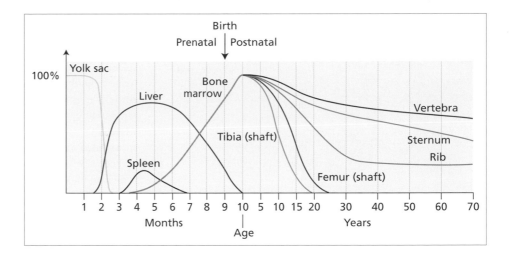

Figure 20.1 Site of erythropoietic tissue in fetus and throughout life.

its length is 8–13 cm, width 4.5–7.0 cm, surface area 45–80 cm² and volume less than 275 cm³. Interestingly, up to 10% of people have accessory spleens, normally as a single piece of tissue that can be found in a variety of sites either locally or more distantly in the abdomen. A spleen greater than 14 cm long is usually palpable (see later). It enlarges in a wide range of diseases and has been measured at up to a massive 2 kg or more in some blood disorders.

The spleen has a complicated structure and several different functions. Essentially, it is enclosed by a connective tissue framework that extends inwards to form a fibrous network. Blood enters at the pelvis and the majority of vessels open into these open networks (the *red pulp*) before re-entering the closed venous system. There is no afferent lymphatic to the spleen and the efferent lymphatic system leaves along the route of the splenic vein. The spleen contains a large amount of lymphatic tissue that is mostly concentrated in concentric rings around the arterioles (*white pulp*). Between the red pulp and white pulp is an *intermediate marginal zone*, which lies at the periphery of the white pulp, blending into the red pulp.

Splenic blood flow and the red pulp

The circulation within the spleen is illustrated in Figure 20.2. Blood is brought to the spleen via the splenic artery, which branches into the trabecular arteries and then arborizes in a pattern that lacks interarterial connections and thus effectively generates end arteries. The central arteries acquire a coaxial sheath of lymphocytes containing lymphoid follicles and this together constitutes the white pulp (see below). These central arteries then split into many arterioles and capillaries, some of which terminate in the white pulp while others go on to enter the red pulp.

In the red pulp there are two major forms of blood circulation: a *closed system*, typical of the rest of the vascular system, in which arteries and veins communicate through endothelial-lined vessels; and an *open circulation*, in which arterioles terminate in free endings on *splenic cords* (also known as the cords of Billroth) and from which cells must subsequently cross an endothelial layer to re-enter the circulation. The cords consist of a fibroblast-like reticular meshwork containing numerous macrophages and erythrocytes and they are critical to the filtration function of the spleen. Red cells in the cords need to gain entry to a venous sinus if they are to be allowed to re-enter the systemic circulation. The sinuses, 20–40 mm in diameter, are lined by endothelial and adventitial cells with a basement membrane and possess narrow interendothelial spaces in the sinus wall through which flexible red cells may pass. Red cells with inflexible membranes, mostly elderly, are not able to pass through these gaps and are ingested by macrophages in the cords. The great majority of blood flows in this unique open system and only a minority of arteries enter the sinuses and connect directly via the collecting vein to the trabecular vein in a typical vascular closed system.

There is thus both a rapid and a slow transit component in the splenic circulation. The rapid transit is of the order of 1–2 min, whereas the open circulation has a circulation time of 30–60 min or even longer. In normal subjects, the blood flows through the spleen as rapidly as through other organs, at a rate of about 5% of blood volume per minute, so that each day the blood has repeated passages through the spleen. During the flow, by a process called *plasma skimming*, the plasma and the leucocytes pass preferentially to the white pulp, while the red cells remain in the axial stream of the central artery. The passage of cells into the sinuses is controlled by their ability to squeeze through the interendothelial spaces, assisted by contraction of the reticular cells.

Blood pooling

The normal red cell content of the spleen is 30–70 mL, which represents less than 5% of the total red cell mass. When the

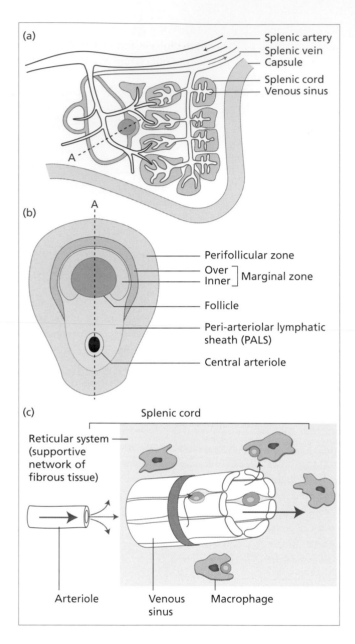

(a)
- Splenic artery
- Splenic vein
- Capsule
- Splenic cord
- Venous sinus

A

(b)
A
- Perifollicular zone
- Over
- Inner] Marginal zone
- Follicle
- Peri-arteriolar lymphatic sheath (PALS)
- Central arteriole

(c)
Splenic cord
- Reticular system (supportive network of fibrous tissue)
- Arteriole
- Venous sinus
- Macrophage

Figure 20.2 The vascular and lymphatic organization of the spleen. (a) Schematic representation of blood flow in the spleen. Blood enters through the splenic artery and then breaks up into splenic arterioles. The white pulp is an aggregation of lymphoid tissue around these vessels. The arterioles then open into splenic cords lined with macrophages. Blood must then re-enter the circulation by passing into a venous sinus. (b) Cross-section of white pulp at section A–B in (a). The central arteriole is surrounded a periarteriolar lymphoid sheath of T lymphocytes and occasional follicles that are rich in B cells. The marginal zone is divided into an inner and outer zone around which there is a large perifollicular zone. (c) Schematic representation of the organization of the red pulp. Blood cells are released by a splenic arteriole into a reticulum-lined splenic cord. Red cells that have flexible membranes are able to gain entry into the venous sinus by passing through gaps in the endothelial lining. Cells that are unable to achieve this are 'filtered' from the blood through ingestion by macrophages. (Adapted from Mebius & Kraal 2005 with permission.)

spleen is enlarged, expansion of the vascular bed occurs. This results in a considerable pool with a high haematocrit and only a slow exchange of red cells with the general circulation. In states of massive hypersplenism, such as myelofibrosis, as much as 40% of the red cell mass may be pooled in the spleen. This pooling will functionally exclude a relatively large volume of red cells from the main arteriovenous circulation, and thus be an important cause of anaemia. In such cases, it should be noted that the red cell mass, as measured by a radionuclide labelling technique, may give a misleadingly normal result, whereas the peripheral blood packed cell volume will give a more reliable measurement of the effectively circulating red cell mass. In

splenomegaly due to cellular infiltration, the pool is less prominent. Conversely, in the congestive splenomegaly of portal hypertension, spleen size with an increased red cell pool is a dominant feature.

The normal spleen contains a reservoir of granulocytes that is in dynamic equilibrium with the circulating granulocytes. It represents 30–50% of the total marginating pool, with a mean transit time through the spleen of about 10 min. Splenic sequestration of granulocytes is thought to be responsible for the neutropenia that often occurs in patients with splenomegaly. Platelets have also been shown to have a significant reservoir in the spleen and are rapidly interchangeable with the circulation. In normal subjects 20–40% of the total platelet mass is pooled in the spleen and the platelets spend up to one-third of their lifespan there. The pool increases when the spleen is enlarged. This pooling and temporary sequestration must be distinguished from the destruction of platelets in the spleen that occurs in many cases of thrombocytopenia.

There is no evidence that the normal spleen is involved in the regulation of plasma volume but splenomegaly is frequently associated with an increased plasma volume that may lead to a dilutional pseudo-anaemia. The mechanism of this effect is uncertain but may include expansion to fill the additional intravascular space, activation of neurohumoral regulation, or protein alterations resulting in an change in colloid cellular osmotic pressure. The clinical importance is that in splenomegaly the blood count may give an exaggerated impression of anaemia and measurement of red cell and plasma volumes can be valuable.

Role of the spleen in ensuring quality control of red cells

The spleen is the body's largest filter of blood and a major function of the spleen is the quality control of red cells. Red cells are normally flexible, whereas cells with abnormal membranes, or those with inclusions that render them relatively inflexible, remain in the cords where they either become conditioned for later transit or are destroyed. *Sequestration* is a reversible process whereby cells are temporarily trapped by adhesion to the reticular meshwork of the cords on their passage through the spleen. Phagocytosis is the irreversible uptake by macrophages of particulate matter, non-viable cells and viable cells that have been damaged by prolonged sequestration or by antibody coating.

In the presence of metabolically active macrophages, the densely packed red cells are deprived of oxygen and glucose. This stress increases membrane rigidity and reduces the natural deformability of the biconcave cell. This effect is particularly marked if there is an underlying abnormality of the red cell metabolic system, if cells are coated with antibody or if they are fragmented or misshapen in other ways. In these situations they remain trapped in the cord space and undergo phagocytosis. Siderotic granules, Howell–Jolly (DNA) bodies, nuclear remnants and Heinz bodies are removed by culling or pitting during temporary sequestration. After removal of the inclusions the red cells return to the circulation. Reticulocytes may be retained in the splenic cords for a considerable proportion of the 2–3 days of their maturation period and during this time they lose their intracellular inclusions, alter the lipid composition of their surface and become smaller in size. It is not clear whether the spleen has any special role in the removal of normal aged red cells and it seems more likely that such cells are removed by the general reticuloendothelial system, which includes both the spleen and the bone marrow.

Immunological function

The spleen is the largest single accumulation of lymphoid tissue in the body and is estimated to contain 25% of the T-lymphocyte pool and 10–15% of the B-lymphocyte pool. T cells, mainly of the CD4$^+$ subtype, are found predominantly in the periarteriolar lymphatic sheath, whereas B cells are located in the follicles and marginal zones of the white pulp. There is also an abundance of macrophages and dendritic cells and the architecture is maintained through a complex anatomical organization that includes a tubular conduit system that transports a range of chemokines and other molecules. The spleen has a unique role in acting as an immunological filter for the bloodstream. Lymphocytes and dendritic cells enter the splenic tissue by initial entry into the marginal zone, and from there can pass into the periarteriolar lymphatic sheath by crossing a lining of sinus cells. There is a constant flow of both T and B cells through the spleen, with T cells typically staying in the spleen for a few hours whereas B cells stay in the follicle and marginal zone for prolonged periods. At present it is not certain how lymphocytes exit the white pulp.

One interesting feature of the immunological function of the spleen is that it is able to act as an important site for both innate and adaptive immune responses. The marginal zone acts as the site for both of these processes, whereas the white pulp is restricted to adaptive immunity. Blood is filtered directly into the marginal zone and here the predominant cell populations are macrophages and marginal-zone B cells. The macrophages express a range of pattern-recognition receptors that recognize bacterial molecules such as lipopolysaccharide, as well as proteins such as SIGNR1 and MARCO that bind directly to both bacteria and viruses. These cells thus act as an important filter for the clearance of blood-borne pathogens. The marginal-zone B cells are a unique B-cell subset that bridges the innate and adaptive immune responses. They are able to recognize bacterial pathogens without the help of T cells and this T-independent antibody response consists largely of low-affinity IgM and can play an important role in limiting bacterial replication. In addition, these B cells can act as antigen presenting cells and are able to migrate to the periarteriolar lymphatic sheath where they present antigen to T cells and facilitate the production of high-affinity IgG antibody. B-cell maturation and clonal expansion occurs in the follicles and plasmablasts, and plasma cells subsequently migrate to the red pulp where they are retained through their expression of CXCR4, which binds to CXCL12 in red pulp tissue.

The T-cell-independent antibody response produces a spectrum of low-affinity IgM antibody clones that provide a first line of immune defence against bacterial sepsis, especially from *Streptococcus pneumoniae*, *Haemophilus influenzae* type b and *Neisseria meningitidis*. The spleen also appears to act as a defence against viral infections and intraerythrocyte parasitic infections such as *Plasmodium* and *Babesia*. The singular role of the spleen in this regard is shown in the immunization of splenectomized individuals with T-independent antigens and in this case antibody titres are typically only 10% of those seen in control subjects.

Given these unique features it is perhaps no surprise that splenectomy is associated with a degree of relative immunosuppression. This deficiency is not profound but there is a small but definite increase in susceptibility to infection with encapsulated bacterial species.

Extramedullary haemopoiesis

As indicated above, the spleen is an important site of haemopoiesis *in utero* and retains the ability to reactivate this process after birth. This can occur as a compensatory erythroblastic hyperplasia in severe anaemia, such as chronic haemolysis, megaloblastic anaemia and thalassaemia major, or as a more generalized haemopoiesis often seen in myelofibrosis or other malignant disorders in the bone marrow. The mechanisms involved in this extramedullary haemopoiesis are poorly understood. It is not clear if pluripotent stem cells are present in the spleen or migrate from the bone marrow. It is even conceivable that changes in the stroma or primary haemopoietic cells that arise due to the underlying pathological process are involved in favouring initiation of the haemopoietic process.

Splenomegaly and hypersplenism

Spleen size

An enlarged spleen is a frequent and important clinical sign. It is thus essential to have a reliable picture of the presence and extent of splenomegaly. In the adult, an enlarged spleen is usually palpable when its length exceeds 14 cm. However, the measurement of spleen size by means of a physical examination of the abdomen is unreliable, as minor enlargement is often undetected by palpation and even a grossly enlarged spleen may be missed in an obese person. Conversely, a lax phrenic–colic ligament or loss of tone of the abdominal wall may give rise to a 'wandering spleen' which will be palpable, as will one that is pushed downwards by a flattened diaphragm in obstructive airways disease.

Reliable information is obtained by radiology through ultrasonic imaging, magnetic resonance imaging (MRI) and computed tomography (CT), all of which give an accurate representation of the anatomy of the spleen and its position in relation to adjacent organs (Figure 20.3). PET-CT may be used to detect tumours, e.g. lymphoma in the spleen (Figure 20.3c). Another method of scanning the spleen is by means of a scintillation camera following radiolabelling of red cells with ^{51}Cr, ^{111}In or ^{99m}Tc (Figure 20.4). Although laborious, it does provide information on the functional size of the spleen, and functional asplenia or atrophy is well demonstrated by this procedure. It is also useful in identifying abnormally positioned and accessory splenic tissue. It is, however, not widely available.

Pathological basis of splenomegaly

Most of the clinical interest in splenomegaly is related to the secondary effects or the underlying aetiology. However, the pathological basis of enlargement can be of value to the histopathologist and may prove valuable in making a diagnosis:

1 reactive increase of white pulp in inflammation and infection;

2 congestive expansion of the red pulp compartment;

3 increased blood pool;

4 increased macrophage function;

5 proliferative cellular infiltration;

6 extramedullary haemopoiesis;

7 storage disease;

8 cysts;

9 solid tumours.

As examples, the characteristic feature of autoimmune red cell haemolysis is intrasinusoidal red cell phagocytosis, whereas hereditary spherocytosis demonstrates red cell sequestration.

Causes of splenomegaly

Splenomegaly is a frequent and important clinical sign. The diseases in which it occurs are listed in Table 20.1. The relative incidence of each cause of splenomegaly is subject to geographical variation. In Western countries, leukaemia and lymphomas, myeloproliferative disorders, haemolytic anaemias, glandular fever and portal hypertension account for most cases. In tropical countries, however, the incidence of these haematological causes of splenomegaly is overtaken by the preponderance of splenic enlargement caused by the parasitic tropical infections: malaria, leishmaniasis and schistosomiasis.

Specific causes of splenomegaly

Malaria

Malaria demonstrates how several pathogenetic mechanisms may be involved in splenomegaly. There are reactive lymphoid changes and the red pulp sinuses dilate with expanded phagocytic activity. The tropical splenomegaly syndrome, associated with recurrent malaria, is particularly common in New Guinea and Central Africa.

Haemoglobin disorders

Splenomegaly is associated with HbC disease in West Africa, with HbE disease in the Far East and with thalassaemia syndromes, which have a wide distribution throughout the tropics. HbSS sickle cell disease is usually associated with splenic atrophy, but the spleen usually remains enlarged in adults with HbS/C and HbS/β-thalassaemia syndromes.

Malignant haematological disorders

In primary proliferative polycythaemia, the increase in spleen size is mainly due to vascularity, with expansion of the red pulp and an increased red cell pool. In myelofibrosis, the red cell pool is remarkably increased and the spleen size is further augmented by myeloid metaplasia and expansion of the reticular elements. In contrast, in chronic myeloid leukaemia and lymphoproliferative disorders the increase in size is attributed mainly to cellular infiltration, while vascularity and red cell pooling have only a minor influence.

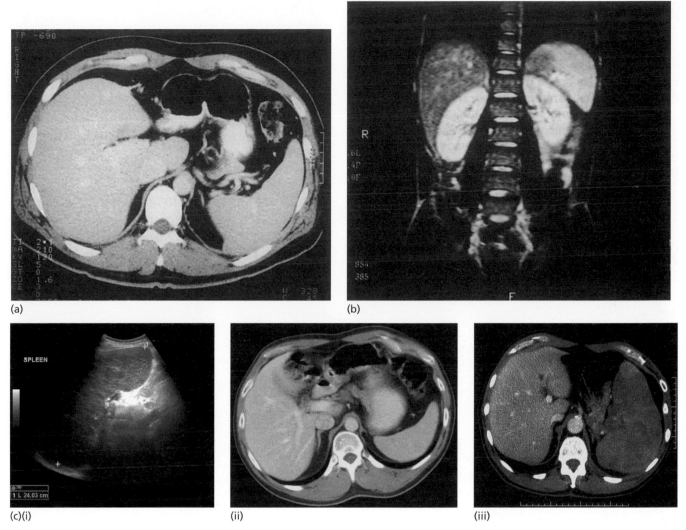

Figure 20.3 Imaging of the spleen by various methods. (a) CT: transverse section showing liver (left) and spleen (right). (b) MRI: coronal (longitudinal) section showing liver, spleen and kidneys. (c, i) Ultrasound of spleen showing splenomegaly (15.3 cm). (ii) Normal spleen (10 cm) on computed tomography (CT) scan. (iii) CT scan: the spleen is enlarged and shows multiple low density areas. A diagnosis of diffuse large cell B lymphoma was made histologically after splenectomy. (d) Ultrasound scan of enlarged spleen. (Figures (c, i) and (c, ii) courtesy of Dr T. Ogunremi).

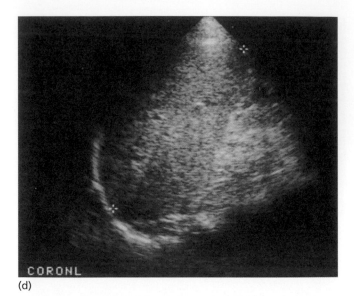

(d)

Figure 20.3 *Continued*

Primary splenic tumours

Primary splenic tumours are rare. Metastatic carcinoma, such as from the breast or lung, is also a rare event.

Portal hypertension

This may be both a cause and a consequence of splenomegaly. In a spleen that is massively enlarged from any cause, the huge increase in blood flow can lead to an increased portal pressure that leads to back-pressure on the spleen and a spiral of compression leading to widening and fibrosis of the red pulp cords. On the other hand, portal vein obstruction due to liver disease can also enlarge and damage the spleen.

Hypersplenism

Hypersplenism is a clinical syndrome and does not imply a specific causal mechanism. It has the following characteristic features:
1 enlargement of the spleen;
2 reduction in one or more of the cell lines in the peripheral blood;
3 normal or hyperplastic cellularity of the bone marrow;
4 premature release of cells into peripheral blood, resulting in reticulocytosis and/or large immature platelets;
5 increased splenic red cell pool, decreased red cell survival and increased splenic pooling of platelets with shortening of their lifespan.

It is not possible to determine all these criteria in each case and the diagnosis of hypersplenism is ultimately confirmed by the response to splenectomy. Most of the diseases listed in Table 20.1 can give rise to secondary hypersplenism. In these conditions, the haematological features of hypersplenism may be obscured or dominated by the primary disease, especially if it

Table 20.1 Causes of splenomegaly.

Haematological
Acute leukaemia
Chronic myeloid leukaemia*
Chronic lymphocytic leukaemia
Malignant lymphomas (some cases present as 'non-tropical primary splenomegaly')*
Chronic (primary) myelofibrosis*
Polycythaemia vera
Essential thrombocythaemia (some cases)
Hairy cell leukaemia*
Gaucher disease*, Niemann–Pick disease, Langerhans cell histiocytosis X*
Primary splenic hyperplasia
  'Non-tropical splenomegaly'
  Splenic anaemia/neutropenia
Thalassaemia
Sickle-cell disease, HbSC disease and other haemoglobinopathies
Haemolytic anaemias
Acute anaemia (rare)
Megaloblastic anaemia (rare)

Systemic
Acute infections: septicaemia, typhoid, infectious mononucleosis, cytomegalovirus
Subacute and chronic infections: tuberculosis, syphilis, brucellosis, subacute bacterial endocarditis, AIDS
Tropical parasitic infections (tropical splenomegaly*): malaria*, leishmaniasis*, schistosomiasis*, trypanosomiasis
Collagen diseases: systemic lupus erythematosus, rheumatoid arthritis (Felty)
Sarcoidosis
Amyloidosis
Cysts
Haemangiomas
Carcinoma (rare)
Congestive splenomegaly
  Portal hypertension
  Cirrhosis
  Splenic/portal/hepatic vein obstruction
  Congestive cardiac failure

*Common causes of splenomegaly.

involves the marrow. Hypersplenism also occurs rarely as a primary event, due to an unknown pathogenetic stimulus, and is sometimes termed *primary splenic hyperplasia*.

Splenectomy

Surgical excision of the spleen has been a standard treatment for the diagnosis and management of a number of disorders associated with an enlarged or hyperactive spleen and also when an otherwise normal spleen mediates the clinical problems associated with an extrasplenic defect such as hereditary spherocytosis or autoimmune acquired haemolytic anaemia. Splenic rupture may also occur from trauma, glandular fever or, rarely, use of colony-stimulating factors such as G-CSF. Splenectomy may also be valuable in making the diagnosis of organomegaly and can bring about significant disease control in some malignant conditions, such as splenic marginal zone lymphoma, where the bulk of the tumour population is located in the spleen. Finally, the spleen is often removed incidentally as part of another surgical procedure. At a surgical level, laparoscopic splenectomy has become the treatment of choice in the absence of portal hypertension or significant medical comorbidity.

Concern about the risks of sepsis after splenectomy in both children and adults has led to a search for alternative procedures for controlling hypersplenism while preserving some degree of splenic function. These include (i) partial arterial embolization; (ii) partial surgical amputation in selected patients in whom some splenic function may be preserved; (iii) localized irradiation; and (iv) immunosuppressive and cytotoxic drugs.

The role of splenectomy in individual diseases is discussed in the relevant chapters but when splenectomy is contemplated for any reason, the preoperative evaluation of the patient requires close cooperation between the surgeon and the haematologist. Vaccinations should be performed and it is valuable to check liver function, obtain appropriate imaging and potentially evaluate the hepatic and portal blood flow by Doppler ultrasound examination.

Complications of splenectomy

Immediate postoperative complications
These are dominated by bleeding, particularly when there is thrombocytopenia and subphrenic abscess. Haemorrhage usually comes from the peritoneal and diaphragmatic surfaces rather than from identifiable blood vessels. Frequently, no specific bleeding source is found at reoperation. The incidence of subphrenic abscess is variable, and appears more likely to occur when adjacent organs are injured either by trauma or during surgery. Infection is also liable to occur following embolization.

Delayed complications
These include overwhelming post-splenectomy infection and a tendency to develop thrombocytosis with a risk of thromboembolic incidents.

Thrombocytosis
In the immediate postoperative period in uncomplicated splenectomy patients, the platelet count rises steeply to a maximum of usually $600-1000 \times 10^9/L$, with a peak at 7–12 days. In a number of patients, the thrombocytosis persists indefinitely after splenectomy. This usually appears to be a consequence of continuing anaemia with a hyperplastic marrow; an inverse relationship exists between the severity of the anaemia and the height of the platelet count. Although a reactive thrombocytosis is not usually associated with thromboembolic problems, the high platelet count may have contributed to the serious and sometimes fatal episodes of pulmonary embolism that have occurred following splenectomy. Mesenteric infarction secondary to portal vein occlusion is more common in patients with myeloproliferative disorders who undergo splenectomy. Postoperative prophylaxis with heparin is usually needed. It is advisable to give antiplatelet therapy (e.g. aspirin 75 mg daily) as long as thrombocytosis is present.

Overwhelming postoperative infection
This may occur in adults as well as in children but it is in children, especially in the first few years of life, that splenectomy is more frequently associated with overwhelming bacterial infections. *Streptococcus pneumoniae* is the most common cause of infection but while *H. influenzae* type B, *N. meningitidis*, *E. coli* and *Pseudomonas* are much less common, they are also associated with serious infection. Death is usually due to septicaemia or meningitis and typically occurs within 5 days of the onset of infection. The vulnerability of young children and their dependence on the spleen to deal with blood-borne infection can be explained by the general immaturity of their lymphoreticular systems. In the absence of the spleen, the defective reticuloendothelial clearance of an encapsulated rapidly growing organism such as pneumococcus may lead to a dangerous bloodstream concentration in too short a time for immunological defence to be mounted. Splenectomy should therefore be postponed until after the age of 5 wherever possible.

When splenectomy is being planned, the patient should be immunized against pneumococcal pneumonia, *H. influenzae* type B (HIB) and meningococcal infection. However, while pneumococcal vaccine contains antigens to a number of strains of *Streptococcus pneumoniae*, it does not give complete protection because some strains are not covered and antibody response to the different antigens is variable. To obtain the maximum immune response, patients should, if possible, be immunized 2–3 months before splenectomy, and a booster dose should be given 5 years later. Most children will have received HIB vaccine but this should be checked; booster doses are not necessary for those who received the full course of three injections. Meningococcal vaccines are effective against types A and C but not against type B, the most prevalent in the West. The patient should also receive meningococcal C conjugate vaccine at a 6-month interval as this gives a higher and more lasting immunization against type C organism. Influenza vaccine is also recommended for asplenic or hyposplenic patients.

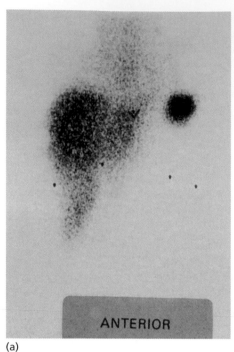
(a)

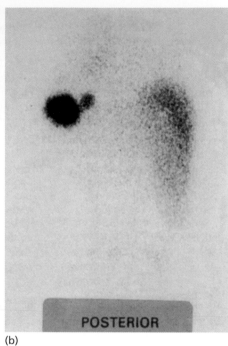
(b)

Figure 20.4 Demonstration of residual splenunculus by a scan of heat-damaged isotope-labelled red cells: (a) anterior view; (b) posterior view. Uptake is predominantly in the liver.

Postoperatively, lifelong prophylactic antibiotics should be advocated in all cases but if this is not possible, antibiotics should be administered at least for the first 2 years after splenectomy for all children up to 16 and when there is underlying impaired immune function. Oral penicillin 250 mg b.d. is usually recommended and patients who are allergic to penicillin should be offered erythromycin 250 mg b.d. When away from home, patients not allergic to penicillin should take a supply of amoxicillin to be used immediately if infective symptoms (pyrexia, malaise, shivering) develop; penicillin-sensitive patients should increase their dose of erythromycin or change to a broader-spectrum preparation. In all such cases, the patient should seek immediate medical help. When travelling to tropical areas, asplenic patients should be advised of the increased risk of severe *Plasmodium* infection and must adhere scrupulously to antimalarial prophylaxis. *Neisseria meningitidis* and *H. influenzae* type B vaccines are also recommended for those travelling abroad. Education of patients or parents is perhaps the most important aspect of management to ensure that they are alert to the possibility of infection and know how to react appropriately. A card indicating that a splenectomy has been carried out should be carried.

Recurrence of symptoms

Accessory splenic tissue may be overlooked at operation; after splenectomy, it may enlarge and cause a recurrence of the symptoms for which the original operation was carried out. The haematological features of hyposplenism (see below) such as Howell–Jolly bodies and increased pitting may be absent; CT or radionuclide scanning (Figure 20.4) will demonstrate the presence of a 'splenunculus' and identify its location for subsequent surgical removal should this be required.

Hyposplenism

Hyposplenism (excluding that induced by medical or surgical intervention) occurs in a wide range of conditions. In some disorders such as sickle cell disease, gluten-induced enteropathy (coeliac syndrome) and dermatitis herpetiformis, hyposplenism occurs frequently; it is seen less frequently in Crohn's disease, ulcerative colitis and essential thrombocythaemia, and it occurs only occasionally in the other conditions listed in Table 20.2. Congenital absence of the spleen is rare and may be associated with organ transposition and with severe malformations of the heart and lungs.

After the age of 65–70 years there is evidence of a decrease in splenic function. In old age, there is a rapid decrease in the weight of the spleen, together with increasing atherosclerotic vascular obstruction and fibrosis.

Patients with functional hyposplenism have impaired immunity to blood-borne bacterial and protozoal infections, and persistent thrombocytosis. Management is similar to that required after splenectomy. It includes prophylactic antibiotics and vaccines (see above) and advice to the patient to seek medical attention immediately in the event of illness or fever. Antiplatelet therapy is advisable when the platelet count is high.

Table 20.2 Causes of hyposplenism.

Congenital aplasia syndrome
Ageing
Haematological disorders
    Sickle cell disease
    Thrombocythaemia
    Myelofibrosis
    Malaria
    Lymphomas
Circulatory
    Splenic arterial/venous thrombosis
Autoimmune disease
    Systemic lupus erythematosus
    Rheumatoid arthritis
    Hyperthroidism
    Sarcoidosis
    Chronic graft-versus-host disease
    Combined immunodeficiency
Gastrointestinal (? immune basis)
    Gluten-induced enteropathy
    Dermatitis herpetiformis
    Crohn's disease
    Ulcerative colitis
    Tropical sprue
Infiltrations
    Lymphomas
    Sézary syndrome
    Myelomatosis
    Amyloidosis
    Secondary carcinomas, especially breast
    Cysts, e.g. hydatid
Nephrotic syndrome
Drugs
    Methyldopa
    Intravenous gammaglobulin
    Corticosteroids
Irradiation
Splenectomy and splenic embolization

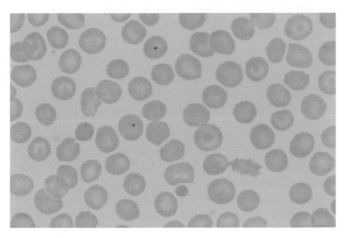

Figure 20.5 Blood film showing features of hyposplenism: Howell–Jolly bodies, target cells and contracted cells.

thocytic forms are also a feature (Figure 20.5). There is usually an increase in the number of reticulocytes in the circulation and occasionally isolated erythroblasts are seen. However, there is no alteration in red cell survival.

Because the number of cells with siderotic granules that enter the circulation is related to the sideroblastic percentage in the bone marrow, the siderocyte count in the peripheral blood is increased in haemolytic anaemias, thalassaemia and sideroblastic anaemia. The number of Howell–Jolly bodies is also variable and is most marked in conditions characterized by dyserythropoiesis. Other red cell inclusions may be prominent in the hyposplenic state: Heinz bodies are found following oxidative injury by drugs and in patients who have glucose-6-phosphate dehydrogenase deficiency or an unstable haemoglobin; precipitated β-chains are found in α-thalassaemia; and crystalline deposits of haemoglobin C in HbC disease.

Leucocyte changes

After splenectomy, there is a rise in the total leucocyte count. A neutrophil leucocytosis in the immediate postoperative period is later replaced by a significant and permanent increase in both lymphocytes and monocytes. Usually the total white cell count stabilizes at between 10 and 15×10^9/L but occasionally it may rise to twice this level. Minor increases in blood eosinophils and basophils have been noted after splenectomy but this is not a regular feature.

In response to infection, splenectomized subjects produce a much greater leucocytosis than persons with intact spleens. Often there is a marked left shift in the differential leucocyte count, with myelocytes and occasionally more primitive cells.

Platelet changes

As indicated above, the thrombocytosis after splenectomy is usually transitory and falls to normal or near-normal values over the following 1–2 months. However, even if the platelet

Haematological effects of splenectomy or splenic atrophy

Characteristic blood changes occur following splenectomy. Similar changes are seen with atrophy of the spleen to less than 20% of normal size and when there is functional asplenia, with or without reduction in the size of the organ.

Red cell changes

The changes in red cell morphology include the presence of Howell–Jolly bodies, siderotic granules and target cells. In a proportion of subjects, irregularly contracted or crenated acan-

count has returned to normal values, occasional large and bizarre platelets can be seen in the blood films of many splenectomized subjects. Their presence suggests that these particular platelets are normally removed by the spleen.

Immunological effects

The spleen plays an important role in immunoglobin synthesis; a fall in the IgM fraction of the serum immunoglobulins is commonly found after splenectomy. IgG levels do not change while IgA and IgE increase. The removal of an organ with a unique ability to recognize and phagocytose circulating particulate antigens would be expected to have serious consequences. Despite this, splenectomy in adults without complicating disease is not usually associated with a substantially increased incidence of infection. It must be assumed therefore that an increase in activity of other lymphoreticular organs compensates for any defects in the immunological defence mechanisms that result from this operation.

Acknowledgement

This chapter was modified from the text prepared by Mitchell Lewis for the fifth edition of *Postgraduate Haematology* and his contribution is gratefully acknowledged.

Selected bibliography

Amlot PL, Hayes AE (1985) Impaired human antibody response to the thymus-independent antigen, DNP-Ficoll, after splenectomy. Implications for post-splenectomy infections. *Lancet* **i**: 1008–11.

Bratosin D, Mazurier J, Tissier JP *et al.* (1998) Cellular and molecular mechanisms of senescent erythrocyte phagocytosis by macrophages. *Biochimie* **80**: 173–95.

Brendolan A, Rosado MM, Carsetti R, Selleri L, Dear TN (2007) Development and function of the mammalian spleen. *Bioessays* **29**: 166–77.

Cadili A, de Gara C (2008) Complications of splenectomy. *American Journal of Medicine* **121**: 371–5.

Corazzo R, Bullen AW, Hall R *et al.* (1981) Simple method of assessing splenic function in coeliac disease. *Clinical Science* **60**: 109–13.

Crane CG (1981) Tropical splenomegaly. Part 2: Oceania. *Clinics in Haematology* **10**: 976–82.

Davies JM, Barnes R, Mulligan D (2002) Update of guidelines for the prevention and treatment of infection in patients with an absent or dysfunctional spleen. British Committee for Standards in Haematology Working Party of the Haematology/Oncology Task Force. *Clinical Medicine* **2**: 440–3.

Ebaugh FG Jr, McIntyre OR (1979) Palpable spleens: ten-year follow-up. *Annals of Internal Medicine* **90**: 130–1.

Fakunle YM (1981) Tropical splenomegaly. Part 1: Tropical Africa. *Clinics in Haematology* **10**: 963–75.

Giebink GS (2001) The prevention of pneumococcal disease in children. *New England Journal of Medicine* **345**: 1177–83.

Green JB, Shackford SR, Sise MJ, Fridlund P (1986) Late septic complications in adults following splenectomy for trauma: a prospective analysis in 144 patients. *Journal of Trauma* **26**: 999–1004.

Groom AC, Schmidt EE, MacDonald IC (1991) Microcirculatory pathways and blood flow in spleen: new insights from washout kinetics, corrosion casts, and quantitative intravital videomicroscopy. *Scanning Microscopy* **5**: 159–73.

Habermalz B, Sauerland S, Decker G *et al.* (2008) Laparoscopic splenectomy: the clinical practice guidelines of the European Association for Endoscopic Surgery (EAES). *Surgical Endoscopy* **22**: 821–48.

Jonasson O, Spigos DC, Moyes MF (1985) Partial splenic embolization: experience in 136 patients. *World Journal of Surgery* **9**: 461–7.

Lowenthal MN, Hutt MS, Jones IG, Mohelsky V, O'Riordan EC (1980) Massive splenomegaly in Northern Zambia. I. Analysis of 344 cases. *Transactions of the Royal Society of Tropical Medicine and Hygiene* **74**: 91–8.

Mebius RE, Kraal G (2005) Structure and function of the spleen. *Nature Reviews. Immunology* **5**: 606–16.

Messinezy M, Macdonald LM, Nunan TO *et al.* (1997) Spleen sizing by ultrasound in polycythaemia and thrombocythaemia: comparison with SPECT. *British Journal of Haematology* **98**: 103–7.

Morinis J, Dutta S, Blanchette V, Butchart S, Langer JC (2008) Laparoscopic partial vs total splenectomy in children with hereditary spherocytosis. *Journal of Pediatric Surgery* **43**: 1649–52.

Musser G, Lazar G, Hocking W *et al.* (1984) Splenectomy for haematologic disease: the UCLA experience with 306 patients. *Annals of Surgery* **200**: 40–5.

Osler W (1908) Discussion on splenic enlargements other than leukaemic. *British Medical Journal* **ii**: 1151–8.

Pickering J, Campbell H (2000) An audit of the vaccinations and antibiotic prophylaxis practices amongst patients splenectomized in Lothian. *Health Bulletin* **58**: 390–5.

Pillai S, Cariappa A, Moran ST (2005) Marginal zone B cells. *Annual Review of Immunology* **23**: 161–96.

Pitchappan R (1980) Review on the phylogeny of splenic structure and function. *Developmental and Comparative Immunology* **4**: 395–416.

Pozo AL, Godfrey EM, Bowles KM (2009) Splenomegaly: investigation, diagnosis and management. *Blood Reviews* **23**: 105–11.

Rescorla FJ, West KW, Engum SA, Grosfeld JL (2007) Laparoscopic splenic procedures in children: experience in 231 children. *Annals of Surgery* **246**: 683–7.

Sampath S, Meneghetti AT, MacFarlane JK, Nguyen NH, Benny WB, Panton ON (2007) An 18-year review of open and laparoscopic splenectomy for idiopathic thrombocytopenic purpura. *American Journal of Surgery* **193**: 580–3.

Schilling RF (2009) Risks and benefits of splenectomy versus no splenectomy for hereditary spherocytosis – a personal view. *British Journal of Haematology* **145**: 728–32.

Schilling RF, Gangnon RE, Travers MI (2008) Delayed adverse vascular events after splenectomy in hereditary spherocytosis. *Journal of Thrombosis and Haemostasis* **6**: 1289–95.

Showalter SL, Hager E, Yeo CJ (2008) Metastatic disease to the pancreas and spleen. *Seminars in Oncology* **35**: 160–71.

Spielmann AL, DeLong DM, Kliewer MA (2005) Sonographic evaluation of spleen size in tall healthy athletes. *AJR American Journal of Roentgenology* **184**: 45–9.

Steiniger B, Rüttinger L, Barth PJ (2003) The three-dimensional structure of human splenic white pulp compartments. *Journal of Histochemistry and Cytochemistry* **51**: 655–64.

Tham KT, Teague MW, Howard CA *et al.* (1996) A simple splenic reticuloendothelial function test. *American Journal of Clinical Pathology* **105**: 548–52.

William BM, Corazza GR (2007) Hyposplenism: a comprehensive review. Part I: basic concepts and causes. *Hematology* **12**: 1–13.

Working Party for the British Committee for Standards in Haematology Clinical Haematology Task Force (1996) Guidelines for the prevention and treatment of infection in patients with an absent or dysfunctional spleen. *British Medical Journal* **312**: 430–4.

Zhang B, Lewis SM (1989) A study of the reliability of clinical palpation of the spleen. *Clinical and Laboratory Haematology* **11**: 7–10.

CHAPTER 21

The molecular basis of leukaemia and lymphoma

George S Vassiliou[1] and Anthony R Green[2]

[1]Wellcome Trust Sanger Institute, Wellcome Trust Genome Campus, Cambridge, UK
[2]Department of Haematology, University of Cambridge, Cambridge Institute for Medical Research, Cambridge, UK

Introduction

Cancer is proving to be more complex and molecularly diverse than we ever imagined, yet the present era is one of optimism that its conquest may be approaching. This apparent oxymoron has come about as a result of dramatic advances in our understanding of carcinogenesis, many derived from research into the pathogenesis of haematological malignancies.

The standard model of leukaemogenesis posits the stepwise acquisition of genetic mutations in a susceptible cell and its progeny, leading to the development of an autonomous clone that expands enough to cause a clinical syndrome. The phenotype of the resulting malignancy is dependent on the nature of the specific mutations and the ontogeny of the host cells. The crux of this model remains largely unchallenged, although the discovery of identical mutations in phenotypically diverse malignancies and the flexibility of the leukaemic stem cell compartment have added new layers of complexity.

This chapter describes the basic concepts of leukaemogenesis and then discusses the types of oncogenic mutations encountered in leukaemia and lymphoma before reviewing selected groups of mutant genes and pathways.

Postgraduate Haematology: 6th edition. Edited by A. Victor Hoffbrand, Daniel Catovsky, Edward G.D. Tuddenham, Anthony R. Green.

Basic concepts in leukaemogenesis

Genes and environment

Most haematological malignancies are sporadic and not attributable to identifiable genetic or environmental risk factors. Nevertheless, the risk of developing these neoplasms is higher in individuals with certain uncommon inherited syndromes, in those exposed to specific environmental agents and in people with acquired preleukaemic disorders (Table 21.1).

Genetic predisposition to cancer operates through inherited genetic variants that are either oncogenic themselves or which accelerate the rate of acquisition of somatic oncogenic mutations. Although uncommon among haematological malignancies, familial cases can offer important insights into the pathogenesis of these neoplasms. Familial acute myeloid leukaemia (AML), albeit very rare, is one of the better understood forms of familial haematological malignancies. In particular, mutations in the haemopoietic transcription factor genes *RUNX1* and *CEBPA* have been identified in rare families with incompletely penetrant autosomal dominant AML syndromes. *RUNX1* mutations are associated with familial platelet syndrome with predisposition to AML, and *CEBPA* mutations with isolated AML. Somatic mutations in *RUNX1* and *CEBPA* are well known to occur in sporadic AML, but their occurrence in familial cases offers strong additional evidence of their leukaemogenic pedigree and argues that although not sufficient to cause AML, they have a primary role in its pathogenesis. Recent dramatic advances in sequencing and genomic technologies are

Table 21.1 Risk factors for the development of leukaemia and lymphoma.

Congenital and inherited syndromes
Inherited bone marrow hypoplasia syndromes
    Fanconi anaemia
    Schwachman–Diamond syndrome
    Dyskeratosis congenita
DNA repair defects
    Bloom syndrome (DNA helicase mutations)
    Ataxia telangiectasia
Inherited predisposition to haematological malignancies
    Chronic lymphocytic leukaemia
    Acute myeloid leukaemia
    Lymphoma
    Myeloma
    Polycythaemia vera
    Essential thrombocythaemia
    Down syndrome

Environmental risk factors
Exposure to genotoxic mutagens
    Atomic bombs
    Chemotherapy
    Radiotherapy
    Benzene
Infections
    HTLV-I
    HIV
    Epstein–Barr virus
    Helicobacter pylori
Immunosuppressive drugs

Acquired preleukaemic disorders
Myelodysplastic syndromes
Myeloproliferative disorders
Acquired aplastic anaemia

---

likely to identify the molecular lesions behind many other forms of familial haematological neoplasms and this is in turn likely to inform our understanding of the sporadic forms of these diseases.

Clonality

Studies of haematological malignancies have been instrumental in establishing the clonal nature of cancer. Three main lines of evidence serve to establish the fact that haematological malignancies are clonally derived from a single ancestral cell.

First, in nearly all lymphoproliferative disorders the malignant cells carry a unique rearrangement in their immunoglobulin or T-cell receptor (TCR) genes. In contrast, proliferating normal lymphocytes show polyclonal and therefore diverse pat-

terns of antigen receptor rearrangements, each with a different antigenic specificity. This offers strong evidence for a clonal origin of lymphoid malignancies and suggests that clonal expansion occurs after antigen receptor rearrangement has been completed.

Second, acquired cytogenetic abnormalities that arise during the development of a malignancy are usually found in all cells of the clone. These microscopically visible clonal markers do not only offer further support to the concept of clonality but in most cases also harbour causative mutations. This is exemplified by the original paradigm, the Philadelphia (Ph) chromosome.

Third, studies of X-chromosome inactivation patterns (XCIPs) in female patients offer a distinct type of evidence in support of clonality. X-inactivation is the physiological process of random inactivation of either the maternal or the paternal X chromosome in all cells of the early female embryo. Once this pattern is set in a cell, it remains fixed in all its subsequent progeny. As a result, normal adult female tissues are mosaics composed, in approximately equal numbers, of cells with one or other X chromosome inactivated. In contrast, neoplastic cells, being derived from a single cell, all have the same X chromosome inactivated and therefore exhibit clonal XCIP, a feature that can be determined by standard molecular tests. One caveat in interpreting apparently clonal XCIPs is that they can sometimes be due to a phenomenon known as skewing. Acquired skewing is thought to arise with advancing age in some normal females as a result of a proliferative difference between cells with one X chromosome inactivated over those with the other (Figure 21.1). This phenomenon can limit the utility of XCIPs as a clonality marker in clinical diagnosis.

Establishing that cancers are clones derived from a single cell sets the framework for understanding carcinogenesis. The next question that needs to be addressed is how a single cell is able to overcome physiological checks to produce a progeny of trillions of cells and what factors dictate the nature of that progeny and by extension its clinical phenotype.

Clonal evolution

Carcinogenesis starts with the acquisition of an advantageous mutation in a single cell through which the cell enters a premalignant phase. Somatic mutations happen at a set frequency in adult cells and although most of them have no biological effects, some do. It is axiomatic that these mutations lead the host cell down the path of carcinogenesis, but it is also firmly established that entering this process does not inevitably lead to cancer.

The process that follows the acquisition of the first precancerous mutation has often been thought to represent a cellular equivalent of Darwinian evolution and recent scientific advances offer support to this dictum. Current evidence suggests that the founding cell establishes a small clonal progeny that remains fairly stable in size until one of its cells acquires an additional

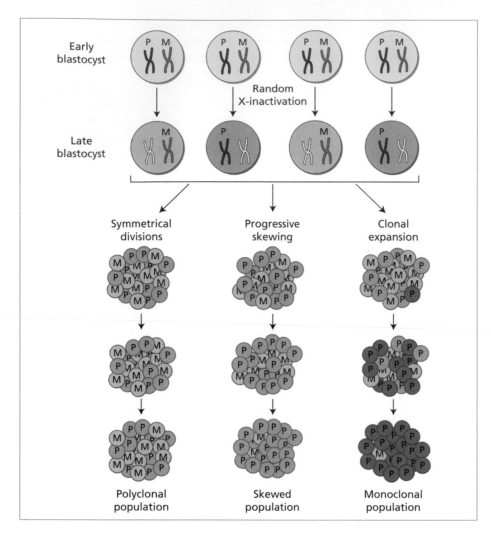

Figure 21.1 X-inactivation and clonality. Both the paternal (Xp or P) and maternal (Xm or M) X chromosomes are active in cells of the early female embryo. However, during the early blastocyst phase, each cell inactivates one or other X chromosome at random. As a result approximately half the cells will have an active Xp (light blue) and half an active Xm (pink). Normally this is followed by symmetrical cell divisions such that this polyclonal population of cells is maintained during life. In some females, one of the two populations of cells slowly outgrows the other as a result of genetic differences between their active X chromosome leading to a skewed population. Alternatively, a single cell (dark blue) acquires an advantageous or cancerous mutation and produces a monoclonal population of cells that outgrows both types of normal cells.

advantageous mutation and establishes a new subclone that expands more aggressively than the original. This *clonal evolution* continues with further subclones emerging harbouring mutations that accelerate their growth, often at the expense of their ability to function normally (Figure 21.2). Eventually, a 'visible' clone emerges whose clinical manifestations are determined by its cellular phenotype, in turn dictated by the nature of the host cell, the type of somatic mutations, or both.

Recent scientific developments, particularly those pertaining to the systematic study of cancer genomes, are revealing that different types of cancer harbour mutations in characteristic combinations of cellular pathways. Mutations in genes within each of these pathways are thought to represent the steps taken during clonal evolution. However, two important aspects of the process remain incompletely understood: first, which cell types within a tissue are susceptible to malignant transformation and, second, whether the mutations are acquired in a specific order or not.

Leukaemia stem cells

Several lines of experimental data suggest that a variable proportion of cells in a given cancer are more primitive compared with the bulk of tumour cells and demonstrate stem cell properties, i.e. self-renewal and differentiation, as well as tumour-initiating properties.

Myeloid maligancies

The similarities between normal and cancer stem cells led scientists to propose that normal stem cells are the cellular targets of cancerous mutations. In this context, oncogenic mutations exploit the self-renewal properties of a normal stem cell to turn it into a cancer-initiating cell. Studies of myeloid malignancies were the first to give credence to this theory beginning with the demonstration that the *BCR–ABL1* fusion gene could be detected in cells of several different lineages, suggesting that the transformed cell had stem cell properties. Subsequently, studies

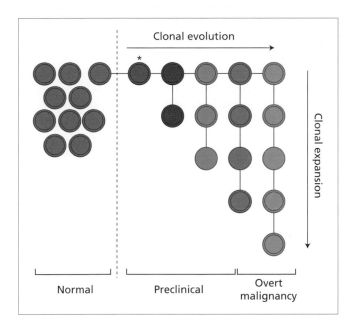

Figure 21.2 Clonal evolution in cancer. The process starts with the acquisition of an advantageous somatic mutation in a single cell (*). Subsequently, the progeny of this cell acquire additional mutations in a stepwise manner that increase their survival advantage leading to enlarging clone sizes until an overtly malignant clone emerges. It is worth noting that the majority of somatic mutations do not give cells any survival advantage and only those that do so are depicted here.

of AML went on to show that blast cells with an immunophenotype similar to that of haemopoietic stem cells (HSCs) could act as leukaemia stem cells (LSCs), while slightly more mature cells could not.

However, the theory that HSCs are the unique hosts of leukaemogenic mutations has recently been challenged with the demonstration that some mutations have the ability to transform maturing haemopoietic progenitors into LSCs (Figure 21.3). It is also worth noting that the ability to impart 'stemness' is not unique to such oncogenes or to haemopoietic cells. In fact the most striking example of dedifferentiation is the recent demonstration that, after the transient ectopic expression of as few as three key normal genes, mature skin fibroblasts can be transformed into induced pluripotent stem cells capable of differentiation to all normal lineages.

Lymphoid malignancies

Unlike many other cancers, mature lymphoid malignancies do not appear to result from transformation of normal stem cells. In contrast, it appears that these malignancies routinely arise in maturing lymphoid cells and that oncogenic mutations such as chromosomal translocations are often attributable to errors made during antigen receptor rearrangement. During normal B-cell development, the immunoglobulin heavy chain (*IGH*) locus undergoes sequential V(D)J recombination, somatic hypermutation and class switching. Therefore, in B-cell malignancies, the timing of an associated translocation can be inferred

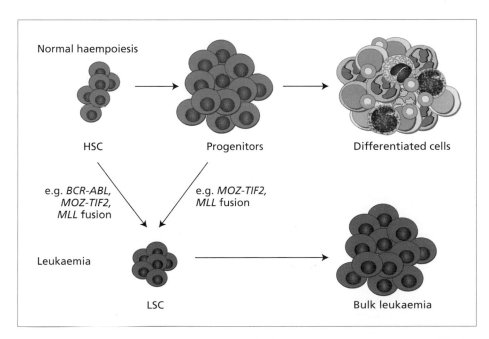

Figure 21.3 Leukaemia stem cells and oncogenes. Oncogenes such as the *BCR–ABL* fusion gene are able to transform normal haemopoietic stem cells (HSC) to leukaemia stem cells (LSC). Strikingly, some other fusion oncogenes, such as the acute leukaemia oncogenes *MOZ–TIF2* and fusions involving the *MLL* gene, are not only able to transform HSCs to LSCs, but are also able to transform committed progenitors to LSCs.

from analysis of the immunoglobulin locus adjacent to the breakpoint.

The cell of origin for mantle cell lymphomas and follicular lymphomas may well be a pre-germinal or germinal centre B cell undergoing immunoglobulin gene rearrangement. The breakpoints of the t(11;14) and t(14;18) translocations tend to occur between the D and J segments of the *IGH* locus, suggesting that they arise from mistakes in DJ recombination. In Burkitt lymphoma, the c-*MYC* gene is frequently juxtaposed with a fully V(D)J rearranged and hypermutated *IGH* variable region in the t(8;14) translocation. Breakpoints are found clustered in the VJ sequences that are particular targets for somatic hypermutation, suggesting that the double-stranded DNA breaks that occur during hypermutation may cause the translocations. Class switch recombination appears to be responsible for many of the translocations that occur in multiple myeloma, because the breakpoints are found in immunoglobulin heavy-chain switch regions (Figure 21.4).

These observations provide evidence that the translocations associated with different B-cell malignancies occur at distinct times within B-cell ontogeny. However, two caveats should be emphasized. First, *IGH* translocations may not represent initiating events. It remains formally possible that an unknown earlier lesion precedes the translocation and occurs in a more primitive cell. Second, transformed cells undergo partial differentiation even after acquiring an *IGH* translocation. For example, follicular lymphoma cells have both the histological appearances and gene expression signatures of germinal centre cells. For this continued differentiation to occur, the pre-germinal centre cell with the t(14;18) translocation must have been able to participate in an antigen-driven germinal centre response. Consistent with this idea, there is evidence that somatic hypermutation can occur within the tumour clone.

Finally, despite their likely origin in maturing cells, at least some of these lymphoid malignancies also appear to harbour cancer stem cell compartments. This has been very clearly demonstrated for multiple myeloma but may also be true of other lymphoid disorders.

The existence of leukaemic stem cells has significant implications for the treatment of malignant haematological disorders. A curative strategy must eliminate all malignant cells with the ability to self-renew and hence the capacity to re-establish the malignancy. Moreover, like their normal counterparts, a fraction of leukaemic stem cells reside within the G_0/G_1 phase of the cell cycle so that many conventional cell treatments are not able to eliminate them.

Phenotype–genotype correlations

A conspicuous feature of haematological malignancies is the close relationship between certain cytogenetic or molecular abnormalities and unique morphological and clinical features. For example, the cells of Burkitt lymphoma are characterized by a very distinctive morphological appearance and are almost universally associated with translocations involving the *MYC* gene. Similarly, acute myelomonocytic leukaemia with abnormal eosinophil precursors (AML M4Eo) is strongly associated with the inv(16) abnormality and acute promyelocytic leukaemia (APL) with the *PML–RARA* fusion gene. Furthermore, many myeloproliferative disorders are specifically connected to particular tyrosine kinase mutations, as is the case for systemic mastocytosis and KIT Asp816Val (*KIT* D816V), eosinophilic leukaemia and *FIP1L1–PDGFRA*, and others (discussed later in this chapter).

There are two potential mechanisms for such associations: first, that the nature of the mutation may determine the phenotype of the resultant leukaemia/lymphoma or, second, that a specific chromosome rearrangement may only provide a selective advantage for progenitor cells committed to a particular lineage. In fact it appears that the former model is operative in many myeloid disorders where targeting of the same or similar stem/progenitor cell leads to different disorders depend-

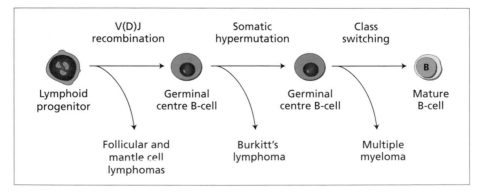

Figure 21.4 The cellular origin of B-cell malignancies. Normal B-cell maturation involves rearrangement and class switching of the immunoglobulin genes. Mistakes occurring during these DNA recombination events can result in chromosomal translocations. Analysis of sequences adjacent to the translocation breakpoints identifies the cell of origin of the translocation.

ing on the nature of the mutation. It is interesting to note, for example, that in systemic mastocytosis the KIT Asp816Val can be detected in cells other than mast cells (e.g. neutrophils), yet it is mast cells that are dramatically increased in number and that generate the clinical features. In contrast, several translocations involving the *IGH* or TCR loci are restricted to lymphoid tumours because sequences adjacent to the oncogenes mimic sequences involved in *IGH* rearrangement and are thus subjected to erroneous DNA recombination events. The translocations may therefore only occur in cells at particular stages of lymphoid differentiation. Another fact relevant to the ontogeny of lymphoid tumours is that lymphoid cells uniquely harbour very potent regulatory elements driving the expression of immunoglobulin loci, which can be recruited by oncogenes as a result of chromosomal rearrangements. This limits the type of oncogenes that can exploit this mechanism to those genes that can transform cells by overexpression, rather than those that need to be activated by other types of mutation such as point mutation or formation of a fusion gene (see later).

Types of somatic mutations

Cancer is a product of somatic mutations, which can be large-scale (e.g. chromosomal translocations, inversions and numerical aberrations) or small-scale (e.g. point mutations, microdeletions and epigenetic changes).

Chromosomal translocations

Chromosomal translocations are probably the most extensively studied genetic abnormalities in haematological malignancies. Balanced translocations involve a reciprocal exchange of genetic material between two chromosomes and may result in aberrant function of genes adjacent to the breakpoint. Two common mechanisms have been described (Figure 21.5).

First, a fusion gene may be generated encoding a fusion protein with oncogenic properties. This mechanism is seen in many of the translocations associated with myeloid malignancies and some associated with acute lymphoblastic leukaemia (ALL). Fusion genes can also result from interstitial deletions (such as deletion of chromosome 4 giving rise to the *FIP1L1–PDGFRA* fusion gene in chronic eosinophilic leukaemia) or intrachromosomal inversions (such as inversion 16 in AML M4Eo). Fusion proteins contain a combination of functional modules donated by the two partner proteins. As a consequence, the fusion protein is endowed with novel functions. For example, in fusion proteins that involve a tyrosine kinase, the partner protein contributes a homotypic interaction domain that leads to spontaneous dimerization or oligomerization of

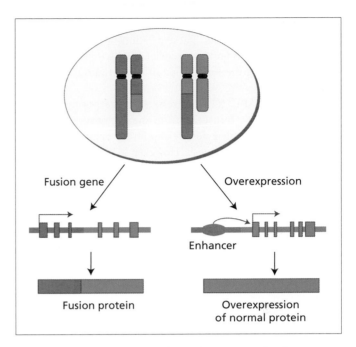

Figure 21.5 Common mechanisms of gene activation by chromosomal translocations: (i) formation of a chimeric gene by fusion of the two genes spanning the chromosomal breakpoints; and (ii) overexpression of an intact gene through the action of a potent enhancer translocated upstream.

the fusion protein, thus resulting in constitutive activation of the kinase moiety (discussed later in this chapter).

The second category of translocations results in a structurally intact gene being placed next to regulatory elements from a gene on the partner chromosome. This scenario is frequently observed in lymphoid malignancies in which a malfunction in the normal process of antigen receptor rearrangement results in translocations involving immunoglobulin or TCR loci. For example, in some B-cell tumours, genes such as *MYC* and *BCL2* are aberrantly expressed in B-cell precursors because they have been placed under the control of the strong enhancers of one of the immunoglobulin loci. Similarly, in some cases of T-cell ALL (T-ALL), the *SCL* (*TAL1*) and *HOX11* (*TLX1*) genes are ectopically expressed in T-cell precursors as a result of translocating next to enhancers from the TCR loci. Transcriptional dysregulation can also occur as a consequence of deletions, such as chromosome 1 deletions resulting in dysregulation of the *SCL* gene in T-ALL.

Balanced translocations give rise to two abnormal derivative chromosomes, one of which usually harbours the main pathogenetic event, although the other may also have a role. For example, in chronic myeloid leukaemia (CML) associated with t(9;22), it is clear that the Ph (derivative 22) chromosome carries the *BCR–ABL1* fusion gene, which is central to the development of this leukaemia. However, in a subset of patients, the derivative 9 chromosome also carries a deletion adjacent to the translocation breakpoints. These deletions arise at the time of the Ph translocation and are associated with a poor prognosis, perhaps reflecting the loss of one or more tumour-suppressor genes.

Similarly, in APL, t(15;17) results in the production of a *PML–RARA* fusion transcript from the derivative 15 chromosome and considerable evidence supports a pivotal role for this transcript in leukaemogenesis. However, in 70–80% of patients, the derivative 17 chromosome also expresses a *RARA–PML* transcript, which encodes a fusion protein with p53-binding domains that influences the development of leukaemia in a mouse model.

What causes translocations to occur in the first instance? In the case of lymphoid tumours, genomic rearrangements and (hyper)mutation are features of normal lymphocyte development. Normal rearrangements of the immunoglobulin and TCR genes require a series of double-strand DNA breaks, with loss of intervening sequences and religation. Oncogenic translocations are likely to represent rare mistakes that arise during this process and there may be several reasons why certain genes are preferentially involved in these translocations. First, motifs similar to those recognized by the immunoglobulin or TCR recombinase have been found adjacent to the *BCL2* and *SCL* genes, which are involved respectively in the t(14;18) translocation of follicular lymphoma and the t(1;14) translocation associated with T-ALL. Second, it is probable that there are only a limited number of genes that, when dysregulated, can transform lymphoid progenitors. Third, physical proximity may play a role, as genes such as *MYC*, *BCL1* and immunoglobulin loci, which are recurrently involved in B-lymphoid translocations, are preferentially positioned in close physical proximity relative to each other in normal B-cell interphase nuclei.

For most myeloid malignancies, the mechanism of translocation is poorly understood. However, double-strand breaks in genomic DNA are thought to be essential and although these can occur spontaneously, their frequency is increased by exposure to ionizing radiation and other DNA-damaging agents known to increase the risk of leukaemia. Normal repair mechanisms, such as homologous recombination or non-homologous end joining, are then recruited to join the broken ends of DNA. However, these mechanisms are not infallible, and it is conceivable that they could misrepair two simultaneous breaks on different chromosomes to generate a translocation. Germline mutations in DNA repair genes (such as Bloom syndrome, Fanconi anaemia and ataxia telangiectasia genes) increase the frequency of chromosome rearrangements as well as the incidence of many cancers, including haemopoietic ones. It may also be relevant that Alu repeat sequences appear to cluster at or near translocation breakpoints in CML and other malignancies, as it has been suggested that the Alu core sequence acts as a binding site for proteins mediating homologous recombination and DNA repair.

Consensus sites for topoisomerase II binding may play a role in some translocations, particularly those involving the *MLL* locus. Topoisomerase inhibitors, such as etoposide and anthracyclines, are well-recognized causes of therapy-related leukaemia, often associated with translocations involving the *MLL* gene on chromosome 11q23. Topoisomerase II creates double-strand breaks during execution of its function of relaxing overwound DNA, and it appears that topoisomerase II inhibitors may stabilize complexes that are formed between the enzyme and free DNA ends, thus increasing the likelihood that those ends might participate in a translocation. It remains controversial whether naturally occurring topoisomerase II inhibitors have any role in infant or childhood leukaemia.

Large deletions and aneuploidy

Chromosome deletions and disorders of chromosome number (aneuploidy) are frequently seen in haematological malignancies. It is thought that quantitative chromosomal changes of this sort contribute to tumorigenesis by altering the expression levels of key oncogenes or tumour-suppressor genes. However, it is likely that in many cases such chromosomal changes may not be directly pathogenic in themselves, but simply a consequence of genomic instability.

Hyperdiploidy is the most frequent cytogenetic abnormality in childhood ALL and can involve any chromosome; thus it may not have a specific pathogenetic function in this disease. Trisomy 8 is the most common numerical abnormality of clonal myeloid disorders and can be seen in AML, myelodysplasia and myeloproliferative disorders. It has been shown that trisomy 8 is associated with increased expression of chromosome 8 genes, but it is not known which, if any, of these genes may have a pathogenetic role.

Cytogenetically visible chromosomal deletions are large and frequently involve several megabases encompassing numerous genes. Identifying the relevant molecular consequences of a deletion is therefore difficult. Classic studies of retinoblastoma demonstrated that deletions act to remove the second copy of the tumour-suppressor gene *RB1*, the other allele of which was inactivated by mutation. This *two-hit model* operates for different tumour-suppressor genes in several solid tumours and may also apply to a subgroup of mantle cell lymphoma, in which 11q deletions remove one copy of the *ATM* gene in up to 50% of cases. The remaining *ATM* allele carries inactivating mutations in virtually all such cases, revealing the key role of inactivating both copies of the gene in this disease.

However, the two-hit model does not apply to many of the deletions associated with haematological malignancies. An alternative model was recently shown to operate in the myelodysplastic 5q– syndrome, where previous studies had failed to identify biallelic inactivation of any of the 40 or so genes within the common deleted region (CDR, the minimal region that is deleted in all cases). Recent advances show that loss of just one copy of the CDR gene *RPS14* may be responsible for many of the features of his disease, while other features may be secondary to the loss of two non-coding microRNAs also within the CDR. The finding that loss of one copy of a gene can be sufficient to affect cellular behaviour is termed *haploinsufficiency*. Additionally, this example suggests that it may be necessary for a deletion to remove more than one critical target gene in order to exert its full tumorigenic effect. Indeed, different combinations of critical genes may be removed by overlapping deletions of varying sizes that affect a similar genomic region.

Submicroscopic mutations

Much of our initial understanding of the molecular pathogenesis of haematological malignancies came from studies of cytogenetically visible chromosomal abnormalities. However, it has since become clear that submicroscopic mutations also play a similarly critical role in many malignancies. Small-scale mutations such as small deletions can disrupt two or more genes; however, most mutations in this group affect single genes by disrupting their coding sequence, which in turn enhances, attenuates or entirely alters the function of the coded protein. Many of these mutations have been described, but it is widely agreed that many examples are yet to be identified.

Activating mutations commonly involve oncogenes encoding tyrosine kinases and members of the RAS pathway and are usually missense mutations or tandem duplications. For example, around 90% of cases of systemic mastocytosis, particularly those with bone marrow involvement, have an activating point mutation in the *KIT* (c-*KIT*) gene, most frequently Asp816Val. This mutation replaces aspartate with the hydrophobic residue valine in the activation loop of the kinase domain of KIT, leading to activation of its kinase activity. *FLT3*, which encodes another receptor tyrosine kinase, is activated by internal tandem duplications, which are seen in 20% of cases of AML. Although the length of DNA duplicated varies, it is always transcribed in-frame and leads to constitutive activation of the kinase, conferring a growth advantage to the cells and translating into a poor prognosis for the patient. In a further 7% of AMLs, constitutive activation of *FLT3* occurs through a single amino acid substitution of Asp835 for a hydrophobic residue, analogous to the *KIT* mutations in systemic mastocytosis.

Activating mutations in genes of the RAS family, comprising the highly homologous proto-oncogenes *HRAS*, *KRAS* and *NRAS*, are among the commonest somatic aberrations in human cancers of all cell types. Up to 20% of all cancers, including haemopoietic malignancies, have mutations in a RAS family member, most commonly *KRAS* or *NRAS*. The RAS family members are critical components of multiple signal transduction networks, especially those that transmit extracellular growth signals to the nucleus. Oncogenic mutations, such as Gly12Val, render the GTPase domain of RAS insensitive to inactivation signals and thus the protein is stuck in a permanent 'on' state and generates a constitutive growth signal. Several related genes such as *BRAF*, as well as genes belonging to related signalling pathways such as *NF1*, are also targets of carcinogenic mutations. As a result the pathway is being targeted by rationally designed drugs, albeit with limited success so far.

Inactivating point mutations are less commonly seen than is the case for solid tumours. Nevertheless, important cell cycle regulators such as the p53 and retinoblastoma genes are not infrequently inactivated by mutation in lymphomas. However, these are thought to be secondary events, occurring during clinical progression and their presence usually correlates with poor prognosis, transformation to higher-grade disease and/or drug resistance. While such tumour-suppressor genes generally require biallelic inactivation to promote tumorigenesis, heterozygous inactivating point mutations of the *CEBPA* gene encoding the transcription factor C/EBPα are found in 20% of cases of M2 AML. Within the haemopoietic system, this gene is expressed exclusively in, and is critical to, the differentiation of myelomonocytic cells. The mutation leads to truncation of the normal protein, but allows the translation of a smaller protein initiated downstream of the mutation. The smaller protein then acts in a *dominant-negative* manner to block the function of the wild-type protein translated from the intact allele, leading to a differentiation block in myelomonocytic cells. Hence, although heterozygous, mutations of this sort can be functionally equivalent to homozygous loss-of-function mutations.

Finally, some mutations appear to alter the function of their target gene/protein in a way which cannot be described as activating or inactivating. Perhaps the best examples of this are mutations in the gene for nucleophosmin (*NPM1*), which are usually in the form of a 4-nucleotide duplication/insertion within its last exon. This leads to a frameshift in the mRNA code and the creation of a novel 13-amino-acid sequence at the C-terminal of the protein. This novel sequence behaves as a nuclear export signal and transforms nucleophosmin from a mainly nucleolar protein to a principally cytoplasmic protein. It is not clear how this leads to leukaemogenesis, but it may be partly due to novel actions of the displaced protein within the cytoplasm or codisplacement of other proteins bound to nucleophosmin out of the nucleus.

Epigenetic effects

In a normal cell, epigenetic mechanisms control several important functions including gene transcription, DNA replication, imprinting and X-inactivation. Somatically acquired epigenetic changes affecting these processes can, without altering nucleotide sequence, alter gene expression and thus have a role in tumorigenesis just as genetic mutations can.

Methylation of DNA sequences within regions involved in the regulation of gene expression is generally associated with transcriptional silencing of the associated genes. Disordered patterns of DNA methylation have been found in a wide variety of haematological malignancies. For example, there is global genomic hypomethylation in chronic lymphocytic leukaemia (CLL) lymphocytes and AML blasts compared with normal haemopoietic cells. In addition, certain candidate genes implicated in neoplasia can be either hypermethylated or hypomethylated compared with their status in normal cells. DNA hypomethylation has been identified at a number of loci implicated in haematological malignancies, including BCL2 in CLL, LTA (the gene encoding tumour necrosis factor β) in CML and AML, and others. Given that hypomethylation generally promotes transcriptional activity, it can cause overexpression of these oncogenes, as has been shown for BCL2. Conversely, DNA hypermethylation of several tumour-suppressor genes, such as p16INK4A (also called CDKN2A), E-cadherin (CDH1) and HIC1, has been described in CLL and AML, as has hypermethylation of SOCS1, an inhibitor of cytokine signalling in many malignancies including AML, CML, myelodysplastic syndrome, lymphoma and myeloma.

It is therefore clear that, as in other cancers, epigenetic modifications are widespread in haematological malignancies. However, most are unlikely to represent initiating lesions and probably reflect downstream consequences of genetic changes. Nonetheless, they still represent pertinent targets for therapeutic intervention, as reflected in the effectiveness of the DNA methyltransferase inhibitor 5-azacytidine and its analogue decitabine in myelodysplastic syndromes.

Molecular basis of malignant transformation

This section illustrates the mechanisms by which acquired genetic changes may result in malignancy. Four specific examples have been chosen to illustrate how distinct cellular processes may be corrupted: tyrosine kinase signalling (the myeloproliferative disorders); intracellular signal transduction (juvenile myelomonocytic leukaemia); regulation of gene transcription (AML); cell cycle control and apoptosis (mantle cell and follicular lymphomas).

Tyrosine kinases and myeloproliferative disorders

Tyrosine kinases are critical for the response of haemopoietic progenitor cells to external growth stimuli. The binding of a ligand to the extracellular surface of a receptor tyrosine kinase (RTK) promotes receptor dimerization, which in turn stimulates autophosphorylation of specific tyrosine residues within the intracellular aspect of the protein. The dimerization and the associated increase in kinase activity result in recruitment of effector molecules and activation of downstream signalling

pathways. Many cytoplasmic tyrosine kinases are also thought to be activated by phosphorylation and dimerization.

Individual myeloproliferative disorders are specifically associated with activation of different tyrosine kinases (Figure 21.6). In some of these diseases, activation of the tyrosine kinase stems from formation of a fusion protein, which undergoes spontaneous dimerization (Figure 21.7a). However, kinase activity can also be increased by more subtle mutations (e.g. JAK2 Val617Phe in polycythaemia vera and KIT Asp816Val in systemic mastocytosis). As a consequence of these changes, the corresponding signalling pathway is activated and this provides the transformed cell with a proliferative or survival advantage.

In CML, the BCR gene becomes fused in-frame with the ABL1 tyrosine kinase gene as a consequence of the Ph translocation (Figure 21.7b). This usually results in the formation of a fusion protein of 210 kDa (hence p210$^{BCR-ABL}$). The fusion protein affects multiple different cellular processes, including intracellular signalling, apoptosis, transcriptional regulation and cellular adhesion. Transgenic mouse models have demonstrated that BCR–ABL is capable of inducing dramatic expansion of myeloid precursors in vivo and can produce a phenotype that resembles the human form of the disease.

Several critical domains in the fusion protein have been mapped, and have provided important insights into its biological activity (Figure 21.7b). The coiled-coil domain of the BCR protein provides a dimerization motif, which promotes spontaneous BCR–ABL1 dimerization leading to constitutive ABL kinase activity. Other domains implicated in oncogenicity are the SH2 domain and the C-terminal actin-binding domain, both in the ABL1 portion; these domains appear to be important for interaction with regulatory molecules and subcellular localization of the fusion protein. Numerous downstream pathways are activated by the BCR–ABL1 protein, including the RAS, phosphatidylinositol 3-kinase, STAT and MAP kinase signalling cascades. The breadth of the pathways perturbed explains the protean effects of the fusion protein. For example, activation of the RAS pathway is thought to contribute to the increased cell division and proliferation seen in CML cells; altered interaction with the actin cytoskeleton and adhesion complexes may underlie the diminished adhesion to inhibitory bone marrow stromal cells; and STAT5-dependent upregulation of BCL-XL is implicated in the reduced apoptosis of CML progenitors.

As shown in Figure 21.7b, two other versions of the BCR–ABL1 protein exist in which the breakpoint occurs in different introns of the BCR gene than that usually seen in CML. The smaller protein, p190$^{BCR-ABL}$, is found in Ph-positive ALL and has a higher level of constitutive tyrosine kinase activity than the p210$^{BCR-ABL}$ protein. This is thought to contribute to the more aggressive behaviour of the ALL. A p230$^{BCR-ABL}$ isoform is also found rarely in patients with CML. In some cases, it is associated with a morphological picture resembling chronic neutrophilic leukaemia and possibly a lower rate of blast trans-

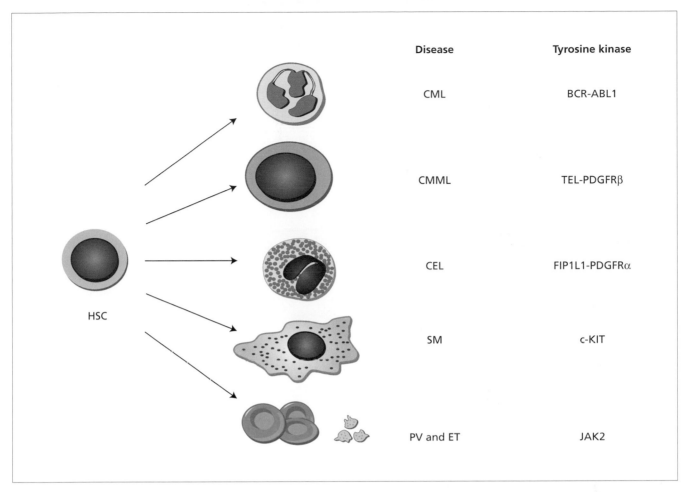

Disease	Tyrosine kinase
CML	BCR-ABL1
CMML	TEL-PDGFRβ
CEL	FIP1L1-PDGFRα
SM	c-KIT
PV and ET	JAK2

HSC

Figure 21.6 Tyrosine kinase mutations in the myeloproliferative disorders. Each disease is associated with a specific activating mutation in a tyrosine kinase gene and this leads to preferential expansion of specific haemopoietic cell progeny. CEL, chronic eosinophilic leukaemia; CML, chronic myeloid leukaemia; CMML, chronic myelomonocytic leukaemia; ET, essential thrombocythaemia HSC, haemopoietic stem cell; PV, polycythaemia vera; SM, systemic mastocytosis.

formation. These variants illustrate how small structural differences in a fusion protein can cause significant differences in disease phenotype.

A group of related tyrosine kinase fusion genes (*PDGFRA*, *PDGFRB* and *FGFR1*) are associated with eosinophilic myeloproliferative disorders. A striking feature of these syndromes is the large number of fusion partners for these kinases, with eight partners currently known for *FGFR1*, six for *PDGFRA* and 17 for *PDGFRB*. As with *BCR* in *BCR–ABL*, most of these partners harbour dimerization domains that facilitate constitutive activation of the tyrosine kinase. However, reflecting their molecular heterogeneity, these disorders exhibit significant clinical diversity. For example, cases associated with the *FIP1L1–PDGFRA* fusion exhibit marked eosinophilia, while those associated with *ETV6–PDGFRB* often show dysplastic features and a lesser degree of eosinophilia. Additionally, cases involving *FGFR1,* collectively known as the 8p11 myelo-proliferative syndrome, are usually associated with a coexisting non-Hodgkin lymphoma. Notably, cases associated with rearrangements of the *PDGFR* genes respond well to imatinib, while those associated with *FGFR1* fusions do not.

RAS family signalling and juvenile myelomonocytic leukaemia

Juvenile myelomonocytic leukaemia (JMML) is a rare disorder of childhood characterized by a marked expansion of both myeloid and monocytic lineages, with varying degrees of dysplasia and exquisite sensitivity to granulocyte/macrophage colony-stimulating factor (GM-CSF) in colony assays. These features reflect the fact that components of the GM-CSF receptor signalling pathway are frequently mutated in JMML (Figure 21.8).

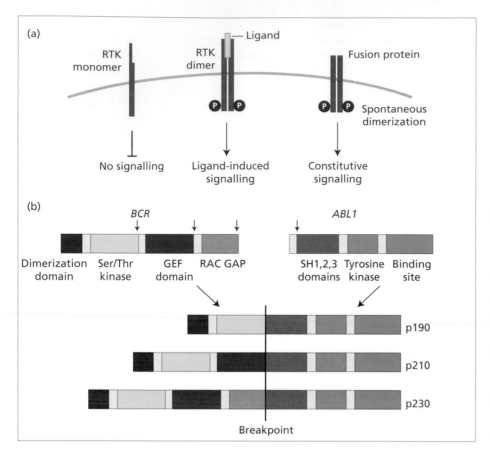

Figure 21.7 Fusion tyrosine kinases. (a) In normal cells, receptor tyrosine kinases (RTK) exist as inactive monomers which, upon ligand binding, become activated by dimerization and autophosphorylation. In contrast fusion tyrosine kinases dimerize spontaneously and are constitutively active. (b) Different forms of *BCR–ABL1* fusion genes containing varying lengths of *BCR* as a result of different breakpoints (arrowheads). These are associated with different molecular effects (see text).

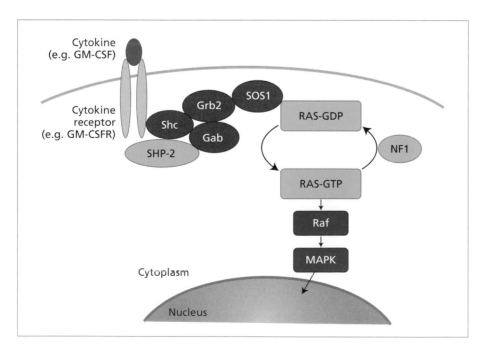

Figure 21.8 The RAS pathway and juvenile myelomonocytic leukaemia (JMML). The Ras pathway mediates many of the downstream effects of cytokine receptor activation. In most cases of JMML, the pathway is activated by mutations in one of three genes depicted in black text: *PTPN11*, the gene coding for the protein SHP-2 (35% of cases), *RAS* (25% of cases) or *NF1* (15% of cases). As a result JMML cells are extremely sensitive to GM-CSF.

Mutations in the *NRAS* or *KRAS* genes are seen in many haematological malignancies, including AML, myelodysplastic syndrome and chronic myelomonocytic leukaemia, especially in subtypes with a monocytic component. Analyses of samples from patients with JMML show point mutations in *NRAS* and *KRAS* in approximately 25% of cases. The point mutations cause single amino acid substitutions, which result in constitutively active forms of the protein and thus mimic markedly amplified signalling from the GM-CSF receptor.

The neurofibromin (*NF1*) gene is also a target for mutations in JMML, but in this case the result is loss of NF1 activity. The incidence of JMML is increased in neurofibromatosis type 1, an autosomal dominant disorder caused by inactivating mutations in the *NF1* gene. This gene encodes a protein that directly interacts with, and inhibits the activity of, RAS proteins. Patients who have both neurofibromatosis type 1 and JMML have a high frequency (60%) of inactivating mutations of the second *NF1* allele in the leukaemic cells. Furthermore, inactivating *NF1* mutations are found in 15% of sporadic cases of JMML without the clinical syndrome of neurofibromatosis. It appears therefore that *NF1* acts as a tumour-suppressor gene, and that inactivation of both alleles allows unchecked signalling through the RAS pathway.

A similar story holds true for *PTPN11*, the gene that encodes the tyrosine phosphatase SHP2. Germline mutations of this gene can cause a developmental disorder, Noonan syndrome, which is associated with an increased incidence of JMML. Up to 35% of non-syndromic patients with JMML have somatic mutations of *PTPN11* in the leukaemic cells. The mutations all cause amino acid substitutions clustering in the N-terminal SH2 domain of the protein, which are thought to result in enhanced phosphatase activity and activation of the downstream RAS pathway that give the host cells a growth advantage over their normal counterparts.

Thus, within the GM-CSF receptor signalling pathway, activation of an activating component (such as *RAS*) has the same pathological consequences as inactivation of an inhibitory component (*NF1*). Moreover, the mutations in *RAS*, *NF1* and *PTPN11* are mutually exclusive. In other words, individual patients carry mutations in only one of these genes, suggesting that mutation of just one component is sufficient to activate the signalling pathway and that additional mutations in the pathway offer no further advantage. This phenomenon, of mutations in the same pathway being mutually exclusive in any one tumour, is increasingly recognized for various different pathways in other haematological and solid tumours.

The core-binding factor complex and acute myeloid leukaemia

Genes encoding transcription factors are common targets for rearrangements or mutations in acute leukaemia. Many of these genes have been found to play important roles in regulating the behaviour of normal haemopoietic stem or progenitor cells, implying that perturbation of normal transcription programmes can be leukaemogenic. Individual transcription factors usually function as part of a multiprotein complex and it has become clear that different components of a given complex may be involved in distinct forms of acute leukaemia.

These principles are exemplified by the core-binding factor (CBF) complex, comprising RUNX1 (also known as AML1 or CBFα) and CBFβ. The normal CBF dimer recognizes and binds specific DNA sequences through the RUNX1 subunit and regulates the expression of many genes important for the differentiation of haemopoietic cells, such as interleukin (IL)-3, GM-CSF and the enhancer for immunoglobulin heavy chain (Figure 21.9a). Adjacent binding sequences in the DNA are important for other transcription factors, and it seems that the CBF dimer acts as a transcriptional organizer by recruiting other transcription factors into a large multimeric complex that regulates expression of target genes. Mice lacking RUNX1 have a complete failure of blood formation, confirming its critical importance for normal haemopoiesis.

The genes for the two CBF subunits represent the most commonly involved genes in acute leukaemia translocations, with t(12;21) (*ETV6–RUNX1*) found in 25% of childhood ALL, t(8;21) (*RUNX1–ETO*) in 15% of AML, and inv(16) (*MYH11–CBFB*) in 10% of AML. It appears that the leukaemogenic effects of these fusion genes are mediated in large part through dominant-negative inhibition of CBF function. For example, *in vitro* experiments confirm that binding of wild-type *RUNX1* to gene enhancers is inhibited in the presence of *RUNX1–ETO*. Moreover, mice carrying the *RUNX1–ETO* fusion gene and a wild-type *RUNX1* allele have exactly the same embryonic lethal phenotype as mice completely lacking *RUNX1*.

The mechanisms by which the fusion genes exert their dominant inhibitory effects are beginning to be understood. The fusion partners of the *CBF* genes appear to recruit nuclear corepressor complexes, leading to transcriptional inhibition of target genes. In fact, in the case of the *RUNX1–ETO* fusion, the *ETO* moiety recruits a complex comprising three proteins, NcoR, SIN3 and a histone deacetylase, resulting in histone deacetylation, a change in chromatin structure and target gene repression (Figure 21.9b). Similarly, the CBFβ–MYH11 fusion protein of inv(16) forms a complex with the normal RUNX1 subunit through the CBFβ moiety, and recruits several transcriptional repressors via the MYH11 component (Figure 21.9c). The end result is similar for both fusion genes, namely transcriptional silencing of genes required for normal differentiation and a consequent maturation arrest.

However, in keeping with the multistep theory of tumorigenesis discussed above, rearrangement of an individual transcription factor gene is not sufficient to give rise to acute leukaemia. Instead, there is mounting evidence for a model in which development of AML requires both a block of differentiation, fre-

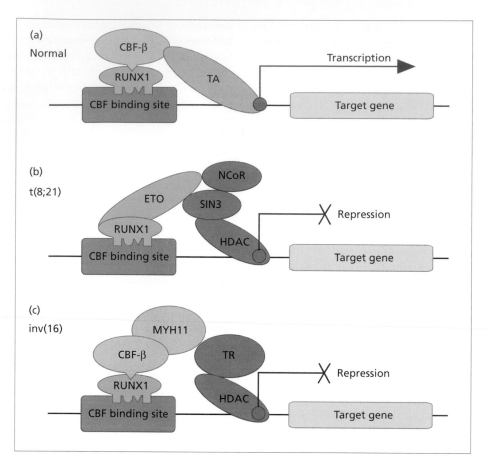

Figure 21.9 Core-binding factor gene fusions, transcriptional repression and acute leukaemia. (a) The normal CBF dimer (composed of RUNX1 and CBFβ) binds specific DNA sequences through the RUNX1 subunit and recruits transcriptional activators (TA) that upregulate the expression of many genes important for haemopoietic cell differentiation. (b) In leukaemic cells carrying the *RUNX1–ETO* fusion gene, the ETO moiety recruits a corepressor complex comprising NcoR, SIN3 and a histone deacetylase (HDAC). This leads to histone deacetylation and inhibition of the expression of haemopoietic differentiation genes. (c) Similarly, the CBFβ–MYH11 fusion binds to normal RUNX1 through its CBFβ moiety and recruits different transcriptional repressors (TR) via MYH11 with analogous effects.

quently provided by subversion of a transcription factor gene (type II mutation), and a proliferative signal, frequently provided by an altered tyrosine kinase (type I mutation). For example, the *FLT3* gene, coding for a receptor tyrosine kinase, is activated in 25% of AML and has been shown to cooperate with *PML–RARA* in a mouse model of APL. In fact most cases of AML harbour both a type I and a type II mutation, and there are several well-characterized examples of both mutation types (Figure 21.10).

Cell cycle control, apoptosis and lymphoma

There is an intimate relationship between the cell cycle and apoptosis. Each phase of the cell cycle is tightly controlled by specific molecular checkpoints, which monitor for DNA damage and mitotic spindle formation before permitting cell cycle pro-

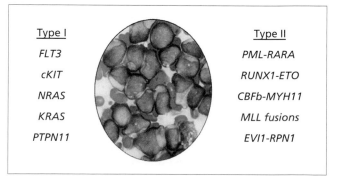

Type I	Type II
FLT3	PML-RARA
cKIT	RUNX1-ETO
NRAS	CBFb-MYH11
KRAS	MLL fusions
PTPN11	EVI1-RPN1

Figure 21.10 Cooperating mutations in acute myeloid leukaemia (AML). The majority of cases of AML harbour at least two types of mutations, a type I mutation which increases proliferation and a type II mutation that blocks haemopoietic differentiation. Some of the most common mutations in each group are listed.

gression. If a checkpoint recognizes damage to the DNA or the mitotic apparatus, this triggers programmed cell death (apoptosis). The enzymes involved in cell cycle control and apoptosis are among the commonest targets of mutation in all cancers, including haematological ones.

Figure 21.11 summarizes some of the main components controlling cell cycle progression and apoptosis, many of which are known to be corrupted in different types of lymphoma. The characteristic chromosomal abnormality associated with mantle cell lymphoma is the t(11;14) translocation, leading to juxtaposition of the cyclin D1 gene (also known as *BCL1*) to an *IGHJ* segment. Cyclin D1 functions in G_1 phase, binding and activating two kinases, CDK4 and CDK6. The cyclin–CDK complex then phosphorylates and inactivates the retinoblastoma (Rb) protein, which is then unable to repress transcription of genes (e.g. E2F) important for the transition to S-phase. Experimental evidence confirms that forced overexpression of cyclin D1 similar to that seen in mantle cell lymphoma leads to a shortened G_1 phase, although overexpression in itself is not sufficient to induce lymphoma in transgenic mice.

Cooperating mutations and epigenetic changes have been found in other genes in the cyclin D1–CDK4–Rb pathway in patients with mantle cell lymphoma. In one study, deletions of

p16INK4A (*CDKN2A*), which codes for an inhibitor of the cyclin D1–CDK4 complex, were seen in 40% of mantle cell lymphomas, and deletions of Rb were present in a further 40% of cases. These additional mutations in genes of the cyclin D1 pathway correlated with markers of active cell proliferation and more aggressive clinical behaviour. Furthermore, epigenetic modifications have been found, such as hypermethylation of *p16INK4A*, which may also reflect gene inactivation. This pattern of several coexisting and synergistic mutations in the same pathway contrasts with the situation in JMML, in which mutations in different components of the RAS–MAP kinase pathway tend to be mutually exclusive. A possible explanation for this discrepancy is that several genes need to be disrupted to overcome the multiple cell cycle checkpoints.

Up to half of all mantle cell lymphomas also exhibit deletions of 11q and the deleted region includes the locus of the *ATM* gene. The *ATM* gene is essential for checkpoint controls at the G_2–M transition in particular, and is activated by double-strand breaks in DNA (Figure 21.11). The remaining *ATM* allele in patients with 11q deletions is almost invariably affected by inactivating mutations, associated with aberrant splicing, truncation or abnormal structure of the protein. Similarly, in the absence of 11q deletions, biallelic point mutations in *ATM* have

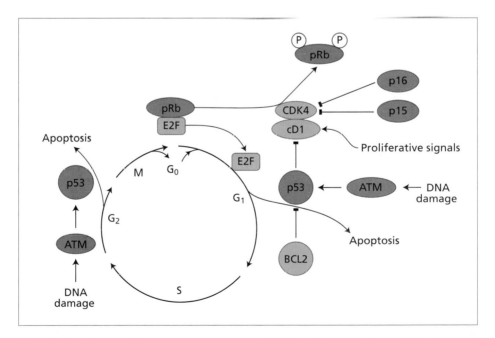

Figure 21.11 Apoptosis and cell cycle control in lymphomagenesis. Proliferative signals activate cyclin D1 (cD1 or BCL1), which complexes with and activates the kinases CDK4 and CDK6. The complex then phosphorylates (P) the retinoblastoma protein (pRb), which is then unable to repress cell cycle progression proteins such as E2F. The proteins p16 and p15 antagonize this process by inhibiting CDK4 and CDK6. Another important cell cycle checkpoint involves activation of ATM signalling secondary to DNA damage. This activates p53, which in turn inhibits cell cycle progression and promotes apoptosis. BCL2 can inhibit the actions of p53 and other apoptotic signals. These genes are frequently mutated in different types of lymphoma (see text). Genes that promote growth are depicted in green and those that inhibit growth or promote apoptosis in red.

been found in mantle cell lymphoma, and patients with a germline mutation in the *ATM* gene (heterozygote carriers for ataxia telangiectasia) have a marked increase in incidence of lymphoma. Taken together, these observations support the hypothesis that *ATM* functions as a tumour-suppressor gene in mantle cell lymphoma.

Follicular lymphoma is characterized by overexpression of the anti-apoptotic protein BCL2 (Figure 21.11), as a result of translocation t(14;18) in which the *BCL2* gene is placed under control of an *IGH* enhancer. Increased levels of BCL2 protein protect the lymphoma cells from a range of apoptotic signals, suggesting a model whereby cells do not have a proliferative advantage as such but accumulate through lack of cell death. BCL2 overexpression also reduces the ability of chemotherapeutic agents to induce apoptosis, and this may explain why it is difficult to cure patients with follicular lymphoma. Transgenic mice in which *BCL2* is placed under the control of an *IGH* enhancer show an accumulation of mature B cells, a propensity to autoimmune diseases and follicular hyperplasia. Malignant lymphomas only develop in these mice after a long latency, and tend to be associated with disruption of other key genes, such as the proto-oncogene *MYC*.

Follicular lymphoma may transform into an aggressive, chemotherapy-resistant, diffuse large B-cell lymphoma. Numerous second hits have been associated with this transformation, and these mutations preferentially involve cell cycle regulators such as those involved in mantle cell and other lymphomas. In particular, deletions involving *p16INK4a* (also called *CDKN2A*) and *p15INK4b* (*CDKN2B*) are found in 70% and mutations in *TP53* (coding for the transcription factor p53) in up to 30% of transformed follicular lymphomas. Presumably these additional mutations confer a proliferation advantage on the cells, resulting in the more aggressive growth.

Summary

Our understanding of the molecular foundations of haematological malignancies has advanced spectacularly in the last two decades. Having established many fundamental principles underpinning leukaemogenesis, we are systematically exposing the key molecular events involved in the process and identifying targets for therapeutic intervention. This progress is steadily transforming the practice of clinical haematology at all levels from diagnosis to treatment and most importantly it is benefiting patients. The introduction of the first molecularly targeted treatments in the form of imatinib for CML and all-*trans* retinoic acid for APL is being followed by the development of an increasing number of therapeutic agents against different diseases and molecular targets. Over the next few years we can expect to witness a revolution in the practice of malignant haematology and hope to harvest the benefits of decades of progress in leukaemia research.

Selected bibliography

Baxter EJ, Scott LM, Campbell PJ *et al.* (2005) Acquired mutation of the tyrosine kinase JAK2 in human myeloproliferative disorders. *Lancet* **365**: 1054–61.

Chen GL, Prchal JT (2007) X-linked clonality testing: interpretation and limitations. *Blood* **110**: 1411–19.

Cross NC, Reiter A (2008) Fibroblast growth factor receptor and platelet-derived growth factor receptor abnormalities in eosinophilic myeloproliferative disorders. *Acta Haematologica* **119**: 199–206.

Ebert BL (2009) Deletion 5q in myelodysplastic syndrome: a paradigm for the study of hemizygous deletions in cancer. *Leukemia* **23**: 1252–6.

Falini B, Mecucci C, Tiacci E *et al.* (2005) Cytoplasmic nucleophosmin in acute myelogenous leukaemia with a normal karyotype. *New England Journal of Medicine* **352**: 254–66.

Frohling S, Dohner H (2008) Chromosomal abnormalities in cancer. *New England Journal of Medicine* **359**: 722–34.

Greaves MF, Wiemels J (2003) Origins of chromosome translocations in childhood leukaemia. *Nature Reviews. Cancer* **3**: 639–49.

Hartmann EM, Ott G, Rosenwald A (2008) Molecular biology and genetics of lymphomas. *Hematology/Oncology Clinics of North America* **22**: 807–23, vii.

Herman JG, Baylin SB (2003) Gene silencing in cancer in association with promoter hypermethylation. *New England Journal of Medicine* **349**: 2042–54.

Huntly BJ, Gilliland DG (2005) Leukaemia stem cells and the evolution of cancer-stem-cell research. *Nature Reviews. Cancer* **5**: 311–21.

Koike K, Matsuda K (2008) Recent advances in the pathogenesis and management of juvenile myelomonocytic leukaemia. *British Journal of Haematology* **141**: 567–75.

Krivtsov AV, Armstrong SA (2007) MLL translocations, histone modifications and leukaemia stem-cell development. *Nature Reviews. Cancer* **7**: 823–33.

Levine RL, Pardanani A, Tefferi A, Gilliland DG (2007) Role of JAK2 in the pathogenesis and therapy of myeloproliferative disorders. *Nature Reviews. Cancer* **7**: 673–83.

Ley TJ, Mardis ER, Ding L *et al.* (2008) DNA sequencing of a cytogenetically normal acute myeloid leukaemia genome. *Nature* **456**: 66–72.

Quintas-Cardama A, Cortes J (2009) Molecular biology of bcr-abl1-positive chronic myeloid leukaemia. *Blood* **113**: 1619–30.

Speck NA, Gilliland DG (2002) Core-binding factors in haematopoiesis and leukaemia. *Nature Reviews. Cancer* **2**: 502–13.

CHAPTER 22

Laboratory diagnosis of haematological neoplasms

Barbara J Bain[1] and Torsten Haferlach[2]

[1]St Mary's Hospital, London, UK
[2]MLL Münchner Leukämielabor GmbH, München, Germany

Introduction

The diagnosis of a haematological neoplasm usually starts from a clinical suspicion, although for chronic leukaemias the diagnosis is sometimes an incidental one. A blood count and blood film is an essential first step whenever leukaemia, lymphoma or other haematological neoplasm is suspected. The next step in the diagnostic process depends on the clinical features and the specific condition that is suspected. In this chapter we discuss the laboratory techniques that are available and how they are integrated into an efficient diagnostic pathway (Figure 22.1). It is of crucial importance that all laboratory investigations are done with an awareness of the medical history and physical findings. It is also essential that a conclusion as to diagnosis is based on integrating the results of all laboratory investigations and imaging in the context of the clinical features. Achieving this can be a challenge if investigations are done in different laboratories on different sites. One possible solution, if all procedures are not performed in a single laboratory, is that a haematologist/haematopathologist should take the lead in making a final diagnosis when the diagnosis depends primarily on the blood and bone marrow and that a haematopathologist/histopathologist should take the lead when the diagnosis depends primarily on a biopsy of another tissue. Three important factors contribute to accurate diagnosis:

Postgraduate Haematology: 6th edition. Edited by A. Victor Hoffbrand, Daniel Catovsky, Edward G.D. Tuddenham, Anthony R. Green
© 2011 Blackwell Publishing Ltd.

1 the provision of very detailed clinical information to laboratories;
2 the correct sample, e.g. blood or bone marrow aspirate specimen (anticoagulated with EDTA or heparin), blood and bone marrow films, trephine or fine-needle biopsy specimen, should all be sent to the laboratory in the shortest possible time;
3 the integration of information technology across different sites dealing with diagnostic samples from a single patient.

Consideration should also be given to the need for centralized diagnosis by a panel of experts when experience has shown that misdiagnosis is common, as for example in lymphoma. It is also necessary to ensure that a diagnosis is achieved in a timely manner, particularly when treatment may be urgent, as in acute leukaemias and aggressive lymphomas.

Blood count and blood film

The most important information that must be extracted from the blood count is the white cell count, the haemoglobin concentration and the platelet count. The red cell indices should also be noted since macrocytosis and, less often, microcytosis can occur in haematological neoplasms. The automated instrument will generally provide a differential count and 'flags' indicating the likely presence of blast cells, abnormal lymphocytes or granulocyte precursors. An abnormal total or differential count should always be verified on a blood film and a blood film should also be examined when there are relevant 'flags'. Even if the blood count is normal, a blood film should be examined for the presence of abnormal cells in any patient with

Morphology   Cytogenetics   Immunophenotyping

Cytochemistry   FISH   Molecular biology

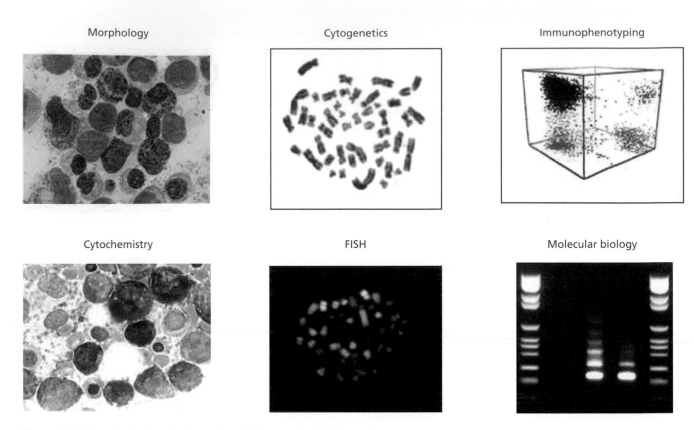

Figure 22.1 The principal methods employed in hematological diagnosis.

lymphadenopathy, splenomegaly, skin infiltration or any other reason to suspect a haematological neoplasm.

The blood film has two major roles. In some circumstances it provides strong evidence of a specific diagnosis that can be confirmed on further testing. In others it suggests a differential diagnosis and indicates the appropriate direction of further tests. A blood film also has the advantage that a rapid provisional diagnosis can be made, something that is important when treatment is urgent. For example, when there are circulating neoplastic cells, a rapid provisional diagnosis of Burkitt lymphoma (Figure 22.2) and acute hypergranular promyelocytic leukaemia (Figure 22.3) can be made from the blood film. Acute microgranular/hypogranular promyelocytic leukaemia (Figure 22.4) should also be suspected from the blood film. Even very infrequent neoplastic cells can suggest the correct diagnosis, for example in hairy cell leukaemia. Other diagnoses that may be strongly suggested by the blood film include most subtypes of acute myeloid leukaemia (AML), chronic lymphocytic leukaemia (CLL) (Figure 22.5), chronic myelogenous leukaemia (CML) (Figure 22.6), follicular lymphoma, splenic marginal zone lymphoma (when the cytological features of splenic lymphoma with villous lymphocytes are present), large granular lymphocyte leukaemia and plasma cell leukaemia.

Sometimes the blood film suggests only a differential diagnosis. Although the cytological features of the previously used FAB

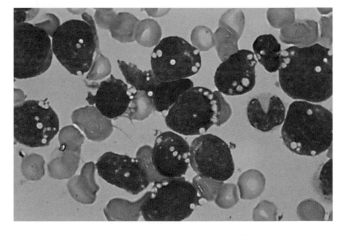

Figure 22.2 Burkitt lymphoma showing blast-like cells with strongly basophilic, heavily vacuolated cytoplasm. The cytological features were once designated 'FAB L3 ALL' but the immunophenotype is that of a mature B cell. Bone marrow film, May–Grünwald–Giemsa (MGG).

(French–American–British) L1 category of acute lymphoblastic leukaemia (ALL) (Figure 22.7) are very likely to indicate that the diagnosis is ALL, this is not so of FAB L2 type (Figure 22.8), which can be cytologically very similar to AML of FAB M0 or

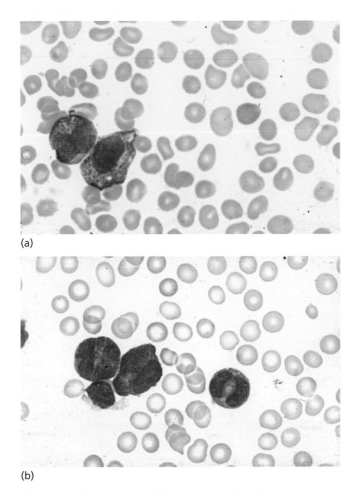

(a)

(b)

Figure 22.3 Two patients with acute promyelocytic leukaemia: (a) acute hypergranular promyelocytic leukaemia; (b) hypogranular/microgranular variant of promyelocytic leukaemia showing typical bilobed nuclei. These two subtypes of AML fall into the single category 'AML with recurrent genetic abnormalities' in the 2008 WHO classification. Peripheral blood films, MGG.

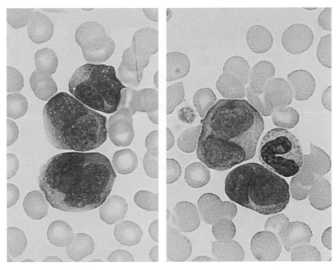

Figure 22.4 Acute hypogranular/microgranular variant of promyelocytic leukaemia showing a range of nuclear forms but note the typical bilobed nucleus in which the two lobes are joined by an isthmus. Bone marrow film, MGG.

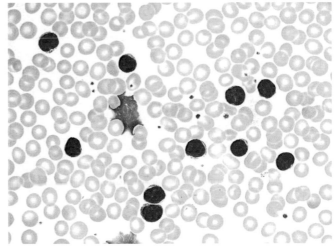

Figure 22.5 Chronic lymphocytic leukaemia showing mature small lymphocytes and a smear cell. Peripheral blood film, MGG.

M1 types (Figures 22.9 and 22.10). Similarly, acute monoblastic leukaemia (Figure 22.11) can be cytologically indistinguishable from large-cell lymphoma or even plasma cell leukaemia.

In suspected myeloid malignancy the blood film is important for the detection of myelodysplastic features, particularly hypogranular and pseudo-Pelger–Huët neutrophils (Figure 22.12). Sometimes the blood film shows only non-specific but nevertheless useful features, for example eosinophilia, rouleaux formation, red cell agglutinates or cryoglobulin deposition.

Whatever the findings on the blood count and film, confirmatory tests are needed. The nature of these will vary according to circumstances but several useful algorithms are guided by information that can be gained from the peripheral blood.

Bone marrow aspirate

A bone marrow aspirate is indicated in virtually all patients with suspected ALL, AML (Figure 22.13), CML, myelodysplastic syndrome (MDS) (Figure 22.14) or multiple myeloma (Figure 22.15). However, a bone marrow aspirate is not necessary for the diagnosis of CLL. The diagnosis of promyelocytic leukaemia may be more readily made on an aspirate than on the peripheral blood since, particularly in the hypergranular form, there may be few leukaemic cells in the blood and in the microgranular/

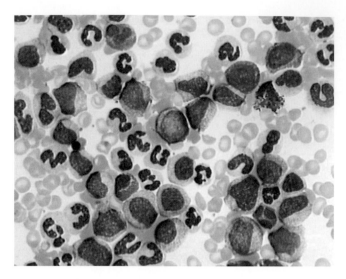

Figure 22.6 Chronic myelogenous leukaemia showing the typical spectrum of granulocytic cells from immature to mature, and including a basophil and some eosinophils.

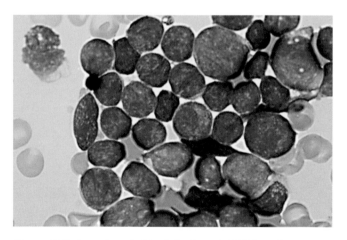

Figure 22.7 Acute lymphoblastic leukaemia FAB L1 subtype showing blast cells that vary in size but which otherwise have fairly uniform cellular characteristics; the nucleocytoplasmic ratio is high and there are small inconspicuous nucleoli. Bone marrow film, MGG.

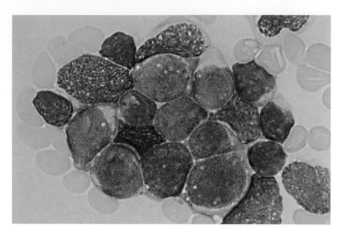

Figure 22.8 Acute lymphoblastic leukaemia FAB L2 subtype showing medium-sized and large pleomorphic blast cells with one or two prominent nucleoli; there are no characteristics that identify the lineage. Bone marrow film, MGG.

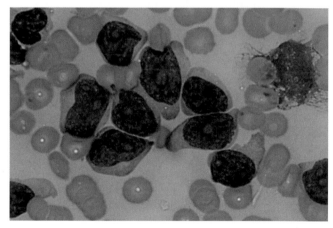

Figure 22.9 Acute myeloid leukaemia FAB M0 subtype showing large blast cells with large prominent nucleoli; there are no cytological features that identify the lineage and Sudan black B and myeloperoxidase cytochemical stains were negative. On immunophenotyping, all B and T lineage markers were negative but there was expression of CD13 and CD33. Without immunophenotyping such a case could not be distinguished from acute lymphoblastic leukaemia L2 subtype. Bone marrow film, MGG.

hypogranular form there may be more hypergranular cells in the bone marrow, thus facilitating the diagnosis. The characteristic cytological features of AML with inv(16) or t(16;16) are apparent in the bone marrow (Figures 22.16 and 22.17) but not usually in the peripheral blood. In the acute leukaemias and in CML and other myeloproliferative neoplasms, a bone marrow aspirate provides material for cytogenetic analysis as well as for morphological assessment (Figure 22.18). Successful cytogenetic investigations from peripheral blood are only worth considering if immature leukaemic cells are present or, particularly when investigating suspected myeloproliferative neoplasms, if

the white cell count is at least 10×10^9/L, as mature cells will not enter metaphase.

Bone marrow aspiration may also be indicated in patients with unexplained cytopenia or a leucoerythroblastic blood film. An aspirate can be useful in lymphoma diagnosis, particularly if accompanied by a trephine biopsy, and can provide suitable material for immunophenotyping and for fluorescence *in situ* hybridization (FISH).

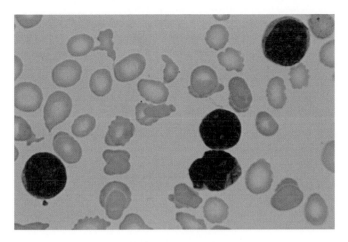

Figure 22.10 Acute myeloid leukaemia FAB M1 subtype showing small to medium-sized blast cells with a high nucleocytoplasmic ratio; one contains an Auer rod. Sudan black B and myeloperoxidase were positive. In the absence of Auer rods and granules, M1 acute myeloid leukaemia may be indistinguishable from acute lymphoblastic leukaemia without the aid of cytochemistry. Peripheral blood film, MGG.

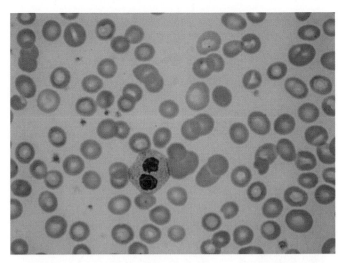

Figure. 22.12 A pseudo-Pelger–Huët anomaly in a neutrophil of a patient with myelodysplastic syndrome. Peripheral blood film, MGG.

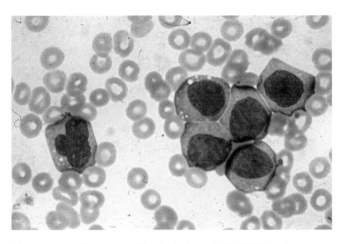

Figure 22.11 Acute monoblastic leukaemia FAB M5a subtype associated with t(9;11)(p22;q23) showing large cells with plentiful cytoplasm; one cell shows nuclear lobulation (defining it as a promonocyte in the WHO classification). In the WHO classification this type of acute myeloid leukaemia is a specific entity within the group 'AML with recurrent genetic abnormalities'. Bone marrow film, MGG.

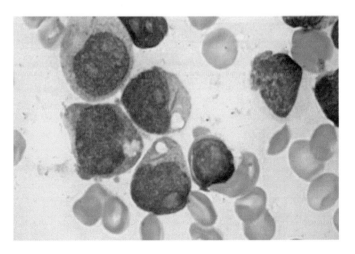

Figure 22.13 Acute myeloid leukaemia showing leukaemic blast cells, several with Auer rods. Bone marrow film, MGG.

Bone marrow trephine biopsy

A bone marrow trephine biopsy is indicated whenever there is a 'dry tap' or the aspirate obtained is aparticulate or dilute. A core biopsy is often necessary in hairy cell leukaemia, acute panmyelosis with myelofibrosis, acute megakaryoblastic leukaemia (Figure 22.19) and in patients being investigated for pan-

cytopenia or a leucoerythroblastic blood film. If the bone marrow is being examined for suspected non-Hodgkin lymphoma (NHL), a trephine biopsy is always indicated since an aspirate may be normal cytologically and immunophenotypically despite there being focal infiltration readily detectable on a core biopsy. Hodgkin lymphoma is very rarely detected in an aspirate whereas a trephine biopsy specimen may provide the primary diagnostic material, particularly in patients with HIV infection who often present with widespread disease. A trephine biopsy should be part of the initial investigation of suspected multiple myeloma; sometimes this confirms the diagnosis when the aspirate findings are equivocal and, even when this is not so, it is useful to have a baseline biopsy to compare with

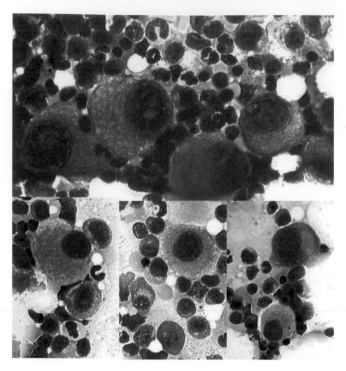

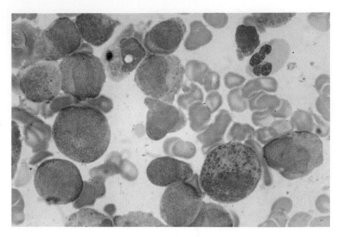

Figure 22.16 Acute myeloid leukaemia (AML) associated with inv(16)(p13.1q22) showing myelomonocytic leukaemia with an abnormal eosinophil precursor that has pro-eosinophilic (purple-staining) granules. This subtype of AML is often referred to, using an adaptation of FAB terminology, as M4Eo. In the WHO classification this subtype of AML, together with similar cases with t(16;16), constitutes a specific entity within the category 'AML with recurrent genetic abnormalities'. Bone marrow film, MGG.

Figure 22.14 Composite image of myelodysplastic syndrome showing the hypolobulated megakaryocytes characteristic of the 5q– syndrome; myelodysplastic syndrome with isolated del(5q) is a specific category in the WHO classification. Bone marrow film, MGG.

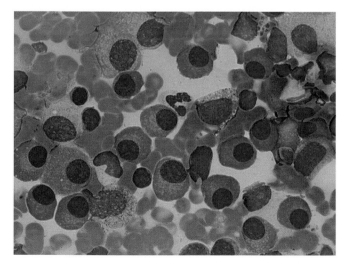

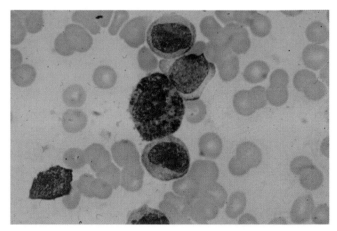

Figure 22.15 Multiple myeloma (plasma cell myeloma) showing virtual effacement of the marrow by myeloma cells. Bone marrow film, MGG.

Figure 22.17 Acute myeloid leukaemia (AML) associated with t(16;16)(p13.1;q22) showing blast cells and an abnormal eosinophil precursor with pro-eosinophilic granules. In the WHO classification this subtype of AML, together with similar cases with inv(16), constitutes a specific entity within the category 'AML with recurrent genetic abnormalities'. Bone marrow film, MGG.

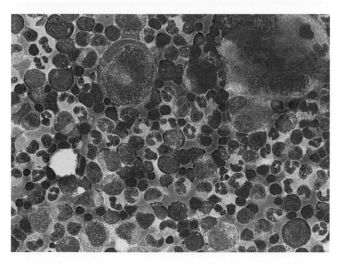

Figure 22.18 Polycythaemia vera with a *JAK2* V617F mutation showing panmyelosis; the large hyperlobulated megakaryocyte (top right) shows emperipolesis. Bone marrow film, MGG.

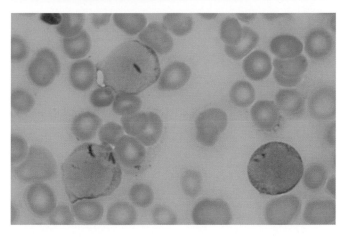

Figure 22.20 Acute myeloid leukaemia (AML) FAB M1 subtype showing Auer rods. This patient had the translocation t(8;21) (q22;q22), identifying a specific entity within the WHO category 'AML with recurrent genetic abnormalities'. Peripheral blood film, myeloperoxidase reaction.

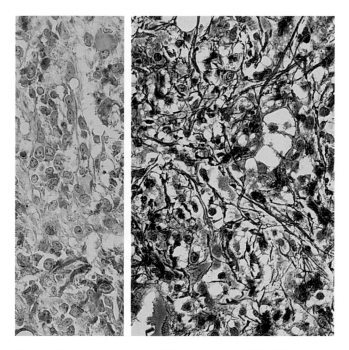

Figure 22.19 Acute megakaryoblastic leukaemia FAB M7 subtype. Bone marrow trephine biopsy shows blast cells (left) and increased reticulin deposition (right).

post-treatment investigations. A trephine biopsy is not generally necessary in CML or CLL whereas it is diagnostically important in suspected essential thrombocythaemia and polycythaemia vera and is essential in primary myelofibrosis and systemic mastocytosis.

There are other indications for trephine biopsy that are more controversial. This procedure may be necessary in ALL or AML

if no aspirate or a poor aspirate is obtained. However, if there are numerous circulating neoplastic cells and if a cellular aspirate is obtained, it does not yield any important extra information. In suspected MDS useful extra information that may contribute to the diagnosis is more likely since marrow architecture is often abnormal and immature (CD34⁺) cells may be detected only on histology or immunohistochemistry.

Cytochemistry

With advances in immunophenotyping and other techniques the role of cytochemistry in haematological diagnosis has declined considerably. A limited role remains. In acute leukaemia, cytochemistry is indicated if there is limited access to immunophenotyping or if delay in obtaining results is expected. For example, FAB M1 AML (and the 2008 WHO category of AML without maturation) can be distinguished from ALL by means of a Sudan black B or myeloperoxidase stain (Figure 22.20) and acute monoblastic/monocytic leukaemia can be distinguished from large-cell lymphoma by means of a non-specific esterase stain (Figure 22.21). Careful attention to cytological detail usually permits the distinction between FAB M3 variant and M5b AML but if there is any doubt the former diagnosis is supported by strong reactions for Sudan black B, myeloperoxidase and chloroacetate esterase and the latter by a positive non-specific esterase reaction. Rarely, a specific diagnosis of a subtype of AML is aided by demonstration of blast cells of basophil lineage showing metachromatic staining with a toluidine blue stain (Figure. 22.22). Perls stain for iron remains a very important cytochemical stain in suspected MDS (Figure 22.23).

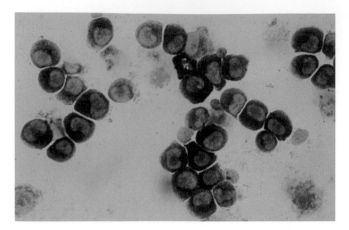

Figure 22.21 Acute monoblastic leukaemia FAB M5a subtype showing strong reaction for non-specific esterase, which confirms the monocytic differentiation. Cytospin preparation, α-naphthyl-acetate esterase.

Periodic acid–Schiff and acid phosphatase reactions can help in the diagnosis of ALL (Figures 22.24 and 22.25) but reactions are not specific and we do not recommend their continued use in a routine diagnostic setting if there is any possibility of carrying out immunophenotyping. A neutrophil alkaline phosphatase score is likewise redundant in the diagnosis of CML, which now depends on cytogenetic and molecular genetic analysis. A tartrate-resistant acid phosphatase reaction can confirm a diagnosis of hairy cell leukaemia but is no longer necessary as long as the immunophenotyping laboratory has an appropriate range of antibodies for this purpose or if immunohistochemistry can be performed in the case of a 'dry tap'.

Histology

Microscopic examination of sections of tissues other than bone marrow remains an essential technique for the diagnosis of many lymphomas. It may also be necessary for the diagnosis of myeloid sarcoma. Immunohistochemistry (see below) is an essential part of histological assessment for haematological neoplasms.

Flow cytometric immunophenotyping

Immunophenotyping can be based on flow cytometry, immunohistochemistry (on tissue sections) or immunocytochemistry (on cytospin preparations or films). The first two of these techniques are of major importance in haematological diagnosis. Flow cytometry is now carried out using multichannel instruments that permit the simultaneous assessment of forward light scatter (indicative of cell size), sideways light scatter (indicative

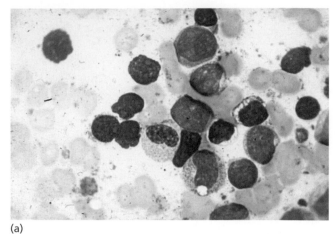
(a)

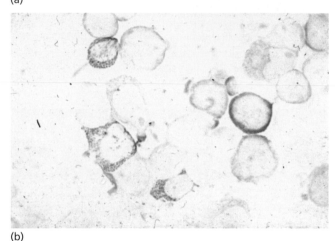
(b)

Figure 22.22 Acute myeloid leukaemia (AML) associated with t(6;9)(p23;q34): (a) MGG-stained bone marrow film shows blast cells and two degranulated basophil precursors; (b) toluidine blue-stained bone marrow film demonstrates metachromatic granules and confirms basophilic differentiation. In the 2008 WHO classification, this subtype of AML constitutes a specific entity within the category 'AML with recurrent genetic abnormalities'.

of granularity and cell complexity) and the expression of up to 10 surface membrane antigens, all simultaneously in one vial (Figure 22.26). With the addition of techniques to 'permeabilize' the cells, cytoplasmic and nuclear antigens can also be studied. When there are numerous circulating neoplastic cells, immunophenotyping is conveniently done on a peripheral blood sample. Otherwise it can be done on a bone marrow aspirate or on a cell suspension from any infiltrated tissue. The main indications for immunophenotyping are as follows.

1 Confirmation of a diagnosis of ALL and its subclassification and identification of an aberrant immunophenotype (leukaemia-associated immunophenotype) that can be used to monitor minimal residual disease (MRD).

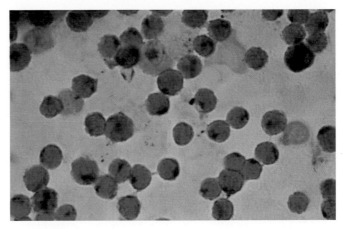

Figure 22.25 T-lineage acute lymphoblastic leukaemia showing focal (Golgi zone) positivity to acid phosphatase in lymphoblasts. Cytospin preparation, acid phosphatase reaction.

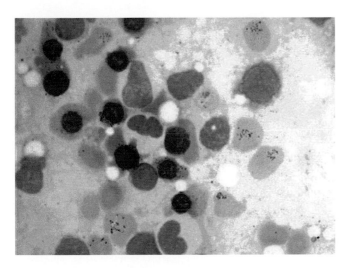

Figure 22.23 Ring sideroblasts and Pappenheimer bodies in erythrocytes in myelodysplastic syndrome. Bone marrow aspirate, Perls stain.

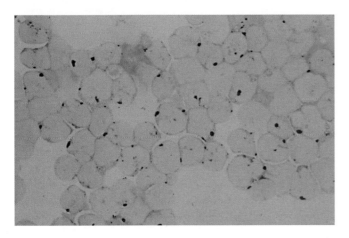

Figure 22.24 Acute lymphoblastic leukaemia showing block positivity to periodic acid–Schiff (PAS) stain. Cytospin preparation of cerebrospinal fluid, PAS stain.

2 Confirmation of a diagnosis of FAB M0 and M7 AML (WHO 2008 classification: AML with minimal differentiation and acute megakaryoblastic leukaemia) and, if not already confirmed by cytochemistry, confirmation of a diagnosis of FAB M5a AML (acute monoblastic leukaemia); support for a diagnosis of acute promyelocytic leukaemia (either hypergranular or hypogranular) by demonstration of lack of expression of CD34 and especially HLA-DR and by non-specific background autofluorescence observed in the isotype controls; identification of leukaemia-associated immunophenotype that can be used to monitor MRD.

3 Identification of mixed-lineage acute leukaemia.

4 Demonstration of light chain restriction, providing presumptive evidence of monoclonality, in B-lineage disorders.

5 Confirmation of a diagnosis of CLL, assessment of prognosis by quantification of CD38 and ZAP70 expression (both prognostically adverse) and monitoring of MRD.

6 Confirmation of a diagnosis of NHL rather than CLL, and support for specific diagnoses such as follicular lymphoma (CD10 often positive) or mantle cell lymphoma (CD5 and nuclear cyclin D1 positive) (see also Chapter 33).

7 Confirmation of a diagnosis of hairy cell leukaemia by demonstration of expression of all or most of CD11c, CD25, CD103 and CD123 (see also Chapter 29).

8 Confirmation of a diagnosis of multiple myeloma or monoclonal gammopathy of undetermined significance (MGUS) by demonstration that plasma cells (identified by expression of CD138 and strong CD38) have light chain-restricted cytoplasmic immunoglobulin and often aberrant expression of CD56 together with failure to express CD19 and CD45 (see also Chapter 31).

9 Support for monoclonality of a T-lymphocyte population by demonstration of a uniform aberrant immunophenotype and restricted expression of CD158 (KIR) epitopes and support for specific diagnoses such as T-prolymphocytic leukaemia (CD7 often positive), adult T-cell leukaemia lymphoma (CD25 positive), large granular lymphocyte leukaemia (usually CD8$^+$CD4$^-$), and hepatosplenic T-cell lymphoma, which is usually T-cell receptor (TCR)-γδ positive and TCR-αβ negative.

10 Confirmation of a diagnosis of blastic plasmacytoid dendritic cell neoplasm by demonstration of expression of CD4, CD56, CD123 and possibly CD7 in the absence of expression of other lineage-specific markers.

11 Demonstration of an antigen that is a potential target of monoclonal antibody therapy, such as CD20, CD33 or CD52.

12 Diagnosis of paroxysmal nocturnal haemoglobinuria by demonstrating that a subpopulation of neutrophils, monocytes

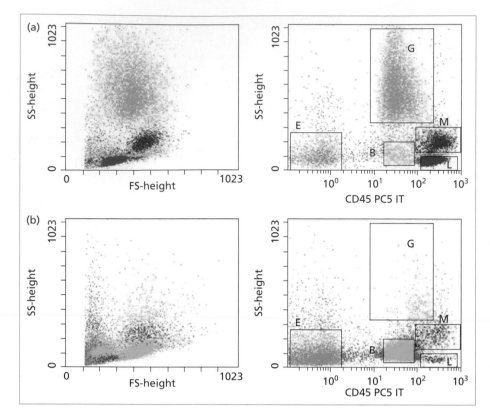

Figure 22.26 Flow cytometry immunophenotyping showing improvement of separation of populations by CD45 and sideways light scatter (SSC) gating. Forward light scatter (FSC) is also shown. (a) Normal bone marrow (left, SSC–FSC plot; right, SSC–CD45 plot); (b) acute myeloid leukaemia bone marrow (left, SSC–FSC plot; right, SSC–CD45 plot). G, granulocytes; M, monocytes; L, lymphocytes; E, erythrocytes; B, blasts. SSC–CD45 gating permits isolation of bone marrow blasts from all other populations, which is not possible by SSC–FSC gating.

or erythrocytes fails to express antigens, such as CD55 and CD59, that are bound to glycosylphosphatidylinositol.

13 Detection and quantification of fetomaternal haemorrhage.

14 Quantification of lymphocyte subpopulations.

15 Support for a diagnosis of MDS based on quantification of blasts and detection of aberrant antigen expression.

16 Assessment of infiltration of body fluids (cerebrospinal fluid, pleural effusion) by leukaemia and/or lymphoma.

Immunohistochemistry

Immunohistochemistry for haematological diagnosis is carried out on tissue sections, particularly from lymph nodes or trephine biopsy specimens. It is an essential part of the diagnostic procedure in haematological neoplasms, particularly lymphoma but also myeloid neoplasms. Examples that illustrate its value in lymphoma diagnosis include the following.

1 Confirmation of follicular lymphoma by demonstration that cells forming neoplastic follicles express CD10 and BCL2 (whereas follicles of reactive follicular hyperplasia are BCL2 negative).

2 Confirmation of mantle cell lymphoma by demonstration of CD5-positive B cells with nuclear expression of cyclin D1.

3 Confirmation of a diagnosis of classical Hodgkin lymphoma (CD15 usually positive, CD30 positive) and its distinction from

nodular lymphocyte-predominant Hodgkin lymphoma (CD15 and CD30 negative and more likely to express B cell-associated antigens such as CD20 and CD79a).

4 Confirmation of Burkitt lymphoma by demonstration of BCL2-negative BCL6-positive B cells with a very high proliferative fraction (approaching 100%) shown using Ki-67 or an equivalent monoclonal antibody.

5 Division of diffuse large B-cell lymphoma (DLBCL) into prognostic groups (see below).

6 Confirmation of hairy cell leukaemia by showing that B cells express CD25, CD72 (DBA44) and annexin A1.

7 Confirmation of clonality in suspected MGUS or multiple myeloma by demonstration of light chain restriction of cytoplasmic immunoglobulin.

8 Confirmation of infiltration in a trephine biopsy specimen in non-Hodgkin and Hodgkin lymphoma (particularly important in patients in whom no neoplastic cells are detected in the bone marrow aspirate and for detection of subtle interstitial or intravascular infiltration in NHL).

DLBCL has been demonstrated by microarray analysis (see below) to be divisible into three major groups with different patterns of gene expression: (i) germinal centre cell; (ii) activated B-cell-like; and (iii) other or indeterminate (see also Chapter 33). Lymphomas showing the gene expression pattern of germinal centre B cells were found to have a better prognosis than activated B-cell-like DLBCL. It is now possible to assign DLBCL to these two major groups on the basis on immunohistochemistry. The germinal centre group express CD10 or, if they do not, they express BCL6 in the absence of MUM1 expression. DLBCL of the activated B-cell-like group are either negative for both CD10 and BCL6 or are CD10 negative but express both BCL6 and MUM1. The prognostic significance is seen clearly in patients treated with CHOP (cyclophosphamide, doxorubicin, vincristine and prednisolone) but may no longer reach statistical significance in those treated with R-CHOP (CHOP plus rituximab). In R-CHOP-treated patients, prognostic significance is shown by the demonstration of BCL2 expression, the best prognosis being in those with a germinal centre phenotype but without BCL2 expression, whose survival curves separate from the other three groups. However, it must be noted that scoring of these immunohistochemical markers is inconsistent between laboratories unless many technical factors are standardized; use of the assignment to germinal centre or non-germinal centre phenotypes to aid treatment decisions would be premature.

In ALL, it is usually possible to perform immunophenotyping on either peripheral blood or a bone marrow aspirate; immunohistochemistry is therefore usually redundant. In AML, immunohistochemistry should be viewed as supplementary to flow cytometric immunophenotyping. It is often unnecessary. However, in the absence of peripheral blood blast cells and if a bone marrow aspirate cannot be obtained, it becomes essential for diagnosis. It can thus be important for the diagnosis of acute megakaryoblastic leukaemias, acute panmyelosis with myelofibrosis and some cases of acute erythroleukaemia, when bone marrow fibrosis may prevent an adequate aspirate being obtained. It is needed for the diagnosis of myeloid sarcoma and blastic plasmacytoid dendritic cell neoplasm (which shows expression of CD4, CD56 and CD123). Immunohistochemistry can be a useful way to demonstrate the presence of an *NPM1* mutation in AML, cytoplasmic rather than nuclear expression being a surrogate marker for these mutations.

Immunohistochemistry for mast cell tryptase is important in confirming a diagnosis of systemic mastocytosis. Aberrant expression of CD2 and CD25 by the mast cells is also useful (although this pattern of reactivity is not specific for systemic mastocytosis). Immunohistochemistry is much less often needed in other myeloproliferative neoplasms.

Cytogenetic analysis

Cytogenetic analysis refers to study of chromosomes by recognition of their morphology and their characteristic banding pattern, demonstrated by staining with a Giemsa stain (for viewing by light microscopy) (Figure 22.27) or a quinacrine stain (for viewing as fluorescent bands under UV illumination). Chromosomes or specific genes of interest in either interphase or metaphase can also be studied by FISH analysis; this technique is both a cytogenetic and molecular genetic technique since the morphology of the chromosomes can be recognized to some extent, at least in metaphase cells, but the probes used are dependent on hybridization to specific DNA sequences. Cytogenetic, FISH and molecular techniques are complementary and which of these is most useful in an individual patient depends on the suspected diagnosis and the aberrations likely to be present. Classical cytogenetic analysis (chromosome banding analysis) requires cells in metaphase so that for conditions with a low mitotic rate, such as CLL and low-grade NHL, FISH or molecular analysis may be preferred. However, with the newer techniques it is possible to achieve metaphases in more than 90% of cases of CLL. Cytogenetic analysis can (i) provide evidence of clonality and thus confirm that a condition is neoplastic when other evidence is absent or equivocal (e.g. in chronic eosinophilic leukaemia, myeloproliferative neoplasms or NK cell leukaemia/lymphoma); (ii) confirm a specific diagnosis (e.g. CML, AML with recurrent translocations or Burkitt lymphoma); and (iii) give prognostic information (e.g. in CLL,

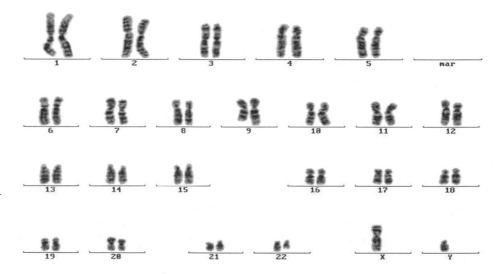

Figure 22.27 A karyogram of Giemsa-stained chromosomes showing t(9;22) (q34;q11.2). The derivative chromosome 22 is the Philadelphia chromosome.

AML, ALL, MDS and multiple myeloma) or indicate that a neoplasm is therapy-induced (t-AML and t-MDS).

It is particularly important that cytogenetic or molecular genetic analysis is performed whenever there is a specific treatment available for patients with a particular genetic abnormality. This includes the following.

1 Conditions sensitive to tyrosine kinase inhibitors (with either *BCR–ABL1* or rearrangement of *PDGFRA* or *PDGFRB*).

2 Acute promyelocytic leukaemia with *PML–RARA* (sensitive to all-*trans* retinoic acid and As_2O_3).

3 MDS with 5q– (sensitive to lenalidomide).

4 MDS with monosomy 7 (sensitive to azacytidine).

5 Burkitt lymphoma with juxtaposition of *MYC* to the immunoglobulin heavy chain, κ or λ locus (responsive to intensive chemotherapy incorporating certain specific agents plus monoclonal antibody treatment).

Table 22.1 The 2008 WHO classification of acute myeloid leukaemia (AML), with categories where genetic analysis is, or may be, essential for categorization shown in blue.

Therapy-related myeloid neoplasms

De novo **myeloid neoplasms**

AML with recurrent genetic abnormalities*

    AML with t(8;21)(q22;q22); *RUNX1–RUNX1T1*

    AML with inv(16)(p13.1q22) or t(16;16)(p13.1;q22); *CBFB–MYH11*

    AML with t(15;17)(q22;q12); *PML–RARA*

    AML with t(9;11)(p22;q23); *MLLT3–MLL*

    AML with t(6;9)(p23;q34); *DEK–NUP214*

    AML with inv(3)(q21q26.2) or t(3;3)(q21;q26.2); *RPN1–EVI1*

    AML with t(1;22)(p13;q13); *RBM15–MKL1*

    Provisional entity: AML with mutated *NPM1*

    Provisional entity: AML with mutated *CEBPA*

AML with myelodysplasia-related changes†

AML not otherwise categorized

Myeloid sarcoma

Myeloid proliferation related to Down syndrome‡

    Transient abnormal myelopoiesis

    Myeloid leukaemia associated with Down syndrome

Blastic plasmacytoid dendritic cell neoplasm

---

*Either cytogenetic or molecular genetic analysis essential for classification.

†Meeting cytogenetic criteria for myelodysplastic syndrome (MDS)-associated cytogenetic abnormalities permits assignment of a case to this category (assignment can also be on the basis of multilineage dysplasia or a previous diagnosis of MDS).

‡Cytogenetic analysis may be necessary to confirm the diagnosis of Down syndrome, particularly in mosaic Down syndrome; an acquired *GATA1* mutation is also present.

Cytogenetic analysis can be considered appropriate whenever it contributes to diagnosis, indicates the prognosis or guides the selection of treatment. It can therefore be considered indicated in the following.

1 All cases of AML: essential for application of the WHO classification, indicates prognosis and is thus relevant to treatment choice (Table 22.1).

2 All cases of ALL: essential for application of the WHO classification, indicates prognosis and is thus relevant to treatment choice; necessary for detection of *BCR–ABL1*-positive cases, although for this purpose FISH and molecular analyses are alternatives (Table 22.2).

3 All cases of mixed-phenotype acute leukaemia: essential for detecting *BCR–ABL1*-positive cases.

4 All cases of suspected CML: essential to confirm *BCR–ABL1*, although FISH or molecular analyses are alternatives.

5 All cases of suspected MDS: necessary for application of the WHO classification including identification of the 5q– syndrome (Figure 22.28) and essential for application of the International Prognostic Scoring System (IPSS) and WHO classification-based Prognostic Scoring System (WPSS).

6 All cases of suspected chronic eosinophilic leukaemia: necessary for detection of translocations that lead to *PDGFRB* rearrangement (imatinib sensitive) and *FGFR1* rearrangement.

7 All cases of suspected NK leukaemia/lymphoma: can demonstrate clonality and thus confirm the diagnosis.

If resources permit, cytogenetic analysis can also be useful in other myeloproliferative and myelodysplastic/myeloproliferative neoplasms. Cytogenetic analysis can be used for the confir-

Table 22.2 The WHO classification of acute lymphoblastic leukaemia, with categories where genetic analysis is essential for categorization shown in blue (see also Chapter 25).

B lymphoblastic leukaemia/lymphoma

B lymphoblastic leukaemia/lymphoma, not otherwise specified

B lymphoblastic leukaemia/lymphoma with recurrent genetic abnormalities

    With t(9;22)(q34;q11.2) and *BCR–ABL1*

    With t(4;11)(q21;q23) and *MLL–MLLT2* or other 11q23 and *MLL* rearrangement

    With t(12;21)(p13;q22) and *ETV6–RUNX1**

    With hyperdiploidy (>50 chromosomes)

    With hypodiploidy (<46 chromosomes)

    With t(5;14)(q31;q32) and *IL3–IGH*

    With t(1;19)(q23;p13.3) and *TCF3–PBX1*

T lymphoblastic leukaemia/lymphoma

---

*Molecular genetic analysis is needed since the translocation is cryptic.

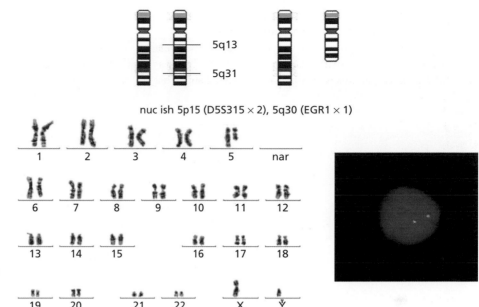

nuc ish 5p15 (D5S315 × 2), 5q30 (EGR1 × 1)

Figure 22.28 An explanatory diagram (top), karyogram of Giemsa-stained chromosomes showing del(5)(q13q31) (bottom left), and FISH showing retention of signal for 5p15 and loss of signal for 5q31 (bottom right) in a patient with 5q– syndrome.

mation of a diagnosis of Burkitt lymphoma, follicular lymphoma or mantle cell lymphoma but FISH may be preferred. Use of the two techniques may give complementary information. Prognostically relevant information is also obtained in multiple myeloma. However, this is best done with preliminary magnetic activation cell sorting using CD138-positive antibodies, as plasma cells may be low and FISH performed on direct bone marrow films may result in insufficient cells for analysis and give misleading results.

Fluorescence *in situ* hybridization

FISH uses labelled oligonucleotide probes that bind to specific DNA sequences. These may be locus-specific probes (including those detecting oncogenes and tumour-suppressor genes), centromeric probes, telomeric probes and whole chromosome paints. Centromeric probes can be used for the detection of monosomies and trisomies. Otherwise, locus-specific probes are those most widely used. By labelling two probes with different fluorochromes it is possible to study two genes that are involved in a specific translocation or other rearrangement. If the probes span the breakpoint, both will be disrupted by the translocation and signals will be adjacent or optically fused on the derivative chromosomes, a double-colour double-fusion technique. Often one probe gives a green signal and the other a red signal so that the fusion signal is yellow. Alternatively, two probes that span the 5′ locus and 3′ locus and overlap can be used in a double-colour break-apart technique; this can be

useful when a single gene, such as *MLL*, is involved in rearrangements with a large number of other genes. FISH is applicable to both metaphase cells and interphase cells (Figure 22.29).

FISH is particularly useful in the following circumstances.

1 Screening for *BCR–ABL1* fusion (peripheral blood cells are suitable whereas cytogenetic analysis is better done on bone marrow) (Figure 22.30).

2 Confirming a specific lymphoma diagnosis by demonstration of *BCL2–IGH* in follicular lymphoma, *CCND1–IGHG1* in mantle cell lymphoma or *MYC–IGHG1* in Burkitt lymphoma (Table 22.3).

3 Detection of translocations or inversions or aneuploidy that was not detected on metaphase cytogenetic analyses because the leukaemic cells did not enter mitosis or the metaphases were of too poor quality, e.g. detection of t(8;21)(q22;q22), t(15;17)(q22;q12), inv(16)(p13.1q22) or *MLL* rearrangement in AML (Figure 22.31) or detection of high hyperdiploidy in ALL (by using centromeric probes for the chromosomes that are most often triplicated).

4 Screening for a cryptic *FIP1L1–PDGFRA* fusion (by detection of loss of *CHIC2*) in chronic eosinophilic leukaemia.

5 Producing prognostically relevant information in CLL by investigation for trisomy 12, del(6)(q21), del(11)(q22–23), del(13)(q14.3) (Figure 22.32) and del(17)(p13).

Spectral karyotyping, also known as 24-colour FISH, is a modification of FISH that permits visualization of each pair of chromosomes in a unique colour. It can be used as a supplement to metaphase cytogenetics to clarify the nature of complex rearrangements (Figure 22.33). Inversions are not detected.

Interphase

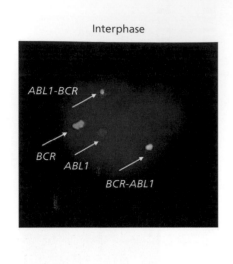

Metaphase

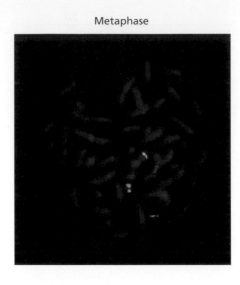

Figure 22.29 Locus-specific probes for *BCR* (green) and *ABL1* (red) applied to an interphase cell and to a metaphase of a patient with chronic myelogenous leukaemia after hybridization with probes for *ABL1* (red) and *BCR* (green) showing *BCR–ABL1* colocalization signals (yellow) on the Philadelphia chromosome and *ABL1–BCR* colocalization signals on derivative chromosome 9.

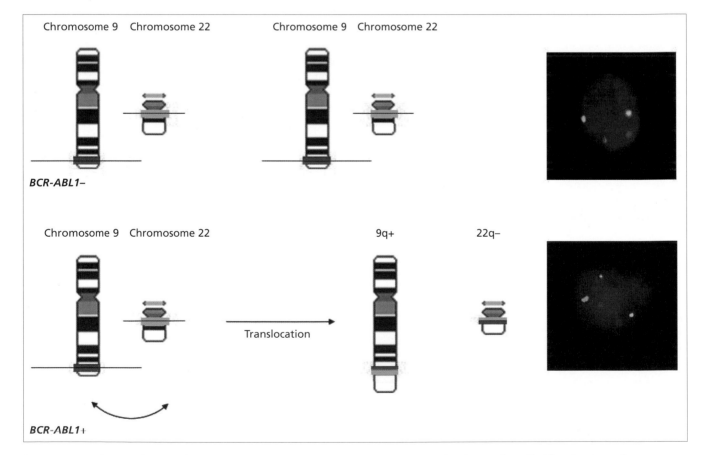

Figure 22.30 Diagram showing the principle of fluorescence *in situ* hybridization for detection of *BCR–ABL1*. Locus-specific probes for *BCR* (green) and *ABL1* (red) have been applied to interphase cells. The normal cell (top) shows two red signals and two green signals, whereas the cell with *BCR–ABL1* shows two normal signals and two fusion signals (*BCR–ABL1* and *ABL1–BCR*).

Table 22.3 Cytogenetic/molecular genetic abnormalities that are incorporated into the 2008 WHO classification of neoplasms of mature T and B cells.

Genetic abnormality	Gene dysregulated	Diagnosis*
t(14;18)(q32;q21) or t(2;18)(p12;q21) or t(18;22) (q21;q11.2)	BCL2	Follicular lymphoma
t(11;14)(q13;q32) or, rarely, t(11;22)(q13;q11)	CCND1	Mantle cell lymphoma
t(8;14)(q24;q32) or t(2;8)(p12;q24) or t(8;22) (q24;q11.2)	MYC	Burkitt lymphoma
inv(14)(q11q32) or t(14;14)(q11;q32) or, less often, t(X;14)(q28;q11)	TCL1	T-prolymphocytic leukaemia
t(2;5)(p23;q35) or one of at least five variant translocations with a 2p23 breakpoint	NPM1–ALK fusion or other fusion gene incorporating part of ALK	Anaplastic large-cell lymphoma, ALK positive

*The genetic abnormality confirms the diagnosis only in an appropriate cytological/histological and immunophenotypic setting.

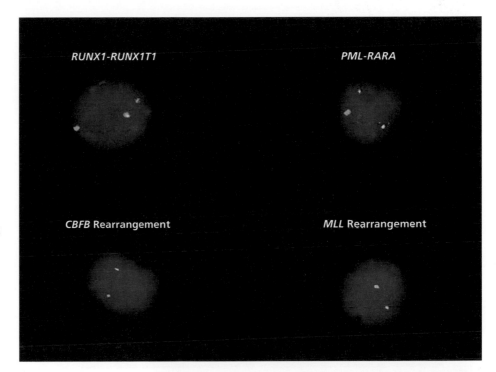

Figure 22.31 Fluorescence *in situ* hybridization in four different patients with acute myeloid leukaemia showing four major cytogenetic/genetic categories of AML: *RUNX1–RUNX1T1* fusion indicative of t(8;21) (top left); *PML–RARA* fusion indicative of t(15;17) (top right); *CBFB* rearrangement, which is likely to indicate *CBFB–MYH11* (bottom left); *MLL* rearrangement (bottom right).

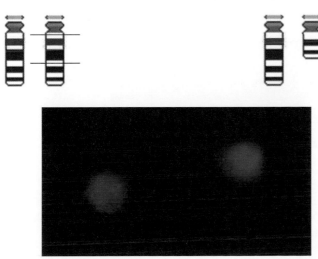

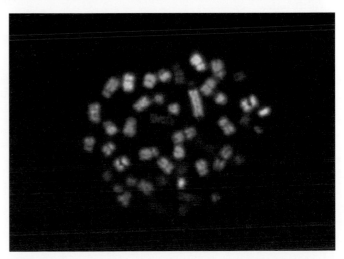

Figure 22.32 Explanatory diagram and fluorescence *in situ* hybridization showing interstitial deletion of 13q14.3 in a patient with chronic lymphocytic leukaemia.

Figure 22.33 Metaphase of a patient with acute myeloid leukaemia and a complex aberrant karyotype after 24-colour fluorescence *in situ* hybridization.

Molecular genetic analysis

Molecular genetic analysis includes Southern blotting (now little used in routine diagnosis), the polymerase chain reaction (PCR) to study genomic DNA (Figures 22.34 and 22.35), and reverse transcriptase polymerase chain reaction (RT-PCR) to study RNA after its reverse transcription. A PCR reaction can also be made quantitative, as in real-time quantitative PCR, an important technique for monitoring MRD (Figure 22.36). PCR and RT-PCR can be alternatives to metaphase cytogenetic anal-

ysis in several subgroups of leukaemia and lymphoma. However, unlike metaphase cytogenetic analysis but similar to FISH, this is a targeted investigation so that only the abnormality that is specifically sought will be detected. Thus, in some diseases additional diagnostic or prognostic information will be found only by using metaphase cytogenetics. On the other hand, PCR has the advantage that only a small amount of DNA is needed and there is no need for dividing cells. Molecular analysis permits the detection of prognostically and therapeutically relevant cryptic rearrangements, such as the *ETV6–RUNX1* rearrange-

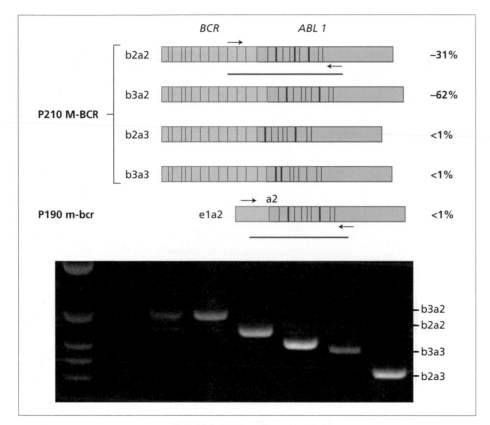

Figure 22.34 An explanatory diagram and a PCR gel showing the various *BCR–ABL1* transcripts that can be identified by PCR.

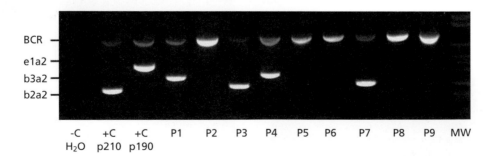

Figure 22.35 *BCR–ABL1* multiplex PCR containing different oligonucleotide ('oligo') combinations. –C, negative control sample containing water instead of a nucleic acid template; +C, positive controls for p210 and p190 fusion types. P, patient samples: P1 and P4 are positive for b3a2 fusion types, P3 and P7 are positive for b2a2 fusion types, P2, P5, P6, P8 and P9 are *BCR–ABL1* negative patient samples. MW, molecular weight standard; BCR, amplification of the non-rearrangend *BCR* gene as internal quality control reaction.

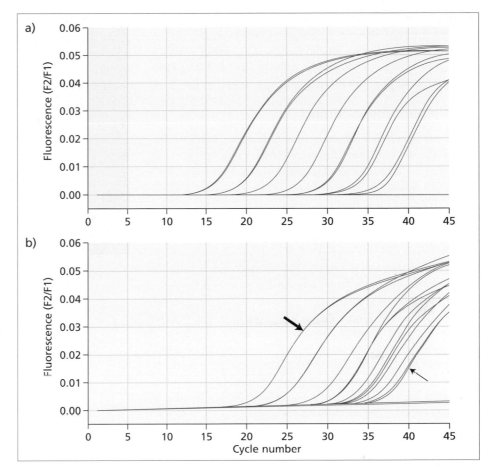

Figure 22.36 Real-time quantitative PCR. Fluorescence is plotted against PCR cycle number. (a) A 10-fold limited dilution series of a *BCR–ABL1*-containing plasmid showing high sensitivity of the PCR. It also serves as a calibration curve for subsequent *BCR–ABL1* calculations. (b) Run with chronic myeloid leukaemia follow-up samples: the large arrow shows a sample with high *BCR–ABL1* load, the small arrow low *BCR–ABL1* load.

ment associated with a cryptic t(12;21)(p13;q22) in ALL. Genomic PCR can be applied to stored samples.

The roles of genomic PCR and RT-PCR include the following.

1 Detection of rearrangement of immunoglobulin heavy and light chain loci and TCR loci, providing evidence of a clonal disorder if a monoclonal rather than an oligoclonal or polyclonal pattern is detected.

2 Detection of leukaemia-related and lymphoma-related chromosomal rearrangements by demonstration of gene juxtaposition or fusion in order to confirm a diagnosis, for example detection of *CCND1–IGHG1* indicative of t(11;14)(q13;q32) to confirm suspected mantle cell lymphoma or detection of *BCL2–IGH* indicative of t(14;18)(q32;q21) to confirm suspected follicular lymphoma. Note that neither of these rearrangements is absolutely specific for the disease in question since *CCND1–IGHG1* also occurs in multiple myeloma and *BCL2–IGH* also occurs in DLBCL, but in the context of appropriate cytology or histology they do permit confirmation of a diagnosis.

3 Detection of gene mutations relevant to diagnosis, for example *KIT* D816V in systemic mastocytosis or either *JAK2* V617F or *JAK2* exon 12 mutation in polycythaemia vera (*JAK2* V617F also occurs in many patients with essential thrombo-

cythaemia or primary myelofibrosis but its detection in a patient with a high haemoglobin concentration confirms the diagnosis of polycythaemia vera and since it is present in the great majority of patients with this diagnosis, measurement of the total red cell mass and plasma volume is generally rendered unnecessary).

4 Prognostic stratification, for example in ALL detection of *ETV6–RUNX1* associated with cryptic t(12;21)(p13;q22) (good prognosis), *TCF3–PBX1* associated with t(1;19)(q23;p13.3) (good prognosis), *MLL–MLLT2* associated with t(4;11) (q21;q23) (poor prognosis) and *BCR–ABL1* associated with t(9;22)(q34;q11.2) (poor prognosis); multiplex PCR, combining a number of primer pairs in a single reaction, is useful for screening simultaneously for more than one rearrangement.

5 Prognostic stratification in AML with normal karyotype, for example *FLT3* internal tandem duplication (ITD) (poor prognosis), *MLL* partial tandem duplication (PTD) (poor prognosis), *NPM1* mutation (good prognosis if not associated with *FLT3* ITD), *CEBPA* mutation (good prognosis if not associated with *FLT3* ITD).

6 Prognostic stratification in CLL: somatic hypermutation, defined as *IGHV* showing less than 98% homology with germline, is found in 50–60% of all cases and correlates with a better prognosis than is found in patients with unmutated *IGHV* genes.

7 MRD detection using *RUNX1–RUNX1T1*, *CBFB–MYH11*, *PML–RARA*, *MLL* rearrangement, *MLL* PTD, *FLT3* ITD, *NPM1* mutation or *CEBPA* mutation.

Whole-genome scanning

There are a number of molecular techniques available for whole-genome scanning. Thus far, these have mainly been used to address research topics, but it is likely that they will soon find a place in routine diagnostic work. These techniques include comparative genomic hybridization (CGH), in which labelled test DNA is hybridized to normal metaphase preparations, and microarray analysis, in which there is hybridization of the labelled test DNA of interest to probes positioned in high density on a microarray surface. Microarray analysis includes CGH arrays and, more frequently used, genome-wide single-nucleotide polymorphism (SNP) arrays. CGH is labour-intensive, less sensitive for the detection of small regions harbouring copy number alterations and likely to remain a research technique. Microarray analysis has a greater potential for diagnostic application since it has a much higher resolution for the detection of genomic aberrations, requires a low amount of starting material and has the potential to be developed as a fully automated molecular laboratory assay.

In CGH assays, test and reference DNAs are labelled with different fluorochromes before being hybridized to microarrays of either oligonucleotides or bacterial artificial chromosome (BAC) probes. CGH microarray analysis is used for the detection of under-representation or over-representation of specific genomic regions in the test DNA. Deletions and amplifications can thus be detected, for example deletion of 13q14 and 11q22 in CLL or intrachromosomal amplification of 21q in ALL.

In SNP array analysis, genomic DNA of a sample of interest is digested by restriction enzymes, amplified, labelled and hybridized to oligonucleotide probes. Probes are either bound to microbeads or are synthesized *in situ* in high density on a microarray surface (Figure 22.37). SNP analysis can be applied to genotyping and is able to distinguish heterozygosity from homozygosity. It can thus be used to detect both loss of heterozygosity and alterations of copy numbers of a genomic region, i.e. gains and losses (Figure 22.38). Acquired somatic uniparental disomy can be detected by comparison of tumour DNA with constitutional DNA. Sensitivity for the detection of a clonal population is similar to that of metaphase cytogenetics. With SNP array technology it is possible to identify uniparental disomy for chromosomal regions that include mutated genes such as *JAK2*, *CEBPA*, *FLT3* and *RUNX1*.

Microarray analysis of gene expression

Microarray analysis was initially applied to the study of cellular gene expression by hybridization of test and control RNA speci-

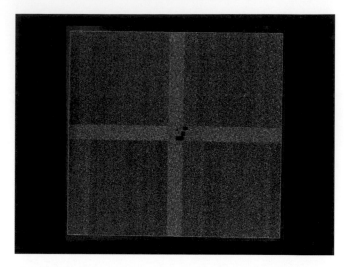

Figure 22.37 High-density single-nucleotide polymorphism (SNP) microarray scan showing the surface of a high-density SNP microarray (Affymetrix SNP 6.0). This chip was designed as hybrid genotyping array to simultaneously measure 906 600 SNPs and copy number alterations at approximately 1.8 million genomic locations.

mens, processed and labelled with different fluorochromes, to single-stranded DNA. The DNA probes were either complementary (c)DNA or synthetic oligonucleotides, arrayed in multiple rows of dots on a microarray surface with each dot interrogating a fragment of a single gene. High-density gene expression profiling (GEP) is a well-established molecular method and has been demonstrated to yield information of both diagnostic and prognostic value.

Primary mediastinal B-cell lymphoma can be distinguished from both DLBCL and Hodgkin lymphoma by its molecular signature. Burkitt lymphoma has a distinctive pattern of gene expression, which can help in making a distinction with DLBCL with *MYC* overexpression. Similarly, small lymphocytic lymphoma, marginal zone B-cell lymphoma and mantle cell lymphoma can be characterized by their differential gene expression signatures.

Prognostic information is provided in DLBCL. Microarray studies have shown that this diagnostic category encompasses at least two molecularly distinct diseases, differing in differentiation stage (i.e. cell of origin), oncogenic mechanisms and clinical outcome. Microarray analysis can also divide mantle cell lymphoma into groups with very different prognosis.

From a diagnostic perspective, GEP has been demonstrated to offer a robust technology platform. For multiple categories of acute leukaemias, for example based on immunophenotype (B-cell and T-cell lineages), chromosomal aberrations (translocations and inversions) or molecular mutations (*NPM1*, *CEBPA*), characteristic gene expression signatures have been identified (Figure 22.39). Moreover, international multicentre studies have demonstrated high intra- and inter-laboratory pre-

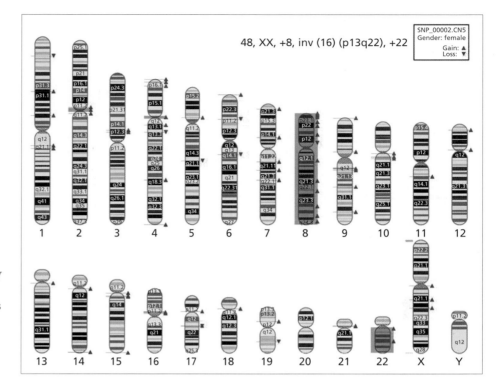

48, XX, +8, inv (16) (p13q22), +22

Figure 22.38 Molecular karyotype based on high-density SNP microarray analysis. Alterations are given by arrows indicating either gains or losses of chromosomal material. The karyotype using conventional chromosome banding techniques is given for comparison.

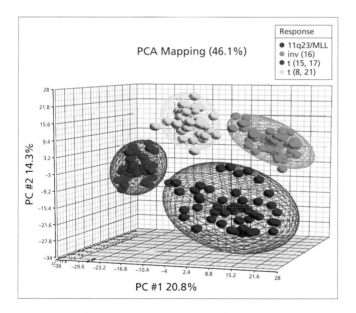

PCA Mapping (46.1%)

Response
- 11q23/MLL
- inv (16)
- t (15, 17)
- t (8, 21)

Figure 22.39 Principal components analysis of various subtypes of acute leukaemia. Patient samples are plotted in a three-dimensional space using the three components capturing most of the variance in the microarray dataset. Each patient sample is represented by a single colour-coded sphere. Adult acute myeloid leukaemia samples from the entities t(8;21)(q22;q22), t(15;17) (q22;q12), inv(16)(p13.1q22) and t(11q23)/*MLL* can clearly be distinguished based on the differential expression of signature genes.

cision in the performance of gene expression analyses, underlining that array-based GEP is a promising molecular assay that could be applied in the diagnosis of haematological malignancies.

Laboratory techniques and the WHO classification of tumours of haemopoietic and lymphoid tissues

The 2008 WHO classification is based on the integration of clinical and pathological features. Among the pathological features, morphology (cytology and histology) is fundamental but there is an increasing use of immunophenotyping for classification of lymphoid, mixed lineage and some myeloid neoplasms and of cytogenetic and molecular genetic information for classification of both lymphoid and myeloid neoplasms. Tables 22.1 and 22.2 illustrate how cytogenetic and molecular genetic information is integrated into the classifications of AML and B-lineage ALL respectively. Two categories of acute leukaemia of ambiguous lineage are also defined by the presence, in addition to the required immunophenotypic characteristics, of t(9;22)(q34;q11.2)/*BCR–ABL1* and 11q23/*MLL* rearrangement respectively. The 2008 WHO classification has also introduced a new genetically defined categorization for lymphoid and myeloid neoplasms associated with rearrangement of *PDGFRA*, *PDGFRB* or *FGFR1*; these categories encompass cases of *BCR–ABL1*-negative chronic myeloid leukaemia (often with eosinophilic differentiation), AML, ALL and lymphoid or myeloid transformation of a myeloproliferative neoplasm.

Otherwise, among the myeloproliferative neoplasms, only the demonstration of t(9;22)(q34;q11.2)/*BCR–ABL1* to confirm or exclude a diagnosis of CML is essential for classification. However, the demonstration of the *JAK2* V617F mutation or a somatic *MPL* mutation is important for making a diagnosis of a myeloproliferative neoplasm rather than a secondary or familial disorder. A *JAK2* exon 12 mutation similarly confirms that polycythaemia is polycythaemia vera rather than a familial or secondary condition.

Cytogenetic and molecular genetic abnormalities are critical in the diagnosis of certain neoplasms of mature lymphocytes (Table 22.3). However, for the majority of cases of CLL and NHL, such analysis is not needed for diagnosis and classification, although it may provide information of prognostic value.

Conclusions

Modern diagnosis, classification and monitoring of haematological neoplasms require integration of multiple diagnostic tools in a systematic manner in order to provide all the information necessary for optimal management of the patient. In addition, application of new diagnostic tools is constantly increasing our understanding of these disorders. New research tools not only give new information but are often rapidly integrated into diagnostic practice. Classifications of lymphoid and myeloid neoplasms increasingly incorporate, and depend on, immunophenotypic and genetic analysis.

Selected bibliography

Alcalay M, Tiacci E, Bergomas R et al. (2005) Acute myeloid leukaemia bearing cytoplasmic nucleophosmin (NPMc+ AML) shows a distinct gene expression profile characterized by up-regulation of genes involved in stem-cell maintenance. *Blood* **106**: 899–902.

Bacher U, Kohlmann A, Haferlach T (2009) Current status of gene expression profiling in the diagnosis and management of acute leukaemia. *British Journal of Haematology* **145**: 555–68.

Bain BJ (2010) *Leukaemia Diagnosis*, 4th edn. Wiley-Blackwell, Oxford.

Bain BJ, Clark DM, Wilkins BS (2009) *Bone Marrow Pathology*, 4th edn. Wiley-Blackwell, Oxford.

Cools J, DeAngelo DJ, Gotlib J et al. (2003) A tyrosine kinase created by the fusion of the PDGFRA and FIP1L1 genes as a therapeutic target of imatinib in idiopathic hypereosinophilic syndrome. *New England Journal of Medicine* **348**: 1201–14.

de Jong D, Xie W, Rosenwald A et al. (209) Immunohistochemical prognostic markers in diffuse large B-cell lymphoma: validation of tissue microarray as a prerequisite for broad clinical applications. *Journal of Clinical Pathology* **62**: 128–38.

Dicker F, Haferlach C, Kern W, Haferlach T, Schnittger S (2007) Trisomy 13 is strongly associated with *AML1/RUNX1* mutations and increased *FLT3* expression in acute myeloid leukaemia. *Blood* **110**: 1308–16.

Falini B, Mecucci C, Tiacci E et al. (2005) Cytoplasmic nucleophosmin in acute myelogenous leukaemia with a normal karyotype. *New England Journal of Medicine* **352**: 254–66.

Gleissner B, Küppers R, Siebert R et al. (2008) Report of a workshop on malignant lymphoma: a review of molecular and clinical risk profiling. *British Journal of Haematology* **142**: 166–78.

Haferlach C, Dicker F, Schnittger S, Kern W, Haferlach T (2007) Comprehensive genetic characterization of CLL: a study on 506 cases analysed with chromosome banding analysis, interphase FISH, IgV(H) status and immunophenotyping. *Leukemia* **21**: 2442–51.

Haferlach T, Kohlmann A, Schnittger S et al. (2005) Global approach to the diagnosis of leukaemia using gene expression profiling. *Blood* **106**: 1189–98.

Haferlach T, Kohlmann A, Klein HU et al. (2009) AML with translocation t(8;16)(p11;p13) demonstrates unique cytomorphological, cytogenetic, molecular and prognostic features. *Leukemia* **23**: 934–43.

James C, Ugo V, Le Couédic JP et al. (2005) A unique clonal JAK2 mutation leading to constitutive signalling causes polycythaemia vera. *Nature* **434**: 1144–8.

Kohlmann A, Schoch C, Schnittger S et al. (2003) Molecular characterization of acute leukaemias by use of microarray technology. *Genes Chromosomes and Cancer* **37**: 396–405.

Lenz G, Wright G, Dave SS et al. (2008) Stromal gene signatures in large B-cell lymphomas. *New England Journal of Medicine* **359**: 2313–23.

Maciejewski JP, Mufti GJ (2008) Whole genome scanning as a cytogenetic tool in hematologic malignancies. *Blood* **112**: 965–74.

Rosenwald A, Wright G, Chan WC et al. (2002) The use of molecular profiling to predict survival after chemotherapy for diffuse large B-cell lymphoma. *New England Journal of Medicine* **346**: 1937–47.

Schlenk RF, Döhner K, Krauter J et al. (2008) Mutations and treatment outcome in cytogenetically normal acute myeloid leukaemia. *New England Journal of Medicine* **358**: 1909–18.

Schoch C, Kern W, Kohlmann A, Hiddemann W, Schnittger S, Haferlach T (2005) Acute myeloid leukaemia with a complex aberrant karyotype is a distinct biologic entity characterized by genomic imbalances and a specific gene expression profile. *Genes Chromosomes and Cancer* **43**: 227–38.

Song MK, Chung J-S, Shin D-H et al. (2009) Prognostic significance of the Bcl-2 negative germinal centre in patients with diffuse large B lymphoma treated with R-CHOP. *Leukemia and Lymphoma* **50**: 54–61.

Vardiman JW, Thiele J, Arber DA et al. (2009) The 2008 revision of the World Health Organization (WHO) classification of myeloid neoplasms and acute leukaemia: rationale and important changes. *Blood* **114**: 937–51.

Walker J, Flower D, Rigley K (2002) Microarrays in haematology. *Current Opinion in Hematology* **9**: 23–9.

CHAPTER 23

Acute myeloid leukaemia

Alan K Burnett[1] and Adriano Venditti[2]

[1]School of Medicine, Cardiff University, Cardiff, UK
[2]Policlinico Tor Vergata, Rome, Italy

Epidemiology of disease

Acute myeloid leukaemia (AML) has an incidence of 2–3 per 100 000 per annum in children, rising to 15 per 100 000 in older adults. It can occur at all ages but has its peak incidence in the seventh decade (Figure 23.1). The incidence does not appear to be increasing beyond that expected in an ageing population, which in itself will considerably increase the burden of the disease to healthcare systems in future years. The fact that most cases occur in older patients has important implications for treatment strategies, in that biological variation associated with chemoresistance and comorbidity, which limits treatment options, increases with age.

Pathophysiology

The more carefully AML is studied, the clearer it becomes that there is considerable heterogeneity between cases with respect to morphology, immunological phenotype, associated cytogenetic and molecular abnormalities and, more recently, patterns of gene expression. This is reflected in the substantially different responses to treatment. Some entities are becoming so distinct that they are regarded as different diseases with specific approaches to treatment.

AML is a malignant clonal disorder of immature cells in the haemopoietic hierarchical system. Leukaemic transformation is assumed to occur in many cases at, or near, the level of the haemopoietic stem cell before it has embarked on any lineage commitment. Some cases may originate at a slightly later stage in cells that are committed to lineage differentiation. These cells

have abnormal function characterized by failure to progress through the expected differentiation programme and/or to die by the process of apoptosis. Associated with this may be retention of the stem cell characteristic of self-renewal. This leads to the accumulation of a clone of cells, which dominates bone marrow activity and leads to marrow failure. The potential for arrest of haemopoiesis at different time points partially explains why there can be such variation in the leukaemic or 'blast' population characterizing the individual case. Adenopathy or organomegaly can occur but are not usual features. Extramedullary disease can occur, including cerebrospinal infiltration, but this is not usual, unlike in lymphoblastic leukaemias. Similarly, most patients present with low peripheral blood counts. While in the majority of cases no direct cause is found, there is an association with irradiation, smoking, some rare congenital abnormalities, chemical exposure and obesity. Perhaps the most frequently identified cause is progression from other myeloproliferative disorders, e.g. myelodysplasia, or as a consequence of prior chemotherapy for another malignancy.

Non-random chromosome abnormalities are found in the majority of cases. These may be structural (gain or loss of material) or reciprocal balanced translocations. The significance of these changes is developing at a steady pace and is discussed below as far as the clinical implications are concerned.

Several molecular changes have also been discovered, either by association with the known cytogenetic abnormalities or somewhat by chance (Table 23.1). There is a variable level of proof at this stage as to whether the recognized molecular abnormalities are sufficient in themselves to cause leukaemia. The most common molecular mutation associated with AML has been found in the FLT receptor.

FMS-like tyrosine (FLT)-3 is a member of the platelet-derived growth factor receptor (PDGFR) subfamily of receptor kinases and is most similar to FMS, KIT and the PDGF receptors. The receptor is expressed in haemopoietic cells restricted to the

Postgraduate Haematology: 6th edition. Edited by A. Victor Hoffbrand, Daniel Catovsky, Edward G.D. Tuddenham, Anthony R. Green

415

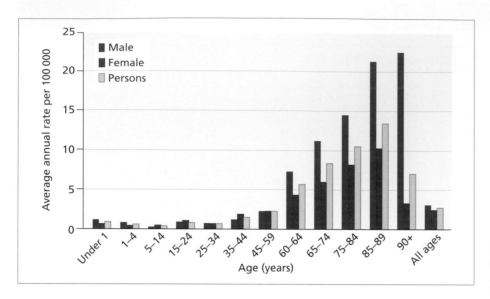

Figure 23.1 Age distribution of AML in the population of Wales: a population study.

CD34-positive fraction and a CD34-negative subfraction of dendritic cell precursors. It is also expressed on neural tissues. Normal FLT-3 receptor is expressed on AML blasts in most cases and can be overexpressed or asynchronously expressed in that it can be expressed not strictly in association with CD34 expression. Most mutations are present in the juxtamembrane domain of the receptor and comprise internal tandem duplications (ITDs) of variable size that are always in-frame and therefore expressed. Such mutations are found in approximately 25% of younger AML cases. Additional point mutations have been found on the activation loop of the interrupted kinase domain, usually at aspartate 835. The consequence of these mutations are activation of the receptor by phosphorylation, which promotes proliferation and resistance to apoptosis. Not only is the mutation the commonest mutation in AML but a large clinical experience confirms that it is strongly predictive of relapse, although it has no implications for the achievement of remission. Mutations are associated with high white cell counts and blast percentage at diagnosis. They are not uniformly distributed across the FAB or cytogenetic subgroups, being rare in FAB M0, M6 and M7 and most common in M3. The incidence is highest in patients with t(15;17), trisomy 8 and normal karyotype and uncommon in other favourable groups and in virtually all poor-risk cytogenetic groups.

There is an increasing belief that most tumours are a result of multiple 'hits' or molecular changes and that a single change may be insufficient to cause the full leukaemic phenotype. In AML, the phenotype is a consequence of both a proliferative lesion and a failure of differentiation, and it seems probable that molecular abnormalities which affect both functions are required. This understanding is now leading to the testing of therapeutic agents which inhibit the molecular consequences of these abnormalities.

Disease classification

The disease is confirmed by an excess of primitive 'blast' cells in the bone marrow, originally in the FAB classification required to be at least 30%. The French–American–British (FAB) morphological classification has been useful in developing a common vocabulary, but has little predictive value with the widespread use of genetic markers. Quality cytochemistry can provide valuable additional diagnostic information. Further precision can be added by immunophenotyping. Although widely used, in many cases where high-quality morphology and cytochemistry is available it is not strictly required to confirm the diagnosis as AML. A revised classification devised under the auspices of the World Health Organization (WHO) recognizes accumulating knowledge of the cytogenetic and molecular characteristics. As discussed later, the leukaemic blasts may demonstrate an 'aberrant' immunophenotype, which together with molecular characterization of cloned breakpoints or mutations has potential use in monitoring response to treatment.

Cytogenetics

The recognition of non-random chromosome abnormalities associated with the various types of AML has had a major impact on understanding of the disease, opening the way for the molecular genetic defects to be unravelled and aiding in the appropriate choice of treatment. A typical range of the more common abnormalities is shown in Figure 23.2. Some of the consequential molecular changes have been carefully investigated and, in the case of some of the reciprocal translocations,

Table 23.1 Examples of genes involved in the cytogenetic abnormalities found in AML.

Cytogenetic abnormality	Genes involved (gene activation)	Protein	FAB type
inv(3)(q21;q26)	Ribophorin 1 (*RPN1*) (3q21) *EVI1* (3q26)	RER transmembrane glycoprotein Multiple zinc fingers	MDS, M0, M1, M2, M4, M5, M6, M7
t(3;3)(q21;q26)	Ribophorin 1 (*RPN1*) (3q21) *EVI1* (3q26)	RER transmembrane glycoprotein Multiple zinc fingers	MDS, M1, M2, M4, M6
t(1;11)(p32;q23)	*AF1P* (1p32) *ALL1* (11q23)	Murine eps 15 homologue *Drosophilia* trithorax homologue	M0, M5
t(1;11)(q21;q23)	*AF1Q* (1q21) *ALL1* (11q23)	No homology to any known protein *Drosophilia* trithorax homologue	M4
t(3;21)(q26;q22)	*EVI1* (3q26) *AML1* (21q22)	Multiple zinc fingers CBF-α*Drosophilia* runt homologue	MDS
t(3;21)(q26;q22)	*EAP* (3q26) *AML1* (21q22)	Ribosomal protein L22 *Drosophila* runt homologue	MDS
t(6;9)(p23;q34)	*DEK* (6p23) *CAN* (9q34)	Nuclear protein Nucleoporin	MDS, M1, M2, M4
t(6;11)(q27;q23)	*AF6* (6q27) *ALL1* (11q23)	GLGF motif *Drosophilia* trithorax homologue	M4, M5
t(7;11)(p15;p15)	*HOXA9* (7p15) *NUP98* (11p15)	Class I homeobox Nucleoporin	MDS, M2, M4
t(8;21)(q22;q22)	*ETO* (8q22) *AML1* (21q22)	Zinc finger CBF-α*Drosophilia* runt homologue	MDS, M2
t(9;11)(p22;q23)	*AF9* (9p22) *ALL1* (11q23)	Nuclear protein, ENL homology *Drosophilia* trithorax homologue	M4, M5
t(10;11)(p12;q23)	*AF10* (p12) *ALL1* (11q23)	Leucine zipper; zinc finger *Drosophila* trithorax homologue	M4, M5
+11	*ALL1* (11q23)	*Drosophila* trithorax homologue	M1, M2
t(11;17)(q23;q21)	*ALL1* (11q23) *AF17* (17q21)	*Drosophila* trithorax homologue Leucine zipper; zinc finger	M5
t(11;19)(q23;p13.1)	*ALL1* (11q23) *ELL* (19p13.1)	*Drosophila* trithorax homologue Transcription enhancer	M4, M5
t(11;19)(q23;p13.3)	*ALL1* (11q23) *ENL* (19p13.3)	*Drosophila* trithorax homologue Transcription factor	M4, M5
t(12;22)(p13;q11)	*TEL* (12p13) *MN1* (22q11)	ETS-related transcription factor Nuclear protein	MDS, M1, M4, M7
t(15;17)(q22;q11–12)	*PML* (15q21) *RARA* (17q21)	Zinc finger Retinoic acid receptor-α	M3
inv(16)(p13;q22)	*MYH11* (16p13) *CBFB* (16q22)	Smooth muscle myosin heavy chain Heterodimerizes with AML1	M4Eo
t(16;16)(p13;q22)	*MYH11* (16p13) *CBFB* (16q22)	Smooth muscle myosin heavy chain Heterodimerizes with AML1	M4Eo
t(16;21)(p11;q22)	*FUS* (16p11) *ERG* (21q22)	RNA-binding protein ETS-related transcription factor	M1, M2, M4, M5

Source: adapted from Caligiuri *et al.* (1997) with permission.

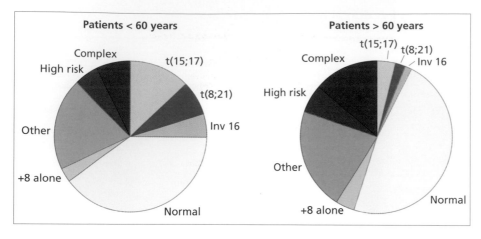

Figure 23.2 Distribution of common cytogenetic abnormalities in patients aged less than or more than 60 years. (Data derived from UK Medical Research Council Database, after Grimwade *et al.* 1998, 2001 with permision.)

Table 23.2 The association of morphology (FAB group) with cytogenetics and immunophenotype in AML.

MIC group	FAB	Immunological markers						Karyotype
		CD7	CD19	CD13	CD33	GPA	CD41	
M2/t(8;21)	M2	−	−	+	+	−	−	t(8;21)(q22;q22)
M3/t(15;17)	M3, M3v	−	−	+	+	−	−	t(15;17)(q22;q12)
M5a/del(11q23)	M5a (M5b, M4)	−	−	+	+	−	−	t/del(11)(q23)
M4Eo/inv(16)	M4Eo	−	−	+	+	−	−	del/inv(16)(q23)
M1/t(9;22)	M1 (M2)	−	−	+	+	−	−	t(9;22)(q34;q11)
M2/t(6;9)	M2 or M4 with basophilia	−	−	+	+	−	−	t(6;9)(p21–22;q34)
M1/inv(3)	M1 (M2, M4, M7) with thrombocytosis	−	−	+	+	−	−	inv(3)(q21;q26)
M5b/t(8;16)	M5b with phagocytosis	−	−	+	+	−	−	t(8;16)(p11;p13)
M2Baso/t(12p)	M2 with basophilia	−	−	+	+	−	−	t/del(12)(p11–13)
M4/+4	M4 (M2)	−	−	+	+			+4

+, Positive; −, negative; no symbol, not specified by MIC Workshop.
FAB, French–American–British classification; GPA, glycophorin A.

the molecular breakpoints have been cloned. Some of these are illustrated in Table 23.1.

The morphological, cytogenetic, immunological and molecular abnormalities are frequently associated as illustrated in Table 23.2 and Figure 23.3. This, together with clinical response data, has led to a recognition that a predominantly morphological classification is no longer adequate to define some subsets which are better recognized as distinct clinically relevant entities based on cytogenetics and molecular characteristics. The previous WHO classification introduced a lower marrow blast threshold of 20% to define the disease, but this is relatively arbitrary and many patients enter treatment with 10% marrow blasts, i.e. high-risk myelodysplastic syndrome.

Treatment

Aspirations for treatment

Given the age distribution of patients who will present with the disease, it must first be decided what the goals of treatment are in an individual patient. In young people, there is little doubt that there is the prospect of significant benefit to be gained from an intensive approach. With increasing age, which is often associated with comorbidity and less responsive disease, the balance of benefit changes to a more palliative approach. Much of what is known about the prospects of successful treatment is derived

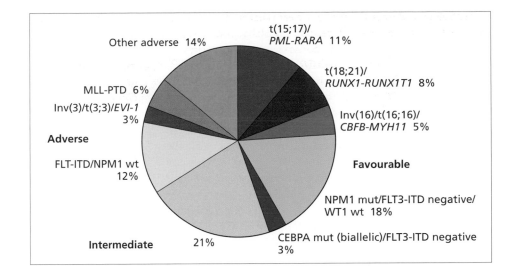

Figure 23.3 Cytogenetics and molecular characteristics of AML. (After Grimwade & Hills 2009 with permission.)

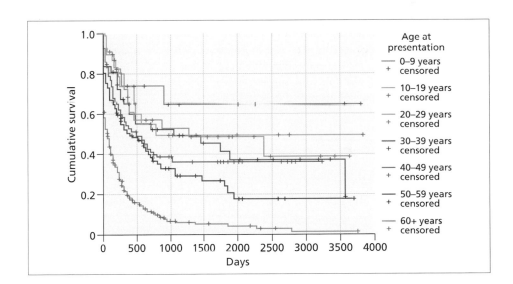

Figure 23.4 Survival of AML in relation to patient age. Data from a Welsh population database.

from large clinical trials. In young patients, these results are usually representative of what can be expected for any age-matched patients. However, only a selected minority of older patients (>60 years) will enter trials, so trial-derived information may be less transferable to the whole population in this age group. A substantial majority of older patients are not considered fit for the usual intensive approach and the priority for such patients is palliative care, optimization of quality of life and minimal hospitalization. Examination of survival in population studies illustrates the dominant effect of age (Figure 23.4); indeed, a substantial proportion of patients over the age of 60 years do not receive more than a palliative treatment approach.

Treatment strategy

The initial clinical priority is to apply chemotherapy to improve marrow function by inducing complete remission (CR). Conceptually, this means an approximate 2-log reduction in tumour burden. This becomes compatible with a bone marrow that appears normal morphologically and is functionally able to produce normal numbers of circulating cells. The traditional consensus definition of CR is based on these premises: less than 5% blast cells in a cellular marrow durable for at least 28 days with a peripheral neutrophil count of 1.5×10^9/L and platelet count above 100×10^9/L, and absence of extramedullary disease. In some cases, these criteria may be met but the morphology is dysplastic. It is not clear whether this is associated with a greater risk of relapse. Similarly, some patients meet the marrow criteria but do not achieve full peripheral count regeneration, now called CRi, i.e. either the neutrophil or platelet count has failed to reach the level required for the definition of CR. This subgroup tends to have a poorer overall survival. In some circumstances, these features may represent a pre-existing dysplastic state; in others it may represent the effects of over-treatment of that particular individual. In the former case, this may have adverse connotations while in the latter it represents optimum treatment. As more sophisticated molecular techniques have become available, it is clear that it is still possible to detect residual disease when all morphological and functional criteria are met. Techniques such as real-time quantitative polymerase chain reaction (RQ-PCR) are capable of detection at a level of 1 in 10^4 or 1 in 10^5 residual cells, but such markers are available for only a minority of cases in which the molecular lesion has been characterized. When it is possible (i.e. in an individual who is heterogeneous for an X-linked marker) to use molecular markers of clonality, it has been noted that in some cases marrow remissions are clonal when they would be expected to represent both alleles of the clonal marker. Sometimes the molecular signature is that of the same clone as the leukaemic cells, suggesting that what the remission represents is a precursor or differentiated state of the malignant clone. It has also been noted that clonal remissions may be derived from the uninvolved allele. As discussed below, there is now intense interest in using validated molecular markers and leukaemia-associated immunophenotypes to predict imminent relapse before this becomes apparent clinically.

Clinical experience has demonstrated that further intensive post-remission treatment is required to 'consolidate' CR. This is delivered at the same intensity as induction in order to achieve further cytoreduction. Under these circumstances, it is possible to achieve disease levels that are beyond the level of molecular detection. It is not clear how many intensive consolidation courses are required, but two or three are generally used in younger patients, and stem cell transplantation may be included. Where intensive induction and consolidation can be given, for example in younger patients, maintenance chemotherapy is not required. A pictorial description of treatment is shown in Figure 23.5.

Treatment details

Induction of remission

The backbone of treatment for 30 years has been the combination of daunorubicin and cytarabine. Usually daunorubicin is given for 3 days in a dose of 45–50 mg/m². Cytarabine is given

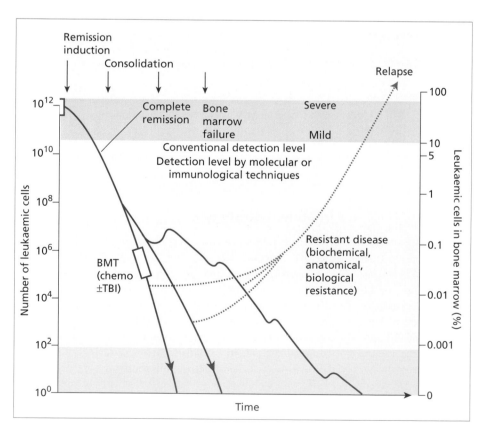

Figure 23.5 Diagnostic presentation of treatment strategy.

Table 23.3 Relationship between complete remission rate and patient age. Patients were all given intensive chemotherapy.

Age (years)	<35	35–55	55–60	61–65	66–70	71–75	75+
Complete remission (%)	88	82	77	62	63	48	59

Source: data derived from the UK Medical Research Council AML Trial database.

for 7–10 days as a continuous infusion or by bolus doses of 100–200 mg/m² daily. Many clinical trials have been conducted that have tested variations of this standard of care. Alternatives to daunorubicin (doxorubicin, mitoxantrone, idarubicin, aclarubicin) or different doses have not yet been shown to be superior overall, although recent studies that have explored higher anthracycline doses may improve the remission rate in older patients. Idarubicin may achieve a better quality of remission, as reflected in a reduced relapse risk in younger patients, but it is more myelosuppressive and limits the intensity of consolidation treatment. In general, on a dose-equivalent basis, daunorubicin remains the anthracycline of choice. Higher doses of cytarabine (3 g/m²) in induction have been tested in recent years, with mixed results and no convincing evidence of overall benefit. Intermediate doses (400 mg/m² daily vs. 200 mg/m² daily) have been tested in younger patients without demonstrating a difference.

Comparison of induction treatment is not simply measured by the rate of remission. By achieving a greater degree of cytoreduction, without necessarily getting more patients into CR, one treatment may be superior because it results in less subsequent relapses. The beneficial effect of the addition of a third drug to the induction combination has some evidence to support it. This will usually be etoposide or thioguanine. A large comparative study did not show any difference between these two drugs when used as the third drug in combination with daunorubicin and cytarabine. The majority of patients who are going to enter remission will do so after one course of treatment. If an incomplete response is obtained, then a second course of the same combination is indicated. A further group will enter remission but these patients have thus shown themselves to have less sensitive disease, and this is reflected in a modestly increased risk of relapse later. If patients fail to achieve a substantial reduction in marrow blasts in the first course or fail to enter CR with a second course, they should be considered refractory to the drugs used up to that point and transferred to an alternative treatment schedule where they can still have a prospect of achieving CR, even though they tend to have a higher risk of rapid relapse.

Results of induction treatment

With this approach to treatment, 50–85% of patients will achieve remission. Of those who do, about 70% will require one course. A number of factors influence the prospects of achieving remission. Age is a dominant and independent risk factor and

a continuous variable; 80% of patients under 60 years will achieve CR, but this prospect diminishes with age (Table 23.3). Clinical performance score at diagnosis is also highly predictive. In younger patients, fewer tend to present with poorer performance scores so this prognostic factor does not move the overall remission rate to any great extent. A larger proportion of older patients will have a poorer risk score and therefore the score has more predictive impact. The distribution of cytogenetic subtypes is related to age, with more-responsive subtypes frequently seen in younger patients and less-responsive subtypes aggregating in older patients. Tumour burden at diagnosis, as represented by white blood count, serum albumin or lactate dehydrogenase levels, will adversely impact on response to induction treatment. It is now possible to measure a number of proteins involved in drug efflux in leukaemic blasts. These 'resistance' proteins, for example P-glycoprotein (see below), tend to be more frequent in older patients and to correlate with a lower remission rate. If patients have had an antecedent haematological disorder, e.g. myelodysplasia, the remission rate will be about 20% lower than in age-matched groups. About 10–25% of older patients embarking on intensive induction chemotherapy will die during the aplastic phase from non-leukaemic causes, which is essentially a failure of supportive care. Induction deaths tend to be associated with the adverse features already mentioned.

Supportive care

It is unusual for induction chemotherapy not to clear most of the leukaemic blasts, however, this is at a cost of 3–4 weeks of severe pancytopenia. Supporting patients through the period of marrow suppression is crucial to treatment outcome; indeed many hold the view that the main reason that treatment has improved is due to improvements in supportive care. It is therefore important that patients are treated in an environment where all necessary supportive facilities are available. Several components of supportive care have to be in place during this period. Careful monitoring of biochemical parameters of renal and hepatic function and coagulation is required. Central venous access is now considered essential, together with high-quality and readily available blood product support.

A priority is the prevention and management of infection. Most patients will receive prophylactic oral antibiotics and antifungals to minimize the risk of infection during the neutropenic period, although routine use of the latter can still be debated. Since hospital-acquired infections are becoming an increasing problem, it can be safer for the patient to be at home provided that close monitoring can be undertaken in the day hospital and that rapid readmission to specialist care is available.

Despite prophylactic measures, most patients will become febrile during neutropenia. This must be considered an indication of a serious, and potentially fatal, infection. The common pathogens are staphylococcal, caused by the use of central catheters, and, increasingly, fungal infections (*Candida* and *Aspergillus*), which are related to the duration of severe neutropenia that results from the more intensive chemotherapy now used. Particular patterns of infection will be determined within individual institutions and will dictate the specific approach to empirical antimicrobial intervention. Fungal infections are a particular problem, not only related to more intensive treatment but also because of the continuous construction that is such a feature of hospital environments. Guidance on intervention should not only be based on evidence from the literature but should also incorporate local microbiological issues (exemplified in Figure 23.6). Nursing expertise is an essential component. It seems probable that improvements in remission rates

in recent years can largely be attributed to better supportive care and nursing skills, which have enabled more intensive treatment to be given safely.

Recombinant growth factors such as granulocyte colony-stimulating factor (G-CSF) or granulocyte/macrophage colony-stimulating factor (GM-CSF) have potential use in two respects. First, if they could curtail the duration of neutropenia, there would be less risk of death during the aplastic phase following induction chemotherapy; this may increase the rate of remission. Second, as many leukaemia cells exhibit receptors for these growth factors, it may be possible to pretreat the patient with growth factor to bring the leukaemic cells into cycle and thereby make them more susceptible to chemotherapy. Extensive studies using G-CSF or GM-CSF to curtail neutropenia have been carried out and some general conclusions can be made. The duration of neutropenia can be reduced by a few days, but it is less easy to demonstrate a reduction in episodes of febrile neutropenia. There is generally no improvement in remission rate. Growth factor use has not increased leukaemic growth or involved relapse.

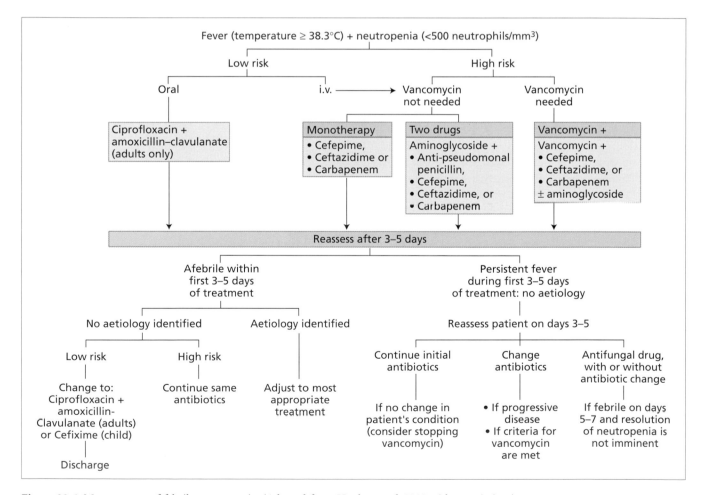

Figure 23.6 Management of febrile neutropenia. (Adapted from Hughes *et al.* 2002 with permission.)

It is primarily a health economics decision that determines whether growth factors are incorporated into routine practice or not. Their use may enable patients to leave hospital earlier. If the local policy is to hospitalize patients during neutropenia, this may save resources. Fewer studies have been carried out to see whether growth factor 'priming' of the leukaemic population would be advantageous. These have generally been unsuccessful but a recent positive study may rekindle interest in this approach, particularly because newer mobilizing agents such as CXCR4 antagonists may soon become available.

Consolidation treatment

Having achieved remission, the priority is to prevent relapse. Optimization of induction treatment is still required as it will influence the quality of remission and thereby the subsequent rate of relapse. Preliminary data suggest that the risk of relapse can be reduced by the addition of the immunoconjugate gemtuzumab ozogamicin (Mylotarg) to induction treatment but it does not change remission rate. Three options are available for younger patients once remission has been achieved: further chemotherapy at induction level of intensity, chemotherapy with autologous stem cell transplantation, or allogeneic stem cell transplantation with or without prior chemotherapy. Chemotherapy will usually involve a further two or three chemotherapy courses. At this point in the treatment, there is a theoretical logic in using different drugs to minimize the

risk of selecting chemoresistant leukaemic clones. Combinations, using cytarabine at increased dosage, amsacrine, etoposide and alternative anthracyclines, are often used (Figure 23.7). Few studies have made direct comparisons between specific combinations, but rather try to work out how many consolidation courses are needed. Two or three courses that are intensive enough to induce 3–4 weeks of neutropenia appears to be achievable but is reaching the limit of tolerability and compliance. High-dose cytarabine ($3\,g/m^2$ on alternative days over 5 days) has been shown to be superior to lower doses ($400\,mg/m^2$ or $100\,mg/m^2$), but only in patients with more sensitive disease. Trials have also shown that intermediate cytarabine doses may be just as effective with less toxicity. It has been suggested that high-dose cytarabine is more effective in the most responsive subtypes of disease (i.e. those with lower-risk disease) based on cytogenetic prognostic markers. Overall, 50–55% of younger patients who enter remission will relapse, usually within the first 2 years. In older patients, the risk is much higher (80%).

Allogeneic stem cell transplantation

There is little doubt that the most effective way to prevent leukaemic relapse in younger patients is allogeneic transplantation from an HLA-compatible sibling donor. Most of the extensive data available are derived from patients in whom the graft was of bone marrow. In these circumstances, the relapse risk will be

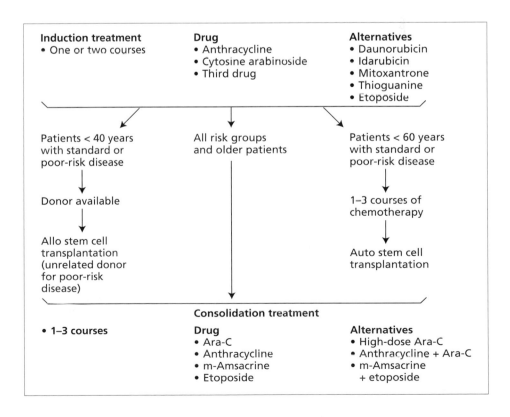

Figure 23.7 Treatment options in AML.

reduced from 45% to about 20%. As there are non-leukaemic causes of death, the overall expectation of cure for recipients of allogeneic bone marrow transplantation is around 60% from the time of transplantation. Some of these survivors will have morbidities that survivors of chemotherapy will avoid, and this needs to be taken into account when advising patients. As the risk of transplant complications, graft-versus-host disease (GVHD) and infections, in particular, increases with age, this approach is normally limited to patients under 45 years, although the precise age cut-off remains controversial and will be a matter of the relative risk of the transplant and of disease recurrence.

Some transplant-related factors may predict for a more favourable outcome, such as a male donor, a cytomegalovirus (CMV)-negative donor when the host is CMV negative and a higher cell count in the graft, and so influence the decision to undergo the treatment, but these seem to be less powerful than disease characteristics in predicting outcome. The extent to which the high-dose preparative regimen necessary to ensure engraftment or the immunological reactivity of the donor marrow via donor T cells eliminates residual leukaemia has been debated extensively. It is assumed that at least some (and probably a major) contribution comes from the immunological graft-versus-leukaemia (GVL) effect. Experience with donors who are mismatched at more than one HLA locus has not been encouraging, but using fully matched unrelated donors has become more reliable, particularly with the development of molecular methods of tissue typing. In expert hands, in carefully selected young patients, this approach may be equivalent to having a sibling donor.

Once remission has been achieved, there is probably no definite requirement to administer more than one course of consolidation chemotherapy before the allograft; however, because of the time required to identify a donor and make the necessary arrangements for the transplant more than one course is usually necessary. It appears that variations in transplantation protocols do not have a major effect on overall survival, for example choice of myeloablative schedule, GVHD prophylaxis or whether bone marrow or peripheral blood is the source of stem cells. However, it may be that the level of immunosuppression with ciclosporin can be manipulated to influence the risk of relapse.

Because the applicability of transplantation is limited, by treatment-related complications, to younger patients, and yet has a very powerful antileukaemic effect, there is recent interest as to whether non-ablative allogeneic transplantation will have a role in older patients. This approach does not require the traditional intensive treatment to ablate the host marrow but provides enough immunosuppression to enable the donor stem cells to engraft. Over a period of weeks, the host haemopoiesis becomes donor, i.e. changes from host to mixed to donor chimerism. It is now clear that that full chimeric engraftment in older patients can be achieved with treatment modalities that are not ablative to the bone marrow. The hope is that this provides sufficient GVL effect. In AML, in a conventional allogeneic transplant, it is not clear how important the GVL effect is, so it remains to be seen whether non-ablative transplantation has a role in consolidation of AML in older patients. However, the preliminary results have shown that this is a viable approach and that over the 2–4 year term the outcomes are encouraging. The reason why use of this procedure in first remission is still debated is that the risk of relapse is highly variable, and because the encouraging results are distorted by the fact that patients who actually receive the transplant have been selected by surviving in remission until the transplant is performed. The assessment of disease-free survival as the measure of comparison ignores the prospect of rescuing patients who relapse by deploying the transplant in second remission.

Autologous stem cell transplantation

Harvesting of stem cells from the bone marrow or peripheral blood during remission and using them after a period of cryopreservation for haematological rescue after myeloablative chemoradiotherapy has been widely used for younger patients who lack donors. This approach has also been shown to be a more effective way of preserving remission compared with chemotherapy. The treatment-related mortality is lower (5–10%) than with allogeneic transplantation, but it lacks a GVL mechanism so the relapse risk is higher (around 35–40%). This results in an overall survival of 50–55% of those who receive this approach. Because the complications are not particularly age related, patients up to their mid-fifties can safely undergo this procedure, but the results of autologous transplantation in older patients (>60 years) is not encouraging.

Patients who receive the autograft early in remission (e.g. within 3 months) do less well than those treated at 3–6 months because of a higher relapse rate. This may reflect patient selection, but it has also been interpreted to mean that, for an autograft to be successful, consolidation chemotherapy beforehand has an important role in cytoreduction of leukaemia cells before the marrow is harvested, so-called *in vivo* purging of disease. Initially there was concern that returning stem cells to patients would be illogical unless efforts were made to eliminate contaminating leukaemia cells first, so-called *ex vivo* purging. Various chemical, cellular and immunologically based techniques were used without clear evidence of benefit. Most clinical experience was gained using 'unpurged' bone marrow supporting myeloablative chemoradiotherapy, which usually comprised cyclophosphamide with total body irradiation or busulfan with cyclophosphamide.

One of the problems with the use of autologous bone marrow has been delayed peripheral blood count recovery, particularly of platelets. This seems to be a feature of AML and is less obvious in other disease indications. Current practice uses peripheral blood or combines peripheral blood and marrow stem cells to ameliorate this problem. This has improved haemopoietic recovery but may be associated with an increased risk of relapse, thus giving no overall survival advantage.

Comparison of consolidation options

For patients under 55 or 60 years, all three treatment options are available, so the dilemma is which treatment approach to take. About 45% of patients entering remission will survive with chemotherapy alone. Of those who receive an allogeneic or autologous stem cell transplant, 55–60% and 50%, respectively, will survive. Patients who receive a transplant are not equivalent to patients receiving chemotherapy alone. They have survived long enough to receive the transplant, whereas those who could not have the transplant may not have done so because they relapsed. Some studies demonstrate that 40% of patients with a donor do not receive an allograft.

Another less frequently considered option is to delay the transplant until there is disease recurrence. Primary treatment of relapse with transplantation is associated with a high rate of failure, so it is necessary to establish a second remission first. However, it is possible to salvage overall about 15% of patients who relapse from chemotherapy. Based on risk factors, it is possible to define those patients who, if they relapse, are likely to enter second remission. In this subgroup the transplant can therefore be delayed because, if first-line treatment does fail, a second CR can be reliably obtained and a transplant delivered. If there is a low chance of second remission, there is a stronger case for transplantation as part of first-line treatment.

Several prospective randomized trials have compared chemotherapy with autologous transplantation and allotransplantation with chemotherapy. In the latter case, these comparisons are not truly randomized but rather compare patients found to have donors, and assumed to be intended to receive an allograft, with those for whom no donor is found. This 'donor versus no-donor' comparison is a substitute for randomization. Although the conclusions are not universal, and despite the superior ability of allograft to reduce the risk of relapse and in some studies to improve the disease-free survival, there have been no differences in survival between these approaches. When those with donors are then compared overall there is only a modest but statistically significant survival benefit in favour of allotransplantation; this may, however, be less clinically significant. When the cytogenetic risk of relapse is taken into account (discussed below), it would appear that transplantation is not required for good-risk patients, and in the absence of an emerging improvement for poor-risk patients, allogeneic transplantation including from unrelated donors is the chosen approach. There is a prospect that chemotherapy may continue to improve so the question of whether allotransplantation will continue to be the best option for standard-risk patients remains a matter of considerable debate, particularly with the emergence of several new prognostic markers. The evidence continues to evolve and the challenge is to apply it to individual patients in daily clinical practice. Part of the problem is that there is a lack of allograft data in the setting of powerful prognostic information.

Factors influencing the risk of relapse

As treatment of disease in younger patients has improved, so the heterogeneity of disease has also become apparent with respect to differences in relapse risk. On multivariate analysis a number of factors have emerged that can predict the risk of relapse irrespective of treatment schedules used, including stem cell transplantation.

Cytogenetics

Patients with t(8;21) and inv(16) have a high remission rate, a lower risk of relapse and a higher rate of second remission, and have a 5-year survival of 65–75%. These patients tend to have lower expression of the 'resistance proteins' and a low frequency of *FLT3* mutations (described below). Acute promyelocytic leukaemia (APL) is now regarded as a separate entity that is uniquely responsive to retinoic acid. In most cases, the disease is characterized by t(15;17), which predicts sensitivity for a differentiation and apoptotic response to retinoic acid. These abnormalities are frequently associated with additional abnormalities such as –X or Y or 9q– in the case of t(8;21), and trisomy 8 in the case of t(15;17). These additional changes do not adversely affect the favourable prognosis. Similarly, the *FLT3* mutation is expressed in about 35% of APL cases but does not affect prognosis in this group of patients. Together, these good-risk patients comprise about 25% of patients under 60 years (Figure 23.2), with a tendency to accumulate in the younger age groups. When good-risk patients occur in the older group, they continue to represent a more favourable group, with a survival of 35% compared with an overall survival of 15–20% in that age group in those treated with intensive chemotherapy.

About 15% of younger patients have cytogenetic abnormalities that are associated with a lower remission rate and a relapse risk on conventional chemotherapy of 85%. These can be identified as –5, del(5q), –7, abnormal 3q, t(9;22), and complex (more than three unrelated changes). Such patients need to be identified early because, even if a remission is achieved, it will be short-lived. Currently, transplantation represents the only viable treatment, but even that is associated with a high relapse risk. There is little evidence that the outlook for this high-risk group has improved over the last 20 years.

Patients who do not fall into the categories described are regarded as standard risk. They have a 5-year survival of 40–45% (Figure 23.8). The impact of this risk stratification is apparent irrespective of chemotherapy used or whether patients receive an allograft or autograft. There are some minor discrepancies between published series, for example trisomy 8 and 11q23 are regarded as poor risk in some series. In larger series, it emerges that patients with 11q23 and a t(10;11) rearrange-

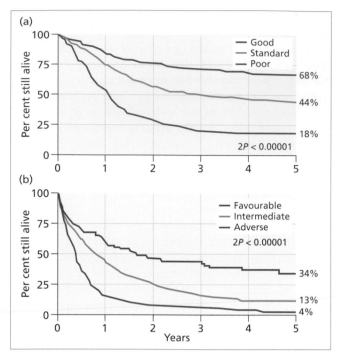

Figure 23.8 The impact of cytogenetic risk groups on treatment outcome. (a) The survival of patients aged under 60 years with good-risk abnormalities – t(8;21), inv (16), t(15;17) – with or without other abnormalities. Poor risk is associated with changes involving chromosome 5 or 7, del 3q or complex abnormalities (more than three abnormalities). The standard-risk group comprises patients who do not have the abnormalities included in the good- or poor-risk categories. (b) The outcome for patients over 60 years old with these abnormalities who were treated with intensive chemotherapy. The relative proportion of the abnormalities in each age group is shown in Figure 23.2.

ment are poor risk (17% survival), whereas other series show in excess of 50% survival in younger patients. As larger data-bases are accumulated it will be possible to allocate less-frequent abnormalities to risk groups.

In older patients, the overall survival of chemotherapy is around 15–20% at 5 years; it is therefore less easy to delineate cytogenetic risk subgroups. Adverse groups are more frequent, and favourable subgroups are less common. This partly accounts for the poorer prognosis of AML in older patients. It is still possible to derive a hierarchical risk stratification in the older patients based on similar criteria already described for younger patients. Some extremely poor subgroups can be identified (Figure 23.8b).

Age

Increasing age, from children to the elderly who are given intensive chemotherapy, is associated not only with a poorer chance of achieving remission but also with an increasing risk of

Table 23.4 Relationship between blast status and cytogenetic group after course 1.

Cytogenetic group	CR (%)	PR (%)	RD (%)
Favourable	77	68	76
Standard	49	41	16
Poor	26	24	4

CR, complete remission; PR, partial remission; RD, resistant disease.

relapse, even allowing for obvious differences in comorbidities and distribution of cytogenetic risk groups. Leukaemias in the elderly more frequently express the drug transport proteins associated with chemoresistance (discussed below).

Response to induction chemotherapy

Patients who enter remission with the first course will have a lower relapse risk than those who require a further course. This has been recognized in various ways. For example, the presence of residual blasts in the bone marrow on day 14 can be used as a reason to give additional treatment. The blast percentage in the bone marrow assessed on recovery from the first treatment course has been shown to be highly predictive, i.e. patients who have more than 20% blasts, even though remission is subsequently achieved, will have a high relapse risk. Both cytogenetics and age are related to this response. When the morphological appearances are related to cytogenetic risk group, it is clear that, for good-risk patients, failure to clear the marrow with the first course is not an adverse feature, whereas in poor-risk patients even those who clear blasts in the first course will have a poor prognosis. In standard cytogenetic risk patients, it is those who fail to clear the marrow that have an adverse risk. From such data, a risk definition incorporating cytogenetics and marrow response can be obtained and this identifies those in the standard cytogenetic risk group who fail to clear the marrow and are thus poor-risk (Table 23.4). This can be further related to age, which suggests that the impact of older age is clearest in the standard-risk patients who clear marrow blasts.

FLT3 mutations

Not only has this mutation emerged as the most frequent in AML but several large series conclude that it is also a major prognostic factor, not for the achievement of remission but particularly for predicting relapse. It provides additional refinement to cytogenetic predictive groups (Figure 23.9). The question of whether *FLT3* status should be used to direct patients' treatment remains unclear, with studies supporting both sides of the argument. As discussed below, *FLT3* mutation is of interest as a potential therapeutic target. Mutations of the activation loop, which occur in 7–10% of patients, have not been shown to be adverse in all studies and may even be favourable, which might be explained by the different methods of detection used. *FLT3* mutation status is complicated by the requirement for rigorous definition of meaningful mutation and a knowledge of the mutant to wild-type ratio, where a high ratio has a more negative impact.

Other molecular abnormalities

The discovery that the nucleophosmin 1 (*NPM1*) gene was mutated in around 50% of cases, usually in those with a normal karyotype, stimulated considerable effort to further subdivide the prognostic groups using molecular information. Overall,

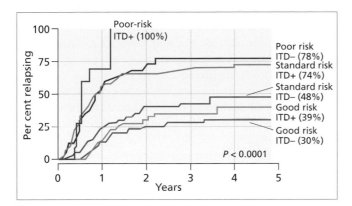

Figure 23.9 The impact of the presence of *FLT3* mutation on relapse risk in each of the risk groups shown in Figure 23.8a. The presence of a mutation in good-risk patients is predominantly in the t(15;17) group but does not significantly change the relapse risk in good-risk patients.

the presence of an *NPM1* mutation confers a favourable outcome. However, it frequently coexists with a *FLT3* mutation, where it modulates the negative effects of *FLT3*. In a large UK study on patients in MRC trials, the prognostic implications of the four possible combined genotypes is clear (Figure 23.10). While it is tempting to suggest that the poor outcome for patients with a *FLT3*-positive *NPM1*-negative genotype could be improved by transplantation, so far there are insufficient data to confirm that this is the case.

About 10% of cases, usually those with a normal karyotype, have a mutation of the CCAAT/enhancer-binding protein α (*CEBPA*) gene. This can occur as a single mutation in about half of cases, which does not influence prognosis, or as two mutations, which confer a favourable prognosis equivalent to patients with favourable cytogenetics. Mutations of c-*KIT* have been reported in 20–30% of patients within the core binding factor (CBF) subset of favourable cases, where it identifies a subset who have a higher risk of relapse.

Mutations of the Wilms tumour (*WT1*) gene have recently been identified, and it is generally agreed that they predict for an increased risk of treatment failure. The use of gene overexpression is a little more problematic because of the need to standardize methodology, but proteins in this category include EVI1 and BAALC, which have been reported to predict poorer survival if overexpressed.

The addition of the molecular subdivision to the prognostic assessment adds considerable complexity for prospective validation and for assessing whether any specific treatment is beneficial, or indeed whether the molecular characteristics add prognostic information to that which is already available, or simply identifies the same patient groups.

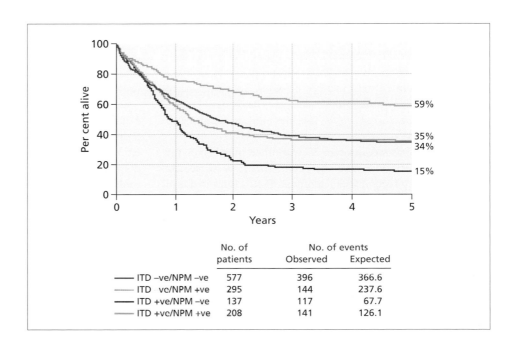

Figure 23.10 The impact of *FLT3/NPM1* genotypes on survival. (After Gale *et al.* 2008 with permission.)

	No. of patients	No. of events	
		Observed	Expected
ITD –ve/NPM –ve	577	396	366.6
ITD –ve/NPM +ve	295	144	237.6
ITD +ve/NPM –ve	137	117	67.7
ITD +ve/NPM +ve	208	141	126.1

Performance score

In older patients, standard assessments of performance vary considerably. These scores are highly predictive for induction treatment success, and will also inevitably relate to which patients are considered candidates for an intensive approach to treatment.

White cell count

High tumour load is an adverse feature for both induction and relapse risk. The threshold for risk is not definitive. A white cell count of 50×10^9/L is often quoted. In subgroups, a prognostic influence is apparent at much lower counts, for example in APL a white cell count at diagnosis of greater than 10×10^9/L is usually agreed as predictive of a higher relapse risk. The impact of a high white cell count is less than that of cytogenetics but may have isolated value when cytogenetics is not available.

Resistance proteins

One of the important biological differences between disease in older patients and that in younger ones is the increased frequency in older patients of the expression of proteins involved in drug transport. These are associated with chemoresistance to some of the drugs used in AML, such as anthracyclines and etoposide. Expression also tends to be associated with a stem cell phenotype and adverse cytogenetics. The most widely studied is P-glycoprotein (P-gp), an energy-dependent transporter protein product of the *MDR1* gene on chromosome 7 and which belongs to the ATP-binding cassette (ABC) transporter family. AML in older patients frequently overexpresses this protein, which has been shown to be predictive for inferior rates of remission and remission duration. The expression levels reported may vary in different series because of differences between measurement techniques. Quantitative flow cytometry has brought a degree of consistency to measurement, but a functional assessment (of dye efflux) and blockade with a P-gp inhibitor is also recommended. *In vitro* preclinical studies have demonstrated that agents such as ciclosporin or its analogue PSC-833 can block P-gp function; however, only one trial to date has so far shown that using such agents has clinical benefit. This may be because P-gp is not the only mechanism of chemoresistance.

Multidrug resistance protein 1 is another member of the ABC transporter family and the gene (*MRP1*) is located on chromosome 16. Lung resistance protein (LRP) is a subunit of the major vault protein, which has been identified in some anthracycline-resistant cell lines and appears to be involved in drug transport. LRP expression has been reported in 30–50% of AML cases in different series, but the majority of studies have been unable to show a correlation with response. Above-normal MRP expression can be found in 50% of patients with untreated AML, but there is no consensus about its impact on survival.

Detection of minimal residual disease

Modern treatments of AML ever more frequently apply the concepts of risk-adapted intensification. An additional, equally crucial, objective is to deliver effective therapies that avoid under- or over-treatment; achieving this has prompted precise measurements of persisting disease, or minimal residual disease (MRD), beyond the threshold of light microscopy. Recently, a significant correlation has been shown between MRD quantified by RQ-PCR or multiparametric flow cytometry and outcome. Therefore, the assumption behind the assessment of MRD is that it will add greater definition to risk prediction by the prognostic factors already recognized. In particular, four major areas of application to the post-remission decision-making process have been identified and are being evaluated: (i) assessment of the quality of response to improve risk stratification and enhance post-consolidation choice (e.g. transplant vs. no transplant); (ii) post-treatment serial monitoring to anticipate overt relapse and plan pre-emptive therapy; (iii) post-stem cell transplantation monitoring to assess the risk of relapse and decide the use of donor lymphocyte infusions; and (iv) identification of markers to pinpoint in the context of targeted-therapy approaches.

Because of the relative insensitivity of techniques such as cytogenetics and fluorescence *in situ* hybridization, molecular and flow cytometry approaches have become the most popular laboratory tests for detecting residual disease. Nucleic acid-based approaches involving RT-PCR have been used particularly in APL. The cloning of a number of breakpoints (Table 23.1) provides the opportunity to utilize a PCR-based approach. Most experience has been gained in APL cases using the PML–RARα hybrid protein as the target, with assays with a sensitivity of 1 in 10^4. A number of conclusions have emerged that currently influence clinical practice. If RQ-PCR remains positive after consolidation chemotherapy, the risk of relapse is high (>70%). However, most of the relapses that subsequently occur are in patients who were found to be negative after consolidation. The majority of patients are molecularly negative at this time, but 20% will nevertheless relapse.

A strategy of regular monitoring of bone marrow (e.g. 3-monthly) is capable of detecting the reappearance of molecular positivity about 3–6 months before haematological relapse. No randomized studies have compared the strategy of retreatment at the time of molecular relapse with intervention at the time of haematological relapse. As the risk of haematological relapse in a patient who was RQ-PCR negative but who then becomes positive is very high, early intervention in this disease seems justified.

Anecdotal evidence suggests that intervention at molecular relapse has a better outcome than intervention at haematological relapse. Less information is available about monitoring of the *AML–ETO* or *CBFB–MYH11* fusion genes associated with t(8;21) and inv(16). Longitudinal studies using the *AML–ETO* fusion have demonstrated that patients in long-term remission may have molecularly detectable 'disease'. This has been attributed to the presence of transcript in other lineages (e.g. monocytes). It seems probable that molecular data will have to be accumulated for each transcript before firm clinical decisions can be based on this information. The transcripts most amenable to monitoring occur in 20–25% of cases which have favourable-risk cytogenetics with fewer relapses, so large prospective trials will be required to accumulate enough patients and enough events to clarify the situation. More sensitivity may be added to this approach using RQ-PCR.

Although several other molecular targets are available, they individually represent small numbers of patients. It may be possible to use a more ubiquitously available molecular target. The *WT1* gene is overexpressed in the majority of AML cases compared with normal haemopoiesis and has been reported to have potential for molecular monitoring in the majority of cases. Mutations of the *RAS* or *FLT3* genes are not likely to be useful in this context because some cases that have the mutation at diagnosis lose it at relapse and vice versa. Conversely, *NPM1* mutations have promise as a stable MRD target. Initial attempts at MRD monitoring have suggested that the *NPM1* mutant allele level reveals residual disease and predicts relapse.

Quantification of MRD by flow cytometry requires the identification at diagnosis of leukaemia-associated aberrant immunophenotypes. These are absent or very infrequent in normal bone marrow but, using a large panel of monoclonal antibodies, can be described in up to 85% of AML cases at diagnosis. These leukaemia-associated immunophenotypes include overexpression of an antigen, coexpression of antigens normally associated with different stages of maturation but which does not occur in novel haemopoiesis, the absence of myeloid antigen expression or the expression of non-myeloid antigens.

The need to test as comprehensive a panel of monoclonal antibodies as possible makes immunological MRD monitoring a quite expensive technology. However, the major impulse for using it derives from its applicability to the vast majority of AML cases, with a sensitivity of 1 in 10^4 or 1 in 10^5. Although this sensitivity is at least 1-log below that of molecular techniques, improvements are expected using six to eight colour technology. Since most published data have been based in single laboratories, additional concerns pertain to lack of common standard operating procedures in order to generate comparable results. From a clinical point of view, several published studies have demonstrated that the immunophenotypic detection of MRD, at post induction or post consolidation, is independently associated with the risk of relapse. There is also evidence that in MRD-positive patients, the use of allogeneic stem cell transplantation confers a superior outcome whereas autologous stem cell transplantation does not alter the unfavourable course dictated by MRD positivity.

The contribution of molecular biology and flow cytometry to the delivery of MRD-directed therapy in AML may be relevant. In fact, given the broad applicability of flow cytometry and the ever rising number of molecular targets identified, one can expect that virtually every patient with AML will be suitable for MRD monitoring and then for individualized management of disease. There is also demand for establishing whether determination of MRD can enhance current risk-stratification strategies based on pretreatment parameters. All these issues can be addressed in the context of large prospective and cooperative studies including parallel determination of MRD by RQ-PCR and flow cytometry.

Impact of prognostic factors on treatment choice

It is becoming routine to take into account the risk of relapse, as defined by some of the factors described, in order to target treatment. The most obvious example is the growing acceptance that transplantation is not required for patients with good-risk disease. Poor-risk patients must be identified promptly and offered either transplantation or some experimental approach since currently available chemotherapy is inadequate. Further data regarding whether transplantation (sibling or unrelated) significantly benefits high-risk patients are needed. Similar information is also required about the significance of *FLT3* status and associated genotypes with respect to the impact of transplantation. Children respond very well to intensive chemotherapy, with the majority enjoying prolonged remissions. Only the small number of children with high-risk features require first-line transplantation.

In older patients (>60 years), either patients or doctors make a judgement at diagnosis as to whether intensive chemotherapy will be beneficial. Prognostic factors such as cytogenetics and performance score can inform this choice. Very poor-risk cytogenetics (e.g. complex changes) carries such a low prospect of success that the question arises as to whether such patients should receive intensive treatment even if considered sufficiently fit.

Acute promyelocytic leukaemia

APL is a special case in which the presence of t(15;17) predicts sensitivity to treatment with all-*trans* retinoic acid (ATRA). It has been recognized for more than 20 years that this leukaemia subtype is sensitive to anthracyclines. Recent experience has clearly demonstrated that the combination of ATRA and chemotherapy has made a dramatic improvement, with survival now expected to exceed 80%. Even better prospects are becoming apparent when the combination of an anthracycline (idarubicin) and ATRA form the backbone of treatment. Simple maintenance with courses of ATRA and orally available agents such as methotrexate and 6-mercaptopurine has been shown in some studies to provide additional benefit. Since the molecular consequences of t(15;17) are known, evaluation of the role of molecular monitoring is most developed in APL and provides a model for disease monitoring in AML.

Treatment in the older patient

Improvement in survival in older patients over the last 20 years has been much more elusive. With better supportive care, intensive chemotherapy can expect to achieve remission in 50–60% of cases. However, 80% of cases will relapse by 2 years. This result has been achieved with various combinations of induction and consolidation schedules and is not improved by maintenance to any great extent. There will be a greater interest in maintenance in future studies. Because the outcome is poor, two issues arise. Are there prognostic factors that confirm which patients will benefit from an intensive treatment approach? The data are less convincing than in younger patients, but younger age (60–70 years), higher performance score and favourable cytogenetic risk group can identify a minority of patients with a better than average outcome. However, several patients have adverse factors: older age, poorer performance score, complex cytogenetics or a chemoresistant phenotype. These patients will have a worse prognosis, which raises the issue of whether they should receive palliative care from the start. One modestly sized study compared a palliative treatment approach with conventional chemotherapy and demonstrated that the use of intensive chemotherapy, because it achieved remission, was more beneficial in older patients; however, no study has yet been large enough to ask that question within the risk groups.

One strategy for improvement is to target the function of P-gp. Only one of several studies using ciclosporin or its analogue has managed to improve survival in relapsed disease, but other studies combining it with first-line treatment have been unsuccessful. This may be because P-gp is not the only resistance mechanism present in leukaemic cells, and once a cell has become resistant by one mechanism there are already other resistance routes.

Management of relapse

The majority of patients will relapse. If this happens after stem cell transplantation, the benefit of further therapy is questionable. However, this is dependent on when the relapse occurs. Within 1 year, further treatment is unlikely to have sustained benefit and retransplantation is usually associated with a very high complication rate. If the relapse occurs later, further chemotherapy with retransplantation may save a few patients. The development of donor lymphocyte infusions has been a very effective approach for the treatment of post-allograft relapse in chronic myeloid leukaemia, but has a low rate of success in AML.

For patients who relapse after chemotherapy, three factors dictate the clinical outcome: duration of first remission, age and cytogenetic risk group. Patients with good-risk disease have a high (75–80%) rate of second remission. Patients who are young with a long CR1 will have a reasonable survival, whereas

Table 23.5 Outcome of relapse in patients over 60 years receiving reinduction treatment ($N = 1529$).

5	CR1 (months)		
	<6	6–12	>12
Remission rate			
15–59 years (%)	15	33	56
60–69 years (%)	11	29	67
>70 years (%)	13	26	53
Survival from relapse at 2 years			
<35 years (%)	10	16	41
35–60 years (%)	7	14	27
60+ years (%)	4	8	16

older patients with a short CR1 will do poorly (Table 23.5). Since the second remission rate in good-risk disease defined by cytogenetics is relatively good, transplantation is usually delayed until second remission. There is no clear 'best choice' chemotherapy for other risk groups, so this is often the setting for experimental therapy development.

APL is again a special case. Patients can respond again to retinoic acid and chemotherapy, but recently arsenic trioxide and the CD33-directed immunoconjugate gemtuzumab ozogamicin have been found to be effective. Remission rates above 80% have been reported; interestingly, following consolidation therapy, a similar proportion can be returned to RQ-PCR negativity. This permits the opportunity for autologous transplantation, the successful outcome of which depends on the autograft and, preferably, the patient being molecularly negative. For patients who remain molecularly positive after reinduction, allogeneic transplantation is indicated.

For non-APL patients, whatever treatment is used to re-establish remission, it is unlikely to be durable without a transplant. Although prospective studies are rare, transplant registry data suggest that about 30% of patients can be salvaged with a transplant with little overall difference whether the source of stem cell is allogeneic or autologous.

Future developments

Classification

The classification of this disease will no doubt continue the trend of taking into account molecular, genetic and clinical features as well as morphology. The technology could eventually allow subgroups to be identified on the basis of a gene expression signature, as shown in Figure 23.11. High-density microarray gene chips can already distinguish major cytogenetic and FAB groups and the presence of an *FLT3* mutation,

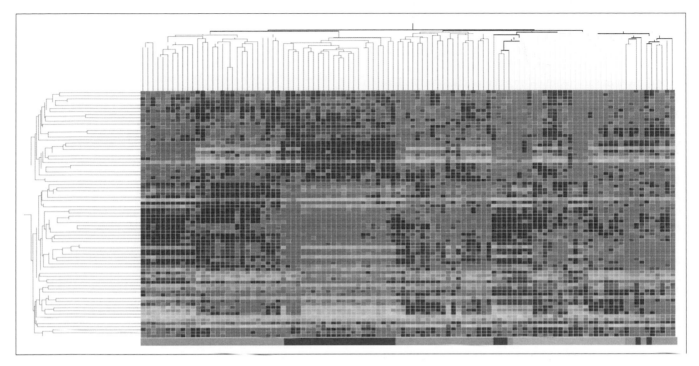

Figure 23.11 A gene cluster of AML samples. A gene list was identified from the 22 283-gene probe set on the Affymetrix U133A gene chip, which was capable of predicting cytogenetic risk group. This list was used to cluster the samples into similar groups and cluster genes showing similar expression profiles (within the cluster, red indicates high expression whereas green is low or absent expression). One group for each of the good- and poor-risk groups was obtained, but several clusters of standard-risk patients were identified, which may correlate with the diverse nature of this subgroup. Blue, good-risk patients; pink, standard-risk patients; yellow, poor-risk patients. Note that the right-hand cluster contains patients with good, standard and poor risk.

and using this information up to 16 subtypes have been proposed. This technology offers no advantage over currently available methods but is at the developmental stage. It will throw light on associated molecular abnormalities that may eventually become targets for drug design and which may be capable of predicting disease or toxicity response. The bioinformatics challenges are considerable given the enormous amount of information that these methods produce.

Therapeutics

There is general acceptance that little further progress will be made by simply shuffling currently available drugs with respect to either scheduling or dosage. There may still need to be refinements with respect to toxicity. There is much interest in targeting treatment, either by matching the treatment approach to the patient based on prognostic factors or by immunologically directing treatment to leukaemic cells and thereby enhancing the selectivity of treatment. Gemtuzumab ozogamicin is an immunotoxin that is being extensively explored in this respect. This is an immunoconjugate combining an IgG4 anti-CD33 humanized monoclonal antibody with the highly potent anti-tumour antibiotic calicheamicin. The key to its utility is that when the antibody combines with CD33 antigen, the complex is rapidly internalized to the cell, where the chemical linker between drug and antibody is lysed. A crucial property is that the linker is lysed only intracellularly and not in the circulation. Although expressed in 90% of cases of AML, CD33 is not leukaemia specific. There is expression on haemopoietic precursors but not on stem cells or, as far as is known, other tissues. The conjugate is clearly active. As a single agent, it can achieve CR in relapse or as first-line treatment in older patients. Pancytopenia is not avoided and transient hepatotoxicity will be seen in some patients. It does not result in the alopecia or mucositis usually associated with chemotherapy. Its use in AML is under investigation in a number of areas, for example in induction in older patients before chemotherapy; for induction in patients unfit for chemotherapy; as maintenance of remission; as first-line and relapse treatment in APL; as part of transplant conditioning; and in simultaneous combination with conventional chemotherapy. All these approaches are still experimental.

Allogeneic transplantation has proved over the years to be a highly effective immunological approach. However, as previously pointed out, the overall survival advantage is not always clear. Part of the reason is that because it is only safely applicable to younger patients, it is competing with the group of patients with the most favourable responses to chemotherapy. Non-intensive transplants have demonstrated that it is feasible to achieve full chimeric status, i.e. 100% donor cells in the bone marrow, without using intensive chemoradiotherapy. This can be done safely in older patients, but there remain concerns about the balance between avoiding relapse on the one hand and GVHD on the other. This could represent a consolidation option for older patients for whom conventional chemotherapy is less successful and where there is an antileukaemic effect of standard allograft. The approach presumes that there will be a significant GVL effect operating in AML. There are only preliminary data on this approach in AML, which is still experimental; assessment in a prospective clinical trial is required.

Many small molecules, particularly tyrosine kinase inhibitors, are becoming available for cancer treatment. So far none has matched the impact of Glivec in chronic myeloid leukaemia. The recognition of the *FLT3* mutation as a common mutation in AML has led to the discovery of several powerful, but not specific, inhibitors of the receptor tyrosine kinase FLT-3, which autophosphorylates the receptor and downstream molecules. Preclinical models provide considerable encouragement for efficacy. Initial clinical studies show a response in about 50% of patients with relapsed disease, with only occasional CRs; the duration of any responses tended to be short. Because of lack of specificity, it is likely that these agents will need to be used in combination with each other, or with chemotherapy. Inhibitors of RAS pathway molecules have also undergone preliminary assessments. Some responses have been seen, but it is also clear that the agents tested are not specific.

Newer more conventional agents (e.g. clofarabine, cloretazine, tipifarnib and demethylation agents) hold promise from unrandomized trials. Since many new treatments will be available, novel approaches to clinical trial design will need to develop to make more rapid progress. Much greater international collaboration is needed to provide sufficient numbers of the patient subgroups or different statistical methods will be required.

Selected bibliography

Adès L, Guerci A, Raffoux E *et al.* (2010) Very long-term outcome of acute promyelocytic leukaemia after treatment with all-*trans* retinoic acid and chemotherapy: the European APL Group experience. *Blood* **115**: 1690–6.

Appelbaum FR, Gundacker H, Head DR *et al.* (2008). Age and acute myeloid leukemia. *Blood* **107**: 3481–3485.

Bullinger L, Dohner K, Bair E *et al.* (2004) Use of gene-expression profiling to identify prognostic subclasses in acute myeloid leukaemia. *New England Journal of Medicine* **350**: 1605–16.

Burnett AK (2002) Acute myeloid leukaemia: treatment of adults under 60 years. *Reviews in Clinical and Experimental Haematology* **6**: 26–45.

Burnett AK (2002) Transplantation in adults with AML: a clinician's perspective. *British Journal of Haematology* **118**: 1–8.

Caligiuri MA, Strout MP, Gilliland G (1997) Molecular biology of acute myeloid leukaemia. *Seminars in Oncology* **24**: 32–44.

Cornelissen JJ, van Putten WL, Verdonck LF *et al.* (2007) Results of a HOVON/SAKK donor versus no-donor analysis of myeloablative HLA-identical sibling stem cell transplantation in first remission acute myeloid leukaemia in young and middle-aged adults: benefits for whom? *Blood* **109**: 3658–3666.

Estey E, Dohner H (2006) Acute myeloid leukaemia. *Lancet* **368**: 1894–1907.

Freeman SD, Jovanovic JV, Grimwade D (2008) Development of residual disease-directed therapy in acute mycloid leukaemia. *Seminars in Oncology* **35**: 388–400.

Gale RE, Green C, Allen C *et al.* (2008) The impact of FLT3 internal tandem duplication mutant level, number, size, and interaction with NPM1 mutations in a large cohort of young adult patients with acute myeloid leukaemia. *Blood* **111**: 2776–2784.

Grimwade D, Haferlach T (2004) Gene-expression profiling in acute myeloid leukaemia. *New England Journal of Medicine* **350**: 1676–8.

Grimwade D, Hills RK (2009) Independent prognostic factors for AML outcome. *Hematology. American Society of Hematology Education Program* 385–95.

Grimwade D, Walker H, Harrison G *et al.* (2001) The predictive value of hierarchical cytogenetic classification in older adults with AML: analysis of 1065 adults entered ino the MRC AML11 Trial. *Blood* **98**: 1312–20.

Hughes WT, Armstrong D, Bodey G *et al.* (2002) 2002 Guidelines for the use of antimicrobial agents in neutropenic patients with cancer. *Clinical Infectious Diseases* **34**: 730–51.

Kern W, Haferlach C, Haferlach T, Schnittger S (2008) Monitoring of minimal residual disease in acute myeloid leukaemia. *Cancer* **112**: 4–16.

Kottaridis PD, Gale RE, Frew ME *et al.* (2001) The presence of a FLT3 internal tandem duplication in patients with acute myeloid leukaemia (AML) adds important prognostic information to cytogenetic risk group and response to the first cycle of chemotherapy: analysis of 854 patients from the United Kingdom Medical Research Council AML 10 and 12 Trials. *Blood* **98**: 1752–9.

Levis M, Small D (2003) FLT3: ITDoes matter in leukaemia. *Leukemia* **17**: 1738–52.

Lowenberg B, Burnett AK, Downing JR (1999) Acute myeloid leukaemia. *New England Journal of Medicine* **341**: 1051–62.

Maurillo L, Buccisano F, Del Principe MI *et al.* (2008) Towards optimization of postremission therapy for residual disease-positive patients with acute myeloid leukaemia. *Journal of Clinical Oncology* **26**: 4944–4951.

Schlenk RF, Dohner K, Krauter J (2008) Mutations and treatment outcome in cytogenetically normal acute myeloid leukaemia. *New England Journal of Medicine* **358**: 1909–1918.

Sonneveld P, List AF (2001) Chemotherapy resistance in acute myeloid leukaemia. *Clinical Haematology Best Practice and Research* **14**: 211–33.

Valk PJM, Verhaak RGW, Beijen MA *et al.* (2004) Prognostically useful gene-expression profiles in acute myeloid leukaemia. *New England Journal of Medicine* **350**: 1617–28.

Adult acute lymphoblastic leukaemia

24

Nicola Gökbuget and Dieter Hoelzer

JW Goethe University Hospital, Medical Clinic II, Frankfurt, Germany

Diagnosis

The classification of blast cell phenotype in adult acute lymphoblastic leukaemia (ALL) requires morphological and cytochemical evaluation, immunophenotyping, cytogenetic and molecular genetic analysis. Morphology remains the method by which acute leukaemia is initially detected and, together with cytochemical reactions, is the major aid in distinguishing between ALL and acute myeloid leukaemia (AML). For more precise subclassification of ALL into B or T lineages, immunological techniques must be used to detect lineage-specific antigens as well as surface or intracytoplasmic molecules (see also Chapter 22). Cytogenetic analysis is generally part of the diagnostic evaluation of ALL because it may have prognostic value, but molecular genetic techniques for identification of particular subsets of ALL (e.g. BCR–ABL-positive ALL) are even more important. Molecular markers and cell surface markers are presently used to evaluate therapeutic efficacy in individual patients by detecting minimal residual disease (MRD).

Morphology

Leukaemic blast cells were formerly divided into L1 to L3 according to the French–American–British (FAB) classification. The subtype L3, observed in approximately 5% of adult ALL patients, was the only one with clinical relevance because it is indicative of mature B-cell ALL, which is subject to different treatment. The diagnosis should be confirmed by surface marker analysis.

According to the new World Health Organization (WHO) classification, ALL is summarized together with lymphoblastic lymphoma under the heading of precursor lymphoid neoplasms, with the major subgroups comprising B lymphoblastic leukaemia/lymphoma not otherwised specified, B lymphoblastic leukaemia/lymphoma with recurrent genetic abnormalities, and T lymphoblastic leukaemia/lymphoma. Mature B-ALL is not mentioned as a separate entity and is included as Burkitt lymphoma under the heading of mature B-cell neoplasms. The WHO classification for ALL is based on cytogenetic aberrations, which may be of limited relevance for clinical management and risk stratification.

Cell surface marker analysis

Acute lymphoblastic leukaemia is divided into subtypes by immunological criteria based on the presence of specific

Table 24.1 Immunological classification, corresponding cytogenetic and molecular aberrations and frequencies in adult ALL.

	Adults (%)*	Surface marker	Cytogenetics†	Molecular genetics†
B-lineage		HLA-DR+, TdT+, CD19+ and/or CD79a+ and/or CD22+		
Pro B-ALL	11	No further differentiation markers	t(4;11)	ALL1(MLL)–AF4
Common-ALL	50	CD10+	t(9;22)	BCR–ABL
Pre B-ALL	12	CD10+/–, cyIgM+	t(9;22), t(1;19)	BCR–ABL, E2A–PBX1
B-ALL	5	CD10+/–, sIgM+	t(8;14)	MYC–IGH
T-lineage		TdT+, cyCD3+ or sCD3+		
Early T-ALL	6	cyCD3+, CD7+, CD5+/–, CD2+/–	t(11;14)	LMO1–TCRα/δ
Cortical T-ALL (Thy ALL)	10	cyCD3+, CD7+, CD1a+, sCD3+/–	t(10;14)	HOX11–TCRα/δ
Mature T-ALL	6	sCD3+, CD1a–		

*Frequencies according to central immunophenotyping of the GMALL Study Group; personal communication of Professor E. Thiel and Dr S. Schwartz, Free University of Berlin, Germany.
†Most frequent, typical aberrations.
cyIgM, cytoplasmic IgM; sIgM, surface IgM; cyCD3, cytoplasmic CD3; sCD3, surface CD3; TdT, terminal deoxynucleotidyltransferase.

receptors or antigens on the cell surface of leukaemic blast cells. Within B- or T-lineage ALL, the subtypes are defined according to their stage of differentiation. For more details on the immunological classification of ALL, see Chapter 22. The frequency and definition of subtypes in adult ALL is given in Table 24.1. The European Group for the Immunological Characterization of Acute Leukaemia (EGIL) has proposed a unified classification for ALL immunophenotypes.

B-lineage ALL

Pro-B ALL, also termed *pre-pre-B ALL* or early pre-B, is CD10 negative and lacks specific B- or T-cell differentiation markers but expresses human leucocyte antigen (HLA)-DR, terminal deoxynucleotidyltransferase (TdT) and CD19, and has rearranged immunoglobulin genes. It occurs in approximately 9–11% of adult ALL.

Common ALL (c-ALL) is the major immunological subtype in adult ALL. It constitutes more than 50% of cases of adult ALL. c-ALL is characterized by the presence of CD10. Blast cells do not express markers that characterize relatively mature B cells such as cytoplasmic or surface membrane immunoglobulins. The blast cells are positive for CD19 and TdT.

Pre-B ALL is characterized by the expression of cytoplasmic immunoglobulin, which is absent in c-ALL, but is identical to c-ALL with respect to the expression of all other cell markers.

Mature B-cell ALL is found in approximately 5% of adult ALL patients. The blast cells express surface antigens of mature B cells, including surface membrane immunoglobulin. CD10 may be present, as well as, occasionally, cytoplasmic immunoglobulin.

T-lineage ALL

Approximately 22% of adult ALL cases have blast cells with a T-cell phenotype. All cases express the T-cell antigen gp40 (CD7) and they may, according to their degree of T-cell differentiation, express other T-cell antigens, for example the E rosette receptor (CD2) or the cortical thymocyte antigen T6 (CD1) (Table 24.1). A minority of T-cell ALL blast cells expresses CD10 together with T-cell antigens. In most cases of T-cell ALL, one or more of the T-cell receptor (TCR) genes are rearranged. These properties make it possible to classify T-cell ALL according to their stage of differentiation.

Early T-precursor ALL accounts for 6% of adult ALL. It shows characteristic T-cell markers (cyCD3 and CD7) but no further differentiation markers.

Thymic (cortical) T-ALL is the most frequent subtype of T-ALL (10%). It is characterized particularly by the expression of CD1a. Surface CD3 may be present. Since this subtype is associated with a better prognosis, its identification is of particular importance.

Mature T-ALL has a frequency of 6%. The blast cells do not express CD1a but they are positive for surface CD3.

Cytogenetic and molecular genetic analysis

Cytogenetic abnormalities are independent prognostic variables for predicting the outcome of adult ALL. In several multicentre studies, clonal chromosomal aberrations could be detected in approximately 62–85% of adult ALL patients.

The Philadelphia (Ph) chromosome, t(9;22)(q34;q11), results from a translocation involving the breakpoint cluster region of the *BCR* gene on chromosome 22 and the *ABL* gene on chromosome 9 (see also Chapters 22 and 27). Polymerase chain reaction (PCR) analyses has revealed that *BCR–ABL*-positive ALL occurs in 20–30% of adults compared with 3% of children. One-third of adult ALL patients with a Ph chromosome show M-*BCR* rearrangements (resulting in a 210-kDa protein), similar to patients with chronic myeloid leukaemia (CML), whereas two-thirds have m-*BCR* rearrangements (resulting in a 190-kDa protein). It is noteworthy that the molecular aberration *BCR–ABL* is more frequently detected than the corresponding chromosome abnormality t(9;22) because of occasional difficulties in obtaining adequate material for cytogenetic analysis (see also Chapter 22). The most frequent form of 11q23 abnormality in ALL is t(4;11)(q21;q23). The translocation is frequently detected in infant leukaemia and in patients with the pro-B ALL subtype (CD10 negative). The overall incidence in adults is approximately 5%. Typical molecular aberrations in ALL with associated cytogenetic translocations and immunological subtypes are summarized in Table 24.1.

The role of cytogenetic analysis in adult ALL has to be re-evaluated critically. The most frequent cytogenetic aberrations and those with the largest prognostic impact can also be detected by the corresponding molecular genetic abnormalities, as mentioned above. These techniques are more reliable and have a greater sensitivity, for example a detection level of more than 10^{-6} for *BCR–ABL*. They are therefore more useful for initial detection of the aberrations and for follow-up analysis of MRD (see below). In addition, the observed incidence of the majority of cytogenetic aberrations is very low and therefore correlation to clinical outcome, and especially therapeutic consequences, are limited. Nevertheless, cytogenetic analysis is still recommended as a routine diagnostic method in ALL.

Minimal residual disease

The detection of blast cells by cytological analysis of bone marrow smears has a sensitivity of 1–5%. More sensitive methods of blast cell detection are available for the identification of MRD. Sensitivity reaches 10^{-4} or more, corresponding to 0.01% blast cells (one leukaemia cell within 10 000 normal cells). MRD evaluation allows quantitative follow-up of individual response after achievement of complete remission detected by bone marrow cytology.

Quantitative PCR can be directed to fusion genes associated with ALL-type translocations such as *BCR–ABL*. These markers are available in 30–40% of adult ALL patients. The detection of individual clonal rearrangements of immunoglobulin (*IGH*, *IGK*) and TCR-β, TCR-δ and TCR-γ genes is more broadly applicable. For this method a high level of standardization regarding methodology and interpretation of results has been achieved (see also Chapter 22). The individual marker can only be detected in blast cells and therefore diagnostic material

is required. With multiparameter flow cytometry, individual leukaemia-specific phenotypes, i.e. characteristic constellations of surface antigens, can be detected with high specificity and sensitivity. MRD detection with any method should be restricted to experienced laboratories that participate in quality control rounds taking place on an international level in Europe.

Clinical features

Most adult ALL patients initially present with clinical symptoms resulting from bone marrow failure. Physical findings such as pallor, tachycardia, weakness and fatigue are due to anaemia; petechiae or other haemorrhagic manifestations are attributable to thrombocytopenia; infectious complications are due to neutropenia. Clinical signs of leukaemia related directly to infiltration of typical organs with leukaemic blasts, such as lymphadenopathy, splenomegaly and hepatomegaly, are present in most patients but are infrequently the reason for which the patient first seeks medical advice.

Symptoms and clinical manifestations of adult ALL patients, aged 15–65 years, entering two consecutive German multicentre trials are given in Table 24.2 according to their classification into the different immunological subtypes. One-third had infection or fever at presentation, and one-third presented with haemorrhagic episodes. Approximately half of the patients presented at diagnosis with lymphadenopathy, splenomegaly and hepatomegaly, and hilar lymph node enlargement or a thymic mass (detected on chest radiography or computed tomography) in approximately 14% of patients. Most patients (85%) with mediastinal masses had T-cell ALL. Massive thymic enlargement can cause dyspnoea, especially when associated with pleural effusions. Although 7% of ALL patients at presentation had central nervous system (CNS) involvement (as demonstrated by leukaemic blast cells in the cerebrospinal fluid), only 4% of these initially had CNS symptoms such as headache, vomiting, lethargy, nuchal rigidity and cranial or peripheral nerve dysfunction.

Virtually any organ can be infiltrated by ALL blast cells, and approximately one-tenth of the patients had such organ involvement but with wide variation between subtypes (Table 24.2). Most often a pleural effusion was observed, and this occurred almost exclusively in those patients with mediastinal enlargement and T-cell ALL. Some of these patients also had a pericardial effusion. Bone or joint pain was rarely observed compared with childhood ALL; bone lesions could be found in only 1% of cases. Initial involvement of the testis was very rare (<1%). Leukaemic infiltration of retina, skin, tonsils, lung or kidney was observed only occasionally, particularly in mature B-cell ALL and to a lesser extent in T-cell ALL, all of them associated with a poorer outcome.

	T-lineage (%)	B-precursor (%)	Mature B (%)
Gender			
Male	73	54	78
Female	27	46	22
Age			
15–20 years	22	19	8
20–50 years	67	58	64
>50 years	11	24	27
Bleeding	28	28	30
Infections	22	29	37
Lymphadenopathy	77	40	61
Hepatomegaly	45	41	56
Splenomegaly	55	43	47
Mediastinal tumour	62	1	5
CNS involvement	8	3	13
Other organ involvement	15	4	32

Table 24.2 Symptoms and clinical signs at diagnosis in adult ALL patients.*

*$N = 640$ patients of GMALL studies 03/87 and 04/89.

Laboratory evaluation

The peripheral blood cell counts at diagnosis of the same cohort of patients are given in Table 24.3, which again shows differences between the subtypes of adult ALL. Overall, the leucocyte count was elevated in 59% of the cohort, 14% had normal counts and 27% had leucopenia. In 92% of the patients, leukaemic blast cells were seen in the blood film. Thus, 'aleukaemic' leukaemias account for only a small proportion of cases of adult ALL. With automated blood counting, the diagnosis may be missed in patients with normal or decreased white blood cell (WBC) counts and with low or zero blast cells in peripheral blood. Regardless, microscopic examination of blood films in people suspected of having acute leukaemia is an absolute requirement. A blood count above 100×10^9/L was observed in 16% of the patients, and occasionally WBC counts above 500×10^9/L occurred. In general, a high WBC count is found more frequently in patients with T-cell ALL compared with those with B-lineage ALL (Table 24.3).

Neutrophils below 0.5×10^9/L were seen overall in 23% of the patients. Severe neutropenia at diagnosis is observed more often in B-precursor ALL (28%). Thrombocytopenia below 25×10^9/L occurred in one-third of adult ALL patients, corresponding roughly with the symptoms of infection and bleeding present at diagnosis. Anaemia at diagnosis is observed in most adult ALL patients, but only in a small proportion is it severe, with haemoglobin under 8 g/dL (Table 24.3).

Bone marrow aspiration or biopsy is mandatory for diagnosis. In less than 15% of patients, the bone marrow cannot be aspirated and a biopsy must be performed. Dry taps are due to densely packed blast cells, fibrosis or inadequate technique; the first two resolve after therapy. Most patients have more than 50%, or even more than 90%, of blast cells in the bone marrow. In under 3% of cases, the blast cells constitute less than 50% of the nucleated marrow cells.

A lumbar puncture should be done to determine whether the CNS is involved. If there is a risk of bleeding as a result of a very

Table 24.3 Blood counts at the time of diagnosis in adult ALL.*

	T-lineage (%)	B-precursor (%)	Mature B (%)
Leucocytes or WBC			
<10×10^9/L	18	40	37
$10–50 \times 10^9$/L	36	31	42
>50×10^9/L	46	29	20
Granulocytes			
<0.5×10^9/L	13	28	3
>0.5×10^9/L	87	72	97
Platelets			
<25×10^9/L	21	32	29
>25×10^9/L	79	68	71
Hb			
<8 g/dL	16	29	17
>8 g/dL	84	71	83

*$N = 640$ patients of GMALL studies 03/87 and 04/89.

low platelet count, or of blast cell contamination due to a very high leukaemic blast content in the peripheral blood, lumbar puncture should be postponed. When the leucocyte count in the spinal fluid is low or the morphological detection of blasts is inconclusive, demonstration of an immunologically defined blast cell population can confirm a diagnosis of CNS involvement.

The most frequent metabolic abnormality is an increased serum uric acid level in approximately half of the patients; hypercalcaemia is rare. Serum lactate dehydrogenase (LDH) is often elevated as a result of cell destruction in patients with a large tumour mass. In a small proportion of patients, the initial fibrinogen level was less than 1 g/L. Disseminated intravascular coagulation in ALL was rarely observed at diagnosis.

Differential diagnosis

Difficulty is rarely experienced in establishing the diagnosis of ALL. The differentiation from lymphocytosis, lymphadenopathy and hepatosplenomegaly in viral infections and other acute or chronic leukaemias can usually be done by lymphocyte surface markers.

Aleukaemic pancytopenic ALL without blast cells in peripheral blood (<10%) has to be distinguished from aplastic anaemia, which may also be a preleukaemic syndrome. In contrast to ALL, in aplastic anaemia the bone marrow is hypocellular. In rare cases with low bone marrow infiltration, an arbitrary distinction between ALL and lymphoblastic non-Hodgkin lymphoma is usually chosen according to the degree of infiltration (above or below 25%).

Mixed or hybrid leukaemias are those in which blast cells express lymphoid as well as myeloid antigens; they may also be described as biphenotypic or bilineage leukaemias. Biphenotypic leukaemias are defined as those in which markers of lymphoid and myeloid lineages are coexpressed on the same leukaemic cells. EGIL has suggested a scoring system that is helpful for definition of biphenotypic leukaemia depending on the type and degree of expression of lymphoid and myeloid markers. Bilineage leukaemias are those with two populations of blast cells that have either lymphoid or myeloid antigens and which might be allocated to an ALL or AML treatment strategy. After the start of therapy with either regimen, one population may disappear whereas the other is maintained and may require a shift of therapy.

Occasionally, difficulties can occur in distinguishing Ph/BCR–ABL-positive ALL from primary lymphoid blast crisis of CML. Sometimes the final diagnosis can be done only after treatment initiation. In ALL patients achieving complete clinical remission (CR), the peripheral blood count shows normal values, whereas in CML it may revert to a chronic phase picture showing leftshift.

Initial evaluation and supportive therapy

Speed in clinical evaluation and diagnosis is important in order to initiate supportive measures and to decide on appropriate therapy. In only a few cases is the leukaemic process so advanced that immediate treatment is necessary (e.g. in patients with symptoms due to a large mediastinal mass and pleural effusion, a very high WBC count or a rapidly progressing B-cell ALL).

A few general measures should be initiated at once. Sufficient fluid intake to guarantee urine output of 100 mL/hour throughout induction therapy should be maintained to reduce the danger of uric acid formation. Patients should also receive allopurinol to reduce the risk of the latter and avoid the danger of urate nephropathy. Allopurinol blocks the enzyme xanthine oxidase, which mediates the generation of uric acid from xanthine as a product of purine catabolism. Allopurinol should be given at a dose of 300 mg/day, which may be increased to 600 mg/day if high leucocyte counts or organomegaly persist. The dose of allopurinol has to be reduced when 6-mercaptopurine is given because it potentiates the action of this drug. Rasburicase is a new recombinant uratoxidase enzyme that catalyses the oxidation of uric acid to allantoin. Rasburicase can reduce high uric acid faster and more safely than allopurinol, thereby preventing tumour lysis syndrome in almost all cases. It might therefore be an alternative in patients with high risk of tumour lysis syndrome.

Parenteral fluid administration may be required when the patient's oral intake is inadequate because of nausea or difficulty in swallowing. Placement of an implantable port system is advantageous when anticipating a long period of induction therapy (see also Chapter 26).

Blood substitution (see also Chapter 26)

In general, platelet transfusions should be given in response to bleeding episodes and to prevent bleeding according to standard recommendations. HLA-matched platelets are given to patients who become refractory to random donor platelets. Red cell transfusions have a lower priority than platelet substitution. They should be given according to haemoglobin values but depending on age, comorbidity (e.g. cardiac) and clinical symptoms.

Infection management

Infection management is of increasing importance in adult ALL. Infections are the major cause of early death (2–20% depending on age), with equal contributions of fungal and bacterial pathogens. Antifungal prophylaxis during vincristine therapy in induction is a problem since azoles may enhance neurotoxic effects. There are also no standards for antibacterial prophylaxis. Moreover, the parallel application of chemotherapy, antifungals and antibiotics may enhance the risk of toxicities (e.g. liver toxicity, nephrotoxicity) and thereby contribute to treatment delays. The optimization of supportive care is a major goal in treatment of adult ALL since early complications not only lead to early death but also to treatment delays and thereby compromise outcome.

Long-term neutropenia is the most important risk factor, but CD4 lymphopenia, antibody deficiency and multiple immunosuppression in allogeneic stem cell transplantation also lead to severe and lethal infections. Whereas formerly Gram-negative microorganisms were the leading cause of febrile neutropenia, in the last decade Gram-positive bacterial infections, mostly caused by staphylococci, have increased and are frequently correlated with indwelling central venous access. However, invasive fungal infections are the most dangerous development, with increasing frequency particularly of mould infections.

The successful management of febrile neutropenia is based on hygienic procedures including body hygiene, germ-reduced food, reverse isolation or high-efficiency particulate air filtration, antibiotic prophylaxis, sufficient diagnostics, and consequent empirical antimicrobial therapy. Prophylaxis and treatment of bacterial, viral and fungal infections should be performed according to published standards as well as institutional guidelines.

Haemopoietic growth factors

The use of haemopoietic growth factors such as granulocyte colony-stimulating factor (G-CSF) is a valuable component of supportive therapy during the treatment of ALL. There is no indication that these CSFs stimulate leukaemic cell growth in a clinically significant manner. Most clinical trials have demonstrated that the prophylactic administration of G-CSF significantly accelerates neutrophil recovery, and several prospective randomized studies have also shown that this is associated with a substantially reduced incidence and duration of febrile neutropenia and of severe infections and reduced induction mortality.

The scheduling of G-CSF is of great importance. When G-CSF is first given at the end of a 4-week induction chemotherapy regimen, potential benefits are limited. Therefore, it is noteworthy that G-CSF may even be given in parallel with chemotherapy without aggravating the myelotoxicity of these specific regimens and that this scheduling is an important determinant of clinical efficacy. On the other hand, after short consolidation cycles, G-CSF is probably more effective if given after the cycle.

Closer adherence to the dose and schedule of chemotherapeutic regimens should be theoretically possible with the use of G-CSF. A benefit in terms of long-term outcome due to increased dose intensity achieved by using G-CSF has not yet been demonstrated in any trial.

Chemotherapy

Chemotherapy of ALL is usually divided into several phases, beginning with remission induction. The objective of induction chemotherapy is to achieve CR, i.e. eradication of leukaemia as determined by morphological criteria and, more recently, also by molecular markers. Post-remission therapy usually consists of intensification or consolidation cycles and maintenance treatment. Most often, specific prophylactic CNS treatment is added.

Remission induction therapy

Correct diagnosis and management of the initial complications are the prerequisites for successful induction therapy. A cautious cell reduction phase is often recommended for patients with a large leukaemic cell burden or a high leucocyte count. Patients with extreme leucocytosis ($>100 \times 10^9$/L) have been treated initially with leucapheresis, but these patients can generally be managed with steroids alone or in combination with vincristine or cyclophosphamide. For mature B-cell ALL, initial treatment with cyclophosphamide and prednisone for 1 week usually results in safe reduction of large tumour masses, in most cases without tumour lysis syndrome.

Standard induction therapy for ALL includes prednisone, vincristine, anthracyclines (mostly daunorubicin) and also L-asparaginase. Further drugs, such as cyclophosphamide, cytarabine (either conventional or high dose), mercaptopurine and others, are added in many protocols, sometimes termed 'early intensification'.

Prednisone and prednisolone have been most frequently administered, although dexamethasone shows higher antileukaemic activity *in vitro* and better penetration of the cerebrospinal fluid. However, extensive use of dexamethasone may be associated with an increased risk of septicaemias and fungal infections, which may be circumvented if treatment time and dose is reduced.

Anthracycline dose intensity and schedule may play an important role in induction therapy of adult ALL. In the past daunorubicin was mostly administered as a weekly schedule, but recently many trials include dose intensification with doses of 30–60 mg/m^2 on a 2–3 day schedule. Intensive anthracycline therapy may be associated with a higher induction mortality. Therefore, intensive supportive care and probably the use of growth factors is recommended with these protocols.

Asparaginase does not affect CR rate but improves leukaemia-free survival (LFS). If not used during induction therapy, it is often included as part of consolidation treatment. Three different asparaginase preparations with significantly different half-lives are available: native *E. coli* asparaginase (1.2 days), *Erwinia* asparaginase (0.65 days) and asparaginase bound to polyethylene glycol (pegaspargase, 5.7 days). Availability may vary between different countries. In order to reach equal efficacy, the application schedule has to be adapted and is generally daily for *Erwinia* asparaginase, every second day for *E. coli* asparaginase and every 1–2 weeks for pegaspargase. Pegaspargase has the advantage of less frequent administration and even more activity distribution.

The role of cyclophosphamide, generally administered at the beginning of induction therapy, has been evaluated in several studies. A randomized study by the Italian GIMEMA group comparing a three-drug induction with or without cyclophosphamide did not show a difference in terms of CR rate (81% vs. 82%). However, in several non-randomized trials, high CR rates (85–91%) were achieved with regimens including cyclophosphamide pretreatment, particularly in adult T-ALL.

High-dose chemotherapy with cytarabine or methotrexate has no role during induction with the exception of a few trials.

Failure of induction therapy

With current regimens the remission rate in ALL is 85–90% (Table 24.4) with low failure rates and a variable early mortality up to 11%, increasing with age from less than 3% in adolescents to 20% in patients over 60 years of age. The main cause of death in approximately two-thirds of the patients is infection, in part fungal infection. Besides mortality, morbidity (e.g. due to

extended cytopenias, subsequent infections such as fungal pneumonias) also has to be considered, which may compromise further treatment and dose intensity. The remaining non-responders may achieve a partial remission or may be refractory to standard treatment. These patients have an extremely poor prognosis. They are therefore candidates for experimental treatment approaches or consideration for stem cell transplantation (SCT), even if not in CR but in good partial remission.

Consolidation therapy

Consolidation therapy refers to high-dose chemotherapy, to the use of multiple new agents or to readministration of the induction regimen. These measures are aimed at eliminating residual leukaemia after induction chemotherapy and thereby preventing relapse as well as emergence of drug-resistant cells.

Intensive consolidation is standard in the treatment of ALL, although consolidation cycles in large studies are very variable and it is impossible to evaluate their individual efficacy. In general it seems that intensive application of high-dose methotrexate is beneficial. However, in adults dosages are probably limited at $1.5–2\,g/m^2$ if given as a 24-hour infusion. Otherwise toxicities, particularly mucositis, may lead to subsequent treat-

Table 24.4 Overall treatment results in adult ALL in larger studies.

Study	N	Median age (range)	SCT	CR (%)	Early death (%)	Survival
LALA 87, France (Thiebaut *et al.* 2000)	572	33 (15–60)	PO	76	9	27% at 10 years
NILG 08/96, Italy (Bassan *et al.* 2001)	121	35 (15–74)	PR	84	8	48% at 5 years
GMALL 05/93, Germany (Gökbuget *et al.* 2001)*	1163	35 (15–65)	PR	83	NR	35% at 5 years
JALSG-ALL93, Japan (Takeuchi *et al.* 2002)	263	31 (15–59)	PO	78	6	30% at 6 years
UCLA, USA (Linker *et al.* 2002)	84	27 (16–59)	PR	93	1	47% at 5 years
Sweden (Hallbook *et al.* 2002)	153	42 (16–82)	PR	75	NR	28% at 5 years
GIMEMA 0288, Italy (Annino *et al.* 2002)	767	28 (12–60)	NR	82	11	27% at 9 years
MD Anderson, USA (Kantarjian *et al.* 2004)	288	40 (15–92)	Ph+	92	5	38% at 5 years
EORTC ALL-3, Europe (Labar *et al.* 2004)	340	33 (14–79)	PO	74	NR	36%[†] at 6 years
LALA 94, France (Thomas *et al.* 2004)	922	33 (15–55)	PR	84	5	36% at 5 years
GOELAL02, France (Hunault *et al.* 2004)	198	33 (15–59)	HR	86	2	41% at 6 years
MRC XII/ECOG E 2993, UK–USA (Rowe *et al.* 2005)	1521	15–59	PO	91	NR	38% at 5 years
GIMEMA 0496, Italy (Mancini *et al.* 2005)*	450	16–60	NR	80	NR	33% at 5 years
Pethema ALL-93, Spain (Ribera *et al.* 2005)	222	27 (15–50)	HR	82	6	34% at 5 years
JCOG-9004 (Tobinai *et al.* 2007)	143	41 (<64)	PO	83	10	32% at 5 years
GMALL 07/03 (Gökbuget *et al.* 2007)*	713	34 (15–55)	PR	89	5	54% at 5 years
NILG 09/00 (Bassan *et al.* 2009)	280	38 (16–66)	PR	84	8	34% at 5 years
Weighted mean	7405			84	7	35%

*Abstract.
[†]Survival of patients in CR.
PO, prospective stem cell transplantation (SCT) in all patients with donor (type a); Ph+, SCT in Ph-positive ALL (type b); PR, SCT according to prospective risk model (type c); HR, prospective SCT in a study for high-risk patients only; NR, not reported.

ment delays and decreased compliance. From paediatric ALL trials there is increasing evidence that intensified application of asparaginase leads to improved overall results. In adult ALL this approach appears to be useful particularly in consolidation, where less toxicity can be expected compared with induction. Several studies have also demonstrated that a modified induction (reinduction) improves outcome. The role of high-dose anthracylines, podophyllotoxins and high-dose cytarabine in consolidation remains open. Overall, in adult ALL stricter adherence to protocols with fewer delays, dose reductions and omission of drugs due to toxicities would be an important contribution to therapeutic progress.

Maintenance therapy

Maintenance even after intensive induction and consolidation is still standard for ALL patients since all attempts to omit it led to inferior long-term outcome. Therefore some groups even prolong maintenance therapy beyond 2 years of total treatment duration. Methotrexate preferably given intravenously and mercaptopurine given orally are the backbone of maintenance. The role of intensification cycles during maintenance remains to be determined. The aim is to eliminate MRD. The optimal form and duration of maintenance therapy remains open but can hopefully be better defined by tailoring according to MRD, to ALL subtype (e.g. none for mature B-ALL) and including new therapeutic options (e.g. a tyrosine kinase inhibitor for *BCR–ABL*-positive ALL).

Prophylaxis of CNS leukaemia

CNS leukaemia occurs in 6% (range 1–10%) of patients with adult ALL at diagnosis, with a higher incidence in T-cell ALL (8%) and mature B-cell ALL (13%). Treatment and prophylaxis of CNS leukaemia may consist of intrathecal methotrexate alone or in combination with cytarabine or prednisone, systemic treatment with high-dose cytarabine or high-dose methotrexate and/or cranial irradiation.

Adult ALL patients who did not receive specific prophylactic CNS treatment in earlier trials have a CNS relapse rate of 30% (range 29–32%). With intrathecal chemotherapy alone, the rate of isolated and combined CNS relapses could be reduced to 13% (range 8–19%). In many adult ALL trials, additional prophylactic CNS irradiation (24 Gy) has been included. Long-term toxicities are apparently less severe than in paediatric patients. This combined approach further reduced the CNS relapse rate to 9% (range 3–19%). There is some evidence that early irradiation after remission induction is superior to delayed irradiation during consolidation treatment.

In many recent trials, combined treatment approaches have shown high efficacy. For high-dose chemotherapy with intrathecal therapy, the rate of CNS relapses was 7% (range 2–16%); with additional CNS irradiation, the relapse rate was 6% (range

1–13%). Several more recent trials have omitted prophylactic CNS irradiation or restricted irradiation to patients with high-risk features.

Because the risk for CNS relapse is associated with other prognostic factors, such as T-cell ALL, B-cell ALL, extreme leucocytosis, high leukaemia cell proliferation rate, high serum LDH level and extramedullary organ involvement, a risk-adapted CNS prophylaxis has been suggested. However, this approach, in contrast to childhood ALL, is not widely used in adults.

Therapy for relapsed and resistant leukaemia

Patients who fail to achieve CR or those who relapse subsequently have been treated with a variety of protocols. The use of regimens including vincristine, anthracyclines and steroids, similar to standard induction treatment, led to CR rates of approximately 60% in earlier studies but these patients generally had no intensive first-line treatment.

High-dose cytarabine has been extensively studied in relapsed adult ALL. From several small pilot studies comprising less than 100 patients, the weighted mean CR rate was 37%. Higher CR rates (50–60%) were achieved with combination regimens that included high-dose cytarabine and mitoxantrone, amsacrine or vincristine plus steroids. Because high-dose cytarabine is increasingly administered during front-line treatment, its efficacy during relapse treatment may be impaired. Therefore, new combinations with idarubicin (CR rate 46–64%) or fludarabine (CR rate 67–83%) or other agents have been evaluated. Nelarabine is a promising new drug for treatment of relapsed T-ALL.

The most significant predictive factor for treatment response in relapsed patients is the duration of first remission. Patients with longer previous remission (>18 months) have a higher CR rate and longer remission duration than those with a short previous remission (<18 months). Therefore in patients with early relapse and also in patients with molecular non-response (MRD persistence), high chemotherapy resistance has to be expected and experimental treatments should be considered for remission induction if available.

For all chemotherapy regimens, the duration of second remission is usually short (<6 months), and the long-term survival rate with chemotherapy alone is less than 5%. Thus, the only cure for adult patients with relapsed or resistant ALL is SCT, and the major aim of relapse treatment is the induction of a second remission with sufficient duration to prepare for SCT.

Stem cell transplantation

Stem cell transplantation from peripheral blood, and to a lesser extent from bone marrow, is an important post-remission strategy for eradication of residual disease in adult ALL. Despite a great number of trials, the indications for SCT in first CR, scheduling and procedures are still not defined satisfactorily. The potential advantages of SCT (short treatment duration, favourable outcome in some trials) must be balanced against the disadvantages (mortality of 20–30%, morbidity, late complications, reduced quality of life) and assessed in relation to the improving outcome of conventional and targeted chemotherapy regimens.

Allogeneic SCT from sibling donors

The outcome of allogeneic SCT from sibling donors for ALL depends on age and remission status of the patient. The best results have been obtained with patients transplanted during first remission, among whom the probability of survival is approximately 50% (Table 24.5). Relapse rate (RR) and transplant-related mortality (TRM) both range between 25 and 30%. Although TRM is strongly correlated with age, the upper age limit for sibling donor SCT has increased continuously up to 50–55 years. After sibling donor SCT in second remission the LFS rate is 34%, and in advanced ALL (refractory or in relapse) it results in an 18% long-term survival rate (Table 24.5).

There is evidence that a graft-versus-leukaemia (GVL) effect is also present in ALL, as indicated by several observations, such as lower RR in patients with acute and/or chronic graft-versus-host disease, lower RR after matched unrelated donor SCT, and induction of remission by withdrawal of prophylaxis against graft-versus-host disease or donor lymphocyte infusions in single patients with relapsed ALL.

Matched unrelated donor SCT

The role of matched unrelated donor SCT has become more important since only one-third of patients have a sibling donor.

The survival in first CR is around 42–45%, with lower RR and higher TRM compared with sibling donor SCT. The results are similar in large prospective trials, with higher RR for sibling donor SCT and higher TRM for matched unrelated donor SCT. The ECOG/MRC study reported an overall survival (OS) of 55% for sibling donor SCT and 46% for matched unrelated donor SCT (restricted to Ph/*BCR–ABL*-positive ALL); in the German Multicenter Study Group for Adult ALL (GMALL) study 06/99, OS was 53% for sibling donor SCT and 44% for matched unrelated donor SCT. TRM reaches 25–35% in matched unrelated donor SCT, particularly in patients older than 35–40 years. Nevertheless, improved results of matched unrelated donor SCT can be expected in the future due to better supportive care, donor selection and extension of indications beyond very high-risk patients.

Cord blood or haploidentical SCT in adult ALL is still experimental and an option only for rare cases; it has been explored by a few very experienced SCT centres.

Autologous SCT

According to published studies, OS after autologous SCT in first CR is 42%. This type of SCT is associated with a higher RR (>50%) because of the risk of reinfusing residual leukaemic cells and even more so because of the lack of a GVL effect. Several randomized studies have shown a similar or poorer outcome for autologous SCT compared with chemotherapy.

The intensity of pretreatment has an important impact on outcome in autologous SCT, since it leads to reduction of tumour load. Thus autologous SCT may be an option in MRD-negative high-risk patients without a donor. Maintenance therapy after autologous SCT, for example with mercaptopurine and methotrexate, or imatinib in Ph-positive ALL (particularly in MRD-positive patients), is also a useful approach.

Table 24.5 Recent results of stem cell transplantation in adult ALL.

Stem cell transplant	Disease stage	N	LFS/OS* (%)	Relapse incidence* (%)	TRM* (%)
Allogeneic	CR1	1100	50 (21–71)	24 (10–50)	27 (12–42)
	CR2	1019	34 (13–60)	48 (62–71)	29 (40–75)
	Relapsed/refractory	216	18 (8–33)	75 (60–77)	47 (46–47)
Autologous	CR1	1369	42 (15–65)	51 (27–68)	5 (0–8)
	CR2	258	24 (20–27)	70 (59–75)	18[†]
Matched unrelated donor	CR1	318	39 (32–51)	10 (6–19)	47 (32–54)
	≥CR2	231	27 (17–28)	8[‡]	75[‡]
	Relapsed/refractory	47	5[‡]	31[‡]	64[‡]
Non-myeloablative	All stages	132	23 (0–50)	47 (30–56)	42 (10–72)

*Weighted mean and range of published studies.
[†]One study.
[‡]One study (Cornelissen *et al.* 2001).
LFS, leukaemia-free survival; OS, overall survival; TRM, transplant-related mortality.

Non-myeloablative SCT

Non-myeloablative SCT or reduced-intensity conditioning regimens are new approaches that deserve evaluation in ALL and which may lead to an extension of indications for allogeneic SCT (see Chapter 38). In contrast to conventional SCT, which mainly relies on cell kill by high-dose chemotherapy and total body irradiation, non-myeloablative SCT relies on the GVL effect. Immunosuppression, for example with purine analogues, other cytostatic drugs and/or low-dose total body irradiation, is followed by the infusion of donor stem cells from a sibling or a matched unrelated donor with adapted immunosuppression to establish host tolerance.

First results indicate that in first CR stable remissions can be achieved in some patients. Literature results show an LFS rate of 23% for patients in all stages, with TRM of 42% and RR of 47%. According to an analysis by the European Group for Blood and Marrow Transplantation, the LFS in 91 adult ALL patients with a median age of 40 years was 18%, with TRM of 24% and RR of 58%. LFS in both studies was considerably higher if non-myeloablative SCT was conducted in first remission.

Indications for SCT in adult ALL

An evidence-based review has underlined the finding that SCT offers an advantage compared with chemotherapy in high-risk patients and in second remission. Other aspects of the review are summarized in Table 24.6. According to a meta-analysis of seven studies, OS for SCT was superior to chemotherapy with

Table 24.6 Evidence-based recommendations for stem cell transplantation (SCT) in adult ALL.

Decision	Recommendation
CR1: allogeneic SCT vs. chemotherapy	Comparable results
	SCT probably superior in high risk
	No SCT in standard risk
CR2: allogeneic SCT vs. chemotherapy	SCT superior
Autologous SCT vs. chemotherapy	Comparable results
Sibling donor vs. matched unrelated donor	Comparable results
Conditioning regimen	Data insufficient
	Advantage for TBI-based regimens
Allogeneic vs. autologous SCT	Advantage for allogeneic SCT

TBI, total body irradiation.

a particular advantage in high-risk patients. Thus the role of allogeneic SCT in standard-risk ALL remains unclear.

The indications for SCT in first remission are not uniformly defined. The major question is whether all patients with a sibling donor should be transferred to SCT or only those with specific risk factors. Currently, in the majority of trials, at least in Europe, SCT indications are based on the presence of adverse prognostic factors including MRD. Allogeneic sibling and matched unrelated donor SCT are considered in a similar way. The status of MRD is of increasing importance in the indications for SCT.

There is general agreement that all patients in second or later remission are candidates for SCT. Depending on donor availability and general condition, experimental procedures such as non-myeloablative SCT, cord blood SCT and haploidentical SCT may be considered.

Outcome of ALL subtypes and prognostic factors

The outcome of adult ALL varies strongly according to age and prognostic factors. Appreciation of the impact of such risk factors (Table 24.7) can result in the generation of risk-adapted treatment protocols for adult ALL.

Age

Age is the most important prognostic factor for ALL. There is a continuous decrease in outcome with increasing age from childhood to elderly patients. It is difficult to define an age limit where a change in prognosis occurs, but in almost all studies the LFS rate is inferior in patients older than 50–60 years. This age limit seems to be practical because patients below this age are candidates for intensified treatment approaches such as SCT, whereas for the older age group new strategies need to be explored, carefully weighing the gain in survival against quality of life. There is increasing evidence that with age-adapted moderate-dose chemotherapy, at least in some of the older patients, long-term remission can be achieved. Patients over 50–55 years of age with high-risk features who have achieved a CR and are in good clinical condition are potential candidates for autologous SCT or non-myeloablative SCT.

Adolescent patients (15–20 years) with ALL are treated either according to protocols for paediatric ALL or in adult ALL trials. Generally, more dose-intensive chemotherapy is applicable in young adults and may contribute to better results.

White blood cell count

An elevated WBC count at diagnosis (above $30–50 \times 10^9$/L) has been confirmed in various trials as a poor prognostic feature. The biological reason for the highly resistant behaviour of

Table 24.7 Adverse prognostic factors for adult ALL.

Factor	All subtypes	B-precursor	T-ALL
At diagnosis			
High WBC count		>30 (range 20–50) × 10^9/L*	>100 × 10^9/L‡
Subtype		Pro-B ALL or CD20-negative pre-B ALL†	Early T† Mature T†
Cytogenetics/molecular genetics	Complex karyotype†	t(9;22)/*BCR–ABL** t(4;11)/*ALL1–AF4** t(1;19)/*PBX1–E2A*†	*HOX11L2*‡ *BAALC*‡
Age	>35, >55, >60*		
During treatment			
Individual response	Steroid response† Late CR (>3–4 weeks)* MRD persistence >10^{-4} for 3–4 months*		

*Established prognostic factors.
†Prognostic factors used by several groups.
‡Rarely used prognostic factor.

B-precursor ALL with high WBC count is unclear. Probably in the future additional molecular markers will help to clarify the underlying mechanisms. Because of the high relapse rate, evaluation of MRD and use of experimental drugs and SCT modalities seem particularly important.

Immunophenotype and cytogenetics

The immunophenotype is an important independent prognostic variable in ALL. In ongoing trials, it is used to adjust treatment regimens accordingly, for example separate regimens for mature B-cell ALL. A further example for clinical application is the identification of patients for antibody therapy, for example anti-CD20 (rituximab) in CD20-positive B-lineage ALL.

T-lineage ALL

The outcome of T-lineage ALL is generally considered superior compared with B-lineage ALL. It comprises the subtypes early T-ALL, thymic (cortical) T-ALL and mature T-ALL, with LFS rates of 25%, 63% and 28%, respectively. Subtype was the most relevant prognostic factor for T-ALL in GMALL studies, with poorer outcome for early and mature T-ALL, whereas high WBC count (>100 × 10^9/L) had no prognostic impact.

The biological relevance of immunophenotype is underlined by the fact that overexpression of HOX11, HOX11L2, SIL-TAL1 and CALM-AF10 is associated with subtypes (i.e. maturation states) of thymocytes. A number of other protential poor-prognosis molecular markers have been reported for T-ALL. The variety of new prognostic markers does not allow integration into current risk models but may serve to identify pathogenetic mechanisms and therapeutic targets. With current

treatment regimens, CR rates of more than 90% and an LFS rate of 40–60% can be achieved in T-ALL.

B-precursor ALL

Pro-B ALL and/or t(4;11)-positive ALL is considered high risk in nearly all trials. It appears to be particularly susceptible to high-dose cytarabine-based regimens and SCT as reported from the GMALL studies. Common ALL/pre-B ALL has a large proportion of Ph-positive ALL. Based on prognostic factors (WBC count and time to achievement of CR) it can be subdivided into standard- and high-risk groups, with significantly different OS rates of 50–60% and 30–40%, respectively. The difference in OS between paediatric and adult ALL is mainly due the poorer outcome of B-precursor ALL.

Ph-positive ALL

The translocation t(9;22) and the respective fusion gene *BCR–ABL* until recently marked the most unfavourable subgroup of adult ALL. Ph/*BCR–ABL*-positive ALL occurs almost exclusively in conjunction with B-precursor ALL (c-ALL, pre-B ALL). The incidence increases with age. In Ph-positive leukaemia, the *BCR–ABL* fusion gene is causally involved in leukaemogenesis and is considered to be essential for leukaemic transformation. Using an inhibitor of the ABL tyrosine kinase (imatinib, Gleevec), cellular proliferation of *BCR–ABL*-positive CML and ALL cells can be prevented selectively (see Chapter 27).

A combination of imatinib with chemotherapy leads to remission rates of 90% and molecular remission even in 50% of patients. In addition, the OS rate is improved to 55–65% compared with 15% in historic trials and the proportion of patients transferred to SCT is increased. Compared with chemotherapy (all combination regimens), no increased toxicity has been described. Furthermore, there have been no reports of unfavourable influence on subsequent SCT, which is still considered the best curative option in Ph-positive ALL.

Results after SCT may be improved by the use of imabinib. A GMALL study showed that the majority of patients with persistent MRD after SCT who achieve molecular remission with imatinib have long-term survival. Thus post-transplant imatinib, either up-front or after detection of MRD, can reduce the relapse rate. In patients undergoing chemotherapy and SCT, it remains open whether and when treatment with imatinib can be stopped.

Older patients with Ph-positive ALL do not have the option of SCT and because of the extremely unfavourable results with chemotherapy, imatinib was evaluated as single-drug treatment for induction. A randomized trial compared imatinib monotherapy with dose-reduced chemotherapy for remission induction. After induction, all patients received imatinib in combination with consolidation chemotherapy. The remission rate for monotherapy was 93% compared with 54% for chemotherapy. OS was improved compared with a historic cohort but in both arms the relapse rate was high and no difference in terms of survival was detected. Therefore optimal remission induction and consolidation for elderly Ph-positive ALL remains to be defined.

Close monitoring of MRD allows the early detection of molecular resistance or molecular relapse. Thereby relapse treatment may be introduced earlier, before detection of cytological relapse. One reason for relapse is probably the development of resistance caused by kinase domain mutations. Therefore, before relapse treatment is started, bone marrow analysis for resistance-inducing mutations should be performed. The efficacy of imatinib treatment, and also of second-generation tyrosine kinase inhibitors such as dasatinib or nilotinib, may be impaired by these mutations. The aim of relapse treatment is achievement of second CR and SCT. For salvage therapy, second-generation inhibitors with or without additional chemotherapy may be considered. Dasatinib and nilotinib have increased efficacy compared with imatinib and are active in the majority of mutations, except the T315I mutation. The remission rates achieved with these drugs in patients failing to respond to imatinib are approximately 30%. They are currently being evaluated in relapse treatment, but trials for *de novo* Ph-positive ALL are starting.

Mature B-ALL

Mature B-ALL is grouped with Burkitt lymphoma according to the WHO classification and is treated according to a specific concept. Treatment is based on childhood B-cell ALL studies that significantly improved outcome. The drugs responsible for the improvement were high doses of fractionated cyclophosphamide, ifosfamide, high-dose methotrexate ($0.5-8\,g/m^2$) and high-dose cytarabine in conjunction with the conventional drugs for remission induction in ALL, given in short cycles at frequent intervals over a period of 6 months.

The application of these childhood B-cell ALL protocols in original or modified form also brought a substantial improvement for adult patients with B-cell ALL. CR rate was increased to approximately 75% (range 62–83%) and LFS rate to 55% (range 20–71%). More than 80% of the cases of mature B-ALL or Burkitt lymphoma express CD20 on their surface. Further significant improvement in survival rates to 80–90% was achieved by the use of rituximab in combination with chemotherapy.

B-cell ALL has a higher incidence of CNS involvement at diagnosis, and of CNS relapse. Therefore, effective measures against CNS disease, such as high-dose methotrexate and high-dose cytarabine, as well as intrathecal therapy, are important components of treatment regimens. On the other hand, maintenance treatment has been omitted. Because relapses occur almost exclusively within the first year in childhood as well as adult B-cell ALL, patients thereafter can be considered cured.

Response to treatment and minimal residual disease

Beside age, the most relevant prognostic factor in ALL is still the achievement of CR. Further prognostic factors related to treatment response are delayed time to CR or response to prednisone therapy. A more accurate approach for assessing individual response is MRD evaluation since this is an independent prognostic factor that reflects primary drug resistance and unknown host factors. There are two major aims of longitudinal MRD evaluation in adult ALL.

1 *Identification of high-risk patients as candidates for SCT or experimental therapy.* After the start of consolidation, high MRD ($>10^{-4}$) at any time is associated with a high relapse risk of 66–88%. In the GMALL studies, patients with high MRD ($>10^{-4}$) after induction and first consolidation are identified as high risk and are candidates for SCT in CR1. Persistent MRD thereby becomes an important new indication for SCT in CR1. However, outcome after SCT is also influenced by MRD status and patients with high MRD before SCT or persisting MRD after SCT have a poorer outcome. However, the optimal treatment of persistent MRD remains to be defined.

2 *Identification of low-risk patients in whom treatment reduction may be justified.* This is an aim that is more difficult to reach. An early and rapid decrease of MRD during induction is associated with a relapse risk of only 8%. However, this is observed in only 10% of patients. Overall, it is difficult to identify adult low-risk patients in whom reduction of therapy would be justified.

Furthermore, MRD evaluation offers a new refined definition of response to treatment, namely molecular CR (defined as MRD level $< 10^{-4}$) and molecular relapse (defined as reappearance of MRD > 10^{-4}). Molecular CR is the aim of induction therapy. During treatment and follow-up molecular relapse is highly predictive of cytological relapse. Molecular bone marrow relapse is also often present in patients with apparently isolated extramedullary relapse. In clinical trials molecular relapse should be treated similarly to cytological relapse.

New integrated risk classification

Prognostic factors are the basis for risk-adapted treatment regimens, with treatment intensity and combination defined according to risk of relapse. The main purpose is to identify patients with a high risk of relapse in order to treat them with the most intensive available therapy, i.e. SCT. However, this is not applicable for all factors. Thus higher age is associated with poorer prognosis but is not an indication for SCT because older patients also have a worse prognosis after transplantation. For other subgroups with originally poor prognosis, improvement was achieved by subgroup-specific treatment, such as for mature B-ALL or Ph-positive ALL. Finally, MRD evaluation allows the assessment of individual response and relapse risk. The majority of adult ALL study groups in Europe use MRD for risk stratification (www.leukaemia-net.org) and most of them combine MRD-based and conventional risk factors. In the past decade a large number of molecular factors with potential correlation to prognosis have been reported. Each new candidate prognostic factor should be evaluated prospectively within specific treatment protocols. Currently agreed poor-prognosis features are summarized in Table 24.7.

Overall outcome of adult ALL

In more than 7000 patients treated in prospective clinical trials the CR rate was 84% (range 74–93%), with 7% (range 1–11%) early death. The OS was 35% (range 27–54%). One major question in the treatment of adult ALL is the role of SCT in post-remission therapy. Notably, no difference is evident in studies focused on SCT ($N = 2696$), with a weighted mean of 84% for CR and 35% for OS, and in studies using risk-adapted approaches ($N = 2443$), with mean CR rates of 83% and OS of 36%. For specific subgroups there is a wide range, from 30–40% for high-risk ALL to 50–60% for standard-risk ALL and 80–90% for mature B-ALL. Outcome is strongly correlated with age.

New treatment approaches for adult ALL

Risk and subtype-adjusted treatment strategies have led to considerable improvement in outcome in mature B-ALL, T-ALL and Ph-positive ALL but less so in adult B-precursor ALL. The poorer outcome of B-precursor ALL is also the major factor contributing to the poorer overall outcome in adults compared with paediatric patients. The most promising new treatment options are based on targeted and subtype-specific approaches with preferably alternative mechanisms of action in order to avoid chemotherapy-induced toxicity.

Antibody therapy

ALL blast cells express a variety of specific antigens, such as CD20, CD19, CD22, CD33 and CD52, which may serve as targets for treatment with monoclonal antibodies. Monoclonal antibody therapy is an attractive approach since it is targeted, subtype specific and, compared with chemotherapy, has different mechanisms of action and side-effects. Their use may be most promising in relation to MRD status and in combination with chemotherapy. The anti-CD20 antibody has been successfully integrated in the therapy of mature B-ALL. It is now also being explored in several studies for CD20-positive B-precursor ALL. Studies with anti-CD52 are ongoing, either in relapse or according to MRD. Single cases showing efficacy of anti-CD33 or anti-CD22 have been reported. Another new promising approach is the use of bispecific T-cell engager antibodies targeted to CD19.

Successful chemotherapy approaches from paediatric protocols

Most of the adult ALL trials are originally based on paediatric protocols. In contrast to adult study groups, which to some extent are focused on high-dose therapies as used in AML and extensive use of SCT, in paediatric trials the major focus has been placed on optimization of intensive chemotherapy regimens. This is one important aim of several planned trials for adult ALL, aiming at intensification of vincristine, steroids, asparaginase, reinduction cycles and maintenance as in paediatric trials. Intensive chemotherapy should be complemented by targeted and individualized treatment elements. Furthermore, better adherence to protocols and encouragement of patients to improve their compliance (e.g. psychosocial counselling, documentation of compliance) are warranted in adult ALL.

Stem cell transplantation

SCT offers an advantage in adult high-risk patients and has contributed to improved outcome. However, procedures need to be optimized, including age limits for dose-reduced conditioning. In younger patients the rate of SCT may be reduced as soon as adaptation of paediatric treatment elements improves survival with chemotherapy only.

Risk-adapted treatment

Optimization of management needs to consider additional factors, such as the availability of a stem cell donor, patient-related factors, disease markers, treatment response and availability of targeted drugs. Prognostic factors and patient characteristics therefore no longer only serve for identification of candidates for SCT in first CR but to define individualized, flexible and patient-specific treatment approaches.

New drugs

Finally, a number of new drugs are under evaluation for treatment of ALL, including antibodies, purine analogues and related drugs such as nelarabine, clofarabine, kinase inhibitors and liposomal preparations of vincristine and cytarabine for intrathecal use. After proof of efficacy these drugs can be integrated in risk- and subgroup-adjusted treatment regimens.

Clinical trials

A standard treatment for adult ALL has so far not been defined. Therefore as many patients as possible should be treated within clinical trials in order to contribute to further treatment optimization. New end points for clinical trials are needed, such as molecular CR, molecular relapse, evaluation of SCT and quality of life. Despite these short-term end points, improvement in OS of the total patient population including all risk groups is the final proof for all new risk-adapted treatment approaches.

Selected bibliography

Annino L, Vegna ML, Camera A et al. (2002) Treatment of adult acute lymphoblastic leukemia (ALL): long-term follow-up of the GIMEMA ALL 0288 randomized study. Blood 99: 863–71.

Apostolidou E, Swords R, Alvarado Y, Giles FJ (2007) Treatment of acute lymphoblastic leukaemia: a new era. Drugs 67: 2153–71.

Arnold R, Massenkeil G, Bornhauser M et al. (2002) Nonmyeloablative stem cell transplantation in adults with high-risk ALL may be effective in early but not in advanced disease. Leukemia 16: 2423–8.

Arnold R, Beelen D, Bunjes D et al. (2003) Phenotype predicts outcome after allogeneic stem cell transplantation in adult high risk ALL patients. Blood 102: Abstract 1719.

Bachanova V, Weisdorf D (2008) Unrelated donor allogeneic transplantation for adult acute lymphoblastic leukemia: a review. Bone Marrow Transplantation 41: 455–64.

Bassan R, Pogliani E, Casula P et al. (2001) Risk-oriented postremission strategies in adult acute lymphoblastic leukemia: prospective confirmation of anthracycline activity in standard-risk class and role of hematopoietic stem cell transplants in high-risk groups. Hematology Journal 2: 117–26.

Bassan R, Spinelli O, Oldani E et al. (2009) Improved risk classification for risk-specific therapy based on the molecular study of MRD in adult ALL. Blood 113: 4153–62.

Bene MC, Castoldi G, Knapp W et al. (1995) Proposal for the immunological classification of acute leukemias. Leukemia 9: 1783–6.

Bruggemann M, Raff T, Flohr T et al. (2006) Clinical significance of minimal residual disease quantification in adult patients with standard-risk acute lymphoblastic leukemia. Blood 107: 1116–23.

Chaidos A, Kanfer E, Apperley JF (2007) Risk assessment in haemotopoietic stem cell transplantation: disease and disease stage. Best Practice and Research. Clinical Haematology 20: 125–54.

Gökbuget N, Hoelzer D (2006) Rituximab in the treatment of adult ALL. Annals of Hematology 85 (Suppl. 1): 117–19.

Gökbuget N, Hoelzer D (2009) Treatment of adult acute lymphoblastic leukemia. Seminars in Hematology 46: 64–75.

Gökbuget N, Arnold R, Buechner Th et al. (2001) Intensification of induction and consolidation improves only subgroups of adult ALL: analysis of 1200 patients in GMALL study 05/93. Blood 98: Abstract 802.

Gökbuget N, Raff R, Brugge-Mann M et al. (2004) Risk/MRD adapted GMALL trials in adult ALL. Annals of Hematology 83 (Suppl. 1): S129–S131.

Gökbuget N, Arnold R, Böhme A et al. (2007) Improved outcome in high risk and very high risk ALL by risk adapted SCT and in standard risk ALL by intensive chemotherapy in 713 adult ALL patients treated according to the prospective GMALL Study 07/2003. Blood 110: Abstract 12.

Goldstone AH, Lazarus HJ, Richards SM et al. (2004) The outcome of 551 1st CR transplants in adult ALL from the UKALL XII/ECOG 2993 Study. Blood 104: 615.

Grabher C, von BH, Look AT (2006) Notch 1 activation in the molecular pathogenesis of T-cell acute lymphoblastic leukaemia. Nature Reviews. Cancer 6: 347–59.

Hagedorn N, Acquaviva C, Fronkova E et al. (2007) Submicroscopic bone marrow involvement in isolated extramedullary relapses in childhood acute lymphoblastic leukemia: a more precise definition of 'isolated' and its possible clinical implications. A collaborative study of the Resistant Disease Committee of the International BFM study group. Blood 110: 4022–9.

Hahn T, Wall D, Camitta B et al. (2006) The role of cytotoxic therapy with hematopoietic stem cell transplantation in the therapy of acute lymphoblastic leukemia in adults: an evidence-based review. Biology of Blood and Marrow Transplantation 12: 1–30.

Hallbook H, Simonsson B, Ahlgren T et al. (2002) High-dose cytarabine in upfront therapy for adult patients with acute lymphoblastic leukaemia. British Journal of Haematology 118: 748–54.

Hoelzer D, Thiel E, Löffler H et al. (1988) Prognostic factors in a multicenter study for treatment of acute lymphoblastic leukemia in adults. Blood 71: 123–31.

Hunault M, Harousseau JL, Delain M et al. (2004) Better outcome of adult acute lymphoblastic leukemia after early genoidentical allogeneic bone marrow transplantation (BMT) than after late high-dose therapy and autologous BMT: a GOELAMS trial. Blood 104: 3028–37.

Kantarjian H, Thomas D, O'Brien S et al. (2004) Long-term follow-up results of hyperfractionated cyclophosphamide, vincristine, doxorubicin, and dexamethasone (Hyper-CVAD), a dose-intensive regimen, in adult acute lymphocytic leukemia. *Cancer* **101**: 2788–801.

Labar B, Suciu S, Zittoun R *et al.* (2004) Allogeneic stem cell transplantation in acute lymphoblastic leukemia and non-Hodgkin's lymphoma for patients ≤50 years old in first complete remission: results of the EORTC ALL-3 trial. *Haematologica* **89**: 809–17.

Larson RA, Dodge RK, Linker CA *et al.* (1998) A randomized controlled trial of filgrastim during remission induction and consolidation chemotherapy for adults with acute lymphoblastic leukemia: CALGB study 9111. *Blood* **92**: 1556–64.

Linker C, Damon L, Ries C, Navarro W (2002) Intensified and shortened cyclical chemotherapy for adult acute lymphoblastic leukemia. *Journal of Clinical Oncology* **20**: 2464–71.

Loberiza F (2006) Summary Slides 2003: part III. *IMBTR/ABMTR Newsletter* **10**: 6–9.

Mancini M (2001) An integrated molecular–cytogenetic classification is highly predictive of outcome in adult acute lymphoblastic leukemia (ALL): analysis of 395 cases enrolled in the GIMEMA 0496 Trial. *Blood* **98**: Abstract 3492.

Mancini M, Scappaticci D, Cimino G *et al.* (2005) A comprehensive genetic classification of adult acute lymphoblastic leukemia (ALL): analysis of the GIMEMA 0496 protacol. *Blood* **105**: 3434–41.

Mohty M, Labopin M, Tabrizzi R *et al.* (2008) Reduced intensity conditioning allogeneic stem cell transplantation for adult patients with acute lymphoblastic leukemia: a retrospective study from the European Group for Blood and Marrow Transplantation. *Haematologica* **93**: 303–6.

Ottmann OG, Pfeifer H (2009) First-line treatment of Philadelphia chromosome-positive acute lymphoblastic leukaemia in adults. *Current Opinion in Oncology* **21** (Suppl. 1): S43–S46.

Ottmann OG, Wassmann B, Pfeifer H *et al.* (2007) Imatinib compared with chemotherapy as front-line treatment of elderly patients with Philadelphia chromosome-positive acute lymphoblastic leukemia (Ph+ALL). *Cancer* **109**: 2068–76.

Pfeifer H, Wassmann B, Pavlova A *et al.* (2007) Kinase domain mutations of BCR–ABL frequently precede imatinib-based therapy and give rise to relapse in patients with de novo Philadelphia-positive acute lymphoblastic leukemia (Ph+ ALL). *Blood* **110**: 727–34.

Pui CH, Jeha S (2007) New therapeutic strategies for the treatment of acute lymphoblastic leukaemia. *Nature Reviews. Drug Discovery* **6**: 149–65.

Raff T, Gökbuget N, Luschen S *et al.* (2007) Molecular relapse in adult standard-risk ALL patients detected by prospective MRD monitoring during and after maintenance treatment: data from the GMALL 06/99 and 07/03 trials. *Blood* **109**: 910–15.

Ribera JM, Oriol A, Bethencourt C *et al.* (2005) Comparison of intensive chemotherapy, allogeneic or autologous stem cell transplantation as post-remission treatment for adult patients with high-risk acute lymphoblastic leukemia. Results of the PETHEMA ALL-93 trial. *Haematologica* **90**: 1346–56.

Rowe JM, Buck G, Burnett AK *et al.* (2005) Induction therapy for adults with acute lymphoblastic leukemia: results of more than 1500 patients from the international ALL trial: MRC UKALL XII/ECOG E2993. *Blood* **106**: 3760–7.

Swerdlow SH, Campo E, Harris NL *et al.* (eds) (2008) *WHO Classification of Tumours of Haematopoietic and Lymphoid Tissues.* IARC, Lyon.

Szczepanski T (2007) Why and how to quantify minimal residual disease in acute lymphoblastic leukemia? *Leukemia* **21**: 622–6.

Takeuchi J, Kyo T, Naito K *et al.* (2002) Induction therapy by frequent administration of doxorubicin with four other drugs, followed by intensive consolidation and maintenance therapy for adult acute lymphoblastic leukemia: the JALSG-ALL93 study. *Leukemia* **16**: 1259–66.

Thiebaut A, Vernant JP, Degos L *et al.* (2000) Adult acute lymphocytic leukemia study testing chemotherapy and autologous and allogeneic transplantation. A follow-up report of the French protocol LALA 87. *Hematology/Oncology Clinics of North America* **14**: 1353–66.

Thomas X, Boiron JM, Huguet F *et al.* (2004) Outcome of treatment in adults with acute lymphoblastic leukemia: analysis of the LALA-94 trial. *Journal of Clinical Oncology* **22**: 4075–86.

Tobinai K, Takeyama K, Arima F *et al.* (2007) Phase II study of chemotherapy and stem cell transplantation for adult acute lymphoblastic leukemia or lymphoblastic lymphoma: Japan Clinical Oncology Group Study 9004. *Cancer Science* **98**: 1350–7.

van der Velden VH, Cazzaniga G, Schrauder A *et al.* (2007) Analysis of minimal residual disease by Ig/TCR gene rearrangements: guidelines for interpretation of real-time quantitative PCR data. *Leukemia* **21**: 604–11.

Yanada M, Matsuo K, Suzuki T, Naoe T (2006) Allogeneic hematopoietic stem cell transplantation as part of postremission therapy improves survival for adult patients with high-risk acute lymphoblastic leukemia: a metaanalysis. *Cancer* **106**: 1657–63.

Childhood acute lymphoblastic leukaemia

25

Dario Campana and Ching-Hon Pui

St Jude Children's Research Hospital, Memphis, Tennessee, USA

Introduction

Leukaemia is the most common childhood cancer and acute lymphoblastic leukaemia (ALL) is the most common subtype, accounting for 75–80% of all cases. Childhood ALL comprises different biological subtypes defined by cell morphology, immunophenotype, gene expression features and genetic abnormalities, some of which are associated with disease aggressiveness and treatment response.

Progress in the treatment of childhood ALL over the last four decades has been steady, with cure rates (i.e. no evidence of disease for 10 years or more) now surpassing 80%. This advance can be attributed to three main factors: recognition of reliable prognostic factors leading to increasingly refined risk-directed therapies, development of clinical trials designed to gain substantial increments in knowledge, and improvements in supportive care. In this chapter, we review the current status of the biological studies and treatment of childhood ALL and discuss future directions for research and treatment.

Postgraduate Haematology: 6th edition. Edited by A. Victor Hoffbrand, Daniel Catovsky, Edward G.D. Tuddenham, Anthony R. Green
© 2011 Blackwell Publishing Ltd.

Epidemiology

The median age at diagnosis for ALL is 13 years and approximately 60% of cases are diagnosed under the age of 20. ALL is the most common malignancy diagnosed in patients younger than 15 years, accounting for 23% of all cancers and 76% of all leukaemias in this age group. In general, the incidence is higher in boys than in girls (four times for T-cell ALL), except that girls have a slightly higher (1.5 times) incidence of leukaemia in the first year of life. The reported incidence of ALL is higher in northern and western Europe, North America and Oceania, and lower in Asia, South America and Africa. In industrialized countries, the incidence is higher among children of European descent than among those of African descent. For example, the annual rate (per million population) of childhood ALL from birth to 19 years of age is 29.7 in the UK and 11.0 in India; in the USA, it is 32.9 for white people and 14.8 for African-Americans.

In developed countries, the incidence of ALL is highest between ages 2 and 5 years. This age peak is accounted largely by ALL with hyperdiploidy (>50 chromosomes) or *ETV6–RUNX1* (also known as *TEL–AML1*) gene fusion. The incidence of childhood ALL is higher among white people than among those of African descent, especially among children 2–5 years of age. T-cell ALL and pre-B leukaemia with t(1;19)/*TCF3–PBX1* (also known as *E2A–PBX1*) fusion are more prevalent among African-American children, who are less likely to have hyperdiploid ALL with more than 50 chromosomes.

Only a small proportion (<5%) of patients with childhood ALL have underlying hereditary genetic abnormalities. Children with Down syndrome have a 10- to 30-fold increased risk of developing ALL. Mutations in the *JAK2* gene, generally found in higher-risk ALL, are frequent in ALL cells of Down syndrome children. Other genetic disorders associated with an increased incidence of ALL include ataxia telangiectasia and Bloom syndrome. The association between leukaemia and congenital immunodeficiencies such as X-linked agammaglobulinaemia and common variable immunodeficiency is not well supported.

Fraternal twins and siblings of affected children are at a twofold to fourfold greater risk of leukaemia during the first decade of life than are unrelated children. In the case of identical twins, when leukaemia occurs in one twin, there is a 20% probability that it will also occur in the other twin, owing to ALL transfer *in utero* via the shared placental circulation. When leukaemia is diagnosed before 1 year of age it almost invariably develops in the other twin, generally within a few months. In identical twins with t(4;11)/*MLL–AF4*, the concordance rate is nearly 100%, with a short latency period (weeks to a few months). In contrast, the concordance rate in twins with the *ETV6–RUNX1* fusion or T-cell phenotype is lower and the postnatal latency period longer, in keeping with the requirement for additional genetic events for leukaemic transformation in these subtypes of ALL. Hyperdiploid ALL also appears to arise before birth but requires postnatal events for full malignant transformation. In contrast, t(1;19)/*TCF3–PBX1* ALL appears to have a postnatal origin in most cases.

Aetiology

Ionizing radiation and chemical mutagens have been implicated in the induction of leukaemia but clear aetiological factors for ALL cannot be identified in nearly all cases. *In utero* exposure to diagnostic X-rays is associated with a slightly increased risk of ALL, proportional to the number of exposures. The association between leukaemia and maternal exposure to potential mutagens, neonatal administration of vitamin K, parental use of medications and drugs, proximity to electromagnetic fields, and exposure to other potential mutagens has been studied but no definitive conclusions reached. A case–control study identified a significantly increased risk of leukaemia among the offspring of men employed in occupations with increased exposure to electromagnetic fields or radiation, a finding that warrants further studies. Industralization, higher socioeconomic status and social isolation appear to be associated with an increased risk of childhood B-lineage ALL, and occasional clustering of

childhood ALL appears to be associated with rural–urban population mixing. Greaves has postulated that absence or diminution of infections early in life might predispose the immune system to aberrant responses to subsequent exposures which in turn might precipitate ALL development from a preleukaemic clone through proliferative or apoptotic stress.

A case–control study found that *in utero* exposure to DNA-damaging drugs, herbal medicines or pesticides was significantly associated with infant leukaemia with *MLL* rearrangements. Deficiency of the detoxifying enzymes glutathione *S*-transferase (GST)-M1 and GST-T1 is associated with infant leukaemia without *MLL* rearrangement, and with ALL in black children, and polymorphisms of NADPH:quinone oxidoreductase have been associated with the development of ALL. Cytochrome P450 CYP1A1*2A and NQO1*2 variant genotypes have also been linked to an increased risk of childhood ALL, and a report has indicated an association between a polymorphism on intron 4 of the gene for aldo-keto reductase 1C3 (*AKR1C3*) and the development of leukaemia. There are also data suggesting that variable expression levels of cell-cycle inhibitor genes *CDKN2A*, *CDKN2B* and *CDKN1B* due to regulatory polymorphisms could contribute to leukaemogenesis. These studies implicate host pharmacogenetics in the development of ALL, a notion that warrants further study.

It has been reported that children diagnosed with ALL had significantly more clinically diagnosed infectious episodes in infancy than did controls; the average number of episodes was 3.6 (95% confidence interval 3.3, 3.9) versus 3.1 (2.9, 3.2). This difference was most apparent in the neonatal period, suggesting that a dysregulated immune response to infection in the first few months of life might promote transition to overt ALL.

Pathogenesis

Genetic changes are central to the development of leukaemia. The dysregulation of genes encoding transcription factors and the resulting subversion of transcriptional pathways that regulate haemopoietic cell homeostasis provides a mechanistic explanation for leukaemogenesis. Haemopoiesis can also be altered by the dysregulated activity of tyrosine kinases, as in the case of the *BCR–ABL1* fusion gene. Alternatively, activating mutations in tyrosine kinase receptors for growth factors may confer a growth advantage to leukaemic cells. This mechanism is exemplified by mutations of *FLT3*, which encodes a receptor tyrosine kinase expressed by immature haemopoietic cells that acts synergistically with other growth factors to stimulate proliferation of haemopoietic progenitor cells. These mutations typically involve small tandem duplications of amino acids that result in constitutive tyrosine kinase activity. Activating mutations of *NOTCH1*, a gene encoding a transmembrane receptor that regulates normal T-cell development, are frequently detected in T-cell ALL. Activating mutations of *NOTCH1* produce constitutive NOTCH1 signalling, which is sufficient to induce T-cell ALL in experimental models, and appears to be an early event in leukaemogenesis. A multicomponent membrane-associated enzyme, γ-secretase, is required for NOTCH1 signalling through mutant NOTCH receptors in T-cell ALL, a finding that provided a rationale for the clinical testing of γ-secretase inhibitors in T-cell ALL. An initial trial with such an agent was disappointing and revealed intolerable gastrointestinal toxicity; more recent data from a murine model suggest that the combination of γ-secretase inhibitors with high-dose glucocorticoids may enhance antileukaemic activity while diminishing toxicity.

A recent large-scale study of DNA single-nucleotide polymorphism (SNP) analysis examined 242 cases of paediatric B-cell precursor ALL and identified lesions in genes encoding key regulators of B-cell differentiation in 40% of the cases. Most prominent were deletions and cryptic translocations involving the *PAX5* gene, which was altered in almost one-third of cases and which would be predicted to block normal B-progenitor cell differentiation prior to immunoglobulin heavy-chain gene rearrangement. Other mutated genes were found in concert with several of the more common translocation-induced chimeric oncogenes, such as *TCF3–PBX1* and *ETV6–RUNX1*, including the essential B-cell developmental genes *TCF3*, *EBF*, *LEF1*, *IKZF1* (Ikaros) and *IKZF3* (Aiolos). A subsequent study showed deletion of *IKZF1* in 83.7% of *BCR–ABL1*-positive ALL; the deletion was also found in chronic myelogenous leukaemia (CML) in blast crisis but not in chronic phase. The *IKZF1* deletions resulted in haploinsufficiency, expression of a dominant-negative Ikaros isoform, or the complete loss of Ikaros expression. Together, these findings suggest that genetic lesions resulting in the loss of Ikaros function are an important event in the development of *BCR–ABL1*-positive ALL.

Clinical and laboratory features

Table 25.1 summarizes clinical and laboratory features of children with newly diagnosed ALL. On physical examination, children with ALL frequently present with pallor, petechiae and ecchymoses, and occasionally mucosal bleeding. Because of anaemia, they may have fatigue and lethargy, dyspnoea, angina and dizziness. Neutropenia may lead to severe infection. Bone pain and arthralgia caused by leukaemic infiltration and, less frequently, haemorrhage or infection can be especially severe in young children. Fever can be caused by infection or by pyrogenic cytokines such as interleukin (IL)-1, IL-6 and tumour necrosis factor released from the leukaemic cells. Liver, spleen, thymus, lymph nodes and central nervous system (CNS) are common sites of extramedullary involvement. An anterior mediastinal mass is typical of T-cell ALL. Painless enlargement of the scrotum can be a sign of testicular leukaemia or hydrocele resulting from lymphatic obstruction. Very rarely, ALL is

Table 25.1 Presenting clinical and laboratory features of children with newly diagnosed ALL.

Feature	Percentage of white children (SJCRH)	Percentage of total (BFM)
Age (years)		
≤1	2.7	2.7
2–9	71.6	79.6
≥10	25.7	17.7
Male	56.0	57.9
Liver edge below costal margin >4 cm	31.6	30.9
Spleen edge below costal margin >4 cm	30.4	27.0
Mediastinal mass	10.4	8.1
Central nervous system leukaemia (CNS3)*	2.7	2.5
Leucocyte count ($\times 10^9$/L)		
<10	46.2	45.9
10–50	29.3	31.8
≥50	24.5	22.3
Haemoglobin <8 g/dL	51.8	53.7
Immunophenotype		
Early pre-B	53.7	69.3
Pre-B	28.9	17.0
T-cell	15.4	13.5
B	2.0	
DNA index ≥1.16	22.1	25.7
t(1;19)/*TCF3–PBX1*	2.9	2.1
t(9;22)/*BCR–ABL1*	2.4	2.2
t(4;11)/*MLL–AFF1*	3.0	2.9
t(12;21)/*ETV6–RUNX1*	18.9	

*CNS3 status denotes the presence of leukaemic cells in a cerebrospinal fluid that contains ≥ 5 leucocytes/μL.
BFM, Berlin–Frankfurt–Münster 90 (1990–95, not including B-ALL) (Schrappe et al. 2000); SJCRH, St Jude Children's Research Hospital (1979–2002).

detected during routine examination in the absence of signs or symptoms.

Blood examination typically reveals anaemia, neutropenia and thrombocytopenia, due to bone marrow replacement and suppression of normal haemopoiesis by leukaemic cells. Haemoglobin is commonly below 8 g/dL. Profound neutropenia (<0.5 × 10^9/L) occurs in 40% of patients, rendering them at high risk of infection. Initial leucocyte counts may range from 0.1 to 1500 × 10^9/L (median 12 × 10^9/L); they are greater than 10 × 10^9/L in slighty over half of patients and greater than 100 × 10^9/L in 10–15% of patients. Most patients have circulating leukaemic blast cells but in cases with low initial counts ($<2 \times 10^9/L$) lymphoblasts are often absent in blood smears. Hypereosinophilia, generally reactive, may be present at diagnosis. Coagulopathy, usually mild, may occur in T-cell ALL and is only rarely associated with severe haemorrhage. A large leukaemic cell burden is commonly accompanied by elevated serum lactate dehydogenase activity and elevated uric acid and phosphorus concentration. An enlarged kidney can be detected in 30–50% of patients but has no prognostic or therapeutic implications. Liver dysfunction due to leukaemic infiltration occurs in 10–20% of patients, is usually mild and has no important clinical or prognostic consequences. Abnormalities of the bone, such as metaphyseal banding, periosteal reactions, osteolysis, osteosclerosis or osteopenia, can be revealed by radiography in half of the patients. As these changes do not affect treatment and outcome, routine diagnostic imaging studies (except for chest radiography to rule out mediastinal mass) is not necessary.

Leukaemic blast cells are identified morphologically at diagnosis in the cerebrospinal fluid (CSF) of approximately one-third of children with ALL, most of whom have no neurological symptoms. Although CNS leukaemia is defined by the presence of at least five leucocytes per microlitre of CSF and the detection of leukaemic blast cells, or by the presence of cranial nerve palsy, the presence of any leukaemic cells in CSF (even from iatrogenic introduction due to a traumatic lumbar puncture) predicts an increased risk of ALL relapse.

Differential diagnosis

The acute onset of petechiae, ecchymoses and bleeding may suggest idiopathic thrombocytopenic purpura (often associated with a recent viral infection, large platelets in blood smears and no evidence of anaemia). Like ALL, aplastic anaemia may also present with pancytopenia and complications associated with bone marrow failure but hepatosplenomegaly and lymphadenopathy are rare, and the skeletal changes associated with ALL are absent.

Infectious mononucleosis and other viral infections can be confused with ALL. Detection of atypical lymphocytes or elevated viral titres aid in the diagnosis. Patients with pertussis or parapertussis may have marked lymphocytosis, but the affected cells are mature lymphocytes rather than lymphoblasts. Bone pain, arthralgia and occasionally arthritis may mimic juvenile rheumatoid arthritis, rheumatic fever, other collagen diseases or osteomyelitis.

Childhood ALL should also be distinguished from paediatric small round cell tumours that involve the bone marrow, including neuroblastoma, rhabdomyosarcoma and retinoblastoma. Generally, in such cases, a primary lesion can be found by routine diagnostic studies, and disseminated tumour cells often form clumps.

Morphology and cytochemistry

Morphological analysis of leukaemic cells distinguishes three subtypes of ALL (L1, L2 and L3) as classified by the French–American–British (FAB) schema. This classification cannot accurately distinguish between ALL and non-lymphoid acute leukaemia, and has no prognostic or therapeutic relevance with contemporary therapy. Cytochemical stains such as periodic acid–Schiff reacts positively with cells in over 70% of ALL cases, while myeloperoxidase, Sudan black and non-specific esterases, including α-naphthyl butyrate and α-naphthyl acetate esterase, are typically negative. Neveretheless, classification of acute leukaemias is currently based on immunophenotypic and genetic analyses.

Immunophenotypic classification

Early pre-B ALL

Leukaemic blast cells of early pre-B ALL resemble normal marrow B-cell precursors. The leukaemic cells always express CD19 and almost all cases have cytoplasmic CD22 and CD79α; surface CD22 expression is also evident in most cases. CD10 and terminal deoxynucleotidyltransferase (TdT) are expressed in 90% of cases, and CD34 in more than 75% of cases. The CD20 antigen is present on a minor proportion of blast cells in half of cases but its intensity might increase during treatment. Early pre-B ALL cells lack expression of surface and cytoplasmic immunoglobulins.

ALL with rearrangement of the *MLL* gene typically has an early pre-B ALL phenotype with distinctive features such as expression of CD15, CD65 and chondroitin protoglycan sulphate, and absence of CD10. Hyperdiploidy (chromosome number >50) is typically associated with weak or undetectable CD45 expression.

Pre-B ALL

The pre-B immunophenotype is defined by the accumulation of cytoplasmic immunoglobulin μ heavy chains with no detectable surface immunoglobulins and is found in approximately 20–25% of cases. Leukaemic cells that express both cytoplasmic and surface immunoglobulin μ heavy chains without κ or λ light chains, a rare finding, have been designated transitional pre-B ALL. Pre-B ALL expresses CD19, CD22 and CD79α and, usually, CD10 and TdT but only two-thirds express CD34. In many cases of pre-B ALL, surface CD20 is absent or is weakly expressed. ZAP-70 expression is more prevalent in cases with a pre-B phenotype. Between 20 and 25% of pre-B ALL cases have either t(1;19)(q23;p13) or der(19)t(1;19)(q23;p13).

B-cell ALL

In 2–4% of childhood ALL cases, cells express surface immunoglobulin μ heavy chains plus either κ or λ light chains. Commonly, cells have L3 morphology according to the FAB classification and express CD19, CD22, CD20 and frequently CD10; CD34 is negative. The less common subtype of B-cell ALL is characterized by blast cells with L1 or L2 morphology, and expression of TdT and/or CD34.

T-lineage ALL

T-lineage ALL cells express CD7 and CD3, the latter most commonly only in the cytoplasm. Other markers commonly expressed include CD2, CD5 and TdT; CD1a, surface CD3, CD4 and CD8 are detected in fewer than 45% of cases. HLA-DR expression is uncommon, and 40–45% of cases are positive for CD10 and/or CD21. CD79α is also weakly expressed in approximately one-third of cases.

T-lineage ALL has been divided into three stages of immunophenotypic differentiation: early (CD7$^+$, cCD3$^+$, surface CD3$^-$, CD4$^-$ and CD8$^-$), mid or common (cCD3$^+$, surface CD3$^-$, CD4$^+$, CD8$^+$ and CD1a$^+$) and late (surface CD3$^+$, CD1a$^-$ and either CD4$^+$ or CD8$^+$). However, many cases have immunophenotypic patterns that do not fit these thymic maturation stages. T-cell receptor (TCR) proteins are heterogeneously expressed in T-lineage ALL. In approximately two-thirds of cases, membrane CD3 and TCR proteins are absent. In half of these cases, however, TCR proteins (TCR-β, TCR-α, or both) are present in the cell cytoplasm. Most cases with membrane CD3 and TCR chains express the αβ form of the TCR, whereas a minority express TCR γδ proteins.

Several studies have yielded conflicting conclusions about the prognostic significance of the expression of surface CD3 and the absence of CD2, CD5 or CD10. We recently identified a subtype of T-ALL, named early thymic precursor (ETP) ALL, which exhibits the gene expression profile of normal ETP cells, a population of recent immigrants from the bone marrow to the thymus that retains multilineage differentiation potential. These leukaemias are positive for CD7 and CD3, lack CD1a and CD8 expression, have weak or absent CD5 expression and express at least one stem cell or myeloid-associated antigen (e.g. CD34, CD117, CD13, CD33, CD11b). These cases are characterized by a dismal response to therapy and a high rate of relapse.

Cytogenetic and molecular classification

Hyperdiploid and hypodiploid ALL

In approximately half of ALL cases, leukaemic cells are hyperdiploid. Hyperdiploid cases with a chromosome number of 51–65 represent a distinct biological subset of B-lineage ALL with an excellent prognosis. Leukaemic lymphoblasts with this karyotype have a marked propensity to undergo apoptosis, and accumulate greater quantities of methotrexate and its active polyglutamate metabolites. These features help to explain the relatively low leukaemic burden at presentation and the favourable prognosis of this ALL subtype. Among chromosomes that are over-represented, only the trisomies of chromosome 4, 10 and 17 were associated with a favourable prognosis in some studies.

In contrast to the overall favourable prognosis of cases with 51–65 chromosomes, ALL cases with near-triploidy (69–81 chromosomes) have a response to therapy similar to that of non-hyperdiploid ALL; cases with near-tetraploidy (82–94 chromosomes) have a high frequency of T-cell immunophenotype. Hypodiploidy (<45 chromosomes) occurs in less than 2% of ALL cases and is associated with a poor outcome.

ALL with *TEL–AML1* (*ETV6–RUNX1*) rearrangements

The t(12;21)(p12;q22) translocation brings together the 5′ portion of the *TEL* (*ETV6*) gene and the nearly complete *AML1* (*RUNX1*) gene. This translocation can usually be detected only by fluorescence *in situ* hybridization (FISH) or reverse-transcriptase polymerase chain reaction (RT-PCR). The non-translocated *ETV6* allele is frequently deleted. This gene fusion is found in approximately 20% of ALL cases. In some series, the *TEL–AML1* abnormality was not significantly associated with outcome, but in most studies it defined a subgroup with excellent prognosis. ALL cells bearing this abnormality reportedly have increased *in vitro* sensitivity to L-asparaginase, as well as to doxorubicin, etoposide, amsacrine and dexamethasone. Similar to T-cell ALL, blast cells with *ETV6–RUNX1* accumulate significantly lower levels of methotrexate polyglutamates than do those with other genetic abnormalities, suggesting that patients with this leukaemia subtype might benefit from an increased dose of methotrexate.

The *ETV6* gene belongs to the Ets family of transcription factors. It is widely expressed and appears to have an essential role in haemopoiesis. *RUNX1* encodes a transcription factor that binds DNA as a heterodimer with core-binding factor (CBF)-β and is essential for the development of definitive haemopoiesis. Transduction of murine bone marrow cells with *ETV6–RUNX1* is associated with a higher frequency of leukaemia resembling ALL. It was recently shown that the ETV6–RUNX1 protein binds to Smad3, a transforming growth factor (TGF)-β signalling target, and alters its capacity to activate target promoters, resulting in reduced sensitivity to TGF-β-mediated inhibition of proliferation. Expression of ETV6–RUNX1 in human cord blood progenitor cells led to the expansion of a candidate preleukaemic population that had a growth advantage in the presence of TGF-β.

ALL with *E2A–PBX1* (*TCF3–PBX1*) rearrangements

Approximately 20–25% of pre-B ALL cases have the t(1;19) (q23;p13) translocation abnormality that juxtaposes the *E2A* (*TCF3*) gene on chromosome 19 and the *PBX1* gene on chromosome 1. The resulting E2A–PBX1 fusion protein contains the transcriptional activation domains of E2A linked to the DNA-binding domain of PBX1 and the encoded protein inappropriately activates the transcription of genes normally regulated by PBX1. Expression of E2A–PBX1 in mice leads to the development of lymphomas and myeloid leukaemias. Another *E2A* fusion gene is created by t(17;19)(q22;p13), in which *E2A* is fused to the gene that encodes the transcription factor hepatic leukaemia factor (*HLF*). Patients with ALL and this gene fusion frequently present with hypercalcaemia and coagulopathy, and have poor prognosis.

The t(1;19) abnormality was associated with an unfavourable outcome in earlier trials. With contemporary treatment protocols, however, patients with this leukaemia subtype have excellent response to initial therapy, and a favourable overall outcome although they still have increased risk of leukaemia relapse in the CNS.

ALL with *MLL* gene rearrangements

Structural alterations involving band 11q23 of chromosome 11 are the most frequent cytogenetic abnormality in infant ALL. In most cases, the target is the *MLL* gene (for mixed-lineage leukaemia; also known as *HRX*, *ALL-1* and *TRX1*). The most common 11q23 abnormality in ALL is t(4;11)(q21;q23), which produces a chimeric protein that contains the N-terminal portion of MLL linked to the C-terminal portion of *AFF1*, but *MLL* has been reported to be linked to more than 50 other genes. The *MLL* gene encodes a DNA-binding protein that regulates the expression of many genes including multiple *HOX* genes. *MLL* is crucial for embryonic development and haemopoiesis, and MLL fusion proteins can transform haemopoietic cells into leukaemia-initiating cells.

Treatment outcome of ALL with an *MLL* gene rearrangement differs by age group, with infants having the worst outcome. Infant ALL with the *MLL–AFF1* gene fusion also has a high prevalence of immature, non-productive and/or oligoclonal antigen-receptor gene rearrangements. Several genes normally expressed in non-lymphoid haemopoietic lineages are overexpressed in *MLL*-rearranged ALL, including *FLT3*, *LMO2*, and *HOX* genes such as *HOXA9*, *HOXA5*, *HOXA4* and *HOXC6*.

ALL with *BCR–ABL1* rearrangements

The t(9;22)(q34;q11) translocation encodes a chimeric gene consisting of the 5′ portion of *BCR* fused to the 3′ portion of *ABL1*, whereby N-terminal sequences of *ABL1* are replaced by *BCR* sequences. In ALL, breaks tend to occur in the minor breakpoint cluster regions, forming a 190-kDa BCR–ABL. This alteration results in a constitutively active ABL tyrosine kinase that induces aberrant signalling and activates multiple cellular pathways. Expression of the BCR–ABL1 chimeric protein results in malignant transformation of haemopoietic cells and causes leukaemia in murine experimental systems. In mice, aggressiveness of *BCR–ABL1* leukaemias is enhanced if the activity of the Arf tumour suppressor is compromised. Genome-wide analysis of *BCR–ABL1* ALL samples revealed deletions of *IKZF1* in 84% of cases whereas deletions were not found in chronic-phase CML samples. Moreover, deletion of *IKZF1* appeared to be a lesion acquired at the time of transformation from CML to lymphoid blast crisis.

BCR–ABL1 ALL has poor prognosis with standard chemotherapy. The development of the tyrosine kinase inhibitor imatinib mesylate has provided a way to disable the molecular mechanisms that drive leukaemic cell growth, and patients with *BCR–ABL1* ALL show dramatic responses. In a recent report, combination chemotherapy together with imatinib yielded an excellent 3-year event-free survival (EFS) exceeding 80% in childhood cases. The development of resistance due to the outgrowth of clones with mutations in the *BCR–ABL1* kinase domain led to the development of newer and more potent inhibitors, such as nilotinib and dasatinib.

Genetic abnormalities in T-cell ALL

Genes that are dysregulated in T-cell ALL include *SCL* (*TAL-1*), *LMO1* (*TTG-1*), *LMO2* (*TTG-2*) and *HOX11*. In a small fraction of cases, *SCL* (a gene involved in early haemopoiesis located on chromosome 1) is inserted into the TCR-δ locus on chromosome 14. Much more frequent (approximately 25% of cases) is the internal deletion in the 5′ untranslated region of *SCL*, which juxtaposes a locus called *SIL* with the *SCL* coding region, resulting in the expression of a fused *SIL–SCL* transcript that encodes a normal SCL protein. *LMO1* is inserted into the TCR-α/δ locus in t(11;14)(p15;q11), while *LMO2* is inserted into this locus in t(11;14)(p13;q11). Activation of *LMO2* by retroviral insertion in its proximity has been implicated in the development of T-cell leukaemia in patients with X linked severe combined immunodeficiency treated with gene therapy. An additional alteration found in T-cell ALL is the deletion from chromosome 9p21 of the *CDKN2A* (*INK4A*) and *CDKN2B* (*INK4B*) genes, which encode p16INK4a and p15INK4b, inhibitors of the Cdk4 cyclin D-dependent kinase. This locus, which is deleted in more than 50% of T-lineage cases, also encodes another important regulator of cell cycle and apoptosis, p19ARF.

Levels of *HOX11*, *TAL1* and *LYL1* mRNA expression have been used to recognize distinct subtypes of T-ALL. Overexpression of *LMO1* or *LMO2* was observed in most samples also overexpressing *TAL1*, and high levels of *LMO2*, but not *LMO1*, were found in cases with high *LYL1* expression.

Table 25.2 Biological features of leukaemic lymphoblasts in T-ALL and prognosis.

Parameter	Prognostic impact	Reference
↑*TAL1*, *LYL1* or *HOX11L2*	Unfavourable	Ferrando *et al.* (2000)
↑*HOX11L2*	None	Cavé *et al.* (2004)
↑*HOX11L2*	Unfavourable	Ballerini *et al.* (2008)
↑*HOX11L2*	Unfavourable	van Grotel *et al.* (2008)
NOTCH1 mutations	None	van Grotel *et al.* (2008); Larson Gedman *et al.* (2009)
NOTCH1 mutations	Favourable	Breit *et al.* (2006); Park *et al.* (2009)
ETP signature	Very unfavourable	Coustan-Smith *et al.* (2009)

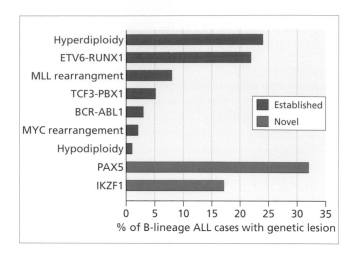

Figure 25.1 Prevalence of genetic abnormalities in newly diagnosed childhood B-lineage ALL. The prevalence of established abnormalities (discovered by conventional karyotyping and fluorescence *in situ* hybridization) and novel abnormalities (discovered by genome-wide analysis with SNP arrays) is shown. Deletions and mutations of *PAX5* and *IKZF1* may occur in cases with established genetic abnormalities. Hyperdiploidy, >50 chromosomes; hypodiploidy, <45 chromosomes.

High expression of *HOX11L2*, a transcriptional regulator closely related to *HOX11*, is frequent and has been associated with poor outcome in some studies (Table 25.2). Activating mutations of *NOTCH1* are frequently found in T-ALL and have been implicated in its pathogenesis. Although there has been some discussion on their prognostic significance, most studies showed either a favourable or no prognostic impact (Table 25.2). Among cases of T-ALL, those bearing the gene expression profile of ETP have a dismal outcome.

Novel subtypes of ALL identified by genome-wide gene expression studies

In early studies using microarray methods for measuring gene expression, profiles that distinguished B-lineage ALL from T-lineage ALL were identified. Moreover, among cases of B-lineage ALL, those with hyperdiploidy (>50 chromosomes), *BCR–ABL1*, *TCF3–PBX1*, *ETV6–RUNX1* or *MLL* gene rearrangement could be clearly distinguished. Subsequent studies have confirmed that gene expression profiling can recognize known subtypes of ALL with accuracy, a capability that may improve risk classification in ALL. To this end, a subset of ALL, identified by hierarchical cluster analysis of gene expression data, comprised many cases that clustered with *BCR–ABL1*-positive cases and had unfavourable outcome. The majority of cases with *BCR–ABL1*-like disease also had deletions in genes involved in B-cell development such as *PAX5* and *IKZF1* (Figure 25.1). Another study showed that *IKZF1* deletions and mutations were associated with a *BCR–ABL1*-like gene expression profile and strongly predicted poor response to chemotherapy and relapse. Finally, it was recently shown that the *P2RY8–CRLF2* fusion (resulting from a recurring interstitial deletion of

the pseudoautosomal region 1 of chromosomes X and Y) is present in 53% of ALL occurring in patients with Down syndrome.

Prognostic factors

Presenting features

Presenting clinico-biological features are commonly used to define subtypes of ALL with different risk or relapse. Presenting age and leucocyte count have prognostic strength in B-lineage but not T-lineage ALL. However, as many as 20% of patients with B-lineage ALL who are considered at lower risk of relapse by these criteria (e.g. age 1–9 years with leucocyte count $<50 \times 10^9$/L) may relapse. Moreover, cases with a very high risk of relapse cannot be reliably distinguished by these criteria. For unclear reasons, boys have worse outcome than girls in many treatment protocols. In some studies, patients of African-American and Hispanic origin had a significantly worse outcome but this was not the case in our single-institution protocols, a finding that might be attributed to equal access to effective contemporary treatment to all patients.

As discussed earlier, primary genetic abnormalities of leukaemic cells are excellent predictors of outcome but correlations are not perfect. For example, as many as 15% of children with favourable genetic features (*ETV6–RUNX1* fusion and hyperdiploidy >50 chromosomes) will eventually relapse, while approximately one-third of those with unfavourable genetic abnormalities (*BCR–ABL1* or *MLL–AF4*) can be cured with chemotherapy alone. It was shown that among patients with *BCR–ABL1*-positive ALL, age over 10 years or a high leucocyte count was associated with a poor outcome; in those with *MLL–AF4*-positive ALL, infant age group (<12 months) conferred a particularly poor outcome. Patients with ETP ALL have a dismal outcome with contemporary therapy irrespective of other presenting features.

Minimal residual disease

A slow reduction of the leukaemic cell burden by remission induction therapy is associated with a poor treatment outcome. Response to therapy, as assessed by morphological examination of bone marrow and peripheral blood smears, has limited sensitivity and accuracy. The advent of methods for detecting minimal residual disease (MRD), which are at least 100 times more sensitive than conventional morphological techniques, has introduced a profoundly new way to monitor response to treatment. The most reliable methods for measuring MRD include flow cytometric profiling of aberrant immunophenotypes, PCR amplification of fusion transcripts and chromosomal breakpoints, and PCR amplification of antigen-receptor genes.

The prognostic importance of MRD in childhood ALL has been unequivocally established by the results of numerous correlative studies. In our studies, patients who had MRD of 0.01% or more in bone marrow during or at the end of remission induction therapy had a significantly higher risk of relapse, while those with MRD of 1% or more at the end of remission induction therapy and those with MRD of 0.1% or more during continuation therapy had an extremely high relapse hazard. In contrast, patients with undetectable MRD on day 19 had a particularly favourable outcome. Investigators of the International Berlin–Frankfurt–Münster (I-BFM) Study Group found that the combined information about MRD on days 33 and 78 could identify three groups of patients with a significantly different outcome: 10-year EFS was 93% for patients who were MRD negative at both time points, 16% for patients with MRD of 0.1% or more at both time points, and 74% for the remaning patients. Investigators of the Dana–Farber Cancer Institute ALL Consortium reported a 5-year risk of relapse of 5% for patients with no detectable (<0.01%) MRD at end of remission induction and 44% for those with detectable MRD. An MRD cut-off level of 0.1% was the best predictor of 5-year relapse hazard in this series: 72% for patients with higher levels of MRD and 12% for those with lower levels. Investigators of the Children's Oncology Group reported that the presence of MRD (0.01% or higher) at the end of remission induction (day

29) was the strongest prognostic indicator, superior to other commonly used prognostic parameters in childhood ALL, and predicted both early and late relapses. Examples of risk classification schema that combine presenting features and MRD assessments are shown in Table 25.3. The prognostic value of MRD in childhood ALL also extends to specific subsets of patients with presenting features traditionally used for risk assignment, and to infants.

Pharmacogenetic variables

Mutations and polymorphisms of genes encoding several drug-metabolizing enzymes have been associated with reponse to therapy. The best-established association regards the thiopurine *S*-methyltransferase gene, which encodes the enzyme that catalyses the inactivation of mercaptopurine. Approximately 1 in 300 patients have an inherited homozygous deficiency of thiopurine *S*-methyltransferase and are therefore extremely sensitive to mercaptopurine. Patients who are heterozygous for this mutation (approximately 10%) have intermediate levels of enzyme activity. Both homozygous and heterozygous deficiencies are associated with a better EFS, likely due to higher dose intensity of mercaptopurine, but they also carry the increased risk of acute toxicities and a higher rate of irradiation-induced brain tumours and therapy-related acute myeloid leukaemia. Hence, mercaptopurine dosages must be carefully adjusted in these patients, an approach that abrogated the clinical impact of these mutations.

The null genotype for the glutathione S-transferase genes *GSTM1* or *GSTT1* and for *GSTP1* V105/V105 is also associated with increased treatment-related toxicity and a lower risk of relapse, perhaps because of reduced detoxification of cytotoxic chemotherapy. In one study, 16 polymorphisms in genes involved in drug metabolism, including *GSTM1* and *TYMS* (thymidylate synthetase), were associated with treatment outcome, while polymorphisms in genes involved in folate metabolism, including those for methylenetetrahydrofolate reductase (*MTHFR*) and methionine synthase reductase (*MTRR*), affected methotrexate sensitivity *in vitro*. A study comparing the polymorphisms of 16 genes with functions related to treatment response to MRD levels on day 8 in blood and on day 28 in bone marrow found that the G allele of a common polymorphism in the gene for the chemokine receptor 5 (*CCR5*) was associated with better MRD clearance than the A allele; the molecular mechanisms underlying this association are unclear. Another study identified 102 SNPs associated with MRD, including 21 in genes associated with antileukaemic drug disposition and five in the *IL15* gene. The mechanisms linking alterations in IL-15 and poor response to chemotherapy are also unclear but recall findings that IL-15 overexpression is associated with increased CNS involvement at diagnosis and CNS relapse in childhood ALL. Significantly higher concentrations

Table 25.3 Current risk classifications of childhood ALL.

Risk group	Features
St Jude Children's Research Hospital	
Low	B-cell precursor immunophenotype and age 1–9 years with leucocyte count <50 × 10^9/L, DNA index ≥1.16 and <1.60, or *ETV6–RUNX*; without CNS (CNS1)* or testicular leukaemia, or t(1;19), t(4;11), t(9;22), *MLL* rearrangement or hypodiploidy <44 chromosomes; MRD <1% at day 15 or remission induction and <0.01% at the end of 6-week remission induction
Standard	T-cell phenotype (except ETP ALL) and B-cell precursor cases not classified as low or high risk
High	ETP ALL phenotype, induction failure, or MRD ≥1% at the end of 6-week remission induction
Children's Oncology Group (B-lineage cases)	
Standard risk – low	1–9 years with leucocyte count <50 × 10^9/L, trisomy 4, 10 or 17 or *ETV6–RUNX1*, no CNS leukaemia (CNS1), or *BCR–ABL1* or *MLL* rearrangement or hypodiploidy; rapid early response (day 15), MRD <0.1% on day 29
Standard risk – average	1–9 years with leucocyte count <50 × 10^9/L, CNS1 or 2, no *BCR–ABL1* or *MLL* rearrangement or hypodiploidy, rapid early response, MRD <0.1% on day 29
Standard risk – high	1–9 years with leucocyte count <50 × 10^9/L; no *BCR–ABL1* or hypodiploidy; slow early response or MRD ≥0.1% on day 29 or *MLL* rearrangement and rapid early response
High	≥10 years or leucocyte count ≥50 × 10^9/L or 1–9 years with leucocyte count <50 × 10^9/L with testicular leukaemia; no *BCR–ABL1* or hypodiploidy
Very high risk	t(9;22)/*BCR–ABL1* or hypodiploidy or *MLL* rearrangement with slow early response or induction failure or MRD ≥1%
Berlin–Frankfurt–Münster Consortium	
Standard	Prednisone good response; no t(9;22)/*BCR–ABL1* or t(4;11)/*MLL–AF4*; MRD negative on days 33 and 78
Medium	Prednisone good response; morphological remission on day 33; no t(9;22)/*BCR–ABL1* or t(4;11)/*MLL–AFF1*; do not fulfill other standard- or high-risk criteria
High	Prednisone poor response; M2 or M3 marrow on day 33; presence of t(9;22)/*BCR–ABL1* or t(4;11)/*MLL–AFF1*; MRD ≥0.1% on day 78

*CNS1, absence of leukaemic blasts in cytocentrifuge preparations of cerebrospinal fluid; CNS2, presence of blasts but leucocytes <5/μL; CNS3, presence of leukaemic cells in a cerebrospinal fluid that contains ≥5 leucocytes/μL.

of methylmercaptopurine nucleotides were found in patients with a non-functional allele of the gene for inosine triphosphate pyrophosphatase, which were associated with a higher probability of severe febrile neutropenia.

Treatment

Overview

The more successful contemporary clinical trials for children with newly diagnosed ALL have resulted in 5-year EFS rates ranging from 75 to 87% (Table 25.4). The general treatment approach relies on three main phases: remission induction, intensification (consolidation) therapy, and continuation treatment. In patients with mature B-cell ALL, regimens of intensive chemotherapy are typically shorter and based primarily on cyclophosphamide, methotrexate and cytarabine, resulting in cure rates of 74–87%. All patients require treatment for sub-clinical leukaemia of the CNS, which should be initiated early in the form of intrathecal therapy.

Remission induction

Rates of complete remission (i.e. absence of leukaemic cells detectable morphologically and restoration of normal haemopoiesis) currently range from 96 to 99%. Remission induction regimens typically include a glucocorticoid (prednisone, prednisolone or dexamethasone), vincristine and asparaginase, with or without one or more additional drugs (e.g. an anthracycline, cyclophosphamide). Intensification of induction therapy may achieve a more effective clearance of leukaemic cells but it might not be necessary for patients lacking unfavourable prognostic features and having a good early response, particularly if they receive post-induction intensification therapy. Intensified induction therapy may increase early morbidity and mortality.

Table 25.4 Results of selected clinical trials in patients with acute lymphoblastic leukaemia.

Study	Years	No. of patients	Age (years)	Percentage 5-year EFS (± SE)	Reference
BFM 95	1995–2000	2169	0–18	78.6 ± 0.9*	Moricke *et al.* (2008)
CCG-1961	1996–2002	2078	0–21	71.3 ± 1.6[†]	Seibel *et al.* (2008)
COALL-97	1997–2003	667	1–18	77 ± 2	Escherich *et al.* (2010)
DFCI-95-01	1996–2000	491	0–18	82 ± 2	Moghrabi *et al.* (2007)
NOPHO ALL-2000	2000–2007	1023	0–15	79.4 ± 1.5	Schmiegelow *et al.* (2010)
SJCRH XV	2000–2007	498	1–18	85.6 ± 2.9	Pui *et al.* (2009)

*6-year event free-survival is reported.
[†]Standard deviation instead of SE is reported.
BFM, Berlin–Frankfurt–Münster; CCG, Children's Cancer Group; COALL, Cooperative Study Group of Childhood Acute Lymphoblastic Leukaemia; DFCI, Dana-Farber Cancer Institute; NOPHO, Nordic Society of Paediatric Haematology and Oncology; SJCRH, St Jude Children's Research Hospital.

Because of its reported longer half-life and increased penetration into CSF, dexamethasone may be more effective than prednisone or prednisolone. Its use yielded an improved outcome in some trials but resulted in excessive life-threatening infections and septic deaths in another study. A small randomized study showed that an increased dose of prednisone produced results comparable to those achieved with dexamethasone in the context of other intensive treatment, suggesting dose rather than type of glucocorticoid influences treatment outcome.

Most remission induction regimens include asparaginase. However, clinical trials limiting that use of asparaginase to the post-induction period yielded low morbidity (especially in terms of thrombotic complications) and excellent overall outcome. The currently available asparaginase for newly diagnosed patients is derived from *Escherichia coli* and there is a polyethylene glycol-bound form of the *E. coli* product (pegaspargase); asparaginase derived from *Erwinia chrysanthemi* is typically used in patients who have hypersensitivity reactions to *E. coli* product. Each type has a different half-life, pharmacokinetics and immunogenicity. In terms of antileukaemic activity, the key issue is the amount of asparagine depletion achieved. Because of lower immunogenicity and less frequent administration, pegaspargase has become the first-line treatment in the USA and is also increasingly used in other childhood ALL trials worldwide. Patients with allergic reactions to either *E. coli* preparation should be treated with *Erwinia* asparaginase.

Intensification (consolidation)

Patients who achieve remission typically receive intensification (also called consolidation) therapy. This consists of the same drug schema used in the remission induction regimen or of a combination of drugs not previously used. Patients with different subtypes of leukaemia may respond particularly well to certain intensification regimens. For example, patients with *ETV6–RUNX1* had an especially good outcome in clinical trials featuring intensive post-remission treatment with glucocorticoids, vincristine and asparaginase, while a very high dose of methotrexate ($5\,g/m^2$) improved treatment outcome of patients with T cell ALL. Other regimens have not proven to be advantageous, such as high-dose intravenous mercaptopurine and high-dose cytarabine.

Delayed intensification (or reinduction), first introduced by investigators of the I-BFM Study Group, is a widely used approach consisting of a repetition of the first remission induction therapy 3 months after the end of remission induction. Investigators at the Children's Cancer Group and of the Associazione Italiana Ematologia ed Oncologia Pediatrica (AIEOP) group reported that double delayed intensification improved patient outcome in patients with intermediate risk. Extended and stronger intensification therapy also significantly benefited patients with high-risk ALL and slow response to initial induction therapy. While reinduction or delayed intensification therapy is probably beneficial to all patients, double or prolonged intensification appears to be beneficial primarily to those with features predicting a higher risk of relapse.

Continuation therapy

With the exception of patients with B-cell (surface immunoglobulin positive) ALL, all children with ALL require prolonged continuation treatment, which typically lasts for 2–2.5 years. Attempts to shorten its duration have led to inferior outcomes, although it should be noted that up to two-thirds of patients could be cured with only 12 months of treatment in one trial. Continuous uninterrupted therapy appears to be more effective than high-dose pulse therapy with prolonged rest periods to recover from myelosuppression.

The classical components of continuation therapy are methotrexate and mercaptopurine, administered weekly and daily, respectively. Low systemic exposure to methotrexate and low dose intensity of mercaptopurine have been associated with an inferior outcome. Conversely, administration of doses gauged to produce the lowest tolerable neutrophil counts reportedly improved outcomes. However, following such an approach too strictly may be counterproductive, resulting in dose interruption and reduction of the overall dose intensity. Parenteral administration of methotrexate circumvents problems of decreased bioavailability and poor compliance associated with oral administration, especially in adolescents. In contrast, mercaptopurine is most effective when it is given orally daily; weekly intravenous administration at a higher dose was shown to be ineffective. In some studies, thioguanine appeared to have a superior antileukaemic effect than mercaptopurine but its use at a daily dose above $40\,mg/m^2$ was associated with a higher rate of toxicities, such as profound thrombocytopenia and hepatic veno-occlusive disease. Intensive treatment with mercaptopurine and methotrexate maintenance therapy has been related to the occurrence of second malignancies, especially in patients with thiopurine methyltransferase deficiency.

Studies have shown that adding intermittent pulses of vincristine and a glucocorticoid (prednisone or dexamethasone) to the methotrexate/mercaptopurine combination is beneficial. Whether this pulse therapy is necessary in contemporary regimens featuring early intensification of therapy remains to be determined.

Prevention and therapy of CNS leukaemia

The infiltration of the leptomeninges by leukaemic cells poses a challenge because the blood–brain barrier provides a pharmacological sanctuary for leukaemic cells and protects them from systemic therapy. Hence, cranial irradiation (12–24 Gy) and methotrexate administered intrathecally after induction of complete remission as a prophylactic measure to prevent CNS leukaemia has become a key feature of childhood ALL treatment since the 1970s. Cranial irradiation can cause serious side-effects and a reduction of the radiation dose to a less harmful 12 Gy appeared to provide adequate protection against CNS relapse. Complete omission of cranial irradiation as tested in early clinical trials also resulted in an acceptable rate of CNS relapse but produced low overall survival rates. A recent study at St Jude Children's Research Hospital tested the feasibility of total omission of prophylactic cranial irradiation. The 5-year survival rate for the 498 patients enrolled was 93.5% and the cumulative risk of an isolated CNS relapse rate was only 2.7%, demonstrating that cranial irradiation can be avoided in the context of effective risk-adapted intrathecal and systemic chemotherapy. Intensive systemic and intrathecal treatment, without cranial irradiation, appears to provide adequate CNS prophylaxis even in infants who have CNS leukaemia at diagnosis. Therefore, most investigators now treat infants (a group of patients particularly vulnerable to CNS irradiation toxicities) without cranial irradiation. Importantly, patients with an isolated CNS relapse have a very high retrieval rate if they did not receive cranial irradiation as CNS prophylaxis.

Systemic treatment including high-dose methotrexate, intensive asparaginase, and dexamethasone as well as optimal intrathecal therapy are essential to control CNS leukaemia. Triple intrathecal therapy with methotrexate, cytarabine and hydrocortisone is more effective than intrathecal methotrexate alone in preventing CNS relapse. Intrathecal therapy should be intensified in patients with detectable ALL blasts in the CSF (even because of traumatic lumbar puncture) as this finding carries an increased risk of CNS relapse and inferior overall outcome.

Allogeneic haemopoietic stem cell transplantation

Patients with the BCR–ABL1 gene fusion, ETP ALL, poor early response or early haematological relapse are the more frequent candidates for transplantation. Nevertheless, the indications for transplantation should be continuously reviewed as treatment improves and new agents become available. For example, the use of imatinib and other tyrosine kinase inhibitors has dramatically improved early treatment response in patients with BCR–ABL1-positive ALL, questioning whether transplantation in first remission should be recommended in these cases. Transplantation has not been shown to improve outcome of other subtypes of very high risk leukaemia, including infant cases and those with MLL rearrangement.

Levels of MRD prior to transplant predict the risk of relapse after transplant. In patients receiving T-cell-depleted grafts, high levels of MRD PCR positivity (0.1–1%) before transplant were consistently associated with relapse after transplant, and patients with lower levels of MRD had a 2-year EFS of 35–50% compared with 70% for MRD-negative patients.

Treatment sequelae

Improvements in supportive care have reduced the early death rate to less than 2%. Remission induction therapy including prednisone, vincristine and asparaginase causes hyperglycaemia in 10–20% of patients, particularly adolescents and patients with obesity, a family history of diabetes mellitus or Down syndrome. The same induction regimen can also lead to a hypercoagulable state in 3–5% of patients, promoting cerebral and/or peripheral vein thromboses. The intensified use of methotrexate and glucocorticoids has been associated with an increased frequency of neurotoxicity and osteonecrosis. High cumulative doses of anthracyclines can produce severe cardiomyopathy, especially in young children. Cranial irradiation may cause second neoplasms within the irradiated field, as well as neuropsychological deficits and endocrine abnormalities, leading to obesity, short stature, precocious puberty and osteoporosis.

Relapse

Leukaemia relapse may occur during or after treatment, usually within 2 years after cessation of therapy but occasionally later (relapses occurring as late as 10 years after diagnosis have been reported). The bone marrow remains the most common site of relapse, while the frequency of relapse in extramedullary sites, such as the CNS and testes, has steadily decreased. Even when extramedullary relapse appears to be an isolated event, it is often associated with submicroscopic residual disease in the bone marrow.

There have been reports of leukaemias morphologically and immunophenotypically characterized as ALL that relapse as acute myeloid leukaemia while retaining the karyotypic and molecular features of the original clone. More insights on the genetic evolution of ALL at relapse were revealed by a recent study where genome-wide DNA copy number analyses were performed on matched diagnosis and relapse samples from 61 children with ALL, indicating that most relapse samples lacked some of the genetic abnormalities present at diagnosis. Backtracking studies revealed that cells corresponding to the relapse clone were often present as minor subpopulations at diagnosis.

Bone marrow relapse, with or without extramedullary involvement, is associated with a poor outcome. Paradoxically, patients with isolated bone marrow relapse generally do worse than those with combined bone marrow and extramedullary relapse. In children with relapsed ALL, adverse risk factors include short initial remission, T-cell immunophenotype, BCR–ABL1 ALL, presence of circulating blast cells or a high leucocyte count at relapse. The presence of MRD at the end of second remission induction is a strong adverse prognostic indicator. Chemotherapy may be sufficient to induce prolonged second remissions in patients without high-risk features but allogeneic haemopoietic stem cell transplantation is a reasonable treatment option for the remaining patients, particularly those who experience haematological relapse during therapy or shortly thereafter, those with T-cell ALL, and those with persistent MRD. The Acute Lymphoblastic Leukaemia Relapse Berlin–Frankfurt–Münster Study Group recently reported the results of a prospective trial including 91 children with relapsed ALL receiving stem cell transplantation. The probability of EFS after transplantation was significantly associated with MRD burden before transplantation, and MRD was the only independent predictive parameter.

Concluding remarks

The current cure rates for children with ALL demonstrate the remarkable progress that has been made in treating this disease through improvements in risk classification, chemotherapy, transplantation and supportive care. Classification of ALL into prognostically meaningful subtypes defined by clinical presenting features and genetic abnormalities of the leukaemic cells is well established. The uncovering of new genetic lesions in leukaemic lymphoblasts using novel screening techniques and the definition of their prognostic significance should further improve risk classification. Genome-wide expression profiling studies may also facilitate the discovery of molecules that critically influence drug resistance. This is shown by studies that established the association of gene expression in leukaemic lymphoblasts with response to treatment in vitro.

The development of robust MRD assays and the understanding of the clinical significance of MRD have opened a new approach to monitoring the response to treatment and have introduced a new concept of 'remission'. MRD assays have been incorporated into many major treatment protocols and are now an integral part of the modern management of childhood ALL. Simplification of MRD methods should widen the application of this powerful prognostic parameter, and extend its potential benefits to most patients, including those living in areas with limited resources. Further progress in optimizing intensity of treatment for each patient is coming from a better understanding of the relation between pharmacogenomic features and responses to chemotherapy, which should lead to significant refinements of treatment schedules and dosages.

Despite these remarkable improvements, standard chemotherapy still produces low cure rates for patients with some subtypes of ALL, such as infants with MLL rearrrangement and those with ETP ALL; for these patients, substantial improvements can only come from the development of new treatment modalities. Imatinib mesylate and other ABL kinase inhibitors are the paradigm of molecular therapy of leukaemia. Other novel agents include inhibitors of FLT3, farnesyltransferase, proteasome, DNA methylation and histone deacetylase. Moreover, there are new formulations of existing agents that may improve efficacy and decrease toxicity. To this end, nucleoside analogues of more recent generation, such as gemcitabine, clofarabine and nelarabine, have shown promise. The application of gene expression-based drug screening might facilitate the identification of new effective compounds, while the detailed understanding of the cooperating genetic abnormalities associated with ALL could identify new targets.

Immunotherapeutic options are progressively emerging. Rituximab (anti-CD20), gemtuzumab ozogamicin (anti-CD33), alemtuzumab (anti CD52) and epratuzumab (anti-CD22) have already been incorporated into some clinical trials;

recombinant immunotoxins and bispecific antibody derivatives have also been developed and are being tested. In the context of haemopoietic stem cell transplantation, donors can be selected so that their natural killer (NK) cells can exert maximum cytotoxicity against the leukaemic cells of the host, and infusions of haploidentical NK cells are being evaluated. Chimeric receptors, composed of single-chain variable domain of murine antibodies and human signalling molecules, can redirect the specificity of autologous or allogeneic immune cells against ALL cells and may therefore enhance the effectiveness of T and NK cell infusions.

For many decades, oncologists have been familiar with the concept that pharmacological sanctuaries (e.g. the CNS) contribute to protect leukaemic cells from chemotherapy. More recent evidence indicates that the bone marrow microenvironment can also anatagonize the effects of chemotherapy. For instance, we found that bone marrow mesenchymal cells protect ALL cells from asparaginase cytotoxicity by forming an asparagine-rich microenvironment, suggesting a scenario whereby ALL cells that reside in mesenchymal cell niches become relatively resistant to chemotherapy. Because agents that interfere with the interaction between ALL and mesenchymal cells are available for clinical use, it should be possible to design protocols that attempt to improve chemotherapy effectiveness by mobilizing ALL cells.

Acknowledgements

Supported by the National Institutes of Health grants P30 A21765, RO1 CA60419, RO1 CA115422, and RO1 CA113482, and by the American Lebanese Syrian Associated Charities (ALSAC).

Selected bibliography

Bader P, Kreyenberg H, Henze GH et al. (2009) Prognostic value of minimal residual disease quantification before allogeneic stem-cell transplantation in relapsed childhood acute lymphoblastic leukemia: the ALL-REZ BFM Study Group. *Journal of Clinical Oncology* **27**: 377–84.

Ballerini P, Landman-Parker J, Cayuela JM et al. (2008) Impact of genotype on survival of children with T-cell acute lymphoblastic leukemia treated according to the French protocol FRALLE-93: the effect of TLX3/HOX11L2 gene expression on outcome. *Haematologica* **93**: 1658–65.

Bercovich D, Ganmore I, Scott LM et al. (2008) Mutations of JAK2 in acute lymphoblastic leukaemias associated with Down's syndrome. *Lancet* **372**: 1484–92.

Borowitz MJ, Devidas M, Hunger SP et al. (2008) Clinical significance of minimal residual disease in childhood acute lymphoblastic leukemia and its relationship to other prognostic factors. a Children's Oncology Group study. *Blood* **111**: 5477–85.

Breit S, Stanulla M, Flohr T et al. (2006) Activating NOTCH1 mutations predict favorable early treatment response and long-term outcome in childhood precursor T-cell lymphoblastic leukemia. *Blood* **108**: 1151–7.

Campana D (2008) Status of minimal residual disease testing in childhood haematological malignancies. *British Journal of Haematology* **143**: 481–9.

Campana D (2008) Molecular determinants of treatment response in acute lymphoblastic leukemia. *Hematology. American Society of Hematology Education Program* 366–73.

Cavé H, van der Werff ten Bosch J, Suciu S et al. (1998) Clinical significance of minimal residual disease in childhood acute lymphoblastic leukemia. European Organization for Research and Treatment of Cancer Childhood Leukemia Cooperative Group. *New England Journal of Medicine* **339**: 591–8.

Cavé H, Suciu S, Preudhomme C et al. (2004) Clinical significance of HOX11L2 expression linked to t(5;14)(q35;q32), of HOX11 expression, and of SIL–TAL fusion in childhood T-cell malignancies: results of EORTC studies 58881 and 58951. *Blood* **103**: 442–50.

Coustan-Smith E, Behm FG, Sanchez J et al. (1998) Immunological detection of minimal residual disease in children with acute lymphoblastic leukaemia. *Lancet* **351**: 550–4.

Coustan-Smith E, Mullighan CG, Onciu M et al. (2009) Early T-cell precursor leukaemia: a subtype of very high-risk acute lymphoblastic leukaemia. *Lancet Oncology* **10**: 147–56.

Davies SM, Borowitz MJ, Rosner GL et al. (2008) Pharmacogenetics of minimal residual disease response in children with B-precursor acute lymphoblastic leukaemia: a report from the Children's Oncology Group. *Blood* **111**: 2984–90.

den Boer ML, van Slegtenhorst M, de Menezes RX et al. (2009) A subtype of childhood acute lymphoblastic leukaemia with poor treatment outcome: a genome-wide classification study. *Lancet Oncology* **10**: 125–34.

Escherich G, Horstmann MA, Zimmermann M, Janka-Schaub GE (2010) Cooperative study group for childhood acute lymphoblastic leukaemia (COALL): long-term results of trials 82, 85, 89, 92 and 97. *Leukemia* **24**: 298–308.

Evans WE, Relling MV (2004) Moving towards individualized medicine with pharmacogenomics. *Nature* **429**: 464–8.

Ferrando AA, Neuberg DS, Staunton J et al. (2002) Gene expression signatures define novel oncogenic pathways in T cell acute lymphoblastic leukaemia. *Cancer Cell* **1**: 75–87.

Flohr T, Schrauder A, Cazzaniga G et al. (2008) Minimal residual disease-directed risk stratification using real-time quantitative PCR analysis of immunoglobulin and T-cell receptor gene rearrangements in the international multicenter trial AIEOP-BFM ALL 2000 for childhood acute lymphoblastic leukaemia. *Leukemia* **22**: 771–82.

Flotho C, Coustan-Smith E, Pei D et al. (2007) A set of genes that regulate cell proliferation predicts treatment outcome in childhood acute lymphoblastic leukemia. *Blood* **110**: 1271–7.

Ford AM, Palmi C, Bueno C et al. (2009) The TEL–AML1 leukemia fusion gene dysregulates the TGF-beta pathway in early B lineage progenitor cells. *Journal of Clinical Investigation* **119**: 826–36.

Greaves M (2006) Infection, immune responses and the aetiology of childhood leukaemia. *Nature Reviews. Cancer* **6**: 193–203.

Hagedorn N, Acquaviva C, Fronkova E *et al.* (2007) Submicroscopic bone marrow involvement in isolated extramedullary relapses in childhood acute lymphoblastic leukemia: a more precise definition of 'isolated' and its possible clinical implications. A collaborative study of the Resistant Disease Committee of the International BFM study group. *Blood* 110: 4022–9.

Hijiya N, Hudson MM, Lensing S *et al.* (2007) Cumulative incidence of secondary neoplasms as a first event after childhood acute lymphoblastic leukemia. *Journal of the American Medical Association* 297: 1207–15.

Holleman A, Cheok MH, den Boer ML *et al.* (2004) Gene-expression patterns in drug-resistant acute lymphoblastic leukemia cells and response to treatment. *New England Journal of Medicine* 351: 533–42.

Hong D, Gupta R, Ancliff P *et al.* (2008) Initiating and cancer-propagating cells in TEL–AML1-associated childhood leukemia. *Science* 319: 336–9.

Imai C, Iwamoto S, Campana D (2005) Genetic modification of primary natural killer cells overcomes inhibitory signals and induces specific killing of leukemic cells. *Blood* 106: 376–83.

Iwamoto S, Mihara K, Downing JR, Pui CH, Campana D (2007) Mesenchymal cells regulate the response of acute lymphoblastic leukemia cells to L-asparaginase. *Journal of Clinical Investigation* 117: 1049–57.

Krivtsov AV, Armstrong SA (2007) MLL translocations, histone modifications and leukaemia stem-cell development. *Nature Reviews. Cancer* 7: 823–33.

Larson Gedman A, Chen Q, Kugel Desmoulin S *et al.* (2009) The impact of NOTCH1, FBW7 and PTEN mutations on prognosis and downstream signaling in pediatric T-cell acute lymphoblastic leukemia: a report from the Children's Oncology Group. *Leukemia* 23: 1417–25.

Moghrabi A, Levy DE, Asselin B *et al.* (2007) Results of the Dana-Farber Cancer Institute ALL Consortium Protocol 95-01 for children with acute lymphoblastic leukemia. *Blood* 109: 896–904.

Moricke A, Reiter A, Zimmermann M *et al.* (2008) Risk-adjusted therapy of acute lymphoblastic leukemia can decrease treatment burden and improve survival: treatment results of 2169 unselected pediatric and adolescent patients enrolled in the trial ALL-BFM 95. *Blood* 111: 4477–89.

Mullighan CG, Goorha S, Radtke I *et al.* (2007) Genome-wide analysis of genetic alterations in acute lymphoblastic leukaemia. *Nature* 446: 758–64.

Mullighan CG, Miller CB, Radtke I *et al.* (2008) BCR–ABL1 lymphoblastic leukaemia is characterized by the deletion of Ikaros. *Nature* 453: 110–14.

Mullighan CG, Phillips LA, Su X *et al.* (2008) Genomic analysis of the clonal origins of relapsed acute lymphoblastic leukemia. *Science* 322: 1377–80.

Mullighan CG, Collins-Underwood JR, Phillips LA *et al.* (2009) Rearrangement of CRLF2 in B-progenitor- and Down syndrome-associated acute lymphoblastic leukemia. *Nature Genetics* 41: 1243–6.

Mullighan CG, Su X, Zhang J *et al.* (2009) Deletion of IKZF1 and prognosis in acute lymphoblastic leukemia. *New England Journal of Medicine* 360: 470–80.

Mullighan CG, Zhang J, Harvey RC *et al.* (2009) JAK mutations in high-risk childhood acute lymphoblastic leukemia. *Proceedings of the National Academy of Sciences USA* 106: 9414–18.

Oudot C, Auclerc MF, Levy V *et al.* (2008) Prognostic factors for leukemic induction failure in children with acute lymphoblastic leukemia and outcome after salvage therapy: the FRALLE 93 study. *Journal of Clinical Oncology* 26: 1496–503.

Park MJ, Taki T, Oda M *et al.* (2009) FBXW7 and NOTCH1 mutations in childhood T cell acute lymphoblastic leukaemia and T cell non-Hodgkin lymphoma. *British Journal of Haematology* 145: 198–206.

Pui CH, Howard SC (2008) Current management and challenges of malignant disease in the CNS in paediatric leukaemia. *Lancet Oncology* 9: 257–68.

Pui CH, Jeha S (2007) New therapeutic strategies for the treatment of acute lymphoblastic leukaemia. *Nature Reviews. Drug Discovery* 6: 149–65.

Pui CH, Cheng C, Leung W *et al.* (2003) Extended follow-up of long-term survivors of childhood acute lymphoblastic leukemia. *New England Journal of Medicine* 349: 640–9.

Pui CH, Robison LL, Look AT (2008) Acute lymphoblastic leukaemia. *Lancet* 371: 1030–43.

Pui CH, Campana D, Pei D *et al.* (2009) Treating childhood acute lymphoblastic leukemia without cranial irradiation. *New England Journal of Medicine* 360: 2730–41.

Raetz EA, Cairo MS, Borowitz MJ *et al.* (2008) Chemoimmunotherapy reinduction with epratuzumab in children with acute lymphoblastic leukemia in marrow relapse: a Children's Oncology Group Pilot Study. *Journal of Clinical Oncology* 26: 3756–62.

Real PJ, Tosello V, Palomero T *et al.* (2009) Gamma-secretase inhibitors reverse glucocorticoid resistance in T cell acute lymphoblastic leukemia. *Nature Medicine* 15: 50–8.

Ribeiro RC, Pui CH (2005) Saving the children: improving childhood cancer treatment in developing countries. *New England Journal of Medicine* 352: 2158–60.

Schmiegelow K, Forestier E, Hellebostad M *et al.* (2010) Long-term results of NOPHO ALL-92 and ALL-2000 studies for childhood acute lymphoblastic leukaemia. *Leukemia* 24: 345–54.

Schrappe M, Reiter A, Zimmermann M *et al.* (2000) Long-term results of four consecutive trials in childhood ALL performed by the ALL-BFM study group from 1981 to 1995. *Leukemia* 14: 2205–22.

Schultz KR, Bowman WP, Aledo A *et al.* (2009) Improved early event-free survival with imatininb in Philadelphia chromosome-positive acute lymphoblastic leukemia: a Children's Oncology Group study. *Journal of Clinical Oncology* 27: 5175–81.

Seibel NL, Steinherz PG, Sather HN *et al.* (2008) Early postinduction intensification therapy improves survival for children and adolescents with high-risk acute lymphoblastic leukemia: a report from the Children's Oncology Group. *Blood* 111: 2548–55.

Sorich MJ, Pottier N, Pei D *et al.* (2008) In vivo response to methotrexate forecasts outcome of acute lymphoblastic leukemia and has a distinct gene expression profile. *PLoS Medicine* 5: e83.

van Dongen JJ, Seriu T, Panzer-Grumayer ER *et al.* (1998) Prognostic value of minimal residual disease in acute lymphoblastic leukaemia in childhood. *Lancet* 352: 1731–8.

van Grotel M, Meijerink JP, van Wering ER *et al.* (2008) Prognostic significance of molecular–cytogenetic abnormalities in pediatric T-ALL is not explained by immunophenotypic differences. *Leukemia* **22**: 124–31.

Yang JJ, Cheng C, Yang W *et al.* (2009) Genome-wide interrogation of germline genetic variation associated with treatment response in childhood acute lymphoblastic leukemia. *Journal of the American Medical Association* **301**: 393–403.

Yeoh EJ, Ross ME, Shurtleff SA *et al.* (2002) Classification, subtype discovery, and prediction of outcome in pediatric acute lymphoblastic leukemia by gene expression profiling. *Cancer Cell* **1**: 133–43.

Zhou J, Goldwasser MA, Li A *et al.* (2007) Quantitative analysis of minimal residual disease predicts relapse in children with B-lineage acute lymphoblastic leukemia in DFCI ALL Consortium Protocol 95-01. *Blood* **110**: 1607–11.

CHAPTER 26

Supportive care in the management of leukaemia

26

Archibald G Prentice[1] and J Peter Donnelly[2]

[1]Royal Free Hospital, London, UK
[2]University Hospital Nijmegen, Nijmegen, The Netherlands

Introduction

The outlook for patients with acute and chronic leukaemias has improved considerably in the past 40 years, mainly because of more effective therapy. Better understanding and management of the complications have also improved survival and quality of life. These complications vary with the pace of the disease (acute or chronic), with specific subtypes of myeloid and lymphoid leukaemias, and with the intensity and duration of therapy.

The effectiveness of support depends on the coordinated work of specialist doctors, nurses, therapists and pharmacists and laboratories, working in facilities dedicated to the care of these patients. In the intensive care of patients with acute leukaemia, it is especially important that there should be clear rules about when and why nurses should ask medical staff to review their observations and equally clear rules about the doctors' responses. Timely and accurate communication between professional groups is essential, and all should be working to agreed written standards. Management of all the complications requires careful and regular recording of basic observations by nurses,

most of whom should be registered and experienced in leukaemia care. This team needs a high skill mix and an overall nurse–patient ratio above 1 to allow internal shift rotation that provides a continuous level of expertise. Whatever the type of leukaemia, patients should be treated according to protocols as part of well-designed controlled clinical trials.

The management of each group of complications is described both in general and with reference to specific types of leukaemia and forms of therapy. Complications requiring supportive care can be classified as follows.

1 Psychological: due to loss of performance and self-determination and protracted treatment-related complications, such as the need for isolation as protection against infection.

2 Reproductive: due to the need to prevent pregnancy in female patients during intensive cytotoxic exposure and to preserve fertility in patients of childbearing age.

3 Anaemia: due to failure of red cell production, bleeding or haemolysis.

4 Bleeding: due to thrombocytopenia and lack of clotting factors, through either failure of production or excessive consumption (disseminated intravascular coagulation).

5 Infections: due to failure of production of adequate numbers of functionally normal neutrophils, and monocytes/macrophages, immune dysregulation and failure of the innate immune response, including the gut mucosal barrier.

Postgraduate Haematology: 6th edition. Edited by A. Victor Hoffbrand, Daniel Catovsky, Edward G.D. Tuddenham, Anthony R. Green
© 2011 Blackwell Publishing Ltd.

6 Metabolic: due to disturbances in fluid and electrolyte and acid–base balance, related to the disease or the treatment or both.

7 Nutritional: when oral intake fails and loss of lean body mass is significant.

8 Nausea and vomiting: due to chemotherapy and other drugs.

9 Pain: due to involvement of specific anatomical sites in the disease or as a result of specific therapies.

10 Palliative supportive care: necessary when cytotoxic therapy fails to induce or maintain lasting complete remission; this does not exclude further cytotoxic therapy as part of other efforts to control distressing symptoms.

Psychological support

Regardless of the subtype of disease and form of therapy, this support starts with an explanation of the diagnosis and treatment by a senior haematologist accompanied by a specialist nurse, both of whom should be active and experienced in this type of care and communication. It is essential to gain the trust of patients and their immediate families or partners from the outset so that they can understand and accept the need for the proposed intensity and duration of treatment and the risks of complications. As well as needing support for their distress on learning the diagnosis, most will also ask for detailed information including prognosis. Any relevant clinical trial can be described, and informed consent can be obtained for enrolment and randomization between different treatment options. A relationship of mutual and complete openness should be established as soon as possible, and questions and discussion encouraged.

Most patients may appear to be psychologically able to deal with these illnesses and all their complications. However, many patients find that loss of control of their normal daily activity is difficult to manage, particularly prolonged stays in hospital, including periods in protective isolation. Nearly all will suffer some loss of self-assurance and self-esteem, particularly if they fall ill at the peak of their responsibilities and abilities in their domestic and working lives. Fear of failure of therapy may be lessened if remission is achieved, but patients' anticipation of the complications of subsequent cycles of therapy may add to their psychological problems.

Having little control over this cumulative experience, patients can develop significant neurotic or psychotic pathology, sometimes well after therapy is finished and as they attempt to resume a normal life. The clinical team must be alert to the development of any signs that such problems are impending and deal with them before patients suffer significant and lasting harm. In dealing with these problems, it is difficult for professional carers to maintain a balanced approach that suits each patient. It is as easy to be too intrusive with those patients who can cope without help as it is to fail to detect psychopathology

in those who cannot. This area of supportive care underlines the need for integrated teamwork.

Regardless of age and subtype, patients with acute leukaemias present with a short history, are often seriously unwell due to acute marrow failure and require immediate admission to a haematology unit for intensive therapy. Their psychological complications are often more intensely expressed and require equally intensive support because their loss of function is so acute and severe. This type of supportive care should be an integral part of any therapy, whether it is given with the intention to achieve complete remission in younger patients or as palliation in the elderly and frail.

Reproductive issues

Before any chemotherapy is given to adolescents and young men, they should be counselled about the possibility of loss of fertility and offered the opportunity to store sperm. If therapy cannot be delayed, sperm should be collected as soon as possible to minimize the risk of damage to sperm already formed and stored and because of the potential infertility induced by any cytotoxic therapy, particularly intensive chemotherapy. Patients who opt to store sperm need expert counselling in all the associated ethical issues before collection, particularly their wish to destroy or preserve the collection should the patient die. They and their partners may wish to conserve the sperm for future fertilization after the patient's death. Loss of fertility due to chemotherapy is much less likely in women, who should avoid falling pregnant while receiving such therapy because of likely damage to the embryo and fetus. Preservation *in vitro* of unfertilized ova is not yet possible and not undertaken routinely.

Impaired sexual function can be a problem in both sexes following intensive chemotherapy. Patients and their partners are often reluctant to discuss these problems with their specialist carers and are more likely to discuss them with nursing colleagues. Expert counselling or psychological care can be effective in restoring potency.

Anaemia and thrombocytopenia

In all types of leukaemias, and with all types of treatment, there is a risk of marrow failure leading to anaemia and thrombocytopenia. The pace at which they develop and their severity vary with the type of leukaemia and therapy, and many of the complications are seen whatever the intensity of therapy. As these causes and effects are most marked in the acute leukaemias, the support needed in that context is described in greater detail. By the time most patients present, their ability to produce red cells and platelets will be severely impaired and they will need regular and frequent transfusions of both. Administration of a wide

Table 26.1 Ten rules for transfusion and coagulation failure in acute leukaemia.

Rule	Reason	Exceptions
1 In younger patients use CMV-negative blood until CMV status known	High transplant-related CMV death risk	No transplant planned
2 Transfuse if Hb <8 g/dL	Symptom control	Cardiac failure
3 Delay if white count >100 × 10⁹/L	Hyperviscosity risks bleeds and clots	None
4 Give platelets priority	Red cells dilute low count	Big bleeds; give both
5 Big volumes need diuretics	Circulatory overload	None but plan K^+ and Na^+ infusions too
6 Keep platelets >10 × 10⁹/L	Prevent bleeding	>20 × 10⁹/L during sepsis
7 Use ABO-identical platelets	Maximize effect	No clinical harm if only non-identical available
8 HLA-restricted platelets if refractory to donations	Loss of effect	May resolve allowing use of non-restricted donations
9 Use pethidine for allergic/febrile reactions	Avoid undetected cumulative steroid immunosuppression	None
10 Use only ABO-compatible plasma-derived products to correct clotting times	Avoid ABO haemolytic reactions	None; therapy determined by specific bleeding problems

range of intravenous therapies, including blood products, may be necessary simultaneously. Long-lasting, tunnelled, multilumen, central venous catheters (CVCs) facilitate rapid intravenous access for such multiple therapies, and also reduce the risk of blood-borne infection by reducing the need for multiple and repeated peripheral venous access. Sterile handling of these lines is therefore essential at all times. It is not necessary to transfuse either whole or fresh blood but there are some simple basic rules that should be followed regarding red cell and platelet transfusion (Table 26.1).

Cytomegalovirus-negative blood products

As transfusion of both red cells and platelets may be required at the outset, it is important to establish immediately whether elective allogeneic stem cell transplantation (SCT) is likely as part of the care plan. If it is, those patients should always be transfused with blood products that are less likely to increase the risk of cytomegalovirus (CMV) transfusion, using leucodepleted or filtered donor blood or blood only from known CMV-negative donors until the patient's own CMV status is known. This applies to all patients under the age of 55 years who have potential sibling donors. CMV infection is a major cause of morbidity and mortality in allogeneic SCT and prevention is more effective than treatment.

Acute anaemia

Onset of anaemia is often rapid in patients with acute leukaemia so they are unable to compensate haemodynamically as in anaemia of slower onset. Because of their acutely reduced red cell mass and hence oxygen-carrying capacity, they are likely to be symptomatic and should be transfused as soon as they have been assessed clinically and the result of their blood count is known. This rule may need to be modified in the presence of symptomatic or treated cardiac disease (see section Planning large-volume transfusions). With chemotherapy, red cell production remains suppressed and the patient remains dependent on repeated transfusions.

Conventional teaching is to try to maintain the haemoglobin level above 10 g/dL. This has been challenged recently and it is possible to lower the threshold of haemoglobin at which red cell transfusion is indicated. There is evidence that patients in other critically ill categories will tolerate much lower levels (as low as 6 g/dL) and that transfusing at higher levels may be harmful. In practice, many leukaemia and transplant units already withhold red cell transfusion until the haemoglobin drops to 8 g/dL depending on other factors such as the degree of compromise of cardiorespiratory function.

Excessive red cell transfusion may lead to alloimmunization, with red cell blood group and white cell HLA antigens potentially creating difficulties for future transfusion and SCT. In the transplant patient (autologous and allogeneic), there is also the risk of iron overload, but this appears unlikely to be a problem with conventional chemotherapy.

Hyperviscosity of high white cell counts

Patients who present with acute leukaemias with very high white blood cell (WBC) counts, particularly over 100 × 10⁹/L, should be given blood only if it is not possible to wait for reduction of the WBC count by either leucapheresis or chemotherapy. These patients are already at risk of thrombotic and haemorrhagic events due to hyperviscosity, and transfusion will increase that risk, even if it is slow. It is probably safe to allow such patients to start their chemotherapy with a haemoglobin level as low as 8 g/dL. Patients with high WBC counts in chronic myeloid leukaemia (CML) may develop hyperviscosity problems, but these are rare in chronic lymphocytic leukaemia (CLL).

Planning large-volume transfusions

When planning a large red cell transfusion, it is essential to estimate in advance the total intravenous fluid load these patients will receive over any following 24-hour period. Most patients with acute leukaemia are elderly and will already have some degree of cardiovascular pathology. Some chemotherapy, such as the anthracyclines commonly used in remission induction of acute myeloblastic leukaemia (AML) and acute lymphoblastic leukaemia (ALL), are also unpredictably cardiotoxic below a total cumulative dose in individual patients. If a large intravenous fluid load is unavoidable and intravascular overload is likely, elective diuretic therapy should be prescribed, usually with small doses (20 mg) of intravenous furosemide (frusemide) at planned intervals throughout a prolonged infusion. The use of diuretics in this way may lead to electrolyte depletion, which requires correction (see section Metabolic support). Careful observation of basic vital signs, more simply daily weights, will indicate whether there is an excessive intravascular fluid load contributing to compromised cardiac and respiratory function.

Platelets take priority

When these patients require both red cell and platelet transfusions, platelets should always be given first. Platelet production is compromised to such a degree that a large red cell transfusion will dilute the platelet count to a potentially dangerous lower level. Platelets for transfusion are provided in single packs known as an adult therapeutic dose, which contains approximately 10^{11} platelets. These are obtained either by apheresis from a single donor or by pooling platelets harvested from the buffy coats of packs of blood from six donors.

Platelets can be given so quickly through a CVC that even with sudden and heavy bleeding it is seldom necessary to give red cells first, and red cells and platelets can be given simultaneously.

Minimum platelet level

There is good evidence to suggest that the previous threshold for the transfusion of platelets (20×10^9/L) was overcautious and a threshold of 10×10^9/L is equally unlikely to lead to significant bleeding. Platelet transfusions may also alloimmunize against red cell and HLA antigens.

In general, platelets are not given until the count falls below the lower limit, but there are exceptions to this rule. It is important to remember that a count just over this lower threshold is often obtained early in the morning and that the count may drop below it within the following 24 hours before a further count is undertaken. Thus the rate of fall in previous counts should prove a useful guide as to when platelet concentrate should be infused. Platelet function and survival may both be compromised in the presence of sepsis and some systemic antibiotics (particularly penicillins in high dose), so the higher threshold of 20×10^9/L should be used in patients with these risk factors. Whenever possible, platelet infusions should not be given temporally close to infusions of amphotericin (see section Infections) because of the evidence that this drug will interfere with platelet function and thus reduce the effectiveness of the donation. This may not be the case with liposomal amphotericin given in conventional doses.

It has been suggested that patients who are stable and not infected may tolerate platelet counts as low as 5×10^9/L, provided the count is unlikely to fall further. This policy requires considerable faith in the accuracy and reproducibility of the laboratory technology for counting platelets.

'Compatible' platelets

Whenever possible, platelet concentrate of a red cell ABO group identical to that of the patient should be transfused. If non-identical platelets are used, there may be loss of platelet function and an inferior increment in the recipient's count. Whether this technical benefit is ever clinically significant has never been proven conclusively, but it seems reasonable to give patients the theoretical best possible donation if they need platelets at all, especially if one applies the policy of only transfusing at the lower count of 10×10^9/L.

Platelet 'increments'

Regular platelet counts are needed to plan platelet transfusions and will also reveal failure to obtain a satisfactory increment in the patient's platelet count following transfusion of an adult therapeutic dose. Such patients are described as 'refractory' to platelet transfusion because of the development of alloantibodies to the HLA antigens borne by platelets, and may manifest bleeding or bruising even before a failure of increment is detected. This refractory state should be confirmed with two platelet counts, one before transfusion and one taken 30 min after transfusion. On confirmation of this problem, the patient's HLA type should be determined immediately if this has not already been performed for the purposes of subsequent transplantation. The National Blood Service will then supply HLA-restricted, if not HLA-identical, platelet donations until such time as a trial of HLA-unrestricted donations can be safely given again. Platelet refractoriness need not be permanent but can recur and is not necessarily heralded by a febrile reaction to transfusion.

Febrile reactions

During the course of treatment, patients will experience many episodes of fever for which there will be many potential explanations. Febrile reactions to blood and blood products are usually easy to identify as they occur during or immediately after the transfusion and should not be confused with the fever of infection (see section Infections). If the reaction occurs during transfusion, transfusion should first be slowed, but if this does not reduce the severity of symptoms and signs then transfusion should be stopped. If this fails to abort the first febrile reaction, only then should a single intravenous injection of an antihistamine, such as chlorpheniramine 25 mg, be given. If that is insufficient, many haematologists will give intravenous hydrocortisone 100 mg, and some will give both hydrocortisone and chlorpheniramine simultaneously.

The frequency and severity of these reactions may lead to the prescription of these two drugs either 'as required' or as prophylaxis for these reactions, which leads in turn to their uncontrolled use by inexperienced junior doctors and nurses. The total cumulative dose of immunosuppressive steroids may go unseen, and the use of hydrocortisone in the management of these febrile reactions should be discouraged. Whether these reactions are due to blood products or drugs such as amphotericin, the most effective treatment or prophylaxis is intravenous pethidine 12.5 mg. This drug is not immunosuppressive and this dose is neither sedating nor, on repetition, addictive, but it should not be used in fever that is probably due to infection.

Specific bleeding problems

In addition to the risk of bleeding because of low platelets, there are further specific coagulation problems that require early detection and planned management. Patients should be monitored for evidence of failure of coagulation, even when they are receiving regular platelet infusions. Clinical observation should include regular fundoscopy for retinal bleeding and testing for haematuria. During remission induction and consolidation therapy for acute leukaemia, platelet transfusion is unavoidable. Fresh-frozen plasma and cryoprecipitate are needed infrequently and should only be used for specific indications and in the absence of virally inactivated products. When correcting coagulation deficiency with plasma-derived products, red cell ABO group-compatible donations should be used to avoid ABO haemolytic reactions. The use of any blood products should follow best practice guidelines provided at present.

Asparaginase in the remission induction phase of the treatment of ALL can inhibit synthesis of coagulation factors, particularly fibrinogen, which should be replaced using fresh-frozen plasma or cryoprecipitate. Very rarely, asparaginase may cause superior sagittal vein thrombosis without warning, but especially in children with unsuspected genetic thrombophilia, for example factor V Leiden.

The hypergranular variant of acute promyelocytic leukaemia (M3) carries a very high risk of bleeding because of disseminated intravascular coagulation (DIC) or fibrinolysis. This can be present at diagnosis or is precipitated by chemotherapy, in either case because of the systemic prothrombotic action of the cytoplasmic granules released by the malignant blasts. The treatment, as in all cases of DIC, is to deal with the primary cause, in this case to lower the blast count as soon after diagnosis as possible. It may be accompanied by microangiopathic haemolytic anaemia. All-*trans* retinoic acid is now a standard part of initial chemotherapy for these patients, as it induces maturation of granulocytes, reducing release of the prothrombotic contents of their granules and lowering the risk of DIC.

Many older adult patients are now anticoagulated with warfarin, aspirin and clopidogrel, or a combination of these, to lessen their risk of acute myocardial infarction or stroke. The physician who initiated this therapy should be identified, if possible, to discuss the risks of stopping these immediately after diagnosis and throughout the treatment of the leukaemia. All antiplatelet therapy should be stopped because protracted and severe thrombocytopenia will recur during the course of therapy. The long action of aspirin and clopidogrel make rapid reversal of their antiplatelet effect impossible if the platelet count drops suddenly. Low-molecular-weight heparin should replace warfarin in those patients who have a high risk of arterial or venous thrombosis, and should be stopped once the platelet count falls below 50×10^9/L. Long-term anticoagulation should not be restarted until all chemotherapy is finished and the patient is in a stable remission with a platelet count above 100×10^9/L.

In patients with chronic and relapsed or refractory leukaemia, there may be chronic mucosal blood loss due to persistent and severe thrombocytopenia, which may be refractory to donor platelet transfusions. Oral tranexamic acid can reduce such blood loss and hormonal suppression can prevent endometrial bleeding. Persistent marrow failure without overt blood loss may require repeat red cell transfusions in patients with chronic leukaemias, particularly CLL. These should be given to relieve symptoms and not according to any set level of haemoglobin. Red cell alloantibodies and iron overload complicate repeated transfusion. Patients with CLL can develop autoimmune haemolysis and thrombocytopenia. The management of these complications is described in Chapter 29.

In all SCT patients, all blood products must be irradiated before transfusion to avoid the risk of graft-versus-host disease (GVHD) mounted by donor lymphocytes against the immunocompromised host. Irradiated blood products are also required in patients having chemotherapy with the aim of early SCT and in those treated with a purine analogue (e.g. fludarabine) to prevent GVHD. The risk of transfusion-related GVHD is much lower in autografts than in allografts. Any transfusion given to those patients whose peripheral blood stem cells (PBSCs) are to be collected within the subsequent 2–3 weeks must also be irradiated, as transfused donor lymphocytes in the PBSC collection may remain alloreactive until after the autograft and lead to clinically significant GVHD.

Growth factor support for anaemia

The most comprehensive reviews of the evidence for the use of granulocyte colony-stimulating factor (G-CSF) and erythropoietin in cancer care are available from the US National Comprehensive Cancer Network (www.nccn.com). The recommendations for the use of erythropoietin are summarized below but these guidelines should be read in full to assess their applicability to the care of individual patients with haematological tumours.

Although it is difficult to define a level of anaemia at which intervention is needed, NCCN emphasizes the need to assess all causes of anaemia (haemoglobin <11.0 g/dL) in cancer patients (tumour-related, chemotherapy-related and all other causes) before correction with either red cell transfusion or erythropoietins. A recent meta-analysis has shown increased mortality associated with the use of erythropoietins in solid tumours and they are not recommended from 6 weeks onwards following the end of cancer treatment. In patients with previous venous thromboembolic episodes, they are also associated with an increased risk of further venous and arterial events, particularly in the presence of ongoing concomitant thrombogenic risk factors, because of either an increased haematocrit (to $42 \pm 3\%$) or as potentially thrombogenic in their own right. In all cases the relative risks and benefits of erythropoietins versus red cell transfusion should be discussed with the patient. Despite the recent Cochrane meta-analysis, there is some uncertainty about the efficacy of erythropoietins in improving quality of life. During initiation and subsequently, the blood pressure should be carefully monitored because of the risk of hypertension associated with erythropoietins.

In solid tumours, NCCN has a level 1 recommendation for the use of erythropoietins in symptomatic patients with chemotherapy-induced anaemias (haemoglobin <10.0 g/dL); however, if the haemoglobin is between 10.0 and 11.0 g/dL, the recommendation to use erythropoietins drops to a level 2b, and in both cases only if there is likely benefit to cancer treatment goals or relief of symptoms. In asymptomatic patients with a haemoglobin of less than 10.0 g/dL, a clear recommendation is not possible and the risks and benefits of both erythropoietins and red cell transfusion should be discussed with the patient. In patients with cancer-related anaemia outside the treatment period, erythropoietins are not recommended. In the treatment of myelodysplastic syndrome (MDS), erythropoietin is recommended by NCCN where intrinsic erythropoietin levels are below 500 mU/mL with or without synergistic G-CSF.

Erythropoietins are not recommended in the treatment of acute leukaemias.

NICE guidance issued in May 2008 is unhelpfully much more prescriptive, recommending the use of erythropoietins only in women with a haemoglobin of 8.0 g/dL or less treated for ovarian carcinoma with platinum-based therapies or those with very severe anaemia who cannot be transfused.

Infections

Some infections occur with all types of leukaemia and therapy, whereas others show more specific associations. As a general rule, the greater the duration and severity of immunosuppression, the greater the risk of life-threatening infection with a bigger range of organisms. During chemotherapy, patients with acute leukaemia have a high risk of life-threatening infections because of neutropenia due to the disease and the chemotherapy, combined with damage to the mucosal barrier and impairment of the innate immune system induced by chemotherapy. The risk is greatest with the profound and protracted immunosuppression required in allogeneic SCT from an unrelated donor.

Infectious agents can be viewed either as professional pathogens (group A streptococci, *Salmonella typhi*) or opportunistic pathogens as depicted in Table 26.2. This limited range of bacteria accounts for most of the opportunistic infections identified during the course of neutropenia, despite the fact that the

Table 26.2 Origins of common potential bacterial pathogens.

	Endogenous	Exogenous
Gram-negative bacilli	Escherichia coli	Pseudomonas aeruginosa
	Klebsiella pneumoniae	Enterobacter cloacae
Gram-positive bacilli	Corynebacterium spp.	Bacillus spp.
	Clostridium spp., e.g. C. septicum	
Gram-positive cocci	Staphylococcus aureus	Enterococcus faecium
	Coagulase-negative staphylococci, e.g. Staphylococcus epidermidis	
	Viridans streptococci, e.g. Streptococcus mitis	
	Enterococcus faecalis	
	Stomatococcus mucilaginosus	

body is colonized with so many more. Strictly anaerobic bacteria are rarely the cause of systemic infection, although they outnumber other bacteria by several billion. Fungal infections tend to occur later during therapy than bacterial infections. The body's surfaces, particularly the oral cavity and gut, are inhabited by billions of bacteria comprising many hundreds of genera, and the environment contains hundreds more bacteria and fungi. Most remain harmless and are never shown to be causes of fever during profound immunosuppression, despite the patient's close encounter with them.

All protocols for prophylaxis, investigation and treatment of infection should be agreed by haematologists and microbiologists and contain all the elements of an integrated plan to reduce morbidity and mortality arising from infection. All protocols should be complemented with regular discussion of individual patients' investigations and results, and by audits of responses to results and of effectiveness of the protocols.

Fever as evidence of infection during chemotherapy and SCT

Most patients with acute leukaemia will be repeatedly neutropenic for prolonged periods and therefore are at risk of becoming febrile at some point. A minority of these episodes will be accompanied by symptoms and signs of localizing infection, such as dysuria and urinary frequency or inflammation around the CVC exit site or tunnel. Because of the perceived need to treat presumed bacteraemia promptly in most cases, the fever will be, at least initially, of unknown origin. This empirical approach has proven of immense value in reducing mortality attributed to Gram-negative bacillary infection but may have some unfavourable consequences including undue reliance on drugs at the expense of microbiological diagnosis, more adverse

drug reactions, emergent bacterial resistance and increased costs. There are indeed many other causes of fever in these patients, including blood products, drugs (chemotherapy and antibiotics), tumour lysis syndrome, DIC and, in SCT, total body irradiation and GVHD. It is sometimes possible to identify one or more of these as the cause(s) of fever and thus avoid unnecessary antibiotic therapy. It has also become clear that fever may arise from the tissue damage associated with mucosal barrier injury induced by certain chemotherapeutic agents, including melphalan, cyclophosphamide, anthracyclines and cytarabine. The initial phase of mucosal barrier injury is characterized by an inflammatory response. Infection cannot be easily and reliably ruled out so fever should always be assumed to herald infection unless there is clear evidence to the contrary.

Infections can go unnoticed because the inflammatory response is muted and pus cannot be formed because of neutropenia. Foci of infections can also be easily overlooked unless physical examination is frequent and thorough. Infections may start as fever with or without bacteraemia, followed by clinical evidence of localized infection, and constant vigilance is needed to detect the sequential development of systemic infection (Figure 26.1). Despite the meagre signs and symptoms of infection in an immunocompromised patient, it is still essential to conduct a careful physical examination, paying particular attention to the oropharynx, including the dentition, the lungs, the skin, nails and exit sites of venous access devices, and the perianal region. Rectal examination is inadvisable in the severely neutropenic and thrombocytopenic patient because of the risk of bacteraemia. The most common sites of infection when present are the oral cavity, the lung and the skin, with its underlying soft tissues. Clinically detectable sources of infections occur in up to one in five cases and tend to be those in the skin

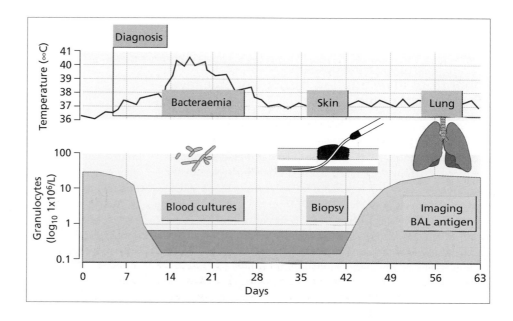

Figure 26.1 Common infections during neutropenia.

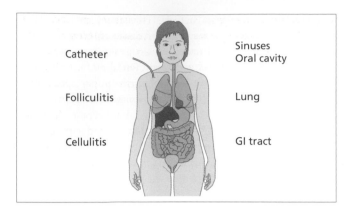

Figure 26.2 Sources of infection.

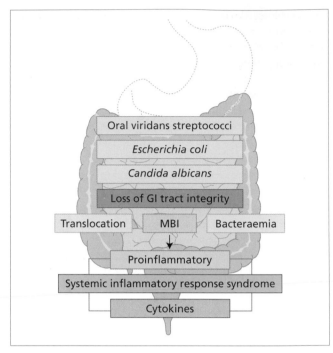

Figure 26.3 Mucosal barrier injury (MBI: the role of mucositis), the systemic inflammatory response and bacteraemia.

Table 26.3 Blood cultures.

When	At onset of fever
How	A sample of 20 mL blood from a peripheral vein and, when present, samples of 20 mL from each lumen of an indwelling vascular catheter
Method	Each sample divided between an aerobic and an anaerobic bottle
Time to positivity	Most organisms are detected within 24 hours and 50% within 12 hours
Time to identity	24–48 hours, i.e. within the empirical phase
Utility	Identifies cause of fever in 20–30% of cases

and its structures or in the mucosal barrier, including the respiratory tract (Figure 26.2). Microbiological proof of infection is found in only 20–30% of cases of neutropenic fever and a further 10–20% of cases can be defined as clinical infections.

All units treating these patients must have a clear written protocol that balances the risks and benefits of exact diagnosis against empirical therapy by making good use of all available evidence at the onset of fever. This protocol must include a description of the specimens to be obtained by the microbiology laboratory. Many diagnostic opportunities are missed if the laboratory is not clear about what is to be done with samples from these patients, and how results should be interpreted and reported. Obtaining specimens from some infectious foci may be difficult if this requires aspiration or biopsy during severe thrombocytopenia. Even when a specimen is obtained from a normally sterile site, the yield of pathogens is usually low, interpretation is difficult and the results may not influence management. Failure to identify a focus of infection and to obtain appropriate samples may leave the fever unexplained. In most cases, microbiological diagnosis depends on identification of pathogens in blood cultures.

Laboratory investigation of neutropenic fever of unknown origin

Blood cultures

The utility of blood cultures depends on adherence to a few simple rules (Table 26.3). The specificity of blood cultures is increased if samples are taken from at least two separate sites, preferably including all lumina of a CVC. Ideally blood should be drawn from a peripheral vein and from the CVC to confirm the significance of growing skin commensals such as the Gram-positive coagulase-negative staphylococci. Other isolates including Gram-negative bacilli and viridans streptococci seldom if ever colonize the lumen of a CVC because they normally originate from the oral cavity and gut in the setting of

mucosal barrier injury, better known by mucositis, its clinical counterpart (Figure 26.3). The fever associated with mucositis may originate from the mucosal damage induced by chemotherapy, and the loss of mucosal integrity that results may permit bacterial translocation leading to systemic infection. Even coagulase-negative staphylococcal bacteraemia may originate in some cases from the gastrointestinal tract or thromboses and may not represent catheter colonization.

The total amount of blood sampled at any one time constitutes a single blood culture. In adults, sensitivity and specificity are increased if at least 20 mL, and preferably 30 mL, of blood taken from each sampling site at each time is divided between an aerobic and an anaerobic bottle to detect the majority of common pathogens.

Oral/rectal swabs

Viridans streptococci of the *mitis* group (*Streptococcus mitis* and *Streptococcus oralis*) are universal residents of the oral cavity and, with the exception of bacterial endocarditis, are seldom associated with infectious diseases. However, in the last two decades, these bacteria have been causing bacteraemia regularly in patients with severe oral mucositis. Similarly, *Clostridium* spp., for example *C. septicum*, are also normal commensal bacteria of the large bowel but can cause bacteraemia in patients suffering from a particularly severe form of gut mucositis, namely neutropenic enterocolitis (typhlitis). Given their presence in most individuals as part of the normal flora, it is pointless to obtain specimens from the oral cavity or rectum to detect these bacteria.

Specimens for pulmonary infection

Investigating pulmonary infection has become more demanding and involves obtaining blood samples as well as specimens from the respiratory tract. Bronchoalveolar lavage (BAL) specimens are advised for patients with pulmonary infiltrates and can yield the pathogen in 30–50% of cases. There are no standards for handling such specimens in the laboratory or in the diagnostic tests themselves. The residue of BAL samples after centrifugation is examined for *Pneumocystis jirovecii* (formerly *carinii*), the acid-fast bacilli and *Nocardia* spp., common bacteria, and moulds (*Aspergillus* spp.) and is subjected to culture for fungi and bacteria, including *Legionella* spp. and *Mycobacterium* spp. BAL should also be examined for the presence of *Aspergillus* galactomannan antigen, which is found frequently in cases of invasive pulmonary aspergillosis, and microbial DNA may be detected by polymerase chain reaction (PCR) techniques.

Standards for virological investigations vary, but the influenza and parainfluenza viruses, adenovirus, respiratory syncytial virus and CMV may also be detected. When superficial pulmonary lesions are present, specimens might be obtained by percutaneous or open lung biopsy, provided that the benefit outweighs the risk, diagnosis is uncertain and treatment is clearly not working. Although neutropenic patients do not produce sputum, they frequently expectorate mucous secretions, which should be sent for microscopy and culture. Recovery of moulds including *Aspergillus* on two or more consecutive occasions increases the likelihood of their being involved in invasive fungal diseases (IFDs) in the presence of pulmonary infiltrates on computed tomography (CT) consistent with invasive aspergillosis. The common practice of microbiology laboratories in discarding expectorated secretions without pus cells should not apply to these patients.

Skin lesions

Identifying the cause of a skin or soft-tissue infection is difficult because culturing superficial swabs of lesions rarely discriminates between pathogens and commensal flora. Culture and histological examination of skin punch-biopsy specimens is very helpful in diagnosing disseminated infections due to *Candida* spp., *Trichosporon* spp. and *Fusarium* spp. To achieve this it is important to ensure that the specimen is actually sent to histopathology *and* microbiology and not assume that it will be. In contrast, aspiration of skin lesions is seldom successful as pus is usually absent.

Gut investigations

In oesophagitis, endoscopy occasionally distinguishes infection due to herpes simplex from that due to *Candida* spp. but clinical suspicion of infective oesophagitis rarely leads to endoscopy because appearances are usually non-specific and the procedure is hazardous. Persistent diarrhoea or abdominal pain requires a cytotoxicity assay on a stool sample for *Clostridium difficile* toxin, and patients with right lower quadrant pain suggestive of typhlitis should have blood cultures taken to exclude the presence of *C. septicum* or *C. tertium*, as recovery of these bacteria usually indicates neutropenic enterocolitis. Although infections due to *Candida* spp., the Gram-negative bacilli, *Escherichia coli*, *Klebsiella pneumoniae*, *Pseudomonas aeruginosa*, *Clostridium* spp. and enterococci, including vancomycin-resistant enterococci (VRE), usually originate from the large bowel, there is no value in culturing faeces as, not surprisingly, there are many more patients colonized than infected.

Urinary tract

Urine should be obtained as cleanly as possible for standard culture when there are signs or symptoms of a urinary tract infection but not otherwise. Urine from SCT recipients with haemorrhagic cystitis should be tested for adenovirus and BK virus.

Non-cultural techniques

The role of non-cultural methods for diagnosis is small but expanding. *Legionella* antigen detection in urine is specific but detects only *L. pneumophila* type 1. Detection of CMV DNA by quantitative PCR may replace detection of the pp65 antigen in peripheral blood neutrophils among SCT recipients, and there is increasing expertise in using PCR to detect fungal DNA in blood and urine, but these remain investigational as there is no standard at present. Kits for the detection of *Aspergillus* antigen in serum, plasma and other sterile body fluids using an enzyme-linked immunosorbent assay (ELISA) are commercially available and can be used to screen patients at risk of aspergillosis. The specificity is generally high but the sensitivity has varied considerably, depending on the nature of the specimen (blood, bronchial material, cerebrospinal fluid), the threshold employed

(0.5–1.5), the characteristics of the population (age, underlying disease), the frequency of sampling (once or twice weekly or less) and the prevalence of the disease in the population under study. The manufacturer now recommends a cut-off of 0.5, which increases sensitivity at the expense of specificity. The sampling frequency of two to three times weekly appears optimal to screen for galactomannan, and detection of the substance in BAL fluid is considered sufficient to upgrade a case of possible invasive pulmonary aspergillosis to the level of probable IFD. There is also a test for detecting the fungal cell wall component β-D-glucan, which shows promise as it detects *Candida* and *Aspergillus* as well as other less frequently encountered moulds including *Fusarium*. However, experience is limited and the optimal positioning of this test for screening and confirming a diagnosis remains to be established. While the detection of the *Aspergillus* antigen and of β-D-glucan is considered equivalent to recovery by culture as mycological evidence, the detection of DNA by PCR is not until, and unless, a standard is established and the test is formally validated.

Surveillance cultures

There is no point in undertaking surveillance cultures unless the results are used to guide therapeutic or prophylactic choice. Obtaining nasal swabs to detect *Staphylococcus aureus* is useful as there is a strong association between carriage and subsequent bacteraemia. Once identified, a carrier can be treated with mupirocin. Carriers of methicillin-resistant *Staphylococcus aureus* (MRSA) should be managed according to local practice but should normally remain isolated from other patients until shown to be free of the bacterium. Surveillance cultures of faeces are used if there is a risk of emergent ciprofloxacin-resistant *E. coli* or *P. aeruginosa* when the drug is being used for prophylaxis. Testing faeces for carriage of these bacteria is a prudent form of surveillance to permit early detection of rising resistance before there is a corresponding rise in the infections caused by resistant bacteria. Detection of *Candida* carriage can be used to start prophylaxis; conversely, failure to detect the yeast or opportunistic Gram-negative bacilli in oral samples or faeces indicates that infection is highly unlikely as the negative predictive value of these cultures exceeds 95%.

Proven systemic infection during neutropenia

Surveys show that the rate of proven bacteraemia during periods of neutropenia has remained between 20 and 25% over many years. In adults, the range of bacteria identified has also altered very little, although the ratio of Gram-positive to Gram-negative organisms has varied. In the 1970s, there were two to three times as many Gram-negative as Gram-positive infections, in the late 1980s and early 1990s this ratio was reversed and now the risks of Gram-negative and Gram-positive infection are approximately equal. It is not entirely clear why this has happened, and individual units can have a pattern of causative organisms that is unique and unlike that found elsewhere. Therefore, it is important for each unit to monitor local rates of isolation of bacterial and other pathogens and their patterns of antibiotic susceptibility in liaison with the microbiologists, who should be active members of the multidisciplinary team.

There have been changes in practice that have been widely applied and are blamed for the changing Gram-negative and Gram-positive rates. For example, in the management of adult acute leukaemia there has been a trend towards more intensity of therapy, with an increasing risk of gut mucositis. In the presence of this complication, blocking gastric acid production increases the risk of viridans streptococcal bacteraemia. The widespread use of indwelling CVCs provides another portal of entry for Gram-positive staphylococci, and to a lesser extent *Candida parapsilosis*, as the microorganisms often colonize the surfaces of the skin in that area. The cause of greatest concern has been the indiscriminate use of oral quinolone antibacterials (ofloxacin, ciprofloxacin, levofloxacin) as prophylaxis against Gram-negative bacteraemia, which has not reliably reduced the overall risk but simply shifted the common causes of bacteraemia towards the Gram-positive organisms. Such prophylaxis is justifiable in allogeneic SCT recipients prepared by myeloablative therapy and in those receiving intensive chemotherapy to induce remission of AML and MDS, but is seldom appropriate in lower-risk patients who are receiving chemotherapy.

Recent studies suggest that the risk of Gram-negative bacteraemia has not diminished in many single centres and is on the increase in some that have never used quinolones as prophylaxis, in those which have recently discontinued this use and even in those in which this use continues (Figure 26.4). The risk of proven bacteraemia fluctuates but may be as high as one in three of febrile episodes, mainly due to a significant doubling of the risk of Gram-negative infections.

It is difficult to reconcile these data with a unifying explanation. However, it does seem clear that despite a relatively high risk of bacteraemia, there is insufficient evidence to support continuous prophylaxis against bacterial infections with broad-spectrum antibiotics during conventional chemotherapy. It is also doubtful that this will substantially reduce the risk of such infections and may actually compromise the efficacy of these antibiotics when they are needed.

In bacteraemia associated with onset of fever, the most commonly identified Gram-negative bacilli are *E. coli*, *P. aeruginosa*, *Klebsiella* and *Enterobacter* spp. and the Gram-positive cocci *Staphylococcus epidermidis*, the viridans streptococci belonging to the *mitis* group *S. mitis* and *S. oralis* and *Staph. aureus* (increasingly the methicillin-resistant strains, i.e. MRSA). Bacteraemia due to other species such as *Enterococcus faecalis* and *Clostridium* spp. tends to occur only after 7–10 days' therapy with broad-spectrum antibiotics, in association with gut mucositis, including neutropenic enterocolitis (typhlitis).

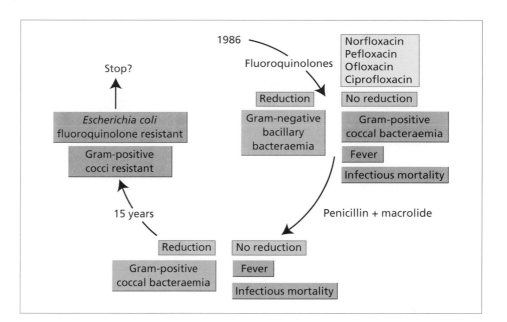

Figure 26.4 The life cycle of fluoroquinolone prophylaxis.

The reported incidence of proven IFD is 5–15% among allogeneic SCT patients, and the risk rises in severe chronic GVHD requiring prolonged immunosuppression with steroids. The majority of these infections are now due to *Aspergillus* spp. and about one in three are seen more than 100 days after engraftment. The mortality rate of IFD remains high in these patients. The rate of IFD during conventional chemotherapy is equally high among those given remission induction chemotherapy for AML and MDS but is less clear among other patients groups. IFD appears to be a significant risk for patients treated for a long time with corticosteroids and also when T-cell suppression is induced by potent purine analogues such as fludarabine and high-dose cytarabine. Patients receiving allogeneic SCT after non-myeloablative therapy may be at greater risk but the data are sparse. The risk is low in the predictably brief duration of neutropenia with autologous SCT.

In allogeneic SCT, the rate of CMV seropositivity and clinical CMV infection vary according to the pretransplant status of the donor and recipient. The post-transplant CMV-associated fatality rate is around 40%. Other herpesviruses may also reactivate including Epstein–Barr virus (EBV), which is associated with lymphoproliferative disorders, and HHV-6 which is associatied with fever.

Prophylaxis of infections

Given that some infections occur frequently and arise from body sites harbouring an abundant normal commensal flora, it is not surprising that antimicrobial prophylaxis is advocated and adopted by many centres treating patients with acute leukaemia. Essentially, when adopted, prophylaxis is started just before chemotherapy is begun with the aim of suppressing or eradicating potentially opportunistic pathogens ahead of the anticipated neutropenia (Figure 26.5).

The early cocktails of non-absorbable antibiotics, such as framycetin, colistin and nystatin (FRACON) or gentamicin, vancomycin and nystatin (GVN), were superseded by co-trimoxazole and colistin and later by the fluoroquinolones norfloxacin, pefloxacin, ofloxacin, ciprofloxacin and levofloxacin. The need for antibacterial prophylaxis is still in doubt. As described above, antibacterial prophylaxis had no impact on the overall incidence of fever or mortality over many years, and almost all patients given such prophylaxis will also be given further broad-spectrum antibiotics for unexplained fever. Some institutes are now faced with patients harbouring fluoroquinolone-resistant *E. coli*, causing them to abandon prophylaxis altogether. Recent meta-analysis confirms a reduction in bacteraemia due to Gram-negative bacilli and even an impact on mortality. However, this should be seen in the context of prevalence, risk and the numbers needed to treat. Patients most likely to benefit are those likely to experience at least 10 days of neutropenia induced by chemotherapy that also causes marked damage to the mucosa of the alimentary tract. These are still patients treated for AML-MDS with intensive chemotherapy and those receiving myeloablative therapy for SCT.

The risk of IFD varies with the intensity of therapy and its complications and is greatest in SCT patients with protracted GVHD. Non-absorbable polyenes, such as amphotericin and nystatin, do not provide systemic protection. Fluconazole reduces the risk of *C. albicans* significantly in SCT, but not in conventional chemotherapy; it is not effective in suppressing certain yeasts, including *C. krusei* and *C. glabrata*, and of course there is no activity against moulds (e.g. *Aspergillus* spp.). In contrast, itraconazole, voriconazole and posaconazole are active

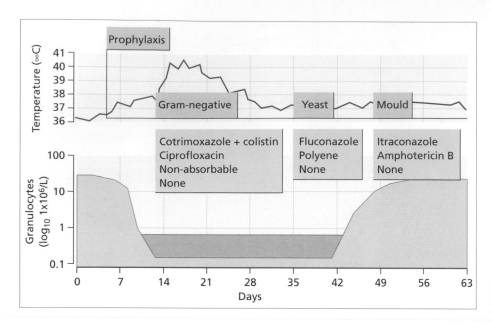

Figure 26.5 Antibiotic choices for prophylaxis during neutropenia.

against a wide range of yeasts and moulds. With the availability of interchangeable oral solution and intravenous formulations, itraconazole is more effective than fluconazole in preventing a range of infections due to *Candida* spp. and *Aspergillus* in SCT and conventional chemotherapy, provided that sufficient drug is given to achieve protective systemic levels. The newer triazole posaconazole has been shown to be effective as prophylaxis for patients given chemotherapy for AML and MDS and for those suffering GVHD. Liposomal amphotericin has been shown to reduce the incidence of IFD when given as an aerosol. There are no data on voriconazole as prophylaxis. This patchy picture has led to considerable confusion that various guidelines have struggled to clarify. Once again the difficulty lies in transplanting trial results to one's own practice. One rule of thumb is to estimate the numbers needed to treat in order to achieve the reported reduction. So, for instance, if the prevalence of invasive aspergillosis in a given centre is around 5%, to reduce this by half would require 20 patients to be treated to prevent a case of invasive aspergillosis. Also, it is proper for any centre with long experience of an effective strategy to critically examine whether the incidence of IFD can be further reduced cost-effectively by adopting prophylaxis with posaconazole or aerosolized liposomal amphotericin. Every centre should have a fairly accurate estimate of the incidence of IFD before making informed decisions about when and what prophylaxis to use.

There is no evidence to support antiviral prophylaxis during neutropenia that is induced by conventional chemotherapy, except in patients with CLL and a strong past history of herpes infection if they are given fludarabine. In allogeneic SCT, all patients are given aciclovir or its equivalent as prophylaxis to reduce their risk of infection with herpes viruses, There is no specific prophylaxis for CMV infection, which carries a high fatality rate. Post-SCT CMV is best prevented by transplanta-

tion from a negative donor to a negative recipient, with exclusive use of leucodepleted blood products. Prophylaxis against EBV infection is also lacking.

Empirical therapy of fever of unknown origin

In the 1960s, the combined mortality rate from Gram-negative and Gram-positive bacteraemia during neutropenia induced by therapy for acute leukaemia was estimated at 90%. The introduction of the prompt empirical use of broad-spectrum antibiotics at the onset of fever was a major advance in supportive care. This routine practice (usually with a β-lactam and an aminoglycoside or else a β-lactam alone; Figure 26.6) has resulted in a mortality rate due to proven bacterial infections of 7% overall, 10% for Gram-negative organisms and 6% for Gram-positive organisms, at 30 days from onset of fever.

Each unit should establish and audit the application of rules for using these antibiotics in the treatment of fever. Other causes of fever have been described above and the likelihood of them explaining a new episode of fever should be carefully considered before antibiotics are given. There should be a working definition of when fever is likely to be due to bacteraemia or other systemic infection to justify systemic antibiotic therapy, including the degree of neutropenia, the day of onset in relation to chemotherapy, whether the temperature has suddenly become elevated, and height and duration of fever. A review of the literature shows wide variation in such definitions as they are applied to clinical trials. For patients receiving conventional chemotherapy for acute leukaemia, one practical suggestion is that once the neutrophil count drops below 0.5×10^9/L and the temperature reaches 38°C twice in 1 hour despite the use of paracetamol, empirical antibiotic therapy should be given. Alternatively, a single temperature exeeding 38°C is also

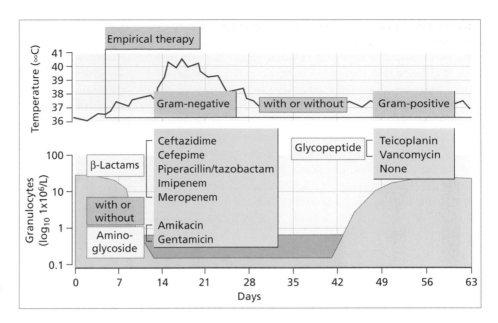

Figure 26.6 Initial empirical antibiotic options during neutropenia.

taken to indicate fever. Clearly, if the patient is in shock or shows early signs of haemodynamic and respiratory instability, a single temperature reading of 38°C is sufficient. The peripheral temperature may be normal or the patient may even be hypothermic on development of shock due to sepsis. Blood cultures should always be taken from both a CVC and a peripheral vein, and always before antibiotics are started. With the increasing use of multilumen CVCs, blood should be taken from more than one lumen, which increases the sample size and also allows identification of possible colonization.

Despite the dramatic reduction in mortality associated with the use of broad-spectrum antibiotics, they have their limitations: they exhibit relatively poor activity against staphylococci (including MRSA) and some streptococci, may provide inadequate coverage when the rate of Gram-negative bacteraemia is increasing, and β-lactams must be given in several daily infusions occupying considerable CVC access time. Infections due to extended-spectrum β-lactamase-producing Gram-negative bacilli should prompt reappraisal of the regimens used for empirical therapy. Similarly, with VRE being associated with increased use of third-generation cephalosporins (e.g. ceftazidime), this class of antibiotics may not be appropriate for empirical therapy in centres facing infections due to these enterococci. The toxicity of the aminoglycosides requires proper monitoring of levels and adjustment of dose or timing of administration.

Meta-analysis of randomized controlled trials confirms that the rate of response of unexplained fever is around 50%, whether an aminoglycoside is used in addition to a β-lactam or not, suggesting that monotherapy using ceftazidime, cefepime, piperacillin–tazobactam, imipenem or meropenem is adequate. There is also no need to add vancomycin or teicoplanin to the initial empirical regimen as there is no measurable benefit in

outcome nor in reducing the rate of defervescence, subsequent infections, use of additional antimicrobial agents or mortality.

Subsequent antimicrobial therapy

When fever persists and no microbiologically or clinically defined infection has been identified, there may be no need to switch to an alternative regimen provided the patient's condition is stable. When a CVC is in place the assumption is often made that CVC-related staphylococcal infection may explain persistent fever, prompting the addition of vancomycin or teicoplanin empirically. However, randomized placebo-controlled trials have shown that there is no impact on response rates or mortality. This practice also encourages the emergence of VRE, so such 'second-line' antibacterial empirical therapy is only justifiable when there is clinical evidence of infection around the exit site or along the track of the CVC or evidence of an infected thrombus related to the location of the catheter in the vein.

Subsequently, antibiotic therapy may be modified, depending on whether a microbiologically defined infection or a clinically defined infection has been identified or the development of a new infection is defined clinically or microbiologically. The empirical regimen should be continued and complemented with other drugs such as a glycopeptide (e.g. vancomycin) or an antifungal agent. There are individual infections that may be proven microbiologically (e.g. *Candida* in blood cultures) or which may be suggested clinically or radiologically (e.g. invasive pulmonary aspergillosis or *Pneumocystis jirovecii* pneumonitis), and these justify switching to alternative therapies or complementing the existing regimen. A readiness to perform early CT of the chest may shorten the time to starting systemic antifungal therapy when invasive pulmonary aspergillosis is suspected. Plain chest radiography is notoriously unreliable and should not be used to confirm or exclude this diagnosis. The use of galactomannan detection in plasma or serum should also be incorporated into the algorithm of management. The relatively high sensitivity that results from the lower threshold of 0.5 means that a positive result can be taken to support antifungal therapy, especially when a CT scan shows lesions consistent with the diagnosis.

Each unit should devise a protocol in which the criteria for adding subsequent therapy are clearly defined, based on clinical and microbiological findings (Table 26.4), either given on the basis of the organism causing a microbiologically defined infection (Figure 26.7) or on the basis of the site involved in a clinically defined infection (Figure 26.8). There is little evidence to

Table 26.4 Rules for additional therapy.

Related to primary infective event
Clinical deterioration
Progression or persistence
Initial bacterial pathogen resistant
Non-bacterial infection
More than 5 days' fever

Related to subsequent infective event
New microbiologically defined infection: bacterial, fungal, viral
New clinically defined infection
New fever

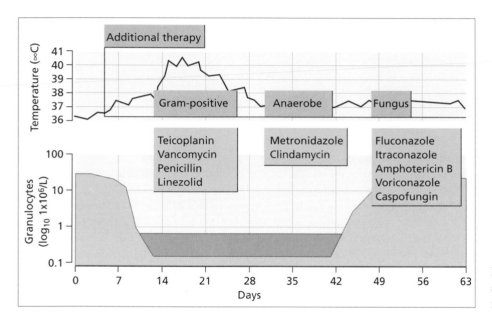

Figure 26.7 Microbiologically directed antibiotic treatment during neutropenia.

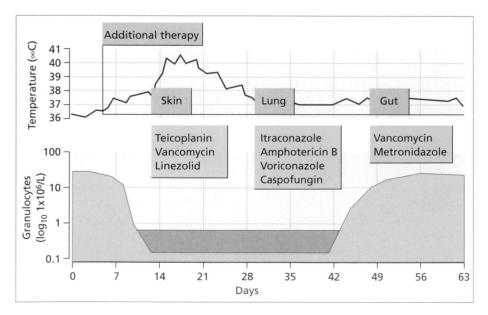

Figure 26.8 Clinically directed antibiotic treatment during neutropenia.

support precise times when additional or substitute antibiotics should be introduced and the automatic rotation or modification of antibiotics should be discouraged. The superiority of any one therapeutic agent over any other active against proven *Aspergillus* spp. IFD or probable or possible IFD is based on relative toxicity. In presumed or proven *Pneumocystis* pneumonitis, the drug of choice is high-dose co-trimoxazole, with steroids to reduce the risk of post-infective fibrosis.

Allogeneic stem cell transplantation patients

The febrile SCT recipient represents a special case of neutropenic fever because of the increased risk of opportunistic infection with viruses, particularly those of the herpes group, herpes simplex and CMV and, increasingly, EBV. The procedures involved in SCT are broadly similar across units and can be divided into myeloablative conditioning therapy or reduced-intensity conditioning. The infective risks and related prophylaxis are also very similar, for example valaciclovir or aciclovir for herpesviruses and a fluoroquinolone to suppress infections due to Gram-negative bacilli.

An alternative approach is to only use these agents prophylactically when the patient is known to be a carrier of the particular organism. SCT recipients predictably develop fever shortly after the time of transplant, typically within a week, and it is essential not to treat the immediate fever of total body irradiation with broad-spectrum antibiotics. There is disagreement about whether broad-spectrum therapy should be started at a predetermined time after transplant on the assumption that fever is imminent, or empirically at the onset of fever. Whichever approach is followed, the pattern of infection during the neutropenia of SCT is fairly predictable, justifying screening for CMV using a pp65 antigen ELISA or PCR, and *Aspergillus* infection using a galactomannan ELISA or PCR, although the latter still lacks standardization. Treatment may be pre-emptive if infection due to either CMV or *Aspergillus* spp. is detected.

In contrast with other neutropenic patients, the risk of infection to SCT recipients extends long after the neutropenia has resolved, particularly with chronic and severe GVHD treated with corticosteroids. These are now the major risk factors for IFD due to *Aspergillus fumigatus*, with perhaps as many as two-thirds of cases occurring after 100 days, with a high case fatality rate, justifying prolonged prophylaxis. Bacteraemia due to certain Gram-negative bacilli, including *P. aeruginosa*, also occurs at this late stage. In addition, the hypogammaglobulinaemia of SCT persists for months or years after transplant, with an increased risk of infection by the encapsulated bacteria *S. pneumoniae* and *Haemophilus influenzae*. During the post-transplant period, prolonged prophylaxis against these bacteria may be justified as diagnosis and appropriate treatment may come too late, but there is limited evidence that prophylaxis is cost-effective. Immunization with a polyvalent pneumococcal vaccine is also recommended. These patients also need to be seen regularly and frequently, and have to be clear about when to report to the transplant or follow-up unit if they are unwell.

Stopping antibiotics after an episode of fever when neutropenic

Antibacterial therapy can be stopped if there there is no evidence of a microbiologically or clinically defined infection provided that fever has resolved and the temperature has been normal for at least 5 days. However, antibiotics should be given for at least 10 days after the onset of bacteraemia. Infections (bacterial or yeast) related to colonization or infection of a CVC or the adjacent tunnel may require removal of the device to reduce the risk of recurrence. Bacteraemia that persists after catheter removal may indicate an infected thrombus which, if confirmed by ultrasound, should be treated with vancomycin and thrombolytic agents for at least a week until blood cultures become sterile. It is less clear when systemic antifungal therapy can be safely stopped for invasive aspergillosis, as radiological changes may persist well after eradication of the causative organism. Typically therapy is given for 4–6 weeks.

Infections specific to childhood and adult ALL

The significant additional risk in these patients is *Pneumocystis jirovecii* pneumonitis, which may be lessened by co-trimoxazole 960 mg b.d. orally twice weekly or 480 mg orally every day. The infection has a characteristically rapid onset and presentation with marked hypoxia, relatively few abnormal physical signs apart from increased respiratory effort and extensive pulmonary shadowing on chest radiography. Confirmation of the diagnosis is difficult as there are no reliable objective tests.

Growth factors and granulocyte infusions

The most comprehensive reviews of the evidence for the use of G-CSF in cancer care are available from the NCCN. The recommendations for the use of growth factors are summarized below but these guidelines should be read in full to assess their applicability to the care of individual patients.

Guidelines from the American Society for Clinical Oncology (ASCO) and European Organization for Research and Treatment of Cancer (EORTC) classify patients according to the rates of febrile neutropenia or, more correctly, fever and neutropenia. If the rate of febrile neutropenia is greater than 20% (previously described as >40%) for any chemotherapy regimen, intermediate risk at 10–20% and low risk at less than 10%, NCCN classify therapy as 'with curative intent' or as 'adjuvant therapy' for the highest level of risk, as 'with the intention to prolong survival' for the next level, and as 'with the intention of symptom control' only for the lowest risk level. In solid tumours they make a level 1 recommendation for the prophylactic use of G-CSF in chemotherapy aimed at cure or prolongation of survival for the end points of risk of febrile neutropenia, hospitalization, use of intravenous antibiotics and the support of intended dose intensity. Some factors that lead to high risk have been identified in a validated study, such as the use of more than two myelosuppressive agents, certain types of drugs (e.g. anthracyclines), more than 85% of planned dose intensity, certain cancer types and no G-CSF use. The guideline recommends evaluation of the patient after each cycle of therapy. If there has been no episode of febrile neutropenia, then G-CSF may not be needed subsequently. If febrile neutropenia has occurred without G-CSF support, it should be considered for subsequent cycles. If febrile neutropenia occurs despite G-CSF support, then dose intensity should be reduced.

Use of G-CSF should be considered on an individual patient basis for intermediate-risk regimens (10–20%); for low-risk regimens (<10%) it is declared unnecessary unless treatment is with curative intent and there is significant risk of serious medical consequences of febrile neutropenia for other reasons. Use of G-CSF in therapy aimed at symptom control depends on the intensity of the therapy so that the combination of a patient at high risk plus a regimen of high intensity may sometimes justify G-CSF support. Alternative less myelosuppressive or dose-reduced therapy, if of comparable benefit, may be preferable.

The British Committee for Standards in Haematology (www. bcshguidelines.com) issued guidelines in 2003 for the use of G-CSF in acute leukaemia, with a level 1a recommendation for its use following intensive consolidation (post-remission) chemotherapy for AML, following intensive chemotherapy for ALL and following intensive chemotherapy for MDS and a level 1b recommendation for its use in accelerating neutrophil recovery after autologous or allogeneic SCT. G-CSF is used routinely to mobilize stem cells for harvesting from peripheral blood. G-CSF may also exert a synergistic effect with erythropoietin in the treatment of anaemia in MDS.

Recombinant human G-CSF may reduce the severity and duration of neutropenia after chemotherapy or SCT, but only if the patient has sufficient stem cells to be stimulated. The response will not be immediate and it remains unclear, despite all the evidence referred to above, that this reduces the risk of serious systemic infection, the mortality rate from these infections or the mortality rate overall. Infusion of high-dose granulocyte collections from donors stimulated by G-CSF may be indicated if infection is resistant to antimicrobials and delayed neutrophil recovery is expected. However, there is little evidence to support their use, and they should be avoided in patients with pre-existing HLA alloimmunization or in those requiring mechanical ventilation.

Infection risks in chronic leukaemias

In the CLLs there is a wide range of suppression of both humoral and cell-mediated immunity and consequently a wide spectrum of potential infecting organisms, from the relatively low-risk superficial herpetic infection to potentially fatal bacterial pneumonia. These risks increase with progression of disease and intensity of therapy. The use of the more potent purine analogues, fludarabine and cladribine, intensify these risks not only by inducing short-term neutropenia but also by profound suppression of T-cell function. Atypical infections such as *Pneumocystis jirovecii* pneumonitis, *Listeria* and fungal infections have been reported, and prophylactic co-trimoxazole is indicated during and for 6 months after these drugs are given in order to allow sufficient recovery of T-cell function. In CLL patients treated with the anti-CD52 antibody alemtuzumab (Campath), there is a high risk of reactivation of CMV infection. In hairy cell leukaemia, there is often combined neutropenia and monocytopenia with a major bacterial infection at presentation. These patients require the same prophylaxis as other CLLs if treated with purine analogues.

The infection risks of CML are similar to those of the acute leukaemias, although less severe in chronic stable phase. Since the introduction of imatinib, which induces rapid, smooth and lasting control of the disease, the risk of infection has been greatly reduced.

Metabolic complications

Fluid balance

Fluid intake and output must be monitored carefully in patients treated intensively. Accurate observation and recording of these data is the task of specialist nurses, and medical staff must review these regularly. Maintenance of fluid balance is a continuous problem in these patients, particularly the elderly, who have an increased risk of renal and congestive heart failure. The delivery of chemotherapy, blood and blood products, antibiotics and parenteral feeding needs large volumes that may exceed physiological requirements without oral intake. Fluid overload happens relatively quickly if monitoring is overlooked and it should be anticipated and avoided (see sections Anaemia and thrombocytopenia, Planning large-volume transfusions).

Vomiting, diarrhoea, sweating and insensible respiratory loss may singly, or in combination, lead steadily, sometimes rapidly, to dehydration. The vasodilatation and hypotension of sepsis will exacerbate hypovolaemia, which should be anticipated. Replacement of volume is achieved with normal saline solution alternating with 5% dextrose solution. Acute onset of these complications can require rapid infusion of colloid (polysaccharide solutions such as gelofusin) for expansion of intravascular volume, particularly when a shift of body fluid from the intravascular space into tissues is suspected as can occur in septic shock. However, polysaccharide solutions are metabolized quickly and solutions of albumin are preferable when loss of plasma osmotic pressure is due to chronic hypoalbuminaemia. Fresh-frozen plasma should not be used for this indication. Prolonged hypovolaemia will result in acute renal tubular necrosis (ATN) and therefore an early decision is needed about the likely cause of oliguria, in case this is due to a 'renal' rather than the 'prerenal' hypovolaemic cause of acute renal failure (ARF). Supporting a balanced throughput of fluid volume is complicated by a number of electrolyte and metabolic problems.

Hyperuricaemia and tumour lysis syndrome

The rapid rate of cell proliferation and death in acute leukaemia increases the catabolism of nucleic acids, which terminates with the excess production of uric acid. Therefore, patients may present with biochemical hyperuricaemia or its clinical consequences or develop these once treatment starts. The most extreme form of this is tumour lysis syndrome (TLS), in which severe hyperuricaemia, hyperphosphataemia, hyperkalaemia and hypocalcaemia are associated with supersaturation of the urine with uric acid, which is then deposited in crystals in the renal tubules and distal collecting system. These biochemical abnormalities result in a major increase in the morbidity and mortality of patients, including ARF, which requires haemodialysis.

TLS is a frequent complication of advanced-stage Burkitt lymphoma and B-cell ALL in childhood and of any adult leukaemia with a very high presenting blast count; despite attempts to manage the metabolic problems, as many as 25% of such children develop ARF on starting chemotherapy. The precise incidence of clinical and subclinical TLS is not known. Subclinical TLS could cause unrecognized morbidity and adversely affect the efficacy and safety of other therapies, some of which are also nephrotoxic.

Standard management for hyperuricaemia is allopurinol (300 mg daily orally), hydration and attempted urinary alkalinization. Hydration is technically easy with CVCs, but the complexities of maintaining fluid balance and avoiding overload are described above. Urinary alkalinization is achievable but complicates the management of fluid and electrolyte balance and, in practice, it is difficult to maintain the urinary pH above 8. Allopurinol blocks the formation of uric acid by inhibition of xanthine oxidase, increasing plasma and urinary concentrations of hypoxanthine and xanthine. Xanthine is less soluble than uric acid in urine and occasional cases of nephropathy are described as a consequence of this therapy. Patients have a backlog of excess uric acid that they must excrete, particularly those with a high tumour burden, and allopurinol has no effect

on that. Hypersensitivity to allopurinol is well recognized, especially in the elderly, and causes distressing allergic dermatitis that may exfoliate. Interaction with other medications (warfarin, thiazide diuretics, antibiotics such as ampicillin and amoxicillin, and chemotherapy such as mercaptopurine and azathioprine) is well described. Many patients have difficulty taking the drug orally; this may not be widely recognized and the alternative intravenous formulation is not sufficiently prescribed. Allopurinol reduces or normalizes the serum uric acid level in the great majority of adult and paediatric patients. The recombinant enzyme rasburicase produces a fall in uric acid concentrations within 1 hour and is a safe and effective alternative for those patients who require rapid control of hyperuricaemia or who cannot tolerate allopurinol. At present, recommended dosage schedules may be excessive and the drug is expensive, but rasburicase also avoids the need for hyperhydration and urinary alkalinization.

Abnormalities of renal function and electrolyte balance

The hyperphosphataemia, hyperkalaemia and hypocalcaemia associated with TLS are described above, but other electrolyte problems occur more commonly. Hypokalaemia and hyponatraemia are the most frequent, and require regular intravenous supplements. Prolonged and copious diarrhoea will also result in hypokalaemia. Both hypokalaemia and hyponatraemia are also intrinsic to the acute leukaemias because of the high plasma levels of lysozyme (particularly in the monocytic FAB subtypes M4 and M5), which interferes with proximal tubular function. Intravenous amphotericin also induces renal tubular wasting of potassium and magnesium. This can be at least partially blocked by the diuretic amiloride (20 mg daily orally) but intravenous supplements of potassium, and less often of magnesium, are usually also required in patients receiving intravenous conventional amphotericin. Oral replacement of these electrolytes is ineffective. Liposomal amphotericin is less likely to create these electrolyte problems.

It is common practice to estimate urea and electrolyte levels daily during the aplastic phase of intensive chemotherapy, and magnesium levels should be estimated twice weekly. Otherwise, hypomagnesaemia may not be appreciated as the cause of confusion, neuropathy assumed to be due to hypocalcaemia and unexplained arrhythmia. Aminoglycosides and vancomycin are also toxic to renal tubules and can exacerbate these problems. Ciclosporin therapy in SCT is also nephrotoxic. Regular and frequent monitoring of the levels of all these drugs will reduce the risk of renal damage.

The same problems with electrolyte balance may occur in the ATN that results from hypotension due to sepsis, major blood loss and pulmonary capillary leak syndrome in acute respiratory distress syndrome. ATN is accompanied by failure of glomerular filtration, with oliguria or anuria, and a rise in the levels of serum creatinine and urea. In these patients, if the primary insult is treated successfully, then ATN resolves with a compensatory diuretic phase and full recovery of renal function. It is important to keep pace with the diuresis with adequate fluid replacement.

Amphotericin is also toxic to glomeruli and it should be discontinued or switched to the liposomal form once the creatinine has exceeded twice the level on starting the drug, assuming that was a normal value. The renal toxicity of amphotericin is almost always reversible and should not exclude its use if there is no pre-existing renal pathology or toxicity related to another drug. Before liposomal preparations were available, intravenous sodium loading was recommended to lessen the renal and electrolyte problems of amphotericin. This is seldom used now although it has never been compared prospectively against liposomal amphotericin.

Liver function abnormalities

In patients presenting with acute leukaemia, raised levels of lactate dehydrogenase are common because this is derived from bone marrow as well as liver. Some will also have nonspecific elevation of alkaline phosphatase and transaminase levels. About half will develop abnormally high levels of one or all of these measures of liver function owing to the direct hepatocellular toxicity of chemotherapy, with increased levels of serum bilirubin sufficient to cause clinical jaundice. It is seldom necessary to modify doses of remission induction drugs because of these abnormalities but recently there has been some concern about the hepatotoxicity of the antimetabolite purine analogue thioguanine, which is no longer available. Cytarabine, another purine analogue, also induces cholestasis and this hepatotoxicity may have been underestimated in the past.

Hyperbilirubinaemia with clinical jaundice is a frequent and sometimes overlooked complication of red cell transfusion that does not of itself indicate liver disease but is more obvious if liver function is impaired for any other reason. The hepatotoxicity of most chemotherapy is transient and resolves spontaneously with regeneration of normal marrow and induction of remission. It is usually asymptomatic and seldom progresses to severe liver failure, ascites, cirrhosis or portal hypertension except in specific cases described below. However, even minor impairment of liver function will affect other drugs that are dependent on liver metabolism to a degree that may require modification of doses.

Severe and fatal liver damage may occur with veno-occlusive disease in allogeneic SCT, described in detail in Chapter 38. This is thought to be a complication of preparatory or conditioning therapies prior to infusion of stem cells. A similar syndrome is seen with the new drug Mylotarg, which is now part of remission induction in the latest MRC AML 15 trial in adults.

Mylotarg, now commonly used in trials of therapy for acute myeloblastic leukaemia, consists of the cytotoxic antibiotic ozogamicin linked to the anti-CD33 monoclonal antibody gemtuzumab and is activated by hydrolysis once it is internalized following attachment of the antibody to leukaemic myeloblasts. This compound has dose-limiting hepatotoxicity. As with the simultaneous use of nephrotoxic drugs, careful monitoring of all potentially hepatotoxic drugs or any drugs that are metabolized by the liver will be necessary if they are used simultaneously. These drugs include the triazole antifungal group (fluconazole, itraconazole, voriconazole, posaconazole and ravuconazole), all of which impair liver function to variable degrees.

Chronic liver damage, including cirrhosis and the greatly increased risk of hepatocellular carcinoma, is now a well-recognized late effect of blood transfusion owing to infection with hepatitis C virus. Attempts to eradicate or reduce the viral load of these patients, using ribavarin and interferon, have met with limited success. As UK blood donors are routinely screened for this virus, the problem should become less prevalent in the future among multiply transfused patients.

The iron overload of multiple transfusion during therapy for acute leukaemias appears to cause clinical liver problems only in transplanted patients and can be reduced subsequently by venesection with or without iron chelation. In patients who are transfusion dependent due to marrow failure associated with chronic leukaemias, myelodysplasia or failure of therapy for any form of leukaemia, the inconvenience and side-effects of iron chelation usually outweigh any potential benefit, especially when life expectancy is short.

Nutritional support

During intensive therapy, anorexia persists, even if nausea and vomiting and the pain of mucositis can be controlled. Loss of total body mass is inevitable, the extent of which depends on the duration of anorexia and the impact of additional catabolic insults such as severe infection. All dietary supplementation should be managed by dietitians and pharmacists in order to calculate accurately the contents of the supplements, on the basis of regular blood results. Oral supplementation may be sufficient to maintain an adequate caloric intake in less severe cases. For patients with a predictable or actual 10% or greater reduction in pretreatment weight, total nutrition is indicated. This is likely in the majority of patients receiving myelo-ablative allogeneic SCT. This can be given through a nasojejunal fine silastic tube, provided that this is inserted before the onset of mucositis, otherwise nutritional support must be given by indwelling intravenous catheter. As soon as patients recover the will to eat, all such dietary supplements can be cautiously withdrawn.

Nausea and vomiting

There is a high risk of severe and acute emesis with intensive chemotherapy. Every effort should be made to prevent this distressing complication and to avoid the development of anticipatory emesis should prophylaxis be ineffective. If control fails early, then the chances of later successful control are reduced. It must be remembered that emesis may be due to other drugs (e.g. analgesics and antimicrobials), to acute infection and to other complications of leukaemia and its treatment such as meningeal relapse, intestinal obstruction (e.g. secondary to hypokalaemia and gut or retroperitoneal bleeding) or intracranial bleeding.

There are three major groups of antiemetic drugs: the serotonin antagonists (e.g. ondansetron, granisetron), the steroids (mainly dexamethasone) and a wide range of drugs that are sedative as well as antiemetic (e.g. metoclopramide, domperidone, haloperidol, lorazepam, cannabinoids and phenothiazines). Of these three classes, the serotonin antagonists will control emesis induced by intensive chemotherapy completely in about two-thirds of patients. Additional dexamethasone may benefit a further 10–20% of patients. All the sedating antiemetic agents are of second choice in intensive therapy. Their dosage, route of administration and scheduling should be strictly controlled and they should not be given on an uncontrolled or as-required basis. Cumulative oversedation is a major risk in these patients, particularly if they need simultaneous opiates for mucositis and antihistamines for allergic reactions to blood and drugs and develop hypoxia of infection or heart failure. Many of these drugs can also cause distressing dyskinesias.

For nausea due to less intensive oral therapy of CLL, oral busulphan or hydoxyurea for CML metaclopramide may suffice and many patients do not need any antiemetic drug. There is a very low risk of nausea with imatinib.

Pain

Bone pain is an uncommon presenting feature of acute leukaemia, is due to an expanded marrow cavity packed with blasts and can occur or recur on relapse. Such pain is relieved by remission induction but may need temporary control with opiates. G-CSF and granulocyte/macrophage colony-stimulating factor (GM-CSF) can cause the same problem by expansion of normal marrow cells due to excessive stimulation.

Avascular necrosis of bone is seen in less than 5% of patients with ALL and lymphomas, particularly in association with high-dose steroids and cyclophosphamide. It usually affects younger patients, involves the ends of long bones and can cause permanent bone death requiring subsequent joint replacement. The diagnosis is elusive and requires magnetic resonance imaging. The pain is often severe enough to need relief with opiates.

High-dose cytarabine can cause a painful vasculitis severe enough to lead to necrosis of soft tissue and skin. The neuropathy of the vinca alkaloids (usually vincristine but occasionally vinblastine) may present as limb pain or as painful constipation. The serotonin antagonists may cause headache in susceptible individuals and headache may also be due to intracranial bleeding or infection. Any bleed in any confined compartment will be painful, for example chest wall pain following haemorrhagic insertion of a CVC.

In SCT, the use of total body irradiation and high-dose chemotherapy make gut mucositis inevitable. The extent, duration and severity vary but most patients will need some level of opiate relief. In most patients, this starts in the second week after therapy and resolves spontaneously without lasting sequelae from the third to fourth week onwards. As with all causes of pain, this requires whatever level of controlled drug analgesia is necessary to make the symptoms bearable without inducing brain or respiratory failure. Continuous intravenous infusion of an opiate is often required in severe mucositis and additional continuous antiemetic may be needed in the same infusion. Palifermin (recombinant human keratinocyte growth factor) has been shown to reduce oral mucositis after intensive chemotherapy. All units should have a written protocol for pain control similar to that used by the local palliative care team.

Palliation

The above account of supportive care of the patient with leukaemia describes a holistic approach. It is common for patients who have experienced this to wish to remain with the same haematology team for their terminal care when there is no further prospect of control of their underlying disease. There should be choices at this stage, which include the transfer of the patient to the palliative care team and joint management by them with haematology in whichever unit the patient and family feel most suits the patient's needs. These choices should include dying at home, an option that requires some help from the acute care unit to mobilize the resources available in some communities to support this option. Most of the issues which arise in this palliative phase of care are described above. There can be much more flexibility in the frequency and choice of blood support, in pain control and in the use of antibiotics. Wherever palliative care is given, the patient and family should not feel abandoned by the team who supported them during previous periods of treatment.

Selected bibliography

Bow EJ, Laverdiere M, Lussier N, Rotstein C, Cheang MS, Ioannou S (2002) Antifungal prophylaxis for severely neutropenic chemotherapy recipients: a meta analysis of randomized-controlled clinical trials. *Cancer* **94**: 3230–46.

Caillot D, Casasnovas O, Bernard A *et al.* (1997) Improved management of invasive pulmonary aspergillosis in neutropenic patients using early thoracic computed tomographic scan and surgery. *Journal of Clinical Oncology* **15**: 139–47.

Cometta A, Calandra T, Gaya H *et al.* (1996) Monotherapy with meropenem versus combination therapy with ceftazidime plus amikacin as empiric therapy for fever in granulocytopenic patients with cancer. The International Antimicrobial Therapy Cooperative Group of the European Organization for Research and Treatment of Cancer and the Gruppo Italiano Malattie Ematologiche Maligne dell'Adulto Infection Program. *Antimicrobial Agents Chemotherapy* **40**: 1108–15.

Cometta A, Kern WV, De Bock R *et al.* (2003) Vancomycin versus placebo for treating persistent fever in patients with neutropenic cancer receiving piperacillin-tazobactam monotherapy. *Clinical Infectious Diseases* **37**: 382–9.

Cruciani M, Rampazzo R, Malena M *et al.* (1996) Prophylaxis with fluoroquinolones for bacterial infections in neutropenic patients: a meta-analysis. *Clinical Infectious Diseases* **23**: 795–805.

De Pauw B, Walsh TJ, Donnelly JP *et al.* (2008) Revised definitions of invasive fungal disease from the European Organization for Research and Treatment of Cancer/Invasive Fungal Infections Cooperative Group and the National Institute of Allergy and Infectious Diseases Mycoses Study Group (EORTC/MSG) Consensus Group. *Clinical Infectious Diseases* **46**: 1813–21.

DesJardin JA, Falagas ME, Ruthazer R *et al.* (1999) Clinical utility of blood cultures drawn from indwelling central venous catheters in hospitalized patients with cancer. *Annals of Internal Medicine* **131**: 641–7.

Donnelly JP (2001) Infection in bone marrow transplant patients. In: *Pathology and Immunology of Transplantation and Rejection* (S Thiru, H Waldmaan, eds), pp. 526–66. Blackwell Science, Oxford.

Engels EA, Lau J, Barza M (1998) Efficacy of quinolone prophylaxis in neutropenic cancer patients: a meta-analysis. *Journal of Clinical Oncology* **16**: 1179–87.

Feusner J, Farber MS (2000) Role of intravenous allopurinol in the management of acute tumour lysis syndrome. *Seminars in Oncology* **28** (Suppl. 5): 13–18.

Furno P, Bucaneve G, Del Favero A (2002) Monotherapy or aminoglycoside–containing combinations for empirical antibiotic treatment of febrile neutropenic patients: a meta-analysis. *Lancet Infectious Diseases* **2**: 231–42.

Gafter-Gvili A, Fraser A, Paul M, Leibovici L (2005) Meta-analysis: antibiotic prophylaxis reduces mortality in neutropenic patients. *Annals of Internal Medicine* **142**: 979–95.

Glasmacher A, Prentice AG, Gorschluter M *et al.* (2003) Itraconazole prevents invasive fungal infections in neutropenic patients treated for haematological malignancies; evidence from a meta-

analysis of 3597 patients. *Journal of Clinical Oncology* **21**: 4616–26.

Goldberg E, Gafter-Gvili A, Robenshtok E, Leibovici L, Paul M (2008) Empirical antifungal therapy for patients with neutropenia and persistent fever: systematic review and meta-analysis. *European Journal of Cancer* **44**: 2192–203.

Imran H, Tleyjeh IM, Arndt CA *et al.* (2008) Fluoroquinolone prophylaxis in patients with neutropenia: a meta-analysis of randomized placebo-controlled trials. *European Journal of Clinical Microbiology and Infectious Disease* **27**: 53–63.

McClelland B (2001) Effective use of blood components. In: *Practical Transfusion Medicine* (MF Murphy, DH Pamphilon, eds), pp. 65–76. Blackwell Science, Oxford.

Maertens J, Van Eldere J, Verhaegen J *et al.* (2002) Use of circulating galactomannan screening for early diagnosis of invasive aspergillosis in allogeneic stem cell transplant recipients. *Journal of Infectious Diseases* **186**: 1297–306.

Minton O, Richardson A, Sharpe M, Hotopf M, Stone P (2008) A systematic review and meta-analysis of the pharmacological treatment of cancer-related fatigue. *Journal of the National Cancer Institute* **100**: 1155–66.

Minton O, Stone P, Richardson A, Sharpe M, Hotopf M (2010) Drug therapy for the management of cancer related fatigue. *Cochrane Database of Systematic Reviews* (1): CD006704. Available at http://www.cochrane.org/reviews/en/ab006704.html

Murphy MF (2001) Haematological disease. In: *Practical Transfusion Medicine* (MF Murphy, DH Pamphilon, eds), pp. 108–18. Blackwell Science, Oxford.

National Comprehensive Cancer Network. NCCN Clinical Practice Guidelines in Oncology, particularly Cancer- and Chemotherapy-induced Anemia, Myelodysplastic Syndrome, and Myeloid Growth Factors. Available at http://www.nccn.org/professionals/physician_gls/f_guidelines.asp guideline

National Institute for Health and Clinical Excellence. Anaemia (cancer-treatment induced): erythropoietin (alpha and beta) and darbepoetin. Technology appraisals TA142. Available at http://guidance.nice.org.uk/TA142

Paul M, Soares-Weiser K, Leibovici L (2003) Beta lactam monotherapy versus beta lactam–aminoglycoside combination therapy for fever with neutropenia: systematic review and meta-analysis. *British Medical Journal* **326**: 1111.

Pui C-H, Mahmoud HH, Wiley JM *et al.* (2001) Recombinant urate oxidase for the prophylaxis and treatment of hyperuricaemia in patients with leukaemia and lymphoma. *Journal of Clinical Oncology* **19**: 697–704.

Spielberger R, Stiff P, Bensinger W *et al.* (2004) Palifermin for oral mucositis after intensive therapy for hematalogic cancers. *New England Journal of Medicine* **351**: 2590–8.

Twycross R, Wilcock A (eds) (2001) *Symptom Management in Advanced Cancer*. Radcliffe Medical Press, Oxford.

Chronic myeloid leukaemia

27

John M Goldman[1] and Tariq I Mughal[2]

[1]Imperial College School of Medicine, Hammersmith Hospital, London, UK
[2]Guy's Hospital, London, UK

Introduction

The term 'myeloproliferative neoplasm' has recently been introduced by the panel of experts convened by the World Health Organization (WHO) to classify tumours of the haemopoietic and lymphoid systems and chronic myeloid leukaemia (CML) is the most common subtype (Table 27.1). This chapter covers CML, chronic neutrophilic leukaemia, chronic eosinophilic leukaemia and some other variants, but the other myeloproliferative neoplasms are described elsewhere in this book.

Chronic myeloid leukaemia (also known as chronic myelogenous leukaemia and chronic granulocytic leukaemia) is a clonal disease that results from an acquired genetic change in a pluripotential haemopoietic stem cell. This altered stem cell proliferates and generates a population of differentiated cells that gradually displaces normal haemopoiesis and leads to a greatly expanded total myeloid mass. One important landmark in the study of CML was the discovery of the Philadelphia (Ph) chromosome in 1960, the next was the characterization in 1973 of the t(9;22)(q34;q11) translocation, a third was the identification in the 1980s of the BCR–ABL (now renamed BCR–ABL1) chimeric gene and associated oncoprotein, and a fourth was the demonstration that introducing the BCR–ABL gene into murine stem cells in experimental animals caused a disease that simulated human CML.

Until the 1980s, CML was generally assumed to be incurable and was treated palliatively, in the early days with radiotherapy and later with alkylating agents, notably busulfan. We now know that CML can be permanently eradicated in the majority of patients who survive haemopoietic stem cell transplantation (SCT), but the proportion of patients eligible for SCT is still relatively small. The introduction into clinical practice in 1998 of the original tyrosine kinase inhibitor (TKI) imatinib mesylate was an extremely important therapeutic advance, as with this agent most patients achieve a complete cytogenetic response and may expect substantial prolongation of survival compared with earlier methods of treatment. Current data suggest that the second-generation TKIs, dasatinib, nilotinib and bosutinib, may be more effective than imatinib.

Epidemiology, aetiology and natural history

The incidence of CML appears to be constant worldwide. It occurs in about 1.0–1.5 per 100 000 of the population per annum in all countries where statistics are adequate. CML is rare below the age of 20 years but occurs with increasing frequency with each decade of life. Currently, the median age of onset is 50–60 years. The incidence is slightly higher in males than in females.

Postgraduate Haematology: 6th edition. Edited by A. Victor Hoffbrand, Daniel Catovsky, Edward G.D. Tuddenham, Anthony R. Green
© 2011 Blackwell Publishing Ltd.

Table 27.1 Myeloproliferative neoplasms (WHO classification).

Chronic myelogenous leukaemia, *BCR–ABL1* positive
Chronic neutrophilic leukaemia
Polycythaemia vera
Primary myelofibrosis
Essential thrombocythaemia
Chronic eosinophilic leukaemia
Mastocytosis
Myeloproliferative neoplasm unclassifiable

Source: Swerdlow *et al.* (2008).

Table 27.2 Sokal index for predicting survival prognostic indices.

Good prognosis	<0.8
Moderate prognosis	0.8–1.2
Poor prognosis	>1.2

Mathematical expression

$\text{Exp}[0.0116(\text{age} - 43.4)] + 0.0345(\text{spleen size} - 7.51) + 0.188[(\text{platelet count}/700)^2 - 0.563] + 0.0887(\text{percentage of blasts} - 2.10)$

The risk of developing CML is slightly but significantly increased by exposure to high doses of irradiation, as occurred in survivors of the atomic bombs exploded in Japan in 1945, and in patients irradiated for ankylosing spondylitis and malignant diseases but, in general, almost all cases must be regarded as sporadic without identifiable predisposing factors. In particular, there is no familial predisposition and no definite association with HLA genotypes. No contributory infectious agent has been incriminated.

Clinically, CML is classically a biphasic or triphasic disease that is usually diagnosed in the initial 'chronic', 'indolent' or 'stable' phase. Until 10 years ago the disease evolved spontaneously after some years into an advanced phase, which could often be subdivided into an earlier accelerated phase and a later acute or blastic phase. This pattern has altered fundamentally since the introduction of TKIs and today the majority of patients may never progress beyond the chronic phase. There has been much debate about the duration of the leukaemia before the diagnosis is established, a question that is essentially unanswerable. If it is assumed that the disease starts with a transforming event in a single stem cell, it could be 5–10 years before the disease becomes clinically manifest. This estimate depends on the assumption that the leucocyte doubling time before diagnosis is not fundamentally different from the doubling time after diagnosis (which may not be the case), and on the observation that the latent interval between exposure to irradiation from atomic bombs and the earliest identifiable increased incidence of CML was about 7 years. One study concluded that a routine blood count might have identified CML on average 6 months before it was actually diagnosed in individual patients.

Patients are usually in the chronic phase when CML is diagnosed. This chronic phase used to last about 2–7 years and these figures may still be valid for the 20% of patients who fail treatment with TKIs; however, for most patients who respond well to TKIs, survival is likely to exceed 20 years and some could have a normal lifespan. In about 50% of the patients who fail TKI treatment the chronic phase transforms unpredictably and abruptly to a more aggressive phase that used to be referred to as 'blastic crisis' and is now usually described as acute or blastic transformation, which may have myeloblastic or lymphoblastic features; in the other half of cases, the disease evolves somewhat more gradually through an intermediate phase described as the accelerated phase, which may last for months or years, before frank blastic transformation supervenes. Occasional patients have a disease that progresses gradually to a myelofibrotic or osteomyelosclerotic picture that is characterized by extensive marrow fibrosis and sometimes gross overgrowth of bony trabeculae; the clinical problems are then usually due to failure of haemopoiesis rather than to blast cell proliferation, but a predominantly blastic disease can still supervene. The duration of survival after onset of transformation is usually 3–9 months.

Classification

The majority of patients with CML have a relatively homogeneous disease characterized at diagnosis by splenomegaly, leucocytosis and the presence of the *BCR–ABL1* fusion gene in all leukaemic cells. The presence of this fusion gene is regarded today as the *sine qua non* for diagnosis of CML. A minority of patients have less typical disease that may be classified as atypical CML, chronic myelomonocytic leukaemia or chronic neutrophilic leukaemia (CNL). Children may have a disease referred to as juvenile chronic myelomonocytic leukaemia. In none of these variants (other than extremely rare variants of CNL) is there a *BCR–ABL1* fusion gene or a Ph chromosome.

Staging

Many attempts have been made to subclassify or 'stage' chronic-phase CML at diagnosis, in a manner that would permit some prediction of the duration of chronic phase in individual patients. The most commonly used classification, devised by Sokal and colleagues in 1984, is based on a formula that takes account of the patient's age, blast cell percentage, spleen size and platelet count at diagnosis (Table 27.2) (http://oncopda.com/sokal.htm). A similar classification, which may or may not prove more useful than that of Sokal, was introduced by Hasford

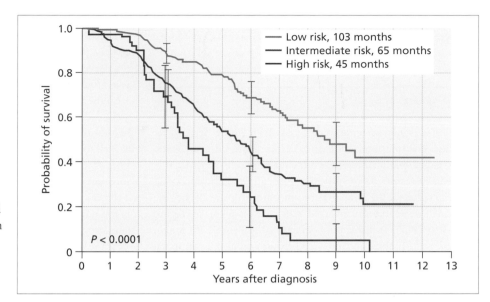

Figure 27.1 Probability of survival and median survival values for a population of CML patients classified into three prognostic categories according to the Euro score devised by Hasford *et al.* (1998).

in 1998 and called the Hasford or Euro score (Figure 27.1); it makes use of eosinophil and basophil numbers in addition to the values included in the Sokal system.

In practice, patients who have a low leucocyte doubling time probably survive longer than those with more rapid doubling times. Moreover, the patient's response to initial treatment does give some information about duration of survival; for example, a complete cytogenetic response to interferon alfa or rapid reduction in *BCR–ABL1* transcript numbers in patients starting treatment with imatinib are both good prognostic factors. Conversely, other possible adverse prognostic factors, such as those that predict a poor response to TKI, may in the future be integrated into systems for staging patients with CML. However, it is likely that the results of gene expression profiling or characterization of genome-wide aberrations will eventually be the most informative approach for predicting overall duration of disease.

Cell biology

It is presumed that the leukaemic stem cell replicates and that its progeny give rise to increased numbers of myeloid progenitor cells and also of differentiated progeny. Thus, the normal marrow is gradually replaced by a leukaemic myeloid mass that expands to fill normal fat spaces and encroaches on areas of long bones that are normally devoid of haemopoiesis in the adult. The increased myelopoiesis involves primarily the granulocyte series, but megakaryocyte and platelet numbers are also usually increased. Obvious erythroid hyperplasia and polycythaemia occur only rarely.

In the absence of a convincing assay for human haemopoietic stem cells, a number of efforts have been made to quantify *in*

vitro its nearest counterpart, variously designated 'long-term culture-initiating cells', 'high-proliferative capacity progenitor cells' or 'blast colony-forming cells'. In general, the numbers of such cells seem to be moderately increased (threefold to tenfold) in CML marrow compared with normal marrow, but results are inconsistent. In contrast, the numbers of committed progenitors (i.e. CFU-GEMM, BFU-E and CFU-GM) are greatly increased compared with normal, and this increase is proportionately much larger in the blood than in the marrow of untreated CML patients. BFU-E and CFU-GM numbers in the blood are significantly correlated with the leucocyte count; their numbers are restored to normal or subnormal levels by appropriate treatment.

Theoretically, an apparently autonomous proliferation of myeloid progenitors could be due to increased responsiveness to one or more physiological stimulators of haemopoiesis or to loss of sensitivity to a normal inhibitor. As a consequence of this, many efforts have been directed to assessing the response of CML progenitors to haemopoietic growth factors, notably granulocyte colony-stimulating factor (G-CSF), granulocyte/macrophage colony-stimulating factor (GM-CSF), interleukin (IL)-3, stem cell factor and erythropoietin. There is some evidence that the autonomous proliferation could be due to an autocrine loop involving G-CSF and IL-3. It may also be due to increased production of elastase by the leukaemia cells that inhibits the response of normal but not leukaemia cells to G-CSF.

CML progenitors in *in vitro* culture systems adhere less well to preformed marrow stromal layers than their normal counterparts. This may be due to an abnormality of an integrin or absence of a glycosylphosphatidylinositol-anchored protein that has not yet been defined. Thus, it is possible that the excessive proliferation of CML progenitors is due partly to their premature escape from physiological inhibitory influences in the stem cell niche.

Cytogenetics

The Philadelphia (originally designated Ph[1], now der22q– or Ph) chromosome (see Chapter 29) is an acquired cytogenetic abnormality that characterizes all leukaemic cells in CML. It is formed as a result of a reciprocal translocation of chromosomal material between the long arms of one chromosome 22 and one chromosome 9, an event referred to as t(9;22)(q34;q11) (Figure 27.2). The (9;22) translocation generates the BCR–ABL1 fusion gene on the Ph chromosome (see below) and also a reciprocal fusion gene, designated ABL1–BCR, on the derivative 9q+ chromosome. Such translocations involving just two chromosomes are described as simple, whereas about 10% of patients have complex translocations involving chromosomes 9, 22 and one or sometimes two other chromosomes.

In CML patients, the Ph chromosome is present in all myeloid cell lineages, in some B cells and in a very small proportion of T cells. It is found in no other cells of the body. This distribution is not altered by traditional treatment with busulfan or hydroxycarbamide (hydroxyurea). Although valuable since the 1960s as a marker of the leukaemic cell, its true pathogenetic signifi-

cance remained uncertain until the identification of the BCR–ABL1 chimeric gene on the Ph chromosome in the 1980s. About 15% of patients have small deletions of chromosomal material on der9q+, which usually include the reciprocal ABL1–BCR gene. Such deletions are thought to occur contemporaneously with the formation of the BCR–ABL1 gene on the Ph chromosome and denoted a relatively poor overall prognosis in the era before imatinib; however, patients with 9q+ deletions respond as well to TKIs as those lacking such deletions. A small proportion of patients with clinically classical CML lack the Ph chromosome and have a normal karyotype; however, these do have a typical BCR–ABL1 gene expressed as a p210 oncoprotein (see below) on a normal-appearing chromosome 22 (or very occasionally on a normal chromosome 9).

Some, but not all, patients acquire additional clonal cytogenetic abnormalities during the course of the chronic phase. There was suspicion that some such changes might be caused in part by administration of alkylating agents, but they can undoubtedly occur spontaneously. The observation of non-random changes, typically +8, +Ph, iso-17q or +19, sometimes means that such new clones will expand and that blastic transformation will manifest itself within weeks or months, but these new clones (other than iso-17q) can remain clinically unimportant for many years. In overt blastic transformation, 80% of patients have clonal cytogenetic changes in addition to the Ph translocation.

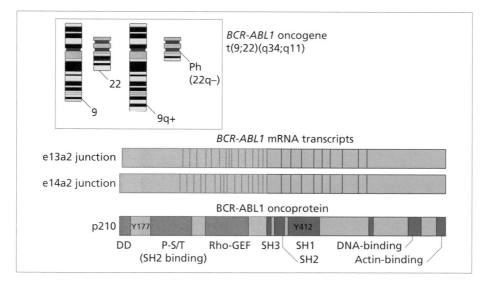

Figure 27.2 The t(9;22) translocation and its products: the BCR–ABL1 oncogene on the Ph chromosome and the reciprocal ABL1–BCR gene on the derivative 9q+ chromosome. In classic CML, BCR–ABL1 is transcribed into mRNA molecules with e13a2 or e14a2 junctions, which are then translated into the p210[BCR–ABL1] oncoprotein. This oncoprotein is a hybrid containing functional domains from the N-terminal end of BCR (dimerization domain, DD), SRC-homology 2 (SH2)-binding and the Rho GTP–GDP exchange factor (GEF) domains and the C-terminal end of ABL1. [Only SRC-homology regions 2, 3 and 1 (SH2, SH3 and SH1 respectively) and the DNA- and actin-binding domains are shown.] Tyrosine 177 (Y177) in the BCR portion of the fusion oncoprotein and tyrosine 412 (Y412) in the ABL1 portion are important for the docking of adapter proteins and for BCR–ABL1 autophosphorylation respectively. P-S/T denotes phosphoserine and phosphothreonine.

Table 27.3 Definitions of cytogenetic and molecular responses.

Cytogenetic response

Designation	Percentage of Ph-positive marrow metaphases	Molecular response (BCR–ABL1 transcript numbers expressed on the international scale)
Complete	0	Baseline, 100%
Partial	1–35	Cytogenetic response, ~1%
Minor	36–65	Major molecular response, 0.1%
Minimal	66–95	Complete molecular response, ~0.001%
None	>95	

Note: The term 'major cytogenetic response' is used to refer to the sum of patients who achieve complete cytogenetic response and those who only achieve a partial cytogenetic response. The level of complete molecular response must depend on the sensitivity of the assay and the term 'BCR–ABL1 transcripts undetectable' is formally more precise.

In the majority of patients at diagnosis all marrow metaphases show the Ph chromosome. In the past treatment with interferon alfa reduced the proportion of Ph-positive metaphases in a minority of patients. Since the introduction of TKIs, serial measurement of the percentage of Ph-positive marrow metaphases has become an important tool in assessing the level of response in individual patients (Table 27.3).

Molecular biology

It was shown in the early 1980s that the *ABL1* proto-oncogene, which encodes a non-receptor tyrosine kinase, was normally located on chromosome 9 but was translocated to chromosome 22 in CML patients. In 1984 the precise positions of the genomic breakpoint on chromosome 22 in different CML patients were found to be clustered in a relatively small 5.8-kb region to which the name 'breakpoint cluster region' (BCR) was given. Later, it became clear that this region formed the central part of a relatively large gene now known as the *BCR* gene, whose normal function is not well defined, and the breakpoint region was renamed 'major breakpoint cluster region' (M-BCR) (see Table 27.3). In contrast, the position of the genomic breakpoint in the *ABL* gene (now often referred to as the *ABL1* gene to distinguish it from the ABL1-related gene, *ARG* or *ABL2*) is very variable, but it always occurs upstream of the second (common) exon (a2). Thus, the Ph translocation results in juxtaposition of 5′ sequences from the *BCR* gene with 3′ *ABL1* sequences derived from chromosome 9 (Figure 27.3). It produces a chimeric gene,

designated *BCR–ABL*, or better *BCR–ABL1*, that is transcribed as an 8.5-kb mRNA and encodes a protein of 210 kDa. This p210$^{BCR–ABL1}$ oncoprotein has far greater tyrosine kinase activity than the normal *ABL1* gene product.

In CML, there are two variants of the *BCR–ABL1* transcript, depending on whether the break in M-BCR occurs in the intron between exons e13 and e14, or in the intron between exons e14 and e15. A break in the former intron yields an e13a2 mRNA junction and a break in the latter intron yields an e14a2 junction. (It should be noted that exon e13 was previously termed exon b2 and exon e14 was previously b3; thus the two RNA junctions were known until recently as b2a2 and b3a2 respectively.) Most patients have transcripts with features of either e13a2 or e14a2, but occasional patients have both transcripts present in their leukaemia cells. The precise type of *BCR–ABL1* transcript has no prognostic significance for CML patients. Moreover, the reciprocal *ABL1–BCR* gene on der9q+ is expressed in about 70% of patients, but its expression or lack of expression does not have prognostic significance.

A minority of patients with Ph-positive acute lymphoblastic leukaemia (ALL), more often adults than children, also have *BCR–ABL1* fusion genes in their leukaemia cells (see Chapters 29 and 31). In about one-third of Ph-positive ALL patients, the molecular features of the *BCR–ABL1* gene are indistinguishable from those of CML; in the remaining two-thirds the genomic breakpoint occurs in the first intron of the *BCR* gene (a zone designated 'minor breakpoint cluster region' or m-BCR) and the *BCR–ABL1* gene results from fusion of the first exon (designated e1) of the *BCR* gene with the second exon (a2) of the *ABL1* gene. The mRNA is designated e1a2 and encodes a protein of 190 kDa (p190$^{BCR–ABL1}$). Very rare patients with CML have a p190 protein instead of the usual p210. Equally rare is the finding of a Ph chromosome in association with chronic neutrophilic leukaemia. Such patients may have an mRNA formed from an e19a2 fusion gene associated with a p230$^{BCR–ABL1}$ oncoprotein.

The *BCR–ABL1* gene has been cloned and inserted into a retroviral vector that has been used to transfect murine haemopoietic stem cells; these transduced stem cells can generate a disease resembling human CML in mice. Thus, the *BCR–ABL1* gene is thought to play a pivotal role in the genesis of chronic-phase CML.

The mechanism by which the BCR–ABL1 oncoprotein alters stem cell kinetics remains ill-defined. It undoubtedly aberrantly autophosphorylates and also phosphorylates a wide range of intracellular proteins that would not normally be phosphorylated, including Crkl, Mek 1/2, Rac and Jnk. It may act by activating the RAS or STAT signal transduction pathways. Alternatively, it may activate the phosphatidylinositol 3-kinase/AKT pathway involved in facilitating apoptosis (Figure 27.4). As an activated ABL1 opposes cellular apoptosis, the *BCR–ABL1* gene might act by impeding programmed cell death in target stem cells.

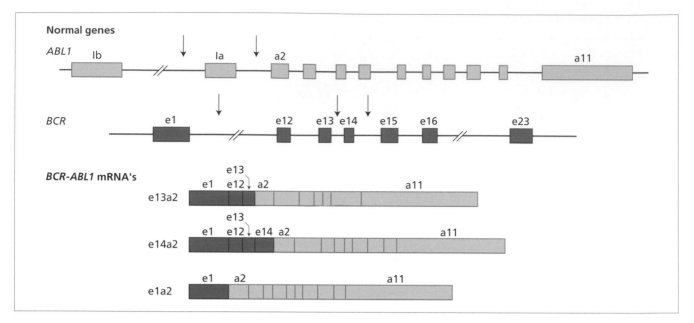

Figure 27.3 The structure of the normal *BCR* and *ABL1* genes and the fusion transcripts found in CML and Ph-positive ALL. The *ABL1* gene contains two alternative 5′ exons (named Ib and Ia) followed by 10 'common' exons numbered a2–a11 (orange boxes). Breakpoints in CML and Ph-positive ALL usually occur in the introns between exons Ib and Ia or between exons Ia and a2 (as shown by vertical arrows). The *BCR* gene comprises a total of 23 exons, 11 exons upstream of the M-BCR region, five exons in the M-BCR that were originally termed b1–b5 and now renamed e12–e16, and seven exons downstream of M-BCR. For convenience, only exons e1, e12–e16 and e23 are shown. Breakpoints in CML usually occur between exons e13 (b2) and e14 (b3) or between exons e14 (b3) and e15 (b4) of the M-BCR (as shown by two vertical arrows placed centrally). The majority of patients with Ph-positive ALL have breakpoints in the first intron of the gene, between e1 and e2 (not shown) (arrow at left). Three possible *BCR–ABL1* mRNA transcripts are shown below. The first two (e13a2 and e14a2 respectively) are characteristic of CML. The bottom mRNA (e1a2) is found in the majority of patients with Ph-positive ALL (see text).

The molecular basis of disease progression is still obscure, but it seems reasonable to infer that one or, more probably, a series of additional genetic events occurs in the Ph-positive clone. When the critical combination of additional events is achieved, clinically definable transformation ensues. At this stage, the leukaemia cells usually harbour one or other of the additional cytogenetic changes referred to above. About 20% of patients with CML in myeloid transformation have point mutations or deletions in the coding sequence of the *TP53* tumour-suppressor gene, a gene implicated in progression of a variety of solid tumours, notably colonic carcinoma. The retinoblastoma (*RB*) gene is deleted in rare cases of CML in megakaryoblastic transformation, and changes in the *LYN*, *EVI1* and *MYC* genes are described. About half of the patients with lymphoid blast transformations have homozygous deletions in the p16 (*CDKN2A*) gene, whose normal function is to inhibit cyclin-dependent kinase 4, and others have deletions of the *IKZF1* (Ikaros) gene. Molecular changes underlying the non-random cytogenetic changes described above have not been identified.

Clinical features

In the past, the majority of patients presented with symptoms, usually attributable to splenomegaly, haemorrhage or anaemia. In recent years, CML has been diagnosed in almost 50% of patients before the onset of symptoms as a result of routine blood tests performed as part of medical examinations in healthy persons, for pregnancy, before blood donation or in the course of investigation for unrelated disorders. When present, symptoms may include lethargy, loss of energy, shortness of breath on exertion or weight loss or haemorrhage from various sites. Increased sweating is characteristic. Spontaneous bruising or unexplained bleeding from gums, intestine or urinary tract are relatively common. Visual disturbances may occur. Fever and lymphadenopathy are rare in chronic phase. The patient may have severe pain or discomfort in the splenic area, often associated with splenic infarction, or may have noticed a lump or mass in the right upper abdomen. Visual disturbances may

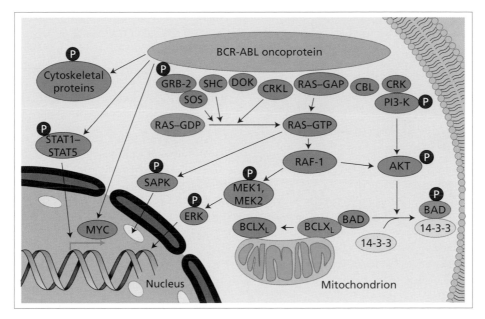

Figure 27.4 Signal transduction pathways affected by BCR–ABL1. The cellular effects of BCR–ABL1 are exerted through interactions with various proteins that transduce the oncogenic signals responsible for the activation or repression of gene transcription, of mitochondrial processing of apoptotic responses, of cytoskeletal organization and of the degradation of inhibitory proteins. The key pathways implicated so far are those involving RAS, mitogen-activated protein kinases, signal transducers and activators of transcription (STAT), phosphatidylinositol 3-kinase (PI3-K) and MYC. Most of the interactions are mediated through tyrosine phosphorylation and require the binding of BCR–ABL1 to adapter proteins such as growth factor receptor-bound protein 2 (GRB-2), DOK, CRK, CRK-like protein (CRKL), SRC homology-containing protein (SHC) and casitas B-lineage lymphoma protein (CBL). As we start to dissect these various interactions, we can design drugs aimed at disrupting specific branches of these pathways in an attempt either to kill the CML cell or to cause its phenotype to revert to normal. It is obvious that the best target is BCR–ABL1 itself, as this is the only protein that is exclusive to the leukaemic clone. The second-best approach is to target key downstream effectors of BCR–ABL1; however, this approach might, in principle, adversely affect normal haemopoiesis as well. P, phosphate.

be due to retinal haemorrhages. Sudden hearing loss occurs very rarely. Patients may present with features of gout or priapism in males, both of which are also rare.

At diagnosis, 50–70% of patients have splenomegaly. The spleen varies from just palpable to being so large that it occupies all the left side of the abdomen and is palpable also in the right iliac fossa. The liver is frequently also enlarged but with a soft edge that is difficult to define. There may be no other abnormal findings. Ecchymoses of varying sizes and ages may be present and may form discoloured subcutaneous lumps. Some patients have asymptomatic retinal haemorrhages. Patients with very high leucocyte counts may have features of leucostasis, with retinal vein engorgement and respiratory insufficiency.

Patients presenting with more advanced disease nearly always have some of the features described above. In addition, they may have bone tenderness or signs of infection. In established blastic transformation, the spleen is frequently enlarged and may be painful. The liver may become very large. Patients may develop fever, lymphadenopathy or very rarely lytic lesions of bone.

Laboratory haematology

Chronic phase

Patients with splenomegaly are usually anaemic, while the haemoglobin concentration may be normal in patients with 'early' disease. The leucocyte count at diagnosis is usually in the range $20–200 \times 10^9$/L, but the diagnosis of CML can be established by appropriate investigations in patients with persistent leucocytosis in the range $10–20 \times 10^9$/L; at the other extreme, occasional patients may present with leucocyte numbers in the range $200–800 \times 10^9$/L. The blood film shows a full spectrum of cells in the granulocyte series, ranging from blast forms to mature neu-

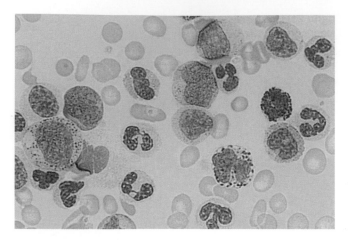

Figure 27.5 Peripheral blood appearances of a patient with CML at diagnosis. Note increased numbers of leucocytes including immature granulocytes and occasional blast cells.

Table 27.4 Criteria for distinguishing the chronic, accelerated and blastic phases of CML based on proposals published by WHO (2001).

Chronic phase
Ability to reduce spleen size and restore and maintain a 'normal' blood count with appropriate therapy

Accelerated phase (defined by one or more of the following features)
Blasts 10–19% of white blood cells in peripheral blood and/or of nucleated bone marrow cells
Peripheral blood basophils ≥20%
Persistent thrombocytopenia (<100 × 10⁹/L) unrelated to therapy, or persistent thrombocytosis (>1000 × 10⁹/L) unresponsive to therapy
Increasing spleen size and increasing white blood cell count unresponsive to therapy
Megakaryocyte proliferation in sheets or clusters in association with marked reticulin or collagen fibrosis

Blastic phase (defined by one or more of the following features)
Blasts >20% of peripheral blood leucocytes or of nucleated bone marrow cells
Extramedullary blast proliferation
Large foci or clusters of blasts in the bone marrow biopsy

Note: In this classification, unlike some other classifications, the acquisition of new cytogenetic abnormalities in addition to the Ph chromosome is not by itself a criterion for 'promoting' a chronic-phase patient to accelerated phase.

trophils, with intermediate myelocytes and neutrophils predominating (Figure 27.5). The percentage of blast cells is loosely related to the absolute number of leucocytes, but a value higher than 12% suggests that the patient may already be in acceleration or transformation. The percentages of eosinophils and basophils are usually increased, and the absence of basophilia casts doubt on the diagnosis. Absolute numbers of lymphocytes and monocytes are slightly increased, but both are reduced as percentages in the differential count. Platelet numbers are usually increased in the range 300–600 × 10⁹/L but may be normal or even reduced. Occasional nucleated red cells are present in the circulation in some patients. The alkaline phosphatase content of the neutrophil cytoplasm is diminished or absent. *BCR–ABL1* transcripts can be demonstrated in the blood with ease, using real-time quantitative polymerase chain reaction (RQ-PCR). In a minority of patients, the leucocyte count, if left untreated, shows cyclical variation, but the overall trend is upwards.

Examination of the bone marrow by aspiration or trephine biopsy is not necessary to confirm the diagnosis of CML, but is usually carried out to assess the degree of marrow fibrosis, perform cytogenetic analysis on marrow cells and exclude incipient transformation. The marrow aspirate may show multiple small hypercellular fragments but is often so hypercellular that fragments cannot easily be discerned. When spread on a glass slide, the trails show a cellular composition resembling that of CML blood. Blast cells in chronic phase number 2–10%. Eosinophils and basophils are usually prominent; megakaryocytes are small, hypolobated and very numerous. Occasionally, Gaucher-like cells are present. The marrow biopsy shows complete loss of fat spaces with dense hypercellularity. The reticulin content may be normal or modestly increased.

Advanced phases

The haematological picture in acceleration is very variable. It may differ little from chronic phase but blast cell numbers may be increased disproportionately (Table 27.4). There may be anaemia in the presence of a normal leucocyte count. Platelet numbers may be greatly increased (>1000 × 10⁹/L) or reduced (<100 × 10⁹/L) in a manner not accounted for by treatment. The marrow also shows a picture no longer consistent with chronic-phase disease, often with increased numbers of blast cells or promyelocytes and/or increased fibrosis.

Blastic transformation is defined by the presence of more than 20% blasts or blasts plus promyelocytes in the blood or marrow. Frequently, this criterion is irrelevant because blast cell numbers in both sites have risen abruptly to exceed 80%. Their morphology is very variable. About 70% of patients have blasts classifiable generally as myeloid, which resemble to a degree the cells that characterize acute myeloid leukaemia (AML) (see Chapter 29). Such cells may be predominantly myeloblastic, monoblastic, erythroblastic or megakaryoblastic, and blast cells of different myeloid lineages frequently coexist. These cells are best defined by their cytochemical and immunophenotypic

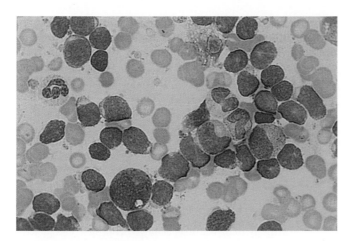

Figure 27.6 Peripheral blood appearances of a patient with CML in lymphoid blast cell transformation.

characteristics, although they do not usually fit neatly into the French–American–British (FAB) classification for AML. About 20% of patients have lymphoid blast cells; these may resemble the FAB L1 cells that typify childhood ALL or, more commonly, have L2 appearances (Figure 27.6). Immunophenotyping shows the typical membrane markers of a precursor B-cell ALL, namely CD10 (CALLA) and CD19 positivity, and further studies may show nuclear positivity for terminal deoxynucleotidyltransferase. Molecular studies show clonal rearrangement of immunoglobulin chains and occasionally of T-cell receptor genes. The remaining 10% of blast cell transformations have mixed myeloid and lymphoid characteristics.

The clinical features associated with advanced disease are quite variable. In some cases, the patient is initially completely asymptomatic and the diagnosis is based entirely on blood and marrow findings. In other cases, the patient may develop fevers, excessive sweating, anorexia and weight loss or bone pain. Rarely, there are localized lytic lesions of bone, which may be single or multiple. Occasionally, patients present with generalized lymphadenopathy; biopsy shows nodal infiltration with blast cells that may be myeloid or lymphoid. Localized skin infiltrates may be seen. Discrete masses of immature leukaemia cells may develop at almost any site; these are sometimes referred to as chloromas or granulocytic sarcomas. Patients with lymphoid blast cells in the blood and marrow may have involvement of the cerebrospinal fluid at the same time, or central nervous system (CNS) involvement may become symptomatic only at a later stage.

Biochemical changes

The biochemical changes seen in CML are non-specific. Patients diagnosed in chronic phase may have a slightly raised serum uric acid but the level is frequently normal. The serum alkaline phosphatase is usually normal or slightly raised. Lactate dehydrogenase is usually raised. Serum K^+ may be spuriously raised due to leakage of intracellular potassium from platelets or, less commonly, from leucocytes after the blood is drawn. In such cases, the K^+ level in freshly drawn citrated blood is usually normal, as is the electrocardiogram. The serum vitamin B_{12} and B_{12}-binding capacity are greatly increased due to raised levels of transcobalamin I.

In transformation, the serum uric acid may be raised, sometimes substantially, and tests of liver function are usually moderately abnormal. Hypercalcaemia is present occasionally and is usually due to bone destruction; very rarely, it may be attributable to a parathormone-like material ectopically produced by the blast cells.

Management of chronic myeloid leukaemia in chronic phase

The management of the newly diagnosed CML patient has changed very greatly in the last decade. In the 1970s, it was conventional for the physician to start treatment soon after diagnosis with busulfan and then to await further developments. The patient received little information about prognosis. Today, in most, but not all, countries, the patient is informed of the diagnosis and given as much information as possible about the disease and its prognosis. The various options for treatment are usually discussed at this stage, which for the younger patient include the possible need for allogeneic SCT at some stage in the disease. This means that the patient, all siblings and other family members should be HLA typed. The issue of gonadal function is important and men who have not completed their families should be offered semen cryopreservation before any treatment is started.

There is no urgency to start treatment immediately in asymptomatic patients with leucocyte counts below 100×10^9/L. This means that leucapheresis with cryopreservation of blood stem cells can be performed before anti-leukaemia treatment is instituted. Such stored cells may be used for autografting at a later date. However, drug treatment should ideally be started soon after the diagnosis is confirmed. The best single agent for patients in chronic phase who are not enrolled in a Phase III study is imatinib. Hydroxycarbamide is a reasonable alternative in the very short term if imatinib is not immediately available. Interferon alfa, until the advent of TKIs the treatment of choice, and busulfan should both be reserved for special indications.

Imatinib mesylate

Imatinib mesylate (Glivec or Gleevec; previously known as STI571), a 2-phenylaminopyrimidine compound, is an ABL1 tyrosine kinase inhibitor that entered clinical trials in 1998. It was thought originally to act by occupying the ATP-binding pocket of the ABL1 kinase component of the BCR–ABL1 onco-protein, thereby blocking the capacity of the enzyme to phosphorylate downstream effector molecules; it is now thought to act also by binding to an adjacent domain in a manner that holds the ABL1 component of the BCR–ABL1 oncoprotein molecule in an inactive or 'closed' conformation (Figure 27.7). The drug rapidly reverses the clinical and haematological abnormalities and induces major cytogenetic responses in over 80% of previously untreated chronic-phase patients. It is usually administered orally at a dose of 400 mg daily, although pilot studies suggest that initial treatment with 600 mg or even 800 mg daily gives more rapid responses.

Side-effects include nausea, headache, rashes, infraorbital oedema, bone pains and, sometimes, more generalized fluid retention. The rashes can from time to time be treated by temporarily interrupting imatinib and then reinstituting it under short-term corticosteroid cover. Hepatotoxicity characterized by raised serum transaminases is occasionally seen and may necessitate stopping the drug. Some caution must also be exercised in the light of very rare reports of potentially fatal cerebral oedema. Patients with black skin may sustain areas of depigmentation. An interesting non-sinister effect, repigmentation of grey hair, has been reported in a small group of responders. The toxicity in general seems to be appreciably less than that associated with interferon alfa.

A significant minority of patients experience neutropenia and/or thrombocytopenia within the first few months of starting treatment with imatinib at standard dosage (400 mg daily).

In some cases, isolated neutropenia may be managed simply by adding G-CSF (300–480 μg subcutaneously on alternate days or less often) for a finite period, after which it may be possible to reduce or stop the drug. In other cases, G-CSF works less well and it may be necessary to reduce or stop imatinib. If thrombocytopenia develops, it may be necessary to reduce the dose, although some believe that the drug may expedite development of resistance at daily doses below 300 mg. Conversely, thrombocytosis sometimes persists in a patient whose leucocyte count is well controlled by imatinib; in such cases, the addition of hydroxycarbamide or anagrelide usually controls the platelet count.

The issue of how long to continue imatinib remains unresolved. For the patient who has achieved complete cytogenetic remission, stopping the drug usually leads to recurrence of Ph positivity and eventually leucocytosis in the majority of cases, although on occasion the cytogenetic remission continues without treatment for many months or even longer. A small proportion of the patients who achieved a complete molecular response that lasted more than 2 years have stopped taking imatinib without evidence of subsequent relapse, an interesting observation that raises the possibility that imatinib may have the capacity to eradicate CML in some cases. At present, the best advice for the responding patient is to continue the drug indefinitely.

A prospective randomized Phase III trial (the IRIS trial) designed to compare imatinib as a single agent with the combination of interferon alfa and cytarabine in previously

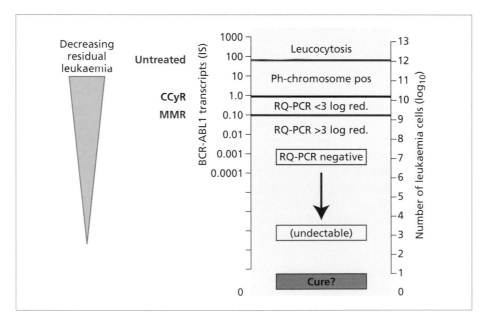

Figure 27.7 Schematic representation of the relationship between measurable parameters (blood leucocyte numbers, Ph-positive marrow metaphases and *BCR–ABL1* transcript numbers) and presumed number of residual leukaemia cells in a patient responding to treatment with a tyrosine kinase inhibitor. CCyR, complete cytogenetic response; MMR, major molecular response.

untreated patients started in June 2000. Analysis after 6 years of follow-up showed that 74% of the patients treated with imatinib achieved complete cytogenetic remission compared with 14% of those in the control arm. The cumulative best complete cytogenetic response rate was 82%, and 63% of all patients randomized to receive imatinib were still on study and in complete cytogenetic remission. The event-free survival was 83% and overall survival 88%. A substantial proportion of the patients in complete cytogenetic remission also achieved a major molecular response (equivalent to a 3-log reduction in *BCR–ABL1* transcript numbers) and this proportion has continued to increase steadily with time on imatinib. A large proportion of the patients in the control arm discontinued interferon alfa and cytarabine for various reasons and thus a formal comparison of survival in the two arms could not be performed. However, comparison of survival of patients treated with imatinib with that of historical control patients treated predominantly with interferon-containing regimens showed highly significant superiority for those who received imatinib.

Predicting response to imatinib

Efforts are now being made to predict an individual patient's response to imatinib 400 mg daily but results are not yet totally reliable. This said, patients whose leukaemia cells tested *in vitro* have a low IC_{50} for imatinib seem to respond better than those with higher IC_{50} values. Patients with normal or high levels of the human organic cation transporter (hOCT)-1, which is responsible for cellular influx of imatinib, also seem to fare better than those with lower levels. Efforts have been made to predict response to imatinib on the basis of gene expression profiling but the results of the different studies are somewhat inconsistent and this method is not yet suitable for clinical application. It is interesting that the Sokal score based on a population of patients treated with busulfan more than 25 years ago still has predictive value for response to imatinib.

Monitoring responses to treatment

The quantity of leukaemic cells remaining in a patient's body while responding to treatment with TKIs can be monitored with considerable precision by use of three modalities in sequence, namely examination of the peripheral blood, bone marrow metaphase cytogenetics and the number of *BCR–ABL1* transcripts in the circulation. Thus for an individual patient the first target is normalization of the blood count, the second elimination of dividing cells in the bone marrow that show Ph-positive metaphases and finally elimination of *BCR–ABL1* transcripts in the blood or marrow. *BCR–ABL1* transcript numbers are usually measured by RQ-PCR and the results may be expressed either as a ratio of *BCR–ABL1* copy numbers to copy numbers of a control gene (×100% on a log scale) or as a log_{10} reduction from standardized value of 0 for untreated patients. In practice the recommended way to express the results is to use a laboratory-specific conversion factor to convert the value obtained in

a given laboratory to a value on the International Scale where 100% is the value for a specific cohort of untreated patients studied in 2002. Patients who achieve a transcript number of 0.1% on the International Scale, equivalent to a 3-log reduction from the baseline for untreated patients, are said to have achieved a major molecular response, while those without detectable transcripts have achieved a complete molecular response (Figure 27.8). The use of fluorescence *in situ* hybridization to detect a *BCR–ABL1* gene in interphase cells is more sensitive than metaphase cytogenetics but much less sensitive than RQ-PCR.

Defining response and failure to respond to imatinib

In 2005 a group of haematologists convened under the aegis of the European LeukemiaNet produced a series of recommendations designed to help clinicians identify patients with newly diagnosed CML in chronic phase started on imatinib 400 mg daily and subsequently judged to have achieved only a suboptimal response or to have failed treatment. The implication was that patients who failed should have their treatment changed and those satisfying criteria for suboptimal response should be monitored closely with the expectation that they too might fail. These original recommendations were updated in 2009 (Table 27.5).

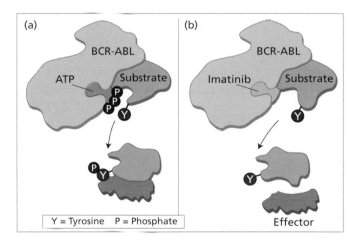

Figure 27.8 The presumed mechanism of action of imatinib. (a) The phosphorylation of a substrate is shown schematically. ATP occupies the pocket in the ABL1 component of the BCR–ABL1 oncoprotein, whence it donates a phosphate (P) group to a tyrosine (Y) residue on an unspecified substrate. The substrate then detaches itself from the BCR–ABL1 oncoprotein and makes functional contact with a further downstream effector molecule. (b) Imatinib occupies the ATP-binding site and thereby prevents phosphorylation of the substrate. This molecule in turn fails to make contact with the effector protein and the signal transduction pathway that would otherwise transmit the 'leukaemia signal' is interrupted.

Table 27.5 Evaluation of overall response to front-line imatinib in early chronic-phase CML.

	Optimal response	Suboptimal response	Failure	Warnings
3 months	CHR and at least minor cytogenetic response (Ph$^+$ ≤ 65%)	No cytogenetic response (Ph$^+$ > 95%)	Less than CHR	NA
6 months	At least partial cytogenetic response (Ph$^+$ < 35%)	Less than partial cytogenetic response (Ph$^+$ > 35%)	No cytogenetic response (Ph$^+$ > 95%)	NA
12 months	Complete cytogenetic response	Partial cytogenetic response (Ph$^+$ ≤ 35%)	Less than partial cytogenetic response (Ph$^+$ > 35%)	Less than major molecular response*
18 months	Major molecular response	Less than major molecular response	Less than complete cytogenetic response	NA
Any time	Stable or improving major molecular response	Loss of major molecular response Mutations†	Loss of CHR Loss of complete cytogenetic response Mutations‡ Additional chromosome abnormalities in Ph-positive cells§	Any rise in transcripts level Other chromosome abnormalities in Ph-negative cells

*Major molecular response denotes *BCR–ABL1/ABL1* or other housekeeping genes ≤0.1% on the international scale.
†*BCR–ABL1* kinase domain mutations highly insensitive to imatinib (see Table 27.3).
‡*BCR–ABL1* kinase domain mutations still sensitive to imatinib (see Table 27.3).
§Additional chromosome abnormalities in Ph-positive cells are a warning factor at diagnosis, while their occurrence during treatment (clonal progression) is a marker of failure. Two consecutive cytogenetic tests are required, showing the same additional chromosome abnormalities in at least two Ph-positive cells.
CHR, complete haematological response; NA, not applicable.

Resistance to imatinib

Resistance to imatinib may be primary or secondary. A very small proportion of patients with newly diagnosed chronic-phase CML fail to achieve a haematological response and a small proportion never achieve a complete cytogenetic response. In these cases the resistance seems to be primary. A larger proportion of patients respond initially at the haematological or cytogenetic level and then lose their responses; such secondary resistance occurs most commonly in the first 2 years after starting treatment and appears to be increasingly rare in patients who have taken imatinib for more than 2 years. The cause of primary resistance is essentially unknown but is likely to reflect the underlying heterogeneity of CML at diagnosis. Similarly, the cause of secondary resistance is poorly defined. It has been associated with a variety of diverse mechanisms, including overexpression of the BCR–ABL1 oncoprotein and overexpression of P-glycoprotein, which expedites efflux of the drug from individual cells, and the acquisition of point mutations in the ABL1 kinase domain. Thus far, Ph-positive subclones with at least 50 different point mutations have been identified in leukaemia cells obtained from patients with variable degrees of resistance to imatinib, and some of these, but by no means all,

are clearly the cause of the resistance. Each mutation encodes a different amino acid substitution in the ABL1 kinase component of the BCR–ABL1 oncoprotein. Cells with one such substitution, the replacement of threonine by isoleucine at position 315 (referred to as the T315I mutation), seem to be especially resistant to the inhibitory action of imatinib and all other TKIs. Cells with other substitutions are relatively less resistant. It is probable that some of these subclones exist before the administration of imatinib but are allowed to expand when the unmutated oncoprotein molecule is inhibited by imatinib; in other cases the mutation may develop *de novo* after initiation of imatinib.

Second-generation tyrosine kinase inhibitors

The remarkable success of imatinib in chronic-phase CML led rapidly to development of other TKIs, notably dasatinib, nilotinib and bosutinib, all of which are clearly more potent than the original TKI. With each of these drugs the largest experience has been gained in treating patients who have failed imatinib, but all are now being tested as up-front treatment for newly diagnosed individuals with promising early results.

Dasatinib

Dasatinib (Sprycel) was first used to treat CML in 2003. Somewhat surprisingly it bears little chemical resemblance to imatinib but acts, like imatinib, by occupying the phosphate-binding pocket and blocking access for ATP. Unlike imatinib it is active with the kinase activation loop in both closed and open configurations. It differs also from imatinib in being active against a wide range of tyrosine kinases in addition to ABL1, of which the most notable are SRC and so-called SRC family kinases. It has therefore been termed a dual inhibitor, on the assumption that its value in CML could be based on its relatively wide spectrum of activity. The original dose was 70 mg twice daily but the recommended dose for patients is now 100 mg once daily. For patients who have failed imatinib, dasatinib induces complete cytogenetic responses in about 50% of patients and some of these responses seem very durable. It is definitely more myelosuppressive than imatinib and treatment must occasionally be interrupted or dosage reduced on account of neutropenia or thrombocytopenia Other side-effects observed include nausea, gastrointestinal disturbances, rashes and pleural effusions, which may or may not be asymptomatic. The latter usually resolve on stopping the drug.

Nilotinib

Nilotinib (Tasigna) was developed by chemical modification of imatinib with the intention of increasing its activity. Nilotinib is about 30 times more active *in vitro* but the recommended oral dose, 400 mg twice daily, does not reflect the *in vitro* ratio. Like dasatinib, it induces complete cytogenetic responses in about 50% of patients who fail imatinib. It is usually well tolerated but side-effects have included headaches, nausea, gastrointestinal disturbances, pancreatitis, raised levels of bilirubin, and abnormal liver function tests. Prolongation of the QT interval has been observed in rare instances.

Bosutinib

The third second-generation TKI in clinical practice is bosutinib, which also targets a relatively wide spectrum of tyrosine kinases. It is also active in patients deemed to have failed imatinib and is being tested in a Phase III study of previously untreated chronic-phase patients. It principal toxic effect is diarrhoea, which may be severe but usually responds to standard antidiarrhoeal agents.

Hydroxycarbamide

Hydroxycarbamide (also known as hydroxyurea) is a ribonucleotide reductase inhibitor that targets relatively mature myeloid progenitors in proliferative cycle. Its pharmacological action is rapid and readily reversible. Treatment for patients in chronic phase usually starts with 1.0–2.0 g daily by mouth and continued indefinitely. The leucocyte count starts to fall within days and the spleen reduces in size. It is usually possible to reverse all features of CML within 4–8 weeks of starting treatment with hydroxycarbamide. The dosage can then be titrated against the leucocyte count, the usual maintenance dose being 1.0–1.5 g daily. In a patient whose leucocyte count is controlled, any reduction in the dose leads to a rapid increase in leucocyte numbers, a phenomenon that disturbs the patient but has no ominous significance. The drug has relatively few side-effects. At high dosage it may cause nausea, diarrhoea or other gastrointestinal disturbance. Some patients get ulcers of the buccal mucosa. Skin rashes are seen. Most patients develop megaloblastic changes in the marrow with macrocytosis in the blood. The drug remains useful today for rapid cytoreduction in the newly diagnosed patient and may also be useful in patients unable to tolerate imatinib, but it rarely causes any degree of reduction in Ph-positive cells in the bone marrow and must therefore be regarded as second- or third-line therapy.

Interferon alfa

Interferon alfa, like hydroxycarbamide, can no longer be regarded as first-line therapy for CML, but may still have a role in management of patients who have failed TKIs. It is a member of a large family of glycoproteins of biological origin with antiviral and antiproliferative properties. Studies in the early 1980s using material purified from human cell lines showed that it was active in reducing the leucocyte count and reversing all features of CML in 70–80% of CML patients. Of particular interest at the time was the observation that 5–15% of patients achieved major reduction in the percentage of Ph-positive marrow metaphases with restoration of Ph-negative (putatively normal) haemopoiesis. It raised the important question of whether these 'cytogenetic responders' would have their life prolonged by treatment with interferon alfa, and prospectively randomized controlled studies were initiated. Compared with hydroxycarbamide, interferon alfa offered a survival advantage that was maximal for those who achieved complete cytogenetic remissions. These observations meant that interferon alfa replaced hydroxycarbamide and busulfan in the 1980s as primary treatment for CML in chronic phase, and remained so until the introduction of imatinib.

Interferon alfa must be administered by subcutaneous injection at daily doses ranging from 3 to 5 million units/m^2. There is no good evidence that the higher doses are clinically superior. Toxicity is common in older patients, but is generally mild and reversible. Almost all patients experience fevers, shivers, muscle aches and general flu-like features on starting the drug; these last usually 2–3 weeks but may be alleviated by paracetamol. They recur when dosage is increased. A significant minority of patients cannot tolerate the drug on account of lethargy, malaise, anorexia, weight loss, depression and other affective disorders or alopecia. Autoimmune syndromes, such as thyrotoxicosis, may also occur. A long-acting form of interferon alfa, peginterferon alfa, has been introduced recently, but other than ease of administration it seems to have little advantage over conventional formulations.

Busulfan

Busulfan (1,4-dimethanesulfonyloxybutane) is a polyfunctional alkylating agent that is now infrequently used (except as conditioning before transplant procedures). It targets a relatively primitive stem cell and the effects of administration are prolonged for some weeks after stopping the drug. It was the mainstay of treatment for CML in the period 1960–80. Treatment was conventionally started with 8 mg daily by mouth and the dosage was reduced as the leucocyte count began to fall. It was essential to reduce the dosage substantially or to stop the drug before the leucocyte count fell below 20×10^9/L because profound and prolonged leucopenia might otherwise be produced.

Busulfan could be administered either in finite courses lasting up to 4 weeks or continuously at a maintenance dose between 0.5 and 2.0 mg daily. Occasional patients were hypersensitive to the effects of busulfan and developed severe, sometimes irreversible, pancytopenia with marrow hypoplasia on standard dosage. Overdosage could achieve the same effect in any patient. Gonadal failure (as mentioned above) invariably occurred within a few months of starting treatment and was almost always irreversible. Other toxic effects included cutaneous pigmentation, pulmonary fibrosis and a wasting syndrome resembling hypoadrenalism. These points notwithstanding, the drug may be useful in older patients whose compliance is uncertain as it can also be given orally in the clinic as a single dose of 50 or 100 mg, to be repeated as necessary after 4 weeks or longer.

Homoharringtonine

Another drug of interest for CML in chronic phase is homoharringtonine (omecetaxine), a semisynthetic plant alkaloid that enhances apoptosis of CML cells. It produces haematological responses in 60–70% of patients and major cytogenetic responses in 25% in small series of patients in chronic phase. The results appear to improve with the addition of interferon alfa. For the moment, it remains an investigational agent.

Allogeneic stem cell transplantation

Younger patients with suitable stem cell donors who fail treatment with TKIs may be offered the option of allogeneic SCT (see Chapter 24). Most specialist centres exclude from consideration patients who are over the age of 50 or 55 years. The major factors influencing survival are patient age, disease phase at time of SCT, disease duration, degree of histocompatibility between donor and recipient, and gender of donor. In general, patients are 'conditioned' for transplant with cyclophosphamide at high dosage followed by total body irradiation, or with the combination of busulfan and cyclophosphamide at high dosage. If all goes well, reasonable marrow function is achieved in 3–4 weeks after the infusion of donor haemopoietic stem cells and the patient leaves the hospital.

The possible major complications include graft-versus-host disease (GVHD), reactivation of infection with cytomegalovirus or other viruses, idiopathic pneumonitis and veno-occlusive disease of the liver. For patients with CML treated by SCT with marrow from HLA-identical siblings, the overall leukaemia-free survival at 5 years is now 60–80% (Figure 27.9). There is a roughly 20% chance of transplant-related mortality and a 15%

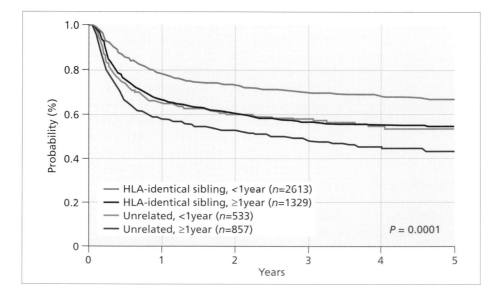

Figure 27.9 Probability of survival for patients with CML in chronic phase who received allogeneic stem cell transplants from an HLA-identical sibling or matched unrelated donor according to whether or not the transplant was performed within 1 year of diagnosis. (Data reproduced from the International Bone Marrow Transplant Registry, Milwaukee, Wisconsin, USA, with permission.)

chance of relapse. Patients surviving without haematological evidence of disease can be monitored by serial cytogenetic studies and by use of the much more sensitive RQ-PCR, which can detect very low numbers of BCR–ABL1 transcripts in the blood or marrow. These studies suggest (but do not prove) that in the majority of long-term survivors the CML may truly have been eradicated.

The recognition that the graft-versus-leukaemia (GVL) effect plays a major role in eradicating CML after allografting led to the concept that the toxicity of the transplant procedure could be substantially reduced by decreasing the intensity of pretransplant conditioning. The strategy is thus to focus predominantly on the use of immunosuppressive rather than myeloablative agents in order to maximize the numbers of haemopoietic stem cells transfused and to exploit the GVL effect mediated by donor alloreactive immunocompetent cells to eliminate the leukaemia cells. Such procedures have been termed variously non-myeloablative SCT, reduced-intensity conditioning SCT or mini-SCT, and reflect advances in our understanding of how SCT actually works (see Chapter 24). It is still too early to say whether non-myeloablative SCT will prove superior to conventional transplantation in the longer term for the younger patient, but the technique could make SCT more widely available to higher risk and perhaps also to older patients.

The qualified success of conventional SCT using matched siblings led in the late 1980s to increasing use of matched unrelated donors for SCT for patients with CML. At present, serologically matched unrelated donors can be identified for about 50% of white patients and for lower percentages of patients of other ethnic origins. However, molecular methods for typing HLA class I and II have now largely superseded serological techniques, and complete matches for a given patient for five gene pairs (HLA-A, -B, -C, -DR and -DQ) are relatively rare. Thus, in the absence of a perfect match the clinician has to decide what degree of mismatch may be acceptable for a given transplant. In general, the results of transplants using such unrelated donors are less good at present than results using HLA-identical siblings, but some patients will probably prove to be cured.

About 10–30% of patients submitted to allogeneic SCT relapse within the first 3 years after transplant. The relapse is usually insidious and characterized first by rising levels of BCR–ABL1 transcripts, then by increasing numbers of Ph-positive marrow metaphases and, finally (if untreated), by haematological features of chronic-phase disease. This provides some rationale for the recommendation that patients should be monitored after transplant by regular RQ-PCR and cytogenetic studies. Rare patients in cytogenetic remission relapse directly to advanced-phase disease without any identified intervening period of chronic-phase disease.

There are various options for the management of relapse to chronic-phase disease, including use of interferon alfa, hydroxycarbamide, imatinib, a second transplant using the same or another donor, or lymphocyte transfusions from the original donor. Such donor lymphocyte infusion (DLI) has gained popularity in recent years, and is believed to reflect the capacity of lymphoid cells collected from the original transplant donor to mediate a GVL effect, even though they may have failed to eradicate the leukaemia at the time of the original transplant. In practice, mononuclear cells are collected from the transplant donor in one or two leucapheresis procedures and transfused to the patient (who receives no other conditioning and usually no prophylaxis for GVHD). Within 3–6 months the leukaemia is restored to complete cytogenetic remission in about 80% of CML patients treated in this way and these responders also achieve PCR negativity. Some responding patients sustain marrow aplasia, which can be reversed by transfusion of marrow cells from the donor. However, severe GVHD may occur and can, on rare occasions, prove lethal. However, the incidence and severity of GVHD can be greatly reduced by starting the lymphocyte transfusions at relatively low cell dose and repeating the transfusion with a higher cell dose at intervals of 4–12 weeks as required, a technique usually referred to as 'escalating-dose' DLI.

At present, opinions are evenly divided on the optimal management of the patient who relapses with increasing BCR–ABL1 transcript numbers or increasing Ph positivity after allogeneic SCT. Some feel that escalating-dose DLI is the best approach, whereas others prefer to resume treatment with imatinib. It may be possible to resolve this issue with a suitably designed prospective study.

Treatment decisions for newly diagnosed patients in chronic phase

Whereas until recently there was still controversy about whether a newly diagnosed chronic-phase patient should be treated initially with a TKI or by allogeneic SCT if he or she had a suitable donor, there is now general agreement that such new patients should first receive treatment with a TKI. There are perhaps two exceptions to this general rule. First, some paediatricians feel that the results of allogeneic SCT in children are so comparatively good that it is reasonable to offer children with matched donors an allograft as initial treatment or after cytoreduction for a finite period with imatinib. Others feel that a child responding well to imatinib should be continued indefinitely on this agent. For treating children there seems at present no general consensus. Second, a case can be made for transplantation as initial therapy in patients for whom the cost of imatinib continued over many years would be totally prohibitive. For such patients a one-off procedure involving allografting might be a better option (Figure 27.10).

For an adult the question whether to start treatment with imatinib 400 mg daily or to embark on treatment with a second-generation TKI cannot currently be resolved. We have more than 10 years' experience with imatinib and 65% of patients

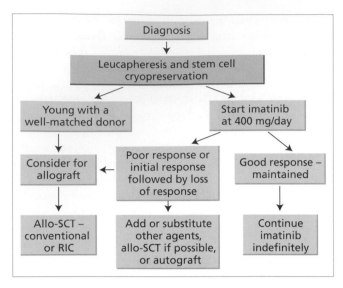

Figure 27.10 Algorithm showing a possible approach to the management of a patient with newly diagnosed CML in chronic phase. Children with HLA-identical siblings (or possibly well-matched unrelated donors) may be eligible for initial treatment by allografting. The great majority of newly diagnosed patients should be treated first with imatinib. Those who respond well and maintain their response should continue on the drug indefinitely. Patients who respond less well or who lose their response should be considered for other therapy including SCT. SCT, stem cell transplantation; RIC, reduced-intensity conditioning.

appear to be doing remarkably well. We have only very limited experience with use of the second-generation TKIs as initial therapy but preliminary results seem to be somewhat superior to those of imatinib. Would it be beneficial to start all new patients on a second-generation TKI? A number of Phase III studies are now in progress to address this question and the answer should become clear in the foreseeable future.

The decision-making process is especially complicated when CML is diagnosed in an asymptomatic patient presenting to an antenatal clinic. For a woman in the first trimester of pregnancy it is probably best to delay treatment, avoiding if possible all forms of chemotherapy, including imatinib. Leucapheresis and/or blood transfusion could be undertaken if essential. The same might apply to patients in the second trimester of pregnancy, but administration of interferon alfa is probably safe at this stage. It is clear that for the patient who conceives while taking imatinib, there is a low but finite risk that the fetus will sustain congenital abnormalities, such as hypospadias, defects in bone formation and exomphalos. The issue whether to recommend termination of pregnancy or to permit the pregnancy to continue will challenge the prospective mother and her medical adviser.

Experimental approaches

Immunotherapy

The demonstration of a powerful GVL effect in CML has renewed interest in the possibility that some form of immunotherapeutic manipulation could be effective in CML. Some evidence suggests that patients vaccinated with peptides corresponding to the junctional region of the BCR–ABL1 protein may generate immune responses that may be of clinical benefit. Other targets for vaccine therapy now under study include Wilms tumour (WT)1 protein, proteinase-3 (PR1) and PRAME, all of which are overexpressed in CML cells. Studies have been initiated in which two vaccines, WT1 and PR1, are combined.

Autografting in chronic phase

Because only a minority of patients are eligible for allogeneic SCT, much interest has focused on the possibility that life may be prolonged and some cures effected by autografting CML patients still in chronic phase. It is possible that the pool of leukaemic stem cells can be substantially reduced by an autograft procedure, and autografting may confer a short-term proliferative advantage on Ph-negative (presumably normal) stem cells. In practice, some patients have achieved temporary Ph-negative haemopoiesis after autografting. Preliminary studies have been reported in which patients have been autografted with Ph-negative stem cells collected from the peripheral blood in the recovery phase following high-dose combination chemotherapy; some such patients achieved durable Ph negativity.

Management of chronic myeloid leukaemia in advanced phase

Accelerated-phase disease

It is difficult to make general statements about the optimal management of patients in accelerated-phase disease as the criteria for this diagnosis are so very varied. Some patients can be managed merely with a minor alteration in their cytotoxic drug regimen. Those who have not been treated previously with imatinib may obtain benefit from the introduction of this agent. Other patients may benefit from splenectomy or regular red cell transfusion. Patients whose disease seems to be moving towards overt blastic transformation may benefit from appropriate cytotoxic drug combinations. Allogeneic SCT should certainly be considered for younger patients if suitable donors can be identified. Reduced-intensity conditioning allografts are probably not indicated, as the efficacy of the GVL effect in advanced-phase CML is not clearly established.

Blastic transformation

Patients in blastic transformation may be treated with combinations of cytotoxic drugs in the hope of prolonging life but cure can no longer be a realistic objective. Conversely, it is not unreasonable to use a relatively innocuous drug such as hydroxycarbamide at higher dosage to restrain blast cell numbers and maintain the patient at home for as long as possible. If the patient has a myeloid transformation, he or she can be treated with drugs that are appropriate to the induction of remission in AML, namely daunorubicin and cytarabine with or without other agents. Blast cell numbers will be reduced substantially in most cases but their numbers usually increase again within 3–6 weeks. Perhaps 20% of patients are restored to a situation resembling chronic-phase disease and this benefit may last for 3–6 months. A very small minority, probably less than 10%, may achieve substantial degrees of Ph-negative haemopoiesis. This is most likely in patients who entered blastic transformation very soon after diagnosis.

Patients in lymphoid transformation may be treated, with a little more optimism, with drugs applicable to the management of adult ALL (e.g. prednisolone, vincristine, daunorubicin and methotrexate with or without L-asparaginase). More than 50% of patients will be restored to 'second' chronic phase, at which point this status can be maintained with daily 6-mercaptopurine and weekly methotrexate. Because leukaemia involving the CNS is so relatively common in responding patients, those who achieve second chronic phase should have neuroprophylaxis with intrathecal methotrexate weekly for six consecutive weeks, but the administration of cranial irradiation is probably excessive. Some patients treated for lymphoid transformation of CML may sustain long periods of apparent 'remission'.

Imatinib may be remarkably effective in controlling the clinical and haematological features of CML in advanced phases in the very short term. In some patients in established myeloid blastic transformation, who received 600 mg daily, massive splenomegaly was entirely reversed and blast cells were eliminated from the blood and marrow, but such responses are almost always short-lived. Thus, imatinib should be incorporated into a programme of therapy that also involves use of conventional cytotoxic drugs and possibly also allogeneic SCT.

Allogeneic SCT using HLA-matched sibling donors can be performed in accelerated phase; the probability of leukaemia-free survival at 5 years is 30–50%. SCT performed in overt blastic transformation is nearly always unsuccessful. The mortality resulting from GVHD is extremely high and the probability of relapse in those who survive the transplant procedure is very considerable. The probability of survival at 5 years is consequently 0–10%. However, patients who can be restored to 'second' chronic phase by combination chemotherapy or by imatinib may have a relatively low risk of transplant-related mortality and may therefore be considered for allogeneic SCT with a view to eliminating both chronic disease and residual blastic disease provided that a suitable donor can be identified.

Variants of chronic myeloid leukaemia (see also Chapter 28)

Ph-negative chronic myeloid leukaemia

About 6% of patients with haematologically acceptable CML lack the Ph chromosome (see above). About half of these patients have a BCR–ABL1 gene that is molecularly identical to the BCR–ABL1 gene of Ph-positive CML; this gene is usually on the morphologically normal chromosome 22q but may occasionally be found on chromosome 9q. Such patients have a clinical course similar to those with Ph-positive disease. Conversely, patients with no BCR–ABL1 gene frequently have haematological features that are subtly different from Ph-positive disease. They may lack basophilia, lack blast and myelocyte peaks in the leucocyte differential, or show dysplastic features. They are more likely to have some degree of monocytosis. These patients respond poorly to imatinib, interferon alfa or hydroxycarbamide, and overall their survival is inferior to that of Ph-positive patients.

Chronic myelomonocytic leukaemia

This is a rare myeloproliferative condition affecting predominantly elderly men but found at all ages (see Chapter 28). The patient may present with features of anaemia or haemorrhage. The spleen is typically enlarged and thus the clinical picture superficially resembles CML. However, the blood and marrow are quite different. Marrow cells lack a Ph chromosome. Blood monocytosis is prominent and monocyte numbers may be as high as $50 \times 10^9/L$. Thrombocytopenia is common. Basophilia and eosinophilia are absent. Dysplastic changes are usually present in the granulocyte and erythroid series. Consequently, the disease is included in the FAB classification of the myelodysplastic syndromes (see Chapter 28).

Very rare patients have been described with a chronic myelomonocytic leukaemia-like blood picture associated with cytogenetic abnormalities in their leukaemia cells other than t(9;22). Most of these patients have either t(5;12) associated with fusion of the ETV and PDGFRB genes or t(8;13) associated with fusion of ZNF198 and FGFR1 genes, but in fact other fusion partners have also been reported (Table 27.6). PDGFRB and FGFR1 both encode receptor tyrosine kinases and are presumably 'activated' by mechanisms analogous to those that activate the ABL1 gene in BCR–ABL1-positive CML. The t(5;12) and t(8;13) leukaemias are both characterized by prominent eosinophilia but basophilia is usually absent. The t(5;12) leukaemias respond

Cytogenetic abnormality	Fusion protein	Leukaemia
t(9;22)(q34;q11)	BCR–ABL1	CML or acute lymphoblastic leukaemia
t(8;22)(p11;q11)	BCR–FGFR1	*BCR–ABL1*-negative CML
t(4;22)(q12;q11)	BCR–PDGFRA	Atypical CML
t(8;13)(p11;q12)	ZNF198–FGFR1	8p Myeloproliferative syndrome
t(6;8)(q27;p11)	FOP–FGFR1	8p Myeloproliferative syndrome
t(8;9)(p12;q33)	CEP110–FGFR1	8p Myeloproliferative syndrome
t(8;19)(p12;q13)	HERV/K–FGFR1	8p Myeloproliferative syndrome
t(5;12)(q31–33;p13)	TEL–PDGFRB	CMML/atypical CML
t(5;7)(q33;q11)	HIP1–PDGFRB	CMML/atypical CML
t(5;17)(q33;p13)	RAB5–PDGFRB	CMML/atypical CML
t(5;10)(q33;q21)	H4–PDGFRB	CMML/atypical CML
t(9;12)(q34;p13)	TEL–ABL1	Atypical CML/*BCR–ABL1*-negative CML
t(9;12)(p24;p13)	TEL–JAK2	Atypical CML/*BCR–ABL1*-negative CML
t(9;22)(p24;q11)	BCR–JAK2	Atypical CML/*BCR–ABL1*-negative CML
del(4)(q12)	FIP1L1–PDGFRA	Hypereosinophilic syndrome

Table 27.6 Cytogenetic abnormalities associated with deregulated tyrosine kinases in chronic myeloproliferative disorders.

CML, chronic myeloid leukaemia; CMML, chronic myelomonocytic leukaemia.

extremely well to low doses of imatinib but the t(8;13) leukaemias do not.

Chronic neutrophilic leukaemia

This is an exceedingly rare disorder that is usually diagnosed incidentally. The patient has a raised blood neutrophil count, often with band forms but without more immature granulocytes, and without basophilia or eosinophilia. The marrow is hypercellular with neutrophil proliferation. The diagnosis is based largely on exclusion of other identifiable causes for the leucocytosis. Marrow cytogenetics are usually normal but clonal abnormality such as +8, +9, del(21q) may be present (see also Chapter 36). Very rare patients have a Ph chromosome and a *BCR–ABL1* fusion gene that codes for an oncoprotein larger than that usually seen in CML, namely 230 kDa (p230$^{BCR–ABL1}$). These cases have been called neutrophilic CML. Most patients have no symptoms referable to the neutrophilia and no physical signs, although some have minor degrees of splenomegaly. Treatment may not be required. Chronic neutrophilic leukaemia is discussed more fully in Chapter 36.

Chronic eosinophilic leukaemia

Most cases of raised eosinophil counts without identifiable primary cause have in the past been classified as examples of

hypereosinophilic syndrome (see Chapter 17). However, it has been shown recently that some such patients respond well to treatment with imatinib, and some of these responding patients have evidence of a new fusion gene designated *FIP1L1–PDGFRA*, resulting from an interstitial deletion on chromosome 4 in their myeloid cells (see Table 27.6). In other cases in which no fusion gene has been identified, the number of immature cells in the blood and marrow is increased and the finding of a clonal cytogenetic abnormality in myeloid cells is strong evidence for a diagnosis of eosinophilic leukaemia or chronic eosinophilic leukaemia. It seems likely therefore that many, if not all, cases previously classified as hypereosinophilic syndrome may turn out to be due to a fusion gene and thus be classified more correctly as examples of eosinophilic leukaemia. Occasional patients with eosinophilic leukaemia progress to blastic transformation in a manner similar to Ph-positive CML. Patients with the *FIP1L1–PDGFRA* fusion gene usually respond well to relatively low doses of imatinib (see Chapters 17 and 36).

Juvenile myelomonocytic leukaemia (see also Chapter 28)

Juvenile myelomonocytic leukaemia (Table 27.7) is a rare disease affecting children under the age of 12 years. It represents about 2% of all childhood leukaemias. It includes a heterogeneous spectrum of myelodysplastic/myeloproliferative diseases

Table 27.7 Diagnostic features of juvenile myelomonocytic leukaemia.

Peripheral blood monocytosis >1 × 10⁹/L

Blasts including promonocytes are <20% of the leucocytes in the blood and <20% of the nucleated cells in the marrow

No Ph translocation of *BCR–ABL1* fusion gene

Plus two or more of the following

Haemoglobin F level increased for patient's age

Immature granulocytes present in the blood

White blood cell count >10⁹/L

Clonal chromosomal abnormality, e.g. monosomy 7

GM-CSF hypersensitivity of myeloid progenitors cultured *in vitro*

that may be difficult to classify. The cause is unknown but there seems to be a genetic predisposition. There is also an important association with neurofibromatosis type 1 with *NF1* mutations and Noonan syndrome characterized by *PTPN11* mutations. Patients usually have symptoms of anaemia with lymphadenopathy and hepatosplenomegaly. There is a variety of skin rashes. Leucocyte numbers are increased with variable numbers of blast cells in the peripheral blood. Such cells are hypersensitive to GM-CSF *in vitro*. The HbF level may be elevated. The marrow is hypercellular but usually lacks chromosomal abnormalities, although monosomy 7 may be present. The disease responds poorly to standard cytotoxic drugs but patients may benefit from allogeneic SCT. Relapse after SCT is relatively common but relapses may be treated successfully with DLI.

Selected bibliography

Arico M, Biondi A, Pui C-H (1997) Juvenile myelomonocytic leukaemia. *Blood* **90**: 479–88.

Arora M, Weisdorf DJ, Spellman SR *et al.* (2009) HLA-identical sibling compared with 8/8 matched and mismatched unrelated donor bone marrow transplant for chronic phase chronic myeloid leukaemia. *Journal of Clinical Oncology* **27**: 1644–52.

Bain B (2003) Cytogenetic and molecular genetic aspects of eosinophilic leukaemias. *British Journal of Haematology* **122**: 173–9.

Baccarani M, Saglio G, Goldman JM *et al.* (2006) Evolving concepts in the management of chronic myeloid leukaemia. Recommendations from an expert panel on behalf of the European Leukaemia-Net. *Blood* **108**: 1809–20.

Baccarani M, Cortes J, Pane F *et al.* (2009) Chronic myeloid leukemia. An update of concepts and management recommendations of the European LeukemiaNet. *Journal of Clinical Oncology* **27**: 6041–51.

Druker BJ, Guilhot F, O'Brien SG *et al.* (2006) Five year follow-up of imatinib therapy for chronic-phase chronic myeloid leukaemia. *New England Journal of Medicine* **355**: 2408–17.

Chronic Myeloid Leukaemia Trialists Collaborative Group (1997) Interferon alfa versus chemotherapy for chronic myeloid leukaemia: a meta-analysis of seven randomized trials. *Journal of the National Cancer Institute* **89**: 1616–20.

Carella AM, Beltrami G, Corsetti MT (2003) Autografting in chronic myeloid leukaemia. *Seminars in Hematology* **40**: 72–86.

Cools J, DeAngelo DJ, Gotlib J *et al.* (2003) A tyrosine kinase created by fusion of the PDGFRA and FIP1L1 genes as a therapeutic target of imatinib in idiopathic hypereosinophilic syndrome. *New England Journal of Medicine* **348**: 1201–14.

de Lavallade H, Apperley JF, Khorashad JS *et al.* (2008) Imatinib for newly diagnosed patients with chronic myeloid leukaemia: incidence of sustained responses in an intention-to-treat analysis. *Journal of Clinical Oncology* **26**: 3358–63.

Goldman JM (2007) How I treat chronic myeloid leukemia in the imatinib era. *Blood* **110**: 2828–37.

Goldman JM, Melo JV (2003) Chronic myeloid leukaemia: advances in biology and new approaches to treatment. *New England Journal of Medicine* **349**: 1449–62.

Goldman JM (2005) Monitoring minimal residual disease in BCR-ABL1-positive chronic myeloid leukaemia in the imatinib era. *Current Opinion in Hematology* **12**: 33–39.

Gratwohl A, Hermans J, Goldman JM *et al.* (1998) Risk assessment for patients with chronic myeloid leukaemia before allogeneic bone marrow transplantation. *Lancet* **352**: 1087–92.

Guilhot F, Chastang C, Michallet M *et al.* (1977) Interferon alfa-2b combined with cytarabine versus interferon alone in chronic myelogenous leukaemia. *New England Journal of Medicine* **337**: 223–9.

Hasford J, Pfirrmann M, Hehlmann R *et al.* (1998) A new prognostic score for survival of patients with chronic myeloid leukemia treated with interferon alfa. Writing Committee for the Collaborative CML Prognostic Factors Project Group. *Journal of the National Cancer Institute* **90**: 850–8.

Hochhaus A, O'Brien SG, Guilhot F *et al.* (2009) Six-year follow-up of patients receiving imatinib for the first-line treatment of chronic myeloid leukaemia. *Leukemia* **23**: 1054–61.

Hughes TP, Kaeda J, Branford S *et al.* (2003) Frequency of major molecular responses to imatinib or interferon alfa plus cytarabine in newly diagnosed chronic myeloid leukaemia. *New England Journal of Medicine* **349**: 1421–30.

Hughes T, Deininger M, Hochhaus A *et al.* (2006) Monitoring CML patients responding to treatment with tyrosine kinase inhibitors: recommendations for 'harmonizing' current methodology for detecting BCR-ABL1 transcripts and kinase domain mutations and for expressing results. *Blood* **108**: 28–37.

Melo JV (1996) The molecular biology of chronic myeloid leukaemia. *Leukemia* **10**: 751–6.

Niemeyer CM, Fenu S, Hasle H *et al.* (1998) Differentiating juvenile myelomonocytic leukaemia from infectious disease: response. *Blood* **91**: 366–7.

O'Brien SG, Guilhot F, Larson RA *et al.* (2003) Imatinib compared with interferon and low dose cytarabine for newly diagnosed chronic-phase chronic myeloid leukaemia. *New England Journal of Medicine* **348**: 994–1004.

Roy L, Guilhot F, Krahnke T *et al.* (2006) Survival advantage from imatinib compared with the combination interferon-α plus cytarabine in chronic-phase chronic myelogenous leukaemia: a historical comparison between two phase 3 trials. *Blood* **108**: 1478–84.

Saglio G, Kim D-W, Issaragrisil S *et al.* (2010) Nilotinib verses imatinib for newly diagnosed chronic myeloid leukemia. *The New England Journal of Medicine* **362**: 2251–9.

Sawyers CL (2010) Even better kinase inhibitors for chronic myeloid leukaemia. *The New England Journal of Medicine* **362**: 2314–15.

Shah NP, Nicholl JM, Nagar B *et al.* (2002) Multiple BCR-ABL1 kinase domain mutations confer polyclonal resistance to the tyrosine kinase inhibitor imatinib (STIS71) in chronic phase and blastic crisis chronic myeloid leukaemia. *Cancer Cell* **2**: 117–25.

Sokal JE, Cox EB, Baccarani M *et al.* (1984) Prognostic discrimination in 'good risk' chronic granulocytic leukaemia. *Blood* **63**: 789–99.

Swerdlow SH, Campo E, Harris NL *et al.* (eds) (2008) *WHO Classification of Tumours of Haematopoietic and Lymphoid Tissues*, 4th edn. IARC, Lyon.

CHAPTER 28

The myelodysplastic syndromes

28

Timothy JT Chevassut[1] and Ghulam J Mufti[2]

[1]Brighton and Sussex Medical School, Royal Sussex County Hospital, Brighton, UK
[2]King's College Hospital and Kings College London, London, UK

Introduction

The myelodysplastic syndromes are a heterogeneous group of clonal stem cell disorders characterized by cytopenias due to impaired blood cell production, a hypercellular and dysplastic bone marrow, and an increased risk of leukaemic transformation. They each exhibit various morphological abnormalities of the blood and bone marrow that are indicative of defective haemopoiesis in one or more lineages. A majority of patients with a myelodysplastic syndrome (MDS) are over the age of 60 years, with the median onset occurring in the seventh decade of life. There is a variable clinical course reflecting the diverse pathobiology of the disease, with some patients having a more indolent progression and longer life expectancy while others present with aggressive disease that evolves rapidly into acute myeloid leukaemia (AML). Overall, approximately 40% of patients will transform to AML during the course of their disease. This broad heterogeneity of clinical course, which is reflected by the diversity of morphological features, provides the basis for the classification schemes and prognostic scoring systems that guide patient management. Recent developments continue to broaden our understanding of the molecular pathogenesis of MDS and provide the rationale for exploring novel therapeutic strategies for patients with this disease.

History

The first description of MDS was in 1900 by Leube who used the term *leukanamie* to describe a patient with severe megaloblastic anaemia that progressed to acute leukaemia. In the 1930s, the term 'refractory anaemia' was coined to refer to a group of patients with a macrocytic anaemia that was unresponsive to iron or other dietary haematinics. While some of these anaemias were apparently attributable to coexisting chronic diseases, others arose *de novo* in otherwise healthy individuals. Bone marrow analysis often revealed a spectrum of abnormalities, notably aberrant maturation of marrow precursors, a variable increase in marrow blasts and, in some patients, the presence of ring sideroblasts. In the 1950s, it was appreciated that AML in the elderly was often preceded by a preleukaemic state characterized by peripheral blood cytopenias and increased numbers of blasts in the marrow. However, the term 'preleukaemia' fell away in the 1970s when it became apparent that many patients never developed leukaemia but died instead of

Postgraduate Haematology: 6th edition. Edited by A. Victor Hoffbrand,
Daniel Catovsky, Edward G.D. Tuddenham, Anthony R. Green
© 2011 Blackwell Publishing Ltd.

complications arising directly from the cytopenias. These included anaemia, infectious problems and bleeding complications. In the 1980s, the term 'myelodysplasia', or more properly *myelodysplastic syndromes* to reflect the heterogeneity of the disease, became more widely used. Indeed, it was the recognition that MDS is a heterogeneous entity of related disorders of haemopoiesis that provided the rational basis for devising diagnostic classification schemes that have evolved over the last three decades.

Incidence

According to European registry data, the overall annual incidence rate for MDS in adults is 3–4 per 100 000. However, this rate increases markedly with age, exceeding 30 per 100 000 for individuals over the age of 80 years. Over 60% of patients are over the age of 70 at diagnosis, with males more likely to be diagnosed with MDS than females by a ratio of 1.4 : 1. MDS in childhood is rare with an annual incidence of 2–3 per million, or less than 5% of paediatric haematological malignancies, tending to occur in children less than 5 years old.

Aetiology

The aetiology of primary MDS remains largely unknown. Various causes have been postulated including ionizing radiation, exposure to benzene, solvents and pesticides, and smoking, but case–control studies are inconsistent. There is some evidence to suggest that polymorphic variation in certain genes may increase susceptibility to MDS, particularly where the role of the encoded protein is to counter environmental insults to the cell. Examples include enzymes responsible for the metabolism of carcinogens, proteins involved with oxidative stress, and the proteins that function to repair damaged DNA.

In approximately 15% of patients, MDS occurs following prior exposure to cytotoxic chemotherapy and/or wide-field radiotherapy, when it is referred to as therapy-related MDS. These cases of MDS typically arise in patients who have received previous cancer treatment or prolonged immunosuppressive therapy. The most commonly implicated cytotoxic agents are the alkylating agents, such as cyclophosphamide, and the topoisomerase II inhibitors, such as etoposide, as well as ionizing radiation and antimetabolite drugs. The latency period between exposure to the mutagenic event and the onset of disease tends to be 5–6 years for the alkylating agents and for radiation but 2–3 years for the topoisomerase II inhibitors, but the range can vary from 1 to 10 years and beyond. The risk increases with age and with prolonged exposure to low-dose chemotherapy, such as prescribed for controlling vasculitic and other autoimmune disorders. The risk of developing therapy-related MDS following autologous transplantation for lymphoma varies widely between series, with some reports as high as 12%. Most cases develop within 5 years of transplantation, with the major risk factors being the duration and amount of pretransplant chemotherapy and whether the patient received total body irradiation. By comparison with primary MDS, these cases of therapy-related MDS are associated with a higher incidence of trilineage dysplasia, genetic abnormalities, evolution to AML and poor response to treatment.

Classification

FAB classification

In 1982, the French–American–British (FAB) group proposed a morphological classification of MDS that divided the disease entity into five subgroups (Table 28.1). The FAB system was based on the percentage of blasts and ringed sideroblasts in the bone marrow and the presence or absence of a peripheral blood monocytosis. Refractory anaemia (RA) was defined as anaemia with a hypercellular marrow exhibiting dyserythropoiesis but minimal granulocytic or megakarocytic abnormalities and a marrow blast count of less then 5%. If the proportion of ring sideroblasts exceeded 15% of erythroid cells, the patient was diagnosed as having refractory anaemia with ring sideroblasts (RARS). Patients with increased numbers of marrow blasts were diagnosed as having refractory anaemia with excess blasts (RAEB) if the blast percentage fell between 5 and 19% or refractory anaemia with excess blasts in transformation (RAEBt) if the blast percentage fell between 20 and 29%. A blast percentage

Table 28.1 The FAB classification of MDS.

Subtype	Blood	Bone marrow
Refractory anaemia (RA)	<1% blasts	Dysplasia <5% blasts
Refractory anaemia with ringed sideroblasts (RARS)	<1% blasts	As for RA and >15% ringed sideroblasts
Refractory anaemia with excess blasts (RAEB)	<5% blasts	Dysplasia 5–19% blasts
Refractory anaemia with excess blasts in transformation (RAEBt)	<5% blasts	Dysplasia 20–29% blasts or Auer rods
Chronic myelomonocytic leukaemia (CMML)	>1 × 10^9/L monocytes	Dysplasia <30% blasts

Table 28.2 The revised WHO classification of MDS.

Subtype	Blood	Bone marrow

Refractory cytopenias with unilineage dysplasia (RCUD)
  Refractory anaemia (RA)
  Refractory neutropenia (RN)
  Refractory thrombocytopenia (RT)
	Unicytopenia or bicytopenia	Dysplasia in >10% of cells of one myeloid lineage only
		<5% blasts
		<15% ring sideroblasts

Refractory anaemia with ring sideroblasts (RARS)	Anaemia	Erythroid dysplasia only >15% ring sideroblasts
Refractory cytopenia with multilineage dysplasia (RCMD)	Cytopenia(s)	Dysplasia in >10% of cells in two or more myeloid lineages <5% blasts <15% ring sideroblasts
Refractory cytopenia with multilineage dysplasia and ring sideroblasts (RCMD-RS)	Cytopenia(s)	Dysplasia in >10% of cells in two or more myeloid lineages <5% blasts >15% ring sideroblasts
Refractory anaemia with excess blasts-1 (RAEB-1)	Cytopenia(s) <5% blasts	Unilineage or multilineage dysplasia 5–9% blasts No Auer rods
Refractory anaemia with excess blasts-2 (RAEB-2)	Cytopenia(s) 5–19% blasts	Unilineage or multilineage dysplasia 10–19% blasts ± Auer rods
Myelodysplastic syndrome – unclassified (MDS-U)	Cytopenia(s) <1% blasts	Dysplasia in <10% of cells in one or more myeloid lineage Cytogenetic abnormality supportive of diagnosis <5% blasts
MDS associated with isolated del(5q)	Anaemia ± thrombocytosis <1% blasts	Prominent megakaryocytes with hypolobated nuclei Isolated del(5q) cytogenetic abnormality <5% blasts

greater than 30% was diagnostic of AML. Finally, chronic mye-lomonocytic leukaemia (CMML) encompassed all cases where the circulating monocyte count exceeded 1×10^9/L. However, this subgroup was particularly heterogeneous, comprising a spectrum of patients whose clinical course varied from more typical MDS to more proliferative states characterized by high monocyte counts and splenomegaly.

WHO classification

The World Health Organization (WHO) classification was first published in 2001 and more recently in a revised form in 2008 (Tables 28.2 and 28.3). It emerged through an international collaborative effort to improve the FAB classification by incor-porating more recent clinical and genetic data. In particular, it recognized the fact that patients with RA but less than 5% marrow blasts had a poorer clinical prognosis if there was evidence of multilineage dysplasia as opposed to unilineage erythroid dysplasia. New diagnoses of refractory cytopenia with multilineage dysplasia (RCMD) and refractory cytopenia with

Table 28.3 Relative frequency of MDS subtypes.

Subtype of MDS	Approximate percentage of MDS cases	Cytogenetic abnormalities	Median survival (months)
RA	10	25	66
RARS	10	<10	72
RCMD	25	50	33
RCMD-RS	10	50	33
RAEB-1	25	30–40	18
RAEB-2	15	40–50	10
Isolated del(5q)	5	100	116

multilineage dysplasia and ring sideroblasts (RCMD-RS) were introduced for patients with bicytopenia or pancytopenia whose marrows exhibited dysplastic features affecting more than 10% of cells in two or more myeloid lineages. Those patients with pure erythroid dysplasia but otherwise lacking evidence of a clonal karyotypic abnormality should be reassessed after 6 months to ensure persistence of these features before making a diagnosis of MDS.

A new subgroup recognized by the WHO classification was MDS with isolated deletion of the long arm of chromosome 5, so-called MDS with isolated del(5q). This was deemed to merit its own separate group based on the consistent clinical and morphological features associated with this cytogenetic abnormality (Figure 28.1). It occurs more usually in elderly women and is characterized by marked macrocytic anaemia and thrombocytosis that is commonly referred to as 5q– syndrome. The bone marrow is typically hypercellular with prominent megakaryocytes that are slightly decreased in size with conspicuously non-lobated or hypolobated nuclei. Erythroid activity is often reduced but dysplasia is generally minimal and myeloblasts comprise less than 5% of cells.

The RAEB entity was also refined to include two subgroups based on the precise percentage of blasts present. The term 'blast cell' here refers to myeloblasts, monoblasts, promonocytes and megakaryoblasts, but not erythroblasts. CD34-positive cells, defined immunophenotypically, are not considered to be synonymous with the blast cell. The two subgroups were denoted as RAEB-1 (blast count <5% in peripheral blood and 5–9% in marrow) and RAEB-2 (blast count 5–19% in peripheral blood and 10–19% in marrow), with the latter having a worse prognosis than the former. The morphological finding of Auer rods is also sufficient for making a diagnosis of RAEB-2. The FAB entity RAEBt, defined originally by a blast count in the marrow of over 20%, was abolished in favour of a diagnosis of AML with multilineage dysplasia that commonly yields poor-risk cytogenetics and refractoriness to chemotherapy. In addition, patients with recurrent leukaemic chromosomal translocations typical of *de novo* AML, namely t(15;17), t(8;21), and inv(16) or t(16;16), are considered to have AML regardless of the percentage of blasts in the bone marrow.

In the revised version of the WHO classification, there has been some refinement of the system to include patients presenting with monocytopenia or bicytopenia and whose bone marrows exhibit dysplasia restricted to a single lineage. This category is denoted refractory cytopenia with unilineage dysplasia (RCUD), which includes RA, refractory neutropenia and refractory thrombocytopenia. There remains the entity of MDS unclassifiable (MDS-U) to denote patients with pancytopenia who fail to fit one of the other categories. Finally, childhood MDS has been incorporated as a separate entity to cover all forms of paediatric myelodysplasia, including a new subgroup of refractory cytopenia of childhood (RCC) to cover cases that fail to meet the criteria for the RAEB subgroups, specifically where there is evidence of dysplasia but fewer than 5% blasts in the marrow.

Finally, the WHO recognizes two additional histological subtypes of MDS, namely hypoplastic MDS and myelofibrotic MDS, each of which account for approximately 10% of cases. Hypoplastic MDS has no independent prognostic significance and may be difficult to distinguish from aplastic anaemia, although both may respond similarly to immunosuppression with antithymocyte globulin. Myelofibrotic MDS, which must be diagnosed from a trephine biopsy that often reveals an excess of blasts, generally follows an aggressive clinical course. Both hypoplastic and myelofibrotic MDS are histological

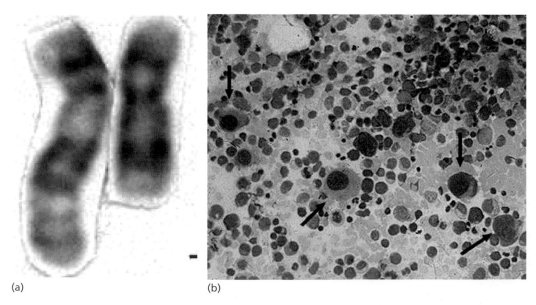

(a) (b)

Figure 28.1 Diagnostic findings in 5q– syndrome demonstrating (a) chromosomal abnormality and (b) typical morphology. Note loss of material from long arm of chromosome 5 and characteristic marrow features (arrows) including hypolobated megakaryocytes with occasional blasts.

entities based on trephine findings rather than diagnostic entities per se.

Pathogenesis

MDS is a complex disease and its pathogenesis is poorly understood. Many molecular abnormalities have been identified from genetic, cytogenetic and epigenetic analyses of the dysplastic cells and these are discussed in the following section. There are also important functional abnormalities relating to the haemopoietic stem cell, its microenvironmental niche, the propensity for apoptosis and the role of host immunity, all of which are undoubtedly relevant to the emergence and progression of the disease.

MDS: a stem cell disorder

In trying to understand the pathogenesis of MDS, most attention has focused on identifying defects in the haemopoietic stem/progenitor compartment. This largely reflects the fact that MDS is a clonal disorder which commonly affects all three myeloid lineages (i.e. megakaryocytic, erythroid and granulocytic/monocytic). Indeed, the presence of trilineage dysplasia and cytogenetic abnormalities provides irrefutable evidence for a multipotent stem/progenitor cell origin. However, whether this is a true haemopoietic stem cell or a myeloid progenitor cell, or indeed a lineage-committed cell in cases of unilineage dysplasia, is not entirely clear. Irrespective of the cell of origin, it is clear that these cells must be capable of sufficient self-renewal in order to perpetuate the disease. Studies using interphase fluorescence *in situ* hybridization (FISH) analysis have recently yielded some insights into the nature of the target cell in MDS and shown, perhaps unsurprisingly, that the situation is complicated and varies from one type of MDS to another. Thus, in 5q– syndrome, the cytogenetic abnormality can be found in both $CD34^+CD38^-$ myeloid progenitors and $CD34^+CD19^+$ pro-B cells, indicative of a true haemopoietic stem cell origin, while in patients with trisomy 8 the cytogenetic abnormality is often absent from the $CD34^+CD38^-$ fraction suggesting that there might be a different initiating event occurring within the haemopoietic stem cell. If so, then this would support the multistep theory of disease progression by which the dysplastic clone evolves over time through acquisition of additional mutational hits, allowing selection of more proliferative subclones.

If indeed the cell of origin in MDS is an aberrant stem or progenitor cell with the capacity for indefinitely perpetuating the dysplastic clone, then no less important is the bone marrow microenvironment in which the cells live. This is termed the stem cell niche, which comprises the stromal, endosteal and vascular environment responsible for maintaining the stem cell through intimate cell–cell contact. In many regards, the stem cell niche is a restatement of the 'seed and soil' hypothesis proposed many years ago to explain how the cellular microenvironment plays a vital role in the pathogenesis of diseases such as MDS. Interfering with this niche by targeting the molecular interactions between the stem cell and its microenvironment represents a novel therapeutic strategy. Such targets include homing molecules such as CD44 or the ligand–receptor interactions between CXCR4 on stem cells and its chemokine ligand SDF-1 (CXCL12) and between Tie-2 on stem cells and angiopoietin-1 on osteoblasts. Murine models of MDS and xenograft transplantation may shed light on the role of the stem cell niche and how it might be disrupted.

Immunological abnormalities in MDS

Immunological abnormalities are commonly encountered in MDS, suggesting that they may play a role in the aetiology and pathogenesis of the disease. This is particularly apparent in cases of hypoplastic MDS that share a number of features in common with aplastic anaemia, notably clinical presentation with macrocytosis and varying levels of dyserythropoiesis. A hypocellular bone marrow is encountered in approximately 10% of cases of MDS and may indeed represent one end of the MDS spectrum that overlaps biologically with aplastic anaemia. Both disorders are characterized by a clonal expansion of T cells that are antigen driven, and there is also an association with HLA-DR15. While the full pathogenesis of hypoplastic MDS and aplastic anaemia remains unknown in detail, both these entities appear to be characterized by a pathological immune response triggered by abnormal haemopoietic stem cells that results in the autoimmune destruction of normal stem cells and/or their niche. In addition, acquired mutations in the *PIGA* gene characteristic of paroxysmal nocturnal haemoglobinuria (PNH) are also encountered, presumably through expansion of small clones in an otherwise hypoplastic marrow, suggesting that PNH similarly is part of this spectrum. Conversely, dysplastic clones carrying cytogenetic abnormalities can emerge in both aplastic anaemia and PNH after treatment and can evolve into frank MDS over time.

A role for the immune system in the pathogenesis of MDS is also borne out by the higher incidence of autoimmune disease in these patients. T-cell-mediated inhibition of haemopoiesis appears to be an important aspect of this mechanism, with oligoclonal $CD8^+$ cytotoxic T cells being found in many patients. However, the antigens produced by the MDS cells that lead to these T-cell responses are largely unknown although, interestingly, WT1-specific $CD8^+$ cells are often detectable in the peripheral blood of MDS patients with trisomy 8. Sometimes, the expanded T cells in MDS can themselves become neoplastic, resulting eventually in the diagnosis of T-cell large granular lymphocytic leukaemia that also falls into this overlap spectrum of bone marrow failure states. Recently, analysis of self-reactive T cells in MDS has focused on the regulatory T cells that play a central role in maintaining immune tolerance. This has revealed a correlation between expanded numbers of CD4+CD25^{high}FoxP3+ regulatory T cells and more aggressive forms of MDS as defined by their blast cell percentage, possibly due to suppression of host antitumour mechanisms. However, the most persuasive evidence for immune dysregulation in MDS arguably comes from the recognition that some forms of the disease, notably hypocellular MDS, like aplastic anaemia can respond well to immunosuppressive therapy with antithymocyte globulin and/or ciclosporin resulting in durable haematological recovery and abrogation of T-cell clones.

Apoptosis in MDS

One of the defining, albeit paradoxical, features of MDS is the presence of cytopenias despite a typically hypercellular bone marrow. For those patients undergoing leukaemic transformation, the cytopenias arise due to maturation block of the malignant cells. However, in cases of MDS that lack an excess of blasts, the cytopenias are a reflection of the ineffective haemopoiesis that is a hallmark of the disease. The mechanism appears to be one of increased apoptosis of haemopoietic precursors in the marrow, as demonstrated using *in situ* end-labelling of fragmented DNA to reveal cells undergoing programmed cell death. Apoptosis is more prominent in early MDS, such as RA and RARS, than in advanced MDS with excess myeloblasts. Indeed, for the blasts to overcome this apoptotic tendency indicates that they have lost their G_2/M checkpoint control that appears to be a necessary requirement for progression to leukaemia. This progression is accompanied by a change in favour of pro-apoptotic proteins such as c-Myc in CD34-positive precursors at diagnosis to anti-apoptotic proteins such as Bcl-2 in leukaemic blasts at time of transformation. Moreover, patients with higher rates of apoptosis have a considerably better overall survival than patients with lower rates of apoptosis, likely reflecting the clonal evolution of the MDS towards AML. This finding is corroborated by flow cytometry analysis of MDS marrow samples to measure relative levels of apoptosis (by annexin V staining) versus proliferation (by Ki67) that demonstrates a shift from apoptosis to proliferation as the disease progresses. These findings underpin the theory that apoptosis plays a major role in the pathophysiology of MDS.

Apoptosis can be initiated by various cytokines, notably tumour necrosis factor (TNF)-α, Fas-ligand, and TNF-related apoptosis inducing ligand (TRAIL). Indeed, all these cytokines and related other ones are typically upregulated in the marrow in MDS, serving as negative regulators of haemopoiesis. Apoptosis can also be triggered by cytotoxic T cells and by signals from marrow stromal cells, probably via activation of similar pathways, and intrinsically following DNA damage and mitochondrial dysfunction that leads in turn to cytochrome *c* release and caspase activation. This balance of pro-apoptotic to anti-apoptotic signals swings in favour of the latter as the MDS

evolves towards AML, with upregulation of NF-κB, altered expression of adapter molecules such as Flice inhibitory protein (FLIP), and enhanced activity of members of the BCL-2 and IAP (inhibitors of apoptosis protein) families. This is borne out by a murine model of MDS/AML in which BCL-2 is conditionally overexpressed alongside an activating *NRAS* mutant gene resulting in a disease entity reminiscent of MDS. In this model, using a stronger promoter to drive BCL-2 gene expression leads to more rapid AML progression, providing experimental insight into the process of leukaemogenesis.

Molecular basis of MDS

Despite the fact that the molecular basis of MDS is poorly understood, recent discoveries have provided important insights into the pathogenesis of the disease. MDS is a preleukaemic disorder characterized by impaired cellular differentiation that has the potential to transform to AML if this abnormality is coupled to enhanced survival and proliferation. Conversely, the myeloproliferative syndromes, including the myelodysplastic–myeloproliferative overlap, are characterized by enhanced survival and proliferation that has the potential to transform to AML if coupled to a block in differentiation. Thus, conceptually at least, both MDS and myeloproliferative disorders represent different routes to acquiring the multiple hits necessary for development of AML.

Cytogenetic abnormalities

Cytogenetic analysis of marrow samples plays an important role in the evaluation of MDS with regard to establishing clonality and determining prognosis. Clonal abnormalities are observed in approximately half of all primary MDS cases and in up to 90% of cases of secondary therapy-related MDS (Table 28.4). Defining such abnormalities and their clonal evolution over

Table 28.4 Cytogenetic abnormalities in MDS with approximate frequency.

Abnormality	Primary MDS (%)	Therapy-related MDS (%)
Complex karyotype	15–20	80–90
del(5q)/monosomy 5	15–20	30–40
del(7q)/monosomy 7	10–15	40–50
Trisomy 8	10–15	10–15
del(20q)	5–10	–
del(17p)	<5	–
del(13q)	<5	–
del(11q)	<5	–
del(12p)	<5	–

time has contributed to our broader understanding of the mechanistic basis of MDS and how it transforms into AML. However, apart from the 5q– syndrome, cytogenetic abnormalities are not specific for particular clinico-morphological subtypes of MDS. Generally, the loss or gain of genetic material, through chromosomal deletions, unbalanced translocations and aneuploidy, is more characteristic of MDS than AML. Conversely, balanced translocations that are typical of *de novo* AML are rarely seen in MDS.

The common chromosomal abnormalities found in MDS include loss of Y, 5q– or monosomy 5, 7q– or monosomy 7, trisomy 8, 20q–, abnormalities of 11q23, and deletions of 17p, 12p, 13q and 11q among others. None of these is specific for MDS as they can also occur in AML and myeloproliferative states. Cytogenetic analysis is required for calculating a risk score according to established prognostic scoring systems, with normal, –Y, del(5q) and del(20q) recognized as good-risk karyotypes while chromosome 7 anomalies, complex (more than three abnormalities) and very complex (more than five abnormalities) are recognized as poor-risk karyotypes. For the three chromosomes (5, 7 and 20) that are commonly wholly or partially lost in MDS, it remains unknown whether the dysplastic phenotype arises due to a haploinsufficient dosage reduction of one or more genes or the complete functional loss of a key tumour-suppressor gene. Similarly, for trisomy 8, it is not clear if this simply causes a dosage increase of a number of normal genes or the gain of function of a mutant oncogene.

5q– syndrome

The 5q– syndrome was originally described in 1974 by Van den Berghe and was the first entity within the group of refractory cytopenias to be associated with a consistent chromosomal aberration, namely the interstitial deletion of 5q. The syndrome is associated with macrocytic anaemia, thrombocytosis, unilobular megakaryocytes and a low propensity to develop into AML. It is more common in females than males. However, not all patients with 5q abnormalities have this syndrome since del(5q), and indeed monosomy 5, are also found in more typical cases of MDS, frequently as part of a complex karyotype with other cytogenetic abnormalities.

The 5q– syndrome, with del(5q) as the sole cytogenetic abnormality, has provided an opportunity to define precisely the molecular defect(s) underlying the pathogenesis of this disease. The search for a minimal common deleted region on the long arm of chromosome 5 has spanned three decades and relied on physical mapping methods. Using FISH analysis, this region has been narrowed down to a 1.5-Mb interval located on 5q32. The advent of high-resolution single-nucleotide polymorphism (SNP) arrays has provided greater refinement of the limits of this deleted region. The search for a tumour-suppressor gene located within this region has involved many different approaches over recent years and resulted in numer-

ous candidate genes. However, it was not known whether 5q– syndrome required the loss of heterozygosity for a particular gene locus or could arise through haploinsufficiency alone of a particular gene.

The best candidate gene for 5q– syndrome was recently identified by way of a functional screening study that used RNA interference (RNAi) to systematically 'knock down' expression of 40 genes in the 5q32 region in normal CD34-positive cells. These cells were cultured in conditions promoting either erythroid or megakaryocytic differentiation. Partial RNAi knockdown of the ribosomal protein S14 gene (*RPS14*) was found to cause a block in erythroid differentiation but preservation of megakaryocytic differentiation that recapitulates the phenotype of 5q– syndrome. Moreover, *RPS14* was able to rescue the 5q– phenotype by re-expression in CD34-positive cells from 5q– syndrome patients. If this result is confirmed, then there would appear to be a remarkable similarity between 5q– syndrome and the congenital bone marrow disorders of Diamond–Blackfan anaemia and Schwachman–Diamond syndrome that arise due to inherited abnormalities of related ribosomal protein genes, namely *RPS19* and *SBDS* respectively. However, while haploinsufficiency of *RPS14* may indeed explain the key clinical features of the 5q– phenotype, this hypothesis fails to account for the growth advantage of the 5q– clone and therefore may not represent the complete genetic pathogenesis of the disease. Nonetheless, with the discovery that the immunomodulatory drug lenalidomide is an effective treatment in 5q– syndrome, studies are ongoing to see whether this drug works by correcting the ribosomal defect caused by deficiency of *RPS14*.

Chromosome 7 abnormalities

Monosomy 7 is the second most common chromosomal abnormality, occurring in up to 20% of MDS cases overall. It can present as a total or partial monosomy and may be an isolated abnormality or part of a complex karyotype. Clinically, monosomy 7 MDS is characterized by a lower median age of affected patients compared with deletions of 5q, severe refractory cytopenias, and tendency to life-threatening infections. Monosomy 7 confers a poor prognosis that ranges from 14 months as an isolated abnormality down to 7 months if the karyotype is complex and involves other abnormalities. At least two distinct regions of common deletions have been identified: the band 7q22 and the more telomeric regions of 7q31–32 and 7q36. This suggests the presence of more than one gene having tumour-suppressive functions located within these disparate regions of 7q. Whether the monosomy 7 MDS phenotype arises due to functional deletion through loss of heterozygosity of a particular gene locus or simply due to genetic haploinsufficiency is not known. There are a number of candidate genes within this region such as *MLL5*, a member of the Hox family, and genes involved with DNA repair. In addition, microRNAs involved in regulation of signalling pathways have been implicated as have associated mutations in *RAS* and *AML1* that commonly coexist with monosomy 7. However, the precise mechanism relating monosomy 7 to MDS remains obscure.

Genetic abnormalities in MDS

Recurrent abnormalities in a large number of genes have been identified in MDS and continue to provide important insights into the disease. These include genes coding for cell surface molecules, signal transduction proteins, transcriptional factors, epigenetic modifiers, protein degradation pathways and many genes of unknown function (Table 28.5).

Mutations of the *AML1* gene (also known as *RUNX1*) have recently been recognized to occur in MDS, particularly where it is treatment-related or radiation-induced. In contrast with the mutations of *AML1* found in M0 AML that are often biallelic, those found in MDS are generally monoallelic and result in *AML1* haploinsufficiency rather than a dominant-negative protein. Moreover, while the mutations in AML tend to occur in the Runt domain and affect DNA binding, mutations in MDS occur more frequently in the C-terminus of the protein causing truncation and loss of its transactivating domain. Interestingly, individuals who inherit one abnormal copy of the *AML1* gene commonly exhibit congenital thrombocytopenia with a propensity to develop AML, suggesting the gene might be acting as a tumour suppressor in this setting.

The *AML1* gene is also involved in one of the few examples of a recurrent MDS-associated chromosomal lesion to be molecularly deciphered, namely the t(3;21) translocation found in some cases of MDS (and in blast crisis in chronic myeloid leukaemia). This translocation rearranges the *AML1* and *EVI1* (also known as *MDS1*) genes, fusing the N-terminus of AML1 with a small portion of MDS1 and nearly all of EVI-1 and resulting in a fusion protein that appears to deregulate normal haemopoiesis. EVI-1 is a zinc finger protein that when overexpressed can block erythroid differentiation and promote transformation. Translocations that involve only chromosome 3, namely t(3;3) and inv(3), both cause overexpression of *EVI1* and are associated with MDS and AML with abnormal megakaryocytes.

Table 28.5 Recurrent mutated genes in MDS according to their major function.

Gene function	Abnormal gene
Cell surface receptor	KIT, FMS, PDGFRB, GCSFR, MPL, FLT3
Signal transduction	NRAS, JAK2
Transcription factor	AML1, GATA-1, PU.1, CEBPA, TP53
Epigenetic factor	MLL, ATRX
Protein degradation	CBL
Unknown function	TET2

Another recurrent cytogenetic abnormality in MDS that is associated with characteristic morphological features is isolated del(20q), which typically involves erythroid and megakaryocytic lineages. Deletions of 20q generally carry a favourable prognosis although the implicated gene, which is likely to reside within the commonly deleted region 20q12, remains unknown.

Activating mutations of *RAS*, usually involving *NRAS*, are found in up to 20% of cases of MDS, especially CMML, and are often associated with *AML1* point mutations. Other genes occasionally found to harbour mutations in MDS include those encoding various cell-surface receptors with kinase activity such as *FMS* (now called *CSF1R*), *KIT*, *FLT3*, *PDGFRB* and *GCSFR*, and those encoding transcription factors such as *GATA1*, *PU.1* (*SPI1*), *CEBPA*, *MLL* and *TP53*. Mutations of the *ATRX* gene located on the X chromosome are associated with the rare phenomenon of acquired HbH disease, also termed acquired α thalassaemia in MDS, in which the dysplastic red cells are markedly microcytic and hypochromic with HbH inclusions.

Recently, the V617F mutation of the *JAK2* gene has been demonstrated in up to 50% of patients with the overlap condition of RARS with thrombocytosis (denoted RARS-T) that exists as a provisional new entity in the updated WHO classification. This mutation, which is more commonly associated with the myeloproliferative disorders, causes constitutive activation of the JAK2 protein and downstream signalling. Similarly, mutations of the *MPL* gene, which are described in essential thrombocythaemia, have also been identified in patients with RARS-T.

A number of state-of-the-art techniques are increasingly being used to further refine our understanding of the molecular pathogenesis of MDS. These include gene expression profiling to identify expressed transcripts and comparative genomic hybridization (CGH) to identify small regions of DNA gain or loss. More recently, high-resolution SNP genotyping microarrays have been used to detect cytogenetically cryptic genomic aberrations (Figure 28.2). These SNP microarrays use chromosomal markers to identify regions of loss of heterozygosity, which occurs either through genetic deletion or functionally via copy-neutral uniparental disomy (UPD), leading to regions of hemizygosity or homozygosity respectively. One study of 119 low-risk MDS patients revealed that UPD occurs in 46% of cases, while deletions and amplifications occur in 10% and 8% of cases respectively. A number of state-of-the-art techniques are increasingly being used to further refine our understanding of the molecular pathogenesis of MDS. These include gene expression profiling using cDNA microarray analysis to identify expressed transcripts, and comparative genomic hybridization (CGH) to identify small regions of DNA gain or loss. More recently, high-resolution single-nucleotide polymorphism (SNP) genotyping microarrays have been used to detect cytogenetically cryptic genomic aberrations (Figure 2). These SNP microarrays use chromosomal markers to identify regions of

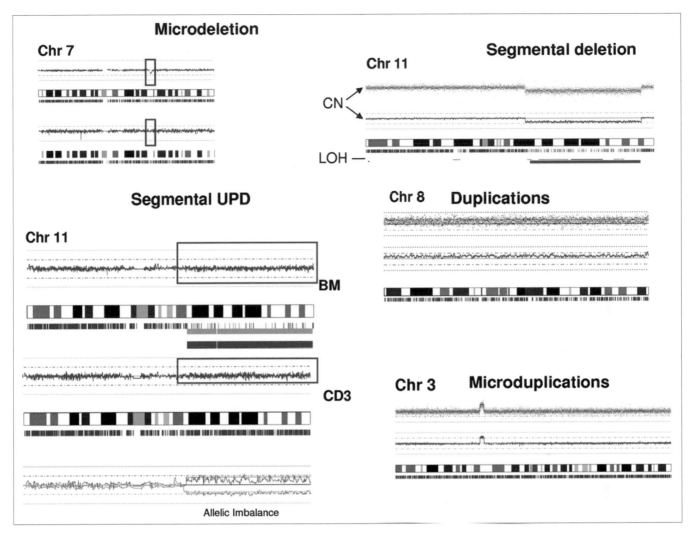

Figure 28.2 Representative examples of genomic mutations identified in MDS patients using single-nucleotide polymorphism analyses with high-density microarrays. BM denotes bone marrow cells and CD3 denotes T lymphocytes. CN, copy number; LOH, loss of heterozygosity; UPD, uniparental disomy. (From Maciejewski & Mufti 2008 with permission.)

loss of heterozygosity, which occurs either through genetic deletion or functionally via copy-neutral uniparental disomy (UPD), leading to regions of hemizygosity or homozygosity, respectively. One study of 119 low-risk MDS patients revealed that UPD occurs in 46% of cases, whereas deletions and amplifications occur in 10% and 8% of cases, respectively. This approach has been used to identify a number of recurrent mutations involving various genes not previously implicated in the pathogenesis of MDS. Most notable amongst these is the *TET2* gene which is located within a region of UPD at chromosomal position 4q24 and is a candidate tumour suppressor gene mutated in 19% of patients with MDS. Importantly, *TET2* has also been shown to be defective in patients with other myeloid malignancies, including CMML (22%), secondary AML (24%) and myeloproliferative disorders (12%). *TET2* shares sequence homology with *TET1*, a fusion partner of the MLL oncogene in

AML that has recently been shown to catalyse the conversion of 5-methylcytosine to 5-hydoxymethylcytosine. However, unlike *TET1*, *TET2* lacks a DNA binding domain and its function remains largely unknown, although it is clearly implicated in the control of normal myelopoiesis. Of particular interest is the fact that the *TET2* mutation appears to be an early genetic lesion identifiable in haematopoietic stem cells that is generally acquired before other mutations, such as the *JAK2* V617F mutation, as evidenced by the fact that *TET2*+ve/*JAK2*+ve myeloproliferative states frequently transform into *TET2*+ve/*JAK2*-ve AML.

The *CBL* gene at chromosomal position 11q23.3 is another candidate tumour suppressor gene recently implicated in MDS. It was identified through demonstration of a recurrent UPD at 11q in 12 of 301 patients (4%) with various myeloid malignancies, including MDS/MPN, CMML and related disorders. Of these, seven patients were found to carry mutations of the *c-CBL* gene, which functions as an E3 ubiquitin ligase involved with ubiquitination and degradation of active protein tyrosine kinases. Interestingly, mutations involving *CBL* appear to be particularly common in myeloproliferative states, showing features of transformation. Finally, one additional gene, the polycomb gene *ASXL1*, has also been shown to be mutated in 4 out of 35 patients with MDS (11%) and 17 out of 39 patients with CMML (43%) in one study and 2 out of 20 patients with RARS-T (10%) in another study. Although the specific function of *ASXL1* remains largely unknown, it appears to be a chromatin-binding protein important for regulating gene expression through epigenetic transcriptional control.

Epigenetic abnormalities

Epigenetics refers to various molecular modifications of chromatin that, without altering the DNA sequence, play a critical role in genomic regulation and control of gene expression. There are two important epigenetic modifications relevant to MDS, namely DNA methylation and histone modification. DNA methylation refers to the addition of a methyl group to cytosine, which can occur wherever this is followed by a guanine within a CpG dinucleotide pair. Such CpG pairs are underrepresented in the human genome but cluster together within so-called CpG islands that tend to be located in the proximity of gene promoter regions. In normal cells, these CpG islands are typically unmethylated, allowing genes to be expressed. However, if a CpG island is methylated, then transcriptional activity at the promoter is impeded and the gene becomes silenced. Thus, aberrant promoter methylation leads to inactivation of the gene, thereby providing an alternative mechanism whereby tumour-suppressor genes can be functionally deleted. This is the paradigm that underpins the rationale for using hypomethylating agents as a novel therapeutic strategy in MDS.

The other major epigenetic control mechanism that works in conjunction with DNA methylation is histone modification. Histones form the chromatin scaffold and closely regulate whether the DNA exists locally in a repressed or permissive state. Biochemical alterations to the tails of the histone molecules influence the degree of compaction of the nucleosomes and hence the level of transcriptional activity of nearby genes. Unlike DNA methylation, which is largely irreversible, histone modifications are more dynamic, particularly acetylation/deacetylation of lysine residues of histones H3 and H4. Moreover, there is a close and cooperative interplay between these two epigenetic control mechanisms that together can render a gene permanently silenced. The significance of this is that combination epigenetic therapies that comprise a hypomethylating agent with a histone deacetylase inhibitor may be more effective than single agents in reawakening silenced tumour-suppressor genes.

Diagnosis

Clinical features

Approximately 20% of cases of MDS are detected incidentally in patients who have a routine blood count taken for unrelated reasons that reveals unexpected cytopenia or dysplasia. The majority of the remainder present with symptoms and signs of bone marrow failure, notably fatigue due to anaemia in up to 80% and infections or bleeding in up to 20%. Among the most common infections are bacterial pneumonias and skin abscesses, occurring particularly in patients with a neutrophil count of less than 1×10^9/L. Features of lymphadenopathy, splenomegaly and hepatomegaly are rarely found. There is a recognized association between MDS and several rare disorders that seem to have an immunological basis, including neutrophilic dermatosis (Sweet syndrome), pyoderma gangrenosum and cutaneous vasculitis.

Blood count

Anaemia is the predominant finding in most patients at presentation, occurring as pancytopenia in 30–50% or in combination with neutropenia or thrombocytopenia in 20–30%. Isolated neutropenia or thrombocytopenia is rarer, accounting for 5–10% of presentations. Occasionally, the blood count is normal and the diagnosis is suggested by abnormal parameters generated by automated cell counters that reflect aberrant morphology, such as the erythrocyte distribution width that can itself become a useful marker of MDS.

Peripheral blood morphology

Morphological abnormalities in the peripheral blood, while generally non-specific for MDS, can nonetheless be very helpful in arriving at a diagnosis. There is commonly marked anisocytosis/poikilocytosis and the red cells tend to be macrocytic and oval-shaped. In sideroblastic anaemia, the blood film is classically dimorphic, containing a minority population of hypochromic microcytic cells; Pappenheimer bodies, which can be confirmed with an iron stain, and basophilic stippling may also be seen. Microcytosis is present in the rare variant of acquired HbH disease. Some patients have occasional circulating erythroblasts in the peripheral blood that are often dysplastic or megaloblastic.

Neutropenia is common and neutrophils often exhibit reduced granulation and the acquired Pelger–Huët anomaly. Hypogranular neutrophils arise due to defective formation of secondary granules, with the agranular ones being highly specific for MDS. The pseudo-Pelger–Huët neutrophil is one that exhibits dense clumping of the chromatin and hypolobulation of the nucleus that is classically bilobed (resembling a pair of spectacles) or even non-lobed (resembling a dumb-bell). This acquired abnormality, which resembles the inherited Pelger–Huët anomaly, is sufficiently characteristic of MDS to be almost pathognomonic.

Monocytosis is present, by definition, in CMML and monocytes can often be morphologically abnormal. While often reduced in MDS, basophils and eosinophils might also be raised in the proliferative overlap syndromes. Circulating blasts may be found in all categories of MDS but if present in significant numbers are more usually indicative of RAEB. Finally, the platelet count is often reduced and platelets may show dysplasia such as hypogranulated and giant forms.

Bone marrow morphology

The ability to diagnosis MDS according to the presence of dysplastic morphology is critically dependent on optimal staining of the marrow slides with a Romanowsky stain (Figure 28.3). Ideally, only a small volume of marrow should be aspirated to avoid excess dilution with peripheral blood. There is often considerable interobserver variation, particularly where the dyserythropoiesis or neutrophil hypogranularity is subtle, but better consistency among observers in identifying frankly abnormal cells such as ring sideroblasts, pseudo-Pelger–Huët cells, micromegakaryocytes and increased blasts.

The bone marrow is hypercellular in the majority of patients, due to erythroid and/or granulocytic hyperplasia, but can be normocellular or, in 10–20% of cases, hypocellular. Dysplastic features can be recognized in any number of lineages and a minimum of 500 cells should be scrutinized to gain an accurate and representative differential of cells present.

Erythropoiesis is usually normoblastic but may exhibit megaloblastic-like features. In patients with sideroblastic anaemia, the erythroblasts are often poorly haemoglobinized or show cytoplasmic vacuolation. The list of dysplastic features is considerable and may include binuclearity and multinuclearity, internuclear bridging, nuclear budding and fragmentation, increased pyknosis, and basophilic stippling. Cytochemical iron staining should be performed in all cases of suspected MDS in order to quantify iron stores and to detect and enumerate ring sideroblasts and pathological non-ring forms.

Granulopoiesis is usually hyperplastic. Dysplasia of the granulocytic series is often quite difficult to appreciate and includes defective granulation and nuclear lobulation. There may be prominent basophilic and eosinophilic differentiation and increased numbers of blasts may be present.

Megakaryopoiesis is commonly dysplastic, of which the most specific feature is the micromegakaryocyte. This is typically the size of a myeloblast with an ill-defined or blebbed periphery and a single monolobed nucleus. Other megakaryocytes may exhibit hypolobulation or contain multiple disparate nuclei due to aberrant maturation. In the acquired 5q– syndrome, there are often increased numbers of megakaryocytes that are variably sized and contain a large non-lobulated nucleus.

Bone marrow histology

Histological analysis of the bone marrow can yield diagnostic information not apparent by morphology, particularly regarding architectural disorder, and should be undertaken routinely whenever a biopsy is being taken in suspected cases of MDS. The majority of patients with MDS will have hypercellular marrows but a significant minority will have a hypocellular marrow. Cytological evidence of dysplasia can be found in all lineages but is most easily detected in the erythroid precursors. Abnormal clustering of megakaryocytes is often seen as are micromegakaryocytes that can be more easily detected by immunohistochemical staining. Reticulin can be modestly increased. Abnormal localization of immature precursors is a much-debated finding that refers to the clustering of promyelocytes and myelocytes in an intertrabecular position. Their presence tends to correlate with the blast percentage in MDS and as such they may signify propensity to leukaemic transformation, but this finding is inconsistent.

Other investigations

Immunophenotyping does not play a major role in the diagnosis of MDS and need not be routinely performed. However, various abnormalities are sometimes discernible, notably low side-scatter, reduced expression of normal myeloid markers, and aberrant patterns of expression of other markers. CD34 expression, and to a lesser degree CD117, often correlates with the blast percentage, while coexpression of CD7 is significant for conferring a worse prognosis.

There are a number of further laboratory tests that are commonly abnormal in MDS but which are rarely indicated for purposes of diagnosis. These include the following.
- Granulocyte function tests to demonstrate defective phagocytosis, cell killing and motility.
- Platelet function tests to demonstrate reduced aggregation and prolonged bleeding time.
- Haemoglobin electrophoresis, or HPLC, to detect HbH (raised in acquired HbH disease) and HbF (raised in juvenile myelomonocytic leukaemia).
- Ferrokinetics to assess erythropoiesis.
- Autoantibodies (found in up to 50% of CMML patients).
- Serum protein electrophoresis to assess immunoglobulins and detect paraprotein.
- Lymphocyte populations to detect altered numbers of T-cell subsets and natural killer cells.

Natural history and prognostic factors

Natural history

The natural history of MDS is highly variable due to the considerable biological heterogeneity of the disease. The median

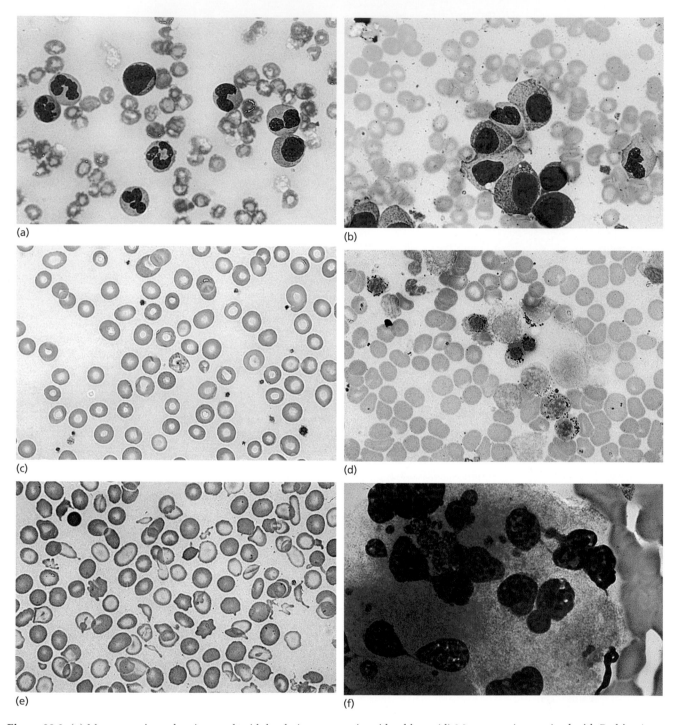

Figure 28.3 (a) Marrow aspirate showing erythroid dysplasia (nuclear irregularity, binucleate pro-erythroblast) and myeloid dysplasia (neutrophil hypogranularity, pseudo-Pelger–Huët cell). (b) Marrow aspirate from a patient with CMML showing monocytes, promonocytes and blast cells. (c) Marrow aspirate stained with Perls stain from a patient with RARS showing ring sideroblasts. (d) Marrow aspirate stained with Perls' stain from a patient with RARS, showing ring sideroblasts. (e) Peripheral blood from a patient with RAEB, ring sideroblasts and acquired haemoglobin H, showing a grossly dimorphic picture. (f) Dysplastic megakaryocyte with widely separated nuclei.

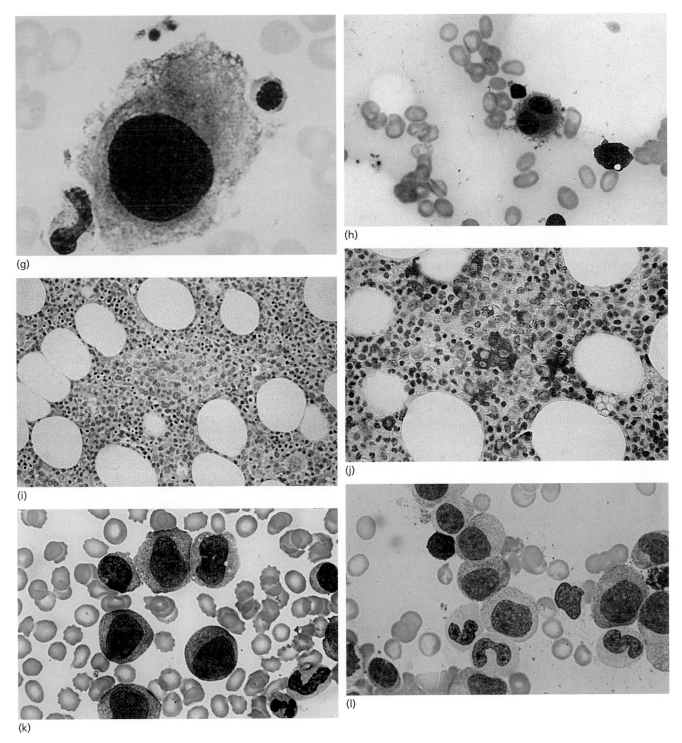

Figure 28.3 *Continued* (g) Large mononuclear megakaryocyte. (h) Micromegakaryocyte. (i) Marrow trephine biopsy showing an abnormal localization of immature precursors (ALIP) (courtesy of Dr Bridget Williams, Department of Histopathology, Royal Victoria Infirmary, Newcastle upon Tyne). (j) Marrow trephine stained for neutrophil elastase showing a 'true ALIP' (courtesy of Dr Bridget Wilkins, Department of Histopathology, Royal Victoria Infirmary, Newcastle upon Tyne). (k) Peripheral blood from a patient with CMML showing monocytes and promonocytes. (l) CMML marrow showing immature myeloid and monocytic cells.

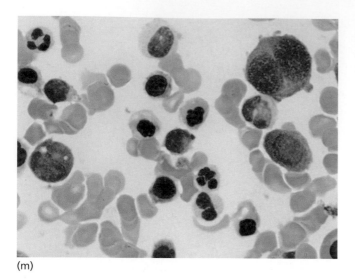

(m)

Figure 28.3 *Continued* (m) Marrow aspirate showing erythroid dysplasia (nuclear irregularity, binucleate pro-erythroblast) and myeloid dysplasia (neutrophil hypogranularity, pseudo-Pëlger cell) from a patient with RCMD.

survival of adult patients with primary MDS is approximately 20 months but this varies from only a few months for patients with high-risk disease up to nearly 12 years for patients with low-risk disease. At one end of the MDS spectrum are patients whose disease rapidly transforms into AML, while at the other end are patients with modest levels of anaemia not requiring transfusion support. Many factors influence the clinical course of the disease, including the subtype of MDS, the levels of dysplasia and blast percentage, and the number of cytopenias present. The biology of the disease, which dictates the rates of clonal expansion and leukaemic evolution, clearly involves genetic and epigenetic abnormalities, although these are difficult to identify in individual patients.

Cytogenetic analysis represents the most important investigation at diagnosis, both for understanding the biology of the disease and for making prognostic recommendations for the patient. Indeed it is possible to construct a prognostic scheme in MDS based solely on the cytogenetic abnormalities. This was recently carried out by the German–Austrian MDS Study Group using data generated from 1202 patients treated with supportive care only. Their analysis was based on a total of 24 different karyotypic abnormalities, ranked according to the median survival of patients with each abnormality, that were then grouped into four risk subgroups. The most common cytogenetic abnormality in each of the four karyotypic subgroups, along with their respective median survival, were as follows: 5q– in good-risk group (55 months); trisomy 8 in intermediate I risk group (29 months); chromosome 7 anomalies in intermediate II risk group (15 months); and complex (more than three anomalies) in poor-risk group (8 months). However, normal karyotype accounted for just over 50% of all the cases

studied and these fell collectively within the good-risk group. For these patients, alternative techniques will be required to further delineate the genetic abnormalities, for instance high-resolution SNP microarrays. One such study of low-risk MDS patients with normal karyotypes identified UPD in 46% of cases analysed compared with deletions in 10%, both of which result in cryptic loss of heterozygosity and potential predisposition to development of MDS. In the future new analytical tools, including matrix CGH, microarray gene expression analyses, proteomics and methylation profiling, will no doubt add further to our understanding of the pathogenesis of MDS, identification of therapeutic targets, and individualization of prognosis and therapy. Until such time, we are left with a long list of clinical and laboratory criteria by which to determine prognosis and optimal management for an individual diagnosed with MDS.

International Prognostic Scoring System

The International Prognostic Scoring System (IPSS) was published in 1997 by an International MDS Risk Analysis Workshop (Tables 28.6–28.8). It was based on the retrospective evaluation of a clinical, morphological and cytogenetic dataset obtained from 816 patients with MDS that was compiled from seven large risk-based studies. These patients were either untreated or had received only short courses of low-dose oral chemotherapy or haemopoietic growth factors. The study included those patients diagnosed with MDS according to the FAB criteria, except for those patients with proliferative CMML defined as having a white cell count greater than 12×10^9/L. A global analysis was performed and critical prognostic variables were evaluated to generate a consensus prognostic scheme, particularly using more refined bone marrow cytogenetic information. In addition to patient age, univariate analysis indicated that the major variables having an impact on disease outcome for evolu-

Table 28.6 International Prognostic Scoring System (IPSS).

Variable	Score value				
	0	0.5	1.0	1.5	2.0
Bone marrow blasts (%)	<5	5–10	–	11–20	21–30
Karyotype*	Good	Intermediate	Poor	–	–
Cytopenias†	0/1	2/3	–	–	–

*Karyotype status: good category includes normal, –Y, del(5q), del(20q); poor category includes complex (three or more) abnormalities, chromosome 7 anomalies; intermediate category includes other abnormalities.
†Cytopenias defined as haemoglobin <10 g/dL, neutrophils <1.8 × 10⁹/L and platelets <100 × 10⁹/L.

Table 28.7 Prognostic outcomes of MDS patients according to IPSS risk score.

Outcome measure	IPSS risk category			
	Low	Intermediate-1	Intermediate-2	High
Combined score	0	0.5–1.0	1.5–2.0	2.5
Leukaemic death	19%	30%	33%	45%
Median time to AML (years)	9.4	3.3	1.1	0.2
Median survival (years)	5.7	3.5	1.2	0.4

The median survival for each of these groups is stratified according to age at diagnosis but broadly ranges from 4 to 12 years for low risk, 2 to 4 years for intermediate-1, 1 to 2 years for intermediate-2, and to <1 year for high risk across all age groups.

Table 28.8 Median survival of MDS patients according to IPSS risk score and age.

Risk group	IPSS score	Median survival (years)			
		<60 years old	>60 years old	<70 years old	>70 years old
Low	0	11.8	4.8	9	3.9
Intermediate-1	0.5–1.0	5.2	2.7	4.4	2.4
Intermediate-2	1.5–2.0	1.8	1.1	1.3	1.2
High	2.5	0.3	0.5	0.4	0.4

tion to AML were cytogenetic abnormalities, percentage of myeloblasts in the marrow, and number of cytopenias.

The IPSS generates an overall score using three criteria, namely blast percentage, number of cytopenias and karyotype risk. Based on this score, patients are allocated into one of four risk groups, namely low, intermediate-1, intermediate-2 or high. The median survival for each of these groups is stratified according to age at diagnosis, but broadly ranges from 5–7 years for low risk, 3–5 years for intermediate-1, 1–2 years for intermediate-2, to 4–8 months for high risk. The value of such a prognostic scoring system is clearly dependent on the type of treatment that a patient receives. The IPSS has been validated in patients undergoing allogeneic transplantation, but the outcome of patients receiving intensive chemotherapy is more dependent on cytogenetic data than the percentage of marrow blasts and the IPSS appears less helpful in this setting. More recently, an alternative prognostic scoring system based on the WHO classification scheme has been promoted to address some of the shortcomings of the IPSS.

WHO Classification-based Prognostic Scoring System

One of the major shortcomings of the IPSS is the fact that the system was designed to be used only at diagnosis and may not be suitable for serial assessment of patients whose disease can evolve over time. In addition, the IPSS pre-dated the revised classification of MDS according to WHO criteria and therefore incorporated some entities, notably CMML, that are now categorized as myeloproliferative overlap disorders. Finally, the IPSS fails to reflect whether or not the patient is dependent on transfusional support, which along with cytogenetics is one of the main prognostic factors affecting survival. For these reasons, the WHO Classification-based Prognostic Scoring System (WPSS) was developed based on the retrospective analysis of 467 Italian patients and validated against 620 German patients (Tables 28.9 and 28.10). All patients had a diagnosis of MDS according to one of the WHO subgroups, but CMML and other overlap disorders were excluded. Analysis of the data showed that the most significant variables for the model were WHO subgroup, the cytogenetic abnormalities and the transfusional requirements of the patient (Figure 28.4). These were incorporated into a scoring system that allowed stratification into five distinct risk groups showing significantly different overall survival and probability of leukaemic progression (Figure 28.5). The median survival (in months) of these five groups was 136 (very low), 63 (low), 44 (intermediate), 19 (high) and 8 (very high). The likelihood of developing leukaemia ranged from a 10-year probability of 7% in the very low risk group to a 50% probability at 8 months in the very high risk group.

The major difference from the IPSS is that the WPSS provides prognostic information from initial evaluation through treatment to follow-up. Thus, the WPSS permits a dynamic estimation of survival and risk of AML transformation at multiple time points during the natural course of MDS and is therefore more versatile than the IPSS in clinical decision-making and

Table 28.9 WHO Classification-based Prognostic Scoring System (WPSS).

Variable	Score value			
	0	1	2	3
WHO category	RA, RARS, 5q–	RCMD, RCMD-RS	RAEB-1	RAEB-2
Karotype*	Good	Intermediate	Poor	–
Transfusion requirement†	No	Regular	–	–

*Karyotype status: good category includes normal, –Y, del(5q), del(20q); poor category includes complex (three or more) abnormalities, chromosome 7 anomalies; intermediate category includes other abnormalities.
†Transfusion dependency defined as having at least one transfusion every 8 weeks over a period of 4 months.

Criteria	WPSS risk category				
	Very low	Low	Intermediate	High	Very high
Combined score	0	1	2	3–4	5–6
Median survival (months)	136	63	44	19	8

Table 28.10 Median survival of MDS patients according to WPSS risk score.

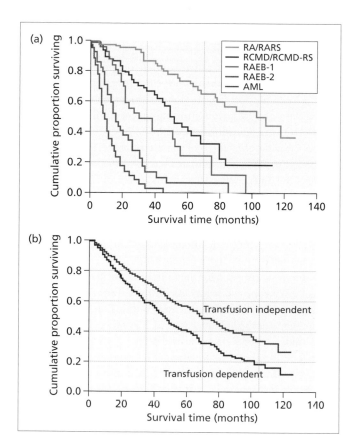

Figure 28.4 Cumulative survival of MDS patients according to (a) WHO subtype diagnosis and (b) transfusion dependence. (From Cazzola *et al*. 2005 with permission.)

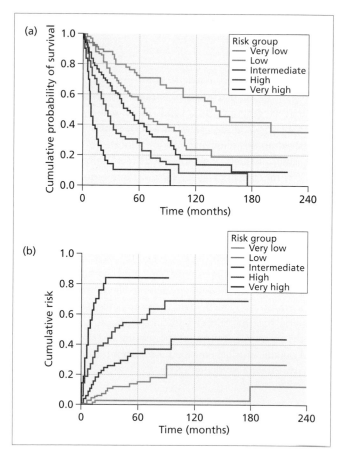

Figure 28.5 (a) Overall survival and (b) cumulative risk of leukaemic transformation in a German cohort of patients with MDS stratified according to WPSS risk categories. (From Malcovati *et al*. 2007 with permission.)

selection of appropriate treatment options. Notably, patients with normal blast counts and those with only erythroid dysplasia have a better prognosis according to the WPSS model but this requires validation. No doubt further revisions will emerge in the future that incorporate additional discriminatory risk factors.

Management and treatment

Traditionally, the management of patients with MDS has been largely unsatisfactory. However, the advent of newer treatment options coupled with better prognostication systems has resulted in some improvements for patients diagnosed with MDS today. Nonetheless, for many such patients who are commonly elderly and with other significant comorbidities, management often consists solely of supportive care, which remains the cornerstone of treatment in MDS. Indeed, for some patients who present with transforming disease or whose health is otherwise very poor, the only realistic option is the palliative relief of their symptoms. On the other hand, some patients may require observation only or may respond to growth factors, thus obviating the need for transfusion support. At the other end of the spectrum are younger fitter patients for whom more intensive treatment options might be considered, including high-dose cytotoxic therapy and stem cell transplantation (SCT). In addition, certain criteria in MDS are now becoming established that predict likelihood of clinical response to newer treatment options including immunosuppression, immunomodulatory drugs and hypomethylating agents.

Three important considerations should be borne in mind in arriving at an appropriate management plan for a patient with MDS: firstly, in asymptomatic patients, a period of observation can be extremely helpful in determining the rate of disease progression; secondly, it can be unwise to base the treatment plan on blood and marrow results during an acute infective episode since neutrophil and blast counts may be transiently increased; and thirdly, the patient's own wishes and expectations, as well as his or her health and social circumstances, should all be part of the overall consideration before arriving at a management plan. The British Committee for Standards in Haematology (BCSH) has produced some consensus guidelines based on an evidence-based review of the published literature to guide optimal treatment of patients with MDS. The management recommendations in this chapter are drawn partly from these guidelines but have also sought to include newer treatment options that have emerged since the guidelines were published.

Supportive care

Patients who exhibit symptoms or signs of clinical anaemia should receive red cell transfusions in order to improve quality of life. However, the potential risks of blood transfusions should always be considered, notably iron overload in multitransfused patients. Therefore, transfusions should only be used to alleviate symptoms of anaemia and not simply to maintain the haemoglobin above an arbitrary level. Other factors that might accentuate anaemia, such as nutritional haematinic deficiencies, haemorrhage, haemolysis or infection, should be sought and treated as appropriate.

Bleeding is a common and potentially serious complication of MDS resulting from both thrombocytopenia and the effect of functionally defective platelets. Platelet transfusions are indicated in MDS patients in the treatment of acute bleeding episodes, or as prophylaxis prior to surgery or following chemotherapy. However, their long-term use, for instance in the prevention of recurrent epistaxis or oral bleeding in elderly patients with persistent thrombocytopenia, presents significant logistical (and financial) issues. Moreover, as for red cell transfusions, platelet transfusions are not without potential complications including allosensitization that can lead to future refractoriness. Antifibrinolytic agents such as tranexamic acid can be useful on occasion but are not routinely recommended.

Chelation therapy

The decision to implement iron chelation in a transfusion-dependent MDS patient is not straightforward. There is a paucity of published literature to suggest that this expensive and inconvenient treatment improves overall survival in MDS. Current BCSH recommendations state that iron chelation should be considered once a patient has received 5 g iron (approximately 25 units of red cells) but only in younger patients for whom long-term transfusion therapy is likely, such as those with sideroblastic anaemia, or in those with good-prognosis disease without significant comorbidities. Desferrioxamine 20–40 mg/kg should be administered by subcutaneous infusion over 10–12 hours for 5–7 days per week with annual audiometry and ophthalmology review. The target ferritin concentration should be below 1000 μg/L and vitamin C 100–200 mg daily can be added after 1 month to enhance chelation. However, these recommendations are likely to be revised in view of the increasing use of the oral iron chelator, deferasirox, in younger transfusion-dependent MDS patients, especially those awaiting allogeneic transplantation for whom iron overload, reflected by a high ferritin level, can adversely influence the outcome of the procedure. Early experience with deferasirox shows that it is well tolerated and controls or reduces iron levels in chronically transfused MDS patients when used at a daily dose of 20–40 mg/kg.

Growth factors

The aim of using recombinant erythropoietin in the treatment of anaemia in MDS is to normalize the haemoglobin level and achieve transfusion independence with enhanced quality of life. However, those patients who stand to benefit the most are also those least likely to respond. Predictors of response include low serum erythropoietin concentration of less than 200 mU/mL (usually raised in MDS) and low transfusion requirements (two or less units per month). In such patients, there is evidence that cytokines can act on haemopoietic progenitor cells to reduce apoptosis and improve erythropoiesis.

Several small studies have demonstrated that erythropoietin is more likely to improve the haemoglobin level in patients with RA or RAEB, while patients with RARS rarely respond unless granulocyte colony-stimulating factor (G-CSF) is also used. A trial of erythropoietin alone at a dose of 10 000 units daily for 6 weeks should be undertaken to determine response. For non-responders, consideration should be given to the addition of daily G-CSF, to doubling the dose of erythropoietin, or both for a further 6 weeks. The synergism achieved by adding G-CSF to erythropoietin can improve response rates in RARS from 8% up to 50%. The precise role of both these cytokines in low-risk MDS patients is currently being assessed in a multicentre randomized trial in the UK to study quality of life, effect on survival and disease progression, and pharmacoeconomics.

The administration of G-CSF to patients with MDS typically results in a dose-dependent improvement in neutrophil numbers and function and is usually reserved for patients with severe sepsis or recovering from intensive chemotherapy. There is insufficient evidence to support its prophylactic use for preventing neutropenic infection, although some patients whose quality of life is compromised by recurrent infective exacerbations may respond to such an approach.

Immunosuppression

The serendipitous discovery that immunosuppression can sometimes yield responses in bone marrow failure states such as aplastic anaemia came from early experience of treating such patients with bone marrow transplantation and observing that some non-engrafters developed autologous haemopoietic recovery. In the case of MDS, there is accumulating evidence to implicate dysfunction of the immune system in the pathogenesis of the disease. Both these reasons provide the rationale for immunosuppression in the treatment of MDS, using either rabbit antithymocyte globulin (ATG) or horse antilymphocyte globulin (ALG), which are both polyclonal immunoglobulin preparations. A number of studies have shown that these treatments can benefit 30–60% of patients with MDS regardless of cellularity. Most clinically meaningful responses are in the erythroid lineage but bilineage and trilineage responses are also seen.

A number of studies have attempted to define key criteria that predict likelihood of response to immunosuppression. One multicentre study that retrospectively analysed 96 patients with MDS treated with ATG demonstrated that low IPSS score and marrow hypocellularity are both associated with better outcomes. Indeed, for young fit patients presenting with hypoplastic MDS, a trial of immunosuppression with ATG should be considered first-line treatment before proceeding to allogeneic transplantation. This conclusion is supported by another study of patients with MDS from the National Institutes of Health cohort, which has demonstrated for the first time that immunosuppressive therapy with ATG and ciclosporin can confer a survival advantage in younger patients with low IPSS scores. Two predictors of response in this study were HLA-DR15 positivity and trisomy 8, with 9 of 12 patients with this cytogenetic finding achieving transfusion independence. Other reports have even documented benefit in some patients to ciclosporin alone, or with corticosteroids, presumably through its immunosuppressive effect, although the benefits appear small and are rarely durable.

Intensive chemotherapy

Treatment of MDS patients with intensive chemotherapy regimens generally yields low remission rates and high relapse rates. AML induction regimens often result in protracted chemotherapy-related hypoplasia with remission rates that are considerably lower than for *de novo* AML. Indeed, marrow samples from patients with AML should be rigorously scrutinized for the presence of morphological dysplasia, which suggests antecedent MDS and predicts poor response to standard chemotherapy. The reasons for this are not clear but may be related to intrinsic drug resistance, lower mitotic rate or expanded pool of malignant stem cells.

Studies from the mid to late 1990s reported remission rates for high-risk MDS of 38–79% but these were generally short-lived, lasting 5–15 months. The karyotype appears to be the major determinant of response to intensive chemotherapy in MDS, with normal karyotype associated with high complete remission (CR) rate and longer remissions while complex karyotypes, particularly loss of chromosome 5 or 7, are associated with low CR rate and shorter remissions. Similarly, patients with therapy-related MDS have a particularly poor prognosis.

There is some evidence from *in vitro* studies that fludarabine is better than daunorubicin when combined with cytarabine. Daunorubicin is a substrate for the P-glycoprotein commonly overexpressed in transforming MDS, resulting in drug resistance. Conversely, fludarabine is an effective DNA terminator that can potentiate the effect of cytarabine by increasing its intracellular concentration. The addition of G-CSF to this regimen in order to sensitize the cells to these drugs has not been shown to confer any significant clinical benefit.

Consolidation of remission by way of autologous SCT is only applicable to a minority of patients due to the difficulty in harvesting CD34-positive progenitors from patients with MDS. Moreover, despite achieving stable engraftment after myeloablative high-dose chemotherapy, the graft is likely to be contaminated with residual disease cells that inevitably compromise any clinical benefit. Data from the European Group for Blood and Marrow Transplantation (EBMT) on 114 patients who received autologous transplantation in first CR have shown a 2-year disease-free survival (DFS) rate of 34% and relapse rate of 64% that is significantly worse than a 2-year DFS rate of 51% for patients with *de novo* AML treated similarly.

Allogeneic stem cell transplantation

Allogeneic SCT represents the only modality of treatment in MDS that has the potential for long-term cure. Historically, busulfan and cyclophosphamide, with or without total body irradiation, were used at high dose to condition the patient by way of total myeloablation allowing disease-free allogeneic stem cells to reconstitute the bone marrow. Over time, it became apparent that the curative potential of the transplant procedure was attributable to not only the toxic conditioning regimen but also the graft-versus-disease effect that clearly suppressed, or even eradicated, residual dysplastic/leukaemic cells. Traditionally, standard allografting was reserved for younger patients with good performance status and high-risk disease whose prognosis was otherwise very poor. Data from both the EBMT and the International Bone Marrow Transplant Registry (IBMT) confirm that at least one-third of patients with MDS are cured by allogeneic SCT from HLA-identical sibling donors. The status of the underlying disease is a major contributing factor in determining DFS at 3 years after transplantation, which according to registry data prior to 1998 is 53–55% for RA/RARS and 28–36% for RAEB/RAEBt/AML. A number of other criteria are recognized as being poor prognostic factors for outcome following allogeneic SCT, including older age, poor-risk cytogenetics, high IPSS score, advanced disease, therapy-related MDS, prolonged disease duration, and marrow fibrosis. However, advances in transplantation and supportive care are leading to a revision of the eligibility criteria for selecting suitable patients with MDS. The major driver for change over the last decade has been to address the extremely high transplant-related mortality (TRM) rate of 37–54% associated with standard allografting and this has resulted in the increasing use of reduced-intensity conditioning (RIC) regimens for MDS patients of all ages.

The optimal timing of transplantation in MDS is influenced by three factors, namely disease state, cytogenetics and age. Patients should be transplanted in a state of remission, after two or three cycles of intensive chemotherapy, since progressive or relapsed disease at time of SCT has a major adverse influence on outcome. Similarly, patients should be transplanted prior to cytogenetic evolution as poor-risk karyotypes are associated with poorer outcomes. Finally, the considerable TRM that accompanies SCT means that survival for older patients is considerably worse than for younger patients. Indeed, much of the

advance in transplantation in MDS has been directed to addressing these issues.

There are three possible sources of stem cells in allogeneic transplantation: sibling donor, volunteer unrelated donor and umbilical cord blood. Approximately one-third of patients receive an HLA-identical sibling donor transplant and this is associated with slightly better survival compared with unrelated donor transplant, with lower rates of TRM and graft-versus-host disease (GVHD). Volunteer unrelated donor transplants do have the advantage of a lower relapse rate compared with sibling donor transplants, illustrating the enhanced graft-versus-leukaemia (GVL) effect that occurs with unrelated donors. As for umbilical cord transplants, these are generally reserved for patients without a suitable HLA-matched donor. They are associated with a lower rate of GVHD and greater tolerance of HLA mismatch but at the expense of possible engraftment failure. However, the use of tandem cord transplants has been found to improve engraftment rates, making this approach a feasible alternative to established SCT procedures.

The major development in allogeneic transplantation that is responsible for expanding the number of eligible patients is the use of RIC regimens. Indeed, the introduction of non-myeloablative RIC has altered the landscape of SCT in MDS and rendered much of the outcome data from the SCT registries largely of historic interest (Table 28.11). Compared with standard conditioning, RIC regimens are characterized by reduced myelosuppression aimed at decreasing toxicity and related mortality. In addition, the RIC regimen must incorporate sufficient immunosuppression to prevent graft rejection by the host. A multitude of RIC protocols have been developed but typically they involve some combination of fludarabine, melphalan or busulfan, and alemtuzumab (Campath-1H) or ATG, occasionally with low-dose total body irradiation also. Alemtuzumab is a humanized IgG1 monoclonal antibody directed against the CD52 antigen expressed on all lymphoid cells, dendritic cells and monocytes, while ATG is directed primarily at T cells. Both alemtuzumab and ATG cause immunosuppression of the host and, because of their long half-lives, also of the donor graft resulting in *in vivo* T-cell depletion. This has the advantage of significantly reducing the incidence of GVHD that remains the major cause of morbidity and mortality following standard conditioning transplants. However, the long-term GVL effect of the transplant is retained, thereby controlling any minimal residual disease but at the expense of increased incidence of life-threatening infections due to delayed immune reconstitution.

A recent single-centre follow-up of allogeneic RIC transplants in 159 patients with MDS/AML (21–72 years, median age 53) reported a TRM rate of 31% and 1-year DFS rates for sibling donor and volunteer unrelated donor transplants of 61% and 59%, respectively. These rates correlated strongly with IPSS risk category, with DFS at 1 year of 86% for intermediate-1 patients, 63% for intermediate-2 patients and 33% for high-risk patients.

Table 28.11 Comparative outcomes from standard myeloablative and reduced-intensity conditioning allogeneic stem cell transplantation in MDS patients from the European registry.

Criteria	Standard myeloablative conditioning (N = 621 patients)	Reduced-intensity conditioning (N = 215 patients)	P-value
Patients over 50 years (%)	28	73	<0.001
Acute GVHD (%)	58	43	<0.001
Chronic GVHD (%)	52	45	Not significant
NRM at 3 years (%)	32	22	0.04
Relapse at 3 years (%)	27	45	<0.01
PFS at 3 years (%)	41	33	Not significant
OS at 3 years (%)	45	41	Not significant

Note that the 3-year progression-free survival (PFS) and overall survival (OS) are comparable between the two groups despite significant age differences, but that the risk of graft-versus-host disease (GVHD) and non-relapse mortality (NRM) are higher for standard transplants while the relapse rate is higher for transplants with reduced-intensity conditioning.

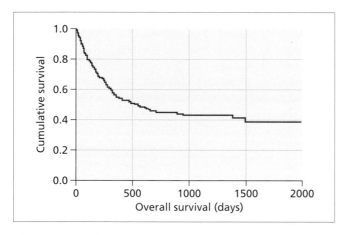

Figure 28.6 Kaplan–Meier survival plot and data for 159 patients with advanced MDS/AML who received a reduced-intensity conditioned allogeneic transplant at King's College Hospital, London. (Figure courtesy of Ziyi Lim.)

In addition, DFS rates correlated strongly with disease status at time of transplantation, with poorer outcomes in patients with relapsed/progressive disease or in partial remission. The survival curve shows evidence of plateau at around 3 years, with overall survival at this time of 46% and a relapse rate of 41%, with 14% of patients experiencing extensive chronic GVHD (Figure 28.6). A more intensive conditioning regimen comprising fludarabine, cytarabine and amsacrine (FLAMSA) combined with ATG, cyclophosphamide and 4-Gy total body irradiation has recently been pioneered by a German group in patients with refractory disease at time of transplantation, with impressive 2-year survival rates of 40%.

The GVL effect that is responsible for much of the therapeutic success associated with allogeneic transplantation can be further harnessed by use of donor lymphocyte infusions in the post-transplant setting. Donor lymphocyte infusions have been used to reinduce remission in patients with clinically relapsed haematological malignancy and to pre-emptively treat patients with molecular/cytogenetic evidence of mixed chimerism or relapsed disease. Durable remissions have been documented in cases of relapsed MDS/AML after transplantation, although results following morphological relapse are often poor. Considerable uncertainty remains regarding the optimal timing and dose of donor lymphocyte infusions in order to maximize the GVL effect while minimizing the risk of precipitating severe GVHD.

Hypomethylating drugs

Promoter hypermethylation leading to epigenetic silencing of tumour-suppressor genes is believed to be a key contributor to the molecular pathophysiology of MDS. This occurs by aberrant cytosine methylation at CpG dinucleotides, leading to inactivation of genes that control cell growth, differentiation and apoptosis. Hypomethylating agents are incorporated into the DNA where they covalently bind to the methyltransferase molecule, thereby inhibiting its function and leading to loss of methylation as DNA is replicated during mitosis. Currently, there are two hypomethylating agents that are approved for use in the treatment of MDS, namely 5-azacytidine (azacitidine) and 5-aza-2′-deoxycytidine (decitabine). Both of these drugs are cytosine nucleoside analogues that were initially developed as cytarabine analogues but had limited activity and unacceptable toxicities when used at high dose. However, at lower doses, they promote myeloid differentiation *in vitro* through gene activation.

The first demonstration of clear therapeutic benefit of hypomethylating agents came from a pivotal Phase III trial of azacitidine in patients with MDS conducted by the Cancer and Leukaemia Group B that has led to its approval by the US Food and Drug Administration (FDA). This study randomized patients to azacitidine 75 mg/m² administered subcutaneously daily for 7 days every 4 weeks or best supportive care with the option of crossover at 4 months. Responses were seen in all FAB subtypes, with 47% of patients achieving CR and 36% demonstrating haematological improvement. The median time to AML transformation or death was 21 months for patients receiving azacitidine compared with 12 months for those receiving best supportive care.

A more recent Phase III trial in MDS patients with intermediate-2 or high-risk disease, the AZA-001 study (Figure 28.7), compared azacitidine with conventional care regimens (best supportive care, low-dose cytarabine or intensive chemotherapy as deemed appropriate) and demonstrated that azacitidine confers a median survival benefit of over 9 months (24.5 vs. 15 months), with almost doubling of the survival at 2 years (51% vs. 26%). Moreover, the haematological improvements seen with azacitidine in this study were of longer duration than those of other care regimens, with higher rates of transfusion independence, fewer infections and overall delay in progression to AML. In addition, subgroup analysis demonstrated that azacitidine is associated with significant benefit in patients with adverse cytogenetics involving chromosome 7, with a 67% reduction in deaths and a survival advantage at 2 years of 33% compared with 8%. This latter finding has been confirmed by another study that found a significant survival advantage in high-risk patients, with median survival of 24.8 months for patients with monosomy 7 or 7q– and 17.3 months for patients with complex cytogenetics. For this challenging group of patients, azacitidine may serve to induce cytogenetic remissions while transplant-eligible patients await donor selection. Current studies are seeking to explore alternative treatment regimens and also to study the role of azacitidine as maintenance therapy to prolong remissions following intensive chemotherapy.

Decitabine has also received FDA approval for the treatment of patients with MDS based on a Phase III evaluation of the drug that demonstrated a 35% overall response rate compared with best supportive care and a significant prolongation of the time to AML or death in the high-risk/intermediate-2 group of patients. However, unlike the azacitidine trial, decitabine failed to produce a statistically significant survival advantage, possibly for dosage reasons, and therefore azacitidine should be considered the preferred therapeutic option. In lower-risk patients a shorter 5-day regimen may yield adequate haematological improvements with acceptable toxicity profile, while in higher-risk patients azacitidine offers an option for individuals who are not suitable for intensive therapy and allogeneic transplantation. Clinical trials are ongoing to study the benefit of other epigenetic modifiers, notably histone deacetylation inhibitors that might enhance the benefit produced by hypomethylation agents.

Lenalidomide

Lenalidomide belongs to a class of compounds termed 'immunomodulatory drugs' that have shown broad activity on the bone marrow microenvironment, including anti-angiogenic activity and cytokine suppression. It has a superior toxicity profile than its predecessor thalidomide, and appears to lack any significant teratogenicity. Moreover, it causes enhancement of erythropoietin receptor signalling, making it an attractive candidate for studying in transfusion-dependent MDS. Lenalidomide was first studied in an open-label single-centre trial in 43 patients with mostly lower-risk MDS; 63% of patients who were transfusion-dependent became independent of transfusion, with the most marked responses observed in those patients with del(5q) compared with normal karyotype or other cytogenetic abnormalities (83% vs. 57% vs. 12%, respectively). A complete cytogenetic response was observed in 10 patients, all but one of whom had del(5q) and this provided the basis for

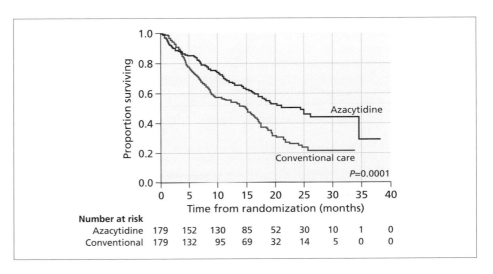

Figure 28.7 Kaplan–Meier plot comparing overall survival for MDS patients randomized to either azacitidine treatment or conventional care regimens (CCR) in the Phase III AZA-001 study. Median survival favours azacitidine over CCR by 9.5 months (24.5 vs. 15 months) with doubling of 2-year survival (51% vs. 26%). (From Fenaux *et al*. 2009 with permission.)

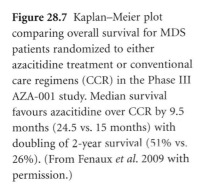

a pivotal Phase II study in 148 transfusion-dependent patients who carried this abnormality. In this larger study, two-thirds of patients became transfusion-independent, with a median time of onset of 4.6 weeks and a median duration that had not been reached at 2 years of follow-up. Cytogenetic response was seen in 73% of patients, of whom 61% had a complete cytogenetic response and this strongly correlated with haematological improvement. No significant difference in response was observed between the two dosing regimens of 10 mg daily or 10 mg daily for 21 days of a 28-day cycle.

Although the precise mechanism of action of lenalidomide in MDS remains unknown, there are a number of hypotheses. The evidence clearly supports the view that the drug directly targets the dysplastic clone given the cytogenetic response and normalization of haemoglobin and platelet levels. One mechanism would be that lenalidomide corrects for the dosage haploinsufficiency caused by the 5q deletion, resulting in normalization of cell cycle arrest and apoptosis. However, lenalidomide is also known to have potent immunomodulatory and anti-angiogenic properties that may clearly be relevant to its therapeutic action. Indeed, clinical benefit from lenalidomide is not only restricted to del(5q) patients, as demonstrated by

another recent study of MDS patients lacking this abnormality that has shown a response rate of 43% with 26% achieving transfusion independence. Thus, lenalidomide represents a promising, albeit expensive, advance in the treatment of some forms of MDS.

Therapeutic strategy

Therapeutic goals

Arriving at the best management plan for an individual patient with MDS can be difficult (Figure 28.8). The initial decision to resolve is whether the goal of treatment should be to extend patient survival or to palliate symptoms with supportive care. This decision is helped by considering prognosis according to the IPSS/WPSS coupled to the patient's age and performance status, always ensuring that any plan is fully in accordance with the patient's own wishes. Treatment of MDS has historically been separated into low-intensity and high-intensity therapies, based on the risk of toxicities. Low-intensity therapies, which include immunosuppressive therapy, biological response modi-

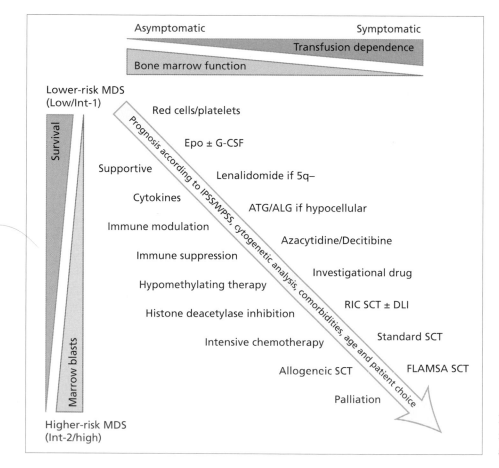

Figure 28.8 Schematic diagram illustrating the treatment options available for patients with MDS.

fiers and cytokines, were reserved for lower-risk patients with the goal of improving cytopenias and quality of life without improving survival. Other low-intensity therapies such as low-dose chemotherapy and methyltransferase inhibitors aim to extend survival, whereas high-intensity therapies such as high-dose chemotherapy and allogeneic SCT aim to alter the course of the disease or even achieve cure.

Many patients with MDS receive supportive care alone, particularly lower-risk patients with chronic cytopenias or patients with higher-risk disease who are unable to tolerate high-intensity therapy. Such patients often become dependent on frequent red cell or platelet transfusions and experience repeated infective and haemorrhagic complications. Regardless of disease status, many patients experience significantly impaired quality of life simply as a consequence of the physical toll caused by frequent laboratory monitoring and transfusions, physician visits, and the fatigue that accompanies this. Thus, improvement in quality of life and alleviation of disease-related symptoms are the key goals of therapy.

Assessing response

In 2000, the International Working Group (IWG) of investigators proposed standardization of response criteria by which to assess the results of different therapies in MDS. These criteria have been widely accepted into clinical practice and were updated in 2006. The investigators grouped patients into IPSS risk categories and recommended that the major goal of therapy for patients with lower-risk disease (low-risk and intermediate-1 categories) is to achieve haematological improvement. For higher-risk patients (intermediate-2 and high-risk categories), the focus turns to altering the natural history of the disease and prolonging life. The IWG criteria define four specific aspects of responses based on treatment goals: haematological improvement, cytogenetic improvement, alteration of disease progression, and quality of life. Haematological improvement is scored for each lineage according to whether there is a major or minor response, while cytogenetic improvement is scored according to whether there is a partial or complete response. Alteration of the natural course of the disease is determined according to various measures of disease progression and survival.

IPSS low

The median survival for low-risk MDS is 4.8 years for those aged over 60 years to 11.8 years for those under 60 years. For this reason, intensive chemotherapy and SCT cannot be justified given their potential for morbidity and mortality. Individuals should be monitored for disease progression and supported as necessary. Where possible, a trial of erythropoietin with or without G-CSF should be undertaken in patients with symptomatic anaemia, while those with del(5q) should ideally receive lenalidomide.

IPSS intermediate-1

For older patients above the age of 65, or less if there are significant comorbidities, supportive care should be offered as for low-risk patients. Immunosuppression with ATG and ciclosporin should be considered for cytopenic patients who are otherwise deemed unfit for intensive chemotherapy, particularly if the marrow is hypocellular with no excess of blasts or adverse cytogenetics. For younger patients below the age of 50 who have either a sibling or unrelated donor available, allogeneic transplantation should be offered as a potentially curative procedure. Whether the conditioning regimen should be myeloablative or non-myeloablative is unclear and should be at the discretion of the local transplant unit. For patients between 50 and 65 years of age, the optimal management is less straightforward given the significant TRM associated with allogeneic SCT and the predicted median survival of 5.2 years for patients less than 60. The impressive data emerging for patients treated with RIC transplantation makes this an attractive treatment option, especially when a sibling donor is available, although unrelated donor transplants are also feasible. While trials demonstrate better outcomes if the transplantation is performed prior to disease progression, this is not always a straightforward decision and some patients may reasonably elect to reserve this option for when there is evidence of clonal evolution or early transformation. Iron overload should be avoided in those patients who remain transplant candidates, either by managing anaemia with erythropoietin with or without G-CSF or by using iron chelation for those who are transfusion-dependent.

IPSS intermediate-2/high

Patients in these poor prognostic categories are known to have median survivals of less than 2 years for intermediate-2 to only a few months for high-risk individuals. Patients below the age of 65 years and without significant comorbidities, particularly where a sibling donor is available, should be offered intensive chemotherapy and RIC transplantation, with myeloablative conditioning reserved for younger fitter patients below 50 years at the discretion of the local transplant unit. However, if the patient fails to achieve at least a good partial remission following intensive chemotherapy, then the prospects of successful outcome from allogeneic transplantation are minimal and palliative treatment with supportive care may be a preferable option, although a FLAMSA-conditioned RIC transplant could be considered in some cases.

For patients over the age of 65 years, the best recommendation is not straightforward. The NCRI AML 16 trial is open for patients over 60 with high-risk MDS and AML, allowing randomization to various treatment options on either intensive or non-intensive arms. However, this will depend on the patient's performance status, comorbidities and own wishes. It is reasonable to await the result of cytogenetic analysis, as patients with poor-risk karyotypes have low response rates to intensive AML-type induction chemotherapy. For such patients, and particularly those with chromosome 7 abnormalities, azacitidine should be considered as an alternative low-intensive treatment option.

With the advent of further novel agents in the future, the most appropriate treatment option is likely to become more complex. However, as with all investigational therapies, patients should be treated within the context of clinical research trials.

Myelodysplastic/myeloproliferative diseases

The WHO classification established a new diagnostic entity for those diseases that share features characteristic of both the myelodysplastic syndromes and the myeloproliferative neoplasms. This overlap category comprises disorders that at the time of initial presentation share clinical, laboratory or morphological findings indicative of underlying dysplastic and proliferative processes. They are usually characterized by hypercellularity of the bone marrow due to proliferation in one or more of the myeloid lineages, with increased numbers of circulating cells that may be morphologically dysplastic. Simultaneously, one or more of the other lineages may exhibit ineffective proliferation so that cytopenias may also be present. The presence of excess blasts is closely correlated with the risk of leukaemic transformation.

The WHO recognizes three distinct entities, namely chronic myelomonocytic leukaemia, atypical chronic myeloid leukaemia and juvenile myelomonocytic leukaemia, and one provisional entity of refractory anaemia with ring sideroblasts and thrombocytosis, with the remainder categorized as myelodysplastic/myeloproliferative neoplasms unclassifiable.

Chronic myelomonocytic leukaemia
(see also Chapter 27)

CMML constitutes 20–30% of cases of MDS. The hallmark feature is peripheral blood monocytosis accompanied by morphological dysplasia of other lineages. CMML is a clonal malignancy that has a male predominance and a median age of presentation of approximately 70 years; only 10% of CMML cases occur in individuals less than 60 years. While the aetiology is largely unknown, therapy-related cases of CMML are very rare.

Clinical and laboratory features

There is a spectrum of clinical and laboratory features found in CMML. The majority of patients present with a leucocytosis that is often accompanied by mild anaemia and thrombocytopenia. Reactive causes due to infection, notably tuberculosis, must be excluded. By definition, the monocyte count must be greater than 1×10^9/L and is usually in the range 2–5 $\times 10^9$/L, but may exceed 80 $\times 10^9$/L. The monocytes generally appear mature and morphologically unremarkable but may have agranular cytoplasm and/or abnormal nuclear lobulation. Promonocytes and monoblasts may also be seen but if they comprise more than 20%, then the diagnosis is AML rather than CMML. Evidence of dysgranulopoiesis is commonly present, including hypogranular and hypolobated neutrophils that are sometimes difficult to distinguish from dysplastic monocytes. The bone marrow is generally hypercellular, usually with striking granulocytic proliferation and invariably monocytic proliferation that can be distinguished using cytochemical studies. Typical features of dysplasia can be identified in all three lineages in over 80% of patients.

Cytogenetic analysis is important for confirming clonality, although abnormalities are only found in 30–40% of cases, notably +8, −7/del(7q) and del(12p), and none is specific for CMML. Up to 40% of patients have point mutations of *RAS* genes, which is higher than for other forms of MDS. Hypermethylation of the *CDKN2B* gene (which encodes the tumour suppressor p15INK4b), resulting in reduced expression, can be demonstrated in approximately 50% of patients. Recently, the *CBL* gene, which encodes the E3 ubiquitin ligase, has been implicated in progressive CMML by its presence within a region of UPD on chromosome 11q. It is important to exclude certain chromosomal translocations, by cytogenetic and polymerase chain reaction (PCR) analysis, that are indicative of alternative diagnoses. These include chronic myeloid leukaemia diagnosed by the *BCR–ABL1* rearrangement and eosinophilia-related disorders associated with abnormalities of *PDGFRA*, *PDGFRB* and *FGFR1*. Mutations of the *JAK2* gene should also be excluded.

Approximately half of patients have splenomegaly, and often hepatomegaly, at diagnosis. Individuals with high monocyte counts may develop a maculopapular skin infiltration, gum infiltration, and monocytic pleural and pericardial effusions. Lymphadenopathy is uncommon but when it occurs it may signal a more acute phase with infiltration of lymph nodes by myeloblasts. Weight loss, fevers and night sweats may occur in symptomatic patients. The number of blast cells plus promonocytes should account for less than 5% of peripheral blood leucocytes and less than 10% of nucleated marrow cells to give a diagnosis of CMML-1. If the blast/promonocyte count is higher than this but less than 20% in either the peripheral blood or bone marrow, or if Auer rods are present, then the diagnosis is CMML-2. This identifies a group of patients who have a worse prognosis and higher risk of transformation to AML, which is diagnosed when the blast/promonocyte count exceeds 20%. Immunophenotyping may be helpful for identifying myelomonocytic populations but can also give prognostic information such as reduced CD14 expression indicating monocytic immaturity, aberrant expression of CD2 and CD56, and the CD34-positive cell percentage.

Natural history and prognosis

The clinical course of CMML is highly variable, with a median survival of approximately 2 years though occasional patients surviving beyond 8 years. There is an age-dependent prognosis that can be calculated using the IPSS according to the blast percentage, number of cytopenias, and karyotypic abnormalities. The distinction between dysplastic and proliferative forms of the disease is unreliable and unhelpful but the separation between CMML-1 and CMML-2, which reflects the marrow blast percentage (<10% and 10–19% respectively), is important and prognostically relevant. Similarly, anaemia and thrombocytopenia are adverse prognostic factors, especially if the patient is transfusion-dependent. A rising lactate dehydrogenase level often reflects a rising blast count, indicating progression to AML with leukaemic transformation occurring in approximately 15–30% of cases.

Management and treatment

Therapy of CMML is unsatisfactory with the vast majority of patients being elderly (>60 years). Supportive care by way of blood transfusions and antibiotics for infections are the mainstay of management. When the proliferative phase prevails, causing symptomatic organomegaly, infiltrative disease or escalating monocytosis, then oral chemotherapy with hydroxycarbamide (hydroxyurea) is the treatment of choice. A European randomized study comparing hydroxycarbamide with etoposide gave a response rate and survival, respectively, of 60% and 20 months for hydroxycarbamide and 36% and 9 months for etoposide. Intensive chemotherapy alone is of little benefit in this age group.

In younger patients, particularly with adverse features, intensive treatment and allogeneic transplantation represent the only possibility of cure. However, the EBMT data for adults with CMML shows poor long-term outcomes with this approach, with 5-year overall survival after transplant (both related and unrelated) of only 21%. As with other forms of MDS, outcomes are better if the patient is transplanted before significant disease progression but this must be weighed against the considerable TRM rate. AML-type induction chemotherapy regimens are unlikely to achieve long-lasting remission on their own unless consolidated with a transplant procedure. A deeper understanding of the biological basis of CMML may lead to targeted therapies analogous to that for chronic myeloid leukaemia and there is a strong case for entering younger patients into clinical trials that seek to test such drugs.

Atypical chronic myeloid leukaemia

Atypical chronic myeloid leukaemia is a poorly defined entity. Importantly, it is negative for the BCR–ABL1 fusion gene associated with the t(9;22) translocation diagnostic of typical chronic myeloid leukaemia (see Chapter 27). It is a leukaemic disorder with myelodysplastic and myeloproliferative features principally involving the neutrophil lineage. Myeloid precur-

sors often comprise more than 10% of cells but blasts are rarely more than 5%. Dysgranulopoiesis is prominent but multilineage dysplasia is also seen.

Patients usually present with anaemia and/or thrombocytopenia that accompany the leucocytosis. Splenomegaly is common and often causes symptoms because of its massive enlargement. Cytogenetic abnormalities can be identified in 80% of cases although none is specific. The outlook is generally poorer for atypical chronic myeloid leukaemia than for CMML, with a median survival of less than 20 months. The response to intensive chemotherapy is poor and the mainstay of management is supportive care and hydroxycarbamide to control proliferative elements of the disease.

Juvenile myelomonocytic leukaemia (see also Chapter 27)

Juvenile myelomonocytic leukaemia (JMML) is a clonal haemopoietic disorder of childhood characterized principally by proliferation of the granulocytic and monocytic lineages. It occurs with an incidence of 1.2 per million, comprising approximately 2–3% of all childhood leukaemias but 40% of childhood MDS. The majority of cases of JMML occur in children under 3 years of age and twice as commonly in boys than girls. There are associations with neurofibromatosis type 1 and Noonan syndrome due to germline mutations in the NF1 and PTPN11 or KRAS genes respectively. There is marked in vitro hypersensitivity of myeloid progenitors to granulocyte/macrophage colony-stimulating factor that is a hallmark feature of JMML and suggestive of defective RAS–MAP kinase signalling that is often attributable to RAS mutations. Monosomy 7 is the most common chromosomal abnormality, found in 25% of cases. A marked increase in the synthesis of HbF is a recurrent finding that has poor prognostic implications.

Clinically, most patients present with constitutional symptoms or evidence of infection and are found to have marked hepatosplenomegaly. Lymphoid and tonsillar enlargement is also common. Typically, there is a leucocytosis comprising neutrophils, myeloid precursors and monocytes, with blasts constituting less than 5% of cells. The marrow is hypercellular and dysplastic features are minimal. The prognosis of JMML is variable with a median survival of 1 year. It is usually rapidly fatal without treatment, causing organ failure, especially respiratory failure due to leukaemic infiltration, while blast transformation occurs infrequently. Although responses are seen to cytarabine-containing regimens, allogeneic transplantation offers the only possibility of cure but with relapse rates of up to 50% in some series.

Refractory anaemia with ring sideroblasts and thrombocytosis

The precise nature of refractory anaemia with ring sideroblasts and thrombocytosis (RARS-T) is a controversial and unresolved issue. These patients meet the criteria for RARS but also have persistently elevated platelet counts over 450×10^9/L. The majority (50–60% of cases) carry the V617F mutation of the *JAK2* gene that is more commonly associated with myeloproliferative disorders. Whether RARS-T represents a *JAK2*-positive myeloproliferative neoplasm with acquired dysplastic features or, conversely, a form of MDS with an acquired proliferative mutation remains partly a question of semantics and partly one of biology. For this reason, RARS-T exists as a provisional entity in the current version of the WHO classification.

Myelodysplasia of childhood

Childhood MDS is recognized as an entity of its own in the current version of the WHO classification but excludes JMML, which is grouped within the myelodysplastic/myeloproliferative category. MDS associated with Down syndrome, which previously accounted for up to 25% of paediatric MDS, is now grouped within a new entity of Down syndrome-related myeloid leukaemia. Most remaining cases of childhood MDS fall within one of the subgroups of conventional MDS, namely RA, RARS, RCMD or RAEB-1/RAEB-2. The term 'refractory cytopenia of childhood' is reserved for cases of MDS associated with persistent cytopenia and less than 5% blasts in the marrow and less than 2% blasts in peripheral blood. About 75% of children with RCC show considerable hypocellularity of the bone marrow, making it difficult to differentiate from congenital bone marrow failure syndromes that can lead to secondary myelodysplasia in affected children. These congenital syndromes include disorders such as Fanconi anaemia, dyskeratosis congenita, Schwachman–Diamond syndrome, amegakaryocytic thrombocytopenia, and pancytopenia with radioulnar synostosis. Understanding the mechanism by which they predispose children to developing MDS has helped shed light on the aetiology of acquired MDS in adulthood. However, a discussion of the biology of these disorders is beyond the scope of this chapter.

Future directions

Traditionally, MDS has been viewed as an awkward collection of biologically related disorders mainly affecting elderly patients for whom treatment options were largely unsatisfactory. The last decade has completely changed this landscape. Today, the molecular pathogenesis of MDS is being revealed through newer technologies that allow better understanding of the biology of this clonal disease and its stem cell origin. The revised WHO classification has helped resolve points of diagnostic ambiguity while large retrospective studies of patients have refined our ability to make accurate predictions about prognosis and survival. As for therapy, two new drug treatments, lena-

lidomide and azacitidine, have shown significant clinical benefit in Phase III trials, including improved survival and quality of life. In addition, increasing numbers of patients are receiving allogeneic transplants made possible through the use of RIC regimens that hold the potential for long-term remission or disease control through donor lymphocyte infusions. We still have a long way to go, but recent developments clearly show that better risk stratification, novel targeted therapies and expanded transplant eligibility are all likely to significantly improve the prospects for patients with MDS in the future.

Selected bibliography

Bowen DT (2005) Chronic myelomonocytic leukaemia: lost in classification? *Hematological Oncology* 23: 26–33.

Bowen D, Culligan D, Jowitt S *et al.* (2003) Guidelines for the diagnosis and therapy of adult myelodysplastic syndromes. *British Journal of Haematology* 120: 187–200.

Cazzola M, Malcovati L (2005) Myelodysplastic syndromes: coping with ineffective hematopoiesis. *New England Journal of Medicine* 352: 536–8.

Delhommeau F, Dupont S, Della Valle V *et al.* (2009) Mutation in TET2 in myeloid cancers. *New England Journal of Medicine* 360: 2289–301.

Ebert BL, Pretz J, Bosco J *et al.* (2008) Identification of RPS14 as a 5q– syndrome gene by RNA interference screen. *Nature* 451: 335–9.

Fenaux P, Mufti GJ, Hellstrom-Lindberg E *et al.* (2009) Efficacy of azacitidine compared with that of conventional care regimens in the treatment of higher-risk myelodysplastic syndromes: a randomized, open-label, phase III study. *Lancet Oncology* 10: 223–32.

Garcia-Manero G (2007) Modifying the epigenome as a therapeutic strategy in myelodysplasia. *Hematology. American Society of Hematology Education Program* 405–11.

Gattermann N (2008) Overview of guidelines on iron chelation therapy in patients with myelodysplastic syndromes and transfusional iron overload. *International Journal of Hematology* 88: 24–9.

Giagounidis A, Fenaux P, Mufti GJ *et al.* (2008) Practical recommendations on the use of lenalidomide in the management of myelodysplastic syndromes. *Annals of Hematology* 87: 345–52.

Greenberg P, Cox C, LeBeau MM *et al.* (1997) International scoring system for evaluating prognosis in myelodysplastic syndromes. *Blood* 89: 2079–88.

Haase D (2008) Cytogenetic features in myelodysplastic syndromes. *Annals of Hematology* 87: 515–26.

Hellström-Lindberg E, Cazzola M (2008) The role of JAK2 mutations in RARS and other MDS. *Hematology. American Society of Hematology Education Program* 52–9.

Hellström-Lindberg E, Malcovati L (2008) Supportive care, growth factors, and new therapies in myelodysplastic syndromes. *Blood Reviews* 22: 75–91.

Ingram W, Lim ZY, Mufti GJ (2007) Allogeneic transplantation for myelodysplastic syndrome (MDS). *Blood Reviews* 21: 61–71.

Kerbauy DB, Deeg HJ (2007) Apoptosis and antiapoptotic mechanisms in the progression of myelodysplastic syndrome. *Experimental Hematology* **35**: 1739–46.

Killick SB, Mufti G, Cavenagh JD *et al.* (2003) A pilot study of antithymocyte globulin (ATG) in the treatment of patients with 'low-risk' myelodysplasia. *British Journal of Haematology* **120**: 679–84.

Kordasti SY, Ingram W, Hayden J *et al.* (2007) CD4$^+$CD25^{high}Foxp3$^+$ regulatory T cells in myelodysplastic syndrome (MDS). *Blood* **110**: 847–50.

Kröger N (2008) Epigenetic modulation and other options to improve outcome of stem cell transplantation in MDS. *Hematology. American Society of Hematology Education Program*, 60–7.

Lim ZY, Ho AY, Ingram W *et al.* (2006) Outcomes of alemtuzumab-based reduced intensity conditioning stem cell transplantation using unrelated donors for myelodysplastic syndromes. *British Journal of Haematology* **135**: 201–9.

Lim ZY, Killick S, Germing U *et al.* (2007) Low IPSS score and bone marrow hypocellularity in MDS patients predict hematological responses to antithymocyte globulin. *Leukemia* **21**: 1436–41.

List A, Kurtin S, Roe DJ *et al.* (2005) Efficacy of lenalidomide in myelodysplastic syndromes. *New England Journal of Medicine* **352**: 549–57.

List A, Dewald G, Bennett J *et al.* (2006) Lenalidomide in the myelodysplastic syndrome with chromosome 5q deletion. *New England Journal of Medicine* **355**: 1456–65.

Maciejewski JP, Mufti GJ (2008) Whole genome scanning as a cytogenetic tool in hematologic malignancies. *Blood* **112**: 965–74.

Malcovati L, Germing U, Kuendgen A *et al.* (2007) Time-dependent prognostic scoring system for predicting survival and leukaemic evolution in myelodysplastic syndromes. *Journal of Clinical Oncology* **25**: 3503–10.

Malcovati L, Porta MGD, Pietra D *et al.* (2009) Molecular and clinical features of refractory anemia with ringed sideroblasts associated with marked thrombocytosis. *Blood* **114**: 3538–45.

Mohamedali A, Mufti GJ (2009) Van-den Berghe's 5q– syndrome in 2008. *British Journal of Haematology* **144**: 157–68.

Mohamedali A, Gäken J, Twine NA *et al.* (2007) Prevalence and prognostic significance of allelic imbalance by single-nucleotide polymorphism analysis in low-risk myelodysplastic syndromes. *Blood* **110**: 3365–73.

Mohamedali AM, Smith A, Gaken J *et al.* (2009) Novel TET2 mutations associated with UPD4q24 in myelodysplastic syndrome. *Journal of Clinical Oncology* **27**: 4002–6.

Mufti GJ, Chen TL (2008) Changing the treatment paradigm in myelodysplastic syndromes. *Cancer Control* **15** (Suppl.): 14–28.

Mufti GJ, Bennett JM, Goasguen J *et al.* (2008) Diagnosis and classification of myelodysplastic syndrome: International Working Group on Morphology of myelodysplastic syndrome (IWGM-MDS) consensus proposals for the definition and enumeration of myeloblasts and ring sideroblasts. *Haematologica* **93**: 1712–17.

Nimer SD (2008) Myelodysplastic syndromes. *Blood* **111**: 4841–51.

Nimer SD (2008) MDS: a stem cell disorder, but what exactly is wrong with the primitive haematopoietic cells in this disease? *Hematology. American Society of Hematology Education Program* 43–51.

Omidvar N, Kogan S, Beurlet S *et al.* (2007) BCL-2 and mutant NRAS interact physically and functionally in a mouse model of progressive myelodysplasia. *Cancer Research* **67**: 11657–67.

Raj K, Mufti GJ (2006) Azacytidine (Vidaza) in the treatment of myelodysplastic syndromes. *Therapeutics and Clinical Risk Management* **2**: 377–88.

Schmid C, Schleuning M, Ledderose G, Tischer J, Kolb HJ (2005) Sequential regimen of chemotherapy, reduced-intensity conditioning for allogeneic stem-cell transplantation, and prophylactic donor lymphocyte transfusion in high-risk acute myeloid leukaemia and myelodysplastic syndrome. *Journal of Clinical Oncology* **23**: 5675–87.

Silverman LR, Demakos EP, Peterson BL *et al.* (2002) Randomized controlled trial of azacitidine in patients with the myelodysplastic syndrome: a study of the Cancer and Leukaemia Group B. *Journal of Clinical Oncology* **20**: 2429–40.

Sloand EM, Wu CO, Greenberg P, Young N, Barrett J (2008) Factors affecting response and survival in patients with myelodysplasia treated with immunosuppressive therapy. *Journal of Clinical Oncology* **26**: 2505–11.

Swerdlow SH, Campo E, Harris NL *et al.* (eds) (2008) *WHO Classification of Tumours of Haematopoietic and Lymphoid Tissues*. IARC Press, Lyon.

Van den Berghe H, Cassiman JJ, David G, Fryns JP, Michaux JL, Sokal G (1974) Distinct haematological disorder with deletion of long arm of no. 5 chromosome. *Nature* **251**: 437–8.

Chronic lymphocytic leukaemia and other B-cell disorders

29

Daniel Catovsky[1] and Emili Montserrat[2]

[1]Institute of Cancer Research, Sutton, Surrey, UK
[2]Institute of Hematology and Oncology, Hospital Clinic, University of Barcelona, Barcelona, Spain

Introduction

Within the broad category of B-cell lymphoproliferative disorders we include a number of disease entities arising from mature B lymphocytes and which involve primarily the blood, bone marrow and other lymphoid organs such as the lymph nodes and spleen. All these disorders are classified by the World Health Organization (WHO) (see Chapter 33) on the basis of their histopathological features. Their clinical course is often chronic and they affect mainly adults. A constant finding in all these entities is the presence in peripheral blood of leukaemic cells in various degrees. Some of these conditions could be considered as primary leukaemias and these are dealt with in this chapter. Others represent the leukaemic phase of indolent non-Hodgkin lymphomas (NHL) and their recognition is important for differential diagnosis and patient management.

The study of lymphoid leukaemias has been enriched with the advent of monoclonal antibodies that define antigenic determinants specific for the B- and T-cell lineages. Characterization of these malignancies is not possible without the use of these reagents, which help define the cell lineage and the maturation stage of the leukaemic cell. DNA analysis for the detection of immunoglobulin and T-cell receptor gene rearrangements has been incorporated as another diagnostic test for cell lineage and clonality and for monitoring minimal residual disease (MRD) after therapy. Chromosome abnormalities that characterize some of the genetic changes in the lymphoid leukaemias are also important for diagnostic and prognostic purposes and are routinely studied by fluorescence *in situ* hybridization (FISH) as it is not easy to obtain metaphases in slowly dividing lymphocytes.

The primary B-cell leukaemias include chronic lymphocytic leukaemia (CLL), which is by far the most common, the rare B-prolymphocytic leukaemia (B-PLL) and hairy cell leukaemia (HCL). The B-cell NHLs that most frequently affect the blood and bone marrow include splenic marginal zone lymphoma (SMZL), mantle cell lymphoma (MCL), particularly the splenomegalic form, and follicular lymphoma which, in its generalized or systemic form, regularly involves the bone marrow and may spill over to the peripheral blood.

Methodology for diagnosis

Examination of the morphology of leukaemic cells in well-prepared peripheral blood and bone marrow films stained with Romanowsky dyes is still the first diagnostic procedure and cannot be replaced by any of the newer, more modern diagnostic techniques.

The second element for the diagnosis of any type of lymphocytosis is to use a small battery of membrane markers to define the immunophenotype (B or T) and whether the process is clonal or polyclonal. Once a monoclonal B-cell proliferation

Postgraduate Haematology: 6th edition. Edited by A. Victor Hoffbrand, Daniel Catovsky, Edward G.D. Tuddenham, Anthony R. Green is established by light-chain restriction (e.g. κ or λ), one can clarify the problem further by using a panel of monoclonal antibodies to define a particular disease immunophenotype. The typical immunophenotype of CLL, as elaborated by the group of one of the authors, is shown in Table 29.1. The original proposal by Matutes and colleagues was revised by replacing CD22 with CD79b, which is one of the components of the B-cell antigen receptor molecule. In Table 29.1, the symbols in parentheses after each of the five markers indicates the expected result in CLL. Figure 29.1 illustrates the contrast between the flow cytometry profile of a case of CLL and one of follicular lymphoma.

Table 29.2 summarizes the results of applying the panel of markers used for the CLL score to the other B-cell disorders in peripheral blood samples. High scores are expected in CLL; low scores are the feature in the other B-cell leukaemias and B-cell NHL. Figure 29.2 illustrates the almost complete lack of overlap between CLL and B-cell NHL evolving with lymphocytosis. However, there are a number of issues that may present problems. First, as shown in Table 29.2, some cases of CLL with atypical morphology (e.g. clefted nucleus, plasmacytoid features) or more than 10% prolymphocytes (CLL/PL) may have scores lower than 4. Rare cases of NHL may approach scores of

Table 29.1 Immunophenotype of CLL: tests used as basis for a scoring system.

Marker (result)	Score
SmIg (weak)	1
CD5 (+)	1
CD23 (+)	1
FMC7 (− or weak)*	1
CD79b (− or weak)	1
Total	5

*Epitope of CD20 but CD20 not useful for scoring.
SmIg, surface membrane immunoglobulin.

Table 29.2 CLL score in B-cell disorders evolving with lymphocytosis.

Disease	Score
CLL	
Typical	4–5
Atypical; CLL/PL	3–5
B-prolymphocytic leukaemia	0–1
Hairy cell leukaemia	0–1
NHL with leukaemia*	0–2

*Follicular lymphoma, MCL, SMZL.

2 or 3; thus reliance only on the immunophenotype may be misleading. Second, the important distinction between CLL and MCL, another CD5-positive disease, may require other tests such as FISH (see below). MCL rarely shows an immunophenotypic score above 2.

An important consideration when using membrane markers is the distinction between CD20 and FMC7. FMC7 has now been recognized as binding to a conformational epitope of CD20, but FMC7 does not correlate with CD20 staining in CLL. Most cases of CLL and other B-cell disorders express CD20, hence its value as a broad B-cell marker and as a target for the monoclonal antibody rituximab. Analysis of the use of CD20 instead of FMC7 for the scoring of CLL in close to 1000 cases has shown that FMC7 is of greater diagnostic value for distinguishing CLL, where it is negative or weak, from the other B-cell disorders, in which it is strongly expressed. The findings with CD20 and FMC7 are similar only in the non-CLL B-cell disorders.

When considering the possibility of a diagnosis of NHL, it is essential to obtain tissue for histology to confirm this suspicion and facilitate the classification of the disease. When the white blood cell (WBC) count is high (e.g. $>50 \times 10^9$/L) and the blood film shows unequivocal features of CLL or B-PLL, lymph node histology is not required.

Bone marrow trephine biopsies are needed to provide important diagnostic and prognostic information (see below) and can confirm a diagnosis of CLL or NHL, provide indications about the mechanism of anaemia or thrombocytopenia and predict the outcome of splenectomy. For disorders with an enlarged spleen, such as B-PLL and HCL, SMZL and some forms of MCL, spleen histology may be of diagnostic value.

The difficulties in eliciting metaphases for cytogenetic analysis in CLL and other small lymphocytic disorders have emphasized the value of FISH analysis, which can be assessed on interphase cells. However, there is no specific genetic abnormality in CLL, but the current FISH studies are valuable as prognostic indicators (see below). FISH is important for excluding the two NHLs that have characteristic abnormalities, MCL with t(11;14)(q13;q32) and follicular lymphoma with t(14;18)(q32;q21).

Chronic lymphocytic leukaemia

Chronic lymphocytic leukaemia accounts for about 25% of all leukaemias. In adults over the age of 50 years it is the most common form, particularly in the West. In the Far East, its incidence is low. CLL affects twice as many males as females, with a peak incidence between 60 and 80 years. The median age of patients at diagnosis is around 70 years. In the MRC CLL trials, 70% of patients entered were aged 60 years or over, and 15% were below 50 years. There is a tendency for older patients to present with less advanced disease. CLL is rarely diagnosed

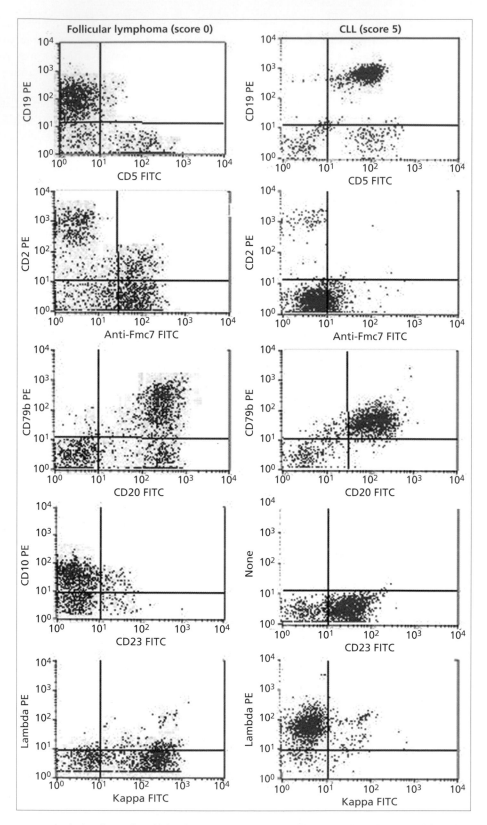

Figure 29.1 Flow cytometry analysis of peripheral blood samples from a case of follicular lymphoma with lymphocytosis (score 0) compared with a case of CLL (score 5) using the antibodies listed in Table 29.1.

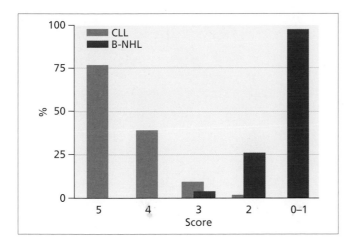

Figure 29.2 Distribution frequency of scores in CLL (high scores) compared with cases of B-cell non-Hodgkin lymphoma (B-NHL) with circulating lymphoma cells (low scores).

Table 29.3 Frequency of *IGHV* usage in CLL by mutation status.

IGHV *gene*	*Unmutated cases (%)*	*Mutated cases (%)*
IGHV1-69	28	1
IGHV3-21	6	19
IGHV4-34	5	13
IGHV3-30	4	10
IGHV1-2	7	4
IGHV3-23	1	10

below the age of 40 years and is even more rare below 30. Of all the leukaemias, CLL has the highest familial incidence, which can be documented in about 10% of patients (see below).

Pioneering work independently developed by Dameshek and Galton in the 1960s introduced the concept of CLL as a progressive accumulation of immunologically incompetent lymphocytes, starting in lymph nodes and/or the bone marrow and gradually expanding to most haemopoietic organs. This concept of slow progression was the basis of the clinical staging systems and explains the gradual abnormalities of the immune system that result in hypogammaglobulinaemia and, not infrequently, autoimmune complications. The bone marrow also reflects the progression of CLL from early interstitial and nodular infiltration to late diffuse lymphocytic replacement of normal haemopoietic elements.

Pathogenesis

Several factors are involved in the pathogenesis of CLL, including antigen stimulation within specific microenvironments and failure to undergo apoptosis. In the past, CLL was considered to be derived from CD5-positive naive B cells. Now there is significant evidence that these B cells are antigen experienced, expressing CD23, CD25, CD27, CD69 and CD71. After VDJ rearrangement the cells may undergo somatic hypermutation, which can be demonstrated by the lack of homology with germline DNA. In half of cases the immunoglobulin variable region heavy chain (*IGHV*) gene is mutated, but in the rest is unmutated. These changes and subsequent complex interactions between the B-cell receptor (BCR), which comprises the immunoglobulin heavy and light chains, and the microenvironment drive the pathogenesis of CLL. The immunoglobulin gene repertoire in CLL shows biased (non-random) V_H usage compared with normal B cells. This restricted V_H usage is linked to the degree of somatic hypermutation. For example, unmutated cases often use *IGHV1-69*, while mutated cases use preferentially *IGHV3-21*, *IGHV4-34*, etc. (Table 29.3). The immunoglobulin repertoire in CLL may be shaped by antigens as yet unknown. This phenomenon, the over-representation of some *IGHV* genes, is not unique to CLL and, in the case of *IGHV1-69* and *IGHV4-34*, is also a feature of other indolent lymphomas.

Approximately 20% of immunoglobulin subsets show similar (homologous) patterns of the complementarity-determining region (CDR)3 in both heavy and light chains, designated 'stereotypes'. These are more common in unmutated cases and provide further evidence for antigen selection in the pathogenesis of CLL. Unmutated cases are associated with autoreactivity and polyreactivity to certain molecules and have a more proliferative pattern of disease with a more aggressive clinical course. Determination of the *IGHV* mutation status as mutated or unmutated is also an important prognostic marker (see below). There are some exceptions, notably *IGHV3-21*, which is more often mutated (see Table 29.3) and is associated with poor outcome (comparable to unmutated cases) and has predominantly light chain expression. The reasons for the different clinical behaviour between unmutated and mutated cases may relate to continuous response to antigen stimulation in the unmutated cases eventually leading to genetic instability, while mutated cases minimize cell division by becoming anergic.

CLL B lymphocytes are long-lived and resistant to apoptosis, as shown by upregulation of the anti-apoptotic proteins BCL2, MCL1, Survivin, Toso. This BCL-2 family of proteins share a BH3 motif that is the target of small molecules currently being tested as new therapies. Gene expression profiling in CLL cells suggests that the disease originates from the transformation of a specific common precursor, likely to be an antigen-experienced memory B lymphocyte. This is supported by the constant expression of CD27. There is no evidence that CLL represents two distinct diseases, although detailed gene expression profiling may show some differences between mutated and unmutated cases, notably, the expression of ZAP-70.

Complex interactions between the BCR and the bone marrow and lymph node microenvironment drive the pathogenesis of CLL. These interactions involve stromal cells, including 'nurse' cells, T cells, cytokines, and pro- and anti-apoptotic factors.

Proliferating centres or pseudofollicles, as seen in histological sections, are the tissue hallmark of CLL and the nerve centre for these interactions. In them, B cells are activated and divide and are in close contact with CD4$^+$ T cells. One important cytokine is tumour necrosis factor (TNF)-α; this is consistently expressed in CLL cells, which also express the TNF-α receptor, suggesting that it may act as a growth factor. Abnormal angiogenesis is also associated with tumour progression and this is modulated by vascular endothelial growth factor. The relevance of the micro-environment is underlined by the therapeutic activity shown recently by immunomodulating and anti-angiogenic agents such as thalidomide and lenalidomide.

Clinical and laboratory features

In at least 50% of patients, the disease is diagnosed by chance, following a routine blood examination. In others, the presentation is prompted by symptoms of anaemia or by the discovery of painless lymph node enlargement. Systemic symptoms such as pyrexia, sweating or weight loss are rare. Not infrequently, a prolonged chest infection or pneumonia is the first manifestation of CLL.

Lymph node enlargement is symmetrical and involves the neck, axillae and inguinal regions. Splenomegaly of variable degree is present in two-thirds of cases. Significant hepatomegaly is less frequent. It is possible to document lymph node enlargement in the hilar regions on routine radiography or in the retroperitoneal regions by ultrasound or computed tomography (CT). Although the latter investigations may not add significant prognostic information and are not used for staging purposes (see below), they are often useful for follow-up after treatment. An abdominal CT scan is important in documenting the extent of abdominal lymphadenopathy in patients presenting with palpable nodes. It is rare to find large para-aortic nodes in patients presenting without peripheral lymphadenopathy. Late in the disease process, however, this is not uncommon, and abdominal CT may be necessary to document progression.

New diagnostic criteria

The International Workshop on CLL (IWCLL) and the WHO recommend that at least 5×10^9/L monoclonal B lymphocytes (CD19$^+$CD20$^+$) should be demonstrated in the blood and that they should fulfil the characteristic CLL phenotype, i.e. CD5$^+$, CD23$^+$, weak or negative staining with FMC7 and CD79b, and weak expression of monoclonal surface membrane immunoglobulin (staining for κ or λ) (see Table 29.1). This, and the characteristic peripheral blood morphology, suffices for the diagnosis of CLL and helps exclude other B-cell disorders, chiefly lymphomas presenting with lymphocytosis (see section Differential diagnosis). A bone marrow aspirate and trephine biopsy is not required for diagnosis if the above findings are typical and the CLL immunophenotypic score is 4–5 (see Table

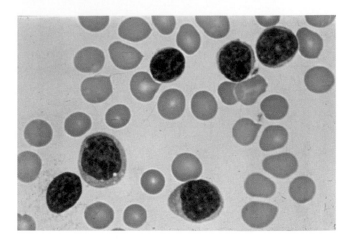

Figure 29.3 Blood film of a typical case of CLL.

29.2). A bone marrow test is required to assess the nature of cytopenias in order to exclude indolent lymphomas in cases scoring 3 or less, and before initiating therapy as a baseline for assessment of response and to interpret the development of cytopenia after therapy. One exception is small lymphocytic lymphoma (SLL), a condition identical to CLL according to the new WHO classification. SLL requires the presence of lymphadenopathy and/or splenomegaly and requires histopathology confirmation by lymph node biopsy. In contrast to CLL, SLL has less than 5×10^9/L B lymphocytes in the peripheral blood. Cases with less than 5×10^9/L B lymphocytes in the peripheral blood and not fulfilling the criteria for SLL are categorized as monoclonal B-cell lymphocytosis (see below).

Morphologically, the lymphocytes in blood films are small and show scanty cytoplasm and a characteristic pattern of nuclear chromatin clumping; the nucleolus is inconspicuous and azurophil granules are seen only in a minority of normal T cells (Figure 29.3). The presence of smudge cells, which correlates with the WBC count, is of diagnostic value. A proportion of prolymphocytes (1–5%) are nearly always seen with counts in excess of 30×10^9/L. If the proportion of prolymphocytes is greater than 10%, it represents a variant designated CLL/PL (Figure 29.4). Some patients have a mixed pattern of small and large cells and others have lymphoplasmacytoid features or even cells with nuclear clefts. These are often associated with other atypical features (see below).

Other haematological features

Anaemia and thrombocytopenia are important prognostic features in CLL and form part of the information used for staging. In advanced CLL, there is heavy lymphocytic infiltration resulting in bone marrow failure. The trephine biopsy shows heavy replacement of fat spaces and haemopoietic cells by lymphocytes (Figures 29.5 and 29.6). In an ageing population it is important always to exclude nutritional deficiencies (iron, folate), which can easily be corrected by appropriate supplements. The possible causes of anaemia in CLL are listed in Table 29.4. The current staging systems do not clearly distinguish the causes of anaemia as having different prognostic significance. This is probably because marrow failure is by far the most common

cause and there is an assumption that most haematologists will be able to detect anaemias not strictly related to the disease.

Hypogammaglobulinaemia is the rule in advanced CLL and is considered to be responsible for the high incidence of upper respiratory tract infections. Small monoclonal bands, often IgM, are seen in less than 10% of cases. The appearance of a monoclonal band during the evolution of the disease or the discovery of free light chains in the urine (Bence Jones proteinuria) may indicate disease transformation (see below, Richter syndrome).

Immune cytopenias

There is evidence that autoimmune complications, e.g. anaemia or thrombocytopenia, which are rare at presentation (10% and 3%, respectively) do not necessarily confer a poor prognosis if adequately treated. It is important always to carry out the direct antiglobulin test (DAT), or Coombs test, at diagnosis in each patient. The importance of the DAT is twofold: to document

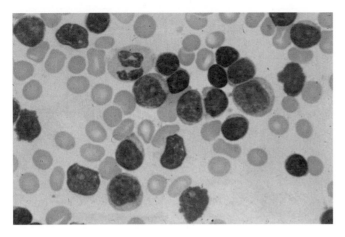

Figure 29.4 Blood film from a case of CLL/PL. Note the dual population of small lymphocytes and larger nucleolated prolymphocytes.

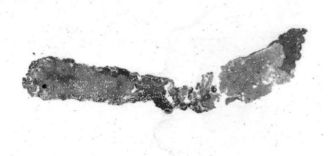

Figure 29.5 Low magnification of a trephine biopsy from a patient with CLL and heavy (packed) lymphocytic infiltration.

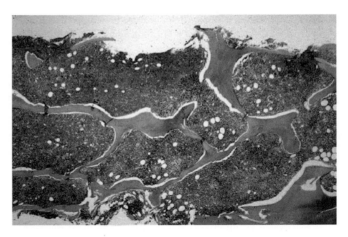

Figure 29.6 Higher magnification of the same case as in Figure 29.5 showing scanty fat spaces and diffuse lymphocytic infiltration.

Table 29.4 Causes of anaemia in CLL and their management.

Cause	Diagnostic test	Treatment	Significance
Bone marrow (BM) failure	BM aspirate and/or trephine biopsy	Corticosteroids, CLL therapy	Advanced CLL: stage III (Rai), stage C (Binet)
Haemolytic anaemia	DAT (Coombs test)	Corticosteroids, immunosuppression, splenectomy	Does not affect prognosis but more frequent in active CLL
Red cell aplasia	BM examination	(See text)	Uncertain
Hypersplenism	BM, spleen size	Splenectomy, CLL therapy	Prognosis depends on stage after splenectomy
Fotate or iron deficiency	Indices, Fe and folate levels	Appropriate supplements	None; restage when anaemia corrected

autoimmune haemolytic anaemia (AIHA) and to detect its triggering after therapy. Not infrequently, patients have a positive DAT at presentation without overt haemolysis (e.g. no reticulocytosis or raised bilirubin).

The LRF CLL4 trial provided an opportunity to examine in detail the clinical significance of a DAT for the development of AIHA. The findings are only applicable to patients who require therapy, i.e. those with Binet stages A-progressive, B and C. At trial entry 14% were DAT positive, and this was associated with Binet stage C and high β_2-microglobulin. A positive DAT was a predictor of the subsequent development of AIHA after treatment in 28%; when negative, it predicted that 93% of patients would not develop AIHA. Those who were DAT positive at entry achieved lower complete remission (CR) rates and had worse progression-free survival (PFS) and overall survival (OS), suggesting indirectly that DAT status may be a useful prognostic factor. Overall, 10% of patients developed AIHA during or after therapy; again, this was linked to stage C, high β_2-microglobulin and positive DAT at entry, and worse outcome. The trial also established that those randomized to fludarabine and cyclophosphamide (FC) had a lower incidence of AIHA (5%) than those randomized to fludarabine alone (11%) and chlorambucil (12%) ($P = 0.01$). Similar data for the comparison between fludarabine and FC were recorded in a German trial. Of note is that AIHA after single-agent fludarabine may be more severe.

The development of autoimmune thrombocytopenic purpura (ITP) is less common and is often associated with positive DAT and AIHA and unmutated *IGHV* genes. The documentation of ITP requires the demonstration of platelet-associated immunoglobulin. If this is not possible, one can still suspect peripheral destruction of platelets by examination of the bone marrow (see below).

A study from the Mayo Clinic which looked retrospectively at the cause of cytopenia in a large cohort showed that those with immune cytopenias did better than those in whom the cytopenia was a result of bone marrow failure, which is not surprising since most of the latter patients would have presented with stage C disease.

Bone marrow examination

Bone marrow aspirates are not as informative as the core biopsy regarding overall cellularity and degree of infiltration. A trephine needs to be at least 2 cm in length (Figure 29.5) to be informative. The value of the biopsy is summarized in Table 29.5. The degree of infiltration provides prognostic information: a densely packed bone marrow (diffuse pattern) with little or no residual fat spaces (Figure 29.6) correlates with advanced CLL: stage C (Binet) or III–IV (Rai). Other bone marrow patterns are interstitial, with relatively abundant fat spaces (Figure 29.7), and nodular (Figure 29.8). Both of these are seen alone or in combination (mixed pattern) in relatively early stages of

Table 29.5 The value of bone marrow trephine biopsies in CLL.*

Prognostic feature
Diffuse pattern: packed bone marrow has poor prognosis

Clarify the nature of cytopenias (before and after therapy)
Low platelets > megakaryocytes
Red cell aplasia
Myelodysplastic changes

Differential diagnosis from low-grade NHL
Paratrabecular pattern not seen in CLL
More proliferation centres in CLL/PL

To assess response to treatment
Nodular partial remission seen only on biopsy (needs immunostaining)
Hypocellular bone marrow, without CLL infiltrates, and low blood counts

*A bone marrow test (aspirate or trephine) is not required for diagnosis.

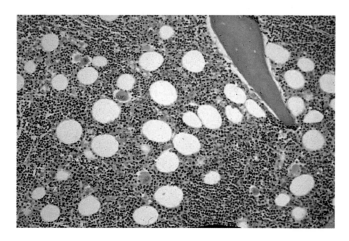

Figure 29.7 Interstitial lymphocytic infiltration in a case of early CLL with preserved haemopoiesis and abundant fat spaces.

the disease. An increased number of megakaryocytes in the presence of low platelets may suggest ITP (Figure 29.9). Absence of red cell precursors and a low reticulocyte count suggest red cell aplasia. When this is due to parvovirus infection, large basophilic erythroid precursors can be seen in the bone marrow aspirates. Paratrabecular deposits are common in follicular lymphoma and may be seen in SMZL and MCL, but not in CLL. Proliferation centres are a unique feature of CLL and SLL. They are seen in lymph node biopsies and, in very active CLL, also in the bone marrow. Proliferating centres have a high labelling index, as detected by immunocytochemistry with Ki-67 or MIB-1, and show prolymphocytes and para-immunoblasts.

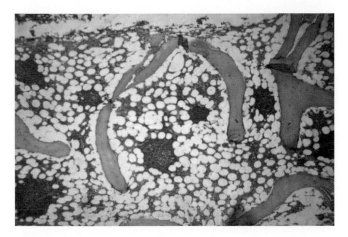

Figure 29.8 Nodular pattern of infiltration in CLL, early in the disease. A similar pattern described as nodular partial remission may be seen after chemotherapy in patients with previously diffuse involvement.

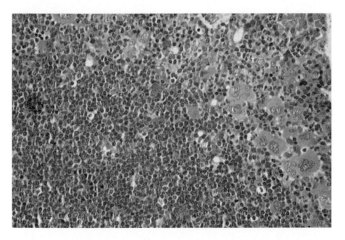

Figure 29.9 Diffuse infiltration in the bone marrow in a patient with CLL, a large spleen and thrombocytopenia. Note the large number of megakaryocytes, which indicated that splenectomy will improve the low platelet count.

There is also a higher expression of CD20 and CD23 in the proliferating centres of lymph nodes and spleen than in the small lymphocytes outside them. This may explain the high levels of soluble CD20 and CD23 in the serum of patients with active CLL.

Bone marrow biopsies are important for assessing response. In particular, a nodular partial remission (PR), which is a good clinical response, can only be defined by a biopsy and not an aspirate. In such cases, the aspirate may show less than 30% lymphocytes which, by the old criteria of response, could have been considered as CR. Immunostaining of the nodules is also important to assess response. If they are composed mainly of B cells (stained with CD20), they reflect residual CLL. If they are mainly T cells (stained with CD3), they may not represent residual CLL and are consistent with a true CR. When assessing responses, it is always useful to compare the pre-treatment bone marrow with the one at the end of therapy.

Staging systems

The two widely accepted systems are those of Rai (1975) and Binet (1981). Rai's staging system takes the view that CLL cells accumulate first in the blood and bone marrow, then in lymph nodes and spleen, finally leading to bone marrow failure. The chances of a patient surviving will depend largely on the stage at which he or she presents to the physician's attention. The original Rai system has five stages: 0, no anaemia, thrombocytopenia or physical signs; I, lymphadenopathy only; II, splenomegaly and/or hepatomegaly with or without lymph node enlargement and without anaemia or thrombocytopenia; III, anaemia (Hb < 11 g/dL), irrespective of physical signs; and IV, thrombocytopenia (platelets < 100×10^9/L), with or without any of the above features. Binet modified this system following extensive multivariate analysis from two French studies. This system has only three stages (A, B and C) and is probably more accurate with respect to prognosis for patients with Rai stages I and II. The Binet system groups together patients with anaemia (Hb < 10 g/dL) and thrombocytopenia (platelets < 100×10^9/L) as group C. The remaining patients are staged according to the number of lymphoid organs involved, considering as one each of the following areas: neck, axillae and inguinal regions, spleen and liver. Group A patients have no organ enlargement or up to two areas; group B patients have three to five involved areas. Thus stage A may correspond to Rai 0, I or II. Recently, the Rai staging has also been simplified and used in trials as follows: stages 0 (low grade), I and II (intermediate), and III and IV (advanced stage). Except for the difference in the level of haemoglobin (10 or 11 g/dL), Rai stages III and IV are the same as Binet C.

In practice, staging is necessary to predict prognosis, make decisions about clinical management and facilitate allocation in randomized trials. Although only patients showing signs of symptoms of disease activity (i.e. upward trend in WBC count, decreasing haemoglobin or platelet levels due to bone marrow infiltration, lymph node or spleen enlargement causing compressive problems, general 'B' symptoms), most stage C and also stage B patients present with some of these features and therefore need therapy.

Because of the increasing practice of routine blood analysis, the presentation patterns of patients with CLL have changed over the last decade. At present, most patients are diagnosed in early phases of the disease (Rai stage 0, Binet stage A), thus undermining the prognostic value of clinical stages as a whole. Moreover, one of the important issues regarding clinical stages, in particular stage A, is that the pace of the disease (i.e. whether it will remain stable or progress) cannot be readily predicted. The Spanish group has shown that a short lymphocyte doubling time (<12 months) in stage A correlates with poor prognosis. Similarly, the French group showed that those with haemoglobin below 12 g/dL and/or lymphocyte count greater than 30×10^9/L fared worse than those with haemoglobin above 12 g/dL and lymphocytes under 30×10^9/L. The MRC examined both these factors in an observational study, MRC CLL3A, and found that both were indicators of prognosis and that the two criteria were independent of each other. As a result, the MRC uses a definition for stage A-progressive for patients with short doubling times, downward trend in haemoglobin and/or platelets, increasing organomegaly and systemic symptoms. Using these criteria, it has been shown in both the CLL3 and CLL4 trials that patients with stage A-progressive disease fared the same as those with stage B, confirming the validity of the clinical criteria used. Patients with both A-progressive and B disease fared better than those with stage C. Using biomarkers such as CD38, ZAP-70 or *IGHV* mutation status, it is possible to predict those patients who will have a short time from diagnosis to progression and will need treatment. However, as advised by the 2008 IWCLL guidelines, these factors should not be used to initiate therapy outside clinical trials.

Numerous new prognostic factors have now emerged in CLL (see below), and these are being tested against the well-established parameters. These are relevant in particular to stage A, but also perhaps for identifying prognosis and good responders in the other stages. While these new tests are incorporated and tested in the clinic, the simple clinical observations, blood counts, symptoms and physical examination will remain as the best guideline on outcome. With the caveat indicated above (i.e. increasing proportion of patients diagnosed in asymptomatic phase of the disease), clinical stages are still very important as a starting point and, when considering the whole population with CLL, remains the best prognostic indicator. However, for randomized trials in which stage A non-progressive patients will not be entered, the prognostic value of staging loses its strength and other measures which assess the biology of the disease have now become more relevant.

Prognostic factors

The median survival of patients with CLL is around 7 years but the individual prognosis is extremely variable. As previously indicated, the clinical staging systems are still the backbone for assessing prognosis. Patients with low-risk disease (Rai 0, Binet A) have a median survival greater than 10 years, those with intermediate-risk disease (Rai I, II; Binet B) have a median survival of 5–7 years, and patients with high-risk disease (Rai III, IV; Binet C) have a median life expectancy of less than 3–4 years. In addition to clinical stages, many other prognostic factors have been proposed, the most extensively investigated and validated being cytogenetics, *IGHV* mutational status, ZAP-70 and CD38 expression in leukaemic lymphocytes, and serum β_2-microglobulin levels.

Once patients require therapy, prognostic factors are overcome by effective treatments. Indeed, response to therapy is, as in all cancers, the most important predictor of survival in patients with CLL. Predictors of response to therapy are being actively investigated. The most reliable are del(17p) and del(11q), reflecting, respectively, abnormalities of the *TP53* and *ATM* genes. Patients with these abnormalities do not respond to conventional fludarabine-based therapy or have a short-lived response. Recently, low expression of the microRNA 34a has also been found to predict poor response. The association between *IGHV* mutations, CD38 and ZAP-70 expression and response is not completely settled, but response duration seems to be shorter in patients with these biomarkers, particularly when they are found together.

Age is relevant in as much as it is associated with causes of death other than the disease itself. The effect of age is greater in stage A, in which up to 50% of patients may die of causes unrelated to CLL, such as other cancers or cardiovascular events. Another adverse prognostic factor that has emerged in all UK CLL trials over the last 30 years is male gender (see below).

Response to treatment has also emerged as an important prognostic variable. However, although it is associated with PFS, an association with OS has not been shown in randomized trials. One reason is that although treatment response matters, a patient not responding to first-line treatment, e.g. chlorambucil, may respond to a second treatment, e.g. FC with or without rituximab (FCR). There is increasing evidence that achieving MRD negativity (see below) is clinically important. Patients in CR with no detectable MRD have a longer PFS and OS than those with persistent MRD. However, MRD negativity is an arbitrary concept that depends on the technique used to assess MRD. In addition, patients who achieve MRD-negative status could be those with biologically less aggressive disease and hence with an intrinsically better prognosis. Another important point is that increasing or prolonging treatment to reach MRD-negative status may convey unnecessary risks such as myelotoxicity and infections. There is also the risk of developing secondary myelodysplastic syndrome (MDS)/acute myeloid leukaemia (AML). Furthermore, patients with aggressive disease, such as those with del(17p), do not usually respond to chemoimmunotherapy, yet these patients are those who could benefit most by achieving MRD-negative CR. Because of all these reasons, MRD eradication as a treatment end point is only justified within clinical trials.

Cytogenetics

There are no specific translocations in CLL. Most abnormalities are deletions, or extra copies such as trisomy of chromosome 12. Translocations have been reported in a few cases, e.g. t(14;19) (see below) or t(14;18), but whether these represent typical cases is equivocal. It was well known that analysis of the karyotype of CLL lymphocytes stimulated to divide by a variety of mitogens elicited positive results in less than 50% of cases.

Table 29.6 Hierarchical model of chromosomal abnormalities in CLL.

Karyotype	Döhner	LRF CLL4
Number of patients	352	579
17p13 deletion	7%	6%
11q22–23 deletion	17%	20%
6q21–23 deletion	8%	8%
12q trisomy	14%	15%
Normal karyotype	18%	15%
13q14 deletion as sole abnormality	36%	36%

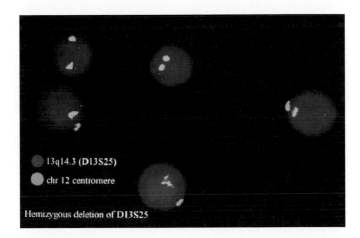

Figure 29.10 FISH analysis with a 13q14 probe showing missing red dots in several cells denoting 13q deletion; all the cells are disomic for chromosome 12 (normal pattern).

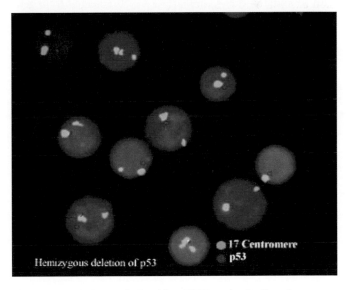

Figure 29.11 FISH analysis with a *TP53* probe (red) and a control 17 probe. Note many cells with only one (instead of two) red dot, indicating *TP53* deletion.

This is due to normal metaphases, which reflected the karyotype of the normal T cells, and the frequent lack of metaphases in cases with high WBC count. Newer techniques are now available that are able to elicit metaphases in a higher proportion of cases. FISH analysis uses specific probes to detect the most common genetic changes on interphase cells. There is now a panel of at least five probes for studying the most frequent abnormalities, which can be detected in 80% of cases. Thus, we are now in a position in CLL similar to that of the acute leukaemias where distinct chromosome abnormalities of prognostic significance can be detected in most patients. However, it is important to state that none of the abnormalities found are unique or specific for CLL and can be found in other B-cell disorders.

The most important contribution to the subject has been that of Dohner, who in 2000 proposed a hierarchical model for prognosis based on the genetic aberrations found in CLL (Table 29.6). This model is based on the prognostic value of such markers and it is necessary because some patients have more than one abnormality, but the one which counts is the one listed higher in Table 29.6. It should be noted that deletions of 13q14 (Figure 29.10) confer a good prognosis (even better than no abnormality), but only provided they are found as the only change. Table 29.6 also shows the incidence of abnormalities in cases from the LRF CLL4 trial.

The 17p deletion (Figure 29.11) has a much higher incidence (three or four times) in patients with advanced CLL, particularly after multiple treatments, than in those requiring treatment for the first time. The result of the 17p13 deletion at the *TP53* locus often correlates with a point mutation in the other allele and this results in total inactivation of the *TP53* suppressor gene, the most common molecular change in cancer. Although the usual method for detecting *TP53* abnormalities is to use FISH to detect deletion of 17p, overexpression of the *TP53* gene can be demonstrated by flow cytometry and immunohistochemistry. The significance of *TP53* overexpression is probably the same, but these methods are often used mainly in histological section of bone marrow and lymph nodes. As

stated above, *TP53* mutations can be detected by polymerase chain reaction (PCR) and carry similar adverse prognosis. A cautionary note was issued in a report from the M.D. Anderson Center and the Mayo Clinic. A study of 99 previously untreated patients with 17p deletion showed significant clinical heterogeneity, with some patients not showing progression for up to 5 years.

The group with deletion of 6q21–23 represents 8% of cases both in Dohner's series and LRF CLL4. These patients tend to present with high lymphocyte counts but apparently have an overall good prognosis. The deletion at 11q22–23 involves the *ATM* gene and it has been suggested that survival in del(11q) cases may depend on whether the gene in the other allele is mutated (seen in 12% of cases). Cytogenetic clonal evolution has been reported in 17% of cases, which tend to be unmutated.

Biological prognostic markers

Numerous biomarkers have emerged in recent studies of CLL. These prognostic factors include genetic markers, mutational status of the *IGHV* gene, V$_H$ gene usage, serum levels of β_2-microglobulin and CD38 and ZAP-70 expression, the latter measured by flow cytometry. A list of these markers is given in Table 29.7. These biological markers have helped to unravel the clinical heterogeneity of CLL. The focus now is on new reproducible markers that relate to the underlying biology, proliferative potential and responsiveness to therapy. Some of these are predictive of time to disease progression from diagnosis; others predict also response to treatment, PFS and OS.

Early work suggested that CD38 expression correlates with unmutated status. Similarly, ZAP-70 emerged from gene expression studies as overexpressed in unmutated cases. The correlation of CD38 and ZAP-70 expression with *IGHV* mutation status is close but not complete and both of these markers assessed by flow cytometry are good predictors of time to disease progression. This may be important information in newly diagnosed patients, especially those with stage A. FISH analysis, which identifies common genetic abnormalities in CLL such as del(6q), trisomy 12, del(13q), del(11q) and del(17p), has been extensively studied in clinical trials, including LRF CLL4 and the German trials. Dohner's hierarchical model for analysis of the cytogenetic abnormalities (see above) has been shown to be reproducible and reliable. FISH has identified two groups of cases associated with aggressive CLL and resistance to conventional chemotherapy. The first group, deletion of 11q22, involves the *ATM* gene and is seen in 20% of those who need

therapy and identifies younger patients, particularly males, who often have significant lymphadenopathy. Although the outcome in del(11q) cases is worse than with other types of cytogenetic abnormality, current combinations such as FC and FCR have significantly improved their response rate and PFS. The other group is defined by the deletion of 17p13, which involves the *TP53* gene and is associated in 85% of cases with a mutation of the *TP53* gene in the other allele. Whether defined by deletion or mutation, the outcome of this group is poor, with a low response rate and very short PFS and OS. A number of recent studies and data from LRF CLL4 suggest that one needs to test for both 17p deletion and mutation to detect all the cases with *TP53* loss of function.

Studies first reported by the group from the M.D. Anderson Center and confirmed in the LRF CLL4 trial have shown the value of measuring β_2-microglobulin, high levels of which are associated with poor treatment response and short PFS. V$_H$ usage has identified the group with *IGHV3-21* as of poor prognosis regardless of their mutational status (mutated in two-thirds of cases). By combining *IGHV* status, V$_H$ usage, FISH results and β_2-microglobulin, it is possible to separate cases that have been entered into LRF CLL4 (therefore requiring therapy, i.e. Binet stage A-progressive, B and C) into three distinct prognostic groups: poor risk (6% of cases), defined by 17p deletion; intermediate risk (72% of cases), defined by unmutated *IGHV* genes or del(11q) or *IGHV3-21* usage or β_2-microglobulin above 4 mg/L; and good risk (22% of cases), defined by mutated *IGHV* genes, but excluding those with *IGHV3-21* usage and/or the other abnormalities that define the intermediate group. These groups are clearly distinguished with respect to PFS and OS.

The IWCLL guidelines do not recommend these tests for diagnosis or for assessment of new patients, but they seem very important once treatment is indicated and for risk assessment when entered into clinical trials.

Table 29.7 Prognostic biomarkers in CLL.

CD38, ZAP-70, CD49b *(flow cytometry)*
IGHV mutational status (PCR)
IGHV usage (PCR)
FISH analysis (four or five probes)
TP53 mutations (DNA based)
Telomere length (DNA based)
CLLU1 (RNA based)
Lipoprotein lipase (RNA based)
Serum factors
   β_2-microglobulin
   Soluble CD23
   Circulating VEGF
   Thymidine kinase

VEGF, vascular endothelial growth factor.

Chromosome translocations involving the *IGH* locus

It is debatable whether translocations of the *IGH* locus are a feature of CLL. Nevertheless, systematic interphase FISH with an *IGH* probe can detect up to 5% of cases with such translocations. Excluding t(11;14), a feature of MCL, some apparently genuine cases of CLL have been reported with t(14;18)(q32;q21) or *IGH/BCL2*, t(14;19)(q32;q13) or *IGH/BCL3*, and very rarely t(8;14)(q24.1;q32) involving the *MYC* gene. The latter cases were described as CLL/PL and some as typical B-PLL. *IGH* translocations have often been described as atypical and associated with poor prognosis. Cases with t(14;19), although rare, have been more extensively characterized. This translocation has been reported in a heterogeneous group of B-cell malignancies including marginal zone lymphomas and, in about half of cases, with a diagnosis of CLL frequently associated with trisomy 12, unmutated *IGHV* genes and low frequency of 13q14 deletion.

IGHV mutation analysis

The most interesting and exciting new findings that relate to prognosis and which may underlie the clinical heterogeneity of CLL are mutational status of the *IGHV* gene and the expression of CD38 and of ZAP-70. Somatic hypermutation is the process by which B cells, after the initial recombination of immunoglobulin genes, undergo further change in order to produce high-affinity antibodies. This event occurs within the germinal centre and gives rise to memory B cells and plasma cells.

CLL was for many years thought to be a disease of early or immature CD5-positive B cells with unmutated *IGHV* genes. More recent studies showed heterogeneity, and this was consolidated by two landmark papers in 1999 by Damle and Hamblin, demonstrating that just over half of the patients had mutated *IGHV* genes (Table 29.8), defined by convention as less than 98% homology to the nearest germline sequence.

Many studies have confirmed the original finding, which suggested initially that there were two forms of CLL: the unmutated type, associated with all the features of poor prognosis; and the mutated type, associated with stable disease and good prognosis (Table 29.8). Of interest is the finding that many of the poor prognostic features, such as stages B and C, male gender, atypical morphology, trisomy 12 and 11q deletion, are seen predominantly in unmutated cases, whereas the opposite is true for the mutated ones.

Data based on gene expression profiling has shown unequivocally that CLL has a characteristic pattern of expression (or signature) that is independent of *IGHV* mutation and is distinct from that of other B-cell lymphomas such as MCL, follicular lymphoma and diffuse large B-cell NHL. The genotype of CLL was defined by a common pattern of expression of 12 000 genes, with only between 23 and 200 differentially expressed in

Table 29.8 Mutational status of *IGHV* genes in CLL (broad differences).

	Unmutated	*Mutated*
Incidence	45%	55%
Male/female ratio	10:1	1.1:1
Trisomy 12	Frequent	Infrequent
Abnormal 13q14	Rare	Common
Stage (Binet)	B and C (2/3)	Stage A (2/3)
Disease course	Progressive	Stable
CD38/ZAP-70	Frequently expressed	More often negative
Therapy*	Often required	Not always needed
Response	Less than optimal	Better
Survival/PFS	Short	Long

*When indicated on clinical grounds.
PFS, progression-free survival.

mutated versus unmutated cases. One notable difference is the high expression (four to five times higher) of ZAP-70 in unmutated cases.

CD38 and ZAP-70

Early studies showed that unmutated cases correlated with higher expression of the transmembrane glycoprotein CD38. This correlation is seen in only two-thirds of cases. Therefore CD38 could not be regarded as a surrogate marker for *IGHV* mutational status. Nevertheless, many studies have now shown that CD38 is an important prognostic marker. Low percentages correlate with stable disease, while a high percentage of CD38-positive cells predicts a short time to disease progression and worse OS.

There are several caveats for the determination of CD38. Although assessed by flow cytometry and simpler than PCR and sequencing, which are used for *IGHV* mutations, CD38 should only be tested on CLL B lymphocytes and should exclude T cells, which strongly express this antigen. This is currently done by triple labelling with CD5, CD19 and CD38 and appropriate gating. Another issue is the best threshold for CD38 positivity. Early reports suggested 30%, but more recent studies recommend a lower figure (7%) as being more likely to be clinically relevant. This relatively simple determination seems to add to the constellation of markers useful for assessing prognosis in individual patients and predicting time to disease progression.

ZAP-70 is a protein tyrosine kinase and is of relevance in T-cell signalling. ZAP-70 can be demonstrated by flow cytometry, immunocytochemistry and Western blotting, and several studies have now shown a high concordance with the mutation status (~90%). Thus, ZAP-70 may be a better surrogate marker than CD38 for establishing *IGHV* mutational status without having recourse to molecular methodology. Studies using ZAP-70 have confirmed its prognostic value, particularly in patients with stage A disease, in whom early assessment of the need for future therapy may be desirable. The assessment of ZAP-70 by flow cytometry (Figure 29.12) requires the exclusion not only of T cells (as for CD38) but also of natural killer (NK) cells, as both cell types express this cytoplasmic protein strongly. Thus, the determination of ZAP-70 requires cell permeabilization procedures and staining for CD3 and CD56 (for T and NK cells), CD19 and CD5 (for CLL cells) and ZAP-70.

Role of microRNAs in CLL

MicroRNAs are a large family of short, non-coding, single-stranded molecules that regulate almost one-third of human genes. They are involved in a variety of normal and pathological processes and have recently been implicated in the pathogenesis of CLL. Two microRNAs, *MIR15* and *MIR16*, are located at 13q14, a region frequently deleted in CLL (see above). Both genes are deleted or downregulated in about two-thirds of cases and have been linked to initiation and progression of the

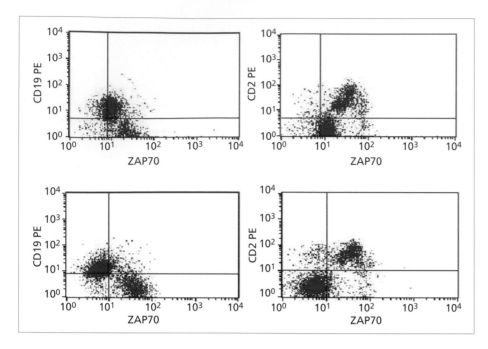

Figure 29.12 Flow cytometry plots of ZAP-70 in CLL. Top left: ZAP-70⁺CD19⁺ lymphocytes. Top right: control ZAP-70⁺ T and NK lymphocytes (CD2⁺). Bottom left: a ZAP-70⁻ case and the positive control T/NK cells (bottom right).

disease. Both microRNAs target *BCL2* which, as a result, is overexpressed in CLL. The expression profiles of microRNAs were investigated by Croce's group in close to 100 cases. They reported a unique microRNA signature that distinguished CLL according to *IGHV* mutation status and ZAP-70 expression. The mouse homologues of *MIR15* and *MIR16* are also deleted in the *TCL1A* transgenic mouse model, which develops a disease very similar to CLL, confirming their relevance in pathogenesis.

Another microRNA that may be important in CLL is *MIR34a*, which has very low expression in cases refractory to chemotherapy and with impaired DNA damage response, irrespective of whether such cases have deletions and/or mutations of *TP53*. If these findings are confirmed, they may provide a new tool for identifying drug-resistant cases and avoiding unnecessary use of non-effective drugs. Other microRNAs that may have relevance to CLL and its prognosis are *MIR29c* and *MIR223*, which were shown to have low expression in poor prognostic cases and to predict treatment-free and overall survival.

Gender differences

In CLL, female patients survive longer than males. The male to female ratio in CLL is 2:1 but in younger patients it is often higher. The proportion of cases with stage A is higher in women than in men, i.e. 40% versus 28%, while in men the proportion with stages B and C is higher. Despite women being older, gender remained an independent prognostic factor for response, PFS and OS in patients entered into UK clinical trials as shown in a number of consecutive MRC trials. This difference might be due at least in part to biological differences since, in a study

of over 900 cases, 51% of men and 37% of women had no *IGHV* mutations; in contrast, 63% of women versus 49% of men did have *IGHV* mutations ($P < 0.0001$).

Differential diagnosis

This has been partly discussed above in the methodology for diagnosis. One problem is when CLL has atypical morphology and another when the CLL immunophenotypic score is below 3. The most common morphological change is the increased proportion of larger nucleolated prolymphocytes. When there are more than 10% of these cells in blood films, the disease is described as CLL/PL.

CLL/PL is a proliferative form of CLL, not infrequently associated with trisomy 12 or *TP53* deletion, high rate of cell divisions (as shown with the antibody Ki-67) and histologically by many proliferating centres in lymph nodes and bone marrow sections. Occasionally, lymph nodes seem totally replaced by prolymphocyte-like cells, a situation that can provisionally be described as 'accelerated' CLL. Peripheral blood films always show a dual population of small lymphocytes and prolymphocytes. CLL does not transform to B-PLL, which is a distinct clinicopathological entity (see below).

When atypical features are present, including those of CLL/PL, it is important to consider the differential diagnosis with NHL evolving with lymphocytosis, notably MCL which, like CLL, is CD5 positive. The best method to exclude (or confirm) MCL is to test for t(11;14) by FISH and/or to demonstrate expression of cyclin D1 by immunohistochemistry. Other NHLs can be excluded by histological criteria (see Chapter 33) and the combination of immunophenotype and peripheral blood morphology (see below).

Genetic predisposition to CLL

Evidence from epidemiological and family studies supports the view that there is inherited susceptibility to CLL in a significant subset of patients. Case reports of leukaemia families and case–control and case cohort studies all showed that the relative risk of developing CLL in patients' relatives is three to eight times higher than in the normal population. The molecular basis of familial CLL is currently being unravelled by means of genome–wide association studies, including both families and sporadic cases. Familial CLL often cosegregates with other B-cell disorders, chiefly Hodgkin lymphoma and lymphoplasmacytic lymphoma, suggesting that the predisposition to CLL is mediated through pleiotropic genes.

The search for the genetic basis of CLL has been active in the last few years with the possibility of collecting DNA samples from familial cases. Figure 29.13 illustrates families with several affected members.. There is a strong rationale for searching for moderate- to high-risk mutations in linkage studies. The largest of these included 206 families and suggested a possible disease locus at 2q21. However, subsequent studies in two large multi-generational families failed to confirm this finding. Therefore the possibility that a single gene mutation is involved in the predisposition to CLL is now considered unlikely, the current hypothesis being that susceptibility to CLL is a consequence of the co-inheritance of several low-penetrance gene variants. This 'common-disease, common-variant hypothesis' concept can only be ascertained by large genome-wide association studies based on the analysis of SNPs. Such a study, conducted at the Institute of Cancer Research, identified for the first time six previously unreported CLL risk loci. The most significant statistical association was at 6p25.3, which is the locus for the gene for interferon regulatory factor 4 (*IRF4*), previously known as *MUM1* (multiple myeloma oncogene 1). *IRF4* is a key regulatory transcription factor involved in lymphocyte development, proliferation and regulation of the immune response.

Monoclonal B-cell lymphocytosis

Recent studies have demonstrated a higher incidence of monoclonal B-cell lymphocytosis (MBL) in 'normal' relatives of patients with familial CLL. Small B-cell clones can be detected by very sensitive flow cytometry assays using CD5, CD19, CD20 and CD79b. The incidence of MBL in these individuals is four times greater than in the general population. The incidence is even higher when looking at people under 40 years of age.

MBL is now defined as the presence of less than 5×10^9/L monoclonal B lymphocytes in the peripheral blood, in the absence of lymphadenopathy, splenomegaly, cytopenias or disease-related symptoms. Patients with MBL may have a moderate absolute lymphocytosis ($>4 \times 10^9$/L) or a completely normal lymphocyte count. In the majority of cases the immunophenotype is identical to that of CLL, i.e. CD5$^+$ and CD23$^+$ monoclonal B lymphocytes. MBL represents either a precursor state for CLL or a distinct entity, in the same way that monoclonal gammopathy of unknown significance (MGUS) relates to myeloma. MBL could be detected in 5% of subjects (aged 60–80 years) with a normal WBC count and in a higher proportion of those presenting with lymphocytosis. MBL may progress to frank CLL at a rate of 1–2% per year. Studies by the Leeds group showed that in those presenting with lymphocytosis, CLL may develop in 15% and that half of them may eventually require treatment. Of interest too is that the 13q14 deletion,

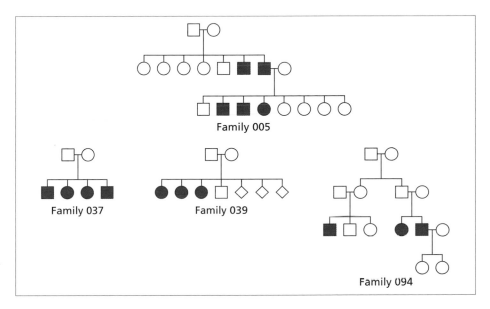

Figure 29.13 Four pedigrees of familial CLL cases with three or more affected per family.

which characterizes benign cases of CLL, is often seen in MBL. Data on *IGHV* usage are still inconclusive but those with higher B-lymphocyte counts tend to show the same biased usage as in CLL.

In a large retrospective study of patients who were found subsequently to have developed CLL (up to 6 years later), a prediagnostic B-cell clone, consistent with MBL, was demonstrated in the majority (98%). This strongly suggests that CLL may always be preceded by MBL, but it does not mean that MBL will always lead to CLL. A Spanish group has shown, using highly sensitive eight-colour flow cytometry instead of the standard four-colour method, that the frequency of MBL (or at least small B-cell clones) was higher than previously reported in healthy individuals, also increasing with age.

Polyclonal B-cell lymphocytosis

In contrast to MBL, a rare abnormality described as polyclonal B-cell lymphocytosis has been recognized. The absolute number of B cells is increased in affected patients, but staining with anti-light chain antibodies shows lack of clonality and normal proportions of κ- and λ-staining cells. For several reasons this entity, which appears not to be malignant, needs to be recognized, not least because in some patients it may mimic CLL or other B-cell disorders. Disease features are median age 40 years, lymphocyte count 3–15 × 10⁹/L (median 6.5), splenomegaly (15%) and mild bone marrow infiltration, sometimes showing intrasinusoidal distribution; 95% of patients are smokers and 90% have HLA-DR7 in their genotype. The cell markers are non-clonal, CD19⁺, FMC7⁺, CD5⁻, CD23⁻, CD27⁺ and the patients have elevated levels of serum IgM (polyclonal). Despite the benign and non-clonal nature, distinct abnormalities have been shown in the B lymphocytes: an extra copy of the long arm of chromosome 3 in the form of iso(3q) and also the presence of *IGH/BCL2* rearrangements. A minority of patients (~3%) may develop NHL. The blood picture is pleomorphic and frequently shows binucleated lymphocytes (Figure 29.14), which are characteristic of this condition. It is important to follow these patients closely and it is even more important not to institute any treatment.

Management

The indications for active treatment depend on the stage of the disease. For patients with stage A (Binet) or stages 0, I and II (Rai), a period of observation may be necessary to decide whether the pattern of the disease is stable or progressive. Most patients with stage B and two-thirds of those with Rai stage II will show progression within the first year or two after diagnosis. This is manifested by further organ enlargement, a downward trend in haemoglobin and/or platelets and a slowly rising WBC count. As responses are better with less disease, some trials have compared early versus delayed therapy to see whether

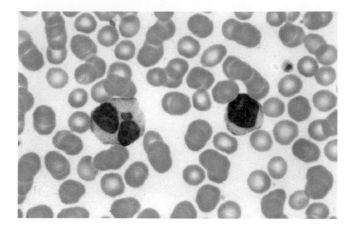

Figure 29.14 Blood film from a case of polyclonal B-cell lymphocytosis showing a binucleated cell characteristic of this condition.

survival improves. A number of trials showed that early treatment with chlorambucil was, if anything, deleterious, with more deaths due to progression in the group treated early. This was confirmed in a large overview. Thus, the old wisdom of watch and wait should continue to prevail for stage A patients, at least for the time being.

Nevertheless, the issue of early treatment in stage A patients may need to be revised, for two main reasons. First, it is now possible to better identify the patients likely to progress using some of the new prognostic factors defined above, for example unmutated *IGHV* genes, CD38/ZAP-70 expression, short lymphocyte doubling time, 17p or 11q deletions. It is in this group that randomized studies are currently being carried out to see whether early therapy may improve survival. Second, the combination of purine analogues with monoclonal antibodies increases the proportion of remitters and the quality of the responses; therefore, there may be of potential benefit early in high-risk cases.

Spontaneous regression

Spontaneous clinical remissions may occur in CLL but these are usually not complete. Based on patients entered in MRC CLL trials, 1.5% of stage A patients may undergo a spontaneous reduction of the lymphocyte count greater than 50%. The remission is rarely complete, most patients having persistent disease by flow cytometry and the remission is usually transient. The mechanisms behind spontaneous remissions are poorly understood but could be triggered by immune-mediated reactions.

Criteria for response

The definitions of response used in the UK for CLL3 and CLL4 trials were broadly similar to the National Cancer Institute (NCI) 1996 guidelines. These definitions have been updated and clarified in the 2008 IWCLL guidelines (see below). A bone marrow biopsy is required to define the category of nodular PR by the presence of discrete or moderately large nodules of residual CLL. In this context, it is important to carry out immunohistochemistry as in some patients the nodules may contain mainly T cells rather than B cells. CR requires normalization of blood counts and the bone marrow, whereas a PR requires the regression of at least 50% of organomegaly and lymphocyte counts. A bone marrow aspirate is required also to assess MRD by flow cytometry (see below).

New IWCLL definition of response

The new IWCLL guidelines include minor changes from the 1996 NCI guidelines. They propose more stringent recommendations for use in clinical trials than in general practice. This is to stress the need to collect useful data in clinical trials rather than to downgrade the care given to patients outside trials. The criteria for CR require less than 4×10^9/L lymphocytes in the peripheral blood and, ideally, without residual CLL cells as tested for MRD by flow cytometry. The definition of CR is otherwise the same as in 1996. For clinical trials the new recommendation is to test for MRD in bone marrow aspirates; thus there are two types of CR: MRD negative and MRD positive (see below). Immunohistochemistry should always be performed if residual nodules are present in the biopsies (see above) and the bone marrow needs to be tested at least 2 months after the end of therapy. CT should be repeated only if it was abnormal at the start of therapy. A new term, incomplete CR, is now used to describe patients with persistent anaemia, thrombocytopenia or neutropenia, due to myelotoxicity, who otherwise fulfil the criteria for CR. If the bone marrow is hypocellular, it is recommended that the biopsy be repeated once the blood counts have recovered.

Assessment of minimal residual disease

Refinements in flow cytometry now contribute to the definition of MRD with the same level of sensitivity as molecular methods. MRD positivity (i.e. >0.05% bone marrow cells) predicts a shorter event-free survival and a shorter remission. The standard method adopted by most international groups is four-colour flow cytometry, which has a level of sensitivity similar to that of allele-specific oligonucleotide PCR (i.e. 1 in 10 000 leucocytes). Thus, CR may now be defined as MRD negative depending on whether there is less than one leukaemic cell per 10 000 leucocytes. Methods have now been standardized and published in a report from the ERIC group. These are based on the CD5/CD19 combination, always with two other reagents such as κ and λ, CD20 and CD38, CD43 and CD79b, CD22 and CD81, and CD45 and CD14. If the first four tubes contain CD5/CD19/κ/λ and all the B cells are CD5$^+$ with restricted light-chain expression, there is no need to test the other MRD combinations. It is likely that the end point of new clinical studies in CLL will be to achieve CR with negative MRD. The sensitivity of the method used to evaluate MRD should always be reported.

MRD should be investigated in the bone marrow, as peripheral blood cells may be MRD negative for some months after treatment using monoclonal antibodies and are thus less reliable at that point.

Treatment

In the last few years, important progress has been made in the treatment of CLL. However, there is not yet a curative therapy for this form of leukaemia. Because of this, and the variable impact of the disease on patient survival, treatment needs to be adapted to the patient's risk. Importantly, the diagnosis of CLL is not equivalent to the necessity for starting therapy. Treatment is only indicated when any of the following features is present: (i) fever without evidence of infection, extreme fatigue, night sweats or weight loss; (ii) increasing anaemia or thrombocytopenia due to bone marrow infiltration by leukaemic cells; (iii) bulky or progressive lymphadenopathy; (iv) massive or progressive splenomegaly; (v) autoimmune cytopenias, which do not respond to corticosteroids; and (vi) rapid lymphocyte doubling time (e.g. <6 months). Hypogammaglobulinaemia or increased WBC counts, in the absence of any of the above criteria, are not enough to initiate treatment. Likewise, younger age, the mere availability of a bone marrow donor, or poor-prognosis biomarkers such as IGHV unmutated status or high ZAP-70 expression are not per se criteria to initiate treatment.

Treatment of patients in early-stage disease (Binet A, Rai 0) with chlorambucil or other alkylating agents delays disease progression rate but does not prolong survival. The impact of recent and more effective therapies in the natural history of patients in early stage as a whole has not been investigated. A proportion of patients in intermediate stage (Rai I and II, Binet B) have indolent disease; these patients may be followed with no therapy, like those in early stage. However, most patients with intermediate-stage disease and nearly all patients with advanced-stage disease (Rai III and IV, Binet C) need therapy.

Factors to be considered before indicating treatment include patient's age, performance status and associated diseases as well as the patient's expectations; also important are the characteristics of the disease, including biomarkers such as del(17p) or del(11q). Corticosteroids as initial treatment for stage C patients have been used in UK trials for many years. These are given at 30 mg/m^2 daily for 3 weeks, and reduced gradually for another week. Platelets rise within 4–6 weeks, as does the haemoglobin, and the WBC count follows a characteristic curve, rising after 3 or 4 weeks, sometimes doubling the initial count and then gradually coming down. This is nearly always accompanied by a decrease in size and softening of lymph nodes and spleen. This effect may facilitate subsequent therapy with agents that affect normal haemopoietic cells, and it seems more important when used before chlorambucil. It is not clear whether steroids are useful before combinations using fludarabine (e.g. FC or FCR).

For many years chlorambucil has been the treatment of choice for CLL. Chlorambucil yields a small proportion of complete responses (5–10%) and although it improves symptoms, survival is only slightly, if at all, affected. Because of this, chlorambucil is usually given to patients not able to tolerate more effective therapies. It should be noted that the doses of chlorambucil (and of cyclophosphamide) have varied widely in different studies and there is a clear indication of a dose–response curve. For example, the CALGB trial and the German CLL5 trial used chlorambucil at a dose equivalent to $40\,mg/m^2$ monthly and the reported CR rates were 3% and 5%, whereas the UK CLL3 and CLL4 trials used $60\,mg/m^2$ and $70\,mg/m^2$ (given as $10\,mg/m^2$ for 7 days every 4 weeks) and the CR rate was higher (7% in CLL4). Chlorambucil is still used as the standard comparator in many current trials. Because of its relative safety it is still recommended for patients over the age of 70 years or those with comorbidities.

A number of randomized studies conducted in the 1970s and 1980s showed that anthracycline-based therapy, such as cyclophosphamide, doxorubicin, vincristine and prednisolone (CHOP), produced a higher response rate than chlorambucil but that survival was not improved. Despite this, CHOP in combination with rituximab (R-CHOP) may be of some efficacy in patients with progressive disease who are poor responders to chlorambucil or fludarabine and, particularly, in those who develop Richter syndrome.

The greatest advance in the treatment of CLL in the last decade has been the development of monoclonal antibodies (Table 29.9) and the advent of the purine analogues (fludarabine, cladribine, pentostatin). Fludarabine's mode of action includes inhibition of DNA synthesis and DNA repair and activation of the apoptotic pathways. These mechanisms significantly enhance the effect of this agent when used in combination with other drugs (e.g. cyclophosphamide and mitoxantrone) and antibodies (e.g. rituximab). Treatment with fludarabine results in a higher CR rate than that achieved with chlorambucil or alkylating-based chemotherapies (20–40% vs. 10%) and a longer disease-free interval, although survival and PFS are not prolonged. The efficacy of fludarabine is improved by combining it with other agents (e.g. cyclophosphamide, mitoxantrone, rituximab). Using fludarabine in combination with other agents the CR rates have increased, for example from 20–35% when used alone in previously untreated patients to 30–45% with cyclophosphamide (FC), 45% with rituximab and 65% with the FCR combination in the experience of the M.D. Anderson Center and confirmed in the CLL4 German trial. FCMR (adding mitoxantrone to FCR) may be an even more powerful combination, currently used in Spanish and UK trials.

The issue of first-line fludarabine and/or its combination with cyclophosphamide has been clarified in randomized controlled trials (Table 29.10). Taken together, current results indicate that FCR not only results in a response rate superior to fludarabine or FC, but a longer freedom from progression. In addition, new evidence from the German CLL8 trial comparing FCR and FC suggests, for the first time in a randomized trial, an improvement in OS. As a result, rituximab-based chemoimmunotherapy is now considered as the best upfront therapy for patients with CLL, particularly for those patients in whom, as discussed above, achieving MRD-negative CR is deemed a worthwhile target.

The FC component of FCR can be given by the intravenous or oral route. Using the intravenous route, fludarabine is given at $25\,mg/m^2$ and cyclophosphamide at $250\,mg/m^2$, both over 3 days. Orally, fludarabine is given at $24\,mg/m^2$ and cyclophosphamide at $150\,mg/m^2$, both over 5 days. Rituximab is given at $375\,mg/m^2$ on day one (or over 2 days) with the first course of FC, and then at $500\,mg/m^2$ on day one for the remaining five courses (courses 2–6), which are given at 4-week intervals.

Two other purine analogues with activity in CLL are cladribine (2-chlorodeoxyadenosine) and pentostatin (2-deoxycoformycin). Cladribine in particular can achieve as good a response as fludarabine and, in previously untreated CLL, the CR rate of the combination cladribine plus cyclophosphamide has been reported as 29% and nodular PR 24%. Although cladribine and fludarabine have not been compared directly, cladribine appears to be the more myelotoxic of the two. Pentostatin has been used

Table 29.9 Monoclonal antibodies in clinical use for CLL.

Alemtuzumab (anti-CD52)
Rituximab (anti-CD20)
Ofatumumab (anti-CD20)
GA101 (anti-CD20)
Lumiliximab (anti-CD23)
Epratuzumab (anti-CD22)

Table 29.10 Results with the combinations FC and FCR in randomized trials.

Study	No. of patients	Therapy	CR (%)	Median PFS (months)
Flinn et al. (US Intergroup Trial E2997)	278	FC	23	32
Catovsky et al. (LRF CLL4)	390	FC	38	43
Eichhorst et al. (German CLL4)	375	FC	24	48
Hallek et al. (German CLL8)	371	FC	27	32
	390	FCR	52	43

in combination with cyclophosphamide (PC) and rituximab (PCR). Another older agent, bendamustine, has rekindled interest because it combines the properties of an alkylating agent and a purine analogue. Bendamustine may be more effective than chlorambucil and is currently undergoing trials in combination with rituximab.

The downside of using combinations with fludarabine or other purine analogues is that they are more myelotoxic (manifested as neutropenia) and immunosuppressive (manifested as lymphopenia) and care should be taken to use prophylactic measures, such as co-trimoxazole to prevent *Pneumocystis jirovecii* pneumonia and aciclovir to prevent herpesvirus reactivations.

The introduction of alemtuzumab (Campath-1H), rituximab and other antibodies (Table 29.9) has opened the door for more targeted biological agents with little or no myelotoxicity. Alemtuzumab (anti-CD52) acts through antibody- and complement-mediated cytotoxicity. It has potent activity in previously untreated CLL but requires prolonged periods (18 weeks) of treatment to achieve CR. In fludarabine-resistant CLL, the CR rate is 2% but 31% achieve a PR. Its role in the management of CLL continues in active investigation, whether as first line, as consolidation to improve the quality of remission and MRD and/or as salvage therapy to rescue resistant cases. Alemtuzumab can be given intravenously or by subcutaneous injection. The standard dose is 30 mg three times a week (normally Monday, Wednesday and Friday), but this dose is reached over 5 days, starting with 5 mg and increasing gradually to 30 mg. The course duration depends on the indication: for eradication of MRD-positive disease it is 4–6 weeks; for the treatment of relapsed/refractory CLL it is 12–18 weeks. Currently, alemtuzumab is being tested in combination with fludarabine, high-dose methylprednisolone and rituximab. Alemtuzumab has activity in del(17p) cases when used alone and in combination with high-dose methylprednisolone. Toxicity of alemtuzumab includes rigors, chills, fever, immunosuppression and lymphocytopenia. Opportunistic infections can be observed. Cytomegalovirus (CMV) reactivation is a problem that deserves close monitoring and pre-emptive therapy. Responses to alemtuzumab vary in different disease sites, being higher in peripheral blood and bone marrow than in spleen or lymph nodes.

Rituximab (anti-CD20) has potent activity in high- and low-grade NHL and CLL when used in combination with fludarabine, FC, FCM, chlorambucil and high-dose methylprednisolone. Its mechanism of action is by complement-dependent cytotoxicity, activation of the intrinsic pathway of apoptosis and membrane-associated kinases. The lack of T-cell immunosuppression and its good tolerability makes it ideal for older individuals. Several studies are ongoing but it is likely that all will be positive, the limiting factor remaining its high cost. Unlike Campath, rituximab has limited activity on its own, unless used in very high doses, therefore remaining as an effective potentiator of apoptosis in combination with cytotoxic drugs.

Of particular interest are other monoclonal antibodies such as ofatumumab (Humax anti-CD20), lumiliximab (anti-CD23) and epratuzumab (anti-CD22) (Table 29.9). Two of the monoclonal antibodies against CD20, ofatumumab and GA101, may have a higher therapeutic index than rituximab. Other new treatments are being actively investigated in CLL, such as the *BCL2* antisense oligonucleotide Genasense (oblimersen). Two new drugs, lenalidomide and flavopiridol, might add to the list of agents active in CLL with del(17p) (such as alemtuzumab and high-dose methylprednisolone), although this notion needs further investigation. At the same time, treatment strategies are becoming more complex, targeting not only leukaemic cells but also the microenvironment, T-cell dysfunction and immune disturbances that are part of the CLL neoplastic process. Lenalidomide (Revlimid; see also Chapter 31) is currently being tested in two Phase III trials: (i) as first-line therapy versus chlorambucil; and (ii) as maintenance after second-line therapy (at least a PR) versus a placebo.

Role of splenectomy

Splenectomy is now rarely indicated for patients with a large spleen and in whom initial treatment achieves only a moderate reduction in spleen size. Patients with features of hypersplenism (peripheral cytopenias and an active bone marrow), as well as those with ITP and AIHA refractory to therapy, may benefit from splenectomy. This has low morbidity and mortality and may benefit patients with a large spleen and low blood counts, even if only as part of a debulking procedure. Prophylaxis with pneumococcal vaccines may not be effective in advanced CLL where antibody formation is reduced; thus patients require long-term penicillin or amoxicillin. Splenectomy may improve quality of life by raising haemoglobin levels and improving platelet counts in about 50% of cases. Although a rise in the lymphocyte count is often seen after splenectomy, one-third of patients still do not require therapy for long periods.

Stem cell transplantation

The number of stem cell transplantation (SCT) procedures for CLL has increased dramatically in Europe in the last decade. Three modalities are currently considered: autologous SCT, conventional allogeneic SCT with high-intensity therapy, and allogeneic SCT with low-intensity procedures or 'mini' allografts.

The necessary condition for the success of an autologous transplant is to achieve CR before the procedure, which is extremely unlikely in patients refractory to the chemoimmuno-therapy regimens. Moreover, unfavourable prognostic factors for response to conventional chemotherapy, for example del(17p) and del(11q), also predict poor results with autologous transplantation. Autologous transplantation does not cure CLL but might prolong survival in selected patients (i.e. those responding to salvage therapy, without unfavourable prognostic factors, and transplanted early in the course of the disease).

The feasibility of autologous SCT in CLL was tested in an MRC pilot study, which registered over 100 patients between 1996 and 2001. After remission with fludarabine and priming with cyclophosphamide, a peripheral blood stem cell harvest was planned in the good remitters (CR, nodular PR). Only two-thirds of patients were transplanted after high-dose cyclophosphamide and total body irradiation. Failure to do so was because of inadequate remission in 20% and failure to harvest enough stem cells (CD34⁺ cells) in those achieving remission. The question of long-term benefits has been tested in a randomized European intergroup study. Preliminary data from this study indicate a prolonged PFS in those who received an autograft, but no difference in OS. A German study showed that patients with unmutated *IGHV* genes do significantly less well than those with mutated *IGHV* genes, but comparison of unmutated cases with a matched group treated without autograft suggests that this therapy may be more beneficial to the unmutated or poor-prognostic cases than to the mutated ones. A problem of major concern with autotransplants is the risk of secondary MDS/AML (2–5%), particularly in patients conditioned with total body irradiation.

Allogeneic transplantation in CLL may offer the chance of cure in a minority of patients. Allogeneic SCT should be particularly considered in those cases refractory to, or who relapse shortly (<12 months) after, modern chemoimmunotherapy. The effect of allografts relies on the graft-versus-tumour effect that notably overcomes poor prognostic features such as 17p deletions. Both family related and unrelated donors are used, the experience with cord blood as a stem cell source being scarce. In unselected registry series, the transplant-related mortality can be as high as 40%, whereas in selected series from experienced centres it is 25–35%. Reduced intensity or 'mini' allografts has lower transplant-related mortality of around 15–25%, but is still higher than with autografts (<5%). In all allograft series there is a plateau in disease-free and overall survival (40–60%), although late relapses (>7 years after transplant) can be observed. Treatment results are better in younger patients, not heavily pretreated and still showing some degree of response to therapy. Allografts should be performed within clinical studies and never as a last desperate attempt in extensively pretreated patients in poor clinical condition, and refractory disease.

Management of autoimmune complications

The most common immune complications in CLL are AIHA, ITP and pure red cell aplasia. Control of haemolysis can be achieved by corticosteroids (prednisolone or dexamethasone), but long-term management requires the DAT to become negative. This can be achieved with the addition of another agent, usually daily cyclophosphamide (100 mg/day), ciclosporin (150 mg twice daily) or mycophenolate mofetil (1 g twice daily). Rarely, in resistant cases, these agents may be used in combina-

tion. The advantage of cyclophosphamide is that it may provide a degree of control of the CLL. Rituximab has been reported to have beneficial effect when used in combination with cyclophosphamide and dexamethasone. AIHA often needs long-term treatment and may require a splenectomy. When the DAT remains positive, the risk of haemolysis continues. Achievement of a CR may be the best way to control AIHA and prevent recurrence. Alemtuzumab has also been shown to be useful for this indication.

ITP, although less common, also requires active treatment, as for AIHA. In those cases not responding to corticosteroids, high-dose γ-globulin infusions over 5 days may improve the platelet count and are often a good guide as to the subsequent benefit of splenectomy. Ciclosporin and rituximab are both effective in refractory ITP. ITP is usually more difficult to manage than AIHA and, more often than in the latter, one needs to resort to splenectomy.

Pure red cell aplasia is an uncommon but well-recognized complication. Some cases are secondary to parvovirus B19 infection. Ciclosporin, with or without courticosteroids, may resolve this complication. Rituximab and alemtuzumab have been reported to be able to reverse this process, which is sometimes very acute. It is paradoxical that rituximab and alemtuzumab have occasionally been reported to facilitate parvovirus infection and cause pure red cell aplasia. Rituximab has also been associated with delayed-onset neutropenia. The exact mechanism of the immune complications in CLL is still poorly understood and this explains the unusual, but well-documented, reports of the same agents causing or correcting these complications.

Richter transformation

'Immunoblastic' or large-cell transformation (Richter syndrome) is the most common form of transformation in CLL. The change occurs usually in one or several lymph nodes which show the features of diffuse large B-cell lymphoma (DLBCL). Richter syndrome is associated with systemic symptoms (fever and weight loss), increased serum lactate dehydrogenase levels and unexpected unilateral lymph node enlargement, not rare in the retroperitoneal area. Richter syndrome occurs in around 7% of CLL cases, but the incidence may be higher if lymph node biopsies are performed when unexplained systemic symptoms (e.g. fever) develop in a patient with previously well-controlled disease. In rare cases, transformation takes place in the bone marrow and is therefore seen in trephine biopsies. In such cases the large blast-like cells spill over to the peripheral blood and the morphology may resemble that of an acute leukaemia (Figure 29.15). Richter syndrome is often associated with monoclonal proteins in the serum or free light chains in the urine. Studies with immunoglobulin gene rearrangements are useful for demonstrating if the new malignant clone arose from a pre-existing CLL B cell or whether it is a new clone. The latter is

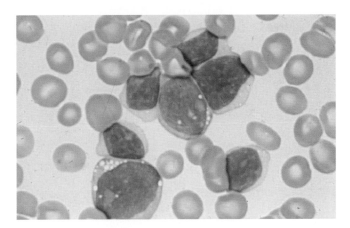

Figure 29.15 Blood film of a patient with Richter syndrome with circulating large blast cells that were positive for surface membrane immunoglobulin.

seen in at least one-third of cases. Genetic imbalances are frequent in Richter syndrome, the most common being *TP53* abnormalities.

Current evidence suggests that intense immunosuppression with agents such as fludarabine and alemtuzumab and the subsequent CD4 lymphopenia may trigger Richter transformation in some cases. Not infrequently, evidence of involvement of Epstein–Barr virus (EBV) in the pathogenesis has been shown by demonstration of EBV latent membrane protein by immunohistology or of EBV-encoded RNA by *in situ* hybridization. A role for EBV in the pathogenesis of Richter syndrome has been reported in close to 15–20% of cases. It is likely that this phenomenon is seen more often in heavily treated patients. In a minority, the large-cell transformation induced by EBV has scattered CD30+CD15+ Reed–Sternberg-like cells, and in others the histology is identical to that of classical Hodgkin lymphoma.

The rare cases of Hodgkin lymphoma are often clonally unrelated to the original CLL clone. Clonally unrelated transformation is more likely to be related to EBV infection. Cases of Hodgkin lymphoma and those with scattered Reed–Sternberg cells show mutated *IGHV* genes, while the majority of DLBCL show identical *IGHV* sequences in the CLL and lymphoma cells. Also, the clonally related DLBCL often carry unmutated *IGHV* genes. It has also been suggested that the risk of Richter transformation is higher in cases using *IGHV4-39* and stereotyped *CDR3* sequences.

Increasingly, positron emission tomography and CT have a role in the diagnosis of Richter syndrome, as in other lymphomas (see Chapters 34 and 35). Similarly, the treatment now involves protocols used in large-cell lymphomas, such as the combination CHOP-R (see also Chapter 35).

Hypercalcaemia with or without obvious osteolytic lesions is a well-recognized but rare finding in very advanced CLL. It does not represent, in itself, transformation to a large-cell lymphoma as the histology is often that of heavy lymphocytic infiltration.

Supportive care

The main objective of treatment for CLL is to prolong survival with a good quality of life; therefore care should be taken to prevent and/or treat promptly any complications arising from the immunodeficiency associated with the disease or its treatment. Thus, prompt antibiotic treatment for seemingly benign upper respiratory tract infections and antiviral measures to prevent the spread of herpetic infections are as important as specific treatment for the disease. Patients with repeated infections and very low serum immunoglobulin levels may benefit from courses of intravenous γ-globulin injections, e.g. 400 mg/kg every 4 weeks, particularly during the winter months. Additional measures are the administration of allopurinol when starting therapy with a WBC count above 50×10^9/L, oral antifungals and histamine H_2 blockers or proton pump inhibitors when using corticosteroids.

Causes of infection in CLL are multifactorial. Neutropenic episodes during chemotherapy require the use of granulocyte colony-stimulating factor (G-CSF). Patients with long-term respiratory infections may require antibiotic prophylactic measures and active physiotherapy programmes. Co-trimoxazole is necessary to prevent infections, particularly *Pneumocystis jirovecii* pneumonia, when fludarabine or alemtuzumab are used. The latter requires regular monitoring for CMV and prompt treatment when such immunosuppressed patients, usually lymphopenic, become symptomatic and positive for CMV. The main factors predisposing to infections in CLL are the number of chemotherapy regimens and the activity of the disease more than the levels of serum immunoglobulins.

Erythropoietin is now an accepted treatment for anaemia associated with cancer therapy. Patients with CLL and persistent anaemia (Hb < 10 g/dL) will benefit from erythropoietin given according to guidelines. There is strong evidence for benefit, particularly an improvement in quality of life. Erythropoietin should be given for a minimum of 4 weeks before deciding that there is no response, and iron deposits need to be adequate. There is no evidence that erythropoietin is useful in pure red cell aplasia. Folic acid supplements are often useful in patients with macrocytic indices resulting from low folate levels. They should always be given in AIHA.

Secondary MDS/AML

The increased intensity of treatments, in particular combinations of alkylating agents and purine analogues, may be responsible for an increased incidence of secondary MDS/AML in CLL. Combinations with mitoxantrone and the use of total body irradiation for SCT are also major risk factors for these secondary events. Single-agent therapy with chlorambucil or fludarabine is rarely associated with MDS/AML.

B-cell prolymphocytic leukaemia

It has become apparent in the last two decades that there are important clinical and laboratory differences between B-PLL and CLL, despite the existence of a group with CLL/PL discussed above. In fact B-PLL is a distinct, but rare, disorder. This is supported by differences in the morphology and cell markers (see Table 29.2) and clinical evolution. Furthermore, recent observations show significant differences in gene expression profiling between these two disorders (see below). The key for diagnosis is the recognition of the prolymphocyte as the predominant cell in well-prepared peripheral blood films. B-PLL is included in the WHO classification (see Chapter 33).

The mean age of patients presenting with B-PLL is 70 years and the main features are splenomegaly without lymphadenopathy and a high WBC count, usually over 100×10^9/L, at the time of presentation. Anaemia and thrombocytopenia are seen in at least 50% of cases. Other laboratory findings are no different from high-count CLL (increased uric acid, low serum immunoglobulins) but the incidence of a monoclonal band appears to be higher than in CLL.

Differential diagnosis

The main diagnostic criterion is the identification of prolymphocytes as the predominant population in blood films. Usually, 55% prolymphocytes is the figure that discriminates B-PLL from CLL and CLL/PL, although the percentage of prolymphocytes in B-PLL is usually greater than 70%. The prolymphocyte is twice the size of a small CLL lymphocyte, has moderately condensed nuclear chromatin, a prominent central nucleolus and a lower nucleus to cytoplasm ratio than CLL cells (Figure 29.16). Using the scoring system described in Table 29.1, most B-PLL score 0–1, rarely 2 or 3. One-third of cases of B-PLL may be CD5+; this and other features may present a diagnostic problem with MCL with leukaemia.

The issue of MCL was revisited by us in eight cases diagnosed in the past as B-PLL but bearing the translocation t(11;14) (q13;32) characteristic of MCL. Detailed histology review and comparison with 13 cases of B-PLL without t(11;14) led us to conclude that the cases with t(11;14) and overexpression of cyclin D1 represent a splenomegalic form of MCL rather than B-PLL.

Molecular studies

The mutational status of *IGHV* genes in B-PLL is heterogeneous, with 53% showing an unmutated pattern. In contrast to

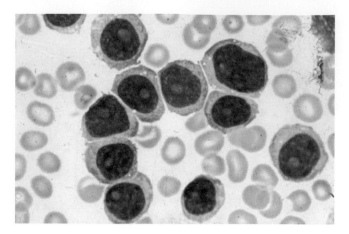

Figure 29.16 Typical blood film from a case of B-prolymphocytic leukaemia with the characteristic large size, abundant cytoplasm and prominent nucleolus.

CLL and CLL/PL, V_H usage involved mainly the V_H3 and V_H4 family, predominantly *IGHV3-23*, *IGHV4-59* and *IGHV4-34*, regardless of mutational status. Another consistent finding in B-PLL is the deletion and/or mutation of *TP53* in just over 50% of cases. This may be one of the factors accounting for the poor prognosis. Gene expression profiling was investigated in 10 cases of B-PLL and compared with 10 cases of CLL (including CLL/PL). Detailed analysis showed significant differences, with close to 6000 genes differently expressed, most of them overexpressed in B-PLL. One of them, *MYC*, is of interest as this gene promotes cell proliferation. Comparison of findings showed a high probability of predicting a difference between CLL and CLL/PL on the one hand and B-PLL on the other, confirming the distinct biology of these two disorders.

Treatment

Alkylating agents are of little value in the management of B-PLL. Response rates (PRs and rare CRs) to splenic irradiation and/or CHOP have been recorded in up to one-third of cases. There are no published data with CHOP-R. Splenectomy is often used to remove a major proliferative focus and tumour bulk in order to relieve hypersplenism and facilitate further therapy. Considering the older age group affected, splenectomy is not a practical proposition in some patients. Some patients may respond to fludarabine, but there are insufficient data in B-PLL on the use of fludarabine combinations, including those using monoclonal antibodies, e.g. FCR, FCMR.

Hairy cell leukaemia

Hairy cell leukaemia is a well-recognized clinicopathological entity that affects males more frequently than females (male to female ratio 4 : 1), usually over the age of 40 years. The disease was first described by Bouroncle and colleagues 50 years ago and has elicited great interest for different reasons: in the 1960s, to establish the diagnostic features of the newly described entity and, in the 1970s and 1980s, advances in immunology led to the identification of the hairy cell as a B cell by the demonstration of heavy- and light-chain immunoglobulin gene rearrangement. In the 1980s and 1990s, there were significant advances in treatment, first with interferon alfa, later with the purine analogues pentostatin and cladribine and, more recently, with the use of rituximab.

Clinical and laboratory findings

The main disease features result from the pancytopenia affecting most patients. Patients with HCL are moderately neutropenic and severely monocytopenic; thus, bacterial and opportunistic infections do occur. There is evidence that the incidence of typical and atypical mycobacterial infections is increased, but this was seen more frequently before the current treatments became available.

The main physical signs are splenomegaly and hepatomegaly. Lymphadenopathy is rare, but this has now been recognized in advanced HCL. Routine CT may show a higher incidence than hitherto suspected of large abdominal nodes. These are more common in relapsed patients and those with long-standing HCL and tend to correlate with bulky disease at presentation.

Anaemia results from reduced bone marrow production and splenic pooling. Haemolysis is exceptional. The WBC count may be low, normal or high (rarely above 20×10^9/L), but neutropenia and monocytopenia are constant. Patients with low WBC count and no circulating hairy cells present diagnostic problems. Platelet counts are below 100×10^9/L in most cases.

Diagnosis

The recognition of typical hairy cells in peripheral blood films is useful for suggesting this diagnosis. Hairy cells are large, twice the size of a normal lymphocyte, and have abundant cytoplasm (low nucleus to cytoplasm ratio) that is characteristically villous in its outline (Figure 29.17). The nucleus is round, oval or slightly indented, and occasionally bilobed. A smooth nuclear chromatin, absence of a visible nucleolus and low nucleus to cytoplasm ratio are hallmarks of typical hairy cells. Cells from the rare HCL variant have similar cytoplasmic features but have a round nucleus with more condensed chromatin and a distinct nucleolus (Figure 29.18).

Bone marrow aspirates are unsuccessful as no fragments and few cells are obtained. Therefore, a trephine biopsy is essential. This shows diffuse interstitial infiltration of variable degree; occasionally the infiltration is focal. A typical feature is the arrangement of the cellular infiltrate, which is loose, leaving plenty of space between cells, often with a clear zone around

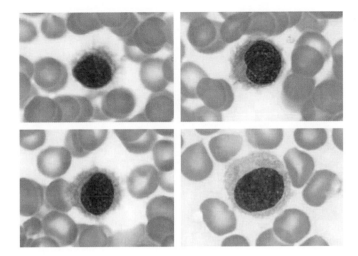

Figure 29.17 Individual hairy cells from blood films from two patients with HCL.

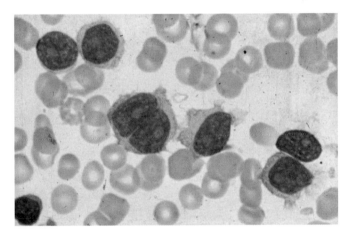

Figure 29.18 Blood film from a case of HCL variant showing large nucleolated villous cells, one of them binucleated.

each cell which is unique to this condition (Figures 29.19 and 29.20). Reticulin is always increased (Figure 29.21) and the cells stain strongly with anti-CD20 (Figure 29.22). The immunocytochemical staining for CD20 is important for demonstrating clusters of hairy cells following therapy, suggesting residual disease. This is otherwise difficult to assess on conventional sections (Figure 29.23). There is now a wider range of reagents that can be used for immunohistochemistry, including annexin A, DBA44 and CD11c.

Spleen histology shows distinct diagnostic features: infiltration by mononuclear cells with a blunt nucleus in the red pulp with little residual white pulp, and formation of pseudosinuses filled with erythrocytes. Tartrate-resistant acid phosphatase (TRAP) demonstrated on hairy cells corresponds to a unique isoenzyme 5 and is specific for HCL. This enzyme is now tested by means of a monoclonal antibody, which can be used in bone

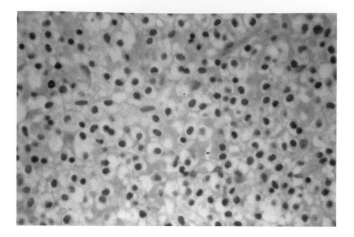

Figure 29.19 Bone marrow trephine section of a case of HCL showing the typical clear zone around the hairy cells in a paraffin-embedded section.

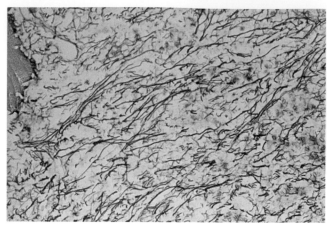

Figure 29.21 Increased reticulin pattern in a case of HCL.

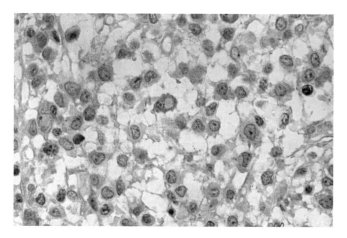

Figure 29.20 Bone marrow trephine from a case of HCL: section embedded in methacrylate giving good morphological detail of the hairy cells.

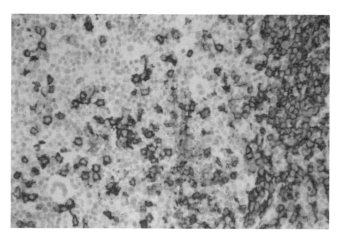

Figure 29.22 Staining for CD20 in a bone marrow section from HCL before treatment.

marrow biopsies. Electron microscopy reveals ribosome–lamella complexes in one-third of cases. Rarely, this intracyto-plasmic inclusion can be seen on light microscopy.

Hairy cells are considered activated B cells with features of late maturation stages. Surface membrane immunoglobulin is usually strong and characteristically shows several heavy-chain isotopes, often including IgA and IgG and sharing a single light chain. The majority show mutated *IGHV* genes. HCL cells are strongly positive for FMC7, CD20 and CD22 but, in contrast to other B-cell disorders, they consistently express CD25, CD103 and CD123. In contrast to CLL, hairy cells are always CD5 negative and their score using the CLL panel is very low (see Table 29.2).

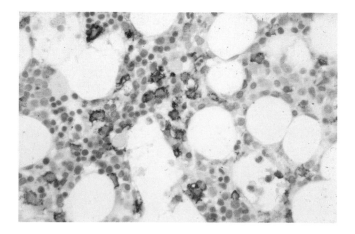

Figure 29.23 Staining for CD20 in a patient treated for HCL showing a cluster of residual CD20+ cells, suggesting that the remission is incomplete.

The HCL variant is very rare and is characterized by high WBC count ($50–80 \times 10^9$/L) and splenomegaly. The cells do not express CD25 and CD123. The main diagnostic difficulty in HCL variant is with SMZL, except for spleen histology, which in the former is mainly red pulp and in the latter predominantly white pulp. HCL variant is now included in the 2008 WHO classification as a splenic B-cell lymphoma/leukaemia unclassifiable, as one of two conditions involving diffusely the splenic red pulp (see also Chapter 33).

Treatment

The prime objectives of treatment should be the normalization of blood counts, as pancytopenia is the main source of complications, and to induce prolonged CR. Two purine analogues, cladribine and pentostatin, are widely used. Other treatments still used but for specific indications are splenectomy and interferon alfa.

Splenectomy is well established and has been shown to improve the quality of life and prolong survival. It should now be reserved for patients with very large spleens and a degree of bone marrow reserve. In about 20% of successfully splenectomized patients, the counts remain normal for many years and no other therapy is indicated; some of them may never relapse although they may remain with some bone marrow involvement.

Interferon alfa has been used widely since the first report by Quesada in 1984. It induces a gradual normalization of blood counts, reduction of hairy cells in the blood and bone marrow, return of monocytes and improvement of neutropenia. The improvements in the blood are not associated with clearance in the bone marrow, and CRs are seen in only 20–30% of cases. The duration of response once interferon alfa is discontinued is relatively short (median 15–18 months), although blood counts may remain normal for well over a year. The tendency once therapy has ceased is to relapse slowly. Interferon alfa is now reserved for problem cases and to help initial treatment in patients with severe cytopenias. Some groups consider that long-term maintenance therapy can be given with benefit to patients in whom purine analogues cannot be used or where they have become ineffective.

The two agents currently used in HCL, pentostatin and cladribine, achieve CR in 80–85% of patients, with the remainder being partial responders. True resistance is seldom seen at first treatment. Long-term results are excellent, with very few patients actually dying of HCL. About 42% relapse by 10 years and 47% by 15 years; 90% of all patients and 95% of those with CR are alive at 10 years if one excludes non-HCL causes of death.

We recently reported the long-term follow-up (median 16 years) of 233 patients treated with either purine analogue. The long-term outcome was similar with both pentostatin and cladribine. The overall CR rate was 80% and the median relapse-

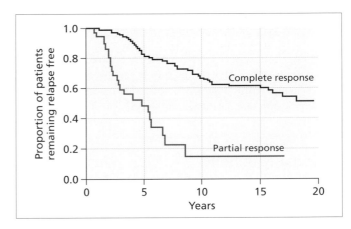

Figure 29.24 Relapse-free survival by response. Complete responders (186 patients) had significantly longer relapse-free survival than partial responders (37 patients) ($P < 0.0001$). (From Catovsky & Else 2009 with permission.)

free survival was 16 years. After relapse, the CR rate decreased with each successive treatment but, when CR was achieved, this was equally as durable as after first-line treatment. Patients with haemoglobin above 10 g/dL and platelets above 100×10^9/L before treatment had the longest relapse-free survival. Patients still in CR at 5 years had only a 25% risk of relapse by 15 years. Complete responders to purine analogues always fare significantly better than partial responders (Figure 29.24). Achievement of CR seems therefore an important therapeutic end point in HCL, as these patients can expect a normal lifespan.

Monoclonal antibodies against CD20 (rituximab) and CD22 (coupled with an immunotoxin) have now shown activity in HCL. Hairy cells strongly express CD20 and CD22, and these antibodies seem to achieve good responses in the group of relapsing patients, although when rituximab is used alone in cladribine relapses the CR rate is low (~15%). Its main role may be, as in other B-cell disorders, when used in combination with one of the purine analogues and this has been our recent experience. Elderly patients may also benefit from antibodies like rituximab as they do not cause myelotoxicity.

Patients with HCL variant respond less well to cladribine and pentostatin and not at all to interferon alfa. Palliation of symptoms and improvement in blood counts can be achieved with splenectomy, which has been the most successful modality in this relatively resistant disease.

Supportive care for HCL is confined to patients undergoing therapy with nucleoside analogues, which can cause transient neutropenia in the early phases and prolonged lymphopenia later on. Long-term co-trimoxazole until lymphocyte counts rise above 1×10^9/L and also long periods on aciclovir are recommended. Major infections are only seen in untreated patients or those responding poorly to therapy.

The leukaemic phase of indolent NHL

There are three types of NHL which not infrequently evolve with lymphocytosis that mimics, and can be confused with, CLL: follicular lymphoma, SMZL (formerly described as splenic lymphoma with circulating villous lymphocytes) and MCL (see also Chapter 33).

Follicular lymphoma

Of patients with follicular lymphoma, 15% may have circulating lymphoma cells (5–20 × 10^9/L), and this correlates with bone marrow involvement. A minority may present with a WBC count in excess of 40 × 10^9/L (up to 200 × 10^9/L) and extensive disease, generalized lymphadenopathy and hepatosplenomegaly. Usually the circulating cells are very small with almost no visible cytoplasm, the nuclear chromatin is smooth without clumps of heterochromatin and no visible nucleolus, and the nuclear shape is angular and has a small cleft (Figure 29.25), seen also at the ultrastructural level (Figure 29.26). The differential diagnosis from CLL is supported by the immunophenotype: follicular lymphoma cells usually score 0 or 1 (see Figure 29.1). Lymph node histology is essential for confirming a diagnosis of follicular lymphoma. Only patients with very high WBC counts may have poor prognosis; cases with a minor degree of spillover respond, as do cases without circulating cells. Late-stage follicular lymphoma may have circulating blasts (centroblasts) characterized by a peripherally located nucleolus and this corresponds with histological transformation to a large-cell lymphoma.

Splenic marginal zone lymphoma

SMZL has been recognized by the WHO classification as a distinct pathological entity (see Chapter 33). Close to two-thirds of patients with this lymphoma have circulating villous lymphocytes. A minority does not have frankly villous cells despite being clonal and in some the diagnosis can be suspected without circulating lymphocytes but can only be established after splenectomy. The true incidence of this condition without circulating villous cells is unknown.

The median age of patients is 69 years and the majority present with splenomegaly. Anaemia and/or thrombocytopenia are seen in 40% of cases. One-third have a serum monoclonal band, usually IgM below 30 g/L. Diagnosis is suspected on a typical blood film (Figure 29.27) showing small lymphocytes with an irregular membrane outline and short villi, often confined to one pole of the cells. The immunophenotype (see Table 29.2) is different from CLL. SMZL cells can be distinguished from HCL and the HCL variant (now separated as a form of splenic lymphoma) because they are negative for CD103 and CD123 but are always positive for CD11c.

Bone marrow aspirates may show the same cells as in the blood, with variable degrees of infiltration. A distinct pattern of intrasinusoidal infiltration (Figure 29.28) is characteristic of SMZL which can be highlighted with anti-B-cell antibodies (CD20, CD79a). This pattern of infiltration is less common in other types of NHL and is not seen in CLL. In addition, the

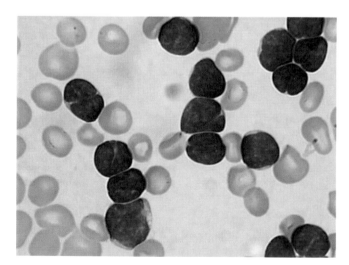

Figure 29.25 Blood film of a patient with follicular lymphoma presenting with significant lymphocytosis (55 × 10^9/L). The cells show a cleaved nucleus, angular shape, homogeneous chromatin pattern, high nucleus to cytoplasm ratio and small size.

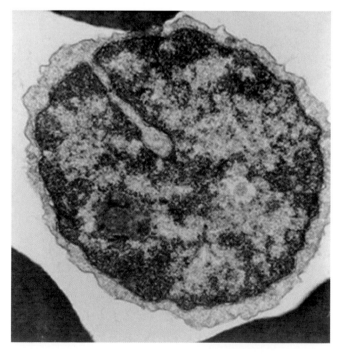

Figure 29.26 Electron microscopy of a circulating follicular centre lymphocyte showing a deep nuclear cleft.

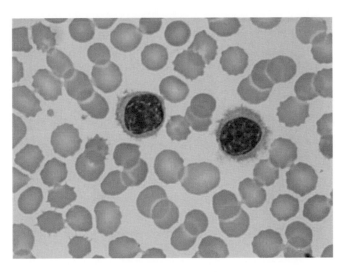

Figure 29.27 Lymphocytes from a case of splenic lymphoma with circulating villous lymphocytes.

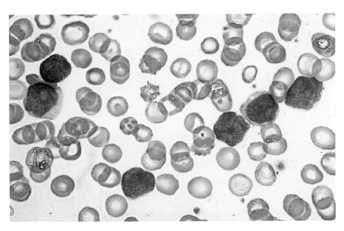

Figure 29.29 Blood film from a patient with mantle cell lymphoma and lymphocytosis. The cells are medium size, slightly irregular in shape and have a speckled nuclear chromatin pattern.

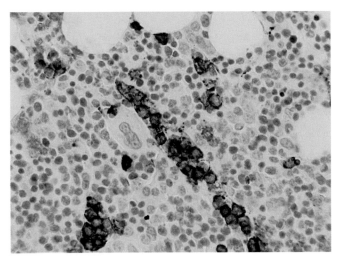

Figure 29.28 Bone marrow trephine biopsy from a case of splenic lymphoma with circulating villous lymphocytes showing the characteristic intrasinusoidal infiltration seen in this disease highlighted by anti-CD20 antibody.

pattern of bone marrow infiltration can be nodular, interstitial and/or paratrabecular.

The spleen histology shows a characteristic bizoned pattern in the white pulp, with a central zone of small lymphocytes with scanty cytoplasm and a peripheral zone of larger cells with more dispersed chromatin and more abundant cytoplasm. The red pulp is always infiltrated by both the smaller and larger cells. Plasmacytic differentiation may be seen.

There is no unique cytogenetic abnormality in SMZL, but unbalanced translocations and deletions of 7q22–32 have been described in about 30%; 50% of cases have a monoallelic deletion at 13q14. Trisomy 3, an abnormality seen in extranodal

marginal zone lymphoma, has been found in 17% of cases. Abnormalities of *TP53* (mainly deletions) are found in 17% and are associated with worse prognosis.

An association with hepatitis C has been reported but the incidence of this is unknown. Of interest is that interferon alfa has been reported to induce CR in some hepatitis C-positive SMZL patients. An association with hyperreactive malaria and tropical splenomegaly has been described in African cases. Large-cell transformation is seen in 10% of cases.

Splenectomy is the treatment of choice when the spleen is a prominent feature. Splenectomized patients fare significantly better than those treated with chemotherapy only. Fludarabine has been reported to induce remissions and recently rituximab has shown beneficial effect (see also Chapter 35). The median survival in our series is 13 years, with 72% of patients alive at 5 years.

Mantle cell lymphoma

Blood and bone marrow involvement are common in MCL. Close to 40% of cases evolving with splenomegaly have significant lymphocytosis, sometimes mimicking CLL, CLL/PL or B-PLL (see above).

Morphologically, the circulating cells are of medium size with a variable amount of cytoplasm, an irregular nucleus with nuclear cleft, a distinctly stippled chromatin pattern and an indistinct nucleolus (Figure 29.29). If small lymphocytes predominate or if there is a mixture of small and large cells, CLL/PL is suspected. A lymphoblastoid form with blast-like cells has been recognized.

Marker studies show that MCL cells are always positive for CD5, CD19 and CD20, thus raising the issue of CLL. In a series of over 60 cases which we studied, the majority (68%) scored 1

(CD5$^+$CD23$^-$, in contrast to CLL), 17% scored 0 (CD5$^-$CD23$^-$) and 15% scored 2 or 3 (CD5$^+$CD23$^+$).

The bone marrow trephine biopsy shows a rather monotonous infiltration by slightly irregular cells. In contrast with CLL, no proliferating centres are seen in MCL. The pattern of bone marrow infiltration is often diffuse in advanced cases, but in other cases is nodular and/or paratrabecular.

The characteristic translocation t(11;14)(q13;q32) is demonstrated in all cases by conventional cytogenetics or by FISH. The rearrangement of the *BCL1/PRAD1* (now called *CCND1*) gene at 11q13 results in the overexpression of cyclin D1, one of the proteins that controls the cell cycle. Cyclin D1 can be demonstrated in histological sections.

Therapy in MCL has been unsatisfactory, although improvements have been reported using fludarabine combinations such as FCMR, as reported by a German study. A significant proportion of MCL patients have *TP53* abnormalities, which underlie their poor response to therapy. New agents such as bortezomib and lenalidomide seem to be active in MCL (see also Chapter 35).

Selected bibliography

Chronic lymphocytic leukaemia

Brenner H, Gondos A, Pulte D (2008) Trends in long-term survival of patients with chronic lymphocytic leukemia from the 1980s to the early 21st century. *Blood* 111: 4916–21.

Catovsky D, Richards S, Matutes E *et al.* (2007) Assessment of fludarabine plus cyclophosphamide for patients with chronic lymphocytic leukaemia (the LRF CLL4 Trial): a randomised controlled trial. *Lancet* 370: 230–9.

Chiorazzi N, Rai KR, Ferrarini M (2005) Chronic lymphocytic leukemia *New England Journal of Medicine* 352: 804–15.

Crespo M, Bosch F, Villamor N *et al.* (2003) ZAP-70 expression as a surrogate for immunoglobulin-variable-region mutations in chronic lymphocytic leukemia. *New England Journal of Medicine* 348: 1764–75.

Crowther-Swanepoel D, Wild R, Sellick G *et al.* (2008) Insight into the pathogenesis of chronic lymphocytic leukemia (CLL) through analysis of IgVH gene usage and mutation status in familial CLL. *Blood* 111: 5691–3.

Dearden C, Wade R, Else M *et al.* (2007) The prognostic significance of a positive direct antiglobulin test in chronic lymphocytic leukemia: a beneficial effect of the combination of fludarabine and cyclophosphamide on the incidence of hemolytic anemia. *Blood* 111: 1820–6.

Delgado J, Matutes E, Morilla AM *et al.* (2003) Diagnostic significance of CD20 and FMC7 expression in B-cell disorders. *American Journal of Clinical Pathology* 120: 754–9.

Del Giudice I, Chiaretti S, Tavolaro S *et al.* (2009) Spontaneous regression of chronic lymphocytic leukemia: clinical and biologic features of 9 cases. *Blood* 114: 638–46.

Del Giudice I, Pileri SA, Rossi M *et al.* (2009) Histopathological and molecular features of persistent polyclonal B-cell lymphocy-

tosis (PPBL) with progressive splenomegaly. *British Journal of Haematology* 144: 726–31.

Di Bernardo MC, Crowther-Swanepoel D, Broderick P *et al.* (2008) A genome-wide association study identifies six susceptibility loci for chronic lymphocytic leukemia. *Nature Genetics* 40: 1204–10.

Dighiero G, Hamblin TJ (2008) Chronic lymphocytic leukaemia. *Lancet* 371: 1017–29.

Eichhorst BF, Busch R, Hopfinger G *et al.* (2006) Fludarabine plus cyclophosphamide versus fludarabine alone in first-line therapy of younger patients with chronic lymphocytic leukemia. *Blood* 107: 885–91.

Flinn IW, Neuberg DS, Grever MR *et al.* (2007) Phase III trial of fludarabine plus cyclophosphamide compared with fludarabine for patients with previously untreated chronic lymphocytic leukemia: US Intergroup Trial E2997. *Journal of Clinical Oncology* 25: 793–8.

Fulci V, Chiaretti S, Goldoni M *et al.* (2007) Quantitative technologies establish a novel microRNA profile of chronic lymphocytic leukemia. *Blood* 109: 4944–51.

Gribben JG, Hallek M (2009) Rediscovering alemtuzumab: current and emerging therapeutic roles. *British Journal of Haematology* 144: 818–31.

Hallek M, Cheson BD, Catovsky D *et al.* (2008) Guidelines for the diagnosis and treatment of chronic lymphocytic leukemia: a report from the International Workshop on Chronic Lymphocytic Leukemia updating the National Cancer Institute Working Group 1996 guidelines. *Blood* 111: 5446–56. Erratum in *Blood* (2008) 112: 5259.

Hallek M, Fingerle-Rowson G, Fink A-M *et al.* (2008) Immunochemotherapy with fludarabine (F), cyclophosphamide (C), and rituximab (R) (FCR) versus fludarabine and cyclophosphamide (FC) improves response rates and progression-free survival (PFS) of previously untreated patients (pts) with advanced chronic lymphocytic leukemia (CLL) [Abstract]. *Blood* 112: 325.

Hamblin TJ (2006) Autoimmune complications of chronic lymphocytic leukemia. *Seminars in Oncology* 33: 230–9.

Hedenus M, Adriansson M, San Miguel J *et al.* (2003) Efficacy and safety of darbepoetin alfa in anaemic patients with lymphoproliferative malignancies: a randomized, double blinded placebo-controlled study. *British Journal of Haematology* 122: 394–403.

Huh YO, Abruzzo LV, Rassidakis GZ *et al.* (2007) The t(14;19) (q32;q13)-positive small B-cell leukaemia: a clinicopathologic and cytogenetic study of seven cases. *British Journal of Haematology* 136: 220–8.

Klein U (2009) Cellular origin of chronic lymphocytic leukemia. *Hematology Education: the Education Programme for the Annual Congress of the European Hematology Association* 3: 55–60.

Landgren O, Albitar M, Ma W *et al.* (2009) B-cell clones as early markers for chronic lymphocytic leukemia. *New England Journal of Medicine* 360: 659–67.

Mao Z, Quintanilla-Martinez L, Raffeld M *et al.* (2007) IgVH mutational status and clonality analysis of Richter's transformation: diffuse large B-cell lymphoma and Hodgkin lymphoma in association with B-cell chronic lymphocytic leukemia (B-CLL) represent 2 different pathways of disease evolution. *American Journal of Surgical Pathology* **31**: 1605–14.

Moreton P, Kennedy B, Lucas G *et al.* (2005) Eradication of minimal residual disease in B-cell chronic lymphocytic leukemia after alemtuzumab therapy is associated with prolonged survival. *Journal of Clinical Oncology* **23**: 2971–9.

Morilla A, Gonzalez de Castro D, Del Giudice I *et al.* (2008) Combinations of ZAP-70, CD38 and IGHV mutational status as predictors of time to first treatment in CLL. *Leukemia and Lymphoma* **49**: 2108–15.

Müller-Hermelink HK, Monserrat E, Catovsky D, Campo E, Harris NL, Stein H (2008) Chronic lymphocytic leukaemia/small lymphocytic lymphoma. In: *WHO Classification of Tumours of Haematopoietic and Lymphoid Tissues* (SH Swerdlow, E Campo, NL Harris *et al.*, eds), pp. 180–82. IARC Press, Lyon.

Murray F, Darzentas N, Hadzidimitriou A *et al.* (2008) Stereotyped patterns of somatic hypermutation in subsets of patients with chronic lymphocytic leukemia: implications for the role of antigen selection in leukemogenesis. *Blood* **111**: 1524–33.

Nicoloso MS, Kipps TJ, Croce CM, Calin GA (2007) MicroRNAs in the pathogeny of chronic lymphocytic leukaemia. *British Journal of Haematology* **139**: 709–16.

Rawstron AC, Villamor N, Ritgen M *et al.* (2007) International standardized approach for flow cytometric residual disease monitoring in chronic lymphocytic leukaemia. *Leukemia* **21**: 956–64.

Rawstron AC, Bennett FL, O'Connor SJ *et al.* (2008) Monoclonal B-cell lymphocytosis and chronic lymphocytic leukemia. *New England Journal of Medicine* **359**: 575–83.

Rosenquist R (2009) Clinical implications of novel biological markers in chronic lymphocytic leukemia. *Hematology Education: the Education Programme for the Annual Congress of the European Hematology Association* **3**: 61–7.

Ruchlemer R, Wotherspoon AC, Thompson JN *et al.* (2002) Splenectomy in mantle cell lymphoma with leukaemia: a comparison with chronic lymphocytic leukaemia. *British Journal of Haematology* **118**: 952–8.

Stamatopoulos K, Belessi C, Moreno C *et al.* (2007) Over 20% of patients with chronic lymphocytic leukemia carry stereotyped receptors: pathogenetic implications and clinical correlations. *Blood* **109**: 259–70.

Stevenson FK, Caligaris-Cappio F (2004) Chronic lymphocytic leukemia: revelations from the B-cell receptor. *Blood* **103**: 4389–95.

Tam CS, O'Brien S, Wierda W *et al.* (2008) Long-term results of the fludarabine, cyclophosphamide, and rituximab regimen as initial therapy of chronic lymphocytic leukemia. *Blood* **112**: 975–80.

Tam CS, Shanafelt TD, Wierda WG *et al.* (2009) De novo deletion 17p13.1 chronic lymphocytic leukemia shows significant clinical heterogeneity: the M. D. Anderson and Mayo Clinic experience. *Blood* **114**: 957–64.

Tobin G (2007) The immunoglobulin genes: structure and specificity in chronic lymphocytic leukemia. *Leukemia and Lymphoma* **48**: 1081–6.

Visco C, Ruggeri M, Laura Evangelista M *et al.* (2008) Impact of immune thrombocytopenia on the clinical course of chronic lymphocytic leukemia. *Blood* **111**: 1110–16.

Wierda WG, Kipps TJ, Mayer J *et al.* (2010) Ofatumumab as single-agent CD20 immunotherapy in fludarabine-refractory chronic lymphocytic leukemia. *Journal of Clinical Oncology* **28**: 1749–55.

Zent CS, Ding W, Schwager SM *et al.* (2008) The prognostic significance of cytopenia in chronic lymphocytic leukaemia/small lymphocytic lymphoma. *British Journal of Haematology* **141**: 615–21.

Zenz T, Mohr J, Eldering E *et al.* (2009) miR-34a as part of the resistance network in chronic lymphocytic leukemia. *Blood* **113**: 3801–8.

Hairy cell leukaemia

Catovsky D, Else M (2009) The treatment of hairy cell leukemia. *Hematology Education: the Education Programme for the Annual Congress of the European Hematology Association* **3**: 137–42.

Else M, Dearden CE, Matutes E *et al.* (2009) Long-term follow-up of 233 patients with hairy cell leukaemia, treated initially with pentostatin or cladribine, at a median of 16 years from diagnosis. *British Journal of Haematology* **145**: 733–40.

Foucar K, Falini B, Catovsky D, Stein H (2008) Hairy cell leukaemia. In: *WHO Classification of Tumours of Haematopoietic and Lymphoid Tissues* (SH Swerdlow, E Campo, NL Harris *et al.*, eds), pp. 188–90. IARC Press, Lyon.

Kreitman RJ, Stetler-Stevenson M, Margulies I *et al.* (2009) Phase II trial of recombinant immunotoxin RFB4(dsFv)-PE38 (BL22) in patients with hairy cell leukemia. *Journal of Clinical Oncology* **27**: 2983–90.

B-cell prolymphocytic leukaemia

Del Giudice I, Osuji N, Dexter T *et al.* (2009) B-cell prolymphocytic leukemia and chronic lymphocytic leukemia have distinctive gene expression signatures. *Leukemia* **23**: 2160–7.

Ruchlemer R, Parry-Jones N, Brito-Babapulle V *et al.* (2004) B-prolymphocytic leukaemia with t(11;14) revisited: a splenomegalic form of mantle cell lymphoma evolving with leukaemia. *British Journal of Haematology* **125**: 330–6.

The leukaemic phase of NHL

Matutes E, Parry-Jones N, Brito-Babapulle V *et al.* (2004) The leukemic presentation of mantle-cell lymphoma: disease features and prognostic factors in 58 patients. *Leukemia and Lymphoma* **45**: 2007–15.

Parry-Jones N, Matutes E, Gruszka-Westwood AM *et al.* (2003) Prognostic features of splenic lymphoma with villous lymphocytes: a report on 129 patients. *British Journal of Haematology* **120**: 759–64.

CHAPTER 30

T-cell lymphoproliferative disorders

30

Estella Matutes

Royal Marsden Hospital and Institute of Cancer Research, London, UK

Introduction and classification

The mature T-cell lymphoproliferative disorders comprise a variety of entities that result from the clonal proliferation of post-thymic T lymphocytes. They should be distinguished from the thymus-derived T-cell neoplasms, i.e. T-cell acute lymphoblastic leukaemia (T-ALL) and lymphoblastic lymphomas, as the disease course and therapeutic approaches are different. The distinction between these two groups of T-cell malignancies is made on clinical grounds, morphology and immunophenotype, i.e. terminal deoxynucleotidyltransferase (TdT)-positive blasts in T-ALL compared with TdT-negative mature T lymphocytes in chronic T-cell disorders.

The incidence of the T-cell disorders varies around the world. Overall they are more common in eastern and rare in western countries, where they account for 15% of lymphoid malignancies. This distribution may relate to host and environmental factors. Advances in immunophenotyping and molecular cytogenetics together with detailed analysis of the morphology and histopathology have contributed to a more precise classification of the T-cell neoplasms. The role of viruses in T-cell malignancies, essentially Epstein–Barr virus (EBV) and human T-cell leukaemia/lymphoma virus (HTLV)-I, has been well recognized. HTLV-I is the aetiological agent of adult T-cell leukaemia lymphoma (ATLL), and EBV has been shown to be involved in the pathogenesis of certain lymphomas such as extranodal T/natural killer (NK) lymphomas.

These advances have shed some light onto the disease pathogenesis and in turn resulted in better therapeutic approaches. Information on gene expression profiling is still in its infancy and is known for few of these diseases. It is likely that in the future this information will have an impact by allowing novel targeted therapies to be devised and by helping to elucidate the genes involved in pathogenesis.

For classification of the T-lymphoproliferative disorders, it is essential to combine the clinical and laboratory features. The latter should include (i) morphology and tissue histology; (ii) immunophenotyping; (iii) molecular genetics using standard techniques such as fluorescence *in situ* hybridization (FISH) or polymerase chain reaction (PCR); (iv) analysis of the T-cell receptor (TCR) chain genes to demonstrate clonality of the T-cell population; and (v) detection of viruses such HTLV-I and EBV. Some of these investigations are key diagnostic tests while others may have prognostic or therapeutic implications. Furthermore, molecular analysis to search for certain oncogenes such as *TCL1* and *TP53*, is relevant by providing clues to the pathogenesis and/or progression of the disease.

On the basis of the clinical manifestations and origin of the neoplasm, the T-lymphoid disorders can be classified into three main groups: (i) primary leukaemias that arise in the bone marrow and evolve with leukaemia; (ii) leukaemia/lymphoma syndromes or the leukaemic phase of T-cell non-Hodgkin lymphomas (T-NHLs) in which the tumour arises in lymphoid tissues but a leukaemic picture is common; and (iii) T-NHLs that originate in lymphoid tissues and rarely involve the blood. Each of these groups includes disease entities distinguishable by their clinical and laboratory features and all have been recognized as such by the WHO classification (Table 30.1).

The disease features of the T-cell malignancies, the basis for diagnosis, their prognosis and management as well as the pathogenic events involved in disease initiation and/or progression are described.

Postgraduate Haematology: 6th edition. Edited by A. Victor Hoffbrand, Daniel Catovsky, Edward G.D. Tuddenham, Anthony R. Green
© 2011 Blackwell Publishing Ltd.

Primary leukaemias

This group includes T-prolymphocytic leukaemia (T-PLL) and T-cell large granular lymphocyte leukaemia (T-LGL leukaemia).

T-prolymphocytic leukaemia

T-PLL was first documented in a patient having clinical features similar to B-prolymphocytic leukaemia (B-PLL) but in whom

Table 30.1 Classification of T-cell lymphoproliferative disorders.

Primary leukaemias
T-cell prolymphocytic leukaemia
T-cell large granular lymphocyte leukaemia

Leukaemia/lymphoma syndromes
Sézary syndrome/mycosis fungoides
Adult T-cell leukaemia lymphoma

Peripheral T-cell lymphomas (T-NHL)
T-NHL not otherwise specified
Specific variants
   Hepatosplenic T-NHL
   Subcutaneous panniculitis like T-NHL
   Angioimmunoblastic T-NHL
   Extranodal T/NK lymphoma, nasal type
   EBV-positive T-cell lymphoproliferative disorders of childhood
   Enteropathy-associated T-NHL
   Anaplastic large-cell lymphoma (cutaneous and systemic)
     (ALK^+ and ALK^-)

the cells had a T-cell phenotype. T-PLL is recognized in the WHO classification as a distinct entity with three morphological variants. Despite the morphological heterogeneity, all these variants have a similar clinical course and identical molecular genetics.

Aetiology

T-PLL is a rare disease accounting for 2% of all mature lymphoid leukaemias and is more frequent than B-PLL. T-PLL has been described in the West and East without geographical clustering. There is no evidence that radiation, carcinogenic agents and/or viruses play a role in its pathogenesis. However, there is a prevalence of T-PLL in patients with ataxia telangiectasia (AT) and it has been speculated, but not yet proven, that the AT mutated gene (*ATM*) may play a role in the development of T-PLL (see section Pathogenesis).

Clinical features

T-PLL affects adults (median age 65 years), predominantly males. Patients manifest with widespread disease and one-third with skin lesions. Main physical signs are hepatosplenomegaly and lymphadenopathy. Effusions are seen in 15% of patients but are frequent during terminal or relapse phases of the disease; central nervous system (CNS) involvement is rare (Table 30.2). Few patients are asymptomatic and they manifest with non-specific symptoms and a slowly progressive lymphocytosis resembling the picture seen in early chronic lymphocytic leukaemia (CLL). This 'smouldering' form of T-PLL progresses in months or rarely years. Lymphocyte counts range from 35 to 1000×10^9/L and one-third of cases have anaemia and/or thrombocytopenia. Serology and/or DNA analysis for HTLV-I/HTLV-II are negative. Liver function tests may be impaired and urate and sodium lactate dehydrogenase (LDH) raised. Bone

Table 30.2 Disease features of mature T-cell disorders.

Disease	Spleen/liver	Nodes	Skin	Others
T-cell prolymphocytic leukaemia	+++/++	++	++	Effusions
T-cell LGL leukaemia	++/+	–	+	Cytopenias, PRCA, autoimmune diseases
Sézary syndrome	–/–	+	+++	
Adult T-cell leukaemia lymphoma	++/++	+++	+	Hypercalcaemia, HTLV-I
Hepatosplenic T-NHL	+++/++	–	+	Extranodal sites
Subcutaneous panniculitis-like T-NHL	–	–	+++	
Angioimmunoblastic T-NHL	++/++	+++	++	AIHA, dysproteinaemia
Extranodal NK/T lymphoma, nasal type	+/+	+	+	Nasal, extranodal sites
Enteropathy-associated T-NHL	–/–	+	–	Bowel
Anaplastic large-cell lymphoma	+/+	++	+	

+++, >70% of cases; ++, 40–70% of cases; +, 20–40% of cases; –, <20% of cases.
AIHA, autoimmune haemolytic anaemia; HTLV, human T-cell leukaemia/lymphoma virus; LGL, large granular lymphocyte; NHL, non-Hodgkin lymphoma; PRCA, pure red cell aplasia.

marrow shows a variable degree of involvement; the pattern of lymphoid infiltration in the trephine biopsy is mixed (interstitial plus diffuse) or diffuse with reticulin fibrosis.

Diagnosis

Morphology and immunophenotyping are the key diagnostic tests. In two-thirds of cases, the lymphocytes have condensed chromatin, regular or irregular nuclear outline, prominent nucleolus and a deeply basophilic cytoplasm with blebs (typical T-PLL) (Figure 30.1). In the remaining, the lymphocytes are smaller in size and the nucleolus is small or not visible by light microscopy (small-cell variant of T-PLL) and/or have a cerebriform nucleus resembling Sézary cells (cerebriform variant). Although small-cell T-PLL has been referred to as 'T-CLL', such designation may lead to confusion as patients with small-cell T-PLL have an aggressive course and the immunophenotype and cytogenetics are similar to typical T-PLL.

Tissue histology is not essential for diagnosis. The spleen histology shows red pulp lymphoid infiltrates with invasion of

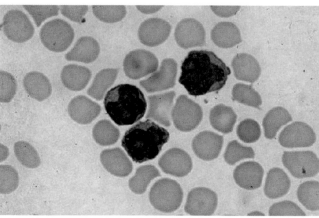

(a)

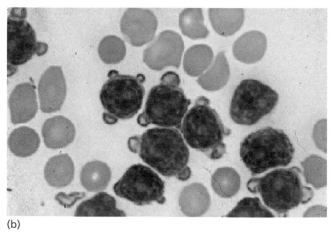

(b)

Figure 30.1 (a, b) Peripheral blood films from two cases of T-PLL showing medium-size lymphoid cells with prominent nucleolus and basophilic cytoplasm.

the white pulp and spleen capsule. Skin histology is different from Sézary syndrome (SS) and shows dermal infiltration preferentially around the appendages without epidermotropism.

Immunophenotyping shows that T-prolymphocytes, unlike T-lymphoblasts, are negative for TdT and the thymic marker CD1a while expressing CD2, CD5 and CD7, the latter with strong intensity. CD3 and anti-TCR-α/β are negative in the cell membrane from 20% of patients but are always expressed in the cytoplasm. The most common phenotype is CD4⁺CD8⁻ (65% of cases); in about 10% the phenotype is CD4⁻CD8⁺, and in 25% it is CD4⁺CD8⁺. CD25 is negative or weak and CD52w (Campath-1H) is strongly expressed (Table 30.3). T-prolymphocytes are negative with monoclonal antibodies against NK cells, TIA-1 and HLA-DR but they may express the lectin NK immunoglobulin receptor CD161.

Cytogenetics and pathogenesis

Chromosomal abnormalities are complex. The abnormality inv(14)(q11;q32) is characteristic of T-PLL and is detected in greater than two-thirds of cases. This juxtaposes the TCR-α gene (*TRA@*, 14q11.2) to the oncogene *TCL1* (14q32.1) resulting in the activation of *TCL1*. Most cases have rearrangement of the *TCL1* gene and overexpression of the TCL-1 protein, supporting the hypothesis that this oncogene plays a role in the pathogenesis of this disease (Table 30.3). In some cases, *TRA@* is juxtaposed to the *MTCP1* gene (Xq28), resulting in the translocation t(X;14)(q28;q11). The *MTCP1* gene has homology with *TCL1* and it has been shown to be expressed in two T-PLL patients who developed the leukaemia following a preceding phase of AT. Transgenic mice with *TCL1* or *MTCP1* develop a T-cell leukaemia similar to T-PLL. Abnormalities of chromosome 8 involving both arms of this chromosome are frequent; although the *MYC* oncogene (8q24) is not rearranged, overexpression of the protein is found in cases with iso(8q). 11q23 abnormalities are rarely detected by cytogenetics, but missense mutations of the *ATM* gene (11q23) are common. There are genetic similarities between the sporadic T-PLL and circulating T lymphocytes from AT patients. These patients are at risk of developing lymphoid malignancies including T-PLL. T-cell clones in AT carry similar abnormalities to leukaemic T-prolymphocytes and expression of *TCL1* transcripts occurs in both the preleukaemic and leukaemic phases in AT patients, as it does in sporadic T-PLL. All these findings stress the relationship between T-PLL and the leukaemia that develops in AT patients. Gene expression profiling in a few T-PLL cases with inv(14) has revealed deregulation of genes involved in the cell cycle, apoptosis and DNA repair that likely play a role in its pathogenesis.

Differential diagnosis

The differential diagnosis of T-PLL arises with B-PLL, T-ALL and other mature T-cell malignancies. Distinction between T- and B-PLL and T-ALL can be made by immunophenotyping.

Table 30.3 Immunophenotype and genotype in T-cell disorders.*

Disease	Immunophenotype	Genotype
T-cell prolymphocytic leukaemia	CD7^{++}, CD4$^+$ or CD4$^+$/CD8$^+$	inv(14), iso(8q), *ATM*, *TCL1*
T-cell LGL leukaemia	CD7$^{+/-}$, CD8$^+$, CD57$^+$, CD16$^+$, CD94$^+$, TIA-1$^+$, granzyme B$^+$, KIRs$^{+/-}$	Deregulation of apoptosis
Sézary syndrome	CD7$^{+/-}$, CD4$^+$, CD8$^-$	Aneuploidy
Adult T-cell leukaemia lymphoma	CD7$^-$, CD4$^+$, CD25$^+$	HTLV-I
Hepatosplenic T-NHL	TCR-γ/δ^+, CD16$^+$, CD56$^+$, TIA-1$^+$ granzyme B$^+$	iso(7q)
Subcutaneous panniculitis-like T-NHL	CD3$^+$, CD8$^+$, TIA-1$^+$, perforin$^+$	Unknown
Angioimmunoblastic T-NHL	CD3$^+$, CD5$^+$, CD10$^+$	+8, +5, del(6q)
Extranodal T/NK lymphoma, nasal type	CD3ε^+, CD56$^+$, LMP-1$^+$, perforin$^+$, TIA-1$^+$, granzyme B$^+$	EBV
Enteropathy-associated T-NHL	CD3$^+$, CD8$^+$, CD103$^+$	?EBV
Anaplastic large-cell lymphoma	CD30$^+$, CD3$^+$, CD25$^+$, EMA$^+$	t(2;5), *NPM–ALK*

*Refers only to the most relevant and distinct features.
ATM, ataxia telangiectasia mutated gene; EBV, Epstein–Barr virus; EMA, epithelial membrane antigen; HTLV, human T-cell leukaemia/lymphoma virus; KIR, killer-cell immunoglobulin-like receptor; LGL, large granular lymphocyte; LMP, latent membrane protein; NHL, non-Hodgkin lymphoma; *NPM–ALK*, nucleolar phosphoprotein–anaplastic lymphoma tyrosine kinase gene.

Distinction between T-PLL and T-cell LGL leukaemia is not problematic except in cases of smouldering small-cell variant T-PLL. Immunophenotype, cytogenetics and morphology distinguish these two conditions. Morphology, clinical features, skin histology and HTLV-I status will differentiate T-PLL from ATLL and SS.

Disease course and therapy

T-PLL has an aggressive course and short survival, estimated to be 7 months in the historical series. Poor predictors for outcome include age, high lymphocyte count, high TCL-1 expression and lack of response to alemtuzumab (Campath-1H) or pentostatin (2′-deoxycoformycin). Patients are resistant or achieve transient responses to most chemotherapies. Pentostatin is effective, with response rates of 45%, 10% of which are complete responses (CRs) with survival improvement. At present, the best front-line treatment is alemtuzumab. Over two-thirds of patients respond to this agent, and most achieve a CR. However, most patients will eventually relapse, and therefore responses need to be consolidated with autologous or allogeneic stem cell transplantation (SCT). Autologous SCT increases disease-free survival, although up to two-thirds of patients will relapse. The chances of cure are higher with allogeneic SCT with non-myeloablative (reduced intensity) conditioning or intensive conditioning but morbidity and mortality are still high. Figure 30.2 illustrates the response to alemtuzumab in a patient with T-PLL.

Large granular lymphocyte leukaemia

LGL leukaemia was first described three decades ago and designated T-CLL to contrast with B-CLL. Names such as Tγ lym-

phoproliferative disorder, chronic T-cell lymphocytosis with neutropenia, T8$^+$/NK, cytotoxic and/or suppressor T-cell CLL were used until 1993 when Loughran coined the term of LGL leukaemia for this disease. Depending on the origin of the LGL cells, LGL leukaemia can be subdivided into two groups: one derived from T cells (CD3$^+$) and another, uncommon, derived from NK cells (CD3$^-$). In the WHO classification, NK-cell LGL is considered separate and designated chronic NK-LGL leukaemia. Here we strictly refer to T-cell LGL leukaemia, which includes cases that result from clonal expansion of a TCR-α/β-positive lymphocyte and a minority from a TCR-γ/δ-positive cell.

Aetiology

The aetiology of T-cell LGL leukaemia is unknown. There is compelling evidence that it results from persistent antigen (auto or foreign) stimulation that leads to the expansion of a memory effector cytotoxic T cell that is not eliminated due to impaired apoptosis. It is frequent in patients with autoimmune diseases, particularly rheumatoid arthritis. These patients, as those with T-cell LGL leukaemia, have a high frequency of the HLA-DR4 haplotype. This suggests a common immunogenetic basis for these two conditions. No infective agent has been shown to be involved in the pathogenesis of the most common form of CD8$^+$ T-cell LGL leukaemia, while recent data indicate that persistent infection by cytomegalovirus (CMV) may be responsible in cases with a CD4$^+$CD8$^{-/+dim}$ phenotype.

Clinical features

T-cell LGL leukaemia affects preferentially adults. Patients are asymptomatic or manifest symptoms derived from cytopenias,

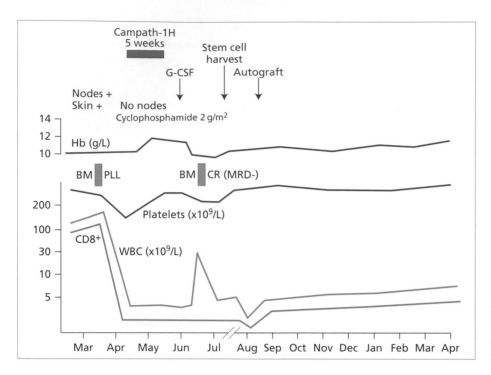

Figure 30.2 Flow chart from a patient with T-PLL illustrating complete response (CR) to alemtuzumab (Campath-1H) and subsequent consolidation with stem cell transplantation.

essentially recurrent infections, autoimmune disease or rarely pure red cell aplasia; it also may be associated with bone marrow failure due to myelodysplasia. The disease may evolve as a pure lymphomatous form in few cases. The CD4+ form is often associated with neoplasms, rarely with autoimmunity. Physical examination shows splenomegaly in two-thirds of patients and hepatomegaly in half; skin lesions may be present but lymphadenopathy is rare (see Table 30.2). The lymphocyte count is normal, low or slightly raised, usually under 15×10^9/L, with most cells being LGLs; neutropenia is common, and one-third of patients have anaemia and/or thrombocytopenia. In a few cases, a Coombs-positive haemolytic anaemia and autoimmune thrombocytopenia is detected. An autoimmune screen may reveal a positive rheumatoid factor, antinuclear antibodies, circulating immune complexes and hypogammaglobulinaemia or hypergammaglobulinaemia. Bone marrow shows mild lymphoid interstitial or intrasinusoidal infiltration; reactive nodules may be present. It is not uncommon that involvement is missed in the aspirates and trephine biopsies unless immunophenotyping or immunohistochemistry are done. There may be erythroid and myeloid hyperplasia with left shift and maturation arrest.

Diagnosis

Morphology, immunophenotyping, and molecular analysis of the configuration of the TCR β- or γ-chain genes are the key diagnostic tests. LGLs are medium in size, have an eccentric nucleus with mature chromatin, no visible nucleolus and abundant cytoplasm with azurophilic granules (Figure 30.3). These contain hydrolases, perforin and cytokines involved in the function of these lymphocytes. At the ultrastructural level, some granules may display a special configuration designated 'parallel tubular arrays'. The lymphocytes in T-cell LGL leukaemia cannot be distinguished morphologically from the minor blood circulating LGL population in normal individuals.

Tissue histology is rarely essential for diagnosis. The spleen histology shows red pulp expansion with an atrophic or reactive white pulp resembling the pattern seen in hairy cell leukaemia; unlike hairy cell leukaemia, the infiltrating cells have a T-cell phenotype and, unlike normal spleen red pulp cells, are CD5−CD45RO−. Sarcoid-like granulomas may be present. The liver shows sinusoidal infiltration extending to the portal tracts.

Immunophenotyping in T-cell LGL leukaemia shows that cells are positive for CD2, CD3, TCR-α/β and rarely TCR-γ/δ; CD5 and CD7 are negative or weakly expressed. Cells negative for CD4 but positive for CD8, CD57, CD16, CD94, TIA-1, granzyme B and perforin is the most common phenotypic profile (Table 30.3 and Figure 30.4). A few cases have unusual phenotypes, i.e. coexpression of CD4 and CD8 or a CD4+CD8−/+dim phenotype with or without coexpression of NK markers such as CD56 or CD161. T-cell activation markers such as HLA-DR determinants and CD38 are variably expressed. Although the p55 α-chain of the interleukin (IL)-2 receptor (CD25) is usually absent in the cell membrane, LGL cells express the p75 intermediate-affinity IL-2 receptor β-chain. A proportion of cases do express one or more killer-cell immunoglobulin-like receptors (KIRs), unlike normal T cells, and their overexpression is considered potentially diagnostic.

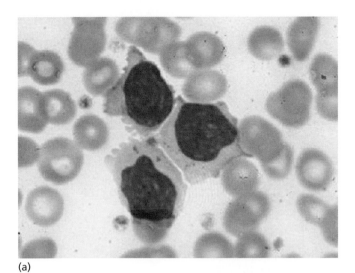

(a)

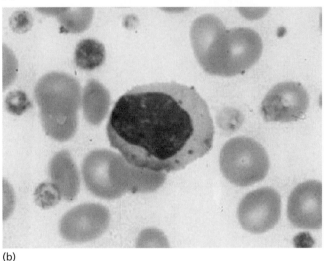

(b)

Figure 30.3 (a, b) Peripheral blood films from patients with T-cell LGL leukaemia showing lymphocytes with an eccentric nucleus, condensed chromatin and abundant pale cytoplasm with azurophilic granules.

Southern blot or PCR studies for the TCR demonstrate the clonal nature of the LGL population and distinguish them from polyclonal LGL proliferations. In T-cell LGL leukaemia, the cells have a rearranged TCR β-chain gene and/or TCR γ-chain gene (Figure 30.5). It is now possible to demonstrate clonality by flow cytometry using a range of monoclonal antibodies against the different variable regions of the TCR β-chain gene. Unlike reactive LGL proliferations, in which different proportions of cells will stain with various monoclonal antibodies, in LGL leukaemia the cells will stain with only one of them.

Pathogenesis

There is no evidence of a recurrent cytogenetic abnormality. It has been postulated that T-cell LGL leukaemia results from the expansion of a terminal memory activated cytotoxic T lymphocyte that is triggered by persistent antigen (auto or foreign) stimulation. This lymphocyte does not undergo activated cell death because of an impaired apoptotic pathway. LGL cells express both Fas (CD95) and its ligand and do not have mutations of the gene. However, gene expression profiling has shown that clonal LGLs have a signature different from normal activated memory cells, with deregulation of genes involved in apoptosis, TCR signalling and immune response. In the group of cases with the phenotype CD4$^+$/CD8$^{-/+dim}$, it has been suggested that CMV is responsible for triggering and maintaining the LGL clone in an individual with a genetic predisposition.

Differential diagnosis

The differential diagnosis of T-cell LGL leukaemia arises with polyclonal T-cell lymphocytosis following splenectomy or as a reaction to viral infections, B-CLL and other T-cell disorders, particularly hepatosplenic lymphoma and T-PLL. DNA analysis allows differentiation between reactive and clonal LGL proliferations, as only in the former will the TCR chain genes be in germline configuration. Morphology and immunophenotyping distinguish T-cell LGL leukaemia from other B- and T-cell disorders.

Prognosis and therapy

The clinical course of T-cell LGL leukaemia is often stable; only few patients present with widespread/progressive disease. It has been suggested that cases whose cells express CD56 or CD26 behave more aggressively. Transformation into a large-cell lymphoma is exceedingly rare.

The prognosis of LGL leukaemia is good compared with other T-cell malignancies. Thus data based on large series of patients show that 80% of them survive at 4 years and the overall median survival is greater than 10 years. The main causes of death are infections and only in few patients is death associated with progressive disease.

A substantial proportion of patients, for example those without cytopenias and with stable blood counts, do not require treatment but only monitoring (i.e. 'watch and wait'), a policy similar to that adopted in stage A CLL. Treatment is indicated in those with severe cytopenias, recurrent infections or progressive lymphocytosis or organomegaly. There is no gold-standard therapy in LGL leukaemia. Therapeutic strategies are based on the use of immunosuppressive agents as there is no evidence that high-dose therapy will benefit these patients by eradicating the clone. These treatments include ciclosporin, low-dose cyclophosphamide (200–300 mg/week) or weekly pulses of methotrexate (10 mg/m^2). Responses are seen in greater than two-thirds of patients. There are no data concerning disease features that will predict response to one or other immunosuppressive drug (Figure 30.6). Corticosteroids and haemopoietic growth factors, such as granulocyte/macrophage colony-stimulating factor, granulocyte colony-stimulating factor or

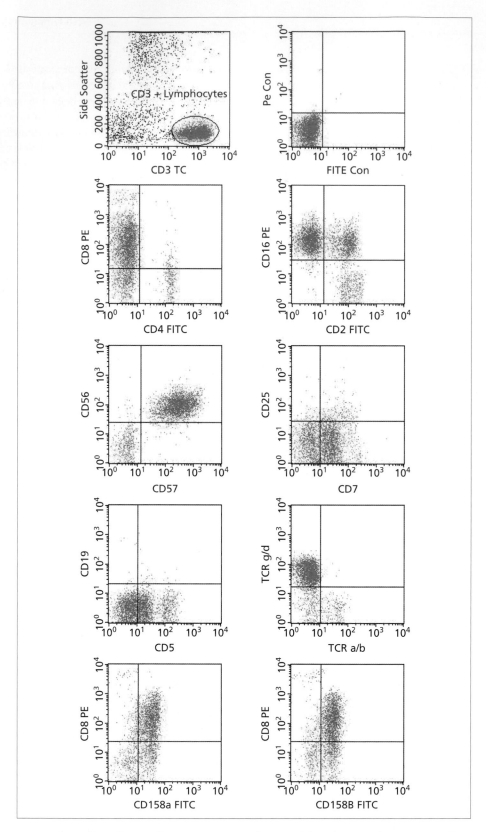

Figure 30.4 Flow cytometry plots of lymphocytes from a γ/δ-positive T-cell LGL leukaemia. The cells have been gated on CD3⁺ cells. The majority of cells express TCR-γ/δ, CD8, CD16, CD56 and CD57 but are negative for TCR-α/β and CD4 and have partial/weak expression of CD5 and CD7. The majority of cells express two killer-cell immunoglobulin-like receptors (CD158a and CD158b), unlike normal LGLs.

erythropoietin, may be useful adjuvants for maintaining or improving the blood cell counts. Few patients respond to pentostatin, although this drug has not been extensively used in LGL leukaemia. Splenectomy does not correct the cytopenias and usually results in an increase in circulating LGLs. Nevertheless, in patients with bulky spleen, this procedure may help by removing tumour burden. Patients with widespread disease (e.g. skin lesions, hepatosplenomegaly, rising white cell count) should be managed with combination chemotherapy. Newer agents such as the monoclonal antibodies anti-CD2 (siplizumab) and anti-CD122, a farnesyltransferase inhibitor and alemtuzumab are being incorporated in the therapeutic scenario.

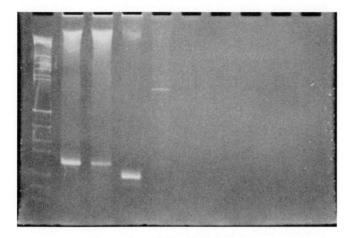

Figure 30.5 PCR analysis of a case of T-cell LGL leukaemia showing a single rearranged band for the TCR γ-chain gene in the blood (second row) and bone marrow (third row). The first row is 1 kb ladder, the fourth a positive control and the fifth a negative control.

Leukaemia/lymphoma syndromes (see Table 30.1)

The leukaemia/lymphoma syndromes comprise neoplasms that arise in peripheral lymphoid tissues but a high frequency present with blood involvement mimicking T-cell leukaemias. These include SS and ATLL.

Sézary syndrome/mycosis fungoides

Aetiology

These are cutaneous T-cell lymphomas (CTCLs), with SS being considered the leukaemic manifestation of mycosis fungoides (MF). Their aetiology is unknown. Although some studies have suggested a link between SS/MF and HTLV-I/II on the basis of the detection of retroviral sequences in the tumour cells, there is no evidence for the involvement of these retroviruses in SS/MF. HTLV-I antibodies are not detected in the patient's serum and clonal integration of HTLV-I in the tumour cells has not been demonstrated in any case with bona fide SS/MF. A cooperative study in more than 100 cases of CTCL using sensitive molecular tests, serology and cell cultures failed to show a single CTCL harbouring HTLV-I/II.

A relationship between MF and other T-cell conditions, chiefly lymphomatoid papulosis, has been entertained. Lymphomatoid papulosis is a recurrent skin eruption characterized by the presence of nodules with evidence by histology of anaplastic Reed–Sternberg-like cells infiltrating the skin; it has a good prognosis. Despite the demonstration of T-cell clonality in two-thirds of the tumours, this condition is not considered malignant in the WHO classification and it is included in the subgroup of primary cutaneous lesions. Lymphomatoid

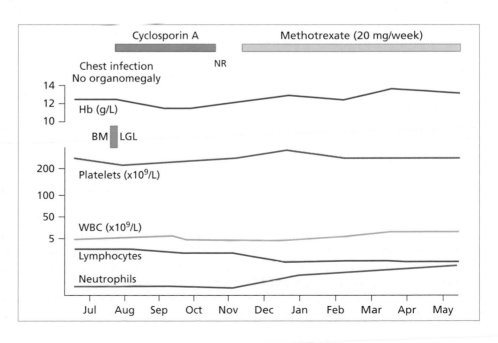

Figure 30.6 Flow chart from a patient with T-cell LGL leukaemia with profound neutropenia (neutrophils 0.1×10^9/L). The patient did not respond to ciclosporin, but the neutropenia improved (neutrophils 1×10^9/L) with weekly pulses of methotrexate.

papulosis may precede not only CTCL but also anaplastic lymphoma and/or Hodgkin disease. The association between lymphomatoid papulosis and CTCL was established in a patient who presented with lymphomatoid papulosis and subsequently developed Hodgkin disease and MF with evidence of the same clone in the three tumours.

Clinical features

SS and MF affect elderly patients and are more common in males. Patients present with pruritus and skin lesions, either localized, e.g. nodules or plaques, or a generalized rash (see Table 30.2). In early-stage disease, the diagnosis is not always made at presentation and the manifestations are considered to be reactive dermatitis. Physical examination shows erythroderma and/or nodules; organomegaly is rare. In SS, the white cell count is normal or raised with circulating atypical lymphocytes. Cytopenias are uncommon and bone marrow is usually not involved. HTLV-I serology is negative even in cases originating from endemic regions for this virus. ISCL-EORTC has proposed a clinical staging system (grades I–IV) based on the extent of the disease, with SS falling into stages III/IV.

Diagnosis

The diagnosis is based on morphology, skin histology and immunophenotyping. The circulating blood lymphocytes are small to large in size and exhibit a cerebriform or hyperchromatic nucleus (Figure 30.7); the cytoplasm is scanty and, in some cases, vacuolation is prominent. According to cell size, two SS variants, small-cell and large-cell, have been recognized. A mixture of small and large cells is the predominant type in the blood. The nuclear configuration of Sézary cells is best defined by ultrastructural analysis, which reveals a serpentine nucleus with multiple indentations.

Skin histology is a key diagnostic test in SS and MF. This shows the presence of dermal lymphoid infiltrates that characteristically extend into the epidermis, a phenomenon designated epidermotropism. Pautrier microabcesses are typical but not unique to these conditions as they may be seen in T-NHL and ATLL.

Histology of other tissues is rarely available at diagnosis. The lymph nodes may show a reactive lymphadenitis or infiltration by lymphoma (Figure 30.8). Bone marrow, when involved, shows a mild interstitial infiltration.

Immunophenotyping demonstrates that circulating Sézary cells are positive for CD2, CD3 and CD5, but CD7 is negative in about 50% of cases (see Table 30.3). The most common phenotype is CD4$^+$CD8$^-$, but other unusual phenotypes, such

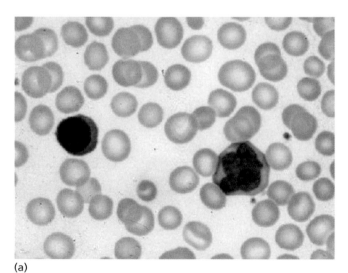

(a)

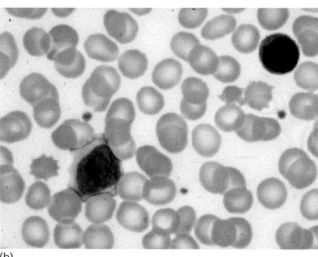

(b)

Figure 30.7 (a, b) Peripheral blood films from a patient with Sézary syndrome showing large and small cells with a convoluted hyperchromatic nucleus.

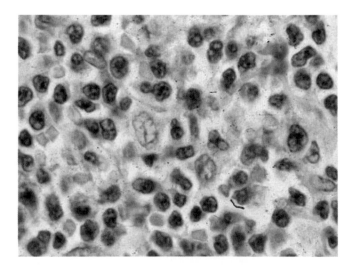

Figure 30.8 Lymph node section from a patient with Sézary syndrome showing diffuse infiltration by lymphoid cells, some with an irregular nucleus.

as CD4$^-$CD8$^+$ or CD4$^+$CD8$^+$, may be seen in rare cases. The neoplastic cells also express the cutaneous lymphocyte antigen (CLA) and the skin homing receptor CCRA. NK-associated markers are usually negative while expression of T-cell activation markers is variable. CD25 may be expressed in Sézary cells but the reactivity is weaker than in ATLL cells. In the skin, the interdigitating Langerhans cells admixed with the neoplastic lymphocytes are positive for CD1a and S-100. Cases transforming into a large T-cell lymphoma display aberrant phenotypes with loss of pan-T markers and often expression of T-cell activation antigens such as CD30, CD25 and HLA-DR.

Cytogenetics

Chromosomal abnormalities are complex and have variable ploidy. Hyperploidy is frequent in the large-cell variant and aneuploidy or hypoploidy in the small-cell form. There are also differences in the DNA content between these two forms when analysed by flow cytometry. There is no evidence for a recurrent chromosomal abnormality in SS, but chromosomes 1, 2, 6 and 17q are the most commonly involved. Clonal evolution may be seen, particularly in cases transforming into large-cell lymphoma. Abnormalities of chromosome 17p have been documented in some cases, as well as p53 protein overexpression and *TP53* gene deletion; however, *TP53* mutations are rare in SS and therefore it has been postulated that the *MDM2* gene may be responsible for *TP53* inactivation in SS.

Differential diagnosis

The differential diagnosis arises with reactive dermatitis, T-PLL presenting with skin lesions, ATLL and other cutaneous lymphomas. Cell morphology and immunological markers allow the distinction between SS and T-PLL and cutaneous B-NHL. HTLV-I serology is the key test for distinguishing SS from ATLL, essentially in cases presenting primarily with cutaneous forms of ATLL. The pattern and extent of skin infiltration and histochemistry allow the differentiation of SS from reactive dermatitis. However, in difficult cases, PCR analysis investigating the configuration of the TCR chain genes is needed; in SS this will show a rearranged T-cell band, unlike reactive dermatitis where the pattern is polyclonal.

Clinical course, prognosis and treatment

The clinical course of MF/SS is usually chronic. Thus, 87% of MF patients survive at 5 years, whereas SS follows a progressive course with shorter survival of around 15% at 5 years. The outcome for patients with abnormal clones seems to be worse than those with random heteroploidy. Transformation of SS or MF into a large-cell T-NHL is uncommon but documented in 8–19% of cases in retrospective studies. Transformation may be localized or systemic and is chiefly associated with advanced stages and a short survival. Only in a few cases has it been demonstrated that the tumour in the phase of transformation arises from the original clone. As SS/MF patients have an increased risk of secondary malignancies, the non-haemopoietic nature of the tumour in these cases needs to be excluded.

A variety of treatments, including topical and systemic agents, have been used in SS/MF. In elderly patients and those with localized skin disease, PUVA (psoralen with UVA irradiation), electron beam irradiation and/or topical carmustine and steroids may alleviate and control the skin symptoms. Local radiotherapy is useful in patients with localized plaques. Systemic therapy is indicated in young patients and/or those with widespread disease. This is based on either single-agent therapy with methotrexate, cyclophosphamide or etoposide or a combination such as CHOP (cyclophosphamide, doxorubicin, vincristine and prednisolone). Over the last decade, new therapies have been employed, such as purine analogues, interferons, retinoids such as bexarotene or etretinate, and immunotherapy with an anti-IL-2 monoclonal antibody conjugated with the diphtheria toxin. Responses to purine analogues (pentostatin, cladribine or fludarabine) range from 30 to 62%. Interferon alfa alone or combined with etretinate appears effective in cases with cutaneous disease but not in systemic disease. Alemtuzumab has been used in some patients with relapsed and refractory disease with encouraging results.

Adult T-cell leukaemia lymphoma

Aetiology and epidemiology

ATLL is a unique malignancy in which the primary aetiological agent has been well established. This disease is caused by a retrovirus, HTLV-I, which is almost universally detected in all patients. ATLL was first described as a clinical entity in 1977. Its association with HTLV-I was demonstrated in the early 1980s almost simultaneously in the USA and Japan, based on seroepidemiological studies and the isolation of HTLV-I from ATLL cells. ATLL is clustered in HTLV-I endemic areas such as Japan, the Caribbean, Africa, South America and the Middle East, and among first/second-generation immigrants from these countries to Europe and the USA. In the UK, this disease is seen in immigrants of Afro-Caribbean descent. Familial cases of ATLL have been documented, and it has been suggested that a shared environment and perhaps a genetic predisposition influence the development of ATLL in these families.

Clinical features

ATLL affects adults without sex predominance. The disease manifests with leukaemia in over two-thirds of cases (leukaemia form), whereas approximately 25% have no blood involvement (lymphoma form). Within the leukaemia form, three subtypes are distinguished: acute, chronic and smouldering. Acute ATLL is the most common, accounting for 65% of cases. Patients present acutely with widespread disease, leucocytosis, opportunistic infections and/or hypercalcaemia. Physical examination shows lymphadenopathy, skin lesions and/or hepatosplenomegaly (see Table 30.2). Chronic ATLL (5% of cases) presents with stable or slowly progressive lymphocytosis with the presence of atypical lymphocytes and minor or no lymphadenopathy or skin involvement. Smouldering ATLL (5% of cases) is characterized by normal blood counts with less than 4% atypical lymphocytes and recurrent skin lesions or lung infiltrates. Hypercalcaemia by definition is not detected in chronic and smouldering ATLL. Both these forms progress in terms of months or rarely years into acute ATLL. A haemophagocytic syndrome preceding this transformation has been documented in smouldering ATLL. A few patients have manifestations of conditions linked to HTLV-I infection such as tropical spastic paraparesis, arthritis and uveitis. These either manifest concomitantly with, or precede the onset of, the T-cell neoplasm. In addition to the symptoms derived from the leukaemia, patients are immunocompromised and develop severe opportunistic infections; infestation by *Strongyloides stercoralis* is frequent and may be fatal. Peripheral blood counts show a raised white cell count with lymphocytosis in the acute and chronic leukaemia forms. Anaemia and thrombocytopenia is seen in close to one-third of cases; eosinophilia and neutrophilia may be present. Biochemistry shows a markedly raised LDH and liver function tests may be abnormal. Hypercalcaemia is the most distinct biochemical abnormality, seen in 50% of cases at presentation and in up to two-thirds during the disease course. Rarely, it is associated with osteolytic lesions. The pathogenesis of hypercalcaemia is described below.

Diagnosis

The diagnosis of ATLL is based on cell morphology, immunophenotype and the demonstration of HTLV-I antibodies in the patient's serum or retrovirus sequences in the cell DNA.

Morphological analysis of peripheral blood films shows a pleomorphic picture with the presence of cells of different size and degree of nuclear irregularities in the acute and chronic leukaemia subtypes. The prototype cell, designated 'flower cell', is a medium-sized lymphocyte with condensed chromatin and a convoluted or polylobated nucleus (Figure 30.9); a few cells may have a cerebriform nucleus and a minority show features of immunoblasts.

Immunological markers show that ATLL cells have a mature activated T-cell phenotype ($CD2^+CD5^+$) and most cases are $CD7^-$. CD3 is expressed in the cytoplasm but, in some cases, cells lack expression of CD3 and TCR-α/β in the membrane. It has been suggested that the decreased numbers of CD3 and TCR molecules in ATLL cells results from cell activation by the retrovirus and that it might play a role in disease pathogenesis. Most ATLL cells have a $CD4^+CD8^-$ phenotype. Uncommon phenotypes such as $CD4^+CD8^+$ or $CD4^-CD8^+$ have been reported in Japan and these cases appear to have a more aggressive course. A distinct feature of ATLL cells is the strong expression of the p55 α-chain of the IL-2 receptor (CD25) in the cell membrane (Figure 30.10). Soluble IL-2 receptors are detected in the patient's serum and the levels correlate with tumour

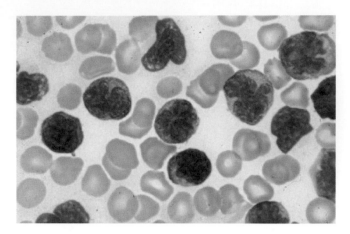

Figure 30.9 Peripheral blood film from a patient with ATLL showing lymphocytes with a polylobed nucleus (flower cells).

burden and response to therapy. Other markers linked to T-cell activation such as HLA-DR determinants and CD38 are expressed in a variable proportion of cases but NK markers are negative.

Tissue histology is not essential for diagnosis in patients presenting with leukaemia. In the lymphoma forms, histology is an important diagnostic test; however, the histological pattern by itself is not sufficient for a diagnosis of ATLL as the pattern of infiltration might be similar in other T-NHLs. Often, there is diffuse infiltration by pleomorphic lymphoid cells of different sizes. ATLL does not fit into a single category in the WHO classification and it is only defined by the presence of HTLV-I. The pattern of skin infiltration is not specific either, as in half the cases it is identical to that in SS, with evidence of epidermotropism. Bone marrow biopsy shows mild or no lymphoid infiltration but bone resorption and proliferation of osteoclasts is not rare, particularly in patients with hypercalcaemia.

Demonstration of HTLV-I is the key test for the definitive diagnosis of ATLL. Serum antibodies to HTLV-I can be detected by ELISA or Western blot in virtually all cases. In a minority of patients who have a clinical and laboratory picture characteristic of ATLL, the retrovirus cannot be detected by either serology or molecular analysis. This suggests that in these cases the initiating event responsible for the development of ATLL is not HTLV-I. When findings are negative for HTLV-I, one should question the diagnosis of ATLL.

Cytogenetics and pathogenesis

ATLL has no distinct chromosomal abnormality but complex karyotypes and clonal evolution are frequent. Common abnormalities include +3, +7, +21, monosomy X, deletion of chromosome Y and rearrangements involving 6q and 14q. Rearrangements of chromosome 14 at breakpoints q11 and q32, characteristic of T-PLL, are rare. Mutations of the tumour-suppressor genes *TP53*, *CDKN2A* (encoding the p16INK4A

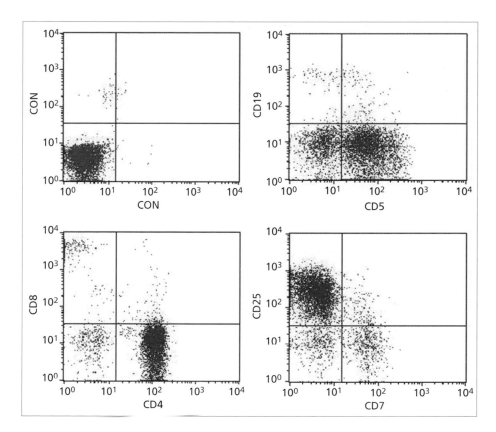

Figure 30.10 Flow cytometry plots of lymphocytes from a patient with ATLL showing reactivity with CD5, CD4 and CD25 while CD7 is negative.

protein) and *CDKN2B* (encoding the p15INK4B protein) have been documented and implicated in development of the disease. In smouldering ATLL, clonal and non-clonal abnormalities have been reported and occasional cases show clonal evolution from the smouldering to the acute phase. Sequential cytogenetic studies during the various phases of HTLV-I infection, from carrier to acute ATLL, might give some clues to the steps involved in leukaemogenesis, as the secondary factors involved in the neoplastic transformation of HTLV-I-infected lymphocytes are largely unknown.

IL-2 and its receptor have been implicated in the pathogenesis on the basis of the independent growth of some HTLV-I-positive cell lines, the continuous transcription of the IL-2 receptor gene, the increased levels of IL-2 receptor mRNA and the fact that HTLV-I induces IL-2 receptor expression in normal T lymphocytes when infected by this retrovirus. However, a role of IL-2 in pathogenesis is uncertain as ATLL cells do not secrete IL-2 nor have increased mRNA levels for this cytokine.

The mechanism of hypercalcaemia seems to relate to the release of cytokines, chiefly a parathyroid-like hormone, IL-1 and tumour necrosis factor (TNF)-β by the tumour cells. These lead to bone resorption and release of calcium into the serum.

It is well established that HTLV-I is the primary aetiological agent of ATLL, shown by the presence of monoclonal/oligoclonal integration of HTLV-I sequences into the leukaemic cell's DNA. Although HTLV-I infection constitutes the first step in the development of ATLL, it is not enough by itself to cause malignancy as only 0.5% of HTLV-I carriers will develop the disease and the life risk of developing ATLL in a carrier is estimated to be around 5%. Infection in early life seems to be a risk factor. HTLV-I does not carry an oncogene and the sites of integration vary from tumour to tumour. However, the retrovirus harbours various regulatory genes (e.g. *tax*) that code for proteins responsible for cell immortalization by activating genes relevant to proliferation and differentiation (*trans*-activation pathway).

Differential diagnosis

The differential diagnosis of ATLL arises with primary T-cell leukaemias and T-NHL not associated to HTLV-I. In addition, smouldering ATLL raises diagnostic problems with carriers of the retrovirus. T-cell leukaemias and T-NHL can be distinguished from ATLL by clinical features, morphology and the presence or absence of HTLV-I. The HTLV-I test is essential, as ATLL-type lymphoma, or its cutaneous form, cannot be distinguished from either T-NHL or MF/SS when only histology is available. In endemic areas and when the picture is not typical of ATLL, DNA analysis is needed in addition to serology to confirm that HTLV-I is clonally integrated in the leukaemic cells. The distinction between smouldering ATLL and carriers of the retrovirus is based on molecular analysis with probes specific for HTLV-I that will show a monoclonal/oligoclonal pattern of retroviral integration in smouldering ATLL versus a polyclonal pattern in the carriers.

Clinical course and therapy

ATLL is an aggressive malignancy for which no successful treatment is yet available, with a median survival of less than 12 months. Patients are refractory or transiently respond to chemotherapy or purine analogues. Smouldering and chronic ATLL pursue an indolent course until the disease progresses and becomes refractory to therapy. The poor outlook of ATLL relates to both chemotherapy resistance and complications (hypercalcaemia and opportunistic infections). Despite advances in disease pathogenesis, management of these patients remains a challenge. Most patients are refractory or achieve transient responses to CHOP, similar schedules and/or immunotherapy with monoclonal antibodies against the IL-2 receptor. Data with alemtuzumab is scanty. A major advance in treatment comes from the use of interferon alfa and the antiretroviral agents zidovudine and lamivudine, either alone or when used after, or combined with, chemotherapy. Following two initial Phase II trials, two prospective studies in France and England confirmed the efficacy of this combination and documented a response rate of 65–92%, of which half were CR, with improved survival. Although the mechanism of action of zidovudine is unknown, *in vitro* studies suggest that the drug inhibits telomerase function and leukaemic cells enter senescence. Consolidation with high-dose therapy and autologous or allogeneic SCT should be considered in young patients.

T-cell non-Hodgkin lymphomas

The tissue-based T-cell NHLs encompass a variety of entities that essentially affect lymphoid tissues and/or extranodal sites. Some of them are frequent in the East but very uncommon in Western countries. A minority of patients may develop or manifest a leukaemic picture and, when the circulating cells are large blasts (Figure 30.11), present problems of differential diagnosis with acute leukaemias. According to the WHO classification, the T-NHLs are classified as shown in Table 30.1.

Peripheral T-NHL not otherwise specified (see also Chapters 33 and 35)

This term includes T-NHL that does not correspond to specific T-NHL entities and most of these are referred to as non-lymphoblastic TdT-negative T-NHL. Patients present with organomegaly, 'B' symptoms and some with extranodal disease; haemophagocytosis and/or impairment of the immune system are not uncommon. Lymph node histology shows diffuse effacement of the architecture by atypical lymphocytes (Figure 30.12), or infiltration may be confined to interfollicular areas (T-zone variant) and/or the paracortical zone. There may be a

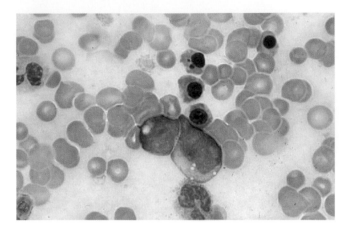

Figure 30.11 Bone marrow aspirate from a patient with T-NHL showing two large blasts.

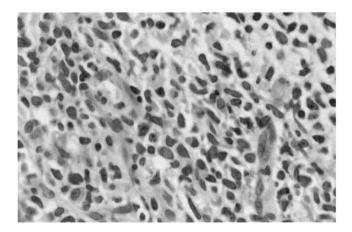

Figure 30.12 Bone marrow trephine biopsy from a patient with peripheral T-cell lymphoma (unspecified) showing diffuse infiltration by pleomorphic lymphoid cells.

background of eosinophils and histiocytes in the lymphoepithelioid variant (Figure 30.13). The neoplastic cells express several T-cell markers (CD2, CD3, CD5, CD7), with variable expression of CD4 and CD8. Aberrant phenotypes with lack of expression of pan-T markers are common. CD52 may be negative in 60% of cases and the proliferative rate is usually high. Bone marrow is rarely involved. There is no consistent chromosomal abnormality but complex karyotypes are common. Gene expression profiling has shown a signature different from other T-NHLs and characterized by deregulation of genes involved in proliferation, apoptosis, transcription, cell adhesion and cytoskeleton organization. Most peripheral T-NHLs should be considered high grade; the 5-year survival is around 20%. Treatments are based on chemotherapy combinations such as intensified CHOP plus etoposide or given at shorter intervals (e.g. every 2 weeks), or gencitabine and platinum schedules followed or not by SCT.

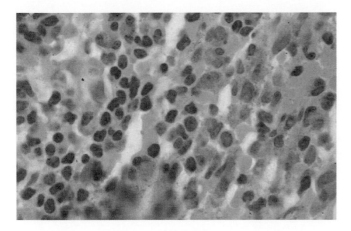

Figure 30.13 Bone marrow trephine showing infiltration by lymphoid cells with marked eosinophilia in a patient with T-NHL.

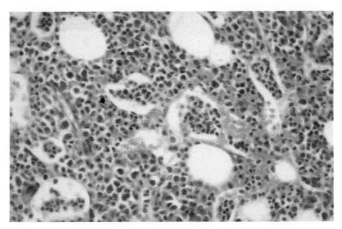

Figure 30.14 Bone marrow trephine section from a patient with hepatosplenic lymphoma showing intrasinusoidal infiltration.

Peripheral T-NHL specific variants (see Table 30.1)

Several specific variants of T-NHL have been considered by the WHO as distinct entities on the basis of the clinical and laboratory features. The most relevant features of these lymphomas are described below.

Hepatosplenic T-NHL

This tumour usually derives from T cells positive for TCR-γ/δ and affects preferentially young males. It is more common in immunocompromised patients. Hepatosplenomegaly is the main feature, but extranodal sites (e.g. skin) may be involved (see Table 30.2). Cytopenias are common but bone marrow involvement is not frequent. A rare form of primary cutaneous γ/δ T-NHL is considered in the WHO classification but should be distinguished from the hepatosplenic T-NHL. The histology is distinct, with an intrasinusoidal pattern of infiltration in all tissues affected such as spleen, liver and bone marrow (Figures 30.14 and 30.15). This mimics the pattern of distribution of normal T γ/δ lymphocytes, which home preferentially in the spleen sinusoids. The neoplastic cells have a CD2$^+$CD7$^+$CD3$^{+/-}$TCR-γ/δ$^+$ phenotype (Figure 30.16) and are usually negative with monoclonal antibodies against TCR-α/β, CD5, CD4 and CD8. Often, the cells are positive for the NK-associated markers CD16 and CD56, the cytotoxic granule-associated proteins TIA-1 and granzyme B, and may aberrantly express multiple KIRs. Molecular studies show rearrangement of the TCR γ- and δ-chain genes while the TCR α- and β-chain genes are in the germline. Cytogenetics have shown that some cases have iso(7q) and it has been suggested that this is a recurrent abnormality in this lymphoma (see Table 30.3). EBV does not play a pathogenic role. The clinical course is aggressive and median survival is less than 2 years. The most effective drugs are pentostatin and platinum-based regimens.

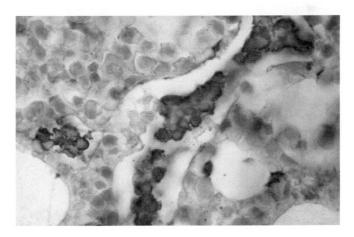

Figure 30.15 Immunohistochemistry of the bone marrow in Figure 30.14 showing that most lymphocytes in the sinusoids express cytoplasmic CD3.

Subcutaneous panniculitis-like T-NHL

This manifests with skin nodules resembling a benign panniculitis; haemophagocytic syndrome is frequent and may be fatal. It may be seen associated with autoimmune diseases, particularly lupus, and it has been speculated that autoimmunity plays a pathogenic role. Skin histology shows lymphoid infiltrates admixed with adipocytes in the subcutaneous tissue with extension to the dermis. Fat and connective tissue necrosis and granulomas are common; vascular invasion may be seen. The mitotic rate is high. The neoplastic cells are positive for CD2, CD3 and often CD8 and express granzyme B, perforin and TIA-1, suggesting that this lymphoma arises from cytotoxic T cells. Molecular analysis shows rearrangement of the TCR β-chain gene. There are limited data on outcome and response to therapy but cases with haemophagocytic syndrome appear to have the worst prognosis. Overall survival at 5 years is 80%.

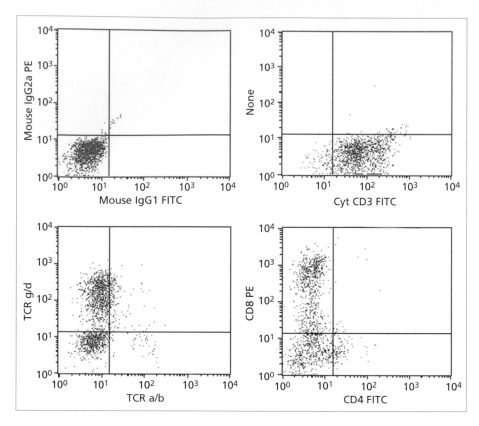

Figure 30.16 Flow cytometry plots of bone marrow cells from a patient with hepatosplenic T-NHL showing that the lymphocytes express membrane TCR-γ/δ, cytoplasmic CD3 and CD8, but are negative for anti-TCR-α/β and CD4.

Angioimmunoblastic T-NHL

Angioimmunoblastic T-NHL had already been described in the 1970s. It affects adults and has an acute onset. 'B' symptoms, pruritus, cutaneous rash, organomegaly, effusions and immune disturbance, comprising autoimmune phenomena, immunodeficiency and/or dysproteinaemia, are common (see Table 30.2). Cases of clonal angioimmunoblastic T-NHL evolving from reactive hyperplasia have been described, and this may correlate with clinical progression. The diagnosis is based on clinical features and histology. The lymph node shows a pleomorphic infiltrate composed of lymphocytes, plasma cells, immunoblasts and eosinophils; proliferation of epithelioid post-capillary venules and increased numbers of follicular dendritic cell meshworks is common. There is obliteration of the follicular structure, described as 'burned-out' follicular centres. The bone marrow is often involved and aspirates may show reactive features with increase in polyclonal plasma cells. The lymphoma cells have a T-cell phenotype ($CD2^+CD5^+CD3^+$) and are often positive for CD4 and CD10; the proliferative rate is high. B immunoblasts may be present but usually are polyclonal. Complex karyotypes with multiple clones involving trisomy 3 or iso(3q), trisomy 5 and del(6q) are common. Most cases have rearrangement of TCR β- and/or γ-chain genes and, in a few cases, both immunoglobulin and TCR chain genes are rearranged; the latter correlates with the presence of an expanded EBV-positive B-cell clone which,

rarely, may progress to a diffuse B-cell lymphoma. The clinical course of angioimmunoblastic T-NHL is acute and prognosis is poor. Although transient spontaneous remissions have been documented, the lymphoma always recurs. Some patients initially respond to corticosteroids or combination chemotherapy but most relapse. Single case reports have documented responses to fludarabine and/or thalidomide. Combinations of gemcitabine and platinum appear to be more effective than CHOP. The median survival ranges from 13 to 17 months. It is likely that more aggressive regimens including SCT and/or combinations of chemotherapy with anti-T-cell monoclonal antibody will improve the dismal outcome of this lymphoma.

Extranodal T/NK lymphoma, nasal type

This type is significantly more frequent in China and Central/South America. Other designations for this lymphoma include lymphomatoid granulomatosis, polymorphic reticulosis, angiocentric immunoproliferative lesion or lethal midline granuloma. Patients are adults and present with systemic symptoms and extranodal disease, frequently involving the aerogastric tract and particularly the nasal cavity; other tissues that may be involved include skin, testes, CNS, lung, bowel and bone. The tumour histology shows lymphoid infiltrates admixed with histiocytes with marked angiocentricity, angiodestruction and ulceration (Figure 30.17).

and/or partial deletion of the *FAS* gene. TCR chain genes are germline in cases with an NK phenotype but rearranged in the minority with a cytotoxic T-cell phenotype. Although the aetiology of this lymphoma is unknown, there is evidence of the pathogenic role of EBV by serology, a high titre of EBV DNA copies in the blood and molecular analysis showing single clonal episomal bands in the tumour cells. Detection of EBV-encoded RNA (EBER) is useful for distinguishing this lymphoma from benign or inflammatory nasal lymphoid infiltrates. The prognosis is variable. Unfavourable factors include advanced stages, high blood EBV copies and disease occurring outside the nasal cavity. Combination chemotherapy, especially including L-asparaginase, together with up-front local radiotherapy seems to be the best approach.

EBV-positive T-cell lymphoproliferative disorders in childhood

These have been incorporated in the new WHO classification. Two forms, systemic and cutaneous, are recognized with a different course and prognosis. They are more frequent in Asian and South American patients and EBV is consistently detected in the lesions, suggesting that the disease is triggered by this virus in an individual with a genetic predisposition. The systemic form corresponds to what was recognized as fatal haemophagocytic syndrome and affects liver, spleen and other organs, while the cutaneous form is confined to the skin particularly in sun-exposed areas. The tissues affected are infiltrated by pleomorphic lymphocytes with a cytotoxic phenotype: CD2$^+$, CD3$^+$, CD56$^-$, TIA-1$^+$ and often CD8$^+$. Haemophagocytosis may be prominent. All cases carry the type A EBV and EBERs can be detected in the neoplastic cells by FISH. The prognosis is poor in the systemic form.

Enteropathy-associated T-NHL

Intestinal lymphomas are often B-cell derived but a minority have a T-cell phenotype and these are designated 'enteropathy-associated T-NHL'. This lymphoma seems to arise from a CD3$^+$CD8$^+$CD103$^+$ T lymphocyte present in the normal epithelial intestinal mucosa. Some patients have a previous history of coeliac disease and/or gluten-sensitive enteropathy. The relationship between enteropathy-type T-NHL and coeliac disease is supported by the higher frequency of this lymphoma in geographical regions where gluten enteropathy is common such as northern Europe; diet may improve symptoms and patients have the HLA genotypes DQA1*0501 and DQB1*0201 seen in coeliac disease. It affects adults and the main manifestations are abdominal pain, chronic diarrhoea and/or weight loss; rarely bowel perforation or obstruction is the first manifestation. In some cases, the diagnosis is made concomitantly with coeliac disease. Histology shows intraepithelial and subepithelial lymphoid infiltration of the mucosa and villous atrophy with reactive eosinophils and histiocytes. Three histological subtypes with regard to the presence or absence of enteropathy have been

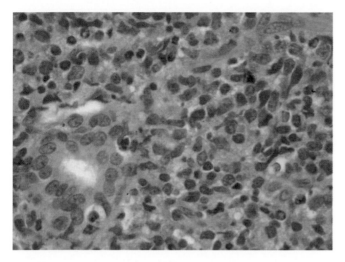

Figure 30.17 Section from a nasal mass of a patient with extranodal T/NK lymphoma, nasal type, showing infiltration by lymphoid cells with angiocentricity.

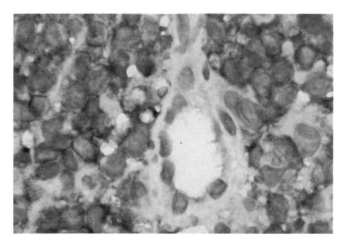

Figure 30.18 Immunohistochemistry of the tissue in Figure 30.17 showing strong reactivity with CD56.

It has been suggested that necrosis relates to the release of TNF overexpressed by the tumour cells and induced by EBV. Immunophenotype shows that most cases have an NK phenotype (CD2$^+$CD3ϵ^+CD56$^+$mCD3$^-$), while a small proportion have a cytotoxic T-cell phenotype (mCD3$^+$) with both subtypes expressing CD56 (Figure 30.18). The neoplastic cells express cytotoxic molecules such as perforin, TIA-1 and granzyme B. HLA-DR determinants, CD38, CD30 and CD25 may be positive, indicating that the tumour cells are activated lymphocytes. The EBV latent membrane protein (LMP)-1 can be demonstrated by immunohistochemistry in most cases. Cytogenetic abnormalities involving iso(6p), del(6q) and iso(1q) are common; some cases may have *TP53* and/or *KIT* mutations documented. These appear to correlate with outcome, which is worst for patients with associated enteropathy. The lymphoma cells express T-cell markers (CD7$^+$CD3$^{+/-}$), cytotoxic granule proteins and rarely are CD8$^+$ or CD4$^+$. The expression of HML-1 (CD103), a marker of normal intestinal lymphocytes, is a consistent finding supporting the theory that this lymphoma arises from intraepithelial mucosa T cells. The TCR β- and γ-chain genes are rearranged. Cytogenetics shows amplification of 9q31 or del(16q) and in some cases *MYC* amplification. A high prevalence of EBV has been documented in Mexican but not European patients. The clinical course is aggressive, with survival estimated to be less than 1 year. Patients with localized bowel disease have longer survival than those with generalized disease. Surgery is often the diagnostic procedure and the first therapeutic approach. Problems in the patient's management include intolerance to chemotherapy due to poor nutrition, low performance status and low albumin.

Anaplastic large-cell lymphoma

Anaplastic large-cell lymphoma (ALCL) is now considered a distinct clinicobiological entity with characteristic molecular features involving the *ALK* gene and expression of Ki-1 (CD30), a marker also present in Reed–Sternberg cells. It has a bimodal age of presentation (childhood and elderly) and shows a male predominance. Lymphadenopathy and cutaneous lesions are the most frequent manifestations but extranodal disease such as bone, lung and liver may be present (see Table 30.2). Systemic symptoms are common and most patients present with advanced stages. There are two forms, systemic and primarily cutaneous, and it is controversial whether these forms are biologically different. In the WHO classification, cutaneous CD30-positive ALCL is considered within the group of primary cutaneous CD30-positive T-cell disorders together with lymphomatoid papulosis and other rare subtypes. In addition, *ALK*-negative ALCL is also considered separately (see also Chapter 33).

Lymph node histology shows lymphoid infiltration of the T zone and paracortical areas, with or without intrasinusoidal involvement. Capsular thickening and fibrous tissue deposition are common. The skin shows infiltration of the dermis and subcutaneous tissue but epidermotropism is rare. Morphologically, ALCL is heterogeneous. The typical morphology is that of very large lymphoid cells, sometimes multinucleated, resembling Reed–Sternberg cells (Figure 30.19). Several morphological variants of ALCL have been recognized: monomorphic, Hodgkin-like, lymphohistiocytic or small cell. Despite this morphological heterogeneity, all these variants bear the t(2;5) translocation and express *ALK*. Most cases have a T-cell phenotype and often lack expression of some T-cell markers, particularly CD3; a few cases have a 'null' (non-B, non-T) phenotype, but molecular analysis demonstrates the T-cell nature of the lymphoma cells.

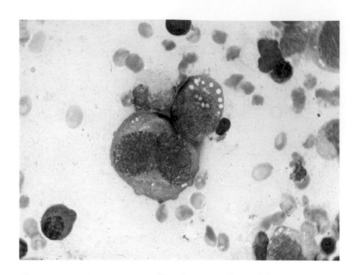

Figure 30.19 Bone marrow film from a patient with CD30-positive ALCL showing infiltration by large bizarre anaplastic cells.

ALCL cells always express CD30 (Ki-1), the hallmark of this lymphoma (see Table 30.3). Lymphocyte activation markers such as CD25, HLA-DR determinants and CD71 and the epithelial membrane antigen (EMA) are often positive while the cells are cytokeratin negative. Unlike Reed–Sternberg cells, ALCL cells are, as a rule, CD15 negative. This is important to consider as diagnostic confusion between this lymphoma and Hodgkin disease frequently arise. Some studies have shown that in most cases ALCL cells express TIA-1, perforin and granzyme B, molecules present in cytotoxic and NK cells, and thus suggested that ALCL cells derive from activated cytotoxic T cells. EBV is consistently negative. The chromosomal abnormality t(2;5)(p23;q35) is characteristic of ALCL. This leads to the rearrangement of the nucleolar phosphoprotein gene (*NPM*) on 5q35 with the anaplastic lymphoma tyrosine kinase (*ALK*) gene on 2p23 (see Table 30.3). This fusion generates a chimeric transcript, *NPM–ALK*, which can be detected by FISH or by reverse transcriptase PCR using specific primers and by immunohistochemistry with an antibody against the *ALK*-encoded p80 protein. A number of variant translocations involving *ALK* with other partner chromosomes have been described and all lead to the deregulation of *ALK*. The expression or absence of p80 protein appears to have prognostic impact. The *NPM–ALK* transcripts are detectable in most cases of nodal Ki-1-positive ALCL, but in only a few with the pure cutaneous form. This reinforces the fact that the latter represent a different entity, as regarded by the WHO classification.

The clinical course of ALCL is variable. Patients with early stages (I/II) and/or primary ALCL fare relatively well compared with those with advanced stages, bulky disease and/or secondary ALCL. The main prognostic factor in multivariate analysis is advanced stage (III/IV). There is no gold-standard therapy for ALCL, which should be tailored according to age, performance status and extent of the disease. Localized skin lesions may respond to radiotherapy but in advanced stages combination chemotherapy should be recommended. Unlike other T-NHLs, patients with ALCL have sensitive disease and usually respond to chemotherapy, with an overall response rate of 55–100% in different series; however, most patients relapse. Autologous SCT has been successful in relapsed or newly diagnosed patients and this is the treatment of choice for young patients with advanced stages.

Differential diagnosis of peripheral T-NHLs

The differential diagnosis arises with (i) T-cell rich B-NHL; (ii) reactive non-neoplastic lymphadenitis; and (iii) rarely, Hodgkin disease or acute leukaemias. In difficult cases, markers should be complemented with TCR and immunoglobulin gene analysis. The latter, in addition, will exclude cases of reactive lymphadenitis with difficult histology. Immunophenotype allows the distinction between large-cell T-NHL and acute myeloid leukaemia.

Diagnostic problems with other diseases may also arise with specific T-NHL subtypes. For instance, subpanniculitis-like T-NHL should be distinguished from benign skin conditions or histiocytosis, angioimmunoblastic T-NHL from reactive disorders, CD30-positive ALCL from Hodgkin disease, and peripheral T-NHL, with marked haemophagocytic component, from histiocytic tumours or a reactive haemophagocytic syndrome. It is important to combine clinical features with histopathology and, if required, with molecular analysis of the TCR chain genes.

Conclusions

The mature or chronic T-cell lymphoproliferative disorders comprise a variety of disease entities with distinct clinical and laboratory features. They can be classified on the basis of the clinical presentation and disease manifestations into primary leukaemias, leukaemia/lymphoma syndromes and T-cell lymphomas. The precise diagnosis is important in terms of patient management, prognosis and therapy. Most of these disorders have an aggressive clinical course and are considered as high- to intermediate-grade lymphomas. The application of molecular techniques together with immunological markers has greatly helped the understanding of their pathogenesis by the identification of genes or oncogenes responsible for disease initiation or progression and has allowed the definition of disease entities. This, in turn, has provided the basis for the development of novel and specific therapies for certain conditions, with improvement in survival. However, further research is needed to define a number of disorders which at present have not emerged as distinct entities.

Acknowledgements

I thank Ricardo Morilla for providing the flow cytometry figures and Lok Lam for providing Figure 30.5.

Selected bibliography

Attygale AD, Kyriakou C, Dupuis J et al. (2007) Histologic evolution of angioimmunoblastic T-cell lymphoma in consecutive biopsies: clinical correlation and insights into natural history and disease progression. *American Journal of Surgical Pathology* **31**: 1077–88.

Beldhadj K, Reyes F, Farcet JP (2003) Hepatosplenic gammadelta T-cell lymphoma is a rare clinicopathologic entity with poor outcome: report on a series of 21 patients. *Blood* **102**: 4261–9.

Brouet JC, Flandrin G, Sasprotes M et al. (1975) Chronic lymphocytic leukaemia of T-cell origin. Immunological and clinical evaluation in eleven patients. *Lancet* **ii**: 890–3.

Chim CS, Ma ES, Loong F et al. (2004) Primary nasal natural killer cell lymphoma: long term treatment outcome and relationship with the International prognostic index. *Blood* **103**: 216–21.

Datta A, Bellon M, Sinha-Datta U et al. (2006) Persistent inhibition of telomerase reprograms adult T-cell leukaemia to p53-dependent senescence. *Blood* **108**: 1021–9.

Dearden CE, Matutes E, Cazin B et al. (2001) High remission rate in T-cell prolymphocytic leukemia with Campath-1H. *Blood* **98**: 1721–6.

Dungarwalla M, Matutes E, Dearden CE (2008) Prolymphocytic leukaemia of B and T cell subtype: a state of the art paper. *European Journal of Haematology* **80**: 469–76.

Herling M, Patel KA, Teitell MA et al. (2008) High TCL1 expression and intact T-cell receptor signalling define a hyperproliferative subset of T-cell prolymphocytic leukaemia. *Blood* **111**: 328–37.

Jaffe ES, Chan JKC, Su I-J et al. (1996) Report of the Workshop on Nasal and Related Extranodal Angiocentric T/Natural Killer Cell Lymphomas. Definitions, differential diagnosis, and epidemiology. *American Journal of Surgical Pathology* **20**: 103–11.

Kchour G, Tarhini M, Kooshyar MM et al. (2009) Phase 2 study of the efficacy and safety of the combination of arsenic trioxide, interferon alpha, and zidovudine in newly diagnosed chronic adult T-cell leukemia/lymphoma (ATL). *Blood* **113**: 6528–32.

Lamy T, Loughran TP Jr (1999) Current concepts: large granular lymphocyte leukemia. *Blood Reviews* **13**: 230–40.

Langerak AW, van den Beemd R, Wolvers-Tettero ILM et al. (2001) Molecular and flow cytometric analysis of the Vβ repertoire for clonality assessment in mature TCRαβ T-cell proliferations. *Blood* **98**: 165–73.

Lundin J, Hagberg H, Repp R et al. (2003) Phase 2 study of alemtuzumab (anti-CD52 monoclonal antibody) in patients with advanced mycosis fungoides/Sézary syndrome. *Blood* **101**: 4267–72.

Matutes E (1999) *T-cell Lymphoproliferative Disorders. Classification, Clinical and Laboratory Aspects.* Harwood Academic Publishers, Amsterdam.

Matutes E (2003) Chronic T-cell lymphoproliferative disorders. *Reviews in Clinical and Experimental Hematology* **6**: 401–20.

Matutes E (2007) Adult T-cell leukaemia lymphoma. *Journal of Clinical Pathology* **60**: 1373–7.

Matutes E (2009) Immunological and clinical features of T-cell LGL disorders. *Hematology Education: the Education Programme for the Annual Congress of the European Hematology Association* **3**: 302–7.

Matutes E, Brito-Babapulle V, Swansbury J *et al.* (1991) Clinical and laboratory features of 78 cases of T-prolymphocytic leukemia. *Blood* **78**: 3269–74.

Matutes E, Taylor GP, Cavenagh J *et al.* (2001) Interferon alpha and zidovudine therapy in adult T-cell leukaemia lymphoma: response and outcome in 15 patients. *British Journal of Haematology* **113**: 779–84.

Matutes E, Wotherspoon AC, Parker NE *et al.* (2001) Transformation of T-cell granular lymphocyte leukaemia into a high grade large T-cell lymphoma. *British Journal of Haematology* **115**: 801–6.

Mercieca J, Matutes E, Dearden C *et al.* (1994) The role of pentostatin in the treatment of T-cell malignancies: analysis of response rate in 145 patients according to disease subtype. *Journal of Clinical Oncology* **12**: 2588–93.

Osuji N, Matutes E, Tjonnfjord G *et al.* (2006) T-cell large granular lymphocyte leukemia: a report on the treatment of 29 patients and a review of the literature. *Cancer* **107**: 570–8.

Osuji N, Beiske K, Randen U *et al.* (2007) Characteristic appearance of the bone marrow in T-cell large granular lymphocyte leukemia. *Histopathology* **50**: 547–54.

Rizvi SA, Evens AM, Tallman MS *et al.* (2006) T-cell non-Hodgkin lymphoma. *Blood* **107**: 1255–64.

Rodriguez-Caballero A, Garcia-Montero AC, Barcena P *et al.* (2008) Expanded cells in monoclonal TCRab⁺/CD4⁺/Nka⁺/CD8⁻/⁺dim T-LGL lymphocytes recognize hCMV antigens. *Blood* **112**: 4609–16.

Shiota M, Nakamura S, Ichinohasama R *et al.* (1995) Anaplastic large cell lymphomas expressing the novel chimeric protein p80 NPM/ALK: a distinct clinicopathologic entity. *Blood* **86**: 1954–60.

Sokol L, Loughran TP Jr (2006) Large granular lymphocyte leukemia. *Oncologist* **11**: 263–73.

Swerdlow SH, Campo E, Harris NL *et al.* (eds) (2008) *WHO Classification of Tumours of Haematopoietic and Lymphoid Tissues.* IARC Press, Lyon.

Taylor GP, Matsuoka M (2005) Natural history of adult T-cell leukemia/lymphoma and approaches to therapy. *Oncogene* **24**: 6047–57.

Thangavelu M, Finn WG, Yelavarthi KK *et al.* (1997) Recurring structural chromosome abnormalities in peripheral blood lymphocytes of patients with mycosis fungoides/Sézary syndrome. *Blood* **89**: 3371–7.

Tien H-F, Su I-J, Tang J-L *et al.* (1997) Clonal chromosome abnormalities as direct evidence for clonality in nasal T/natural killer lymphomas. *British Journal of Haematology* **97**: 621–5.

Willenze R, Jansen PM, Cerroni L *et al.* (2007) Subcutaneous panniculitis T-cell lymphoma: definition, classification and prognostic factors. An EORTC Cutaneous Lymphoma Group study of 83 cases. *Blood* **111**: 838–45.

Yang J, Epling-Burnette PK, Painter JS *et al.* (2008) Antigen activation and impaired Fas-induced death-inducing signalling complex formation in T-large granular lymphocyte leukaemia. *Blood* **111**: 1610–16.

CHAPTER 31

Multiple myeloma

31

Jesús San-Miguel[1] and Joan Bladé[2]

[1]Hospital Universitario de Salamanca, Salamanca, Spain
[2]Hospital Clinic de Barcelona, Barcelona, Spain

Definition

Multiple myeloma (MM) is characterized by the proliferation of a single clone of plasma cells that produce a monoclonal protein. The plasma cell proliferation results in extensive skeletal involvement, with osteolytic lesions, hypercalcaemia, anaemia and/or soft tissue plasmacytomas. In addition, the excessive production of nephrotoxic monoclonal immunoglobulin can result in renal failure and an increased risk of developing potentially life-threatening infections due to the lack of functional immunoglobulins. The clinical and laboratory manifestations of the disease, including their management, are discussed in this chapter.

Epidemiology and aetiology

The annual incidence of MM is 4 per 100 000. It represents approximately 1% of all malignant diseases and 15% of all haematological malignancies. The incidence of MM is lower in Asian populations and in blacks is twice that in whites; MM is slightly more frequent in men than in women. The median age

Postgraduate Haematology: 6th edition. Edited by A. Victor Hoffbrand,
Daniel Catovsky, Edward G.D. Tuddenham, Anthony R. Green
© 2011 Blackwell Publishing Ltd.

at diagnosis is 65–70 years. Only 15% and 2% of the patients are younger than 50 and 40 years, respectively.

The cause of MM is unknown. Radiation may play a role in some cases. An increased risk has been reported in farmers, particularly those who use herbicides and insecticides, and in people exposed to benzene and other organic solvents. However, the number of cases is small and more data are needed to establish a significant relationship. MM and monoclonal gammopathy of undetermined significance (MGUS) have been reported in familial clusters. A relationship between MM and pre-existing inflammatory diseases has been suggested, and plasma cell dyscrasias associated with protracted stimulation of the reticuloendothelial system have been reported in experimental studies. However, more recent case–control studies do not support a role for chronic antigenic stimulation in the aetiopathogenesis of MM.

Pathogenesis

MM is a B-cell malignancy characterized by the accumulation of terminally differentiated clonal plasma cells in the bone marrow, the production of a monoclonal immunoglobulin detectable in serum and/or urine and the presence of lytic bone lesions. In order to understand the pathogenesis of MM, it is important to review not only the molecular changes involved in the development of the malignant clone, but also the mechanisms responsible for the interaction between the malignant plasma cells and their microenvironment, since they play a relevant role in bone destruction, tumour cell growth, survival, migration and drug resistance.

Cellular origin of myeloma cells

Normal differentiation from early B cells to plasma cells is characterized by three B-cell specific DNA remodelling mechanisms that modify immunoglobulin genes: VDJ rearrangement, somatic mutation and class switch recombination. Rearrangements of the immunoglobulin genes of B-cell precursors to form a B-cell receptor (BCR) occur in the bone marrow, while antigen recognition, selection, somatic hypermutation and class switch recombination take place in the germinal centre lymph node. Sequence analysis of the immunoglobulin V_H gene support the post-germinal origin of myeloma cells, which have successfully completed somatic hypermutation (without intraclonal variation) and IgH switching before migrating to the bone marrow, where they will interact with stromal cells before finally differentiating into long-lived plasma cells.

Genetic abnormalities

Molecular cytogenetic investigations of myeloma cells have demonstrated that almost all cases of MM are cytogenetically abnormal. MM is characterized by marked karyotypic instability.

IGH translocations

A primary event in many kinds of B-cell tumour is dysregulation of an oncogene that, as a result of translocation to the *IGH* locus (14q32) or, somewhat less often, the *IGL* locus (κ 2p11 or λ 22q11), is juxtaposed near one of the potent immunoglobulin enhancers. In MM, *IGH* translocation may be classified into primary or secondary. Primary *IGH* translocations occur as initiating events during the pathogenesis of MM, whereas secondary translocations are involved in progression. Most primary *IGH* translocations result from errors in B-cell-specific DNA modification processes, mostly *IGH* switch recombination or less often somatic hypermutation. The breakpoints occur mainly within or immediately adjacent to *IGH* switch regions or J_H regions. In contrast, secondary translocations are mediated by other kinds of recombination mechanism that do not specifically target B-cell specific DNA modification processes. Unlike other B-cell tumours, in MM there is a marked diversity of chromosomal loci involved in *IGH* translocations. About 40% of MM tumours have *IGH* translocations involving five recurrent chromosomal patterns (Figure 31.1): 11q13 (*CCND1*), 4p16 (*FGFR/MMSET*), 16q23 (*MAF*), 6p21 (*CCND3*) and 20q11 (*MAFB*).

The prevalence of t(11;14) according to interphase fluorescence *in situ* hybridization (FISH) analysis is 15–20% and is readily detectable by karyotyping. As result of the translocation, *CCND1* is juxtaposed to the powerful *IGH* 3′ enhancer(s) on der(14), and its expression is dysregulated, as indicated by gene expression profiling and reverse transcriptase polymerase chain reaction (RT-PCR) in 100% of MM cases with t(11;14).

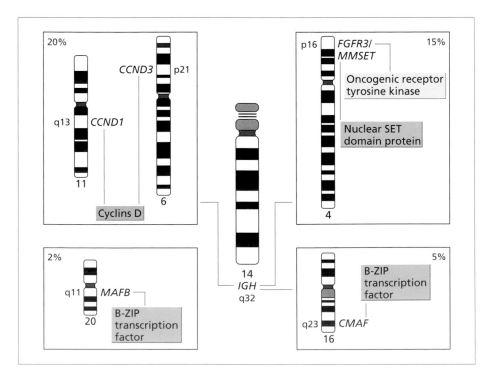

Figure 31.1 *IGH* translocations in multiple myeloma.

The t(4;14) translocation is identified in approximately 15% of MM cases using FISH analysis, but cannot be detected by karyotyping techniques. This translocation results in the simultaneous deregulation of the fibroblast growth factor receptor 3 (*FGFR3*) gene on der(14) and the multiple myeloma SET domain (*MMSET*) gene on der(4). FGFR3 is one of the high-affinity tyrosine kinase receptors for the FGF family of ligands. Both *FGFR3* and *MMSET* genes are not normally expressed in plasma cells but are overexpressed as a result of t(4;14). However, gene expression profiling and RT-PCR analysis have shown that only 75% of MM cases with t(4;14) display simultaneous overexpression of MMSET and FGFR3. In the remaining 25% of cases, only MMSET is upregulated and the lack of FGFR3 expression is linked in most cases to loss of the *FGFR3* gene on der(14). These data suggest that *MMSET* may be the critical transforming event in MM harbouring t(4;14), whereas *FGFR3* could be dispensable. In some cases (10%) the translocated *FGFR3* contains activating mutations that may be involved in MM progression.

The incidence of t(14;16) is 5–10%. The breakpoints on 16q23 occur over a region 550–1350 kb centromeric to *MAF*. Taking into account such a long distance, it is still an open question whether or not *IGH* may act as enhancer for *MAF* in this translocation. Moreover, overexpression of MAF is observed in half of myeloma cases, while the prevalence of t(14;16) is low. The t(6;14) translocation has been found in a low proportion (3%) of MM cases. Using microarray analyses, high levels of cyclin D3 mRNA have been shown in cases with t(6;14) detected by FISH. The t(14;20) translocation leads to deregulation of *MAFB* (20q23), which like *MAF* encodes a B-ZIP transcription factor, but in contrast to t(14;16), *MAFB* translocations have structural features that indicate they are secondary translocations.

It should be noted that several FISH studies have shown that MGUS display similar numerical and structural chromosomal abnormalities to those observed in MM. Thus, the prevalence of *IGH* translocations in MGUS is similar to that in MM, which favours the hypothesis that *IGH* rearrangements are early genetic events in the tumorigenic process leading to MM. Interestingly, the existence of MGUS cases with t(4;14) that remain stable for many years suggests that this chromosomal abnormality would be insufficient for further progression to MM.

Some of these molecular events represent potential therapeutic targets. Thus the t(4;14) translocation generates constitutive activation of the oncogenic receptor tyrosine kinase FGFR3 with subsequent phosphorylation of the anti-apoptotic STAT3 signalling pathway. Therefore, the use of inhibitors of the FGFR3 tyrosine kinase, as well as inhibitors of cyclin-dependent kinases, could be attractive therapeutic targets. Similarly c-Maf, which is overexpressed in MM patients with t(14;16) as well as in some MM cases lacking this translocation, also represents a potential target.

Gains and losses of chromosomal material: monosomy 13, deletion of 17p and gains of 1q

Although *IGH* translocations are a hallmark in many cases of MM, there are other chromosomal abnormalities also involved in pathogenesis and prognosis that result in changes in chromosomal copy number. The loss of chromosome 13 is the most common monosomy in MM (40–50% of newly diagnosed patients). This abnormality shows a strong association with t(4;14) and t(14;16), deletion of 17p and gains on 1q. Chromosome 17p deletion, which includes loss of *TP53*, occurs at a lower frequency (5–10% of newly diagnosed MM), but its prognostic influence seems to be more important. Classical cytogenetics, FISH and comparative genomic hybridization analysis have all demonstrated that gains on 1q are some of the most common abnormalities in MM. Mostly they are the result of tandem duplications and jumping segmental duplications of the chromosome 1q band. The increased expression of *CKS1B* (1q21) detected in MM with gains of 1q has been suggested as the cause of increased proliferation in these cases.

Aneuploidy

Patients with MM may be grouped in two major categories according to ploidy status assessed by karyotyping: the hyperdiploid group (more than 46/47 chromosomes) and the non-hyperdiploid group, composed of hypodiploid (up to 44/45 chromosomes), pseudodiploid (44/45 to 46/47) and near tetraploid (more than 74). Non-hyperdiploid MM is characterized by a very high prevalence of *IGH* translocations involving the five recurrent partners. Likewise, monosomy/deletion 13 and gains on 1q occur predominantly in non-hyperdiploid MM. In contrast, the hyperdiploid group is associated with recurrent trisomies involving odd chromosomes (3, 5, 7, 9, 11, 15 and 19) and with a low incidence of structural chromosomal abnormalities. Similar associations have been observed on analysing DNA content by flow cytometry.

Late genetic events

Some genetic changes in MM, such as secondary translocations, mutations, deletions and epigenetic abnormalities, are considered late oncogenic events and are associated with disease progression. Dysregulation of *MYC* is a paradigm for secondary translocations in MM. Most karyotypic abnormalities involving *MYC* correspond to complex translocations and insertions that often are non-reciprocal and frequently involve three different chromosomes. Activating *RAS* mutations are considered molecular markers of disease progression. Thus, the prevalence of activating *KRAS* and *NRAS* mutations is over 75% in MM cases at relapse. *TP53* inactivation, via either deletion or mutation, seems to be more frequently associated with disease progression. Methylation is an epigenetic change that has been described in MM and acts as an inactivating mechanism of the tumour-suppressor genes *CDKN2B* and *CDKN2A*. Although it has also been detected in MGUS, its prevalence is much higher in advanced MM and extramedullary forms of the disease.

Molecular classification of MM based on gene expression profiling

Gene expression analysis of MM has confirmed the huge genetic diversity of this tumour. Recently, the classification of MM into seven different groups has been proposed. Each group displays a specific genetic signature and some of them are associated with a particular *IGH* translocation or ploidy status and with a characteristic clinical behaviour. Table 31.1 summarizes this classification, which connects genetic abnormalities, cell transcriptome and clinical features of patients.

Dysregulation of cyclin D genes as a potential unifying event in MM pathogenesis

There is no common genetic mechanism to explain the pathogenesis of MM. However, it can be speculated that although *IGH* translocations induce upregulation of different oncogenes, it is possible that all *IGH* translocations involved in MM converge on a common pathway resulting in inhibition of differentiation and an increase in cell survival and proliferation. Gene expression profiling analysis has demonstrated that expression of *CCND1*, *CCND2* and *CCND3* is increased in virtually all MM patients, supporting the recent hypothesis of a potential unifying event in pathogenesis. Approximately 25% of MM cases

display overexpression of one of these cyclins, which may be triggered directly by an *IGH* translocation such as t(11;14) and t(6;14) that dysregulates *CCND1* and *CCND3* respectively, or indirectly by an *IGH* translocation involving *MAF* and *MAFB* genes which encode a transcription factor that targets cyclin D2. Nearly 40% of MM cases express increased cyclin D1 through biallelic dysregulation of *CCND1* and without apparent t(11;14); most of the remaining cases of MM, including those with t(4;14), have increased expression of cyclin D2. The expression level of cyclin D has also been incorporated into the molecular classification (Table 31.1).

Interaction between plasma cells and their microenvironment

As far as the pathogenesis of MM is concerned, interactions between the myelomatous plasma cells and their microenvironment can be as important as the genetic lesions. In the bone marrow, MM cells adhere to extracellular matrix proteins and bone marrow stromal cells through a series of adhesion molecules, for example the β_1 integrin family (VLA-4, VLA-5, VLA-6; also called CD49d, CD49e and CD49f), intercellular adhesion molecule (ICAM)-1 and vascular cell adhesion molecule (VCAM)-1 (Figure 31.2). In addition, bone marrow stromal cells produce a stromal cell-derived factor (SDF)-1 that binds to CXCR4 on the surface of myeloma cells, inducing both

Table 31.1 Molecular classification of multiple myeloma.

Group	Specific translocation	Frequency (%)	Cyclin D expression	Genetic signature	Prognosis	Other characteristics
1 PR	–	12	CCND2	↑CCNB1, ↑CCNB2, ↑MCM2, ↑BUB1, ↑MAGEA6, ↑MAGEA3, ↑GAGE1	Unfavourable	Normal karyotypes
2 LB	–	11	CCND2	↑EDN1, ↑IL6R, ↓DKK1, ↓FRZB	Favourable	Lower number of bone lesions
3 MS	t(4;14) FGFR3/MMSET	18	CCND2	↑FGFR3, ↑MMSET, ↑PBX1, ↑PAX5	Unfavourable	
4 HY	–	26	CCND1	↑TRAIL, ↑DKK1, ↑FRZB, ↓CKS1B	Favourable	Hyperdiploid karyotype, bone lesions
5 CD-1	t(11;14) CCND1 or t(6;14) CCND3	8	CCND1 or CCND3	↑CEBPB, ↑NID2, ↑SET7	Favourable	
6 CD-2	t(11;14) CCND1 or t(6;14) CCND3	17	CCND1 or CCND3	↑MS4A1 (CD20), ↑PAX5, ↑CD27, ↑CXCR4	Favourable	
7 MF	t(14;16) MAF or t(14;20) MAFB	8	CCND2	↑MAF, ↑MAFB, ↑CXCR1, ↑ITGB7, ↓DKK1	Unfavourable	Lower number of bone lesions

PR, proliferation; LB, low bone disease; MS, *MMSET*; HY, hyperdiploid; CD-1: *CCND1/CCND3*; CD-2, *CCND1/CCND3*; MF, *MAF/MAFB*.

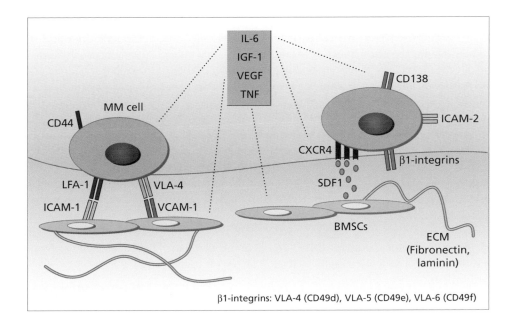

Figure 31.2 Interactions between plasma cells and the microenvironment. See text for definition of abbreviations.

chemotaxis of plasma cells and upregulation of surface adhesion molecules such as VLA-4. Bone marrow homing of plasma cells is likely further facilitated through other adhesion molecules expressed by myeloma cells, such as CD138, CD38, CD44 and CD106.

Adhesion of myeloma cells to the bone marrow microenvironment induces a cell adhesion-mediated drug resistance phenotype via three mechanisms: (i) cell cycle arrest at G_1 (associated with upregulation of p27, an inhibitor of cyclin-dependent kinases); (ii) apoptosis inhibition via upregulation of FLIP-L, an endogenous inhibitor of FAS (CD95); and (iii) protection of tumour cells from initial drug-induced DNA damage (double-strand breaks) by reducing topoisomerase II activity. The binding of MM cells to the bone marrow microenvironment also induces the transcription and secretion of cytokines, such as tumour necrosis factor (TNF)-α, interleukin (IL)-6, insulin-like growth factor (IGF)-1, IL-21, SDF-1α and vascular endothelial growth factor (VEGF), by both the plasma cells and the bone marrow stromal cells; this triggers signalling pathways (e.g. RAF/MEK/MAPK, PI3K/AKT and JAK/STAT) that promote cell proliferation and prevent apoptosis. These pathways are also potential targets for therapeutic intervention (Figure 31.3). In addition, cytokines modulate the production of additional adhesion molecules, which in a vicious circle enhance cell adhesion further.

In summary, it appears that the bone marrow microenvironment provides a sanctuary for myeloma cells by both promoting proliferation and blocking apoptosis, thereby allowing tumour progression and eventual emergence of drug resistance. Interruption by downregulating the interactions between the tumour cell and its microenvironment can potentially halt cell growth and proliferation and be of benefit to patients.

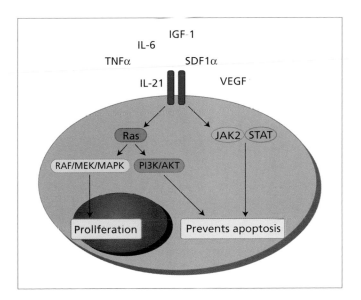

Figure 31.3 Signalling pathways involved in myeloma pathogenesis. See text for definition of abbreviations.

Influence of pathogenesis on the clinical features of MM and the development of bone lesions

The interaction between MM cells and the microenvironment not only favours tumour growth but is also responsible for the final myeloma portrait (see below). This interaction stimulates other cytokine cascades responsible for osteolytic lesions, which can result in bone pain, hypercalcaemia and neurological compression syndromes. Bone marrow infiltration also impairs normal haemopoiesis, leading to anaemia. MM cells secrete monoclonal protein (M-protein) that increases plasma viscosity. In addition, M-protein, and particularly light chains, are responsible for the impairment of renal function, leading ultimately to renal failure. Hypercalcaemia due to osteolytic disease may also contribute to renal failure. Patients are also at increased risk of developing potentially life-threatening infections due to the lack of functional immunoglobulins.

Bone disease is one of the hallmarks of MM (see below). Osteolysis is mediated by an imbalance between osteoclast activity (increased) and osteoblast activity (decreased). Adhesion of MM cells to stromal cells induces the secretion of osteoclast-activating factors such as TNF-α, IL-6, IL-1, matrix metalloproteinases, hepatocyte growth factors, parathyroid hormone-related protein, RANK-L, VEGF, IGF and macrophage inflammatory protein (MIP)-1α. Two of the most important are RANK-L (receptor activator of NF-κB ligand) and MIP-1α.

RANK-L is a transmembrane molecule, and is also called TRANCE (TNF-related activation-induced cytokine) or OPG-L (osteoprotegerin ligand). RANK-L binds to its functional receptor RANK (TNF receptor superfamily) on osteoclasts, stimulating osteoclastogenesis by inducing differentiation and maturation and stimulating resorption activity. Its activity can be blocked by osteoprotegerin (OPG), a receptor for OPG-L, which acts as a decoy receptor for RANK-L. Therefore osteoclastic activity is regulated by a delicate balance between RANK-L and OPG. In fact, under normal physiological conditions the levels of OPG are significantly higher than those of RANK-L. In contrast, in MM this balance is disrupted by increasing expression of RANK-L and decreasing expression of OPG. It has been suggested that the decline in OPG is mediated by myeloma cell uptake and degradation. MIP-1α is a potent stimulator of osteoclast formation through a dual mechanism: (i) it enhances the activity of RANK-L and (ii) it directly stimulates osteoclast precursors to differentiate into mature forms. MIP-1α gene expression is abnormally regulated in MM due to unbalanced expression of the acute myeloid leukaemia (AML)-1A and AML-1B transcription factors. This imbalance also induces IL-3, which stimulates osteoclast formation. In addition IL-3, as mentioned below, indirectly inhibits osteoblast formation.

In MM, in addition to the marked osteoclast activation, there is inhibition of osteoblast function. The WNT signalling pathway is critical for osteoblast differentiation. Indeed, the mesenchymal stem cell requires WNT signalling to differentiate into mature bone-forming osteoblasts. Myeloma cells produce DKK1, which inhibits the WNT pathway, and a soluble WNT inhibitor (sFRP-2) that suppresses osteoblast differentiation. Other relevant factors involved in osteoblast activity are RUNX2 and IL-3. The transcription factor RUNX2 is important in dividing mesenchymal stem cells to differentiated osteoblasts. MM patients with osteolytic lesions show a significant reduction of RUNX2, which may be the result of WNT signalling

inhibition by DKK1. IL-3 leads not only to increased osteoclast formation but also to inhibition of osteoblast differentiation. Bone marrow plasma from multiple myeloma patients, which exhibited high IL-3 levels, blocked osteoblast formation in human cultures, and this inhibition was partially reversed by the addition of a neutralizing antibody to human IL-3.

Differential diagnosis

The diagnostic criteria for the monoclonal gammopathies have been reviewed by the International Myeloma Working Group (IMWG). The main clinical entities are MGUS, primary systemic amyloidosis (see also Chapter 32), smouldering multiple myeloma and symptomatic multiple myeloma.

Monoclonal gammopathy of undetermined significance

MGUS has a high prevalence (3.2% and 5.8% in individuals over 50 and 70 years of age, respectively). MGUS is characterized by the presence of a serum M-protein (<30 g/L) and less than 10% plasma cells in the bone marrow with no evidence of other B-cell lymphoproliferative disorder and no symptoms or organ or tissue impairment due to the monoclonal gammopathy. The transformation rate to a malignant plasma cell disorder is about 1% per year, with an actuarial probability of malignant evolution of 30% at 25 years of follow-up. When the different causes of death are considered, the actuarial probability of malignant transformation at 25 years of follow-up is only 11%, much lower than the actuarial prediction. The main factors associated with MGUS progression include M-protein size, IgA isotype, abnormal free light-chain ratio and the 'evolving type' (rising M-protein during the first years of follow-up), and the presence of more than 95% phenotypically aberrant plasma cells within the bone marrow compartment.

When the proportion of bone marrow plasma cells is consistent with MGUS but the patient has a nephrotic syndrome, congestive heart failure, peripheral neuropathy, orthostatic hypotension or massive hepatomegaly, the most likely diagnosis is primary systemic amyloidosis resulting from the deposition of amyloidogenic light chains. On the other hand, in a patient with constitutional symptoms, lytic bone lesions, a small M-spike and less than 10% plasma cells in the bone marrow, the most likely diagnosis is metastatic carcinoma with coincidental MGUS.

Smouldering multiple myeloma

The term 'smouldering multiple myeloma' was first defined by Kyle and Greipp as the presence of a serum M-protein (>30 g/L) and 10% or more plasma cells in the bone marrow in the absence of lytic bone lesions or clinical manifestations due to

Table 31.2 Myeloma related organ or tissue impairment (end-organ damage) due to the plasma cell proliferative process.

Increased serum calcium
Renal insufficiency
Anaemia: haemoglobin 2 g/dL below the lowest normal limit
Bone lesions: lytic lesions or osteoporosis with compression fractures (possibly confirmed by MRI or CT)
Other: symptomatic hyperviscosity (rare), amyloidosis, recurrent bacterial infections (more than 2 episodes in 12 months), extramedullary plasmacytomas

Table 31.3 Symptomatic multiple myeloma.*

M-protein in serum and/or urine
Bone marrow (clonal) plasma cells or plasmacytoma[†]
Related organ or tissue impairment (end-organ damage, including bone lesions)

*Some patients may have no symptoms but have related organ or tissue impairment.
[†]If flow cytometry is performed, most plasma cells (>90%) will show a 'neoplastic' phenotype.

the monoclonal gammopathy. More recently, the IMWG considered that the term 'asymptomatic myeloma' could be more appropriate. This condition was defined as the presence of an M-protein ($\geq$30 g/L) and/or 10% or greater bone marrow plasma cells in the absence of symptoms or organ or tissue impairment due to the monoclonal gammopathy. About 10% of patients diagnosed with MM have smouldering disease. This situation is clinically and biologically very close to that observed in MGUS. However, the plasma cell mass is much higher and most cases will eventually evolve into symptomatic MM.

The risk of transformation is 10% per year during the first 5 years and then decreases to 3% in the subsequent 5 years, with a cumulative probability of progression of 73% at 15 years. Risk factors for transformation include high M-component, IgA isotype, more than 20% plasma cells in the bone marrow, presence of urinary light chains, immunoparesis, abnormal free light-chain ratio, and the presence of more than 95% phenotypically aberrant plasma cells within the bone marrow compartment.

Symptomatic multiple myeloma

The diagnosis of symptomatic MM requires the presence of an M-protein in serum and/or urine, increased plasma cells in the bone marrow or plasmacytoma, and related-organ or tissue impairment (including bone lesions). The more common symptoms are fatigue from anaemia and bone pain due to the skeletal involvement. Some patients may have no symptoms but they can have related organ or tissue impairment. Clinical and laboratory features may include anaemia, skeletal involvement (lytic lesions and/or severe osteoporosis with or without compression fractures), renal failure, hypercalcaemia, recurrent bacterial infections, extramedullary plasmacytomas or associated amyloidosis (Table 31.2). The criteria agreed by the IMWG for the diagnosis of symptomatic MM are shown in Table 31.3. Of note, no serum or urine M-protein values were included, since about 40% of patients with symptomatic MM have a serum M-protein level lower than 30 g/L and 3% have non-secretory myeloma. In the same sense, no minimal proportion of bone marrow plasma cells was required because about 5% of

Table 31.4 Laboratory work-up for a patient with monoclonal gammopathy.

History and physical examination
Complete blood count and differential peripheral blood film
Chemistry including calcium and creatinine
Serum protein electrophoresis and immunofixation
Nephelometric quantification of immunoglobulins
24-hour urine collection for electrophoresis and immunofixation
Bone marrow aspirate (cytogenetics, immunophenotyping and plasma cell labelling index if available)
Radiological skeletal bone survey: CT or MRI may be helpful
β_2-Microglobulin, C-reactive protein and lactate dehydrogenase
Measurement of free monoclonal light chains if available

patients with well-documented symptomatic MM have less than 10% plasma cells in their bone marrow. Table 31.4 illustrates the laboratory work-up for patients with monoclonal gammopathies.

Other special forms of plasma cell dyscrasia

Plasma cell leukaemia

Plasma cell leukaemia was initially described by Kyle in 1974 as a plasma cell disorder characterized by a relative peripheral blood plasmacytosis of more than 20% of total nucleated cells, or an absolute number of plasma cells greater than 2×10^9/L. There are two forms of plasma cell leukaemia: the *de novo* presentation in leukaemic phase, and secondary cases corresponding to already diagnosed MM that evolve into a leukaemic phase. The clinical course of plasma cell leukaemia is usually very aggressive and resistant to conventional treatment and therefore new agents should be urgently investigated in these patients.

Solitary plasmacytoma of bone

The existence of a solitary plasmacytoma has been recognized in up to 3% of patients with a plasma cell dyscrasia, usually on the vertebral column. The diagnostic criteria require the existence of a solitary plasma cell tumour in which the biopsy confirms plasma cell histology, a negative skeletal survey, absence of plasma cell infiltration in a random bone sample (<10%), as well as no evidence of anaemia, hypercalcaemia or renal impairment. Some groups suggest that patients in whom a paraprotein persists after the eradication of plasmacytoma with local treatment should undergo a review of the diagnosis. The treatment of choice is local radiotherapy, but about two-thirds of patients with solitary bone plasmacytoma develop MM at 10 years' follow-up, with a median time to progression of 2 years.

Extramedullary plasmacytoma

Extramedullary plasmacytoma is a plasma cell tumour that arises outside the bone marrow, most frequently in the upper respiratory tract (nose, paranasal sinuses, nasopharynx and tonsils). Other sites include parathyroid gland, orbit, lung, spleen, gastrointestinal tract, testes and skin. In most cases the lesion is unique, although the presence of more lesions (multiple plasmacytomas) has also been reported. Diagnosis is based on the detection of the plasma cell tumour in an extramedullary site, in the absence of bone marrow plasma cell infiltration, bone lytic lesions and other signs of MM (end-organ damage).

Non-secretory multiple myeloma

This specific type of MM requires particular attention, since it is very difficult to diagnose. The only way to make a definitive diagnosis is to demonstrate the presence of tissue infiltration (usually bone marrow) by cells with plasma cell morphology. However, plasma cell infiltration must be greater than 10% and clonality must be assessed by immunophenotyping (demonstration of cytoplasmic immunoglobulins with restricted light chain: positive production without excretion). In addition, the serum free light chains are abnormal and this is a most useful parameter for the follow-up of these patients. However, exceptional cases exist in which no monoclonal protein can be observed within the plasma cells. In these cases, it is mandatory to demonstrate clonality by the study of the rearrangement status of the immunoglobulin genes. Additional detection of aneuploid DNA content by flow cytometry or an abnormal clone by cytogenetics may be helpful.

IgM multiple myeloma

This exceptional form of myeloma has been reported very rarely and must be distinguished from Waldenström macroglobulinaemia. The morphology and immunophenotype of the infiltrating cells will give the definitive diagnosis, as well as the existence of osteolytic lesions, which are absent in Waldenström macroglobulinaemia.

Osteosclerotic myeloma (POEMS syndrome)

POEMS syndrome is characterized by polyneuropathy, organomegaly, endocrinopathy, M-protein and skin changes. The clinical picture consists of a chronic inflammatory demyelinating polyneuropathy, more motor than sensory, and osteosclerotic lesions. Hepatomegaly is observed in half of the patients. Hyperpigmentation, hypertrichosis, angiomatous lesions on the trunk, gynaecomastia and testicular atrophy may occur. Papilloedema is frequently present. The M-protein is commonly of IgA λ type (<30 g/L) and the bone marrow contains less than 5% plasma cells. Thrombocytosis is common. Castleman disease can be associated and VEGF is universally increased. Biopsy of an osteosclerotic lesion is generally necessary to confirm the diagnosis.

Disease complications and their management

Figure 31.4 illustrates the clinical manifestations of multiple myeloma.

Skeletal involvement

Bone involvement is the most frequent clinical complication in patients with MM. About 70% of patients have lytic bone lesions with or without osteoporosis and another 20% have severe osteoporosis without lytic lesions. The skeletal involvement leads to bone pain and can result in pathological fractures. The pathophysiology of bone disease has been described above. Some patients develop pathological fractures of long bones and require orthopaedic surgery. In the event of extensive lesions, surgery can be followed by radiation therapy. On the other hand, prophylactic orthopaedic intervention must be considered in patients with large lytic lesions at high risk of fracture. It is important to consider that patients with severe back pain due to vertebral compression fractures can benefit from vertebroplasty or kyphoplasty. Spinal cord compression caused by a vertebral fracture is very rare in patients with MM. This complication is usually caused by a plasmacytoma arising from a vertebral body.

Between 15 and 20% of patients with MM have hypercalcaemia at the time of diagnosis. A common complication of hypercalcaemia is renal impairment caused by interstitial nephritis. Treatment of hypercalcaemia with hydration and bisphosphonates is a medical emergency. Zoledronic acid is the bisphosphonate of choice (quicker response and significantly longer time to recurrence compared with pamidronate). With the

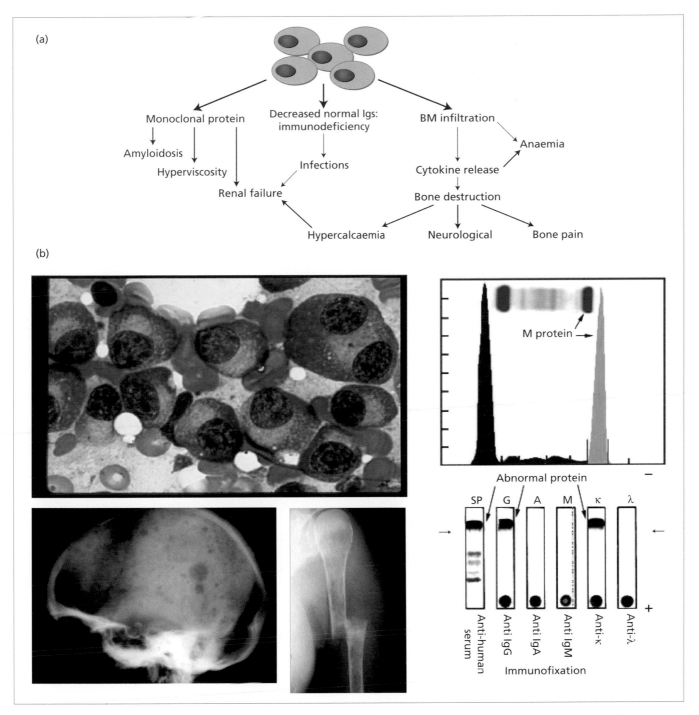

(a)

Monoclonal protein

Amyloidosis

Hyperviscosity

Renal failure

Decreased normal Igs: immunodeficiency

Infections

BM infiltration

Anaemia

Cytokine release

Bone destruction

Hypercalcaemia

Neurological

Bone pain

(b)

M protein

Abnormal protein

SP G A M κ λ

Anti-human serum

Anti IgG

Anti IgA

Anti IgM

Anti-κ

Anti-λ

Immunofixation

Figure 31.4 (a) Clinical manifestations in myeloma and (b) bone marrow infiltration, monoclonal band (IgGK by immunofixation) osteolytic lesions resulting in a pathological fracture.

availability of zoledronic acid, forced diuresis and glucocorticoids are usually no longer necessary.

Oral clodronate and the intravenous agents pamidronate and zoledronic acid are of clinical benefit in the treatment of bone disease in patients with MM. For different reasons clodronate has not been extensively used in clinical practice outside the UK and the Nordic countries. Pamidronate is administered at a monthly dose of 90 mg via a 2-hour intravenous infusion. Zoledronic acid, at a monthly dose of 4 mg, is at least as effective as pamidronate and has the advantage that it can be administered via a 15-min infusion. In patients with renal function impairment, the dose of zoledronic acid must be reduced to a

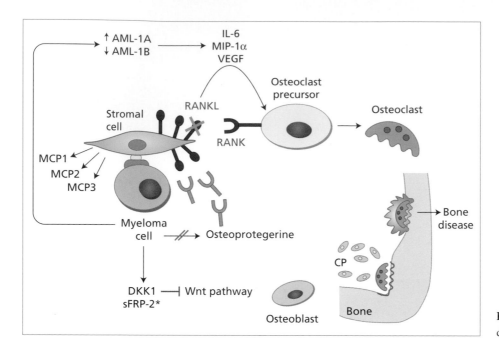

Figure 31.5 Pathogenesis of bone disease. (For abbreviations, see text)

maximum of 3 mg. A panel from the American Society of Clinical Oncology (ASCO) recommended the use of either pamidronate or zoledronic acid in patients with MM with either lytic bone lesions or osteoporosis. It was suggested that bisphosphonates should be used indefinitely once initiated. However, the appearance of severe late complications, such as osteonecrosis of the jaw, related to the duration of bisphosphonate exposure has resulted in a reconsideration of the initial recommendations. Osteonecrosis of the jaw is associated with the duration of bisphosphonate exposure, type of bisphosphonate (higher with zoledronic acid than with pamidronate) and history of recent dental procedure. The current recommendations for treatment with bisphosphonates in MM patients, based on a Mayo Clinic consensus statement as well as consensus panels from both the IMWG and the ASCO, do not recommend the initial use of bisphosphonates for more than 2 years. In relapsed patients treatment with bisphosphonates can be restarted and administered concomitantly with active therapy. Finally, in patients in whom the bone disease is a consequence of excess RANK-L activity, newer molecules such as denosumab might be of benefit. The pathogenesis of myeloma bone disease is summarized in Figure 31.5.

Renal failure

About 20% of patients with MM have a serum creatinine higher than 177 μmol/L (2 mg/dL) at diagnosis. The degree of renal failure is usually moderate, with a serum creatinine lower than 354 μmol/L (4 mg/dL). However, in some series up to 10% of patients with newly diagnosed MM have renal failure severe enough to require dialysis from the time of diagnosis. The main causes of renal failure in MM are (i) light-chain excretion resulting in cast nephropathy (myeloma kidney) and (ii) glomerular deposition of immunoglobulin (light-chain amyloidosis or immunoglobulin deposition disease). In myeloma kidney, the typical feature consists of the presence of myeloma casts, mainly composed of light chains, in the distal tubules and collecting ducts. There is a correlation between the degree of cast formation and the severity of renal failure. Light-chain tissue deposition usually consists of glomerular deposits of immunoglobulins resulting in nephrotic syndrome. The amyloid deposits are fibrillar structures of light chains showing positive Congo red staining. In light-chain deposition disease, the deposit of light-chain immunoglobulins is non-fibrillar (Congo red negative). In contrast with amyloidosis, the light chain is usually of κ type. The characteristic clinical feature is a nephrotic syndrome, but renal function can rapidly deteriorate resembling glomerulonephritis (see also Chapter 32).

The median survival of patients with MM and renal insufficiency is less than 1 year. However, the prognosis mainly depends on the reversibility of renal function. Thus, the median survival of patients with reversible renal failure is similar to that of patients with normal renal function, whereas patients with non-reversible renal failure have a median survival of less than 6 months. The factors associated with renal function recovery include serum creatinine lower than 354 μmol/L (4 mg/dL), 24-hour urinary protein excretion lower than 1 g, and serum calcium higher than 2.875 mmol/L (11.5 mg/dL).

Vincristine, doxorubicin (Adriamycin) and high-dose dexamethasone (VAD), or cyclophosphamide and dexamethasone, or even dexamethasone alone in very fragile patients, appear to be better approaches than melphalan-containing regimens because of both lower myelosuppression and quicker action. Of these, the most frequently used has been VAD. However, it seems that the effect of vincristine and doxorubicin is only marginal, the efficacy of VAD mainly coming from high-dose dexamethasone. In addition, a randomized trial from the Nordic Myeloma Study Group has recently shown that the association of dexamethasone and cyclophosphamide was more convenient and as effective as VAD when given as up-front therapy. The novel drugs introduced for myeloma treatment may also be of great value in patients with renal failure. Taking into account that the action of bortezomib is very quick, it is probably an ideal agent for rapidly decreasing light chains in order to prevent the development of irreversible renal failure by avoiding further tubular light-chain damage. In a retrospective series of 24 patients with relapsed/refractory MM and dialysis-dependent renal failure, the overall response rate (RR) was 75%, with 30% complete remissions (CR) or near-CR. Hopefully, ongoing prospective studies will confirm the benefit of borte-zomib-based therapies in patients with newly diagnosed myeloma and renal failure. The association of lenalidomide and dexamethasone could also be a good treatment option for patients with renal failure. However, the dose of lenalidomide must be adjusted to the degree of renal failure according to the guidelines for the use of lenalidomide in patients with renal function impairment. Although thalidomide has been used for more than 10 years, little information on its efficacy and toxicity in patients with renal failure is available, but it is also probably a useful agent for these patients.

With regard to the use of high-dose therapy/autologous stem cell transplantation (SCT) in patients with MM and renal failure, the largest experience comes from the Arkansas group, with a reversibility of renal failure of 43% but higher morbidity and mortality (6% and 13% after a single or tandem transplant, respectively) than in patients with normal renal function. Chemoresistant disease, low serum albumin and older age were associated with a poorer outcome. According to the results of a Spanish group, patients with serum creatinine above 442 μmol/L (5 mg/dL), haemoglobin below 9.5 g/dL and/or poor perform-ance status should be excluded from autologous SCT because of the high transplant-related mortality (TRM). In patients with no overt myeloma and low plasma cell mass in whom renal function impairment is due to glomerular light-chain deposi-tion (light-chain deposition disease), the likelihood of response is higher than that in MM because of the low plasma cell mass at the time of transplantation. In this situation there is no need for tumour reduction with induction chemotherapy before stem cell mobilization and high-dose therapy.

Theoretically, the removal of nephrotoxic light chains with plasma exchange could avoid further renal failure and hopefully prevent irreversible renal failure. The Mayo Clinic group, in a small controlled trial, compared chemotherapy with chemo-therapy plus plasma exchange and found only a trend in favour of the group including plasma exchange. Similarly, in a large randomized trial there was no conclusive evidence that plasma exchange improved the outcome of patients with MM and acute renal failure. In our experience, patients with renal failure severe enough to require dialysis do not benefit from plasma exchange. However, it is our belief that in non-oliguric patients an early plasma exchange programme along with forced diure-sis and chemotherapy could be of benefit. When excluding the patients who die in this early period, the median survival of patients with MM and non-reversible renal failure needing chronic dialysis is almost 2 years and 30% of them survive for more than 3 years. Thus, long-term dialysis is a worthwhile supportive measure for patients with MM and end-stage renal failure.

Anaemia and bone marrow failure

Approximately 35% of patients with newly diagnosed MM have a haemoglobin lower than 9 g/dL. In addition, severe anaemia is a frequent complication later in the course of the disease due to disease progression. Anaemia is associated with a significant loss in quality of life and poor prognosis. The main causes of anaemia in MM are bone marrow replacement by plasma cells, relative erythropoietin deficiency, renal insufficiency and chem-otherapy with cytotoxic agents.

Severe granulocytopenia and thrombocytopenia at the time of diagnosis are unusual. About 10% of patients have a platelet count of less than 100×10^9/L, but platelet counts lower than 20×10^9/L with risk of severe bleeding are very unusual. The development of an unexplained pancytopenia in patients previ-ously treated with alkylating agents, particularly melphalan, is suspicious of myelodysplasia.

A number of trials have shown the beneficial effect of recom-binant human erythropoietins and darbepoetin alfa in the treatment of myeloma-associated anaemia. The response to erythropoietin is associated with a significant improvement in quality of life. An important aspect is that the most significant improvement in quality of life is reached when the haemoglobin increases from 11 to 12 g/dL, but levels above 14 g/dL should be avoided due to its association with a higher risk of thrombosis. Thus, the goal should be maintenance of the haemoglobin around 12 g/dL, with careful dose tritiation in order to achieve a good quality of life while minimizing severe complications such as thrombotic events. The major cause of erythropoietin failure is iron deficiency. Iron repletion should be indicated when there is evidence of functional iron deficiency measured by an increased soluble transferrin receptor. The efficacy of oral iron is limited. It seems that the best iron supplemental therapy is the administration of iron saccharate. Treatment with granu-locyte colony-stimulating factor (G-CSF) may be required to treat chemotherapy-induced severe granulocytopenia. Patients treated with lenalidomide may occasionally require G-CSF therapy.

Infection

Infectious complications are the major cause of morbidity and mortality in patients with MM. The highest risk of infection is observed during the first 2 months of starting therapy, in patients with severe chemotherapy-induced granulocytopenia and in those with relapsed and refractory disease. The main cause of infection in MM is the impaired antibody production, leading to a decrease in the uninvolved immunoglobulins. Other important causes include chemotherapy-induced granulocytopenia, renal function impairment and glucocorticoid treatment, particularly high-dose dexamethasone. Most infections in newly diagnosed patients and during the first cycles of chemotherapy are caused by *Streptococcus pneumoniae*, *Staphylococcus aureus* and *Haemophilus influenzae*, while in patients with renal failure, as well as in those with relapsed and/or refractory advanced disease, more than 90% of the infectious episodes are caused by Gram-negative bacilli or *Staph. aureus*.

An infectious episode in a patient with MM should be managed as a potentially serious complication requiring immediate therapy. In case of suspected severe infection and before the identification of the causal agent, treatment against encapsulated bacteria and Gram-negative microorganisms should be initiated. Although prophylaxis of infection in patients with MM is a controversial issue, some general guidelines can be offered. Intravenous immunoglobulin prophylaxis is not recommended. Pneumococcal vaccination is recommended, particularly in patients with IgG myeloma with high-serum M-protein levels, which are usually associated with very low levels of uninvolved immunoglobulins. Antibiotic prophylaxis is likely of benefit within the first 2 months of initiation of therapy, especially in patients at high risk of infection (recent past history of serious infections, such as recurrent pneumonia, or renal failure).

Nervous system involvement

Spinal cord compression from a plasmacytoma, which occurs in about 10% of patients, is the most frequent and serious neurological complication in MM. The dorsal spine is the most common site of involvement, followed by the lumbar region. The clinical picture of spinal cord compression consists of back pain and paraparesis. Although it can evolve for several days or even a few weeks, the onset can be abrupt, resulting in severe paraparesis or paraplegia in a few hours. The picture is usually accompanied by a sensitive level. Lumbar involvement can cause a cauda equina syndrome (low back pain with radicular distribution and leg weakness).

Spinal cord compression is an emergency requiring immediate medical action. When suspected, urgent magnetic resonance imaging (MRI) should be performed. If confirmed, treatment with high-dose dexamethasone must be started immediately at a loading dose of 100 mg followed by 25 mg every 6 hours followed by progressive tapering. Local radiation therapy should be started as soon as possible, simultaneously with high-dose dexamethasone. If the spinal cord compression is caused by a vertebral collapse or by spinal instability rather than a plasmacytoma (which is very rare), urgent surgical decompression followed by fixation of a prothesis of bone graft or methacrylate is required.

Nerve root compression can cause back pain that follows a radicular metameric distribution with or without radicular sensory involvement. Treatment with radiation therapy is helpful, allowing time for the action of systemic chemotherapy. Clinically significant peripheral neuropathy is very uncommon in newly diagnosed patients with MM. Leptomeningeal involvement in the central nervous system (CNS) with detection of plasma cells in the cerebrospinal fluid (CSF) is exceedingly rare. The frequency of CNS involvement is roughly 1%, the most frequent presenting features being paraparesis, symptoms from increased intracranial pressure, cranial nerves palsies and confusion. The CSF examination frequently shows plasma cells of plasmablastic morphology as well as an increased protein concentration with positive immunofixation for the myeloma protein. Unfortunately, despite active treatment measures such as intrathecal therapy (methotrexate, cytarabine, glucocorticoids), cranial or even craniospinal irradiation along with systemic therapy, the prognosis is extremely poor with a median survival of 3 months from the diagnosis of CNS involvement.

Prognostic factors

The outcome for patients with MM is highly heterogeneous, with survival duration ranging from a few months to more than 10 years. This heterogeneity relates to (i) specific characteristics of the tumour itself, (ii) host factors and (iii) a series of factors resulting from the interaction between the tumour clone and the host, which mainly reflect tumour burden and disease complications (Table 31.5).

Host factors

The favourable influence of a good performance status (ECOG $\geq$ 2) and young age (<65–70 years) is well established. In contrast, neither sex nor race has prognostic influence. Immune surveillance, by T and natural killer (NK) cells, plays a relevant role in most malignancies, and low numbers of mature NK and CD4 cells have been reported in advanced-stage MM. In addition, patients who develop expanded T-cell clones (CD8$^+$CD57$^+$CD28$^-$), which can recognize autologous idiotypic immunoglobulin structures, display favourable outcome.

Table 31.5 Prognostic factors in MM.

Prognostic factors	Tumour related	Host related	Tumour burden
Essential	Cytogenetics/FISH: t(4;14), t(14;16), TP53, RB	Age Performance status	Internatonal Staging System (β_2-microglobulin/albumin)
Additional	Plasma cell proliferation Immunophenotyping markers		
New and promising	Gene molecular markers: PSMD9 (p27), CKS1B (1q21)	Immune status	Circulating clonotypic plasma cells sRANK-L

Malignant clone factors

The second cohort of prognostic factors are those that reflect specific characteristics of myelomatous plasma cells and include morphology, immunophenotyping, cytogenetics, oncogenes, multidrug resistance and proliferative activity of plasma cells. Immature/plasmablastic morphology is associated with poor outcome. With regard to antigen expression, we have observed that downregulation of CD117 (c-Kit) and CD56, and expression of CD28 and CD19, are associated with poor prognosis. As occurs with acute leukaemia, cytogenetics is emerging as one of the most important prognostic tools for MM. Therefore, investigation of cytogenetic changes (mainly by FISH, since cells from MM patients frequently do not yield mitoses in conventional karyotyping) should be mandatory in all newly diagnosed MM patients. Among IGH translocations, t(4;14) and t(14;16) have been consistently associated with unfavourable prognosis, whereas t(11;14) does not have a negative influence on survival. Initial studies indicated that monosomy 13/del(13) was associated with poor outcome; however, recent analyses based on large series of MM patients have revealed that the presence of monosomy 13/del(13) as a unique abnormality, without concomitant IGH abnormalities, is probably not indicative of unfavourable prognosis. In contrast, del(17p) (with deletion of the TP53 gene) is one of the most, if not the most, adverse prognostic factor in MM. It has also been reported that amplifications on 1q and del(22) are associated with poor outcome, although this requires confirmation in larger series of patients. Moreover, the presence of complex as well as non-hyperdiploid karyotypes also predict treatment failure. Similarly, patients with chromosome losses detected by comparative genomic hybridization display very short survival. In contrast, hyperdiploid tumours with multiple trisomies involving chromosomes 3, 5, 7, 9, 11, 15, 19 and 21 tend to have a favourable prognosis. In line with this latter observation, we have shown that patients with hyperdiploid DNA cell content (defined by flow cytometry) have a favourable outcome. Finally, the proliferative activity of the malignant plasma cells, as assessed either by the labelling index with bromodeoxyuridine or by flow cytometry, is one of the most important prognostic markers.

Tumour burden and disease complications

A high proportion of plasma cells in the bone marrow, diffuse bone marrow infiltration and the presence of circulating plasma cells reflect a high tumour burden, but their prognostic influence is modest. Similarly, the impact of skeletal lesions, evaluated by radiography or bone resorption markers, is not clear. In contrast, disease complications such as anaemia, thrombocytopenia and particularly renal insufficiency have a major influence. Nevertheless, the most important factor is the concentration of β_2-microglobulin, which increases as a result of both growth of tumour burden and deterioration in renal function. The higher the value, the worse the prognosis. In contrast, β_2-microglobulin is not helpful for disease monitoring. C-reactive protein is a surrogate marker for IL-6 (a major plasma cell growth factor), which also correlates with outcome. In contrast to hypoalbuminaemia, neither the amount of paraprotein nor its isotype influences prognosis.

Only a few of the prognostic factors have real independent value. A summary of the most important is shown below.

1 Two host factors (age and performance status) reflect the ability of the patient to tolerate chemotherapy.

2 Two intrinsic characteristics of the malignant clone (cytogenetics and plasma cell proliferative activity).

3 One biochemical marker that reflects tumour burden (β_2-microglobulin).

A new International Staging System (ISS), derived from more than 11 000 patients, has shown that β_2-microglobulin and albumin are the best combination of easily available markers for discriminating prognostic subgroups: stage I (β_2-microglobulin <3.5 mg/dL, albumin >3.5 mg/dL); stage III (β_2-microglobulin >5.5 mg/dL); stage II (the rest). This substitutes for the Durie and Salmon classification, which affords little prognostic information. In the next few years improved staging systems using cytogenetics and S-phase analysis should be developed for use by reference centres and eventually for all patients with myeloma.

Response to therapy as a prognostic factor

In addition to all the variables that can be measured at diagnosis and which have already been mentioned, response to front-line therapy represents one of the most important prognostic factors in most haematological malignancies. In the case of MM there is still open debate about the importance of the depth of response on patient outcome. The reason for this controversy is probably that, historically, until the introduction of high-dose chemotherapy, CR was extremely rare and the only available comparison was between responding patients (achieving partial or minor responses) and non-responding patients, with the former having a better outcome. A recently published meta-analysis including 21 reports with independent datasets for which outcome data were reported has shown a very significant association between the maximal response obtained after treatment and the two main long-term-outcome parameters, i.e. overall survival (OS) and time to progression-related events. However, it is clear that more sensitive techniques (e.g. multiparametric immunophenotyping, molecular analysis of bone marrow plasma cells by PCR, serum free light chain test, and imaging techniques such as MRI or positron emission tomography to detect myeloma activity outside the bone marrow) are needed to evaluate response in MM and these may contribute to a better assessment of the impact of response in final outcome. We have shown that when transplanted MM patients show undetectable residual myelomatous plasma cells by immunophenotyping, progression-free survival (PFS) and OS are significantly longer, and this parameter is significantly more powerful than negative immunofixation.

Criteria of response

Response criteria were initially developed by the Chronic Leukaemia and Myeloma Task Force (CLMTF) in 1968. The main response parameter was a minimum 50% reduction in the M-protein. In 1972 the Southwest Oncology Group (SWOG) defined partial response (PR) as a reduction of at least 75% in the calculated serum paraprotein synthetic rate and/or a decrease of at least 90% in urinary light chain urine protein excretion sustained for at least 2 months. The Medical Research Council (MRC) introduced the concept of plateau phase, defined as a period of stability after chemotherapy in which tumour progression does not occur despite the presence of measurable disease. The minimum period of stability required for definition of plateau phase was 3 months. Since CRs were rarely observed with the classical conventional dose chemotherapy, neither the CLMTF nor the SWOG response criteria included a definition of CR. In addition there were no definitions for relapse and progression.

EBMT criteria for response, relapse and progression

With the introduction of high-dose therapy/SCT, the M-protein disappears in a significant number of patients, a fact that is associated with a significant prolongation of survival. In this context, the European Group for Blood and Marrow Transplantation (EBMT) developed new criteria defining CR (negative immunofixation in serum and urine and less than 5% bone marrow plasma cells), PR ($\geq$50% reduction in serum M-component and $\geq$90% in 24-hour urine Bence Jones proteinuria), minimal response (MR) (25–49% decrease in M-component), as well as criteria for relapse (reappearance of M-protein by immunofixation in patient who had achieved CR, and progression from PR or MR). Any type of response should be maintained for a minimum of 6 weeks. These criteria have been shown to be useful and reproducible in both transplant and non-transplant series as well as in prospective clinical trials.

Uniform response criteria

The IMWG has expanded the EBMT criteria by adding the categories of stringent CR (sCR) and very good partial response (VGPR) (Table 31.6). Patients with negative immunofixation in serum and urine and with a normal free light-chain ratio are considered in sCR. The free light-chain measurement has also been included for the evaluation of response in patients with non-secretory and oligosecretory disease. VGPR requires a decrease in the M-protein size of at least 90%. In addition, time to event, duration of response, clinical relapse and time to

Table 31.6 International uniform response criteria for multiple myeloma (IMWG response criteria).

Response category*	Criteria
Complete remission (CR)	Negative immunofixation (serum and urine)
	<5% bone marrow plasma cells
	No soft tissue plasmacytomas
Stringent CR	As above, *plus*
	Normal free light-chain ratio
	Absence of clonal plasma cells[†]
Very good partial response	$\geq$90% decrease in serum M-protein
	Urine M-protein <100 mg per 24 hours
Partial response	$\geq$50% decrease in serum M-protein
	$\geq$90% decrease in urine M-protein or <200 mg per 24 hours
	$\geq$50% decrease in soft tissue plasmacytomas

*All response categories require two consecutive measurements made at any time.
[†]Determined by immunohistochemistry or immunofluorescence.

alternative therapy are emphasized as critical end points. More recently, the IMWG has considered the possibility of also adding the parameters 'CR by immunophenotyping' and 'CR by molecular techniques', as well as the reintroduction of minor responses for treatment evaluation of relapse/refractory patients.

Treatment

In this section we focus on the treatment of the malignant clone, since the management of disease complications (anaemia, renal insufficiency, bone disease) has been discussed above.

Melphalan–prednisone (MP) was introduced for the treatment of MM in the late 1960s. In the subsequent 30 years treatment improvements remained stagnant, since more complex chemotherapy combinations (e.g. VCMP, VBAD, VAD) only led to small increases in the overall RR but without differences in survival, as assessed in a large meta-analysis that included over 6000 patients. The next step forward was the use of high-dose melphalan followed by stem cell support (autologous SCT) for young mycloma patients, which resulted in a significant improvement in disease-free survival and OS. However, for elderly patients, MP remained the standard of care. From 2000, there was a revolution in the treatment of MM with the availability of new agents with distinct mechanisms of action: the immunomodulatory drugs thalidomide and lenalidomide (Revlimid) and the proteasome inhibitor bortezomib (Velcade).

In this section we first discuss the treatment of newly diagnosed patients stratified according to age (above or below 65–70 years), which categorizes the patients as transplant or non-transplant candidates, and then analyse the options for relapse/refractory patients, as well as emerging novel agents.

Treatment of newly diagnosed transplant candidate patients

Currently, treatment in this setting usually includes three to six cycles of induction therapy, consolidation with autologous SCT and the possibility of maintenance therapy.

Induction

The VAD combination has long been the gold standard as a preparatory regimen for young newly diagnosed MM patients who are candidates for autologous SCT, with PR rates ranging from 52 to 63% and CR rates from 3 to 13%. However, novel drug combinations appear to be superior to VAD-like regimens for decreasing tumour burden before transplantation. As shown in Table 31.7, three randomized trials have compared thalidomide (T)-based regimens (TD or TAD or TVAD) versus either high-dose dexamethasone or VAD as initial therapy in transplant-eligible patients. In all studies, thalidomide combinations

were superior to conventional induction treatment, although the response rate (PR or greater) obtained with thalidomide plus dexamethasone (63%) was lower than that achieved with TAD or TVAD (80%, with CR rates usually <10%). The MRC group has compared cyclophosphamide (C) plus thalidomide and dexamethasone with CVAD as induction regimen before transplantation; the thalidomide arm was significantly superior (RR 87% vs. 75%; CR 20% vs. 12%). In studies evaluating bortezomib combination therapy, data from a French randomized trial that compared bortezomib plus dexamethasone with VAD show the superiority of bortezomib plus dexamethasone, both before and after transplantation (Table 31.7). The Italian group has reported similar results on comparing bortezomib, thalidomide and dexamethasone with thalidomide and dexamethasone (Table 31.7). The high efficacy of bortezomib-based regimens as induction treatment is consistent with several pilot studies using either bortezomib plus dexamethasone alone or in combination with doxorubicin (Adriamycin/Doxil) or thalidomide, with RRs usually over 80% and CR rates of 18–32%. With regard to lenalidomide, two large randomized studies have shown that the majority of patients (>85%) respond to lenalidomide plus dexamethasone induction, but a minimum of four to six cycles would probably be required to achieve a substantial number of CRs. Thalidomide or bortezomib combinations did not affect stem cell collection or granulocyte and platelet recovery after transplantation. For lenalidomide, three recent reports indicate a decrease in CD34-positive cells collected and recommended harvesting early in the course of induction with lenalidomide and/or using cyclophosphamide along with G-CSF. Although these novel induction regimens appear to be clearly superior to VAD, a longer follow-up is still required.

Autologous stem cell transplantation

High-dose therapy (usually melphalan 200 mg/m^2) followed by autologous SCT prolonged OS compared with standard-dose therapy in prospective randomized trials conducted by the French (IFM) and English (MRC) groups and has provided evidence for more than 10-year survivorship in at least a subset of patients. Nevertheless, although the SWOG 9321 study in the USA, the French MAG91 study and the Spanish PETHEMA-94 trial confirmed the benefit of autologous SCT in terms of RR and event-free survival (EFS), they did not find superiority in terms of survival compared with standard-dose therapy. These discrepancies can be partly explained by differences in study design (the Spanish study randomized patients responding to initial therapy, while in the others randomization was performed up-front), differences in the conditioning regimens and, particularly, differences in the intensity and duration of the chemotherapy arm (the dose of alkylating agents and steroids was higher in the SWOG and Spanish trials, which may explain why OS for conventionally treated patients was longer in these two studies compared with the IFM and MRC trials).

Table 31.7 Response to induction treatment in transplant candidate patients: results from Phase III front-line trials.*

Regimen	Patients	PR or better (%)	CR + n-CR (%)	Study
TD vs. D	470	63 vs. 46	7 vs. 2.6	Rajkumar *et al.* (2008)
TD vs. VAD	200	76 vs. 52	10 vs. 8	Cavo *et al.* (2005)
TAD vs. VAD	400	–	35 vs. 13	Macro *et al.* (ASH 2006)
TVAD vs. VAD	230	81 vs. 66	–	Zervas *et al.* (2007)
CTD vs. CVAD	251	87 vs. 75	19 vs. 9	Morgan *et al.* (ASH 2007)
BD vs. VAD	482	80 vs. 63	21 vs. 8	Harousseau *et al.* (ASH 2008)
BTD vs. TD	256	93 vs. 74	36 vs. 9	Cavo *et al.* (ASH 2008)
LD_{high} vs. LD_{low}[†]	445	82 vs. 71	4 vs. 2	Rajkumar *et al.* (ASH 2008)
LD vs. D	198	85 vs. 51	22 vs. 4	Zonder *et al.* (ASH 2007)

*Response after autologous SCT (CR + n-CR): TAD vs. VAD (16% vs. 11%); CTD vs. CVAD (51% vs. 39%); BD vs. VAD (35% vs. 24%); BTD vs. TD (57% vs. 28%).

[†]High-dose dexamethasone (three pulses), low-dose dexamethasone (one pulse).

A, Adriamycin; B, bortezomib; D, dexamethasone; L, lenalidomide; T, thalidomide; V, vincristine; CR, complete remission; n-CR, near complete remission; ASH, American Society for Hematology Annual Meeting.

Table 31.8 Result of randomized trials comparing autologous SCT with chemotherapy.

	Patients	CR (%)	EFS (months)	OS (months)
IFM90 (Attal *et al.* 1996)	200	22/5	28/18	57/44
MRC 03 (Child *et al.* 2003)	401	44/8	31/19	54/42
PETHEMA 95 (Bladé *et al.* 2005)	185	30/11	42/33	61/66
US-Intergroup (Barlogie *et al.* 2006)	516	11/11	25/21	58/53

CR, complete remission; EFS, event-free survival; OS, overall survival.

Despite these discrepancies, high-dose therapy is currently considered standard of care for younger patients with MM, mainly based on the benefit on RR and EFS.

In the setting of novel agents, it is also important to define whether autologous SCT enhances the RRs obtained with these new induction regimens. As mentioned above, studies based on bortezomib combinations, including two randomized trials, have shown that the CR rate was improved following autologous SCT (Table 31.8), suggesting that induction with novel agents and autologous SCT are complementary rather than alternative treatment approaches. Nevertheless, the benefit in terms of EFS and OS remains to be seen. With regard to thalidomide, it appears that the initial advantage of thalidomide-based regimens (TAD) compared with VAD is not so evident after autologous SCT. Data on lenalidomide are very encouraging, though still scanty. Nevertheless, some investigators argue that this approach may be challenged by the optimal results obtained with 'long-term' treatment with novel combinations (i.e. lenalidomide plus dexamethasone). Although a randomized trial comparing these two approaches would be most interesting, the transplant approach induces a very high CR rate (a goal in all haematological malignancies) and patients enjoy a long-term period free of treatment.

With regard to tandem autologous SCT, its use will decrease for two reasons: (i) according to the French and Italian experience, only patients achieving less than a VGPR with the first transplant benefit from the second; and (ii) a similar benefit is obtained on using thalidomide as consolidation/maintenance therapy. In contrast, a second transplant at relapse may be increasingly used, providing that the duration of the response to the first transplant has lasted for more than 2–3 years.

Maintenance

The third step in the sequence of treatment is maintenance. Interferon and/or corticosteroids have shown little benefit and have been abandoned. The availability of novel agents (particularly thalidomide and lenalidomide, which are available in oral formulations) has transformed the concept of maintenance in an attempt to prolong the duration of responses after transplantation. The IFM group has shown that thalidomide maintenance after tandem autologous SCT is significantly superior to no maintenance or pamidronate alone in terms of EFS (52%, 36% and 37% at 3 years) and OS (87% vs. 74% at 4 years). This superiority has been confirmed by an Australian study that compared thalidomide plus prednisone with prednisone alone. Of note, the Arkansas group has also observed that the use of thalidomide as part of the induction and maintenance phases was associated with longer EFS, although this does not translate into a prolonged OS. This raises an important concern about whether the continuous use of novel agents may induce more resistant relapses. Moreover, the benefit of thalidomide maintenance for patients who are already in CR as well as for those with poor cytogenetics is not well established. Accordingly, although randomized trials are required to define the role of long-term maintenance (>1 year), a short treatment with thalidomide would be justified in patients who have not achieved CR after autologous SCT. It is possible that the better tolerance of lenalidomide will facilitate its use in maintenance programmes.

Allogeneic stem cell transplantation

Allogeneic SCT remains the only curative therapeutic approach in MM. However, it is associated with a high TRM (up to 30–50%) and high morbidity mainly due to chronic graft-versus-host disease (GVHD). Accordingly, it should be used in carefully defined situations and preferably within the context of clinical trials. In order to decrease TRM, different reduced-intensity conditioning regimens (allo-RIC), mainly based on fludarabine and melphalan or fludarabine plus radiotherapy (2 Gy) have been introduced. The TRM decreases by 25–25% but this is associated with a higher incidence of relapses. In a prospective randomized trial, the French group compared double autologous SCT with autologous SCT followed by allo-RIC among patients displaying poor prognostic features (high β_2-microglobulin and monosomy 13). Unfortunately, there were no event-free survivors at 5 years after either double autologous SCT or autologous SCT followed by allo-RIC. In contrast, the Italian group, using a similar approach, has described an improvement in terms of OS among patients receiving autologous SCT followed by allo-RIC compared with double autologous SCT. The Spanish group has recently reported a comparison between double autologous SCT and autologous SCT followed by allo-RIC in patients failing to achieve at least near CR after a first autologous SCT. Although there was a higher increase in CR rate and a trend towards a longer PFS in favour of allo-RIC, this was associated with a trend towards a higher TRM (16% vs. 5%; $P = 0.07$) and no statistical difference in EFS and OS. Differences in patient characteristics, GVHD prophylaxis and conditioning regimens could contribute to these discrepant results. Moreover, unfortunately, a high proportion of patients developed extramedullary relapses without bone marrow involvement, indicating that although the disease may be under control in the bone marrow milieu, extramedullary spread may occur.

With regard to the use of allogeneic SCT as rescue therapy, a prerequisite is to obtain a CR or VGPR before the transplant since most patients with active disease will not benefit from this procedure. Once again these transplants should be performed by experienced groups and within clinical trials. Donor lymphocyte infusions given for relapsed myeloma following allogeneic transplantation induce responses in 30–50% of patients, but unfortunately the long-term efficacy is limited.

Treatment of newly diagnosed elderly and non-transplant candidate patients

MP has been the gold standard for over 40 years, although recent results based on the combination of MP with either thalidomide or bortezomib, and probably also with lenalidomide, indicate that there are now new standards of care for elderly MM patients. As shown in Table 31.9, five randomized trials have compared thalidomide plus MP (MPT) with MP. In all studies both the RRs and CRs were significantly higher in the MPT arm (RR 57–76% for MPT vs. 31–48% for MP; CR 7–16% for MPT vs. 1–4% for MP). Moreover, the five studies showed a significant advantage of MPT treatment in terms of PFS/time to progression (TTP) (prolongation in PFS ranging from 2 to 9 months). However, only in the two French studies was MPT treatment associated with a significant prolongation in OS. The toxicity associated with the high dose of thalidomide used in some of these trials may explain the survival discrepancies. Preliminary data from the MRC Myeloma IX trial show that the combination of cyclophosphamide, thalidomide and dexamethasone is superior to MP in terms of RR (82% vs. 49%) and CR (22% vs. 6%). The proteasome inhibitor bortezomib has been tested in combination with MP (BMP) in a pilot study conducted by the Spanish group; the positive results have been recently confirmed in a large (682 patients) randomized study (VISTA) that showed the superiority of BMP over MP (RR 71% vs. 35%; CR 30% vs. 4%). BMP treatment was associated with a 52% reduction in risk of progression, with a median TTP of 24 compared with 16.6 months ($P < 0.0001$) and a 36% reduction in risk of death, which translates into an OS at 3 years of 72% for BMP and 59% for MP. This benefit was present despite 45% of MP patients receiving bortezomib on progression. In addition, time to next therapy and treatment-free interval were significantly prolonged in patients treated with BMP and the benefit of this combination was observed across all patient subgroups, including those with advanced age, renal insufficiency and high-risk cytogenetics.

Lenalidomide has also been combined with MP. A pilot study showed an RR of 81%, a CR of 17% and an EFS of 87% at 16 months, and it is currently being tested in a randomized trial comparing lenalidomide plus MP with MP. Nevertheless, these MP combinations are being challenged by the recent results reported with lenalidomide plus dexamethasone, particularly using low-dose dexamethasone, with a 2-year survival probability of 82% in patients 65 years or older.

A final controversial issue is whether there is a preference for any one of the three novel MP combinations.

Table 31.9 Results from randomized Phase III trials in newly diagnosed elderly patients.

Study	Regimen	No. of patients	CR with negative immunofixation	TTP/PFS (months)	Overall survival
GIMEMA (Palumbo *et al.* 2006, 2008)	MPT	129	15.5%	29.2	NS (45 vs. 47 months)
	MP	126	2.4%	13.6	
IFM 99 (Facon *et al.* 2007)	MPT	125	13%	27.5	51.6 vs. 33.2 months
	MP	196	2%	17.8	HR 0.59, $P = 0.0006$
IFM 01 (Hulin *et al.*, ASH 2007, Abstract 75)	MPT	113	7%	24.1	45.3 vs. 27.7 months
	MP	116	1%	19	HR N/A, $P = 0.03$
NMSG (Gulbrandsen *et al.*, EHA 2008, Abstract 209)	MPT	362	6%	20	29 vs. 33 months
	MP		3%	18	
HOVON (Wijermans *et al.*, ASH 2008, Abstract 649)	MPT	152	1%	TTP, 0.05	NS
	MP	149	1%	PFS, NS	
VISTA (San Miguel *et al.* 2008)	BMP	344	30%	24.0	72% vs. 59% at 3 years
	MP	338	4%	16.6	HR 0.61, $P = 0.0078$

B, bortezomib; M, melphalan; P, prednisone; T, thalidomide; CR, complete remission; TTP, time to progression; PFS, progression-free survival; HR, hazard ratio; ASH, American Society for Hematology Annual Meeting; EHA, European Haematology Association Annual Meeting.

1 The most mature data are with MPT and BMP.
2 For patients with antecedent, or risk of, deep venous thrombosis (DVT), BMP could be the preferred option.
3 In patients with antecedent peripheral neuropathy, lenalidomide plus MP should be the choice.
4 In patients with renal insufficiency, BMP is safe.
5 In patients living long distances from hospital, oral treatment (MPT, or lenalidomide plus MP) would be preferable.
6 In patients with poor compliance with treatment, BMP could be better.
7 If costs are a concern, MPT is less expensive.
An individualized treatment approach would probably be valuable. The toxicity profile of novel agents is discussed at the end of the treatment section.

In patients over 75 years of age or in fragile condition, the recommendation is to use modified regimens, with a lower dose of thalidomide (100 mg) and lenalidomide (15–20 mg) or bortezomib 1 mg/m² (or a weekly schedule). One additional possibility in these patients is to substitute melphalan with cyclophosphamide (50 mg/day or 1 g every 21 days), since this latter agent is less myelotoxic. In very elderly patients, special attention must be paid to infectious episodes (require active treatment) and renal function (appropriate hydration), particularly during the first 3 months of treatment when they are responsible for the high incidence of early deaths.

Treatment at relapse

It is important to separate the young (<55 years) from the elderly (>55 years) patients. In patients relapsing after transplantation, we discriminate three cohorts of patients: early

relapse (<1 year), intermediate relapse (1–3 years) and late relapse (>3 years). If the relapse occurs within the first year after transplantation, patients should be immediately considered high risk and, in order to overcome drug resistance, rescued with either a combination of all potentially effective drugs (e.g. BTD plus cisplatin, Adriamycin, cyclophosphamide and etoposide; or bortezomib, lenalidomide and dexamethasone) or alternating cycles of two combinations of non-cross-resistant agents (BCD alternating with lenalidomide or TAD). Nevertheless, it must be pointed out that these types of combinations should ideally be conducted within controlled clinical trials. If CR is achieved, the patient could proceed to allogeneic SCT with RIC, although this must still be considered an investigational approach.

If relapse occurs 1–3 years after autologous SCT, we would favour rescue with novel agents used in a sequential (not simultaneous) manner, starting with one line of treatment (different from the one used as induction) and shifting to the second and subsequent lines only when disease progression occurs. Within this category of patients, those under 55 years old with an HLA-identical sibling and a suboptimal response to the first line of treatment should be considered for allogeneic SCT with RIC. Finally, if relapse occurs more than 3 years after the first autologous SCT, an attractive possibility is reinduction with the initial treatment or other novel-agent combination followed by a second autologous SCT.

In the elderly patients, treatment decisions at relapse must take into account the general condition of the patient. Once the patient relapses, after up-front treatment, the durations of subsequent responses to rescue therapies are progressively shortened. Therefore, the current goal in relapsed MM is to optimize the efficacy of novel drugs through their most appropriate combinations, to establish optimal sequences of treatment and to promote active clinical research on experimental agents that have already shown promising activity in *in vitro* and animal models.

At first relapse, a regimen based on novel drugs (thalidomide, lenalidomide or bortezomib) and different from that used as

induction should be instituted. Table 31.10 summarizes the most relevant results and combinations reported in relapsed patients. Thalidomide has been widely used, although few randomized studies have been conducted; the RR ranges between 25 and 70% depending on whether it has been used as a single agent or in combination with alkylating agents and corticosteroids. Bortezomib as a single agent has been shown to be

Table 31.10 Relapse/refractory patients: response to thalidomide, lenalidomide and bortezomib: single agents and combinations.

Drug/combination	No. of patients	Response rate		Study
		PR or better (%)	CR (%)	
Thalidomide-based combinations				
T monotherapy (200–800 mg)	169	24	2	Singhal (*N Engl J Med* 1999)
T monotherapy (meta-analysis)	1629	28	1.6	Glasmacher (*Br J Haematol* 2005)
TD	>400	42–58	3–13	Several*
TD vs. placebo-D	116	65 vs. 28	NR	Fermand *et al.* (ASH 2006)
TCD	>200	56–76	5–20	Several†
Lenalidomide-based combinations				
L monotherapy	104	14	4	Richardson (*Blood* 2006)
LD vs. D	175 vs. 176	60 vs. 22	15 vs. 2	Weber & Dimopoulos (*N Engl J Med* 2007)
LAD	69	87	23	Knop (ASH 2007)
Pegylated liposomal doxorubicin + VDL	62	75	29 (CR + n-CR)	Baz (*Ann Oncol* 2007)
LCD	21	65	NR	Morgan (*Br J Haematol* 2007)
Bortezomib-based combinations				
B monotherapy vs. D	669	43 vs. 18	16 vs. 1	Richardson (*N Engl J Med* 2005)
Pegylated liposomal doxorubicin + B vs. B monotherapy	646	48 vs. 43	14 vs. 11	Orlowski (*J Clin Oncol* 2007)
BM	26	47	11	Berenson (*J Clin Oncol* 2006)
BM	21	68	34 (CR + n-CR)	Popat (ASH 2007)
BCP	37	88	40	Reece (*J Clin Oncol* 2008)
BCD	50	82	16	Kropff (*Br J Haematol* 2007)
BCD	47	75	31	Davies (*Haematologica* 2007)
Immunomodulators (thalidomide/lenalidomide) plus bortezomib				
BT ± D	85	55	16 (CR + n-CR)	Pineda-Román (*Leukemia* 2008)
BT + pegylated liposomal doxorubicin	21	56	22 (CR + n-CR)	Chanan-Khan (*Leukemia and Lymphoma* 2005)
BTAD	20	63	24 (CR + n-CR)	Hollmig (ASH 2006)
BTMP	30	67%	14 (CR), 7 (n-CR)	Palumbo (*Blood* 2007)
BTMD	53	60	11	Terpos (*Leukemia* 2008)
BL	27	79	33	Richardson (ASH 2007)

*Weber (*J Clin Oncol* 2003), Dimopoulos (*Ann Oncol* 2001) and Palumbo (*Haematologica* 2001).

†Kropff (*Haematol J* 2003), García-Sanz (*Leukemia* 2004) and Dimopoulos (*Haematol J* 2004).

A, Adriamycin; B, bortezomib; C, cyclophosphamide; D, dexamethasone; L, lenalidomide; M, melphalan; P, prednisone; T, thalidomide; V, vincristine; CR, complete remission; n-CR, near complete remission; ASH, American Society for Hematology Annual Meeting.

significantly superior to high-dose dexamethasone in relapsed/ refractory patients (RR 43% vs. 18%; CR 16% vs. 1%; TTP 6 vs. 3 months). The addition of pegylated doxorubicin increased EFS to 9.3 months. With regard to lenalidomide, a large randomized trial has shown that lenalidomide plus dexamethasone is significantly superior to dexamethasone alone (RR 60% vs. 20%; CR 15% vs. 2%; TTP 11.1 vs. 4.7 months). The most widely used regimens at relapse include:
• thalidomide/dexamethasone or thalidomide/cyclophosphamide/dexamethasone;
• lenalidomide/dexamethasone or lenalidomide/dexamethasone/doxorubicin;
• bortezomib/dexamethasone or bortezomib/liposomal doxorubicin with or without dexamethasone or bortezomib/cyclophosphamide/dexamethasone (Table 31.10).

At second or subsequent relapse, usually after the patient has already failed bortezomib and at least one immunomodulator, a clinical trial with experimental agents should be encouraged. If the patient is not a candidate for active therapy, palliative treatment with oral cyclophosphamide (50 mg/day) and prednisone (30 mg on alternating days) can be considered.

Side-effects associated with novel agents

Because of the previous history of thalidomide a major concern was its toxicity profile. The side-effects are dose related and the most common include constipation, weakness, somnolence and neuropathy. Peripheral neuropathy is a common adverse event with thalidomide therapy and often limits the dose and duration of treatment. The use of combination therapy has raised concern about an increased risk of DVT. Apparently the major risk of DVT occurs when tumour load is high and thalidomide is combined with chemotherapy, especially Adriamycin (30% incidence vs. 4% when thalidomide is used alone). Accordingly, in this setting, anticoagulant prophylaxis with low-molecular-weight heparin (LMWH) or aspirin is mandatory. Current data suggest that lenalidomide is better tolerated than thalidomide in several aspects: it does not usually produce clinically significant somnolence, constipation or neuropathy, although the incidence of myelosuppression is higher, mainly neutropenia (grade 3 in 17–30%) and thrombocytopenia, which are manageable with dose reduction and growth factor support. Similarly to thalidomide, lenalidomide is associated with a higher risk of DVT (5–25%) and the risk increases in patients with comorbidities, previous history of DVT, concomitant use of erythropoietin, high-dose dexamethasone, anthracyclines or high tumour mass. For these reasons, anticoagulant prophylaxis with LMWH or aspirin is mandatory. The most frequent toxicities of bortezomib include fatigue, gastrointestinal symptoms (grade 3 in 15–25%), cyclical thrombocytopenia and, particularly, peripheral neuropathy. This latter side-effect, classified as grade 3 in 9–20% of patients, is the main reason for treatment discontinuation, and the early detection of peripheral neuropa-

thy is most important in order to reduce the dose or frequency of injections. Nevertheless, it resolved or improved in two-thirds of patients after completion or discontinuation of therapy.

Promising new drugs

Some of the molecular events responsible for the transformation of a normal into a malignant plasma cell represent potential therapeutic targets. Thus the t(4;14) translocation leads to constitutive activation of the oncogenic tyrosine kinase receptor FGFR3, with subsequent phosphorylation of the anti-apoptotic STAT3 signalling pathway. Moreover, several *IGH* translocations lead to cyclin D deregulation, and represent a common pathogenic event in MM. Therefore, the use of inhibitors of cyclin-dependent kinases, aurora kinase inhibitors and inhibitors of the FGFR3 tyrosine kinase could be attractive therapeutic targets. Although *in vitro* studies have shown that FGFR3 tyrosine kinase inhibitors such as CHIR-258/TKI or AB1010 inhibit FGFR3 autophosphorylation in cells carrying the translocation, resulting in cell growth arrest and apoptosis, preliminary clinical data show very limited activity as single agents.

The second area of MM pathogenesis that has important implications for treatment is the interaction between the malignant cell and the bone marrow microenvironment, which promotes MM cell growth and proliferation. As mentioned in the section on pathogenesis, adhesion of myeloma cells to bone marrow microenvironment induces a drug-resistant plasma cell phenotype. Moreover, this binding also induces the transcription and secretion of cytokines (TNF-α, IL-6, IGF-1, SDF-1α, VEGF), by both the plasma cells and bone marrow stromal cells, that on interacting with their corresponding receptors trigger signalling pathways (e.g. RAF/MEK/MAPK, PI3K/AKT and JAK/STAT) that promote cell proliferation and prevent apoptosis. Several drugs that affect these pathways are already in the early phases of clinical investigation, including the following.
1 Agents against receptors present in plasma cells, which can be targeted by specific drugs or monoclonal antibodies, including death receptors (e.g. DR4-6 and FAS), tyrosine kinase receptors, VEGF-R, TACI, IL6-R, IGF-1R or the CD56 or CD40 antigens.
2 Several clinical trials are being conducted with inhibitors directed at signalling pathways, including farnesyltransferase (tipifarnib), RAF (RAF 265), STAT3 (atiprimod), mTOR (everolimus) or AKT (perifosine).
3 Drugs that interfere with the unfolded protein response and epigenetics, such as the new proteasome inhibitors (NPI-0052 and carfilzomib), Hsp90 inhibitors or histone deacetylase inhibitors.

Unfortunately, the expectations raised by some of these agents have not been confirmed in the clinic as yet. It is probable that these targeted therapies will be more effective in combinations with other agents that have already shown clear efficacy in MM.

Acknowledgements

This work was partially supported by the following grants: Fondo de Investigación Sanitaria-FIS (RTICC-RD06/0020/0006 and RTICC-RD06/0020/0005) and Junta de Castilla y León (Grupos de Investigación de Excelencia. Ref. GR33).

Selected bibliography

Attal M, Harousseau JL, Stoppa AM et al. (1996) A prospective, randomized trial of autologous bone marrow transplantation and chemotherapy in multiple myeloma. New England Journal of Medicine 335: 91–7.

Attal M, Harousseau JL, Facon T et al. (2003) Single versus double autologous stem cell transplantation for multiple myeloma. New England Journal of Medicine 349: 2495–502.

Attal M, Harousseau JL, Leyvraz S et al. (2006) Maintenance therapy with thalidomide improves survival in patients with multiple myeloma. Blood 108: 3289–94.

Avet-Loiseau H, Attal M, Moreau P et al. (2007) Genetic abnormalities and survival in multiple myeloma: the experience of the Intergroupe Francophone du Myelome. Blood 109: 3489 95.

Barlogie B, Tricot G, Anaissie E et al. (2006) Thalidomide and haematopoietic-cell transplantation for multiple myeloma. New England Journal of Medicine 354: 1021–30.

Barlogie B, Zangari M, Bolejack V et al. (2006) Superior 12-year survival after at least 4-year continuous remission with tandem transplantations for multiple myeloma. Clinical Lymphoma and Myeloma 6: 469–74.

Berenson JR, Anderson KC, Audell RA et al. (2010) Monoclonal gammopathy of undetermined significance: a consensus statement. British Journal of Haematology 150: 28–38.

Bladé J (2006) Monoclonal gammopathy of undetermined significance. New England Journal of Medicine 355: 65–70.

Bladé J, Rosiñol L (2007) Complications of multiple myeloma. Hematology/Oncology Clinics of North America 21: 1231–46.

Bladé J, Samson D, Reece D et al. (1998) Criteria for evaluating disease response and progression in patients with multiple myeloma treated with high-dose therapy and haematopoietic stem cell transplantation. British Journal of Haematology 102: 1115–23.

Bladé J, Rosinol L, Sureda A et al. (2005) High-dose therapy intensification versus continued standard chemotherapy in multiple myeloma patients responding to the initial chemotherapy: long term results from a prospective randomized trial from the Spanish cooperative group PETHEMA. Blood 106: 3755–9.

Brenner H, Gondos A, Pulte D (2008) Recent major improvement in long-term survival of younger patients with multiple myeloma. Blood 111: 2521–6.

Bruno B, Rotta, M, Patriarca F et al. (2007) A comparison of allografting with autografting for newly diagnosed myeloma. New England Journal of Medicine 356: 1110–20.

Cavo M, Zamagni E, Tosi P et al. (2005) Superiority of thalidomide and dexamethasone over vincristine/doxorubicin/dexamethasone (VAD) as primary therapy in preparation for autologous transplantation for multiple myeloma. Blood 106: 35–9.

Chanan-Khan AA, Kaufman JL, Metha J et al. (2007) Activity and safety of bortezomib in multiple myeloma patients with advanced renal failure: a multicenter retrospective study. Blood 109: 2604–6.

Child JA, Morgan GJ, Davies FE et al. (2003) High-dose chemotherapy with haematopoietic stem-cell rescue for multiple myeloma. New England Journal of Medicine 348: 1875–83.

Dimopoulos M, Spencer A, Attal M et al. (2007) Lenalidomide plus dexamethasone for relapsed or refractory multiple myeloma. New England Journal of Medicine 357: 2123–32.

Dispenzieri A, Kyle RA, Katzmann JA et al. (2008) Immunoglobulin free light chain ratio is an independent risk factor for progression of smoldering (asymptomatic) multiple myeloma. Blood 111: 785–9.

Dispenzieri A, Katzmann JA, Kyle RA et al. (2010) Prevalence and risk of progression of light-chain monoclonal gammopathy of undetermined significance: a retrospective population-based cohort study. Lancet 375: 1721–8.

Durie BGM, Harousseau JL, San Miguel JF et al. (2006) International uniform response criteria for multiple myeloma. Leukemia 20: 1467–73.

Facon T, Mary JY, Hulin C et al. (2007) Melphalan and prednisone plus thalidomide versus melphalan and prednisone alone or reduced-intensity autologous stem cell transplantation in elderly patients with multiple myeloma (IFM 99-06): a randomized trial. Lancet 370: 1209–18.

Fermand J-P, Jaccard A, Macro M et al. (2006) A randomized comparison of dexamethasone + thalidomide (Dex/Thal) vs Dex + Placebo (Dex/P) in patients (pts) with relapsing multiple myeloma (MM) [Abstract]. Blood 108: 3563.

Fonseca R, Barlogie B, Bataille R et al. (2004) Genetics and cytogenetics of multiple myeloma: a workshop report. Cancer Research 64: 1546–58.

Garban F, Attal M, Michallet M et al. (2006) Prospective comparison of autologous stem cell transplantation followed by dose-reduced allograft (IFM99-03 trial) with tandem autologous stem cell transplantation (IFM99-04 trial) in high-risk de novo multiple myeloma. Blood 107: 3474–80.

Greipp PR, San Miguel J, Durie BG et al. (2005) International staging system for multiple myeloma. Journal of Clinical Oncology 23: 3412–20.

Gutiérrez NC, García JL, Hernández JM et al. (2004) Prognostic and biologic significance of chromosomal imbalances assessed by comparative genomic hybridization in multiple myeloma. Blood 104: 2661–6.

Hideshima T, Anderson KC (2002) Molecular mechanisms of novel therapeutic approaches for multiple myeloma. Nature Reviews. Cancer 2: 927–37.

International Myeloma Working Group (2003) Criteria for the classification of monoclonal gammopathies, multiple myeloma and related disorders. *British Journal of Haematology* **121**: 49–57.

Kuehl WM, Bergsagel PL (2002) Multiple myeloma: evolving genetic events and host interactions. *Nature Reviews. Cancer* **2**: 175–87.

Kumar SK, Rajkumar SV, Dispenzieri A *et al.* (2008) Improved survival in multiple myeloma and the impact of novel therapies. *Blood* **111**: 2516–20.

Kyle RA, Rajkumar SV (2004) Multiple myeloma. *New England Journal of Medicine* **351**: 1860–73.

Kyle RA, Therneau TM, Rajkumar SV *et al.* (2006) Prevalence of monoclonal gammopathy of undetermined significance. *New England Journal of Medicine* **354**: 1362–9.

Kyle RA, Remstein ED, Therneau TM *et al.* (2007) Clinical course and prognosis of smoldering (asymptomatic) multiple myeloma. *New England Journal of Medicine* **356**: 2582–90.

Lacy MQ, Dispenzieri A, Gertz MA *et al.* (2006) Mayo Clinic consensus statement for the use of bisphosphonates in multiple myeloma. *Mayo Clinic Proceedings* **81**: 1047–53.

Mateo G, Montalban MA, Vidriales MB *et al.* (2008) Prognostic value of immunophenotyping of multiple myeloma: a study on 685 patients uniformly treated with high dose therapy. *Journal of Clinical Oncology* **26**: 2737–44.

Mateos MV, San Miguel JF (2007) Bortezomib in multiple myeloma. *Best Practice and Research. Clinical Haematology* **20**: 701–15.

Orlowski RZ, Nagler A, Sonneveld P *et al.* (2007) Randomized phase III study of pegylated liposomal doxorubicin plus bortezomib compared with bortezomib alone in relapsed or refractory multiple myeloma: combination therapy improves time to progression. *Journal of Clinical Oncology* **25**: 3892–901.

Paiva B, Vidriales MB, Cervero J *et al.* (2008) Multiparameter flow cytometry remission is the most relevant prognostic factor for multiple myeloma patients who undergo autologous stemm cell transplantation. *Blood* **112**: 4017–23.

Palumbo A, Bringhen S, Caravita T *et al.* (2006) Oral melphalan and prednisone chemotherapy plus thalidomide compared with melphalan and prednisone alone in elderly patients with multiple myeloma: randomized controlled trial. *Lancet* **367**: 825–31.

Palumbo A, Bringhen S, Liberati AM *et al.* (2008) Oral melphalan, prednisone, and thalidomide in elderly patients with multiple myeloma: updated results of a randomized controlled trial. *Blood* **112**: 3107–14.

Perez-Persona E, Vidriales MB, Mateo G *et al.* (2007) New criteria to identify risk of progression in monoclonal gammopathy of uncertain significance and smoldering multiple myeloma based on multiparameter flow cytometry analysis of bone marrow plasma cells. *Blood* **110**: 2586–92.

Rajkumar SV, Rosiñol L, Hussein M *et al.* (2008) Multicenter, randomized, double-blind, placebo-controlled study of thalidomide plus dexamethasone compared with dexamethasone as initial therapy for newly diagnosed multiple myeloma. *Journal of Clinical Oncology* **26**: 2171–7.

Richardson PG, Sonneveld P, Schuster MW *et al.* (2005) Bortezomib or high-dose dexamethasone for relapsed multiple myeloma. *New England Journal of Medicine* **352**: 2487–98.

San Miguel JF, Garcia-Sanz R (2005) Prognostic features of multiple myeloma. *Best Practice and Research. Clinical Haematology* **18**: 569–83.

San Miguel JF, Schlag R, Khuageva NK *et al.* (2008) Bortezomib plus melphalan and prednisone for initial treatment of multiple myeloma. *New England Journal of Medicine* **359**: 906–17.

Walker R, Barlogie B, Haessler J *et al.* (2007) Magnetic resonance imaging in multiple myeloma: diagnostic and clinical implications. *Journal of Clinical Oncology* **25**: 1121–8.

Weber DM, Chen C, Niesvizky R *et al.* (2007) Lenalidomide plus dexamethasone for relapsed multiple myeloma in North America. *New England Journal of Medicine* **357**: 2133–42.

Zervas K, Mihou D, Katodritou E *et al.* (2007) VAD-doxil versus VAD-doxil plus thalidomide as initial treatment for multiple myeloma: results of a multicenter randomized trial of the Greek Myeloma Study Group. *Annals of Oncology* **18**: 1369–75.

Zhan F, Huang Y, Colla S *et al.* (2006) The molecular classification of multiple myeloma. *Blood* **108**: 2020–8.

CHAPTER 32

Amyloidosis

32

Simon DJ Gibbs and Philip N Hawkins

National Amyloidosis Centre, Royal Free and University College London Medical School, London, UK

Introduction

Amyloidosis is a disorder of protein folding in which normally soluble proteins are deposited in the extracellular space as insoluble fibrils that progressively disrupt tissue structure and function. Some 25 different unrelated proteins can form amyloid *in vivo*, and clinical amyloidosis is classified according to the fibril protein type (Table 32.1). Of interest, although the term 'amyloid' is derived from the Greek for 'starch-like', the misnomer was recognized over 100 years ago and has remained unchallenged.

Amyloid deposition is remarkable in its diversity; it can be systemic or localized, acquired or hereditary, life-threatening or merely an incidental finding. Clinical consequences are seen when the accumulation of amyloid fibrils is sufficiently substantial to cause structural disruption of tissues or organs, leading to their impairment or failure. The pattern of organ involvement varies within and between fibril types and clinical phenotypes overlap greatly. In systemic amyloidosis, virtually any tissue may be involved and the disease is often fatal, although its prognosis has been improved by increasingly effective treatments for some of the conditions that underlie it. Greater understanding of the pathogenesis of the disease, allowing improved subtyping and appropriate targeted therapies, with improved supportive care including haemodialysis and solid organ transplantation in selected patients have also influenced the prognosis of this disorder. In localized amyloidosis, deposits are confined to a particular organ or tissue and are usually clinically silent, although they can cause serious consequences such

as haemorrhage in local respiratory or urogenital tracts. In addition to the amyloidoses, local amyloid deposition is a pathological feature of uncertain significance in other important diseases including Alzheimer disease, the prion disorders and type 2 diabetes mellitus.

The chapter is devoted mainly to describing the clinical features, diagnosis and management of AL (monoclonal immunoglobulin light chain) amyloidosis, which is the most common and serious form of systemic amyloidosis in industrialized societies. The differential diagnosis and other amyloid fibril types that can mimic AL type, including their diagnosis and management, are also discussed.

Pathogenesis of amyloid

Amyloidosis challenges the dogma that the tertiary structure of proteins is determined solely by their primary amino acid sequence. Amyloid-forming proteins can exist in two completely different stable structures, the transformation evidently involving massive refolding of the native form into one that can autoaggregate in a highly ordered manner to produce the characteristic predominantly β-sheet, rigid, non-branching fibrils of 10–15 nm in diameter and of indeterminate length. Acquired biophysical properties common to all amyloid fibrils include insolubility in physiological solutions, relative resistance to proteolysis, and ability to bind Congo red dye in an ordered manner that gives the diagnostic green birefringence under cross-polarized light.

Amyloid deposition can occur in three circumstances.
1 When there is a sustained abnormally high concentration of certain normal proteins, such as serum amyloid A (SAA) protein in chronic inflammation and β_2-microglobulin in renal

Postgraduate Haematology: 6th edition. Edited by A. Victor Hoffbrand, Daniel Catovsky, Edward G.D. Tuddenham, Anthony R. Green
© 2011 Blackwell Publishing Ltd.

Table 32.1 Classification of amyloidosis.*

Type	Fibril precursor protein	Clinical syndrome
AA	Serum amyloid A protein	Systemic amyloidosis associated with acquired or hereditary chronic inflammatory diseases. Formerly known as secondary or reactive amyloidosis
AL	Monoclonal immunoglobulin light chains	Systemic amyloidosis associated with myeloma, monoclonal gammopathy, occult B-cell dyscrasia. Formerly known as primary amyloidosis
ATTR	Normal plasma transthyretin	Senile systemic amyloidosis with predominant cardiac involvement
ATTR	Genetic variants of transthyretin (e.g. ATTR Met30, Ala60, Ile122)	Familial amyloid polyneuropathy (FAP), with systemic amyloidosis and often prominent amyloid cardiomyopathy
$A\beta_2M$	β_2-Microglobulin	Dialysis-related amyloidosis (DRA) associated with renal failure and long-term dialysis. Predominantly musculoskeletal symptoms
$A\beta$	β-Protein precursor (and rare genetic variants)	Cerebrovascular and intracerebral plaque amyloid in Alzheimer disease. Occasional familial cases
AApoAI	Genetic variants of apolipoprotein A-I (e.g. AApoAI Arg26, Arg60)	Autosomal dominant systemic amyloidosis. Predominantly non-neuropathic with prominent visceral involvement, especially nephropathy. Minor wild-type ApoAI amyloid deposits may occur in the aorta
AApoAII	Genetic variants of apolipoprotein A-II	Autosomal dominant systemic amyloidosis with predominant renal involvement
AFib	Genetic variants of fibrinogen α chain (e.g. AFib Val526)	Autosomal dominant systemic amyloidosis. Non-neuropathic usually with prominent nephropathy
ALys	Genetic variants of lysozyme (e.g. ALys His67)	Autosomal dominant systemic amyloidosis. Non-neuropathic with prominent renal and gastrointestinal involvement
ACys	Genetic variant of cystatin C (Gln68)	Hereditary cerebral haemorrhage with cerebral and systemic amyloidosis
AGel	Genetic variants of gelsolin (e.g. Asn187)	Autosomal dominant systemic amyloidosis. Predominant cranial nerve involvement with lattice corneal dystrophy
AIAPP	Islet amyloid polypeptide	Amyloid in islets of Langerhans in type 2 diabetes mellitus and insulinoma
ALECT2	Leukocyte chemotactic factor II	Systemic amyloidosis with predominant renal involvement

*Amyloid composed of peptide hormones, prion protein and unknown proteins not included.

failure, which underlie susceptibility to AA and β_2-microglobulin amyloidosis respectively.

2 When there is a normal concentration of a normal, but inherently amyloidogenic, protein over a very prolonged period, such as transthyretin (TTR) in senile amyloidosis and β-protein in Alzheimer disease.

3 When there is production of an acquired or inherited variant protein with an abnormal structure, such as amyloidogenic monoclonal immunoglobulin light chains in AL amyloidosis or the hereditary amyloidogenic variants of TTR, lysozyme, apolipoprotein A-I and fibrinogen Aα chain.

The genetic and environmental factors that influence individual susceptibility to and timing of amyloid deposition are unclear, but once the process has begun, amyloid deposition is unremitting as long as the supply of the respective precursor protein remains undiminished.

Amyloid deposits consist mainly of amyloid fibrils but they also contain some common minor constituents, including certain glycosaminoglycans (GAGs) and the normal circulating plasma protein serum amyloid P component (SAP), as well as various other trace proteins. SAP binds in a specific calcium-dependent manner to a ligand that is present on all amyloid fibrils but not on their precursor proteins. This phenomenon is the basis for the use of SAP scintigraphy in some centres for imaging and monitoring amyloid deposits. Studies in knockout mice indicate that SAP contributes to amyloidogenesis.

Amyloid fibril-associated GAGs mainly comprise heparan and dermatan sulphates. Their universal presence, restricted heterogeneity and intimate relationship with the fibrils suggest that they may also contribute to the development or stability of amyloid deposits, a possibility that has lately been supported by the inhibitory effect of low-molecular-weight GAG analogues on the experimental induction of AA amyloidosis in mice.

Many of the pathological effects of amyloid can be attributed to its physical presence. Extensive deposits, which may amount to kilograms, are structurally disruptive and incompatible with normal function, as are strategically located smaller deposits, for example in glomeruli or nerves. Amyloid fibrils may also be directly cytotoxic but they appear to evoke little or no local inflammatory reaction in the tissues. However, the relationship between the quantity of amyloid and degree of associated organ dysfunction differs greatly between individuals, and there is a strong impression that the rate of new amyloid deposition may be as important a determinant of progressive organ failure as the amyloid load itself.

Treatments that substantially reduce the supply of amyloidogenic precursor protein frequently result in stabilization or regression of existing amyloid deposits, and are often associated with preservation or improvement in the function of organs infiltrated by amyloid.

Systemic AL amyloidosis

Systemic AL (formerly known as 'primary') amyloidosis occurs in a small proportion of individuals with monoclonal B-cell dyscrasia. AL fibrils are derived from monoclonal immunoglobulin light chains, which are unique in each patient. It is this uniqueness of an individual's light chains that helps to explain the considerable heterogeneity in the way AL amyloidosis affects individual organs and its clinical outcome. Virtually any organ other than the brain may be directly affected. The kidneys, heart, liver and peripheral nervous system are the organs most often involved and most often associated with clinical consequences. Early symptoms are often non-specific. Screening techniques can fail to detect any underlying monoclonal gammopathy, leading to a delay in diagnosis, by which time the deposits are often extensive and the prognosis poor. This emphasizes the need to consider AL amyloidosis as a potential diagnosis in a range of vague clinical presentations, and the need for prompt appropriate investigations, such as biopsy of the affected organ and serum free light chain (SFLC) analysis.

AL fibrils and monoclonal light chains

AL amyloid fibrils are derived from the N-terminal region of monoclonal immunoglobulin light chains and consist of the whole or part of the variable (V_L) domain. The molecular mass of the fibril subunit protein therefore varies between about 8 and 30 kDa. All monoclonal light chains are structurally unique and the propensity for certain ones to form amyloid fibrils is an inherent property related to their particular structure. Only a small proportion of monoclonal light chains are amyloidogenic, but it is not possible to identify these from their class or abundance. Monoclonal light chains that form amyloid are able to exist in partly unfolded states, involving loss of tertiary or higher order structure. These readily aggregate, with retention of β-sheet secondary structure, into protofilaments and fibrils.

The inherent 'amyloidogenicity' of certain monoclonal light chains has been demonstrated in an *in vivo* model in which purified Bence Jones proteins were injected into mice. Animals receiving light chains from patients with AL amyloidosis developed typical amyloid deposits composed of the human protein, whereas animals receiving light chains from myeloma patients without amyloid did not. AL fibrils are more commonly derived from λ than κ light chains, despite the fact that κ isotypes predominate among both normal immunoglobulins and monoclonal gammopathies. Some amyloidogenic light chains have distinctive amino acid replacements or insertions compared with non-amyloid monoclonal light chains, including replacement of hydrophilic framework residues by hydrophobic ones, changes that can promote aggregation and insolubility. Certain light-chain isotypes, notably $V_{\lambda VI}$, are especially amyloidogenic, and there is a degree of concordance between some isotypes and their tropism for being deposited as amyloid in particular organ systems. For example, the $V_{\lambda VI}$ isotype often presents with dominant renal involvement, whereas the $V_{\lambda II}$ isotype frequently involves the heart.

The plasma cell dyscrasia

Although almost any dyscrasia of differentiated B lymphocytes, including multiple myeloma, Waldenström macroglobulinaemia and other malignant lymphomas/leukaemias, may produce a monoclonal immunoglobulin that can form AL amyloid, well over 80% of cases are associated with low-grade and otherwise 'benign' monoclonal gammopathies. Histological studies indicate that amyloid deposition occurs in up to 15% of cases of myeloma, but usually in small and clinically insignificant amounts, and that it probably occurs in less than 5% of patients with 'benign' monoclonal gammopathy of undetermined significance (MGUS). The cytogenetic abnormalities that commonly occur in multiple myeloma and MGUS, such as 14q translocations and 13q deletion, have also been observed in AL amyloidosis, but their prognostic significance has not been fully elucidated.

Clinical features

AL amyloidosis accounts for 1 in 1500 deaths in the UK and occurs equally in men and women. The age-adjusted incidence of AL amyloidosis in the USA is estimated to be 5.1–12.8 per million persons per year, which is equivalent to approximately 600 new cases per year in the UK. The median age at presentation is 65 years, but it can occur in young adults and is most likely underdiagnosed in the elderly, in whom it would be expected to have the highest incidence. AL amyloidosis is the most serious and commonly diagnosed form of systemic amyloidosis, and presently outnumbers referrals of AA amyloidosis to the UK National Amyloidosis Centre by a factor of 4:1.

Commonly, presenting features are non-specific and can be as vague as decreased exercise tolerance, fatigue, anorexia, weight loss and malaise. Not infrequently, patients are misdiagnosed with cardiac failure with symptoms and signs such as worsening pedal oedema and/or exertional dyspnoea. All these symptoms can be manifestations of amyloid infiltration resulting in nephrotic syndrome with or without renal impairment, cardiac involvement, neuropathy and hepatomegaly. Dysfunction of a single organ may dominate the clinical picture. The heart is affected in more than 50% of patients and in 30% a restrictive cardiomyopathy is a presenting feature. Rarer cardiac presentations include arrhythmias and angina, the latter sometimes due to coronary amyloid angiopathy. Dominant renal amyloid is the presenting feature in one-third of patients, typically presenting with nephrotic syndrome and/or renal impairment. Gut involvement may cause motility disturbances, which can also be secondary to autonomic neuropathy, and malabsorption, perforation, haemorrhage or obstruction. Macroglossia occurs in 5–10% but is almost pathognomonic of AL amyloidosis (Figure 32.1). Hyposplenism is not infrequent in both AA and AL amyloidosis but is rarely documented or clinically significant. Painful sensory polyneuropathy with

changes in pain and temperature sensation followed later by motor deficits occur in 10–20% of cases and carpal tunnel syndrome occurs in 20%. Autonomic neuropathy leading to impotence, orthostatic hypotension and gastrointestinal disturbances may occur alone or together with peripheral neuropathy, and has a poor prognosis. Involvement of dermal blood vessels is common and may cause purpura, most distinctively in a periorbital distribution ('raccoon eyes'). Direct skin involvement takes the form of papules, nodules and plaques, usually on the face and upper trunk. Articular amyloid is rare but the symptoms can be severe and superficially mimic an inflammatory polyarthritis. Soft-tissue infiltration may occur, characteristically involving the submandibular region or the glenohumeral joints and surrounding tissues to produce the 'shoulder pad' sign, or lymph nodes themselves can be infiltrated. Thyroid infiltration with amyloid, occasionally resulting in hypothyroidism, has been reported. An uncommon but serious manifestation of AL amyloidosis is an acquired bleeding diathesis that may be associated with deficiency of factor X and sometimes also factor IX, or with increased fibrinolysis. It does not occur in other amyloidoses, although in both AL and AA disease there may be serious bleeding in the absence of any identifiable factor deficiency.

Diagnosis and investigation of AL amyloidosis

Amyloid should be considered in the differential diagnosis of renal failure, nephrotic syndrome, restrictive cardiomyopathy, peripheral or autonomic neuropathy and hepatomegaly, but early symptoms are often very non-specific and insidious, such as malaise or weight loss. The index of suspicion should be high in patients known to have clonal B-cell dyscrasias, but in practice the diagnosis of amyloidosis is usually an unexpected finding following biopsy of an organ with disturbed function. The approach to diagnosis is outlined in Table 32.2, and essentially comprises confirmation of the presence of amyloid, determination of fibril type, characterization of the underlying plasma cell dyscrasia, and evaluation of the extent, distribution and function of involved organs.

Confirming the presence of amyloid

Histology
In systemic forms of amyloidosis, deposits occur in blood vessels and as small interstitial foci throughout the body. This provides the basis for 'screening' biopsies, such as of the rectum by flexible sigmoidoscopy or of abdominal fat by needle aspiration, both of which are diagnostic in 50–80% of cases. Bone marrow trephine biopsies performed to differentiate MGUS from myeloma in a newly diagnosed plasma cell dyscrasia can also be used to diagnose amyloidosis and are almost pathognomonic of the AL type, hence routine Congo red staining should

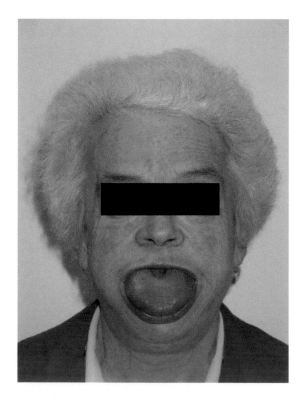

Figure 32.1 Macroglossia in AL amyloidosis.

Table 32.2 Suggested approach to the investigation and monitoring of suspected AL amyloidosis.

	Confirmation of amyloid	Determination of amyloid type	Evaluation of organ involvement	Investigation of plasma cell dyscrasia	Monitoring
Pathology	Biopsy and Congo red histology of affected organ, screening tissue (e.g. rectum or fat aspirate) or any available specimen	Immunohistochemical staining of tissue sections with a panel of antibodies to amyloid fibril proteins (often not definitive in AL amyloidosis)	Biopsy of affected organ (but subsequent biopsies merely to determine the extent of amyloid involvement are not recommended)	Bone marrow aspirate and trephine biopsy with immunophenotyping	Follow-up biopsies usually not helpful in monitoring amyloid load
Haematology, biochemistry, immunology		Identification of a monoclonal gammopathy supports AL type, but may be an incidental finding	Serum creatinine and creatinine clearance, albumin, 24-hour urine protein Liver function tests Coagulation screen NT-pro-BNP, troponin, thyroid function tests	Full blood count, urea and electrolytes, creatinine, calcium Immunoglobulins Electrophoresis and immunofixation of serum and urine Quantitative serum free light chain assay	Quantitative serum free light chain assay (every month or two) NT-pro-BNP (3–6 monthly) Electrophoresis and immunofixation of serum and urine (3–6 monthly)
Imaging	SAP scintigraphy	SAP scintigraphy (evidence of marrow involvement is indicative of AL type)	Echocardiogram, ECG, SAP scintigraphy	Skeletal survey	SAP scintigraphy (6–12 monthly)
Other		DNA analysis for hereditary forms of amyloidosis Amyloid fibril protein sequencing	As otherwise indicated, e.g. nerve conduction studies, cardiac MRI		Serial assessment of organ function, e.g. liver and renal function tests, including 24-hour proteinuria estimations, echocardiography and other investigations as indicated

NT-pro-BNP, N-terminal pro-brain natriuretic peptide.

be considered in these instances. Diffuse parenchymal amyloid deposits may occur in few or many organs, and biopsy of a clinically affected organ, for example the kidney, heart, liver or gastrointestinal tract, is likely to give positive results in more than 95% of cases. The appearance on haematoxylin and eosin-stained tissue of pink amorphous material should raise suspicion of amyloid and prompt further more specific stains. Many cotton dyes, fluorochromes and metachromatic stains are used, but Congo red stains that produce green birefringence under cross-polarized light is generally accepted to be the diagnostic gold standard in amyloidosis (Figure 32.2). False-positive and false-negative interpretation of the Congo red stain is not rare but can be minimized by using the alkaline-alcohol method (described by Puchtler and colleagues), fresh reagents, tissue sections of optimal 5–10 μm thickness, inclusion of positive control tissue and high-quality polarizing filters. Some Congo red techniques stain connective tissues quite strongly and produce white or very pale-green birefringence that can cause diagnostic errors.

The histological appearance of light chain deposition disease (LCDD) can mimic AL amyloidosis and can initially cause a diagnostic challenge. However, unlike AL amyloidosis, LCDD deposits lack the fibrillar configuration, with no affinity for Congo red stain and do not produce the characteristic green birefringence of amyloid under cross-polarized light.

Electron microscopy

Electron microscopy is helpful in distinguishing between AL amyloidosis and LCDD. Amyloid deposits are fibrillar, whereas LCDD deposits are granular. However, amyloid fibrils cannot always be convincingly identified ultrastructurally, and a diagnosis of amyloidosis made through electron microscopy alone should be regarded with caution since other pathological processes involve deposition of fibrillar material.

SAP scintigraphy

Radiolabelled SAP scintigraphy is a specific nuclear medicine imaging technique that demonstrates the presence and distribution of amyloid deposits *in vivo* in a quantitative manner. It was developed, and is used routinely, at the UK National Amyloidosis Centre. ^{123}I-labelled SAP localizes rapidly and specifically to amyloid deposits of all fibril types, in proportion to the amount of amyloid present. SAP scintigraphy confirms the presence of amyloid in most patients with AL type and virtually all with AA type, as well as most hereditary forms. The scans provide information that is different and complementary to biopsy histology, including whole-body and individual organ amyloid load both at diagnosis and in serial follow-up studies, for example following chemotherapy in AL amyloidosis (Figure 32.3). It is a particularly good imaging modality for detecting amyloid deposition in the liver, spleen, kidneys, bone marrow and adrenal glands. The organ distribution of amyloid on SAP scintigraphy can be indicative of the fibril type, for example bone uptake essentially occurs only in AL amyloidosis. Unfortunately, amyloid in the moving heart and in small or diffuse hollow structures such as nerves, the gastrointestinal tract and the lungs is not adequately visualized by SAP scintigraphy. Various other tracers, including conventional bone-seeking agents and radiolabelled aprotinin, sometimes localize non-specifically to amyloid deposits but do not have any defined clinical role.

Identifying fibril type

It has been common practice to diagnose apparently 'primary' cases of amyloidosis as AL in type, especially when a monoclonal gammopathy can be demonstrated. However, the under-

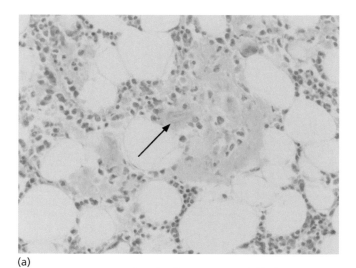
(a)

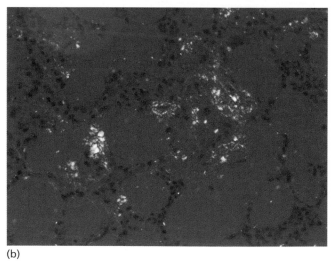
(b)

Figure 32.2 Appearance of amyloid in a bone marrow biopsy (×40, 6-μm section). (a) Congo red stain showing amorphous pink material in the interstitium and small blood vessel (arrow). (b) Same section under high-intensity cross-polarized light showing diagnostic apple-green birefringence.

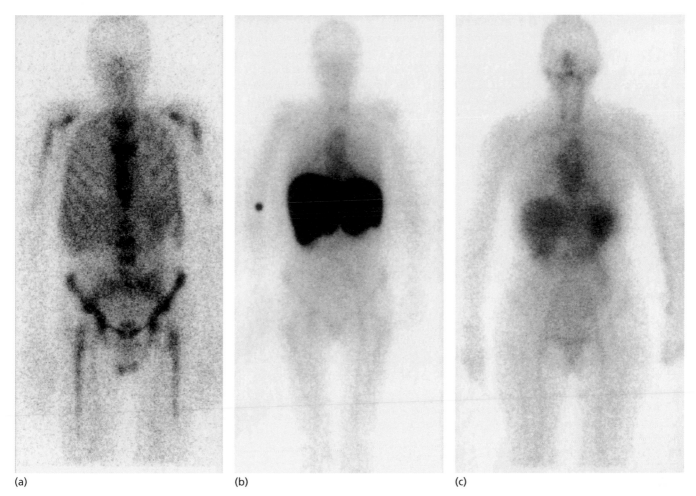

(a)　　　　　　　　　　　　(b)　　　　　　　　　　　　(c)

Figure 32.3 Radiolabelled ^{123}I-SAP whole-body scintigraphy, anterior images. (a) The tracer has localized virtually exclusively to amyloid deposits in the bones in this particular patient, a distribution that is almost pathognomonic for amyloid of AL type. (b, c) Serial scintigraphs in a 56-year-old woman with AL amyloidosis. At presentation in 1998 (b) she had massive uptake in the spleen and liver, obscuring any renal signal. She underwent high-dose chemotherapy, and the follow-up scan in 2002 (c) shows that the deposits have regressed substantially.

lying chronic inflammatory disease process is clinically covert in 5–10% of patients with AA amyloidosis, and a family history is quite often absent in patients with hereditary amyloidosis, due to variable penetrance and late onset of symptoms. The coincidental presence of a monoclonal gammopathy can therefore be gravely misleading and lead to misdiagnosis of AL amyloidosis and inappropriate use of cytotoxic agents. The combination of immunohistochemical staining and DNA analysis is vital to aid confirmation of amyloid fibril type and exclusion of hereditary forms of amyloidosis.

Immunohistochemistry

Immunohistochemical staining of amyloid-containing tissue sections using a panel of antibodies against known amyloid proteins is the most accessible method for characterizing fibril type. However, definitive results are often not obtained in AL amyloidosis due to a combination of background staining of normal immunoglobulin and failure of antibodies to bind to κ or λ light chains in their abnormal amyloid conformation. In contrast, antibodies against serum amyloid A protein can confirm or exclude AA amyloidosis in virtually all cases and, with optimization, immunohistochemical staining is usually definitive in hereditary forms involving TTR, fibrinogen and apolipoprotein A-I. Reliable interpretation of immunohistochemical stains is not possible unless positive and negative controls have been used, and the specificity of staining by absorption with appropriate antigens has been demonstrated in each run.

DNA analysis

The clinical features in hereditary systemic amyloidosis are often indistinguishable from those in AL amyloidosis. Sequencing of the genes associated with hereditary amyloidosis should be performed routinely to exclude hereditary amyloidosis when the AL type cannot be confirmed with absolute certainty by immunohistochemistry as well as in all patients in whom familial disease is suspected. DNA analysis for mutations in the genes coding for TTR, fibrinogen Aα chain, lysozyme, apolipoprotein A-I, apolipoprotein A-II and gelsolin are now available at major amyloid centres, including the UK National Amyloidosis Centre. Importantly, hereditary TTR and fibrinogen Aα chain amyloidosis are much more common than previously thought. Compounding this, a family history of amyloidosis may be absent due to incomplete penetrance. In a British series of 350 cases, 34 patients were initially misdiagnosed as having AL amyloidosis until genetic sequencing demonstrated the alternative hereditary types. Hereditary TTR amyloidosis can present with polyneuropathy and/or amyloid cardiomyopathy, and there should be a low threshold for sequencing the gene for TTR in patients with this phenotype. Hereditary fibrinogen Aα-chain amyloidosis should be considered in any patient with an exclusive renal presentation and has a distinctive appearance on renal biopsy, with extensive glomerular involvement and notable absence of extraglomerular amyloid. Corroboration by immunohistochemistry and clinical features is necessary to confirm that identified mutations are indeed the cause of the amyloid. It is often only possible therefore to be confident of the diagnosis of AL amyloidosis after exclusion of AA and hereditary types by immunohistochemistry and genetic sequencing respectively.

Mass spectrometry

Amyloid fibril proteins can also be characterized by various proteomic analyses including mass spectrometry, although these techniques are not yet routinely available.

Assessment of the plasma cell dyscrasia

A monoclonal whole paraprotein or free light chains can be identified by electrophoresis and immunofixation of serum and urine in only 80% of patients with systemic AL amyloidosis. However, SFLC analysis (Freelite, The Binding Site, Birmingham, UK) can demonstrate a clonal excess of SFLCs in over 90% of cases and can be used to quantitatively monitor the effects of chemotherapy on the underlying plasma cell clone on a frequent basis. Unlike whole intact paraproteins, which have a half-life of 5–20 days, SFLCs have half-lives of only 2–6 hours, which means that they are ideal for gauging response to chemotherapy and have become the standard of care in AL amyloidosis. In patients with renal failure, κ and λ free light chains are retained in the serum, leading to higher than normal individual light chain levels, but the ratio of free κ to free λ continues to enable the clonal disease to be followed.

Bone marrow aspiration and trephine biopsy are required to characterize the underlying B-cell dyscrasia, which comprises a subtle plasma cell infiltrate in about 80% of cases. The presence of amyloid in a bone marrow specimen other than blood vessels

is highly suggestive of AL type. Immunophenotyping and cytogenetic findings in AL amyloidosis are similar to those in myeloma. Immunoparesis occurs frequently in AL amyloidosis. Lytic lesions or hypercalcaemia are diagnostic of myeloma and so skeletal surveys are routinely recommended in new cases of AL amyloidosis to help distinguish myeloma from MGUS.

Assessment of organ involvement

There are now international consensus criteria, detailed by Gertz and colleagues in 2005, for defining organ involvement in AL amyloidosis (Table 32.3). Organ involvement by amyloid is variously defined clinically, histologically, according to organ function and by SAP scintigraphy where available. ECG and two-dimensional Doppler echocardiography are vital tools for evaluating cardiac involvement. In cardiac amyloidosis, ECG may demonstrate reduced QRS voltages in the limb leads and

Table 32.3 Non-invasive diagnostic criteria for amyloid-related major organ involvement.

Heart
Echocardiogram demonstrates mean wall thickness >12 mm, no other cardiac cause found

Kidney
Proteinuria >0.5 g per 24 hours, predominantly albumin

Liver
Total liver span >15 cm in the absence of heart failure or alkaline phosphatase >1.5 times the institutional upper limit of normal

Nerve
Peripheral: clinical; symmetric lower extremity sensorimotor peripheral neuropathy
Autonomic: gastric emptying disorder, pseudo-obstruction, voiding dysfunction not related to direct organ infiltration

Gastrointestinal tract
Direct biopsy verification with symptoms

Lung
Direct biopsy verification with symptoms
Interstitial radiographic pattern

Soft tissue
Tongue enlargement, clinical
Arthropathy
Claudication, presumed vascular amyloid
Skin
Myopathy by biopsy or psudohypertrophy
Lymph node (may be localized)
Carpal tunnel syndrome

Source: Gertz *et al.* (2005) with permission.

poor R-wave progression in the chest leads ('pseudo-infarct' pattern). Echocardiography typically reveals concentrically thickened and echogenic heart valves. Cardiac amyloidosis is a restrictive cardiomyopathy and diastolic dysfunction is easily missed and difficult to quantify. Cardiac magnetic resonance imaging (MRI) is emerging as a useful tool for identifying cardiac amyloidosis and distinguishing it from other restrictive cardiomyopathies. The status of other organs can be assessed either through routine tests of organ function, such as liver function tests, serum creatinine and 24-hour urine measurements, or by specialist investigations as indicated, for example autonomic function and nerve conduction tests and high-resolution pulmonary computed tomography (CT).

Glomerular proteinuria (predominantly albuminuria) is present in about 90% of patients with renal involvement. Abnormalities in liver function tests are unusual and do not occur until liver amyloidosis is substantial, and are most commonly obstructive in nature. Right-sided heart failure due to amyloid cardiomyopathy may cause obstructive liver function tests in the absence of liver involvement by amyloid. Anaemia is uncommon unless amyloidosis is associated with myeloma, bleeding or chronic kidney disease. An abnormal clotting screen is relatively common. A prolonged thrombin time is the most frequent abnormality, but is generally of no clinical consequence. A prolonged prothrombin time due to acquired factor X deficiency is the most likely coagulation abnormality to be associated with clinically significant bleeding.

Elevation of N-terminal pro-brain natriuretic peptide (NT-pro-BNP) and cardiac troponin concentrations occur in a wide variety of cardiac conditions and in chronic kidney disease. However, significant myocardial AL amyloidosis is excluded by NT-pro-BNP concentrations below 30 pmol/L. Cardiac troponin and NT-pro-BNP concentrations appear to be powerful predictors of prognosis and survival after chemotherapy. A staging system for patients with newly diagnosed AL amyloidosis using these two biomarkers has been proposed but requires further validation.

Differential diagnosis

Alternative diagnoses that frequently need to be considered include amyloidosis of non-AL types (principally AA and hereditary forms), localized forms of AL amyloidosis, and non-amyloid diseases such as LCDD and paraprotein-associated neuropathies including POEMS syndrome and treatment-related toxicities.

Natural history

Systemic AL amyloidosis is a progressive systemic disease that left untreated has a prognosis far worse than AA and hereditary amyloidoses. Median survival without treatment in historical series is only 12–15 months. Half of deaths are due to cardiac involvement, and in patients in whom heart failure is evident at presentation, median survival is 6 months.

Until recently, amyloid deposition has been thought to be inexorably progressive and irreversible. It is now clear that amyloid deposits usually exist in a slowly dynamic state, and that they often gradually regress if the supply of amyloid fibril precursor protein can be reduced. However, the turnover of amyloid varies substantially between different individuals and organs and the factors that may influence this are not yet understood. The knowledge that amyloid can regress has encouraged a much more aggressive approach to patient management in recent years.

Prognostic factors

Prognosis varies in AL amyloidosis but is generally poor if the disease is left untreated. With adequate suppression of amyloidogenic light chains, and under favourable circumstances, amyloid may stabilize or regress, organ function may improve gradually and prolonged survival is not infrequent. Proteinuria often improves over 12–24 months with adequate suppression of the underlying clone, but improvement in renal function, soft-tissue involvement including macroglossia, and cardiac amyloidosis is generally very slow indeed after a haematological response. Therefore, patients should be informed that treatment is aimed at preventing disease progression while being encouraged that survival has steadily improved from a median of 1–2 years in the 1980s and 1990s to more than 4 years currently.

Various factors help to predict survival at diagnosis. Symptomatic or substantial echocardiographic evidence of cardiac amyloid is associated with a prognosis of only 6–12 months. Patients with liver involvement and hyperbilirubinaemia (bilirubin > 35 μmol/L) rarely survive more than 4 months. Significant autonomic neuropathy, progressive clonal disease unresponsive to chemotherapy and a bone marrow plasmacytosis of over 20% are also associated with poor outcomes. A large whole-body amyloid load on SAP scintigraphy and evidence of accumulation of amyloid on follow-up SAP scans are also poor prognostic features.

A better prognosis is associated with proteinuria or peripheral neuropathy as the dominant clinical feature, substantial suppression of underlying clonal disease by chemotherapy and regression of amyloid deposits on serial SAP scintigraphy. More recently, NT-pro-BNP concentration has been introduced as a prognostic marker, with raised values at diagnosis associated with a poorer prognosis and a fall in concentration >30% after chemotherapy associated with improved survival.

Management

Specific therapies that inhibit formation of amyloid or enhance its clearance are not yet available, although both strategies are being rigorously pursued. Currently, the objective of treatment in AL amyloidosis is to suppress production of the amyloidogenic monoclonal light chains in the hope that progression of the disease will be slowed, halted or reversed. However, many patients have advanced multisystem disease at diagnosis and tolerate chemotherapy poorly.

Quantitative measurements of SFLCs are usually the most effective means for guiding ongoing treatment in individual patients. Although it is generally desirable to suppress the underlying clonal disease as rapidly and as extensively as possible, reduction in the concentration of the amyloidogenic free light chain by just 50–75% can be sufficient to halt disease progression in the majority of patients and confer substantial survival benefit, regardless of the chemotherapy used. Hence, more intensive suppression of the clonal disease beyond this may be unnecessary. This is particularly important given the broad range of organ involvement and impairment in AL amyloidosis that is associated with higher rates of treatment-related toxicities than in myeloma. Chemotherapy must be tailored to the individual patient, balancing the need for complete remission with the need to minimize treatment toxicity.

Certain organs affected by amyloid tend to fare better than others following treatment. Proteinuria and liver function often improve when the clonal disease is adequately suppressed, whereas cardiac disease, macroglossia and peripheral nerve function tend to improve extremely slowly if at all. International consensus criteria on the definitions of clonal and organ responses and progression were described by Gertz and colleagues in 2005.

Autologous peripheral blood stem cell transplantation

Use of high-dose melphalan therapy and autologous stem cell transplantation (SCT) in AL amyloidosis was first reported in 1996, and several series have reported clinical benefit in up to 80% of patients who survived the procedure. In the largest reported series, consisting of 394 patients, a complete clonal response occurred in 41%. Of those alive and in clonal response 1 year after autologous SCT, median survival has not been reached after 10 years of follow-up. However, treatment-related mortality (TRM) with autologous SCT has been consistently and substantially higher than in multiple myeloma, ranging from 5 to 43%, reflecting the compromised function of multiple organ systems by amyloid. Even stem cell mobilization has significant risks in AL amyloidosis. Causes of death include cardiac arrhythmias, intractable hypotension, multiple organ failure and gastrointestinal bleeding. Patient selection has since been refined and criteria for eligibility for autologous SCT developed, with the main exclusion criteria being overt cardiac involvement, more than two vital organ systems involved, a history of gastrointestinal bleeding and age over 65 years. Improvements in TRM have gradually resulted from better patient selection with improved supportive care and physician experience.

The exact role of SCT in AL amyloidosis remains controversial and its apparently good outcome may reflect selection of fitter good-prognosis patients. Regardless, because of its special problems in AL amyloidosis, it is recommended that such patients are treated in units with expertise in this particular disease. In eligible patients, autologous SCT with melphalan 200 mg/m^2 is often recommended as first-line therapy without induction chemotherapy except in those with underlying myeloma. Lower doses of melphalan appear to compromise the efficacy of transplantation. Stem-cell mobilization is often achieved with the use of granulocyte colony-stimulating factor (G-CSF) alone, as the underlying plasma cell burden is usually relatively small. The French group compared autologous SCT with oral melphalan and dexamethasone in a randomized study and found no difference in response rates between the two arms but a significantly higher TRM for the autologous SCT arm (24%) and a longer overall survival in the melphalan/dexamethasone arm, throwing into question the routine use of autologous SCT in AL amyloiodosis. However, the trial has attracted some controversy, with higher than expected rates of TRM in autologous SCT compared with other case series and the use of lower doses of melphalan (140 mg/m^2) in some of the patients undergoing SCT, prompting calls for further study in this area.

Melphalan and dexamethasone

Since 1999, melphalan and dexamethasone have been widely used in Europe and been found to be a well-tolerated and effective oral chemotherapy, with clonal response rates of 67% including complete responses in 37%, organ response rates of 50% and median overall survival of about 5 years. However, median time to response is slow at 4.5 months, and the problem of stem-cell toxicity makes it a less attractive regimen for patients who may subsequently be eligible for autologous SCT. Renal dose adjustment is required and the long-term leukaemogenesis of this regimen has yet to be established.

Cyclophosphamide, thalidomide and dexamethasone

Thalidomide has been used extensively in combination therapies for plasma cell disorders but doses above 200 mg daily are poorly tolerated in AL amyloidosis. Amyloid-related cardiac involvement or peripheral neuropathy results in increased sensitivity to the adverse effects of thalidomide, such as fluid retention fatigue, constipation and neuropathy. Lower doses of single-agent thalidomide reduce toxicity but also markedly reduce responses rates. The use of thalidomide as maintenance treatment in AL amyloidosis has not yet been established. Addition of dexamethasone to intermediate-dose thalidomide improves the response rate to about 50%, with a median time to response of less than 4 months, but is associated with significant toxicity in 60% of patients. The cyclophosphamide, thalidomide and dexamethasone (CTD) regimen has been used extensively in the treatment of AL amyloidosis in the UK since

2002 and incorporates the addition of weekly oral cyclophosphamide 500 mg to low-dose thalidomide (100–200 mg) and two pulses of dexamethasone over a 21-day cycle. A risk-adapted approach using even lower doses of both thalidomide (50–100 mg) and dexamethasone in high-risk patients maintains good clonal response rates while decreasing the incidence of severe toxicity to around 20%. Overall SFLC response rates are around 75%, with an SFLC clonal response rate of 37%. Organ responses occur in approximately 50%. Median duration of response is 32 months. Fatigue and fluid retention requiring increased diuretic use remain the most troublesome toxicities of this regimen. Patients with severe nephrotic syndrome are at particular risk of venous and arterial thrombosis and should receive thromboprophylaxis. However, CTD has the advantage of being a stem cell-sparing oral regimen that does not require dose adjustment in renal impairment and is rapidly acting, the majority of patients achieving at least a partial (>50%) SFLC response after only 1 month of treatment.

Bortezomib

The proteasome inhibitor bortezomib is emerging as one of the most effective and rapidly acting therapies in the treatment of AL amyloidosis. In a recent multicentre study of 94 patients, most of whom had relapsed following previous treatments, clonal responses with bortezomib-based therapy occurred in 70% including complete remission CR in 25%, and the median time to clonal response was only 1 month. Organ responses occurred in 30%, and median time to progression was 14 months; major toxicities included peripheral and autonomic neuropathy. However, unlike in myeloma, cytopenias were rare with bortezomib, most likely due to the smaller plasma cell burden in the bone marrow. Its optimal dosing, long-term efficacy and use with dexamethasone, alkylators and other agents are the subject of ongoing clinical studies.

Lenalidomide

The thalidomide analogue lenalidomide has lately also been reported in several small studies in AL amyloidosis. Maximum tolerated dose is typically about 15 mg. Efficacy is markedly improved when administered with dexamethasone, and is associated with clonal response rates of about 50%, including complete remission in 20%. Organ responses were reported as approximately 22%. Toxicity from infections, even without neutropenia, appears to be surprisingly high, especially in patients with severe renal or cardiac impairment. Time to response is relatively slow, with a median in one study of 6 months when lenalidomide was used alone. However, lenalidomide remains an attractive treatment option in patients with severe neuropathy in whom thalidomide or bortezomib are relatively contraindicated. Use of lenalidomide in combination regimens and its role as maintenance therapy are currently under investigation.

Vincristine, doxorubicin and dexamethasone

Vincristine, doxorubicin (Adriamycin) and dexamethasone (VAD) and similar regimens have been well established as infusional induction regimens in myeloma (see Chapter 31), associated with response rates of 60–80%, complete response rates of 10–25% and rapid reduction in tumour burden. They do not deplete stem-cell reserve, keeping open the option for subsequent autologous SCT. Problems with the use of VAD in AL amyloidosis include exacerbation of peripheral and autonomic neuropathy by vincristine, and induction or worsening of fluid retention in renal or cardiac amyloidosis by dexamethasone. Doxorubicin has not been shown to exacerbate amyloid cardiomyopathy. The SFLC response rate is approximately 65%, and organ responses are seen in 50%. However, like in myeloma, the inconvenience of this regimen relative to newer oral therapies has led to a decline in its use.

Melphalan and prednisolone

In the early 1990s, cyclical oral melphalan with or without prednisolone was the first chemotherapy to be demonstrated in a randomized controlled trial as effective in the treatment of AL amyloidosis. However, benefits of treatment were typically not observed for at least 6 months and were substantial in only 20% of cases. As such, the use of melphalan was a breakthrough in the treatment of AL amyloidosis, but it is now no longer routinely recommended in low doses either as a single agent or with prednisolone.

Intermediate-dose intravenous melphalan

The variable absorption of melphalan from the gastrointestinal tract led investigators to trial intravenous intermediate-dose melphalan (25 mg/m^2) and oral dexamethasone in patients with untreated multiple myeloma. This regimen has also been used as first-line therapy in patients with AL amyloidosis, who were selected on the basis that they were not fit enough to receive VAD-based treatment because of age, poor performance status, severe amyloid cardiomyopathy or neuropathy. Dexamethasone was omitted in patients with significant fluid retention. Efficacy, in terms of both clonal disease and organ response, was similar to that of VAD. However, this regimen was found to be associated with an unacceptably high rate of TRM (12%) and is now little used.

Allogeneic bone marrow transplantation

A case of successful allogeneic bone marrow transplantation in AL amyloidosis was reported in 1998 and since then a European study has reported on allogeneic and syngeneic haemopoietic cell transplantation in 19 patients with AL amyloidosis. Overall TRM was 40% and haematological response occurred in eight patients, with only one relapse after 31 months of follow-up. This treatment option is thus rarely exercised at present.

Supportive treatment

Supportive therapy remains a critical component of management of AL amyloidosis. For cardiac amyloidosis, the mainstay of treatment is diuretics. Vasodilating drugs and beta-blockers are generally best avoided as they often worsen symptoms significantly. Fluid overload should be treated with fluid restriction, loop diuretics and a low-salt diet. Refractory oedema may respond well to the addition of spironolactone. Salt-poor albumin infusions can occasionally be helpful. Dysrhythmias may respond to amiodarone or to pacing.

In renal amyloidosis, rigorous control of hypertension is vital, and inhibiton of angiotensin-converting enzyme and/or angiotensin II is often recommended in the context of proteinuria. Renal dialysis may be necessary, and is usually both feasible and acceptably tolerated. In autonomic neuropathy, fludrocortisone 100–200 µg/day can be helpful in some patients, but may cause or exacerbate fluid retention. Midodrine is an effective pressor agent, starting at 2.5–15 mg thrice daily. Midodrine causes activation of the α-adrenergic receptors of the arteriolar and venous vasculature, producing an increase in vascular tone and elevation of blood pressure. Its chief adverse effect is supine hypertension, and other pressor agents must be coadministered with caution. Gastroparesis causing symptoms of early satiety and nausea can be managed with prokinetic agents such as metaclopramide, along with advice about small frequent meals that are of soft consistency. Diarrhoea due to amyloid gut involvement or autonomic neuropathy may respond to loperamide and codeine phosphate. Malnutrition is not uncommon and is often underestimated. Significant weight loss should be treated with protein and vitamin supplementation and the patient should be reviewed by an experienced dietitian. Feeding via a percutaneous endoscopic gastrostomy may occasionally be required. Amyloid- and treatment-related peripheral neuropathy can be disabling and difficult to treat. Analgesia including opioids and non-steroidal anti-inflammatory drugs, amitriptyline, venlafaxine, antiepileptics, TENS and/or gabapentin/pregabalin have all been used, although anecdotal reports suggest limited efficacy. Withdrawal or dose reduction of any neurotoxic chemotherapies, such as thalidomide or bortezomib, should be considered.

Surgical resection of amyloidotic tissue is occasionally beneficial but, in general, a conservative approach to surgery, anaesthesia and other invasive procedures is advised. Should any such procedure be undertaken, meticulous attention to blood pressure and fluid balance is essential, especially in patients with renal and/or cardiac involvement. Amyloidotic tissues may heal poorly and are liable to haemorrhage.

Solid organ transplantation

Renal and cardiac transplantation have been used in selected patients with AL amyloidosis for over 25 years. Renal transplantation should be considered in relatively young patients with otherwise well-preserved extrarenal organ function who have chemotherapy-responsive disease. Cardiac transplantation should be considered in patients with isolated end-stage cardiac failure who would otherwise be eligible for autologous SCT. In such patients, cardiac transplantation must be followed by chemotherapy to prevent recurrence of cardiac amyloid or its accumulation in other organ systems. Liver transplantation has been performed in only a very small number of patients with generally disappointing results.

Localized AL amyloidosis

Localized deposits of AL amyloid can occur almost anywhere in the body, with characteristic sites including the skin, airways, conjunctiva and urogenital tract. They may be nodular or confluent and are associated with a usually inconspicuous focal infiltrate of clonal B cell-producing amyloidogenic light chains. Progression of localized AL amyloid into a truly systemic disease is exceedingly rare, and conservative management is usually appropriate. Orbital AL amyloid presents as mass lesions that can disrupt eye movement and the structure of the orbit. Localized laryngeal AL amyloidosis is a well-recognized syndrome that is often amenable to direct or laser excision, but hereditary systemic apolipoprotein A-I amyloidosis can also present in this manner. Amyloidosis in the bronchial tree is virtually always of localized AL type, as are solitary or multiple amyloid nodules within the lung tissue. If accessible, brochoscopic lasering of stenosing lesions can bring symptom relief. In contrast, diffuse alveolar septal parenchymal deposition is commonly a manifestation of systemic AL amyloidosis. There are anectodal reports that inhaled steroids may benefit pulmonary symptoms. Breast amyloidosis has been associated with Sjögren disease in some cases, and mucosa-associated lymphoid tissue (MALT) lymphoma should be excluded. Lichenoid and macular forms of cutaneous amyloid are thought to be derived from keratin or related proteins, whereas nodular cutaneous amyloid deposits are generally of AL type and can sometimes be a manifestation of systemic AL amyloidosis. Localized urogenital AL amyloid deposits are often incidental findings but may present with haematuria or, less commonly, obstruction. They can occur anywhere from the renal collecting system to the urethra, although are most usually identified within the bladder. Management is conservative or with transurethral laser resection when symptoms occur; cystectomy is rarely required.

Other forms of systemic amyloidosis

Among more than 3000 patients with systemic amyloidosis who have been referred for evaluation at the National Amyloidosis

Centre, approximately 55% have had AL type, 15% AA (reactive systemic) type, and the remainder have had a variety of hereditary, localized and other types. Although some features of systemic AL amyloidosis are very characteristic of this particular type, such as macroglossia, periorbital purpura and certain permutations of organ involvement, the clinical phenotypes of AA, AL and hereditary systemic amyloidosis can be indistinguishable. Furthermore, the underlying chronic inflammatory disease process is clinically covert in 5–10% of patients with AA amyloidosis, and a family history is often absent in patients with hereditary TTR and fibrinogen Aα-chain amyloidosis, which are the most common familial forms.

AA amyloidosis

Reactive systemic AA (secondary) amyloidosis occurs in 1–5% of patients with chronic inflammatory diseases that evoke a substantial acute-phase response, after a median latency of about 15–20 years. AA amyloid fibrils are derived from the circulating acute-phase reactant SAA, the serum concentration of which can increase from the healthy reference range of less than 10 mg/L to over 1000 mg/L during active inflammation. The commonest associated diseases in the developed world include rheumatoid arthritis, juvenile idiopathic arthritis and Crohn's disease. Familial Mediterranean fever and other rare periodic fever syndromes can result in AA amyloidosis. Chronic infections remain important causes in some parts of world. Castleman disease of the solitary plasma cell type should be considered among the underlying conditions that remain clinically covert.

Most patients present with nephropathy, particularly proteinuria, but liver and gastrointestinal involvement may occur at a late stage. Clinical involvement of the heart and nerves occurs very rarely. Diagnosis of AA amyloid is usually achieved by renal (or rectal) biopsy, and the AA fibril type can be confirmed immunohistochemically using anti-SAA antibodies in almost all cases. SAP scintigraphy virtually always shows involvement of the spleen and kidneys; hepatic involvement is a late feature associated with a poor prognosis. Treatment in AA amyloidosis should decrease the underlying inflammation so that SAA levels remain well controlled, preferably below 10 mg/L. The exact nature of the treatment will depend on the underlying inflammatory disease, and ranges from inhibitors of tumour necrosis factor in rheumatoid arthritis and colchicine in familial Mediterranean fever to surgical resection of Castleman disease tumours. Any therapy that reduces SAA production to healthy baseline levels prevents further deposition of AA amyloid, frequently leads to the regression of existing amyloid deposits with improvement in amyloid-related organ dysfunction, and significantly improves long-term survival. Kidney transplantation generally has excellent outcomes in AA amyloidosis.

β₂-Microglobulin amyloidosis

β_2-Microglobulin amyloidosis, also known as dialysis-related amyloidosis, occurs because of the accumulation of β_2-microglobulin in renal failure and predominantly affects articular and periarticular structures in patients with end-stage renal failure who have been on dialysis for at least 7–10 years. Susceptibility factors include older age and the use of non-biocompatible dialysis membranes. Carpal tunnel syndrome is often the first clinical manifestation, and large-joint arthralgias, tenosynovitis, spondyloarthropathies and periarticular bone cysts are common. Although β_2-microglobulin amyloidosis is a systemic form of amyloidosis, deposits outside the musculoskeletal system are seldom of clinical significance. The disabling arthralgia may respond partially to non-steroidal anti-inflammatory drugs or corticosteroids, but the only really effective treatment for this condition is normalization of β_2-microglobulin levels through renal transplantation. Carpal tunnel syndrome is amenable to surgery but may recur.

Transthyretin amyloidosis

Normal TTR is inherently but weakly amyloidogenic, and minor TTR amyloid deposits are common in elderly individuals. Clinically significant involvement is almost completely restricted to the heart and carpal tunnel, and senile cardiac amyloid derived from wild-type TTR occurs in up to 25% of subjects over 80 years of age and is most likely under-recognized by physicians. This syndrome is extremely rare before 65 years of age. Patients may survive for many years with reasonably good quality of life managed with diuretics alone; specific therapies are currently being tested.

Hereditary systemic amyloidoses

Hereditary systemic amyloidosis is caused by deposition of genetically variant proteins as amyloid fibrils, and is associated with mutations in the genes for TTR, fibrinogen Aα chain, cystatin C, gelsolin, apolipoprotein A-I, apolipoprotein A-II and lysozyme. These disorders are all inherited in an autosomal dominant manner with variable penetrance, and usually present in adult life.

Familial amyloidotic polyneuropathy (FAP) associated with mutations in the gene for TTR is the most common type of hereditary amyloidosis. It is characterized by progressive and disabling peripheral and autonomic neuropathy, often with cardiac involvement. Vitreous amyloid deposits may also occur and are virtually pathognomonic of the syndrome. Symptoms typically present between the third and seventh decades. More than 100 TTR variants are associated with FAP, the most frequent of which is the substitution of methionine for valine at residue 30 (TTR Met30). There are well-recognized foci of this in Portugal, Japan and Sweden, but FAP has been reported in most ethnic groups. TTR Ala60 is the most frequent cause of FAP in the British and Irish population, typically presenting after 50 years of age and usually with marked cardiac involvement. TTR Ile122 occurs in 3–4% of black Africans and is associated with a phenotype indistinguishable from senile (wild-type) cardiac amyloidosis. The majority of TTR is produced by hepatocytes, and liver transplantation is the only effective treatment for this disorder. Although the visceral amyloid deposits frequently regress following liver transplantation, the neuropathy is often irreversible and established cardiac amyloidosis may paradoxically progress due to ongoing fibril formation by wild-type TTR in this particular organ. Combined heart and liver transplantation has been performed successfully in a small number of cases.

The syndrome of non-neuropathic hereditary systemic amyloidosis is caused by mutations in the genes for fibrinogen Aα chain, lysozyme, apolipoprotein A-I and apolipoprotein A-II. Most such patients present with renal impairment and/or proteinuria, but substantial deposits in the liver and spleen are frequent in hereditary lysozyme and apolipoprotein A-I amyloidosis, and the heart may be involved in hereditary apolipoprotein A-I amyloidosis. Prominent neuropathy occurs in some patients with apolipoprotein A-I Arg26. Although kindreds with hereditary amyloidosis are rare, 5–10% of patients referred to the National Amyloidosis Centre with apparently sporadic amyloidosis do in fact have hereditary forms of the disease. About half of these are associated with TTR mutations, and most of the remainder are associated with variant fibrinogen Aα chain Val526. Penetrance of this particular mutation is extremely low in most families, thus obscuring the genetic aetiology, but the renal histology is characteristic, showing substantial accumulation of amyloid within enlarged glomeruli but none in blood vessels or the interstitium. Renal impairment is often noted in the fourth or fifth decade, and end-stage renal failure is managed with dialysis or renal transplantation. Variant fibrinogen Aα-chain amyloidosis can recur in the transplanted graft and median survival of kidney transplants in patients attending our centre has been 7 years though this can be much longer. Combined liver–kidney transplants have been performed in this condition though with notable mortality. Hereditary cystatin C amyloidosis manifests in Icelandic families as cerebral amyloid angiopathy with recurrent cerebral haemorrhage, and gelsolin variants are associated with corneal lattice dystrophy and cranial neuropathy, most often in Finnish patients.

DNA analysis should now performed routinely on patients with systemic amyloidosis in whom AA or AL fibril type cannot be definitively verified. The newly described leukocyte chemotactic factor II (LECT2) form of amyloidosis can also mimic AL, AA and hereditary forms of amyloid-related kidney disease but usually manifests as isolated, stable or slowly progressive renal impairment, often with positive kidney and adrenal gland

signalling on SAP scintigraphy; currently it can only be reliably identified with mass spectrometry.

Conclusion and future directions

Improved understanding of the aetiology and pathogenesis of amyloid has led to numerous recent advances in the characterization and management of amyloidosis. Chemotherapy in systemic AL amyloidosis can now be guided by its early effect on SFLC concentration, and routine DNA analysis can prevent patients with otherwise unrecognized hereditary amyloidosis from receiving inappropriate cytotoxic treatment. Clinical improvement following successful treatment of the various conditions that underlie amyloidosis is always delayed, and supportive measures are of great importance.

Novel therapeutic strategies include small molecules, monoclonal antibodies, peptides and GAG analogues that bind to fibril precursors and stabilize their native fold, or which interfere with refolding and/or aggregation into the common amyloid conformation or SAP depletion. Immunotherapy approaches are being explored as specific therapies directed at promoting regression of amyloid. Several of these new therapeutic approaches are already being tested in patients with the hope that they may be effective in a diverse spectrum of amyloid-related disorders in the near future.

Selected bibliography

Benson MD, Uemichi T (1996) Transthyretin amyloidosis. *Amyloid: the International Journal of Experimental and Clinical Investigation* **3**: 44–56.

Benson MD, James S, Scott K *et al.* (2008) Leukocyte chemotactic factor 2: a novel renal protein. *Kidney International* **74**: 218–22.

Booth DR, Sunde M, Bellotti V *et al.* (1997) Instability, unfolding and aggregation of human lysozyme variants underlying amyloid fibrillogenesis. *Nature* **385**: 787–93.

Botto M, Hawkins PN, Bickerstaff MCM *et al.* (1997) Amyloid deposition is delayed in mice with targeted deletion of the serum amyloid P component gene. *Nature Medicine* **3**: 855–9.

Comenzo RL, Gertz MA (2002) Autologous stem cell transplantation for primary systemic amyloidosis. *Blood* **99**: 4276–82.

Comenzo RL, Vosburgh E, Falk RH *et al.* (1998) Dose-intensive melphalan with blood stem-cell support for the treatment of AL (amyloid light-chain) amyloidosis: survival and responses in 25 patients. *Blood* **91**: 3662–70.

Dispenzieri A, Lacy MQ, Kyle RA *et al.* (2001) Eligibility for haematopoietic stem-cell transplantation for primary systemic amyloidosis is a favourable prognostic factor for survival. *Journal of Clinical Oncology* **19**: 3350–6.

Drüeke TB (1998) Dialysis-related amyloidosis. *Nephrology, Dialysis, Transplantation* **13** (Suppl. 1): 58–64.

Dubrey SW, Cha K, Anderson J et al. (1998) The clinical features of immunoglobulin light-chain (AL) amyloidosis with heart involvement. *Quarterly Journal of Medicine* **91**: 141–57.

Gertz MA, Lacy MQ, Dispenzieri A et al. (2002) Stem cell transplantation for the management of primary systemic amyloidosis. *American Journal of Medicine* **113**: 549–55.

Gertz MA, Comenzo R, Falk RH et al. (2005) Definition of organ involvement and treatment response in immunoglobulin light chain amyloidosis (AL): a consensus opinion from the 10th International Symposium on Amyloid and Amyloidosis. *American Journal of Hematology* **79**: 319–28.

Gibbs SDJ, Sattianayagam PT, Lachmann HJ et al. (2008) Risk-adapted cyclophosphamide, thalidomide and dexamethasone (CTD) for the treatment of systemic AL amyloidosis: long term outcomes among 202 patients [Abstract]. *Blood* **112**: 611.

Gibbs SDJ, Sattianayagam PT, Hawkins PN, Gillmore JD (2009) Cardiac transplantation should be considered in selected patients with either AL or hereditary forms of amyloidosis: the UK National Amyloidosis Centre experience. *Internal Medicine Journal* **39**: 786–7.

Gibbs SDJ, Sattianayagam PT, Lachmann HJ et al. (2009) Solid-organ transplantation in AL amyloidosis: lessons learned and future directions [Abstract]. *Clinical Lymphoma and Myeloma* **1**: 65–6.

Gillmore JD, Lovat LB, Persey MR et al. (2001) Amyloid load and clinical outcome in AA amyloidosis in relation to circulating concentration of serum amyloid A protein. *Lancet* **358**: 24–9.

Hawkins PN (2002) Serum amyloid P component scintigraphy for diagnosis and monitoring amyloidosis. *Current Opinion in Nephrology and Hypertension* **11**: 649–55.

Hawkins PN, Lavender JP, Pepys MB (1990) Evaluation of systemic amyloidosis by scintigraphy with ^{123}I-labelled serum amyloid P component. *New England Journal of Medicine* **323**: 508–13.

Jaccard A, Moreau P, Leblond V et al. (2007) High-dose melphalan versus melphalan plus dexamethasone for AL amyloidosis. *New England Journal of Medicine* **357**: 1083–93.

Kastritis E, Wechalekar AD, Dimopoulos MA et al. (2010) Bortezomib with or without dexamethasone in primary systemic (light chain) amyloidosis. *Journal of Clinical Oncology* **20**: 1031–7.

Kyle RA, Gertz MA (1995) Primary systemic amyloidosis: clinical and laboratory features in 474 cases. *Seminars in Hematology* **32**: 45–59.

Kyle RA, Gertz MA, Greipp PR et al. (1997) A trial of three regimens for primary amyloidosis: colchicine alone, melphalan and prednisone, and melphalan, prednisone, and colchicine. *New England Journal of Medicine* **336**: 1202–7.

Lachmann HJ, Booth DR, Booth SE et al. (2002) Misdiagnosis of hereditary amyloidosis as AL (primary) amyloidosis. *New England Journal of Medicine* **346**: 1786–91.

Lachmann HJ, Gallimore R, Gillmore JD et al. (2003) Outcome in systemic AL amyloidosis in relation to changes in concentration of circulating free immunoglobulin light chains following chemotherapy. *British Journal of Haematology* **122**: 78–84.

Palladini G, Perfetti V, Obici L et al. (2004) Association of melphalan and high-dose dexamethasone is effective and well tolerated in patients with AL (primary) amyloidosis who are ineligible for stem cell transplantation. *Blood* **103**: 2936–8.

Pepys MB, Herbert J, Hutchinson WL et al. (2002) Targeted pharmacological depletion of serum amyloid P component for treatment of human amyloidosis. *Nature* **417**: 254–9.

Puchtler H, Sweat F, Levine M (1962) On the binding of Congo red by amyloid. *Journal of Histochemistry and Cytochemistry* **10**: 355–64.

Samson D, Gaminara E, Newland A et al. (1989) Infusion of vincristine and doxorubicin with oral dexamethasone as first-line therapy for multiple myeloma. *Lancet* **ii**: 882–5.

Sanchorawala V, Wright DG, Seldin DC et al. (2001) An overview of the use of high-dose melphalan with autologous stem cell transplantation for the treatment of AL amyloidosis. *Bone Marrow Transplantation* **28**: 637–42.

Schey SA, Kazmi M, Ireland R, Lakhani A (1998) The use of intravenous intermediate dose melphalan and dexamethasone as induction treatment in the management of de novo multiple myeloma. *European Journal of Haematology* **61**: 306–10.

Scholand SO, Lokhorst H, Buzyn A et al. (2006) Allogeneic and syngeneic haematopoietic cell transplantation in patients with amyloid light-chain amyloidosis: a report from the European Group for Blood and Marrow transplantation. *Blood* **107**: 2578–84.

Skinner M, Sanchorawala V, Seldin DC et al. (2004) High dose melphalan and autologous stem-cell transplantation in patients with AL amyloidosis, an 8-year study. *Annals of Internal Medicine* **140**: 85–90.

Sunde M, Serpell LC, Bartlam M et al. (1997) Common core structure of amyloid fibrils by synchrotron X-ray diffraction. *Journal of Molecular Biology* **273**: 729–39.

Swerdlow SH, Campo E, Harris NL et al. (eds) (2008) *WHO Classification of Tumours of Haematopoietic and Lymphoid Tissues.* IARC, Lyon.

UK Myeloma Forum AL Amyloidosis Guidelines Working Group (2004) Guidelines on the diagnosis and management of AL amyloidosis. *British Journal of Haematology* **125**: 671–700.

Wechalekar AD, Hawkins PN, Gillmore JD (2007) Perspectives in the treatment of AL amyloidosis. *British Journal of Haematology* **140**: 365–77.

Wechalekar AD, Lachmann HJ, Offer M, Hawkins PN, Gillmore JD (2008) Efficacy of bortezomib in systemic AL amyloidosis with relapsed/refractory clonal disease. *Haematologica* **93**: 295–8.

The classification of lymphomas: updating the WHO classification

33

Elias Campo[1] and Stefano A Pileri[2]

[1]Hospital Clinic, University of Barcelona, Barcelona, Spain
[2]Bologna University School of Medicine, St Orsola Hospital, Bologna, Italy

Introduction

The classification of lymphoid neoplasms in the World Health Organization (WHO) proposal is based on two major principles: stratification of the neoplasms according to their cell lineage and the definition of non-overlapping distinct diseases that are clinically relevant. The identification of these diseases is based on a combination of morphology, immunophenotype, genetic and molecular features and clinical manifestations.

The 2001 WHO classification of lymphoid neoplasms was based on the Revised European–American Classification of Lymphoid Neoplasms (REAL) published by the International Lymphoma Study Group (ILSG) in 1994. The validation of this proposal in a large series of tumours and the publication of the third edition of the WHO classification ended a long history of controversy between different classification schemes that used different terminologies and concepts among pathologists and clinicians in different parts of the world.

The revision of the current WHO classification in 2008 has integrated concepts and criteria developed in the last few years by different working groups (IWCLL, EORTC among others) and has refined definitions of well-established diseases, incorporated new entities and developed new concepts and ideas related to the biology of lymphomas. However, the classification still has contentious aspects, such as provisional entities corresponding to categories for which the WHO Working Group felt there was insufficient evidence to recognize as distinct diseases at this time (Table 33.1).

Mature B-cell neoplasms

Chronic lymphocytic leukaemia/small lymphocytic lymphoma

Chronic lymphocytic leukaemia/small lymphocytic lymphoma (CLL/SLL) is a neoplasm of mature small B-cell lymphocytes that commonly express CD5 and CD23 and have dim expression of surface IgM/IgD. The tumour usually involves the peripheral blood and bone marrow but also lymph nodes, spleen, liver and other extranodal sites. The new WHO classi-

Postgraduate Haematology: 6th edition. Edited by A. Victor Hoffbrand, Daniel Catovsky, Edward G.D. Tuddenham, Anthony R. Green
© 2011 Blackwell Publishing Ltd.

Table 33.1 WHO classification of mature lymphoid neoplasms.

Mature B-cell neoplasms
Chronic lymphocytic leukaemia/small lymphocytic lymphoma
B-cell prolymphocytic leukaemia
Splenic B-cell marginal zone lymphoma
Hairy cell leukaemia
Splenic lymphoma/leukaemia unclassifiable
   Splenic diffuse red pulp small B-cell lymphoma
   Hairy cell leukaemia variant
Lymphoplasmacytic lymphoma/Waldenström
    macroglobulinaemia
Heavy chain diseases
Plasma cell myeloma
Solitary plasmacytoma of bone
Extraosseous plasmacytoma
Extranodal marginal zone lymphoma of mucosa-associated
    lymphoid tissue (MALT lymphoma)
Nodal marginal zone lymphoma
   Paediatric nodal marginal zone lymphoma
Follicular lymphoma
   Paediatric follicular lymphoma
Primary cutaneous follicle centre lymphoma
Mantle cell lymphoma
Diffuse large B-cell lymphoma (DLBCL), not otherwise specified
   T-cell/histiocyte-rich large B-cell lymphoma
   Primary DLBCL of the CNS
   Primary cutaneous DLBCL, leg type
   EBV-positive DLBCL of the elderly
DLBCL associated with chronic inflammation
Lymphomatoid granulomatosis
Primary mediastinal (thymic) large B-cell lymphoma
Intravascular large B-cell lymphoma
ALK-positive large B-cell lymphoma
Plasmablastic lymphoma
Large B-cell lymphomas arising in HHV8-associated multicentric
    Castleman disease
Primary effusion lymphoma
Burkitt lymphoma
B-cell lymphoma, unclassifiable, with features intermediate
    between DLBCL and Burkitt lymphoma

B-cell lymphoma, unclassifiable, with features intermediate
    between DLBCL and classical Hodgkin lymphoma

Mature T-cell and NK-cell neoplasms
T-cell prolymphocytic leukaemia
T-cell large granular lymphocytic leukaemia
Chronic lymphoproliferative disorder of NK cells
Aggressive NK-cell leukaemia
Systemic EBV-positive T-cell lymphoproliferative disease of
    childhood
Hydroa vacciniforme-like lymphoma
Adult T-cell leukaemia/lymphoma
Extranodal NK/T-cell lymphoma, nasal type
Enteropathy-associated T-cell lymphoma
Hepatosplenic T-cell lymphoma
Subcutaneous panniculitis-like T-cell lymphoma
Mycosis fungoides
Sézary syndrome
Primary cutaneous CD30-positive T-cell lymphoproliferative
    disorders
   Lymphomatoid papulosis
   Primary cutaneous anaplastic large-cell lymphoma
Primary cutaneous γδ T-cell lymphoma
Primary cutaneous CD8-positive aggressive epidermotropic
    cytotoxic T-cell lymphoma
Primary cutaneous CD4-positive small/medium T-cell lymphoma
Peripheral T-cell lymphoma, unspecified
Angioimmunoblastic T-cell lymphoma
Anaplastic large-cell lymphoma, ALK positive
Anaplastic large-cell lymphoma, ALK negative

Hodgkin lymphoma
Nodular lymphocyte predominant Hodgkin lymphoma
Classical Hodgkin lymphoma
   Nodular sclerosis classical Hodgkin lymphoma
   Lymphocyte-rich classical Hodgkin lymphoma
   Mixed cellularity classical Hodgkin lymphoma
   Lymphocyte-depleted classical Hodgkin lymphoma

Source: Swerdlow *et al.* (2008) with permission.

fication has adopted the definition of the disease proposed by the International Workshop on CLL (IWCLL): this requires, in the absence of extramedullary tissue involvement, the presence of 5×10^9/L monoclonal B lymphocytes with a CLL phenotype in the blood. The diagnosis of CLL may be established with lower cell counts when the patient has cytopenias or disease-related symptoms. The term 'small lymphocytic lymphoma' refers to non-leukaemic neoplasms with the same morphology

and phenotype. This new definition of CLL expands the number of patients who will be categorized as having monoclonal B-cell lymphocytosis (MBL).

The bone marrow is infiltrated in virtually all cases with an interstitial, nodular or diffuse pattern. The lymph nodes show effacement of the architecture by a diffuse infiltration. Aggregates of prolymphocytes and para-immunoblasts, called proliferation centres, are an almost constant feature in the lymph nodes (Figure 33.1). The proliferative cells tend to accumulate in these areas and are also associated with some follicular dendritic cells and increased numbers of CD4+ T cells. The detection of ZAP-70 by flow cytometry is an important prognostic marker of the disease that correlates well with the mutational status of the immunoglobulin genes. CD38 expression is also considered a prognostic marker (see also Chapter 29).

Molecular studies have recognized two major subtypes based on the mutational status of the immunoglobulin genes. Thus,

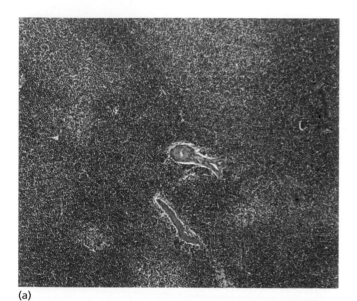
(a)

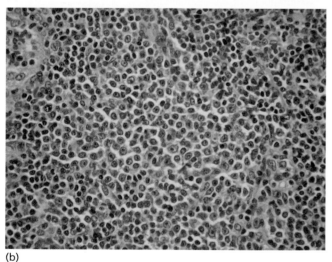
(b)

Figure 33.1 Lymph node involved by chronic lymphocytic leukaemia. (a) At low power the lymph node shows diffuse effacement of the architecture with vaguely nodular pale areas that correspond to the proliferation centres. (b) At higher magnification the proliferation centre contains larger cells with nuclei that have a central nucleolus (prolymphocytes and para-immunoblasts).

40–50% of cases have unmutated immunoglobulin genes (>98% homology with the germline), whereas 50–60% have hypermutated genes. Patients with unmutated CLL have a more aggressive disease. Analysis of immunoglobulin gene sequences has revealed a marked bias in use of the different regions, suggesting an influence of certain antigens in the selection of tumour cells. The most common genetic alterations in CLL are deletions of chromosome 13q (50%), trisomy 12 (20%), 11q deletions (15%) and 17p deletions (10%); 13q deletions are more common in mutated CLL whereas 11q and 17p deletions are more frequent in unmutated CLL and are associated with a worse prognosis.

Transformation into a more aggressive tumour occurs in 2–10% of patients (Richter syndrome). The two most common forms of transformation are diffuse large B-cell lymphoma (DLBCL) and, less frequently, Hodgkin lymphoma (HL). DLBCL arising in unmutated CLL usually corresponds to the clonal evolution of the preceding CLL, whereas in mutated CLL it frequently corresponds to a different lymphoid neoplasm.

B-cell prolymphocytic leukaemia (see also Chapter 29)

B-cell prolymphocytic leukaemia (B-PLL) is a malignancy of B prolymphocytes that affects the blood, bone marrow and spleen and is characterized by more than 55% prolymphocytes in the blood. B-PLL does not include transformed CLL, CLL with increased prolymphocytes, and blastoid mantle cell lymphoma with t(11;14)(q13;q32), which should be excluded. B-PLL is an uncommon disease of old patients (median age 65–69 years) and similar male/female distribution. Patients have 'B' symptoms, massive splenomegaly, absent or minimal lymphadenopathy and a rapidly rising lymphocyte count, usually over 100×10^9/L. Anaemia and thrombocytopenia are seen in 50%.

The cells strongly express surface IgM with or without IgD and mature B-cell antigens. CD5 and CD23 are only positive in 20–30% and 10–20% of cases, respectively. Complex karyotypes are common and 17p deletions associated with *TP53* gene mutations are detected in 50% of cases.

Median survival is 30–50 months. *IGHV* mutations, ZAP-70 and CD38 expression are heterogeneous and, contrary to CLL, lack precise clinical prognostic value.

Splenic marginal zone lymphoma

Splenic marginal zone lymphoma (SMZL) is a B-cell neoplasm composed of small lymphocytes that surround and replace the germinal centres and mantle of the reactive follicles in the white pulp, and merge with a peripheral (marginal) zone of larger cells including scattered transformed blasts. Both small and larger cells infiltrate the red pulp. The patients usually have a leukaemic and splenomegalic presentation with villous lym-

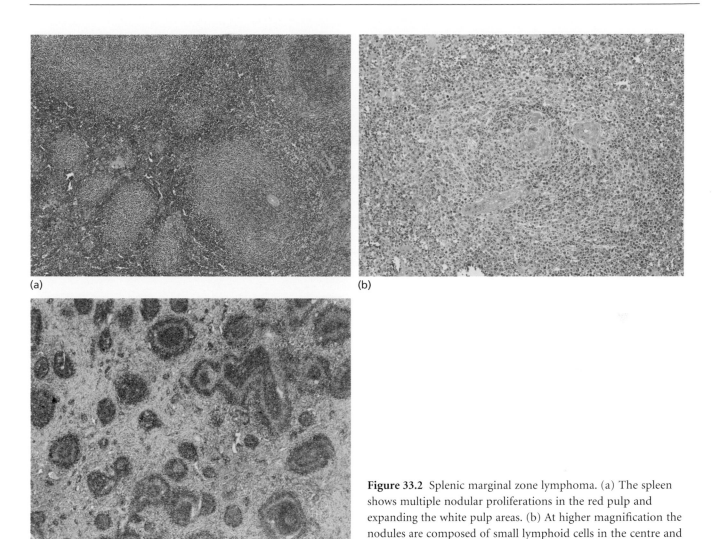

(a)

(b)

(c)

Figure 33.2 Splenic marginal zone lymphoma. (a) The spleen shows multiple nodular proliferations in the red pulp and expanding the white pulp areas. (b) At higher magnification the nodules are composed of small lymphoid cells in the centre and larger cells at the periphery. (c) The tumour cells are IgD positive.

phocytes in the blood. The disease also involves the splenic hilar lymph nodes and bone marrow but extension to peripheral lymph nodes is uncommon (Figure 33.2).

There are no distinctive phenotypic markers for SMZL, whose diagnosis requires the exclusion of other lymphoma types. Most cases exhibit IgM/IgD and a mature B-cell phenotype but other markers are usually negative (Figure 33.2). The immunoglobulin genes are unmutated in approximately half of the cases, which also tend to have deletions of chromosome 7q31–32 and a more unfavourable evolution. Some cases are positive for hepatitis C virus and may respond to antiviral treatment. The clinical course is usually indolent but some patients may have progressive disease and transformation to a large-cell lymphoma may occur. The hairy cell leukaemia variant and lymphomas with a diffuse infiltrate of the red pulp are included in a provisional category termed 'splenic B-cell lymphoma/leukaemia, unclassifiable'.

Lymphoplasmacytic lymphoma/Waldenström macroglobulinaemia

Lymphoplasmacytic lymphoma (LPL) and Waldenström macroglobulinaemia have been redefined in the new classification. LPL is a B-cell neoplasm composed of small lymphocytes, plasmacytoid lymphocytes and plasma cells usually involving the bone marrow and sometimes lymph nodes and spleen that does not fulfil the criteria for any other B-cell neoplasm which may have plasmacytic differentiation. Although the detection of a paraprotein is common, it is not required for the diagnosis. Waldenström macroglobulinaemia is an LPL with bone marrow involvement and an IgM monoclonal gammopathy of any concentration. Because these entities do not have specific markers, it is essential to exclude the presence of any other B-cell neoplasm that may have a plasmacytic differentiation.

Table 33.2 Plasma cell neoplasms.

Monoclonal gammopathy of undetermined significance
Plasma cell myeloma
   Asymptomatic (smouldering) myeloma
   Non-secretory myeloma
   Plasma cell leukaemia
Plasmacytoma
   Solitary plasmacytoma of bone
   Extraosseous (extramedullary) plasmacytoma
Immunoglobulin deposition diseases
Osteosclerotic myeloma (POEMS syndrome)

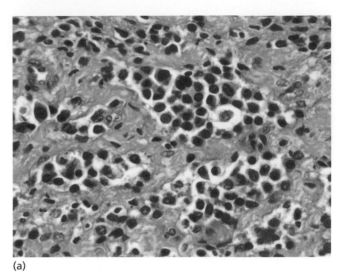

(a)

Plasma cell neoplasms (see also Chapter 31)

Plasma cell neoplasms encompass a spectrum of lesions characterized by the clonal expansion of terminally differentiated B cells that usually secrete a class-switched immunoglobulin (Table 33.2).

Monoclonal gammopathy of undetermined significance

Monoclonal gammopathy of undetermined significance (MGUS) is defined by less than 10% clonal plasma cells in the bone marrow and less than 30 g/L of an M-protein and absence of end-organ damage. This condition is considered a preneoplastic process since evolution to overt plasma cell malignancy does not always occur.

Plasma cell myeloma

Plasma cell myeloma is a bone marrow neoplasm characterized by multifocal proliferation of plasma cells associated with a serum M-protein and symptomatic disease related to different organ dysfunction or lytic bone lesions. The plasma cells in the bone marrow expand in small or large clusters. Some cases may present asymptomatically, whereas in others the tumour cells spread to the peripheral blood in the form of a plasma cell leukaemia. The phenotype of these cells is aberrant, with expression of CD19 and CD56 in 75% of cases and other markers such as CD117, CD20, CD52 and CD10. Chromosomal translocations involving the 14q32 region occur in 40% of cases; the partner translocations include *CCND1* (cyclin D1) at 11q13, *MAF* at 16q23, *FGFR3* at 4p16, *CCND3* (cyclin D3) at 6p21 and *MAFB* at 20q11. Tumours lacking these alterations are usually hyperdiploid.

Plasmacytoma

Plasmacytoma is a solitary tumour lesion composed of clonal plasma cells that may occur in bones or extraosseous tissues (Figure 33.3). Bone plasmacytomas evolve to plasma cell myeloma in two-thirds of patients. In contrast, extraosseous

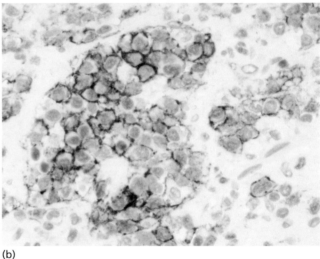

(b)

Figure 33.3 Plasmacytoma of the nasal cavity. (a) Atypical plasma cells embedded in fibrous stroma. (b) Plasma cells are CD138 positive

localized lesions have a relatively indolent behaviour without bone marrow involvement, suggesting a closer relationship to MALT lymphomas than bone marrow plasma cell neoplasms.

Extranodal marginal zone lymphoma of mucosa-associated lymphoid tissue (MALT lymphoma)

MALT lymphomas are extranodal B-cell neoplasms composed of a heterogeneous population of small lymphocytes, marginal zone lymphocytes with cleaved nuclei (centrocyte-like), cells with clear cytoplasm resembling monocytoid B cells, cells with plasmacytic differentiation and occasional large transformed cells. All these cells expand the marginal zone of reactive follicles and in some cases may colonize the germinal centres but preserve the mantle zone area. In epithelial tissues the neoplastic cells infiltrate the epithelium forming lymphoepithelial lesions (Figure 33.4). These tumours occur most commonly in the gastrointestinal tract, salivary gland, lung, head and neck, ocular adnexa, skin and less frequently thyroid and breast.

The lymphoma cells express mature B-cell markers, IgM and less often IgG or IgA, but IgD is usually negative. CD5, CD10 and CD23 are negative, although some CD5-positive cases have been described. Four major translocations have been associated

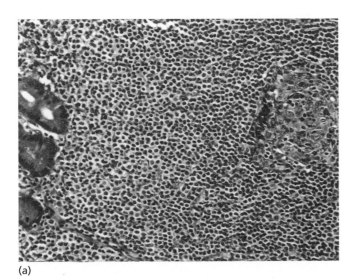

(a)

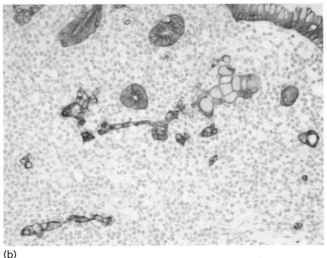

(b)

Figure 33.4 Gastric marginal zone lymphoma of the mucosa-associated lymphoid tissue (MALT lymphoma). The gastric mucosa is infiltrated by a monotonous population of lymphoid cells that surrounds a residual germinal centre (a) and destroys the glands, creating lymphoepithelial lesions clearly observed with cytokeratin staining (Cam 5.2 immunoperoxidase staining) (b).

with these lymphomas, t(11;18), t(1;14), t(14;18) and t(3;14), that generate the chimeric gene *BIRC3–MALT1* or activate *BCL10*, *MALT1* and *FOXP1*, respectively. The t(11;18) translocation tends to occur more frequently in gastric and lung lymphomas, whereas the t(14;18) translocation is more often seen in salivary gland and ocular adnexa tumours. Interestingly, *MALT1* and *BCL10* participate in activation of the same NF-κB pathway.

These lymphomas arise in topographic sites with a pre-existing chronic inflammatory lesion induced by infectious, immunological or unknown stimuli. Thus gastric lesions are associated with *Helicobacter pylori*, *Campylobacter jejuni* is detected in the immunoproliferative small intestinal disease, *Chlamydia psittaci* in ocular adnexa tumours of certain geographic regions, and *Borrelia burgdoferi* in some cutaneous MALT lymphomas. Autoimmune disorders of the salivary gland (Sjögren syndrome) and thyroid (Hashimoto disease) are the preceding lesions of MALT lymphomas in these locations.

The lymphoma responds to control of the underlying infectious disease and local treatments but may relapse in extranodal territories after many years. Nodal dissemination may precede clinically the detection of extranodal involvement. Tumours with the translocations described appear to be resistant to antibiotic therapy. Transformation to large-cell lymphomas may occur.

Nodal marginal zone lymphoma

Nodal marginal zone lymphoma (NMZL) is a primary lymphoma of the lymph nodes that resembles extranodal MALT lymphomas (Figure 33.5). An extranodal or splenic lymphoma should be ruled out before this diagnosis is established. Although the morphology and phenotype is similar to MALT lymphoma, primary NMZL does not exhibit the typical translocations of these tumours. Patients may present with disseminated disease and 60–80% survive more than 5 years. Some cases may evolve to large B-cell lymphomas.

NMZLs in the paediatric age group seem to have distinctive clinical and morphological features. Thus they present predominantly in males as asymptomatic localized tumours and morphologically the residual follicles may have features of progressive transformed germinal centres with eroded mantle zones by the tumour cell infiltration. The prognosis of these patients seems excellent with conservative therapy.

Follicular lymphoma

Follicular lymphoma (FL) is a neoplasm composed of cells of the germinal centres, with different proportions of small centrocytes and large centroblasts, that usually has a follicular growth pattern (Figure 33.6). These tumours are common in Western countries, accounting for around 20–30% of all lymphomas.

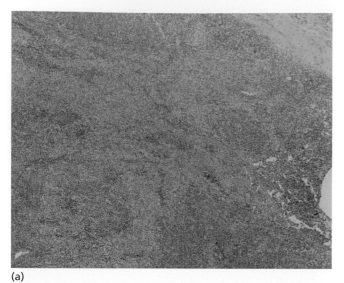
(a)

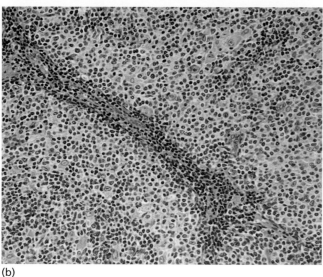
(b)

Figure 33.5 Nodal marginal zone lymphoma. (a) Tumour cells with a clear appearance infiltrate the node, with partial preservation of the architecture. (b) Higher magnification reveals the clear cytoplasm of the tumour cells.

These tumours have been graded according to the number of large cells as follows: grade 1 (0–5 large cells per high-power field), grade 2 (6–15 large cells) and grade 3 (>15 large cells). The new WHO classification considers that grades 1 and 2 represent a morphological continuum that is not associated with relevant clinical or biological differences and therefore this distinction is not encouraged. However, grade 3 tumours are further distinguished into grades 3a and 3b according to the presence of intermingled small centrocytes in grade 3a whereas grade 3b is composed entirely of large cells. According to the genetic and phenotypic features, FL grade 3a seems more related to FL grade 1–2, whereas FL grade 3b may be closer to DLBCL. Any diffuse area composed of more than 15 large cells should

be reported as DLBCL, and the percentage of the respective DLBCL and FL components indicated.

FL has a mature B-cell phenotype with coexpression of the germinal-centre markers CD10 and BCL-6 (Figure 33.6). CD5, CD43 and CD23 are negative. IRF4/MUM1, an antigen related to plasma cell differentiation, is also usually negative. BCL-2 is positive in 85–90% of FL grade 1–2 but only in 50% of grade 3. BCL-2 staining is very useful because reactive germinal centres are negative (Figure 33.6). This expression reflects the presence of the t(14;18) translocation that is the genetic hallmark of this lymphoma and which targets the *BCL2* gene. FL grade 3b is less frequently positive for CD10 and BCL-2 protein and the t(14;18) translocation is only detected in 5–40% of cases. In contrast, these lymphomas express IRF4/MUM1 in 40% of the cases and carry 3q27 and *BCL6* rearrangements in 30–50% of cases, whereas these aberrations are rare in FL grades 1–3a.

The tumour cells are associated with a rich microenvironment of different types of T cells and histiocytes that seem to play a major role in determining the biological behaviour of the lymphoma.

In situ follicular lymphoma or intrafollicular neoplasia

In situ FL or intrafollicular neoplasia is a variant in which the tumour cells are limited to the germinal centres of the follicles. Usually, only a number of the lymph node follicles are involved whereas others are reactive. The tumour cells are recognized by their strong BCL-2 expression inside the germinal centres and absence of CD10- and BCL-6-positive tumour cells outside the follicles. The BCL-2-positive cells in the follicle carry the t(14;18) translocation. Some of these cases may correspond to early involvement of a lymph node by a disseminated tumour. A second group of patients may develop overt FL during follow-up but most patients remain free of lymphoma elsewhere after many years of follow-up.

Paediatric follicular lymphoma

Paediatric FL occurs in children and young adults, usually involving the head and neck region but also the testis with localized disease. The lymphomas are BCL-2 negative, do not carry the t(14;18) translocation and are grade 3. These cases have a relatively good evolution.

Primary intestinal follicular lymphoma

Primary intestinal FL occurs frequently in the duodenum as an incidental finding (Figure 33.7). These cases have a conventional morphology, phenotype and genetic findings. However, the tumours express IgA and remain localized, with an excellent prognosis even without treatment.

Primary cutaneous follicle centre lymphoma

Primary cutaneous follicle centre lymphoma generally presents in the skin of the head and trunk. The tumour cells may grow

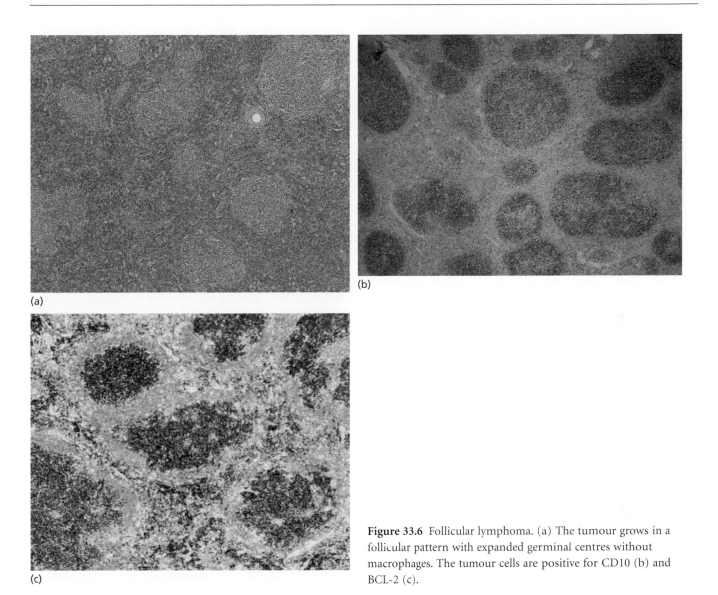

(a)

(b)

(c)

Figure 33.6 Follicular lymphoma. (a) The tumour grows in a follicular pattern with expanded germinal centres without macrophages. The tumour cells are positive for CD10 (b) and BCL-2 (c).

Figure 33.7 Follicular lymphoma of the duodenum.

with a follicular or more diffuse pattern. The cells express B-cell markers and BCL-6, whereas CD10 is positive in cases with a follicular pattern but tend to be lost in the diffuse component. BCL-2 expression and the t(14;18) translocation are usually negative. The tumours may relapse but have a good outcome without extracutaneous dissemination even with only localized therapy.

Mantle cell lymphoma

Mantle cell lymphoma (MCL) is a B-cell neoplasm generally composed of monomorphous small to medium-sized lymphoid cells with irregular nuclear contours and cyclin D1 overexpression secondary to *CCND1* translocation (Figures 33.8 and 33.9). This tumour comprises 3–10% of non-Hodgkin lymphomas and occurs mainly in males, with a median age around 60 years. Most MCLs are diagnosed as disseminated nodal disease but a

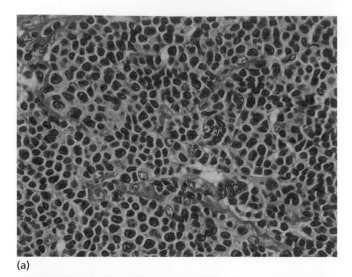

(a)

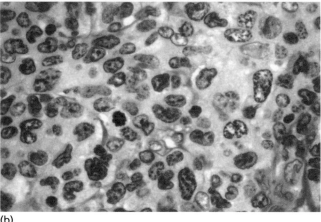

(b)

Figure 33.8 Mantle cell lymphoma with classical (a) and pleomorphic (b) morphology.

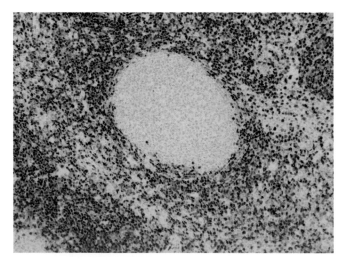

Figure 33.9 Mantle cell lymphoma is positive for cyclin D1.

number of patients are initially seen with leukaemic disease, bone marrow involvement and frequently splenomegaly, but without lymphadenopathy. Extranodal involvement is very common. Some tumours may have a blastoid or pleomorphic cytology resembling lymphoblasts or DLBCL, respectively. These cytological variants are associated with higher proliferative activity, more complex karyotypes and worse prognosis. The tumour cells grow with a vaguely nodular, diffuse or mantle zone pattern. Some cases may show restricted infiltration to the inner mantle zones of otherwise reactive follicles, a situation that has been named *in situ* MCL. The tumour cells express mature B-cell markers, with intense CD20 and surface immunoglobulin, and coexpress CD5 and CD43. CD23 and germinal-centre markers are negative.

MCL exhibits the t(11;14) translocation that targets cyclin D1. Complex karyotypes with many secondary aberrations are common. Cyclin D1-negative cases are exceptional, and their diagnosis requires strict morphological and phenotypic criteria. These cases have high expression of cyclin D2 or cyclin D3 and some of them carry a t(2;12) translocation that fuses cyclin D2 to the κ light chain immunoglobulin gene locus. SOX11, a transcription factor expressed in conventional MCL, is also express in cyclin D1-negative tumours and therefore its detection may be of help in recognizing this variant.

In general MCL has an aggressive clinical course, with poor response to chemotherapy and a median survival of 3–5 years. Proliferation is considered the best prognostic parameter. Patients presenting with disease limited to the blood, bone marrow and sometimes the spleen, without lymphadenopathy, have been reported to have a better prognosis. These tumours seem to have a distinct expression profile and simple karyotypes.

Diffuse large B-cell lymphoma not otherwise specified

DLBCL is a neoplasm of large B lymphocytes with a diffuse growth pattern. These lymphomas are heterogeneous and several morphological variants, phenotypical and molecular subtypes and different entities have been recognized (Table 33.3). DLBCL is very common and accounts for 25–30% of adult non-Hodgkin lymphomas. Usually, these cases present as primary tumours but they can also represent the transformation of a less aggressive B-cell lymphoma.

Morphologically, DLBCL not otherwise specified may have centroblastic, immunoblastic or anaplastic cytology (Figures 33.10 and 33.11). These variants are related to biological and genetic features of the tumour but they have poor reproducibility and broad overlap that prevent their use as major classifiers. Phenotypically, DLBCL not otherwise specified expresses mature B-cell markers. CD5 is detected in a subset of these tumours that seem to have a more aggressive behaviour, particularly in Eastern populations. The expression of the germi-

Table 33.3 Diffuse large B-cell lymphoma (DLBCL): variants, subgroups, subtypes and entities.

DLBCL, not otherwise specified
Common morphological variants
   Centroblastic
   Immunoblastic
   Anaplastic
Rare morphological variants
Molecular subgroups
   Germinal centre B-cell-like
   Activated B-cell-like
Immunohistochemical subgroups
   CD5-positive DLBCL
   Germinal centre B-cell-like
   Non-germinal centre B-cell-like

DLBCL subtypes
T-cell/histiocyte-rich large B-cell lymphoma
Primary DLBCL of the central nervous system
Primary cutaneous DLBCL, leg type
EBV-positive DLBCL of the eldery

Other lymphomas of large B cells
Primary mediastinal (thymic) large B-cell lymphoma
Intravascular large B-cell lymphoma
DLBCL associated with chronic inflammation
Lymphomatoid granulomatosis
ALK-positive large B-cell lymphoma
Plasmablastic lymphoma
Large B-cell lymphoma arising in HHV8-associated multicentric
   Castleman disease
Primary effusion lymphoma

Borderline cases
B-cell lymphoma, unclassifiable, with features intermediate
   between DLBCL and Burkitt lymphoma
B-cell lymphoma, unclassifiable, with features intermediate
   between DLBCL and classical Hodgkin lymphoma

Source: Swerdlow *et al.* (2008) with permission.

nal-centre markers CD10 and BCL-6 has been related to a germinal-centre origin of the tumours, whereas the expression of IRF4/MUM1 antigen has been associated with an origin in non-germinal centre activated B cells (Figures 33.10 and 33.11). These two immunophenotypic subgroups of DLBCL have a clear correlation with the two subtypes of germinal-centre and activated B-cell DLBCL recognized by gene expression profiling. However, the controversial results obtained in different studies on the prognostic significance of these phenotypic subgroups preclude their use in clinical practice.

Genetically, 20–30% of DLBCL not otherwise specified exhibit the t(14;18) translocation and *BCL2* gene rearrange-

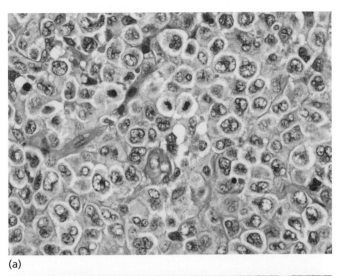

(a)

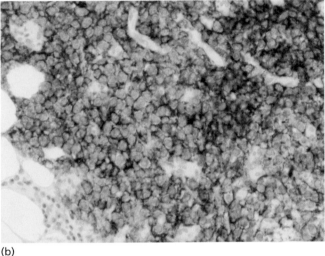

(b)

Figure 33.10 Diffuse large B-cell lymphoma (a) positive for CD10 (b) suggests a germinal centre cell origin.

ment. These cases are associated with CD10 expression and a germinal-centre origin. Translocation of the 3q27 region and *BCL6* rearrangements are found up to 30% of cases. *MYC* translocations have been observed in up to 10% of cases and are usually associated with complex karyotypes. Contrary to Burkitt lymphoma in which *MYC* is rearranged with immunoglobulin genes in virtually all cases, in DLBCL around 40% of these translocations involve a non-immunoglobulin gene.

Gene expression profiling of DLBCL not otherwise specified has identified two major subtypes, germinal-centre B cell-like (GCB) and activated B cell-like (ABC) DLBCL, that express genes related to germinal-centre cells or activated B cells with a secretory function, respectively. ABC but not GCB DLBCL exhibits constitutive activation of the NF-κB pathway. These subtypes of DLBCL differ in genetic and molecular aspects, suggesting that they correspond to different clinical entities.

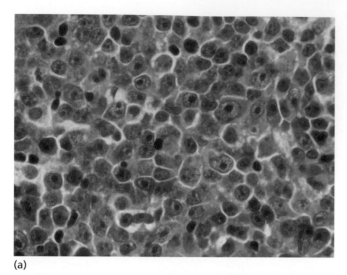

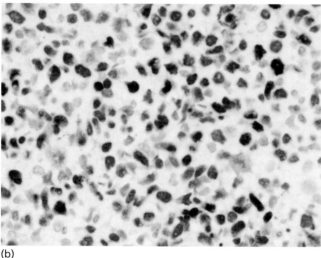

Figure 33.11 Diffuse large B-cell lymphoma with immunoblastic morphology (a) and positivity for MUM1/IRF4 (b) suggesting a non-germinal centre cell origin.

The clinical outcome is also different, with 5-year survival rates of 59% and 30% in GCB and ABC DLBCL, respectively. In addition, the clinical phenomenon of late relapse or relapse as FL occurs in patients with GCB DLBCL. The prognostic value of these molecular subtypes has been retained in patients treated with rituximab-containing regimens.

T-cell/histiocyte-rich large B-cell lymphoma

T-cell/histiocyte-rich large B-cell lymphoma is characterized by a limited number of scattered large B cells immersed in a rich background of T cells and frequently histiocytes. The tumour cells express mature B-cell markers and frequently BCL-2 and EMA, although CD30, CD15 and CD138 are negative. The background is composed of CD3 and CD4 T cells and CD68-

positive histiocytes. T-cell rosettes surrounding tumour B cells are not seen. Cases positive for Epstein–Barr virus (EBV) and a similar morphology would be better classified as EBV-positive DLBCL. This tumour presents with disseminated disease involving lymph nodes but also spleen, liver and bone marrow. Failure to therapy and International Prognostic Index (IPI) score are predictors of survival.

DLBCL with a predominant extranodal location

The WHO classification recognizes a series of DLBCL subtypes and entities characterized by predominantly extranodal presentation (Table 33.3).

Primary mediastinal (thymic) large B-cell lymphoma

Primary mediastinal (thymic) large B-cell lymphoma (PMBL) seems to originate in a thymic B cell and predominates in young women presenting with a large mediastinal mass that frequently invades adjacent structures. Progression outside the mediastinum frequently involves extranodal sites such as kidney, liver, adrenal or central nervous system (CNS). The tumour is mainly composed of large cells with abundant pale cytoplasm that express mature B-cell markers but usually lack surface immunoglobulin. CD30 is positive in 80% of cases, although not as uniformly as in HL. CD15 is negative. Genetically, PMBL has frequent gains and amplifications of 9p24 and inactivating mutations of *SOCS1*. These tumours have a distinctive expression profile relatively similar to that of HL, confirming the pathological evidence of the relationship between these two tumours. In fact, some patients may present with combined HL and PMBL at diagnosis or relapse or have tumours with intermediate features of both (see below). The outcome of these tumours is more favourable than other DLBCL, with a 5-year survival of 65%.

Intravascular large B-cell lymphoma

Intravascular large B-cell lymphoma is a distinctive lymphoma characterized by the growth of large B cells within the lumina of small to medium-sized vessels and capillaries (Figure 33.12). It is relatively rare in Western countries but more common in Eastern populations. This lymphoma is very aggressive and frequently diagnosed only at post-mortem. An isolated cutaneous variant with better prognosis has been identified, mainly in women.

Primary cutaneous DLBCL, leg type

Primary cutaneous DLBCL, leg type, is a primary cutaneous lymphoma composed almost exclusively of atypical large B cells that commonly presents in the lower extremities. These tumours express an activated B-cell phenotype with positivity for IRF4/MUM1 and CD10 negativity. BCL-6 is frequently positive and BCL-2 is strongly expressed. The genetic and molecular profiles are relatively similar to those found in ABC DLBCL. The prog-

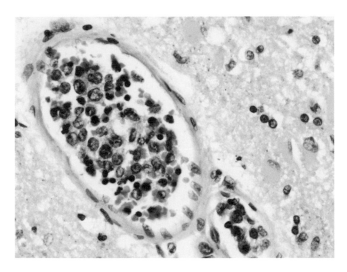

Figure 33.12 Intravascular lymphoma in the brain.

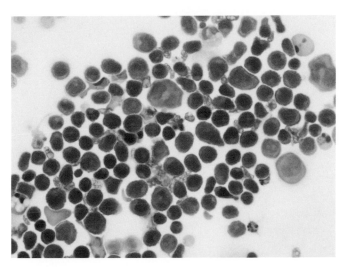

Figure 33.13 Primary effusion lymphoma. The tumour cells were present in the pleura and have a large plasmablastic morphology.

nosis is poor and the tumour tends to disseminate to extracutaneous sites.

Large-cell lymphomas of terminally differentiated B cells

The updated WHO classification has included different lymphoma entities that have in common the proliferation of large lymphoid cells with a terminally differentiated B-cell phenotype characterized by variable or total lack of CD20 expression, and less frequently CD79a, but which express plasma cell-associated antigens such as CD38 and CD138. Most of these tumours are infected with EBV or human herpesvirus (HHV)-8 and occur in patients with a certain immunodeficiency status.

ALK-positive large B-cell lymphoma

ALK-positive large B-cell lymphoma is a distinctive disease characterized by proliferation of large B cells with plasmablastic differentiation that express ALK and which are EBV negative. These tumours present in young immunocompetent patients, usually with nodal involvement and aggressive behaviour. ALK expression is due to *ALK* rearrangements, particularly with clathrin [t(2;17)] or less frequently nucleophosmin [t(2;5)]. Contrary to other lymphomas in this group, viral infection and immunodeficiency are absent.

Plasmablastic lymphoma

Plasmablastic lymphoma is a large B-cell lymphoma with immunoblastic morphology and plasma cell immunophenotype that present mainly in extranodal sites such as oral mucosa and gastrointestinal tract of immunosuppressed patients. HIV infection is the main cause but post-transplant or immunosuppressive treatments are also common causes. Most of the tumours are EBV positive and latent membrane protein (LMP)-

1 negative. The clinical behaviour is aggressive with poor response to therapy.

Primary effusion lymphoma

Primary effusion lymphoma occurs mainly in immunosuppressed patients associated with HHV-8 and, frequently, EBV infection. It is characterized by proliferation of large pleomorphic B cells that lack expression of B-cell markers and immunoglobulin but which express plasma cell-associated antigens and CD30 (Figure 33.13). These tumours usually present as effusion lymphomas with no involvement of tissues. However, some patients may present with, or later develop, a solid tumour in extranodal sites.

Burkitt lymphoma

Burkitt lymphoma (BL) is mainly a tumour of children and young adults and is characterized by monotonous proliferation of medium-sized B cells with a mature B and germinal-centre phenotype, negative or very weak BCL-2 expression, high proliferation (Ki-67 > 95%) and the t(8;14) translocation with *MYC* rearrangement. These tumours occur endemically in equatorial Africa and other geographic areas and sporadically throughout the world. BL is also seen associated with immunodeficiency, particularly HIV infection. The tumour mainly involves extranodal sites, particularly the abdominal cavity, and in endemic areas jaws and facial bones. The tumour may infiltrate the CNS. A leukaemic phase may be seen in patients with bulky disease and occasional patients may present with a pure leukaemic disease (Burkitt leukaemia variant). The tumour is clinically aggressive but potentially curable with current protocols.

Morphologically, the tumour cells are very monomorphic. The high proliferation is typically associated with a 'starry sky'

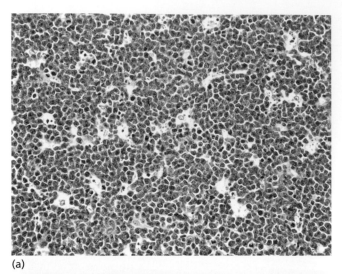

(a)

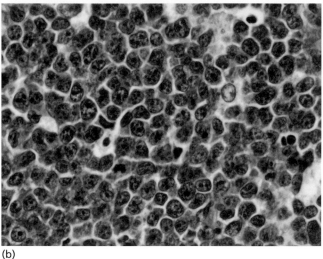

(b)

Figure 33.14 Burkitt lymphoma. (a) 'Starry sky' pattern due to the abundant histiocytes with apoptotic bodies. (b) Monotonous medium-sized cells with high proliferation.

pattern because of the high number of histiocytes phagocytosing apoptotic bodies (Figure 33.14). Genetically, the t(8;14) translocation is found in most tumours with very few if any additional genetic alterations. However, up to 10% of cases with typical morphology and phenotype may lack this translocation. On the other hand, DLBCL may have high proliferation and may also exhibit *MYC* rearrangements that make the differential diagnosis between BL and DLBCL difficult.

Two recent studies using microarray technology have described the gene expression profile of BL that refines the differential diagnosis with DLBCL. This BL signature is composed of a group of genes that are targets of the *MYC* gene, high expression of germinal centre-related genes and low expression of NF-κB target genes and MHC class I genes.

B-cell lymphoma, unclassifiable, with features intermediate between DLBCL and Burkitt lymphoma

Borderline cases between DLBCL and BL comprise tumours with a morphology that resembles BL but which have an atypical phenotype such as strong BCL-2 protein expression, tumours with blastic nuclear morphology but negative for terminal deoxynucleotidyltransferase and cyclin D1, or tumours with a BL phenotype but with more irregular nuclei than acceptable for this lymphoma. Some of these cases were diagnosed previously as Burkitt-like lymphomas. These tumours express a mature B-cell phenotype with a high proliferative index. Strong expression of BCL-2 protein should suggest the presence of t(14;18) in addition to t(8;14) ('double hit'). *MYC* rearrangements may occur with a non-immunoglobulin gene and may be associated with complex karyotypes. Lymphomas with typical morphology of DLBCL with high proliferative activity and/or t(8;14) should not be included in this category. Clinically, the patients are older than those with conventional BL, the disease is usually disseminated and the bone marrow and peripheral blood may be involved. The clinical evolution is very aggressive with poor response to therapy. These cases are not considered a specific entity but a working category. Some cases may represent transformed FL, evolving DLBCL activating particular molecular pathways, and some of them may perhaps represent some specific entity not well recognized yet. However, independent of the possible biological significance, these patients should be recognized and studied separately from conventional DLBCL and BL.

B-cell lymphoma, unclassifiable, with features intermediate between DLBCL and classical Hodgkin lymphoma

These tumours are B-cell lymphomas that have clinical, morphological and/or immunophenotypic features that overlap those of DLBCL, particularly PMBL, and HL. These cases are diagnosed frequently in young men presenting with a large mediastinal mass that is sometimes associated with surpraclavicular lymph nodes. Most of these cases are composed of sheets of large cells with a pleomorphic aspect, sometimes lacunar appearance, associated with some inflammatory infiltrate. The phenotype combines strong expression of a complete B-cell programme (CD20, CD79a, BOB-1, OCT2, PAX5) with CD30 and CD15 positivity. Some cases resembling classical nodular sclerosis HL with uniform expression of CD20 and other B-cell markers and lack of CD15 may also be included in this category. In contrast, cases resembling PMBL that lack CD20 and which are positive for CD15 or EBV may also be diagnosed in this category. Composite lymphomas with clear areas of PMBL and HL should not be included in this group and both components should be mentioned in the diagnosis. The overlapping morphological and phenotypical features of these tumours have been validated as authentic biological characteristics by microarray expression profiling studies that have demonstrated the similarities between PMBL and HL. These tumours probably represent evidence of plasticity in the differentiation pathways of B cells.

Mature NK-cell/T-cell neoplasms

These tumours derive from natural killer (NK) cells and T cells of peripheral lymphoid organs and can be roughly subdivided into three groups: leukaemic, extranodal and nodal. These are discussed in the following sections, with the exception of T-cell prolymphocytic leukaemia, T-cell large granular lymphocyte leukaemia and chronic lymphoproliferative disorders of NK cells, which are considered in Chapter 30.

Aggressive NK-cell leukaemia

This is a rare neoplasm, mainly observed among Asians, and exhibits systemic proliferation of NK cells almost always associated with EBV and an aggressive clinical course. Patients are usually middle-aged of either sex. The most commonly involved sites are the peripheral blood, bone marrow, liver and spleen (Figure 33.15). Fever and constitutional symptoms are common. Frequent complications are coagulopathy, haemophagocytic syndrome (HPS) or multiorgan failure. A specific overlap with extranodal NK/T-cell lymphoma may exist. Circulating leukaemic cells exhibit a morphological spectrum, from 'normal LGL' to elements with atypical infolded nuclei, open chromatin and distinct nucleoli. They express CD2, CD3ε, CD56 and cytotoxic molecules. Surface CD3 is absent. T-cell receptor (TCR) genes

are in germline configuration. Most cases pursue a fulminant clinical course.

EBV-positive T-cell lymphoproliferative disorders of childhood

Systemic EBV-positive T-cell lymphoproliferative disease of childhood and hydroa vaccineforme-like lymphoma are the prototypes of these diseases. Both are prevalent in Asia and Central and South America with no sex predilection. EBV-positive T-cell lymphoproliferative disease of childhood can develop shortly after primary EBV infection or in the setting of chronic active EBV infection. It may have a rapid evolution with fatal outcome. Hydroa vacciniforme-like lymphoma is associated with sensitivity to insect bites and sun exposure and behaves indolently. In both conditions, there is strong suggestion of a genetic defect in the host immune response to EBV. The infiltrating T cells are usually small and lack significant cytological atypia, but at times are pleomorphic, medium/large with irregular nuclei and frequent mitoses (Figure 33.16). They are positive for CD2, CD3, TIA and EBV but negative for CD56, and have monoclonally rearranged TCR genes.

Adult T-cell leukaemia/lymphoma (see also Chapter 30)

Adult T-cell leukaemia/lymphoma (ATLL) is endemic in southwestern Japan, the Caribbean basin and parts of Central Africa, its distribution resembling that of human T-cell leukaemia/lymphoma virus (HTLV)-I. The disease has a long latency with exposure of affected individuals to the virus very early in life. Although causally linked to ATLL, HTLV-I itself is insufficient to cause neoplastic transformation, additional genetic events being required. Most patients present with widespread lymph node and peripheral blood involvement, the skin being affected in more than 50%. ATLL is characterized by variable clinical and histological features. In particular, the behaviour varies from acute (with usual hypercalcaemia and possible lytic bone

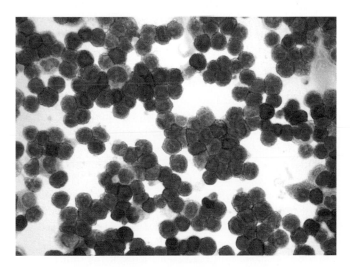

Figure 33.15 Cytospin from the peripheral blood of a patient with aggressive NK-cell leukaemia, stained for CD56 (alkaline phosphatase anti-alkaline phosphatase technique).

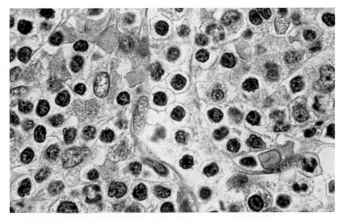

Figure 33.16 Bone-marrow involvement by EBV-positive lymphoproliferative disorder in a 16-year-old boy.

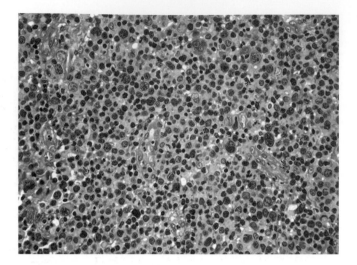

Figure 33.17 Lymph node infiltration in a patient with adult T-cell leukaemia/lymphoma.

lesions) to lymphomatous, chronic or smouldering, while the growth may consist of small to large-sized pleomorphic cells or display anaplastic or even angioimmunoblastic-like morphology (Figure 33.17). Tumour elements are usually $CD2^+CD3^+CD5^+CD25^+CD7^-$. Most cases are $CD4^+CD8^-$, a few $CD4^-CD8^+$ or $CD4^+CD8^+$. CCR4 and FoxP3 are frequently expressed, CD30 may be positive and cytotoxic molecules are absent. TCR genes are clonally rearranged. Clinical subtypes, age, performance status, serum calcium and lactate dehydrogenase levels are major prognostic indicators. The acute and lymphomatous variants have a short survival (2 weeks to more than 1 year), while the chronic and smouldering forms behave more indolently but can progress to an acute phase (see also Chapter 30).

Extranodal NK/T-cell lymphoma, nasal type

Extranodal NK/T-cell lymphoma, nasal type, more often occurs in adult males from Asia, Mexico and Central and South America. The tumour is EBV positive with type II latency, although LMP-1 expression is variable. Usually, these lymphomas affect the nasal cavity, nasopharynx, paranasal sinuses and palate. Extranasal locations include the skin, soft tissue, gastrointestinal tract and testis. Patients with nasal disease suffer from nasal obstruction or epistaxis, or extensive mid-facial destruction (so-called lethal midline granuloma). Irrespective of the site of presentation, the lymphomatous infiltrate is diffuse with angiocentric and angiodestructive features and frequent necrosis. Neoplastic cells may be small, medium-sized, large or anaplastic with numerous mitotic figures and azurophilic granules in Giemsa-stained touch preparations (Figure 33.18). Phenotypically, they are positive for CD2, CD56, CD3ε and cytotoxic markers but negative for CD3. Occasional cases are $CD7^+$ or $CD30^+$. It is noteworthy that CD56 is not specific for these lymphomas, being detected in other peripheral T-cell

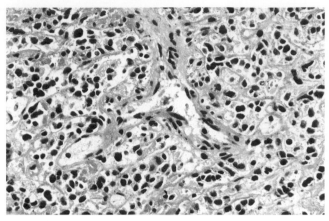

Figure 33.18 Destructive lesion of the nasal cavities in the course of extranodal NK/T-cell lymphoma, nasal type.

lymphomas, mainly carrying γδ-TCR. A diagnosis of extranodal NK/T-cell lymphoma, nasal type should be accepted with scepticism if EBV-encoded RNA *in situ* hybridization is negative. TCR and *IGHV* genes are usually in germline configuration, the former being clonally rearranged in a few instances. The prognosis of extranodal NK/T-cell lymphoma, nasal type is variable, being always poor for cases occurring outside the nasal cavity. It is noteworthy that survival has recently been improved with more intensive regimens including up-front radiotherapy and L-asparaginase.

Enteropathy-associated T-cell lymphoma

Enteropathy-associated T-cell lymphoma (EATL) is an intestinal tumour of intraepithelial T lymphocytes, usually consisting of large lymphoid cells admixed with numerous histiocytes and eosinophils and associated with necrosis. The adjacent small intestinal mucosa shows villous atrophy, crypt hyperplasia, increased lamina propria lymphocytes and plasma cells, and intraepithelial lymphocytosis (Figure 33.19). The disease occurs more often in areas with a high prevalence of coeliac disease (i.e. northern Europe). In 10–20% of cases, EATL is composed of monomorphic medium-sized cells with no inflammatory background and rare necrosis. Such monomorphic variant (type II) EATL may occur sporadically, without risk factors for coeliac disease, and has a broader geographic distribution. Patients (usually adults) present with abdominal pain, frequently associated with intestinal perforation. The tumour forms one or more ulcerating mucosal masses that invade the wall of the intestine (frequently jejunum or ileum). Neoplastic cells are positive for CD3, CD7, CD103, TCR-β and cytotoxic molecules, negative for CD4 and CD5, with variable expression of CD8 and CD30. Type II EATL has a distinctive immunophenotype ($CD3^+CD4^-CD8^+CD56^+TCR-β^+$). TCR β and γ genes are always clonally rearranged. The prognosis is poor, with death frequently resulting from abdominal complications.

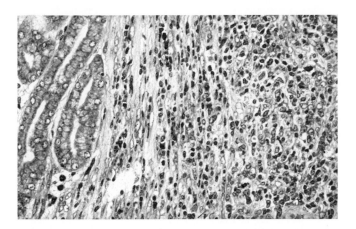

Figure 33.19 Enteropathy-associated T-cell lymphoma. Remnants of the mucosa are seen on the left-hand side.

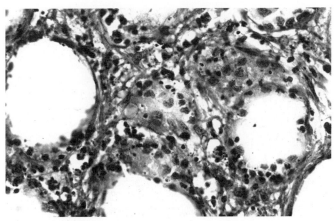

Figure 33.21 Example of subcutaneous panniculitis-like T-cell lymphoma. Features of 'rimming' are easily seen.

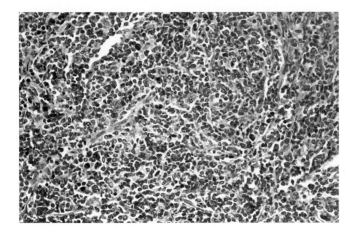

Figure 33.20 Splenic red pulp involvement by hepatosplenic T-cell lymphoma.

Hepatosplenic T-cell lymphoma

Hepatosplenic T-cell lymphoma is a rare neoplasm derived from cytotoxic T cells, mostly of the γδ type. It affects adolescents and young adults, with male predominance. Up to 20% of these lymphomas arise in the setting of chronic immunosuppression, usually for solid organ transplantation or prolonged antigenic stimulation. It may also occur in patients, especially children, treated with azathioprine and infliximab for Crohn's disease. Clinically, it is characterized by hepatosplenomegaly, systemic symptoms and marked thrombocytopenia. Morphologically, neoplastic cells are monotonous, with medium-sized nuclei, loosely condensed nuclear chromatin, inconspicuous nucleoli and a rim of pale cytoplasm. In the spleen, they infiltrate the red pulp cords and sinuses with atrophy of the white pulp, while in the liver and bone marrow they show intrasinusoidal diffusion (Figure 33.20). Phenotypically, most cases are positive for CD3 and TCR-δ1,

partly positive for CD56 and CD8, and negative for TCR-αβ, CD4 and CD5. A minority carries the α/β dimer. The cells express TIA1 and granzyme-M, but not granzyme-B and perforin. They have rearranged TCR-γ genes. Cases of γδ origin show biallelic rearrangement of TCR-δ genes. Isochromosome 7q is present in most instances. Trisomy 8 and loss of a sex chromosome may also be present. The course is aggressive, with initial response to chemotherapy but rapid relapse. The median survival is less than 2 years.

Subcutaneous panniculitis-like T-cell lymphoma

Subcutaneous panniculitis-like T-cell lymphoma is a rare cytotoxic T-cell lymphoma that preferentially infiltrates subcutaneous tissue, is slightly commoner in females and has a broad age spectrum. In the new WHO classification, cases expressing TCR-γδ are classified as primary cutaneous γδ T-cell lymphoma. About 20% of patients have an associated autoimmune disease, mostly systemic lupus erythematosus. Patients present with multiple subcutaneous nodules, usually in the absence of other involved sites. Systemic symptoms are recorded in more than 50% of patients. Cytopenias and elevated liver function tests are common, and frank HPS is seen in 15–20%. The infiltrate involves the fat lobules with riming around individual fat cells and usually spares septa as well as the overlying dermis and epidermis (Figure 33.21). Vascular invasion is seen occasionally, while necrosis and karyorrhexis are common. The cells have a mature αβ T-cell phenotype (βF1+), usually CD8+ with expression of cytotoxic molecules and negative for CD56. The neoplastic cells show rearrangement of TCR genes, and are negative for EBV. Dissemination to lymph nodes and other organs is rare. The 5-year overall survival (OS) is 80%; however, if HPS occurs, the prognosis is poor.

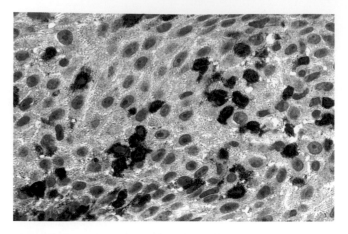

Figure 33.22 Mycosis fungoides. The epidermis is infiltrated by neoplastic T cells with cerebriform nuclei and strong CD3 expression.

Mycosis fungoides and Sézary syndrome (see also Chapter 30)

Mycosis fungoides is the commonest primary cutaneous T-cell lymphoma (CTCL) and is characterized by epidermotropic infiltrates of small to medium-sized T lymphocytes with cerebriform nuclei (Figure 33.22). It usually affects adults or the elderly with a male predominance, but can also occur in children and adolescents. The disease is limited to the skin, with classical evolution of patches, plaques and tumours. Extracutaneous dissemination occurs in advanced stages. Mycosis fungoides slowly progresses over years or sometimes decades. Histological transformation (i.e. >25% blasts in the dermal infiltrates) occurs mainly in the tumour stages. The typical phenotype is $CD2^+CD3^+TCR-\beta^+CD5^+CD4^+CD8^-CD7^-$. TCR genes are clonally rearranged in a proportion of cases. The single most important prognostic factor is the clinical stage. In the more advanced stages, the prognosis is poor as it is in the case of histological transformation. Rare clinical–morphological variants include folliculotropic mycosis fungoides, pagetoid reticulosis and granulomatous slack skin.

Sézary syndrome is defined by erythroderma, generalized lymphadenopathy and presence of neoplastic T cells with cerebriform nuclei (so-called Sézary cells) in skin, lymph nodes and blood. This is a rare disease accounting for less than 5% of CTCLs. It occurs in adults with a male predominance. The histological and phenotypic features in Sézary syndrome may be similar to those of mycosis fungoides. TCR genes are clonally rearranged. The 5-year OS is 10–20%.

Primary cutaneous CD30-positive T-cell lymphoproliferative disorders

These lesions include primary cutaneous anaplastic large-cell lymphoma (C-ALCL) and lymphomatoid papulosis, which form a spectrum with overlapping histopathological and phenotypic features. Their appearance and course are therefore critical for the diagnosis.

Primary cutaneous anaplastic large-cell lymphoma

C-ALCL is composed of large cells with an anaplastic, pleomorphic or immunoblastic morphology, the vast majority of which express CD30. By definition, C-ALCL should not be preceded by or coincide with mycosis fungoides. It must also be distinguished from systemic ALCL, which is a different entity. Most patients present with solitary or localized nodules or tumours, and sometimes papules located on the trunk, face, extremities or buttocks, that often undergo ulceration and sometimes show partial or complete spontaneous regression, as in lymphomatoid papulosis. Besides CD30 positivity, the neoplastic cells display an activated $CD4^+$ T-cell phenotype with variable loss of CD2, CD5 and/or CD3. Unlike systemic ALCL, C-ALCL expresses CLA but not EMA or ALK. Unlike Hodgkin and Reed–Sternberg cells, staining for CD15 is generally negative. Most cases show clonal TCR gene rearrangement. The prognosis is favourable, with a 10-year OS of approximately 90%, although local relapses are frequent.

Lymphomatoid papulosis

Lymphomatoid papulosis is a chronic, recurrent, self-healing skin disease that most often occurs in adults with male preponderance, affects trunk and extremities and is characterized by paradoxical eruptions of papular, papulonecrotic and/or nodular lesions that tend to disappear within 3–12 weeks possibly leaving a scar. The duration of the disease may vary from several months to over 40 years. The prognosis is excellent. Morphologically, the large CD30-positive cells may be intermingled with a variable number of inflammatory cells or predominate as a monotonous population. The phenotype is similar to that of C-ALCL. Clonally rearranged TCR genes are detected in about 60% of lesions.

Primary cutaneous γδ T-cell lymphoma

This tumour consists of a clonal proliferation of activated γδ T cells with a cytotoxic phenotype. A possibly related condition may affect mucosal sites. Primary cutaneous γδ T-cell lymphoma is rare (1% of CTCLs) and more often observed in the extremities of adults with no sex predilection. It may be predominantly epidermotropic with patches/plaques or may give rise to deep dermal or subcutaneous tumours, with or without epidermal necrosis and ulceration. Dissemination to mucosal and other extranodal sites is frequent. HPS may occur. 'B' symptoms are seen in most patients. The tumour cells characteristically exhibit a $\beta F1^-CD3^+CD2^+CD5^-CD7^{+/-}CD56^+$ phenotype with strong expression of cytotoxic proteins. The cells are strongly positive for TCR-δ with appropriate detection methods. The cells show clonal rearrangement of the TCR-γ and TCR-δ genes. TCR-β may be rearranged or deleted, but is not expressed. Primary cutaneous γδ T-cell lymphoma is resistant to multi-agent chemotherapy and/or radiation and has a poor prognosis, with a median survival of approximately 15 months.

Peripheral T-cell lymphoma not otherwise specified

Peripheral T-cell lymphoma not otherwise specified is a heterogeneous group of tumours that corresponds with none of the T-cell entities defined in the WHO classification. It accounts for approximately 30% of peripheral T-cell lymphomas in Western countries. Most patients are adults with a slight male predominance, and show peripheral lymphadenopathy and 'B' symptoms. Generalized disease is often encountered, with bone marrow, liver, spleen and extranodal tissue involvement. Leukaemic spread is uncommon. The cytological spectrum is extremely broad, from highly polymorphous to monotonous. Clear cells and Reed–Sternberg-like elements can be seen and high endothelial venules increased. An inflammatory background is often present (Figure 33.23). The differential diagnosis with angioimmunoblastic T-cell lymphoma may require extensive immunophenotyping. Peripheral T-cell lymphoma not otherwise specified usually displays an aberrant T-cell phenotype, with frequent loss of CD5 and CD7. A CD4$^+$CD8$^-$ profile predominates in nodal cases. CD4$^+$CD8$^+$ or CD4$^-$CD8$^-$ is sometimes seen, as is CD8, CD30, CD56 and/or cytotoxic granule expression. CD52 is absent in 60% of cases. Aberrant CD20 and/or CD79a expression is occasionally encountered. Proliferation is high and Ki-67 rates over 80% are associated with poor outcome. TCR genes are clonally rearranged. Gene expression profiling has revealed deregulation of genes involved in matrix deposition, cytoskeleton organization, cell adhesion, apoptosis, proliferation, transcription and signal transduction. The products of these genes might have therapeutic relevance. EBV integration is found in some cases. Peripheral T-cell lymphoma not otherwise specified is highly aggressive with poor response to therapy, frequent relapses and 5-year OS of 20–30%. The IPI is the only factor consistently associated with prognosis. New scoring systems have recently been proposed.

Angioimmunoblastic T-cell lymphoma

Angioimmunoblastic T-cell lymphoma is characterized by a polymorphous infiltrate constantly involving lymph nodes with prominent proliferation of high endothelial venules and follicular dendritic cells (Figure 33.24). Spleen, liver, skin and bone marrow are also frequently affected. It occurs in middle-aged/elderly individuals of either sex and accounts for approximately 15–20% of peripheral T-cell lymphomas. Virtually all patients present with advanced-stage disease, systemic symptoms, polyclonal hypergammaglobulinaemia, circulating immune

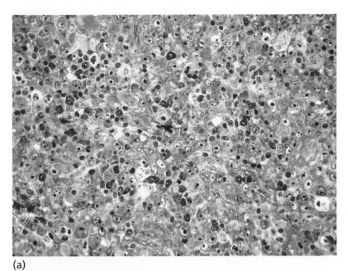

(a)

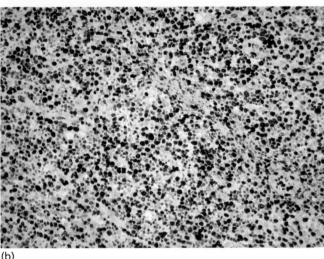

(b)

Figure 33.23 Peripheral T-cell lymphoma not otherwise specified. (a) The tumour consists of large cells with immunoblastic-like appearance. (b) The proliferative rate as shown by Ki-67 marking is very high.

complexes, cold agglutinins with haemolytic anaemia, positive rheumatoid factor and anti-smooth muscle antibodies. Skin rash is frequently observed. Other common findings are pleural effusion, arthritis and ascites. Angioimmunoblastic T-cell lymphoma is characterized by partial effacement of the lymph node architecture with sparing of the peripheral cortical sinuses. The neoplastic infiltrate is composed of small to medium-sized lymphocytes, with clear to pale cytoplasm and mild cytological atypia. They often form small clusters around hyperplastic high endothelial venules and follicular dendritic cells, and are admixed with small reactive lymphocytes, eosinophils, plasma cells and histiocytes. An expansion of EBV-positive B immunoblasts is usually present. The neoplastic cells have the phenotype of follicular T-helper cells positive for mature T-cell markers,

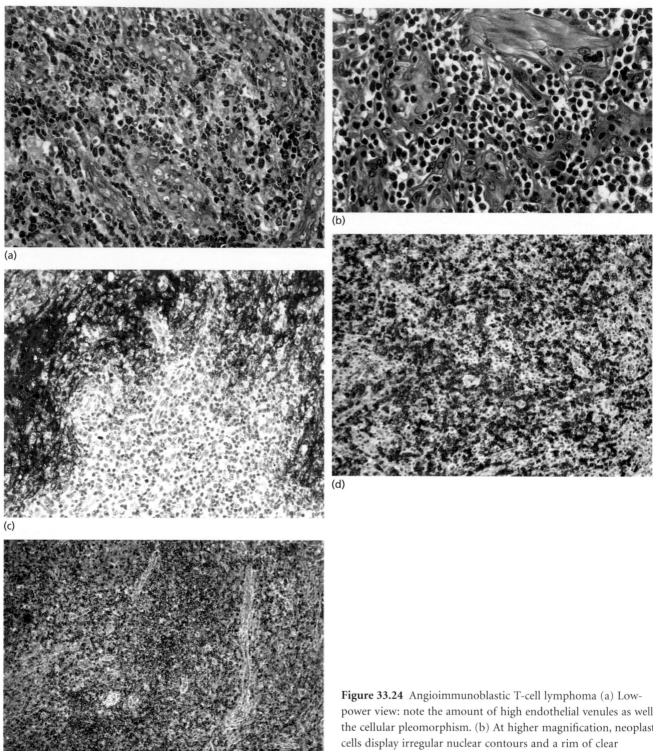

Figure 33.24 Angioimmunoblastic T-cell lymphoma (a) Low-power view: note the amount of high endothelial venules as well as the cellular pleomorphism. (b) At higher magnification, neoplastic cells display irregular nuclear contours and a rim of clear cytoplasm. (c) Hyperplasia of follicular dendritic cells recognized with CD21 staining. The tumour cells are positive for CD10 (d) and CXCL13 (e).

i.e. CD4, CD10, CXCL13, PD1, SAP and ICOS (Figure 33.24). TCR genes are clonally rearranged in most cases. Clonal *IGHV* gene rearrangements are found in about 25–30% of cases, and correlate with expanded EBV-positive B cells. The clinical course is aggressive with a median survival of less than 3 years. Patients often succumb to infectious complications. Supervening large B-cell lymphoma (often but not invariably EBV positive) can occur.

Anaplastic large-cell lymphoma, ALK⁺

ALCL ALK⁺ is characterized by large neoplastic cells with abundant cytoplasm and kidney/horseshoe-shaped nuclei (so-called hallmark cells), with a translocation involving the *ALK* gene and expression of both ALK protein and CD30. ALCL with similar morphology and phenotype, but lacking *ALK* rearrangement and ALK protein, is considered as a separate category (ALCL ALK⁻). ALCL ALK⁺ shows a higher prevalence in the first three decades of life and a male predominance and frequently involves both lymph nodes and extranodal sites. Most patients present with stage III–IV disease and 'B' symptoms. The morphology

may be variable. The 'common' appearance (60% of cases) consists of large tumour cells, frequently with hallmark appearance, that tend to grow within the sinuses, resembling a metastatic tumour (Figure 33.25). Some cases may have a lymphohistiocytic pattern (10%) characterized by few tumour cells overwhelmed by reactive histiocytes. A small-cell variant (5–10%) has been recognized that seems to have a worse prognosis. Some cases (3%) may mimic HL but the cells are ALK positive and CD15 negative. Relapses may reveal morphological features different from those seen initially. The tumour cells are CD30 positive. In cases with t(2;5)/*NPM–ALK* translocation, ALK staining is both cytoplasmic and nuclear. In cases with variant translocations, ALK staining may be membranous or cytoplasmic. Most ALCL ALK⁺ are positive for EMA, express cytotoxic markers and bear one or more T-cell antigens, although some may have null phenotype. EBV is negative. TCR gene is rearranged. The most frequent genetic alteration is t(2;5)(p23;q35) involving the *ALK* and nucleophosmin (*NPM*) genes. Variant translocations lead to fusion of the *ALK* gene with other partners on chromosomes 1, 2, 3, 17, 19, 22 and X. All these aberrations result in upregulation and different subcellular

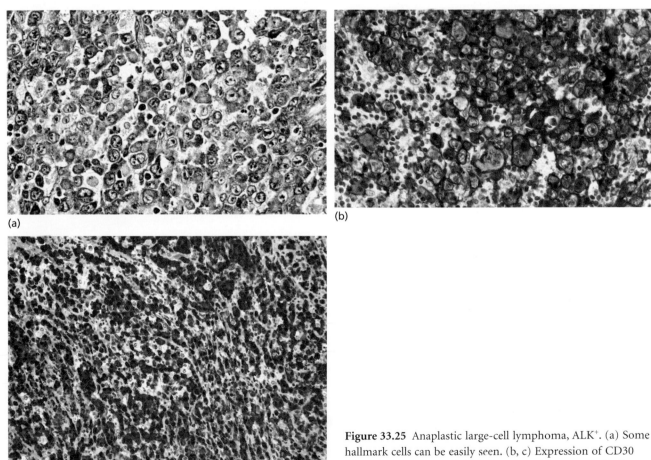

Figure 33.25 Anaplastic large-cell lymphoma, ALK⁺. (a) Some hallmark cells can be easily seen. (b, c) Expression of CD30 (b) and ALK protein (c) (alkaline phosphatase anti-alkaline phosphatase, Gill's counterstain, ×500 and ×250, respectively).

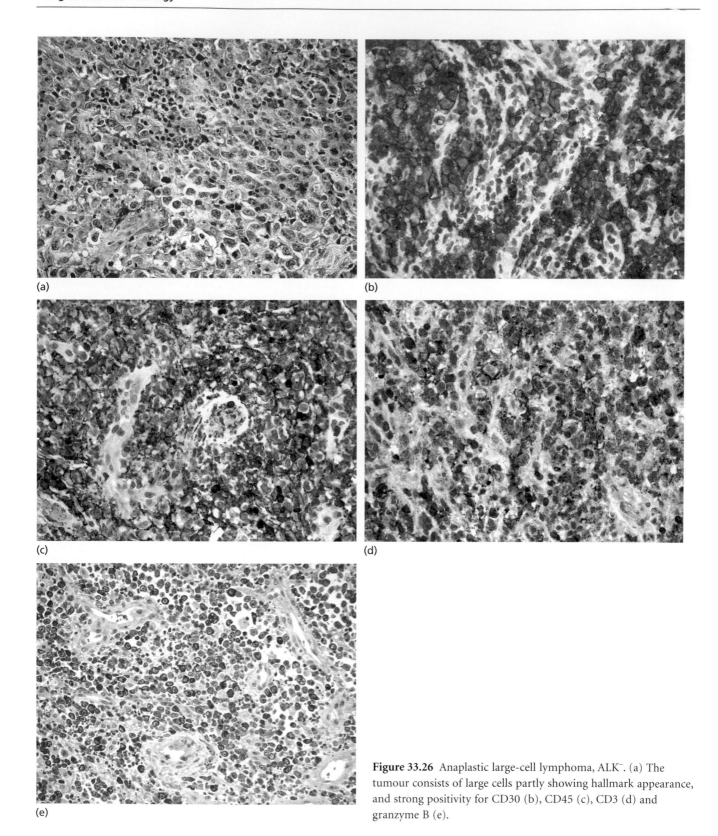

Figure 33.26 Anaplastic large-cell lymphoma, ALK⁻. (a) The tumour consists of large cells partly showing hallmark appearance, and strong positivity for CD30 (b), CD45 (c), CD3 (d) and granzyme B (e).

distribution of ALK protein but do not have clinical relevance. ALCL ALK⁺, ALCL ALK⁻ and peripheral T-cell lymphoma not otherwise specified have different chromosomal and gene expression profiles. The IPI predicts the clinical outcome. The 5-year OS is about 80%.

Anaplastic large-cell lymphoma, ALK⁻

In the new WHO Classification, ALCL ALK⁻ is a provisional entity. Most cases express both T-cell-associated and cytotoxic markers (Figure 33.26). The tumour must be distinguished from C-ALCL, other CD30-positive T- or B-cell lymphomas with anaplastic features, and classical HL. ALCL ALK⁻ affects adults with a slight male predominance, involves lymph nodes and, less frequently, extranodal sites. Most patients are staged III–IV, with 'B' symptoms. Usually, the organ architecture is effaced by solid cohesive sheets of neoplastic cells. In the lymph node, the latter tend to diffuse through sinuses, mimicking metastatic carcinoma. The main differential diagnosis is with peripheral T-cell lymphoma not otherwise specified and classical HL but immunophenotypic and molecular studies can distinguish these entities in most cases. In this regard, BSAP/PAX5 staining is useful: classical HL shows weak positivity in most

cases, a finding not observed in ALCL ALK⁻. In contrast, the distinction between peripheral T-cell lymphoma not otherwise specified and ALCL ALK⁻ is not always clear-cut, although recent gene expression profiling studies have definitely shown distinct signatures. Homogeneous strong CD30 staining on the cell membrane and Golgi area of all neoplastic cells favours the diagnosis of ALCL ALK⁻, as does complete loss of T-cell markers. Most cases show clonal TCR gene rearrangement and EBV is negative. ALCL ALK⁻ has a 5-year OS poorer than that of ALCL ALK⁺ (49% vs. 80%), but definitively better than peripheral T-cell lymphoma not otherwise specified (49% vs. 32%).

Hodgkin lymphoma

HL accounts for about 10% of lymphoid tumours. Irrespectively of the histotype, HL is characterized by the following features: (i) usual onset in the lymph nodes, preferentially cervical ones; (ii) predilection for young adults; and (iii) small number of mononucleated and multinucleated tumour cells (Hodgkin and Reed–Sternberg cells) within an exuberant inflammatory milieu and often ringed by rosettes of T lymphocytes. Biological and clinical studies have shown that HL comprises two disease enti-

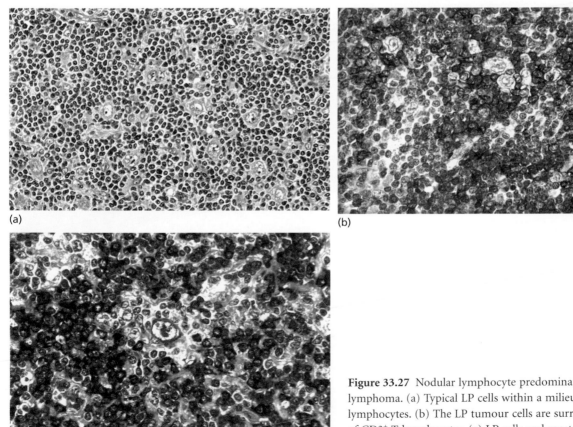

(a)

(b)

(c)

Figure 33.27 Nodular lymphocyte predominant (LP) Hodgkin lymphoma. (a) Typical LP cells within a milieu of small lymphocytes. (b) The LP tumour cells are surrounded by rosettes of CD3⁺ T lymphocytes. (c) LP cells and most small lymphocytes express CD79a.

ties: nodular lymphocyte predominant HL (NLPHL) and classical HL.

Nodular lymphocyte predominant Hodgkin lymphoma

NLPHL is a monoclonal B-cell tumour characterized by a nodular or a nodular and diffuse proliferation of scattered large multilobated neoplastic cells, known as 'popcorn' or LP cells (Figure 33.27). These reside in a follicular background with large follicular dendritic cell meshworks filled with non-neoplastic lymphocytes and histiocytes. One-third of the cases diagnosed in the past as NLPHL were lymphocyte-rich classical HL. It is currently unclear whether a diffuse NLPHL exists, its borders with T-cell/histiocyte-rich large B-cell lymphoma being not always sharp. NLPHL represents approximately 5% of HL cases. Patients are predominantly males in the fourth decade of life. LP cells are regularly positive for CD20, CD79a, EMA, BCL-6 and CD45. In contrast to Hodgkin and Reed–Sternberg cells of classical HL, tumor cells are positive for Oct-2, BOB.1 and immunoglobulin light and/or heavy chains but lack CD15,

CD30 and EBV infection. The tumour cells are ringed by T-follicular helper cells that are positive for CD3, CD4, PD-1 and (to a lesser extent) CD57. LP cells show clonal *IGHV* gene rearrangement, with a high load of somatic mutations that may be ongoing. Aberrant somatic hypermutations of *PAX5*, *PIM1*, *RhoH/TTF* (now called *RHOH*) and *MYC* genes are recorded in 80% of cases. NLPHL is an indolent disease with frequent relapses that usually remains responsive to therapy. Advanced stages have an unfavourable prognosis. Progression to large B-cell lymphoma-like lesions is seen in 3–5% of cases.

Classical Hodgkin lymphoma

Classical Hodgkin lymphoma is a monoclonal lymphoid neoplasm (mostly derived from B cells) composed of Hodgkin and Reed–Sternberg cells within a variable mixture of reactive lymphocytes, eosinophils, neutrophils, histiocytes, plasma cells, fibroblasts and collagen fibres (Figure 33.28). Based on the characteristics of the inflammatory background, and to a certain extent on the morphology of Hodgkin and Reed–Sternberg cells (i.e. lacunar cells), four histological subtypes are distinguished:

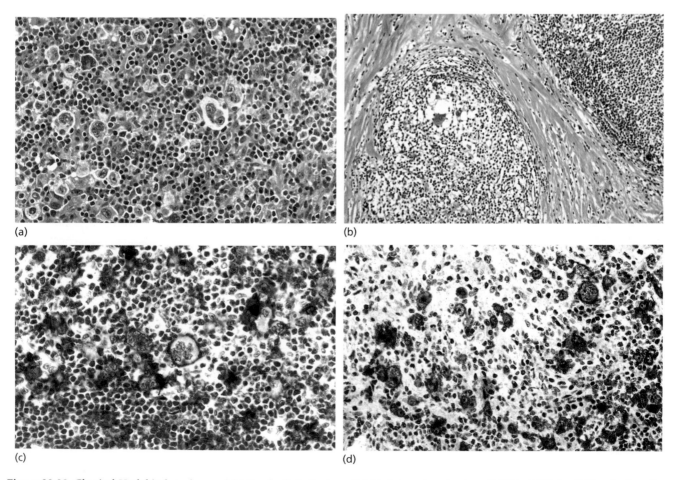

(a) (b) (c) (d)

Figure 33.28 Classical Hodgkin lymphoma. (a) Mixed cellularity type. (b) Nodular sclerosing type (H&E, ×100). (c, d) Neoplastic cells positive for CD30 (c) and CD15 (d).

lymphocyte rich, nodular sclerosis, mixed cellularity and lymphocyte depleted. The immunophenotypic and genetic features of Hodgkin and Reed–Sternberg cells are identical in these histological subtypes, whereas clinical features and EBV association vary. Classical HL accounts for 95% of HLs, with a bimodal age curve in resource-rich countries, showing a peak at 15–35 years and a second peak in late life. Classical HL most often involves cervical lymph nodes and in approximately 60% of patients (usually with the nodular sclerosis subtype) causes a mediastinal mass. Hodgkin and Reed–Sternberg cells typically represent 0.1–10% of the cellular infiltrate. The composition of the reactive milieu varies according to the subtype. Hodgkin and Reed–Sternberg cells are CD30 positive in nearly all cases, and CD15 positive in most. In 30–40% of cases CD20 may be detected, usually of varied intensity and in a minority of Hodgkin and Reed–Sternberg cells. The B-cell nature of neoplastic cells is sustained in about 95% of cases by their expression of BSAP/PAX5, though weaker than that of reactive B cells. EBV-positive Hodgkin and Reed–Sternberg cells show a latency II pattern (LMP1[+], EBNA-2[−]). Characteristically, the transcription factors Oct-2 and BOB.1 are absent in about 90% of cases, while PU.1 is consistently absent. Reed–Sternberg cells contain clonal *IGHV* gene rearrangements in more than 98% of cases, and clonal TCR gene rearrangements in rare instances. The rearranged *IGHV* genes harbour a high load of somatic hypermutations, usually not ongoing.

Selected bibliography

General

Gall EA, Mallory TB (1942) Malignant lymphoma: a clinicopathologic survey of 618 cases. *American Journal of Pathology* **18**: 341–429.

Harris NL, Jaffe ES, Stein H *et al.* (1994) A revised European–American classification of lymphoid neoplasms: a proposal from the International Lymphoma Study Group. *Blood* **84**: 1361–92.

Lennert K (1978) *Malignant Lymphomas other than Hodgkin's Disease*. Springer Verlag, New York.

Lukes RJ, Collins RD (1974) Immunologic characterization of human malignant lymphomas. *Cancer* **34** (4 Suppl.): 1488–503.

Non-Hodgkin's Lymphoma Classification Project (1997) A clinical evaluation of the International Lymphoma Study Group classification of non-Hodgkin's lymphomas. *Blood* **89**: 3909–18.

Non-Hodgkin's Lymphoma Pathologic Classification Project (1982) National Cancer Institute sponsored study of classifications of non-Hodgkin's lymphomas: summary and description of a working formulation for clinical usage. *Cancer* **49**: 2112–35.

Rappaport H (1966) *Tumors of the Haematopoietic System. Atlas of Tumor Pathology*. Armed Forces Institute of Pathology, Washington, DC.

Swerdlow SH, Campo E, Harris NL *et al.* (eds) (2008) *WHO Classification of Tumours of Haematopoietic and Lymphoid Tissues*. IARC, Lyon.

B-cell neoplasms

Campo E, Miquel R, Krenacs L, Sorbara L, Raffeld M, Jaffe ES (1999) Primary nodal marginal zone lymphomas of splenic and MALT type. *American Journal of Surgical Pathology* **23**: 59–68.

Campo E, Raffeld M, Jaffe ES (1999) Mantle-cell lymphoma. *Seminars in Hematology* **36**: 115–27.

Campo E, Chott A, Kinney MC *et al.* (2006) Update on extranodal lymphomas. Conclusions of the Workshop held by the EAHP and the SH in Thessaloniki, Greece. *Histopathology* **48**: 481–504.

Crespo M, Bosch F, Villamor N *et al.* (2003) ZAP-70 expression as a surrogate for immunoglobulin-variable-region mutations in chronic lymphocytic leukaemia. *New England Journal of Medicine* **348**: 1764–75.

Fernandez V, Salamero O, Espinet B *et al.* (2010) Genomic and gene expression profiling defines indolent forms of mantle cell lymphoma. *Cancer Research* **70**: 1408–18.

Hallek M, Cheson BD, Catovsky D *et al.* (2008) Guidelines for the diagnosis and treatment of chronic lymphocytic leukaemia: a report from the International Workshop on Chronic Lymphocytic Leukaemia updating the National Cancer Institute Working Group 1996 guidelines. *Blood* **111**: 5446–56.

Isaacson PG, Du MQ (2004) MALT lymphoma: from morphology to molecules. *Nature Reviews. Cancer* **4**: 644–53.

Jares P, Colomer D, Campo E (2007) Genetic and molecular pathogenesis of mantle cell lymphoma: perspectives for new targeted therapeutics. *Nature Reviews. Cancer* **7**: 750–62.

Karube K, Guo Y, Suzumiya J *et al.* (2007) CD10[−]MUM1[+] follicular lymphoma lacks BCL2 gene translocation and shows characteristic biologic and clinical features. *Blood* **109**: 3076–9.

Le Gouill S, Talmant P, Touzeau C *et al.* (2007) The clinical presentation and prognosis of diffuse large B-cell lymphoma with t(14;18) and 8q24/c-MYC rearrangement. *Haematologica* **92**: 1335–42.

Lenz G, Wright G, Dave SS *et al.* (2008) Stromal gene signatures in large-B-cell lymphomas. *New England Journal of Medicine* **359**: 2313–23.

Lin P, Medeiros LJ (2007) High-grade B-cell lymphoma/leukaemia associated with t(14;18) and 8q24/MYC rearrangement: a neoplasm of germinal centre immunophenotype with poor prognosis. *Haematologica* **92**: 1297–301.

Ott G, Rosenwald A (2008) Molecular pathogenesis of follicular lymphoma. *Haematologica* **93**: 1773–6.

Ott G, Katzenberger T, Lohr A *et al.* (2002) Cytomorphologic, immunohistochemical, and cytogenetic profiles of follicular lymphoma: 2 types of follicular lymphoma grade 3. *Blood* **99**: 3806–12.

Ponzoni M, Ferreri AJ, Campo E *et al.* (2007) Definition, diagnosis, and management of intravascular large B-cell lymphoma: proposals and perspectives from an international consensus meeting. *Journal of Clinical Oncology* **25**: 3168–73.

Rawstron AC, Bennett FL, O'Connor SJ *et al.* (2008) Monoclonal B-cell lymphocytosis and chronic lymphocytic leukaemia. *New England Journal of Medicine* **359**: 575–83.

Shimoyama Y, Yamamoto K, Asano N, Oyama T, Kinoshita T, Nakamura S (2008) Age-related Epstein–Barr virus-associated B-cell lymphoproliferative disorders: special references to lymphomas surrounding this newly recognized clinicopathologic disease. *Cancer Science* **99**: 1085–91.

Taddesse-Heath L, Pittaluga S, Sorbara L, Bussey M, Raffeld M, Jaffe ES (2003) Marginal zone B-cell lymphoma in children and young adults. *American Journal of Surgical Pathology* **27**: 522–31.

Traverse-Glehen A, Pittaluga S, Gaulard P *et al.* (2005) Mediastinal grey zone lymphoma: the missing link between classic Hodgkin's lymphoma and mediastinal large B-cell lymphoma. *American Journal of Surgical Pathology* **29**: 1411–21.

T-cell and NK-cell neoplasms

Agostinelli C, Piccaluga PP, Went Ph *et al.* (2008) Peripheral T-cell lymphoma not otherwise specified: the stuff of dreams, genes and therapies. *Journal of Clinical Pathology* **61**: 1160–7.

Chiarle R, Voena C, Ambrogio C, Piva R, Inghirami G (2008) The anaplastic lymphoma kinase in the pathogenesis of cancer. *Nature Reviews. Cancer* **8**: 11–23.

Cuadros M, Dave SS, Jaffe ES *et al.* (2007) Identification of a proliferation signature related to survival in nodal peripheral T-cell lymphomas. *Journal of Clinical Oncology* **25**: 3321–9.

de Leval L, Rickman DS, Thielen C *et al.* (2007) The gene expression profile of nodal peripheral T-cell lymphoma demonstrates a molecular link between angioimmunoblastic T-cell lymphoma (AITL) and follicular helper T (TFH) cells. *Blood* **109**: 4952–63.

Dunleavy K, Wilson WH, Jaffe ES (2007) Angioimmunoblastic T-cell lymphoma: pathobiological insights and clinical implications. *Current Opinion in Hematology* **14**: 348–53.

Huang Y, de Reyniès A, de Leval L *et al.* (2010) Gene expression profiling identifies emerging oncogenic pathways operating in extranodal NK/T-cell lymphoma, nasal type. *Blood* **115**: 1226–37.

Iqbal J, Weisenburger DD, Greiner TC *et al.* (2010) Molecular signatures to improve diagnosis in peripheral T-cell lymphoma and prognostication in angioimmunoblastic T-cell lymphoma. *Blood* **115**: 1026–36.

Jaccard A, Petit B, Girault S *et al.* (2009) L-Asparaginase-based treatment of 15 western patients with extranodal NK/T-cell lymphoma and leukaemia and a review of the literature. *Annals of Oncology* **20**: 110–16.

Lamant L, De Reynies A, Duplantier MM *et al.* (2006) Gene expression profiling of systemic anaplastic large cell lymphoma reveals differences depending on ALK status and two distinct morphological ALK$^+$ subtypes. *Blood* **109**: 2156–64.

Liang X, Graham DK (2008) Natural killer cell neoplasms. *Cancer* **112**: 1425–36.

Ohshima K, Kimura H, Yoshino T *et al.* (2008) Proposed categorization of pathological states of EBV-associated T/natural killer-cell lymphoproliferative disorder (LPD) in children and young adults: overlap with chronic active EBV infection and infantile fulminant EBV T-LPD. *Pathology International* **58**: 209–17.

Piccaluga PP, Agostinelli C, Califano A *et al.* (2007) Gene expression analysis of peripheral T cell lymphoma, unspecified, reveals distinct profiles and new potential therapeutic targets. *Journal of Clinical Investigation* **117**: 823–34.

Piva R, Agnelli L, Pellegrino E *et al.* (2010) Gene expression profiling uncovers molecular classifiers for the recognition of anaplastic large-cell lymphoma within peripheral T-cell neoplasms. *Journal of Clinical Oncology* **28**: 1583–90.

Savage KJ (2007) Peripheral T-cell lymphomas. *Blood Reviews* **21**: 201–16.

Savage K (2008) Prognosis and primary therapy in peripheral T-cell lymphomas. *Hematology. American Society of Hematology Education Program*, 280–8.

Savage K, Harris NL, Vose JM *et al.* (2008) ALK$^-$ anaplastic large-cell lymphoma is clinically and immunophenotypically different from both ALK$^+$ ALCL and peripheral T-cell lymphoma, not otherwise specified: report from the International Peripheral T-cell Lymphoma Project. *Blood* **111**: 5496–504.

Stein H, Foss DH, Dürkopp H *et al.* (2000) CD30(+) anaplastic large cell lymphoma: a review of its histopathologic, genetic and clinical features. *Blood* **96**: 3681–5.

Tripodo C, Iannitto E, Florena AM *et al.* (2009) Gamma-delta T-cell lymphomas. *Nature Reviews. Clinical Oncology* **6**: 707–17.

Tsukasaki K, Hermine O, Bazarbachi A *et al.* (2009) Definition, prognostic factors, treatment, and response criteria of adult T-cell leukaemia-lymphoma: a proposal from an international consensus meeting. *Journal of Clinical Oncology* **27**: 453–9.

Went P, Agostinelli C, Gallamini A *et al.* (2006) Marker expression in peripheral T-cell lymphoma: a proposed clinical–pathologic prognostic score. *Journal of Clinical Oncology* **24**: 2472–9.

Willemze R, Meijer CJ (2006) Classification of cutaneous T-cell lymphoma: from Alibert to WHO-EORTC. *Journal of Cutaneous Pathology* **33** (Suppl. 1): 18–56.

Willemze R, Jansen PM, Cerroni L *et al.* (2008) Subcutaneous panniculitis-like T-cell lymphoma: definition, classification, and prognostic factors: an EORTC Cutaneous Lymphoma Group Study of 83 cases. *Blood* **111**: 838–45.

Yu H, Shahsafaei A, Dorfman DM (2009) Germinal-centre T-helper-cell markers PD1 and CXCL13 are both expressed in angioimmunoblastic T-cell lymphoma. *American Journal of Clinical Pathology* **131**: 33–41.

Zettl A, deLeeuw R, Haralambieva E, Müller-Hermelink HK (2007) Enteropathy-type T-cell lymphoma. *American Journal of Clinical Pathology* **127**: 701–6.

Hodgkin lymphoma

Gallamini A, Hutchings M, Rigacci L *et al.* (2007) Early interim 2-[^{18}F]fluoro-2-deoxy-D-glusose positron emission tomography is prognostically superior to international prognostic score in advanced-stage Hodgkin's lymphoma: a report from a joint Italian–Danish study. *Journal of Clinical Oncology* **25**: 3746–52.

Küppers R (2009) The biology of Hodgkin's lymphoma. *Nature Reviews. Cancer* **9**: 15–27.

Pileri SA, Falini B, Agostinelli C, Stein H (2008) Pathobiology of Hodgkin's lymphoma. In: *Hoffman's Haematology* (R Hoffman, EJ Benz, SJ Shattil *et al.*, eds), 4th edn, pp. 1220–38. Elsevier Churchill Livingstone, Philadelphia.

Hodgkin lymphoma

34

Jonathan Sive and David Linch

UCM Medical School, London, UK

Introduction

Hodgkin lymphoma is an uncommon tumour, although it is one of the more frequent malignancies in young people. Traditionally, radiotherapy was the primary therapeutic approach, and the first successful combination chemotherapy regimen was introduced in the 1960s. Since then, combined modality therapy has developed allowing reduction of both chemotherapy and radiotherapy doses. The outcome of patients with Hodgkin lymphoma has improved greatly over the last few decades such that it should now be considered curable in the large majority of cases. With the excellent cure rates now attainable, the late effects of treatment have become more apparent. Current therapeutic strategies must aim to maintain these high cure rates while minimizing these late effects.

Epidemiology

Hodgkin lymphoma is a relatively uncommon malignancy, with an incidence in the UK of about 2.4 per 100 000 per annum, and an overall male to female ratio of 1.4 : 1. It is a disease that affects young adults, and is the third most commonly diagnosed cancer in people aged 15–29 years. The previously described second peak in older age groups is partly an artefact, due to

misreporting of non-Hodgkin (mainly anaplastic) lymphomas in this age group. The overall incidence is stable in comparison to that of non-Hodgkin lymphomas, which appears to be rising. Worldwide prevalence rates vary, with more than 5.5 per 100 000 in Yemen and Lebanon and less than 1 per 100 000 in China and Japan. At least some of this variation, and that of the proportions of histological subtypes, appears to relate to the degree of industrialization. As a consequence of the excellent responses to treatment, mortality rates are low (0.4 per 100 000 per annum in the UK). Mortality increases with age and in countries with less access to treatment.

Aetiology

Although no clear-cut aetiological agent has been identified for Hodgkin lymphoma, Epstein–Barr virus (EBV) has long been theorized to play a causative role. EBV nucleic acids and proteins have been detected in 25–50% of cases, and patients with Hodgkin lymphoma have different serological profiles of antibodies to EBV-associated antigens prior to diagnosis compared with healthy controls. However, differences remain between histological subtypes, age groups and geographical locations, and a precise causative role has not been definitively identified. No other infectious agents have shown a consistent association.

Immunosuppression is associated with an increased risk of developing Hodgkin lymphoma, especially in HIV infection, which increases the risk by 7–14 times. However, in contrast to non-Hodgkin lymphomas, the incidence is not directly correlated with a low CD4 count, and the prevalence has actually

Postgraduate Haematology: 6th edition. Edited by A. Victor Hoffbrand, Daniel Catovsky, Edward G.D. Tuddenham, Anthony R. Green
© 2011 Blackwell Publishing Ltd.

Table 34.1 WHO classification of Hodgkin lymphoma.

Nodular lymphocyte-predominant Hodgkin lymphoma
Classical Hodgkin lymphoma
    Nodular sclerosis classical Hodgkin lymphoma
    Mixed-cellularity classical Hodgkin lymphoma
    Lymphocyte-rich classical Hodgkin lymphoma
    Lymphocyte-depleted classical Hodgkin lymphoma

Table 34.2 Immunophenotype of Hodgkin lymphoma.

	Classical Hodgkin lymphoma: presence/absence of Reed–Sternberg cells	*Nodular lymphocyte-predominant Hodgkin lymphoma: presence/ absence of lymphocytic and histiocytic cells*
CD30	Present	Absent
CD15	Usually present	Absent
Immunoglobulin	Absent	Present
CD20	Absent	Present
Other B-cell markers	Ususally absent	Usually present

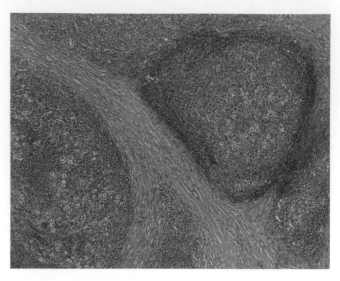

Figure 34.1 Low-power view of lymph node biopsy of classical Hodgkin lymphoma showing nodularity and sclerosis.

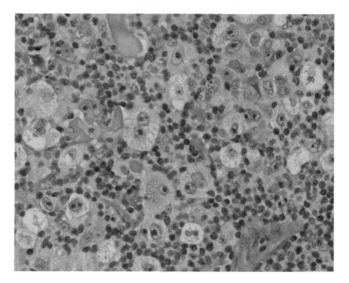

Figure 34.2 High-power view of classical Hodgkin lymphoma showing abundant Reed–Sternberg cells and occasional eosinophils.

increased with better viral control since the introduction of highly active antiretroviral therapy.

Histological classification (see also Chapter 33)

Hodgkin lymphoma is broadly classified into two distinct entities: classical Hodgkin lymphoma (CHL) and nodular lymphocyte-predominant Hodgkin lymphoma (NLPHL). Both types are characterized by the histological appearance of only a small number of neoplastic Hodgkin/Reed–Sternberg (HRS) cells in an inflammatory background of reactive T cells and eosinophils, with varying degrees of fibrosis.

CHL is divided into four subtypes (Table 34.1). In the developed world, nodular sclerosing Hodgkin lymphoma accounts for the majority of cases. Although the HRS cell has now been identified as being of B-cell lineage, the mature B-cell antigen expression pattern is often low or absent (Table 34.2 and Figures 34.1–34.4).

NLPHL has a distinct histological appearance, with HRS cells having a lymphocytic and histiocytic or 'popcorn' appearance. The immunophenotype is more typical for a B cell, being positive for CD20 and immunoglobulin expression (Figures 34.5–34.8).

Pathogenesis

Nature of malignant cell

The pathogenesis of Hodgkin lymphoma is still not completely understood. Indeed, the nature of the underlying neoplastic cell was only confirmed relatively recently, when single-cell studies from microdissected specimens were performed. These confirmed that the HRS cell of CHL is of B-cell origin, probably of a germinal or post-germinal centre type, with clonal rearrange-

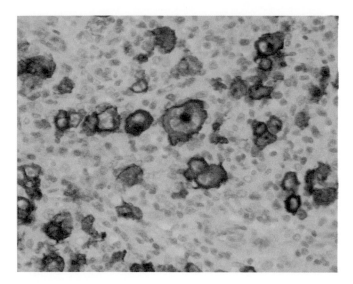

Figure 34.3 CD30 immunostain of classical Hodgkin lymphoma showing clear membranous and Golgi apparatus staining of the Hodgkin/Reed–Sternberg cells.

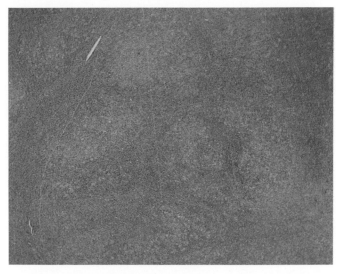

Figure 34.5 Low-power view of lymph node biopsy of nodular lymphocyte-predominant Hodgkin lymphoma showing nodular features and slight mottled appearance of the follicles.

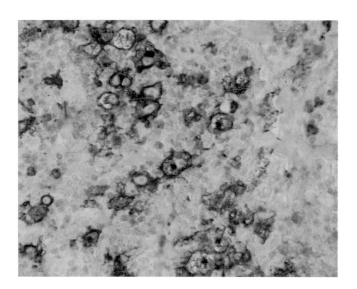

Figure 34.4 CD15 immunostain of classical Hodgkin lymphoma.

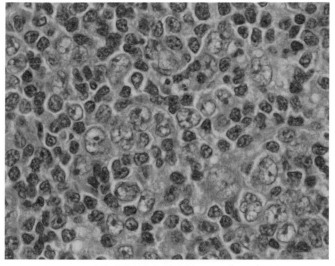

Figure 34.6 High-power view of nodular lymphocyte-predominant Hodgkin lymphoma showing many convoluted lymphocytic and histiocytic or 'popcorn' cells.

ments in the V, D and J segments of the IgH chain locus in the majority of patients. There is absent immunoglobulin expression in HRS cells, indicative of crippling mutations in the immunoglobulin gene or defective expression of the transcription factor(s) that regulate the B-cell differentiation programme. In contrast, the malignant lymphocytic and histiocytic cells of NLPHL have both the genotype and immunophenotype of typical post-germinal centre B cells (Table 34.2). Whereas there is markedly reduced or absent expression of the transcription factor Oct2 or its coactivator BOB1 in HRS cells of CHL, these factors are highly expressed in the malignant cells of NLPHL.

Mechanism of tumorigenesis

Information on the mechanisms leading to development of a malignant phenotype is limited, and the inability to perform functional studies on cells purified from tissue specimens means that almost all data are derived from cultured cell lines.

Several pathways have been identified as being linked to the growth and survival of HRS cells. NF-κB signalling is increased, caused by a number of upstream mechanisms, such as reduced levels of IκB, which normally acts as an inhibitor. The inactiva-

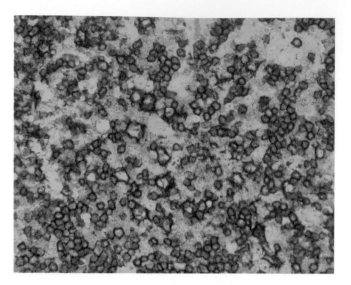

Figure 34.7 CD20 staining of nodular lymphocyte-predominant Hodgkin lymphoma. Note that the lymphocytic and histiocytic cells are typically surrounded by a rosette of CD20-negative reactive T cells.

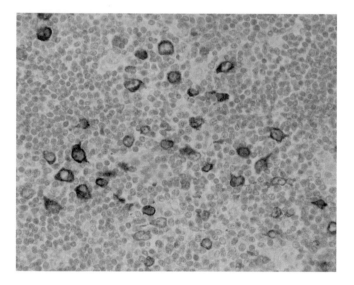

Figure 34.8 J-chain immunostaining of nodular lymphocyte-predominant Hodgkin lymphoma demonstrating immunoglobulin production of lymphocytic and histiocytic cells, a feature not seen in classical Hodgkin lymphoma.

tion of IκB is caused by, among other factors, the EBV-derived latent membrane protein (LMP)-1. This is one of the mechanisms by which EBV may act as a viral aetiological agent for the development of Hodgkin lymphoma. Other pathways implicated in tumorigenesis include activated protein (AP)-1, the JAK/STAT and NOTCH signalling pathway, and autocrine effects from interleukin (IL)-13 activity.

Unlike some other haematological neoplasms, no specific chromosomal translocation has been identified on cytogenetic analysis, but the presence of aneuploidy with widespread chromosomal abnormalities suggests underlying genomic instability.

Mechanism of surrounding tissue reaction

The characteristic surrounding inflammatory tissue of Hodgkin lymphoma is a mixture of T cells (mainly CD4+ T-regulatory cells), histiocytes, plasma cells, eosinophils and neutrophils. The background is thought to be cytokine-induced, for example eotaxin released from fibroblasts causing eosinophil infiltration. This cytokine release may also account for the characteristic blood abnormalities associated with Hodgkin lymphoma, and the systemic 'B' symptoms.

Clinical presentation

Hodgkin lymphoma can present in a variety of ways. Most commonly, however, it arises within a lymph node, presenting as an enlarged but painless lump, usually in the neck or supra-clavicular region. Mediastinal nodes are involved in up to 60% of cases at presentation and retroperitoneal nodes in 25%. Presentation in the subdiaphragmatic nodes alone is less common.

A mediastinal mass detected on chest radiography is also common, either after investigation for pulmonary symptoms (e.g. chest discomfort, cough or dyspnoea) or as an incidental finding (Figure 34.9). Other presentations, such as bone marrow infiltration, cholestasis and autoimmune phenomena, are well documented but much rarer.

An important feature of Hodgkin lymphoma is the initial contiguous pattern of spread through adjacent lymph nodes; only later does haematogenous spread to more distant organs take place. Splenomegaly may occur without direct disease involvement, although hepatosplenomegaly almost invariably indicates disease infiltration. Peripheral blood manifestations are common but non-specific, with lymphocytopenia and anaemia being indicators of advanced disease. The prognostic significance of eosinophilia is unclear.

Systemic 'B' symptoms are found in approximately 25% of patients at presentation. An 'A' staging merely represents the absence of 'B' symptoms. These consist of weight loss, night sweats and fevers. The so-called Pel–Ebstein fever describes a characteristic intermittent fever associated with Hodgkin lymphoma. However, its specificity and indeed existence has been called into question. Other systemic symptoms include pruritus, alcohol-induced pain at the site of affected lymph nodes and skin lesions.

NLPHL tends to present with chronic asymptomatic peripheral lymphadenopathy; 80% of cases present with early-stage

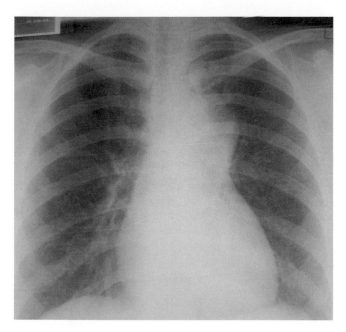

Figure 34.9 Chest radiograph showing enlarged superior mediastinum.

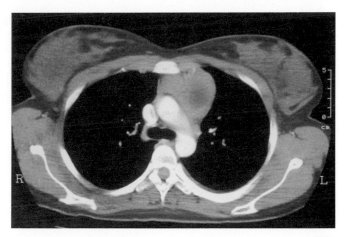

Figure 34.10 CT scan of the chest showing large anterior mediastinal mass with area of probable necrosis.

disease and, compared with CHL, mediastinal involvement and 'B' symptoms are less common. NLPHL tends to relapse late as a large-cell lymphoma, in keeping with its phenotype being more similar to non-Hodgkin lymphomas.

Diagnosis and staging

The diagnosis of Hodgkin lymphoma is made histologically, usually from an affected lymph node. Routine light microscopy is almost always augmented by immunohistochemical staining (see Figures 34.3, 34.4, 34.7 and 34.8).

Once the diagnosis has been confirmed, full staging is carried out by computed tomography (CT) from neck to pelvis, and bone marrow biopsy where indicated. Staging is still based on the Ann Arbor system (Table 34.3), which was developed over 30 years ago primarily to define who would benefit from radiotherapy. The Cotswolds modification, made in 1989, takes into account the importance of bulky disease and the fact that laparotomy and diagnostic splenectomy are no longer recommended due to the associated morbidity and mortality (Figure 34.10).

Functional imaging plays an increasing role, with gallium scanning now effectively superseded by ^{18}F-fluorodeoxyglucose positron emission tomography (FDG-PET) (Figure 34.11). Hodgkin lymphoma is usually FDG-avid, and so is assumed to be positive on presentation. PET is beginning to form part of standard initial staging investigations, especially where FDG-avidity on PET will alter the stage and the treatment strategy employed.

Table 34.3 Ann Arbor staging system with Cotswolds modifications for Hodgkin lymphoma.

Stage	
I	Involvement of a single lymph-node region or lymphoid structure (e.g. spleen, thymus, Waldeyer ring)
II	Two or more lymph node regions on the same side of the diaphragm
III	Lymph nodes on both sides of the diaphragm
III1	With splenic hilar, coeliac or portal nodes
III2	With para-aortic, iliac, mesenteric nodes
IV	Involvement of extranodal site(s) beyond that designated 'E'

Modifying features	
A	No symptoms
B	Fever, drenching night sweats, weight loss >10% in 6 months
X	Bulky disease: more than one-third widening of mediastinum, >10 cm maximum diameter of nodal mass
E	Involvement of single, contiguous or proximal extranodal site
CS	Clinical stage
PS	Pathological stage

Bone marrow infiltration is only found in around 6% of cases (and even less in NLPHL), and bone marrow biopsy is only indicated in advanced-stage disease (IIB to IV), in the presence of cytopenias, or if mandated by a clinical trial. In otherwise localized disease, the pick-up rate for upstaging by bone marrow involvement is very low. PET positivity of infiltrated bone marrow has some concordance with histological analysis but

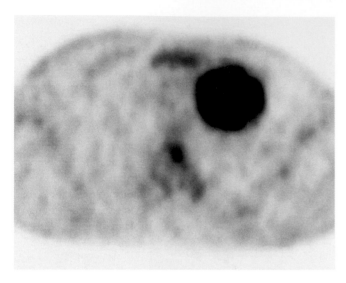

Figure 34.11 FDG-PET scan showing FDG avidity of large mediastinal mass.

has not been shown to correlate strongly enough to supersede its use.

Magnetic resonance imaging (MRI) is largely restricted to the evaluation of specific situations such as bony involvement or spinal cord compression.

Prognostic factors

Several attempts have been made to identify clinically relevant prognostic factors and combine them to allow risk stratification. Limited-stage disease (I and II) has been subdivided into favourable and unfavourable groups by the European Organization for Research and Treatment of Cancer (EORTC) on the basis of the number of nodal areas, age, systemic symptoms and large mediastinal adenopathy (Table 34.4) This stratification was first developed in the era when radiotherapy was the mainstay of treatment, but the EORTC H7 trial on limited-stage disease demonstrated the ongoing validity of this approach in defining favourable and unfavourable patient groups. However, the implications for treatment are still not clear, and in the UK and the USA all early-stage patients are usually managed the same way.

In advanced-stage disease, the International Prognostic Index (IPI) or Hasenclever score was developed based on an analysis of over 5000 patients treated initially with an anthracycline-containing chemotherapy regimen. Seven factors were identified, each of which reduced the 5-year freedom from progression rate by around 8% (Table 34.5).

NLPHL has a slightly better prognosis than CHL, although its potential for late relapse as a large-cell lymphoma necessitates ongoing post-treatment surveillance. A recent retrospec-

Table 34.4 EORTC risk factors in localized disease.

Favourable
Patients must have all of the following features:
 Clinical stage I and II
 Maximum of three nodal areas involved
 Age < 50 years
 ESR < 50 mm/hour without 'B' symptoms or ESR < 30 mm/hour with 'B' symptoms
 Mediastinal/thoracic ratio <0.35

Unfavourable
Patients have any of the following features:
 Clinical stage II with involvement of at least four nodal areas
 Age > 50 years
 ESR > 50 mm/hour if asymptomatic or ESR > 30 mm/hour if 'B' symptoms
 Mediastinal/thoracic ratio >0.35

ESR, erythrocyte sedimentation rate.

Table 34.5 Hasenclever index.

Age > 45 years
Male gender
Serum albumin < 40 g/L
Haemoglobin < 10.5 g/dL
Stage IV disease
Leucocytosis (white cell count $\geq 15 \times 10^9$/L)
Lymphopenia (<0.6 $\times 10^9$/L or <8% of the white cell count)

tive analysis at 4 years showed freedom from treatment failure rates for CHL and NLPHL patients of 88% and 82%, respectively, and overall survival rates of 96% and 92%. Poor prognostic factors in NLPHL have been identified as advanced stage, anaemia and lymphopenia.

Response assessment

Assessment of disease response requires repeat imaging (Figure 34.12) and, if infiltrated on staging investigations, repeat bone marrow biopsy. The utility of PET is increasingly well understood, and in any case of residual disease it can help differentiate between active disease and fibrotic material. In view of this, the previous CR(u) (unconfirmed) classification to describe residual masses of uncertain significance on CT has been eliminated. Responses to treatment are now classified as complete response (CR), partial response (PR), stable disease or progressive/relapsed disease (Table 34.6).

False-positive PET results can occur after treatment, so imaging is recommended at 3 or 6 weeks after chemotherapy

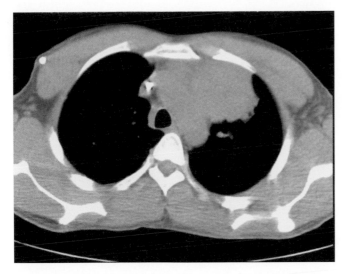

Figure 34.12 CT scan of the chest showing large residual mass at end of treatment.

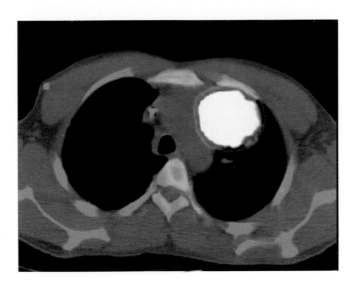

Figure 34.13 PET/CT scan of same patient as in Figure 34.12 showing FDG avidity of large residual mass.

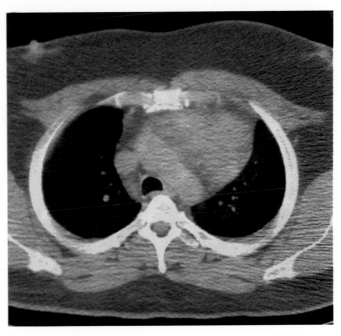

Figure 34.14 PET/CT scan showing FDG-'cold' residual mass.

recent data from non-Hodgkin lymphomas have raised concerns about both the extent of predictive value and the degree of interobserver agreement in the interpretation of scans. Future strategies may employ a more quantitative approach, incorporating standard uptake values rather than qualitative interpretations as simple positive or negative.

At present, PET response-adapted therapies are not recommended outside of clinical trials. Post-remission surveillance with either CT or PET has not been shown to be useful in guiding treatment.

Treatment

The treatment of Hodgkin lymphoma is often called one of the success stories of cancer treatment. What was once an invariably terminal condition is now considered curable in the majority of cases. Early treatment strategies were based exclusively on radiotherapy, and the staging and prognostic systems still reflect this to an extent. Although radiotherapy resulted in high rates of remission in localized disease, relapse rates were high. Subsequent developments in field size have focused on balancing the benefits of lower relapse rates associated with larger fields with the reduced toxicity from smaller ones.

Starting in the 1940s, cytotoxic chemotherapy was introduced, initially with single agents, before the development of combination regimens. The first of these was the MOPP regimen in the 1960s, comprising mustine, vincristine (Oncovin), procarbazine and prednisolone, which was gradually adjusted to maintain efficacy but reduce toxicities. In the 1970s, an

and radiotherapy, respectively. Other causes of false-positive PET results include rebound thymic hyperplasia, infection, inflammation, brown fat and extramedullary haemopoiesis. In the event of uncertainty as to the nature of the PET-positive lesion, biopsy is recommended. PET is also used in NLPHL, but it may be less reliably FDG-avid, making interpretation more difficult (Figures 34.13 and 34.14).

Interim PET to assess response and guide prognosis (e.g. after two to four cycles of treatment, after salvage treatment or before consideration of autograft or allograft) has been assessed for its value in predicting long-term response. There is evidence that negative PET at this stage can be predictive of outcome, but

Table 34.6 Response definitions for clinical trials.

Response	Definition	Nodal masses	Spleen, liver	Bone marrow
CR	Disappearance of all evidence of disease	(a) FDG-avid or PET positive prior to therapy; mass of any size permitted if PET negative (b) Variably FDG-avid or PET negative; regression to normal size on CT	Not palpable, nodules disappeared	Infiltrate cleared on repeat biopsy; if indeterminate by morphology, immunohistochemistry should be negative
PR	Regression of measuable disease and no new sites	≥50% decrease in SPD of up to six largest dominant masses; no increase in size of other nodes (a) FDG-avid or PET positive prior to therapy; one or more PET positive at previously involved site (b) Variably FDG-avid or PET negative; regression on CT	≥50% decrease in SPD of nodules (for single nodule in greatest transverse diameter); no increase in size of liver or spleen	Irrelevant if positive prior to therapy; cell type should be specified
SD	Failure to attain CR/PR or PD	(a) FDG-avid or PET positive prior to therapy; PET positive at prior sites of disease and no new sites on CT or PET (b) Variably FDG-avid or PET negative; no change in size of previous lesions on CT		
Relapsed disease or PD	Any new lesion or increase by ≥50% of previously involved sites from nadir	Appearance of a new lesion(s) >1.5 cm in any axis, ≥50% increase in SPD of more than one node, or ≥50% increase in longest diameter of a previously identifed node >1 cm in short axis Lesions PET positive if FDG-avid lymphoma or PET positive prior to therapy	>50% increase from nadir in the SPD of any previous lesions	New or recurrent involvement

CR, complete remission; CT, computed tomography; FDG, [^{18}F]fluorodeoxyglucose; PD, progressive disease; PET, positron emission tomography; PR, partial remission; SD, stable disease; SPD, sum of the product of the diameters.

alternative regimen comprising doxorubicin (Adriamycin), bleomycin, vinblastine and dacarbazine (ABVD) was developed, originally as salvage treatment for patients who had failed MOPP chemotherapy, and was designed as far as possible to contain non-cross-resistant drugs to those in MOPP. ABVD was subsequently shown to be as effective as MOPP, with lower rates of infertility and secondary leukaemias, and has become the first-line regimen of choice in most situations.

Recent trends in treatment strategy have focused on the combination of chemotherapy and radiotherapy in early-stage disease and better risk stratification in all patients. The aim is to minimize toxicities where possible, but allow escalation of treatment in those in poorer-risk groups. A further factor is that many patients who relapse or fail to respond to initial therapy may be cured with subsequent salvage treatment, such as combination chemotherapy in relapse after radiotherapy or high-dose chemotherapy supported by stem cell autograft. This again raises issues about treatment selection, such as whether it is better to use more aggressive treatment strategies up front to minimize relapse risk or try to minimize toxicities with less intensive treatment, with the expectation that salvage treatment can be used in those who relapse.

Table 34.7 Chemotherapy regimens.

ABVD	Doxorubicin, bleomycin, vinblastine, dacarbazine
BEACOPP	Bleomycin, etoposide, doxorubicin, cyclophosphamide, vincristine, procarbazine, prednisone
BEAM	Carmustine, etoposide, cytarabine, melphalan
ChlVPP	Chlorambucil, vinblastine, procarbazine, prednisolone
ChlVPP/PABlOE	Chlorambucil, vinblastine, procarbazine, prednisone alternating with prednisolone, doxorubicin, bleomycin, vincristine, etoposide
ChlVPP/EVA	Chlorambucil, vinblastine, procarbazine, prednisone, etoposide, vincristine, doxorubicin
ESHAP	Etoposide, cytarabine, cisplatin, methylprednisolone
GEM-P	Gemcitabine, cisplatin, methylprednisolone
ICE	Ifosfamide, carboplatin, etoposide
MOPP	Mechlorethamine, vincristine, procarbazine, prednisone
MOPP/ABV	Mechlorethamine, vincristine, procarbazine, prednisone, doxorubicin, bleomycin, vinblastine
MOPP/EBV/CAD	Mechlorethamine, vincristine, procarbazine, prednisone, epirubicin, bleomycin, vinblastine, lomustine, doxorubicin, vindesine
Stanford-V	Bleomycin, doxorubicin, etoposide, mechlorethamine, prednisone, vinblastine, vincristine

The number of different treatment options (Table 34.7) and ability to treat relapse disease has also made interpretation of trial data more complicated. Risk stratification and treatments vary widely, and long follow-up periods are required to assess long-term advantages in terms of overall survival benefit. Paradoxically, many of the best trials with robust data on long-term outcomes are hampered by the fact that treatments under investigation have often become obsolete by the time of final analysis.

Nodular lymphocyte-predominant Hodgkin lymphoma (Table 34.8)

As discussed above, NLPHL is a distinct entity and needs to be considered separately from a therapeutic standpoint. There are no prospective randomized trials carried out specifically in NLPHL, so treatment recommendations have been more difficult to make.

Its better prognosis and tendency to present in early stage means that local treatment such as radiotherapy or even just surgical resection is often used. Surgery alone has been shown to confer an excellent overall survival rate, but there is a substantial relapse rate necessitating further treatment in many patients. A recent trial of surgery and observation alone produced a 4-year overall survival rate of 100% but progression-free survival of only 57%. Advanced disease is treated in the same way as CHL, with combination chemotherapy.

Use of the anti-CD20 monoclonal antibody rituximab is an attractive therapeutic option, and recent Phase II trials indicate response rates of 94–100% in newly diagnosed, relapsed and refractory disease, with complete response rates of around 50%. Its precise role has yet to be defined, and in the absence of Phase III trial data its use is highly variable from centre to centre.

Classical Hodgkin lymphoma: early stage

As noted above, treatment of Hodgkin lymphoma is constantly developing, and as disease control has improved, much of the emphasis is on reduction of toxicities.

Treatment of early-stage disease was traditionally with radiotherapy, but despite the impressive response rates two important problems were evident. Firstly, even the largest fields were associated with relapse rates of 20–30%, usually outside the treatment field, indicating the presence of occult metastatic disease at the time of presentation. Secondly, there were clinically significant toxicities, particularly secondary cancers and cardiac damage. In view of this, combined modality treatment was developed to try to gain the maximum benefits of both chemotherapy and radiotherapy, while minimizing the toxicities associated with both. Radiotherapy alone is nowadays only recommended for early-stage NLPHL.

Combined modality treatment (CMT) has been shown in a number of trials to give a superior progression-free survival compared with radiotherapy alone. The most recent EORTC H8 trial has also demonstrated an overall survival benefit in favourable-risk patients of 97% at 10 years compared with 92% with radiotherapy alone, albeit with a chemotherapy regimen (MOPP/ABV) that has been superseded by ABVD. Reduced rates of secondary cancers with CMT compared with radiotherapy alone were noted in a retrospective analysis of 181 favourable-group patients. This was assumed to be due to the reduced-dose radiotherapy in the CMT group.

Further trials have attempted to reduce the amount of radiotherapy by reducing dose and field size. Radiotherapy is now usually given as involved fields (as opposed to extended) and at a maximum of 30 Gy in the combined modality setting. Attempts

Table 34.8 Selected randomized trials in early-stage disease.

Study	Disease stage and treatment	Number of patients	Failure-free survival (%)	Overall survival (%)	Time (years)	Conclusion
Radiotherapy (RT) vs. combined modality treatment (CMT)						
GHSG HD7 (Engert *et al.* 2007)	I_A–II_A (favourable risk) A: RT alone B: ABVD ×2 + RT	650	FFTF 67 (A) vs. 88 (B) B better than A*	92 (A) vs. 94 (B) No difference detected	7	CMT (using ABVD) superior to RT alone for early-stage disease
EORTC H8-F (Fermé *et al.* 2007)	I–II (favourable risk) A: MOPP/ABV ×3 + IFRT B: STNI	542	EFS 98 (A) vs. 74 (B) A better than B*	97 (A) vs. 92 (B) A better than B*	5 (FFS) 10 (OS)	CMT superior to RT alone for early-stage disease
Chemotherapy vs. combined modality treatment						
NCIC/ECOG (Meyer *et al.* 2005)	I–II_A A: ABVD ×4 or ×6 (stratified by response) B: STNI ± ABVD ×2 (stratified by risk factors)	399	EFS 86 (A) vs. 88 (B) No difference detected	96 (A) vs. 94 (B) No difference detected	4	No difference between CMT and chemotherapy alone
New York (Straus *et al.* 2004)	I_A–III_A A: ABVD ×6 B: ABVD ×6 + RT	152	FFP 86 (A) vs. 81 (B) No difference detected	97 (A) vs. 90 (B) No difference detected	5	No difference between CMT and chemotherapy alone

*Statistically significant difference ($P < 0.05$).

EFS, event-free survival; FFP, freedom from progression; FFS, failure-free survival; FFTF, freedom from treatment failure; IFRT, involved-field radiotherapy; OS, overall survival; STNI, subtotal nodal irradiation.

are ongoing to define the optimum treatment and to determine whether sites of bulky disease require additional radiotherapy boosts.

Chemotherapy regimens vary, but based on outcomes in trials of patients with advanced disease, ABVD is usually the treatment of choice. The number of cycles used at present is usually three or four, but there may be the potential to reduce this to two. There are also attempts to reduce the toxicity of the drug regimen, for example by omitting dacarbazine.

Trials have examined whether radiotherapy can be omitted completely by treating with chemotherapy alone. In two trials comparing CMT with chemotherapy alone, both following patients for 5 years, freedom from progression and overall survival rates were similar. This has led some to suggest that treating with chemotherapy alone may eventually prove to provide the best results in such patients but, in the absence of clear evidence or expert consensus, CMT remains the most widely used treatment. The ongoing UK-based RAPID trial in early-stage disease should give further guidance on the value of interim PET in guiding treatment.

Classical Hodgkin lymphoma: advanced stage (Table 34.9)

Since it was developed in the 1970s, originally as a salvage regimen for relapsed disease after MOPP, ABVD has remained the treatment of choice for most cases of advanced disease, with eight cycles of treatment standard in Europe. Cannelos and colleagues demonstrated its superiority to MOPP in terms of response rate (82% vs. 67%) and 5-year failure-free survival (61% vs. 50%), although the 5-year overall survival rates were similar (73% vs. 66%). Significantly, long-term serious toxicities such as infertility and secondary cancers were reduced with ABVD, which contains no alkylating agent. ABVD has subsequently been compared with various other treatments, including alternating regimens such as MOPP/ABV, ChlVPP/PABlOE and hybrids such as ChlVPP/EVA and MOPP/EBV/CAD. In all cases, ABVD has been shown superior in terms of the balance of response and treatment toxicities.

Recently, attempts have been made to develop more intensive regimens to improve outcomes in poor-risk disease. The most

Table 34.9 Selected randomized trials in advanced-stage disease.

Study	Disease stage and treatment	No. of patients	Failure-free survival (%)	Overall survival (%)	Time (years)	Conclusion
Chemotherapy alone						
CALGB (Cannellos *et al.* 1992)	III–IV A: MOPP B: MOPP/ABVD C: ABVD	361	FFS 50* (A) vs. 65 (B) vs. 61 (C) B and C better than A* C least toxicities	66 (A) vs. 75 (B) vs. 73 (C)	5	Established ABVD as best-choice regimen for response and toxicities
Stanford (Horning *et al.* 2002)	I_E–IV Stanford V ± radiotherapy	856	FFP 89	96	5	Established efficacy of Stanford V regimen
GHSG HD9 (Diehl *et al.* 2003)	II_B–IV A: COPP/ABVD B: BEACOPP C: Escalated BEACOPP	1201	FFTF 69 (A) vs. 76* (B) vs. 87* (C) B better than A* C better than A and B*	83* (A) vs. 88 (B) vs. 91* (C) C better than A*	5	Escalated BEACOPP gave improved outcomes in advanced disease
Intergruppo Italiano Linfomi (Gobbi *et al.* 2005)	II_B–IV A: ABVD B: Modified Stanford V C: MOPP/EBV/ CAD	355	FFS 78 (A) vs. 54* (B) vs. 81 (C) B worse than A and C* More toxicities in B, more dose reductions in C	90 (A) vs. 82* (B) vs. 89 (C) B worse than A*	5	No benefit of modified Stanford V or MOPP/EVA/ CAD over ABVD
BNLI LY09 (Johnson *et al.* 2005)	I_B–IV A: ABVD B: ChlVPP/ PABlOE and ChlVPP/EVA	807	EFS 75 (A) vs. 75 (B) More toxicities in B	90 (A) vs. 80 (B)	3	No benefit of hybrid regimens over ABVD
Chemotherapy and radiotherapy						
GELA H89 (Ferméet *al.* 2006)	III_B–IV Treated to PR/CR with ABVPP or MOPP/ABV A: Consolidation chemotherapy B: Consolidation radiotherapy	533 (418 to PR or CR)	DFS 73 (A) vs. 78 (B)	84 (A) vs. 79 (B)	10	No advantage to consolidation radiotherapy over consolidation chemotherapy
EORTC 20884 (Aleman *et al.* 2003)	III–IV Treated to CR with MOP/ABV A: Consolidation radiotherapy B: No consolidation radiotherapy	739 (421 to CR)	EFS 79 (A) vs. 84 (B)	85 (A) vs. 91 (B)	5	No advantage to consolidation radiotherapy once CR has been reached

*Statistically significant difference ($P < 0.05$).

BNLI, British National Lymphoma Investigation; CALGB, Cancer and Leukaemia Group B; CR, complete remission; DFS, disease-free survival; EFS, event-free survival; EORTC, European Organization for the Research and Treatment of Cancer; FFP, freedom from progression; FFS, failure-free survival; FFTF, freedom from treatment failure; GELA, Groupe d'Etudes de Lymphomes d'Adulte; PR, partial remission.

promising of these appears to be escalated BEACOPP (bleomycin, etoposide, doxorubicin, cyclophosphamide, vincristine, procarbazine and prednisone). This regimen was developed by the German Hodgkin Lymphoma Study Group, based on mathematical modelling showing a greater benefit from escalating drug doses than reducing the time interval between cycles. Increased myelosuppression was offset by the use of granulocyte colony-stimulating factor (G-CSF). Initial results in trials comparing BEACOPP with COPP/ABVD showed significantly improved outcomes in both freedom from treatment failure and overall survival. Increased toxicities have led to attempts for risk stratification in order to assess which patients required escalated BEACOPP and which could have the less-intensive BEACOPP or ABVD. This approach may well prove to be the most sensible way to proceed, especially using PET to assess initial response, but precise validated risk groups have still to be established.

The role for consolidation radiotherapy in advanced disease remains controversial. The EORTC 20884 trial showed no apparent benefit of adjuvant radiotherapy for patients who have achieved a CR with chemotherapy alone, and direct comparison of adjuvant radiotherapy with two extra cycles of chemotherapy also showed no advantage at 10-year follow-up for both disease-free survival and overall survival (GELA H89 trial). Radiotherapy may well have a role to play after less extensive chemotherapy treatment, and in patients who have only achieved a PR. It should be noted that both escalated BEACOPP and Stanford V (another more intensive regimen) make substantial use of radiotherapy as part of the treatment. For example, 85% of patients in the original Stanford trials received radiotherapy. In the 2003 escalated BEACOPP data, over 60% of all patients received radiotherapy.

The role of interim PET to guide treatment is being increasingly well understood. The German HD15 trial has demonstrated good negative predictive value of interim PET in advanced disease treated with BEACOPP chemotherapy. The impact on overall survival is not yet evaluable, but the authors have suggested that consolidation with radiotherapy could be omitted on the basis of a negative PET scan.

Relapsed and progressive disease

A proportion of patients receiving chemotherapy, either *de novo* or after radiation failure, will have refractory disease or will relapse after remission. Occasional patients can be cured by radiotherapy if the persistent or relapsed disease is localized, but the majority of patients will require systemic therapy. In patients with long first remissions, a significant proportion of patients may be cured by further standard-dose chemotherapy, but the results of such approaches are poor if the remission has been short or the disease was refractory to initial chemotherapy. In the report of the long-term follow-up of the initial cohort of patients treated with MOPP at the National Cancer Institute,

there were no survivors beyond 10 years in those who had not achieved a remission.

High-dose chemotherapy and autologous stem cell transplantation was first pioneered in relapsed Hodgkin lymphoma 50 years ago, but it is only in the last two decades that it has become an established modality of treatment. In the last decade, peripheral blood stem cells have replaced the use of bone marrow as the source of haemopoietic stem cells. In the early 1980s, the procedure-related mortality associated with an autograft was in the order of 10%, but with improved patient selection and better supportive care this has fallen to 3% or less. In large single-centre series and in registry reviews, the overall survival rates of patients receiving autologous transplantation for relapsed or resistant disease are approximately 40–50%. A number of different conditioning regimens have been used, and high-dose chemotherapy is generally preferred to total body irradiation. This is because chemotherapy is logistically easier to administer, appears as effective as total body irradiation and may be associated with less pneumonitis, particularly in patients who have received mediastinal radiation in the preceding year. Following high-dose therapy it is common practice to irradiate persistent masses or sites of previous high-volume disease, although there are no trial data to substantiate this practice.

Prior to high-dose therapy, standard-dose salvage chemotherapy is usually given to reduce disease bulk and demonstrate chemosensitivity. Regimens vary, but will consist of an alkylating agent-containing combination, with different drugs from the initial ABVD treatment (e.g. DHAP, ESHAP, IVE, ICE, GemP). In patients with progressive disease despite standard-dose chemotherapy or who have persistent 'B' symptoms or a raised lactate dehydrogenase, the risks of high-dose therapy are probably too high to justify proceeding to this course of action. However, it must be noted that in some cases a mass will not immediately shrink in size, and failure to achieve a formal response (complete or partial remission) as defined by CT should not automatically disqualify a patient from receiving an autograft.

The British National Lymphoma Investigation (BNLI) carried out a small randomized trial of treatment with carmustine (BCNU), etoposide, cytarabine and melphalan (BEAM) followed by autologous stem cell transplantation or mini-BEAM (the same drugs at lower doses) in patients with refractory or relapsed disease. There was a highly significant progression-free survival advantage in the group receiving high-dose therapy, and similar results have subsequently been reported from a larger German study. Neither study demonstrated an overall survival benefit, and this may be partly due to the small size of the trials, but may also be because some patients failing standard-dose salvage therapy can still be rescued by high-dose therapy at a later time. The raises the issue of the optimal time to consider an autograft procedure. It is widely recommended for all patients below the age of 65 years who fail first-line chemotherapy, although this may not be appropriate if there has been a first complete remission lasting more than 3 years.

The role of allogeneic transplantation has become clearer over the last few years, with much of the evidence suggesting a move from myeloablative to reduced intensity conditioning regimens, which rely heavily on the graft-versus-Hodgkin effect. Transplant-related mortality with reduced intensity conditioning appears to be of the order of 15–25% compared with 40–60% in the older reports of myeloablative treatment. The long-term outcomes are also encouraging, with a 4-year progression-free survival of 39% and overall survival of 55%. There also appears to be a benefit from donor lymphocyte infusions: 56% of patients with progression post allograft showed a response to this treatment. At present an allograft is indicated for patients who have relapsed after an autograft. The possibility has been raised that reduced-intensity allografts should also be considered in those patients predicted to do poorly with an autograft (e.g. those who are PET-positive after salvage therapy). This approach requires further investigation.

Alternative approaches that may prove useful in selected patients are salvage radiotherapy and repeat autologous transplantation.

Treatment of Hodgkin lymphoma in childhood

Hodgkin lymphoma in children and adolescents is curable in over 90% of cases. With rising numbers of long-term survivors, the impact of long-term effects becomes increasingly important. A number of specific childhood regimens have been developed that aim to maintain these excellent remission rates but which reduce the likelihood of developing late effects.

Chemotherapy is usually combined with radiotherapy to minimize the toxicity from either modality, and risk stratification is used to avoid over-treatment of good-risk disease. Fertility can be damaged by both chemotherapy and radiotherapy, and strategies to avoid this include sperm storage (where possible) and avoidance of procarbazine in boys and moving ovaries out of radiation fields by oophoropexy in girls. Radiation can also have direct effects on bone and soft tissue, and minimizing the dose and field size can reduce the impact on growth and on the final height a developing child will reach. Reduction of anthracycline exposure can minimize cardiac toxicity in later life.

Treatment of Hodgkin lymphoma in pregnancy

Hodgkin lymphoma in pregnancy is rare, but the common presentation during adolescence and young adulthood is a sign that cases can and do arise (one estimate is 1 in 6000 pregnancies). Its treatment in pregnancy presents unique challenges in that the well-being of the fetus as well as the mother will be affected. Pregnancy does not seem to affect outcome in treated disease, with 48 cases of Hodgkin lymphoma during pregnancy showing similar 20-year outcomes to matched controls.

Staging investigations should be limited to avoid radiation exposure; abdominal and pelvic CT is avoided if possible and PET is not recommended. All cytotoxic chemotherapy is potentially teratogenic, with the highest risks of fetal malformations in the first trimester. In the second and third trimesters the risk is lower, but there is an increased incidence of fetal or neonatal death, intrauterine growth retardation, preterm delivery and low birth weight. Radiotherapy should also be avoided during the first trimester, with uterine shielding used to reduce fetal radiation exposure.

Presentation during the first trimester is difficult to combine with a risk-free pregnancy. In these cases early delivery or termination is usually recommended, followed by standard treatment. Treatment in the second and third trimesters can be managed with normal treatment regimens, with careful monitoring of the pregnancy and ensuring delivery does not coincide with cytopenias. Occasionally in early-stage or low-risk disease, it may be possible to treat partially during the pregnancy, or even delay treatment until after delivery, to allow adequate disease control and normal pregnancy. Breast-feeding is contraindicated during staging and treatment, as drugs and contrast and nuclear imaging agents can all concentrate in breast milk.

Late effects of treatment

As the cure rate for Hodgkin lymphoma has increased and longer-term follow-up data have become available, the significance of the late effects of treatment have become more apparent. In a study of young adults aged 29 years or less at diagnosis and who achieved a stable complete remission after first- or second-line therapy, the actuarial overall survival at 20 years was 93% and 85% respectively, compared with 98.5% in the age-matched general population. In some patients treated for favourable-risk disease it has been shown that, at 12–15 years after therapy, the mortality risk related to therapy exceeds the risk of dying from Hodgkin lymphoma. The two most frequent causes of excess deaths are second malignancies and ischaemic heart disease. Patients who are hyposplenic following either splenectomy or irradiation should be on a vaccination programme and receive prophylactic antibiotics.

The overall increased risk of secondary cancers in patients with Hodgkin lymphoma is estimated at 0.4–0.7% per year. This cumulative effect explains the cancer risk rising with time after treatment. (The exception to this is secondary myelodysplastic syndrome and acute myeloid leukaemia, which peaks at 5–9 years after exposure to chemotherapy.) The commonest second malignancy is lung cancer. This is mainly attributable to radiotherapy although chemotherapy also contributes to the risk. Patients who have had thoracic irradiation must be warned of the risk of developing secondary lung cancer and should be strongly discouraged from smoking. The risk of developing secondary acute myeloid leukaemia is related to the accumulated dose of alkylating agents received and therefore occurs predominantly in patients who have had a remitting and relapsing disease course.

The risk of secondary breast cancer is greatest in women who have received mediastinal or axillary radiation at less than 35 years of age. The risk of such patients ever developing breast cancer was as high as one in four in some series. There is also a clear dose–response relationship, emphasizing the need to use the minimal radiation dose required for tumour control. Other malignancies that occur in excess in patients treated for Hodgkin lymphoma include non-Hodgkin lymphomas, cancers of the colon, stomach, head and neck and thyroid, and malignant melanoma.

In view of these risks, it is recommended that screening for secondary malignancies is carried out as part of routine post-treatment review. Patients who received radiotherapy or alkylating agents should have annual chest radiography, and younger women should be enrolled on a breast cancer screening programme. In the UK, women who received radiotherapy that impinged on the breasts when they were under the age of 35 years are invited to attend screening from 10 years after the radiotherapy. Mammography is used in most patients but MRI is preferable in younger women and in those with denser breast tissue.

The Stanford group reported a threefold increase in relative risk of cardiac death in Hodgkin lymphoma survivors, representing a major risk given that the incidence of cardiac disease in the general population is already so high. The major contributory factor is mediastinal irradiation, especially if a dose in excess of 30 Gy is used. Chemotherapy is also associated with accelerated coronary artery disease. It is not clear which drugs cause this but anthracyclines and vincristine have both been implicated. Bleomycin exposure (as in ABVD) is associated with an 18% risk of pulmonary fibrosis, and was associated with reduction in overall survival, especially in older patients. Radiotherapy fields that included the lungs are an additional risk factor for lung injury.

The most common endocrine disorders are hypothyroidism following radiotherapy to the lower neck, and infertility. Around half of patients receiving neck irradiation will develop hypothyroidism and will need to be monitored and treated accordingly. Infertility is caused both by irradiation of the gonads and the use of cytotoxic drugs such as procarbazine and alkylating agents. It is their repeated use that is most damaging, and young female patients receiving an autologous transplant will often remain fertile if they are still menstruating prior to high-dose therapy. Sperm cryopreservation prior to chemotherapy should be offered to men who have not completed their families. Of the multidrug regimens, escalated BEACOPP causes

more infertility in both men and women than ABVD. Artificial insemination has a relatively low success rate per cycle, although intracytoplasmic sperm injection may be more successful. Hodgkin lymphoma may be sufficiently slow-growing to allow harvesting of eggs, *in vitro* fertilization and embryo storage in those young women who have an established partner. Oocyte preservation and ovarian tissue banking are currently in development and remain experimental.

The psychological trauma associated with contracting a malignant disease, receiving radiotherapy and chemotherapy, and coping with the risk of eventual relapse is considerable. A significant proportion of patients report lower perceived levels of overall health, dissatisfaction in their personal relationships, and difficulties in obtaining life assurance and financial loans as a result of the disease and its treatment. Chronic fatigue is also increased, with a raised incidence over and above that explicable by cardiovascular or thyroid toxicity.

Novel therapies

Cytotoxic drugs

Gemcitabine, an analogue of cytarabine, has been found to have antitumour activity in Hodgkin lymphoma, and of the cytotoxic drugs appears to have the most potential for augmenting the efficacy of current treatments. It is well tolerated, and response rates in excess of 35% in heavily pretreated patients have been achieved with use as a single agent. Combination regimens have been developed, including GEM-P (gemcitabine, cisplatin and methylprednisolone) which produces response rates of 60–65%.

The proteasome inhibitor bortezomib appears to be a good candidate drug based on *in vitro* studies, although it has not yet demonstrated a significant benefit in clinical trials.

Immunotherapy

As in many fields of cancer treatment, immune modulation has great potential for treatment. Monoclonal antibodies have been developed against the cell membrane proteins CD25 and CD30, including conjugates with radioisotopes (e.g. [131]I). The graft-versus-lymphoma effect of donor lymphocytes seen in allogeneic transplantation has demonstrated the potential benefits of cytotoxic T lymphocytes. Attempts are being made to develop clonal populations of T lymphocytes that would target HRS cells expressing EBV-derived antigens.

Conclusion

Much progress has been made in recent years regarding both the cellular aspects of the HRS cell and the treatment of the resultant tumour. The results of therapy are extremely good, and attention must be paid to minimizing late effects of treatment. In many cases the same ultimate survival outcome can be achieved using different therapeutic approaches. The choice depends on an appreciation of the short-and long-term side-effects, and increasingly the patient must be involved in an informed decision-making process.

Acknowledgements

Acknowledgements are due to the departments of Imaging and Nuclear Medicine at University College London Hospital, London for the radiological slides, and the Department of Histopathology, University College London for the histopathology slides.

Selected bibliography

Aleman BM, Raemaekers JM, Tirelli U et al. (2003) Involved-field radiotherapy for advanced Hodgkin lymphoma. New England Journal of Medicine 348: 2396–406.

Armitage JO (2010) Early-stage Hodgkin's lymphoma. The New England Journal of Medicine 363: 653–662.

Bhatia S, Robison LL, Oberlin O et al. (1996) Breast cancer and other second neoplasms after childhood Hodgkin's disease. New England Journal of Medicine 334: 745–51.

Biggar RJ, Jaffe ES, Goedert JJ et al. (2006) Hodgkin lymphoma and immunodeficiency in persons with HIV/AIDS. Blood 108: 3786–91.

Bonadonna G, Zucali R, Monfardini S, De Lena M, Uslenghi C (1975) Combination chemotherapy of Hodgkin's disease with adriamycin, bleomycin, vinblastine, and imidazole carboxamide versus MOPP. Cancer 36: 252–9.

Bonfante V, Santoro A, Viviani S et al. (1997) Outcome of patients with Hodgkin's disease failing after primary MOPP–ABVD. Journal of Clinical Oncology 15: 528–34.

Canellos GP, Anderson JR, Propert KJ et al. (1992) Chemotherapy of advanced Hodgkin's disease with MOPP, ABVD, or MOPP alternating with ABVD. New England Journal of Medicine 327: 1478–84.

Cheson BD, Pfistner B, Juweid ME et al. (2007) Revised response criteria for malignant lymphoma. Journal of Clinical Oncology 25: 579–86.

Dann EJ, Bar-Shalom R, Tamir A et al. (2007) Risk-adapted BEACOPP regimen can reduce the cumulative dose of chemotherapy for standard and high-risk Hodgkin lymphoma with no impairment of outcome. Blood 109: 905–9.

Devita VT Jr, Serpick AA, Carbone PP (1970) Combination chemotherapy in the treatment of advanced Hodgkin disease. Annals of Internal Medicine 73: 881–95.

Diehl V, Franklin J, Pfreundschuh M et al. (2003) Standard and increased-dose BEACOPP chemotherapy compared with COPP–ABVD for advanced Hodgkin's disease. New England Journal of Medicine 348: 2386–95.

Duggan DB, Petroni GR, Johnson JL et al. (2003) Randomized comparison of ABVD and MOPP/ABV hybrid for the treatment of advanced Hodgkin's disease: report of an intergroup trial. Journal of Clinical Oncology 21: 607–14.

Engert A, Franklin J, Eich HT et al. (2007) Two cycles of doxorubicin, bleomycin, vinblastine, and dacarbazine plus extended-field radiotherapy is superior to radiotherapy alone in early favourable Hodgkin lymphoma: final results of the GHSG HD7 trial. Journal of Clinical Oncology 25: 3495–502.

Fermé C, Mounier N, Casasnovas O et al. (2006) Long-term results and competing risk analysis of the H89 trial in patients with advanced-stage Hodgkin lymphoma: a study by the Groupe d'Etude des Lymphomes de l'Adulte (GELA). Blood 107: 4636–42.

Fermé C, Eghbali H, Meerwaldt JH et al. (2007) Chemotherapy plus involved-field radiation in early-stage Hodgkin disease. New England Journal of Medicine 357: 1916–27.

Gobbi PG, Levis A, Chisesi T et al. (2005) ABVD versus modified stanford V versus MOPPEBVCAD with optional and limited radiotherapy in intermediate- and advanced-stage Hodgkin lymphoma: final results of a multicenter randomized trial by the Intergruppo Italiano Linfomi. Journal of Clinical Oncology 23: 9198–207.

Hasenclever D, Diehl V (1998) A prognostic score for advanced Hodgkin disease. International Prognostic Factors Project on Advanced Hodgkin Disease. New England Journal of Medicine 339: 1506–14.

Horning SJ, Hoppe RT, Breslin S, Bartlett NL, Brown BW, Rosenberg SA (2002) Stanford V and radiotherapy for locally extensive and advanced Hodgkin's disease: mature results of a prospective clinical trial. Journal of Clinical Oncology 20: 630–7.

Johnson PW, Radford JA, Cullen MH et al. (2005) Comparison of ABVD and alternating or hybrid multidrug regimens for the treatment of advanced Hodgkin lymphoma: results of the United Kingdom Lymphoma Group LY09 Trial. Journal of Clinical Oncology 23: 9208–18.

Josting A, Nogová L, Franklin J et al. (2005) Salvage radiotherapy in patients with relapsed and refractory Hodgkin lymphoma: a retrospective analysis from the German Hodgkin Lymphoma Study Group. Journal of Clinical Oncology 23: 1522–9.

Juweid ME, Stroobants S, Hoekstra OS et al. (2007) Use of positron emission tomography for response assessment of lymphoma: consensus of the Imaging Subcommittee of International Harmonization Project in Lymphoma. Journal of Clinical Oncology 25: 571–8.

Linch DC, Winfield D, Goldstone AH et al. (1993) Dose intensification with autologous bone-marrow transplantation in relapsed and resistant Hodgkin's disease: results of a BNLI randomized trial. Lancet 341: 1051–4.

Loeffler M, Brosteanu O, Hasenclever D et al. (1998) Meta-analysis of chemotherapy versus combined modality treatment trials in Hodgkin disease. International Database on Hodgkin Disease Overview Study Group. Journal of Clinical Oncology 16: 818–2.

Longo DL, Young RC, Wesley M et al. (1986) Twenty years of MOPP therapy for Hodgkin disease. Journal of Clinical Oncology 4: 1295–306.

Majolino I, Pearce R, Taghipour G, Goldstone AH (1997) Peripheral-blood stem-cell transplantation versus autologous bone marrow transplantation in Hodgkin's and non-Hodgkin's lymphomas: a new matched-pair analysis of the European Group for Blood and Marrow Transplantation Registry Data. *Journal of Clinical Oncology* **15**: 509–17.

Mauz-Körholz C, Gorde-Grosjean S, Hasenclever D *et al.* (2007) Resection alone in 58 children with limited stage, lymphocyte-predominant Hodgkin lymphoma-experience from the European network group on paediatric Hodgkin lymphoma. *Cancer* **110**: 179–85.

Meyer RM, Gospodarowicz MK, Connors JM *et al.* (2005) Randomized comparison of ABVD chemotherapy with a strategy that includes radiation therapy in patients with limited-stage Hodgkin lymphoma: National Cancer Institute of Canada Clinical Trials Group and the Eastern Cooperative Oncology Group. *Journal of Clinical Oncology* **23**: 4634–42.

Ng AK, Bernardo MP, Weller E (2002) Long-term survival and competing causes of death in patients with early-stage Hodgkin's disease treated at age 50 or younger. *Journal of Clinical Oncology* **20**: 2101–8.

Nogová L, Reineke T, Brillant C *et al.* (2008) Lymphocyte-predominant and classical Hodgkin lymphoma: a comprehensive analysis from the German Hodgkin Study Group. *Journal of Clinical Oncology* **26**: 434–9.

Noordijk EM, Carde P, Dupouy N *et al.* (2006) Combined-modality therapy for clinical stage I or II Hodgkin lymphoma: long-term results of the European Organization for Research and Treatment of Cancer H7 randomized controlled trials. *Journal of Clinical Oncology* **24**: 3128–35.

Peggs KS, Hunter A, Chopra R *et al.* (2005) Clinical evidence of a graft-versus-Hodgkin-lymphoma effect after reduced-intensity allogeneic transplantation. *Lancet* **365**: 1934–41.

Peggs KS, Anderlini P, Sureda A (2008) Allogeneic transplantation for Hodgkin lymphoma. *British Journal of Haematology* **143**: 468–80.

Schellong G, Pötter R, Brämswig J *et al.* (1999) High cure rates and reduced long-term toxicity in paediatric Hodgkin disease: the German-Austrian multicenter trial DAL-HD-90. *Journal of Clinical Oncology* **17**: 3736–44.

Schmitz N, Pfistner B, Sextro M *et al.* (2002) Aggressive conventional chemotherapy compared with high-dose chemotherapy with autologous haemopoietic stem-cell transplantation for relapsed chemosensitive Hodgkin disease: a randomized trial. *Lancet* **359**: 2065–71.

Schulz H, Rehwald U, Morschhauser F *et al.* (2008) Rituximab in relapsed lymphocyte-predominant Hodgkin lymphoma: long-term results of a phase 2 trial by the German Hodgkin Lymphoma Study Group (GHSG). *Blood* **111**: 109–11.

Specht L, Grey RG, Clarke MJ, Peto R (1998) Influence of more extensive radiotherapy and adjuvant chemotherapy on long-term outcome of early-stage Hodgkin disease: a meta-analysis of 23 randomized trials involving 3,888 patients. International Hodgkin Disease Collaborative Group. *Journal of Clinical Oncology* **16**: 830–43.

Steidl C, Lee T, Shar SP *et al.* (2010) Tumor-Associated macrophages and survival in classic Hodgkin's Lymphoma. *The New England Journal of Medicine* **362**: 875–85.

Stein H, Marafioti T, Foss HD *et al.* (2001) Down-regulation of BOB.1/OBF.1 and Oct2 in classical Hodgkin disease but not in lymphocyte predominant Hodgkin disease correlates with immunoglobulin transcription. *Blood* **97**: 496–501.

Straus DJ, Portlock CS, Qin J *et al.* (2004) Results of a prospective randomized clinical trial of doxorubicin, bleomycin, vinblastine, and dacarbazine (ABVD) followed by radiation therapy (RT) versus ABVD alone for stages I, II, and IIIA nonbulky Hodgkin disease. *Blood* **104**: 3483–9.

Swerdlow AJ, Higgins CD, Smith P *et al.* (2007) Myocardial infarction mortality risk after treatment for Hodgkin disease: a collaborative British cohort study. *Journal of the National Cancer Institute* **99**: 206–14.

Viviani S, Bonadonna G, Santoro A *et al.* (1996) Alternating versus hybrid MOPP and ABVD combinations in advanced Hodgkin disease: ten-year results. *Journal of Clinical Oncology* **14**: 1421–30.

Non-Hodgkin lymphoma

35

Kate Cwynarski[1] and Anthony H Goldstone[2]

[1]Royal Free Hospital, London, UK
[2]University College London, London, UK

Epidemiology

Frequency

The incidence of non-Hodgkin lymphoma (NHL) has increased in the Western world over recent decades, rising by 3–5% per annum. The rate of increase exceeds that of most malignancies and the reason for this is unclear. This is partially explained by the higher incidence of NHL in immunosuppressed patients but the role of environmental factors is suggested. NHL has become the fifth most common cancer in the USA, occurring at a frequency of approximately 17.4 per 100 000.

NHL is slightly more common in males than in females, and in the USA it is more common in white people than in black people. Although NHL can occur at any age, the incidence rises considerably with age. As life expectancy increases there is a consequent increased frequency of NHL.

Geographical variations

The proportions of cases in different histological categories vary markedly from one country to another and among different racial groups. Although some of these variations may be spurious, reflecting local medical practice, real differences undoubtedly exist. For example, follicular lymphoma (FL), one of the

Postgraduate Haematology: 6th edition. Edited by A. Victor Hoffbrand, Daniel Catovsky, Edward G.D. Tuddenham, Anthony R. Green
© 2011 Blackwell Publishing Ltd.

most common NHLs in Europe and the USA, is rare in Japan and other Far Eastern countries. In contrast, human T-cell leukaemia/lymphoma virus (HTLV)-I is much more common in the Far East (Japan) and the Caribbean islands than in Western countries.

These differences are perhaps not surprising, given the role of the immune system (from which these neoplasms arise) in constantly monitoring and reacting to antigenic factors in the environment. This must cause variations between different parts of the world in the degree to which individual cell populations in lymphoid tissue are activated, which is likely to be reflected in the frequency variations of different lymphomas.

Aetiology

In the majority of cases of NHL, the cause is not identified, although several factors are known to play a role in lymphomagenesis. A small number of lymphomas originate from chronic antigenic stimulation; for example, *Helicobacter pylori* infection appears to be a possible causative agent for the development of gastric mucosa-associated lymphoid tissue (MALT) lymphoma. Eradication of *H. pylori* with antibiotics appears to be initial effective therapy for localized gastric MALT lymphoma. Similarly, infection with *Campylobacter jejuni* has been suggested recently to be associated with the development of immunoproliferative small intestinal disease.

Viruses

Several viruses have been implicated in lymphoma pathogenesis, although none of them is directly causative in the same way as the oncogenic viruses that induce neoplasia in animals.

Epstein–Barr virus

Epstein–Barr virus (EBV) was first thought to be associated with lymphomagenesis following its isolation from endemic Burkitt lymphoma tissue, but it is now known to be a major factor causing development of NHL in immunosuppressed individuals, for example HIV-infected patients or those recovering after solid-organ/allogeneic haemopoietic stem cell transplantation (allogeneic SCT), in whom it is called post-transplant lymphoproliferative disease (PTLD). There are two forms of cellular infection by EBV: latent and replicative. In latent infection, the virus enters the cell and remains in the DNA; B cells become immortalized and acquire neoplastic potential. In replicative infection, viral particles are released from cells, whereas the cells themselves die.

It is the latent type of infection that transforms infected resting B cells into proliferating blasts. The mechanism of this remarkable effect depends on the expression of several viral latent proteins that are under the control of a master transcription factor, EBV nuclear antigen (EBNA)-2. The pattern of viral gene expression that drives this process is called the growth programme (Table 35.1).

This process can occur in the presence of the following conditions: (i) the EBV-infected cells that express the growth programme must be unable to exit the cell cycle and become resting memory B cells; and (ii) the cytotoxic T-cell response must be impeded, so that lymphoblasts would not be killed. PTLD may therefore develop when B cells (other than naive B cells) become infected and express the growth programme without being able to exit it, and continue to proliferate in the absence of effective cytotoxic T-cell response.

EBV is also associated with the development of the endemic (African) type of Burkitt lymphoma (BL), in which it is expressed by 98%. However, the exact mechanism of EBV involvement in the development of BL is unclear. None of the

Table 35.1 Transcriptional programmes used by EBV to establish and maintain infection.

Type of infected B cells*	Programme	Genes expressed	Function of the programme
Naive cell	Growth	EBNA-1 through EBNA-6, LMP-1, LMP-2A, LMP-3B	Activated B cell
Germinal centre cell	Default	EBNA-1, LMP-1, LMP-2A	Differentiate activated B cells into memory cells
Peripheral blood memory cell	Latency	None	Allows lifetime persistence
Dividing peripheral blood memory cell		EBNA-1 only	Allows viral DNA in latency programme cell to divide
Plasma cell	Lytic	All lytic genes	Replicates virus in plasma cell

*Except where indicated, the types of cell are primarily restricted to the lymphoid tissues of the Waldeyer ring.
EBNA, EBV nuclear antigen; LMP, latent membrane protein.
Source: Thorley-Lawson DA, Gross A (2004) Persistence of the Epstein–Barr virus and the origins of associated lymphomas. *New England Journal of Medicine* **350**: 1328–37 with permission.

Table 35.2 Chromosomal translocations found in non-Hodgkin lymphoma.

Translocation	Gene involved	Type of lymphoma
t(8;14)(q24;q32)	MYC and IgH	Burkitt lymphoma
t(8;2)(p11/2;24)	MYC and Igκ	Burkitt lymphoma
t(8;22)(q24;q11)	MYC and Igλ	Burkitt lymphoma
t(11;14)(q24;q32)	BCL1 (cyclin D1) and IgH	Mantle cell lymphoma
t(14;18)(q32;q21)	BCL2 and IgH	Follicular lymphoma
t(3;4)(q27;q32) and variants	BCL6 and various partners	Large B-cell lymphoma
t(2;5)(p23;q35)	NPM and ALK	T-cell anaplastic large-cell lymphoma

growth-promoting latent genes is expressed, whereas the only detected latent protein of the virus is EBNA-1. BL is characterized by deregulated activation of *MYC* oncogene (Table 35.2), resulting in a sustained proliferation mode in which cells express EBNA-1 only. EBV may therefore have a role in the development of BL. However, given the multistep process of tumorigenesis, it is actually impossible to be sure whether the final cellular or viral phenotype of BL is related to the original infected precursor.

Human T-cell leukaemia/lymphoma virus type I

HTLV-I infection affects 15–20 million individuals worldwide, although 95% of these are likely to remain asymptomatic carriers. Adult T-cell leukaemia lymphoma (ATLL) is a T-cell malignancy that occurs after a 40- to 60-year period of clinical latency in about 3–5% of HTLV-I-infected individuals. ATLL cells are monoclonally expanded and harbour an integrated provirus. Persistent oligoclonal/polyclonal expansion of HTLV-I-bearing cells has been shown to precede ATLL, supporting the fact that in ATLL tumour cells arise from a clonally expanding non-malignant cell (see also Chapter 30).

Human herpesvirus 8
(Kaposi sarcoma-associated virus)

Human herpesvirus (HHV)-8 is the causative agent of both Kaposi sarcoma (KS) and primary effusion lymphoma. It is also detected in 100% and 50% of patients with multicentric Castleman disease who are HIV positive and HIV negative respectively. HHV-8, called also Kaposi sarcoma-associated virus (KSHV), appears to have an important role in the pathogenesis of both KS and primary effusion lymphoma, elaborating

growth factors and cytokines that promote tumour growth. It encodes putative oncogenes and genes that stimulate angiogenesis and cell proliferation, including G protein-coupled receptor promoting cell transformation and angiogenesis and 'interleukin (IL)-6 homologous cytokine', preventing cell apoptosis in IL-6-dependent cell lines.

The KSHV G-protein-coupled receptor (vGPCR) is a homologue of the human IL-8 receptor that signals constitutively, activates mitogen- and stress-activated kinases, and induces transcription via multiple transcription factors, including AP-1 and nuclear factor (NF)-κB. Furthermore, vGPCR causes cellular transformation *in vitro* and leads to KS-like tumours in transgenic mouse models.

KSHV also encodes a cyclin D homologue, K cyclin, which is thought to promote viral oncogenesis. The expression of K cyclin in cultured cells not only triggers cell cycle progression but also engages the p53 tumour-suppressor pathway, which probably restricts the oncogenic potential of K cyclin.

Hepatitis C virus

Hepatitis C virus (HCV) infection is associated with the development of essential mixed cryoglobulinaemia, a low-grade lymphoproliferative disorder that can progress to NHL. HCV may induce lymphoproliferation by binding to the CD81 receptor on the surface of B lymphocytes, which could lower the threshold for antigen response or induce DNA mutations and is associated with markers of lymphoproliferation. Furthermore, HCV-infected individuals have an elevated prevalence of circulating lymphocytes with abnormal chromosomal translocations associated with NHL, e.g. t(14;18).

An association between HCV infection and NHL has been examined in many retrospective case–control studies. Notably, however, there has been substantial heterogeneity in the magnitude of association across studies, with odds ratios (ORs) ranging from 2 to 10. A large cohort study of US military veterans (including 146 394 HCV-infected individuals and 572 293 uninfected individuals) demonstrated that HCV infection precedes the development of NHL and is associated with an increased NHL risk over a period of at least 7 years [hazard ratio (HR) 1.28, 95% CI 1.12–1.45]. Whether HCV is associated with an increased risk of all NHL subtypes or only certain subtypes has not been resolved. A pooled analysis of data from seven case–control studies showed associations between HCV and diffuse large B-cell lymphoma (DLBCL), lymphoplasmacytic NHL and marginal zone NHL.

Among HCV-infected patients with splenic marginal zone NHL, treatment of the HCV infection with interferon alfa-based regimens can lead to resolution of HCV and, simultaneously, regression of NHL. This observation also suggests that HCV directly contributes to lymphoproliferation in at least a subset of NHL cases. Clearance of the virus should be considered in the therapeutic algorithm for this rare lymphoma.

Immunosuppression

HIV-infected patients are at increased risk of developing NHL, and AIDS-related lymphoma is an AIDS-defining illness. This is the second most common tumour in individuals with HIV and although studies show a decline in incidence in the era of highly active antiretroviral therapy (HAART), AIDS-related lymphomas have increased as a percentage of first AIDS-defining illness. The development of AIDS-related lymphoma has been shown to be related to age, low CD4 cell count and no prior treatment with HAART. The pathogenesis is almost certainly multifactorial. The increased risk of infections with viruses such as EBV, chronic antigen exposure and cytokine stimulation arising from repeated infections result in polyclonal B-cell activation and therefore a greater chance of mutations that develop randomly during mitosis. Almost all cases of central nervous system (CNS) lymphomas and Hodgkin lymphoma diagnosed in immunosuppressed patients are EBV positive.

Lymphomas develop in less than 1% of allogeneic SCT recipients, although the risk is higher in patients receiving rigorous T-cell-depleted transplants followed by heavy post-graft immunosuppression, for example with antithymocyte globulins for graft-versus-host disease (GVHD). In heart or lung transplants, the incidence of lymphomas is as high as 4–7%. Most post-transplant lymphomas are EBV related (see above on EBV-related lymphomas). At early stages, they may be polyclonal or oligoclonal and only later become monoclonal, but the clonal nature of the proliferation does not appear to predict closely the response to immunosuppression withdrawal, which may result in spontaneous remission.

Genetic and occupational factors

Several studies have reported an increased risk of NHL in first-degree relatives of lymphoma probands compared with the general population. The temporal proximity of sibling pairs argues for environmental as well as genetic aetiology.

An increased incidence of NHL has been reported in people working in agriculture, forestry and logging industries, as well as in those involved in the metalworking, machinery, printing and publishing industry, motor vehicles and telephone communications. The risk seems to increase with employment duration and vary by histological type.

Personal use of hair dye has been inconsistently linked to risk of NHL. A study of 4461 NHL cases and 5799 controls from the International Lymphoma Epidemiology Consortium 1988–2003 has recently been reported. An increased risk of NHL (OR 1.3, 95% CI 1.1, 1.4) associated with hair-dye use was observed among women who began using hair dye before 1980. Analyses by NHL subtype showed increased risk for FL (OR 1.4, 95% CI 1.1, 1.9) and chronic lymphocytic leukaemia/small lymphocytic lymphoma (OR 1.5, 95% CI 1.1, 2.0). Occupational exposure to specific chemicals, such as benzidine, mineral, cutting or lubricating oil, pesticides, herbicides and wood dust seem to play an important role in the development of NHL. However, the exact impact of these factors is still debated and their contribution to pre-existing genetic factors is not totally clear.

Cytogenetics and oncogenes

Cytogenetic analysis in NHL can be difficult, given the problem of isolating neoplastic cells from tissue biopsy samples for karyotypic analysis. However, several large studies suggest that nearly all cases have a cytogenetic abnormality. It may be either numerical or structural but a number of translocations are particularly interesting because of their association with specific types of lymphoma and the insights they have provided into the process of lymphomagenesis. Rearrangements frequently involve T-cell receptor (TCR) or immunoglobulin genes, which rearrange as part of the normal process of lymphoid differentiation (see Chapter 19). In some cases, the aberrant recombination may be due to structural similarities between the regions close to the breakpoints and the heptamer/nonamer recombinase-recognition sequences bordering the normally rearranging genes. The rearrangements typically cause deregulation (usually upregulation) of oncogenes brought under the influence of immunoglobulin TCR promoter and enhancer sequences (see Table 35.2).

There is some disagreement concerning the frequency of the t(14;18) translocation in FLs, but most studies report its presence in about 85% of patients. Some of the discrepancies may reflect true geographical variation, for instance in Japan the reported incidence is only 33%. The breakpoints on chromosome 18 occur at two sites, approximately 20 kb apart, within or near the transcriptional unit of the *BCL2* gene. Approximately two-thirds of the breakpoints occur within 150 bp, known as the major breakpoint region, in the 5′-untranslated region of the *BCL2* gene, and most of the remaining breakpoints occur 3′ to this in the minor cluster region. The *BCL2* gene codes for a protein localized in the inner mitochondrial membrane, which is involved in the inhibition of apoptosis rather than the induction of proliferation. This blockade of cell death in neoplastic germinal centre cells may account for the fact that the FLs are, at least initially, slow-growing.

The usual cytogenetic abnormality in BL is a translocation involving the *MYC* gene on chromosome 8 and the immunoglobulin heavy-chain gene on chromosome 14, which is found in over 80% of cases. Although both the endemic and sporadic forms of BL have the same gross translocations, there are subtle differences at the molecular level. Variant translocations involve chromosome 8 and either chromosome 2 or 22, where the breakpoints involve, respectively, κ and λ light-chain genes. In all cases, there is upregulation of c-Myc, a nuclear transcription factor involved in cell proliferation and the control of apoptosis.

The t(11;14) translocation is found in mantle cell lymphomas (MCLs). The oncogene on chromosome 11 is known as *BCL1/PRAD1* (now called *CCND1*), and encodes a D-cyclin involved in cell cycle control (Table 35.2).

The *BCL6* gene encodes a transcription factor of the zinc finger family whose precise function is unknown. It has recently been suggested that it maintains B cells in a germinal centre-like state, inhibiting B-cell differentiation. Rearrangements of *BCL6* occur in over one-third of large-cell lymphomas, and in an even higher number of cases mutations within the gene are found. The presence of *BCL6* rearrangement has been suggested to predict favourable prognosis, although not confirmed in all studies (Table 35.2).

T-cell lymphomas are less frequent than B-cell lymphomas and have been less extensively studied at the molecular level. T-cell lymphoblastic lymphomas may have abnormalities similar to those found in T-cell acute lymphoblastic leukaemia (ALL), such as abnormalities of the *TAL1* gene on chromosome 1, the *HOX11* gene on chromosome 10 and the *LMO2* gene on chromosome 11.

Anaplastic Ki-1 (CD30)-positive large-cell lymphomas are usually of T-cell origin, and in at least half of the cases there is a t(2;5)(p23;q35) translocation (see Table 35.2). The genes involved in this translocation encode a receptor tyrosine kinase called anaplastic lymphoma kinase (ALK) on chromosome 2, and nucleophosmin on chromosome 5. The resulting hybrid gene (*NPM–ALK*) encodes a hybrid protein in which about 40% of nucleophosmin is fused to the entire cytoplasmic portion of ALK. The nucleophosmin moiety not only induces ALK expression (as nucleophosmin is a ubiquitously expressed nuclear protein) but also activates the kinase through cross-linking with subsequent mitogenic activity, promoting T-cell transformation and tumour growth.

When a chromosomal translocation is found frequently in a particular lymphoma type, e.g. t(14;18) in FL, and if the break-point falls within a well-defined and limited region(s), polymerase chain reaction (PCR) analysis may be used to either assist in diagnosis or detect minimal residual disease. However, the clinical significance and value of such studies have yet to be determined, as it is not completely clear what the prognostic importance may be of small numbers of cells carrying this translocation in patients who are in clinical remission.

Recently, DNA microarray technology has opened new avenues for the understanding of lymphomas. By hybridization of cDNA to arrays containing more than 10 000 different DNA fragments, this approach allows simultaneous evaluation of the mRNA expression of thousands of genes in a single experiment. These data can then be used for identification of lymphoma subgroups, with a defined gene expression pattern, not previously identified by morphology, cytogenetics or molecular techniques. This approach has already provided novel insights into

different entities of B-cell NHLs; measurement of the expression of only six genes was found to be predictive of OS in DLBCL and the prognosis of FL has been related to the molecular features of tumour-infiltrating cells.

Clinical features

The median age of presentation of low-grade lymphomas and large-cell lymphomas is around 55–60 years, with a slight male predominance. In FL, the marrow is involved in about 50% of cases at diagnosis. BL often presents with extranodal disease, appearing in the jaw in Africa and as gastrointestinal disease or in other intra-abdominal sites in the West. Hypercalcaemia is frequent.

Widespread painless lymphadenopathy is more common at presentation in NHL than in Hodgkin disease and contiguous spread is not so apparent. Superior vena cava syndrome caused by a bulky mediastinal mass is also more frequent in NHL than in Hodgkin lymphoma. Hepatosplenomegaly is frequent at diagnosis.

Patients with indolent histology are less likely to have 'B' symptoms (unexplained fever of 38°C or higher, night sweats and loss of more than 10% of body weight in 6 months) than those with an aggressive histology, but this is not invariable. Some patients present with systemic symptoms without peripheral lymphadenopathy, which can result in considerable delay in diagnosis. Symptoms and signs may be due to the involvement of particular organs (e.g. skin, gastrointestinal tract, salivary glands, lungs, renal tract and CNS).

Lymphoblastic lymphoma usually occurs in children and young adults, often with thymic mass, systemic symptoms and bone marrow failure.

Laboratory investigations

Histological diagnosis from either excision or core biopsy of a lymph node, bone marrow or extranodal mass is essential (Figures 35.1–35.8). Fine-needle aspiration has been used to exclude an infection (i.e. mycobacterial) or suggest lymphoma but can lead to delay in establishing a diagnosis. Fine-needle aspiration should not be performed except in suspected cases of T-lymphoblastic lymphoma or BL, when a diagnosis can be made on the morphology and immunophenotype, and therapy can be urgent. Immunocytochemistry is now performed routinely, with cytogenetic and immunoglobulin or TCR rearrangement analysis and, more recently, DNA microarray testing in specialized units.

Anaemia at diagnosis is usually indicative of widespread disease and may reflect a non-specific manifestation of malignancy. However, it can also be due to hypersplenism or bone marrow infiltration. Occasional patients, most often those with

Figure 35.1 Anaplastic large-cell lymphoma of T-cell type.

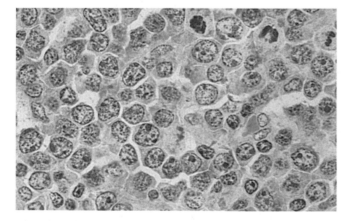

Figure 35.2 Large B-cell lymphoma. The cells are larger than normal lymphocytes and have a round nucleus with prominent nucleoli, some adjacent to the nuclear membrane ('centroblasts').

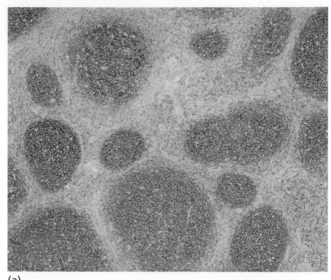

(a)

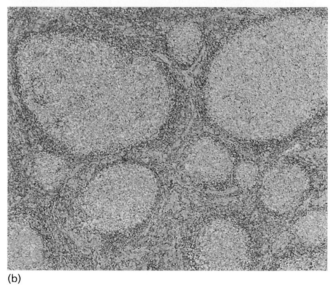

(b)

Figure 35.3 Immunostaining of follicular lymphoma showing its typical nodular appearance: (a) CD20 is expressed by the tumour cells, whereas (b) CD3 is confined to reactive T cells. (Paraffin sections: APAAP immunoalkaline phosphatase stain.)

indolent histology, have an autoimmune haemolysis. The white count is variable. Overspill of lymphoma cells into the blood is relatively frequent in late stages of indolent lymphoma and can infrequently be seen by light microscopy at diagnosis. It can be detected much more frequently using PCR. Hypoalbuminaemia is another non-specific feature associated with a systemic disturbance and is indicative of a poor prognosis. A raised lactate dehydrogenase (LDH) level is usually associated with advanced disease and is an important independent prognostic factor (Tables 35.3–35.5). Paraproteins are found in about 15% of indolent lymphomas and in a little less than 5% of histologically

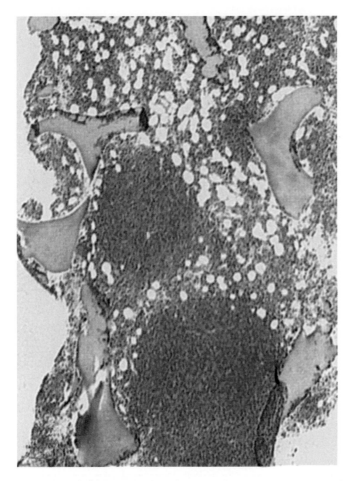

Figure 35.4 Non-Hodgkin lymphoma in the marrow: paratrabecular localization.

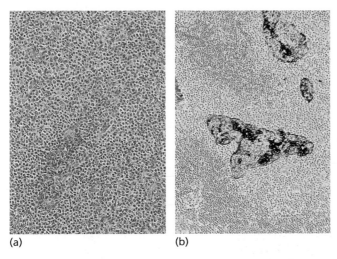

(a)   (b)

Figure 35.5 Marginal zone lymphoma of a salivary gland. (a) Sheets of marginal zone B cells and formation of a lymphoepithelial lesion. (b) Immunoperoxidase stain for low-molecular-weight cytokeratin (MNF116) shows positive staining of normal epithelial cells infiltrated by lymphoma.

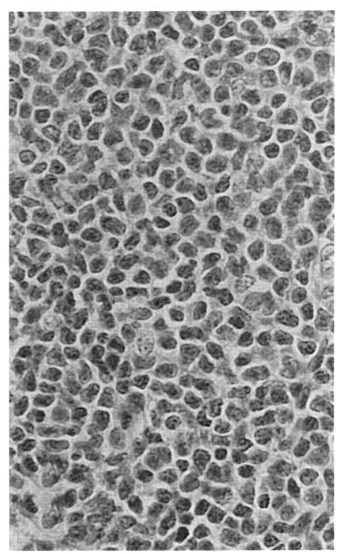

Figure 35.6 Irregular small lymphoid cells (small cleaved cells; centrocytes) typical of mantle cell lymphomas.

Table 35.3 Prognostic factors for aggressive lymphoma: International Prognostic Index (IPI).

Age > 60 years
Ann Arbor stage III or IV
Increased lactate dehydrogenase concentration
Performance score >2
Involvement of more than one extranodal site

Source: The International Non-Hodgkin's Lymphoma Prognostic Factors Project (1993) A predictive model for aggressive non-Hodgkin's lymphoma. *New England Journal of Medicine* **329**: 987–94 with permission.

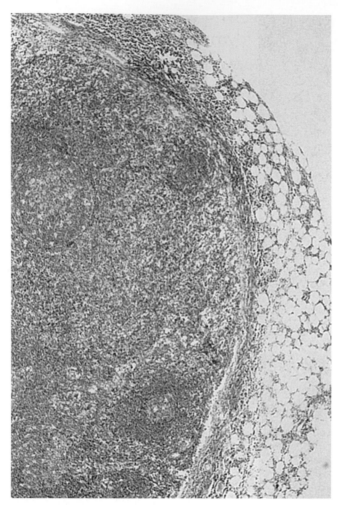

Figure 35.7 Peripheral T-cell lymphoma. Expansion of the paracortical region of a lymph node, with wide separation of germinal follicles.

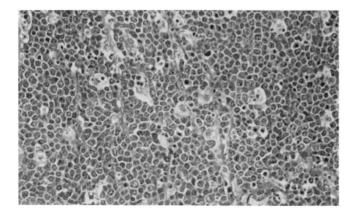

Figure 35.8 Burkitt lymphoma. Sheets of lymphoblasts and 'starry sky' tangible body macrophages.

Table 35.4 Prognostic factors for follicular lymphoma: Follicular Lymphoma International Prognostic Index (FLIPI).

Age > 60 years
Ann Arbor stage III/IV
Haemoglobin <12 g/dL
Serum lactate dehydrogenase elevated
Number of nodal areas involved: more than four sites

Source: Solal-Celigny P, Roy P, Colombat P *et al.* (2004) Follicular lymphoma international prognostic index. *Blood* **104**: 1258–1265 with permission.

Table 35.5 Prognostic factors for mantle cell lymphoma.

Age > 60 years
Performance status
Serum lactate dehydrogenase
Leucocyte count
Ki-67 immunostaining index

Source: Hoster *et al.* (2008) with permission.

aggressive lymphomas. Levels of β_2-microglobulin have been shown to be of prognostic value in some low-grade lymphomas.

Staging

The Ann Arbor staging system, initially developed for Hodgkin disease, is used in adults with NHL (Table 35.6). Inspection of the Waldeyer ring is particularly important, and a bone marrow biopsy should be performed in all patients. Radiography, computed tomography (CT), magnetic resonance imaging (MRI) or positron emission tomography (PET) are used for initial staging of the disease and are of value in monitoring response to therapy and detection of residual disease or relapse. Using PET, fluorodeoxyglucose (FDG)-avid lymphomas include DLBCL, Hodgkin lymphoma, FL and MCL, while variably FDG-avid lymphomas include other aggressive and indolent lymphomas. As treatment differs for patients with stage I disease (DLBCL and FL) and more advanced stages, PET at diagnosis can have significant therapeutic implications. Staging laparotomy is no longer routinely performed. At the end of therapy, PET has been incorporated into the revised response criteria.

Cerebrospinal fluid (CSF) examination should be considered if there are clinical signs of CNS disease, or for patients presenting with high-grade NHL at certain anatomical sites such as paranasal sinus, breast, epidural area or testis. Cytological assessment by cytospin and immunophenotyping should be

Table 35.6 Ann Arbor staging system.

Stage I	Involvement in a single lymph node region or single extralymphatic site
Stage II	Involvement of two or more lymph node regions on the same side of the diaphragm; localized contiguous involvement of only one extralymphatic site and lymph node region (stage IIE)
Stage III	Involvement of lymph node regions on both sides of the diaphragm; may include spleen
Stage IV	Disseminated involvement of one or more extralymphatic organs with or without lymph node involvement

considered. Intrathecal prophylaxis should be administered at the time of first CSF examination in these patients. Serology for HIV and hepatitis B virus (HBsAg, HBcAb and HBsAb) and HCV should be performed in all patients as appropriate concomitant antiviral therapy may be indicated during and after therapy.

Treatment

Treatment of NHL is mainly based on the histological findings, although therapeutic decisions are influenced by the patient's age, performance status and disease extension. The two main subtypes comprise over two-thirds of cases in the Western world: DLBCL, an aggressive lymphoma, and FL, which follows a more indolent course. There are also a number of subtypes of lymphoma with distinct clinical and pathological features and therapeutic strategies that are discussed separately. Some of the NHLs are potentially curable and thus access to timely sophisticated diagnostic services and expert clinical opinion is necessary to ensure accurate diagnosis and tailored therapy.

Particular considerations prior to therapy should include a formal assessment of cardiac function for older patients and those with a previous history of diabetes or cardiac disease if anthracycline therapy is considered. Accurate analysis of renal function is necessary before the administration of high-dose methotrexate and platinum-containing regimens.

Follicular lymphoma

Localized disease

Approximately 10–20% of patients with FL present with non-bulky localized (stage I/IIA) disease. Localized radiotherapy can cure approximately half of patients with stage I and one-quarter of those with stage IIA. Although the addition of chemotherapy may produce better results, local radiotherapy is currently considered an appropriate approach for these cases and represents the treatment of choice in most centres. Accurate definition of the truly localized forms is therefore crucial in ensuring an appropriate treatment design for such patients. PET/CT is increasingly performed at presentation in order to help clarify stage, as FL is uniformly an FDG-avid lymphoma.

Using very sensitive tests such as PCR for the t(14;18) translocation, the majority of patients with localized disease have been shown to have low-level involvement in the bone marrow or peripheral blood. However, after treatment with involved-field radiotherapy, durable disappearance of Bcl-2/IgH-positive cells has been observed in a significant proportion of cases. Patients with localized disease, confirmed on PET/CT (and a negative bone marrow biopsy), should therefore receive involved-field radiation without undue delay, aiming not only to eliminate their symptoms but also to achieve disease cure.

Adding adjuvant chemotherapy to radiotherapy for localized disease

As most relapses following radiotherapy occur outside the radiation field, it has been postulated that a reasonable approach may be to combine radiotherapy with systemic chemotherapy, aiming to reduce relapse risk and improve cure rate.

The British National Lymphoma Investigation (BNLI) prospectively compared the outcome of patients with localized low-grade lymphoma treated with radiotherapy, with or without adjuvant continuous chlorambucil. There were no significant differences in either overall survival (OS) or disease-free survival (DFS) between the two treatment groups (maximal follow-up 18 years). Intensification of chemotherapy (e.g. CHOP; Table 35.7) also failed to improve patient outcome. Although there have been some retrospective and prospective non-randomized trials that have reported improved progression-free survival (PFS) in patients given combined modality treatment compared with radiotherapy alone, at present there are no proven data to support the addition of chemotherapy. Chemotherapy should therefore be used in such patients only after relapse.

Is there any place for radiotherapy in relapsed localized disease?

Low-dose (4 Gy) involved-field radiotherapy appears to provide a high response rate (92% overall response rate, with 61% complete responses) with durable remissions (>1 year) in patients with relapsed disease. Low-dose radiotherapy should therefore be considered in patients with recurrent localized disease, irrespective of their initial presentation.

Advanced disease

Patients with FL tend to have a highly variable outcome. Although some patients experience early progression and die of

Table 35.7 Chemotherapy protocols used in NHL.

CVP	Cyclophosphamide, vincristine, prednisolone
FMC	Fludarabine, cyclophosphamide, mitoxantrone
CHOP	Cyclophosphamide, doxorubicin, vincristine, prednisolone
MACE-CYTABOM	Doxorubicin, etoposide, prednisolone, cytarabine, bleomycin, vincristine, methotrexate
MACOP B	Methotrexate, doxorubicin, cyclophosphamide, vincristine, bleomycin
m-BACOD	Methotrexate, bleomycin, doxorubicin, cyclophosphamide, vincristine, dexamethasone
ESHAP	Etoposide, cytarabine, methylprednisolone, cisplatin
Mini-BEAM	BCNU, etoposide, cytarabine, melphalan
ICE	Ifosfamide, carboplatin, etoposide
DHAP	Dexamethasone, high-dose cytarabine, cisplatin
DVIP	Dexamethasone, etoposide, ifosfamide, cisplatin
CODOX-M/IVAC	Cyclophosphamide, doxorubicin, high-dose methotrexate/ifosfamide, etoposide, high-dose cytarabine
Hyper-CVAD	Hyperfractionated cyclophosphamide, vincristine, doxorubicin, dexamethasone
ACVBP	Doxorubicin, cyclophosphamide, vindesine, bleomycin, prednisolone

their disease in less than 5 years, others may have an indolent course and live for 15 years or longer. Conventional chemotherapy has not been shown to prolong long-term survival compared with observation. For some patients management is mainly targeted to reducing symptoms and prolonging time to progression (TTP) rather than prolonging survival. Previously FL was considered an incurable disease but it is possible that novel approaches (immunochemotherapy, radioimmunotherapy, transplantation strategies) and their combination will lead to prolonged survival and potential cure in some patients.

Patient quality of life and treatment-related side-effects should be carefully considered, especially in the background of a disease with a median survival of 10–15 years and which occurs mainly in elderly patients, whose life expectancy irrespective of disease may be less than 20 years. However, there is a risk of transformation to high-grade lymphoma of approximately 3% per annum that has significant impact on outcome.

Management therefore ranges from a 'watch-and-wait' approach to different kinds of chemotherapy regimens (monoclonal antibodies applied in symptomatic patients) to the experimental intensive therapies considered in younger patients that aim to prolong survival and achieve cure, for example autologous or allogeneic SCT.

What is required is a series of complementary structured randomized studies that will give proper data over a number of years. Unfortunately, newer modalities such as monoclonal antibodies with some sort of SCT will inevitably be introduced during the lifetime of an incidental patient's disease and thus 'skew' the findings. It is almost impossible to study a patient over 10–15 years without allowing him or her to potentially benefit from new treatments emerging during that period.

Patients with the histological subtype FL grade 3b follow a more aggressive course and should be treated according to practice for aggressive large-cell lymphomas.

Chemotherapy for follicular lymphoma

As mentioned above, historically treatment has been unable to prolong long-term survival. Therefore, it is mainly offered to reduce symptoms and signs of the disease and improve quality of life.

A large number of patients are asymptomatic at diagnosis. Deferral of treatment in such patients seems to have no adverse impact on survival. The BNLI reported the outcome of patients with asymptomatic advanced stage III/IV low-grade lymphoma who were randomly assigned to receive oral chlorambucil $10\,mg/m^2$ continuously ($N = 158$) versus observation until disease progression ($N = 151$) (local radiotherapy to symptomatic enlarged lymph nodes was permitted in both arms). There was no significant difference in OS and cause-specific survival between the two arms. However, age below 60 years and stage III versus IV conferred a significant survival advantage. The actuarial chance of not requiring chemotherapy at 10 years was almost 20%, supporting the strategy of 'watch and wait' in these 'advanced' patients. Similarly, the Groupe d'Étude des Lymphomes Folliculaires (GELF) found no differences in OS between patients with low tumour burden randomized to prednimustine/interferon versus observation only. Results from the UK NCRI 'Watch and Wait' study, in which asymptomatic patients with low-volume disease are randomized between rituximab and observation, are awaited. As a rule, conservative management should be considered in asymptomatic patients in order to maintain their quality of life without unnecessary toxicity.

First-line chemotherapy for advanced-stage follicular lymphoma

Those individuals who have symptoms can receive either oral or intravenous therapies. Oral chlorambucil and cyclophosphamide, both alkylating agents, remain good therapies for those who do not need rapid debulking of their tumour mass. The combination chemotherapeutic regimens CVP (cyclophosphamide, vincristine, prednisolone) and CHOP (cyclophosphamide, vincristine, Adriamycin, prednisolone) with rituximab (R-CHOP) are widely used. Rituximab/bendamustine has been shown to be efficacious in a randomized non-inferiority study (vs. R-CHOP) and well tolerated, with similar haematological and infectious complications but without inducing alopecia.

The role of doxorubicin-containing regimens for indolent lymphoma is controversial. There has been no direct randomized comparison between R-CHOP and R-CVP. Comparison of outcome from up-front Phase II/III studies demonstrates prolongation of response duration and higher overall response rate (ORR) and complete responses (CR) following R-CHOP, although it is not known whether this will translate into overall survival benefit. There is some evidence from retrospective studies that risk of transformation may be lower with anthracycline-based therapy though this needs confirmation. However, haematological and non-haematological (alopecia, cardiac) toxicity are greater with R-CHOP.

Nevertheless, there are some patients for whom doxorubicin-containing regimens may be appropriate, although the data to support this approach remain controversial. Grade IIIB FL is a definite indication, while those who present with constitutional symptoms, high tumour burden and elevated LDH (all parameters suggesting more aggressive disease, despite the indolent histology) may be more appropriate for doxorubicin-containing combinations.

Seven randomized controlled trials involving 1943 patients with indolent lymphomas (1480 with FL) have been included in a recent meta-analysis comparing the outcome after radio-chemotherapy with chemotherapy alone. In five of the trials patients had no prior therapy. Patients treated with radiochemotherapy had better OS (HR for mortality 0.65, 95% CI 0.54–0.78), overall response (relative risk of tumour response 1.21, 95% CI 1.16–1.27) and disease control (HR of disease event 0.62, 95% CI 0.55–0.71) than patients treated with chemotherapy alone.

Purine analogues

The more recent purine analogues, fludarabine, 2-chlorodeoxyadenosine (cladribine) and deoxycoformycin (pentostatin), represent a group of potently lymphotoxic antimetabolite agents, non-cross-resistant to alkylating agent therapy. Their activity in the indolent NHLs, particularly in the follicular subtype, may be due to their unique ability as antimetabolites to inhibit resting as well as dividing cells.

Several retrospective studies suggested a higher response rate with single-agent fludarabine compared with alkylating agent-based regimens. However, prospective randomized trials failed to confirm these results, suggesting CVP/CHVP plus interferon to be as good as single-agent fludarabine. Several retrospective/Phase I studies have suggested that fludarabine-containing combinations (e.g. fludarabine/cyclophosphamide, fludarabine/mitoxantrone/dexamethasone) are superior to traditional alkylating agent regimens or fludarabine only, providing a higher CR rate in both therapy-naive and relapsed patients. However, other studies failed to repeat these results, emphasizing the need for prospective randomized trials.

Fludarabine does cause immunosuppression, resulting in increased incidence of opportunistic infection necessitating prophylaxis against *Pneumocystis jirovecii*. It may also cause myelosuppression and adversely affect stem cell harvesting. However, it is usually well tolerated and its use has become much easier since the introduction of an oral formulation. Several studies performed in patients with chronic lymphocytic leukaemia and low-grade lymphoma confirmed oral fludarabine to be as effective as the intravenous formulation.

Side-effects of chemotherapy

Chemotherapy-related side-effects should be considered seriously, taking into account the historical inability of chemotherapy to improve patient survival. Chemotherapy may adversely affect quality of life, causing myelosuppression and immunosuppression with increased risk of infections. Myelodysplastic changes and increased risk of leukaemia were mainly reported with alkylating agents, although these may also be associated with fludarabine. For young patients, infertility may be a primary concern of treatment.

Interferon

Recombinant interferon alfa has been used simultaneously with initial cytotoxic chemotherapy or as maintenance therapy in patients who responded to initial chemotherapy, aiming to enhance immunological response and prolong survival. Interferon has been shown to improve DFS but the benefit did not appear to translate into improved OS, unless an anthracycline regimen was used. Benefit has not been proven in the rituximab era and therefore it is not widely used at present.

Monoclonal antibodies

The addition of the monoclonal antibody rituximab to chemotherapy regimens has been associated with improvements in response rates, PFS and OS, although it is unclear whether advanced indolent NHL can be cured without allogeneic SCT.

Rituximab is an anti-CD20 chimeric monoclonal antibody that was the first approved for NHL treatment. The cell-surface antigen CD20 is in many ways an ideal target as it is expressed by 95% of B cells in NHL but not by haemopoietic stem cells; it has a functional role in B-cell growth and also does not normally circulate as a free antigen in plasma, so the free antigen does not compete for antibody binding. Response is achieved via several mechanisms, including complement-dependent cytotoxicity, antibody-dependent cellular cytotoxicity and induction of apoptosis. Rituximab is also able to sensitize lymphoma cells to the cytotoxic activity of chemotherapy.

Table 35.8 Monoclonal antibodies in NHL.

Antibody	Antigen	Conjugate
Rituximab (IDEC-C2B8, Rituxan)	CD20	None
Alemtuzumab (Campath-1H)	CD52	None
Epratuzumab (hLL2)	CD22	None
Apolizumab (Hu1D10, Remitogen)	HLA-DR	None
Ibritumomab tiuxetan (IDEC-Y2B8, Zevalin)	CD20	^{90}Y
Tositumomab (Bexxar)	CD20	^{131}I
Immunotoxins	CD19, CD22	*Pseudomonas* exotoxin A (PE38), ricin A, Shiga toxin

The efficacy and tolerability of monoclonal antibodies targeted against CD20 and other antigens expressed by lymphoma cells are also being explored (Table 35.8).

Previously untreated low-grade lymphoma

Single-agent therapy with rituximab appears to be effective in previously untreated low-grade NHL, yielding a high response rate of 62–73%, including 20–44% CRs.

A number of Phase II studies have suggested that extending therapy with rituximab maintenance schedules is associated with improved outcomes compared with rituximab induction alone. A Phase III trial comparing rituximab maintenance therapy with observation only (following rituximab induction) showed a significantly improved PFS in those who received rituximab maintenance, with no increase in treatment-related adverse events. Whether maintenance with rituximab to these complete responders can prolong survival remains to be seen and studies are addressing this.

The single-agent activity of rituximab, coupled with its distinct mechanisms of action, non-overlapping toxicity and ability to sensitize lymphoma cells to cytotoxic activity, has encouraged researchers to evaluate its combinations with chemotherapy. In a number of large Phase III trials, rituximab plus chemotherapy (CHOP or CVP) has demonstrated significant activity, achieving improvements in ORR (81% vs. 57%, with CRs of 40% vs. 10% respectively; $P < 0.0001$) and prolongation of time to treatment failure and TTP and OS compared with CVP alone ($P < 0.0001$ for both parameters).

A characteristic chromosomal translocation, t(14;18), leading to overexpression of *BCL2*, an anti-apoptotic gene that may serve as a survival factor for lymphoma cells, is carried by 85% of patients with FL and can be detected by PCR. Achievement of molecular remission after therapy (clearance of *BCL2*-positive cells) appears to be associated with prolonged PFS and may even predict a longer OS. Various chemotherapy regimens (e.g. FND-R, CHOP-R) have yielded similar results, reporting molecular remissions with prolonged PFS. Rituximab-containing chemotherapy regimens appear to increase both clinical and molecular remission rates when compared with those usually achieved with chemotherapy only, giving grounds for optimism.

Relapsed low-grade lymphoma

Single-agent rituximab has limited efficacy in relapsed disease, providing responses in 38–59% of patients, including CR in up to 28%. However, responses are not durable and patients eventually relapse. Many studies now suggest that combination immunochemotherapy may be more effective than single-agent rituximab or chemotherapy alone and thus this treatment may be offered to patients with relapsed disease who can tolerate a combined regimen. However, results of prospective comparative trials are still needed to confirm the superiority of this strategy, especially in the setting of first-line chemoimmunotherapy. Concerns regarding the ability to mobilize stem cells after fludarabine should be taken into account if subsequent autologous SCT is considered.

A study by the German Low-grade Lymphoma Study Group compared the combination of fludarabine, cyclophosphamide and mitoxantrone (FCM) with rituximab plus FCM in patients with relapsed FL and MCL. This study was stopped early after 147 patients had been randomized when R-FCM treatment revealed a significant improvement in response rates, response duration, and survival over that of FCM alone.

Rituximab maintenance

A recent meta-analysis of randomized controlled trials that compared rituximab maintenance therapy with observation or treatment at relapse (no maintenance) has recently been published. Five trials including 1143 adult patients were included in this meta-analysis. Data for 985 patients with FL were available for the meta-analysis of OS. Patients treated with maintenance rituximab had statistically significantly better OS than patients in the observation arm or patients treated at relapse (HR for death 0.60, 95% CI 0.45–0.79). The rate of infection-related adverse events was higher with rituximab maintenance treatment (HR 1.99, 95% CI 1.21–3.27). Patients with refractory or relapsed (i.e. previously treated) FL had a survival benefit with maintenance rituximab therapy (HR for death 0.58, 95% CI 0.42–0.79), whereas previously untreated patients did not (HR for death 0.68, 95% CI 0.37–1.25). Maintenance therapy with rituximab was offered either as four weekly infusions every 6 months or as a single infusion every 2–3 months. Open questions still exist regarding the effect of rituximab maintenance on the outcome of patients with FL, some of which are currently being evaluated in randomized clinical trials. These questions include the effects of rituximab maintenance therapy compared with rituximab at disease progression, effects of rituximab maintenance therapy in previously untreated patients with advanced FL, effects of rituximab maintenance therapy in patients with FL following rituximab and chemotherapy induction, the optimal duration of rituximab maintenance therapy, and the optimal schedule of rituximab maintenance.

Presently it is felt to be reasonable to offer rituximab maintenance to patients responding to reinduction with chemotherapy with or without rituximab regardless of whether they received rituximab with initial chemotherapy. There has been no direct comparison of rituximab maintenance with autologous or allogeneic SCT but any of these treatment options for patients who have responded to second-line chemotherapy may be considered. There are many factors to consider, such as response duration, morbidity, survival, quality of life, potential of 'cure' and financial criteria. The multidisciplinary team meeting is a venue to discuss such options but clearly involving the patient in such treatment choices is recommended.

New unconjugated antibodies and combinations of monoclonal antibodies

New monoclonal antibodies directed at different antigens expressed by lymphoma cells are being investigated, for example anti-CD22 (hLL2, epratuzumab), anti-HLA-DR (Hu1D10, apolizumab, Remitogen) and anti-CD19 monoclonal antibodies (see Table 35.8). New monoclonal antibodies directed against CD20 include ofatumumab (HuMax CD20), IMMU-106 (hA20) which has a greater than 90% humanized framework, and GA-101, a novel third-generation fully humanized and optimized monoclonal antibody. These agents are highly cytotoxic against B-cell lymphoid cells and are currently being evaluated. Veltuzumab is a humanized anti-CD20 monoclonal antibody that has significantly reduced off-rates and increased complement-dependent cytotoxicity in lymphoma cell lines.

Greater efficacy than rituximab *in vivo* has been demonstrated in preclinical lymphoma models and this agent is being assessed clinically. The combination of epratuzumab (anti-CD22) and rituximab has been shown to induce durable responses in patients with recurrent indolent NHL in an international multicenter trial. Apolizumab is a humanized IgG1 antibody specific for a polymorphic determinant found on the HLA-DR β-chain expressed by normal and malignant B cells. It has been shown to be well tolerated and effective in a proportion of patients with rituximab-refractory FL. Alemtuzumab (Campath-1H), directed against CD52, may be used in both T-cell and B-cell NHL. An increased risk of opportunistic infection (related to T-cell depletion) may limit its use and its efficacy is described separately in the relevant sections.

Combinations of monoclonal antibodies directed at different antigens may have a synergistic effect, leading to increased response rates. Various combinations are being investigated (e.g. rituximab and alemtuzumab, rituximab and epratuzumab). Data are still too limited to draw final conclusions about their potential toxicity and efficacy. In summary, there is little doubt about the efficacy of rituximab in FL, but there is still doubt as to whether any treatment significantly modifies the ultimate duration of disease.

Radioimmunoconjugates

FL is a radiosensitive malignancy and a targeted strategy using radiotherapy involves the use of radiolabelled monoclonal antibodies such as ^{131}I-labelled or ^{90}Y-labelled anti-CD20 antibodies. ^{90}Y-ibritumomab tiuxetan (Zevalin; Bayer Schering Pharma AG, Berlin, Germany) is an immunoconjugate comprising murine IgG1 and the anti-CD20 monoclonal antibody ibritumomab covalently bound to the chelator tiuxetan, which provides stable linkage to the radioisotope. Radioimmunoconjugates kill tumour cells predominantly by radioactive emission and can therefore be effective in patients who do not respond to unconjugated antibodies (e.g. rituximab). The most common radioisotopes are ^{131}I (β/γ-emitter) and ^{90}Y (a pure β-emitter) (Table 35.9). The β-particles emitted

Table 35.9 Characteristics of currently available radioimmunoconjugates used in NHL.

Characteristics	^{131}I	^{90}Y
Emission	β and γ	β
Half-life	8 days	2.5 days
Energy	–	×5
Imaging	Can be used for radioimmunoscintigraphy	Cannot be used for radioimmunoscintigraphy by conventional methods*
Stability	Rapid degradation after endocytosis	Retained stable by tumour cells after endocytosis
Hospitalization	Hospitalization	Outpatient*

*As a result of having no γ emission.

Table 35.10 Potential problems when using radioimmunoconjugates.

Requires special knowledge and can be given by an expert only

Treatment with ^{131}I (emitting γ-particles) requires hospitalization for isolation

Accumulative toxicity may limit future stem cell harvesting

Long-term toxicity unknown (possibility of secondary malignancies)

by ^{131}I and ^{90}Y radioisotopes have high penetration (over many cell diameters), allowing eradication of tumour cells that are not expressing the targeted antigen but which are adjacent to target CD20-positive cells; this is known as the 'crossfire' effect. Although ^{131}I is inexpensive and easily conjugated, ^{90}Y has five times more energy, a longer path length and a shorter half-life than ^{131}I (2.5 days vs. 8 days). A potential problem with pure β-emitters such as ^{90}Y is that dosimetry is relatively complicated. However, pure β-emitters can be given to outpatients, as there is no radiation risk for those who come into contact with them. This risk is substantially higher with γ-emitters such as ^{131}I (Table 35.10).

Radioimmunoconjugates in patients with relapsed disease

During the past decade, two products directed against the CD20 antigen, ^{131}I-labelled tositumomab and ^{90}Y-labelled ibritumomab tiuxetan, have been studied. Both products have produced response rates of 70–80% in patients with relapsed/treatment-naive low-grade lymphoma, and 50–60% in low-grade lymphoma that has transformed into an intermediate or high-grade lymphoma. Median duration of response to a single course of treatment approached 1 year. The treatment was well tolerated. However, prolonged myelosuppression with a potential risk of long-term myelodysplastic syndrome/myeloid leukaemia was noted. A Phase III trial comparing rituximab with ^{90}Y-labelled ibritumomab tiuxetan in patients with relapsed/refractory low-grade lymphoma/transformed B-cell NHL confirmed the efficacy of radioimmunoconjugates, showing a higher response rate in those who received ^{90}Y-labelled ibritumomab tiuxetan. There was no difference in median TTP, but durable responses (≥6 months) were more frequent in the radioimmunotherapy arm. A recent meta-analysis demonstrated that response rates, response duration and safety profile of ^{90}Y-ibritumomab tiuxetan in elderly patients (>70 years) were similar to those of younger patients.

These agents have been used in patients prior to transplantation, with the aim of reducing disease bulk, and in some cases establishing CR before consolidation with high-dose therapy. Whether patients can achieve a similar outcome from radioimmunotherapy without proceeding to a transplant procedure is unknown.

Radioimmunoconjugates in therapy-naive patients

Radioimmunoconjugates are particularly effective when used earlier in the disease course and in less bulky (<5 cm diameter) disease. The recently published First-Line Indolent Trial (FIT), an international randomized controlled Phase III trial, evaluated the safety and efficacy of consolidation therapy with a single dose of ^{90}Y-ibritumomab tiuxetan in 414 patients with advanced-stage FL who achieved a partial response (PR) or better with first-line induction treatment. Consolidation of first remission with ^{90}Y-ibritumomab tiuxetan was highly effective with no unexpected toxicities, prolonging PFS by 2 years and resulting in high PR-to-CR conversion rates regardless of type of first-line induction treatment (although only 15% of patients received rituximab-containing chemotherapy). Median PFS with consolidation was prolonged in all IPI risk subgroups. The most common toxicity with ^{90}Y-ibritumomab tiuxetan was haematological, and grade 3 or 4 infections occurred in 8% of patients. Whether such benefit will be seen after radiochemotherapy remains to be evaluated.

Immunotoxins

Immunotoxins are specific antibodies connected to toxins through a linker that is easily cleavable on the malignant cell surface but which is stable while the toxin circulates in the blood. For the immunotoxin to be effective, the antigen should be expressed extensively on the surface of the targeted cell, and should be able to be internalized in response to antibody binding so that the toxin can kill the cell. The most commonly used toxins (ricin A, diphtheria, *Pseudomonas* exotoxin A and Shiga-like toxin-1) kill by inhibiting protein synthesis. The efficacy and safety of most of these immunotoxins have yet to be proven. However, an anti-CD22 immunotoxin called RFB4(dsFv)-PE38 (BL22) has been recently reported to be extremely potent in patients with hairy cell leukaemia who failed cladribine (see also Chapter 29). The CD22 antigen is expressed by other lymphoproliferative disorders (i.e. MCL and DLBCL) and the BL22 immunotoxin may also be applied in these patients.

Stem cell transplantation in low-grade NHL

Autologous stem cell transplantation

Autologous SCT can prolong OS in relapsed disease and can extend PFS in first remission. With more than 10 years of follow-up, the survival curves demonstrate a plateau indicating a potential cure in certain patients. A recently published retrospective analysis by the European Group for Blood and Marrow Transplantation (EBMT) of 693 patients with follicular lymphoma who underwent autologous SCT between 1979 and 1995 reported a 15-year PFS and OS of 27 and 47% respectively. Notably, the PFS curve begins to plateau after 10 years, suggesting that some patients may be cured. Combined data from St Bartholomew's Hospital and the Dana-Farber Cancer Institute in 121 recipients of autologous SCT in second, third or fourth complete remission also support this observation, with a survival plateau after 13 years. At 10 and 15 years, PFS of 48 and 47% and OS of 54 and 44%, respectively, were reported. A comparison of second complete remission age-matched controls showed superior OS with autologous SCT compared with conventional therapy (61% vs. 41% at 10 years; 54% vs. 30% at 15 years).

Second malignancies are the most common cause of late non-relapse mortality after autologous SCT. Although recipient age, number of prior chemotherapeutic regimens, and use of fludarabine, etoposide and alkylating agents may predispose patients to myelodysplastic syndrome (MDS)/acute myeloid leukaemia (AML), it is now clear that haemopoietic SCT independently adds to the overall risk. The inclusion of total body irradiation (TBI) into the conditioning regimen markedly increases the risk of MDS/AML. The EBMT analysis noted a fourfold increased risk of secondary malignancies at 10 years. The Dana-Farber group, who used a TBI-containing conditioning regimen, demonstrated a 16% risk of second malignancy at 10 years, even though patients underwent autologous SCT in first remission and therefore were exposed only to one prior regimen. An increased incidence of hypothyroidism, hypogonadism, infections, anxiety, depression and cardiac dysfunction were also reported.

In contrast, three studies comparing the outcome after TBI-based autologous SCT compared with further conventional-dose chemotherapy in patients responding to first-line induction chemotherapy have shown no difference in OS between the arms. The PFS benefit, seen for patients autografted in two of these studies, is balanced by an increased risk of second cancers in the autograft arm. Autografting in first complete remission is not therefore generally recommended.

Non-conjugated monoclonal antibodies, radioimmunoconjugates and autologous stem cell transplantation

It is well established that conventional chemotherapy does not prolong survival in patients with low-grade lymphoma. However, autologous SCT may improve PFS, and most patients with FL will eventually relapse due to contamination of the harvest product with lymphoma cells or regrowth of malignant cells that survived the transplantation procedure. Molecular remission before transplantation appears to be linked to increased PFS. Therefore, it is tempting to try to purge the stem cells before transplantation in order to minimize harvest contamination and reduce relapse risk. Similarly, it might be a reasonable approach to add rituximab post transplant ('mopping up'), aiming to eradicate residual cells that survived high-dose chemotherapy (ongoing EBMT Lym1 study). The efficacy of both stem cell purging/post-transplant 'mopping-up' is still debated, and results from prospective randomized trials are awaited.

Radioimmunoconjugates may also be used as part of autologous SCT in NHL, enabling the delivery of higher radiotherapy doses without significantly increasing treatment-related toxicity. Phase I and II studies have demonstrated the addition of a radioimmunoconjugate to standard conditioning regimens to be well tolerated and associated with a potential increase in efficacy. Randomized studies are ongoing and long-term follow-up will be important, given the potential for these agents to increase rates of treatment-related MDS and AML.

Allogeneic stem cell transplantation in low-grade lymphoma

Advanced low-grade lymphomas are usually incurable with conventional-dose chemotherapy. It is uncertain whether cures are possible with autologous SCT and bone marrow transplantation from a human leucocyte antigen (HLA)-identical sibling. Earlier studies suggested that allogeneic SCT using myeloablative conditioning was potentially curative, although the transplant-related mortality (TRM) was high. This strategy combines the cytoreductive effect of the conditioning agents with the alloreactive donor T cells to eliminate residual lymphoma. The problems of tumour contamination of the graft and secondary MDS/AML are not concerns compared with autologous SCT.

Reduced-intensity SCT is being increasingly used for various kinds of haematological malignancies, aiming to exploit the curative potential of this modality by inducing a graft-versus-tumour effect without the morbidity and mortality associated with conventional transplantation. Several retrospective studies have suggested this approach to be less toxic and potentially curative in patients with low-grade lymphoma. At 2–5 years of follow-up, OS rates are at least comparable to those obtained with myeloablative regimens. In an Italian multicentre study a relapse risk of 14% and 3-year OS of 88% were observed for patients with FL. This outcome is similar to that described by a UK group, although different rates of acute and chronic GVHD reflect differences in prophylaxis (T-cell depletion).

Treatment of transformed follicular lymphoma

There is approximately a 3% per annum risk of transformation of FL to a more aggressive phenotype. In the pre-rituximab era the outcome after chemotherapy was generally poor, with median survival of 1.2–1.8 years reported. Consideration for autologous SCT after chemotherapy was thus advocated and in small Phase II studies 30% survival at 5 years has been described. Although published data are scant, outcome appears to be improved after rituximab, CHOP or other combination chemotherapy regimens, especially for patients who had received no prior therapy for their low-grade disease and who achieve complete remission following treatment of the transformed disease. Thus autologous SCT is commonly withheld in this subgroup. Allografting using reduced-intensity conditioning is another option and its efficacy described in small series, with a 60% OS at 4 years observed in chemosensitive patients.

Suggested algorithm for therapy of low-grade NHL (mostly follicular lymphoma)

Localized disease
• Use of involved-field radiation

Disseminated disease (stage III/IV)

• *Asymptomatic patient.* In asymptomatic patients a 'watch and wait' policy is generally appropriate. Younger patients with advanced asymptomatic disease may be considered for clinical trials (e.g. BNLI trial: rituximab in patients with stage III/IV asymptomatic low-volume FL).

• *Symptomatic patient.* Use of chemotherapy and/or immunotherapy to relieve symptoms. Treatment regimen should be chosen according to patient's performance status and age. The efficacy of maintenance rituximab is presently being evaluated.

• *Relapsed disease.* At the time of relapse it is important to evaluate the patient's symptoms and rule out biological progression as identified by histological evidence of progression, asynchronous growth in prior disease sites, appearance of 'B' symptoms and high LDH. Patients who have previously achieved a prolonged response to alkylating agents may be retreated, whereas those who failed to respond or progressed quickly may benefit from purine analogue-based therapies, with the concomitant administration of monoclonal antibodies. The addition of maintenance rituximab has improved results even further. Histological evidence of transformation or clinical suspicion of more aggressive disease indicates the need for anthracycline-containing regimens.

• *Further intensification of treatment.* Autologous SCT may be valuable in patients beyond CR1, providing a prolonged DFS and OS. Autologous SCT may be considered for patients who have histological evidence of transformation and who had received prior therapy for low-grade disease. Younger patients with progressive disease may be considered for allogeneic SCT, the only potentially curative therapy for patients with advanced disease. Useful outcomes have been seen in patients undergoing reduced-intensity allogeneic SCT.

Marginal zone B-cell lymphoma

The term 'marginal zone lymphoma' refers to three closely related lymphoma subtypes: nodal, primary splenic and extranodal lymphomas of mucosa-associated lymphoid tissue (MALT) (see Chapter 33). MALT lymphomas are the most common, representing about 7% of NHLs, of which at least one-third present as primary gastric lymphoma. These lymphomas are characterized by mature B cells lacking expression of CD5 and CD10.

MALT lymphoma

Staging
Up to 25% and 46% of patients with gastric and non-gastric MALT lymphoma respectively have disseminated disease at presentation so more extensive staging is indicated, including gastroduodenal endoscopy with multiple biopsies. For patients presenting with gastric MALT lymphoma, consideration should be given to endoscopic ultrasound for evaluation of depth of infiltration if this is not evaluable by CT. It is essential to assess the *H. pylori* status in all cases (see below). Wherever possible, the t(11;18) status, which is positive in about 30–40% of cases, should also be determined as this is of prognostic and therapeutic value.

Treatment
Helicobacter pylori infection appears to be a possible causative agent for development of gastric MALT lymphoma. Eradication of *H. pylori* with antibiotics appears to be initial effective therapy for localized gastric MALT lymphoma. Preliminary analysis of the LY03 trial (International Extranodal Lymphoma Study Group, the United Kingdom Lymphoma Group and the Groupe d'Etude des Lymphomes de l'Adulte) confirmed that at least half of the cases treated with antibiotics achieve histological complete remission. Median time for optimal response is 6 months, but some patients require 24 months to achieve complete remission. Response rate is highest in those whose disease is restricted to the mucosa (78%) and in those who have no nodal involvement by endoscopic ultrasonography. The extent of tumour penetration into the gastric wall is inversely correlated with complete remission rate.

Based on these data it seems reasonable to treat localized disease with antibiotic therapy, followed by strict endoscopic follow-up, including multiple biopsies 2 months after therapy to confirm eradication of bacteria, with repeated endoscopies and biopsies at least twice per year for 2 years to confirm histological regression of the tumour.

Histological complete remission does not necessarily predict cure: PCR for the detection of monoclonality remains positive in approximately half of those who achieve histological complete remission, suggesting suppression but not eradication of the lymphoma clone. In cases of unsuccessful eradication of *H. pylori* (PR/resistance disease), a second-line high-dose antibiotic regimen containing three or four drugs, one of which should be omeprazole (e.g. omeprazole, bismuth citrate, metronidazole, tetracycline), should be administered. Those patients whose tumour fails to regress despite second-line therapy frequently express t(11;18) or t(1;14) and those who present with *H. pylori*-negative localized gastric lymphoma may still respond to chemotherapy (e.g. oral cyclophosphamide/ chlorambucil), immunotherapy (monoclonal antibodies), radiotherapy or more rarely surgery, or combinations of these treatments. Data from small series suggest low-dose radiotherapy to be highly effective for patients with stage I/II disease, providing a 5-year DFS of 93%. At present there are no prospective randomized trials comparing these modalities.

Surgical resection is not recommended because the frequent multicentric nature of MALT lymphomas necessitates radical surgery with its attendant morbidity. Patients with advanced-stage disease are unlikely to be cured with antibiotics only and are therefore treated with systemic chemotherapy/immunotherapy up-front.

Splenic marginal zone lymphoma (with or without villous lymphocytes) and nodal variant

Splenic marginal zone lymphoma (SMZL) often presents as splenomegaly with bone marrow and peripheral blood involvement, with associated cytopenias, whereas lymph nodes/extranodal sites are usually spared. SMZL is characterized by micronodular infiltration of the spleen with marginal-zone differentiation; the immunophenotype usually shows cells positive for IgM and pan B antigens and negative for CD5, CD10, CD23 and cyclin D1, with variable expression of IgD, cytoplasmic immunoglobulin and CD43 (described further in Chapter 33).

It generally tends to have an indolent course; however, autoimmune complications are often associated with tumour progression, with increase of blastic forms and shorter survival. The median survival is around 10 years and more than 60% of patients are alive at 5 years. Approximately 10% of cases undergo transformation to DLBCL. To date no definitive curative therapy has been established and thus therapeutic intervention is generally reserved for patients with symptomatic active disease.

Splenectomy is considered to be the treatment of choice for symptomatic patients (pain, cytopenias), resulting in correction of pancytopenia and improvement in quality of life. Up to half of patients do not require further therapy. Retrospective studies have reported better OS in splenectomized patients than those treated with chemotherapy, although this may reflect selection bias. In the majority of evaluable cases a worsening of both the degree and pattern of bone marrow infiltration after splenectomy has been observed. A change in intrasinusoidal to nodular infiltration has been reported.

The utility of purine analogues with or without anti-CD20 antibodies has to be clarified in prospective trials, although retrospective data suggest these modalities to be effective.

Non-gastric MALT lymphoma

MALT lymphoma can also occur in salivary glands, skin, thyroid, conjunctiva, orbit, larynx, lung, breast, kidney, liver and prostate; in these cases it tends to have an indolent course. Treatment should be tailored to the patient, considering the site of disease and the patient's symptoms. Management therefore ranges from a 'watch-and-wait' policy, through various kinds of therapy, including chemotherapy, monoclonal antibodies (e.g. rituximab) and radiotherapy, to surgery.

A number of reports have suggested an association between ocular adnexal MALT lymphoma and *Chlamydia psittaci*, although this has precipitated much debate. However, there is wide variability (0–80%) in the seroprevalence of *C. psittaci* in series of ocular adnexal lymphomas, which may partly reflect methodological differences among published studies. Reponses to doxycycline have been documented in the treatment of ocular MALT lymphoma and this agent may be considered, although the time to response may be prolonged.

Waldenström macroglobulinaemia

Waldenström macroglobulinaemia (WM) is a clinical syndrome occurring in most patients with a lymphoplasmacytic lymphoma, rather than a specific pathological diagnosis. WM represents a clonal expansion of post-germinal centre lymphoid cells expressing IgM, CD19 and CD20. The morphological, immunophenotypic and genetic features are described in Chapter 33.

High IgM levels may cause hyperviscosity syndrome, manifested as fatigue, headache, blurred vision, mucosal bleeding, impaired cognition or coma. Other clinical manifestations include haemostatic abnormalities, polyneuropathies (which may be related to anti-myelin-associated glycoprotein antibodies), cryoglobulinaemias, cold agglutinin haemolytic anaemia and the consequences of tissue deposition such as amyloidosis. Depending on the degree of marrow infiltration, patients may present with mild anaemia or with severe pancytopenia. Progressive anaemia is the most common indication for initiation of treatment. Approximately one-third of patients present with lymphadenopathy, splenomegaly or hepatomegaly.

Factors predictive of poor prognosis include age over 65 years, anaemia, thrombocytopenia, serum monoclonal protein concentration above 70 g/L and raised levels of β_2-microglobulin. These factors form the basis of the International Prognostic Staging System for WM (IPSSWM).

Patient management ranges from 'watch and wait' for asymptomatic patients, through various types of chemotherapy (e.g. alkylating agents with or without steroids, CHOP, purine nucleoside analogues), monoclonal antibodies (e.g. rituximab) and immunomodulators (e.g. thalidomide), to autologous/allogeneic SCT. Patients presenting with hyperviscosity also need adjuvant plasmapheresis.

Chemotherapy

Alkylating agents (e.g. chlorambucil) with or without prednisolone have been the mainstay of treatment for patients with symptomatic WM, producing remissions in 50–75% of patients. Responses are usually slow and toxicity minimal provided the dose is adjusted for cytopenias. Response rates of 60% and median survival of about 60 months have been observed. Combination chemotherapy (CHOP or CVP) produces comparable response rates to single-agent alkylating agents and more rapid responses, but with greater toxicity. The advantages of regimens such as CHOP include the rapidity of response and the lack of compromise to subsequent stem cell harvesting.

Purine analogues (e.g. fludarabine and cladribine) appear to be active in both previously untreated patients and those who fail to respond to alkylating agents/relapsed disease, providing response rates of 38–85% and 30–50% respectively. One disadvantage of purine analogue therapy is the prolonged lymphopenia that results, with consequent risk of opportunistic infections. Prophylaxis against opportunistic infections (aciclovir and co-trimoxazole or pentamidine) during therapy and for approximately 6 months following completion of treatment is essential. Another concern is the recent reports suggesting an increased incidence of Richter transformation and development of secondary MDS/AML in WM patients treated with nucleoside analogue-containing regimens. These data favour limiting exposure of WM patients to nucleoside analogues, particularly younger patients.

Monoclonal antibodies

Several studies have shown rituximab to be active in WM, providing responses in up to 35% of previously untreated patients. However, rituximab can cause a sudden rise in serum IgM and viscosity in certain patients, which may lead to complications; therefore, close monitoring of these parameters and symptoms of hyperviscosity is recommended during therapy. Similarly, ^{90}Y-ibritumomab tiuxetan (Zevalin) is likely to be effective and a Phase I trial evaluating this monoclonal antibody in patients with WM is ongoing. Rituximab is commonly added to chemotherapy schedules with reported improvement in outcome.

Stem cell transplantation for Waldenström macroglobulinaemia

Several small studies have reported encouraging results with autologous SCT in heavily pretreated patients, providing high response rates (95%), with improved PFS in some patients. However, at least half of these patients relapse, and the impact of this approach on long-term survival is not known. Allogeneic SCT does produce prolonged remissions with potential cures compared with autologous SCT, but TRM approaches 40%. Future strategies in WM will include a plan to evaluate the role of autologous SCT along with biological agents (e.g. rituximab purging), maintenance strategies (including immunotherapy) and evaluation of non-myeloablative regimens containing fludarabine to achieve higher response rates and improve survival.

Novel therapies

Agents with efficacy include bortezomib, immunomodulatory drugs (thalidomide, lenalidomide), sildenafil (Viagra), Akt inhibitors and novel monoclonal antibodies and have been described in a number of small studies. A combination of these agents with chemotherapy may increase treatment efficacy, inhibiting diverse pathways that are important for tumour growth and survival.

Guidelines for Waldenström macroglobulinaemia

The Fourth International Workshop on WM, a consensus panel, published its recommendations for the treatment of patients with WM in 2009.

1 First-line combinations such as rituximab with nucleoside analogues with or without alkylating agents or with cyclophosphamide-based therapies (CHOP) or the combination of rituximab with thalidomide are recommended. Limiting exposure to nucleoside analogues is recommended in younger patients because of the reports of the associated increase in incidence of Richter transformation and development of secondary MDS/AML.

2 Patients with relapsed disease can be treated with an alternative first-line agent or with the same agent again. Thalidomide with or without chemotherapy can also be considered at relapse. In the salvage setting, reuse of a first-line regimen or use of a different regimen should be considered along with bortezomib or alemtuzumab.

3 Autologous SCT may be considered for patients with refractory or relapsing disease. However, patients considered for autologous SCT may fail mobilization following treatment with alkylating agents or nucleoside analogues.

4 Allogeneic transplantation should only be undertaken in the context of a clinical trial.

5 Plasmapheresis should be considered as interim therapy until definitive therapy can be initiated.

6 The panel reaffirmed its encouragement of the active enrolment of patients with WM onto innovative clinical trials whenever possible.

7 Patients should be stratified according to the IPSSWM.

Mantle cell lymphoma

This represents approximately 5–10% of NHLs, with a median age at presentation of 60 years. The majority of patients have advanced-stage disease at the time of diagnosis, with approximately 80% having stage IV disease, 50% having gastrointestinal involvement and 70% bone marrow involvement. The MIPI score (see Table 35.5) is a combined clinical and biological score devised by the European MCL Network after a retrospective analysis of 350 patients.

Typically, patients have a short response to treatment with frequent relapses and a median survival of 3–5 years. However, a minority (10–15%) of patients appear to have more indolent disease and are long-term survivors, suggesting a 'watch-and-wait' approach should be considered at diagnosis.

Conventional chemotherapy regimens do improve PFS, but rarely lead to cure. None of the following chemotherapeutic regimens – CVP, CHOP, MCP, fludarabine, bendamustine – seem to be significantly better than any other, providing an OS of only 3–5 years. The addition of rituximab to these regimens appears to improve remission rates but does not influence PFS or OS. A number of studies are addressing the merit of rituximab maintenance but this is unproven to date.

An alternative approach for patients who are fit for more intensive strategies is the Hyper-CVAD multidrug regimen, which incorporates high doses of methotrexate and cytarabine, and rituximab. Efficacy with this regimen was first described by the group at the M.D. Anderson Cancer Center who have recently reported a 7-year OS of 68% for patients under 65 years. Multicentre Phase II trials using this regimen performed by the Southwestern Oncology Group (SWOG) and researchers in Italy have not reproduced these impressive results, with 22–42% of patients not completing treatment due to toxicity.

The efficacy of another intensive approach has recently been described by the Nordic group in their MCL2 study. This incorporates intensive immunochemotherapy using 'maxi-CHOP', high-dose cytarabine and rituximab, and is consolidated by *in vivo* purged SCT. A 5-year OS of 74% was reported although the follow-up is short. A majority of patients achieved PCR negativity after SCT, which was associated with prolonged response duration.

Similar efficacy of up-front autologous SCT after chemoimmunotherapy (CHOP, high-dose cytarabine and rituximab) and *in vivo* purging has also been described recently in Phase II studies by the Groupe de l'Etude des Lymphomes de l'Adulte (GELA) and an Italian multicentre report. Prolonged follow-up of 10 years in the latter has shown that 71% of 28 patients are alive, with 50% of patients disease-free. A number of groups are also assessing the efficacy of maintenance rituximab after autologous SCT. The European MCL network has also identified that the achievement of molecular remission, after immunochemotherapy with or without autologous SCT, is a strong prognostic factor in patients with MCL.

Allogeneic transplantation is also considered for patients with MCL, although it is not standard practice to perform this up-front and is generally reserved for patients with relapsed disease. A retrospective analysis of reduced-intensity allogeneic SCT for MCL reported to the EBMT identified 279 patients transplanted between 1998 and 2006. At 1 and 3 years OS was 60% and 43% and PFS 49% and 29% respectively. Survival was significantly worse for patients with a poor performance status, refractory disease or those transplanted before 2002. The M.D. Anderson Cancer Center has recently reported the outcome of 30 patients, with disease beyond first remission, undergoing an allograft using fludarabine, cyclophosphamide and rituximab as a preparative regimen. Durable remissions were observed and a PFS of 5–9 years described. Donor chimerism of 95% or more was associated with disease control, while chronic GVHD was a major cause of TRM.

For patients who have previously received standard salvage regimens, novel agents such as mTOR inhibitors, bortezomib, immunomodulatory agents (lenalidomide and thalidomide) and flavopiridol have been used with reports of efficacy. Multicentre Phase II and III studies of the mTOR inhibitor temsirolimus (CCI-779) involving patients with relapsed or refractory MCL have been recently reported. ORRs of 22–38% have been described. Median duration of response of 7.1 months and median OS of 13.6 months were reported. Adverse effects were predominantly haematological and thrombocytopenia was the most frequent cause of dose reduction. Other mTOR inhibitors are being evaluated in Phase II studies. Whether the outcome of patients can be improved by combining an mTOR inhibitor with other agents while maintaining an acceptable safety profile is the subject of ongoing and future clinical trials.

A number of multicentre Phase II studies of bortezomib in patients with relapsed or refractory MCL have reported ORR of 33–47%. A median duration of response of 9 months and median time to progression of 6.2 months have been described. The most common adverse effects are peripheral neuropathy, fatigue and thrombocytopenia. Lenalidomide, an agent with antineoplastic, anti-angiogenic, pro-erythropoietic and immunomodulatory properties, has also been used for patients with relapsed and refractory MCL. A Phase II trial involving 15 MCL patients described an ORR of 53%, median duration of response of 13.7 months and median PFS of 5.6 months. The toxicities of therapy were predominantly haematological, but manageable with dose reduction or dose interruption. Flavopiridol, a cyclin inhibitor, and other specific cyclin-dependent kinase inhibitors have been shown to be biologically active and are being evaluated in MCL patients.

Aggressive B-cell NHL

Treatment of DLBCL is mainly based on anthracycline-containing combinations, with or without adjuvant radiotherapy. However, there are some variations in treatment related to patient age, performance status, stage, disease bulk (<10 cm vs. ≥10 cm), IPI risk group and presence of primary extranodal disease (see Table 35.3). The other histological entities, anaplastic large-cell lymphoma and grade 3b FL, are treated similarly.

A large international trial has suggested that in patients under 60 years of age, the presence of two of the following risk factors – raised LDH, stage III or IV and poor performance status – predicts a lower chance to achieve CR and increased risk of relapse (see Table 35.3).

Localized disease: non-bulky stage I, with no additional risk factors

The BNLI reported a 10-year DFS and OS of 35% and 67%, respectively, in 243 patients who were treated with local radiotherapy for stage I/IE disease. In patients younger than 60 years ($N = 140$), the actuarial cause-specific death approached 80%. It is therefore quite clear that local radiotherapy is insufficient and systemic treatment such as chemotherapy is necessary.

A significantly improved DFS and OS in patients who received combined modality treatment with a brief chemotherapy course (three cycles of anthracycline-containing regimen) followed by radiotherapy has been reported in a prospective randomized trial. Patients with non-bulky stage I disease with no additional risk factors (age >60 years, elevated serum LDH, performance status 2–4) have a 5-year OS of 94%. Patients with at least one of the above adverse risk factors have a 5-year OS of around 70%. One randomized study has shown that the outcome for patients older than 60 years with limited-stage disease and no risk factors is equivalent after four courses of R-CHOP chemotherapy to that after four courses of CHOP chemotherapy and involved-field radiotherapy. Consideration of this approach may be appropriate if radiotherapy is not thought feasible.

Stage II–IV disease

Patients with more advanced-stage disease should receive combination chemotherapy. It is now over 30 years since the doxorubicin-containing CHOP regimen was first introduced. Despite a CR rate of 60–70%, less than 40% remain disease-free at 5 years from diagnosis. Since that time, different chemotherapy regimens have been introduced (e.g. MACOP-B, m-BACOD; see Table 35.7), although none of them has proved superior to CHOP. Several prospective studies have failed to show any advantage of intensified regimens over CHOP, supporting the continued use of CHOP in DLBCL. A collaborative study by SWOG/Eastern Cooperative Oncology Group (ECOG), comparing CHOP with three different intensified regimens (MACOP-B, m-BACOD and Pro-MACECytabom), showed no survival advantage of any of these regimens compared with CHOP. However, it should be noted that most of the Phase III studies have compared CHOP with various chemotherapy regimens that contained a lower dose of doxorubicin and/or cyclophosphamide, two of the most potent drugs in DLBCL

therapy, which may partially explain the inferiority of these combinations.

Adjuvant immunotherapy has been shown to significantly improve patient outcomes. A prospective randomized trial performed by GELA in 399 elderly patients with previously untreated DLBCL demonstrated a significant advantage for CHOP-R over CHOP alone. Patients in the CHOP-R group had a higher CR rate (75% vs. 63%, $P < 0.005$), improved PFS (2-year disease progression of 9% vs. 22%, $P < 0.007$; 2-year relapse rate of 14% vs. 25%, $P = 0.002$) and increased OS (2-year OS 70% vs. 57%, $P < 0.007$), with no significant increase in treatment-related toxicity. This study identified CHOP-R as the gold-standard therapy in elderly patients with DLBCL. These results were corroborated in young patients with good-prognosis DLBCL in the MInT study.

The German High-Grade NHL Study Group (Deutsche Studiengruppe Hochmaligne Lymphome; DSHNHL) also demonstrated the efficacy of shortening intervals between CHOP from 3 weeks to 2 weeks (CHOP-14). This approach was also shown to improve the outcome of patients, notably without relevant additional toxicity. More recently, the RICOVER-60 study, performed by the DSHNHL, demonstrated that six cycles of R-CHOP-14 significantly improved event-free survival (EFS), PFS and OS over six cycles of CHOP-14 treatment for patients over 60 years with DLBCL. No further benefit was observed after eight cycles of chemoimmunotherapy.

Prophylactic therapy to the central nervous system

Patients with DLBCL who present with a high IPI score (particularly those with high LDH and/or extranodal disease) are at higher risk for CNS relapse and should therefore receive CNS prophylactic therapy (see CNS prophylaxis, p. 681).

Adjuvant radiotherapy

The role of adjuvant radiotherapy in DLBCL remains controversial. Although this kind of radiotherapy is recommended at present for patients with stage I/II disease, it is unclear if adjuvant radiotherapy has any benefit in patients with advanced (stage III–IV) bulky disease, who have completed six to eight cycles of systemic combination chemotherapy.

The maximum tumour (bulk) diameter (MTD) has been shown to be an adverse factor affecting outcome in many studies. Arbitrary cut-off points for bulky disease have been set between 5 cm and 10 cm, depending on clinical considerations, although a recent study in the rituximab era has identified a cut-off point of 10 cm to delineate those patients with bulky disease. The addition of rituximab decreased but did not eliminate the adverse prognostic effect of MTD in this study performed in young patients with good-prognosis DLBCL (MInT study).

Radiation may cause short- and long-term side-effects and therefore minimal effective doses should be delivered, aiming to minimize toxicity (e.g. salivary glands, orbital structures, lung, heart).

Up-front autologous stem cell transplantation

The merit of up-front (performed in CR1) autologous SCT is unproven. A meta-analysis of 15 randomized controlled trials including 3079 patients has recently been published. Overall treatment-related mortality was 6% in the group receiving autologous SCT and was not significantly different from that of the group receiving conventional chemotherapy (OR 1.33, 95% CI 0.91–1.93; $P = 0.14$). Thirteen studies including 2018 patients showed significantly higher CR rates in the group receiving autologous SCT (OR 1.32, 95% CI 1.09–1.59; $P = 0.004$). Despite higher CR rates after autologous SCT there was no OS or EFS benefit compared with conventional chemotherapy. The pooled HRs were 1.04 (95% CI 0.91–1.18; $P = 0.58$) and 0.93 (95% CI 0.81–1.07; $P = 0.31$) respectively. Subgroup analysis of prognostic groups according to the IPI did not show any survival difference between those receiving autologous SCT and controls in 12 trials, although there was suggestive but inconclusive evidence that poor-risk patients may benefit from autologous SCT. Whether the response of histological subtypes ('activated B cell subtype' vs. 'germinal centre') is different is unclear at present and may warrant evaluation. Further assessment of the role of autologous SCT for high-risk patients should be conducted in large trials with harmonized procedures and definitions, which would facilitate the comparability of results and improve the assessment of its value.

Autologous stem cell transplantation in relapsed and primary refractory disease

Once a patient has failed initial chemotherapy, the prognosis is poor and long-term OS is less than 10%. The prospective randomized multinational Parma trial demonstrated the superiority of intensified treatment in patients with sensitive relapse, providing a significantly longer EFS than those treated with chemotherapy. However, high-dose therapy followed by autologous SCT is effective only in those who have shown some response to conventional-dose second-line (salvage) chemotherapy prior to autologous SCT (PR or chemoresponsive relapse). A retrospective UK study of 57 lymphoma patients (26 with histologically aggressive NHL) identified that of 16 patients with progressive disease after first-line salvage, only one patient (4%) subsequently responded to second-line salvage regimens. The PFS and OS at 3 years in this subgroup was only 4%. Since patients who progress on first-line salvage therapy have a very low chance of responding to a second-line salvage regimen, they should therefore be considered instead for experimental therapies.

The subgroup of patients that fails to respond to induction is defined as 'primary refractory disease'. Attempts to overcome this biological resistance, by early autologous SCT, have failed to achieve better results than conventional chemotherapy. Autologous SCT should therefore be limited to those who respond to second-line chemotherapy.

The role of PET following second-line chemotherapy prior to autologous SCT has been evaluated in a number of studies. A positive FDG-PET scan before autologous SCT has been correlated with inferior PFS and OS and an increased risk for relapse.

Allogeneic stem cell transplantation in aggressive NHL

Some patients are likely to have a very poor prognosis with conventional therapy, including those who failed autologous SCT, those presenting with a very high IPI and those with special subtypes of aggressive NHL (e.g. γδ T-cell NHL). Such patients may be considered for allogeneic SCT. Several reports have suggested allogeneic SCT to be potentially curative in high-risk patients with chemosensitive disease. There is no certainty regarding the existence of a strong graft-versus-leukaemia effect in intermediate/high grade of the disease, whereas mortality following transplantation remains high, indicating that this treatment should be reserved for selected patients only.

There are scant data available at present regarding the role of low-intensity SCT in aggressive NHL, although a number of recent reports suggest there is a role for this approach. Although a relatively high TRM (32%) and a high relapse rate (33%) have been reported, the 4-year OS was 44% for patients with *de novo* DLBCL that was chemotherapy sensitive before reduced intensity transplantation. Chemotherapy-refractory patients had a poor outcome. The majority of patients included in these studies had very advanced disease, received multiple lines of therapy and failed a prior autologous transplantation procedure, which might have adversely affected results. There is little evidence to support a clinically relevant anti-DLBCL effect secondary to donor lymphocyte infusions from these series. Further studies that explore low-intensity SCT in earlier stages are ongoing.

Primary mediastinal B-cell lymphoma

Primary mediastinal B-cell lymphoma (PMBL) is a discrete clinicopathological entity, representing less than 3% of all non-NHL cases. The disease affects females more frequently than men, and peaks in incidence in the third and fourth decades. Molecular analyses have revealed it to be distinct from other types of large B-cell lymphoma. PMBL typically presents with a bulky mass in the anterior mediastinum and symptoms related to local compressive effects are not uncommon.

Initial therapy is critical in treating PMBL as salvage therapy for recurrence or progressive disease is of limited efficacy. However, this creates a challenge in delivering the most effective therapy while minimizing the long-term sequelae in a young patient population. Retrospective analyses suggest patients with PMBL may respond better to third-generation multiagent chemotherapy regimens (i.e. MACOP-B and VACOP-B) than to CHOP. The addition of rituximab may mitigate such differences and may also diminish the role of consolidation radiotherapy.

Intravascular large B-cell lymphoma

Intravascular large B-cell lymphoma is an extremely rare form of NHL and is characterized by an accumulation of large neoplastic B cells within blood vessel lumina. These lymphomas preferentially affect the elderly and involve the CNS, reported in approximately 30% of patients, lungs and skin. Prognosis is generally poor. Patients presenting with only skin lesions appear to have a significantly better survival than patients with other clinical presentations (3-year OS 56% vs. 22%). Multiagent chemotherapy using agents with higher CNS bioavailability is the preferred mode of treatment. The role of autologous SCT in younger patients with unfavourable features is being explored.

Extranodal lymphomas

At least 25% of NHLs arise from tissues other than lymph nodes, including sites that normally contain no lymphatic tissue. The incidence of NHL, particularly primary extranodal lymphoma, is gradually increasing (e.g. primary CNS/gastrointestinal/breast), most probably due to the increase in viral infections, especially HIV, and exposure to environmental factors.

Primary gastrointestinal lymphoma

Gastrointestinal lymphoma is the most common form of extranodal lymphoma, accounting for 30–40% of cases and 4–20% of all NHL cases.

Diffuse large-cell lymphoma of the stomach
Advanced gastrointestinal DLBCL tends to behave primarily like nodal advanced disease. These tumours were traditionally treated with gastrectomy; however, recent data suggest that this strategy is unnecessary in most cases, where combination chemoimmunotherapy (six to eight courses of R-CHOP) with or without adjuvant radiotherapy provides high response and cure rates. For patients with localized gastric diffuse large-cell lymphoma, short-course chemoimmunotherapy (three to four courses of R-CHOP) followed by involved-field radiotherapy has been shown to be effective.

In some cases, histological transformation of MALT lymphoma may have occurred and therefore it is reasonable to add anti-*H. pylori* therapy, aiming to eradicate the bacteria and avoid potential relapses. Furthermore, anti-*H. pylori* therapy applied in these '*H. pylori*-positive' cases yields a high response rate, suggesting that an antigenic drive may be present in a subset of aggressive gastric lymphomas.

Diffuse large-cell lymphoma of the intestine
At present, there are no studies that demonstrate surgery to be unnecessary, and management is therefore based on surgical resection followed by systemic chemotherapy.

Immunoproliferative small intestinal disease
Immunoproliferative small intestinal disease (IPSID), also known as α-chain disease, arises in small intestinal MALT and is characterized by the expression of a monotypic truncated immunoglobulin α-heavy chain without an associated light chain. IPSID is mostly found in young adults of low socioeconomic class in developing countries. The aetiology of this disease is unclear, although various causative pathogens (e.g. *Campylobacter jejuni*) and genetic and toxic mechanisms have been proposed.

Half of all IPSID patients present with concurrent intestinal B-cell lymphoma, whereas most of the remaining patients develop frank lymphoma within a few years. Whereas patients with early-stage disease may respond to antibiotics, those who present with more advanced disease should be treated with chemotherapy.

Primary CNS lymphoma

Primary CNS lymphoma is defined as lymphoma arising in the craniospinal axis (brain, spinal cord, leptomeninges and eye). It is usually disseminated within the nervous system at presentation (in 50% of immunocompetent patients and in nearly 100% of HIV-positive patients). The histology in most cases is compatible with diffuse large-cell lymphoma (90%) or non-cleaved cell lymphoma. Age, poor performance status, involvement of deep structures, high LDH level and a high protein level in the CSF have been shown to predict poor prognosis.

Previously, the traditional therapy was based on whole-brain irradiation. Unfortunately, the median survival was 12–18 months and 5-year survival less than 10%, suggesting that radiotherapy is insufficient. The combination of high-dose methotrexate (>3 g/m² over 2–3 hours) and radiotherapy appears to be more effective, providing a 5-year OS of 30–50%, but may cause delayed neurotoxicity, especially in patients older than 60 years. Many groups avoid radiotherapy up-front in these older patients and defer radiotherapy until relapse. A recent randomized study has shown that the efficacy of high-dose methotrexate is improved by using it in combination with cytarabine. Other protocols that include combinations of other CNS-penetrating agents have been evaluated but their efficacy has not been directly compared.

Further attempts to reduce long-term neurotoxicity in this group, delivering lower doses of radiotherapy or omitting radiotherapy, by providing intensified chemotherapy regimens such as up-front autologous SCT have been described and are being explored further.

Treatment of secondary CNS lymphoma

Secondary CNS lymphoma may present as cranial nerve palsies, headache, cognitive disturbance or spinal cord compression. It may occur concurrently with a systemic lymphoma, during therapy or may present as a late relapse.

There is no consensus on how best to treat secondary CNS lymphoma and scant data regarding the effects of treatment on survival, quality of life and cognitive function. Whether the CNS relapse is confined to brain parenchyma or the leptomeninges alters the approach. Options for the former include chemotherapy (high-dose methotrexate or combination chemotherapy), immunotherapy, cranial radiotherapy and autologous SCT. These approaches are often combined. A large retrospective analysis of 113 cases with isolated CNS relapse involving brain parenchyma reported a median OS of 1.6 years (95% CI 0.9–2.6 years), although this does not reflect the outcome of all patients. Other studies have described a median survival of less than 6–12 months with no survival difference in patients with leptomeningeal, parenchymal or combined parenchymal/leptomeningeal disease. Treatment of isolated leptomeningeal involvement commonly includes intrathecal methotrexate or cytarabine. The latter agent is also available as a liposomal product and cytocidal levels are maintained for at least 14 days in the CSF.

Nodal peripheral T-cell NHL (see also Chapter 30)

Peripheral T-cell lymphomas (PTCLs) are a biologically and clinically heterogeneous group of rare disorders that result from clonal proliferation of mature post-thymic lymphocytes. There is geographical variation in the frequency of the different subtypes and in Europe, PTCL unspecified, anaplastic large-cell lymphoma (ALCL) and angioimmunoblastic T-cell lymphoma (AITL) account for about three-quarters of all cases. PTCL unspecified, and particularly natural killer (NK)-cell lymphomas, are more common in Asia and the Far East.

Extranodal presentation is common in PTCL. Paraneoplastic features are well described, including eosinophilia, haemophagocytic syndrome and autoimmune phenomena (particularly seen in AITL). Most patients present with unfavourable IPI scores (>3) and poor performance status. A number of T-cell-specific IPI features have been described, including age,

performance status, LDH, bone marrow involvement and Ki-67 expression.

Excluding anaplastic lymphoma kinase (ALK)-positive ALCL, which has a good outcome, 5-year survival for other nodal and extranodal T-cell lymphomas is about 30%. Treatment of T-cell lymphomas is commonly based on multiagent chemotherapy (e.g. CHOP), although patient outcome remains disappointing and the majority of patients die of their disease. A number of small Phase II studies have assessed (and are assessing) the efficacy and toxicity of combining CHOP chemotherapy with alemtuzumab. Whether outcome is improved is unclear although infectious toxicity is greater. CD52 expression in PTCL is unclear, with some groups reporting a high rate of CD52 negativity. Gemcitabine-containing combination chemotherapy regimens (gemcitabine, cisplatin and methylprednisolone: GEM-P, PEGS, CHOP-EG) have been shown to be efficacious, although no comparative study has been performed. At present, no chemotherapy regimens have been found to be superior to CHOP.

The similarity in PFS and OS is an indication of the poor response to second-line therapies. Consideration for up-front autologous SCT (performed in first CR) is recommended (except for ALK-positive ALCL) as improvements in long-term outcome have been reported in prospective and retrospective analyses. However, approximately 25% of patients show disease progression during first-line chemotherapy and thus are not candidates for autologous SCT.

Initial treatment of refractory disease is usually with platinum-based combination chemotherapy prior to consolidation with a transplant. Alternatively, purine analogue or gemcitabine-containing combination chemotherapy regimens may be considered. There are also a number of experimental agents that have shown promise and patients should also be considered for inclusion in suitable clinical trials where available. Early data regarding the efficacy of histone deacetylase inhibitors (Depsipeptide), pralatrexate (a novel antifolate agent) and antibodies to CD52, CD25 and the IL-2–toxin conjugate dinileukin difitox (ONTAK) have been reported. Patients with chemosensitive relapsed disease may be considered subsequently for allograft. In addition, a number of agents, including ciclosporin, thalidomide, rituximab and bevacizumab (MAb to VEGF-A), are being assessed for the treatment of AITL in Phase II trials.

Enteropathy-associated T-cell lymphoma

Enteropathy-associated T-cell lymphoma is an aggressive tumour of the small bowel that is strongly associated with coeliac disease, of which it may be the presenting feature in adults. A gluten-free diet appears to markedly reduce the risk for lymphoma. The outcome is poor, partly due to the biology of the disease and partly the performance status of patients in the setting of malabsorption and malnutrition. Conventional chemotherapy gives poor results but there are some long-term survivors (~10%). Dose intensification is often attempted, using salvage-type chemotherapy with or without high-dose methotrexate, as is up-front autologous SCT but has yet to be confirmed as beneficial in adequate trials and must be seen as experimental.

Anaplastic large-cell lymphoma

The WHO classification recognizes two distinct subtypes of ALCL, primary systemic and primary cutaneous types, which exhibit differences in immunophenotype, genetics and clinical behaviour (see Chapter 33). It is now known that approximately 60% of cases of systemic ALCL express the ALK protein (ALK⁺) and have a significantly superior survival to ALK-negative cases. Since cases of ALK-negative ALCL appear to have a prognosis similar to that of PTCL unspecified, it has been suggested that they should be treated similarly.

Systemic ALK-positive ALCL occurs at a young age (median <30 years) and shows a male predominance. The majority of patients present with 'B' symptoms, advanced-stage disease and involvement of multiple extranodal sites. However, the majority of patients fall into lower IPI categories because of good performance status, younger age and a normal LDH. Combination anthracycline-based chemotherapy (e.g. CHOP) is associated with a 5-year OS of 60–93%. Prognosis is so good in this group of patients that transplantation should only be considered at relapse. Platinum-based chemotherapy is standard for patients with relapsed disease, although monoclonal antibodies directed against CD30 and/or specific inhibitors of NPM–ALK are under investigation. Patients with ALK-positive ALCL autografted at relapse have a 3-year EFS/PFS/OS of 67–100%.

Hepatosplenic T-cell lymphoma

This is a rare entity, affecting mainly younger men. It is a distinctive and aggressive disease with a characteristic presentation (liver, spleen and bone marrow involvement but rarely lymphadenopathy) and clinical course. Most patients exhibit a characteristic phenotype (typical histology showing sinusoidal infiltration with tumour cells in the affected tissues), expression of the γδ TCR and an isochromosome 7q abnormality (described in Chapter 33).

The outlook is very poor with scant data regarding effective therapies and a number of single case reports concerning treatment with CHOP, alemtuzumab, purine analogues (fludarabine, pentostatin or cladribine) or their combination. However, responses are often transient and there is increasing enthusiasm for early allogeneic SCT, although its efficacy is also unclear due to the small number of patients in published reports. A recent literature review identified 7 of 17 (40%) patients who had been treated with allogeneic SCT and who were alive and in CR. Thus

prolonged remission duration is observed in some patients after allogeneic SCT and the outcome appears to be superior compared with chemotherapy.

Extranodal NK/T-cell lymphoma, nasal type

This is an aggressive, largely extranodal lymphoma, usually of NK-cell type but with recognized T-cell phenotypic variants. These are very rare in the Western world but commoner in Asia and South America. It is usually associated with EBV and often presents as localized disease in and around the nasal structures. Local extension and dissemination is frequent, usually to regional nodes and distant extranodal structures such as skin, testis and gut. An association with the haemophagocytic syndrome has been described.

Survival at 5 years ranges from 20 to 35% in different series but most of the cases included in these figures are localized stage I/II nasal presentations, and when considered separately the patients with disseminated disease almost all die, mostly within a few months. Involved-field radiotherapy produces excellent initial control for patients with stage I/II disease, and may be followed by CHOP-based chemotherapy, although its merit is unclear.

Adult T-cell leukaemia lymphoma (see also Chapter 30)

ATLL is divided into four different clinical subtypes, with the acute (leukaemic) and lymphomatous subtypes being more common than the chronic and smouldering forms. Lymphadenopathy, hepatosplenomegaly, skin lesions and hypercalcaemia are observed in the majority of patients. The prognosis for acute and lymphoma subtypes is poor, with a median survival of only 6.2 and 10.2 months respectively. Patients are immunocompromised and opportunistic infections are common, including *Pneumocystis jirovecii* pneumonia, aspergillosis or candidiasis, *Strongyloides stercoralis* and cytomegalovirus.

Despite significant advances in understanding the pathogenesis of ATLL, results of treatment remain disappointing. Responses to conventional chemotherapy are poor. A number of Phase II studies of the combination of the antiretroviral drug zidovudine and interferon alfa have reported significant activity in patients with ATLL and have been administered successively with chemotherapeutic regimens such as CHOP. Conjugated and unconjugated monoclonal antibodies (anti-CD25, anti-CD4, anti-CD52) have all been tested in small numbers of patients. Other agents being evaluated include arsenic trioxide and bortezomib.

There appears to be minimal long-term benefit in autografting patients with ATLL, with the majority of patients relapsing within 1 year of transplantation. Prolonged DFS has been described after allogeneic SCT, with many of the reports derived from retrospective analyses of the Japanese Registry Data. Age and remission status at transplantation have been identified as significant predictors of survival and since the median age at presentation with ATLL is approximately 60 years, reduced-intensity conditioning is generally favoured. The estimated 3-year overall and relapse-free survival rates have been reported as approximately 45% and 35% respectively.

Histiocytic and dendritic cell neoplasms

Precursor haematological neoplasm: CD4⁺CD56⁺ haematodermic neoplasm

The derivation of this clinically aggressive neoplasm (previously called blastic NK-cell lymphoma), with a high incidence of cutaneous involvement and risk of leukaemic dissemination, is thought to be a plasmacytoid dendritic cell precursor. Although patients typically present with cutaneous manifestations, about half have nodal or bone marrow involvement at presentation and many rapidly develop extracutaneous spread. The coexistence of myelodysplasia has been described in approximately 15–20% of cases.

The prognosis is very poor, with most patients dying from their disease within 2 years. Remissions achieved by systemic chemotherapy are rarely maintained and resistance to subsequent chemotherapy is common. Whether patients should be treated with regimens used in acute leukaemias or aggressive lymphomas is unclear.

High-grade lymphoma

Burkitt lymphoma and small non-cleaved Burkitt-like lymphoma

These are highly aggressive forms of NHL, frequently involving extranodal organs (e.g. CNS in 20%) but usually without tumour cells detected in the peripheral blood and characterized by dysregulation of the *MYC* oncogene. BL is a distinct entity that includes endemic and sporadic types and cases associated with immunodeficiency or immunosuppression. Transcriptional and genomic profiling has defined BL, an entity with a favourable outcome, more precisely. Mature aggressive B-cell lymphomas with chromosomal breakpoints at the *MYC* locus but without a gene signature for BL conversely have an adverse clinical outcome.

Effective treatment of patients with BL is based on multidrug combination chemotherapy (e.g. CODOX-M/IVAC, Hyper-CVAD; see Table 35.7) that includes drugs such as methotrexate and cytarabine , which penetrate the CNS extremely well.

Rituximab is commonly added to such regimens, although randomized trials demonstrating its efficacy have not been performed. Approximately 50–80% of adult patients can be cured with these intensive chemotherapy regimens, and in paediatric populations the cure rate is even higher.

The risk of tumour lysis syndrome, especially after initiating chemotherapy, is relatively high, reflecting the high proliferation rate of tumour cells. Vigorous hydration with alkalinization, accompanied by administration of recombinant urate oxidase (rasburicase), or a uric acid synthesis inhibitor such as allopurinol, are very important in preventing/reducing the severity of this complication (see also Chapter 26). Hypercalcaemia is also frequent at presentation and needs appropriate therapy with hydration and bisphosphonates.

Lymphoblastic lymphoma

Lymphoblastic lymphoma is a lymphoproliferative disorder derived from early B/T cells and patients should therefore be treated as for ALL (see Chapters 24 and 25) using protocols such as UKALL 2003, UKALL XII, Hyper-CVAD or German NHL-BFM 90. These generally use multidrug induction followed by high-dose methotrexate, with or without consolidation chemotherapy blocks (depending on stage).

Autologous SCT (with or without TBI) in first remission gives as good an outcome as extended chemotherapy and both treatment modalities are followed. Most adult studies show EFS of 30–50%, which is inferior to outcome in paediatric studies. Allogeneic SCT provides a lower relapse rate compared with autologous SCT; however, long-term survival is not necessarily higher due to increased TRM as observed with allograft. Allogeneic SCT is commonly deferred for the relapsed patients with chemosensitive disease.

Tumour regression in lymphoblastic lymphoma is often incomplete and has not been shown to be predictive for relapse. The role for consolidative mediastinal radiotherapy in those with residual masses is contentious. In children it appears to add to toxicity without leading to improved outcome. Consequently, paediatric studies reserve local radiotherapy for 'high-risk' patients, such as those with suboptimal volume response of a mediastinal mass during induction chemotherapy. In adults, a proportion (12–47%) of patients who subsequently relapse had undergone previous radiotherapy, often to the site of subsequent relapse, suggesting doubtful benefit. One study suggested that higher radiotherapy doses (36 Gy) were associated with reduced local relapse rates but such doses are associated with increased toxicity.

The efficacy of nelarabine, a nucleoside analogue prodrug of 9-β-D-arabinofuranosylguanine, for the treatment of patients with T-cell lymphoblastic lymphoma whose disease has not responded to, or has relapsed after, treatment has been described. The most common adverse events associated with nelarabine are neurotoxic and have been dose-limiting.

Lymphomatoid granulomatosis

Lymphomatoid granulomatosis is a rare angiocentric and angiodestructive lymphoreticular proliferation that usually primarily affects the lungs, although other sites such as skin, CNS and kidney may be involved. The immunophenotype has been described as a T-cell-rich, EBV-associated, B-cell lymphoproliferative disorder. However, primary CNS lymphomatoid granulomatosis appears to be derived from clonal T cells in some cases and appears not to be associated with EBV.

Treatment is currently not well established. Spontaneous remission has been reported. The therapeutic approach ranges from immunomodulatory agents (corticosteroids, interferon, ciclosporin), chemotherapy (cyclophosphamide, CHOP) or immunotherapy (rituximab). A number of case reports have described the efficacy of autografting. The prognosis of this disorder has been considered to be poor, with a 5-year survival in less than 50% of cases and with progression to lymphoma in 13% of cases. Primary CNS lymphomatoid granulomatosis appears to have a better prognosis.

Castleman disease

Castleman disease is a rare atypical lymphoproliferative disorder classified according to the histopathology of the affected lymph nodes as hyaline–vascular, plasma-cell type or a mixed variant of the two (discussed in more detail in Chapter 33). Classification may also be based on whether the disease is localized or multifocal, the latter often associated with systemic features and abnormal laboratory findings.

Localized Castleman disease

Localized Castleman disease is commonly of the hyaline–vascular variant and patients are usually asymptomatic. It usually presents in young adults with isolated masses in the mediastinum (60–75%), neck (20%) or less commonly the abdomen (10%). Excision of the affected lymph node results in subsequent cure in a majority of cases. Patients with the plasma-cell type or the mixed-type variant frequently have systemic manifestations and the disease is multifocal with widespread adenopathy and multiorgan involvement (see below).

Multicentric Castleman disease

Multicentric Castleman disease (MCD) is a relatively rare lymphoproliferative disorder that occurs in the fourth or fifth decade of life but at younger ages in people who are HIV positive. Today, MCD is most commonly diagnosed in individuals infected with HIV, although the effect of HAART on incidence and prognosis is unclear.

MCD typically presents with fevers, multifocal lymphadenopathy, hepatosplenomegaly, polyneuropathies, effusions and weight loss. Laboratory investigations may reveal thrombocytopenia, anaemia, raised serum C-reactive protein, hypoalbuminaemia and hypergammaglobulinaemia. Not only is MCD itself potentially fatal due to organ failure but it is also associated with an increased incidence of NHL. HHV-8 has been found to be present in 100% and 50% of cases of HIV-positive and HIV-negative MCD respectively.

The diagnosis is established on lymph node biopsy and the characteristic features of HIV-associated MCD are interfollicular plasmablasts that express the HHV-8 latent nuclear antigen. These plasmablasts also express high levels of λ light-chain-restricted IgM, but are polyclonal and do not contain somatic mutations in their *IGV* genes, suggesting that they arise from naive B lymphocytes.

There are no definitive gold-standard treatments for MCD. No randomized trials have been conducted on account of the infrequency of the diagnosis and often only case reports have appeared in the literature. Resolution of systemic symptoms can be achieved with chemotherapy (etoposide or vinblastine) but relapse occurs and many patients remain dependent on chemotherapy for life. Lymphoma schedules such as CHOP or immunomodulatory therapy with thalidomide or interferon alfa have also been used, with efficacy described. The initiation of HAART in HIV-positive patients, often in combination with chemotherapy, appears to be well tolerated and is associated with immune reconstitution. The role of antiviral agents (ganciclovir, cidofovir, foscarnet) is unclear. Administration of the humanized anti-IL-6 receptor antibody to patients with MCD has been associated with improvements in inflammatory parameters, fatigue and lymphadenopathy. This likely reflects that dysregulated overproduction of IL-6 underlies at least some of the clinical abnormalities. However, benefit was not sustained and recurrence was observed.

A number of small studies have shown that rituximab can induce impressive clinical, biochemical and radiological sustained response in HIV-related MCD. Its efficacy as initial therapy and for relapsed patients has been described. Exacerbation of Kaposi sarcoma lesions after rituximab has been described.

CNS prophylaxis in aggressive NHL

There is a 5% incidence of CNS relapse in most large studies of aggressive NHL. These include DLBCL, PTCL, the blastoid variant of MCL, ATLL, NK-cell lymphoma and primary mediastinal B-cell lymphoma. The factors of importance include high IPI score, elevated LDH, involvement of more than one

Table 35.11 Risk factors for CNS involvement.

High IPI score
Extranodal sites involved (0 or 1 vs. >1)
Raised LDH level
Age < 60 years
Specific involvement of the following organs: bone marrow,
    testis, paranasal sinuses, Waldeyer ring
Low albumin level
Retroperitoneal glands

extranodal site and specific sites such as bone marrow, testis, breast, epidural space, paranasal sinuses and Waldeyer ring (Table 35.11).

The use of rituximab has recently been shown to be associated with a significantly lower incidence of CNS disease in elderly patients with aggressive CD20-positive lymphoma treated in the RICOVER-60 trial. Patients treated with R-CHOP-14 had a relative risk for CNS disease of 0.58 (95% CI 0.3, 1.0; $P = 0.046$) compared with patients treated with CHOP-14. CNS prophylaxis with intrathecal methotrexate was offered to patients with involvement of bone marrow, testes, upper neck, or head. The estimated 2-year incidence of CNS disease was 6.9% (CI 4.5, 9.3) after CHOP-14 and 4.1% (CI 2.3, 5.9) after R-CHOP-14.

The outcome of those who develop CNS relapse is extremely poor, with a median survival of less than 6 months (discussed later). Thus intrathecal chemotherapy is routinely administered to patients considered at high risk. However, agreement regarding the optimal regimen, the frequency of administration and whether high-dose systemic (methotrexate, cytarabine) chemotherapy should also be offered is lacking.

All patients with BL or lymphoblastic lymphoma should receive CNS prophylaxis with both intrathecal and high-dose systemic chemotherapy, as the observed incidence of CNS relapse without prophylaxis is about 20%. Standard treatment incorporates both intrathecal therapy and high-dose systemic chemotherapy with methotrexate and cytarabine.

There is no evidence to support routine use of CNS prophylaxis in any patient with low-grade lymphoma.

Suggested algorithm for therapy of aggressive NHL

At diagnosis

• Anthracycline-containing combination chemotherapy with rituximab (CHOP-R) is already proven to be superior to CHOP in patients who are more than 60 years old.
• Patients with intermediate-high/high IPI score (particularly those who present with raised LDH and/or extranodal involvement) should receive CNS prophylactic therapy.

• Adjuvant radiotherapy may be considered in patients with bulky disease.
• No clear role for up-front autologous SCT (performed in CR1).

At relapse

• Second-line regimens (e.g. ESHAP, DVIP, DHAP, mini-BEAM), followed by autologous SCT.
• Allogeneic SCT may be considered in patients who have failed autologous SCT or in those with special subtypes of NHL (e.g. γδ lymphoma).

Lymphoma in the immunocompromised patient

Most frequently, the disease is diagnosed in patients with acquired immunodeficiency caused by HIV infection (AIDS-related lymphoma) or immunosuppressive drugs (e.g. PTLD).

AIDS-related NHL

The histological diagnosis in the majority of such patients is diffuse large-cell lymphoma (60%) or BL (30%). Patients tend to present with advanced-stage disease, 'B' symptoms, extranodal sites of disease and bone marrow involvement. Prior to the introduction of HAART (highly active antiretroviral therapy), treatment with standard-dose chemotherapy induced high levels of toxicity and a high incidence of opportunistic infections. Since the regular use of HAART, the immunolgical function and haemopoietic reserve of these patients has improved dramatically. This is associated with a reduction in the incidence of infections and an outcome similar to that of non-HIV-infected patients. Increasingly, similar treatment strategies adopted for HIV-negative patients (e.g. CHOP, m-BACOD, CDE, EPOCH, CODOX-M/IVAC) with or without rituximab are used. The use of rituximab has been associated with a significant reduction in progression of lymphoma on treatment, and in death due to lymphoma. However, an increase in infectious deaths has been described in patients with CD4 cell counts less than 50×10^6/L and thus caution or more vigilant antimicrobial prophylaxis and surveillance is advocated in this cohort.

Improvements in the immune function and haematological reserves of HAART-treated patients, and better supportive care, have made stem cell mobilization and high-dose chemotherapy approaches possible in HIV-infected patients. The feasibility and efficacy of autologous SCT for HIV-positive patients with relapsed lymphoma has been widely described by single centres and cooperative groups. In a recently published retrospective study performed by the EBMT, a similar outcome for HIV-negative and HIV-positive lymphoma patients undergoing autologous SCT has been described.

HIV-positive patients with BL should also receive intensive regimens used in the HIV-negative setting, such as CODOX-M/IVAC with or without rituximab, as the outcome has been shown to be equivalent to that in HIV-negative patients in small studies.

Post-transplant lymphoproliferative disorder

PTLD ranges from polyclonal plasmacytic hyperplasia to monoclonal B-cell proliferation, polymorphic hyperplasia/lymphoma, immunoblastic lymphoma or myeloma. EBV causes the majority of these disorders: impaired T-cell function leads to proliferation of latently EBV-infected polyclonal B cells, whereas subsequent genomic mutations result in monoclonal PTLD. Prevention of EBV infection/reactivation may therefore be essential. Antiviral agents (e.g. aciclovir, ganciclovir), passive immunotherapy and pre-emptive immunotherapy, using cytotoxic T lymphocytes targeted against EBV, are all applied to prevent PTLDs, with variable success.

The optimal treatment of PTLD is still not clearly defined due to lack of randomized Phase III trials. Most published data are in the form of case series. Therapeutic options in PTLD include immunosuppression reduction, transplant organ resection, radiotherapy, chemotherapy and immunotherapy. Patients may respond to reduction in immunosuppressive therapy, especially those who develop PTLD within 1 year from transplant (ORR 80% vs. 10% in patients who developed PTLD beyond 1 year). Case series and Phase II studies of rituximab monotherapy following failure of reduction of immunosuppression have confirmed efficacy in inducing remission in a proportion of patients (44–65%) with PTLD. Toxicity appears to be low, but significant numbers of patients progressed on therapy or relapsed after rituximab, some died of lymphoma and many required intensification to chemotherapy. A risk score for identifying patients with PTLD most likely to respond to rituximab monotherapy has been proposed, using age over 60 years, performance status ECOG 2–4 and raised LDH as poor risk markers. Chemotherapy (i.e. CHOP) is usually reserved for those patients who have failed to respond to previous modalities. Adoptive immunotherapy following allogeneic SCT may also be effective. Donor lymphocyte infusion may cause severe GVHD, limiting its use. In contrast, anti-EBV cytotoxic T lymphocytes do provide a more specific effect, but are less available, being produced over weeks to months by expert laboratories and their infusion is associated with regulatory challenges.

Cutaneous lymphomas

Primary cutaneous T-cell lymphoma

Primary cutaneous T-cell lymphoma (CTCL) comprises a heterogeneous group of extranodal NHLs, of which mycosis fungoides/Sézary syndrome are the most common clinicopathological subtypes (see also Chapter 30). Mycosis fungoides is characterized by distinct clinical stages of cutaneous disease consisting of patches/plaques, tumours and erythroderma in which the whole skin is involved. Sézary syndrome is defined by the presence of erythroderma, peripheral lymphadenopathy and a minimum number of Sézary cells within the peripheral blood. These clinicopathological entities are closely related pathogenetically but are distinct from other less common types of primary CTCL, including primary cutaneous CD30-positive lymphoproliferative disorders, which have an excellent prognosis, and other CTCL variants which generally have intermediate or poor prognosis and are more closely related to peripheral T-cell lymphomas.

For mycosis fungoides, two staging systems are in regular use, including a TNM (primary tumour, regional nodes, metastasis) system and a clinical staging system specifically designed for CTCL. Most cases of primary CTCL are not curable but patients with very early stage disease (IA) are highly unlikely to die of their disease. The 5-year and 10-year OS are 80% and 57%, respectively, with disease-specific survival rates of 89% and 75% at 5 and 10 years respectively. Patients with folliculotropic variants of mycosis fungoides have a worse prognosis. Therapy is based on 'skin-targeted modalities', including PUVA (psoralen with UVA irradiation), electron beam radiation, narrowband UVA (NB-UVA), topical steroids, nitrogen mustard, carmustine and vitamin D. PUVA and NB-UVA remain the gold-standard therapies at early stages (IA/IIA), whereas systemic therapies are reserved for more advanced stages. Treatment options in these cases may include chlorambucil, methotrexate, doxorubicin, etoposide, retinoids, rexinoids, interferon, extracorporeal photopheresis, interferon alfa/gamma, or conjugated monoclonal antibodies (e.g. anti-CD52) and immunotoxins (e.g. IL-2 receptor-specific fusion protein combined with diphtheria toxin, which selectively targets the IL-2 receptor on malignant and activated T cells). Systemic therapies are frequently combined with topical agents. Interferon alfa with or without phototherapy appears to be highly effective in advanced disease, providing responses in up to 80% of patients. Other immunomodulatory agents, such as recombinant human IL-2, anti-idiotype vaccines and gene therapies, are under investigation.

Young patients with biologically aggressive mycosis fungoides who have failed conventional therapies may be considered for allogeneic SCT. There is increasing enthusiasm for reduced-intensity approaches for a number of reasons: the average age of patients with CTCL is 60 years, many patients have chronically infected skin ulcers and the risk of life-threatening sepsis is lower. Efficacy of reduced-intensity allogeneic SCT has been reported by a number of groups.

Sézary syndrome is an aggressive CTCL, characterized by erythroderma, lymphadenopathy and circulating malignant T cells with ceribriform nuclei. Therapy is usually based on a combination of systemic and topical therapy: chemotherapy (e.g. alkylating agents, including temozolomide), IL-2–diphtheria toxin, anti-CD52 monoclonal antibodies, retinoids/rexinoid, accompanied with topical steroids or PUVA. Extracorporeal photopheresis may also be effective, especially in those who present with a low number of circulating Sézary cells. Patients with Sézary syndrome have an 11% 5-year survival, with a median survival of 32 months from diagnosis.

CD30-positive large-cell lymphoma is the most common form of non-mycosis fungoides primary CTLC that appears to have an indolent course, with 5-year survival in 90% of cases. These patients are usually treated successfully with spot radiation or surgical excision, and only those who progress are considered for systemic treatment. On the other hand, patients with CD30-negative large T-cell lymphoma tend to have aggressive disease with poor prognosis and should therefore receive multiagent systemic chemotherapy at diagnosis, irrespective of disease stage.

Cutaneous B-cell lymphoma

Primary cutaneous B-cell lymphoma (CBCL) comprises a group of lymphomas characterized by dominant infiltration of clonal B cells in the skin. Primary cutaneous follicle centre lymphoma, the most frequent CBCL, is characterized by a localized slowly progressive lesion in the neck/head or trunk and is associated with an excellent prognosis (5-year OS >95%). In most cases the tumour cells do not express Bcl-2 and MUM-1. Local radiation remains the preferred therapy for patients with localized disease (localized with regional satellites), whereas those who present with disseminated skin disease may be observed or treated with systemic chemotherapy with or without monoclonal antibodies (e.g. rituximab). Primary cutaneous marginal zone lymphoma, the second most common CBCL, is also considered to have an indolent course, with a 5-year OS approaching 100%. Patient management is similar to that of patients with primary cutaneous follicle centre lymphoma.

A more aggressive type of CBCL, primary cutaneous large B-cell lymphoma leg-type, typically presents with nodules/tumours on one or both legs, although other anatomical sites may be involved. Elderly patients, particularly females, are most commonly affected. The lesions commonly demonstrate strong expression of Bcl-2, MUM-1 and Bcl-6. Despite its less indolent nature, the treatment of choice for early stages remains local (local radiation or excision), whereas those who present with disseminated disease are treated with systemic chemotherapy with or without adjuvant monoclonal antibodies. The 5-year disease-specific survival is approximately 50%. The extent of skin lesions has been associated with prognosis.

In summary, primary cutaneous lymphomas comprise a heterogeneous group of B- and T-cell lymphomas with a variety of clinical presentations and prognoses. Accurate diagnosis and assessment of prognostic factors determine patient management. The majority of patients should be considered for conservative palliative therapy (e.g. local or topical treatments), unless they present with histologically aggressive lymphoma (e.g. large-cell CTCL) or disseminated stage of an 'indolent' disease (extracutaneous involvement), for which they should receive systemic therapy. New emerging therapies (monoclonal antibodies, topical and systemic rexinoids, recombinant toxins and immunomodulators) may succeed in improving long-term outcome, although further studies are needed.

Lymphoma in elderly patients

Diffuse large-cell lymphoma accounts for 50% of lymphomas in patients older than 60 years. Unfortunately, the outcome in this population is worse than that observed in younger adults, partly because of the high incidence of coexisting medical problems affecting organ function. Attempts to improve patient outcome, providing intensified chemotherapy regimens (compared with CHOP), ended with increased toxicity without improvement in survival, whereas less toxic regimens were often less effective. However, the prospective randomized GELA study, comparing CHOP with CHOP plus rituximab (CHOP-R), reported an improved DFS and OS in elderly patients (>60 years) treated with CHOP-R, with no increase in treatment-related toxicity.

The addition of granulocyte colony-stimulating factors can shorten duration of neutropenia, enabling the delivery of chemotherapy at the planned time and dose intensity. Several studies have recently reported encouraging results with autologous SCT in patients older than 60 years (4-year OS in patients with chemosensitive relapsed disease approached 40%), indicating the feasibility of this treatment in selected patients.

Selected bibliography

Al-Tourah AJ, Gill KK, Chhanabhai M et al. (2008) Population-based analysis of incidence and outcome of transformed non-Hodgkin lymphoma. *Journal of Clinical Oncology* **26**: 5165–9.

Ardeshna KM, Smith P, Norton A et al. (2003) Long-term effect of a watch and wait policy versus immediate systemic treatment for asymptomatic advanced-stage non-Hodgkin lymphoma: a randomized controlled trial. *Lancet* **362**: 516–22.

Armitage J, Vose J, Weisenburger D (2008) International peripheral T-cell and natural killer/T-cell lymphoma study: pathology findings and clinical outcomes. *Journal of Clinical Oncology* **26**: 4124–30.

Balsalobre P, Diez-Martin JL, Re A et al. (2009) Autologous stem-cell transplantation in patients with HIV-related lymphoma. *Journal of Clinical Oncology* **27**: 2192–8.

Barr PM, Lazarus HM (2008) Follicular non-Hodgkin lymphoma: long-term results of stem-cell transplantation. *Current Opinion in Oncology* **20**: 502–8.

Bessell EM, Hoang-Xuan K, Ferreri AJ, Reni M (2007) Primary central nervous system lymphoma: biological aspects and controversies in management. *European Journal of Cancer* **43**: 1141–52.

Boehme V, Schmitz N, Zeynalova S, Loeffler M, Pfreundschuh M (2009) CNS events in elderly patients with aggressive lymphoma treated with modern chemotherapy (CHOP-14) with or without rituximab: an analysis of patients treated in the RICOVER-60 trial of the German high-grade non-Hodgkin lymphoma study group (DSHNHL). *Blood* **113**: 3896–902.

Bohlius J, Herbst C, Reiser M, Schwarzer G, Engert A (2008) Granulopoiesis-stimulating factors to prevent adverse effects in the treatment of malignant lymphoma. *Cochrane Database of Systematic Reviews* CD003189.

Bower M, Powles T, Williams S *et al.* (2007) Brief communication: rituximab in HIV-associated multicentric Castleman disease. *Annals of Internal Medicine* **147**: 836–9.

Cheson BD, Pfistner B, Juweid ME *et al.* (2007) Revised response criteria for malignant lymphoma. *Journal of Clinical Oncology* **25**: 579–86.

Dave SS, Wright G, Tan B *et al.* (2004) Prediction of survival in follicular lymphoma based on molecular features of tumour-infiltrating immune cells. *New England Journal of Medicine* **351**: 2159–69.

Dave SS, Fu K, Wright GW *et al.* (2006) Molecular diagnosis of Burkitt's lymphoma. *New England Journal of Medicine* **354**: 2431–42.

Diez-Martin JL, Balsalobre P, Re A *et al.* (2009) Comparable survival between HIV positive and HIV negative non-Hodgkin and Hodgkin lymphoma patients undergoing autologous peripheral blood stem cell transplantation. *Blood* **113**: 6011–14.

Dimopoulos MA, Gertz MA, Kastritis E *et al.* (2009) Update on treatment recommendations from the Fourth International Workshop on Waldenstrom's Macroglobulinemia. *Journal of Clinical Oncology* **27**: 120–6.

Doolittle ND, Abrey LE, Shenkier TN *et al.* (2008) Brain parenchyma involvement as isolated central nervous system relapse of systemic non-Hodgkin lymphoma: an International Primary CNS Lymphoma Collaborative Group report. *Blood* **111**: 1085–93.

Dreyling M, Hiddemann W (2008) Dose-intense treatment of mantle cell lymphoma: can durable remission be achieved? *Current Opinion in Oncology* **20**: 487–94.

Ferrucci PF, Zucca E (2007) Primary gastric lymphoma pathogenesis and treatment: what has changed over the past 10 years? *British Journal of Haematology* **136**: 521–38.

Feugier P, Van Hoof A, Sebban C *et al.* (2005) Long-term results of the R-CHOP study in the treatment of elderly patients with diffuse large B-cell lymphoma: a study by the Groupe d'Etude des Lymphomes de l'Adulte. *Journal of Clinical Oncology* **23**: 4117–26.

Fisher RI, Gaynor ER, Dahlberg S *et al.* (1993) Comparison of a standard regimen (CHOP) with three intensive chemotherapy regimens for advanced non-Hodgkin lymphoma. *New England Journal of Medicine* **328**: 1002–6.

Forstpointner R, Unterhalt M, Dreyling M *et al.* (2006) Maintenance therapy with rituximab leads to a significant prolongation of response duration after salvage therapy with a combination of rituximab, fludarabine, cyclophosphamide, and mitoxantrone (R-FCM) in patients with recurring and refractory follicular and mantle cell lymphomas: results of a prospective randomized study of the German Low Grade Lymphoma Study Group (GLSG). *Blood* **108**: 4003–8.

Greb A, Bohlius J, Schiefer D, Schwarzer G, Schulz H, Engert A (2008) High-dose chemotherapy with autologous stem cell transplantation in the first line treatment of aggressive non-Hodgkin lymphoma (NHL) in adults. *Cochrane Database of Systematic Reviews* CD004024.

Gyan E, Foussard C, Bertrand P *et al.* (2009) High-dose therapy followed by autologous purged stem cell transplantation and doxorubicin-based chemotherapy in patients with advanced follicular lymphoma: a randomized multicenter study by the GOELAMS with final results after a median follow-up of 9 years. *Blood* **113**: 995–1001.

Haioun C, Itti E, Rahmouni A *et al.* (2005) [^{18}F]fluoro-2-deoxy-D-glucose positron emission tomography (FDG-PET) in aggressive lymphoma: an early prognostic tool for predicting patient outcome. *Blood* **106**: 1376–81.

Hoster E, Dreyling M, Klapper W *et al.* (2008) A new prognostic index (MIPI) for patients with advanced-stage mantle cell lymphoma. *Blood* **111**: 558–65.

Illerhaus G, Muller F, Feuerhake F, Schafer AO, Ostertag C, Finke J (2008) High-dose chemotherapy and autologous stem-cell transplantation without consolidating radiotherapy as first-line treatment for primary lymphoma of the central nervous system. *Haematologica* **93**: 147–8.

Ishitsuka K, Tamura K (2008) Treatment of adult T-cell leukaemia/lymphoma: past, present, and future. *European Journal of Haematology* **80**: 185–96.

Kaplan LD, Lee JY, Ambinder RF *et al.* (2005) Rituximab does not improve clinical outcome in a randomized phase 3 trial of CHOP with or without rituximab in patients with HIV-associated non-Hodgkin lymphoma: AIDS-Malignancies Consortium Trial 010. *Blood* **106**: 1538–43.

Kyriakou C, Canals C, Goldstone A *et al.* (2008) High-dose therapy and autologous stem-cell transplantation in angioimmunoblastic lymphoma: complete remission at transplantation is the major determinant of Outcome-Lymphoma Working Party of the European Group for Blood and Marrow Transplantation. *Journal of Clinical Oncology* **26**: 218–24.

Lenz G, Staudt LM (2010) Aggressive lymphomas. *The New England Journal of Medicine* **362**: 1417–29.

Lenz G, Wright GW, Emre NC *et al.* (2008) Molecular subtypes of diffuse large B-cell lymphoma arise by distinct genetic pathways. *Procedings of the National Academy of Sciences USA* **105**: 13520–5.

McMillan A (2005) Central nervous system-directed preventative therapy in adults with lymphoma. *British Journal of Haematology* **131**: 13–21.

Matthews GV, Bower M, Mandalia S, Powles T, Nelson MR, Gazzard BG (2000) Changes in acquired immunodeficiency syndrome-related lymphoma since the introduction of highly active antiretroviral therapy. *Blood* **96**: 2730–4.

Matutes E, Oscier D, Montalban C *et al.* (2008) Splenic marginal zone lymphoma proposals for a revision of diagnostic, staging and therapeutic criteria. *Leukemia* **22**: 487–95.

Montoto S, Davies AJ, Matthews J *et al.* (2007) Risk and clinical implications of transformation of follicular lymphoma to diffuse large B-cell lymphoma. *Journal of Clinical Oncology* **25**: 2426–33.

Morris E, Thomson K, Craddock C *et al.* (2004) Outcomes after alemtuzumab-containing reduced-intensity allogeneic transplantation regimen for relapsed and refractory non-Hodgkin lymphoma. *Blood* **104**: 3865–71.

Morschhauser F, Radford J, Van Hoof A *et al.* (2008) Phase III trial of consolidation therapy with yttrium-90-ibritumomab tiuxetan compared with no additional therapy after first remission in advanced follicular lymphoma. *Journal of Clinical Oncology* **26**: 5156–64.

Navarro WH, Kaplan LD (2006) AIDS-related lymphoproliferative disease. *Blood* **107**: 13–20.

Oksenhendler E, Boulanger E, Galicier L *et al.* (2002) High incidence of Kaposi sarcoma-associated herpesvirus-related non-Hodgkin lymphoma in patients with HIV infection and multicentric Castleman disease. *Blood* **99**: 2331–6.

Parker A, Bowles K, Bradley JA (2010) Diagnosis of post-transplant lymphoproliferative disorder in solid organ transplant recipients – BSCH and BTS guidelines. *British Journal of Haematology* **149**: 675–92.

Pfreundschuh M, Trumper L, Osterborg A *et al.* (2006) CHOP-like chemotherapy plus rituximab versus CHOP-like chemotherapy alone in young patients with good-prognosis diffuse large-B-cell lymphoma: a randomized controlled trial by the MabThera International Trial (MInT) Group. *Lancet Oncology* **7**: 379–91.

Pfreundschuh M, Schubert J, Ziepert M *et al.* (2008) Six versus eight cycles of bi-weekly CHOP-14 with or without rituximab in elderly patients with aggressive CD20+ B-cell lymphomas: a randomized controlled trial (RICOVER-60). *Lancet Oncology* **9**: 105–16.

Rezvani AR, Storer B, Maris M *et al.* (2008) Nonmyeloablative allogeneic haematopoietic cell transplantation in relapsed, refractory, and transformed indolent non-Hodgkin lymphoma. *Journal of Clinical Oncology* **26**: 211–17.

Rodriguez J, Conde E, Gutierrez A *et al.* (2007) The results of consolidation with autologous stem-cell transplantation in patients with peripheral T-cell lymphoma (PTCL) in first complete remission: the Spanish Lymphoma and Autologous Transplantation Group experience. *Annals of Oncology* **18**: 652–7.

Rohatiner AZ, Nadler L, Davies AJ *et al.* (2007) Myeloablative therapy with autologous bone marrow transplantation for follicular lymphoma at the time of second or subsequent remission: long-term follow-up. *Journal of Clinical Oncology* **25**: 2554–9.

Savage KJ, Harris NL, Vose JM *et al.* (2008) ALK⁻ anaplastic large-cell lymphoma is clinically and immunophenotypically different from both ALK⁺ ALCL and peripheral T-cell lymphoma, not otherwise specified: report from the International Peripheral T-Cell Lymphoma Project. *Blood* **111**: 5496–504.

Schulz H, Bohlius J, Skoetz N *et al.* (2007) Chemotherapy plus rituximab versus chemotherapy alone for B-cell non-Hodgkin lymphoma. *Cochrane Database of Systematic Reviews* CD003805.

Sehn LH, Berry B, Chhanabhai M *et al.* (2007) The revised International Prognostic Index (R-IPI) is a better predictor of outcome than the standard IPI for patients with diffuse large B-cell lymphoma treated with R-CHOP. *Blood* **109**: 1857–61.

Thomson KJ, Morris EC, Bloor A *et al.* (2009) Favourable long-term survival after reduced-intensity allogeneic transplantation for multiple-relapse aggressive non-Hodgkin lymphoma. *Journal of Clinical Oncology* **27**: 426–32.

Tsukasaki K, Hermine O, Bazarbachi A *et al.* (2009) Definition, prognostic factors, treatment, and response criteria of adult T-cell leukaemia-lymphoma: a proposal from an international consensus meeting. *Journal of Clinical Oncology* **27**: 453–9.

van Oers MH, Klasa R, Marcus RE *et al.* (2006) Rituximab maintenance improves clinical outcome of relapsed/resistant follicular non-Hodgkin lymphoma in patients both with and without rituximab during induction: results of a prospective randomized phase 3 intergroup trial. *Blood* **108**: 3295–301.

Vidal L, Gafter-Gvili A, Leibovici L *et al.* (2009) Rituximab maintenance for the treatment of patients with follicular lymphoma: systematic review and meta-analysis of randomized trials. *Journal of the National Cancer Institute* **101**: 248–55.

Whittaker SJ, Marsden JR, Spittle M, Russell Jones R (2003) Joint British Association of Dermatologists and UK Cutaneous Lymphoma Group guidelines for the management of primary cutaneous T-cell lymphomas. *British Journal of Dermatology* **149**: 1095–107.

Willemze R, Jaffe ES, Burg G *et al.* (2005) WHO-EORTC classification for cutaneous lymphomas. *Blood* **105**: 3768–85.

Yeo W, Chan TC, Leung NW *et al.* (2009) Hepatitis B virus reactivation in lymphoma patients with prior resolved hepatitis B undergoing anticancer therapy with or without rituximab. *Journal of Clinical Oncology* **27**: 605–11.

CHAPTER 36

Myeloproliferative neoplasms

Peter J Campbell[1] and Anthony R Green[2]

[1]Cancer Genome Project, Wellcome Trust Sanger Institute, Cambridge, UK
[2]Cambridge Institute for Medical Research, Cambridge, UK

Introduction

For the purposes of this chapter, the term 'myeloproliferative neoplasm' (MPN) refers to clonal disorders of haemopoiesis that lead to an increase in the numbers of one or more mature blood cell progeny. The chronic myeloid leukaemias would fit this definition and share pathogenetic features with some of the MPNs, but have historically (since the discovery of the Philadelphia chromosome) been studied separately from the MPNs and are described in another chapter. Myelodysplastic syndrome (MDS) can also, in a minority of cases, fit our working definition of MPN, in being associated with increased numbers of mature cell progeny, but dysplasia is a major feature and there are, usually, coexisting cytopenias. Not surprisingly, a small number of patients do not fit neatly into a single category and exhibit features of both MPN and MDS.

This chapter focuses on the classical MPNs: polycythaemia (rubra) vera (PV), essential thrombocythaemia (ET) and primary myelofibrosis (PMF), three related disorders originally grouped together by William Dameshek in 1951. They share clinical, morphological and molecular features and can transform, in their course, into one another. They are clonal disorders of the pluripotent haemopoietic stem cell and have, to varying degrees, the potential to transform into acute myeloid leukaemia (AML). Secondary (non-clonal) polycythaemias and

thrombocytoses are also discussed in this chapter, as they often enter the differential diagnosis of their clonal counterparts.

In addition, some of the less common MPNs are described, namely mastocytosis and its variants, the clonal eosinophilic syndromes and chronic neutrophilic leukaemia. The ontogeny of the target cell for transformation is less well established in these disorders, but there is accumulating evidence implicating the pluripotent haemopoietic stem cell in at least some cases.

The polycythaemias

True polycythaemia refers to an absolute increase in total body red cell volume (or mass), which usually manifests itself as a raised haemoglobin concentration (Hb) and/or packed cell volume (PCV). A raised Hb (or PCV) can also be secondary to a reduction in plasma volume, without an increase in total red cell volume; this is known as apparent (or relative) polycythaemia.

True polycythaemia is further subdivided into primary polycythaemia (namely PV), a clonal haematological disorder, and secondary polycythaemia, which results from an increased erythropoietin drive, either in the presence or absence of hypoxia (Figure 36.1).

Polycythaemia vera

The central pathological feature of PV is an expansion in the total red cell mass, although elevations in the platelet and/or neutrophil counts are relatively common. The first description

Postgraduate Haematology: 6th edition. Edited by A. Victor Hoffbrand, Daniel Catovsky, Edward G.D. Tuddenham, Anthony R. Green
© 2011 Blackwell Publishing Ltd.

of PV was by Vaquez in 1892. Osler, in 1903, published the first series of patients, identifying salient clinical features setting PV apart from other erythrocytoses. Considerable information has been gathered about PV since the work of these pioneers, much of it due to the work of the Polycythaemia Vera Study Group (PVSG), which was set up in 1967 with the aim of optimizing diagnosis and management of PV. The recent discovery of the V617F mutation in the pseudokinase domain of the tyrosine kinase JAK2, in nearly all cases of PV, represents a major advance in our understanding of this disorder.

Pathophysiology

PV is a stem cell disorder characterized by hyperplasia of all three major myeloid cell lineages. The first line of evidence in support of the stem cell origin of PV came in the form of clonality studies. Using X-chromosome inactivation patterns in the mid-1970s Fialkow and colleagues showed that neutrophils, erythrocytes and platelets originated from the same clone. Large studies have since confirmed these findings.

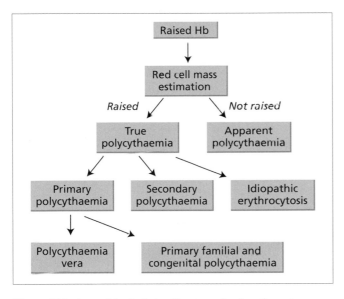

Figure 36.1 An aetiological classification of polycythaemia.

Erythropoiesis in PV is autonomous and does not rely on erythropoietin (Epo). Plasma levels of this hormone are reduced in PV patients, and PV progenitor cells, unlike normal ones, can survive *in vitro* and give rise to erythroid colonies (BFU-E) in the absence of added Epo (endogenous erythroid colonies). PV erythroid progenitors show increased sensitivity to Epo but also to several other growth factors, including insulin-like growth factor (IGF)-1, thrombopoietin, interleukin (IL)-3 and granulocyte/monocyte colony-stimulating factor. Germline mutations in the Epo receptor (EpoR) are known to occur in inherited polycythaemia, but such mutations are absent in patients with PV.

In 2005, several groups identified a unique acquired mutation in the cytoplasmic tyrosine kinase JAK2 in myeloid cells from the great majority of patients with PV. JAK2 lies downstream of several cell surface receptors including EpoR. Upon Epo binding to EpoR, JAK2 becomes phosphorylated and in turn phosphorylates downstream targets, most important of which are the STATs (signal transducers and activators of transcription), leading to stimulation of erythropoiesis. Valine 617 is located in the JH2 domain of JAK2, which acts to repress its kinase activity (Figure 36.2). The V617F mutation leads to increased kinase activity, confers cytokine independence and results in erythrocytosis in a mouse transplant model. The mutation appears to be fairly specific to the classical MPNs and although it has been reported in small numbers of patients with related myeloid neoplasms, it is not present in lymphoid or non-haemopoietic cancers. Intriguingly, the mutation is homozygous in a large proportion of patients with PV and PMF but this is rare in ET. It appears that the moderate familial predisposition to MPNs can be largely attributed to an inherited haplotype block surrounding the *JAK2* gene, although the mechanism underlying this interaction between somatic and germline genetics has not been identified.

When appropriately sensitive methods are used for the detection of the V617F mutation, about 95% of PV patients are positive. Recently, mutations elsewhere in *JAK2* have been described in most of the V617F-negative patients who have PV by strict diagnostic criteria. These mutations cluster in exon 12,

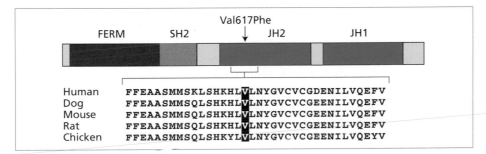

Figure 36.2 Diagrammatic representation of JAK2 indicating the location of valine 617 and the very high degree of cross-species amino acid homology in its JH2 domain. The JH2 domain normally acts to repress the kinase activity of JAK2, but its ability to do so is impaired in the presence of the JAK2 V617F mutation. (Modified from Baxter *et al.* 2005 with permission.)

and can be of several different types, but all seem to affect the pseudokinase domain, leading to constitutive activation of the JAK2 kinase. Interestingly, compared with PV patients with the V617F mutation, those carrying exon 12 mutations tend to be younger and have a more isolated erythrocytosis, with less frequent thrombocytosis and leucocytosis. The molecular basis for these differences in phenotype has not been identified.

Recently, mutations in a novel tumour-suppressor gene, *TET2*, have been identified in myeloid disorders of all types, including MPNs. In particular, 20–25% of patients with MDS, 50% of patients with chronic myelomonocytic leukaemia, 12–15% of patients with MPN and about 20% of patients with AML carry somatically acquired mutations of the gene. Little is known about how the gene functions in normal cells, nor how disruption of the gene promotes myeloid disorders. However, the mutation is found in early haemopoietic progenitors, can either pre-date or post-date *JAK2* V617F mutation, and allows stable engraftment of haemopoietic cells in immunodeficient mice.

Clinical features

Epidemiology
The annual incidence of PV is reported to be around 2–3 per 100 000 population with a male to female ratio of 1.2 : 1. The median age at onset is 55–60 years and although incidence increases with age, PV can occur at any age even, rarely, in childhood.

Thrombotic complications
Thrombosis is the most common serious complication of PV. Untreated PV patients run a greatly increased risk of thrombosis, which can be arterial, venous or microvascular. The increased PCV leads to an increased blood viscosity, rheological abnormalities and abnormal platelet–endothelial contact. Additionally, procoagulant changes in platelets (e.g. decreased response to prostaglandin D_2), thrombocytosis and pre-existing vascular disease can all conspire to dramatically increase thrombotic risk.

Arterial occlusions can lead to myocardial infarcts, strokes, transient ischaemic attacks, amaurosis, scotomata, and mesenteric and limb ischaemia. Less commonly, microvascular occlusions affecting the extremities and erythromelalgia can occur.

In the venous circulation, unusual sites such as the splanchnic vessels can be involved. As a result, mesenteric, splenic and hepatoportal thromboses (Figure 36.3) are recognized presenting features of PV. Recent data indicate that this propensity to venous thrombosis in atypical sites is particularly strongly correlated with presence of the *JAK2* V617F mutation, and indeed patients presenting with otherwise unexplained splanchnic vein thrombosis will often be found to have the mutation, even in the absence of an overt MPN. Superficial thrombophlebitis,

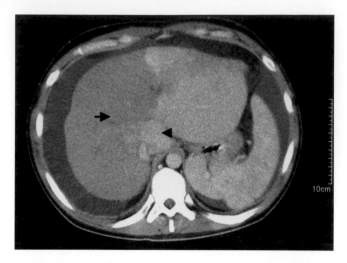

Figure 36.3 Polycythaemia vera presenting with Budd–Chiari syndrome in a 28-year-old man: contrast computed tomography showing reduced enhancement of the right lobe of the liver (arrow) with characteristic sparing of the caudate lobe (arrowhead). On this occasion, the left lobe was also relatively spared. Marked ascites and a bulky spleen are also seen.

conventional deep venous thromboses and pulmonary emboli are also seen.

Neurological features
Over and above the consequences of occlusive vascular lesions, the sluggish cerebral blood flow secondary to the increased PCV is thought to underlie features such as headaches, drowsiness, insomnia, amnesia, tinnitus, vertigo, chorea and even depression. Transient visual disturbances also occur.

Pruritus
This symptom occurs in about one-quarter of PV patients and in some it may be severe. It is characteristically aquagenic, precipitated by warm baths, and can be associated with erythema, swelling or even pain. Pruritus is often relieved by controlling the PCV, but its aetiology remains elusive. Basophilia, hyperhistaminaemia and iron deficiency may have a role and there is an increased incidence in patients with a lower mean corpuscular volume.

Skin
Plethora, dilated conjunctival vessels and rosacea-like facial skin changes are not uncommon at presentation. Brown discoloration of the skin, erythromelalgia and, rarely, Sweet syndrome may be seen.

Splenomegaly
Palpable splenomegaly is seen in 30–50% of cases of PV. It is unclear if its presence affects prognosis, but it may be associated with an increased risk of progression to myelofibrosis.

Hypertension and gout

Hypertension is probably more common in patients with PV as is hyperuricaemia, with gout seen in about 5% of cases.

Leukaemic transformation

This is perhaps the most feared complication of PV, but the risk of developing acute leukaemia in PV patients treated only with venesection is very small (1–3%). However, this risk increases dramatically (more than 10-fold) when radioactive phosphorus (^{32}P), chlorambucil or irradiation are used as treatment. The median time interval between first starting such therapy and developing acute leukaemia is 5–8 years. Interestingly, in about half of patients transforming to acute leukaemia from a preceding *JAK2*-positive MPN, the leukaemia is *JAK2* negative.

Myelofibrosis

Progression to myelofibrosis (Figure 36.4) occurs in around 10–20% of PV cases at 15 years after diagnosis. This figure is approximate, not least because different studies have used distinct criteria to define myelofibrotic transformation. Transformation often occurs gradually over many years and is thought to be associated with an increased risk of leukaemic conversion. The management of these patients is similar to that of PMF.

Investigations

The diagnosis of PV requires both the identification of features in support of this diagnosis and the exclusion of secondary and apparent polycythaemia. The original set of diagnostic criteria was formulated by the PVSG in the 1970s. The British Committee for Standards in Haematology (BCSH) guidelines for diagnosing PV, taking into account the latest advances in the molecular understanding of these disorders, are shown in Table 36.1.

Most patients can now be diagnosed on the basis of a raised haematocrit together with the presence of the *JAK2* V617F mutation. It is also important to emphasize that the V617F mutation has been identified in a small proportion of other hematological malignancies (e.g. AML, chronic myelomonocytic leukaemia and myelodysplasia). However, none of these disorders is associated with a raised red cell mass and clinical distinction from PV is rarely an issue. The role of bone marrow biopsy in the evaluation of PV remains controversial, but it may be useful as a baseline investigation for later comparison in younger patients with the disorder, or if there are atypical clinical and laboratory features at presentation.

A minority of patients with clinical PV is negative for the V617F mutation, even when tested using sensitive detection methods. Many reference laboratories now offer highly sensitive molecular testing for *JAK2* exon 12 mutations, and this should be considered in patients who have a typical clinical and laboratory presentation of PV but who are negative for the V617F mutation. Rarely, patients will be negative for both

Table 36.1 Diagnostic criteria for polycythaemia vera, as recommended in the BCSH guidelines.

JAK2-positive polycythaemia vera	
A1	High haematocrit (>0.52 in men, >0.48 in women) *or* raised red cell mass (>25% above predicted)*
A2	Mutation in *JAK2*

Diagnosis requires both criteria to be present

JAK2-negative polycythaemia vera	
A1	Raised red cell mass (>25% above predicted) *or* haematocrit >0.60 in men, >0.56 in women.
A2	Absence of mutation in *JAK2*
A3	No cause of secondary erythrocytosis
A4	Palpable splenomegaly
A5	Presence of an acquired genetic abnormality (excluding *BCR–ABL1*) in haemopoietic cells
B1	Thrombocytosis (platelet count >450 × 10^9/L)
B2	Neutrophil leucocytosis (neutrophil count >10 × 10^9/L in non-smokers, >12.5 × 10^9/L in smokers)
B3	Radiological evidence of splenomegaly
B4	Endogenous erythroid colonies or low serum erythropoietin

Diagnosis requires A1 + A2 + A3 + either another A or two B criteria

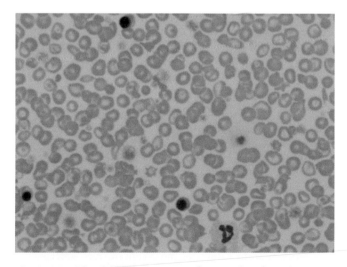

Figure 36.4 Blood film from a case of post-polycythaemic myelofibrosis after splenectomy. Note the presence of nucleated erythrocytes, giant platelets and features of splenectomy including target cells, spherocytes and acanthocytes.

*Dual pathology (coexistent secondary erythrocytosis or relative erythrocytosis) may rarely be present in patients with a *JAK2*-positive MPN. In this situation, it would be prudent to reduce the haematocrit to the same target as for polycythaemia vera.

V617F and exon 12 *JAK2* mutations. In these patients, the diagnosis of PV can be made if the other criteria set out in Table 36.1 are met, but it should be remembered that this group of truly *JAK2*-negative PV is very rare, and secondary erythrocytosis, idiopathic erythrocytosis and relative erythrocytosis are all much more likely diagnoses in this clinical setting.

Treatment

Identification of the *JAK2* V617F mutation has generated much interest in the development of therapeutic JAK2 inhibitors. However, as patients with PV currently have a very good prognosis, new agents will have to display an excellent safety profile. For the time being, the treatment of PV should employ existing treatment modalities whose effectiveness has been validated, as described below.

In the absence of thrombocytosis, regular venesection remains the mainstay of treatment for PV in patients who can tolerate it. A target haematocrit of 0.45 or less is widely used, following the demonstration that in patients with PV, higher haematocrits are associated with a significantly increased risk of thrombosis. Venesection has little impact on the haematocrit in the short term: the purpose of regular venesection is to induce iron deficiency such that the haematocrit remains chronically below the target threshold of 0.45. Thus, typical venesection regimens start with phlebotomy every 2–3 weeks until the haematocrit is controlled, and thereafter phlebotomy is generally needed every 1–3 months, depending of factors such as dietary iron intake and erythropoietic activity.

Cytoreductive therapy is recommended for patients unable to undergo venesection and those with thrombocytosis, in view of the probable increased risk of thrombosis. Hydroxycarbamide (hydroxyurea) is the most commonly used drug. It is orally bioavailable and generally very well tolerated. It will reduce both the haematocrit and the platelet count. The commonest complications are leucopenia or thrombocytopenia, which are dose dependent and can usually be avoided by close monitoring of the blood count when the drug is first introduced. In susceptible patients it can cause photosensitivity, painful leg ulcers and gastrointestinal side-effects. The usual dose is 0.5–2 g daily.

It has been suggested that hydroxycarbamide may increase the inherent leukaemogenic risk associated with PV. This concern is largely based on studies involving small numbers of patients or patients who have also required other cytotoxic agents (and may therefore represent a subgroup with more aggressive disease). At present, there are no convincing data to show that hydroxycarbamide, when used as a single agent, significantly increases the risk of leukaemia, although a small effect cannot be excluded. Preliminary data from studies of hydroxycarbamide in sickle cell disease are reassuring, but longer follow-up is required.

Interferon alfa is effective in controlling both the platelet count and the PCV, and there are some data that it may induce impressive reductions in the burden of V617F-positive cells in the blood. It is not widely used because of its cost, route of administration (subcutaneous injection) and its side-effects (including fatigue, flu-like symptoms and depression). However, it can be useful in young patients who are reluctant to take other cytotoxic agents, in pregnancy and in patients with intractable pruritus. The usual dose range is 3–5 million units three times per week.

Anagrelide is a newer agent that lowers the platelet count by inhibiting megakaryocyte differentiation. It can be useful in controlling the platelet count of patients being treated with venesection and can also be combined with hydroxycarbamide to allow the use of lower doses of both agents. Approximately 10% of patients are completely refractory to anagrelide. The usual dose is 1–2 mg daily, but occasional patients may require doses of up to 8 mg daily. Its side-effects are mainly secondary to its inotropic and vasodilatory properties and include headaches, palpitations and fluid retention.

Busulfan is sometimes used in elderly patients or when all other treatments are not tolerated. It is very convenient as it need only be administered intermittently, but may increase the risk of leukaemia. The usual dosage is 25–75 mg as a single dose every 2–3 months. Low-dose aspirin (75–100 mg daily) reduces thrombotic complications in PV and is used in most patients without contraindications to this drug. Pruritus often improves with control of the PCV but paroxetine, antihistamines and aspirin (in some cases) can help. There is also evidence that interferon can be useful in intractable cases.

In view of the age of most patients and the relatively benign natural history of treated PV, bone marrow transplantation is not advocated for stable disease. The role, if any, of transplantation employing reduced-intensity conditioning regimens is not yet clear.

Prognosis

In the first half of the 20th century, untreated polycythaemia had a dismal prognosis with a 50% survival of less than 2 years. However, adequately treated PV now has a relatively benign natural history with a life expectancy of over 11 years, bearing in mind that the average age of onset is 60 years. Factors predictive of poorer prognosis and increased complication rates in PV include *JAK2* mutation burden and white cell count at diagnosis, both factors probably serving as surrogate markers of disease activity.

Other causes of erythrocytosis

All disorders with an increased red cell mass that are not due to clonal proliferation of haemopoietic progenitors are included under this heading. They are most conveniently subclassified into primary and secondary causes. In primary polycythaemia, the defect is intrinsic to the red cell precursors, which are hypersensitive to Epo. In secondary polycythaemia, the defect is upstream of the red cell precursors. The latter group can be

Table 36.2 Causes of erythrocytosis other than polycythaemia vera.

Primary erythrocytosis
Primary familial and congenital polycythaemia

Secondary erythrocytosis
Erythrocytosis in the presence of systemic hypoxia
Chronic hypoxia
  Lung disease
  Hypopnoea
  High altitude
  Congenital cyanotic heart disease
Defective oxygen transport
  High-affinity haemoglobins
  Red cell metabolic defects (low 2,3-DPG)
  Methaemoglobinaemia
  Heavy smoking (carboxyhaemoglobinaemia)

Erythrocytosis in the absence of systemic hypoxia
Inherited/congenital erythrocytosis
  Chuvash polycythaemia
  Inherited mutations in *EPOR* and oxygen signalling
Abnormal erythropoietin secretion
  Renal tumours
  Cystic/polycystic kidney disease
  Renal transplantation
  Renal hypoxia (e.g. renal artery stenosis)
  Cerebellar haemangioma
  Hepatocellular carcinoma
Endocrine syndromes
  Administration of androgenic steroids
  Cushing syndrome
  Conn syndrome
  Phaeochromocytoma (rarely)
  Bartter syndrome

Idiopathic erythrocytosis

further subdivided into polycythaemias in the presence or absence of systemic hypoxia. A small group of patients do not fall into any of these categories and are given the diagnosis of idiopathic erythrocytosis (Table 36.2). The clinical management of many of these syndromes is not well defined.

The term 'apparent polycythaemia' refers to a raised haematocrit in the absence of a raised red cell mass and is discussed later in this chapter.

Primary erythrocytosis

Inherited/congenital erythrocytosis
Chuvash polycythaemia is an autosomal recessive condition that is endemic in the Russian mid-Volga river region of Chuvashia. Patients have increased levels of circulating Epo but do not carry mutations of EpoR. Chuvash polycythaemia was recently shown to be associated with a C→T mutation at nucleotide 598 (leads to an Arg200Trp substitution) in the von Hippel–Lindau (*VHL*) gene. The *VHL* gene is pivotal for ubiquitination and subsequent degradation of HIF-1 transcription factor, which is central to the oxygen-sensing pathway. This *VHL* mutant leads to a reduced rate of degradation of HIF-1 and upregulation of downstream targets including Epo, leading to polycythaemia. Recently, some of the rare non-Russian families with inherited polycythaemia were also shown to carry *VHL* mutations, and occasional pedigrees with mutations elsewhere in the oxygen-sensing pathway have been described, including the *PHD2* and *HIF2A* genes.

Primary familial and congenital polycythaemia (PFCP) is a rare disorder in which erythropoiesis is intrinsically overactive. The disorder is usually transmitted in an autosomal dominant manner with some cases appearing sporadically. Clinical features include the presence of isolated erythrocytosis without evolution into leukaemia or other MPNs, absence of splenomegaly, normal white blood cell and platelet counts, low or normal plasma Epo levels, normal haemoglobin–oxygen dissociation curve/P_{50}, and hypersensitivity of erythroid progenitors to Epo. Mutations in the gene encoding EpoR have been described in several (but not all) families with PFCP. In most cases, the mutations lead to a C-terminal truncation of the EpoR protein, with increased sensitivity to Epo.

Secondary erythrocytosis

Erythrocytosis in the presence of systemic hypoxia
Chronic lung disease and hypopnoea
Lung disease is the predominant cause of chronic systemic hypoxia at sea level. Hypoxaemic chronic obstructive pulmonary disease is the commonest syndrome, but any lung–airway disease leading to chronic hypoxia could cause polycythaemia. Syndromes such as obstructive sleep apnoea and hypoventilation due to muscle weakness or paralysis can also occasionally be associated with secondary erythrocytosis.

Where possible, hypoxia should be ameliorated by treating the lung disease or with home oxygen therapy. Erythrocytosis has opposing effects on oxygen delivery as it increases the oxygen-carrying capacity while also increasing blood viscosity. Unfortunately, there is little evidence from clinical trials to guide management. In practice, many specialists suggest that venesection should be performed for haematocrits above 0.55.

High altitude
Residents at altitudes above 4000 m compensate for the ambient hypoxia by multisystem adaptation, including mild erythrocytosis, increase in capillary perfusion and lung diffusion capacity as well as biochemical changes in metabolic enzymes and myoglobin. Excessive altitude polycythaemia (PCV ≥ 0.65) is

seen in a proportion of cases and is often accompanied by hyperuricaemia and proteinuria. Some of these individuals eventually decompensate and develop chronic mountain sickness (Monge disease). Such people deteriorate steadily and develop extreme polycythaemia (sometimes PCV ≥ 0.75), arterial desaturation and right heart failure. Resettlement at lower altitudes halts disease progression and can partly reverse it. Treatment with angiotensin-converting enzyme (ACE) inhibitors has been shown in randomized studies to reduce the PCV and proteinuria seen in excessive altitude polycythaemia.

Congenital cyanotic heart disease

Congenital heart defects leading to a right-to-left shunt can cause dramatic erythrocytosis (up to PCV of 0.80). Surgery to correct the cardiac defect should be undertaken when possible. A few inoperable patients survive to adulthood and the management of their erythrocytosis is not straightforward. As in patients with chronic lung disease, the increase in oxygen-carrying capacity afforded by erythrocytosis is countered by an increased viscosity and associated haemodynamic changes. Here, however, we are often dealing with young patients with responsive vasculatures, which can usually accommodate such changes. Some experts advocate venesection when the PCV is greater than 0.60, whereas others allow the haematocrit to rise further and venesect for symptoms such as recurrent haemoptysis, marked fatigue or deteriorating exercise tolerance.

High-affinity haemoglobins

High-affinity haemoglobins release less oxygen for a given oxygen partial pressure, and may thus give rise to tissue hypoxia. This leads to an Epo-driven erythrocytosis, which tends to renormalize Epo levels. The pathognomonic anomaly is a left shift in the oxygen dissociation curve (Figure 36.5). The precise

variant can be identified by mutational screening of DNA or by protein mass spectrometry.

There are over 40 haemoglobin variants with an increased affinity for oxygen, all dominantly inherited. Most are due to mutations in β-globin, with a small number due to mutations in α-globin. Mutations are clustered in regions of the globin chains involved in the regulation of the transition between tense (T) and relaxed (R) states of haemoglobin. Normally, oxy-HbA is in the T state and has low affinity for oxygen, and deoxy-HbA is in the R state and has high affinity for oxygen. Thus, mutations at the αβ contact site (e.g. Hb San Diego), the C-terminus (e.g. Hb Bethesda) and the 2,3-diphosphoglycerate (2,3-DPG)-binding site (e.g. Hb Helsinki) are the commonest.

Most people with a high-affinity haemoglobin are in good health and are either diagnosed coincidentally or after being noticed to be plethoric. Some experience excessive muscle fatigue after vigorous exercise. Hyperviscosity is rarely a problem and surveys have failed to identify increased cardiovascular morbidity or mortality. Pregnancy is not adversely affected, even in mothers with haemoglobin affinity that exceeds that of HbF. Generally, therefore, no management is required, unless symptomatic.

Red cell metabolic defects

Very rare cases of erythrocytosis are due to abnormalities in red cell metabolism that lead to a reduction in intraerythrocytic 2,3-DPG. The best characterized defect is a mutant 2,3-DPG mutase. The only well-characterized family with this disorder showed autosomal recessive inheritance, although heterozygous family members had a decreased P_{50} and, in some cases, a moderate erythrocytosis. This disorder is excluded by the finding of a normal P_{50} in a fresh blood sample.

Methaemoglobinaemia

Oxidation of haem iron converts it from its normal ferrous (Fe^{2+}) to the ferric (Fe^{3+}) form and, correspondingly, haemoglobin (HbA) becomes methaemoglobin (Met-HbA). This constitutes an important antioxidant mechanism for the red cell, and conversion of Met-HbA back to HbA requires the generation of NADH from glycolysis. The rate of HbA auto-oxidation is about 20 times slower under normal circumstances than the rate of Met-HbA reduction, thus preventing Met-HbA accumulation.

Methaemoglobin has an increased affinity for oxygen and a left-shifted oxygen dissociation curve. Pathological acquired methaemoglobinaemia can result from exposure to strong oxidants (e.g. dapsone, paraquat, benzocaine) and can be life-threatening when severe but is rarely sufficiently long-lived to give rise to polycythaemia.

Hereditary methaemoglobinaemias can be due to haemoglobin mutations involving amino acids around the haem pocket (HbM disease), or secondary to enzymatic deficiencies

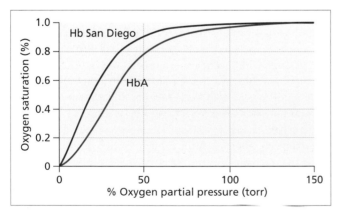

Figure 36.5 Haemoglobin–oxygen dissociation curves from a 27-year-old man with a raised red cell mass and a normal person (HbA) showing the presence of a high-affinity haemoglobin ('left shift'). Mass spectrometric analysis showed the man to be heterozygous for Hb San Diego, a high-affinity β-chain variant.

that interfere with the generation of NADH, which is required for day-to-day methaemoglobin reduction (namely NADH reductase and cytochrome b_5 reductase). In view of the chronic nature of the methaemoglobinaemia in these disorders, secondary erythrocytosis can develop in the same manner as for high-affinity haemoglobin mutants.

Heavy smoking

Heavy smoking can lead to mild polycythaemia in the absence of hypoxic lung disease. The underlying cause of this is a raised carboxyhaemoglobin (CO-Hb) level resulting from chronically raised carbon monoxide (CO) levels. CO-Hb levels in urban dwelling non-smokers are rarely higher than 2%, with levels ranging from 3 to 20% in smokers. The short half-life of CO in the body (3–5 hours) leads, in smokers, to a rise in CO-Hb during the day and a fall during sleep, making it difficult to compare measurements taken at different times. Binding of CO to Hb, as well as displacing oxygen, leads to a conformational change similar to that seen in methaemoglobinaemia, with a similar left shift in the oxygen dissociation curve and a fall in P_{50}.

Erythrocytosis in the absence of systemic hypoxia

Abnormal erythropoietin secretion

Abnormal Epo secretion is a well-recognized cause of secondary erythrocytosis and is most commonly secondary to renal pathologies such as renal tumours (benign and malignant), polycystic kidney disease and diseases associated with local hypoxia such as renal cysts, hydronephrosis and renal artery stenosis. The polycythaemia usually responds to treatment of the underlying renal pathology.

Erythrocytosis occurs in 20–30% of patients after renal transplantation. The biggest risk to such patients is hypertension, strokes and cardiovascular complications. In many cases, the erythrocytosis and associated hypertension respond to ACE inhibitors. Theophylline may also be effective in some cases. Patients who remain polycythaemic despite such therapy should be treated with repeated venesection to maintain their haematocrit below 45%; 30–40% of cases resolve spontaneously.

Non-renal tumours can rarely be associated with polycythaemia. The commonest reported ones are hepatocellular carcinoma, cerebellar and other haemangiomas and large uterine fibromyomas. Polycythaemia responds to removal of the tumour in most of these cases.

Endocrine disorders

The mechanism underlying the development of polycythaemia in most endocrine disorders lies in the overproduction of androgens, which can produce polycythaemia by increasing Epo levels and also, probably, through a direct action on bone marrow progenitors.

Idiopathic erythrocytosis

In a small proportion of patients with polycythaemia the criteria for the diagnosis of PV are not met and no other aetiology for the raised red cell mass can be identified. This group is heterogeneous and likely to include patients with germline mutations causing polycythaemia as well as some that will go on to develop overt PV. With the advent of increasingly sophisticated diagnostic tests and the identification of the molecular lesions in many inherited forms of polycythaemia, idiopathic erythrocytosis is becoming a rare entity.

Apparent polycythaemia

Apparent polycythaemia refers to a raised PCV in the presence of a normal red cell volume (<25% above the predicted mean normal value). The raised haematocrit is due to a reduction in the plasma volume. Smoking, hypertension, obesity, excessive alcohol and diuretic therapy have all been associated with apparent polycythaemia. Pathogenesis is uncertain and almost certainly heterogeneous.

It is not clear whether apparent polycythaemia is associated with increased rates of thrombosis, but it seems sensible to encourage affected individuals to avoid known predisposing factors. There are no convincing data that routine venesection is beneficial.

Essential thrombocythaemia

The fundamental pathological feature of ET is a persistent elevation in the platelet count. However, ET has been poorly understood largely because of a lack of positive diagnostic criteria together with the fact that cases labelled as ET are likely to be pathogenetically heterogeneous. In 1934 Epstein and Goedel first described a patient with persistent elevation of the platelet count in association with megakaryocyte hyperplasia and tendency for venous thromboses and haemorrhage. Subsequently, Ozer and Gunz independently described two series of patients in 1960, thus confirming ET as a specific clinical entity. The recent discovery that approximately half the cases of ET carry the *JAK2* V617F mutation, as do half the cases of PMF and nearly all cases of PV, has enhanced our understanding of the relationship between the three disorders.

Pathophysiology

X-chromosome inactivation patterns provided the first evidence that ET may be a clonal stem cell disorder involving granulocytes, platelets and red cells but not T cells. For about 60% of patients a molecular basis for the clonality can be found, with about 55% of ET patients positive for the *JAK2* V617F mutation, and a further 5% carrying activating mutations near the transmembrane domain of the thrombopoietin receptor gene *MPL*.

Clinical and pathological features vary significantly between patients with ET, suggesting that the disease is heterogeneous. Prospective data from over 800 patients with ET has demonstrated that the presence or absence of the *JAK2* V617F mutation divides ET into two biologically distinct disorders. Mutation-positive ET exists along a continuum with PV as it displays multiple features of the latter, with significantly increased haemoglobin levels, neutrophil counts and bone marrow erythropoiesis, more venous thromboses and a higher incidence of polycythaemic transformation. Mutation-negative patients do nonetheless exhibit many clinical and laboratory features characteristic of an MPN including the presence of endogenous erythroid colonies and a risk of transformation to acute leukaemia. Patients with *MPL*-positive ET appear to have a phenotype that more closely resembles *JAK2*-negative ET, with an isolated thrombocytosis and less hypercellular bone marrow.

Clinical features

Epidemiology

The annual incidence of ET is similar to that of PV at around 1.5–2.0 cases per 100 000 population. The median age at onset is 50–55 years and although it can occur at any age, it is rare in childhood.

Thrombotic complications

As with PV, thrombotic complications are the main cause of morbidity and mortality in ET. Thromboses are present in around 15–20% of patients at presentation and may be arterial or venous. The range of clinical syndromes is similar to PV, but the frequency of splanchnic thromboses is probably lower and strongly correlated with presence of the *JAK2* V617F mutation.

A number of risk factors are associated with an increase in the risk of thrombosis in patients with ET. The best characterized are age over 60 years and a prior history of thrombosis. Other risk factors for thrombosis in ET are likely to include diabetes, hyperlipidaemia, hypertension and cigarette smoking. More recently, it has been reported that white cell count and reticulin levels at diagnosis have predictive value for thrombosis (and indeed other complications) in ET. The exact role these and other predictors have in individualizing treatment regimens remains unclear.

Haemorrhagic complications

Bleeding is less common and less well studied than thrombosis in ET, but can be dramatic when it happens. Efforts to correlate the thrombotic risk with platelet function abnormalities have generally been fruitless and this investigation is also unable to predict haemorrhagic risk. However, bleeding is more common in patients with platelet counts above 1000×10^9/L and, in at least some cases, this is due to acquired von Willebrand disease, with a decrease in circulating high-molecular-weight multimers caused by adsorption to the surface of the excessive platelets.

Splenomegaly and hyposplenism

Splenomegaly is present in about 5% of ET patients at diagnosis and is rarely more than mild. Progressive enlargement of the spleen during the course of ET should raise suspicion of evolving myelofibrosis. It has been suggested that, over time, some patients with ET develop splenic atrophy secondary to silent microinfarcts in the splenic microcirculation. However, frank hyposplenism and its complications are rare.

Transformation to myelofibrosis or polycythaemia vera

Transformation to myelofibrosis and, more rarely, to PV are recognized complications of ET. Some, but not all, cases of apparent polycythaemic transformation may represent resolution of prior iron deficiency, as can happen with iron supplementation and after the menopause. The insidious onset of myelofibrotic transformation and the reluctance to serially study bone marrow trephine biopsies have hampered attempts to define its nature and frequency. Nonetheless, recent studies have shown that progression of reticulin levels over time shows extensive interindividual variability and can be influenced by choice of therapy, being more marked in patients treated with anagrelide (see below). From the available data, myelofibrotic transformation occurs in less than 10% and polycythaemic transformation in less than 1–2% of ET patients over 10 years.

Leukaemic transformation

ET can evolve into MDS or AML even in untreated cases, but only rarely. The presence of cytogenetic abnormalities and treatment with alkylating agents increase this risk. Approximately 3% of patients treated with hydroxycarbamide alone develop MDS or AML if followed for a median time of 8 years. As with PV, there are no data to demonstrate that hydroxycarbamide as a single agent significantly increases the risk of leukaemia inherent to this disease, but a small effect cannot be excluded.

Investigations

The lack of pathognomonic features and the existence of many other causes of a raised platelet count have posed significant hurdles in the diagnosis of ET. The identification of the *JAK2* V617F mutation now provides a very useful positive diagnostic criterion for approximately 50% of ET patients. However, for V617F-negative patients, ET remains a diagnosis of exclusion and can only be made after other clonal blood disorders and reactive thrombocytosis have been ruled out. A proposed diagnostic schema for ET, as outlined by the BCSH guidelines, is given in Table 36.3.

Table 36.3 Diagnostic criteria for essential thrombocythaemia as recommended in the BCSH guidelines.

A1	Sustained platelet count >450 × 10⁹/L
A2	Presence of an acquired pathogenetic mutation (e.g. in the *JAK2* or *MPL* genes)
A3	No other myeloid malignancy, especially PV*, PMF†, CML‡ or MDS§
A4	No reactive cause for thrombocytosis and normal iron stores
A5	Bone marrow aspirate and trephine biopsy showing increased megakaryocyte numbers displaying a spectrum of morphology with predominant large megakaryocytes with hyperlobated nuclei and abundant cytoplasm. Reticulin is generally not increased (grades 0–2/4 or grade 0/3)

Diagnosis requires A1–A3 or A1 + A3–A5

*Excluded by a normal haematocrit in an iron-replete patient.
†Indicated by presence of significant bone marrow fibrosis (≥2/3 or 3/4 reticulin) *and* palpable splenomegaly, blood film abnormalities (circulating progenitors and teardrop cells) or unexplained anaemia.
‡Excluded by absence of *BCR–ABL1* fusion from bone marrow or peripheral blood.
§Excluded by absence of dysplasia on examination of blood film and bone marrow aspirate.

An alternative set of diagnostic criteria, based largely around salient bone marrow morphological features, have been proposed as part of the WHO classification of tumours. Included in these is the concept of 'prefibrotic myelofibrosis', a putative group of patients previously labelled as ET who reportedly have increased rates of transformation to myelofibrosis over time. These proposals remain highly controversial in the MPN literature. In particular, studies of interobserver reliability for the histological component of this classification have shown it to be poorly reproducible, and a prospective multicentre study of the prognostic discrimination achieved by such a label found it to be minimal. Nevertheless, bone marrow histological features such as giant multilobated megakaryocytes and megakaryocyte clustering (Figure 36.6) can be of value in making the diagnosis of ET.

Reactive thrombocytosis

Thrombocytosis is most commonly reactive and secondary to increased levels of circulating cytokines that stimulate thrombopoiesis. Inflammatory, vasculitic and allergic disorders, acute and chronic infections, malignancies, haemolysis, iron deficiency and blood loss can all lead to an increased platelet count (Table 36.4). Reactive thrombocytosis can sometimes be marked and, occasionally, the platelet count can be greater than

Table 36.4 Causes of a reactive thrombocytosis.

Iron deficiency
Blood loss (acute or chronic)
Hyposplenism/splenectomy
Surgery
Acute bacterial infection
    Pneumonia, septicaemia, meningitis, diverticular abscess, etc.
Chronic inflammation
    Vasculitides
    Inflammatory bowel disease
    Connective tissue disorders
    Rheumatoid arthritis
    Chronic infections
Malignancies
Rebound thrombocytosis
    Following treatment of immune thrombocytopenic purpura
    Recovery from chemotherapy
Drugs
    Vincristine

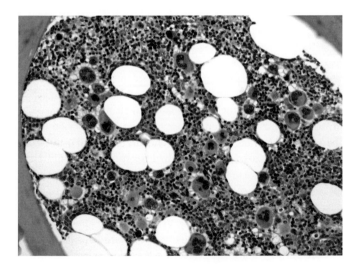

Figure 36.6 Bone marrow trephine section (haematoxylin and eosin, H&E) from a 60-year-old man with essential thrombocythaemia. Note the hypercellularity and marked increase in megakaryocyte numbers, consisting largely of clusters of mature multilobated forms.

1000 × 10⁹/L. There is usually evidence of ongoing inflammation in the form of a raised erythrocyte sedimentation rate or C-reactive protein but this is not always the case.

Other clonal thrombocytoses

A number of other haematological malignancies can be associated with thrombocytosis. Chronic myeloid leukaemia (CML) can be excluded by demonstrating the absence of the

BCR–ABL1 fusion transcript. Iron deficiency can mask the typical raised red cell mass of PV, although the clinical utility of distinguishing iron-deficient PV from ET is probably minimal. Established PMF can be excluded by the absence of significant bone marrow fibrosis and other characteristic laboratory features such as leucoerythroblastic blood film and splenomegaly.

Lastly, MDS can also be associated with a thrombocytosis in a minority of cases, but there are usually coexisting cytopenias, dysplastic features or specific cytogenetic abnormalities (e.g. deletion 5q). Sometimes, refractory anaemia with ringed sideroblasts can be associated with thrombocytosis and the presence of the *JAK2* V617F mutation; this illustrates the overlap among these chronic myeloid disorders.

Treatment

When considering the management of patients with ET, it is helpful to stratify them into risk groups, according to their risk of vascular complications, and take treatment decisions on this basis. Patients may be assigned to a high-, intermediate- or low-risk category.

High-risk patients

High-risk patients are those over 60 years old or those with one or more high-risk features, i.e. a platelet count of 1500×10^9/L or more, a prior history of thrombosis or significant thrombotic risk factors such as diabetes or hypertension. In high-risk patients, control of the platelet count with hydroxycarbamide reduces thrombotic events compared with no cytoreductive therapy. The MRC PT-1 trial has recently compared treatment with hydroxycarbamide plus low-dose aspirin to anagrelide plus low-dose aspirin. Patients receiving anagrelide plus aspirin were significantly more likely to reach the composite primary end point (arterial thrombosis, venous thrombosis or major haemorrhage) and more likely to discontinue their allocated treatment. Compared with hydroxycarbamide plus aspirin, treatment with anagrelide plus aspirin was associated with a significantly increased rate of arterial thrombosis, major haemorrhage and myelofibrotic transformation, but a decreased rate of venous thromboembolism. These results suggest that hydroxycarbamide plus aspirin should remain first-line therapy for high-risk patients. Anagrelide is a useful second-line agent but the decision to use concurrent aspirin should depend on the relative risks of arterial thrombosis and haemorrhage in the individual patient.

Analysis of patients from the PT-1 trial according to *JAK2* status has shown that compared with V617F-negative patients, mutation-positive patients share many features with PV including a higher risk of venous thrombosis. Moreover, V617F-positive patients were more sensitive to hydroxycarbamide than anagrelide, raising the possibility that hydroxycarbamide is particularly effective in these patients.

Interferon alfa can give good control of the platelet count in ET, but as discussed under PV, its significant side-effect profile, subcutaneous administration and cost prevent its widespread use. It has a clearer role in the management of ET in pregnancy (see later) and some favour it in young patients. Busulfan can achieve good control of the platelet count but is only rarely used because of concerns over its long-term leukaemogenic potential. This is true for other alkylating agents and for radioactive phosphorus (^{32}P).

Intermediate-risk patients

Intermediate-risk patients are those between 40 and 60 years old who lack any of the high-risk features listed above. It is not clear whether it is beneficial to lower the platelet count in this group. Most receive either aspirin alone, or hydroxycarbamide and aspirin.

Low-risk patients

Low-risk patients are those younger than 40 years old who lack any high-risk features. Low-risk patients are usually given low-dose aspirin alone unless there is a contraindication such as previous peptic ulceration or allergy to salicylates. Antiplatelet agents such as dipyridamole or clopidogrel should be considered in these cases. In the setting of ET-associated haemorrhage, it is probably best to avoid antiplatelet agents.

Prognosis

Few studies have directly addressed survival in ET and these have reached different conclusions. Some suggest that mortality at 10 years is that of age-matched controls, whereas others found it to be worse. In high-risk patients, hydroxycarbamide reduces vaso-occlusive events from 10.7 to 1.6 per 100 patient-years.

Essential thrombocythaemia and pregnancy

ET is the MPN encountered most frequently in women of childbearing age. In pregnancy, the commonest complication of ET is first-trimester miscarriage, which occurs in up to 30% of pregnancies. This is thought to be secondary to placental microinfarcts and insufficiency. The reported increased incidence of antiphospholipid antibodies in ET may contribute to this. Other less frequent complications include intrauterine death, growth retardation, premature delivery and pre-eclampsia. The risk of maternal thrombosis and haemorrhage is higher than in normal pregnancy, although a successful outcome (live birth) is achieved in around 60% of cases and no maternal deaths were seen in a recent review of 220 pregnancies.

The optimal management of ET in pregnancy has not yet been fully defined. There is conflicting evidence about the effectiveness of aspirin but, given the good documentation of its safety in a large unrelated study of pre-eclampsia, it should probably be given to most patients who are pregnant or planning a pregnancy. Pregnancies deemed at high risk of thrombosis either on the basis of a prior history of thrombosis or a platelet count over $1500 \times 10^9/L$ should be considered for therapy with a combination of interferon and aspirin. Hydroxycarbamide and anagrelide should not be used on account of their teratogenic potential. In addition to lowering the platelet count, cases at the highest risk of thrombosis, such as those with previous thrombosis, hypertension or diabetes, should be considered for antithrombotic prophylaxis, normally in the form of low-molecular-weight heparin.

The platelet count may rise dramatically in the postpartum period but can normally be controlled with hydroxycarbamide or anagrelide. Hydroxycarbamide and anagrelide are excreted in breast milk so that breast-feeding is contraindicated while a patient is receiving either of these agents. Although interferon alfa is also excreted in breast milk, it is unlikely to be absorbed intact by the baby and there are anecdotal reports of successful breast-feeding while the mother was receiving interferon.

Primary myelofibrosis

Also known as agnogenic myeloid metaplasia and idiopathic myelofibrosis, PMF has the poorest prognosis of the MPNs. PV and ET can develop into a condition that resembles PMF, usually after a latency of many years. The first reported case of PMF is probably that described by Hueck in 1879 as a 'peculiar leukaemia'. It was not until Dameshek's seminal work in 1951 that PMF was recognized as an MPN. The identification of the *JAK2* V617F mutation in approximately half the cases of PMF and ET and nearly all cases of PV has revolutionized our understanding of the relationship between the three disorders. In fact, analogous to the concept of chronic and accelerated phase in CML, it may well be that PMF represents an accelerated phase of MPN, associated with the acquisition of further genetic abnormalities. In this model, patients presenting with apparently *de novo* PMF may have had a preceding undiagnosed disorder such as ET or PV.

Pathophysiology

PMF is a clonal MPN of the pluripotent haemopoietic stem cell, in which the proliferation of multiple cell lineages is accompanied by progressive bone marrow fibrosis. This is true for both *JAK2* V617F-positive and -negative cases while the precise effect of the mutation on the PMF phenotype awaits further studies.

Marrow fibrosis is thought to be secondary to the release of proinflammatory cytokines from abnormal clonal cells (primarily megakaryocytes), which act to stimulate fibroblast proliferation and fibrosis. In support of this premise, transgenic mice expressing high levels of thrombopoietin rapidly develop mye-

lofibrosis in association with increased megakaryocyte numbers. Additionally, mice expressing reduced levels of the transcription factor GATA-1, which impairs the ability of their megakaryocytes to differentiate into platelets, also develop myelofibrosis in association with increased expression of cytokines such as transforming growth factor (TGF)-β1, platelet-derived growth factor (PDGF) and vascular endothelial growth factor in the bone marrow.

In the peripheral circulation there is an increase in the number of CD34-positive cells together with increased numbers of progenitors capable of giving rise to a variety of haemopoietic colonies. As with PV and ET, erythroid and megakaryocytic colonies can also be derived in the absence of exogenous growth factors.

The same molecular abnormalities seen in chronic-phase MPNs, such as mutations in *JAK2*, *MPL* and *TET2*, are found in patients with PMF, underscoring the interrelated nature of these disorders. Nonetheless, other mutations and epigenetic abnormalities are more frequently found in PMF, in keeping with the more aggressive phenotype, poorer prognosis and later stage of the disease. For example, cytogenetic abnormalities are found in up to 60% of cases. The commonest are deletions of 20q and 13q, trisomy 8, and abnormalities of chromosomes 1, 5, 7 and 9. Oncogene mutations are not infrequently found, and include point mutations in the *RAS*, *KIT* and *TP53*.

Clinical features

Epidemiology

The estimated annual incidence of PMF is around 0.5–1.5 per 100 000 population, with most patients diagnosed in the sixth decade and roughly equal involvement of the two sexes. Up to one-third of patients are asymptomatic at diagnosis and many of these are discovered after unrelated blood tests show modest abnormalities such as anaemia and thrombocytopenia.

Splenomegaly

An enlarged spleen is found in almost all patients at presentation and splenic pain/discomfort is a common presenting symptom of PMF. Most cases develop moderate to marked splenomegaly during the course of the disease and about 10% of cases develop massive splenomegaly, with the spleen extending to the right iliac fossa (Figure 36.7). This dramatic increase in splenic mass (up to 20–30 times normal) can lead to a substantial increase in splenic blood flow which, in the most severe cases, can lead to portal hypertension with oesophageal varices and ascites. Painful and painless splenic infarcts are common sequelae of splenomegaly in PMF.

Extramedullary haemopoiesis

The spleen is the commonest site of extramedullary haemopoiesis in PMF. The liver is also usually involved and this can lead to significant hepatomegaly. Unusual sites can sometimes be

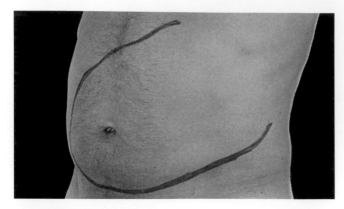

Figure 36.7 Massive splenomegaly in a 53-year-old man with an 8-year history of primary myelofibrosis.

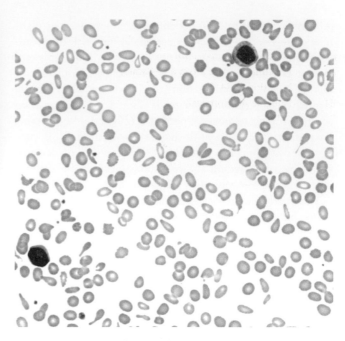

Figure 36.8 Peripheral blood film in primary myelofibrosis showing a blast, an abnormal myelocyte, teardrop red cells and marked anisopoikilocytosis.

affected, leading to haemopoietic tumours surrounded by a capsule of connective tissue. Such sites include lymph nodes, central nervous system, skin, pericardium, peritoneum, pleura, ovaries, kidneys, adrenals, gastrointestinal tract and lungs. Many such cases remain asymptomatic, but involvement of the central nervous system can be a cause of serious morbidity. Treatment with radiotherapy or surgery, when required, almost always leads to resolution of these masses.

Systemic symptoms

A hypermetabolic state presenting with fevers, anorexia, weight loss and night sweats develops in many cases of PMF, sometimes early in the disease. The presence of such symptoms is associated with a poor prognosis.

Anaemia

Mild to moderate anaemia is found in most patients at presentation and worsens as myelofibrosis progresses. The anaemia is in large part due to reduced erythropoiesis, but may be compounded by hypersplenism, bleeding and iron or folate deficiency. Acquired HbH disease is a rare complication.

Platelet abnormalities

Platelet counts are raised in up to half of the cases at presentation and can be associated with thrombotic complications. However, progressive thrombocytopenia is a frequent occurrence and becomes increasingly troublesome as the disease progresses. Dysmegakaryopoiesis and abnormal platelet function further add to the risk of haemorrhagic complications.

White cells and leukaemic transformation

The presence of immature myeloid as well as erythroid progenitors is a characteristic feature of PMF (Figure 36.8). Neutrophilia is common, as are modest elevations in basophil and eosinophil counts. As the disease progresses, leucopenia increases in frequency and is believed to be secondary to progressive hyper-

splenism, dysmyelopoiesis and progressive replacement of the bone marrow by fibrotic tissue. In end-stage PMF, myeloid precursors become increasingly common relative to mature cells, as do circulating blasts. Transformation to AML occurs in 20–30% of cases of PMF and is usually rapidly fatal.

Investigations

Diagnostic criteria for PMF are shown in Table 36.5. Other causes of bone marrow fibrosis are listed in Table 36.6.

Peripheral blood

The presence of myeloid and erythroid precursors in the peripheral blood (leucoerythroblastic blood picture) is common in PMF (see Figure 36.8). Other causes of a leucoerythroblastic blood film include bone marrow infiltration, severe sepsis, severe haemolysis and a sick neonate. Teardrop poikilocytes (dacryocytes), basophilic stippling, macrocytosis (which may or may not be secondary to folate deficiency), giant platelets and megakaryocyte fragments may also be present.

Bone marrow

Attempts at bone marrow aspiration often yield a dry tap or a haemodilute sample, making aspirate morphology of limited diagnostic value. Sufficient material can often be obtained from either bone marrow or peripheral blood to assess the karyotype, which can help exclude diagnoses such as CML. Other chromosomal abnormalities may be found in up to 60% of cases as

Table 36.5 Diagnostic criteria for primary myelofibrosis.

JAK2-positive primary myelofibrosis

A1	Reticulin ≥ grade 3 (on a 0–4 scale)
A2	Mutation in *JAK2*
B1	Palpable splenomegaly
B2	Otherwise unexplained anaemia (Hb < 11.5 g/L for men, < 10 g/L for women)
B3	Teardrop red cells on peripheral blood film
B4	Leucoerythroblastic blood film (presence of at least two nucleated red cells or immature myeloid cells in peripheral blood film)
B5	Systemic symptoms (drenching night sweats, weight loss >10% over 6 months *or* diffuse bone pain)
B6	Histological evidence of extramedullary haemopoiesis

Diagnosis requires A1 + A2 and any two B criteria

JAK2-negative primary myelofibrosis

A1	Reticulin ≥grade 3 (on a 0–4 scale)
A2	Absence of mutation in *JAK2*
A3	Absence of *BCR–ABL1* fusion gene
B1	Palpable splenomegaly
B2	Otherwise unexplained anaemia (Hb < 11.5 g/L for men, < 10 g/L for women)
B3	Teardrop red cells on peripheral blood film
B4	Leuckoerythroblastic blood film (presence of at least two nucleated red cells or immature myeloid cells in peripheral blood film)
B5	Systemic symptoms (drenching night sweats, weight loss >10% over 6 months *or* diffuse bone pain)
B6	Histological evidence of extramedullary haemopoiesis

Diagnosis requires A1 + A2 + A3 and any two B criteria

Table 36.6 Differential diagnosis of marrow fibrosis.

Haematological malignancies
    Primary myelofibrosis
    Chronic myeloid leukaemia
    Acute myelofibrosis (AML M7)
    Myelodysplasia
    Myeloma
    Hairy-cell leukaemia
    Non-Hodgkin lymphoma
    Hodgkin disease
    Systemic mastocytosis
Metastatic carcinoma
Infections
    Tuberculosis
    Leishmaniasis
Drugs/toxins
    Benzene
    Thorotrast
    Irradiation
Bone disease
    Paget disease
    Osteopetrosis
    Hyperparathyroidism
    Hypoparathyroidism
Inflammatory diseases
    Systemic sclerosis
    Systemic lupus
Other
    Grey platelet syndrome

detailed above. Abnormalities of chromosomes 5 and 7 are usually found in patients with prior exposure to genotoxic agents and are associated with a poor prognosis.

Bone marrow trephine biopsy is essential to make a diagnosis of PMF. Initial stages are characterized by an increase in bone marrow cellularity in association with disorganization of marrow architecture and the presence of abnormal large megakaryocytes often occurring in clusters (Figure 36.9). Bone marrow fibrosis becomes increasingly dominant and progressively replaces haemopoiesis. Intrasinusoidal haemopoiesis can sometimes be seen at this stage (Figure 36.10). The degree of fibrosis is best demonstrated using silver impregnation, which stains reticulin fibres (Figure 36.9). Collagen fibres are best demonstrated using a trichrome stain. The degree of fibrosis can be graded from 0 to 4 according to severity. In a minority of cases of advanced PMF, osteosclerosis ensues with thickening of the trabecula and extensive deposition of osteoid. Such changes may be evident on plain radiography.

Treatment

The only curative treatment for PMF is allogeneic stem cell transplantation, but this is only appropriate for a small proportion of patients. In the remaining cases therapy remains supportive and aimed at alleviating symptoms, but has little impact on the relatively poor survival of PMF patients. It is for this reason that the future development of therapeutic JAK2 inhibitors is most eagerly awaited for these patients, rather than for those with PV or ET who have a much better prognosis.

Conventional allogeneic bone marrow transplantation is only a realistic option in young patients, who represent perhaps 10% of all cases. The decision to proceed to transplantation should always be made in light of the patient's specific prognosis, age and general fitness. Only small series have been reported and the long-term survival of patients 45 years and younger is approximately 50%, with a 30% transplant-related mortality. For patients 45 years and older, outcomes are much worse, with long-term survival of 10–20%. Small numbers of reduced-intensity transplants have been reported, which show that this

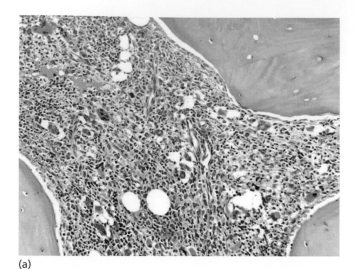

(a)

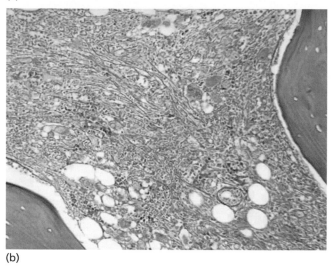

(b)

Figure 36.9 Bone marrow trephine sections from a patient with early-stage primary myelofibrosis. The H&E stain (a) shows hypercellularity, disorganized architecture, increase in megakaryocyte numbers and prominent sinusoids. The silver stain (b) also shows a marked increase in reticulin fibres.

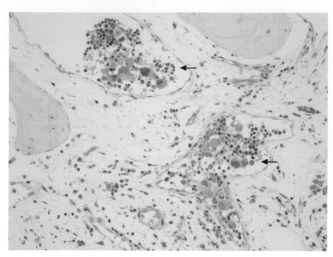

Figure 36.10 Bone marrow trephine section in primary myelofibrosis (H&E). Note the presence of two dilated sinusoids (arrows) containing immature haemopoietic cells, including megakaryocytes.

modality is feasible and safe in patients over 50 years old, although its efficacy is not yet clear.

Anaemia responds to treatment with androgens in up to one-third of cases, with the best responses seen in patients without massive splenomegaly and with a normal karyotype. The drugs most commonly used are oxymetholone (50–150 mg daily) and danazol (400–600 mg daily). Both of these can have virilizing effects and can lead to abnormal liver function. Patients with a reduced red cell survival may respond to treatment with corticosteroids. Human recombinant Epo has recently shown promise in small clinical studies of anaemia in PMF. Splenectomy also has a role (see below). Despite these treatments, most patients become transfusion dependent eventually.

Cytoreductive therapy can be useful in the management of some aspects of PMF, such as hepatosplenomegaly, constitutional symptoms and troublesome thrombocytosis. Hydroxycarbamide is the most widely used agent but anagrelide has also been used for thrombocytosis.

The indications for splenectomy include splenic pain, constitutional symptoms, portal hypertension and transfusion-dependent anaemia. In contrast, there is no good evidence that thrombocytopenia responds to splenectomy. The procedure has significant mortality (around 10%) and morbidity, particularly in elderly patients. Problems include perioperative bleeding, infection and thrombosis as well as rebound thrombocytosis and progressive hepatomegaly. It is particularly important to correct any coagulation abnormalities prior to surgery.

Splenic irradiation is an alternative to splenectomy in some cases and can significantly reduce splenic size, albeit transiently. This procedure is not without complications as it can lead to life-threatening cytopenias. Radiotherapy can also be useful for treating pockets of extramedullary haemopoiesis involving vital organs or body cavities.

The anti-angiogenic drug thalidomide has been reported to improve anaemia, thrombocytopenia or splenomegaly in approximately one-third of patients, but these changes are clinically significant only in a small proportion (20%). Thalidomide is poorly tolerated at conventional doses (>100 mg daily) with more than half of the patients being unable to tolerate it beyond 3 months. Furthermore, thalidomide increases the risk of extreme thrombocytosis and probably that of venous thrombosis, and needs special precautions for use in view of its extreme teratogenicity. Trials of lower doses of the drug alone or in combination with prednisolone suggest that such doses are

Table 36.7 Prognostic scoring systems in myelofibrosis: the Lille scoring system.

Number of adverse prognostic factors	Risk group	Cases (%)	Median survival (months)
0	Low	47	93
1	Intermediate	45	26
2	High	8	13

Adverse prognostic factors: Hb 10 g/dL, WBC < 4 or >30 × 10⁹/L.
Source: Dupriez *et al.* (1996) with permission.

Table 36.8 Prognostic scoring systems in myelofibrosis: the Sheffield prognostic system.

Age (years)	Hb (g/dL)	Karyotype	Median survival in months (95% CI)
<68	>10	Normal	180 (6–354)
		Abnormal	72 (32–112)
	≤10	Normal	54 (46–62)
		Abnormal	22 (14–30)
≥68	>10	Normal	70 (61–79)
		Abnormal	78 (26–130)
	≤10	Normal	44 (31–57)
		Abnormal	16 (5–27)

Source: Reilly *et al.* (1997) with permission.

better tolerated and may be similarly efficacious. Bisphosphonates can help with bone pain.

Prognosis

The median survival is 3–5 years, but the range is very wide. As a result, efforts have been made to devise algorithms to individualize prognosis. The two most widely used algorithms are shown in Tables 36.7 and 36.8. Recently, an elevation in CD34 cell count above 300 × 10⁶/L and the presence of *JAK2* V617F mutation were also identified as adverse prognostic features.

Mastocytosis

Mastocytosis comprises a rare group of disorders characterized by a pathological increase in mast cells in tissues including the skin, bone marrow, liver, spleen, lymph nodes and gastrointestinal tract. Mastocytosis can be an isolated finding or can form part of other haematological disorders, including MDS, MPNs or AML. Some cases involve just the skin (cutaneous mastocytosis) whereas others involve multiple tissues and are associated

Table 36.9 Classification of mastocytosis.

Cutaneous mastocytosis
  Urticaria pigmentosa and variants
  Mastocytoma of the skin
Systemic mastocytosis
  Indolent
  Aggressive
Systemic mastocytosis with associated haematological non-mast cell disorder
Mast cell leukaemia
Mast cell sarcoma

Source: modified from Valent *et al.* (2001) with permission.

with systemic symptoms (systemic mastocytosis). Paediatric mast cell disease is generally a reactive condition rather than a clonal MPN and is not further discussed here. A classification of mast cell diseases has been proposed (Table 36.9).

The first case of urticaria pigmentosa (a form of cutaneous mastocytosis) was described in 1869 by Nettleship, and systemic disease due to increased mast cells was first documented by Ellis in 1949. The observation that stem cell factor (SCF) is an essential growth factor for mast cell development has led to significant advances in our understanding of this group of diseases.

Pathophysiology

After a search for abnormalities of SCF failed to identify any pathological changes, researchers turned to c-Kit, the tyrosine kinase receptor for SCF. A point mutation in the *KIT* gene leading to a single amino acid substitution (Asp816Val) in c-Kit was thus identified. This mutation leads to ligand-independent phosphorylation of c-Kit and consequent clonal expansion of mast cells.

Asp816Val was originally identified in cases of mastocytosis with associated haematological disorders but is now known to be present in the majority of adults presenting with urticaria pigmentosa or indolent systemic mastocytosis. More recently, other activating mutations affecting the same codon have been identified in a minority of adult cases of cutaneous mastocytosis (Asp816Tyr, Asp816Phe). A different mutation has been reported in a small number of cases of paediatric mastocytosis, namely Lys839Glu, which surprisingly gives rise to a dominant-negative (inactivating) form of c-Kit; the significance of this observation remains unresolved.

Recent reports have suggested that in some cases of mastocytosis, the c-Kit mutation is found in other haemopoietic cells such as B cells, myeloid cells and T cells. These results suggest that mastocytosis, as with the classical MPNs, may be a clonal disorder of the haemopoietic stem cell.

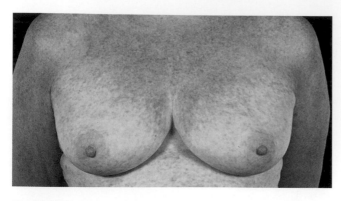

Figure 36.11 Urticaria pigmentosa in a 55-year-old woman. Note the widespread pink or brownish macules that become confluent in areas.

Clinical features

Cutaneous manifestations

Urticaria pigmentosa is the usual presenting feature in children and adults with isolated mastocytosis. Yellowish-brown lesions, usually macular and sometimes papular, appear in a patchy distribution. Less commonly, there is diffuse involvement of the skin, which becomes thickened and darker brown (Figure 36.11). Pruritus is common, as is flushing, and some cases develop haemorrhagic bullous disease. Whealing of lesions on rubbing is known as the Darier sign.

Systemic disease

Systemic manifestations are very heterogeneous and are thought to be largely secondary to mast cell mediator release. Episodes of flushing, angio-oedema, or even anaphylaxis with or without any specific trigger, can arise as a result of systemic histamine release. Gastrointestinal symptoms include abdominal pain, diarrhoea, nausea and vomiting. Gastritis and peptic ulceration may occur secondary to hyperhistaminaemia and severe cases may develop malabsorption. Osteoporosis is well recognized and can sometimes lead to pathological fractures. Peripheral blood cytopenias may arise secondary to mast cell infiltration of the bone marrow. Hepatosplenomegaly is more common in cases associated with another clonal haematological disorder. Fever, fatigue and weight loss can sometimes ensue and may result from the release of cytokines such as tumour necrosis factor (TNF)-α and IL-1.

Symptoms of organ failure due to infiltration are characteristic of aggressive systemic mastocytosis. Depending on the organs involved, cytopenias, pathological fractures, impaired liver function, ascites and malabsorption can all be seen.

Investigations

Clinical features of mastocytosis can be highly suggestive of the disease but diagnosis usually requires histological and biochem-

Table 36.10 Criteria for the diagnosis of systemic mast cell disease.

Major
Multifocal dense infiltrates of mast cells in bone marrow and/or other extracutaneous tissues

Minor
More than 25% of mast cells on bone marrow smears or tissue biopsies are atypical or spindle-shaped
Identification of a codon 816 KIT point mutation in blood, bone marrow or lesional skin
Mast cells in bone marrow, blood or other lesional tissues expressing CD25 or CD2
Baseline total serum tryptase greater than 20 ng/mL

Major and one minor or three or more minor criteria needed for diagnosis

Source: modified from Valent *et al.*(2001) with permission.

ical confirmation. An algorithm has been proposed for the diagnosis of systemic mast cell disease and is shown in Table 36.10.

Routine investigations should include a full blood count, liver function tests and a random serum tryptase. Tests for histamine metabolites in 24-hour urine specimens are probably no more useful than measurements of serum tryptase. Plasma levels of soluble CD25 and CD117 (c-Kit) have shown promise as novel markers of mast cell disease.

Bone marrow aspiration and trephine biopsy allow assessment of bone marrow involvement. Mast cell aggregates can be visualized on conventional haematoxylin and eosin-stained sections (Figure 36.12) but stand out much more clearly with stains such as toluidine blue (Figure 36.13). Immunochemistry using anti-tryptase antibodies can also be very useful, being highly specific for mast cells. Flow cytometry for expression of CD2 and CD25 in bone marrow mast cells may be useful as this phenotype is not seen in normal mast cells.

Abdominal ultrasound or computed tomography should be performed to look for hepatosplenomegaly and lymphadenopathy. Plain radiography and bone densitometry can be used to determine if bone involvement and osteoporosis are present. Endoscopy and biopsy can be useful if gut involvement is suspected.

Treatment

Despite significant advances in the understanding of its pathophysiology, no curative treatment exists for mastocytosis, the management of which remains symptomatic. There are four main components to the management of mastocytosis:
1 avoidance of factors that can trigger mediator release from mast cells;

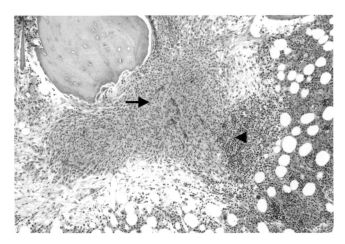

Figure 36.12 Systemic mastocytosis involving the bone marrow (H&E). Malignant whorls of rounded and spindle-shaped mast cells are seen infiltrating the bone marrow in a paratrabecular distribution (arrow). A lymphoid aggregate and areas of hypocellularity are seen interspersed between the mast cell infiltrate and neighbouring haemopoietic islands (arrowhead). (Courtesy of Dr Wendy Erber.)

2 treatment of acute mediator release;
3 treatment of chronic mediator release;
4 reduction of the mast cell burden/organ infiltration.

Avoidance of triggers of mast cell mediator release is primarily an exercise in patient education. Severe reactions due to systemic mast cell mediator release are difficult to predict in patients with mastocytosis and do not correlate well with disease category, mast cell burden or severity of other symptoms. All patients and relevant healthcare workers should be warned of particular triggers, including general anaesthesia, contrast radiography and insect stings. Known mast cell activators such as morphine and dextran should only be introduced with great caution. Patients with previous anaphylaxis or severe hypotension should carry injectable adrenaline and they, their family and friends should be instructed in its intramuscular administration. Local mediator release in cutaneous mastocytosis can be moderated by avoidance of triggering factors such as friction and heat.

Acute systemic mast cell mediator release should be treated in much the same way as other forms of anaphylaxis. Treatment with adrenaline and intravenous fluids should be started as soon as possible, with early involvement of intensive care specialists in severe cases. Antihistamines (H_1 and H_2 blockers) should be introduced and continued long term if the episode is particularly severe or recurrent.

Symptoms of chronic mediator release are the commonest clinical problem in mastocytosis. Symptomatic cutaneous disease should be managed with the help of a dermatologist. Treatments include H_1 and H_2 blockers, topical corticosteroids and PUVA (psoralen with UVA irradiation) for severe disease.

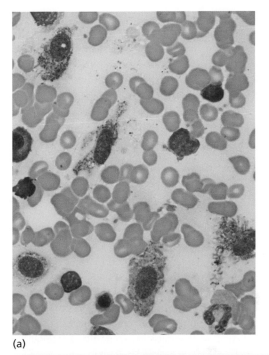

(a)

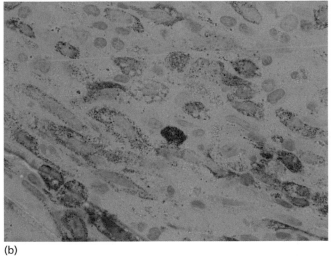

(b)

Figure 36.13 Toluidine blue stain of bone marrow aspirate (a) and trephine biopsy section (b) in systemic mastocytosis. Abnormal spindle-shaped mast cells containing metachromatic granules are seen.

Non-life-threatening systemic symptoms such as flushing, abdominal pain and diarrhoea should be treated with H_1 and H_2 blockers, sodium cromoglycate and corticosteroids. Inhibitors of prostaglandin synthesis, such as aspirin and non-steroidal anti-inflammatory drugs, can also be useful. Aspirin should always be started with caution as it can initially lead to acute mediator release. Such drugs can be used prophylactically if symptoms recur frequently. Gastrointestinal disease usually responds to the drugs used to treat chronic systemic symptoms.

Anecdotally, leukotriene antagonists help with abdominal cramps and diarrhoea. Peptic ulcer and reflux disease should be treated with proton pump inhibitors. Osteoporosis should be treated with bisphosphonates and may be prevented with bisphosphonates or calcium and vitamin D supplementation. Bone density should be recorded and monitored according to the severity of osteoporosis. Radiotherapy can help with severe localized pain.

For patients in whom adequate symptomatic control cannot be achieved and for those with aggressive mastocytosis, interferon alfa, usually given in combination with oral corticosteroids, should be considered. Splenectomy may help reduce the mast cell burden and associated systemic symptoms. Cladribine has been found effective in isolated cases of aggressive systemic mastocytosis.

Treatment with chemotherapy is usually reserved for cases of rapidly progressive aggressive mastocytosis, mast cell leukaemia and mast cell sarcoma, but published data are not encouraging. Mast cell sarcoma may also respond to local radiotherapy when appropriate. Allogeneic bone marrow transplantation should also be considered. Treatment of any associated haematological disorder should be undertaken as appropriate for that disorder and the overall prognosis is usually that of the latter.

Future treatments

Treatments that target the mutant c-Kit tyrosine kinase have attracted a lot of interest recently. Imatinib is known to inhibit wild-type c-Kit *in vitro* and to be active against juxtamembrane mutants of c-Kit found in gastrointestinal stromal tumours. In contrast, the drug does not have the same effect on malignant mast cells carrying codon 816 mutations, probably because the mutant c-Kit does not allow access of imatinib to the site, hence conferring resistance to this drug in a similar way to acquired imatinib resistance in CML. In keeping with this, there have been early reports of its lack of efficacy in the presence of codon 816 mutations. A recent report showing that imatinib was effective in patients with mastocytosis with associated eosinophilia but without demonstrable *KIT* mutations awaits confirmation, particularly as these cases may represent variants of chronic eosinophilic leukaemia (CEL). Novel tyrosine kinase inhibitors that can inhibit the Asp816Val mutant c-Kit *in vitro* are under investigation.

Prognosis

Age and disease category are the most important determinants of outcome. The most benign syndrome is paediatric mastocytoma, which disappears with time in over 50% of cases. Paediatric urticaria pigmentosa also has a good prognosis and resolves in about half of the cases.

In adult mastocytosis, urticaria pigmentosa is usually associated with mast cell deposits in the marrow or other tissues, making this a systemic syndrome. Indolent systemic mastocytosis carries a favourable prognosis and usually persists as a chronic low-grade disorder, although it rarely progresses to aggressive mastocytosis or mastocytosis associated with another haematological malignancy. Aggressive systemic mastocytosis can show a slowly progressive or a rapid clinical course but its overall prognosis has not been well defined in clinical studies. Mast cell leukaemia is rare but has a grave prognosis, with a median survival of less than 6 months.

Clonal hypereosinophilic syndromes

The term 'hypereosinophilic syndrome' (HES) was coined by Hardy and Anderson in 1968, who gave it the definition still in use today. Recently, major progress has been made in elucidating the molecular pathogenesis of clonal eosinophilia as described below.

Pathophysiology

Eosinophilia can be divided into three categories: reactive, idiopathic and clonal (Table 36.11). Reactive eosinophilia, which is by far the most common, is discussed in Chapter 17.

Idiopathic eosinophilias are those in which the cause is obscure. Within this category, HES describes patients with an unexplained elevation of peripheral blood eosinophils ($>1.5 \times 10^9$/L) for more than 6 months associated with end-organ damage (see Chapter 17). Many of these are probably cases of CEL for which the molecular defect has not been identified.

Clonal eosinophilias are those in which the eosinophilia is part of a clonal haematological malignancy. CEL is defined as an eosinophil count in excess of 1.5×10^9/L, with evidence of eosinophil clonality or an increased blast count in blood or bone marrow. The distinction between this entity and HES is blurred as it relies on the availability of a clonal marker. Indeed it has been shown recently that 25–50% of cases labelled as HES in fact have a microdeletion on chromosome 4, which results in the fusion of the *FIP1L1* and *PDGFRA* genes and the generation of a constitutively active tyrosine kinase. Importantly, patients carrying this fusion respond well to the tyrosine kinase inhibitor imatinib. Some patients with HES who do not carry this fusion gene also respond to imatinib, suggesting that in such cases other tyrosine kinases may be dysregulated.

In addition to CEL, a number of other haematological malignancies may be associated with increased numbers of clonal eosinophils, and in many cases this reflects tyrosine kinase dysregulation. *PDGFRA* rearrangements (e.g. *TEL–PDGFRB*) may present as chronic myelomonocytic leukaemia or atypical CML. The 8p11 myeloproliferative syndrome (EMS) is associated with rearrangements in the *FGFR1* gene (e.g. *ZMYM2–FGFR1*) and leads to a chronic MPN that frequently presents with eosinophilia and associated T-cell lymphoblastic lymphoma. CML,

Table 36.11 Causes of eosinophilia.

Reactive eosinophilia
Infections
    Parasitic
    Others (rarely)
Vasculitides
    Polyarteritis nodosa
    Churg–Strauss syndrome
Connective tissue disorders
    Rheumatoid arthritis
    Systemic sclerosis
    Systemic lupus erythematosus
Allergic and inflammatory disorders
    Asthma
    Eczema
    Bullous skin diseases
    Inflammatory bowel disease
Drug reactions
    Hypersensitivity
    L-Tryptophan
Immunodeficiencies
    Wiskott–Aldrich syndrome
    Job syndrome (hyper-IgE)
Neoplasia
    Hodgkin disease
    Non-Hodgkin lymphoma
    Peripheral blood T-cell clones
    Some cases of acute lymphoblastic leukaemia
    Non-haematological cancers (rare)

Clonal eosinophilia
Chronic eosinophilic leukaemia
Atypical chronic myeloid leukaemia (*PDGFRA* fusions)
8p11 Myeloproliferative syndrome (*FGFR1* fusions)
Chronic myeloid leukaemia (*BCR–ABL1* fusion)
Acute myeloid leukaemia, e.g. carrying inv(16)
Acute lymphoblastic leukaemia (occasionally)

Idiopathic eosinophilia
Hypereosinophilic syndrome

a consequence of the *BCR–ABL1* tyrosine kinase fusion protein, may also be associated with clonal eosinophilia.

Eosinophilia as part of the malignant clone also occurs in patients with AML associated with inversion of chromosome 16 and the *SMMHC–CBFB* rearrangement. It has been reported that rare cases of acute lymphoblastic leukaemia may be associated with clonal eosinophilia but in this disease the eosinophilia is more usually secondary to growth factor release. Growth factor release is also believed to underlie the reactive eosinophilia seen in Hodgkin disease and in cases with clonal T cells in the peripheral blood.

Sustained hypereosinophilia can lead to symptomatology and end-organ damage regardless of its aetiology, but does not always do so. The reasons for this are unclear but may lie in the heterogeneity of eosinophilia and genetic differences between individuals that affect the propensity of eosinophils and other granulocytes to inflict tissue damage.

Clinical features (see also Chapter 17)

Much of the tissue damage in eosinophilia is believed to be secondary to eosinophil degranulation and release of mediators such as eosinophil cationic protein and major basic protein. Eosinophil mediators act mainly locally in tissues infiltrated by eosinophils to cause tissue damage. The recent finding that a raised serum tryptase in a subset of cases with clonal eosinophilia hints at a role for other cells (mast cells) in some cases.

Patients can present with constitutional symptoms such as fatigue, muscle aches or fevers. Pruritus, angio-oedema, diarrhoea and cough may also be present. Many tissues can be involved, but cardiac disease is the major cause of mortality. The heart can be affected by endomyocardial fibrosis, pericarditis, myocarditis and intramural thrombus formation. Death is usually due to dilated cardiomyopathy.

Involvement of the central and peripheral nervous systems can result in mononeuritis multiplex, paraparesis, encephalopathy and even dementia. Pulmonary involvement can take the form of pulmonary infiltrates, fibrosis or pleural disease with effusions. Gastrointestinal involvement can manifest as diarrhoea, gastritis, colitis, hepatitis or Budd–Chiari syndrome. The skin can be affected by pruritus, angio-oedema, papules or plaques. Rarely, other tissues such as the kidneys and bones can be involved.

Investigations

There are two aims in the investigation of eosinophilia: one is to establish its aetiology and the other to look for evidence of end-organ damage. As regards the former, given the diverse nature of the aetiologies of eosinophilia, a full history including family history, drug history and travel history can provide valuable clues. Investigations will usually aim to exclude reactive causes and will be guided by the clinical picture.

Bone marrow aspiration will reveal morphological abnormalities associated with haematological malignancies and allows cytogenetic analysis. It is also important to look for clonal T-cell receptor (TCR) gene rearrangements, the *FIP1L1–PDGFRA* and *BCR–ABL1* fusion genes, as well as rearrangements of the *PDGFRB* and *FGFR1* genes. It has been reported that serum tryptase is raised in patients with the *FIP1L1–PDGFRA* fusion.

Investigations to assess end-organ damage will depend on the clinical presentation. However, echocardiography should be

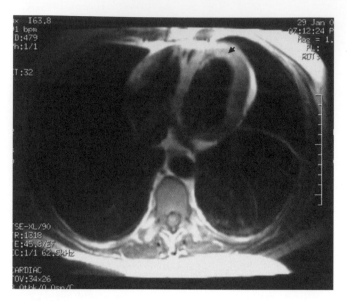

Figure 36.14 Cardiac MRI scan in a 65-year-old man with hypereosinophilic syndrome showing a rim of subendocardial fibrosis (arrow).

performed and repeated annually in patients with sustained eosinophilia, particularly as cardiac disease correlates poorly with the eosinophil count. If there is strong clinical suspicion of cardiac damage, then cardiac magnetic resonance imaging (MRI) can be useful, as this is more sensitive in detecting early disease (Figure 36.14). If there is doubt as to the aetiology of cardiac disease, endomyocardial biopsy may demonstrate eosinophil infiltration. Serial monitoring of pulmonary function may be required if there is evidence of lung involvement.

Treatment

Treatment should be used to halt or reverse organ damage. Eosinophilia without evidence of end-organ damage does not usually require treatment. When underlying clonal or non-clonal disorders are identified they should be treated appropriately.

Patients with rearrangements of the *PDGFRA* or *PDGFRB* genes respond well to imatinib, with normalization of eosinophil counts within weeks. A trial of imatinib is also reasonable in patients with HES who lack a clonal marker, as a proportion of these patients also respond.

For patients who do not respond to imatinib, prednisolone is the initial treatment of choice. Steroids reduce blood eosinophilia and the inflammation resulting from tissue infiltration. Cardiac disease may respond even in the absence of a significant reduction in the eosinophil count. Hydroxycarbamide and interferon alfa may benefit patients resistant to steroids. Cladribine and ciclosporin were also found to be of use in some cases.

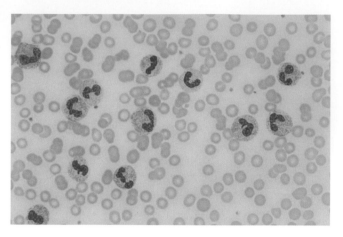

Figure 36.15 Abundance of mature neutrophils and band forms in a blood film from a patient with chronic neutrophilic leukaemia.

Prognosis

The reported prognoses of CEL and HES are highly variable, with estimates of 3-year survival ranging from 23 to 96%. This is likely to reflect heterogeneity within these two categories of patients. In patients with HES, indicators of a poor prognosis include lack of response to steroids, a markedly elevated eosinophil count, normal IgE levels, splenomegaly, dysplastic features and male sex. Many of these adverse prognostic indicators may simply be markers of clonal (versus reactive) eosinophilia.

Chronic neutrophilic leukaemia

Chronic neutrophilia is a very common entity, and is usually secondary to chronic infections, chronic inflammation or malignancy. A very small subgroup of patients with chronic neutrophilia have chronic neutrophilic leukaemia (CNL), a clonal haematological disorder (Figure 36.15). Given the absence of a specific marker for this disease, CNL, like ET, is a diagnosis of exclusion (see also Chapter 27).

Pathophysiology

Cases can be subdivided into two main groups: 'true' CNL and neutrophilic CML. The two groups are only distinguishable by the presence in the latter of a rare type of *BCR–ABL1* rearrangement that produces a 230-kDa fusion protein (p230). In addition, rare patients with MDS can closely mimic CNL but exhibit dysplastic features and there are anecdotal reports of PV evolving into a disorder indistinguishable from CNL. The literature also includes reports of what was thought to be clonal chronic neutrophilia in association with plasma cell dyscrasias. However, data are accumulating that this type of neutrophilia is non-

Table 36.12 Diagnostic features of chronic neutrophilic leukaemia.

Peripheral blood leucocytosis $>25 \times 10^9/L$
Segmented neutrophils and bands $>80\%$ of white blood cells
Immature granulocytes $< 10\%$ of white blood cells
Myeloblasts $< 1\%$ of white blood cells
Hypercellular bone marrow biopsy
Neutrophilic granulocytes increased in percentage and number
Myeloblasts $< 5\%$ of nucleated marrow cells
Normal neutrophil maturation pattern
Hepatosplenomegaly
No identifiable cause of reactive neutrophilia
No evidence of another haematological malignancy
No Philadelphia chromosome or *BCR–ABL1* fusion
No evidence of another myeloproliferative disorder (i.e. normal PCV, platelets $< 600 \times 10^9/L$, no bone marrow fibrosis or other features of PMF)
No evidence of a myelodysplastic syndrome (i.e. no dysplasia, monocytes $< 1 \times 10^9/L$)

Source: modified from Vardiman *et al.*(2001) with permission.

clonal and probably a result of cytokine release from clonal plasma cells.

Diagnostic features of CNL are shown in Table 36.12. Neutrophilic CML usually exhibits these features, save for its association with the p230 *BCR–ABL1* rearrangement.

Clinical features and treatment

A recent review of the literature identified only 33 cases that fulfilled criteria for CNL. These cases exhibited a male to female ratio of 2:1 and a median age at diagnosis of 62.5 years (range 15–86 years). The median survival was 30 months, with only 28% of patients surviving to 5 years. Transformation to AML ensued in 21% (7 of 33) and this was invariably lethal. Other causes of death included sepsis and haemorrhage.

Haemoglobin was normal with platelet counts above $100 \times 10^9/L$ in most cases. The mean leucocyte count at diagnosis was $54.3 \times 10^9/L$ with mature and band forms in the peripheral blood. Vitamin B_{12} levels were raised and neutrophil alkaline phosphatase levels were not low in most cases. Hyperuricaemia and gout were common. The spleen may be moderately enlarged. Bone marrow biopsies were markedly hypercellular and showed marked granulocytic proliferation, as did the bone marrow aspirates. Cytogenetic abnormalities were seen in about one-third, with del(20q), del(11q), del(12p), +8, +9 and +21 being mentioned in the WHO classification of tumours. In a small number of cases, X-chromosome inactivation patterns were used to demonstrate the clonal nature of CNL in patients lacking a cytogenetic marker.

The optimal treatment of CNL remains unclear. Oral cytoreductive agents such as hydroxycarbamide and busulfan can control the neutrophil count, as can interferon. The only potentially curative modality is allogeneic bone marrow transplantation and this option should be considered in younger patients.

Neutrophilic chronic myeloid leukaemia

This entity is probably even more rare than CNL, with only a handful of documented cases in the literature. The reported cases followed a more benign course than conventional CML, with a lower white cell count, lower proportion of immature granulocytes, milder anaemia, less marked splenomegaly and a lower propensity to acute transformation. Given recent advances in the treatment of *BCR–ABL1*-related diseases, it is important to consider and exclude neutrophilic CML during the investigation of chronic neutrophilia.

Transient abnormal myelopoiesis of Down syndrome

Children born with Down syndrome show a 10- to 20-fold increased risk of leukaemia, despite not showing an increased incidence of other cancer types. One haematological disorder, characteristically found only in neonates with Down syndrome, is transient abnormal myelopoiesis (TAM), also known as transient myeloproliferative disorder or transient leukaemia.

Incidence, clinical features and treatment

About 10% of neonates with Down syndrome are thought to develop TAM, although this may be underestimated since many otherwise healthy babies with trisomy 21 do not routinely have blood tests performed. Additional problems with recognition arise from the fact that many normal neonates with Down syndrome show mild abnormalities of blood counts, including polycythaemia and thrombocytopenia. About 25% of neonates with TAM are asymptomatic, with the blood film showing sometimes significantly elevated numbers of circulating immature myeloid cells, including basophilic blasts, nucleated red cells, megakaryocyte fragments and thrombocytosis or thrombocytopenia. In symptomatic babies, the clinical features are variable but can include neonatal jaundice, bleeding problems, respiratory distress and rarely liver failure.

The natural history of TAM is intriguing. In the majority of babies, the disorder resolves spontaneously by 3 months of age, without the need for treatment. Severely symptomatic infants, especially those with respiratory or hepatic dysfunction, can be treated very effectively with low-dose cytarabine chemotherapy. About 20% of neonates with TAM will subsequently develop acute megakaryoblastic leukaemia (AMKL) before the age of 4 years, although sometimes the leukaemia develops without antecedent TAM.

Pathophysiology

The fact that TAM only occurs in neonates points to it being a disorder of fetal haemopoiesis, and this presumably also explains why it is self-limiting in most cases. The characteristic association between TAM and AMKL indicates that a multistep model of mutation is operative in this clinical progression. Firstly, the disorder only occurs in trisomy 21, suggesting that there are genes on this chromosome that somehow predispose to abnormal fetal haemopoiesis. Several ETS family members and *RUNX1* are found on chromosome 21, but the key molecular pathways here have not been identified. Secondly, the development of TAM is tightly linked with the acquisition of characteristic mutations in the gene for the transcription factor GATA-1, located on the X chromosome. These mutations cluster in the first two coding exons of the gene and tend to be disruptive (frameshift insertions or deletions, splice-site and nonsense mutations). They all have the end result of generating a transcript in which protein translation is initiated downstream of the usual start site, leading to a GATA-1 protein lacking the first 84 amino acids. This prevents its interaction with another transcription factor, FOG1, leading to the characteristic phenotype of TAM. Thirdly, the progression to AMKL is probably driven by acquisition of further mutation(s). In particular, *JAK3* activating mutations are found in a small percentage of patients with AMKL in Down syndrome, although the mutations for most cases have not yet been identified.

Selected bibliography

Barbui T, Carobbio A, Rambaldi A, Finazzi G (2009) Perspectives on thrombosis in essential thrombocythemia and polycythemia vera: is leukocytosis a causative factor? *Blood* **114**: 759–63.

Barosi G, Ambrosetti A, Finelli C *et al.* (1999) The Italian Consensus Conference on Diagnostic Criteria for Myelofibrosis with Myeloid Metaplasia. *British Journal of Haematology* **104**: 730–7.

Baxter EJ, Scott LM, Campbell PJ *et al.* (2005) Acquired mutation of the tyrosine kinase JAK2 in human myeloproliferative disorders. *Lancet* **365**: 1054–61.

Campbell PJ, Green AR (2006) The myeloproliferative disorders. *New England Journal of Medicine* **355**: 2452–66.

Campbell PJ, Scott LM, Buck G *et al.* (2005) Definition of subtypes of essential thrombocythaemia and relation to polycythaemia vera based on JAK2 V617F mutation status: a prospective study. *Lancet* **366**: 1945–53.

Dupriez B, Morel P, Demory JL *et al.* (1996) Prognostic factors in agnogenic myeloid metaplasia: a report on 195 cases with a new scoring system. *Blood* **88**: 1013–18.

Finazzi G, Caruso V, Marchioli R *et al.* (2005) Acute leukaemia in polycythemia vera: an analysis of 1638 patients enrolled in a prospective observational study. *Blood* **105**: 2664–70.

Gotlib J, Cross NC, Gilliland DG (2006) Eosinophilic disorders: molecular pathogenesis, new classification, and modern therapy. *Best Practice and Research. Clinical Haematology* **19**: 535–69.

Harrison CN, Gale RE, Machin SJ, Linch DC (1999) A large proportion of patients with a diagnosis of essential thrombocythemia do not have a clonal disorder and may be at lower risk of thrombotic complications. *Blood* **93**: 417–24.

Harrison CN, Bareford D, Butt N *et al.* (2010) Guideline for investigation and management of adults and children presenting with a thrombocytosis. *British Journal of Haematology* **149**: 352–75.

James C, Ugo V, Le Couedic JP *et al.* (2005) A unique clonal JAK2 mutation leading to constitutive signalling causes polycythaemia vera. *Nature* **434**: 1144–8.

Kralovics R, Passamonti F, Buser AS *et al.* (2005) A gain-of-function mutation of JAK2 in myeloproliferative disorders. *New England Journal of Medicine* **352**: 1779–90.

Landolfi R, Marchioli R, Kutti J *et al.* (2004) Efficacy and safety of low-dose aspirin in polycythemia vera. *New England Journal of Medicine* **350**: 114–24.

Levine RL, Wadleigh M, Cools J *et al.* (2005) Activating mutation in the tyrosine kinase JAK2 in polycythemia vera, essential thrombocythemia, and myeloid metaplasia with myelofibrosis. *Cancer Cell* **7**: 387–97.

Levine RL, Pardanani A, Tefferi A, Gilliland DG (2007) Role of JAK2 in the pathogenesis and therapy of myeloproliferative disorders. *Nature Reviews. Cancer* **7**: 673–83.

McMullin MF, Bareford D, Campbell P *et al.* (2005) Guidelines for the diagnosis, investigation and management of polycythaemia/erythrocytosis. *British Journal of Haematology* **130**: 174–95.

McMullin MF, Reilly JT, Campbell P *et al.* (2007) Amendment to the guideline for diagnosis and investigation of polycythaemia/erythrocytosis. *British Journal of Haematology* **138**: 821–2.

Metcalfe DD (2008) Mast cells and mastocytosis. *Blood* **112**: 946–56.

Passamonti F, Cervantes F, Vannucchi AM *et al.* (2010) A dynamic prognostic model to predict survival in primary myelofibrosis: a study by the IWG-MRT (International Working Group for Myeloproliferative Neoplams Research Treatment), *Blood* **115**: 1703–8.

Pikman Y, Lee BH, Mercher T *et al.* (2006) MPLW515L is a novel somatic activating mutation in myelofibrosis with myeloid metaplasia. *PLoS Medicine* **3**: e270.

Reilly JT, Snowden JA, Spearing RL *et al.* (1997) Cytogenetic abnormalities and their prognostic significance in idiopathic myelofibrosis: a study of 106 cases. *British Journal of Haematology* **98**: 96–102.

Scott LM, Scott MA, Campbell PJ, Green AR (2006) Progenitors homozygous for the V617F mutation occur in most patients with polycythemia vera, but not essential thrombocythemia. *Blood* **108**: 2435–7.

Scott LM, Tong W, Levine RL *et al.* (2007) JAK2 exon 12 mutations in polycythemia vera and idiopathic erythrocytosis. *New England Journal of Medicine* **356**: 459–68.

Spivak JL, Silver RT (2008) The revised World Health Organization diagnostic criteria for polycythemia vera, essential thrombocytosis, and primary myelofibrosis: an alternative proposal. *Blood* **112**: 231–9.

Swerdlow SH, Campo E, Harris NL *et al.* (eds) (2008) *WHO Classification of Tumours of Haematopoietic and Lymphoid Tissues*. IARC, Lyon.

Tefferi A, Thiele J, Orazi A *et al.* (2007) Proposals and rationale for revision of the World Health Organization diagnostic criteria for polycythemia vera, essential thrombocythemia, and primary myelofibrosis: recommendations from an ad hoc international expert panel. *Blood* **110**: 1092–7.

Valent P, Horny HP, Escribano L *et al.* (2001) Diagnostic criteria and classification of mastocytosis: a consensus proposal. *Leukemia Research* **25**: 603–25.

Vardiman JW, Pierre R, Thiele J *et al.* (2001) Chronic myeloproliferative disorders. In: *World Health Organization Classification of Tumours. Pathology and Genetics of Tumours of the Haematopoietic and Lymphoid Tissues* (ES Jaffe, NL Harris, H Stein, JW Vardiman, eds), pp. 15–44. IARC Press, Lyon.

Wilkins BS, Erber WN, Bareford D *et al.* (2008) Bone marrow pathology in essential thrombocythemia: interobserver reliability and utility for identifying disease subtypes. *Blood* **111**: 60–70.

CHAPTER 37

Histocompatibility

Ann-Margaret Little[1], Steven GE Marsh[2] and J Alejandro Madrigal[2]

[1]Histocompatibility and Immunogenetics, Gartnavel General Hospital, Glasgow, UK
[2]The Anthony Nolan Research Institute, Royal Free Hospital, London, UK

37

The major histocompatibility complex and human leucocyte antigens

In the 1950s three independent scientists, Jean Dausset, Rose Payne and Jon van Rood, described the presence of alloantibodies in the sera of individuals exposed to genetically non-identical tissues such as the fetus in pregnancy and/or blood cells after transfusion. These alloantibodies were subsequently shown to react against protein antigens, encoded by a genetic region called the major histocompatibility complex (MHC). The MHC had also been independently identified in animal models of skin transplantation and tumour immunology, where genetically different strains of mice were shown to reject transplants from one another. Genetically identical mice could accept such transplants without rejection.

These observations led to theories of self/non-self discrimination, and the elucidation of the genetics of MHC genes encoding the protein 'histocompatibility' (or transplantation) antigens. Analysis of the structure and function of histocompatibility antigens has led to the establishment of routine and successful transplant protocols for both solid organ and haemopoietic stem cells between genetically disparate individuals.

The MHC in humans is located on the short arm of chromosome 6 (6p21.3). This region of the genome has been extensively studied and fully sequenced as part of the Human Genome Project (www.sanger.ac.uk/HGP/Chr6/). The MHC is an extremely gene-dense region of the genome, and it can be divided into 'three' subregions based on the type of genes found.

The genes encoding histocompatibility antigens are located within the MHC class I and II regions (Figure 37.1). These genes are called HLA genes (defined as human leucocyte antigens, although originally called human locus-A). HLA genes found in the class I region differ in structure from those found in the class II region and as a result the encoded proteins also differ. HLA class I genes encode a polypeptide of about 340 amino acids. This polypeptide is found as a cell-surface transmembrane glycoprotein and is associated with the soluble protein β_2-microglobulin encoded by a gene on chromosome 15.

There are three classical class I genes: HLA-A, HLA-B and HLA-C. Their encoded proteins are expressed on virtually all nucleated cells within the body and also on platelets. The expression of HLA class I proteins varies for different types of tissues. For example, expression is high on lymphocytes but low on hepatocytes and tissues comprising the nervous system. In addition there are class I genes encoding non-classical class I molecules called HLA-E, HLA-F and HLA-G. The tissue distribution of these molecules is more restricted than that of HLA-A, -B and -C, and this is a reflection of their differing function. These molecules are not considered as transplantation antigens.

HLA class II molecules are similar in structure to HLA class I molecules. They are composed of two MHC-encoded polypeptide chains (α and β). HLA class II molecules, unlike class I, have a restricted tissue distribution. They are mainly expressed on antigen-presenting cells such as B cells, dendritic cells, macrophages and also activated (but not resting) T cells. There are three classical class II molecules: HLA-DR, HLA-DQ and HLA-DP. In addition, there are other non-classical class II molecules encoded by the HLA-DM and HLA-DO genes. These non-classical class II molecules are not transplantation antigens but do contribute to the antigen-presenting function of class II molecules.

Postgraduate Haematology: 6th edition. Edited by A. Victor Hoffbrand, Daniel Catovsky, Edward G.D. Tuddenham, Anthony R. Green
© 2011 Blackwell Publishing Ltd.

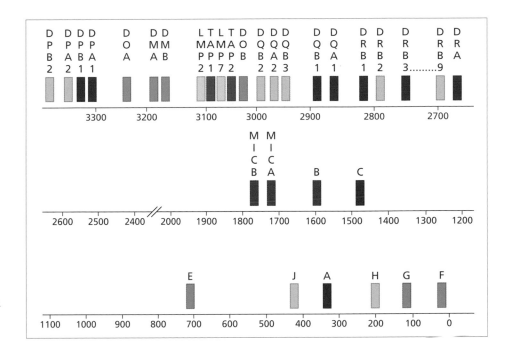

Figure 37.1 Diagrammatic representation of the major histocompatibility complex. Approximate location of HLA-A, -B, -C, -DRA, -DRB, -DQA, -DQB, -DPA and -DPB genes are indicated. Other related genes are also present.

The class III region of the MHC does not contain any HLA genes. This region contains genes encoding proteins with various different functions including proteins involved in the immune response such as tumour necrosis factor (TNF)-α and TNF-β and complement components C2, C4 and Bf.

Structure of HLA proteins

The X-ray crystallographic structure of the extracellular domains of several HLA class I and II proteins has been resolved. The structures are divided into four domains as illustrated in Figure 37.2. The two most membrane-distal domains, $\alpha 1$ and $\alpha 2$ for HLA class I and $\alpha 1$ and $\beta 1$ for HLA class II, form a β-pleated sheet surrounded on both sides by two α-helices. In both class I and II structures a short peptide is found bound in the cleft. Thus both class I and class II proteins can be considered trimolecular proteins consisting of three subunits: HLA heavy chain, β_2-microglobulin and peptide form class I molecules, and HLA α- and β-chains and peptide form class II molecules.

Antigen processing and presentation

Peptide binding to HLA class I and II proteins plays an important role in the function of these molecules. The way in which peptides are derived and the binding procedure differs for the two classes of molecules and this is reflected in their different function.

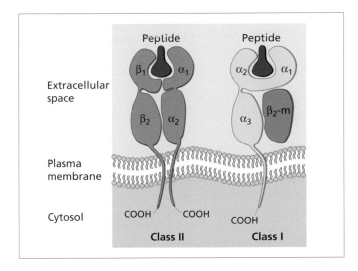

Figure 37.2 Diagrammatic representation of HLA class I and II molecules showing protein domains and bound peptide.

HLA class I molecules are assembled within the endoplasmic reticulum (ER). The heavy chain is directed to the ER via a leader peptide sequence. Within the lumen of the ER, the extracellular domains of the heavy chain associate with β_2-microglobulin. This association is mediated by ER-resident chaperones including calnexin and calreticulum.

Association with peptide also occurs within the ER. Peptides are derived from the cytoplasmic degradation of molecules that takes place in the proteasome, a multicatalytic protein complex. Peptides produced by the proteasome are actively transported into the ER via a transmembrane peptide pump called TAP (transporter associated with antigen processing). Association between HLA class I heavy chain/β_2-microglobulin complex and peptide is catalysed by another ER-resident chaperone called tapasin associated with the thiol oxidoreductase ERp57.

Once the class I trimolecular complex is formed, the molecule can leave the ER and complete its journey to the cell surface via the Golgi apparatus. The journey of a class II molecule differs from that of a class I molecule. Both α- and β-chains are directed to the ER, where a complex of three $\alpha\beta$ chains and three invariant chains is formed. The invariant chain is also a transmembrane protein. Association of HLA class II molecules with the invariant chain effectively blocks the peptide-binding site on the class II molecule, thus preventing binding of ER-resident peptides. Invariant chain cytoplasmic tail sequences direct the class II molecule through the Golgi apparatus, but unlike class I molecules the class II molecules take a detour to endosomal vesicles before arriving at the cell surface. The non-classical HLA-DM and HLA-DO molecules are located within endosomal vesicles and it is here that the invariant chain is cleaved, leaving a peptide, called CLIP, blocking the class II peptide binding cleft. Specific peptide binding is catalysed by HLA-DM, and may also be aided by HLA-DO. The peptides that bind to class II molecules are derived from proteins that have been processed by the endocytic pathway. These proteins can be derived from the internalization of cell surface or extracellular proteins, or from endogenous cytosolic proteins via processes of autophagocytosis. Thus the antigen presentation pathway for HLA class II molecules differs from that of HLA class I molecules by directing the class II molecules to a location where they can bind peptides that are in the majority, differently sourced from those presented by class I molecules.

Peptides derived from exogenous sources may also be presented by HLA class I molecules via cross-presentation pathways. The detailed mechanisms involved in these pathways are not fully elucidated but such events likely play a significant role in ensuring an adequate immune response is elicited by the ability to present antigenic peptides from the same source on both class I and II molecules.

HLA function

Once presented at the cell surface, HLA molecules, together with bound peptide, are subject to surveillance by circulating T cells and natural killer (NK) cells. Both these cell types possess receptors that recognize and interact with HLA molecules. Typically, T cells expressing the CD4 molecule recognize HLA class II molecules and T cells expressing CD8 recognize HLA class I molecules. The specificity of interaction is determined during development of T cells within the thymus, such that circulating T cells should not interact with HLA molecules presenting peptides derived from normally expressed self proteins. However, the presentation of non-self peptides, for example peptides derived from viral or bacterial proteins, or aberrant expression of tumour antigens can initiate, in appropriate conditions, activatory signals mediated by the T-cell receptor and coreceptors, resulting in the generation of an immune response against the cells expressing the target HLA protein–peptide complex.

NK cells have a determining role in the immune response to tumours and viral infections. NK cells function in innate immune responses and also contribute to the development of adaptive immune responses. The interactions between HLA molecules and NK cell receptors also impact on alloimmune responses occurring after transplantation and pregnancy. NK cells express a highly diverse repertoire of receptors, including killer cell immunoglobulin-like receptors (KIRs), that elicit either activatory or inhibitory signals. Some HLA class I molecules have been identified as ligands recognized by KIRs. Thus the interaction between an NK cell and target cell is influenced by the interaction between HLA on the target cell and KIRs on the NK cell. Typically, an interaction between HLA class I molecule and corresponding KIR will result in a negative signal and this will outweigh any additional activatory signals; thus the NK cell will not attack the target cell. However, if a cell has lost expression of HLA molecules as a result of malignancy or viral infection, the absence of the inhibitory signal will result in activatory signals being dominant and allow NK cell-mediated attack on the target cell. Interactions between HLA and KIR have been implicated in various medical conditions, including infectious disease, autoimmunity, cancer, reproduction and transplantation. KIRs are encoded within a multigene complex on chromosome 19, the gene organization of which varies within different haplotypes. KIR genes are also functionally polymorphic, thus making analysis of KIRs as challenging as that of HLA, if not more so.

HLA polymorphism

The outstanding feature of HLA genes and the proteins encoded is the extensive polymorphism exhibited. At each of the genes there are multiple possible variants (Table 37.1). The variants are called alleles. The nucleotide sequence differences between HLA alleles at a given locus can be translated into the protein sequence and analyses of the polymorphism has demonstrated that most variation exists within the peptide-binding domains. Experimental data support this by showing that different HLA proteins bind peptides with different sequences. Thus one of the functions of HLA polymorphism is to allow the presentation of numerous different peptides to the immune system. As there are six antigen-presenting 'classical' HLA molecules (HLA-A, -B, -C, -DR, -DQ, -DP) and most individuals are heterozygous for these loci, potentially each individual has 12 different HLA molecules, each of which can bind thousands of different peptides. The existence of a polymorphic polygenic

Table 37.1 Number of HLA alleles and serologically defined antigens by April 2010.

HLA gene	No. of alleles	No. of antigens
A	1001	24
B	1605	50
C	690	9
DRA	3	–
DRB1	785	20
DRB3	52	1
DRB4	14	1
DRB5	19	1
DQA1	35	–
DQB1	108	7
DPA1	28	–
DPB1	133	–

antigen-presenting system gives each individual the capacity to elicit immune responses against a wide variety of protein antigens. A complete listing of currently defined HLA alleles is given at www.ebi.ac.uk/imgt/hla/.

HLA polymorphism also varies within different populations. Variation in climate, geography and infectious pathogens are factors considered to have influenced the evolution of HLA polymorphism. It is therefore not surprising to find that HLA allele frequencies vary for different ethnic groups. This has an impact on unrelated donor transplantation: an HLA-matched donor is most likely to be found within a donor pool of the same ethnicity as the patient.

HLA polymorphism therefore functions as an advantage at the level of both a single individual and a population in terms of defence against pathogens. The extreme diversity found makes it very likely that someone somewhere possesses an HLA molecule that can be effective in generating an immune response against any infectious agent. However, HLA polymorphism is a significant obstacle to finding a matched unrelated donor for transplantation.

HLA associations with disease

Because both HLA class I and class II molecules control the positive and negative selection of T-cell receptors in the thymus and modulate the activity of NK cells, it is not surprising to find many associations between HLA and immune system disorders such as autoimmune disease. The first strong association described was that of HLA-B27 with ankylosing spondylitis and related seronegative spondylarthropathies, where over 95% of affected individuals possess an HLA-B*27 allele. Despite tremendous effort to discover the immunological basis for the association between B27 and ankylosing spondylitis, the answer

is still unknown. Other factors must also be involved because only 3–4% of individuals with HLA-B27 will develop disease. HLA type has also been associated with susceptibility to, and protection from, infectious diseases. Individuals possessing *HLA-B*53:01*, an allele prevalent within African populations, are more likely to be resistant to severe malaria. This association is supported by experiments showing that the B53 allotype can present a peptide derived from the malaria parasite. With HIV infection, the HLA type of the infected individual can influence the rate of disease progression. HLA-B35 is associated with more rapid progression to AIDS, whereas HLA-B27 and HLA-B57 are associated with slower disease progression. These associations reflect the function of different HLA molecules in the presentation of HIV peptides to CD8$^+$ T cells in order to evoke an immune response against HIV-infected cells.

HLA class II molecules are restricted in their tissue distribution. However, appropriate stimulation can induce the expression of class II molecules on tissues where they are not normally expressed. This aberrant HLA class II expression may contribute to an autoimmune reaction by providing HLA–peptide complexes not encountered during T-cell receptor education in the thymus. Among the many associations between HLA class II molecules and autoimmune and/or inflammatory disease is that between rheumatoid arthritis and HLA-DR4. This association has been linked to the presence of an epitope contributed by residues 67, 70, 71 and 74 of the β-chain that contributes to a pocket (P4) in the peptide-binding site, thus supporting the role of peptide binding in the disease.

For other associations between HLA and disease, the answer has been found. Haemochromatosis has been associated with haplotypes possessing *HLA-A*03*. Genetic mapping has identified the gene, *HFE*, responsible for this association. Thus associations between HLA and disease may not be directly related to the HLA allotype but may be due to the presence of other genes that are closely linked or which are hitch-hiking within particular HLA haplotypes.

Associations between HLA type and hypersensitivity to drugs have also been reported, leading to the application of HLA typing to patient treatment. *HLA-B*57:01* typing is used to identify HIV-infected patients at risk from life-threatening hypersensitivity to the drug abacavir, an inhibitor of HIV-1 reverse transcriptase. The mechanism of this interaction is thought to involve an interaction between the drug and a peptide normally presented by the *HLA-B*57:01* encoded protein, resulting in a highly immunogenic CD8$^+$ T-cell immune response.

HLA nomenclature

The naming of HLA specificities falls under the remit of the WHO Nomenclature Committee for Factors of the HLA System. The Committee names HLA genes, alleles and serologically defined antigenic specificities. The names of the antigens, which were originally defined using either serological or cellular techniques, are a combination of letters which indicate the gene encoding the antigen, and numbers assigned in chronological order of their description. An example of an individual's HLA type determined by cellular and serological methods is A1, A2; B7, B13; Cw6, Cw7; Dw1, Dw13; DR1, DR4; DR53; DQ5, DQ8; DPw1, DPw4.

The numbering of antigens encoded by HLA-A and -B genes is in a single series for historical reasons, as these antigens were originally believed to represent the products of a single gene. The use of a lower case 'w' between the gene name and antigen number indicates a provisional specificity, although in most cases these have been removed. The exceptions are Bw4 and Bw6, which represent public epitopes rather than distinct antigens, HLA-C antigens (e.g. Cw1), to distinguish them from complement factors, and the HLA-D and HLA-DP antigens defined by cellular techniques.

Many HLA antigens have been characterized by serological methods into two or more subtypes, which are called 'splits', with the parent antigen called 'broad'. Thus both A23 and A24 are splits of the broad antigen A9. It is convention to indicate the broad antigen specificity in parentheses following the designation of the split, for example A23(9) or A24(9). A full listing of all the serologically and cellularly defined HLA antigens is given in Table 37.2.

Since 1987 the WHO Nomenclature Committee for Factors of the HLA System has assigned official names to HLA allele sequences. It was recognized that a single antigenic specificity, such as HLA-A2, defined by serology could be subdivided still further by DNA sequencing. Each allele is given a numerical designation that may be up to eight digits in length. The gene name is followed by an asterisk (*) and then the numerical designation. Each allele name consists of at least two, and maximally four, fields. The first field indicates the allele group, which often corresponds to the broad serological antigen encoded by the allele. The second field is used to list subtypes, numbers

assigned in the order in which the DNA sequences have been determined. Alleles whose numbers differ in the first two fields must differ in one or more nucleotide substitutions that change the amino acid sequence of the encoded protein. The third field is used to name alleles that differ only by synonymous nucleotide substitutions (also called silent or non-coding). The fourth field is used to name alleles that differ in either intron, or 3' or 5' regions of the gene. Lastly, an allele may have a suffix indicating aberrant expression; for example N indicates that it is a null allele with no protein being expressed, L indicates low cell surface expression and S indicates that the molecule is expressed only in a soluble form. For example, the $A*24:02:01:01$ and $A*24:02:01:02L$ alleles differ only by a single nucleotide which lies within an intron at a splice site. $A*24:02:01:01$ is expressed at normal levels on the cell surface, whereas $A*24:02:01:02L$ is expressed at very low levels on the cell surface due to the splice mutation.

Many new HLA alleles are reported each year (Figure 37.3). Details of the most recent advances in HLA nomenclature can be found in the latest WHO Nomenclature Committee for Factors of the HLA System Report or by accessing the IMGT/HLA Sequence Database, the official database of the Nomenclature Committee (www.ebi.ac.uk/imgt/hla).

HLA matching in transplantation

The benefits of HLA polymorphism in allowing the generation of immune responses against a wide range of antigens is completely negated when transplantation of organs and cells between genetically disparate individuals is considered. Typically, an individual will possess T cells capable of reacting against a foreign antigen at a frequency of 1 in 10^4–10^5. However, if cells from two HLA disparate individuals are mixed, the frequency of responding cells can be as high as 1–10%. These responding cells are called alloreactive cells.

Table 37.2 Complete listing of recognized serological and cellular HLA specificities.

A	B	C	D	DR	DQ	DP
A1	B5	Cw1	Dw1	DR1	DQ1	DPw1
A2	B7	Cw2	Dw2	DR103	DQ2	DPw2
A203	B703	Cw3	Dw3	DR2	DQ3	DPw3
A210	B8	Cw4	Dw4	DR3	DQ4	DPw4
A3	B12	Cw5	Dw5	DR4	DQ5(1)	DPw5
A9	B13	Cw6	Dw6	DR5	DQ6(1)	DPw6
A10	B14	Cw7	Dw7	DR6	DQ7(3)	
A11	B15	Cw8	Dw8	DR7	DQ8(3)	
A19	B16	Cw9(w3)	Dw9	DR8	DQ9(3)	
A23(9)	B17	Cw10(w3)	Dw10	DR9		
A24(9)	B18		Dw11(w7)	DR10		
A2403	B21		Dw12	DR11(5)		
A25(10)	B22		Dw13	DR12(5)		

Table 37.2 *Continued*

A	B	C	D	DR	DQ	DP
A26(10)	B27		Dw14	DR13(6)		
A28	B2708		Dw15	DR14(6)		
A29(19)	B35		Dw16	DR1403		
A30(19)	B37		Dw17(w7)	DR1404		
A31(19)	B38(16)		Dw18(w6)	DR15(2)		
A32(19)	B39(16)		Dw19(w6)	DR16(2)		
A33(19)	B3901		Dw20	DR17(3)		
A34(10)	B3902		Dw21	DR18(3)		
A36	B40		Dw22	DR51		
A43	B4005		Dw23	DR52		
A66(10)	B41		Dw24	DR53		
A68(28)	B42		Dw25			
A69(28)	B44(12)		Dw26			
A74(19)	B45(12)					
A80	B46					
	B47					
	B48					
	B49(21)					
	B50(21)					
	B51(5)					
	B5102					
	B5103					
	B52(5)					
	B53					
	B54(22)					
	B55(22)					
	B56(22)					
	B57(17)					
	B58(17)					
	B59					
	B60(40)					
	B61(40)					
	B62(15)					
	B63(15)					
	B64(14)					
	B65(14)					
	B67					
	B70					
	B71(70)					
	B72(70)					
	B73					
	B75(15)					
	B76(15)					
	B77(15)					
	B78					
	B81					
	B82					
	Bw4					
	Bw6					

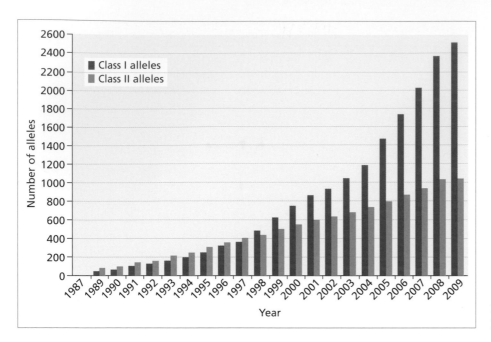

Figure 37.3 Increase in number of HLA alleles identified by year.

Alloreactions are responsible for the inability to transplant organs and cells between genetically different individuals. To overcome alloreactivity, it is necessary to define the HLA type of donor and recipient and to select an HLA-matched donor wherever possible. In solid organ transplantation, HLA matching is encouraged for kidney transplants, where outcome data support a beneficial role of HLA matching. However, immunosuppressive therapy is extremely effective in renal transplantation and this allows for imperfect matching to be performed and optimum usage of all available organs. Nevertheless, it is critical to avoid transplantation of mismatched donor kidneys possessing HLA types against which the patient has raised alloantibodies as a result of a previous mismatched transplant, pregnancy or blood transfusion. The presence of such alloantibodies can lead to hyperacute rejection, but immunodepletion protocols may be used to remove such donor-specific antibodies. HLA matching for other solid organs such as liver and heart and lung is not usually performed. The liver is an immunoprivileged site that tolerates HLA mismatches, whereas heart and lung transplants are usually performed on patients for whom no other chance of life is possible, thereby disallowing selection of HLA-matched donors. Alloreactions mediated following solid organ transplantation are usually only directed at the transplanted organ and with effective post-transplant immune monitoring can be managed with appropriate immunosuppression.

Patients receiving blood products, for example random pooled platelets, can produce antibodies against the HLA molecules present on transfused platelets. The presence of HLA-specific antibodies can lead to platelet refractoriness, and for these patients it is advisable to seek HLA-matched platelet donors.

Alloreactions occurring after haemopoietic stem cell transplantation (SCT) can result in failure of the cells to engraft or graft-versus-host disease (GVHD), in which donor cells mediate attack on various tissues within the host's body. The risks of graft rejection and GVHD are significantly reduced if the donor cells are histocompatible with the patient. The perfect donor is an identical twin. However, this will only be the case for very few patients. The chances of finding an HLA-matched sibling donor for a patient is theoretically one in four (25%). Therefore, again, the majority of patients will not be able to find a suitable donor within their family.

Another source of HLA-matched donors are the various volunteer donor registries that exist throughout the world. The first volunteer donor register, the Anthony Nolan Trust, was established in London in 1974 at a time when unrelated donor transplants were viewed as experimental. Since this time, the outcome of unrelated donor transplantation has vastly improved and the use of unrelated volunteer donors is now accepted practice. There are now over 60 volunteer donor registers throughout the world. In addition, the successful use of cord blood-derived stem cells for transplantation has driven the establishment of cord blood banks in many countries. An advantage of using cord blood cells in clinical transplantation is that a reduced degree of HLA matching is acceptable. Thus patients who fail to find a matched unrelated donor may receive mismatched cord blood stem cells. There are a number of factors that may negate the use of cord blood stem cells, such as the number of nucleated cells to be infused, particularly for adult patients, as these may be insufficient to enable engraftment, and the inability to obtain donor cells for future donor lymphocyte infusion. However, the use of double cord units in adults can overcome the problem of cell numbers and it is certain that cord blood will be an important player in widening the application of haemopoietic SCT.

There are over 13 million potential volunteer adult donors and cord blood units registered for use in haemopoietic SCT worldwide. Unrelated adult and cord blood donations take place as a result of the successful international networking of the worldwide adult donor registries and cord blood banks, under the auspices of the World Marrow Donor Association. In 2007, 42% of haemopoietic stem cell donations were sourced in a country different to that of the patient. Details on both volunteer donor and cord blood registries can be found on www.bmdw.org.

HLA matching required for haemopoietic stem cell transplantation

The importance of HLA matching in haemopoietic SCT is well accepted. However, the degree of resolution required at each locus for an optimum match is not fully understood. Data obtained from large multicentre registry studies support the importance of optimum matching, which consists of allele-level matching for HLA-A, HLA-B, HLA-C and HLA-DRB1. The role of HLA-DQB1 is still not defined. Mismatching for HLA-DQB1 does not appear detrimental in studies published by the National Marrow Donor Program; however, an HLA-DQB1 mismatch with another HLA mismatch (HLA-A, -B or -C) was more detrimental than a single HLA-A, -B or -C mismatch. Furthermore, a hierarchy of beneficial mismatching has not been proven in terms of antigen-level mismatching over allele-level mismatching. Any type of mismatch can have a negative effect on transplant outcome. Because HLA-B and HLA-C are in linkage disequilibrium (i.e. matching for HLA-B increases the chance that HLA-C will also be matched), it is more difficult to mismatch for one and not the other. Similarly, HLA-DRB1 and -DQB1 genes are in linkage disequilibrium. HLA-A is the most telomeric of the HLA genes and in less linkage disequilibrium with other HLA class I genes; therefore, when selecting an HLA-mismatched donor, HLA-A is usually the easiest locus to mismatch. Therefore most mismatching targets HLA-DQB1 and then HLA-A. However there are no data to support HLA-A mismatching as being clinically more acceptable than mismatching for other single loci. The role of HLA-DPB1 is emerging in analysis of large patient and donor cohorts, including the International Histocompatibility Workshop studies. In these studies, HLA-DPB1 mismatching is associated with reduced disease relapse, together with an increase in acute GVHD. The association between HLA-DPB1 and disease relapse suggests that HLA-DP molecules may mediate a functional role in a graft-versus-leukaemia response.

Histocompatibility testing procedures

Detection of HLA polymorphisms can be performed by either targeting the DNA sequence of the HLA gene or by analysis of the expressed protein.

Serology

Serology describes the use of antibodies to detect epitopes on target antigens. HLA polymorphism results in the presence of different antigenic epitopes on the protein molecule. Antibodies used to define these antigenic epitopes are usually obtained from multiparous women, and can also be created using monoclonal antibody technology. The latter has the advantage of being available in unlimited supply. Serology involves the incubation of peripheral blood mononuclear cells (PBMCs), or separated T and B cells for distinguishing HLA class I from class II, with serum containing antibodies of known anti-HLA specificity. If the PBMCs express the appropriate HLA molecules, then binding between the antibodies in the serum and the PBMCs will occur. This binding will result in lysis of the PBMCs after the addition of complement components. The cells can be stained in order to detect which cells are alive (no reaction) and which cells are dead (positive reaction). The pattern of positive and negative reactions is then interpreted to give an HLA type.

In order to obtain a full HLA type, panels of antisera have to be screened to cover the range of recognized HLA specificities. Despite the number of serological reagents that have been analysed, there are many HLA class I and II polymorphisms which remain undetected by serology (see Table 37.1). Many of these polymorphisms are not present on the surface of the HLA molecules but are found within the peptide-binding site, and could alter the peptide-binding specificity of the HLA molecule and hence the antigen presentation function of the molecule. Thus serological typing does not detect all the functional polymorphisms of HLA molecules.

DNA-based methods

The introduction of the polymerase chain reaction (PCR) for analysis of DNA has led to the establishment of rigorous DNA-based methodologies that can be applied for genetic diagnostics. DNA-based methods are now used routinely for histocompatibility typing.

The most frequent HLA class I antigen in white populations and the first HLA antigen to be defined, HLA-A2, encompasses three serological variants. Sequencing analyses have shown that at least 199 alleles encode the HLA-A2 specificity. Of these 199 alleles, 155 differ by substitutions that are predicted to influence the antigen presentation function of the HLA-A2 molecule, and 10 alleles (A*02:15N, A*02:32N, A*02:43N, A*02:53N, A*02:82N,

A*02:83N, A*02:88N, A*02:94N, A*92:13N and *A*92:25N*) contain mutations which prevent expression of the HLA-A2 antigen.

For HLA class I molecules the polymorphism is mostly localized within the α1 and α2 domains, which are encoded by exons 2 and 3 respectively of the class I gene. For HLA class II, the α1 domain of the β-chain, encoded by exon 2, is most polymorphic for DRB1, whereas for DQ and DP, the polymorphism extends to both the α1 and β1 domains. Thus DNA methods for HLA class I typing focus predominantly on exons 2 and 3, whereas for HLA class II exon 2 is targeted.

Sequence-specific oligonucleotide and sequence-specific primer methods

The most widely used DNA-based methods for HLA typing are PCR sequence-specific primers (PCR-SSP) and PCR sequence-specific oligonucleotides (PCR-SSO). These methods use DNA primers (SSP) or DNA probes (SSO) that react with polymorphic sequence motifs present within the nucleotide sequence of HLA alleles. The presence of a positive reaction indicates that the polymorphism defined by the primer or probe is present in the DNA sample, whereas a negative reaction defines the absence of that particular sequence polymorphism.

For PCR-SSO typing, the target DNA molecule is amplified by locus-specific PCR (e.g. all HLA-A alleles are amplified in one PCR) or by group-specific PCR (e.g. all DRB1*04 alleles are amplified in one PCR). The PCR product is immobilized directly onto a solid-phase matrix containing pre-immobilized HLA-specific oligonucleotide probes, for example nylon membrane or Luminex xMAP microspheres. Interaction between the immobilized probes and HLA PCR product is measured as positive, whereas no binding between probe and PCR product is measured as negative. Most methods utilize specific software to measure positive and negative reactions and to assign the interpreted HLA type.

PCR-SSP typing (Figure 37.4) utilizes multiple PCR primer pairs all tested independently on the same sample DNA. The primer pairs are designed such that the 3′ end defines the specificity of the primer with the target sequence. To obtain a full HLA type requires numerous primer pairs which have been designed to operate under identical PCR amplification conditions. If the target sequence for a primer pair is present in the sample DNA, a PCR product will be produced, whereas if the target sequence is not present there will be no PCR product. The presence and absence of PCR products can be visualized after agarose gel electrophoresis. Because of the extensive HLA polymorphism, specialized software is usually required to interpret results. PCR-SSP can be used to perform a full HLA type or to target a particular group of HLA alleles to obtain a high-resolution type (e.g. subtype A*02).

The resolution of the typing results obtained by PCR-SSO and PCR-SSP methods can vary depending on the number of probes or primer mixes utilized, with an increasing number required for higher resolution. As SSO methods utilize less PCR steps, this method is more useful for high-throughput HLA genotyping, for example as required by laboratories with large sample numbers, including unrelated haemopoietic donor registry laboratories. SSP methods are more suitable for smaller volumes and are reserved for quick turnaround typing or for achieving higher resolution on particular samples.

Regardless of the number of typing reagents used with PCR-SSP and PCR-SSO methods, the end result is the presence or absence of a reaction between a probe or primer of a known sequence and the target HLA sequence. Thus the data generated can be directly related to the DNA sequence of the HLA alleles possessed by an individual.

Direct sequencing

The generation of a database of known nucleotide sequences of HLA alleles has had a tremendous impact on the transfer of

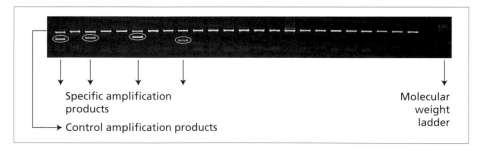

Figure 37.4 Example of PCR-SSP test. Photograph of an ethidium bromide-stained agarose gel containing electrophoresed PCR products. In this example, 24 PCR primer mixes have been utilized to determine HLA-*DRB1*11* subtype. Each lane on the gel contains the product from amplification of a non-polymorphic region of the genome. The presence of this product indicates successful amplification. A second band is observed in lanes 1, 3, 6 and 9, where specific amplification of a polymorphic region from an HLA gene is achieved. If no second band is present, then the individual being tested does not possess the complementary HLA polymorphism. The pattern of positive and negative reactions (presence and absence of second bands) is interpreted to give the HLA type. (Courtesy of Franco Tavarozzi, The Anthony Nolan Trust.)

methodologies from serology to DNA-based techniques. Improvements in automated instrumentation for DNA sequencing has also made this methodology an affordable alternative for HLA typing. The sequencing techniques utilized for HLA typing involve PCR amplification and direct sequencing of the PCR product. The strategies developed have focused on the amplification of DNA fragments containing the polymorphic exons, which for the majority of class I alleles extends to a fragment containing exons 2 and 3 at a minimum. The overall size of an HLA class I gene is about 3.2 kb and therefore it is feasible to target all exons (and introns) within the gene to define the polymorphisms present; this additional information greatly increases the resolving power of sequencing methods.

HLA class II genes are much larger than HLA class I genes and the amount of sequence information available for exons outside exon 2 is limited. HLA class II sequencing methods minimally target exon 2, with additional data sought from exon 3 to resolve some exon 3 known polymorphisms. HLA-DQB1 also benefits from analysis of both exon 2 and exon 3.

As most loci are heterozygous, assignment of HLA type is dependent on the use of software capable of assigning heterozygous positions. In addition an up-to-date database of all known HLA sequences is required (Figure 37.5).

The advantages of DNA-based methods over serology are numerous and include the ease with which typing reagents (primers, probes) can be synthesized and the interpretation of the data as directly relating to nucleotide sequence, whereas the data obtained with polyclonal antisera requires extensive knowledge of cross-reactivities of sera with different HLA antigens. In addition, the storage of material is simplified for DNA typing, as live cells are not required.

Ambiguities

DNA typing methods can generate ambiguous results when both alleles in a heterozygous combination are analysed together. Therefore it can be difficult to determine whether a sequence motif is in the *cis* or *trans* orientation compared with a different motif. This problem is overcome by performing allele-specific amplifications on samples with ambiguities prior to analysis, usually by SSO or sequencing. Alternatively, sequencing primers can be designed to target particular polymorphisms, allowing separation of the two alleles in a heterozygous sample. Fewer ambiguities are obtained using PCR-SSP as the PCR primers used link *cis* polymorphisms.

Cellular assays

Cellular methods for assessing potential alloreactivity between patient and donor can also be utilized for the selection of the most appropriate stem cell donor. The mixed lymphocyte culture (MLC) assay has been used since the 1960s. MLC meas-

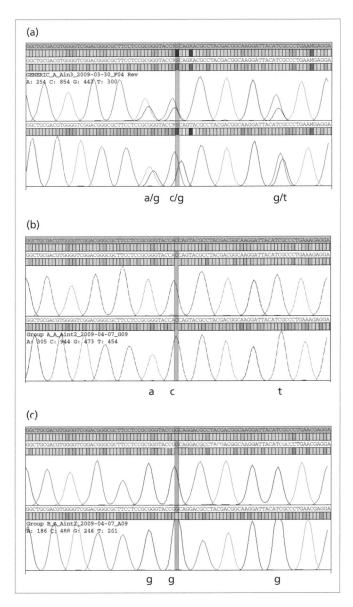

Figure 37.5 HLA sequencing electropherogram. The electropherograms are from ASSIGN software analysis of sequencing performed on an HLA-A PCR product containing exons 2, 3 and 4. (a) Heterozygous loci. The sequence is read from left to right. For this short stretch of nucleotides (12 from 822 analysed for HLA-A), eight different results are possible for the heterozygous nucleotides: ACG, ACT, AGG, AGT, GCG, GCT, GGG and GGT. Overall analysis of all 822 nucleotides gives an ambiguous result of A*03:01, *24:02 or A*03:07, *24:56 or A*03:08, *24:07 or A*03:15, *24:53 or A*03:17, *24:21. (b, c) Separated loci. By sequencing the two HLA-A alleles after separation using allele-specific PCR primers, the heterozygous ambiguities are resolved. The result for (b) gives ACT and for (c) gives GGG. The final result for this ambiguity, after analysis of all 822 nucleotides sequenced, is HLA-A*03:01, *24:02. (Courtesy of Shem Wallis-Jones, The Anthony Nolan Trust.)

ures the reactivity of donor T cells against alloantigens expressed by patient cells, i.e. graft versus host direction. By mixing both donor and patient cells together, any alloreactions that occur will cause the responding donor cells to proliferate and incorporate ^{3}H-thymidine, which can be measured. The patient cells are prevented from proliferating by being gamma-irradiated prior to the mixing of cells. However, since the introduction of DNA-based methods for HLA class II typing, the MLC reaction is infrequently used. Indeed studies have indicated that positive MLC reactions in the absence of detectable HLA class II mismatches are not predictors of the development of GVHD after bone marrow transplantation.

More sensitive cellular assays have been developed to measure HLA disparity. The cytotoxic T-lymphocyte precursor (CTLp) assay uses limiting dilution analysis to measure the frequency of donor CTLs responding to predominantly HLA class I mismatches on patient cells. High frequencies of CTLp have been shown to be strongly associated with HLA class I mismatches, which may have escaped detection by the low to medium level of resolution of conventional typings that were widely used for class I matching prior to the use of allele-level DNA typing. Similarly, the helper T-lymphocyte precursor (HTLp) assay measures the HTL response of the donor to HLA class II mismatches, with HLA-DR mismatches associated with high HTLp frequencies with no apparent contribution from HLA class I mismatches. Both CTLp and HTLp assays can be combined in a single limiting dilution analysis, thus minimizing the use of often valuable material.

The drawback of cellular assays is that they take up to 2 weeks to perform, and they require viable cells from both donor and patient. With more widespread use of high-resolution HLA typing techniques, the number of laboratories performing cellular assays has decreased significantly.

Other genetic polymorphisms

HLA polymorphisms clearly play an important role in determining the outcome of haemopoietic SCT. There are also other genetic polymorphisms that have been demonstrated to influence outcome. Minor histocompatibility antigens (mHA) are alloantigens that are also capable of initiating an immune response when their genes are mismatched for patient and donor, despite the presence of HLA matching. Minor histocompatibility antigens are peptides derived from normal self proteins that possess polymorphisms. A donor and patient may share HLA type, but differ in the polymorphism found in the mHA gene. Several human mHA have been defined, for example HA1, HA2, HA3. The genes encoding several of these mHA have been described and this has allowed the development of typing procedures for these genes using techniques such as PCR-SSP.

Single-nucleotide polymorphisms (SNPs) in other genes, particularly cytokines, have also been shown to have an impact on the outcome of SCT. Recent studies have described the significant correlation between transplant outcome in patients suffering from acute leukaemias and three SNPs in the *CARD15* (caspase recruitment domain 15) gene, now called *NOD2* (nucleotide-binding oligomerization domain 2). These may be defined by a variety of techniques that are able to target single mutations within a gene.

There is therefore a choice of techniques that may be used for optimum donor selection for patients requiring SCT. Each methodology has its advantages and disadvantages. It is now accepted practice that DNA-based typing should be performed on all related and unrelated donors and patients. Serology and cellular assays may be used to complement the outcome of DNA typing. A major challenge for the future of histocompatibility typing for SCT will be to acquire a greater understanding of what types of mismatches are acceptable in that they do not result in adverse alloreactions, and also to know which mismatches are detrimental. It is likely that more sensitive and reproducible cellular assays may play a role in determining these mismatches. The use of ELISPOT assay and real-time PCR methods for detecting low numbers of cytokine-producing cells may in the future become additional tools for the histocompatibility laboratory, especially for the selection of best mismatched donors when no optimum matched donor is available.

Selected bibliography

History
Klein J (1986) *Natural History of the Major Histocompatibility Complex.* John Wiley & Sons, New York.

HLA molecular structure
Bjorkman PJ, Saper MA, Samraoui B *et al.* (1987) Structure of the human class I histocompatibility antigen, HLA-A2. *Nature* **329**: 506–12.

Brown JH, Jardetzky TS, Gorga JC *et al.* (1993) Three-dimensional structure of the human class II histocompatibility antigen HLA-DR1. *Nature* **364**: 33–9.

HLA and KIR
Kulkarni S, Martin MP, Carrington M (2008) The Yin and Yang of HLA and KIR in human disease. *Seminars in Immunology* **20**: 343–52.

Parham P (2006) Taking license with natural killer cell maturation and repertoire development. *Immunological Reviews* **214**: 155–60.

HLA nomenclature
Holdsworth R, Hurley CK, Marsh SGE *et al.* (2009) The HLA Dictionary 2008: a summary of HLA-A, -B, -C, -DRB1/3/4/5, -DQB1 alleles and their association with serologically defined HLA-A, -B, -C, -DR and -DQ antigens. *Tissue Antigens* **73**: 95–170.

Marsh SGE, Albert ED, Bodmer WF *et al.* (2010) Nomenclature for factors of the HLA system, 2010. *Tissue Antigens* **75**: 291–455.

Marsh SGE, Parham P, Barber LD (2000) *The HLA Facts Book.* Academic Press, London.

Robinson J, Waller MJ, Fail SC *et al.* (2009) The IMGT/HLA database. *Nucleic Acids Research* **37**: D1013–D1017.

HLA polymorphism

Little A-M, Parham P (1999) Polymorphism and evolution of HLA molecules. *Reviews in Immunogenetics* **1**: 105–23.

HLA matching in haemopoietic stem cell transplantation

Bray RA, Huryley CK, Kamani NR *et al.* (2008) National Marrow Donor Program HLA matching guidelines for unrelated adult donor hematopoietic cell transplants. *Biology of Blood and Marrow Transplantation* **14**: 45–53.

Lee SJ, Klein J, Haagenson M *et al.* (2007) High-resolution donor–recipient HLA matching contributes to the success of unrelated donor marrow transplantation. *Blood* **110**: 4576–83.

Petersdorf EW (2008) Optimal HLA matching in hematopoietic cell transplantation. *Current Opinion in Immunology* **20**: 588–93.

Shaw BE, Gooley TA, Malkki M *et al.* (2007) The importance of HLA-DPB1 in unrelated donor hematopoietic cell transplantation. *Blood* **110**: 4560–6.

Minor histocompatibility antigens

Spaapen R, Mutis T (2008) Targeting haematopoietic-specific minor histocompatibility antigens to distinguish graft-versus-tumour effects from graft-versus-host disease. *Best Practice and Research. Clinical Haematology* **21**: 543–57.

Histocompatibility testing procedures

Beksac M (2007) *Bone Marrow and Stem Cell Transplantation.* Humana Press, Totowa, NJ.

Bidwell JL, Navarrete C (2000) *Histocompatibility Testing.* Imperial College Press, London.

Powis SH, Vaughan RW (2003) *MHC Protocols.* Humana Press, Totowa, NJ.

Useful URLs

IMGT/HLA Database: www.ebi.ac.uk/imgt/hla/

HLA Nomenclature: hla.alleles.org

World Marrow Donor Association: www.worldmarrow.org

HLA population data: www.allelefrequencies.net

CHAPTER 38

Stem cell transplantation

38

Charles Craddock[1] and Ronjon Chakraverty[2]

[1]Centre for Clinical Haematology, Queen Elizabeth Hospital, Birmingham, UK
[2]Royal Free and University College Medical School, London, UK

Introduction

Haemopoietic stem cell transplantation (SCT) represents an important and increasingly utilized curative therapy in haematological malignancies and has an emerging role in the management of patients with haemoglobinopathies and bone marrow failure. Improvements in supportive care and treatment of post-transplant complications, a greater availability of alternative donors and advances in tissue typing have simultaneously improved transplant outcome and patient eligibility. The realization that an immunologically mediated graft-versus-leukaemia (GVL) effect makes a major contribution to the curative effect of an allograft has underpinned the concept that allogeneic transplantation can be used as a platform for antitumour immunotherapy. These advances have coincided with the advent of reduced-intensity conditioning (RIC) regimens, which have substantially reduced the morbidity and mortality of allografting and resulted in a marked increase in the number of stem cell transplants, particularly allografts, performed over this period in Europe and worldwide (Figure 38.1).

Postgraduate Haematology: 6th edition. Edited by A. Victor Hoffbrand, Daniel Catovsky, Edward G.D. Tuddenham, Anthony R. Green
© 2011 Blackwell Publishing Ltd.

Immunological basis of stem cell transplantation

The major complications of allogeneic SCT are caused by the immunological responses triggered by the infusion of donor haemopoietic progenitors and lymphocytes into an immunosuppressed host. These can take the form of either a host-versus-graft (HVG) or a donor-derived graft-versus-host (GVH) response. Clinically, the HVG response can result in graft rejection, while a GVH response may manifest itself as either graft-versus-host disease (GVHD) or a GVL reaction. It is now possible to blunt the HVG reaction by optimizing the immunosuppressive properties of the conditioning regimen and consequently graft rejection is rare in most clinical settings. In contrast, GVHD and disease relapse remain the major complications of allogeneic transplantation and novel approaches that permit the induction of GVL without inducing host injury are required. Conversely, autologous SCT is a relatively unremarkable immunological event in which these allogeneic responses are absent.

Antigens and cellular effectors

The antigens against which HVG and GVH responses are directed include the products of highly polymorphic genes lying

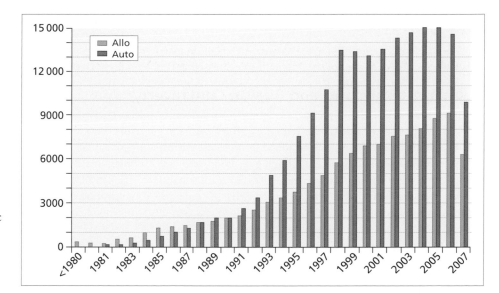

Figure 38.1 Numbers of (a) allogeneic and (b) autologous stem cell transplants performed within Europe. (From Ljungman *et al.* 2010 with permission.)

within the major human leucocyte antigen (HLA) complex on chromosome 6 and minor histocompatibility antigens (minor H antigens) encoded by a number of disparate genes lying outside the HLA system. These antigens and the methods employed to identify them have been reviewed in Chapter 37.

In very general terms, the degree of difference or 'incompatibility' between the donor and recipient will define the risk of graft rejection and/or GVHD. Thus, in situations where the donor is genetically identical to the recipient (syngeneic transplantation), graft rejection or significant GVHD is not observed. For patients undergoing allogeneic transplantation using an HLA-identical sibling, the relevant antigens are minor H antigens, which are polymorphic proteins recognized by T cells as processed peptides in the context of a 'self' HLA molecule. To date, just over 20 such antigens have been identified and include antigens that are ubiquitously expressed on host tissue (e.g. HY antigens encoded by genes on the Y chromosome) or which have restricted tissue distribution (e.g. HA-1 or HA-2, which are only expressed by the haemopoietic system). Female donors, specifically multiparous individuals who have had male infants, may have been primed against HY antigens and as a consequence have circulating T cells that recognize male patient cells expressing these proteins. This is likely to underlie the increased risk of GVHD in male recipients of female grafts.

Where a patient has no HLA-identical sibling donor, an alternative donor may be considered. In this case, the transplant centre will generally seek a donor who is matched with the recipient at each of the HLA-A, -B, -C, -DRB1 and -DQB1 loci (the so-called '10/10 match'). Even with a complete 10/10 match, the risk of GVHD is higher than for an HLA-identical sibling, presumably because the number of polymorphic minor H antigen differences is likely to be greater. In the situation where the donor and recipient are mismatched for one or more class I or II HLA antigens, the risk of transplant complications

is higher since the adult T-cell repertoire contains a very high frequency of cells (~5%) with the potential to react or cross-react with mismatched HLA molecules. Although single HLA mismatches can be reasonably well tolerated clinically, greater degrees of mismatch are associated with increased rates of graft rejection or GVHD. There is a great deal of interest relating to the possibility of 'permissive' HLA mismatches that do not result in a worse transplant outcome. For example, it has been proposed recently that mismatches at HLA-DPB1 (a locus not usually considered in matching with unrelated donors) may actually be associated with an improved outcome because of a lower risk of disease relapse. The degree of HLA mismatch that can be tolerated is greater in patients transplanted using umbilical cord blood (UCB), possibly as a result of the cotransfer of naive donor T cells with less potential for cross-reactivity against HLA antigens.

More extensive HLA disparity, following for example haploidentical transplantation, is only feasible under conditions in which the patient receives highly immunosuppressive conditioning and high doses of haemopoietic progenitor cells (to offset the risk of graft rejection) and where T cells are almost completely depleted from the graft (to prevent prohibitive rates of GVHD). In this setting, certain HLA class I mismatches may play an important role in activating donor natural killer (NK) cells. NK cells express inhibitory killer immunoglobulin-like receptors (inhibitory KIRs) that recognize certain classes of 'self' HLA class I molecules. Upon KIR interaction with a cognate class I ligand, NK functions are inhibited. Conversely, NK-mediated lysis will be triggered if the appropriate inhibitory KIR ligand (an HLA-C or HLA-B molecule) is not presented on the target cell (so-called 'missing self recognition'). While this is not sufficient to induce GVHD, it may result in killing of tumour cells in certain cancers such as acute myeloid leukaemia (AML).

Acute graft-versus-host disease

GVHD is a complex immunological disorder in which donor T cells with specificity for recipient antigens not expressed in the donor initiate tissue damage. The recipient, as a result of immunosuppression or immunodeficiency, is incapable of rejecting the T cells mediating the alloreactive response. Conditioning-induced tissue injury leads to the release of proinflammatory cytokines and altered chemokine or adhesion molecule expression. These changes impact on the developing GVH response leading to cytokine dysregulation and enhanced trafficking of cellular effectors to the organs targeted in GVHD.

Induction of GVHD (Figure 38.2) requires the interaction of donor T cells with host antigen-presenting cells (APCs), most probably dendritic cells within secondary lymphoid organs such as lymph nodes and gut-associated lymphoid tissue. Host APCs are activated by proinflammatory cytokines, such as tumour necrosis factor (TNF)-α or interleukin (IL)-1β, which are released following tissue damage induced by the conditioning regimen. Activated APCs upregulate surface expression of HLA molecules and costimulatory (e.g. B-7 family) molecules and demonstrate increased secretion of inflammatory mediators (e.g. cytokines and inflammatory chemokines). Donor CD4 and CD8 T cells with anti-host specificity, activated on interaction with host APCs, proliferate and develop effector functions that lead to the secretion of effector cytokines (e.g. TNF-α, interferon-γ, IL-2, IL-17) or the induction of perforin/granzyme B pathways required for cellular cytotoxicity. 'Imprinting' of tissue-specific homing molecules (integrins or chemokine receptors) by APCs within certain locations (e.g. gut-draining lymph nodes) permits trafficking of alloreactive T cells from secondary lymphoid tissue to inflamed peripheral tissues. At these sites, T cells aid recruitment of other cellular effectors such as neutrophils, eosinophils, macrophages and NK cells, which together cause the epithelial injury resulting in the clinical manifestations of GVHD in gut, skin and liver. Importantly, GVHD at its initiation is an antigen-specific adaptive immune response but as the immune response develops it becomes less specific so that cells lacking the relevant antigens are targeted in the ensuing response. It follows that efforts designed to prevent or treat GVHD are likely to be more successful prior to, or at the point of induction of, the alloreactive response.

Chronic graft-versus-host disease

Chronic GVHD is a disorder associated with continuing host injury and profound immunodeficiency. The pathogenesis of this disorder is less well defined, partly as a result of the lack of preclinical models that fully recapitulate its onset and clinical features. However, it is clear that at least a component of the inflammatory process observed results from impairment of negative selection of auto-aggressive T cells within the thymus.

This may be consequent upon previous damage to the thymus as a result of acute GVHD and leads to a situation in which autoreactive T cells can enter the periphery and lead to tissue injury. This may help to explain why individuals with chronic GVHD develop some clinical features normally associated with autoimmunity (e.g. immune cytopenias). In contrast to acute GVHD, where CD8 cells are regarded as the most relevant effectors, CD4 cells are thought to be more important for the development of chronic GVHD. CD4 cells might provide helper functions for B cells leading to the production of antibodies against alloantigens or autoantigens or enhance macrophage generation of transforming growth factor (TGF)-β that leads to increased collagen deposition by fibroblasts.

Graft-versus-leukaemia effect

The importance of an immunologically mediated GVL effect in contributing to the curative effect of allogeneic SCT is supported by the observations that T-cell depletion (TCD) increases the risk of relapse and that patients who develop GVHD have a lower risk of disease relapse. Conclusive evidence was provided by the demonstration that infusion of donor lymphocytes can produce durable remissions in patients who have relapsed after allogeneic SCT. It has subsequently been shown that donor lymphocyte infusion (DLI) is a remarkably effective salvage therapy in chronic myeloid leukaemia (CML), with more than 80% of patients achieving a sustained molecular remission. Durable responses can also be achieved in patients transplanted for indolent lymphoma and Hodgkin lymphoma, with responses being observed less commonly in patients with aggressive lymphoma, myeloma or acute leukaemias. As would be predicted, DLI can be complicated by the development of GVHD, although the risk of this life-threatening complication is reduced if the lymphocytes are infused following a significant delay (>12 months) after transplantation or by using an escalating dose schedule rather than a single 'bulk' infusion. For the most part, the antigens recognized in a GVL reaction overlap with those recognized during GVHD. Clinical separation of GVL and GVHD may reflect increased sensitivity of normal or malignant haemopoietic tissue to an emerging GVH reaction compared with epithelial cells. Selective expression of antigenic targets of a GVH reaction on haemopoietic tissues (e.g. the minor H antigen HA-1, proteinase 3 or WT1) or leukaemic blasts (e.g. the product of the *BCR–ABL1* fusion gene) may also underlie the development of a GVL reaction in the absence of GVHD. This concept forms the basis of novel strategies to deliver a GVL effect without a concomitant risk of GVHD, such as peptide vaccination or gene transfer of T-cell receptors (TCRs) specific for leukaemic antigens.

Immune reconstitution

Allogeneic SCT is followed by a prolonged period of cellular and humoral immunodeficiency while donor-derived immune

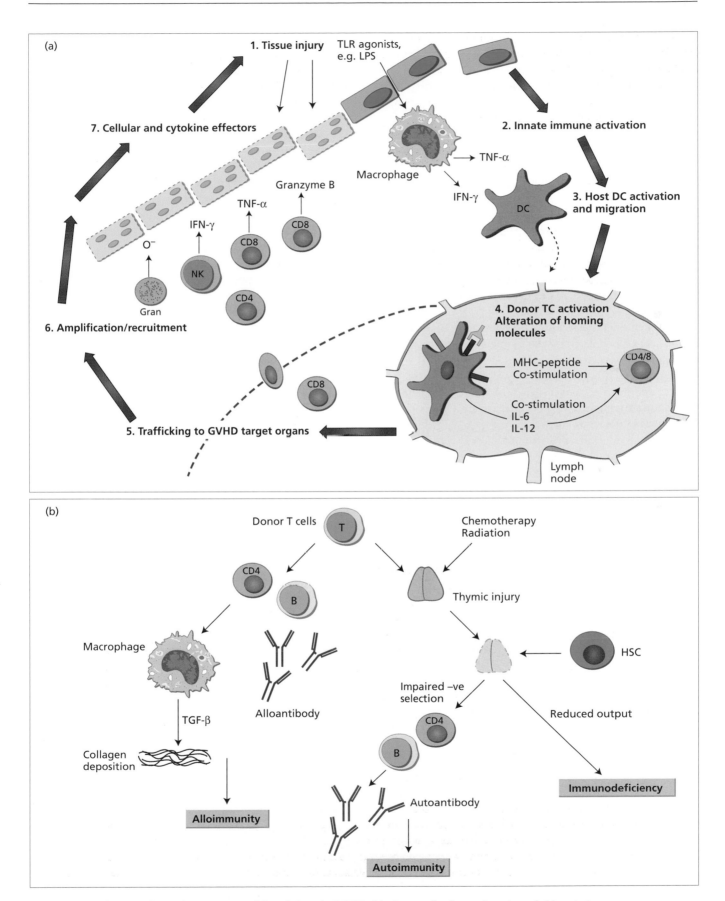

Figure 38.2 Pathophysiology of acute GVHD (a) and chronic GVHD (b). See text for for explanation of abbreviations.

recovery occurs. Reconstitution of an immune response after transplantation can be evaluated in the clinic by monitoring the absolute numbers of T (CD4, CD8), B and NK cell numbers. NK cell numbers recover most rapidly while other subsets (especially CD4 cells and B cells) recover more slowly. In patients who have received a T-cell-depleted graft, T-cell recovery is substantially delayed. Analysis of thymic function after transplantation can be evaluated by measuring the episomal DNA excision circles of the TCR δ locus deleted during recombination of the TCR in functional $\alpha\beta$ T cells (known as TREC, for T-cell receptor excision DNA circles). TREC levels are low for the first 6 months following transplantation and recover thereafter. As a consequence, the T-cell repertoire is limited and mostly dependent on expansion of donor memory T cells. Thymic function is reduced in adults and may be further compromised by the effects of chemoradiotherapy and GVHD. Significant HLA mismatching between donor and recipient may also lead to 'holes' within the T-cell repertoire due to perturbations in thymic selection. These defects reflect a failure of donor-derived thymic emigrants to interact with peptides presented in the context of 'foreign' host HLA molecules.

Quantitative B-cell deficiency is present in virtually all patients in the first months after transplantation and may persist for a number of years post transplantation as a consequence of reductions in the number of marrow B-cell precursors, particularly in patients with chronic GVHD. This defect in B-cell production has multifactorial causes, including damage to the bone marrow stroma, the deleterious effect of inflammatory cytokines and the lympholytic effects of glucocorticoid therapy.

The source of stem cells also influences the kinetics of immune reconstitution. Thus, peripheral blood stem cell (PBSC) grafts, which contain higher numbers of haemopoietic progenitors and mature T cells, are associated with more rapid immune reconstitution than bone marrow grafts. Cord blood transplantation may be affected by poor immune reconstitution in adults since the number of haemopoietic progenitors is often limited and the transferred T cells are naive. Thus, patients are at heightened risk of reactivation of cytomegalovirus (CMV) or Epstein–Barr virus (EBV).

Stem cell engraftment

Biology of stem cell engraftment

The establishment of durable donor haemopoiesis after SCT depends on the engraftment of long-term reconstituting haemopoietic stem cells (HSCs) (see Chapter 1). These cells, defined by their capacity for self-renewal as well as their ability to differentiate into all haemopoietic lineages, are normally resident in the bone marrow at low frequency but can be mobilized into the peripheral blood by cytokines or chemotherapy. A high frequency of haemopoietic stem and progenitor cells is also present in UCB. The cell surface glycoprotein CD34 is expressed on haemopoietic progenitors and HSCs and is currently widely used as a stem cell marker in clinical transplantation. However, it is important to remember that xenograft studies have demonstrated that HSCs reside within a CD34$^+$CD38$^-$ subpopulation and that many of the cells within the CD34$^+$ population lack the properties of a long-term reconstituting stem cell.

Murine transplant studies have established that in a syngeneic setting, where there is no HVG reaction, transplantation of very small numbers of HSCs can result in durable engraftment of lethally irradiated recipients. In contrast, host immunosuppression is required to blunt an HVG reaction capable of rejecting the transplanted stem cell inoculum when there is donor–host HLA disparity, whether the donor is an HLA-identical sibling or an alternative donor.

Clinical factors determining stem cell engraftment

The sole determinant of durable engraftment after an autologous or syngeneic transplant is stem cell number and graft failure is exceedingly rare providing at least 2×10^6 CD34$^+$ cells per kilogram are transplanted. Clinically durable engraftment in allograft recipients is determined by the degree of HLA disparity, the number of transplanted T cells and the size of the stem cell inoculum (Table 38.1). The immunosuppressive properties of the conditioning regimen play a critical role in blunting the HVG response and incorporation of total body irradiation (TBI) or drugs such as cyclophosphamide or fludarabine are highly effective in facilitating HSC engraftment. Historically, high rates of graft failure were observed when TCD was introduced as a form of GVHD prophylaxis in the late 1980s. However, the recognition that donor T cells play a critical role in facilitating engraftment led to redesign of conditioning regimens in patients receiving T-cell-depleted grafts so that their immunosuppressive properties were optimized. The widespread availability of PBSCs from sibling or unrelated donors (see below) allows transplantation of five to ten times more CD34-positive cells than if harvested bone marrow were used. Consequently, the use of PBSCs has played an important role in optimizing engraftment in settings such as TCD or trans-

Table 38.1 Factors determining stem cell engraftment.

Autologous transplantation
Stem cell dose

Allogeneic transplantation
Intensity of host immunosuppression delivered by the conditioning regimen
Numbers of donor T cells in the stem cell inoculum
Degree of genetic disparity between donor and host

plantation of a mismatched donor where a significant risk of graft failure rate would be expected were bone marrow to be used as the stem cell source. Incorporating these principles into clinical practice has markedly reduced the risk of graft failure such that it occurs in fewer than 1% of patients undergoing an HLA-identical sibling allograft and fewer than 5% of those transplanted from an unrelated donor. For a long time graft failure was a major complication of cord blood transplantation (CBT), particularly in adult recipients, and this likely reflected the low stem cell dose. The recent demonstration that the simultaneous transplantation of two cord blood units delivers durable rates of engraftment in the region of 95% has dramatically improved outcome of UCB transplants in adults.

Stem cell mobilization

Biology of stem cell trafficking

In steady-state haemopoiesis only very small numbers of haemopoietic stem and progenitor cells are present in the peripheral blood. The localization of haemopoietic stem and progenitor cells within the bone marrow cavity is mediated through the binding of a range of adhesion molecules, including CXCR4 and VLA4, with their cognate ligands on bone marrow stroma. Recent studies have demonstrated that administration of haemopoietic growth factors such as granulocyte colony-stimulating factor (G-CSF) disrupts the adhesion of progenitors to the bone marrow stroma resulting in their mobilization into the peripheral blood in large numbers. This has had a dramatic impact on transplant practice, resulting in peripheral blood replacing bone marrow as the commonest source of haemopoietic progenitors in both autologous and, more recently, allogeneic transplants. Antagonists to CXCR4 have now been shown to have the potential to significantly augment G-CSF-mediated stem cell mobilization and this promises to increase further the effectiveness of cytokine-mediated stem cell mobilization. Adhesive interactions between haemopoietic progenitors and the bone marrow stroma also play a critical role in the homing of transplanted HSCs and stem cell engraftment can be augmented in animal models by manipulation of the levels of adhesion molecule expression on haemopoietic progenitors and bone marrow stroma. As yet these observations have not been translated into clinical practice.

Stem cell mobilization in clinical practice

In patients undergoing autologous SCT, G-CSF administered alone or after myelosuppressive chemotherapy represents the commonest method of stem cell mobilization. Until recently G-CSF was only administered in conjunction with myelosuppressive doses of salvage chemotherapy or cyclophosphamide. While this represents a highly effective method of stem cell mobilization in the majority of patients, it is now clear that administration of G-CSF alone, albeit at somewhat higher doses, can be equally effective and is substantially less toxic. As a result many units now utilize four daily subcutaneous injections of G-CSF, with stem cell harvesting on days 5 and 6. The minimum target cell dose of 2×10^6 CD34$^+$ cells per kilogram can be harvested from more than 90% of patients using either G-CSF alone or G-CSF in combination with salvage chemotherapy or cyclophosphamide. In patients who fail to mobilize the target number of CD34$^+$ cells, a number of possibilities exist. A second mobilization procedure can be performed using higher doses of G-CSF or, where appropriate, an additional chemotherapeutic drug such as cyclophosphamide or etoposide. Alternatively, the CXCR4 antagonist plerixafor can be used in conjunction with G-CSF. In the small minority of eligible patients who fail to mobilize adequate numbers of PBSCs using this approach, allogeneic transplantation should be considered.

G-CSF-mobilized PBSCs are increasingly used as a stem cell source in allogeneic SCT. The apparent safety of G-CSF doses in the range routinely used for autologous stem cell mobilization ($10–15 \, \mu g/kg$ for 4–6 days) has resulted in all major unrelated donor panels offering this as an alternative to bone marrow harvest. However, it is important that all donors are counselled about the attendant side-effects in the form of myalgia, bone pain and headache. Other reactions are less common, and there are rare reports of splenic rupture. Consequently, donors should be advised to report immediately any pain in the left upper quadrant or shoulder tip. Although the effects of G-CSF on the fetus are not known, all female donors of childbearing age should have a negative pregnancy test prior to its administration. Donors also need to be aware of the 2–3% chance that an additional bone marrow harvest will be required if G-CSF fails to mobilize sufficient PBSC.

Choice of stem cell source and dose

Autologous transplantation

The use of PBSCs as a stem cell source is associated with more rapid engraftment than would be observed with harvested bone marrow and this, coupled with their ease of procurement, has secured their role as the standard stem cell source in autologous transplants. The generally accepted minimum number of haemopoietic progenitors required for engraftment after autologous SCT is 2×10^6 CD34$^+$ cells per kilogram. While increasing the number of CD34$^+$ cells transplanted hastens neutrophil and platelet engraftment, there is little evidence that transplantation of more than 5×10^6 CD34$^+$ cells per kilogram is beneficial and there remain concerns that higher stem cell doses may be associated with an increased risk of tumour contamination. In patients with myeloma, many centres aim to harvest a minimum of 4×10^6 CD34-positive cells per kilogram in order that sufficient cells are available so that a tandem transplant, or second autograft at the time of relapse, is possible.

Sibling and unrelated donor transplantation

PBSCs are the most frequently used stem cell source for patients undergoing a sibling allograft and are increasingly used in unrelated donor transplant recipients. While PBSCs are established as the preferred stem cell source in reduced-intensity allografts, for the reasons discussed above, the relative merits of PBSCs and bone marrow in patients transplanted using a myeloablative regimen remains a matter of debate. Thus while transplantation of PBSCs results in earlier neutrophil and platelet engraftment, which may reduce transplant-related mortality (TRM), particularly in patients with advanced leukaemia, there are emerging registry data that demonstrate an increased incidence of chronic GVHD compared with patients transplanted with bone marrow. This is likely to be consequent on the five- to tenfold greater dose of T cells in a PBSC harvest compared with bone marrow (Table 38.2). As yet it remains unclear whether the increased risk of chronic GVHD associated with the use of PBSC results in a reduction in relapse rate. Thus while PBSCs are routinely used as a stem cell source in patients being allografted for advanced leukaemia, where TRM is a major cause of treatment failure, bone marrow is still preferred in diseases such as aplastic anaemia where chronic GVHD is an important cause of treatment failure. Long-term follow-up studies comparing the outcome of patients transplanted using bone marrow and PBSCs will clearly be important in order to define the optimal stem cell source in standard-risk leukaemias. In paediatric transplantation, bone marrow remains the preferred stem cell source and the use of PBSCs is less common.

Cell dose is an important factor determining outcome after both matched sibling and unrelated donor transplants and this effect is noted in recipients of both bone marrow and PBSCs. This effect is primarily mediated through a reduction in TRM consequent on accelerated immune reconstitution in recipients of a higher stem cell dose. The lowest acceptable stem cell dose to secure engraftment in an allogeneic setting is considered to be 2×10^6 CD34-positive cells per kilogram (2×10^8 mononuclear cells per kilogram if bone marrow is being used), although in practice the majority of patients transplanted using in excess of 1×10^6 CD34-positive cells per kilogram will engraft. Since outcome is improved with higher doses, most centres aim for a

dose in the region of 4×10^6 CD34-positive cells per kilogram. In patients transplanted from an HLA-identical sibling using a T-replete myeloablative regimen, there is some evidence that the incidence of chronic GVHD is increased if the stem cell dose exceeds 8×10^6 CD34-positive cells per kilogram. In this setting it may therefore be reasonable to have a target dose of $4–8 \times 10^6$ CD34-positive cells per kilogram. However, there is no evidence, as yet, that there should be an upper limit on cell dose in patients transplanted using an RIC regimen or from an unrelated donor.

Cord blood transplantation

UCB contains a high proportion of haemopoietic progenitors and HSCs and is an increasingly important stem cell source in paediatric and adult transplantation. Importantly, HLA disparity appears better tolerated in recipients of UCB and as a consequence the incidence of severe GVHD is lower with mismatched UCB than would be expected using a comparably mismatched unrelated donor. This has important implications in terms of donor identification in patients with uncommon HLA types for whom a suitably matched unrelated donor cannot be readily identified. A major factor limiting the uptake of CBT has been delayed or failed engraftment, which has been a common problem particularly in adult recipients. The two most important factors determining the likelihood of neutrophil and platelet engraftment after CBT are nucleated cell dose and HLA disparity. More recently, it has been shown that transplantation of two cord blood units, harvested from two separate donors, increases the speed of engraftment and is associated with a decreased risk of primary graft failure. This observation has substantially increased the number of CBT procedures performed in adults and encouraging results have been reported in patients with high-risk leukaemia using both myeloablative and, more recently, RIC regimens. Selection of cord blood units remains a complex area and consideration must be given to both stem cell dose and HLA disparity in identification of suitable unit(s) (Figure 38.3). Immune reconstitution is markedly delayed after CBT and viral infections, particularly CMV and adenovirus, coupled with fungal infections result in a substantial TRM. For all these reasons it is recommended that cord blood unit selection and transplantation should be performed by physicians with experience in this field.

Stem cell manipulation and expansion

Immunophenotypic characterization of haemopoietic stem and progenitor cells has permitted the development of strategies by which PBSC grafts can be manipulated *ex vivo*. By conjugating antibodies that recognize CD34 with magnetic beads it is possible to achieve highly efficient enrichment of CD34$^+$ cells from a PBSC or bone marrow harvest. This technology also allows, as a consequence of passive depletion of CD34$^-$ cells, effective depletion of donor T cells in allogeneic stem cell harvests and

Table 38.2 Comparison of the cellular composition of a typical bone marrow harvest compared with G-CSF-mobilized in a peripheral blood stem cell (PBSC) (after two aphereses).

	CD34 cells ($\times 10^6$)	CD34 cells ($\times 10^6$/kg)	CD3 cells ($\times 10^6$)	CD3 cells ($\times 10^6$/kg)
PBSCs	240	3.4	11 519	156
Bone marrow	105	1.5	1400	20

Data courtesy of Ginny Turner.

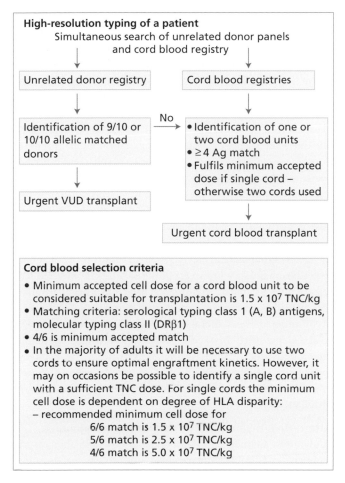

High-resolution typing of a patient
Simultaneous search of unrelated donor panels and cord blood registry

Unrelated donor registry

Cord blood registries

Identification of 9/10 or 10/10 allelic matched donors

No

• Identification of one or two cord blood units
• ≥ 4 Ag match
• Fulfils minimum accepted dose if single cord – otherwise two cords used

Urgent VUD transplant

Urgent cord blood transplant

Cord blood selection criteria

• Minimum accepted cell dose for a cord blood unit to be considered suitable for transplantation is 1.5 x 10^7 TNC/kg
• Matching criteria: serological typing class 1 (A, B) antigens, molecular typing class II (DRβ1)
• 4/6 is minimum accepted match
• In the majority of adults it will be necessary to use two cords to ensure optimal engraftment kinetics. However, it may on occasions be possible to identify a single cord unit with a sufficient TNC dose. For single cords the minimum cell dose is dependent on degree of HLA disparity:
  – recommended minimum cell dose for
    6/6 match is 1.5 x 10^7 TNC/kg
    5/6 match is 2.5 x 10^7 TNC/kg
    4/6 match is 5.0 x 10^7 TNC/kg

Figure 38.3 Possible algorithm for identification of alternative donors in patients requiring urgent allogeneic transplantation who lack a sibling donor. TNC, total nucleated cell dose; VUD, volunteer unrelated donor.

can be used to provide an effective form of GVHD prophylaxis. The importance of cell dose in determining engraftment and outcome after SCT has led to studies aimed at expanding either the stem cell or progenitor population prior to transplantation. In the autologous setting this strategy has not been widely adopted, if only because collection of adequate numbers of cells to ensure rapid engraftment can now be reliably achieved in the great majority of patients. There is, however, significantly more interest in allografting, particularly in CBT, where engraftment can be delayed because of suboptimal stem cell or progenitor numbers.

Conditioning regimens: basic principles

The combination of drugs and radiotherapy administered prior to stem cell infusion is termed the conditioning or preparative regimen. In autologous SCT, where there is no alloreactive

response, the sole purpose of the conditioning regimen is disease eradication. The most common conditioning regimens used in autologous transplantation utilize alkylating agents alone or in combination and other chemotherapeutic drugs.

In the setting of allogeneic SCT the conditioning regimen has conventionally served two purposes: immunosuppression designed to abrogate an HVG reaction thereby preventing graft rejection, and myeloablation in order to achieve tumour eradication. A number of refinements have been made over the past three decades to the design and delivery of myeloablative conditioning regimens. However, they are still associated with significant toxicity which precludes their use in patients older than 50–55 years (45–50 years for recipients of unrelated donor transplants). The recent demonstration that durable donor engraftment can be reliably achieved using a non-myeloablative preparative regimen, coupled with increased awareness of the potency of the GVL reaction, has led to the development of a range of reduced intensity regimens. These protocols are associated with a substantially reduced TRM, allowing allogeneic transplantation to be safely performed in patients in whom it would previously have been contraindicated on the grounds of age or comorbidity. However, experience with RIC regimens is still relatively limited and longer follow-up and, where possible, randomized trials are required before their role in the management of older patients with haematological malignancies can be defined with precision. The encouraging results to date in older patients suggest that there may potentially be a role for their use in younger patients in preference to myeloablative regimens because of their reduced early mortality and possible longer-term benefits such as preserved fertility.

Conditioning regimens in autologous SCT

Conditioning regimens in autologous SCT are designed with dose intensification in mind and are limited mainly by considerations of extramedullary toxicity. High-dose melphalan (200 mg/m²) is the standard conditioning regimen in myeloma autografts. BEAM (carmustine, etoposide, cytarabine, melphalan) is widely used in patients with lymphoma. Autologous transplants are rarely indicated in the management of AML and acute lymphoblastic leukaemia (ALL) but both busulfan/cyclophosphamide and cyclophosphamide/TBI are effective preparative regimens in these diseases. A number of other drug combinations incorporating melphalan, busulfan and thiotepa are used in solid tumours. The major extramedullary toxicities of these regimens are mucositis and gastrointestinal toxicity. Disappointingly, there are few prospective randomized data on which to base the choice of conditioning regimen in autologous SCT. In myeloma a randomized comparison between a TBI-containing regimen and high-dose melphalan alone demonstrated that no benefit was associated with the use of TBI. However, there are no large randomized studies of preparative regimens in lymphoma.

Myeloablative conditioning regimens in allogeneic SCT

The two commonest myeloablative conditioning regimens used in allogeneic SCT employ combinations of cyclophosphamide and either TBI or busulfan.

TBI/cyclophosphamide

Cyclophosphamide is an alkylating agent that, when administered in the doses routinely used in myeloablative conditioning regimens (120–200 mg/kg), has both immunosuppressive and antileukaemic properties. It is a prodrug that must be metabolized by the cytochrome P450 system in the liver to produce metabolically active derivatives, principally phosphoramide mustard, which exert their cytotoxic activity through the production of interstrand DNA links. The two major complications of cyclophosphamide at the doses employed in allogeneic transplantation are haemorrhagic cystitis and cardiac toxicity. Haemorrhagic cystitis results from the toxic effects of a cyclophosphamide metabolite, acrolein, on the uroepithelium and can be reduced by use of sodium 2-mercaptoethanesulfonate (MESNA), while cardiac toxicity is very rare at doses of cyclophosphamide below 150 mg/kg.

TBI has dual immunosuppressive and antileukaemic properties when administered in myeloablative doses (typically 12–14.4 Gy). Radiobiological principles predict that the toxicity of TBI can be reduced by either decreasing the overall dose of radiation or, as is now common, by giving it in fractionated form over a number of days (e.g 14.4 Gy divided into eight fractions over 4 days). The degree of immunosuppression produced by TBI-containing regimens is related to the total dose of irradiation delivered. The use of higher TBI doses is therefore an effective method of optimizing engraftment in myeloablative allografts where there is use of TCD or an alternative donor and consequently an increased risk of graft failure. Haematological malignancies are highly radiosensitive and the risk of disease relapse is reduced if a higher dose of TBI is used, although this benefit is blunted by increased transplant toxicity (see below). Early complications associated with the use of TBI include nausea, vomiting, diarrhoea and parotitis which can usually be managed symptomatically. Increased doses of TBI are also associated with pneumonitis and veno-occlusive disease (VOD) of the liver, both of which may be life-threatening. Long-term complications include cataract formation, hypothyroidism, infertility and, in children, growth retardation.

Busulfan/cyclophosphamide

Busulfan/cyclophosphamide is a myeloablative preparative regimen that has the practical advantage of not requiring the presence of irradiation facilities on site. Busulfan is an alkylating agent with potent activity against leukaemic progenitors and is a core component of both allogeneic and autologous transplant regimens. Historically, busulfan has only been available as an oral preparation, used at a dose of 14–16 mg/kg delivered 6-hourly over a period of 4 days. In this formulation, VOD and pulmonary and central nervous system (CNS) toxicity represent major complications. The pharmacokinetics of oral busulfan are highly variable because it undergoes first-pass metabolism in the liver and there is therefore substantial interpatient variability in plasma drug levels using a standard dosing schedule. Because the incidence of VOD is closely correlated with higher plasma busulfan levels and patients with low busulfan levels also have an increased risk of relapse, oral preparations of busulfan are far from ideal. Two approaches have been used to overcome this problem. A number of groups use frequent (6-hourly) measurement of plasma busulfan levels during the first 24 hours of administration of an oral preparation followed by dose adjustment over the following 3 days in order to achieve a therapeutic busulfan level. Using such a targeted approach the Seattle group have achieved excellent results using busulfan/cyclophosphamide with a very low risk of VOD and reduced relapse rates compared with those achieved using oral busulfan. Alternatively, a recently developed intravenous formulation of busulfan delivers therapeutic drug levels predictably and is associated with markedly reduced toxicity. It should be remembered that with both preparations prophylactic phenytoin or clonazepam should be used to prevent seizures, a complication associated with the administration of high doses of busulfan.

Alternative myeloablative conditioning regimens

Fludarabine augments alkylator-induced cell killing *in vitro* and regimens combining fludarabine with intravenous busulfan appear to be active and well tolerated. Of note, the incidence of VOD using this combination appears to be low and further studies of this regimen are indicated. In patients undergoing a sibling allograft for ALL, etoposide is often substituted for cyclophosphamide and a TBI/etoposide regimen has been shown in some studies to be associated with improved outcome.

In non-malignant disorders, such as aplastic anaemia, cyclophosphamide alone can be used as a conditioning regimen and is sufficiently immunosuppressive to permit engraftment of allogeneic stem cells provided an adequate stem cell inoculum is transplanted. Addition of fludarabine is increasingly used in conjunction with cyclophosphamide in patients with sickle cell disease and thalassaemia.

Comparison of myeloablative conditioning regimens

Sibling allografts

There are two central questions in the design of myeloablative conditioning regimens: is there any survival benefit to be gained from intensifying the conditioning regimen and are cyclophosphamide/TBI and busulfan/cyclophosphamide equally effective preparative regimens?

Prospective randomized trials in patients undergoing a sibling allograft for AML have failed to show any improvement in survival using an increased dose of TBI. Studies performed in the past two decades have shown that while increasing the TBI dose reduces the risk of leukaemic relapse, this benefit is offset by a concomitant increase in TRM. Similarly, there is no evidence that addition of busulfan to a cyclophosphamide/TBI regimen has any impact on disease-free survival.

The decision to use cyclophosphamide/TBI or busulfan/cyclophosphamide as a conditioning regimen in sibling allografts has been studied in a number of randomized studies, all of which used oral busulfan without plasma level targeting. Given the substantial toxicity associated with the use of oral busulfan, the results of these studies need to be interpreted with caution since they may well underestimate the potential benefit of a busulfan/cyclophosphamide regimen utilizing targeted or intravenous busulfan. However, it is of interest that both regimens appeared equally effective for patients undergoing a sibling allograft for CML in first chronic phase, while there appeared to be some benefit attached to the use of a TBI-based regimen in patients with advanced leukemia. The advent of new delivery strategies for busulfan makes it important to re-examine the optimal myeloablative preparative regimen in patients with AML and myelodysplastic syndrome (MDS) and such studies are underway. As noted above, preliminary results with a combination of fludarabine and intravenous busulfan are also promising.

Unrelated donor transplants

The optimal conditioning regimen in patients undergoing an unrelated donor transplant has not been determined and there are few randomized trials in this setting. The greater degree of HLA disparity associated with the use of an unrelated donor results in a higher risk of graft failure than that observed using an HLA-identical sibling. For this reason many groups elect to use a cyclophosphamide/TBI-based regimen, with its greater immunosuppressive properties, although it should be noted that equivalent results have been reported in a number of large series using a busulfan/cyclophosphamide regimen. The other important factor determining the choice of conditioning regimen in unrelated donor transplant is whether TCD is employed. Regimens utilizing rigorous *ex vivo* TCD are associated with a higher risk of graft failure and the use of *in vivo* approaches, using antithymocyte globulin (ATG) or alemtuzumab, is preferred if TCD is to be used. In all patients receiving a TCD unrelated donor transplant, it is important to ensure that the conditioning regimen is sufficiently immunosuppressive if primary graft failure is to be avoided.

Cord blood transplants

The increased HLA disparity and high rates of primary graft failure in CBT makes it critical to optimize the immunosuppressive properties of the preparative regimen. In adults undergoing transplantation using a myeloablative regimen, engraftment rates in the region of 90–95% can be achieved by the addition of fludarabine to a cyclophosphamide/TBI regimen, providing an adequate stem cell inoculum is used. ATG was initially used as additional GVHD prophylaxis in myeloablative CBT but is less commonly used now because of delayed immune reconstitution and an increased risk of post-transplant lymphoproliferative disorders.

Strategies for GVHD prophylaxis in myeloablative regimens

Post-transplant immunosuppression using various combinations of ciclosporin, methotrexate, prednisolone and mycophenolate mofetil represent the commonest forms of GVHD prophylaxis in patients after a myeloablative sibling or unrelated donor transplant. Randomized trials from the Seattle group established the use of intravenous ciclosporin (2.5–5 mg/kg daily) and short-course methotrexate (administered on days 2, 4, 8 and 12 post transplant) as the most effective form of GVHD prophylaxis in patients transplanted undergoing a T-replete allograft using either an HLA-identical sibling or volunteer unrelated donor.

Rates of chronic extensive GVHD are in the region of 30% and 66% for recipients of T-replete sibling and unrelated donor transplants despite the use of ciclosporin/methotrexate GVHD prophylaxis. TCD is an additional, and highly effective method of reducing the risk of both acute and chronic GVHD. TCD can be achieved either by manipulating the stem cell inoculum *ex vivo* or by the *in vivo* administration of T-cell-depleting antibodies such as ATG or alemtuzumab (a humanized monoclonal antibody that recognizes CD52). Although a highly effective method of GVHD prophylaxis, TCD is associated with an increased risk of relapse and graft failure and delays immune reconstitution, increasing the risk of post-transplant infections such as CMV. There have been no randomized studies demonstrating a survival benefit for TCD. Clearly, the form of GVHD prophylaxis used for any particular patient should be selected with their individual risk of both GVHD and relapse in mind. Thus it may be desirable to avoid the use of TCD in patients with advanced leukaemia in whom the risk of relapse is high. In contrast, patients with a low risk of disease recurrence may benefit from more intensive GVHD prophylaxis. However, there remains no consensus concerning the use of TCD in allogeneic transplantation. Many UK and European groups, while performing T-replete sibling allografts, would choose to use *in vivo* TCD in unrelated donor transplant recipients. Compromise strategies in which TCD is used at the same time as further intensifying the conditioning regimen are of interest.

Reduced-intensity conditioning regimens in malignant and non-malignant disease

As recently as 10 years ago it was believed that a myeloablative conditioning regimen was essential if durable engraftment of donor stem cells was to be achieved. A decade's experience has confirmed that reduced-intensity regimens that incorporate either fludarabine or low-dose (200 cGy) TBI as a core immunosuppressive component consistently result in long-term donor stem cell engraftment with a remarkable reduction in toxicity, particularly in older patients or patients with significant comorbidities. At the same time there is now convincing evidence that such regimens provide a platform for a potentially curative GVL effect. As a result, numerous Phase II trials have demonstrated long-term disease-free survival after RIC allografts in patients whose outcome with conventional chemotherapy would be extremely poor. Currently the most important unresolved questions are, firstly, whether low-dose TBI/fludarabine or fludarabine in combination with an alkylating agent represents the optimal conditioning regimen and, secondly, whether a T-replete stem cell inoculum or some form of TCD should be used. Although there is no universally accepted definition of what constitutes an RIC regimen, the European Group for Blood and Marrow Transplantation (EBMT) definition of a regimen incorporating fludarabine with low-dose TBI (4 Gy or less) or other immunosuppressive or chemotherapeutic drug such as cyclophosphamide or melphalan is generally accepted.

Choice of RIC regimen

Low-dose (200 cGy) TBI-based regimens

Pioneering work in a canine model by Storb's group demonstrated that durable engraftment could be achieved with a non-myeloablative conditioning regimen that used immunosuppressive doses of TBI (200–450 cGy) in conjunction with post-transplant immunosuppression in the form of ciclosporin and mycophenolate mofetil. In the late 1990s the Seattle group confirmed these results in patients with high-risk haematological malignancies and noted a substantial reduction in transplant toxicity compared with a myeloablative regimen. Early results from this group demonstrated a small but significant risk of graft failure with this regimen and fludarabine is now routinely incorporated into low-dose (200 cGy) TBI regimens. Accumulating data in the last decade confirms that this regimen now reliably achieves high rates of engraftment and full donor chimerism and is associated with a substantially reduced TRM compared with myeloablative preparative regimens. Its main drawback is a significant risk of acute and chronic GVHD. Recent data demonstrate that up to 66% of patients experience chronic extensive GVHD, the management of which is often very challenging, particularly in elderly and more frail patients.

Non-TBI-based regimens

At the same time as low-dose TBI regimens were being developed in Seattle, groups at the M.D. Anderson Cancer Center, Bethesda and Jerusalem demonstrated that durable engraftment of sibling and unrelated donor stem cells could be achieved with a similar reduction in transplant toxicity using a combination of fludarabine and an alkylating agent such as melphalan,

busulfan or cyclophosphamide. All groups reported a significant risk of severe acute and extensive chronic GVHD using ciclosporin with or without methotrexate as the sole form of GVHD prophylaxis. There are currently no data comparing the outcome of different RIC regimens. Given the significant risk of GVHD associated with the use of both regimens, a major area of research has focused on defining the optimal form of GVHD prophylaxis.

Strategies for GVHD prophylaxis in RIC regimens

Currently, two contrasting approaches are used for GVHD prophylaxis in patients undergoing an RIC allograft. The first uses combinations of ciclosporin, methotrexate and mycophenolate mofetil as the sole form of GVHD prophylaxis and is used in patients transplanted using a T-replete stem cell inoculum. The alternative approach uses ciclosporin alone and is most common in patients transplanted using either ATG or alemtuzumab as *in vivo* TCD. Supporters of a T-depleted approach argue that the incidence of acute, and particularly chronic, GVHD is otherwise unacceptably high, particularly in older patients transplanted using an unrelated donor. It can also be argued that this strategy generates an effective platform for the subsequent delivery of DLI with less GVHD-related toxicity. They point to the effectiveness of ATG and alemtuzumab in reducing the risk of GVHD while at the same time securing high rates of durable donor engraftment. Those favouring a T-replete strategy highlight potential abrogation of a GVL effect by TCD. They also cite the delay in immune reconstitution associated with the use of TCD and consequent increased risk of viral, particularly CMV, infection. As with many debates in transplantation there are no randomized data to support either approach. Substantial numbers of patients achieve durable remissions with both T-replete and TCD regimens. While there may be an increased risk of disease relapse with a T-cell-depleted regimen, much would appear to depend on the intensity of TCD and the form of post-transplant immunosuppression employed.

Clinical management of patients undergoing stem cell transplantation

The use of PBSCs coupled with improved supportive care has decreased the 100-day TRM of autologous transplantation to 1–3% in most centres. The morbidity and mortality of allogeneic SCT has also continued to fall over the last two decades but the 100-day TRM remains in the region of 10–20% depending on patient age, donor type, disease status and stem cell source. This progress reflects advances in supportive care and, in patients undergoing an unrelated donor transplant, more accurate tissue typing. Despite this organ toxicity, acute GVHD and infections consequent on delayed immune reconstitution still represent major causes of morbidity and mortality in the first few months after allogeneic transplantation (Figure 38.4). In addition, chronic GVHD remains an increasing burden for patients and transplant services alike with the increasing use of mismatched unrelated and cord blood donors. The long-term complications of allogeneic transplantation, which can signifi-

cantly compromise a patient's quality of life, are also increasingly recognized and have led to the introduction of specific late-effects clinics where multidisciplinary input from transplant physicians, endocrinologists, gynaecologists, ophthalmologists and psychologists can be provided.

Practicalities of stem cell infusion and blood product support

Stem cell products are infused in the same way as other blood products except for the fact that online blood filters should not be used. Stem cell products must not be irradiated. They may either be infused once collected or, in the case of cryopreserved products, be infused immediately after being unfrozen, at the patient's bedside. The most common side-effect of the cryopreservative (dimethyl sulphoxide, DMSO) is nausea but since it is excreted by the lungs, a garlic-like odour is also observed for 2–3 days after stem cell infusion. Damage to red blood cells releases free haemoglobin, which can precipitate acute renal failure, and thus patients should be adequately hydrated prior to stem cell infusion and for the following hours. In all patients urine output must be monitored closely.

Patients will require red cell and platelet support during the immediate post-transplant period. In allograft recipients, particularly cord blood transplants and patients receiving myelotoxic drugs such as ganciclovir, platelet transfusion may be required for a number of months after transplantation. All cellular blood products should be irradiated (25 Gy) prior to administration in order to prevent transfusion-related GVHD (see Chapter 26). This should be commenced 6 weeks prior to transplant and is continued for 6 months after an autologous transplant or indefinitely for allogeneic transplants. In patients undergoing allogeneic SCT where there is a major ABO incompatibility between donor and recipient (e.g. a group O recipient receiving group A bone marrow), the graft must be depleted of red cells prior to administration unless PBSCs are being transplanted in which case red blood cells are usually effectively depleted during leucapheresis. The subsequent choice of blood group for platelets or red cells depends on the precise nature of the ABO incompatibility, the time from SCT and the results of blood grouping. Delayed erythroid engraftment or haemolysis caused by continuing synthesis of isohaemagglutinins by host lymphocytes may occur several weeks after stem cell infusion and is associated with the presence of a positive direct antiglobulin test and anti-donor red cell antibodies in serum or red cell eluates.

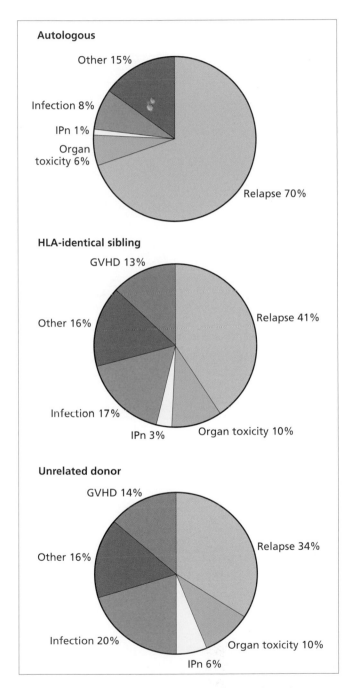

Figure 38.4 Causes of death after stem cell transplantation 2001–2006. (Courtesy of the International Bone Marrow Transplant Registry.)

Complications of allogeneic SCT

Early complications (days 0–90)

Graft failure

Primary graft failure is defined as failure to achieve a neutrophil count above 0.5×10^9/L within 28 days of stem cell infusion and in the great majority of cases is caused by failure of the conditioning regimen to blunt an HVG reaction. It is rare unless there is marked donor–host HLA disparity, such as the use of a mismatched unrelated or family donor, or *in vitro* TCD has been deployed. Primary graft failure should be suspected in patients who fail to demonstrate any evidence of neutrophil engraftment by day +21 and should be investigated urgently with a bone marrow aspirate and trephine (which must be processed urgently), chimerism studies and virology to exclude parvovirus B19 or human herpesvirus (HHV)-6 infection. Patients with no morphological evidence of engraftment and an absence of donor chimerism require urgent intervention in the form of a second transplant, from the same donor if available. Such patients require further conditioning, and fludarabine with or without low-dose TBI provides potent immunosuppression in this setting. If there is no evidence of engraftment but peripheral blood lymphocytes type as donor, then an infusion of CD34-positive selected PBSCs may be employed without prior conditioning therapy. Alternatively, cryopreserved autologous stem cells, if available, can be infused. The mortality of primary graft failure is in excess of 50% and it is therefore important to consider performing an autologous harvest in patients, such as unrelated donor recipients, where there is a significant risk of graft failure.

Secondary graft failure is defined as the occurrence of sustained neutropenia and thrombocytopenia after donor engraftment. It is rare after sibling allografts and occurs predominantly in recipients of mismatched or unrelated donor transplants. The aetiology of secondary graft failure is often complex but causes that need to be considered include late graft rejection, drugs (co-trimoxazole and ganciclovir), viral infection (CMV, HHV-6 and parvovirus B19), disease relapse and rarely hypersplenism. Secondary graft failure is associated with significant mortality related to fungal infections and must be investigated urgently with a bone marrow aspirate and trephine and urgent chimerism studies. In patients with a hypocellular marrow and evidence of donor T-cell engraftment, a second infusion of donor stem cells is required.

Acute graft-versus-host disease

Acute pattern GVHD usually occurs within the first 3 months post transplant, at or near the time of engraftment, and is characterized by the presence of rash, diarrhoea or abnormal liver function tests. Depending on the type of protocol employed, between 20% and 70% of patients will develop this disorder. Acute pattern GVHD occurring after 3 months, with no features of chronic GVHD, is also increasingly recognized in patients receiving RIC transplants, often following withdrawal of immunosuppression. Risk factors for the development of acute GVHD include increased recipient age, unrelated or HLA-mismatched donor transplantation and the use of a female donor. Children have a lower risk of acute GVHD and recipients of CBT may have a lower incidence of GVHD compared

with adult bone marrow transplantation with similar degrees of HLA disparity.

Skin GVHD typically presents as a maculopapular rash involving the face, neck, palms and soles but may extend to involve the whole body (Figure 38.5). In the worst cases it progresses to erythroderma, with bullae formation and painful blistering. Histology shows apoptosis at the base of dermal crypts, dyskeratosis, and evidence of lymphocytes in a perivas-

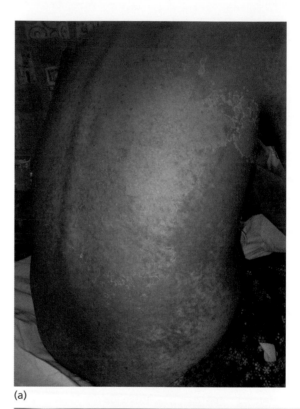

(a)

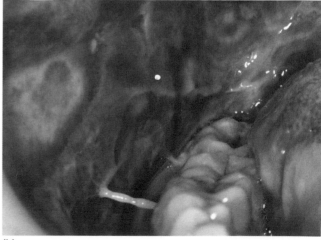

(b)

Figure 38.5 Acute skin GVHD: (a) acute cutaneous GVHD; (b) chronic oral GVHD.

cular distribution or adjacent to dyskeratotic keratinocytes. Gastrointestinal involvement presents with nausea, vomiting, secretory diarrhoea and/or abdominal pain. In more advanced disease, severe abdominal pain and distension in associated with voluminous, occasionally bloody, diarrhoea may occur. Gastric, antral and rectal biopsies have a high diagnostic yield, with diagnostic features including the presence of apoptotic cells in the base of crypts and a lymphocytic infiltrate. A well-defined manifestation of upper gut GVHD is the development of anorexia and nausea, both of which usually resolve rapidly if treated with low-dose methylprednisolone (1 mg/kg). A rising bilirubin and raised alkaline phosphatase are the initial features of liver GVHD, which typically develops later than skin or gut GVHD. Liver histology is diagnostic and demonstrates a portal tract lymphocytic infiltration, pericholangitis and bile duct loss.

Accurate and early diagnosis of acute GVHD is essential for effective management of this potentially life-threatening disorder. Where possible diagnostic biopsies should be taken to both confirm the presence of GVHD and assist in the exclusion of other aetiologies. It is also important to stage GVHD accurately and the criteria devised by Glucksberg (and recently updated by the International Bone Marrow Transplant Registry) are widely used (Table 38.3). This staging system is a reliable indicator of prognosis and guides the intensity of treatment required. Grade 2–4 acute GVHD should be treated with high-dose methylprednisolone (typically 2 mg/kg daily), which is tapered according to response. In the setting of limited skin GVHD and upper gut GVHD, topical or oral steroids (1 mg/kg) coupled with optimization of ciclosporin levels may be sufficient to control symp-

toms. Approximately 70% of patients will improve significantly with oral or intravenous corticosteroid therapy, but a number will either fail to respond or relapse when immunosuppression is tapered. Failure to respond to 7 days of intravenous corticosteroid therapy defines steroid-resistant acute GVHD and these patients require the use of second-line therapies. Unfortunately, individuals with steroid-refractory acute GVHD have a poor prognosis, with a non-relapse mortality in excess of 70% secondary to persistent GVHD or as a result of infectious complications. Currently, robust evidence supporting efficacy of second-line treatments is lacking. Some patients with acute pattern GVHD affecting skin may respond to phototherapy. Patients with predominant gut involvement may respond to oral non-absorbable steroids or the monoclonal antibody infliximab. In other patients, treatment with other monoclonal antibodies such as daclizumab or pentostatin may be of benefit. More recently, encouraging results have been reported with the use of donor or third-party mesenchymal stromal cells, with a response rate of 60–70%. Application of this approach will require evaluation in prospective randomized studies. Patients with acute severe GVHD often require intensive supportive measures including replacement of gastrointestinal losses, parenteral nutrition, pain control and infectious prophylaxis.

Infectious complications

Bacterial, fungal, protozoal and viral infections are a major cause of morbidity and mortality after allogeneic transplantation. Host factors include neutropenia, post-transplant immunosuppression and acute or chronic GVHD requiring steroid therapy. Numerous additional factors contribute to delayed

Table 38.3 Glucksberg staging of acute GVHD: (a) clinical staging; (b) clinical grading.

(a)

Stage	Skin	Liver bilirubin	Gut
+	Maculopapular rash <25% body surface	34–51 μmol/L	Diarrhoea 500–1000 mL/day or persistent nausea
++	Maculopapular rash 25–50% body surface	51–102 μmol/L	Diarrhoea 1000–1500 mL/day
+++	Generalized erythroderma	102–255 μmol/L	Diarrhoea >1500 mL/day
++++	Desquamation and bullae	>255 μmol/L	Pain ± ileus

(b)

Overall grade	Skin	Liver	Gut	Functional impairment
0 (none)	0	0	0	0
I (mild)	+ to ++	0	0	0
II (moderate)	+ to +++	+	+	+
III (severe)	++ to +++	++ to +++	++ to +++	++
IV (life-threatening)	+ to ++++	++ to ++++	++ to ++++	+++

Source: from Blume KG, Forman SJ, Appelbaum FR, eds (2004) *Thomas' Hemopoietic Stem Cell Transplantation*, 3rd edn. Blackwell Science, Oxford, with permission.

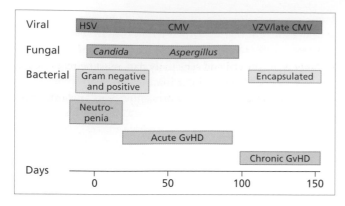

Figure 38.6 Temporal pattern of infectious complications after allogeneic stem cell transplantation.

immune reconstitution after an allograft and include thymic atrophy in adults, the use of TCD and a suboptimal stem cell inoculum. Infectious complications are a particular challenge after CBT. The temporal pattern of infectious complications after allogeneic SCT is shown in Figure 38.6.

Considerable progress has been made in the development of strategies to reduce the risk of infection after allogeneic SCT. All patients should be nursed in single rooms, preferably with laminar airflow or high-efficiency particulate air filtration. Evidence supports the use of triazole antifungals, such as fluconazole 400 mg daily, as an effective means of reducing *Candida* infection. Aciclovir (200–400 mg four times daily) is usually administered to prevent herpes simplex virus (HSV) reactivation. Quinolone antibiotics (e.g. ciprofloxacin 500 mg twice daily) are used by some units to reduce the risk of severe Gram-negative infections, although the evidence supporting this measure is inconclusive and practice should be guided by advice from local microbiologists concerning the prevalence and sensitivity of drug-resistant organisms. Patients should receive co-trimoxazole (480 mg twice daily three times per week) at the time of neutrophil engraftment (neutrophils >1.0 × 10^9/L) to prevent *Pneumocystis jirovecii* infection. If allergic to co-trimoxazole, nebulized pentamidine (300 mg monthly) can be substituted, although it should be remembered that this provides incomplete protection from *Pneumocystis* pneumonia and for this reason some units prefer to use dapsone.

Allogeneic transplants, particularly recipients of TBI-containing regimens, continue to be at long-term risk from infections caused by encapsulated bacteria such as *Streptococcus pneumoniae* and *Haemophilus influenzae* and require lifelong prophylaxis with penicillin (250 mg twice daily) or erythromycin (250 mg twice daily) if allergic to penicillin. Antibody titres to diseases for which childhood vaccination is performed decline after SCT. Revaccination is therefore recommended, particularly in allograft recipients, and most centres commence such a programme 12 months after transplantation.

Herpesvirus infection: CMV, HSV and varicella zoster

Human CMV is a ubiquitous herpesvirus present in up to 60% of the general population, which reactivates after allogeneic SCT giving rise to either asymptomatic infection or, less commonly, end-organ damage (CMV disease) and death. Patients at the highest risk of CMV reactivation are seropositive recipients, especially those who receive TCD or unrelated donor grafts, and patients who develop GVHD requiring steroid therapy. CMV reactivation occurs in 40–80% of at-risk patients and until recently a substantial number of such patients developed CMV disease. CMV disease most commonly manifests as pneumonitis but can rarely cause gastrointestinal ulceration, hepatitis and retinitis. Until recently CMV was the commonest cause of infectious death after allogeneic transplantation. It is now possible to detect low levels of CMV infection after transplantation, using either polymerase chain reaction (PCR)-based detection of CMV or detection of pp65 antigen in peripheral blood leucocytes (CMV antigenaemia). The introduction of these sensitive diagnostic techniques coupled with the development of effective antiviral drugs has markedly reduced the incidence of CMV disease. Primary infection of seronegative patients may occur as a result of the infusion of stem cell or blood products from a CMV-positive donor but is rare. For this reason seronegative transplant recipients should receive CMV-negative or leucodepleted blood products to limit the possibility of primary infection.

All patients at risk of CMV infection (all CMV-seropositive patients and any patient with a seropositive donor) should undergo weekly PCR or CMV antigenaemia testing from engraftment until 100 days after transplantation. Patients with CMV reactivation should be treated promptly with ganciclovir (5–10 mg/kg daily adjusted according to renal function), a nucleoside analogue that inhibits viral thymidine kinase. The major side-effect of ganciclovir is myelosuppression, which is especially problematic in patients transplanted using an unrelated or cord blood donor. Randomized studies have confirmed that this pre-emptive treatment strategy reduces the risk of CMV disease and death after sibling allogeneic transplantation. The use of prophylactic ganciclovir, which is administered regardless of whether there is evidence of CMV infection, does not improve outcome and is associated with significant bacterial and fungal infections consequent on high rates of myelotoxicity. For this reason a pre-emptive approach to prevention of CMV disease is generally preferred. Foscarnet, a DNA polymerase inhibitor, has less myelotoxicity than ganciclovir and is effective as part of a pre-emptive approach, although it is associated with significant nephrotoxicity.

The incidence of CMV pneumonitis after allogeneic transplantation has substantially reduced since the advent of effective screening and pre-emptive treatment strategies. It occurs in patients with evidence of CMV reactivation within the first 100 days after transplantation and typically presents with dyspnoea, hypoxaemia and pulmonary infiltrates. Ganciclovir and foscarnet are often ineffective in patients with established CMV pneumonitis. However, recent studies have demonstrated significant activity of cidofovir, which is considered in some units as first-line treatment in all patients with CMV pneumonitis. Cidofovir is nephrotoxic but can usually be safely administered if attention is paid to adequate hydration and other nephrotoxic drugs, particularly foscarnet, are discontinued. The role of high-titre CMV immunoglobulin in the treatment of CMV pneumonitis remains unclear, although it is still widely used, if available. The effective treatment of CMV infection delays the development of an immune response to CMV and as a result late (beyond 100 days post-transplant) CMV reactivation and disease is increasingly observed. Risk factors for late CMV infection include previous CMV reactivation, lymphopenia and the presence of active GVHD.

Other members of the herpesvirus family have the potential to cause significant morbidity after allogeneic SCT. The incidence of HSV, which used to be very common in the first 30 days after SCT, has been sharply reduced by the use of prophylactic aciclovir. Reactivation of varicella zoster virus (VZV) occurs in up to 50% of at-risk patients after allogeneic SCT and typically presents as shingles with severe pain and a dermatomal vesicular eruption. Less commonly, VZV reactivation presents with atypical pain (headache or undiagnosed abdominal pain) in the absence of a rash. Prompt treatment of VZV infections with high-dose intravenous aciclovir is indicated after allogeneic SCT to prevent dissemination but also to reduce the severity of post-herpetic neuralgia. HHV-6 is also increasingly being reported in association with a syndrome variously associated with delayed engraftment, encephalitis and hepatitis.

Fungal infections

Fungal infections remain a major complication after SCT, reflecting the absence of accurate diagnostic tests and the inadequacy of current therapies. A high index of clinical suspicion is therefore required in transplant patients, particularly allografts, and most units administer systemic antifungal therapy early in the management of neutropenic fever. Risk factors for the development of fungal infection include prolonged neutropenia after SCT, the use of high-dose corticosteroids for treatment of GVHD and a history of prior fungal infection.

Effective strategies exist for the prophylaxis and treatment of infection with yeasts (*Candida* spp.) but are lacking for infection with moulds such as *Aspergillus* spp. *Candida* infections typical manifest as oral thrush and less commonly as oesophageal candidiasis. Hepatosplenic candidiasis is seen occasionally, presenting with high spiking fevers at the time of engraftment in association with abnormal liver function tests. Ultrasound or computed tomography (CT) of the liver and spleen will confirm the diagnosis. Prophylactic use of fluconazole (400 mg daily) has proved effective in reducing the incidence of both superficial and invasive candidiasis. Patients who develop either hepatosplenic candidiasis or candidaemia should be treated with systemic antifungals, usually liposomal amphotericin. All indwelling catheters must be removed. Emergence of fluconazole-resistant *Candida* species such as *Candida kruseii* or *Candida glabrata* is of concern and sensitivity data must be requested in any patient with *Candida* infection.

Aspergillus infections usually present prior to or shortly after engraftment. The most common manifestation is as invasive pulmonary aspergillosis (IPA), which typically presents with an antibiotic-resistant fever, a significantly raised C-reactive protein, and abnormal chest radiography or high-resolution CT, often in the absence of respiratory symptoms. Rarely invasive *Aspergillus* infections can present with cerebral or hepatic disease. Accurate diagnosis of *Aspergillus* infections remains problematic since spores are only rarely cultured from lavage fluid or infected tissues and the sensitivity and specificity of other currently available diagnostic techniques is low. Contradictory results have been obtained using galactomannan detection assays and the initially encouraging results with PCR technology have not been confirmed by all groups. Operationally, the most helpful test in deciding whether IPA is a clinical possibility is high-resolution CT of the chest, which should be obtained in all patients with a neutropenic fever that has persisted for more than 72 hours. While the characteristic radiographic features of peripheral nodular shadows, with or without evidence of cavitation or a 'halo' sign, may take weeks to develop, the presence of any significant pulmonary infiltrate substantially increases the likelihood of *Aspergillus* infection and is an indication for the consideration of treatment doses of liposomal amphotericin or voriconazole. Importantly, the liklihood of IPA in a patient with a normal chest on high-resolution CT is low. Improved antifungal drugs now make it possible to contemplate allogeneic transplantation in patients with a previous proven or suspected invasive fungal infection. Risk factors for recrudescence of fungal disease in this setting include a short period (<6 weeks) of antifungal treatment prior to transplant, the use of bone marrow or cord blood cells as opposed to PBSCs, occurrence of grade 2 or greater acute GVHD, and CMV reactivation.

Organ toxicity
Gastrointestinal toxicity

Mucositis is frequently observed in patients transplanted using a myeloablative conditioning regimen but is less common in patients transplanted using an RIC regimen. Symptoms of oral pain and pain on swallowing typically develop in the first few days after stem cell infusion and peak approximately 8 days post transplant. The severity of mucositis is closely correlated with the intensity of the conditioning regimen, the use of higher doses of fractionated TBI and the inclusion of methotrexate as a component of the GVHD prophylaxis regimen. Patients with severe mucositis should receive adequate (often opiate) analgesia and be monitored for evidence of airway obstruction. In patients who develop symptoms of severe oesophagitis, the possibility of superadded infection with *Candida albicans* or HSV must be considered, the latter typically being associated with intractable vomiting.

Diarrhoea and/or abdominal pain are common manifestations of conditioning toxicity. Alternative causes of diarrhoea in the first 4 weeks after transplantation include enteritis due to *Clostridium difficile*, rotavirus or CMV, acute GVHD and pancreatitis. VZV reactivation can occasionally present with severe abdominal pain, often in association with markedly deranged liver function tests sometimes days in advance of, or even in the absence of, the development of classic vesicles.

Liver toxicity

Abnormalities in liver function tests are commonly observed after allogeneic SCT and causes include VOD, drugs, infectious complications, cholelithiasis, acute GVHD and transfusional iron overload (Table 38.4). VOD is a clinical syndrome characterized by a triad of hyperbilirubinaemia (bilirubin >34 μmol/L), weight gain (>5% over baseline), and painful hepatomegaly. It is associated with evidence of damage to sinusoidal endothelial cells and hepatocytes and subsequent damage to the central veins in zone 3 of the hepatic acinus. In severe cases hepatic venular occlusion and widespread zonal disruption may lead to portal hypertension, hepatorenal syndrome, multiorgan failure and death. Risk factors for the development of VOD include the use of conditioning regimens containing busulfan or higher doses of TBI, pretransplant abnormalities of liver function tests, previous abdominal irradiation and recent exposure to the anti-CD33 antibody gemtuzumab ozogamicin (Mylotarg). A diagnosis of VOD is most commonly made on clinical criteria.

Table 38.4 Causes of abnormal liver function tests after allogeneic SCT.

Precipitant	Clinical presentation
Veno-occlusive disease	Hyperbilirubinaemia associated with weight gain, ascites and painful hepatomegaly
Drugs	Ciclosporin (hyperbilirubinaemia), azole antifungals (raised AST)
Haemolysis	Fall in Hb associated with unconjugated hyperbilirubinaemia and positive Coombs test
Biliary obstruction	Dilated biliary tree associated with gallbladder 'sludge' or cholelithiasis
Infection	Viral hepatitis, fungal infection (disseminated aspergillosis or candidiasis), cholangitis lenta (progressive development of obstructive picture occurring days after an episode of sepsis)

Hepatic Doppler studies demonstrating evidence of reversal of portal flow support the diagnosis. Definitive diagnosis requires transjugular venous liver biopsy, which has significant morbidity in the early post-transplant period and is therefore often avoided. It is important to exclude other causes of hyperbilirubinaemia, particularly ciclosporin toxicity (which can present with a very similar clinical picture), haemolysis (typically consequent on donor–recipient ABO mismatch or transplantation-associated microangiopathic haemolytic anaemia) and the hepatitis of sepsis (cholangitis lenta). Management is supportive, consisting of careful fluid balance, the judicious use of diuretics and, where necessary, haemofiltration. There is now convincing evidence that defibrotide can effectively treat severe VOD. Because of the clinical similarities between VOD and ciclosporin toxicity, it is wise to discontinue ciclosporin for at least 48 hours in any patient in whom a diagnosis of VOD is suspected.

Renal toxicity

The importance of the daily monitoring of weight, fluid balance and renal function in the effective management of patients after SCT cannot be overestimated. Impairment of renal function is frequently observed after allogeneic SCT unless careful attention is paid to fluid balance and the nephrotoxic potential of drugs commonly used during SCT, especially ciclosporin, amphotericin, aminoglycosides and loop diuretics. Ciclosporin-related renal toxicity is usually easily reversible by temporary omission and dose reduction. Occasionally, ciclosporin toxicity manifests itself as a microangiopathic haemolytic anaemia with features of thrombotic thrombocytopenic purpura/haemolytic–uraemic syndrome. Withdrawal of the drug is mandatory. There is no convincing evidence that plasmapheresis is beneficial. Introduction of an alternative immunosuppressant (e.g. mycophenolate mofetil) should be considered. Late renal toxicity is observed in patients on long-term ciclosporin and patients who have undergone a TBI-based allograft.

Pulmonary infections and non-infectious complications

A range of pulmonary infections occurs after allogeneic SCT. In the first month after transplantation bacterial and fungal pneumonias are common. CMV, respiratory syncytial virus, influenza and parainfluenza are important causes of pneumonitis and typically occur in the first 90 days after transplantation. *Pneumocystis* pneumonia and *Toxoplasma* infection are still seen occasionally in the first few months after transplantation in patients who do not receive, or who are not compliant with, co-trimoxazole prophylaxis.

Non-infectious pulmonary complications occurring after allogeneic transplantation can be reversible but demand prompt diagnosis if treatment is to be effective. Pulmonary oedema consequent on either increased capillary hydrostatic pressure caused by fluid overload or increased capillary permeability due to irradiation or sepsis is frequently seen in the post-transplant period. Idiopathic pneumonia syndrome, defined as diffuse lung injury occurring after SCT for which no infectious or non-infectious aetiology can be identified, typically occurs 30–50 days after transplantation. The classic presentation includes dyspnoea, non-productive cough, hypoxaemia and non-lobar infiltrates on chest radiography and can progress rapidly to acute respiratory distress syndrome. Treatment is supportive but frequently unsatisfactory, and steroids have little effect on outcome. Diffuse alveolar haemorrhage is seen predominantly in patients undergoing autologous SCT but can also be seen in allogeneic recipients. This complication usually occurs within the first 2–3 weeks of transplantation and presents with dyspnoea, non-productive cough and hypoxaemia. Radiographic changes include interstitial or alveolar shadowing. Definitive diagnosis requires bronchoscopy, which shows fresh blood on repeated lavage. Early recognition of this disorder is essential since early intervention with high-dose steroids may significantly improve survival.

Post-transplant lymphoproliferative disease

Post-transplant lymphoproliferative disease (PTLD) includes a spectrum of EBV-driven B-cell hyperproliferative states that range from polyclonal benign proliferations to life-threatening neoplastic disease. Most cases of PTLD involve EBV-seropositive donors and present with lymphadenopathy and fever. In contrast to the PTLDs that develop following solid organ transplantation, the majority of cases after SCT are of donor origin and arise as a result of inadequate T-cell control of proliferation of EBV-infected B cells. Risk factors for the development of PTLD include TCD, particularly the use of ATG, and increased HLA disparity. Recent reports suggest that the use of alemtuzumab for TCD may now also be associated with an increased risk of PTLD. Weekly PCR quantitation of EBV viraemia is indicated in patients undergoing allogeneic transplantation that incorporates ATG or alemtuzumab and in all CBT procedures. Patients with a rising EBV load may be managed by a reduction in immunosuppression or treated with pre-emptive anti-CD20 monoclonal antibody (rituximab), although the triggers for intervention have not been precisely defined. In patients with a documented PTLD, early treatment with rituximab and, where possible, cessation of immunosuppressive therapy are the key to treatment. DLI using EBV-specific cytotoxic T lymphocytes has also been used with effect.

Intensive care support

The likelihood of developing organ failure requiring admission to the intensive therapy unit (ITU) after SCT varies widely according to stem cell source (autologous vs. allogeneic), the intensity of the conditioning regimen and the presence of pretransplant comorbidities. While recent studies suggest a reduction in the proportion of transplant recipients requiring ITU admission, it remains the case that at least 10% of allografted patients, and in some institutions significantly more,

will require ITU admission at some stage during their treatment.

Analysis of outcome in patients admitted to ITU has identified factors determining survival at varying stages after transplantation, allowing rational decisions about the likelihood of benefit of sustained intensive care in patients with multiorgan failure. Further sophistication in defining who will benefit from admission to ITU has been provided by the application of scoring systems. These include the Acute Physiology and Chronic Health Evaluation (APACHE) II and III mortality prediction models and Simplified Acute Physiology Score (SAPS) prognostic systems. Application of these scores prior to admission to ITU and, where appropriate, after a 72-hour period on ITU is helpful in identifying patients who will benefit from institution or continuation of intensive support. A number of studies have indicated that the development of progressive organ failure or the presence of multiorgan failure 72 hours after admission to ITU predicts an extremely poor outcome. The careful integration of these data into discussion with relatives and, where possible, patients can spare many the indignity of prolonged and futile intervention.

Late complications

As the results of allogeneic SCT have improved, its long-term complications have come to be better recognized. Chronic GVHD, secondary malignancies, and growth and fertility disorders represent an increasingly important cause of morbidity in patients who have been cured of their underlying disease.

Chronic GVHD

Chronic GVHD refers to a complex syndrome occurring more than 3 months following allogeneic transplantation and is its commonest long-term complication. There is increasing recognition that its onset can be variable and that patients may present features of both acute and chronic GVHD (often referred to as overlap syndrome). Registry data show that chronic GVHD occurs in approximately one-third of patients undergoing T-replete transplants from HLA-identical siblings, rising to two-thirds of patients receiving T-replete grafts from unrelated donors. Risk factors for the development of chronic GVHD include increased recipient age, the use of PBSCs as opposed to bone marrow as stem cell source, transplantation from an unrelated or HLA-mismatched donor, the use of a T-replete stem cell inoculum and the presence of prior acute GVHD. Chronic GVHD may develop directly from acute GVHD (progressive), after the resolution of an episode of acute GVHD, or *de novo* in patients with no history of chronic GVHD. The clinical manifestations are characterized by features of both immunodeficiency and 'autoimmunity' (Figure 38.7). Previous grading systems for chronic GVHD have classified its severity as limited or extensive (Table 38.5), although the utility of this staging system has been questioned. Patients with progressive-type onset, extensive skin involvement, throm-

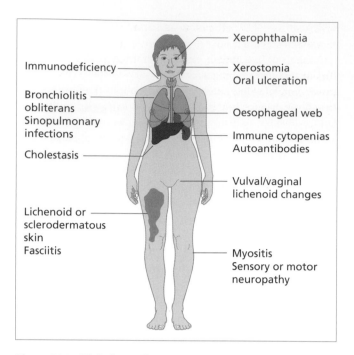

Figure 38.7 Clinical manifestations of chronic GVHD

Table 38.5 Classification of chronic GVHD.

Limited chronic GvHD
Either or both
Localized skin involvement
Hepatic dysfunction as a result of chronic GVHD

Extensive chronic GvHD
Either
Generalized skin involvement
or
Localized skin involvement and/or hepatic dysfunction as a result
  of chronic GVHD
plus
Liver histology showing chronic aggressive hepatitis bridging
  necrosis or cirrhosis
or
Involvement of eye (Schirmer test with <5 mm wetting)
or
Involvement of minor salivary glands or oral mucosa
  demonstrated on labial biopsy
or
Involvement of any other target organ

Source: from Blume KG, Forman SJ, Appelbaum FR, eds (2004)
Thomas' Hemopoietic Stem Cell Transplantation, 3rd edn.
Blackwell Science, Oxford, with permission.

bocytopenia or bronchiolitis obliterans have a particularly poor prognosis. A new scoring system based on the number of organs involved and the severity within each affected organ is likely to be adopted, particularly in trials of novel therapies.

Current treatment options are unsatisfactory and in the first instance involve immunosuppression with ciclosporin or prednisolone prior to the institution of a gradual reduction in responding patients. In patients, who fail to respond or who show steroid dependency, second-line therapies including extracorporeal photopheresis, sirolimus and rituximab can be effective. Extracorporeal photopheresis is particularly beneficial in patients with sclerodermatous involvement and appears to be less effective in patients with visceral disease. Rituximab has been employed successfully in some patients, with responses observed particularly in patients with musculoskeletal involvement. Other treatments suggested include non-absorbable steroids for those with gut involvement, tacrolimus (FK506), thalidomide and imatinib. Definitive prospective randomized data supporting any of these strategies are lacking.

Secondary malignancies
The incidence of solid tumours in recipients of allogeneic SCT is increased compared with control populations and includes a higher rate of skin or buccal cavity squamous cell carcinoma and melanoma. In the largest study to date, the cumulative incidence of all solid tumours was 2.2% at 10 years and 6.7% at 15 years, although the latter figure may represent an overestimate. Risk factors for the development of secondary malignancies include the use of TBI in the conditioning regimen and the presence of chronic GVHD.

Growth, puberty and fertility
Retarded growth is seen predominantly in children who receive transplants at a younger age (<10 years) and in those who have received irradiation, particularly cranial irradiation. Growth retardation is multifactorial and although growth hormone levels may be diminished as a consequence of hypothalamic or pituitary irradiation, this does not entirely account for the observed reduction in height. Gonadal failure (both testicular and ovarian) is a common consequence of myeloablative conditioning regimens, particularly those which contain TBI or busulfan. While prepubertal females receiving cyclophosphamide alone (as for transplantation in severe aplastic anaemia) have a high probability of experiencing a normal puberty, most receiving other preparative regimens will fail to regain normal ovarian function and will require sex hormone replacement therapy for the induction of puberty. Thereafter sex hormone replacement is indicated to maintain the menstrual cycle and normal bone turnover/mineralization, but the optimal duration of therapy and the potential long-term risks of hormone replacement therapy in this setting are unknown. Although about 10% of women who receive TBI-containing regimens

Table 38.6 Immediate complications of autologous SCT.

Organ	Complications
Lung	Diffuse alveolar haemorrhage, interstitial pneumonitis especially in recipients of bleomycin/carmustine- and TBI-containing regimens
Gastrointestinal	Mucositis, nausea, diarrhoea
Hepatic	Asymptomatic elevation of bilirubin or AST, veno-occlusive disease (especially recipients of busulfan-containing regimens)
Renal	Prerenal acute renal failure, renal toxicity (nephrotoxic antibiotics), interstitial nephritis
Cardiac	Arrhythmias, cardiac failure (cyclophosphamide)

Table 38.7 Impact of pretransplant patient and donor characteristics on outcome after allogeneic SCT.

Patient age
Donor match (sibling vs. unrelated donor)
Donor sex (female; male is associated with worse outcome)
Disease stage
Time from diagnosis to transplant (applies to patients with CML in first CP)
Patient CMV serostatus (if undergoing volunteer unrelated donor transplant)

may have some recovery of gonadal function, the overall incidence of pregnancy is very low. The advent of RIC raises the prospect that some women may remain fertile after transplantation and in this case prior therapies and age will be additional factors determining fertility. In males, cryopreservation of sperm should be performed at diagnosis since chemotherapy and transplantation both result in a high rate of male infertility.

Complications of autologous SCT

The morbidity and mortality of autologous SCT is much lower than that observed in allogeneic transplantation. The major toxicities relate to immediate or delayed organ failure caused by the conditioning regimen or complications consequent on neutropenia or thrombocytopenia (Table 38.6). The major infectious complications are bacterial and fungal and occur in the main in the first 28 days after transplantation. Late complications are rare but include pulmonary fibrosis in patients who have received busulfan and carmustine and gonadal failure in recipients of TBI or busulfan-containing regimens. Female recipients of BEAM chemotherapy may recover some gonadal function. The development of myelodysplasia is a well-recognized late complication, particularly in patients transplanted using a TBI-based regimen. In general, treatment-related MDS or AML occurs within 12 months of transplantation and is most frequently associated with abnormalities of chromosome 5 or 7 or a complex karyotype. It appears that prior chemotherapy is the most important factor in the development of MDS or AML since the leukaemia-associated cytogenetic abnormality can be detected in the infused stem cell inoculum.

Patient factors determining outcome after allogeneic stem cell transplantation

The major causes of treatment failure after allogeneic transplantation are organ toxicity, infectious complications, GVHD and disease relapse (see Figure 38.4). TRM after allografting is determined by specific patient and donor characteristics and these can be used to calculate transplant risk, providing useful information in assessing whether an individual patient is likely to benefit from allogeneic transplantation (Table 38.7). The advent of RIC regimens and alternative stem cell sources has increased the importance of developing a robust estimate of TRM. Recent studies in patients allografted using an RIC regimen have allowed the development of a comorbidity scoring system that assists in prediction of TRM and overall survival. These important studies require validation in specific RIC regimens, particularly those incorporating alternative donors or TCD, but offer the prospect of developing a more rational basis of selecting candidates for allogeneic transplantation.

Indications for transplantation

SCT is now an essential constituent of the treatment strategy for many haematological malignancies. In the case of autologous transplantation current practice has been informed by the results of randomized controlled trials comparing the outcome of transplanted patients with those who have received standard chemotherapy. However, methodological challenges have made it much more challenging to perform randomized trials in the setting of allogeneic transplantation. Obstacles not only include randomization biases introduced because of the fixed perceptions of either physicians or patients but also the very real problem that the allograft arm may include a smaller proportion of patients with high-risk disease given the propensity of such patients to relapse before they reach transplantation. The only effective approach that allows these biases to be removed is the use of a 'donor versus no-donor' analysis, which exploits

Table 38.8 Indications for SCT.

| | Autologous SCT | Allogeneic SCT | |
		Sibling transplant	VUD transplant
AML first CR			
Good-risk cytogenetics	NR	NR	NR
Standard-risk cytogenetics	R	R	NR
Poor-risk cytogenetics	R	R	R
AML second CR	R	R	R
ALL (normal cytogenetics) first CR	D	R	NR
ALL t(9;22) first CR	R	R	R
ALL second CR	R	R	R
CML first CP	NR	R (after trial of imatinib)	R (after trial of imatinib)
MDS	NR	R	R
Myeloma	R	R	D
Hodgkin disease first CR	NR	NR	NR
Hodgkin disease relapsed	R	R	D
NHL DLBCL first CR	D	D	D
NHL DLBCL relapse	R	R	D
NHL follicular	D	R	D
Aplastic anaemia	NR	R	D
Haemoglobinopathies	NR	R	D

ALL, acute lymphoblastic leukaemia; AML, acute myeloid leukaemia; CML, chronic myeloid leukaemia; CR, complete remission; D, developmental; DLBCL, diffuse large B-cell lymphoma; MDS, myelodysplastic syndrome; NHL, non-Hodgkin lymphoma; NR, not recommended; R, recommended; VUD, volunteer unrelated donor.

the availability of an HLA-identical sibling donor as a form of biological randomization. However, such an approach is hard to apply in rarer diseases and difficult to apply to recipients of alternative donor transplants. Consequently, many of the recommendations concerning the role of allogeneic transplantation in specific diseases will continue to be based on registry data or institutional Phase II studies.

In order to provide a robust framework for SCT, the EBMT publishes a regularly updated summary of indications for transplantation (Table 38.8), allowing a consistent approach to be adopted. This categorizes specific diseases according to whether autologous or allogeneic SCT is accepted as standard therapy, is a promising treatment modality requiring further evaluation, or is not indicated.

Factors determining the choice of an allogeneic stem cell donor: the donor algorithm

An HLA-identical sibling donor can be identified in fewer than one-third of patients eligible for an allogeneic transplant. In older patients, where potential sibling matches may have medical conditions precluding stem cell donation, the likelihood of locating a suitable matched donor is significantly lower. Two potential donor options now exist for adults lacking a suitable sibling donor in the form of either an unrelated or cord blood donor.

Thanks to the rapid expansion of unrelated donor registries, approximately 12 million unrelated donors are now registered worldwide. As a result it is possible to identify a suitable donor in up to 70–80% of Caucasians, although this figure is much lower in other ethnic groups. Preferably the donor should be matched for HLA A, B, C; DRB1, and DQB 1 (10/10). Initial results with unrelated donor transplantation were associated with a high TRM and an increased incidence of severe GVHD. In the last decade there has been a marked improvement in outcome of unrelated donor SCT because of the availability of molecular typing at class I and II loci of the HLA complex. It is now clear that the presence of multiple disparities at class I or II loci are associated with a worse transplant outcome (see Chapter 37). As yet we lack sufficient information to allow us to identify whether specific allelic mismatches are of particular clinical significance. Although the recent growth in the size of unrelated donor registries internationally has increased the availability of volunteer unrelated donors, their unrepresentative ethnic composition limits the availability of donors for ethnic minorities. Consequently, the timely identification of a suitable alternative donor remains a challenge for a significant number of patients, particularly those with high-risk acute leukaemia who require urgent transplantation.

UCB has long been known to be a rich source of haemopoietic progenitors and recent results have demonstrated that high rates of durable engraftment can be achieved in adults, comparable to those achieved in children, providing the cell dose is optimized. Importantly, it appears that greater degrees of HLA mismatch can be tolerated using UCB than with a volunteer unrelated donor. As a result it is possible to transplant a cord blood unit mismatched at two or fewer HLA-A, -B or -DRB1 antigens as long as an adequate cell dose is available. This, coupled with the speed of procurement of UCB units, has resulted in the emergence of cord blood as an increasingly important alternative stem cell source in both adults and children. Although initial results using UCB in adults were compromised by delayed engraftment and a high rate of primary graft failure, these problems have largely been overcome by ensuring the use of a high total nucleated cell dose or two cord blood units. As a result UCB is increasingly recognized as an important stem cell source in adults with high-risk leukaemia lacking a suitable unrelated donor, providing strict matching and cell dose requirements are adhered to, although its precise role needs to be defined in prospective clinical trials.

Until recently, haploidentical transplants were associated with unacceptable rates of graft failure and GVHD because of the presence of HLA disparity at all major HLA antigens. However, the ability to maximize the stem cell dose, using G-CSF-mobilized progenitors, coupled with the development of efficient methods of TCD, has significantly improved outcome and it is now an important treatment option in children lacking an unrelated donor. In adults many allograft centres now prefer UCB as a stem cell source in adults without an unrelated donor but a number of European centres now also report encouraging results in adults using haploidentical donors.

Management of disease relapse

Disease relapse remains a major cause of treatment failure after allogeneic transplantation and is caused by either resistance of tumour cells to the conditioning regimen or failure of the donor immune system to eradicate residual malignant haemopoiesis. Possible mechanisms for tumour cells evading a GVL effect include downregulation of HLA class I or II expression or absence of costimulatory molecules on leukaemic blasts or location of residual cells in privileged sites such as the CNS or testes. While it is possible to reduce the risk of disease relapse after a myeloablative allograft by increasing the intensity of the preparative regimen, this approach does not translate into improved overall survival because of the increased TRM associated with a more intense conditioning regimen. Consequently, optimization of the GVL effect represents the only mechanism by which

the antileukaemic activity of a myeloablative allograft can be augmented. In routine clinical practice the options for manipulating a GVL effect are limited and are restricted to modifying the intensity of post-transplant immunosuppression, for example through the institution of a rapid ciclosporin taper in patients at a high risk of disease relapse. While the prophylactic use of DLI in patients deemed at high risk of relapse is an attractive option, such an approach is difficult to effect in practice because many patients will relapse early while still on immunosuppression and before DLI can be administered. In those patients in whom a course of prophylactic DLI can be commenced before disease relapse, the risk of severe GVHD associated with its use in the first 12 months after transplantation represents a significant problem.

In patients transplanted using an RIC regimen, there is limited room for increasing the intensity of the conditioning regimen without increasing transplant toxicity. Maximizing a GVL effect can be achieved by limiting post-transplant immunosuppression. There remains considerable debate as to whether the presence of mixed T-cell chimerism after an RIC allograft is associated with an increased risk of disease relapse. On the basis that it is an indicator of bidirectional tolerance and therefore permissive for disease relapse, a number of units administer prophylactic DLI in patients who have been transplanted using an RIC regimen in whom mixed T-cell chimerism persists after the withdrawal of post-transplant immunosuppression. Definitive data concerning the effectiveness of this approach in improving outcome are not yet available.

The management of patients who relapse after allogeneic transplantation is complex and in many patients should probably be palliative. This particularly applies to patients transplanted for acute leukaemia who relapse within the first 12–18 months post transplant or patients with a history of severe acute or chronic extensive GVHD. However, there is now a significant population of patients in whom DLI or a second transplant should be considered. Two factors determine the use of DLI in clinical practice. Firstly, the ability of DLI to deliver durable remissions is highly dependent on the underlying haematological malignancy. Thus up to 80% of patients who have relapsed after an allograft for CML will achieve a durable molecular remission with DLI in contrast to patients transplanted for acute leukaemia or myeloma where response rates are much lower. Prior cytoreduction appears to increase the likelihood of patients with relapsed acute leukaemia achieving a durable response to DLI. The major complications of DLI are myelosuppression and GVHD. Myelosuppression is most commonly observed in patients with overt haematological relapse and may require treatment with G-CSF and occasionally transfusion of donor CD34-positive selected PBSCs. In early studies DLI was administered as a single bulk infusion and was associated with a significant risk of severe GVHD. However, the recognition that use of an escalating schedule of administration substantially reduces the risk of severe GVHD without compromising its efficacy has markedly reduced the toxicity of DLI. The explanation why early DLI is associated with such a high risk of severe GVHD is unclear but may relate to more rapid expansion of donor alloreactive T cells in the profoundly lymphopenic environment present in the first few months after transplantation. An alternative approach in patients who relapse late and in whom there was no evidence of either acute or chronic GVHD is a second allograft using an RIC regimen. Although associated with an increased TRM, a number of studies now show a significant chance of long-term disease-free survival after a second allograft in a significant proportion of such patients.

Relapse after autologous SCT is caused by either resistance of the underlying haematological malignancy to the myeloablative conditioning regimen or infusion of contaminating tumour cells at the time of transplantation. Patients with myeloma in whom the duration of response to the first transplant was greater than 18 months may benefit from a second autograft, although whether this is superior to the outcome of treatment with one of the newer agents such as bortezomib or lenalidomide is unknown. Allogeneic transplantation using an RIC regimen is an important treatment option in patients with Hodgkin disease or non-Hodgkin lymphoma who have relapsed after an autologous transplant.

Future developments in stem cell transplantation

Autologous SCT

Relapse remains the commonest cause of treatment failure in patients after autografting. It is likely that the most important cause of disease recurrence after an autologous transplant is caused by tumour chemoresistance or radioresistance. Most of the drugs contained in preparative regimens are already administered at close to the limit of extramedullary toxicity and there is therefore little room for further dose escalation. Consequently, efforts to reduce relapse rate will depend on either altering the mode of delivery of currently used agents or the development of new forms of chemotherapy or radiotherapy. The recent advent of an intravenous preparation of busulfan is an example of how improved drug delivery can improve the pharmacokinetic profile of an antitumour agent, thereby reducing toxicity and increasing activity. Many haematological malignancies are highly radiosensitive and there is interest in the possibility of increasing the effective dose of irradiation delivered to the marrow without increasing organ toxicity using radiolabelled immunoconjugates. Early-phase clinical studies using α (^{131}I) or β (^{90}Y) emitters conjugated to haematopoietic antigens, such as CD45 or CD66, demonstrate that such an approach is feasible and Phase II studies in myeloma and lymphoma are ongoing. Alternatively, drugs that disrupt tumour cell binding to the bone marrow microenvironment, such as the CXCR4 antago-

nist plerixafor, may overcome cytoadhesion-mediated drug resistance and increase the activity of drugs such as melphalan. Although contamination of PBSC grafts by malignant cells can undoubtedly contribute to disease relapse after an autologous transplant, there is no evidence that purging of stem cell collections reduces relapse risk.

Allogeneic SCT

The major advances in allogeneic transplantation in the past decade have been the introduction of RIC regimens and the increased availability of alternative donors. As a result allogeneic transplantation is increasingly employed as a treatment option in patients with haematological malignancies. However, the challenges of allografting remain substantially unchanged: GVHD, infection and disease relapse. Since all three, to a greater or lesser extent, are consequent on a failure to regulate or harness the donor immune response appropriately, advances in their management are rarely made alone but are interlinked.

The development of novel strategies to prevent GVHD are dependent on whether they are to be employed in the context of TCD or not. In patients transplanted using a T-replete stem cell inoculum, drugs such as mycophenolate mofetil and sirolimus are being actively considered as alternatives for GVHD prophylaxis. In the setting of TCD, where the risk of GVHD is low, the emphasis is on minimizing the impairment in immune reconstitution and increased infectious complications caused by depletion of donor T cells. One promising approach by which this might be achieved is through the use of 'add backs' of antigen-specific T cells recognizing common post-transplant viral pathogens such as CMV, EBV or adenovirus. Such cells can be generated either by coculturing donor lymphocytes with APCs primed with candidate antigens followed by expansion or by early selection on the basis of interferon-γ secretion (a technique termed 'IFN-γ capture'). Alternatively, antigen-specific cells might be selected directly from peripheral blood using immunomagnetic techniques based on labelling of antigen-specific cells using HLA class I–peptide multimers. In situations where a donor has no relevant immunity (e.g. where a CMV-seropositive patient is transplanted from a seronegative donor), gene transfer of a TCR specific for the relevant viral antigen is under investigation. In order to improve coverage against multiple pathogens, infusion of donor lymphocytes from which alloreactive T cells have been depleted may hasten immune reconstitution without incurring the risk of GVHD normally associated with DLI. Such an 'allodepletion' strategy can be achieved by either directly removing donor CD8 cells from the infusion, given that CD8 cells are postulated to be the major effectors of GVHD, or alloreactive T cells can be depleted from the graft by incubating cells *ex vivo* with recipient APCs. Activated T cells capable of mediating

GVHD can be identified by their expression of CD25 or other activation markers and removed using magnetic selection techniques or an immunotoxin. Preclinical models have suggested that transfer of memory phenotype T cells may also permit more rapid immune recovery without inducing GVHD, although whether such cells are truly representative of human memory T cells remains to be determined. There is also substantial interest in the feasibility of transferring naturally occurring or *ex vivo* expanded CD4$^+$FoxP3$^+$ or IL-10-producing regulatory T cells as a means of preventing conventional T cells from inducing GVHD. The best approach for isolating and expanding these regulatory populations remains unknown, but the results from ongoing trials are keenly awaited.

From first principles, reducing the risk of relapse can be achieved by increasing the intensity of the conditioning regimen (ideally without increasing transplant toxicity), administering antileukaemic therapies in the post-transplant period or by optimizing the GVL effect. Incorporating radioimmunotherapy (e.g. with antibodies directed at antigens specific for haemopoietic cells or malignant cells) into the preparative regimen shows promise in the setting of allogeneic as well as autologous SCT and may prove of value in patients with advanced leukaemia, where relapse is the most important cause of treatment failure. Alternatively, patients judged to be at high risk of relapse may benefit from administration of adjunctive therapies after transplantation (e.g. tyrosine kinase inhibitors or demethylating agents), reducing the residual disease burden while a GVL response is established. Prophylactic DLI might be administered in high-risk patients following TCD transplantations with the aim of boosting a GVL response. Given the high rate of GVHD associated with this approach, particularly if an unrelated donor has been used, there has been interest in the use of CD8 depletion or allodepleted DLI. Alternatively, the use of donor T cells that have been expanded selectively to recognize tumour-associated antigens or lineage-restricted minor H antigens (e.g. by expanding donor cells in the presence of peptide mixes) may prove effective. Early clinical studies examining the use of lymphocytes generated against minor H antigens or leukaemia-specific antigens such as WT1 and proteinase 3 are currently ongoing. Gene transfer of TCRs specific for such antigens is also of promise. If successful such an approach, coupled with a TCD transplant, may offer the prospect of disassociating GVHD from GVL.

Selected bibliography

Appelbaum FR (2000) Is there a best transplant conditioning regimen for acute myeloid leukemia? *Leukemia* **14**: 497–501.

Appelbaum FR (2007) Hematopoietic-cell transplantation at 50. *New England Journal of Medicine* **357**: 1472–5.

Boeckh M, Ljungman P (2009) How we treat cytomegalovirus in hematopoietic cell transplant recipients. *Blood* **113**: 5711–19.

Deeg HJ (2007) How I treat refractory acute GVHD. *Blood* **109**: 4119–26.

Ferrara JL, Levine JE, Reddy P, Holler E (2009) Graft-versus-host disease. *Lancet* **373**: 1550–61.

Finke J, Bethge WA, Schmoor C *et al.* (2009) Standard graft-versus-host disease prophylaxis with or without anti-T-cell globulin in haematopoietic cell transplantation from matched unrelated donors: a randomised, open-label, multicentre phase 3 trial. *Lancet Oncology* **10**: 855–64.

Gluckman E, Rocha V (2009) Cord blood transplantation: state of the art. *Haematologica* **94**: 451–4.

Gratwohl A, Hermans J, Goldman JM *et al.* (1998) Risk assessment for patients with chronic myeloid leukaemia before allogeneic blood or marrow transplantation. Chronic Leukemia Working Party of the European Group for Blood and Marrow Transplantation. *Lancet* **352**: 1087–92.

Gratwohl A, Baldomero H, Schwendener A *et al.* (2009) The EBMT activity survey 2007 with focus on allogeneic HSCT for AML and novel cellular therapies. *Bone Marrow Transplantation* **43**: 275–91.

Hegenbart U, Niederwieser D, Forman S *et al.* (2003) Hematopoietic cell transplantation from related and unrelated donors after minimal conditioning as a curative treatment modality for severe paroxysmal nocturnal hemoglobinuria. *Biology of Blood and Marrow Transplantation* **9**: 689–97.

Ljungman P, Bregni M, Brune M *et al.* (2010) Allogeneic and autologous transplantation for haematological diseases, solid tumours and immune disorders: current practice in Europe 2009. *Bone Marrow Transplantation* **45**: 219–34.

Petersdorf EW (2008) Optimal HLA matching in hematopoietic cell transplantation. *Current Opinion in Immunology* **20**: 588–93.

Schmitz N, Linch DC, Dreger P *et al.* (1996) Randomised trial of filgrastim-mobilised peripheral blood progenitor cell transplantation versus autologous bone-marrow transplantation in lymphoma patients. *Lancet* **347**: 353–7.

Schmitz N, Beksac M, Bacigalupo A *et al.* (2005) Filgrastim-mobilized peripheral blood progenitor cells versus bone marrow transplantation for treating leukemia: 3-year results from the EBMT randomized trial. *Haematologica* **90**: 643–8.

Sierra J, Storer B, Hansen JA *et al.* (1997) Transplantation of marrow cells from unrelated donors for treatment of high-risk acute leukemia: the effect of leukemic burden, donor HLA-matching, and marrow cell dose. *Blood* **89**: 4226–35.

Socie G, Salooja N, Cohen A *et al.* (2003) Nonmalignant late effects after allogeneic stem cell transplantation. *Blood* **101**: 3373–85.

Sorror ML, Maris MB, Storb R *et al.* (2005) Hematopoietic cell transplantation (HCT)-specific comorbidity index: a new tool for risk assessment before allogeneic HCT. *Blood* **106**: 2912–19.

Urbano-Ispizua A, Schmitz N, de Witte T *et al.* (2002) Allogeneic and autologous transplantation for haematological diseases, solid tumours and immune disorders: definitions and current practice in Europe. *Bone Marrow Transplantation* **29**: 639–46.

CHAPTER 39

Normal haemostasis

39

Keith Gomez[1], Edward GD Tuddenham[1] and John H McVey[2]

[1]Haemophilia Centre and Thrombosis Unit, Royal Free and University College London Medical School, London, UK
[2]Molecular Medicine Thrombosis Research Institute, London, UK

Introduction

Haemostasis is one of a number of protective processes that have evolved in order to maintain a stable physiology. It has many features in common with (and to some extent interacts with) other defence mechanisms in the body, such as the immune system and the inflammatory response. These links are most clearly seen in ancient species such as the horseshoe crab (*Limulus polyphemus*), where a primitive 'coagulation' pathway is initiated by entry of endotoxin into the haemolymph. Vestiges of this process still exist in humans and may give rise to serious clinical consequences. For example, disseminated intravascular coagulation (DIC) can be initiated by Gram-negative septicaemia. However, consequent upon the development of a high-pressure blood circulatory system, extra components have evolved and have resulted in a complex, highly integrated process in all vertebrates (Figure 39.1). Indeed, analysis of the haemostatic network in bony fish suggests that the network in its entirety evolved over 430 million years ago, prior to the divergence of bony fish from tetrapods.

The high blood pressure generated on the arterial side of the vertebrate circulation requires a powerful, almost instantaneous but strictly localized procoagulant response in order to minimize blood loss from sites of vascular injury without compromising blood flow generally. Systemic anticoagulant and clot-dissolving components have also evolved to prevent extension of the procoagulant response beyond the vicinity of vascular injury resulting in unwanted thrombus formation in the slow, sometimes intermittent, blood flow in the veins. The resultant haemostatic system is thus a complex mosaic of activating or inhibitory feedback or feed-forward pathways that integrates its five major components (blood vessels, blood platelets, coagulation factors, coagulation inhibitors and fibrinolytic elements). Furthermore, links between haemostasis and other elements of the body's overall defence response, such as the complement and kinin-generating processes and inflammation, must also be considered.

This chapter reviews current concepts of haemostasis in humans and is aimed at providing a background for the understanding of the haemostatic disorders described in succeeding chapters. Attempting to understand these complex events is a considerable task, even to the expert; for the relative newcomer to the subject, it may first be useful to present an overview of events that follow damage to a blood vessel and which lead to effective haemostasis and subsequent restoration of vessel patency. Following this introduction, each of five main areas will be examined in relative isolation, while at the same time acknowledging points of interaction and overlap.

Postgraduate Haematology: 6th edition. Edited by A. Victor Hoffbrand,
Daniel Catovsky, Edward G.D. Tuddenham, Anthony R. Green
© 2011 Blackwell Publishing Ltd.

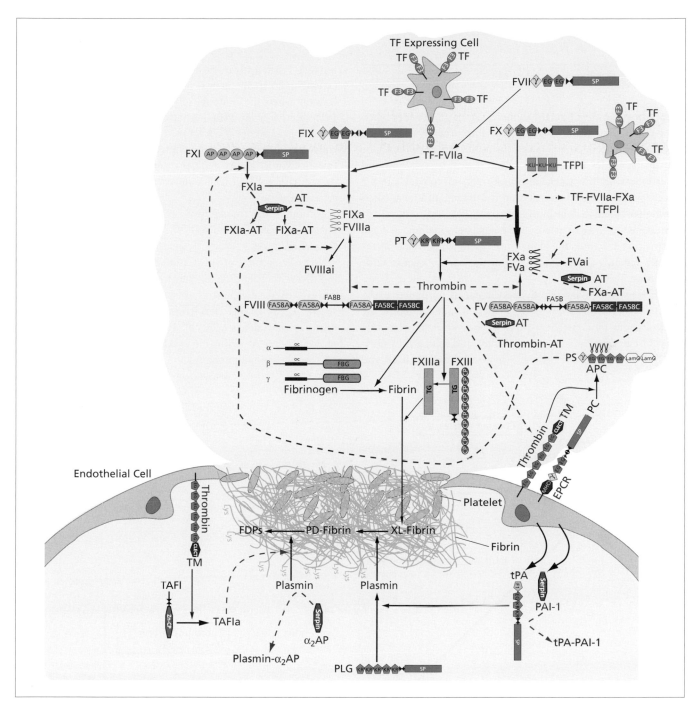

Figure 39.1 The haemostasis network. The network includes elements of coagulation initiation via TF–FVIIa interaction, amplification via the tenase (FVIIIa–FIXa) and prothrombinase (FVa–FXa) complexes, feedback inhibition through specific inhibitors, and clot dissolution by fibrinolysis. Module organization of proteins is indicated (see Figure 39.8) and all abbreviations are given in the text. Protein names are coloured as follows: functionally active proteins, red; inactivated or inhibited proteins, blue; precursors and fibrinogen-derived components, black. Lines and arrows are coloured as follows: dashed red lines, positive procoagulant feedback loops; dashed blue lines, negative feedback and inhibitory loops; solid black lines, interactions or processes. Cream boxes indicate assembly of macromolecular complexes on a cellular phospholipid surface. The process of blood coagulation is initiated by the exposure of cells expressing TF to flowing blood. Thrombin generation is propagated by a series of positive feedback loops, leading to fibrin deposition. This process is controlled by a series of negative feedback steps: the initiation complex is inhibited by the formation of the quaternary complex TF–FVIIa–FXa–TFPI and the active proteases FIXa, FXa and thrombin are inactivated by the serpin AT. In addition, thrombin initiates a negative feedback pathway by activating PC, leading to the inhibition of FVa and FVIIIa. The generation of fibrin leads to activation of the fibrinolytic pathway through binding of tPA, which leads to plasminogen activation and fibrin degradation. This pathway is also subject to inhibition through the binding of the serpins PAI-1 and α_2-antiplasmin (α_2AP) to tPA and plasmin respectively. All these processes, plus platelet activation, occur simultaneously or with short lag times. (From McVey JH, Tuddenham EGD (2007) Genomics of haemostasis. In: *Genomics and Clinical Medicine* (D Kumar, ed.). Oxford University Press, Oxford with permission.)

Overview of haemostasis

In the most simplistic terms, blood coagulation occurs when the enzyme thrombin is generated and proteolyses soluble plasma fibrinogen, forming the insoluble fibrin polymer, or clot; this provides the physical consolidation of vessel wound repair following injury. 'Haemostasis' refers more widely to the process whereby blood coagulation is initiated and terminated in a tightly regulated fashion, together with the removal (or fibrinolysis) of the clot as part of vascular remodelling; as such, haemostasis describes the global process by which vessel integrity and patency are maintained over the whole organism, for its lifetime.

Although it is pedagogically convenient to present the subsystems of haemostasis as if they operate independently, the whole haemostatic mechanism is integrated *in vivo* so that thrombin generation is localized, limited and followed by fibrinolysis and tissue remodelling, which are also localized and limited. Furthermore, thrombin generation is not a simple exponential cascade as was originally envisaged by Davie and Ratnoff when the 'waterfall' hypothesis was described in the 1950s. Rather, it is a complex network of interactions with positive and negative feedback loops. Thus the effects of varying the concentration of any component in such a system are not intuitively obvious. Figure 39.2 presents a version of the earlier cascade concept for intrinsic and extrinsic pathways of thrombin generation.

Although a tremendous improvement over previous ideas, obvious deficiencies of such a scheme include the following.
• No explanation for the variation in clinical phenotype resulting from deficiencies of the components of the intrinsic pathway. While deficiencies of factor (F)VIII and FIX can cause severe bleeding, FXI deficiency is generally a much milder disorder and deficiencies of FXII, prekallikrein and high-molecular-weight kininogen (HMWK) are not associated with any clearly defined phenotype.

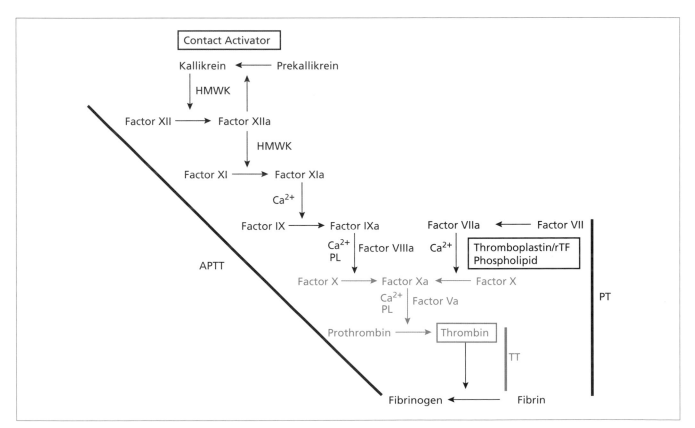

Figure 39.2 The coagulation cascade. The traditional concept of blood coagulation with separate intrinsic (red) and extrinsic (blue) pathways converging on the common pathway (green) with the generation of FXa. The activated partial thromboplastin time (APTT) is initiated by the addition of a contact activator (e.g. kaolin or silica) and tests for deficiencies in the intrinsic pathway. The prothrombin time (PT) is initiated by addition of thromboplastin and phospholipids and tests for deficiencies in the intrinsic pathway. The thrombin time (TT) is initiated by addition of thrombin and tests for an inhibitor of thrombin (most commonly heparin) or a problem with fibrin cleavage. HMWK, high-molecular-weight kininogen; PL, phospholipid.

• No explanation for the variation in the rate of thrombin generation observed experimentally.

• Implies that clot formation can occur as a result of two independent pathways. In fact it is clear that the interaction between FVII and tissue factor (TF) is the initiator of all coagulation processes, both in normal haemostasis and pathological situations such as thrombosis.

• No recognition of the complex role of platelets in clot formation (see Chapter 40).

Despite these faults the waterfall hypothesis remains a valuable tool for understanding the common coagulations tests that are used in clinical practice today.

Tissue factor initiates blood coagulation

A major development over the past 10 years has been the realization that exposure of blood to cells expressing TF on their surface is both necessary and sufficient to initiate blood coagulation *in vivo*. The contact system (intrinsic pathway; see Figure 39.2) therefore does not appear to have a physiological role in haemostasis. Table 39.1 presents some other putative roles for the contact factors in body defence. TF is constitutively expressed at biological boundaries such as skin, organ surfaces, vascular adventitia and epithelial–mesenchymal surfaces, where it functions as a 'haemostatic envelope'. This ensures that following disruption of vascular integrity blood is immediately exposed to cells expressing TF, leading to the initiation of blood coagulation. The primary control of haemostasis is therefore the anatomical segregation of cells expressing functional TF from other components of the coagulation network present in blood.

Table 39.1 Role of contact factors in integrating body defence mechanisms.

Pathway involved	Function	Comment
Coagulation	Prevention of blood loss	Not essential for normal haemostasis
Fibrinolysis	Maintenance of vessel patency	May be important
Complement	Contribution to immune response	Not essential
Kinin generation	Pain, capillary permeability, cardiovascular effects	May be important *in vivo*
Renin–angiotensin system	Blood pressure control	No demonstrated role *in vivo*
Chemotaxis	Phagocytosis, bactericidal activity	May be important *in vivo*

Amplification of the initial stimulus

An updated concept of TF-initiated thrombin generation, including the important feedback reactions of thrombin, is shown in Figure 39.3. As stated above, it is now clear from various *in vitro* and *in vivo* experiments that the physiological initiator of blood coagulation is exposure of the circulating zymogen FVII to membrane-bound TF. Activation of FVII to the protease FVIIa and formation of a very high affinity complex of TF with FVIIa results in the activation of FIX and FX by the TF–FVIIa complex. In the absence of its activated cofactor FVa, FXa generates only trace amounts of thrombin from prothrombin. Although insufficient to initiate significant fibrin polymerization, thrombin formed in this initiation stage of coagulation is able to back-activate FV, FVIII and FXI by limited proteolysis. In the amplification phase of coagulation, FXIa activates FIXa which forms a complex with FVIIIa. This is the tenase complex (FVIIIa–FIXa) that activates sufficient FXa to form a complex with FVa, the prothrombinase complex (FVa–FXa). This results in the explosive generation of thrombin that ultimately leads to generation of a fibrin clot.

A key feature of these processes is the assembly of multimolecular complexes on a phospholipid surface provided *in vivo* by cell membranes. For procoagulant complexes such as tenase and prothrombinase, this surface is provided by activated platelets. Each of these complexes consist of a cofactor (TF, FVa, FVIIIa), an enzyme (FVIIa, FIXa, FXa) and a substrate that is a zymogen (FIX, FX and prothrombin) of a serine protease. The product of one reaction becomes the enzyme in the next complex. The cofactors FV and FVIII are themselves activated by limited proteolytic digestion.

Feedback inhibition of the procoagulant response

The process of amplification occurs independently of the TF–FVIIa complex, which is rapidly inactivated by tissue factor pathway inhibitor (TFPI), released from thrombin-activated platelets or found on the surface of endothelial cells, by the formation of a quaternary inhibited complex (Figure 39.4). This explains the requirement for further activation of FX via FIXa–FVIIIa, and back-activation of FXI by thrombin, to permit further activation of FIX. Figure 39.4 also indicates the role of one of the other important inhibitors of the network, antithrombin (AT), which damps down thrombin generation by forming inactive complexes with FIX, FX, FXI and thrombin. The rate of inhibition by AT is substantially increased by binding a variety of polysulphated mucopolysaccharides known as glycosaminoglycans (GAGs) on the surface of endothelial cells.

Thrombin also proteolytically activates an anticoagulant pathway, the protein C (PC) pathway (Figure 39.4). Thrombomodulin (TM), an endothelial cell surface receptor,

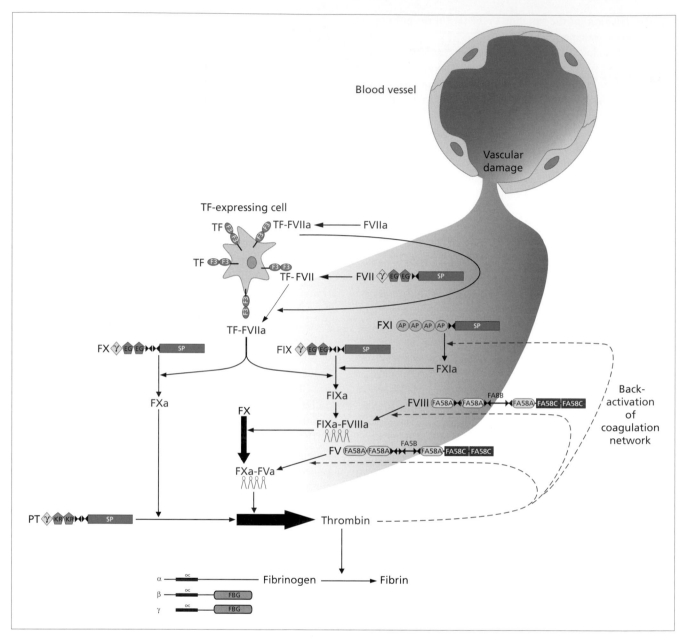

Figure 39.3 The haemostasis network: fibrin generation. Following vascular damage blood coagulation is initiated by exposure of FVII to cells expressing the integral membrane protein TF. Activation of FVII to the protease FVIIa results in the activation of FIX and FX by the TF–FVIIa complex. In the absence of its activated cofactor FVa, FXa generates only trace amounts of thrombin. Although insufficient to initiate significant fibrin polymerization, trace amounts of thrombin formed in this initiation stage of coagulation are able to back-activate FV and FVIII by limited proteolysis. In the amplification phase of coagulation, FVIIIa forms a complex with FIXa, activating sufficient FXa that (in complex with FVa) leads to the explosive generation of thrombin, ultimately leading to generation of a fibrin clot. The tenase (FVIIIa–FIXa) and prothrombinase (FVa–FXa) complexes assemble on phospholipid surfaces. Colours and symbols as in Figure 39.1.

plays a pivotal role in the activation of this anticoagulant pathway. TM binds thrombin and, by an allosteric mechanism, alters its substrate specificity. The procoagulant substrates of thrombin, including FV, FVIII and fibrinogen, are no longer efficiently proteolysed. The preferred substrate of the thrombin–TM complex is PC, a zymogen that is proteolysed to activated PC (APC). The activation of PC can be augmented by another cellular receptor, endothelial cell protein C receptor (EPCR),

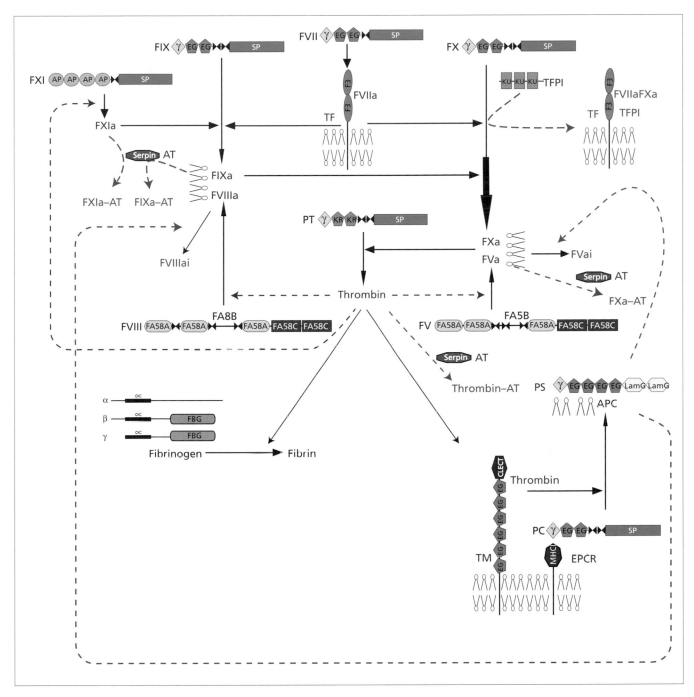

Figure 39.4 The haemostasis network: inhibition of thrombin generation. The initiation of blood coagulation via generation of FIXa and FXa by TF–FVIIa is shut down by the action of TFPI, which forms a quaternary complex with TF–FVIIa–FXa. Further generation of FIXa occurs following back-activation of FXI by thrombin. The serine proteases FIXa, FXa, FXI and thrombin are all inhibited by AT. At the endothelial cell surface thrombin bound to TM activates PC bound to its receptor EPCR. APC in complex with its cofactor PS inactivates FVa and FVIIIa by further proteolytic cleavages Colours and symbols as in Figure 39.1.

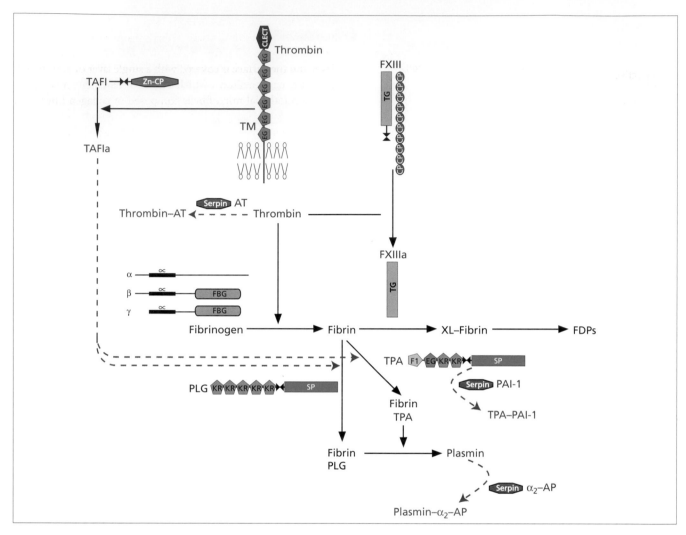

Figure 39.5 The haemostasis network: fibrinolysis. Both PLG and tPA bind to polymerized fibrin, promoting the cleavage of PLG by tPA to active plasmin, which then degrades cross-linked fibrin to soluble FDPs. Modulation of fibrinolysis is achieved by serpin inhibition: PAI-1 inactivates tPA, while α_2-antiplasmin (α_2AP) inhibits plasmin. In addition, TAFIa removes Lys residues from fibrin, removing PLG and tPA binding sites. Colours and symbols as in Figure 39.1.

which provides a direct endothelial cell binding site for PC and thus increases the apparent affinity of the thrombin–TM complex for PC; however, not all endothelial cells coexpress TM and EPCR. In complex with its cofactor, protein S (PS), APC rapidly inactivates the procoagulant cofactors FVa and FVIIIa by specific proteolysis, forming a negative feedback loop. The PC pathway is most active in the microvasculature, where the relative concentration of EPCR is highest.

Fibrinolysis

The final step in the regulation of fibrin deposition is the prevention and/or rapid removal of insoluble fibrin by the fibrinolytic system (Figure 39.5) described more fully later in the chapter. Briefly, once sufficient fibrin is generated it binds tissue plasminogen activator (tPA), leading to the increased activation of plasminogen (PLG). This results in the formation of plasmin at the site of the fibrin clot, which breaks down fibrin into soluble fibrin degradation products. The fibrinolytic system is also subject to inhibition through the action of inhibitors of tPA and plasmin, namely plasminogen activator inhibitor (PAI)-1 and α_2-antiplasmin respectively.

Blood vessels

Blood vessel structure

The basic structure of blood vessels comprises three layers (Figure 39.6a): the intima, the media and the adventitia. It is

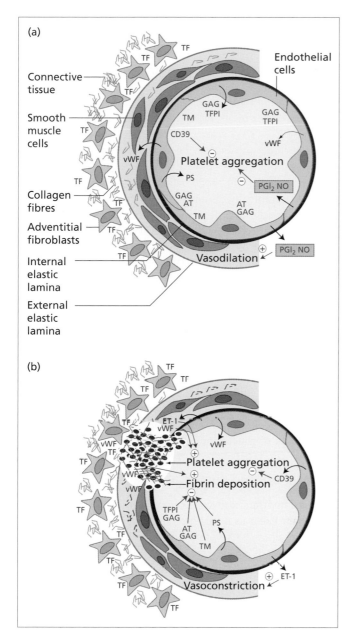

Figure 39.6 Blood vessel architecture and functions in haemostasis. (a) The anatomy of a generic vessel in the resting state. The layer thicknesses vary widely between arterial and venous circulation and between large and small vessels. In the absence of vessel damage, cells expressing TF are anatomically separated from components of the blood coagulation network, preventing initiation of coagulation. In addition, coagulation inhibitors present on the endothelial surface and inhibitors of platelet aggregation maintain vessel patency. (b) The localized haemostatic response to vessel injury: initiation of coagulation by TF exposure and platelet activation/aggregation by exposure of extravascular collagen to plasma VWF. Procoagulant responses away from lesion site are damped down by anticoagulant and antiplatelet factors derived from endothelium.

the components of these layers and the size of these layers themselves that differentiate arteries from veins, and indeed arteries or veins of different sizes. The intima is the innermost layer and the surface is covered with a single layer of endothelial cells (the endothelium), which rest on a basement membrane of subendothelial microfibrils composed of collagen fibres and some elastin. The media or middle layer contains mainly circularly arranged smooth muscle cells and collagen fibres, and is divided from the outer adventitia by the external elastic lamina. Contraction and relaxation of smooth muscle cells regulates intravascular pressure and the rate of blood flow. The elastin allows vessels to stretch and recoil, maintaining vascular tone. The adventitia or outermost layer is composed of collagen fibres and fibroblasts that protect the blood vessel and anchor it to surrounding structures.

The endothelium

The endothelium functions in a multitude of physiological processes including intracellular transport, the regulation of vasomotor tone and maintenance of blood flow. Endothelial cells possess surface receptors for a variety of physiological substances, for example thrombin and angiotensin II, which may influence vascular tone directly or indirectly through various haemostasis-related events. Once activated, endothelial cells express at their surface, and in some cases release into the plasma, a variety of intracellular adhesion molecules, for example vascular cell adhesion molecule (VCAM), E-selectin, P-selectin and von Willebrand factor (VWF), which modulate leucocyte and platelet adhesion, inflammation, phagocytosis and vascular permeability.

However, the endothelium should not be regarded as a simple homogeneous cell type. It would appear that endothelial cell phenotypes are differentially regulated. At any given point in time, structural and functional phenotypes may vary between segments of the vascular tree, and at any given location the endothelial phenotypes may change from one moment to the next. Endothelial cell heterogeneity occurs between different organs, within the vasculature of a given organ, and even between neighbouring endothelial cells of a single vessel.

The platelet–vessel wall interaction

Healthy unperturbed endothelial cells exert a powerful inhibitory influence on haemostasis by virtue of the factors they release or express on their surface (see Figure 39.6a). Two of these, prostaglandin (PG)I$_2$ (or prostacyclin) and nitric oxide (NO), also known as endothelium-derived relaxing factor, have powerful vasodilator activity, acting on smooth muscle cells in the vessel wall (basal-directed secretion) and hence modulating blood flow. Both substances inhibit aggregation of platelets and leucocytes (luminal-directed secretion) by raising intraplatelet levels of cyclic adenosine monophosphate (cAMP) and cyclic guanosine monophosphate (cGMP) respectively (see below).

PGI_2 is the major prostaglandin synthesized by endothelial cells, a small amount also being produced by fibroblasts and smooth muscle cells. Its action on platelets involves binding to a specific G protein-coupled receptor (PTGIR) that activates adenylate cyclase, thus increasing the intraplatelet cAMP concentration. This promotes Ca^{2+} uptake into the dense tubular system and inhibits phosphatidylinositol metabolism, both of which prevent platelet aggregation and the consequent release of storage granules containing procoagulant molecules such as VWF and FV. The precursor of PGI_2 is arachidonic acid, derived from endothelial cell membrane phospholipids by phospholipases. Arachidonic acid is first converted to PGG_2 and PGH_2, the so-called cyclic endoperoxides, by cyclooxygenase, and then to PGI_2 by prostacyclin synthetase. Thrombin, and other agents (see above) that are generated at the site of injury, stimulate the synthesis of PGI_2 by adjacent endothelial cells, which counteracts the platelet-aggregating activity of the protease and thereby helps to localize platelet plug formation. Elevation of intravascular pressure and trauma, including venepuncture, also increase PGI_2 production and may be a source of artefactually high plasma levels. PGI_2 is rather unstable, with a half-life of only a few minutes in whole blood, and degrades spontaneously to 6-keto-$PGF_{1\alpha}$. This degradation product is biologically inert, but in some tissues a variable proportion of PGI_2 may be enzymatically converted to 6-keto-$PGF_{1\alpha}$ or $6,15$-diketo-$13,14$-dihydro-$PGF_{1\alpha}$, which retain some platelet-inhibitory activity.

The once-held belief that PGI_2 is a circulating hormone that limits platelet–platelet interactions within the bloodstream is probably false, as plasma levels of PGI_2 are at least two orders of magnitude below that needed to inhibit platelet aggregation. Although in some settings, such as following severe trauma, it is possible that markedly raised systemic levels could occur transiently, it is more likely that PGI_2 serves mainly as a local hormone, principally concerned with vascular tone, but possibly also inhibiting the extension of the platelet plug beyond the immediate vicinity of any endothelial damage.

NO is synthesized in smooth muscle cells, macrophages and activated platelets, as well as by endothelial cells. Its synthesis and secretion may be constitutive (when it serves as a local hormone to 'fine tune' blood flow). Stimulated (inducible) synthesis of NO also occurs in endothelial cells exposed to cytokines such as interleukin (IL)-1, tumour necrosis factor (TNF) or endotoxin. This produces a slower but longer-lasting rise in NO and can have undesirable side-effects such as inflammation, cytotoxicity or prolonged hypotension. Like PGI_2, it has a very short half-life (3–5 s) and is rapidly oxidized to the inactive nitrite (NO_2^-) or nitrate (NO_3^-) forms.

In addition to PGI_2 and NO, endothelial cells also express an ecto-ADPase (CD39) on their cell surface, which rapidly metabolizes ATP and ADP released from activated platelets to AMP, thereby drastically reducing or abolishing platelet recruitment and aggregation in response to thrombin.

The 21-amino-acid peptide endothelin (ET)-1 is the predominant isoform of the endothelin peptide family, which includes ET-2, ET-3 and ET-4. It exerts various biological effects, including vasoconstriction and the stimulation of cell proliferation in tissues both within and outside the cardiovascular system. In the endothelium, ET-1 is predominantly released abluminally towards the vascular smooth muscle, where it acts as a potent vasoconstrictor and mitogen for smooth muscle cells. In addition, ET-1 stimulates the production of cytokines and growth factors. Furthermore, it stimulates neutrophil adhesion and platelet aggregation and is chemotactic for macrophages.

Thrombospondin (TSP)-1 is an abundant constituent of the α-granules of platelets and Weibel–Palade bodies of endothelial cells. TSP-1 was first identified as a thrombin-sensitive protein that was released in response to activation of platelets by thrombin. Upon release from platelets, TSP-1 binds to the platelet surface in a Ca^{2+}-dependent manner and interacts with integrins $\alpha_{IIb}\beta_3$ and $\alpha_v\beta_3$, CD36 and the integrin-associated protein (IAP), integrin-bound fibrinogen and fibronectin. TSP-1 activates $\alpha_{IIb}\beta_3$ through its binding to IAP. This results in spreading of platelets and aggregation.

von Willebrand factor

VWF is a multimeric glycoprotein that plays an important role in primary haemostasis by promoting platelet adhesion to the subendothelium at sites of vascular injury under high shear-rate conditions. It is also a carrier of FVIII and this association protects FVIII from rapid proteolysis. Failure of FVIII to bind VWF, as occurs in type 2N von Willebrand disease (see Chapter 41), leads to its rapid turnover and resulting FVIII deficiency. VWF is synthesized by endothelial cells, megakaryocytes and platelets. In endothelial cells VWF may be secreted directly into the circulation or stored in Weibel–Palade bodies. The VWF produced in megakaryocytes and platelets is not secreted but stored in α-granules. Release of VWF from these stores occurs following activation of endothelial cells or platelets. Some therapeutic products, such as desmopressin, may work by stimulating release of stored VWF.

Mature VWF is composed of disulphide-linked subunits, each comprising 2050 amino acid residues and up to 22 carbohydrate side-chains. Each subunit has a molecular mass of approximately 278 kDa, of which 10–19% is carbohydrate. Two subunits joined at their C-termini by a disulphide bridge form a dimer. Additional disulphide bridges between dimers lead to the formation of larger multimers that range in size from

500 kDa to in excess of 10 000 kDa (Figure 39.7). The ultra-large VWF multimers are predominantly stored but when secreted by endothelial cells may appear as globular molecules or as thin filaments that are several microns long. These ultra-large VWF multimers can only be detected transiently in normal plasma because they are cleaved by a plasma metalloproteinase (ADAMTS-13). Deficiency or inhibition of ADAMTS-13 results in accumulation of ultra-large VWF multimers in plasma, leading to enhanced shear-induced platelet aggregation and microvascular thrombosis as seen in thrombotic thrombocytopenic purpura (TTP) (see Chapter 44).

VWF contains binding sites for collagen, fibrinogen and the platelet receptor, glycoprotein (GP)Ib. When vascular injury exposes subendothelial collagen, VWF binds and becomes unwound from its globular form (Figure 39.7c). This exposes more binding sites and allows the capture of platelets from the circulation. Thus VWF, and to some extent fibrinogen, act as bridges between the platelet and the injured vascular wall. Mutations in the genes encoding the GPIbα complex that lead to loss of function cause the bleeding disorder Bernard–Soulier syndrome. Conversely, gain-of-function mutations in either VWF or GPIb that increase the interaction lead to type 2B von Willebrand disease or pseudo (platelet-type) von Willebrand disease (see Chapter 41).

Endothelial cell anticoagulant activities

Endothelial cells regulate coagulation by a number of mechanisms. The activity of the PC pathway is promoted by expression of two cellular receptors. TM is constitutively expressed on all endothelial cells with the exception of the brain. EPCR is expressed strongly in the endothelial cells of arteries and veins in heart and lung, less intensely in capillaries in the lung and skin, and not at all in the endothelium of small vessels of the liver and kidney. In addition, endothelial cells synthesize and secrete PS, the cofactor for APC in the inactivation of FVa and FVIIIa.

Endothelial cells regulate the initiation of coagulation by synthesizing and secreting the main physiological inhibitor of the FVIIa–TF initiating complex, namely TFPI. This is described in greater detail below. Endothelial cell-surface GAGs are important in binding TFPI and also modulate the activity of AT, which inhibits thrombin and FXa and to a lesser extent FIXa and FXIa.

Endothelium and vessel injury

Disruption of the vessel wall following injury leads to exposure of procoagulant stimuli (see Figure 39.6b). Cells of the adventitia or epithelial cells of the surrounding tissues express TF constitutively on their surfaces. Formation of a complex between TF and FVII present in blood flowing from the injured vessel initiates coagulation, resulting in fibrin generation. Exposure of collagen within the subendothelial layers of the vessel wall leads to immobilization of plasma VWF, triggering platelet adhesion, aggregation and activation. Release of the contents of platelet α-granules increases the local VWF concentration and activation of endothelial cells results in release of Weibel–Palade bodies, further increasing the local concentration of VWF and expression of the cell adhesion molecule P-selectin, leading to further recruitment of platelets. In addition, release of ET-1 from the endothelium stimulates platelet aggregation and vasoconstriction, limiting blood loss. The anticoagulant activities of the endothelial cells discussed above serve to limit fibrin deposition and prevent vascular occlusion.

Endothelial cell-derived fibrinolytic factors

Three important fibrinolytic factors are detectable in the vessel wall: tPA and PAI-1 are synthesized primarily by endothelial cells, whereas urinary plasminogen activator (uPA, urokinase) is mainly derived from fibroblast-like cells in the kidney and gut. Unlike VWF and P-selectin, tPA and PAI-1 are not stored in Weibel–Palade bodies and, in the resting state, synthesis and secretion are slow, resulting in low circulating levels. However, stimulated synthesis and release occur in response to a variety of stimuli.

Platelets

Platelets play a vital role in the formation of an aggregate or primary plug that stems blood loss at the site of injury, but also by supplying a cellular surface tailored to the assembly of procoagulant complexes such as tenase and prothrombinase. Chapter 40 gives details of platelet biogenesis and function, including their specific roles in haemostasis.

Coagulation factors

Table 39.2 provides a summary of the characteristics of the proteins discussed, including gene location, number of exons, molecular mass, circulating concentration, plasma half-life and presumed function. The domain structure and modular nature of the proteins is shown in Figure 39.8. This demonstrates the similarity between coagulation factors that belong to the same protein family, such as the serine proteases (e.g. compare FVII, FIX, FX and PC).

Tissue factor

The formation of the FVIIa–TF complex is unambiguously regarded as the sole initiator of coagulation in both normal and

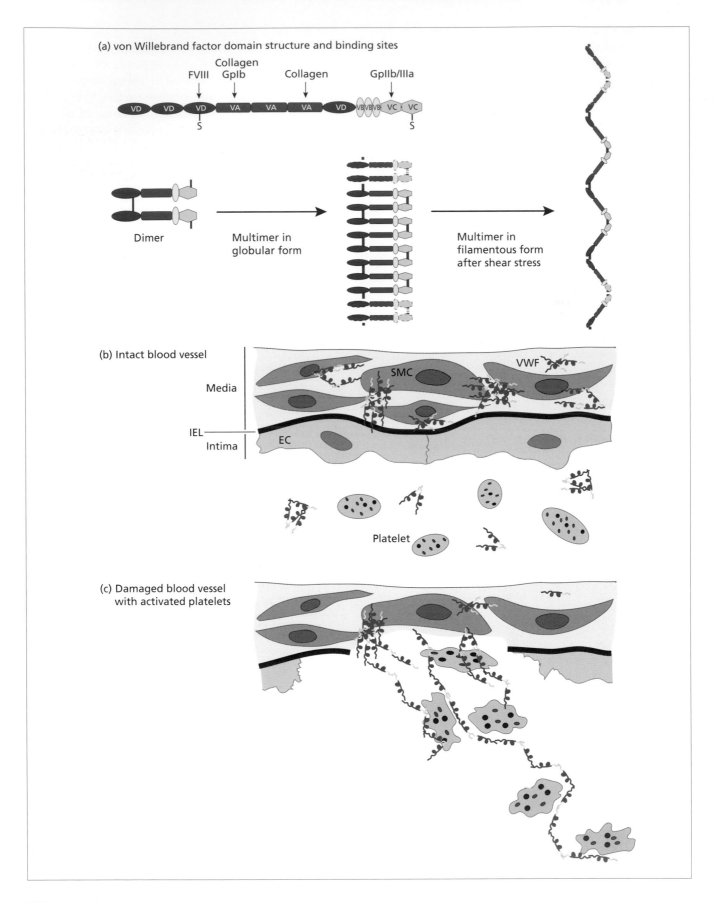

(a) von Willebrand factor domain structure and binding sites

FVIII

Collagen
GpIb

Collagen

GpIIb/IIIa

VD VD VD VA VA VA VD VB VB VB VC VC
S   S

Dimer

Multimer in
globular form

Multimer in
filamentous form
after shear stress

(b) Intact blood vessel

Media

IEL

Intima

SMC

VWF

EC

Platelet

(c) Damaged blood vessel
with activated platelets

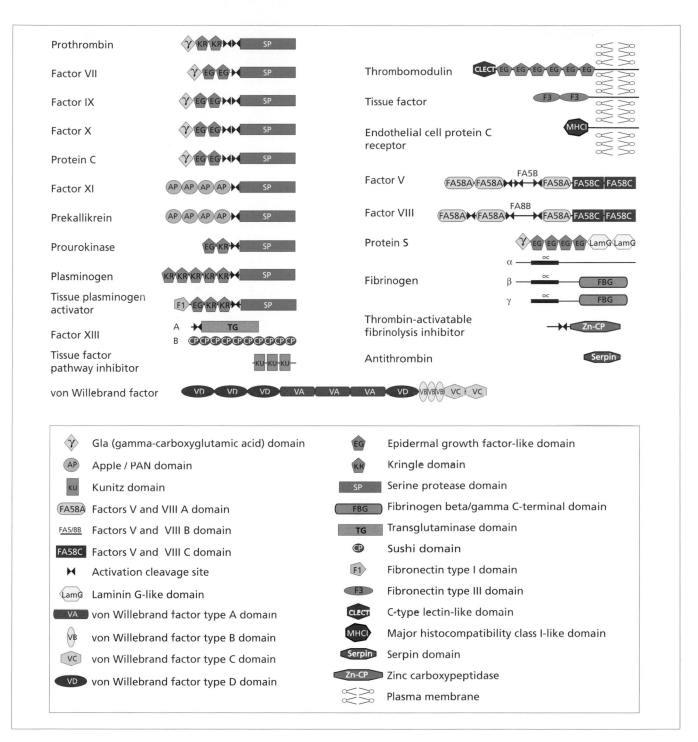

Figure 39.8 Modular organization of haemostasis proteins. The evolutionary relationship of many factors is suggested by their modular organization, represented as proposed by Bork and Bairoch (available at www.bork.embl-heidelberg.de/modules/).

Figure 39.7 Role of von Willebrand factor (VWF) in haemostasis. (a) VWF domain structure with important binding sites. Dimers are formed when individual monomers become joined through disulphide bonds at the C-terminus. Multiple dimers are then joined at the N-terminus to form high-molecular-weight multimers that take on a globular shape. When exposed to flowing blood under high shear stress the multimers become filamentous, exposing their binding sites. (b) In normal vasculature the ultra-high-molecular-weight VWF multimers required for full VWF function are found only in the subendothelium. The circulation contains lower-molecular-weight multimers. After disruption of the endothelium (c), exposure of high-molecular-weight multimers to flowing blood applies shear stress, causing the multimers to unravel and capture activated platelets. The coagulation cascade forms on the surface of these platelets. Thus VWF acts to localize the process of clot formation to the site of vascular damage. EC, endothelial cell; IEL, internal elastic lamina; SMC, smooth muscle cell.

Table 39.2 Key proteins involved in the haemostatic network.

Common name	Abbreviation	Subunit	Gene symbol	Gene location	No. of exons	Amino acids (mature)	M_r of monomer (kDa)	Plasma level ($\mu g/mL$)	Plasma level ($nmol/L$)	$t_{1/2}$ (hours)	Main action
Tissue factor	TF		F3	1p22–p21	6	263	44	NA	NA	NA	Cofactor for FVII/FVIIa
Prothrombin	FII		F2	11p11.1	14	579	72	90	1400	65	Clots FBG, activates PC, FXI, TAFI
Factor V	FV		F5	1q23	25	2196	330	10	30	15	Cofactor for FXa
Factor VII	FVII		F7	13q34	8	416	50	0.5	10	3	Activates FIX and FX
Factor VIII	FVIII		F8	Xq28	26	2332	330	0.1	0.3	10	Cofactor for FIXa
Factor IX	FIX		F9	Xq27	8	415	56	5	90	25	Activates FX
Factor X	FX		F10	13q34	8	445	59	8	135	40	Activates prothrombin
Factor XI	FXI		F11	4q35	15	607	80*	5	30	45	Activates FIX
Prekallikrein	PK		KLKB1	4q35	15	638	86	50	580	35	Anti-angiogenic, profibrinolytic
Factor XIII[†] (A chain)	FXIII	A	F13A1	6p25.3–p24.3	15	731	75[†]	10	30	200	Cross-links fibrin
Factor XIII[†] (B chain)	FXIII	B	F13B	1q31	12	641	80[†]	10	30	200	Cross-links fibrin
Fibrinogen (α-chain)[‡]	FGN	α	FGA	4q28	6	866	68[‡]	3000	9000	90	Mechanical stabilization of clot
Fibrinogen (β-chain)[‡]	FGN	β	FGB	4q28	8	491	52[‡]	3000	9000	90	Mechanical stabilization of clot
Fibrinogen (γ-chain)[‡]	FGN	γ	FGG	4q28	10	453	49[‡]	3000	9000	90	Mechanical stabilization of clot
von Willebrand factor	VWF		VWF	12p13.3	52	2050	255	10	40	12	Cell adhesion and FVIII carrier
Thrombomodulin	TM		THBD	20p11.2	1	557	60	NA	NA	NA	Cofactor in PC/TAFI activation

Name	Abbreviation	Gene	Location							Function
Endothelial protein C receptor	EPCR	PROCR	20q11.2	7	220	27	NA	NA	NA	Cofactor in PC activation
Protein C	PC	PROC	2q13–14	9	419	62	4	65	6	Inactivation of FVa and FVIIIa
Protein S	PS	PROS1	3q11.2	15	676	69	10 (free)	145	?	Inactivation of FVa and FVIIIa
Tissue factor pathway inhibitor	TFPI	TFPI	2q32	12	304	42	0.08	2.5	?	Inhibition of coagulation initiation
Antithrombin	AT	SERPINC1	1q23–q25.1	9	464	58	140	2400	5	Inhibits thrombin, FIX, FX, FXI
Heparin cofactor II	HCII	SERPIND1	22q11.21	5	499	66	90	1200	60	Prevention of arterial thrombosis?
Plasminogen	PLG	PLG	6q26	14	791	92	200	2000	50	Dissolution of clot in wound repair
Tissue plasminogen activator	tPA	PLAT	8p12	14	562	69	0.005	0.07	0.03	Plasma activator of plasminogen
Prourokinase	UK	PLAU	10q24	11	431	54	0.0015	0.04	0.03	Tissue activator of plasminogen
Plasminogen activator inhibitor 1	PAI-1	SERPINE1	7q21.3–q22	9	379	52	10	200	0.1	Inhibition of tPA and uPA
α_2-Antiplasmin	α_2-AP	SERPINF2	17p13	9	452	67	70	1000	72	Inhibition of plasmin
Thrombin-activatable fibrinolysis inhibitor	TAFI	CPB2	13q14.11	11	401	60	5	75	0.2	Inhibition of fibrinolysis

*FXI circulates as a 160-kDa homodimer of two 80-kDa monomers.
†FXIII circulates as a 326-kDa tetramer of two A- and two B-chains.
‡Fibrinogen circulates as a 340-kDa complex of two each of A-, B- and C-chains.

pathological coagulation. The processed mature TF protein is 263 amino acids in length after signal peptide cleavage. The 219-residue extracellular region consists of two fibronectin type III domains anchored into the cell membrane by a 23-residue transmembrane sequence. The extracellular region binds tightly to FVIIa to form a highly active procoagulant complex after exposure of cell surface TF to plasma FVII. The 21-residue cytoplasmic domain has been implicated in intracellular signalling; however, transgenic experiments in mice have shown that this domain is not required for either development or coagulant function, so its role is still unclear.

Vascular adventitial cells, neuroglia, vascular smooth muscle and epidermal cells express TF constitutively. It therefore forms a protective envelope around blood vessels and organs, ready to initiate clotting as soon as blood leaks out of vessels. TF is also expressed by monocytes and endothelium after activation by inflammatory cytokines or by endotoxin, as occurs in sepsis, and on cancerous tissues. Intravascular exposure of TF by any route, but particularly after atherosclerotic plaque rupture, can result in pathological thrombosis. Recent work has also focused on the novel hypothesis that functionally active TF can circulate in flowing blood on small procoagulant particles (microparticles), which may also be transferred from one blood cell type to another via specific receptor-mediated interactions.

Factor VII

Plasma FVII binds to TF, for example after vessel trauma or plaque rupture, to form a complex that initiates coagulation by directly activating FX and to a lesser extent FIX. The FVII gene (*F7*) lies adjacent to the factor X gene (*F10*), suggesting gene duplication during evolution, and close to that of protein Z (*PZ*) at 13q34. In common with the other serine proteases of the coagulation network (FIX, FX, prothrombin, PC), as well as PS and PZ, FVII has an N-terminal domain that contains a number (9–12) of glutamic acid residues that are post-translationally modified by the addition of a carboxyl group to the γ-carbon by a vitamin K-dependent carboxylase. This γ-carboxyglutamic acid (GLA) domain confers affinity to negatively charged phospholipid membranes such as those of activated platelets or endothelial cells, promoting the assembly of functional multiprotein complexes on these surfaces. Proteins containing GLA modules are commonly referred to as 'vitamin K-dependent factors' as this vitamin is a cofactor in the carboxylation reaction. Blocking this post-translational modification with coumarin derivatives such as warfarin represents the current therapy for the long-term treatment and prevention of thromboembolic events. FVII in common with other GLA domain-containing proteins has a primary translation product that contains a propeptide sequence encoded by exon 2 that directs the γ-carboxylation at 10 Glu residues within the GLA domain encoded by exon 3. The GLA domain is followed by

two epidermal growth factor (EGF)-like domains encoded by exons 4 and 5. Exon 6 encodes the connecting or activation peptide, and exons 7 and 8 the serine protease domain. FVII is activated by cleavage between residues Arg152 and Ile153, yielding a two-chain disulphide-linked FVIIa molecule; however, this has little catalytic activity until it is bound to TF. The half-life of FVII zymogen in plasma is 3 hours and, remarkably, the half-life of the FVIIa enzyme is 2.5 hours, probably because there is no plasma inhibitor capable of effectively neutralizing free FVIIa. In recent years, recombinant FVIIa has entered clinical use as a treatment, first, for haemophiliacs with inhibitors to exogenous FVIII and, second, for a wider range of bleeding problems and general surgical intervention.

Factor X

The gene and protein structures of FX closely resemble those of FVII. Unlike FVII, zymogen FX circulates as a two-chain disulphide-linked heterodimer due to excision of a tribasic peptide (Arg-Lys-Arg) at residues 139–141 during synthesis. The light chain of FX therefore consists of the GLA domain with 11 γ-carboxyglutamic acid residues, the amphipathic helix and two EGF-like domains. The half-life of FX in plasma is 36 hours. FX is activated by either FIXa–FVIIIa or TF–FVIIa on phospholipid surfaces in the presence of Ca^{2+} ions. FXa forms a phospholipid-bound complex with FVa, which efficiently activates prothrombin (prothrombinase complex).

Factor IX

The FIX gene (*F9*) is located at Xq26, about 15.2 Mb from the FVIII gene (*F8*); thus deficiencies of both factors are X-linked disorders. Deficiency of either FVIII or FIX results in clinical haemophilia (A or B respectively), as the main function of FIX is to participate in the tenase complex (FIXa–FVIIIa). The FIX promoter has been extensively studied and includes sites for liver-specific transcription factors and an androgen-responsive promoter element, which accounts for the haemophilia B Leiden phenotype (FIX deficiency which corrects spontaneously at puberty). The plasma half-life of FIX is 18 hours.

The mature protein is a single-chain molecule consisting of 415 amino acids and the GLA domain contains 12 γ-carboxyglutamic acid residues. Either TF–FVIIa or FXIa cleaves FIX within the connecting peptide (between residues 145–146 and 180–181). Unlike FVII and FX, FIX requires two proteolytic cleavages, releasing an activation peptide, in order to achieve full activation.

Factor XI

FXI is a zymogen of a serine protease that has four Apple (PAN1–4) domains and a serine protease domain in each monomer. The protein circulates as a homodimer, with the two monomer subunits linked via a series of interactions between the two Apple four domains that includes a disulphide bridge. Activation of FXI is by a single cleavage performed by thrombin. It is clear that dimerization is required for full function of this factor presumably due to obstruction of essential binding sites in the monomer form. FXIa then activates FIX directly in free solution. FXI activation by the contact protein FXIIa was originally thought to be a relevant step in intrinsic or contact-activated coagulation (see Figure 39.2), but it is now considered that the feedback activation of FXI by trace thrombin provides a physiologically relevant route for generation of increased amounts of FIXa to assemble tenase during the amplification of the initial TF stimulus (see Figure 39.3).

Factor XIII

FXIII circulates as a tetramer of two A-chains and two B-chains. The B-chains function as carrier for the A-chains which, after activation by thrombin, function as a transglutaminase to cross-link fibrin and other proteins in the clot, resulting in a stable structure. FXIIIa contains a free sulphydryl group at the active site. Platelets also contain FXIII A-chain dimers, which are fully functional after thrombin activation.

von Willebrand factor

The primary translation product of the VWF mRNA is a 2813 amino acid polypeptide that includes a 22 amino acid signal peptide and a 741 amino acid propeptide that is essential for multimerization. The mature protein contains four repeating domains termed A, B, C and D. During post-translational processing, monomer subunits dimerize and then multimerize with excision of the propeptide. VWF is synthesized in endothelial cells (where it is stored in Weibel–Palade bodies) and in megakaryocytes, where it is stored in the α-granules of platelets. Both Weibel–Palade body and α-granule VWF are released on stimulation by various agonists, including thrombin. Plasma also contains VWF, which is released from endothelial cells via a constitutive pathway. VWF serves two unique functions in haemostasis: as a carrier for FVIII and as the ligand mediating binding between platelets and the subendothelium.

Factor VIII

The FVIII gene (*F8*) spans 187 kb of the X chromosome (Xq28) and encodes a protein of 2351 amino acids. After removal of the 19 amino acid signal sequence, a single chain of 2332 amino acids is transiently formed but is subsequently further processed prior to release as a series of heterodimers, due to variable cleavage within the B-domain sequence. Because of internal homology, the FVIII domain structure can be represented as A1–A2–B–A3–C1–C2. The B domain is not necessary for procoagulant function as B domain-deleted FVIII has

full activity. The B-domain sequences of FV and FVIII share little sequence identity, although their lengths are similar and both are heavily glycosylated. It is likely that the glycosylated B domain functions in promoting endoplasmic reticulum/Golgi transport since deficiency of LMAN1 (also known as ERGIC 53), a mannose-binding protein, results in combined deficiency of FV and FVIII. FVIII also has three short acidic interdomain peptides (a1, a2 and a3) that are closely implicated in FVIII function.

FVIII is the essential cofactor for activation of FX by FIXa in the tenase complex. It has no function until proteolysed to FVIIIa by thrombin or FXa at Arg372-Ser373 and Arg1689-Ser1690. FVIIIa is directly inactivated by APC cleavage at Arg336-Ser337 and Arg562-Ser563; however, functional activity of FVIIIa also decays rapidly by dissociation of the A2 subunit from FVIIIa. The crystal structure of FVIIIa has recently been solved by two groups.

Factor V

The mature protein product is 2196 amino acids in length after cleavage of a 28 amino acid signal peptide. The structure of FV, like that of FVIII, can be represented as A1–A2–B–A3–C1–C2. In contrast with FVIII the B domain is required for full procoagulant function. FV also differs from FVIII in that it lacks the three short acidic interdomain peptides (a1, a2 and a3) implicated in FVIII function.

FV is the cofactor for the activation of prothrombin by FXa. It has no cofactor activity until proteolysed by thrombin or FXa at Arg709-Ser710, Arg1018-Thr1019 and Arg1545-Ser1547. FVa is inactivated by APC through cleavages at Arg506-Ser507 and Arg1765-Leu1766. The initial (and rate-limiting) cleavage is at Arg506. This is the site of the mutation in FV Leiden (FV Arg506Gln) that is resistant to APC, leading to the most common form of familial thrombophilia.

Fibrinogen

The fibrinogen gene cluster is located on chromosome 4q32 in the order β–α–γ, with β transcribed in the opposite direction to α and γ. The three chains of fibrinogen are disulphide cross-linked and folded together in an intricate manner. The overall structure of fibrinogen is a symmetrical dimer, $\alpha_2\beta_2\gamma_2$. Viewed by electron microscopy, the molecule is trinodular, with the outer two globular domains (fragments D) containing the C-termini of all three chains connected to the central globular domain (fragment E), which contains the N-termini of all six chains tethered together by disulphide bonds. Coiled regions, forming α-helical ropes, connect the lateral and central globular domains.

Polymerization of fibrinogen occurs when thrombin cleaves two short negatively charged fibrinopeptides A and B from the N-termini of the α- and β-chains respectively. This reveals new

N-terminal sequences in the fragment E region (called knobs) that fit into holes in the fragment D regions. Polymerization then occurs spontaneously in a staggered half-overlap array, which can elongate indefinitely in either direction. Electron microscopy studies were and still are important in resolving the molecular architecture of fibrillar fibrin formation, but from 1997 elegant crystal structures of parts of the fibrin(ogen) molecule were successfully produced in a number of laboratories. These structures reveal the elegant mechanisms of fibrin polymerization.

Prothrombin

The mRNA encodes a preproleader sequence similar to that found in other vitamin K-dependent proteins, followed by a GLA domain, two kringle domains, an activation peptide and a serine protease domain. FXa complexed with FVa activates prothrombin zymogen to thrombin on a phospholipid surface (prothrombinase) on cleavage of two peptide bonds. The first, between Arg271 and Thr272, releases the protease domain from the GLA and kringle domains; the second, between Arg320 and Ile321, generates the catalytic site of thrombin by a typical trypsin-like conformational rearrangement. Cleavage at Arg320 yields the protease (meizothrombin) that retains membrane-binding properties. Cleavage at Arg271 yields thrombin and severs covalent linkage with the N-terminal domain known as fragment 1.2. Fully cleaved thrombin is termed α-thrombin, and is rapidly released from its site of production to participate in numerous haemostatic functions free in solution: acting as a procoagulant against many substrates including fibrinogen, FV, FVIII and FXI; acting in complex with TM as an anticoagulant against PC; and acting to activate cellular transmembrane protease-activated receptors. Thrombin also activates thrombin-activatable fibrinolytic inhibitor (TAFI), in complex with TM, inhibiting fibrinolysis.

Naturally occurring inhibitors of blood coagulation

In common with other defence mechanisms, such as those resulting in kinin release and complement activation, the blood coagulation process can be activated very rapidly when the need arises. This involves the generation of proteolytic enzymes, such as thrombin, that are potentially lethal if their action is not limited. For example, 10 mL of plasma can generate, in theory, sufficient thrombin to clot all of the fibrinogen in the body in 30 s. That it does not normally do so is due partly to the fact that the procoagulant response is most pronounced in the vicinity of the platelet plug forming at the point of vascular injury, while elsewhere coagulation is inhibited by substances in plasma or on the vascular surface that exhibit anticoagulant activity.

Classification of physiological anticoagulants

Physiological anticoagulants fall into two main groups: those that inhibit the serine proteases of the coagulation cascade (both Kunitz-type and serpins) and those involved in destruction of the activated coagulation cofactors FVa and FVIIIa (components of the PC system). These inhibitors assume great physiological significance: relatively minor deficiencies (50–70% of average levels) of some of these inhibitors, such as might be found in individuals heterozygous for a genetic defect, are associated with an increased incidence of thrombosis. Homozygous deficiencies are frequently either fatal in the first few years of life unless prophylactic replacement therapy is instituted, or are not found in nature, suggesting early fetal loss.

In addition to the specific inhibitors, there are some other inhibitory mechanisms that do not fit into either of the above categories, one of these being the detoxifying property of the liver, which plays an important role in removal of activated clotting factors, both directly and after their combination with natural inhibitors. Furthermore, the removal of free thrombin occurs as a result of its adsorption onto fibrin or onto fibrin(ogen) degradation products. The latter, which cannot themselves take part in a clot, may interfere with normal fibrin polymerization. Although less well defined than the others, this group appears to be physiologically important, as qualitative defects of fibrinogen (dysfibrinogenaemias) that result in reduced thrombin binding may be associated with a thrombotic disorder (see Chapter 45).

Tissue factor pathway inhibitor: a Kunitz-type inhibitor

The various serpins found in blood (see below) probably play no physiological role in the inhibition of FVIIa in the initiating TF–FVIIa complex. Instead, the action of this serine protease–cofactor complex is modulated by TFPI, which is located on the endothelial cell surface, within platelets, in plasma and on monocytes. Two alternatively spliced isoforms of TFPI (α and β) have been identified in humans that differ in their domain structure and mechanism of cell surface binding. TFPIα has an acidic N-terminal region followed by three Kunitz-type protease inhibitory domains (K1–K3) and a basic C-terminal region. K2 is responsible for binding and direct inhibition of FXa and K1 inhibits FVIIa in a FXa-dependent manner. K3 and the C-terminal region do not directly inhibit proteolysis but they are necessary for rapid inhibition of FXa by K2. Recent data intriguingly suggest that this may be mediated through an interaction with PS acting as a cofactor in the formation of the TFPI–FXa complex. TFPIα indirectly associates with the endothelial cell surface through a non-covalent association with a glycosylphosphatidylinositol (GPI)-anchored coreceptor. It can also bind non-specifically to endothelial cell GAGs via the basic C-terminal region; it is thought that this interaction is responsible for the twofold to fourfold increase in plasma TFPI following infusion of heparin. TFPIβ has the N-terminal acidic region followed by K1 and K2 but lacks K3 and the C-terminal region of TFPIα. Instead it has a different C-terminal region encoding a GPI-anchor attachment sequence that allows it to directly associate with the cell surface.

Most TFPI in the vasculature (~ 85%) is associated with endothelial cells, particularly in the microcirculation, with a smaller amount (5–10%) being found in platelets and the rest in plasma. Virtually all circulating TFPI is associated with lipoproteins and has undergone variable amounts of proteolytic degradation within its C-terminal region. As a result plasma TFPI has reduced anticoagulant activity and is unlikely to play an important role as an *in vivo* inhibitor of blood coagulation.

Disruption of the murine *TFPI* gene is incompatible with normal development, suggesting that a deficiency of functional TFPI might lead to clinical thrombosis. However, as the bulk of intravascular TFPI is associated with the endothelial cell surface, simple measurement of plasma TFPI levels is not a clear indicator of a deficiency state. Moderately low plasma levels can occur in DIC, septicaemia and following major surgery, possibly due to increased utilization, but heparin infusion increases plasma TFPI in such patients. Whether congenital deficiency of TFPI is a risk factor for thrombosis remains uncertain: after several negative studies in this area, recently a case–control study found a relationship between low levels of free plasma TFPI (non-lipoprotein bound) and enhanced risk of deep vein thrombosis and myocardial infarction.

Serine protease inhibitors (serpins) and heparin

Human plasma contains at least seven inhibitors of serine protease coagulation factors. Apart from α_2-macroglobulin, all are single-chain serpins of molecular mass 40–65 kDa. Specificity is imparted by their tertiary structure, which engenders high affinity for a defined substrate or small range of substrates. Of this group, only AT and heparin cofactor II (HCII) assume haemostatic significance, acting predominantly on proteases generated late in the coagulation cascade (i.e. thrombin and FXa). A deficiency of any of the other serpins (although sometimes giving rise to a clinical disorder due to the failure of neutralization of a serine protease not involved in coagulation pathways) is asymptomatic in terms of haemostasis.

Several serpins contain GAG-binding sites that, particularly in the case of AT and HCII but to a lesser extent for PAI-1 and APC inhibitor, greatly enhance the rate of interaction with (although not the affinity for) their specific protease(s). Since a major source of heparin-like material is heparan sulphate on the endothelial cell surface, another possible function of the heparin-binding site of these inhibitors (especially AT and

HCII) might be to allow them to exert a general and constitutive anticoagulant effect on intact vessels; this may also act to prevent extension of a procoagulant response beyond an area of damaged endothelium.

Antithrombin

AT (formerly ATIII) is a 58-kDa serpin that is synthesized principally in the liver, with a high plasma concentration of 2.4 μmol/L. The turnover of AT *in vivo* is complex, with a rapid initial clearance ($t_{1/2}$ 10 min) due to equilibration with endothelial cell-bound AT, a slower clearance ($t_{1/2}$ 3 hours) due to equilibration with the extravascular compartment, and a much slower linear phase with an overall $t_{1/2}$ of 90 hours.

Disruption of the murine AT gene results in death of all embryos shortly before birth due to severe cardiac and hepatic thrombosis. In humans, AT deficiency is associated with familial thrombosis.

AT forms a stable 1:1 complex with several serine protease coagulation factors, predominantly thrombin but also to some extent FIXa, FXIa, FXIIIa and kallikrein. Initially, the serine at the active centre of the protease cleaves a peptide bond (involving Arg393) in the 'reactive centre loop' near the C-terminus of AT: a conformational change in the serpin ensues resulting in irreversible trapping of the protease against the inhibitor. The inactivated enzyme–serpin complex is then cleared rapidly. Complex formation is progressive and only with thrombin and FXa is it rapid enough to be of physiological significance. In purified *in vitro* systems, the $t_{1/2}$ is around 30 s for free thrombin, 90 s for FXa and 10–25 min for the other enzymes. In each case, the inhibitor–protease complex is rapidly cleared ($t_{1/2}$ 3 min) from the circulation by the liver.

Heparin, without altering the stoichiometry, induces a more than 2000-fold increase in the rate of thrombin inactivation by AT, such that its action becomes almost instantaneous ($t_{1/2} < 0.01$ s). The unique mechanism of this activation involves release of the reactive centre loop from partial insertion in the β-sheet core of AT following heparin binding. Heparin also strongly enhances AT neutralization of FXa and, to a lesser extent, FIXa, particularly in the presence of Ca^{2+}. The enhancement of AT inhibition of thrombin and FXa by heparin is the basis of its use as a therapeutic anticoagulant to prevent thromboembolism. At therapeutic concentrations there is no significant effect on AT inhibition of FXIa and FIXa.

Anti-angiogenic and antitumour activities have also been described for the cleaved serpin in mouse models. This finding provides further evidence for the interrelationship of coagulation and angiogenic pathways.

Heparin cofactor II

This 65-kDa serpin is present in plasma at the high concentration of 90 mg/L (1.2 μmol/L). It appears to be a specific 1:1 inhibitor of thrombin and to have little or no anti-FXa activity. The rate of thrombin neutralization by HCII is increased approximately 1000-fold by heparin, although because of its lower heparin affinity it requires five to ten times more heparin than does AT. Interaction seems to depend largely on the high anionic charge of heparin and related GAGs. Details of the molecular mechanism of HCII interaction with thrombin have recently been elucidated by X-ray crystallography.

That HCII has some physiological significance is suggested by the fact that it falls in parallel with AT in DIC. However, as AT is in twofold molar excess over HCII, the latter cannot altogether compensate for a deficiency of AT, which, as stated above, is a well-established cause of a thrombotic tendency. Whether HCII deficiency leads to a similar clinical picture remains to be established, as few cases have yet been described and only occasionally has concomitant thrombotic disease been present. Mice with HCII knockout develop normally and do not show spontaneous thrombosis; however, they show an enhanced propensity to carotid occlusion after deliberate injury to the endothelium, corrected by infusion of purified HCII, suggesting that HCII has a role in prevention of arterial thrombosis.

Heparin and heparin-like substances in plasma

Although the term 'heparin' implies a single compound, it in fact refers to a heterogeneous mixture of sulphated polysaccharides that are all members of the GAG group. The major pharmaceutical source is porcine intestinal mucosa. By virtue of its strong positive charge, heparin combines non-specifically with a number of cationic proteins such as albumin and reacts in a highly specific way with β-lipoproteins, fibrinogen, HCII and AT. It also mobilizes platelet factor (PF)4 and TFPI, which are bound to GAGs on the surface of endothelial cells, and releases lipoprotein lipase into plasma.

Unfractionated heparin (UFH) is an extremely heterogeneous polymer, being composed of between 10 and 100 saccharide units. Only about one-quarter of the polysaccharides has any anticoagulant activity *in vitro*. The pharmaceutical properties of heparin are unpredictable, because of its heterogeneity, with marked variation in pharmacokinetics and side-effects, the most serious of which is heparin-induced thrombocytopenia (see Chapter 46). The realization that the anticoagulant action of UFH was mostly delivered by short pentasaccharides has led to the use of more efficient fractionation procedures (including cleavage by nitrous acid, heparinase and oxidizing agents), yielding a number of low-molecular-weight heparin (LMWH) preparations. LMWHs contain 10–20 saccharide units (4–6 kDa) and because of their more uniform composition have much better pharmacokinetics and fewer side-effects. More recently, a synthetic pentasaccharide has come into therapeutic use, although whether this has any clear benefits over LMWH remains to be established.

UFH and the various LMWHs differ in their affinities for the plasma factors with which they interact and in the specific serine proteases that they inhibit. This, together with the timing of blood samples in relation to dosage interval, is critically important in laboratory monitoring of the therapeutic effect (see Chapter 47). The major anticoagulant activity of both UFH and LMWH is attributed to the pentasaccharide sequence containing at its centre a 2,3,6-(SO_3) trisulphated glucosamine group. It is this that binds to lysine or tryptophan residues in AT in the region of the D helix, inducing the conformational change in the inhibitor. A second anticoagulant action of UFH (at least 20 saccharide units are required) involves direct binding between thrombin (but not FXa or other proteases) and a heparin sequence adjacent to the pentasaccharide. This brings thrombin and AT into close proximity and is necessary for the antithrombin activity. As LMWHs generally have fewer than 20 saccharide units, they have little or no antithrombin action and their anticoagulant action is mediated through inhibition of FXa. This explains why LMWHs have little effect on the activated partial thromboplastin time and are measured using an anti-FXa assay.

There is of course no detectable heparin in normal plasma. However, endogenous heparin-like molecules (e.g. dermatan sulphate and heparan sulphate) are present on the surface of endothelial cells and, by enhancing the action of AT and HCII, these would have antithrombotic effects. Such mechanisms seem to be of clinical importance, as recurrent thromboses have been reported in association with several dysfunctional AT molecules that inhibit thrombin normally in the absence of heparin but which do not show enhanced reactivity in its presence, presumably due to defects at the heparin-binding sites. At points of vascular injury, local accumulation of activated platelets provides a source of heparin-neutralizing activity that could overcome the anticoagulant effects of endothelial cell-bound heparinoids and permit the procoagulant response to proceed.

Protein Z and protein Z-dependent inhibitor

PZ is a 62-kDa vitamin K-dependent plasma protein that serves as a cofactor for the inhibition of FXa by PZ-dependent protease inhibitor (ZPI). Although PZ was first described in the 1970s, ZPI is a recently identified 72-kDa member of the serpin superfamily.

The organization of the PZ gene and the structure of the molecule are very similar to those of coagulation factors FVII, FIX, FX and PC; however, the PZ 'serine protease' domain lacks the canonical active-site His and Ser residues and therefore cannot function as a protease. PZ circulates in plasma in a complex with ZPI. Inhibition of FXa by ZPI in the presence of phospholipid and Ca^{2+} ions is enhanced 1000-fold by PZ, but ZPI also inhibits FXIa in a process that does not require PZ, phospholipid or Ca^{2+}. ZPI activity is consumed during coagulation through proteolysis mediated by FXa (with PZ) and FXIa. PZ may serve to dampen the procoagulant response *in vivo* as PZ deficiency dramatically increases the severity of the prothrombotic phenotype of FV Leiden mice. Studies to determine the potential roles of PZ and ZPI deficiency in human thrombosis are in progress.

α₁-Antitrypsin

This is a serpin whose primary targets are pancreatic and leucocyte elastases. In coagulation the major inhibitory activity is directed against FXIa and FXa, although the chief physiological inhibitor of FXIa is probably protease nexin 2. It has little effect on overall thrombin inhibition and a straightforward deficiency of α₁-antitrypsin is not associated with hypercoagulability.

An abnormal molecular form of α₁-antitrypsin in which there is a Met→Ser substitution at the active centre (antitrypsin Pittsburgh) has been described, resulting in a higher affinity for thrombin. At a plasma concentration of 25 µmol/L, the variant circulates at a 10-fold higher level than AT and gives rise to a clinical bleeding tendency. However, it is unaffected by heparin.

Protease nexin 2

This is a Kunitz-type serine protease inhibitor that is found in the α-granules of platelets. Normally, there is very little in plasma but it is released at sites of platelet activation, following which the single Kunitz domain enters into a tightly bound inhibitory complex with FXIa. It is one of several isoforms of Alzheimer β-amyloid protein precursor present in platelets. Deficiency of protease nexin 2 has not been described.

C1-esterase inhibitor

The primary target of this serpin is the activated form of the first component of complement, but it also contributes in a minor way to the neutralization of FXIa and plasmin. Deficiency of C1-esterase inhibitor, although of no haemostatic consequence, causes angioneurotic oedema, the characteristic lesions of which may sometimes be confused with haematomas.

α₂-Antiplasmin

This serpin is the principal inhibitor of the fibrinolytic enzyme plasmin. It also has weak activity against several coagulation proteases, especially the contact factors. However, any anticoagulant action against proteases late in the coagulation cascade (e.g. FXa) is only apparent at concentrations well in excess of those in normal plasma. Its mechanism of action and clinical importance are discussed further in the section on fibrinolysis.

α₂-Macroglobulin

α₂-Macroglobulin is composed of four identical chains and has a molecular mass of 740 kDa. It is not a member of the serpin superfamily and its effects are not restricted to serine proteases. It binds to coagulation factors at a site away from the active site, the interaction involving the formation of a bond between cysteine and glutamate residues in the inhibitor and a lysine residue in the protease. Inhibition is produced by stearic hindrance rather than by active site inactivation and indeed the proteases retain some esterolytic and amidolytic activity, particularly against small peptides, a fact that should be borne in mind when using chromogenic substrates to assay coagulation inhibitors. It is responsible for approximately 50%, 20% and 10% of the inhibition of kallikrein, thrombin and FXa respectively.

Deficiency of α₂-macroglobulin is not associated with a thrombotic tendency. However, it is an acute-phase reactant and it is possible that, when elevated under conditions of stress or when the other major antithrombins or antiplasmins are overwhelmed, it might become a significant inhibitor of coagulation or fibrinolysis. Moreover, it has been suggested that the raised level of α₂-macroglobulin that exists in children (150–200% of adult values) may compensate for a low level of AT, and explain why thrombotic episodes do not usually occur before puberty in congenitally AT-deficient patients.

The protein C pathway: inhibition of cofactors FVa and FVIIIa

The activated forms of coagulation cofactors FV and FVIII (FVa and FVIIIa) are potent procoagulants that enormously enhance the activity of serine protease factors in the tenase and prothrombinase complexes (see above). It is not unexpected that these cofactors should be subject to a negative feedback mechanism that limits their procoagulant activity. This is achieved by a complex series of reactions collectively referred to as the protein C pathway. Four key factors are now known to be involved, and their role in the haemostatic network is shown in Figure 39.4.

Protein C

This vitamin K-dependent serine protease has an identical modular composition to the procoagulant factors FVII, FIX and FX. It circulates in blood as a two-chain disulphide-linked molecule. During biosynthesis, the primary translation product is proteolytically processed releasing the dipeptide Lys156Arg157. In order to exert its anticoagulant effect, PC must first be activated to APC. This is achieved by the action of thrombin, which cleaves the heavy chain to release a 12-residue (Gly158–Arg169) activation peptide, revealing the active site by the usual chymotrypsin-like mechanism. Thrombin activation of PC is slow in free solution but is markedly accelerated by specific endothelial cell receptors for both thrombin (TM) and PC (EPCR), which coordinate the assembly of a membrane complex for PC activation.

APC interacts with PS bound to the phospholipid surface of activated platelets, enhancing the anticoagulant activity of APC (see below) against FVa and FVIIIa. These procoagulant cofactors are inactivated by APC on the platelet surface by specific cleavage in their A domains, terminating the activity of the tenase and prothrombinase complex by disrupting their binding sites for FIXa and FXa respectively. In the absence of PS, this reaction is inefficient. The most common form of familial thrombosis is FV Leiden, which is caused by mutation of Arg506 to Gln, which makes the molecule resistant to cleavage by APC.

It appears that APC inactivation of FVa is a prerequisite for efficient inactivation of FVIIIa *in vivo*, as FVIIIa inactivation is also impaired in these patients, although there is no abnormality in the FVIII molecule. Since the discovery of FV Leiden other less common FV mutants have been found with a similar phenotype. None of the mutations reported in the FVIII molecule have been shown to cause a similar prothrombotic phenotype. PC is synthesized in the liver, and, being vitamin K dependent, is often low in the newborn. Even though its substrates (FV and FVIII) are normal at birth, this deficiency is compensated for by the reduction in plasma of the vitamin K-dependent procoagulant factors (prothrombin, FVII, FIX and FX). Because warfarin treatment initially decreases PC levels faster than FVII, FIX, FX and prothrombin levels, it can paradoxically increase the procoagulant tendency when anticoagulant treatment is first begun (many patients starting on warfarin are given heparin in parallel to combat this). Disruption of the murine PC gene results in lethal perinatal consumptive coagulopathy, whereas in humans homozygous PC deficiency is associated with lethal purpura fulminans (in the absence of PC replacement therapy) and heterozygous individuals have a high risk of venous thrombosis. There is increasing appreciation of the role of the PC pathway in regulation of inflammation and the concept of signalling mechanisms allowing 'cross-talk' between the haemostatic and inflammatory networks. This is well demonstrated by the protective effect of administration of APC concentrate to animals with induced sepsis. The survival benefits that APC concentrate provides in this situation has subsequently been seen in patients with sepsis and multiorgan failure. Recently, variant recombinant PC molecules have been produced that appear to have either anticoagulant or anti-inflammatory effects independent of each other.

Thrombomodulin

TM is an integral transmembrane receptor found on endothelial cells in virtually all body tissues. It appears to be absent in the brain vasculature and in hepatic sinusoids and lymph node venules. TM is essential for normal fetal development as shown by mouse knockout studies, although TM$^{+/-}$ heterozygous mice appear to be completely healthy.

The protein has an extracellular region composed of an N terminal lectin-like or CLECT domain, six EGF-like domains, a transmembrane sequence and a small cytoplasmic region. TM forms a 1:1 complex with thrombin (via the protease's anion-binding exosite I and TM's EGF-like domains 4–6), preventing binding of the protease to its various procoagulant substrates (fibrinogen, FV, FVIII, FXIII and protease-activated receptors involved in platelet aggregation). TM also plays a part in binding of PC zymogen and, after formation of the TM–thrombin complex on the cell surface, there is a 20 000-fold increase in the rate of activation of PC, so that thrombin effectively becomes an anticoagulant. Binding of PC to TM is also enhanced by EPCR.

The TM–thrombin complex is short-lived, being endocytosed by endothelial cells, where the thrombin is taken up and degraded by lysosomes while TM recirculates to the cell membrane.

Endothelial protein C receptor

EPCR was cloned in 1994 as a novel transmembrane receptor on endothelial cells that was able to bind PC and promote its activation by the thrombin–TM complex. The extracellular portion of EPCR is related to the MHC class I/CD1 proteins; however, it lacks the α3 domain found in the extracellular portion of most of the family: there is good evidence that the α1 and α2 extracellular domains of EPCR interact with the GLA domain of PC. EPCR may function by localizing the PC molecule to the endothelial cell surface, moving laterally on the cell surface to locate a thrombin–TM complex, then presenting the PC molecule optimally for thrombin cleavage to form APC.

The essential role of EPCR was demonstrated recently by targeted deletion of the murine EPCR gene, resulting in early fetal death with evidence of thrombosis at the maternal–fetal interface. Abrogation of EPCR function *in vitro* reduces the rate of PC activation by thrombin–TM. In contrast, inhibition of EPCR action by a specific anti-EPCR monoclonal antibody in baboons given thrombin resulted in reduced APC levels amid evidence of excessive coagulopathy. Blockade of EPCR on challenge with *Escherichia coli* also led to worse outcomes in an animal model of sepsis, whereas administration of APC improved survival in experimental sepsis.

Protein S and C4b-binding protein

PS is a single-chain vitamin K-dependent glycoprotein chiefly synthesized in the liver by endothelial cells. Unlike the other vitamin K-dependent coagulation proteins it is not a serine protease, having two C-terminal LamG domains rather than a serine protease domain, and the N-terminal GLA domain is followed by four EGF-like domains rather than the two usually seen in the serine proteases (see Figure 39.8). About 40% of the PS in plasma is in the free form, whereas the remaining 60% is associated in a 1:1 complex with C4b-binding protein (C4bBP). Both forms bind strongly via the PS GLA domain to negatively charged phospholipids exposed on the surface of activated platelets. Free PS (although having no strong inhibitory effect on FVa or FVIIIa itself) forms a Ca^{2+}-dependent complex with APC, helping to orient the APC active site above the phospholipid surface and enhancing its anticoagulant activity against both proteins. However, C4bBP-bound PS does not enhance PC function against FVa, suggesting a role for C4bBP in modulation of the APC pathway. Free thrombin cleaves PS N-terminal to the GLA domain, removing its ability to bind to both phospholipid and PC and thereby abolishing its PC cofactor activity.

C4bBP is a large molecule containing seven α-chains (each of which binds one molecule of the C4b component of comple-

Table 39.3 Haemostasis changes during pregnancy.

Platelet count	No consistent change but often falls
Platelet aggregation	Progressive enhancement
Fibrinogen	Progressive rise up to 400% basal
Prothrombin	No consistent change
Factor V	No consistent change
Factor VII	Progressive rise up to 300% basal
Factor VIII	Progressive rise up to 200% basal
von Willebrand factor	Progressive rise up to 250% basal
Factor IX	Variable, no consistent change
Factor X	No consistent change
Factor XI	Variable, no consistent change
Factor XIII	Progressive fall to 50% basal
Antithrombin	No consistent change
Tissue factor pathway inhibitor	Progressive rise
Protein C	No consistent change, but APC resistance increases
Protein S	Progressive fall to 50% basal
Plasminogen	Progressive rise up to 300% basal
tPA	No consistent change
α_2-Antiplasmin	Progressive rise up to 300% basal
PAI-1	Progressive rise up to 300% basal
PAI-2	Progressive marked rise

ment) and a single β-chain (to which one molecule of PS attaches). It is an acute-phase reactant, which can increase by up to fourfold in severe inflammatory states. It is likely that such raised levels would disturb the equilibrium between free and bound PS, and result in a fall in the free (biologically active) form, predisposing to a hypercoagulable state.

Many haemostatic factors change during pregnancy. Free PS falls during pregnancy (Table 39.3) and to a lesser extent in women receiving estrogen supplements, but it is disputed whether this results from altered reactivity with C4bBP or if it contributes to hypercoagulability in pregnancy or during estrogen therapy. Total PS, like other vitamin K-dependent factors, is reduced in the newborn; levels as low as 20% of adult values can occur. However, this is compensated for by a marked reduction in C4bBP at birth (5–20% of adult levels), so that a relatively normal level of functional (free) PS is maintained.

The possibility that PS might have PC-independent functions in coagulation has been raised by the recent finding that PS binds to the K3 domain of TFPI. The full relevance of this finding is not yet known.

Protein C inhibitors

As with other serine proteases, APC is subject to inhibition by serpins (half-life of APC in plasma is 15–20 min), including APC inhibitor (PCI), PAI-1 and α_1-antitrypsin. The relative contributions of these *in vivo* are difficult to assess. PCI slowly but progressively blocks the action of APC (and, to a much lesser extent, thrombin and FXa), in each case forming a 1:1 complex: in addition PCI action is enhanced 20-fold by heparin and more weakly by other GAGs, but the physiological significance of this is uncertain. Despite the name, disruption of the murine PCI gene leads not to coagulopathy but to infertility due to lack of inhibition of another protease target of the serpin, the sperm protein acrosin.

Fibrinolysis

It is widely acknowledged that the principal functions of the fibrinolytic system are to ensure that excess fibrin deposition is either prevented or rapidly removed (i.e. that a localized procoagulant response is achieved without compromising blood circulation generally) and, following re-establishment of haemostasis, the fibrin mesh is removed during wound healing. The system of profibrinolytic and antifibrinolytic factors that has evolved to meet these requirements is closely coupled to that which results in fibrin clot formation. Fibrinolysis is essentially a localized, surface-bound phenomenon, with most events being catalysed by the presence of cross-linked fibrin itself, i.e. 'fibrin orchestrates its own destruction'. For this reason, the assays of fibrinolytic factors carried out in the soluble phase, in particular in systemic blood, may be misleading and should be interpreted with great caution.

Components of the fibrinolytic system

These include PLG and plasmin, several endogenous (tissue or plasma derived) or exogenous (e.g. bacterial or venom derived) PLG activators, and a number of inhibitors of plasmin or of the PLG activators. Some basic features of the endogenous factors are shown in Table 39.2, and a simplified representation of their interaction in Figure 39.5. Both endogenous and exogenous fibrinolytic factors have been used clinically to treat venous and arterial thrombosis, with varying degrees of success (see Chapter 47).

Plasminogen and plasmin

PLG is a single-chain glycoprotein zymogen of the serine protease plasmin, which carries out the enzymatic degradation of cross-linked fibrin. Besides its active site serine, plasmin contains five kringle domains, four of which have a lysine-binding site, through which the molecule interacts with lysine residues in its substrates (e.g. fibrin), its activators (e.g. tissue PLG activator and urinary PLG activator) and its inhibitors (principally PLG activation inhibitor type 1). In its native form, it has a glutamic acid residue at its N-terminus and is known as

Glu-PLG. Conversion of PLG to plasmin can proceed via two routes. Most PLG activators (see below) cleave the Arg561–Val562 bond to form Glu-plasmin, a disulphide-linked two-chain molecule. The heavy chain is derived from the N-terminal region and bears the lysine-binding sites, whereas the C-terminal light chain contains the serine active centre. Glu-plasmin, despite being a serine protease, is functionally ineffective as its lysine-binding sites remain masked. It is converted autocatalytically to Lys-plasmin by N-terminal cleavage, chiefly between Lys76 and Lys77, which exposes the lysine-binding sites and thus markedly enhances its interaction with fibrin.

Both Glu- and Lys-plasmin also attack the same Lys76–Lys77 bond in Glu-PLG to form the zymogen Lys-PLG. This binds to fibrin before activation to the protease and is thus brought into close proximity with the physiological PLG activators (which also bind to fibrin) that convert it to Lys-plasmin. As a consequence, the conversion of PLG to plasmin by tPA is enhanced by two to three orders of magnitude; this serves to localize the fibrinolytic response to the fibrin clot, where plasmin is to some extent protected from the effects of circulating antiplasmins, which (as indicated below) would otherwise neutralize plasmin extremely rapidly (< 50 ms). The fact that Lys-PLG is potentially a much more effective agent in fibrinolysis than Glu-PLG is reflected in its half-life, which is around 20 hours compared with 50 hours for the latter.

Action of plasmin on fibrin and fibrinogen

Plasmin can hydrolyse a variety of substrates including FV and FVIII, but its major physiological targets are fibrin and fibrinogen, which are split progressively into a heterogeneous mixture of small soluble peptides (plasmin attacks at least 50 cleavage sites in fibrinogen) known collectively as fibrin degradation products (FDPs). The first stage in the proteolysis of fibrinogen involves the removal of several small peptides (fragments A, B and C) from the C-terminus of the A α-chains, each involving cleavage after a lysine residue. This is rapidly followed by removal of the first 42 amino acids from the N-terminal end of the B β-chain (the Bβ1–42 fragment). The large residual portion, which is known as fragment X, and which still contains fibrinopeptide A, remains thrombin-clottable and will agglutinate some *Staphylococcus* spp. Assay of the Bβ1–42 fragment released from fibrinogen by plasmin gives a sensitive index of fibrinogenolytic activity.

Asymmetrical digestion of all three pairs of chains of fibrin or fibrinogen then occurs with the release of the D fragment, in which the chains remained linked by disulphide bonds. The residue, known as fragment Y, is again attacked by plasmin, cleaving a second fragment D and leaving the disulphide-linked N-terminal ends of all six chains, which are referred to as fragment E. Fragments Y, D and E are not thrombin-clottable and do not agglutinate staphylococci. Their presence can be detected immunologically using an antibody-coated latex bead agglutination assay, which provides a simple test for most FDPs, although carefully prepared serum must be used to prevent cross-reactivity of the antibody with fibrinogen in plasma. These assays detect the degradation products of both fibrin and fibrinogen indiscriminately.

Following thrombin generation and consequent activation of FXIII, intermolecular or intramolecular transamidation of the α- or β-chains by FXIIIa occurs and then the action of plasmin yields characteristic D-dimer, D-dimer–E fragments and oligomers of fragments X and Y (collectively known as cross-linked FDP or XDP), in addition to X, Y, D and E. These XDPs can be detected very simply using monoclonal antibody-coated latex beads. Because the monoclonal antibodies to XDPs do not cross-react with fibrinogen, they can be detected directly in citrated plasma. The presence of D-dimers in blood samples can be used in a clinical algorithm that predicts the likelihood of the presence of venous thrombosis (see Chapter 47).

Furthermore, plasmin-induced cleavage of the N-terminal end of the β-chain of fibrin (the Bβ1–14 fibrinopeptide B fragment having been removed by thrombin) produces a β15–42 fragment, the detection of which indicates fibrin (as opposed to fibrinogen) degradation. Consequently, assays for the Bβ1–42 and β15–42 fragments used in combination may be clinically useful by indicating whether fibrinogen or fibrin has been degraded, and thus whether fibrinolytic activity is primary or secondary to fibrin formation. However, clinically, FDP assays are used to detect DIC, when mixed fibrin/fibrinogen degradation products appear in the circulation.

Plasminogen activators

Tissue plasminogen activator

tPA is a serine protease secreted by endothelial cells. It is not synthesized by the liver or kidney but is found in most extravascular body fluids, including saliva, milk, bile, cerebrospinal fluid and urine. Intravascular tPA is quickly cleared by the liver or inactivated by the fast-acting tPA inhibitor (see below), the half-life of tPA in plasma being approximately 2 min. The resting level of tPA in plasma is around 70 pmol/L, most of which is in an inactive complex with tPA inhibitors (see below).

Several physical and biochemical stimuli, including venous occlusion, strenuous exercise, thrombin, adrenaline and vasopressin or its analogues such as DDAVP (see Chapter 41), markedly increase the rate of tPA release, although its biological activity remains negligible until it becomes bound to fibrin, whereupon its affinity for and action upon PLG is greatly potentiated. The activity of tPA is further enhanced by plasmin itself, which cleaves tPA at Arg275-Ile276 into a two-chain molecule, whose binding sites are exposed, thus enabling it to form a complex with PLG and fibrinogen more readily. The ability of venous occlusion to stimulate tPA release from endothelial cells forms the basis of a test of fibrinolytic activity known as the 'cuff test'.

Both single-chain tPA and the two-chain form possess very little serine protease activity until they bind to fibrin, whereupon tPA affinity for, and activation of, fibrin-bound PLG is increased at least 100-fold. The principal interactions involve binding between the second kringle domain of tPA and lysine residues on the α- and β-chains of fibrin (in particular Lys157 on the α-chain of partly degraded fibrin). This association enhances cleavage of the Arg561–Val562 bond in adjacent PLG molecules, forming active plasmin.

Urinary plasminogen activator

So called because it was first extracted from urine, uPA is synthesized chiefly by the tubules and collecting ducts in the kidney and by fibroblast-like cells in the gastrointestinal tract. It is a serine protease secreted as an inactive single-chain zymogen (prourokinase) that is cleaved by activators in plasma (including kallikrein and plasmin) at Lys158-Ile159 to produce active two-chain uPA. The protease activity of uPA is associated with the heavy chain, which may dissociate from the light chain carrying the PLG-binding site. The isolated heavy chains, which are also known as low-molecular-weight urokinase, are therefore poorer PLG activators than the two-chain form.

uPA cleaves the same Arg561–Val562 bond in PLG as tPA. Although uPA contains a kringle domain, this does not impart high affinity for fibrin and it binds instead (via its EGF-like domain) to its cell-associated receptor. Thus it has been proposed that uPA may be preferentially involved in cellular events (such as differentiation and mitogenesis) rather than with dissolution of fibrin clots.

Exogenous plasminogen activators

These are derived from non-human sources, including animals (e.g. vampire bat saliva and some snake venoms) and certain plants and microorganisms. The best known of these is streptokinase (SK), which is derived from some strains of β-haemolytic streptococci and which has for many years been used, with moderate success, as a fibrinolytic agent for the treatment of life-threatening thrombotic states. SK is a non-enzymatic polypeptide that forms a stable 1:1 complex with PLG, as a result of which the latter undergoes a conformational change, unmasking its serine-active centre. The 'plasmin' that is formed remains associated with SK but can convert free PLG to plasmin.

Inhibitors of fibrinolysis

The plasmin-generating potential of plasma is sufficient to completely degrade all the fibrinogen in the body in a very short period of time. It is prevented from doing so by the PLG activa-

tor inhibitors or PAIs, most of which belong to the serpin family, and by a number of circulating inhibitors of plasmin itself (the antiplasmins).

Inhibitors of plasminogen activation

Plasminogen activator inhibitor type 1

PAI-1 is an important fast-acting serpin inhibitor of tPA, uPA and, to a small extent, plasmin, and is secreted by endothelial cells. It is also found in platelet α-granules. In plasma, it occurs in two forms: a functionally active 'free' form (that is stabilized by association with vitronectin) and as an inactive complex with tPA. Basal PAI-1 concentration in plasma is low at 0.5 nmol/L, of which at least 80% is in complex with tPA or uPA. It follows a diurnal rhythm, with an early morning peak that is around twice that in the late afternoon, and its activity is also increased by heparin. There is growing evidence that elevated levels of PAI-1 are associated with an increased incidence of venous and arterial thrombosis, and there is a suggested association between the early morning peak level of PAI-1 and a higher incidence of myocardial infarction at that time, the extent of this diurnal variation being associated with polymorphisms in the PAI-1 gene (SERPINE1).

The three main profibrinolytic serine proteases (tPA, uPA and plasmin) all cleave the same bond (Arg346–Met347) in the reactive centre loop of PAI-1, and are thus inhibited in the same way as described in the section on AT. PAI-1 binds non-covalently to fibrin, but although it can then complex with and inhibit fibrin-bound tPA (with most of the complexes remaining bound to the fibrin), it does so less effectively than with free tPA. Soluble tPA–PAI-1 complexes are rapidly removed by the liver ($t_{1/2}$ 4 min), as are uPA–PAI-1 complexes that have dissociated from fibrin.

Plasminogen activator inhibitor type 2

This serpin inhibitor of tPA is mainly produced by the placenta and may thus contribute to the inhibition of fibrinolysis that occurs during pregnancy. It is also synthesized in monocytes and epidermal cells, but is not usually found in the plasma of non-pregnant subjects. It is detectable in plasma from about the eighth week of pregnancy, rising to a peak at around 33 weeks and falling only slowly after delivery, the half-life being around 24 hours. Paradoxically, levels are often low in pre-eclampsia due to placental insufficiency. The inhibitory action of PAI-2 involves its Arg380-Thr381 residues and it is more effective against uPA than tPA, although for both the potency is at least 10-fold less than that of PAI-1.

Similarly, other protease inhibitors such as α_1-antitrypsin, C1-esterase inhibitor, α_2-antiplasmin (see below), α_2-microglobulin and protease nexin 1 (one of a group of cell membrane-bound heparin-potentiated serpins) also neutralize tPA, but at a rate that is probably too slow to be of physiological significance. However, α_2-microglobulin is thought to be the major inhibitor of the SK–PLG complex.

Inhibitors of plasmin

As they do with thrombin and tPA, a number of the broad-spectrum inhibitors contribute to neutralization of plasmin. By far the most potent plasmin inhibitor is the serpin α_2-antiplasmin, a single-chain glycoprotein synthesized by the liver, which has a half-life of about 60 hours and shows considerable sequence identity with AT and α_1-antitrypsin. Its physiological importance is supported by the fact that a congenital deficiency (known as Miyasato disease) is associated with a clinically significant bleeding disorder due to uncontrolled fibrinolytic activity, and that levels are reduced in DIC and during thrombolytic therapy.

α_2-Antiplasmin

This serpin is the predominant plasmin inhibitor. It forms a stable 1:1 complex with plasmin, in which the protease is completely inactivated. The reaction appears to involve the cleavage by plasmin of a specific Leu–Met bond in the inhibitor, exposing the reactive loop Arg364–Met365 peptide bond to the serine active centre on the light chain of plasmin. Plasmin-modified α_2-antiplasmin can also bind to native Glu-PLG and to fibrin, the latter reaction being mediated by FXIIIa-mediated cross-linking. Thus, in addition to inactivating preformed plasmin, α_2-antiplasmin retards fibrinolysis by reducing PLG activation and by 'masking' the lysine-binding sites through which plasmin(ogen) interacts with fibrin. However, these subsidiary mechanisms for inhibiting fibrinolysis are to some extent overcome by any Lys-plasmin(ogen) present, which has a higher affinity than Glu-PLG for fibrin, and is thus less susceptible to the action of α_2-antiplasmin.

In plasma (as opposed to on fibrin strands), although the concentration of PLG ($\sim 2\,\mu$mol/L) exceeds that of α_2-antiplasmin ($\sim 1\,\mu$mol/L), basal fibrinogenolytic activity is minimal because the tiny amounts of plasmin normally generated under physiological conditions are rapidly neutralized by the inhibitor. However, in certain pathological conditions (e.g. obstetric emergencies or snake bite) where extreme activation of fibrinolysis occurs, the latter may be swamped. Under these circumstances, other inhibitors, in particular α_2-microglobulin and histidine-rich glycoprotein, may become clinically important. The action of α_2-microglobulin on plasmin is similar to its effect on thrombin. Following the plasmin-induced cleavage of a specific Arg–Leu bond in the inhibitor, the latter forms a 1:1 complex with the light chain of plasmin. The serine active site of plasmin is not involved and the complex retains weak biological activity, albeit only briefly, until it is removed in the liver. Histidine-rich glycoprotein inhibits fibrinolysis by blocking the lysine-binding sites of PLG, thus preventing its interaction with fibrinogen.

Lipoprotein A

The protein portion of lipoprotein A is termed apo(a). It is synthesized in the liver and circulates in plasma. There is considerable structural homology with PLG, as it possesses both serine protease and kringle domains. It can compete with PLG for binding sites on fibrin(ogen) or tPA, and may also increase PAI-1 expression, both actions potentially inhibiting fibrinolysis. That lipoprotein A has some clinical importance is indicated by the finding that raised levels are associated with an increased incidence of thrombosis.

Thrombin-activated fibrinolytic inhibitor

In the presence of thrombomodulin, thrombin activates carboxypeptidase B, also called TAFI, and TAFIa in turn inhibits fibrinolysis; this provides another link between coagulation and the fibrinolytic pathway. TAFI removes the C-terminal lysine residues formed by limited plasmin proteolysis of fibrin, removing the binding sites for PLG and tPA. Thus the fibrin cofactor function in PLG activation is reduced, downregulating fibrinolysis. Mice with TAFI knockout have defective wound repair, and data from backcrossing against heterozygous PLG-deficient mice showed that TAFI modulates both fibrinolysis and cell migration *in vivo*.

Selected bibliography

Aird WC (2003) Endothelial cell heterogeneity. *Critical Care Medicine* **31**: S221–S230.

Bajaj MS, Birktoft JJ, Steer SA *et al.* (2001) Structure and biology of tissue factor pathway inhibitor. *Thrombosis and Haemostasis* **86**: 959–72.

Bouma BN, Meijers, JC (2003) Thrombin-activatable fibrinolysis inhibitor (TAFI, plasma procarboxypeptidase B, procarboxypeptidase R, procarboxypeptidase U). *Journal of Thrombosis and Haemostasis* **1**: 1566–74.

Caen J, Wu Q (2010) Hageman factor, platelets and polyphosphates: early history and recent connection. *Journal of Thrombosis and Haemostasis* **8**: 1670–4.

Colman RW (1999) Biologic activities of the contact factors *in vivo* potentiation of hypotension, inflammation, and fibrinolysis, and inhibition of cell adhesion, angiogenesis and thrombosis. *Thrombosis and Haemostasis* **82**: 1568–77.

Dahlback B, Villoutreix BO (2003) Molecular recognition in the protein C anticoagulant pathway. *Journal of Thrombosis and Haemostasis* **1**: 1525–34.

Esmon CT (2000) The endothelial cell protein C receptor. *Thrombosis and Haemostasis* **83**: 639–43.

Gomez K, McVey JH, Tuddenham EG (2005) Inhibition of coagulation by macromolecular complexes. *Haematologica* **90**: 1570–6.

Huntington JA (2003) Mechanisms of glycosaminoglycan activation of the serpins in hemostasis. *Journal of Thrombosis and Haemostasis* **1**: 1535–49.

Morrissey JH (2001) Tissue factor: an enzyme cofactor and a true receptor. *Thrombosis and Haemostasis* **86**: 66–74.

Ngo JC, Huang M, Roth DA, Furie BC, Furie B (2008) Crystal structure of human factor VIII: implications for the formation of the factor IXa–factor VIIIa complex. *Structure* **16**: 597–606.

Ruggeri ZM (2003) Von Willebrand factor, platelets and endothelial cell interactions. *Journal of Thrombosis and Haemostasis* **1**: 1335–42.

Saenko EL, Ananyeva NM, Tuddenham EG *et al.* (2002) Factor VIII: novel insights into form and function. *British Journal of Haematology* **119**: 323–31.

Schmaier AH (2000) Plasma kallikrein/kinin system: a revised hypothesis for its activation and its physiologic contributions. *Current Opinion in Hematology* **7**: 261–5.

Shen BW, Spiegel PC, Chang CH *et al.* (2008) The tertiary structure and domain organization of coagulation factor VIII. *Blood* **111**: 1240–7.

Weiler H, Isermann BH (2003) Thrombomodulin. *Journal of Thrombosis and Haemostasis* **1**: 1515–24.

CHAPTER 40

The vascular function of platelets

Stephen P Watson[1] and Paul Harrison[2]

[1]Centre for Cardiovascular Sciences, Institute for Biomedical Research, College of Medical and Dental Sciences, University of Birmingham, Birmingham, UK
[2]Oxford Haemophilia and Thrombosis Centre, The Churchill Hospital, Oxford, UK

Introduction

Platelets are small anucleate cells that play a critical role in haemostasis and thrombosis. Platelets ordinarily circulate in the bloodstream in a quiescent state but undergo 'explosive' activation following damage to the vessel wall, leading to the rapid formation of a platelet aggregate or vascular plug and occlusion of the site of damage. From a pragmatic viewpoint, the more rapid that vascular plug formation occurs, the lower the amount of blood that is lost. To facilitate a rapid response, platelets are enriched in signalling proteins and surface receptors, and activation is associated with the generation of the positive feedback or amplification mediators ADP and thromboxane (Tx)A$_2$, and release of the adhesion proteins fibrinogen and von Willebrand factor (VWF), which support aggregate formation and the generation of thrombin through the coagulation cascade. The importance of platelets in haemostasis is illustrated by the excessive bleeding associated with defects in platelet function or platelet number. On the other hand, the activation of platelets in diseased blood vessels (e.g. at sites of plaque rupture) can lead to arterial thrombotic disorders such as stroke and myocardial infarction, two of the major causes of morbidity and mortality in the Western world.

It is essential that platelets circulate in the bloodstream in a quiescent state but that they undergo rapid activation as and when necessary. To achieve this balance, endothelial cells constitutively release nitric oxide (NO) and generate prostacyclin to inhibit platelet activation through elevation of the cyclic nucleotides cGMP and cAMP, respectively. In addition, endothelial cells express the ecto-ADPase CD39, which removes the feedback mediator ADP, and thrombomodulin, which converts the procoagulant action of thrombin to an anticoagulant action. Under normal circumstances, platelets are unable to form stable contacts on endothelial cells, but this can occur on diseased or activated endothelial cells or at sites of disturbed flow, including arterial bifurcations where plaques are commonly formed. Adhesion of platelets to endothelial cells promotes local inflammatory events that can initiate plaque formation, endothelial activation and damage. Lesions in the endothelial layer lead to exposure of subendothelial matrix proteins, particularly collagens and membrane surface-expressed tissue factor, which can initiate powerful platelet activation and coagulation, respectively.

Platelets have a wider role than solely supporting platelet aggregation (Figure 40.1). Platelet dense granules and α-granules are packed with a rich diversity of small molecules and proteins that play fundamental roles in many aspects of haemostasis, including vessel constriction, leucocyte recruitment and vessel repair. The ability to release such a diverse library of biological molecules may reflect the evolutionary relationship of the platelet to the haemocyte in lower organisms, which is

Postgraduate Haematology: 6th edition. Edited by A. Victor Hoffbrand, Daniel Catovsky, Edward G.D. Tuddenham, Anthony R. Green
© 2011 Blackwell Publishing Ltd.

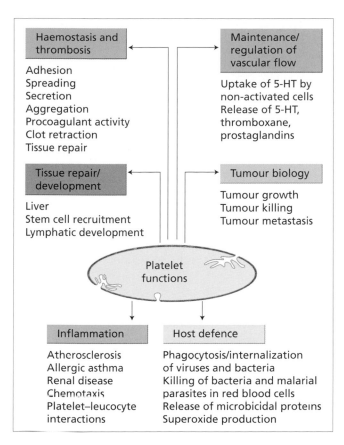

Figure 40.1 Functional roles of the platelet in the vasculature.

involved in both the innate defence system and the prevention of excessive blood loss. In higher organisms, two distinct sets of cells perform these functions, namely thrombocytes (or platelets) and leucocytes, and of course the function of the platelet has evolved to prevent excessive blood loss in a high-pressure arterial system. The contribution of platelets to many vascular responses is an area that is gaining increasing recognition, but one that is challenging to investigate because many mediators are released from other vascular cells.

Platelets are a major target in the treatment of individuals at risk of thrombosis. However, careful consideration is required as to whether a patient should receive antiplatelet therapy and for how long, bearing in mind that such treatment always carries a risk of increased bleeding. For the majority of individuals receiving the orally active antiplatelet drugs aspirin or clopidogrel this risk is extremely low, but it is not zero. In this context, the increasing tendency of otherwise healthy passengers to take aspirin as an antiplatelet therapy in long-haul flights should be viewed with concern as the major risk is venous thrombosis, which is minimally inhibited by treatment with aspirin. The small increase in risk of bleeding may therefore exceed any potential benefit.

The decision on whether a patient should receive antiplatelet therapy is based on the net sum of risk factors for arterial thrombosis, such as age, stress, weight, sex, lifestyle, cholesterol level, blood pressure, smoking and previous thrombotic history, and the potential risk from excessive bleeding. It is now accepted that individuals judged to be at medium to high risk of thrombosis should receive some form of antiplatelet therapy (unless otherwise contraindicated), usually low-dose aspirin or clopidogrel, and nearly always in combination with other treatments such as statins and blood pressure-lowering drugs. There is also a small but significant advantage in using clopidogrel and aspirin in combination for the treatment of patients at high risk of thrombosis, although this also leads to an increase in significant bleeds. Stronger inhibitors of platelet function, namely blockers of the major platelet integrin $\alpha_{IIb}\beta_3$, are used only in acute situations of thrombotic risk in the clinic, for example in cases of unstable angina or angioplasty and stenting, because of their narrow therapeutic window.

The aim of this short review is to describe the features of platelets that enable them to perform their physiological roles in the vasculature. More extensive information on all aspects of platelet function in health and disease can be found in the second edition of the excellent textbook *Platelets*, edited by Alan Michelson.

Platelet structure and organelles

Platelets have several unique features that enable them to efficiently perform their primary function, namely the rapid formation of a vascular plug following vessel injury. Platelets are extremely small and discoid in shape, with dimensions in the human of approximately $3.0 \times 0.5\,\mu m$ and a mean volume of 7–11 fL. This shape and small size enables platelets to be 'marginated' by the red blood cells to the edge of the vessel, placing them next to the endothelial cells and therefore in the correct position to respond to vascular damage. Platelets are abundant in the circulation, with numbers in humans usually in the range $150–400 \times 10^9$/L. This relatively high count represents a considerable degree of redundancy, as individuals with platelet counts as low as 20×10^9/L often exhibit only occasional major spontaneous bleeds, although they are at increased risk of excessive bleeding during major trauma and surgery.

The discoid shape of the platelet is formed by the platelet cytoskeleton, which consists of a spectrin-based membrane skeleton, circumferential bands of a single microtubule that lie beneath the plasma membrane and a rigid actin filament network that fills the cytoplasm of the cell. The disc shape is not essential for platelet function as mouse platelets that lack β_1-tubulin, the major component of the microtubules, are spherical and yet undergo normal aggregation and secretion. The rigid structure and platelet strength is supported by 2 million copies of actin per platelet, of which approximately 40% in a non-stimulated cell are assembled into actin polymers. These polymers connect with each other and with the cyosolic tail of the membrane glycoprotein (GP)Ibα via filamin in a lattice-like structure that gives the platelet its discoid shape.

Platelets lack a nucleus, which is consistent with their short lifespan of 10 days and their acute role in haemostasis. Platelets exhibit a very limited and specific degree of protein synthesis, as the result of residual mRNA that has been carried over from their precursor cell, the megakaryocyte, although interestingly the number of platelet/megakaryocyte genes is higher than any other blood cell lineage. However, although there is little historical evidence to suggest that the general capacity to synthesize new proteins is of major relevance, more recent evidence suggests that activated platelets can synthesize a small number of key proteins that may be of functional significance. The presence of low levels of platelet mRNA also provides an opportunity to perform a limited number of genetic studies, although concern over contamination from nucleated cells, which express several orders of magnitude higher levels of mRNA, necessitates the need for direct confirmation of protein expression. Potentially, many of these issues can be addressed at the level of the platelet precursor cell, the megakaryocyte, but these are present at low copy number in bone marrow and access to tissue is a problem particularly in humans. Despite these concerns, the application of both genomic and proteomic approaches have given an unprecedented insight into the protein composition of the platelet, although the challenge remains to identify the function and interplay of the key proteins, as many may be vestigial or have been carried over from the megakaryocyte.

Platelets contain four main types of storage granule, dense granules, α-granules, lysosomes and peroxisomes, although the significance of the latter two is unclear. There are between five and nine dense granules in platelets and these contain high levels of ADP, ATP, polyphosphates, 5-hydroxtryptamine (5-HT; also known as serotonin) and Ca^{2+}. There are about 80 α-granules per platelet and these contain a rich diversity of proteins and membrane receptors that support haemostasis, vascular repair, inflammation and host defence (Table 40.1). Many of these proteins are made *de novo* in the megakaryocyte, such as platelet factor (PF)4 and VWF, whereas others are taken up from the plasma by receptor-mediated endocytosis, including fibrinogen. The major components of α-granules include fibrinogen and VWF, which support platelet adhesion and aggregation; factor (F)V, protein S and tissue factor pathway inhibitor (TFPI), which play key roles in regulating coagulation and fibrinolysis; the chemokines SDF-1α, PF4, β-thromboglobulin, ENA-78 and RANTES, which attract haemopoietic stem cells and leucocytes; and the growth factors platelet-derived growth factor (PDGF) and vascular endothelial growth factor (VEGF) A and C, which support vessel repair and angiogenesis. Platelet α-granules also express key transmembrane proteins that become exposed on fusion with the plasma membrane and support platelet aggregate formation and leucocyte recruitment, including the major platelet integrin $\alpha_{IIb}\beta_3$, P-selectin (CD62) and CD40L. The expression of

Table 40.1 Platelet α-granule constituents.

Physiological role	Constituent
Angiogenesis	VEGF-A, VEGF-C, PDGF
Antibodies	IgG
Coagulation cascade	Factor V, fibrinogen, tissue factor pathway inhibitor
Endothelial cell activation	TGF-β
Fibrinolysis	Plasminogen, PAI-1, α_2-antiplasmin
Growth factors	PDGF, FGF, HGF, IGF-1, EGF
Leucocyte recruitment	Chemokines: PF4, RANTES, β-thromboglobulin, ENA-78, SDF-1α
Matrix breakdown	Hydrolytic enzymes MMP-2, MMP-9
Membrane proteins	$\alpha_{IIb}\beta_3$, P-selectin, CD40L
Bacterial killing	Microbicidal proteins
Miscellaneous	Amyloid β-protein precursor, Gas6
Proteases	Protease nexin II
Platelet aggregation	Fibrinogen, fibronectin, VWF
Irreversible aggregation	Thrombospondin (locks fibrinogen bridges between $\alpha_{IIb}\beta_3$)

Examples of platelet α-granule constituents and their physiological roles are shown. Several other molecules have also been reported to be present in α-granules and to be released on activation.

P-selectin is used to monitor platelet α-granule secretion by flow cytometry.

Platelets are enriched in signalling proteins, which facilitate the rapid switch from quiescence to activation, and have a high cytoskeletal protein content that gives rise to the dramatic changes in morphology and which enables the platelet aggregate or thrombus to withstand the very high shear forces that exist in the arteriolar system. Platelets have a network of intracellular membranes known as the dense tubular system (part of the endoplasmic reticulum) that release intracellular Ca^{2+} in response to the second messenger inositol 1,4,5-trisphosphate (IP3). Platelets have a network of invaginations of the surface membrane, known as the surface-connected canalicular system, which increase the surface area of the plasma membrane during platelet spreading and thereby provide more sites for release of intracellular granules. The surface-connected canalicular system also gives rise to membrane tethers that play a vital role in supporting adhesion. Platelets contain several mitrochondria that generate energy during their short lifespan.

Animal models

Genetically modified mice and other organisms, notably zebrafish, are being increasingly used to address the *in vitro* and *in vivo* function of specific genes and proteins in platelets (and thrombocytes), but with the caveat of a number of differences to human platelets with regard to rheology and protein composition. For example, the mouse genome lacks the gene for the only Fc receptor found on human platelets, FcγRIIA, and mouse platelets do not express one of the major receptors for thrombin on human platelets, PAR-1. There are also important differences in participation of protein isotypes in signalling cascades and various responses. Moreover, the relevance of many of the *in vivo* models (such as tail bleeds and vessel wall injury by ferric chloride or laser ablation) to haemostasis and thrombosis in humans is uncertain and fails to mimic the conditions that give rise to arterial thrombosis, which typically occurs on ruptured atherosclerotic plaques. Nevertheless, despite these concerns, the processes that govern platelet activation in mice and other species appear to be shared with humans, and the value of animal models in analysing platelet activation and *in vivo* haemostasis and thrombosis, and thereby establishing a foundation for ongoing and future clinical trials, is immense.

Platelet formation

Platelets are formed from megakaryocytes, one of the largest cells in the bone marrow, reaching more than 50 μm in diameter. The nucleus of the megakaryocyte undergoes a process known as endomitosis that involves nuclear replication without cellular division, giving rise to DNA ploidy values that range from 4n to 128n. The reason why endomitosis occurs is not fully understood, but it may simply reflect the need to increase the DNA content to enable the cell to expand its protein synthetic capacity to generate 2000–3000 platelets per megakaryocyte. In addition, it allows cell growth and differentiation to occur without interruption by nuclear and cell divisions.

The differentiation of bone marrow progenitor cells into megakaryocytes is regulated by the cytokine thrombopoietin (TPO), which was first identified in the mid 1990s. The TPO receptor, c-Mpl, expressed on stem cells, megakaryocytes and platelets, signals via the JAK/STAT family of kinases and transcription factors, respectively. An acquired mutation in JAK2 (valine to phenylalanine residue at position 617) leads to an increase in JAK2 activity and accounts for approximately 50% of patients with essential thrombocythaemia and almost 100% of patients with polycythaemia vera, which are associated with an increase in either platelet or red blood cell counts respectively. The same mutation also underlies myelofibrosis, which often occurs as a late-stage progression of these two myeloproliferative disorders. TPO is synthesized at a constant rate in the liver and its circulating free levels are largely controlled by binding and internalization mediated through c-Mpl on the platelet surface. This provides a simple and elegant means of tightly controlling the platelet count. Thus, if the platelet count decreases, the free level of TPO rises and there is an increase in

megakaryocytopoiesis and platelet formation. Two TPO mimetics (eltrombopag and romiplostim) have recently entered clinical use for treatment of immune thrombocytopenia.

One of the outstanding questions in this field over the years has been the events underlying platelet formation. There is now a growing consensus that megakaryocyte differentiation occurs in a defined compartment of the bone marrow known as the osteoblastic niche and that megakaryocytes subsequently migrate and adhere to sinusoidal endothelial cells through a process that is regulated by the chemokine SDF-1α and its receptor CXCR4. At this vascular niche, the megakaryocytes generate long thin processes known as proplatelets, which form platelets at their terminals. The proplatelet arms protrude between bone marrow sinusoidal endothelial cells and release platelets directly into the bloodstream. This carefully orchestrated process ensures that platelets are not released into the bone marrow. Megakaryocytes also undergo chemotaxis into the bloodstream where they can also form platelets. Dynamic visualization of the events underlying thrombopoiesis within bone marrow has recently been captured *in vivo* by Junt and colleagues. To maintain a normal platelet count, approximately 1 million new platelets are released into the blood every second but this can dramatically increase by a factor of 10 in severe haemorrhage.

Thrombus formation

The events that underlie platelet adhesion and aggregation, and which eventually lead to thrombus formation, at the intermediate to high rates of shear (1000–5000/s) of the arteriolar system are discussed below and depicted in Figure 40.2.

Platelet capture and stable adhesion

The initial event that takes place on damage to the vasculature is the tethering or capture of platelets through the interaction of VWF with the GPIb–IX–V complex. VWF and GPIb do not interact unless a conformational change is induced in VWF as a consequence of its binding to collagen and/or elevated shear. The fast on-rate of association between VWF and GPIbα enables binding to take place at the intermediate to high shear forces of the arteriolar system. However, a fast off-rate of association means that this interaction alone is not sufficient to give rise to rapid stable adhesion. Thus, platelets translocate in the direction of flow on a surface of VWF or when they first come into contact with a damaged vessel wall. Application of high-resolution imaging technology has revealed that most platelets translocate in a stop–start manner through sliding rather than rolling and thus this serves to minimize the drag forces on adhesive bonds. Furthermore, the capture of platelets is facilitated by the formation of membrane tethers, thin processes of lipid bilayer that are pulled away from the platelet

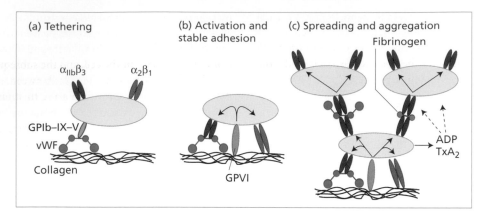

Figure 40.2 Thrombus formation at arteriolar rates of shear. Platelets are tethered by VWF bound to immobilized collagen, which then activates the low-affinity receptor GPVI leading to activation of integrins $\alpha_{IIb}\beta_3$ and $\alpha_2\beta_1$, which bind to VWF/fibrinogen and collagen, respectively. This mediates stable adhesion and further activation of GPVI. The signals from GPVI and the two platelet integrins induce spreading of platelets on the matrix and release of the feedback messengers ADP and TxA$_2$. VWF and fibrinogen, in combination with ADP, TxA$_2$ and thrombin, mediate thrombus formation (aggregation) and stabilization (clot retraction). The formation of a procoagulant surface also supports formation of thrombin (not shown).

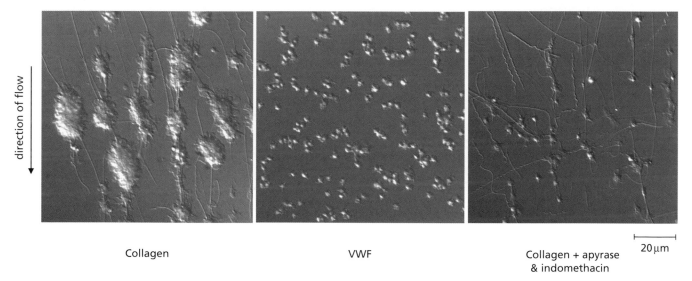

direction of flow

Collagen

VWF

Collagen + apyrase & indomethacin

20 μm

Figure 40.3 Platelet adhesion and aggregation at arteriolar shear. Human blood, anticoagulated with 40 μmol/L P-PACK, was flowed over collagen or VWF at a shear rate of 1000/s for 4 min and rinsed with Tyrode buffer for 5 min. Differential interference contrast images of adherent platelets were recorded. Where indicated, blood was pretreated with indomethacin (10 μmol/L) and apyrase (5 U/mL) to reduce the secondary mediators, TxA$_2$ and ADP respectively, prior to flow.

surface under the influence of haemodynamic force. These highly dynamic structures can extend as far as 30 μm in length, or ten times the size of a platelet, with much of their length being derived from the surface-connected canalicular system. The formation of membrane tethers helps to sustain adhesion within high-shear environments by minimizing the drag on captured platelets.

The conversion to stable adhesion is primarily dependent on activation of β_1 and β_3 integrins by other receptors, most notably the collagen receptor GPVI and vessel wall-generated thrombin. This transition can be readily demonstrated *in vitro* by comparing adhesion and aggregate formation when blood flows over immobilized VWF or collagen, as illustrated by the static records shown in Figure 40.3. The majority of platelets translocate on a surface of VWF and form small stable aggregates only after several minutes, presumably as a result of weak activation of platelet integrins by GPIb–IX–V. In comparison, platelets undergo rapid stable adhesion and form large aggregates on collagen. This process is critically dependent on the binding of plasma-derived VWF to collagen through its A3 domain, unmasking the binding site for GPIb within the VWF A1 domain, and the release of the positive feedback mediators ADP and TxA_2. Dynamic imaging is required to observe this train of events in full.

The integrins that mediate stable adhesion on collagen are $\alpha_{IIb}\beta_3$ (GPIIb/IIIa) and $\alpha_2\beta_1$ (GPIa/IIa), which bind to immobilized VWF and collagen, respectively. The role of $\alpha_2\beta_1$ in this process is masked by the 50 times higher level of $\alpha_{IIb}\beta_3$, which is expressed at approximately 80 000 copies per platelet, with a further 40 000 copies on intracellular α-granules that become exposed on activation. Platelets express three other integrins that have the potential to mediate stable adhesion *in vivo*, $\alpha_5\beta_1$, $\alpha_6\beta_1$ and $\alpha_v\beta_3$, which bind to fibronectin, laminin and vitronectin, respectively. The two β_1 integrins are expressed at 1000 copies per platelet and $\alpha_v\beta_3$ at a tenfold lower level, and therefore their actions are also masked by the much greater level of $\alpha_{IIb}\beta_3$.

The capture and recruitment of circulating platelets onto a growing aggregate occurs in a similar way but in this case β_1 and β_3 integrin activation is mediated by the release of ADP and TxA_2, and the local formation of thrombin. Binding of VWF to integrin $\alpha_{IIb}\beta_3$ on the surface of activated platelets mediates tethering of non-activated platelets through GPIb–IX–V. High-resolution imaging studies have revealed that the initial stage involves discoid-shaped platelets and is reversible and independent of ADP and TxA_2. This initial phase therefore serves to recruit platelets into the growing aggregate. This is followed by an irreversible phase that is associated with a marked change in platelet morphology and platelet activation, and which is dependent on released secondary mediators and localized thrombin formation.

There are important differences in the mechanisms that give rise to adhesion and aggregation at the low and very high rates of shear found in the venous system and in stenosed arteries, respectively. At the relatively low flow that exists in venules and larger veins, which generate shear forces of less than 500/s, platelets are able to adhere directly to exposed subendothelial matrix proteins and undergo stable adhesion independent of VWF and GPIb–IX–V, although this interaction is thought to contribute to this response. Release of secondary mediators and generation of thrombin is also sufficient to enable aggregate growth to occur independent of VWF and GPIb–IX–V. At shear rates of 10 000/s and above, which are found in stenosed vessels, adhesion and aggregation are mediated entirely by the interaction of soluble and immobilized VWF with GPIb–IX–V, and are independent of platelet activation and integrin $\alpha_{IIb}\beta_3$.

Spreading

Platelets undergo a characteristic set of morphological changes on contact with a surface, known collectively as spreading, the pattern of which is agonist dependent, as illustrated in Figure 40.4. Initial shape change or rounding is followed by the generation of finger-like projections known as filopodia, which grow from the periphery of the cell, and the subsequent formation of lamellipodia, which fill in the areas between adjacent filopodia. Actin–myosin stress fibres then serve to strengthen the spread platelets. As these events proceed, granules and organelles are squeezed into the centre of the cell, resulting in a characteristic 'fried egg' appearance. These dramatic changes in morphology are brought about by a powerful severing and reassembly of the actin cytoskeleton. The spreading of platelets and formation of stress fibres helps to secure the platelet and thrombus against the flow and shear forces of the vascular system.

Granule secretion and TxA_2 formation

The secretion of ADP from dense granules and the *de novo* generation of TxA_2 from arachidonic acid, liberated by the action of cytosolic phospholipase (PL)A_2, play a critical feedback role in mediating platelet activation. In nearly all cases, activation of platelets by low concentrations of agonists is potentiated by the release of the two feedback agonists, and only high concentrations of powerful stimulants such as thrombin are able to induce full aggregation (measured in a Born aggregometer) in the presence of inhibitors of the two feedback stimuli. The major physiological role of the two feedback mediators, along with thrombin, is to generate a platelet aggregate on the monolayer of cells that have adhered to subendothelial collagen (see Figure 40.3).

Secretion from platelet α-granules usually occurs concomitantly with that from dense granules, although there is evidence for subtle differences in their regulation. The α-granules contain a wide variety of protein constituents that play various roles in haemostasis, host defence and wound repair, including VWF and fibrinogen, which together with their plasma counterparts support aggregate formation. Fusion of α-granules with the platelet plasma membrane has the potential to increase the expression of $\alpha_{IIb}\beta_3$ to over 120 000 copies per platelet. This is of relevance in the use of membrane-impermeable $\alpha_{IIb}\beta_3$ blockers, as these can only reach α-granule-localized integrin following degranulation or through internalization. Fusion of α-granules also leads to expression of P-selectin on the platelet surface, which is the major ligand for P-selectin glycoprotein ligand (PSGL)-1 on circulating tissue factor-rich microparticles and leucocytes. The capture of microparticles provides a mechanism for further activation of the coagulation cascade on a growing thrombus, while binding to leucocytes contributes to inflammatory events at the vessel wall.

Aggregation

Aggregation is the specific term used for the cross-linking of activated platelets through binding of bivalent or multivalent

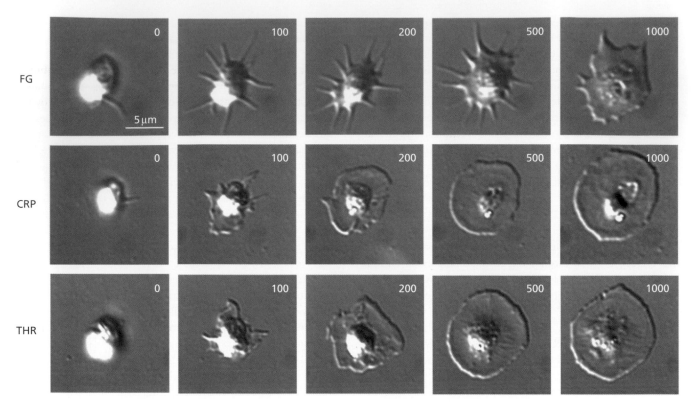

Figure 40.4 Distinct morphological changes in washed human platelets exposed to fibrinogen (FG), collagen-related peptide (CRP) or thrombin (THR). Representative morphology of a single platelet on each surface at specific time points (seconds) are shown. (From Thornber K, McCarty OJ, Watson SP, Pears CJ (2006) Distinct but critical roles for integrin αIIbβ3 in platelet lamellipodia formation on fibrinogen, collagen-related peptide and thrombin. *FEBS Journal* **273**: 5032–5043 with permission.)

ligands to integrin $\alpha_{IIb}\beta_3$. It should not be confused with agglutination, which refers to the passive cross-linking of non-activated platelets. The latter describes the response to high concentrations of the antibiotic ristocetin for example, which induces cross-linking of VWF to GPIb–IX–V. Ristocetin is used in the clinical testing laboratory to investigate possible defects or gain-of-function mutations in either plasma VWF or GPIb.

The integrin $\alpha_{IIb}\beta_3$ is present in a low-affinity form on non-stimulated platelets but undergoes a conformational change to a high-affinity form in response to 'inside-out' signals. The subsequent binding of bivalent ligands to platelets mediates platelet aggregation and adhesion. In turn, these interactions lead to clustering of $\alpha_{IIb}\beta_3$ on the platelet surface and the generation of 'outside-in' signals that regulate actin polymerization (and therefore platelet spreading) and other responses in synergy with other platelet receptors.

Fibrinogen, VWF and fibronectin have similar affinities for integrin $\alpha_{IIb}\beta_3$ but under low shear conditions, fibrinogen is considered to be the major ligand because of its much higher concentration in plasma. On the other hand, as discussed above, the importance of the interaction of VWF with integrin $\alpha_{IIb}\beta_3$ increases with shear. For many years the role of fibronectin in

supporting aggregation was considered to be minor, in part because standard Born aggregation assays are not altered in the absence of the matrix protein. However, more recent studies in fibronectin-deficient mice and in *in vitro* flow assays have emphasized an important, albeit poorly understood, role for fibronectin in the initiation, growth and stabilization of platelet aggregates. Indeed, the importance of fibronectin may be related to its ability to bind to additional proteins such as fibrinogen and thrombospondin, and in this way contributes to the stability of the platelet aggregate. Overall, however, we have a relatively poor understanding of the interplay between fibrinogen, VWF and fibronectin, and are still unable to explain why a combination of $\alpha_{IIb}\beta_3$ ligands is more effective in supporting aggregation and thrombus formation.

Thrombus stabilization

There is increasing recognition of the significance of so-called 'late events' that help to stabilize the platelet aggregate or thrombus in the high shear environment of the arterial circulation. These events involve remodelling of the actin cytoskeleton and the interaction of several platelet membrane proteins with themselves or with each other. The affinity of the latter interactions is low and so these only occur when platelets are brought into close contact with each other.

The ability of blood clots to retract over a course of minutes to hours has been known for over 200 years and is termed clot retraction. The platelets are the force-generating components of this response, with integrin $\alpha_{IIb}\beta_3$ playing a fundamental role both by linking cytoplasmic actin filaments to surface-bound fibrin polymers and by generating intracellular signals that, together with those from other receptors, enable myosin to serve as a motor and drive the process. A novel actin-dependent, but fibrin-independent, mechanism of retraction has been recently described that brings newly captured platelets into the aggregate and presumably also strengthens the aggregate by reducing the shear forces at the aggregate edge.

Through the work of Brass and others, it is now recognized that the aggregate is consolidated by the binding of a number of platelet membrane proteins to themselves (homophilic interactions) or to other surface receptors on adjacent platelets (heterophilic interactions). Examples of such interactions include the binding of ephrins and Eph kinases to each other, the homophilic binding of PECAM-1, the interaction of the immunoglobulins, JAM-A, JAM-C, ESAM and CD226 with each other and possibly other ligands, and the binding of semaphorin 4D with its ligand plexin-B1. Studies using blocking antibodies and mutant mice have provided evidence that these interactions contribute to the stability of the thrombus, although in many cases it is unclear if this is through the generation of intracellular signals or by strengthening platelet–platelet interaction. There is also evidence that some of these interactions inhibit aggregate growth, such as those involving PECAM-1 and ESAM, and it is possible that these help to limit the degree of thrombus formation.

Many of the adhesion proteins that mediate platelet formation become shed during activation, including GPVI, GPIbα, GPV, P-selectin, and semaphorin 4D, and potentially this may serve to limit thrombus growth. On the other hand, in the case of CD40L, which becomes exposed on platelet activation, there is evidence that its shedding and subsequent binding to integrin $\alpha_{IIb}\beta_3$ via a KGD motif stabilizes thrombus formation.

Further research is urgently required to establish the contribution of many of these interactions and events to thrombus formation.

Procoagulant activity

The classic cascade model of blood coagulation has been replaced by a cell-based model of haemostasis in which coagulation takes place on different surfaces, in overlapping steps – initiation, amplification and propagation – such that thrombin is generated at the very sites that it is required. Activated platelets provide a negatively charged phospholipid surface for the assembly of two multiprotein complexes that form part of the intrinsic and amplication pathway of coagulation, namely

the tenase and prothrombinase complexes. A complex of FIXa and FVIIIa on the negatively charged lipid surface converts FX to FXa (tenase complex), which in turn forms a complex with FVa on the same surface to efficiently convert prothrombin to thrombin (prothrombinase complex). In this way, a large amount of thrombin is generated in the vicinity of the growing aggregate that serves to enhance platelet activation and convert fibrinogen to fibrin.

The platelet procoagulant response, which is mediated by exposure of phosphatidylserine, is elicited only by very powerful platelet agonists or combinations of agonists, and requires sustained entry of Ca^{2+} across the plasma membrane. However, the molecular basis of this response awaits identification of the 'scramblase' that promotes translocation of phosphatidylserine to the outer leaflet. Five patients have been described with a mild bleeding disorder linked to defective procoagulant activity, a condition known as Scott syndrome, and this provides evidence that this pathway plays an important role in thrombus formation, although the identification of further patients is required to consolidate this. Procoagulant activity can be monitored by flow cytometry in the presence of external Ca^{2+} through the binding of fluorescently labelled annexin A5, FXa and other ligands.

The activation of platelets by powerful agonists and entry of Ca^{2+} is associated with formation of microparticles and these too have been proposed as providing a massive increase in the surface area for binding of the tenase and prothrombinase complexes. However, although microparticles are a highly active area of research in the context of thrombotic disorders, it is one that is severely hampered by technical limitations due to their small size and heterogeneity, especially as microparticles are also formed by other blood cells, including leucocytes and megakaryocytes.

Stimulatory receptors and their signalling pathways

The major physiological agonists that mediate platelet activation can be divided according to whether they signal primarily through single transmembrane proteins that regulate Src and Syk family tyrosine kinases or via seven-transmembrane-spanning proteins that are coupled to heterotrimeric G proteins. The former group includes the adhesion molecules collagen, VWF and fibrinogen, and the latter the so-called 'soluble' agonists thrombin, ADP and TxA_2 (Figure 40.5).

The collagen receptor GPVI is the most powerful of the adhesion receptors, signalling through tyrosine phosphorylation of an immunoreceptor tyrosine-based activation motif (ITAM) in its associated FcR γ-chain, leading to formation of an LAT signalosome and activation of PLCγ2. Integrin $\alpha_{IIb}\beta_3$ and GPIb–IX–V generate much weaker signals independent of LAT that

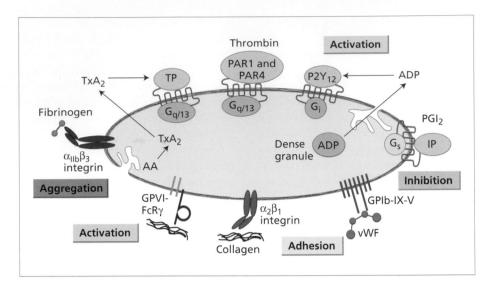

Figure 40.5 Schematic of the major tyrosine kinase-linked and G protein-coupled receptors regulating platelets. The major receptors regulating platelet activation and inhibition are shown. The major signalling receptors that mediate platelet activation are the tyrosine kinase-linked receptor GPVI and the G protein-coupled receptors for TxA$_2$, thrombin and ADP. Of this group, the P2Y$_{12}$ ADP receptor is unique in that it synergizes with the receptors for the other agonists to mediate powerful activation. The GPIb–IX–V complex is critical for platelet tethering and integrins α$_2$β$_1$ and α$_{IIb}$β$_3$ for stable adhesion and, in the case of the latter, platelet aggregation. All three of these adhesion receptors also generate weak tyrosine kinase-based intracellular signals of uncertain significance. The prostacyclin receptor (IP) elevates cAMP and, in combination with nitric oxide which elevates cGMP (not shown), mediates powerful platelet inhibition.

nevertheless mediate spreading and activation in synergy with other receptors. Signalling by GPVI and integrin α$_{IIb}$β$_3$ occurs in distinct regions of the platelet membrane, with the former signalling in cholesterol-rich membrane domains known as lipid rafts (Figure 40.6). Importantly, GPVI, GPIb–IX–V and integrin α$_{IIb}$β$_3$ are expressed only on platelets and their precursor cell, the megakaryocyte.

The heterotrimeric G proteins are composed of α and βγ subunits, and take their name from the α subunit, although both subunits regulate effector proteins. Thrombin and TxA$_2$ receptors activate both G$_q$ and G$_{13}$, which regulate PLCβ and Rho kinase, respectively, whereas the P2Y$_1$ ADP receptor is coupled only to G$_q$. Both G proteins pathways have been shown to play important roles in mediating aggregation, although G$_{13}$ is only able to induce shape change in the absence of other G$_q$. The P2Y$_{12}$ ADP receptor is unique among this group of receptors in that it is coupled to the G$_i$ family of G proteins. On its own, the P2Y$_{12}$ receptor induces very weak activation of platelets, but mediates powerful activation in synergy with Ca^{2+}-mobilizing receptors.

Tyrosine kinase-linked receptors

GPIb–IX–V

The GPIb–IX–V is unique to platelets and consists of four subunits, GPIbα, GPIbβ, GPIX and GPV, at a ratio of 2:2:2:1. It is estimated that there are 25 000 copies of the complex on the platelet surface. The principal ligand for GPIb–IX–V is VWF, which consists of a series of multimers that vary in size from 500 to more than 20 000 kDa and which give rise to the characteristic VWF ladder when analysed by gel electrophoresis. The larger multimers of VWF are more effective in mediating platelet tethering and platelet activation. VWF is stored and released from endothelial cell Weibel–Palade bodies as an ultra-large multimer and is broken down into the smaller multimers observed in the circulation by the specific metalloproteinase ADAMTS-13. Deficiencies in ADAMTS-13 lead to the persistence of ultra-large VWF multimers in the circulation and a life-threatening thrombotic microangiopathy known as thrombotic thrombocytopenic purpura (TTP), which is characterized by VWF-rich platelet aggregates in the skin and vital organs. Multimeric VWF also interacts and stabilizes FVIII.

At high rates of shear, multimeric VWF undergoes a change from a globular to an extended form that can reach several microns in length and which has multiple platelet and collagen binding sites. VWF can also self-associate when extended to form very large filaments on the surface of endothelial cells and on collagen. In this extended form, VWF is able to tether to platelets through the GPIb–IX–V complex and thereby support adhesion and aggregation. This extended form of VWF is also induced by the bacterial antibiotic ristocetin or the snake venom toxin botrocetin, which are therefore frequently used as experi-

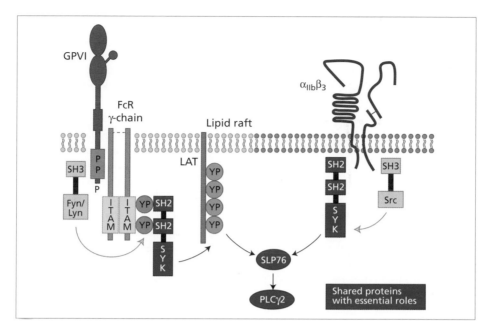

Figure 40.6 Schematic of GPVI and $\alpha_{IIb}\beta_3$ signalling. Activation of the collagen receptor GPVI leads to tyrosine phosphorylation of the FcR γ-chain ITAM by the two Src kinases, Fyn and Lyn. This leads to recruitment of the tandem SH2 domain-containing tyrosine kinase Syk, which mediates tyrosine phosphorylation of the adapter proteins LAT and SLP-76, and PLCγ2. Signalling occurs in cholesterol-rich membrane domains known as lipid rafts. The integrin $\alpha_{IIb}\beta_3$ also signals through Src and Syk tyrosine kinases leading to activation of PLCγ2. However, there are a number of differences to the GPVI signalling cascade, including (i) Src and Syk binding directly to the β3 cytoplasmic tail independent of an ITAM; (ii) the integrin uses Src; (iii) signalling occurs outside of lipid rafts; and (iv) is independent of LAT. These differences may account for the much weaker signal from the integrin relative to that from GPVI.

mental tools to promote binding to GPIbα in a low-shear environment.

The critical role of extended VWF in mediating platelet tethering is dependent on the fast on-rate of association of its A1 domain to GPIbα. However, as discussed above, other agonists such as collagen are required to mediate *rapid* activation of platelet integrins leading to stable adhesion and aggregation. This two-stage process may have evolved to help prevent adhesion and aggregation occurring when platelets are exposed to VWF in the absence of other stimuli, such as may occur on the surface of endothelial cells during release of the adhesive protein.

GPIbα generates weak intracellular signals through Src and Syk tyrosine kinases that mediate platelet spreading and integrin $\alpha_{IIb}\beta_3$ activation. It is speculated that this plays an important role in mediating platelet activation *in vivo* in synergy with other receptors, although studies using mice with a selective defect in signalling by GPIbα are required to test this.

GPIb–IX–V binds to several other cell surface and plasma proteins, including integrin $\alpha_M\beta_2$ (also known as Mac-1 or CR3) and P-selectin of leucocytes. The storage of platelets at 4°C has been shown to lead to clustering of GPIb–IX–V and it is believed that this leads to binding to $\alpha_M\beta_2$ and clearance of

platelets by the reticuloendothelial system, thus preventing their storage at this temperature and limiting their shelf-life. The interaction with $\alpha_M\beta_2$ and P-selectin contributes to attachment and transmigration of leucocytes through a mural thrombus. Binding to P-selectin has also been reported to support rolling of platelets on activated endothelium in low-pressure vessels.

Mutations in GPIbα, GPIbβ and GPIX give rise to the bleeding disorder Bernard–Soulier syndrome, which is characterized by macrothrombocytopenia. Bernard–Soulier syndrome is a rare disorder, with only a few hundred cases described worldwide. The reduction in platelet count and increase in platelet size in this condition is due to the pivotal role of GPIb–IX–V in supporting platelet formation via the interaction of the GPIbα cytoplasmic tail and the platelet cytoskeleton.

GPVI and integrin $\alpha_2\beta_1$

Collagen is recognized as the most thrombogenic component of the subendothelial matrix. Nine forms of collagen have been described within the vessel wall, with types I and III being the predominant ones in the deeper layers of the vessel wall and type VI in more superficial layers. The major receptors for collagen on platelets are the immunoglobulin GPVI and the integrin $\alpha_2\beta_1$, which are expressed at 4000–6000 and 1500–2500 copies per platelet, respectively. There are reports of additional receptors for collagen, although these need to be confirmed and their role determined. The majority of vascular collagens activate GPVI and integrin $\alpha_2\beta_1$, with the possible exception of collagen type IV in the basement membrane which forms a lattice rather than a fibrillar structure.

Collagen is composed of three helical chains, which interact to form a superhelical structure that is interrupted by non-helical regions. The presence of glycine (G) at every third position is essential to form the helical structure. In addition, the amino acids proline (P) and hydroxyproline (O) make up approximately 10% of the helical backbone. Synthetic collagen peptides based on these three amino acids have been shown to bind selectively to GPVI or integrin $\alpha_2\beta_1$. Peptides that are specific to GPVI have a backbone of GPO residues, whereas peptides that bind to $\alpha_2\beta_1$ have a backbone of GPP residues interspersed with at least one or more GER-containing motifs, such as GFOGER. The GER sequence confers binding to the Mg^{2+} ion present in the I-domain of $\alpha_2\beta_1$. GPP is unable to bind to $\alpha_2\beta_1$ or GPVI but is required to present GER in a helical conformation that is necessary for it to bind to the integrin. Many snake toxins target GPVI, including the C-type lectin convulxin, which is a tetramer of α and β subunits and induces powerful activation through clustering.

GPVI forms a complex with the FcR γ-chain and is the major signalling receptor for collagen. The FcR γ-chain contains an ITAM, defined by the sequence $YXXLX_{6-12}YXXL$. ITAMs play a critical role in signalling by a variety of immune receptors, including T- and B-cell antigen receptors, and several Fc receptors, including the FcεRI mast cell receptor and the low-affinity immune receptor FcγRIIA, which is the only Fc receptor on human platelets. ITAM receptors signal through sequential activation of Src, Syk and Tec family kinases. Src family kinases, including Fyn and Lyn, mediate phosphorylation of the conserved tyrosines in the ITAM that enables binding of the tandem SH2 domain containing Syk family kinase and initiation of a downstream signalling cascade that culminates in Tec kinase-mediated phosphorylation and activation of PLCγ2. The adapter proteins SLP-76 and LAT form an intracellular scaffold in this cascade that facilitates activation of PLCγ2. Although the essential features of signalling by all ITAM-associated receptors are conserved, the individual proteins that make up an ITAM signalling pathway are cell specific.

Although GPVI is primarily known as a receptor for collagen, it is also activated by laminin and by globular adiponectin. Because of the low affinity for GPVI, the interaction with laminin requires prior binding to the integrin $\alpha_6\beta_1$. Laminin is a major component of the basement membrane and may therefore mediate platelet activation following minor injuries that fail to expose subendothelial collagen or tissue factor. The significance of the interaction with globular adiponectin is unclear, especially as low levels are associated with type 2 diabetes and metabolic syndrome.

The primary role of integrin $\alpha_2\beta_1$ is to support platelet adhesion to collagen at sites of damage to the vasculature and to cause a net increase in binding to GPVI in view of the modest affinity of collagen for the immunoglobulin receptor. Integrin $\alpha_2\beta_1$ also mediates weak activation of PLCγ2, although the physiological significance of this is unclear due to the more powerful action of GPVI and the redundancy in signalling with other receptors. The physiological significance of $\alpha_2\beta_1$ in supporting thrombus formation *in vivo* is masked by the much greater level of expression of integrin $\alpha_{IIb}\beta_3$.

Several patients have been described with acquired disorders that lead to reduction or abrogation of expression or signalling by GPVI. In general, these patients exhibit mild bleeding, but the presence of additional complications means that it is unclear if this is due solely to the defect in GPVI. Only three patients have been described with an acquired deficiency of $\alpha_2\beta_1$ and they too have other vascular complications. Polymorphisms in the non-coding region of the α_2 subunit lead to a threefold to fivefold increase in expression of the integrin. A weak correlation has been found between the high-expressing polymorphic forms and thrombotic disease.

Integrin $\alpha_{IIb}\beta_3$

Integrin $\alpha_{IIb}\beta_3$ is the most abundant protein on the platelet surface and is estimated to comprise approximately 15% of surface proteins, with less than 20 nm between individual receptors. As discussed above, $\alpha_{IIb}\beta_3$ binds to several bivalent ligands in the vasculature including fibrinogen, VWF, fibronectin and vitronectin. Although all of these are capable of supporting platelet aggregation, fibrinogen is considered to be the major ligand because of its much higher concentration in plasma. In all cases, the binding of these soluble ligands requires 'inside-out' activation of integrin $\alpha_{IIb}\beta_3$ to a high-affinity conformation in the presence of divalent cations.

The clustering of $\alpha_{IIb}\beta_3$ generates weak 'outside-in' signals that have been shown to induce platelet spreading, clot retraction and secretion in combination with other platelet agonists such as ADP. The integrin signals through at least two and possibly more pathways. The most thoroughly characterized of these is the activation of Src and Syk tyrosine kinases by direct interaction with the β3 cytosolic tail. The sequential activation of these two kinases leads to actin polymerization and activation of PLCγ2. In addition, the β3 cytosolic tail has been shown to bind and activate cytosolic PLA_2 independent of the former pathway. Although the work of Shattil and others has established that $\alpha_{IIb}\beta_3$ regulates Syk independent of an ITAM, there is recent evidence that the integrin signals in human platelets through the low-affinity immune receptor FcγRIIA, despite the fact that it is expressed at 3000–5000 copies per platelet (i.e. ~ 4% of the level of $\alpha_{IIb}\beta_3$). The challenge therefore is to establish the relative importance of all these pathways in $\alpha_{IIb}\beta_3$ signalling, although this is particularly difficult as FcγRIIA is not expressed in the mouse genome.

The discovery that the Arg-Gly-Asp (RGD) sequence in fibronectin mediates its interaction with integrin $\alpha_5\beta_1$ led to the unexpected discovery that small peptides or snake toxins containing this sequence could also inhibit binding of fibronectin to integrin $\alpha_{IIb}\beta_3$. This subsequently resulted in the realization that other matrix proteins use RGD to bind to integrin $\alpha_{IIb}\beta_3$, including VWF, vitronectin and CD40 ligand. Paradoxically, however, the major site of interaction of fibrinogen with the integrin is via a KQAGDV sequence at the C-termini of its two γ-chains, even though it has two pairs of RGD sequences and the binding of fibrinogen can be blocked by synthetic RGD-containing peptides.

The critical role of integrin $\alpha_{IIb}\beta_3$ in aggregation, coupled with the fact that the other antiplatelet agents available at the time (namely aspirin and ticlopidine, which has been superseded by clopidogrel) are not completely effective in preventing cardiovascular events, encouraged the groups of Coller and Phillips to develop inhibitors of integrin $\alpha_{IIb}\beta_3$ as novel antiplatelet agents. A chimeric Fab molecule, abciximab, was introduced into the clinic in 1994 and was later followed by two RGD-based peptide inhibitors, eptifibatide and tirofiban. The three inhibitors have been approved for use in patients undergoing percutaneous coronary interventions involving stenting and in patients with unstable angina. Excessive bleeding and thrombocytopenia are major side-effects for all three of these $\alpha_{IIb}\beta_3$-blocking agents and thus limits their use to patients considered to be at high risk of thombosis within a hospital setting. Unexpectedly, clinical trials with orally active $\alpha_{IIb}\beta_3$ antagonists were associated with increased mortality, increased bleeding and occasional severe thrombocytopenia. The reason for the lack of efficacy is partly due to induction of conformational changes in the integrin that expose neoepitopes and can therefore lead to platelet activation through the low-affinity immune receptor FcγRIIA, as recently demonstrated by Newman's group.

G protein-coupled receptors

P2Y$_1$ and P2Y$_{12}$ ADP receptors

ADP was reported to activate platelets in the early 1960s but it has only been within the last decade that its critical role as a positive feedback agonist has finally been established. This delay in recognition arose because ADP is a weak platelet agonist, and it is only through its ability to mediate powerful platelet activation in synergy with Ca^{2+}-mobilizing receptors via the P2Y$_{12}$ receptor that its critical role in thrombus formation is achieved. The latter is illustrated by the clinical efficacy of the P2Y$_{12}$ receptor antagonist, the thienopyridine clopidogrel (Plavix), in the long-term prevention of thrombosis. Clopidogrel is a prodrug that is metabolized by the liver to generate an active metabolite that covalently modifies, and therefore irreversibly inhibits, the P2Y$_{12}$ ADP receptor. The related thienopyridine prasugrel, which is at an advanced stage of clinical development, is metab-

olized more rapidly to the same active metabolite as clopidogrel and therefore has a faster onset of action. Two competitive P2Y$_{12}$ receptor antagonists that are analogues of ADP are also in clinical development, cangrelor (AR-C69931MX) and ticagrelor (AZD6140). Competitive antagonists have the advantage of a faster onset of action as well as increased safety due to their reversible nature. Ticagrelor, but not cangrelor, is available after oral administration and so has potential in the long-term treatment of patients at risk of thrombosis.

ADP stimulates sustained platelet aggregation in platelet-rich plasma through the synergy between the P2Y$_{12}$ receptor, which is coupled to the G$_i$ family, and the P2Y$_1$ receptor, which is coupled to G$_q$. In contrast, each receptor stimulates only weak partial aggregation, which in the case of P2Y$_1$ is not sustained. There are about 150 copies of P2Y$_1$ per platelet and it has been proposed that its role is to support rapid platelet activation in synergy with P2Y$_{12}$. At later times, its action is masked by the activation of thrombin and TxA$_2$ receptors, which are expressed at five to ten times higher levels and which signal through G$_q$ and G$_{13}$. Consistent with this, arterial but not venous thrombus formation is reduced in mice deficient in the P2Y$_1$ receptor or which have been pretreated with a P2Y$_1$ receptor antagonist. However, it is unclear whether the P2Y$_1$ receptor performs a similar function in humans, as patients with a bleeding disorder associated with a defect in P2Y$_1$ have not been described. A striking feature of the P2Y$_1$ receptor is its ability to undergo rapid desensitization and this, together with its low level of expression, may serve to prevent activation of platelets following exposure to ADP in the absence of other platelet stimuli. This may occur, for example, following damage of other vascular cells.

The P2Y$_{12}$ ADP receptor activates the G$_i$ family of G proteins, predominantly G$_{i\alpha2}$, leading to inhibition of adenylyl cyclase and activation of phosphatidylinositol 3-kinase (PI3K). It is the latter, and possibly other pathways, that underlies its ability to synergize with Ca^{2+}-mobilizing receptors, whereas inhibition of adenylyl cyclase on its own is insufficient to mediate activation. Eight gene mutations in P2Y$_{12}$ have been identified in patients with a mild bleeding disorder, consistent with its critical role in supporting platelet activation. This number is likely to rapidly increase as testing and sequencing procedures are refined.

TxA$_2$ receptor

TxA$_2$ signals through a single G protein-coupled receptor, the TP receptor, which is coupled to G$_q$ and G$_{13}$ heterotrimeric G proteins, which activate PLC and Rho kinase, respectively. The TP receptor is alternatively spliced in its C-terminus to two isoforms, TPα and TPβ, which have the same pharmacology and signal in the same way. The consensus is that platelets express only the TPα isoform and certainly the field assumes that the platelet has a single TP receptor. TxA$_2$ has a very short half-life and is rapidly metabolized to the inactive metabolite TxB$_2$, which prevents its use in functional studies, where the stable mimetic, U46619, is preferred. TxB$_2$ is routinely used to monitor formation of TxA$_2$ by radioimmunoassay and U46619 is sometimes used in the clinical evaluation of patients with suspected thromboxane receptor defects. Arachidonic acid, which is a direct substrate for cyclooxygenase, is used to check for activity of the TxA$_2$ pathway.

The clinical importance of the TxA$_2$ pathway in platelet activation is illustrated by the antithrombotic action of aspirin, which inhibits platelet cyclooxygenase. The irreversible nature of the acetylation induced by aspirin, in combination with the inability of platelets to synthesize significant levels of new proteins, means that the effective antithrombotic concentration of aspirin is considerably lower than that required to target cyclooxygenase in other cells. Large-scale clinical trials have shown that aspirin reduces the mortality of myocardial infarction by approximately 25% and the number of major vascular events in individuals at risk by about one-third. The clinical effectiveness of low-dose aspirin is similar to that of the P2Y$_{12}$ receptor antagonist clopidogrel. An Arg→Leu mutation in the first extracellular loop of the TP receptor has been linked to a mild bleeding syndrome in two unrelated families, although 'aspirin-like' defects are frequently seen in patients with mild platelet-based bleeding disorders, suggesting that the number of mutations in this receptor is likely to increase.

PAR-1 and PAR-4 thrombin receptors

Thrombin is among the most powerful of all platelet agonists and induces activation of human platelets through the proteolytic cleavage of PAR-1 and PAR-4, and of mouse platelets through binding to PAR-3 which facilitates cleavage and activation of PAR-4. Thrombin releases a short peptide from the N-terminal region of PAR-1 and PAR-4 to expose a sequence that functions as a tethered ligand by binding to the receptor and promoting activation. Synthetic peptides corresponding to the newly exposed receptor-specific sequences induce activation in the absence of receptor cleavage. These thrombin receptor-activating peptides can be used to selectively activate the individual PAR receptors. In humans, it is believed that PAR-1 mediates rapid activation in response to low concentrations of thrombin, whereas PAR-4 is activated by higher concentrations of the protease. PAR-1 and PAR-4 signal through G$_q$ and G$_{13}$ heterotrimeric G proteins, activating PLCβ and Rho kinase, respectively. Patients with defects in either of the thrombin receptors have yet to be identified, possibly because defects in thrombin-mediated platelet activation are not routinely investigated in a clinical setting.

The GPIbα subunit of the GPIb–IX–V expresses a high-affinity binding site for thrombin that is believed to position the protease in the vicinity of the PAR-1 and PAR-4 receptors in order to facilitate activation, in line with increasing evidence that the various actions of thrombin are achieved through binding to proteins that localize the protease to specific sites. There is limited and controversial evidence to suggest that

binding of thrombin to GPIbα generates weak signals, but the major pathway of platelet activation is believed to be mediated through the PAR-1 and PAR-4 receptors. Several direct inhibitors of thrombin are used in the clinic as anticoagulants in patients at risk of heparin-induced thrombocytopenia. To our knowledge, there is no direct evidence indicating that their clinical efficacy is also mediated through inhibition of platelet activation.

Other platelet receptors and their ligands

Platelets express a large number and diversity of receptors for a variety of ligands, including adhesive proteins, amines, chemokines, cytokines, lipids, nucleotides, proteases and transmembrane proteins. Many of the receptors are present at such a low level, or are not ordinarily exposed to their ligand, that their physiological role in mediating or potentiating activation may be minimal, although they could potentially play a role in disease. Examples include regulation of human platelets by endothelin-1, Gas6, insulin-like growth factor, leptin, vasopressin, platelet-activating factor and PDGF. In some cases, expression of a receptor on the platelet surface appears to reflect a role in megakaryocyte development/platelet formation rather than in regulating platelet activation. Examples include the SDF-1α receptor, CXCR4, and the TPO receptor c-Mpl. SDF-1α plays a key role in supporting migration of megakaryocytes to the vascular niche in bone marrow and TPO is the major regulator of megakaryocyte growth and development. Both receptors also mediate weak potentiation of platelet activation, although the physiological significance of this is unclear. As discussed above, there is also increasing evidence for the role of a number of surface proteins in mediating 'late events' that serve to consolidate the growing thrombus. The function of a number of the other platelet receptors is discussed below.

5-HT$_{2A}$ receptors

Platelets contain very high levels of 5-HT, which is taken up by an active transport mechanism and stored in dense granules. Release of 5-HT induces powerful vasoconstriction, thereby limiting blood loss. 5-HT mediates weak platelet activation through the 5-HT$_{2A}$ receptor, which is coupled to G$_q$, but there is little evidence to suggest that this plays a major role in supporting thrombus formation.

α$_{2A}$-Adrenoceptor

Adrenaline activates the α$_{2A}$-adrenoceptor, which is coupled to the G$_i$ family of proteins, predominantly G$_z$. As is the case for the P2Y$_{12}$ ADP receptor, the α$_{2A}$-adrenoceptor is able to induce powerful platelet activation in synergy with Ca^{2+}-mobilizing receptors. Platelet dense granules contain a very low level of adrenaline and the catecholamine is also present in plasma. Recent studies in α$_{2A}$-adrenoceptor knockout mice have provided evidence for a minor physiological role of adrenaline in supporting haemostasis, although it is not clear if this is also the case in humans, even though platelet function tests frequently use adrenaline as a co-agonist.

P2X$_1$ ATP receptor

P2X$_1$ is a receptor for ATP, which is released alongside ADP from dense granules. It is the only known ligand-gated ion channel on the platelet surface. Binding of ATP promotes direct entry of Ca^{2+} into the platelet, which occurs over a much more rapid time course than IP3-mediated Ca^{2+} mobilization and subsequent entry of extracellular Ca^{2+} via store-operated Ca^{2+} entry. The P2X$_1$ receptor has been shown to induce platelet shape change but requires the presence of other receptors to mediate aggregation. The physiological role of P2X$_1$ may therefore be to facilitate rapid activation of platelets in synergy with other agonists, including ADP, in a similar way to that proposed for P2Y$_1$. In this context, it is intriguing that P2X$_1$ also undergoes extremely rapid desensitization and this too may serve to prevent 'unwanted' activation. There is evidence from studies in mutant mice that the P2X$_1$ receptor contributes to, but is not essential for, thrombus formation, and as yet no patients have been identified with a mild bleeding disorder attributed solely to a mutation in the ion channel.

FcγRIIA

Clustering of the low-affinity immune receptor FcγRIIA by immune complexes or via primary and secondary antibodies mediates powerful activation through an ITAM-based pathway that is believed to be similar to that used by the collagen receptor GPVI. FcγRIIA is not thought to have a physiological role in supporting thrombus formation, but it mediates activation by immune complexes and is the causative receptor in heparin-induced thrombocytopenia. It is intriguing that FcγRIIA is absent from the mouse genome and that mice platelets do not appear to express an Fc receptor.

CD36

The scavenging receptor CD36 is among the most highly expressed of platelet surface glycoproteins being present at approximately 20 000 copies per platelet. Despite the fact that it was first identified on platelets more than 30 years ago, it is only within the last 2 years through the work of Eugene Podrez and colleagues that it has been implicated as a major player in mediating the increased platelet responsiveness seen in patients with dyslipidaemia. Oxidized choline glycerophospholipids are present at sufficiently increased levels in the plasma of humans with low levels of high-density lipoprotein to potentiate activation of platelets by threshold concentrations of ADP and other agonists. Moreover, this potentiation is not seen in individuals who do not express CD36 on their platelets, suggesting that they may be protected against the dyslipidaemia-induced prothrombotic state. However, further research is required to evaluate the contribution of platelet CD36 to cardiovascular disease.

CLEC-2

The C-type lectin receptor CLEC-2 has recently been shown to mediate powerful activation of platelets in response to the snake venom toxin rhodocytin, or its endogenous ligand podoplanin. The latter is expressed on lymphatic endothelial cells, renal epithelial cells, type I lung alveolar cells and on the leading edge of tumours, where it is implicated in cancer metastasis. Mice deficient in CLEC-2 or podoplanin die shortly after birth, and embryos at mid- to late gestation from both sets of mice have blood-filled lymphatics and severe oedema due to defective separation of lymphatic vessels from the blood vasculature. CLEC-2 signals through an ITAM-like pathway similar to that used by GPVI and FcγRIIA, although intriguingly it uses a single rather than a tandem YXXL motif to activate Syk.

Second messenger pathways underlying activation

The activation of PLCγ2 and PLCβ (predominantly β2) isotypes by tyrosine kinase-linked or G protein-coupled receptors, respectively, generates IP3 and 1,2-diacylglycerol (DG), which mobilize Ca^{2+} and activate protein kinase C (PKC), respectively. The G protein α-subunit G$_{13}$ regulates the GTP exchange factor (GEF), p115Rho, to form active Rho, a small G protein that regulates a number of effectors, including inhibition of myosin light chain phosphatase thereby inducing phosphorylation of myosin light chains leading to shape change and actin-stress fibre formation. G$_i$-coupled receptors inhibit adenylyl cyclase and activate PI3K, the latter underlying the remarkable synergy with Ca^{2+}-mobilizing receptors. These second messenger pathways are discussed in further detail.

Calcium

The divalent cation Ca^{2+} plays a critical role in mediating platelet activation, usually in combination with other signalling pathways. An increase in Ca^{2+} is brought about by its release from intracellular stores by the action of IP3 and by entry through the plasma membrane, predominantly through store-operated Ca^{2+} entry. The latter has recently been shown to occur via binding of the transmembrane protein STIM-1, which is localized to intracellular stores, to the surface membrane Ca^{2+} channel, Orai-1, with the trigger for entry being the release of Ca^{2+} from the store. The entry of Ca^{2+} through Orai-1 is critical for procoagulant activity and possibly other responses, but interestingly is not required for aggregation. The released Ca^{2+} is efficiently removed from the cytosol by Ca^{2+}-ATPases in the endoplasmic reticulum (SERCA) and in the plasma membrane (PMCA).

Diacylglycerol and protein kinase C

PKC refers to a family of structurally similar lipid-regulated protein kinases that is divided into *classical* isotypes regulated by Ca^{2+} and DG, *novel* isotypes regulated by DG, and *atypical* isotypes regulated independently of the two messengers. Human platelets express two classical isotypes, α and β, and three novel isotypes, δ, θ and η. The novel isotype PKCε is also expressed in mouse platelets. PKCα is the major isoform regulating dense granule and α-granule platelet secretion in mouse platelets, with increasing evidence suggesting that the other PKCs have isotype-specific inhibitory and activatory roles.

DG, together with Ca^{2+}, regulates the Rap1 (also known as Rap1b) GTP exchange factor, CALDAG-GEF1. Rap1 plays a critical role in mediating activation of integrin $\alpha_{IIb}\beta_3$, although this role can be bypassed by high concentrations of powerful ligands. CALDAG-GEF1-deficient mice and patients with defective expression of the exchange factor (leucocyte adhesion deficiency type III) have defective Rap1 activation and a bleeding diathesis.

Phosphatidylinositol 3-kinase

PI3K generates from phosphatidylinositol 4,5-bisphosphate the 3-phosphorylated lipid second messenger phosphatidylinositol 3,4,5-trisphosphate, which is rapidly hydrolysed to phosphatidylinositol 3,4-bisphosphate, which is also believed to be a messenger. The two 5-phosphorylated lipids mediate translocation of proteins containing one or more pleckstrin homology (PH) domains to the membrane, including PLCβ and PLCγ isoforms, protein kinase B (Akt) and the Tec family kinases Btk which mediates phosphorylation of PLCγ2. Platelet express several regulatory and catalytic subunits of PI3K, although p110β and p85α are believed to the major catalytic and regulatory subunits supporting activation downstream of both G protein-coupled and tyrosine kinase-linked receptors.

The molecular basis of platelet activation

The physiological end points of platelet activation are stable adhesion, aggregation, granule secretion, TxA_2 formation, spreading with stress fibre formation, clot retraction and procoagulant activity. These responses are regulated by a bewildering interplay between tyrosine kinase- and G protein-regulated signalling pathways, with evidence of considerable redundancy in their actions. Here we provide brief details on the major mechanisms that underlie each of these events.

Stable adhesion and aggregation

Both of these responses are mediated through activation of integrin $\alpha_{IIb}\beta_3$ by 'inside-out' signals from tyrosine kinase and G protein receptors. Activation of the integrin is brought about by the binding of talin to the β3 cytoplasmic tail via a FERM domain in its head region. Platelet activation is associated with the recruitment of talin from the cytoplasm to the β3 tail via a

process that remains poorly understood but which is regulated in part by binding of Rap1 to its effector protein RIAM. The interaction of talin with the β3 tail leads to separation of a salt bridge between the α_{IIb} and β_3 subunits, and a resulting conformational change in the extracellular region of the integrin from a bent to an extended conformation. Recently, the FERM domain-containing protein kindlin-3 has also been shown to bind to the β3 tail and to mediate activation in combination with talin, although the precise details of this interaction remain to be established. Ligand engagement of the integrin leads to clustering and generation of 'outside-in' signals that stimulate actin polymerization and PLCγ2, which support many aspects of platelet activation including spreading and granule secretion.

Secretion

Platelet dense granule and α-granule secretion is triggered through a synergistic interaction between Ca^{2+} and PKC-regulated pathways, with both arms being critical for secretion to occur. Granule fusion is orchestrated by a superfamily of proteins termed SNAREs (soluble N-ethylmaleimide-sensitive attachment protein receptors) that form a universal membrane fusion machine. The activity of SNARE proteins is regulated by a series of chaperone proteins that facilitate membrane fusion. PKC phosphorylates several SNARE and chaperone proteins, including Munc-18, syntaxin-4 and SNAP-23, altering their affinity for their binding partners. For example, phosphorylation of Munc-18 interferes with its ability to bind to syntaxin-4 and phosphorylation of syntaxin-4 by PKC inhibits its ability to bind SNAP-23. This allows syntaxin-4 to interact with SNARE proteins on the opposing membrane, promoting fusion and granule secretion. There is evidence for differential regulation of the two sets of granules, although the molecular basis of this is not known and in general dense granule and α-granule secretion occur together.

TxA₂ formation

Cytosolic PLA_2 liberates arachidonic acid from membrane phospholipids and is regulated by Ca^{2+} and serine phosphorylation downstream of mitogen-activated protein kinases. Ca^{2+} is critical for activation whereas phosphorylation causes a relatively small increase in activity and on its own is insufficient to mediate activation. The liberated arachidonic acid is metabolized by cyclooxygenase and thromboxane synthase to PGG_2/PGH_2, which immediately convert into TxA_2, and by lipoxygenase enzymes to leukotrienes.

Actin polymerization

Activation of platelets leads to a series of dramatic changes in platelet morphology that helps to secure the thrombus at the site of injury in the high-pressure arteriolar system. In addition, actin polymerization plays an important but poorly understood role in signalling by platelet surface glycoprotein receptors, including GPVI and integrin $\alpha_{IIb}\beta_3$. Actin is assembled into a number of morphological distinct structures, including filopodia, actin nodules, lamellipodia and stress fibres downstream of small GTP-binding proteins. For example, the small G protein Rac1 drives formation of lamellipodia in platelets through the Arp2/3 complex, while the small G protein Rho regulates formation of actin–myosin stress fibres. Mice deficient in Rac1 or treated with inhibitors of Rho kinase have unstable aggregates, emphasizing the importance of actin polymerization in generating and strengthening the thrombus. The small G protein(s) that regulates formation of filopodia and actin nodules in platelets, and the significance of these structures, is yet to be clarified.

Inhibitory agonists and their receptors

It is essential for platelets to have powerful inhibitory mechanisms that prevent activation in intact healthy vessels and which limit thrombus growth during haemostasis. The prevention of platelet activation in the intact circulation is ordinarily achieved by the antithrombotic nature of the endothelial cell surface, which has effective mechanisms for removal of platelet stimulatory agonists by endothelial cells, most notably ADP and thrombin, and by the release of NO and prostacyclin from endothelial cells. The endothelial cell surface expresses the ecto-ADPase CD39, which removes circulating ADP, and thrombomodulin, which regulates the level of thrombin. The role of CD39 in removing ADP is critical given the ability of the nucleotide to induce activation in synergy with other agonists.

The major direct mechanism of inhibition of platelet function is through elevation of the cyclic nucleotides cGMP and cAMP by NO and prostacyclin, respectively. The two cyclic nucleotides mediate their effects in platelets through regulation of cGMP-dependent protein kinase (PKG)-1 and cAMP-dependent protein kinase (PKA). In addition, cGMP regulates the three major platelet phosphodiesterases (PDEs), including inhibition of PDE3, thereby leading to an increase in the level of cAMP. There is therefore cross-talk between the two cyclic nucleotides even though many of the targets for PKG-1 and PKA are believed to be distinct. This is illustrated by the demonstration that PKG-1 but not PKA mediates inhibition of platelet activation through phosphorylation of the IP3 receptor-associated cGMP kinase substrate (IRAG), which is expressed in a macromolecular complex with PKG-1 and the IP3 receptor type 1. Phosphorylation of IRAG by PKG-1 inhibits IP3-induced Ca^{2+} release and, importantly, targeted deletion of the IP3-binding region of IRAG prevents NO-mediated inhibition of platelet activation, whereas the inhibitory effect of cAMP is retained. In contrast, elevation of cAMP has been shown to lead to inhibition of activation of PLC. The two cyclic nucleotides induce phosphorylation of many substrates in platelets, including VASP, and it is likely that phosphorylation of several of these mediates platelet inhibition.

There is evidence that a family of platelet glycoproteins, characterized by the presence of tandem immunoreceptor tyrosine-based inhibitory motifs (ITIMs) in their cytosolic tails, mediate weak inhibition of activation by both tyrosine kinase-linked and, to a lesser extent, G protein-coupled receptors. PECAM-1 is the most characterized of this family of proteins and is expressed at a level of approximately 10 000 copies per platelet. Two further inhibitory ITIM-containing transmembrane proteins have recently been identified, G6b-B and CEACAM-1, although paradoxically a further ITIM protein that becomes exposed on activation, TREM-like transcript (TLT)-1, supports weak activation. It has been proposed that the inhibitory ITIM proteins mediate their effects through binding to the tandem SH2 domain-containing protein tyrosine phosphatases SHP-1 and SHP-2, but as yet there is no direct evidence for this. The functional significance of this relatively weak effect is unclear, and perhaps a more intriguing proposal is that ITIM receptors help to dampen down constitutive signalling by tyrosine kinases in non-stimulated platelets, thereby helping to prevent unwanted platelet activation.

The endothelial surface also plays a significant role in preventing excessive thrombus growth, again through removal of ADP and thrombin, by release of NO and prostacyclin, and by activation of the fibrinolytic pathway. Additional mechanisms also help to limit excessive growth, including shedding of platelet surface glycoprotein receptors, cleavage of intracellular proteins through calpain, and removal of intracellular messengers and reversal of phosphorylation by the action of tyrosine and serine/threonine phosphatases.

Nitric oxide

NO is the most important inhibitor of platelet function. It is constitutively released from endothelial cells and can also be inducibly upregulated. NO has a short half-life in the vasculature, of the order of 3–5 s, which results in the highest concentration of the gaseous transmitter being found in the vicinity of the endothelial cell, a key site of inhibition of platelet function. NO mediates powerful inhibition of platelet activation and promotes vasodilatation. These effects are mediated through direct activation of guanylyl cyclase, leading to the generation of cGMP and activation of protein kinase G (PKG). The substrates for PKG in platelets include PDE3, which hydrolyses cAMP as described above. Thus, NO mediates inhibition through elevation of both cAMP and cGMP. Phosphorylation of the combined PKA/PKG substrate VASP, an actin-binding protein, is often used to assess activation of inhibitory pathways and be achieved by both Western blotting and flow cytometry.

Prostacyclin

Prostacyclin (PGI_2) is the major prostaglandin released by endothelial cells. It is synthesized in stimulated endothelial cells from arachidonic acid through the sequential actions of cyclooxygenase and prostacyclin synthetase. Prostacyclin activates the seven-transmembrane-spanning IP receptor on platelets, which is coupled to G_s and thereby activates adenylyl cyclase. Prostacyclin exerts a powerful inhibitory effect on platelets and also promotes vasodilatation through elevation of cAMP. Prostacyclin also has a short half-life in the vasculature and so its primary action is believed to occur in the vicinity of the vessel wall when the growing thrombus comes into contact with the endothelium. This action is facilitated by the liberation of arachidonic acid from the platelet, which is converted to prostacyclin by the endothelial cells.

Adenosine

Platelets express the adenosine A_{2A} receptor, which is also coupled to G_s. However, the A_{2A} receptor is expressed at a low level and is not considered to be a major route of inhibition. However, increased adenosine levels induced by dipyridamole may contribute to its antithrombotic action.

Platelet-based bleeding problems

Bleeding can be due to abnormalities in platelet function/ number or to extensive antiplatelet medication. Abnormalities in either platelet function and/or number are associated with an increased risk of classical bleeding symptoms and clearly demonstrate the importance of platelets in haemostasis. Patients with platelet disorders present with a typical mucocutaneous bleeding pattern of variable severity and are often prone to bleeding during surgery and trauma. However, inherited platelet defects are an uncommon cause of bleeding and are difficult to diagnose and manage, with wide variation in practices between laboratories. Before any platelet function test is requested, a full clinical and family history is taken to determine the underlying cause of the bleeding problem. This includes studying the pattern of bleeding, whether it is lifelong or recent, triggered by trauma (e.g. dentistry, surgery or accident), is present within other family members and associated with any medication the patient may be taking. As von Willebrand disease is the most commonly inherited bleeding disorder but presents with a platelet-like bleeding pattern, many patients including those with potential coagulation defects usually undergo a series of investigations for a bleeding disorder that includes platelet function and coagulation testing. Although bleeding histories are subjective and can vary within a lifetime, they remain an important screening method for diagnosing a potential platelet defect. However, it is also important to exclude acquired defects of platelet function, including those caused by antiplatelet drugs and other clinical disorders. A complete drug history is therefore important as aspirin and non-steroidal anti-inflammatory drugs are the commonest causes of an acquired platelet defect and testing may have to be deferred and repeated. Some patients are also screened before surgery to exclude the presence of either an inherited or acquired platelet defect because of the associated increased risk of bleeding. Inherited platelet defects can be classified according to the severity of bleeding, with severe disorders such as Glanzmann thrombasthenia and Bernard–Soulier syndrome usually being detected very early in life, while more mild bleeding disorders (e.g. due to $P2Y_{12}$ deficiency) often not being detected for many years until the patient is exposed to surgery or trauma. Indeed, there is overlap between symptoms in milder platelet defects and the normal population, which may be partly related to varying levels of plasma VWF, making the former group difficult to diagnose. Further information on inherited platelet bleeding disorders is given in Chapter 48.

Platelet function testing

Platelet function tests are primarily used to aid in the diagnosis and management of patients presenting with bleeding problems. If a platelet defect is suspected, then there is a variety of tests available that can be used to diagnose any underlying cause of the bleeding problem. The investigation of platelet function is often affected by the collection and processing of blood samples. Platelets are prone to not only artefactual *in vitro* activation but also desensitization. Normal platelet function is highly dependent on extracellular Ca^{2+} and Mg^{2+} concentrations and so the choice of anticoagulant is important even though citrate remains the most widely used traditional anticoagulant. Most current testing is still performed on citrated blood within a few hours of sampling.

Global tests of platelet function are often initially used as screening tests during the laboratory investigation of individuals with suspected haemostatic defects. Since global tests of platelet function do not enable specific diagnosis of platelet disorders, they are normally performed as the first part of a two-step strategy that requires further testing with more specialized assays of platelet function to confirm or refute any clinical diagnosis. The most commonly proposed rationale for testing global platelet function as a first-line investigation is exclusion of a platelet function disorder so that further specialized testing can be avoided. For this reason, global platelet function tests are usually initially performed at the same time as global assays of coagulation pathway function (prothrombin time and activated partial thromboplastin time), VWF screening tests (VWF:Ag, VWF:RCo and FVIII:C) and measurement of platelet number with a full blood counter. The most widely performed tests for initially screening platelet function disorders are currently the template bleeding time, light transmission aggregometry (LTA) and the closure time within the platelet function analyser (PFA)-100.

The bleeding time was the first *in vivo* test of platelet function and is performed by timing the arrest of bleeding from standard-sized cuts made in the skin of the forearm. Although the test has been refined, most clinicians consider the test to be poorly reproducible, invasive, insensitive (particularly to mild platelet defects) and time-consuming. Despite these drawbacks, the test is surprisingly still widely used as a first-line screening tool and can identify patients with severe platelet defects. However, given the problems faced with the *in vivo* bleeding time, a number of *in vitro* tests that attempt to accurately simulate platelet function have been developed. These include the PFA-100 and cone and plate(let) analyser (CPA) devices. These simulate high-shear platelet adhesion to foreign surfaces (e.g. collagen) and either monitor the drop in flow rate as an aperture is closed by platelet adhesion/aggregation or study the degree of platelet aggregation and surface coverage respectively. The PFA-100 instrument has been widely used for the last 10 years and provides optional replacement of the bleeding time as a limited screening test, as it is more sensitive to many platelet defects and von Willebrand disease. Although the instrument therefore has good negative predictive value for eliminating severe platelet defects and von Willebrand disease, it is very important that further diagnostic tests are still performed if clinical suspicion of a platelet defect is strong. The CPA has also been commercialized recently as the IMPACT device, which may also have potential as a screening tool, although it is still under development as a clinical test. The IMPACT-R or research version of the instrument is currently available and is not suitable for routine clinical use. However, it is highly likely that these types of instruments will be increasingly used in the future and may prove to be useful as aids in screening and diagnosing platelet defects, monitoring antiplatelet therapy and predicting bleeding and thrombosis in various patient groups.

Automated cell counting of whole blood in the modern full blood count investigation is an essential screening test in patients with abnormal bleeding. Modern blood counters can rapidly detect abnormalities in platelet number, platelet size distribution and mean platelet volume (MPV) and provide a reliable method for screening samples from patients provided good quality control procedures are followed within the laboratory. Normal results will therefore rapidly eliminate thrombocytopenia and anaemia as potential causes of bleeding and ensure that any platelet function tests that are being performed will not be affected by low platelet counts. If any abnormalities in platelet count, MPV or distribution are flagged by the instrument, then a blood smear should be examined to confirm defects in platelet number, size and granule content. Whole-blood morphology may also assist in the diagnosis of platelet

disorders by indicating abnormalities such as red cell schistocytes in TTP or neutrophil inclusions and giant platelets in MYH-9-related disorders.

Depending on the results of clinical and laboratory screening of patients, a series of diagnostic platelet function tests are usually performed. Since the 1960s, platelet aggregometry has quickly become the gold standard of platelet function testing and has revolutionized our ability to identify and diagnose a wide variety of platelet defects. Conventional Born aggregometers monitor the changes in light transmission that occur in a suspension of platelets in plasma or a physiological buffer that are stimulated with different concentrations of various agonists (e.g. ADP, collagen, adrenaline, ristocetin). Whole-blood impedance base aggregometers are now also common and measure the changes in electrical resistance between two electrodes caused by platelet adhesion and aggregation after addition of agonists. Typical parameters recorded from LTA tracings include shape change, lag phase, rate of aggregation, and maximal and final extent of aggregation. These parameters, coupled with the pattern of primary and secondary aggregation responses obtained with different dosages of different agonists, enable the experienced operator to diagnose specific signalling defects. Modern aggregometers are now multichannel, fully computerized, easy to use compact instruments and some can also simultaneously measure ATP secretion levels by luminescence (Figure 40.7). Measurement of the storage and release of the dense granular nucleotides can also be performed by a variety of alternative methods for confirming either storage and/or release defects, although recent surveys suggest that this is underused. The interpretation of aggregation traces remains challenging due to the feedback actions of ADP and TxA$_2$, as illustrated in Figure 40.7 for a 10-μmol/L concentration of ADP.

The introduction of flow cytometry into haematology laboratories provided an exquisite, sensitive and powerful tool for studying and diagnosing various platelet defects. Flow cytometric analysis of platelets is performed in fresh whole blood or in platelet-rich plasma, and the technique can be used with very small fluid volumes, even in thrombocytopenia. This technique is used to determine the copy density of platelet membrane glycoproteins and receptors, and is therefore useful for confirming the absence of various glycoproteins or receptors in disease. Platelet function testing can also be performed and the ability of platelets to degranulate, express activation markers (e.g. P-selectin) and expose procoagulant phospholipids can also be diagnostically useful. A major limitation of the above tests is that they are performed at low shear conditions and therefore do not mimic accurately many of the important physiological processes of platelet adhesion, activation and aggregation that occur at higher shear rates *in vivo*. Development of new tests that attempt to accurately simulate primary haemostasis has therefore become a growth industry (e.g. PFA-100, IMPACT and Placor PRT).

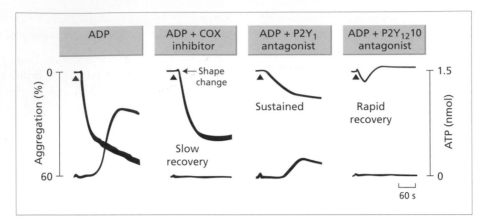

Figure 40.7 The effect of pharmacological inhibitors on ADP-induced platelet aggregation and secretion. ADP (10 μmol/L) stimulates rapid sustained aggregation and ($\alpha_{IIb}\beta_3$-dependent) ATP secretion as measured using Born lumiaggregometry. In the presence of the cyclooxygenase inhibitor indomethacin (10 μmol/L), ADP stimulates marked aggregation that slowly (minutes) decays, whereas secretion is abolished. Aggregation is preceded by a small increase in optical density (shape change) that is inhibited in the presence of the P2Y$_1$ antagonist MRS2179 (100 μmol/L). Aggregation and ATP secretion are partially reduced in the presence of MRS2179 (100 μmol/L). In contrast, ADP stimulates a small transient aggregation response in the presence of the P2Y$_{12}$ receptor antagonist AR-C67085 (1 μmol/L), whereas secretion is abolished. (From Dawood *et al.* 2007 with permission.)

There is clearly still no gold standard for platelet testing, and indeed there may never be, and LTA remains the most widely used test. However, a variety of screening and diagnostic tests coupled with an accurate bleeding history will always be required to confirm a platelet-based bleeding disorder, simply because of the heterogeneity in the range of disorders encountered coupled with the cross-talk between receptors. Specialist test centres will therefore still be required for the identification of rare and new platelet-based defects.

Platelets and thrombosis

There is also much recent interest in the possibility of using platelet function tests to reliably detect platelet hyperreactivity in patients with arterial thrombosis (e.g. myocardial infarction, unstable and stable angina, stroke, transient ischaemic attacks and peripheral vascular disease). This could potentially allow patients to be risk stratified and their treatment adjusted accordingly to potentially improve their clinical outcomes. The increasing interest in this area and clinical discussion of aspirin or clopidogrel 'resistance' has also resulted in the development of a variety of instruments that can be useful for preclinical testing (e.g. Platelet Mapping System, VerifyNow, Plateletworks, Aspirinworks, Placor PRT). The VerifyNow test was originally developed as a whole-blood cartridge-based test to monitor $\alpha_{IIb}\beta_3$ blockade because of the narrow therapeutic window and increased bleeding risk associated with these types of drugs. The test has also been adapted to measure aspirin and P2Y$_{12}$ block-ade with two other cartridge formulations. Platelet responsiveness to antiplatelet drugs can now also be easily monitored by the tests mentioned as well as by LTA, whole-blood aggregometry, PFA-100 and IMPACT. Poor responders or 'resistant' individuals can therefore be identified, although it is still unclear how to manage them and whether there is a clinically relevant relationship between poor response and outcome. Emerging evidence suggests that the true incidence of so-called aspirin resistance is probably very low (when noncompliance is accounted for) and that many studies are measuring platelet hyperreactivity and not blockade of cyclooxygenase type 1. Although recent meta-analyses suggest that this could nevertheless be clinically informative, it is still unclear how to reliably identify these patients, with which test and cut-off (as different tests give different results) and then actually how to manage these patients. Testing is therefore still very much in the clinical research setting. Indeed, recent International Society for Thrombosis and Haemostasis (ISTH) Scientific and Standardization Committee guidelines suggest that aspirin resistance should still not be routinely monitored and the wider question remains whether routine testing of platelet hyperreactivity and/or drug responsiveness is actually clinically necessary. Certainly there is a spectrum of platelet responsiveness within the normal population and those individuals with a stable or even an acquired hyperreactive phenotype could theoretically be at higher risk of thrombosis.

Clopidogrel resistance is a totally different phenomenon as this is a prodrug that requires metabolism by liver cytochrome P450. This results in the generation of an active metabolite that irreversibly inhibits the P2Y$_{12}$ receptor. Differences in the efficiency of metabolism between individuals (related to their P450 genotype) taking standard clopidogrel dosing results in a spectrum of responsiveness and recent meta-analysis suggests that poor responders are indeed prone to increased risk of thrombosis, especially when undergoing angioplasty. Again, there is a variety of tests available to monitor the efficacy of clopidogrel, including LTA, VASP phosphorylation and VerifyNow. One of the problems facing the investigator is not only which test to use but also the definition of a suitable cut-off defining a non-response and how to effectively manage these individuals. Although there are emerging clinical cardiology guidelines, as yet they do not include routine monitoring of clopidogrel responsiveness, but further research is required in this important area. This problem could potentially be eliminated by prasugrel (which is metabolized efficiently in clopidogrel non-responders) and the emerging direct P2Y$_{12}$ inhibitors cangrelor and AZD6140 (Ticagrelor), providing the risk of bleeding is within acceptable limits.

It is clear that large well-designed prospective trials are required in this area where patients with hyperreactive platelets and/or a poor response to aspirin/clopidogrel are randomized to different treatments based on a platelet function test result. Only with this type of data will personalized platelet function testing perhaps become a reality in the future.

Conclusions and future developments

Given that platelets were considered to be just pieces of circulating dust about 150 years ago, they are now one of the most important cells in pathology. Now that the megakaryocytic/platelet genome and proteomes are being defined, many new platelet proteins have been discovered and exact roles in haemostasis and thrombosis will shortly be defined. Nevertheless, with all these developments and information, the individual is left with a bewildering complexity and a feeling of 'where will it all end?' In considering this, it is important to recognize that, perhaps surprisingly, many of the proteins in platelets appear to have minor or negligible roles in regulating activation. The number of proteins and pathways that play major roles in regulating platelet activation is apparently much smaller.

The ultimate goal of most platelet research remains the development of improved antithrombotic agents that provide effective treatment without an increased risk of bleeding. Although it may never be possible to fully attain this goal, as we begin to understand more about the events that underlie thrombus formation, there will be increased opportunity for discovery of more rational forms of therapy. New medicines targeted to the very early stages of platelet activation or the amplification phase (as proven with aspirin and clopidogrel) may be more effective in preventing thrombosis without significantly disturbing normal haemostasis.

Acknowledgements

S.P.W. is a British Heart Foundation Chair. The authors gratefully acknowledge the support of the British Heart Foundation, Wellcome Trust and BBSRC, and all the past and present members of their laboratories who have significantly contributed to the ideas and thoughts that have formed the basis of this chapter. We are extremely grateful to Hans Deckmyn, Johan Heemskerk and Ban Dawood for careful reading of a near-final version and their constructive comments.

Selected bibliography

General
Michelson A (2007) *Platelets*, 2nd edn. Academic Press, San Diego.

Clinical conditions, evaluation and guidelines
Bolton-Maggs PBM, Chalmers EA, Collins PL *et al.* (2006) A review of inherited platelet disorders with guidelines for their management on behalf of the UKHCDO. *British Journal of Haematology* **135**: 603–33.

Chen ZM, Jiang LX, Chen YP *et al.* (2005) Addition of clopidogrel to aspirin in 45,852 patients with acute myocardial infarction: randomized placebo-controlled trial. COMMIT (ClOpidogrel and Metoprolol in Myocardial Infarction Trial) collaborative group. *Lancet* **366**: 1607–21.

Dawood B, Wilde J, Watson SP (2007) Reference curves for aggregation and ATP secretion to aid diagnose of platelet-based bleeding disorders: effect of inhibition of ADP and thromboxane A$_2$ pathways. *Platelets* **18**: 329–45.

Gao C, Boylan B, Bougie D *et al.* (2009) Eptifibade-induced thrombocytopenia and thrombosis in humans require FcγRIIA and the integrin β3 cytoplasmic domain. *Journal of Clinical Investigation* **119**: 504–11.

Harrison P, Frelinger AL III, Furman MI, Michelson AD (2007) Measuring antiplatelet drug effects in the laboratory. *Thrombosis Research* **120**: 323–36.

Hayward CP, Harrison P, Cattaneo M, Ortel TL, Rao AK (2006) The Platelet Physiology Subcommittee of the Scientific and Standardization Committee of the International Society on Thrombosis and Haemostasis. Platelet function analyzer (PFA)-100 closure time in the evaluation of platelet disorders and platelet function. *Journal of Thrombosis and Haemostasis* **4**: 312–19.

Levine RL, Gilliland DG (2008) Myeloproliferative disorders. *Blood* **112**: 2190–8.

Linden MD, Jackson DE (2010) Platelets: Pleiotropic roles in atherogenesis and atherothrombosis. *International Journal of Biochemistry & Cell Biology* [Epub ahead of print].

Michelson AD, Cattaneo M, Eikelboom JW *et al.* (2005) Platelet Physiology Subcommittee of the Scientific and Standardization Committee of the International Society on Thrombosis and Haemostasis; Working Group on Aspirin Resistance. *Journal of Thrombosis and Haemostasis* **3**: 1309–11.

Reviews

Battinelli EM, Hartwig JH, Italiano JE Jr (2007) Delivering new insight into the biology of megakaryopoiesis and thrombopoiesis. *Current Opinion in Hematology* **14**: 419–26.

Bhatt DL, Topol EJ (2003) Scientific and therapeutic advances in antiplatelet therapy. *Nature Reviews. Drug Discovery* **2**: 15–28.

Brass LF, Zhu L, Stalker TJ (2008) Novel therapeutic targets at the platelet vascular interface. *Arteriosclerosis, Thrombosis and Vascular Biology* **28**: s43–s50.

Coller BS, Shattil SJ (2008) The GPIIb/IIIa (integrin αIIbβ3) odyssey: a technology-driven saga of a receptor with twists, turns, and even a bend. *Blood* **112**: 3011–25.

Cosemans JM, Iserbyt BF, Deckmyn H, Heemskerk JW (2008) Multiple ways to switch platelet integrins on and off. *Journal of Thrombosis and Haemostasis* **6**: 1253–61.

Gachet C (2008) P2 receptors, platelet function and pharmacological implications. *Thrombosis and Haemostasis* **99**: 466–72.

Gawaz M, Langar H, May AE (2005) Platelets in inflammation and atherogenesis. *Journal of Clinical Investigation* **115**: 3378–84.

Harrison P, Goodall AH (2008) 'Message in the platelet': more than just vestigial mRNA! *Platelets* **19**: 395–404.

Hartwig J, Italiano J Jr (2003) The birth of the platelet. *Journal of Thrombosis and Haemostasis* **1**: 1580–6.

Haslam RJ, Dickinson NT, Jang EK (1999) Cyclic nucleotides and phosphodiesterases in platelets. *Thrombosis and Haemostasis* **82**: 412–23.

Italiano JE Jr, Shivdasani RA (2003) Megakaryocytes and beyond: the birth of platelets. *Journal of Thrombosis and Haemostasis* **1**: 1174–82.

Jackson SP (2007) The growing complexity of platelet aggregation. *Blood* **109**: 5087–9.

Jackson SP, Schoenwalder SM (2003) Antiplatelet therapy: in search of the magic bullet. *Nature Reviews. Drug Discovery* **2**: 775–89.

Kaushansky K (2005) The molecular mechanisms that control thrombopoiesis. *Journal of Clinical Investigation* **115**: 3339–47.

Kaushansky K (2008) Historical review: megakaryopoiesis and thrombopoiesis. *Blood* **111**: 981–6.

Mackman N (2008) Triggers, targets and treatments for thrombosis. *Nature* **451**: 914–18.

Nieswandt B, Watson SP (2003) Platelet–collagen interaction: is GPVI the central receptor? *Blood* **102**: 449–61.

Ouwehand WH (2007) Platelet genomics and the risk of atherothrombosis. *Journal of Thrombosis and Haemostasis* **5**: 188–95.

Patel SR, Hartwig JH, Italiano JE Jr (2005) The biogenesis of platelets from megakaryocyte proplatelets. *Journal of Clinical Investigation* **115**: 3348–54.

Prevost N, Mitsios JV, Kato H *et al.* (2009) Group IVA cytosolic phospholipase A2 (cPLA2α) and integrin αIIbβ3 reinforce each other's functions during αIIbβ3 signalling in platelets. *Blood* **113**: 447–53.

Ruggeri ZM (2002) Platelets in atherothrombosis. *Nature Medicine* **8**: 1227–34.

Sachs UJ, Nieswandt B (2007) *In vivo* thrombus formation in murine models. *Circulation Research* **100**: 979–91.

Shattil SJ, Newman PJ (2004) Integrins: dynamic scaffolds for adhesion and signalling in platelets. *Blood* **104**: 1606–15.

Varga-Szabo D, Pleines I, Nieswandt B (2008) Cell adhesion mechanisms in platelets. *Arteriosclerosis, Thrombosis and Vascular Biology* **28**: 403–12.

Watson SP (2009) Platelet activation by extracellular matrix proteins in haemostasis and thrombosis. *Current Pharmaceutical Design* **15**: 1358–72.

Watson SP, Auger JM, McCarty OJ, Pearce AC (2005) GPVI and integrin αIIbβ3 signalling in platelets. *Journal of Thrombosis and Haemostasis* **3**: 1752–62.

Weyrich AS, Schwertz H, Kraiss LW, Zimmerman GA (2009) Protein synthesis by platelets: historical and new perspectives. *Journal of Thrombosis and Haemostasis* **7**: 241–6.

Woulfe DS (2005) Platelet G protein-coupled receptors in hemostasis and thrombosis. *Journal of Thrombosis and Haemostasis* **3**: 2193–200.

Research papers

Avecilla ST, Hattori K, Heissig B *et al.* (2004) Chemokine-mediated interaction of hematopoietic progenitors with the bone marrow vascular niche is required for thrombopoiesis. *Nature Medicine* **10**: 64–71.

Inoue O, Suzuki-Inoue K, McCarty OJ *et al.* (2006) Laminin stimulates spreading of platelets through integrin alpha6beta1-dependent activation of GPVI. *Blood* **107**: 1405–12.

Italiano JE Jr, Lecine P, Shivdasani RA, Hartwig JH (1999) Blood platelets are assembled principally at the ends of proplatelet processes produced by differentiated megakaryocytes. *Journal of Cell Biology* **147**: 1299–312.

Junt T, Schulze H, Chen Z *et al.* (2007) Dynamic visualization of thrombopoiesis within bone marrow. *Science* **317**: 1767–70.

Ono A, Westein E, Hsiao S *et al.* (2008) Identification of a fibrin-independent platelet contractile mechanism regulating primary hemostasis and thrombus growth. *Blood* **112**: 90–9.

Podrez EA, Byzova T, Febbraio M *et al.* (2007) Platelet CD36 links hyperlipidemia, oxidant stress and a prothrombotic phenotype. *Nature Medicine* **13**: 1086–95.

Ruggeri ZM, Orje JN, Habermann R, Federici AB, Reininger AJ (2006) Activation-independent platelet adhesion and aggregation under elevated shear stress. *Blood* **108**: 1995–2002.

CHAPTER 41

Inherited bleeding disorders

Michael A Laffan[1] and K John Pasi[2]

[1]Imperial College School of Medicine, Hammersmith Hospital, London, UK
[2]Centre for Haematology, Institute of Cell and Molecular Science, Barts and The London School of Medicine and Dentistry, London, UK

Introduction

The existence of lifelong bleeding disorders and their familial occurrence was noted in the medical literature as early as the 16th century. No doubt this was because the clinical syndrome of haemophilia is highly distinctive: early writers were impressed by the helplessness of the physician in the face of haemophilic bleeding. A full understanding of the pathophysiology and genetics of these disorders was long delayed because of the complexities of the clotting mechanism. Advances in protein chemistry and recombinant DNA technology have now produced a comprehensive account of normal coagulation, the coagulation defect in haemophilia and the underlying molecular genetics. An earlier chapter outlines the coagulation mechanism. In this chapter, the clinical features of the most common inherited bleeding disorders, haemophilia and von Willebrand disease (VWD), are described, together with a summary of the genetic lesions identified in their various deficiency states.

Advances in molecular biology have enabled more precise diagnosis and reduced the dependence on plasma-derived concentrates, at least in the economically rich countries. Direct identification of the mutation responsible for the factor deficiency in individual kindreds has provided a better understanding of structure–function relationships and the pathophysiology of the bleeding disorder. It has also superseded the use of

restriction fragment length polymorphisms (RFLPs), thus removing the uncertainty from carrier detection in the vast majority of cases.

Haemophilia A

Pathophysiology

Haemophilia A and B are caused by deficiency of factor (F)VIII and FIX respectively. FVIII and FIX are the two components of the intrinsic tenase (see Chapter 39) and so not surprisingly their absence causes virtually identical patterns of bleeding. Combined with the fact that they are both encoded on the long arm of the X chromosome (Xq28ter) they present almost indistinguishable sex-linked clinical syndromes and laboratory tests are required to determine which is present. In both cases, failure to form the intrinsic tenase complex results in failure to produce the thrombin burst characteristic of normal coagulation. As a result a loose friable fibrin mesh is produced that is mechanically easily dislodged and which has increased susceptibility to fibrinolysis. Fibrinolytic breakdown of the clot is also favoured by the failure of the weak thrombin burst to activate the thrombin-activatable fibrinolysis inhibitor (TAFI). The consequent failure to consolidate the primary haemostatic (platelet) plug results in the characteristic bleeding pattern of haemophilia, which is delayed after trauma but much prolonged. Replacement by intravenous infusion of the deficient factor can normalize the haemostatic mechanism of the haemophilic individual.

Postgraduate Haematology: 6th edition. Edited by A. Victor Hoffbrand, Daniel Catovsky, Edward G.D. Tuddenham, Anthony R. Green
© 2011 Blackwell Publishing Ltd.

Table 41.1 Haemophilia A*: clinical severity.

FVIII (units/dL)	Bleeding tendency	Relative incidence (%)
< 1	Severe: frequent spontaneous[†] bleeding into joints, muscles and internal organs	50
2–5	Moderate: some 'spontaneous' bleeds, bleeding after minor trauma	30
> 5–45	Mild: bleeding only after significant trauma, surgery	20

*This table is also applicable to FIX, FX and FII deficiences, but not to FVII, FXI, FV, FXIII or von Willebrand factor deficiencies (see text).

[†]'Spontaneous' bleeding refers to those episodes in which no obvious precipitating event preceded the bleed. No doubt, minor tissue damage consequent on everyday activities actually initiates bleeding.

Clinical features

Haemophilia A affects approximately 1 in 10 000 live births and is equally common in all ethnic groups. The vast majority of patients are male, but haemophilia can occur very rarely in females (see below). The severity and frequency of bleeding in X-linked FVIII deficiency are inversely correlated with the residual FVIII level. Table 41.1 summarizes this relationship and gives the relative frequency of the categories, based on UK national data. The main load- or strain-bearing joints (ankles, knees and elbows) are most affected but any joint can be the site of bleeding. If untreated, this intracapsular bleeding causes severe swelling, pain, stiffness and inflammation, which gradually resolves over days or weeks. It is not clear why bleeding in haemophilia shows a predilection for joints, but it has been suggested that low levels of tissue factor (TF) expression in synovial tissue may be at least part of the explanation.

Blood is highly irritating to the synovium and causes an immediate inflammatory reaction in the joint. In the longer term, blood and particularly increased iron deposition promote a chronic proliferative synovitis resulting in overgrowth of friable and highly vascular synovium that has an increased tendency to further bleeding, thus setting up a vicious circle. As a result of the vicious circle of bleeding and synovial hypertrophy, a particular joint frequently becomes the 'target joint' in an individual, whereas other joints may be relatively spared. Blood also has a rapid destructive effect on cartilage that is evident after only a single haemarthrosis. Accumulation of iron in chondrocytes may also contribute to the multifactorial degenerative arthritis, resulting in irregularity of articular contour,

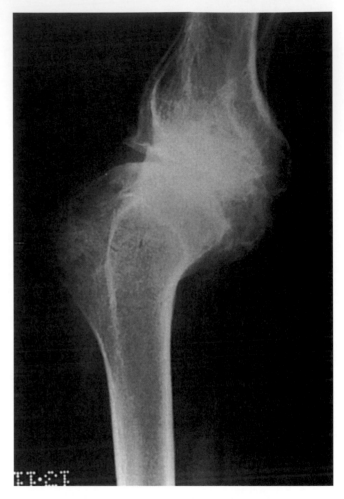

Figure 41.1 Radiograph of knee joint showing advanced haemophilic arthropathy. Note the loss of cartilage, eburnation, deformity subluxation, osteophytes, subchondral cysts and irregularity of joint contours.

thinning of the cartilage, bony overgrowth and subchondral cysts, and finally ankylosis (Figure 41.1).

Muscle bleeding can be seen in any anatomical site, but it most often presents in the large load-bearing groups of the thigh, calf, posterior abdominal wall and buttocks. Local pressure effects often cause entrapment neuropathy, particularly of the femoral nerve with iliopsoas bleeding. This causes a common symptom triad of groin pain, hip flexure and cutaneous sensory loss over the femoral nerve distribution. Bleeding into the calf, forearm or perineal muscles can lead to ischaemic necrosis and contracture.

Haematuria is less common than joint or muscle bleeding in individuals with haemophilia, but severely affected patients have one or two episodes per decade. These may be painless and resolve spontaneously, but, if bleeding is heavy, it can produce clot colic. Usually, no anatomical abnormality is found to account for the haematuria on radiological investigation.

Central nervous system bleeding is uncommon but can occur after a slight head injury and remains a significant cause of death in haemophilia A. Intestinal tract bleeding usually presents as obstruction due to intramural haemorrhage, but haematemesis and melaena also occasionally occur and should be routinely investigated, as they may be due to peptic ulcer or malignancy.

Oropharyngeal bleeding, although uncommon, is clinically dangerous, as extension through the soft tissues of the floor of the mouth can lead to respiratory obstruction. Bleeding from the tongue after laceration can be very persistent and troublesome due to fibrinolytic substances in saliva and the impossibility of immobilizing the tongue.

Surgery and open trauma invariably lead to dangerous haemorrhage in the untreated individual with haemophilia. There may be persistence of haemorrhage, often after an initial short-lived period of haemostasis. Clots, if formed, are bulky and friable and break off, with renewed haemorrhage occurring intermittently over days and weeks. Today this is only seen in patients who are resistant to conventional replacement therapy due to the presence of inhibitors (see below) or when patients with mild or moderate haemophilia present after their first surgical or dental procedure.

Bruising is a feature of haemophilia A but is usually only of cosmetic significance as it remains superficial and self-limiting. Large extending ecchymoses may occasionally require treatment.

Presentation

When a woman is known to be a carrier or at high risk, the cord blood FVIII level will establish the diagnosis in the infant. However, haemophilia may be sporadic and in approximately one-third of cases there is no family history. In such cases, haemophilia may come to light in the neonatal period with cephalohaematoma or other bleeding resulting from the trauma of birth. In cultures where early circumcision is the rule, this will cause prolonged haemorrhage, as was noted in the Babylonian Talmud almost 2000 years ago. Quite often, the diagnosis is delayed until it is noticed that the infant has many large bruises from hand pressure when being picked up or from minor knocks on the cot. These sometimes cause diagnostic confusion and the erroneous label of 'non-accidental injury' may be applied, with needless psychological trauma to the parents. As soon as the infant starts to walk actively, joint bleeding begins to appear. In other children, excessive bleeding from the eruption of primary dentition, or from lacerations, leads to the performance of diagnostic tests. In patients who have some functional FVIII, even 1 or 2% (moderate haemophilia) may be sufficient to largely prevent spontaneous bleeding and delay diagnosis until bleeding occurs after trauma or surgery. Mild cases may only present in adulthood when severe trauma or surgery provokes unusual bleeding.

Investigation of coagulation defects and haemophilia

Investigation of a suspected inherited bleeding disorder usually begins with the global tests of coagulation. These tests reflect the history of coagulation investigation. Thus they force the coagulation system to function in a way that has been useful in the laboratory but which is considerably removed from normal physiology. As a result we routinely use tests such as the activated partial thromboplastin time (APTT) which, when abnormal, may indicate the presence of a severe disorder such as haemophilia or an irrelevant one such as FXII deficiency. Nonetheless, once this is understood, these tests remain extremely useful in detecting and diagnosing coagulation disorders. The principal routine tests in common use are the prothrombin time (PT) and the APTT, also known as the partial thromboplastin time with kaolin (PTTK) or the kaolin cephalin clotting time (KCCT). These tests require the activity of all the conventional procoagulant factors except FXIII; however, they do not require the presence of platelets (they are performed using platelet-poor plasma and exogenous phospholipid) and do not activate the protein C/protein S system.

Prothrombin time
In the PT, coagulation is triggered using a thromboplastin, i.e. tissue factor (TF) plus phospholipid, which may be derived from animal tissue (typically rabbit brain) or increasingly is relipidated recombinant human TF. The plasma is recalcified and the clotting time recorded. The PT will be prolonged by deficiencies of FVII, FX, FV, FII or fibrinogen.

Activated partial thromboplastin time
The APTT is triggered using a negatively charged surface (e.g. kaolin or silica) to initiate contact activation. Further progression requires the addition of phospholipid (partial thromboplastin) and calcium. It is thought that activation of coagulation rarely proceeds by this route *in vivo* and consequently deficiency of the contact factors is not associated with any increased tendency to bleeding. The APTT will be prolonged by deficiencies of FXII, FXI, FIX, FVIII, FX, FV, FII, fibrinogen, prekallikrein and high-molecular-weight kininogen. It is therefore abnormal in haemophilia A and B.

Thrombin time
The thrombin time is performed simply by adding a dilute preparation of thrombin to citrated platelet-poor plasma and recording the clotting time. Recalcification and phospholipid are not required. Prolongation of the thrombin time therefore implies that there is either an inhibitor of thrombin present (most commonly the effect of heparin) or that there is a problem with fibrin cleavage or polymerization. It is extremely sensitive to the presence of unfractionated heparin but is also prolonged by low or abnormal fibrinogen and hypoalbuminaemia.

Inhibitors

The simplest interpretation of a prolonged test of coagulation is that one or more of the factors required for its execution is deficient in the patient's plasma. A frequently encountered alternative is that an inhibitor of coagulation, usually an antibody, is present. The presence of an inhibitor is typically demonstrated by a mixing test in which normal and the test plasma (with a prolonged clotting time) are mixed in equal proportions. Correction of the prolonged clotting time by the normal plasma indicates a coagulation factor deficiency and failure to correct indicates the presence of an inhibitor.

When an inhibitor is detected, further tests are performed to determine whether it has specificity for a particular clotting factor or not. Non-specific inhibitors usually fall into the class of antiphospholipid antibodies and are paradoxically associated with thrombosis rather than bleeding (see Chapter 46). Specific inhibitors are most commonly directed against FVIII, resulting in an 'acquired' haemophilia.

Specific factor assays

When initial tests or clinical history suggests single factor deficiency, then specific factor assays are performed to determine which is affected. This is most usually done by performing a bioassay in which the ability of the test plasma to correct the defect in plasma lacking a specific factor is measured. Bioassays have the advantage of directly measuring the biological activity of the factor in question but because they also utilize other plasma components, they are susceptible to numerous interferences and confounding effects. This can be avoided in some cases by using artificial small substrates (chromogenic substrates). This aids automation and avoids interference but often does not capture all aspects of the molecule's biological activity. Finally, the physical amount of the factor present can be assessed immunologically. Immunological assays are accurate and precise, but of course do not give information about the functional activity of the molecules that have been measured.

Laboratory diagnosis of haemophilia

Initial tests show a prolonged APTT, normal PT and thrombin time (if performed) and a normal platelet count. This will usually prompt specific factor assays of FVIII, FIX and FXI and, in the case of haemophilia A, results shows FVIII clotting activity below 50 units/dL, with all other factors normal. Von Willebrand factor (VWF) antigen and activity (ristocetin cofactor) are also normal.

FVIII assays

In most laboratories the FVIII assay is a modified APTT and is often referred to as a 'one-stage assay' because the activation of FVIII and coagulation are performed in a single step. However, it is also possible to construct a 'two-stage assay' in which the FVIII is activated in a first step and then the activity is measured in a second separate step. Chromogenic FVIII assays use a two-stage procedure. The two assays normally give similar results but the distinction is important because some defective FVIII molecules give different results in the two assays. Most commonly in these cases, the one-stage assay gives a higher result than the two-stage but the patient's bleeding phenotype is more in keeping with the latter (lower) result. Thus the assessment of the severity (and sometimes even the diagnosis) of the haemophilia can be mistaken if the two assays are not carried out and compared.

Treatment

Clotting factor concentrates

The discovery in the early 1960s that FVIII was concentrated in cryoprecipitate and the subsequent description of the production of antihaemophilic globulin in a closed bag system revolutionized treatment for haemophilia. Home treatment for the majority of patients became feasible and with the advent of lyophilized concentrates prepared from cryoprecipitate made from the plasma from many thousands of donors, the prospect of a normal life for the severely affected haemophilic individual was brought very close. However, use of such plasma-derived concentrates was associated with the transmission of hepatitis C virus (HCV), hepatitis B virus (HBV) and HIV. Although these infections were present at only low frequency in the donor population, concentrates were made from many thousands of donations and so most, if not all, batches of concentrate were infected, particularly with HCV. Since 1985 virucidal methods have been rigorously applied (such as terminal dry heat treatment, solvent/detergent treatment, nanofiltration and pasteurization) in conjunction with donor selection and plasma pool screening and quarantining. As a result of these measures, plasma-derived concentrates are now very safe such that the risk of HIV, HBV or HCV transmission is close to zero. However, there remains the problem of transmission of non-lipid-coated viruses (such as hepatitis A and parvovirus), which can survive solvent/detergent sterilization, and the possibility that new viruses will emerge. For these reasons, products are required to undergo more than one inactivation process. For FIX concentrate, the process of nanofiltration has been used, which can prevent transmission of non-lipid-coated viruses.

It has recently transpired that the prion protein responsible for variant Creutzfeldt–Jakob disease (vCJD) may be transmitted via pooled plasma concentrates, although only a single case has been reported to date. With the ongoing concern about prion transmission through blood and blood products, concentrates are no longer produced from plasma drawn from countries with notable vCJD in the donor population.

The plasma-derived clotting factor concentrates in use at present are high-purity products with a high specific activity. They are prepared chromatographically, which results in an end product of high specific activity. The advent of recombinant clotting factor concentrates has further enhanced safety of replacement therapy.

Recombinant FVIII

The structure of the FVIII gene and the isolation of cDNA clones encoding the complete FVIII sequence were described in 1984. This has allowed the manufacture of FVIII in cell culture, which therefore eliminates the risk of disease transmission from donors. Progressive refinements have in some cases eliminated all additional animal protein from the cell culture medium and any protein added as stabilizer in the lyophilized product. Recombinant FVIII can be made either from the wild-type 'full-length' cDNA or from cDNA that has the large B domain deleted. The B domain has been shown to be completely dispensable for the procoagulant function of FVIII and its absence does not change the half-life of the molecule. It is therefore curious that one B domain-deleted product has shown a marked discrepancy between one-stage and two-stage assays. Subsequent developments suggest that the origin of the discrepancy in this concentrate may be post-translational modification rather than the absence of the B domain.

Recombinant technology may allow the development of modified bioengineered FVIII molecules with enhanced pharmacokinetics, specific activity or reduced immunogenicity. A prolonged half-life may also be achieved by coupling FVIII to other molecules such as polyethylene glycol, to liposomes or by altering glycosylation. Fusion of FVIII with Fc or albumin has also been achieved, with a markedly enhanced half-life in preclinical studies. Although there is enthusiasm for these approaches, which are all under active development, clinical trials will decide which if any are effective and safe.

Assay of recombinant clotting factors

In pharmacokinetic studies, it was found that the chromogenic assay produced considerably higher levels than one-stage assays.

The influence of phospholipids on these discrepancies was studied. It was found that when the APTT reagent was replaced by platelets in the one-stage assay, the results of the chromogenic assay and the one-stage assay were similar. Furthermore, using the principle of 'like versus like', this discrepancy between chromogenic and one-stage methods could be eliminated by using the recombinant product diluted in haemophilic plasma as a standard reference. In this case it is the standard calibration against reference plasma that is adjusted.

Treatment of haemophilia

Since the development of replacement therapy, the goal of treatment for haemophilia patients has been the prevention of haemorrhagic episodes. Based on studies from haemophilia carriers and patients with mild haemophilia, we can deduce that a level of 5–30% is adequate to arrest minor bleeds, but inadequate for major surgery or trauma. At least 60% sustained throughout the healing period is needed for normal wound healing to occur. The severity and the frequency of haemarthrosis is directly related to the degree of deficiency of the clotting factor, but the precise plasma level needed to prevent haemarthrosis is still unknown.

After trauma or at the onset of bleeding, therapeutic infusion of replacement factor should be administered as early as possible and to a haemostatic level to stop or prevent haemorrhage. The dosing of factor replacement is still based on theoretical calculations and clinical experience. Guidelines for the treatment of haemorrhagic episodes in haemophilia are given in Table 41.2, with the estimated likely effective level required for haemostasis. If sufficient FVIII is available, it is physiological to restore the FVIII level into the normal range and maintain it there by continuous infusion or frequently repeated infusion.

Formulae based on plasma volume and expected recovery give a rough guide to dosage required to achieve a given level,

Table 41.2 Indications and guidelines for factor replacement in haemophilia A and B.

Site of haemorrhage	Optimal factor level (%)	Dose (units/kg body weight)		Duration (days)
		FVIII	FIX	
Joint	30–50	20–30	30–50	1–2
Muscle	30–50	20–30	30–40	1–2
Gastrointestinal tract	40–60	30–40	40–60	7–10
Oral mucosa	30–50	20–30	30–40	Until healing
Epistaxis	30–50	20–30	40–60	Until healing
Haematuria	30–100	25–50	70–100	Until healing
Central nervous system	60–100	50	80–100	7–10
Retroperitoneal	50–100	30–50	60–100	7–10
Trauma or surgery	50–100	30–50	60–100	Until healing

Source: Escobar (2003) with permission.

but where the level is critical, as for surgery or when there is serious bleeding, it should always be checked by assay after infusion. On average, FVIII infusion produces a plasma increment of 2 units/dL per unit infused per kilogram body weight. From this, a simple formula can be derived:

Dose to be infused (units)

= [weight (kg) × increment needed (units/dL)]/2

Assessing the period of treatment required is a matter of clinical judgement of the individual episode or lesion.

Cover for surgery, other than very minor procedures, requires maintenance of normal FVIII levels for at least 1 week, followed by a period at reduced dosage during convalescence. This can be achieved either by repeated bolus injections every 8–12 hours (paying particular attention to trough levels, which should not fall below 50 units/dL) or by continuous infusion. The half-life of FVIII varies considerably and may be particularly short in children, requiring more frequent dosing. It should also be noted that the doses required during the immediate postoperative period may be considerably more than expected.

Prophylaxis

There is a long tradition of giving prophylaxis to young boys with haemophilia; prophylaxis was developed as early as 1958 in Malmö, Sweden. The rationale for the prophylactic model was the observation that chronic arthropathy was seen less frequently and less severely in individuals with a FVIII level of 1–4 units/dL.

Today prophylaxis is regarded as the standard of care for all boys with severe haemophilia. Regular prophylactic treatment is begun at 1–1.5 years before the onset of joint bleeds, so-called primary prophylaxis. Ideally, FVIII is administered every second day at a dose of 25–40 units/kg. The goal is to maintain a trough level of 1 unit/dL or more, which may require individual adjustment of size and frequency of dosing, and so to avoid all bleeds. Evidence from trials indicates that the risk of bleeding rises as the duration of FVIII levels below 1 unit/dL increases. There is good historic evidence that the Malmö model is effective in preventing haemophilic arthropathy. For the youngest cohort of boys born in 1981–90, who began prophylaxis between 1 and 2 years of age with 4000–9000 units/kg annually, both the orthopaedic and radiological scores were zero (Figure 41.2). More recently, a large randomized study comparing prophylaxis with enhanced on-demand therapy showed that after 6 years of therapy, 93% of those on primary prophylaxis had a normal joint score on magnetic resonance imaging (MRI) compared with only 55% on intensive on-demand regimens.

Use of the peripheral vein is the preferred approach when beginning prophylactic treatment. However, if this is not possible then the implantation of an indwelling venous access device (e.g. Port-a-Cath) may be necessary. Substantial experience with Port-a-Cath has been published. Although the advan-

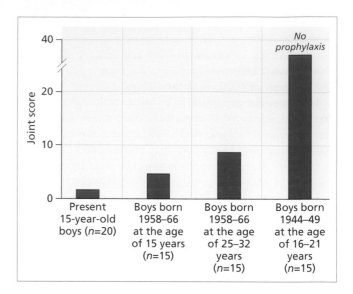

Figure 41.2 Orthopaedic joint scores for patients intensively treated in the present. A group of 15-year-old boys compared with a less intensively treated group at different ages and with patients not receiving prophylaxis (historical control subjects). (From United Kingdom Haemophilia Centre Doctors' Organisation 2003 with permission.)

tages of such devices are recognized, septic complications remain a challenge. A number of studies have been published that show an infection rate ranging from 0.2 to 3.4 infections per 1000 catheter-days but increasing with frequency of use. Another alternative is the fashioning of a small arteriovenous fistula in the arm.

In older patients who have established joint disease or have had previous joint bleeds, prophylaxis is also effective in reducing bleeding episodes and/or slowing progression of joint disease. This 'secondary' prophylaxis may be used continuously or for a limited period to allow the synovial hypertrophy in a target joint to regress or be targeted to periods when bleeding is more likely (such as sporting activity).

Desmopressin

A non-blood-derived alternative to FVIII concentrate, desmopressin (1-deamino-8-D-arginine vasopressin) can be used to treat mild haemophilia. Desmopressin acts via the V_2 receptors on endothelial cells to stimulate exocytosis of Weibel–Palade bodies, the endothelial storage organelles that contain primarily VWF and, in some tissues, also FVIII. In practice, this effect can be used to elevate the plasma FVIII level twofold to fourfold above baseline. Desmopressin is a synthetic analogue of vasopressin and retains the antidiuretic action of the natural hormone but not its vasopressor activity. Patients are advised to restrict their fluid intake after desmopressin. This is especially important in young children in whom unrestricted fluid intake may result in hyponatraemia and convulsions. Desmopressin is contraindicated in elderly patients and those with vascular disease, because arterial thrombosis has been reported following desmopressin in these circumstances.

Desmopressin can correct the haemostatic defect in mild haemophilia A or VWD sufficiently to cover minor surgery or treat a minor bleeding episode. A typical regimen would be to give 0.3 µg/kg body weight either by slow intravenous infusion over 20 min or by subcutaneous injection. Desmopressin also releases tissue plasminogen activator and so tranexamic acid is frequently given as well. A high-concentration nasal spray is also available that delivers 150 µg per actuation. The effect is maximal at 30 min after an intravenous dose and 1 hour following a subcutaneous or intranasal dose. The FVIII level rises threefold on average. The half-life of the endogenously released FVIII is about 8 hours but may be shorter in some cases and the fall-off should be documented. The dose can be repeated and although tachyphylaxis occurs such that the second dose may produce a rise only 30% of the first, there is often no further drop with succeeding doses. If repeated doses are given over a short interval (e.g. 48–72 hours), the FVIII response to desmopressin injection should be assayed to ensure that the reserves are not exhausted.

Complications of therapy

Inhibitors

Antibodies to FVIII (inhibitors) are most common in patients with severe rather than mild haemophilia. They are most likely to develop during childhood within the first 25 exposures to FVIII after which they are infrequent, but do rarely develop after years of treatment. Prospective studies have shown that in the past the incidence of inhibitors in patients with haemophilia has generally been underestimated. Studies to determine the true incidence are fraught with difficulty owing to bias in patient selection, frequency and sensitivity of testing and previous treatment. When studied closely, inhibitors have been detected in around 25–30% of patients with severe haemophilia at some stage in their treatment. However, many of these are low-level transient inhibitors that are not a long-term problem for treatment. The cumulative incidence of high-responding inhibitors is in the region of 10–15%. The likelihood of an individual developing an inhibitor is strongly dependent on the genetic lesion responsible for the FVIII deficiency. Patients with large deletions or stop codons in the light chain appear to be particularly prone to inhibitor development. However, some missense mutations causing mild to moderate haemophilia, particularly those in the light chain, are also associated with a high frequency of inhibitor development. Approximately 25% of patients with the common intron-22 inversion develop inhibitors. There is also evidence that when FVIII is adminis-

tered in large amounts (e.g. severe bleeds) or in association with inflammatory stimuli (e.g. surgery), this increases the likelihood of inhibitor development. As more is learned of the molecular bases for FVIII deficiency, it should be possible, perhaps in association with human leucocyte antigen typing, to define more precisely the individual risk. Because the development of inhibitors is unpredictable, it is important to test for their emergence at clinic visits and before operations.

Antibodies to FVIII frequently have a time-dependent component in their action and therefore an incubation time of 2–4 hours is required to reliably measure the full effect of the antibody. Inhibitors usually inactivate FVIII in a predictable linear manner (type 1 kinetics) but they may have complex equilibria and not inactivate all available FVIII (type 2 kinetics) and these are seen particularly in mild to moderate and acquired haemophilia. Inhibitors are most commonly measured using the Bethesda assay where 1 Bethesda unit (BU) is the amount of antibody that reduces the FVIII activity in pooled normal plasma by 50% after 2 hours incubation. Some inhibitors are 'low-responding' and remain at a low or moderate level (< 5–10 BU) after further FVIII exposure, whereas in high responders treatment with FVIII elicits a sharp anamnestic rise after 5–8 days and inhibitor levels may reach hundreds or thousands of BU. Low responders can be treated repeatedly with high doses of FVIII concentrate. However, high responders are refractory to treatment with FVIII concentrate and therefore alternative therapies are required.

Inhibitors: treatment of bleeding

Porcine FVIII functions well in human plasma but is frequently neutralized less efficiently by the anti-FVIII antibodies produced in humans with haemophilia. This has made it a useful alternative treatment in patients with inhibitors. However, it is not free of the problems associated with plasma-derived products and so recombinant porcine FVIII is in development and entering clinical trials.

At present the most common approach to achieving haemostasis in patients with inhibitors is to use a 'bypassing agent' that promotes thrombin generation without depending on the intrinsic tenase. The currently available bypassing agents are human recombinant FVIIa and a plasma-derived prothrombin complex concentrate that contains activated coagulation factors (factor eight inhibitor bypassing activity, or FEIBA). Human FVII was cloned in the mid-1980s and recombinant FVIIa was developed specifically as treatment for bleeding episodes in individuals with haemophilia complicated by inhibitory antibodies. Activated FVII is an inefficient enzyme when not complexed with TF and does not therefore produce systemic activation of coagulation when infused. Its mechanism of action in haemophilia has been the subject of much debate. It seems most likely that FVIIa binds to the surface of activated platelets at the site of injury and promotes FXa formation there. Recent evidence suggests that platelets may be able to synthesize TF or at least acquire it from circulating microparticles. High concentrations (30–90 nmol/L) are required to generate sufficient FXa and FIIa to achieve haemostasis.

The advantages of recombinant FVIIa include viral safety, low systemic activation of coagulation, effectiveness independent of inhibitor titre and an excellent overall safety profile allowing home use and ease of administration. The main disadvantage is the short half-life and therefore the need for frequent administration. Recent studies suggest that this can be overcome by using a single very large dose for mild to moderate bleeds.

Both native and activated prothrombin complex concentrates appear to be able to bypass FVIII and have a role in the treatment of patients with FVIII antibodies. The substance(s) responsible for the FVIII bypassing activity are undefined but their efficacy appears to derive from a combination of activated clotting factors and the elevation of prothrombin concentration, which is a major determinant of thrombin generation. The activated prothrombin complex concentrates contain more of the FVIII bypassing activity and are designed specifically for use in patients with FVIII inhibitors. Activated prothrombin complex concentrates have proved efficacious in controlling bleeding in many situations. The problems with FEIBA are that is of plasma origin and it contains some FVIII, which may cause an anamnestic rise in inhibitor titre. On the other hand, its longer dosage interval (given once or twice daily) makes it more suitable for prophylactic use. A major problem with both bypassing agents is that there is no reliable laboratory measure of their haemostatic effect.

Treatment of inhibitors: immune tolerance

Bypassing agents are considerably less effective than FVIII at achieving haemostasis and cannot yet provide reliable prophylaxis. It is therefore highly desirable to eliminate a FVIII inhibitor, a process referred to as immune tolerance induction (ITI). Basic ITI regimens involve the continued administration of FVIII, and both low-dose (25 units/kg alternate days) or high-dose (order of 100 units/kg twice daily) FVIII regimens have been used. Neither regimen has been conclusively shown to be superior and either may need to be continued for 12 months or more. Overall, the success rate is approximately 70%, after which prophylaxis must be maintained to prevent re-emergence of the antibody. The success is greatest in younger patients (< 7 years), with a historic peak titre below 200 BU, and when treatment is begun after allowing the inhibitor to fall to below 5 BU by avoiding further FVIII exposure. For resistant cases the use of a FVIII concentrate containing VWF may be more successful or the regimens may be combined with anti-CD20, or corticosteroids, alkylating agents, plasmapheresis and immunoglobulin (Malmö regimen). Success is defined as normalization of the FVIII recovery and a FVIII half-life greater than 6 hours.

Molecular genetics of haemophilia A

The FVIII gene (Figure 41.3) spans 190 kb of the X chromosome. The protein-coding regions (exons) are separated by 25 introns, some of very large size (e.g. intron 22 is over 35 kb). FVIII is synthesized in the liver, spleen and lymph nodes but also in some endothelial cells (probably in the lung), which creates the desmopressin-releasable pool. The amino acid sequence contains a triplicated region (A1, A2, A3 in Figure 41.4), whose elements are more than 30% homologous with each other. A second duplicated homology region (C1, C2) is responsible for the phospholipid-binding properties of the molecule. The third type of sequence in the protein is the heavily glycosylated B domain, which is coded entirely within exon 14, connects A2 and A3, and is removed on thrombin activation of FVIII.

The processed mRNA specifies a protein of 2351 amino acids, from which a 19-amino-acid N-terminal leader sequence is cleaved on secretion. The mature plasma protein initially consists of a single chain of 2332 amino acids, but as a result of proteolysis circulates as a series of light-chain and heavy-chain heterodimers with B domains of varying length.

The vast majority (> 90%) of FVIII circulates in complex with VWF, in the absence of which its half-life is extremely short. Studies of FVIII have identified the A3 (1648–1689), C1 and C2 domains as important for VWF binding but it is uncertain how many of these interact directly with VWF because in isolation the recombinant fragments have a much lower affinity. After thrombin activation, the cofactor consists of a heterotrimer: the N-terminal heavy chain corresponding to region A1 and the A2 domain isolated by cleavages at 372/373 and 740/741, which is held by a divalent cation-dependent linkage to the C-terminal light chain corresponding to part of A3 plus C1 and C2 (see Figure 41.4). The B domain is discarded by cleavages at 740/741 and 1689/1690. Thrombin cleavage also results in release of FVIII from VWF.

Protein C cleaves FVIIIa at 336/337 and 562/563, totally inactivating the cofactor. The crystal structure of FVIII has recently been reported and several of the interactions mapped including the FIX-binding site on the A2 and A3 domains. The C domains appear to be responsible for phospholipid binding.

Thanks to the development of polymerase chain reaction (PCR)-based rapid screening and sequencing methods, the mutations in nearly all patients with haemophilia A can be identified (Table 41.3). Consequently, a large database of mutations has accumulated and is maintained at http://hadb.org.uk. These include large deletions and missense mutations, as well as nonsense, frameshift, splicing (affecting mRNA processing) and insertional mutations. Surprisingly, about half of all severe haemophilia A is due to a major inversion (Figure 41.4) that occurs quite frequently during male gametogenesis (approximately 1 in 10 000 spermatozoa).

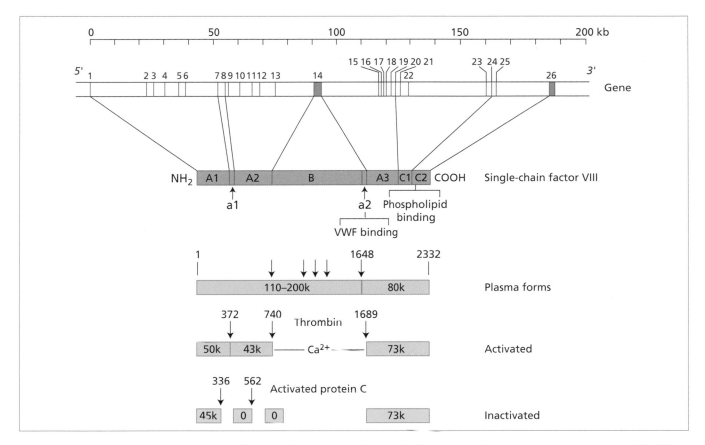

Figure 41.3 The FVIII gene and protein. Top line, scale for gene in kilobase pairs of DNA; second line, location of exons (protein-coding segments) of the FVIII gene shown as solid bars; second to third line, corresponding domains of FVIII gene and protein; fourth line, plasma FVIII is heterogeneous due to cleavage at various points within the B domain during synthesis and secretion, yielding heterodimers in which the heavy chain (N-terminal segment) pairs from 740 to 1648 amino acids; fifth line, thrombin activation releases the a2 segment from the light chain, the B domain from the heavy chain and cleaves between the A1 and A2 domains; bottom line, inactivation of factor VIIIa by activated protein C is accompanied by cleavages at 336, releasing the a1 domain and 562 in the middle of the A2 domain.

Haemophilia A in females

True homozygous haemophilia A is rare, but well described, being due to the marriage of a carrier to an affected male, often a cousin. Severe menstrual haemorrhage occurs but responds to FVIII infusion. Haemophilia A has been described in a female with Turner syndrome. The random process of X-chromosome inactivation allows only one FVIII gene to function in each female cell. Thus carriers of haemophilia A have on average 50% of the mean normal level of the clotting factor (or its antigen FVIII:Ag). However because the process is random, skewing of the inactivation towards the X chromosome containing the abnormal or the normal FVIII gene may occur, resulting in a FVIII level that is either well within the normal range or low enough to produce a mild haemophilia phenotype. By measuring the level of VWF antigen (VWF:Ag), the autosomally coded carrier protein for FVIII, it is possible to improve discrimination as carriers will tend to have lower levels of FVIII than VWF. Even so, there is still some overlap (about 15%) where the carriers have a normal ratio. It is therefore important to note that while a low level of FVIII strongly implies carriership, a normal FVIII level by no means excludes it.

Translocation through the FVIII locus has given rise to severe haemophilia in an affected female due to exclusive inactivation of the normal X chromosome. Due to sperm mutation in the father, especially in the prevalent inversion, a carrier can present *de novo* with no family history of haemophilia. The most usual reason for finding a low FVIII in a female if the above has been excluded is VWD. This should usually be evident from assays of VWF. Of course, VWD and haemophilia A can coexist in the same family, which makes carrier detection difficult. Type 2N VWD (see below) may also be confused with mild haemophilia A.

Table 41.3 Mutations responsible for haemophilia A.

Mutation type	No. of mutations observed	Percentage
Intron 22 inversion		
Distal	260	30.7
Proximal	37	4.4
Rare	5	0.6
Total	302	35.7
Intron 1 inversion		
Total	8	1.0
Point mutations		
Missense	323	38.2
Nonsense	79	9.3
Total	402	47.5
Small deletions or insertions		
Small deletions	63	7.5
Small insertions	22	2.6
Combination of insertions and deletions	1	0.1
Total	86	10.2
Large deletions (> 50 bp)		
Total	25	3.0
Splice-site mutations		
Intronic	20	2.4
Cryptic	2	0.2
Total	22	2.6

Source: Graw *et al.* (2005) with permission.

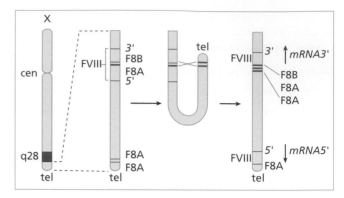

Figure 41.4 How the tip flips: the mechanism of inversion through intron 22. The mutation is responsible for up to half of all cases of severe haemophilia A. During spermatogenesis, at meiosis the single X pairs with the Y chromosome in the homologous regions, but there is nothing to pair with most of the long arm of X. Unfortunately, the possibility of intrachromosomal pairing and crossover exists because there are three copies of a gene designated *F8A*, one lying within intron 22 and two in the opposite orientation situated 400 kb telomeric to the FVIII gene. Crossover with either the distal or the proximal *F8A* copy divides the FVIII gene in two, such that separately transcribed mRNAs are produced, neither of which encodes functional FVIII.

Isolated FIX deficiency is always hereditary and the clinical severity of haemophilia B generally shows the same relationship with the residual factor level as for FVIII in haemophilia A, although recent data suggest that on average the phenotype might be slightly less severe.

Haemophilia B

Inheritance and diagnosis

Haemophilia B is an X-linked deficiency of FIX and the clinical manifestations are essentially the same as for haemophilia A. It is less common than haemophilia A and has an incidence of approximately 1 in 50 000 live births. FIX is responsible for the activation of FX in the presence of activated FVIII, calcium and phospholipid. FIX is synthesized in the liver and is a vitamin K-dependent protease that is similar to prothrombin, FVII, FX and protein C. The FIX gene is located on the long arm of the X chromosome and contains eight exons encoding a protein of 454 amino acids. The complete sequence of the gene has been determined and in virtually all cases of haemophilia B genetic mutations have been identified, the vast majority of mutations being missense. A haemophilia B database is also available at http://www.kcl.ac.uk/ip/petergreen/haemBdatabase.html.

Treatment

The mainstay of treatment is FIX concentrate. Previously, intermediate-purity prothrombin complex concentrates containing all the vitamin K-dependent factors were used. However, these concentrates were associated with a risk of thrombosis, particularly when used repeatedly, for example in surgery. This was probably due to accumulation of high levels of FX and FII, which have longer half-lives than FIX. Subsequently, high-purity FIX concentrates have been developed produced by either monoclonal antibody or affinity chromatography methods. FIX concentrates are prepared from the same screened plasma pools as FVIII and undergo similar viral inactivation procedures Although the FIX gene was cloned in 1982, the development of recombinant FIX was hampered by the post-translational modification that it requires. Recombinant FIX is now widely used and although it is clinically effective, the recovery is only about 80% of that observed with plasma-derived FIX.

Dosage calculation in the treatment of haemophilia B follows the same principles as set out for FVIII deficiency, except that a higher initial dosage is required because of lower recovery:

Dose to be infused (units) = [weight (kg) × increment needed (units/dL)]/0.9 (or 0.8 for recombinant FIX)

Also, the longer half-life (18 hours) means that daily infusions often suffice to maintain good levels after surgery, but as with FVIII the half-life may be much shorter in children and more frequent dosing required. Severely affected patients are usually maintained on twice-weekly prophylaxis to prevent spontaneous bleeds. This is practicable because of the longer half-life of the factor.

Complications of therapy

Inhibitors

Inhibitors in haemophilia B are much less common than in haemophilia A. Only about 2–3% of patients with severe haemophilia B will develop inhibitors, but interestingly many of these inhibitors present with anaphylaxis to infusions of FIX concentrate. Unlike FVIII inhibitors, FIX inhibitors are not time dependent, but can be similarly quantitated by a modified Bethesda assay. The majority of patients who develop inhibitors have large gene deletions or nonsense mutations occurring in the first 20% of the FIX gene. Acute management of bleeding can be achieved with recombinant FVIIa (as with haemophilia A). However, immune tolerance is frequently far less successful and can be complicated by the development of nephrotic syndrome.

Gene therapy for haemophilia

Haemophilia is an excellent model for gene therapy because the clinical manifestation is the result of a deficiency of the single gene product and only a small amount of protein is required to ameliorate symptoms.

Although preliminary data from Phase I trials were encouraging, the plasma levels of FVIII or FIX attained were notably less than in the animal models and certainly insufficient to free patients from treatment with clotting factor concentrates. Also, there has been a universal short duration of transgene activity. Although no inhibitors have been documented, this remains a theoretical risk. Furthermore, the detection of small amounts of viral vector genome in the semen continues to raise the possibility of the risk of germline integration. Insertional mutagenesis has occurred in a Phase I trial of Moloney retrovirus carrying the interleukin receptor, and this has been a cause for concern but was partly the result of the selection pressures applied to the transduced cells. New vectors, particularly modified serotypes and engineered self-complementary adeno-associated virus, which rarely integrates into the host genome,

will form the next generation of gene therapeutics and are about to enter clinical trials.

The ethics of gene therapy for haemophilia are complex: it could be argued that for young patients with haemophilia, regular prophylactic factor infusions already deliver a near-normal life. Gene transfer in haemophilia has played an integral role in furthering the science of gene therapy in general but it is still likely to be a long time before it becomes routine therapy for children with haemophilia.

General organization of haemophilia care

As these are relatively uncommon disorders, with many and varied effects on patients and families at all stages of life who require care and support services across the whole field of medicine and social services, it is now accepted that this care can best be delivered comprehensively by referral centres. The staff of a major comprehensive care centre will include physicians, nurses, social workers, laboratory scientists and physiotherapists, devoting all or a substantial part of their time to haemophilia care. An orthopaedic surgeon or musculosketal rheumatologist prepared to see haemophilic patients regularly in a clinic set aside for their problems is a valuable addition to this team. In the UK, there is now a national service specification produced by the Haemophilia Alliance for Haemophilia and related conditions, which sets out the standards of care to be provided through the haemophilia centre network originally set up in the 1960s and early 1970s. It is recognized that not every centre can provide every facility and that there should be a fairly wide distribution according to population density, which determines numbers of patients. As defined by the national specification, the functions of a centre are to provide 24-hour emergency treatment for haemophilic patients and their families and a full range of diagnostic tests for identifying new patients and monitoring treatment. Full records should be kept of all treatments, whether given in hospital or as home therapy. Progress should be monitored through regular follow-up, with paediatric, dental and orthopaedic referrals being organized by the centre as necessary. (Many centres are indeed in paediatric departments or run by paediatricians.) Genetic counselling, including carrier detection and antenatal diagnosis, must be available for families of patients with haemophilia. Large centres providing all these facilities and treating at least 40 patients with severe haemophilia will be designated comprehensive care centres. It is envisaged that all patients will have access to a comprehensive care centre, either directly or via their smaller local centre. A part-time or full-time social worker should be part of the team, able to review the wider problems of living that affect the haemophilic patient at school, home and work. Centres provide access to specialized care for monitoring patients with HIV and HCV infection. On diagnosis, all patients are issued with a special medical card indicating

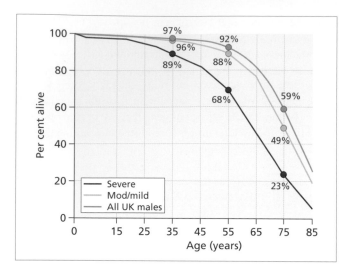

Figure 41.5 Survival in men in the UK with haemophilia who were not infected with HIV and in the general male population of the UK in 1999. Note that these data still include deaths related to hepatitis C infection. (From Darby *et al.* 2007 with permission.)

laboratory test results, inhibitor status, main centre and local centre for treatment.

Caring for haemophilic patients and their families is demanding but rewarding. Despite the setbacks in the 1980s due to virus transmission, the trend continues to be an ever-improving life expectancy and social participation, based on continuing medical progress and multiprofessional input into patient care. It is both tragic and ironic that the main foundation on which this progress rested (factor concentrate) has also been the route by which life-threatening infections have been introduced to about half of the most severely affected patients with haemophilia A. However, there are now effective therapies for both HIV and HCV infection. The younger generation of haemophiliacs is now treated with virus-safe or recombinant concentrates and has escaped both HIV and liver disease, and lead virtually normal lives (Figure 41.5).

Acquired haemophilia

This chapter is devoted primarily to the inherited form of haemophilia arising from mutations in the FVIII and FIX genes but haemophilia can also arise as a result of autoantibodies that neutralize FVIII cofactor activity. The incidence is approximately 1.5 per million per year and it tends to occur predominantly in older patients, although there is also an increased frequency after pregnancy and in association with other autoimmune disorders. The antibodies usually show time-dependent (type 2) neutralization of FVIII and a residual FVIII level is often detectable. The pattern of bleeding is distinct from that

in inherited haemophilia, with a much greater incidence of soft tissue and mucosal bleeding, often out of proportion to the FVIII level. Treatment for bleeding is the same as for inhibitors in hereditary haemophilia and suppression of the inhibitor requires immunosuppressive therapy (e.g. corticosteroids, cyclophosphamide and anti-CD20 antibody).

von Willebrand disease

Although described in 1926, our understanding of this complex and variable bleeding disorder remains far from complete. The basic defect common to all variants is a deficiency of one or more aspects of VWF functional activity. The abnormality may be quantitative and/or qualitative.

von Willebrand factor

VWF is encoded by a gene on chromosome 12, which was cloned simultaneously by several groups in 1986. The pre-pro-VWF primary translation product comprises a 22-amino-acid signal peptide, a 741-amino-acid propeptide and the 2050-amino-acid mature subunit. The pro-VWF monomer is composed of four types of domains (A–D) arranged as follows: NH_2–D1–D2–D′–D3–A1–A2–A3–D4–B1–B2–B3–C1–C2–CK–COOH. VWF is produced predominantly in vascular endothelial cells and also in megakaryocytes, although plasma VWF derives entirely from endothelial cell production. After translation the monomer enters the endoplasmic reticulum and the signal peptide is removed. The monomers then dimerize via the C-terminal cysteine knot domain before leaving the endoplasmic reticulum to the Golgi, where the dimers are joined via their N-termini to form a series of multimers with molecular masses ranging from 1000 to 20 000 kDa. During this process the molecule is extensively glycosylated with N- and O-linked glycans that form 20% of its final molecular weight. Importantly, approximately 13% of the N-linked glycans terminate in an ABO blood group antigen. In endothelial cells, multimerized VWF is then transferred into Weibel–Palade bodies, some of which pass directly to the cell surface to release their contents (constitutive pathway) while others remain in the cell for release when needed (regulated pathway). Platelet VWF does not contribute significantly to plasma VWF and is stored in the α-granules of platelets prior to release after platelet activation. During synthesis, the VWF propeptide, which is essential for multimerization, is cleaved from the mature molecule, stored with VWF in the Weibel–Palade bodies and released with it into plasma but is not known to have any further function thereafter. Some VWF is also secreted ablumenally from the base of the endothelial cell where it binds directly to collagen in the subendothelial matrix.

Rapid release of VWF from the endothelial Weibel–Palade storage granules can be induced via the regulated pathway by a number of agonists including thrombin, adrenaline, histamine and vasopressin. This can be used to advantage by using desmopressin to treat mild forms of VWD. Elevation of plasma VWF due to increased synthesis and secretion occurs as part of the acute-phase response to injury, inflammation, infection and neoplasia, and in pregnancy and hyperthyroidism. These responses are presumed to be physiological in promoting enhanced haemostasis but could reach pathological expression in being associated with an increased risk of thrombosis. The confounding effects of stress and inflammation need to be taken into account when measuring VWF levels in attempting to diagnose VWD.

An appreciation of the complex structure–function relationship of VWF is essential in order to understand the classification of VWD. The two principal functions of VWF are (i) binding to matrix molecules, particularly collagen, at sites of vascular injury and subsequent capture of platelets to form the primary haemostatic plug and (ii) the stabilization of FVIII in the circulation. The adhesive function of FVIII requires functional binding sites for collagen and the platelet glycoproteins GPIb

and GPIIb/IIIa (also known as integrin $\alpha_{IIb}\beta_3$). The VWF released from endothelial cells into plasma is in the form of ultra-large multimers, which are subsequently cleaved into smaller forms by the action of the plasma metalloprotease ADAMTS-13. This is of critical importance because it is the high-molecular-weight multimers that have the greatest collagen- and platelet-binding activity: absent cleavage results in formation of platelet microthrombi and vascular occlusion and excessive cleavage results in increased bleeding.

Although FVIII and VWF are entirely distinct entities with separate functions (Figure 41.6), they circulate together as a complex in which VWF protects FVIII from degradation, so that a deficiency of VWF or a reduction in its ability to bind FVIII may also result in a low plasma level of FVIII. Therefore, deficiency of VWF can give rise to a dual haemostatic defect: reduced plasma levels of FVIII (due to its shorter half-life in the absence of VWF) and a defect in primary haemostasis because of the failure in assisting platelets to adhere to the cut edges of small blood vessels (see Chapters 39 and 40). Clearly, the multistep synthesis, assembly and secretion of VWF and its multiple

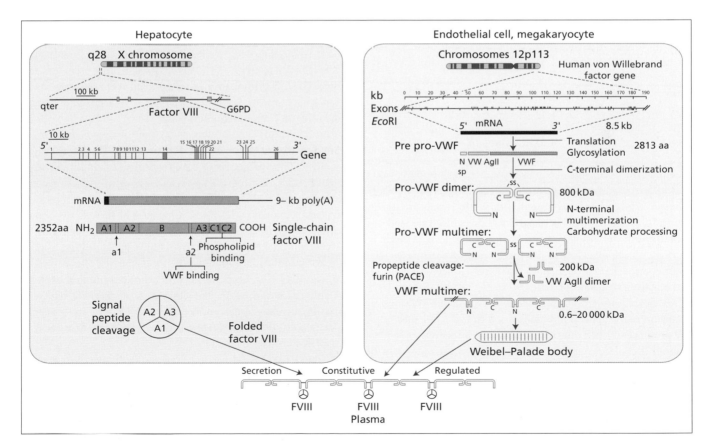

Figure 41.6 Assembly of FVIII–VWF complex. FVIII synthesized by hepatocytes as a single chain is partially proteolysed and (possibly) complexed with VWF prior to release. VWF is synthesized as a single-chain precursor, which dimerizes with disulphide bond formation, then multimerizes with further disulphide exchange, with concomitant loss of a large propeptide segment. The propeptide is essential for multimer formation and probably functions as an acidic disulphide isomerase.

binding interactions provide many ways in which mutations of the VWF gene can give rise to varying types of disease. In particular, the multimeric structure is susceptible to dominant-negative effects of mutant alleles. The diagnosis of VWD is based on the recognition that for normal VWF function it must be (i) present in adequate amounts, (ii) have a normal multimeric structure, and (iii) have intact functional domains (binding sites). When any of these properties is only slightly reduced, the presence or absence of a bleeding tendency may also depend on the quality and quantity of the other components, particularly platelets and collagen, with which VWF must interact.

Clinical features

The clinical features vary according to the severity of the deficiency. The most common clinical picture is of an autosomal dominant, mild to moderately severe bleeding tendency. However, we now understand that the inheritance of VWD may be more complex than a simple autosomal dominant pattern (see below). Patients suffer from bruising, epistaxes, prolonged bleeding from minor cuts, menorrhagia and excessive, but not often life-threatening, bleeding after trauma or surgery. Patients often present for investigation in the second or third decade after prolonged bleeding from dental extraction or surgery has aroused clinical suspicion. Menorrhagia, unexplained by local or hormonal factors, can also be the presenting symptom: an estimated 20% of women with menorrhagia have VWD. The distribution of bleeding in VWD can be explained on the basis that VWF is required for platelet adhesion at high shear rate, which is the condition of flow found in the smallest blood vessels exposed to trauma in skin and mucous membranes. Haemarthroses do not occur in typical mild dominant VWD. Much less common is autosomal recessive (type 3) VWD, where VWF is completely absent and FVIII:C levels are usually around 1 or 2 units/dL. These patients have a bleeding tendency that clinically resembles severe haemophilia A, with haemarthroses, muscle bleeds and life-threatening haemorrhage after trauma, as well as proneness to small-vessel bleeding, which is not a feature of haemophilia A.

Mild bleeding symptoms of the type typical of VWD are very common in the general population and thus are not specific for the presence of a bleeding disorder. It is now recommended that a simplified bleeding score (e.g. Bowman) is used to assess the likelihood of a significant defect in haemostasis and that the result is borne in mind when interpreting the results of laboratory investigations.

Laboratory diagnosis

Preliminary diagnosis

After obtaining a suggestive personal history and a family history, the preliminary tests required are a full blood count, coagulation screen, FVIII assay, VWF:Ag and a measure of VWF activity, usually ristocetin cofactor activity (VWF:RCo).

The laboratory diagnosis of VWD rests on assessing both the amount of VWF present (VWF:Ag) and its functional capacity. At present, it is generally possible to assess three important functions.

1 *FVIII binding.* Assessed first by a FVIII assay and then if this is reduced, by an assay of VWF FVIII-binding capacity using a modified ELISA-based technique.
2 *Platelet-dependent function.* The standard assessment of VWF adhesive functional activity remains the ristocetin cofactor assay (VWF:RCo). In this assay, dilutions of patient plasma are tested for their ability to promote platelet agglutination in the presence of the antibiotic ristocetin.
3 *Collagen-binding function (VWF:CB).* This recently introduced measurement is performed in an ELISA-based assay in which a well coated with collagen is used to capture VWF.
Measures of VWF:RCo and VWF:CB are both sensitive to the loss of high-molecular-weight multimers, but measure different binding properties of VWF. Thus they should be seen as complementary rather than alternative assays.

In addition, a global measure of primary haemostasis is also useful. Traditionally this was provided by the template bleeding time but this has a poor sensitivity for VWD and has largely been replaced by devices such as the PFA-100. The PFA-100 has very good sensitivity for VWD, although obviously does not distinguish it from platelet disorders and will not detect collagen abnormalities. Repeatedly normal PFA-100 results make a disorder of VWF function unlikely.

Secondary tests for classification of VWD

If a deficiency suggestive of VWD is detected then further tests, in particular multimeric analysis and ristocetin-induced platelet aggregation (RIPA), are recommended to allow accurate subtyping of the VWD. The most important of these is VWF multimer size analysis, which will demonstrate the distribution of VWF multimers and the pattern of flanking bands (Figure 41.7) adjacent to the main multimer bands. Using the tests described above, VWD can be classified into a limited number of types (Tables 41.4 and 41.5). The classification of VWD has been examined many times and extensive guidelines are available, detailed in the bibliography. What follows is necessarily a limited summary of much work.

Type 1 VWD is defined as a simple quantitative deficiency of VWF and the VWF present should be functionally normal. This means that the VWF:Ag and VWF:RCo should be concordant and the VWF should have an essentially normal multimeric pattern. In practice it is acceptable that the ratio of antigen to function should be in excess of 0.7 and there should be no significant loss of high-molecular-weight multimers, although on close inspection many subtle abnormalities of multimer pattern can be discerned.

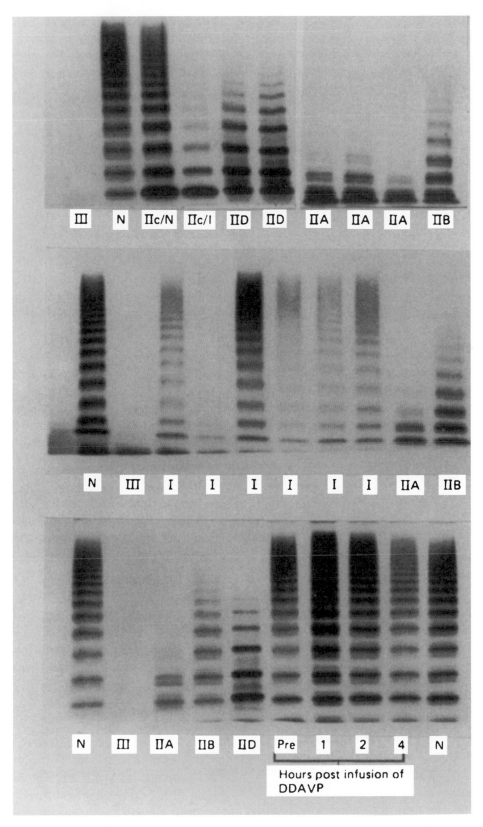

Figure 41.7 Multimer analysis of VWF from patients with VWD and normal control subjects. Note that many cases classified at present as type 2A were previously subdivided according to the details of the abnormality of triplet pattern.

The characteristic of the 2A, 2B and 2M variants is a functional deficiency of VWF activity, which is reduced to below 0.7 of the antigenic measure. In type 2A, this results from a lack of high- and intermediate-size VWF multimers, whereas in type 2M a similar loss of platelet-binding activity is seen despite the presence of normal VWF multimeric composition and is caused by mutations in the VWF GPIb-binding site. Loss of high-molecular-weight multimers in type 2A may arise from failures of intracellular processing or from accelerated proteolysis in the circulation due to mutations close to the ADAMTS-13 cleavage site. VWD due to an isolated collagen-binding defect without loss of high-molecular-weight multimers is rare, although a handful of cases have been reported. The associated bleeding disorder is mild, perhaps because VWF contains two collagen-binding sites.

In type 2B, VWF binds prematurely with platelets in the circulation and in the laboratory will agglutinate platelets at a low concentration of ristocetin (0.5 mg/mL) that has no effect with normal VWF (i.e. positive RIPA). If normal washed platelets are resuspended in the patient's plasma, the phenomenon is reproduced, demonstrating that the abnormality is in the plasma. Studies with purified type 2B VWF show that, unlike normal VWF, it binds directly to platelets without prior activation. *In vivo* this results in the loss of high-molecular-weight multimers and platelets from the circulation due to *in vivo* formation of platelet aggregates and also to increased cleavage of VWF by ADAMTS-13. Thus routine platelet aggregation studies with a range of ristocetin dosages should be performed

as part of the diagnostic work-up, as it is important to detect this variant (see below), which does not always show up in the other tests. Indeed a recent analysis showed that many patients with type 2B VWD have normal platelet counts and VWF multimer patterns.

A fourth type 2 variant, called type 2N (for Normandy), has been described. This is characterized by reduced affinity for FVIII but it is normal in other respects. Thus, laboratory investigations reveal only a reduced FVIII level (5–35%), which is easily mistaken for mild haemophilia. A clue to the correct diagnosis may come from the family history, and confirmation requires an assay of VWF FVIII-binding capacity or genetic analysis of FVIII and the VWF FVIII-binding site in the D' domain. The majority of patients are found to be type 1, which accounts for 75% of kindreds. Types 2A and 2B are fairly common, together accounting for about 15% of kindreds. Although classification has proved useful in understanding VWD and can help in planning treatment, some forms remain difficult to classify and may show features of more than one type.

Problems in diagnosis of type 1 VWD

The diagnosis of type 1 VWD implies that the patient has a significantly low level of VWF, which is responsible for an increased tendency to bleed. It is often not easy to be certain of this conclusion for the following reasons.

1 Slightly low levels of VWF are common in the population. Although the lower end of the normal range for VWF in the general population is approximately 50 units/dL, most of the 2.5% of the population who have levels below this have normal haemostasis. In particular, individuals with blood group O have VWF levels on average 30% lower than those with non-O blood groups and the lower end of a 'blood group O normal range' is approximately 35 units/dL. Thus the lower limit of the normal range is not the minimum level required for normal haemostasis (Table 41.6). Nonetheless, individuals with blood group O are over-represented in the group with type 1 VWD and there is a continuous relationship between bleeding tendency and VWF level that extends into the normal range without a clear cut-off between normal and abnormal.

2 A history of minor bleeding episodes (e.g. easy bruising, epistaxes) is very common in the population and is not a good

Table 41.4 Primary classification of von Willebrand disease.

Subclassification	Type of VWF deficiency	VWF protein function
Type 1	Quantitative partial deficiency	Normal
Type 2	Qualitative functional deficiency	Abnormal
Type 3	Quantitative complete deficiency	Undetectable

Table 41.5 Secondary classification of type 2 von Willebrand disease.

Subtype	Platelet-associated function	FVIII-binding capacity	High-molecular-weight VWF multimers
2A	Decreased	Normal	Absent
2B	Increased affinity for GPIb	Normal	Usually reduced/absent
2M	Decreased	Normal	Normal and occasionally ultra-large forms
2N	Normal	Markedly reduced	Normal

Table 41.6 Influence of ABO blood group on VWF:Ag values (u/dl) in volunteer blood donors.

ABO type	N	VWF:Ag geometric mean	VWF:Ag geometric mean ± 2SD
O	456	74.8	35.6–157.0
A	340	105.9	48.0–233.9
B	196	116.9	56.8–241.0
AB	109	123.3	63.8–238.2

Note the significantly lower levels in donors of blood group O compared with non-O donors.

Source: Gill *et al.* (1987) with permission.

predictor of bleeding in other circumstances such as operations. Equally, the patient may not yet have been exposed to a significant test of haemostasis.

3 As a result of the two points above, a history of, say, easy bruising and slightly low VWF levels will often be found together. However, this does not mean that the patient has VWD and caution should be exercised in drawing this conclusion as it has many consequences for the patient.

4 Intercurrent events such as stress, exercise, illness and pregnancy may all elevate the VWF level, making it difficult to be certain that a representative measure of VWF levels has been obtained. It is therefore necessary to perform carefully standardized sets of assays with concordant results on at least two occasions to be sure of the diagnosis and its severity.

5 The family history is often unhelpful, particularly in mild cases where penetrance is weak or variable. This is probably the result of the modifying effects alluded to in (1) above. It is now evident that in some families, VWD does not segregate with the VWF gene. By inference, therefore, some of the mutations responsible for the type 1 phenotype will occur at loci other than the VWF gene, although what these are remains to be determined.

6 Finally, review of many cases previously diagnosed as type 1 VWD has concluded that many are in fact better categorized as type 2M after better assessment of the VWF antigen-activity ratio.

When there is a clear bleeding history and FVIII, VWF:Ag and VWF:RCo are all clearly reduced (e.g. < 25 units/dL) and the platelet count is normal, the diagnosis is easily made (see Tables 41.4 and 41.5). However, in the absence of a clear bleeding history, individuals with VWF activity in the range 25–50 units/dL are best regarded as simply being at slightly increased risk of bleeding. When VWF levels in the range 25–50 units/dL are associated with bleeding, it is very likely that other factors such as mildly impaired platelet function play a contributory role. This is especially true of the milder cases of type 1 VWD (see below).

Treatment

Patients with mild or moderate VWD attend infrequently for treatment. The first-line treatment for minor bleeding after local measures have failed in type 1 VWD is desmopressin. This will produce a brisk rise in VWF and FVIII levels (30 min after intravenous infusion) and a shortening of the bleeding time (for details of therapy see discussion of mild haemophilia A; see p. 800). Desmopressin is much less effective in types 2A and 2M, presumably because the patient's released VWF is highly abnormal and still unable to promote platelet adhesion. Desmopressin is generally regarded as contraindicated in type 2B VWD, as the released abnormal VWF will cause circulatory platelet aggregates to form, with a further fall in the platelet count. Before relying on desmopressin for therapy, patients should be given a test dose of DDAVP in order to determine the response at 30–60 min because it varies considerably. In addition, the duration of the response is also variable and further samples at 6–8 hours should be taken: some forms of type 1 VWD (e.g. VWF Vicenza) are characterized by a much shortened survival of VWF. A therapeutic trial may also be worthwhile in type 2A as some families do respond. In type 2N, the FVIII response is of normal magnitude but is of limited efficacy due to its short duration, emphasizing the importance of making the correct diagnosis. It may still be useful for minor procedures. Desmopressin is best avoided in small children (< 2 years) as there is a risk of hyponatraemia and consequent seizures. It is also contraindicated in elderly patients or those with arterial disease as there is a risk of arterial thrombosis. Desmopressin therapy is often combined with tranexamic acid. However, tranexamic acid may be effective on its own in some circumstances such as menorrhagia or as a mouthwash for oral cavity bleeding.

In patients in whom desmopressin is ineffective or contraindicated, the next line of treatment is a concentrate containing adequate amounts of functionally active VWF with preservation of the high-molecular-weight multimers. As with all concentrates, the source of plasma and viral inactivation are also important. Recombinant VWF concentrate is not yet licensed but is in early clinical trials. Cryoprecipitate has been used in these circumstances but cannot be subjected to viral inactivation procedures and is therefore not recommended as first-line therapy. Factor concentrates will always be required for treatment of type 3 VWD. Depending on the responses obtained with desmopressin, the duration of treatment and the presence of other contraindications, they may also be required in other type 2 and type 1 variants. FVIII concentrates vary considerably in the amount of VWF they contain and in the extent to which this is degraded or remains in the form of functionally active high-molecular-weight multimers. Those that contain significant amounts of VWF that were effective in treating VWD were initially of intermediate purity, but high-purity more specifically designed VWF concentrates are now available that contain well-preserved VWF protein. The composition and VWF/FVIII ratio varies considerably between products. It is important to remember that following infusion of some high-purity VWF with low FVIII content there is a delay of approximately 12 hours before the level of FVIII rises substantially and, if rapid correction is required, FVIII concentrate should also be given. In general, none of these replacement treatments is reliable in correcting the bleeding time, but this is not necessarily a bar to effective haemostasis. This seemingly paradoxical result may be because they do not correct the deficiency of intraplatelet VWF or because the largest high-molecular-weight multimers are not present. In situations when concentrates fail to stop bleeding, cryoprecipitate and platelet concentrates may prove effective.

Clinical course and complications

Patients with types 1 and 2 VWD lead relatively normal lives, with normal life expectancy. Menstruation is seldom a cause of severe blood loss, although menorrhagia is common. This can usually be managed satisfactorily with antifibrinolytics or by oral contraceptive estrogen/progesterone combinations. The Mirena coil is also effective. If these are not effective, then self-administration at home of desmopressin by intranasal or sub-cutaneous routes can be useful. In later years, some patients require hysterectomy. During pregnancy, the VWF levels rise spontaneously to the normal or low-normal range in most patients with type 1 VWD. In type 2, the response is unpredictable and should be closely monitored: because of increased production of abnormal VWF, VWF:Ag may rise to normal levels but with VWF:RCo still significantly low. Type 2B is particularly complicated in pregnancy because the rise in endogenous VWF production exacerbates the thrombocytopenia. Patients with severe type 3 disease have a clinical course resembling severe or moderately severe haemophilia A, including the development of joint damage. A small number of patients with type 3 disease develop antibodies to VWF, which inhibit its platelet adhesion-promoting property and cause rapid removal from the circulation of infused material. Unlike anti-FVIII antibodies, some anti-VWF antibodies may mediate anaphylactic shock.

Molecular genetics

The cloning of VWF cDNA and its gene has led to progress in identifying the underlying mutations responsible for the various phenotypes (Figure 41.8). As with the FVIII gene, the sheer size of the DNA region involved presents some problems of localization, but these are being overcome by powerful screening methods. A database of mutations responsible for VWD has been established at http://www.shef.ac.uk/vwf/vwd.html.

Type 1

In the last few years there have been extensive studies to determine the molecular basis of type 1 VWD and a number of important points have emerged. Firstly, in about 35% of cases, the disorder does not segregate with the VWF locus and is therefore presumably the result of the combination of other modifying genes, in particular the ABO locus. This phenomenon is most common in individuals diagnosed with VWD and VWF levels above 30 units/dL and involves a disproportionate number of blood group O individuals. The likelihood of the disorder segregating with the VWF gene and of a causative mutation being identified increases significantly as the VWF level falls and a mutation is found in all cases where the VWF multimer pattern is abnormal. Among those with type 1 VWD and an identified mutation, mutations are widely scattered throughout the molecule. Similarly, in the more severe cases a typical autosomal dominant pattern of inheritance with strong penetrance is seen, whereas in milder cases this is often not apparent.

Type 2

Mutations responsible for type 2 VWD affect the relevant functional site in the molecule and the corresponding portion of the gene. Mutations causing types 2M and 2B both affect the binding site for platelet GPIb on VWF and are found within the A1 domain of the molecule. They are inherited dominantly. As discussed above, type 2A may arise from increased susceptibility to proteolysis by ADAMTS-13 and this type is associated with mutations in the A2 domain. Otherwise, type 2A mutations are scattered throughout the gene but particularly in the propeptide, D'–D3 and the cysteine knot. In general, type 2A is dominant but occasional recessive forms occur. Mutations causing type 2N are found in the FVIII-binding site in the D' domain but because the binding capacity of VWF greatly exceeds the FVIII concentration, the inheritance is recessive.

Type 3

Type 3 is characterized by the complete absence of VWF and so arises from inactivating or null mutations in both VWF alleles and is inherited in an autosomal recessive manner. The rare patients who develop antibodies to VWF nearly all have large deletions of their VWF gene.

Pseudo von Willebrand disease (platelet-type)

Several families have been described with a disorder closely resembling type 2B VWD, but in whom mixing experiments show the defect to be in their platelets rather than their plasma. Patients with pseudo VWD have moderately reduced levels of VWF:Ag and platelets, with an enhanced response of their platelet-rich plasma to low levels of ristocetin (0.5 mg/mL). The addition of normal cryoprecipitate to their washed platelets

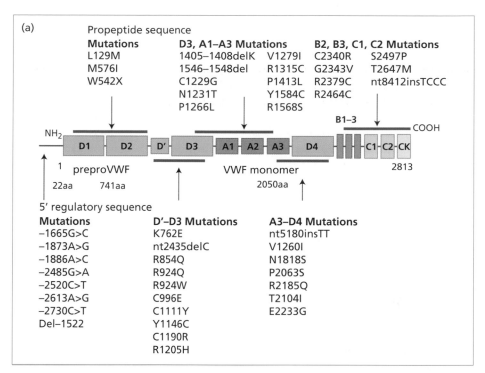

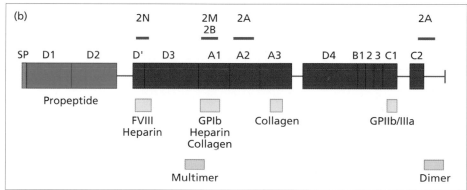

Figure 41.8 (a) Mutations found in patients diagnosed with type 1 VWD in the Canadian and European studies. Note that not all these mutations have been shown to be causal and that classification as type 1 may sometimes be contentious. (From James *et al.* 2007 with permission.) (b) Distribution of mutations responsible for type 2 VWD. The domain structure of the monomer is shown, as well as the regions in which the mutations cluster in relation to the functional domains of the molecule. (From Goodeve *et al.* 2007 with permission.)

Table 41.7 Disorders associated with acquired von Willebrand syndrome and mechanism responsible.

Disorder	Mechanism	Treatment
Hypothyroidism	Reduced synthesis	Correct thyroid status
Aortic stenosis	Shear stress	Replace aortic valve
Myeloproliferative	Adherence to platelets and increased cleavage	Restore platelet count to normal
IgG paraprotein	Immune	IVIG, chemotherapy to reduce paraproteins
IgM paraprotein	Immune	Chemotherapy (IVIG ineffective)
Wilms tumour	Adsorption	Tumour removal if possible

IVIG, intravenous immunoglobulin.

causes spontaneous aggregation, whereas the reverse experiment is without effect (compare with type 2B). Missense mutations in platelet membrane GPIb, such that it spontaneously binds higher multimers of VWF, have been shown to be the underlying cause of this autosomally dominant mild bleeding syndrome. Treatment has not been extensively evaluated, but it should probably be with normal platelet concentrates, rather than desmopressin or cryoprecipitate. Thus this syndrome should be excluded by mixing tests as above or by genetic analysis before diagnosing type 2B VWD.

Acquired von Willebrand syndrome

In a number of circumstances patients may acquire a deficiency of VWF function that is not inherited. The commonest association is with a paraprotein that binds to VWF and accelerates clearance, producing a type 2A or type 3 pattern. It is also associated with myeloproliferative disease when thrombocytosis is present and in hypothyroidism (Table 41.7). Severe aortic stenosis can cause sufficient shear damage to VWF to cause an acquired von Willebrand syndrome that resolves after valve replacement. In the long term, treatment of the underlying disorder will improve the syndrome. If urgent treatment is required, then replacement therapy may be necessary (taking into account accelerated clearance) or IgG paraproteins will usually respond to intravenous immunoglobulin.

Selected bibliography

Darby SC, Kan SW, Spooner RJ et al. (2007) Mortality rates, life expectancy, and causes of death in people with hemophilia A or B in the United Kingdom who were not infected with HIV. *Blood* **110**: 815–25.

Escobar MA (2003) Treatment on demand: *in vivo* dose finding studies. *Haemophilia* **9**: 360–7.

Gill J, Endres-Brooks PJ, Bauer WJ et al. (1987) The effect of ABO blood group on the diagnosis of von Willebrand disease. *Blood* **69**: 1691–5.

Goodeve A, Eikenboom J, Castaman G et al. (2007) Phenotype and genotype of a cohort of families historically diagnosed with type 1 von Willebrand disease in the European study, Molecular and Clinical Markers for the Diagnosis and Management of Type 1 von Willebrand Disease (MCMDM-1VWD). *Blood* **109**: 112–21. Erratum appears in *Blood* (2008) **111**: 3299–300.

Graw J, Brackmann H-H, Oldenburg J, Schneppenheim R, Spannagl M, Schwaab R (2005) Haemophilia A: from mutation analysis to new therapies. *Nature Reviews. Genetics* **6**: 488–501.

Haemophilia Alliance. A national service specification for haemophilia and related conditions. Available at www.haemophiliaalliance.org.uk

Hay CR, Brown SA, Collins PW et al. (2006) The diagnosis and management of factor VIII and IX inhibitors: a guideline from the UK Haemophilia Centre Directors' Organization. *British Journal of Haematology* **133**: 591–605.

James PD, Notley C, Hegadorn C et al. (2007) The mutational spectrum of type 1 von Willebrand disease: results from a Canadian cohort study. *Blood* **109**: 145–54.

Keeling DM, Tait C, Makris M (2008) Guideline on the selection and use of therapeutic products to treat haemophilia and other hereditary disorders. *Haemophilia* **14**: 671–84.

Laffan MA, Brown SA, Collins PW et al. (2004) The diagnosis of von Willebrand disease. A guideline from the UK Haemophilia Centre Doctors' Organization. *Haemophilia* **10**: 199–217.

Lillicrap D (2009) Genotype/phenotype association in von Willebrand disease: is the glass half full or empty? *Journal of Thrombosis and Haemostasis* **7** (Suppl. 1): 65–70.

Manco-Johnson MJ, Abshire TC, Shapiro AD et al. (2007) Prophylaxis versus episodic treatment to prevent joint disease in boys with severe hemophilia. *New England Journal of Medicine* **357**: 535–44.

Mannucci PM (2003) Haemophilia: treatment options in the twenty-first century. *Journal of Thrombosis and Haemostasis* **1**: 1349–55.

Mannucci PM, Schutgens RE, Santagostino E, Mauser-Bunschoten EP (2009) How I treat age-related morbidities in elderly persons with hemophilia. *Blood* **114**: 5256–63.

Mikaelsson M, Oswaldsson U, Sandberg H (1998) Influence of phospholipids on the assessment of FVIII activity. *Haemophilia* **4**: 646–50.

Ngo JCK, Huang M, Roth DA, Furie BC, Furie B (2008) Crystal structure of human factor VIII: implications for the formation of the factor IXa–factor VIIIa complex. *Structure* **16**: 597–606.

NHS Management Executive (1993) *Health Service Guidelines: Provision of Haemophilia Treatment and Care.* BAPS, Heywood.

Nichols WL, Hultin MB, James AH et al. (2008) von Willebrand disease (VWD): evidence-based diagnosis and management guidelines. The National Heart, Lung, and Blood Institute (NHLBI) Expert Panel report (USA). *Haemophilia* **14**: 171–232.

Pasi KJ, Collins PW, Keeling D et al. (2004) Management of von Willebrand disease. A guideline from the UK Haemophilia Centre Doctor's Organization. *Haemophilia* **10**: 218–31.

Rodriguez-Mercham EC, Lee CA (2003) *Inhibitors in Patients with Haemophilia.* Blackwell Science, Oxford.

Sadler JE, Budde U, Eikenboom JC et al. (2006) Update on the pathophysiology and classification of von Willebrand disease: a report of the Subcommittee on von Willebrand Factor. *Journal of Thrombosis and Haemostasis* **4**: 2103–14.

United Kingdom Haemophilia Centre Doctors' Organisation (2003) Guidelines on the selection and use of therapeutic products to treat haemophilia and other heritary bleeding disorders. *Haemophilia* **9**: 1–23.

von Willebrand Disease Database. Available at http://www.shef.ac.uk/vwf/vwd.html

CHAPTER 42

Rare bleeding disorders

42

Flora Peyvandi and Marzia Menegatti

A. Bianchi Bonomi Hemophilia and Thrombosis Center, IRCCS Cà Granada, Ospedale Maggiore, Milan, Italy

Introduction

The rare bleeding disorders (RBDs), including the inherited deficiencies of such coagulation factors as fibrinogen, factor (F) II, FV, combined FV and FVIII, FVII, FX, FXI, FXIII and of multiple deficiency of vitamin K-dependent factors, are usually transmitted in an autosomal recessive manner. The prevalence of RBDs in the general population is low, and homozygous or double heterozygous deficiencies vary from 1 in 500 000 for FVII deficiency to 1 in 2 million for prothrombin and FXIII deficiencies (Table 42.1). The prevalence of RBDs is also strongly influenced by ethnicity and is significantly increased by a high rate of consanguinity in the population.

Until 1980, only sparse information on RBDs was available, but in the last decade the number of reported studies has considerably increased, particularly pertaining to the molecular aspects of RBDs. At the same time, interest in the worldwide distribution of RBDs led to the creation of large databases aimed at collecting epidemiological data and at providing information to haemophilia organizations and treatment centres involved in reducing or preventing complications of bleeding. Two recent large data collections have helped to derive the worldwide distribution of RBDs (Figure 42.1), one by the World Federation of Haemophilia (WFH, http://www.wfh.

org/) and the other by the International Rare Bleeding Disorders Database (RBDD, www.rbdd.org). The WFH started collecting information on haemophilia care throughout the world in 1998, but collection of data on RBDs only started in 2004. The current global survey includes basic demographic information, data on care resources and treatment products, and information on the prevalence of infectious complications such as HIV and hepatitis C in individuals with haemophilia, von Willebrand disease, platelet disorders and other RBDs. The RBDD, developed in 2004, has spearheaded the development of an international network of care providers to work together to discuss prevalence, clinical manifestations, and need for coordinated and consistent data collection. The goal of this international community effort is to better identify the number of affected individuals throughout the world, to define the clinical manifestations and sequelae associated with these disorders, and to share diagnostic and treatment expertise. Comparison of the data obtained by the two surveys shows similar results, confirming that FVII and FXI deficiencies are the most prevalent RBDs (representing about 29–33% of the total number of affected patients), followed by deficiencies of fibrinogen, FV and FX (8–9%), FXIII (~ 6%) and combined FV and FVIII (~ 5%), while the rarest disorder was FII deficiency with a prevalence of 2%.

It is not possible to define a clear bleeding pattern among patients with RBDs, as symptoms are varied and heterogeneously distributed, but on the whole bleeding that endangers life, such as central nervous system (CNS) and musculoskeletal bleeding, appears to be less frequent than in haemophilia.

Postgraduate Haematology: 6th edition. Edited by A. Victor Hoffbrand, Daniel Catovsky, Edward G.D. Tuddenham, Anthony R. Green
© 2011 Blackwell Publishing Ltd.

Table 42.1 General features of autosomal recessive deficiency of coagulation factors.

Deficiency	Estimated prevalence*	Gene (chromosome)
Fibrinogen	1 in 1 million	FGA, FGB, FGG (all on 4q28)
Prothrombin	1 in 2 million	F2 (11p11–q12)
Factor V	1 in 1 million	F5 (1q24.2)
Combined factor V and VIII	1 in 1 million	LMAN1 (18q21.3–q22) MCFD2 (2p21–p16.3)
Factor VII	1 in 500 000	F7 (13q34)
Factor X	1 in 1 million	F10 (13q34)
Factor XI	1 in 1 million	F11 (4q35.2)
Factor XIII	1 in 2 million	F13A1 (6p24–p25) F13B (1q31–q32.1)
Vitamin-K dependent coagulation factors	Reported in about 30 families	GGCX (2p12) VKORC1 (16p11.2)

*Including dysfunctional proteins.

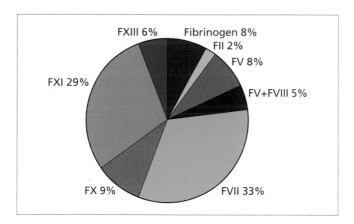

Figure 42.1 Worldwide distribution of rare bleeding disorders derived from two main large data collections (WFH and RBDD).

The laboratory diagnosis of RBDs is currently carried out by means of coagulation screening tests, such as the activated partial thromboplastin time, the prothrombin time and the thrombin time, applied to subjects reporting a clinical and family history of bleeding. Abnormal results of screening tests should be followed by specific coagulation assays in order to make the specific diagnosis of an RBD. Molecular diagnosis is based on a search for mutation in the genes encoding the corresponding coagulation factors. Exceptions are combined deficiency of FV and FVIII, caused by mutations in genes encoding proteins involved in FV and FVIII intracellular transport

(MCFD2 and LMAN1), and combined deficiency of vitamin K-dependent proteins (FII, FVII, FIX and FX), caused by mutations in genes that encode enzymes involved in post-translational modification and in vitamin K metabolism (GGCX and VKOR). Genetic analysis is also important for prenatal and preimplantation genetic diagnosis, especially in those countries with a high rate of RBDs and consanguinity, particularly where genetic prevention by premature termination of pregnancy is not allowed. Since mutation detection became a relatively easy and available strategy in different laboratories worldwide, and it is not always clear whether the identified mutation could be the cause of the severe deficiency of a specific clotting factor, family history associated with allele frequency in the genetic population are important to determine if the identified mutations are common polymorphisms.

Treatment of RBDs is a difficult task, since information on the clinical management of RBDs is often scarce and replacement therapy of coagulation factors may require the prescription of unlicensed products that are not readily available. A patient's personal and family history of bleeding are important guides for management. Dosages and frequency of treatment depend on the minimal haemostatic level of the deficient factor, its plasma half-life and the type of bleeding episode. The main treatments in RBDs are represented by non-transfusional adjuvant therapies (antifibrinolytic amino acids, estrogen/progestogen) and replacement therapy of the deficient coagulation factor. Unfortunately, information on the safety and efficacy of the few available products is scarce and experience in their optimal use significantly more limited than that available for haemophilia.

Particular care should be paid to women affected by RBDs. Since the latter are inherited in an autosomal recessive manner, roughly about 50% of patients are women. This implies that the global distribution of RBDs also reflects the global distribution of affected women, posing important social and medical problems, such as excessive menstrual bleeding (or menorrhagia) and bleeding during pregnancy and childbirth. Affected women also suffer the secondary consequences of such events, such as chronic iron-deficiency anaemia and a significantly reduced quality of life, due mainly to a complicated reproductive life but also to limitations in social activities and work. Postpartum bleeding often occurs if replacement therapy is not administered after delivery. Recurrent miscarriages are also described, but only in afibrinogenaemic and FXIII-deficient women. In the end, pregnancy is not contraindicated in patients with RBDs but requires a multidisciplinary approach: the best management of pregnancy should be decided through the coordinated action of a team composed of paediatricians, haematologists and obstetricians. In addition to female healthcare, the same team should ensure investigation and management of potentially affected newborns, particularly in families already having one affected child, because severe FVII, FX and FXIII deficiencies present with a high risk of intracranial haemorrhage during the first week of life.

Fibrinogen deficiency

Fibrinogen deficiency is heterogeneous and two main phenotypes can be distinguished: plasma and platelet levels of the protein are not measurable or very low, leading to afibrinogenaemia and hypofibrinogenaemia. In other cases, low clottable fibrinogen contrasts with normal or moderately reduced fibrinogen antigen leading to dysfibrinogenaemia and hypodysfibrinogenaemia. Fibrinogen is produced in the hepatocyte from three homologous polypeptide chains, Aα, Bβ and γ, which assemble to form a 340-kDa hexamer. The three genes encoding fibrinogen Bβ (*FGB*), Aα (*FGA*) and γ (*FGG*), ordered from centromere to telomere, are clustered in a region of approximately 50 kb on chromosome 4 in humans.

Experimental disruption of the α-chain gene makes mice completely deficient in all the fibrinogen chains. There is no evidence of defective embryonic development, but the importance of fibrinogen in pregnancy is demonstrated in studies with fibrinogen knockout mice, which cannot maintain gestation to term. Both arterial and venous thromboembolic complications have been reported in afibrinogenaemic patients.

However, in the majority of patients no traditional thrombotic risk factors are present: one explanation for this predisposition is that even in the absence of fibrinogen, platelet aggregation is possible due to the action of von Willebrand factor and, in contrast to haemophiliacs, afibrinogenaemic patients are able to generate thrombin, both in the initial phase of limited production and also in the secondary burst of thrombin generation. In an *in vivo* thrombosis model, the number of embolized thrombi was sixfold higher in fibrinogen knockout mice than in wild-type mice, with large emboli very often leading to vessel occlusion (Table 42.2).

Clinical manifestations and treatment

Dysfibrinogenaemic and hypofibrinogenaemic patients are usually asymptomatic, while those with afibrinogenaemia have a bleeding tendency that usually manifests in the neonatal period, with 85% of cases presenting umbilical cord bleeding. Bleeding may also occur in the skin, gastrointestinal tract, genitourinary tract or the CNS, while persistent damage to the musculoskeletal system and resulting handicap is less frequent. A milder symptom such as epistaxis is also frequent. Women may suffer from menometrorrhagia, but some have normal menses. First-trimester abortion is common in women with afibrinogenaemia but less common in those with dysfibrinogenaemia and

Table 42.2 Knockout mouse models of coagulation factors and vitamin K dependent proteins.

Coagulation factor	Embryonic lethality	Compatible with survival to adulthood	Murine phenotype
Fibrinogen	No	Yes	Normal embryonic development, bleeding events in one-third of newborns, females with deletion of both alleles do not support pregnancy due to vaginal bleeding
FII	Partial	No	Neonatal haemorrhage, no survival beyond several days, loss of vascular integrity
FV	Partial	No	Death caused by haemorrhage in neonates, no survival beyond 2 hours, vascular defects
FVII	No	No	Normal embryonic development, death caused by haemorrhage in neonates, no survival beyond 24 days, no vascular defects
FX	Partial	No	Death caused by haemorrhage in neonates, no survival beyond 20 days, no vascular defects
FXI	No	Yes	Normal life, no tendency to spontaneous bleeding
FXIII	No	Yes	Reproduction impaired and bleeding episodes associated with reduced survival
Vitamin K dependent (*GGCX*)	Partial	No	Massive intra-abdominal haemorrhage
Vitamin K dependent (*VKORC1*)	No	No	Death caused by predominantly intracerebral haemorrhage 2–20 days after birth

has not been reported in hypofibrinogenaemia. Postpartum bleeding is relatively frequent when no prophylactic replacement therapy is given.

The conventional treatment is episodic and on-demand, in which fibrinogen is administered as soon as possible after onset of bleeding; however, effective long-term secondary prophylaxis with administration of fibrinogen every 7–14 days (particularly after CNS bleeds) has recently been described. Replacement therapy is effective in treating bleeding episodes in congenital fibrinogen disorders but, depending on the country of residence, patients receive fresh-frozen plasma (FFP), cryoprecipitate or fibrinogen concentrate. The latter is the treatment of choice because it is virally inactivated and thus safer than cryoprecipitate or FFP. In many countries fibrinogen concentrates remain inaccessible due to the cost of production.

Molecular defects

In 1999, a homozygous deletion of approximately 11 kb in the *FGA* gene was first identified as a cause of inherited afibrinogenaemia in four members of a Swiss family by Neerman-Arbez and colleagues. Since this report many other mutations, the majority in *FGA*, have been identified in patients with afibrinogenaemia (in homozygosity or compound heterozygosity) or hypofibrinogenaemia. The relatively high number of mutations located in *FGA* led to the hypothesis that mutations tend to cluster in this gene, resulting in complete lack of production of fibrinogen Aα chain or of a severely truncated protein. Of particular interest are missense mutations that lead to complete fibrinogen deficiency. These are clustered in the highly conserved C-terminal globular domains of the Bβ and γ chains. Recent functional studies of these mutations in transfected cells have demonstrated either impaired assembly or impaired secretion of the fibrinogen hexamer, demonstrating the importance of these globular structures in quality control of fibrinogen biosynthesis. To date only two missense mutations, p.Cys64Phe and p.Met70Arg (Cys45Phe and Met51Arg, numbering without the signal peptide) located at the start of the coiled-coil in *FGA*, have been found in fibrinogen deficiency.

Among the large number of mutations identified in patients with congenital afibrinogenaemia, two common mutations were found in individuals of European origin, both in *FGA*: the Asp153SerfsX4 mutation (or c.510+1G→T according to the nomenclature guidelines of the Human Genome Variation Society, www.hgvs.org) and the *FGA* 11-kb deletion, both found on multiple haplotypes. Accordingly, the Asp153SerfsX4 should be the first mutation to be screened in all new patients of European origin. Figure 42.2 shows the mutations accounting for afibrinogenaemia and hypofibrinogenaemia identified so far. Two further residues of prime interest in screening for dysfibrinogenaemia are residue Arg16 in exon 2 on *FGA*, which is part of the thrombin cleavage site in the fibrinogen Aα chain,

and residue Arg275 in exon 8 on *FGG*, which is important for fibrin polymerization.

Prothrombin deficiency

Prothrombin deficiency is perhaps the rarest inherited coagulation disorder, with a prevalence of about 1 in 2 million. Based on the measurement of prothrombin (FII) activity and antigen level, two main phenotypes can be distinguished: hypoprothrombinaemia (both levels are concomitantly low) and dysprothrombinaemia (normal or near-normal synthesis of a dysfunctional protein); hypoprothrombinaemia associated with dysprothrombinaemia was also described in compound heterozygosity. FII, a vitamin-K dependent glycoprotein synthesized by liver, is the zymogen of the serine protease α-thrombin and is encoded by a gene of approximately 21 kb located on chromosome 11. No living patient with undetectable plasma prothrombin has been reported so far, consistent with the demonstration that in mice complete prothrombin deficiency obtained by gene knockout is incompatible with life, resulting in embryonic or neonatal lethality (see Table 42.2).

Clinical manifestations and treatment

Hypoprothrombinaemia, with plasma levels below 10%, is characterized by severe bleeding manifestations such as spontaneous haematomas and haemarthroses, intracerebral bleeding and gastrointestinal haemorrhages. Clinically, dysprothrombinaemia manifests as a variable bleeding tendency that is usually less severe than true deficiency, while heterozygote subjects are usually asymptomatic although, occasionally, excessive bleeding after surgical procedures can be observed. In homozygous women menorrhagia is frequent.

Replacement therapy is needed only in homozygous patients, in case of bleeding or to ensure adequate prophylaxis before surgical procedures. Since no FII concentrate exists, FFP, prothrombin complex concentrate (PCC) or both are used for treating patients. In severe clinical settings, higher levels of prothrombin may be achieved with PCCs without the risk of potential volume overload induced by FFP. However, most PCCs contain other vitamin-K dependent coagulation factors, which could potentially induce thrombotic complications.

Molecular defects

Genetic variants have been identified all along the prothrombin gene, although frequently they involve the catalytic area, consistent with the fact that they affect the enzymatic activity of the protein. Mutations in different exons may cause similar phenotypic expression of prothrombin. Most of the natural mutants derive from missense mutations (80%), although insertion/deletions (10%), nonsense mutations (6%) and splice-site

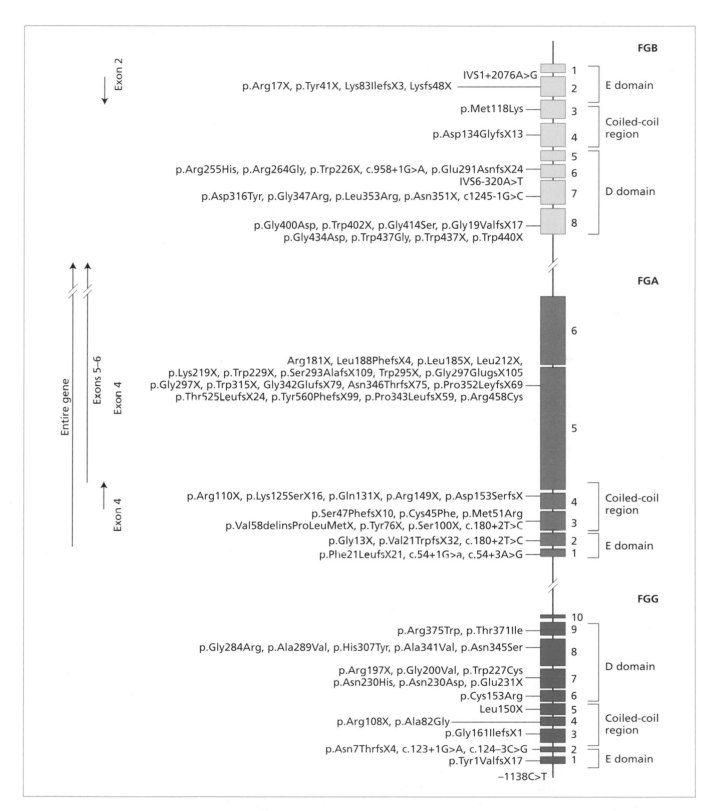

Figure 42.2 Schematic representation of the localization of the main mutations along the human fibrinogen genes, projected onto the exons encoding the domains of the protein. Exons (rectangles) are drawn to scale while introns (lines) are not to scale. Gross deletions are indicated by arrows.

mutations (4%) have also been described. The abnormalities may be classified according to the site of the defect, i.e. in the activation mechanism or in the protease activity of thrombin. The latter group can be subdivided into two subtypes: one in which there is defective amidolytic activity and another where there is defective interaction of thrombin with substrates because of mutations in the molecular recognition domains. Other mutations indirectly affect the catalytic activity of thrombin, as they cause perturbation of the Na^+-binding site of the enzyme. However, while *in vitro* Na^+ binding seems to play a major role in thrombin activity, the natural prothrombin mutants with altered Na^+ binding described so far (Arg517Gln and Lys556Thr, in exons 13 and 14, respectively) had only a mild haemorrhagic phenotype. To date several functional studies have been performed to elucidate the structure–function relationship. However, recent biochemical characterization of natural prothrombin mutants (Des-Lys9/10 and Phe299(7)Val) has revealed an important role of the A-chain for correct function of the catalytic B-chain of thrombin. These natural mutations could affect the interaction of divalent metals with thrombin, recently localized at the interface between the A and B chains, which seem to stabilize the active conformation of thrombin. Figure 42.3 shows the mutations identified so far.

Factor V deficiency

FV has a double role in the coagulation process: it is a protein cofactor required by the prothrombinase complex for thrombin generation, but also contributes to the anticoagulant pathway by downregulating FVIII activity, so that FV deficiency may result in either haemorrhagic or thrombotic tendency. The majority of individuals with FV deficiency are characterized by concomitant deficiency of FV activity and antigen levels (type I deficiency), but approximately 25% have normal antigen levels, indicating the presence of a dysfunctional protein (type II deficiency). FV is mainly secreted by hepatocytes, but there is evidence that it can also be synthesized *in vivo* in the megakaryocyte/platelet lineage. FV is encoded by a large (80 kb) and complex (25 exons) gene located on chromosome 1. Experimental deficiency of FV in gene knockout mice leads to defective embryonic development and early haemorrhagic death. However, mice expressing minimal FV activity below the sensitivity threshold of the detection assay (< 0.1%) differ from the complete knockout mice because they do survive (see Table 42.2).

Clinical manifestations and treatment

Symptomatic patients usually present with skin and mucous membrane bleeding; epistaxis and menorrhagia are relatively frequent, even in patients with measurable FV levels. Typically, FV-deficient patients are difficult to diagnose and often come to medical attention because of a positive family history or abnormal preoperative laboratory screen. On the whole, it appears that the clinical phenotype of patients with FV deficiency is completely different from that seen in the mouse knockout model. Haemarthroses and haematomas occur in only 25% of patients, and life-threatening bleeding episodes in the gastrointestinal tract and the CNS are rare. There are no published data on management of pregnancy in women with FV deficiency. Postoperative and oral cavity haemorrhages are common, but not fully predictable, as these symptoms also occur with plasma levels as high as 5–10%. This discrepancy is likely to be explained by the relatively poor sensitivity of FV bioassays, which do not measure those small amounts of the factor that are probably sufficient to make the deficiency compatible with life and a mild clinical phenotype. Replacement therapy with FV can be administered only through FFP, preferably virus inactivated, because no FV concentrate is available and FV is not contained in significant amount in cryoprecipitate or PCCs.

Molecular defects

Among rare coagulation disorders, FV deficiency is one of the least characterized from the molecular point of view, with only 56 genetic defects hitherto described, the majority of them identified in the last 4 years (Figure 42.4). A total of 48 mutations seem to be responsible for the type I deficiency, only one being recurrent (Tyr1702Cys, repeatedly found in Italian individuals), confirming the remarkable allelic heterogeneity of the disease. A mild type I deficiency (decrease in FV levels) has also been associated with two FV variants: the functional Met2120Thr polymorphism, demonstrated to cause about 25% reduction in FV levels, and the HR2 haplotype defined by a group of more than 10 polymorphisms; among these, the dominant contribution of the Asp2194Gly variant was demonstrated by expression experiments in eukaryotic cells. Only one genetic defect, Ala221Val, associated with type II deficiency has so far been reported. Mutations causing FV deficiency do not cover the full spectrum of possible genetic lesions, since mutations located in the promoter as well as large deletions are absent. Missense mutations are completely absent in the large exon 13, coding for the whole B domain. This can probably be explained by an increased tolerance of this domain to variations, as suggested by the fact that it is highly polymorphic and not evolutionarily conserved. Finally, no clear genotype–phenotype correlation emerges between the clinical phenotype, plasma FV levels and the corresponding associated mutations in FV deficiency. In fact, despite carriership of the same mutations, some patients often present with a more severe bleeding pattern than others. Recently, the possibility that the severe FV-deficient phenotype may be modulated by a concomitant procoagulant defect was investigated by Duckers and colleagues, who showed that congenital FV deficiency associated with reduced plasma levels of

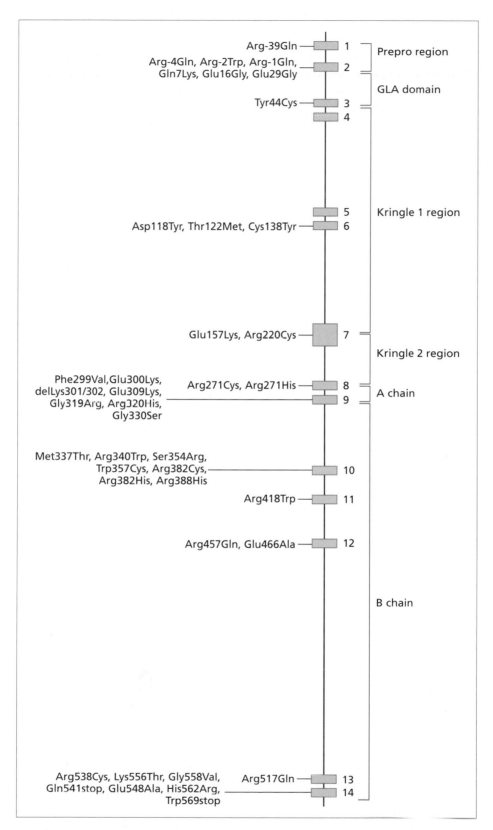

Figure 42.3 Schematic representation of the localization of the main mutations along the human prothrombin gene, projected onto the exons encoding the domains of the protein. Exons (rectangles) are drawn to scale while introns (lines) are not to scale.

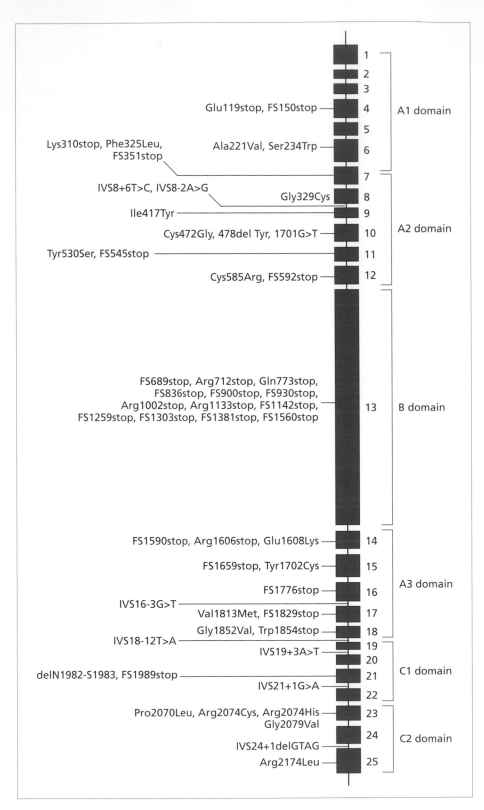

Figure 42.4 Schematic representation of the localization of the main mutations along the human FV gene, projected onto the exons encoding the domains of the protein. Exons (rectangles) are drawn to scale while introns (lines) are not to scale.

tissue factor pathway inhibitor, which decreases the FV requirement for minimal thrombin generation to less than 1%, probably protects patients from severe life-threatening bleeding.

Combined deficiency of factor V and factor VIII

For many years the molecular mechanism for combined deficiency of these two factors, each transmitted with different patterns of inheritance (autosomal recessive for FV, X-linked for FVIII) and involving proteins encoded by different genes, was not understood. Finally, in 1998 combined FV and FVIII deficiency (F5F8D) was causally associated with mutations in the *LMAN1* gene, encoding lectin mannose-binding protein (previously named *ERGIC-53*), a 53-kDa type 1 transmembrane protein that acts as a chaperone in the intracellular transport of both factors. More recently, in 2003, another locus associated with the deficiency was identified in about 15% of affected families with no mutations in *LMAN1*; this was named the *MCFD2* gene, encoding multiple coagulation factor deficiency (MCFD)2 protein, which acts as a cofactor for LMAN1, specifically recruiting correctly folded FV and FVIII in the endoplasmatic reticulum. Recent studies have failed to identify additional components of the LMAN1–MCFD2 receptor complex, supporting the idea that F5F8D might be limited to *LMAN1* and *MCFD2*.

Clinical manifestations and treatment

F5F8D is characterized by concomitantly low levels (usually 5–20%) of the two coagulation factors, both as coagulant activity and as antigen. It appears that the concomitant presence of two coagulation defects does not enhance the haemorrhagic tendency observed in each defect separately (see section on FV deficiency). The phenotypes associated with mutations in *MCFD2* and *LMAN1* are indistinguishable and manifested only by deficiencies of FV and FVIII, although a selective delay in secretion of the cargo protein procathepsin C has been observed in HeLa cells overexpressing a dominant-negative form of LMAN1.

Symptoms are usually mild, with a predominance of easy bruising, epistaxis, and bleeding after dental extractions. Menorrhagia and postpartum bleeding have also been reported in affected women. More severe symptoms, such as haemarthroses and umbilical cord bleeding, are observed very seldom and gastrointestinal and CNS bleeding have been reported in only a few patients. Soft-tissue haematomas are unusual. Because of the mild clinical pattern, bleeding episodes are usually treated on demand and do not require regular prophylaxis. Sources of both FV and FVIII are needed and their differential plasma half-lives (FV 36 hours, FVIII 10–14 hours) have to be taken into consideration.

As there are no FV concentrates available and there is little or no FV present in cryoprecipitate or PCCs, replacement of FV can currently be achieved only through the use of FFP, preferably with virus-inactivated plasma. For FVIII replacement, a large number of products are available: the synthetic hormone desmopressin (DDAVP) can be successfully used for minor bleeding episodes to raise FVIII. However, the chemical efficacy of DDAVP needs to be tested in each patient and more than three to four consecutive treatments should be avoided. For severe bleeding, plasma-derived FVIII or recombinant FVIII concentrates are the treatments of choice and include FFP, plasma-derived concentrates and recombinant FVIII.

Molecular defects

F5F8D is caused by mutations in LMAN1 or MCFD2 proteins. The first is encoded by a gene of approximately 29 kb located on chromosome 18 and containing 13 exons, while the latter is encoded by a shorter gene of approximately 19 kb located on chromosome 2 and containing four exons. To date, a total of 48 mutations (Figures 42.5 and 42.6) have been described (32 in *LMAN1* and 16 in *MCFD2*; http://www.med.unc.edu/isth/mutations-databases/FVandVIII_2006numbers.htm). All the *LMAN1* mutations reported so far are null mutations, with the exception of a Cys→Arg mutation that disrupts a disulphide bond required for oligomerization and which also destabilizes the protein. In contrast, both null and missense mutations have been identified in *MCFD2*; in particular, five of six missense mutations reported (Asp81Tyr, Asp89Ala, Asp122Val, Asp129Glu and Ile136Thr) disrupt LMAN1 binding, indicating that LMAN1 and MCFD2 must function as a unit to transport FV and FVIII. Recently, Zhang and colleagues have performed a genotype–phenotype analysis to evaluate if mutations in the two different genes are associated with differences in FV and FVIII plasma levels. Mean plasma levels of FV and FVIII in patients with *MCFD2* mutations were significantly lower than those in patients with *LMAN1* mutations. These data suggest that MCFD2 may play a primary role in the export of FV and FVIII from the endoplasmatic reticulum.

Some mutations in both *LMAN1* and *MCFD2* recurred in more than one family, for example Met1Thr, 89insG and Lys302stop on *LMAN1* or IVS2+5G→A and Ile136Thr mutations on *MCFD2*. In particular, the *MCFD2* IVS2+5G→A appears to be one of the most common mutations causing F5F8D and it has now been identified in at least 13 unrelated families from different geographic regions (India, Italy, USA, Serbia and Germany).

Factor VII deficiency

FVII deficiency is the most common autosomal recessive coagulation disorder (1 in 500 000). A typical feature of this disease

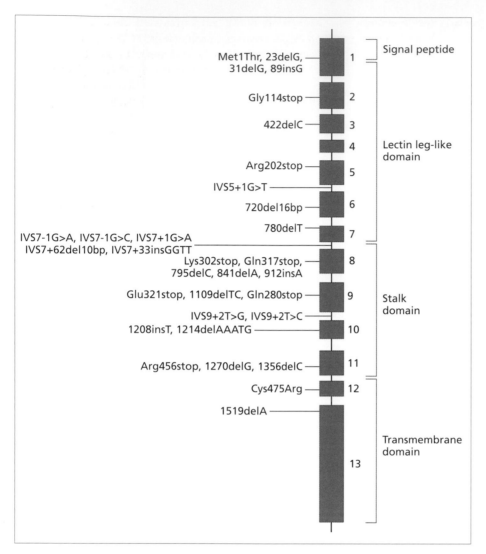

Met1Thr, 23delG, — 1
31delG, 89insG

Gly114stop — 2

422delC — 3

4

Arg202stop — 5

IVS5+1G>T —

720del16bp — 6

780delT — 7

IVS7-1G>A, IVS7-1G>C, IVS7+1G>A
IVS7+62del10bp, IVS7+33insGGTT

Lys302stop, Gln317stop, — 8
795delC, 841delA, 912insA

Glu321stop, 1109delTC, Gln280stop — 9

IVS9+2T>G, IVS9+2T>C —
1208insT, 1214delAAATG — 10

Arg456stop, 1270delG, 1356delC — 11

Cys475Arg — 12

1519delA —

13

Signal peptide

Lectin leg-like
domain

Stalk
domain

Transmembrane
domain

Figure 42.5 Schematic representation of the localization of the main mutations along the human *LMAN1* gene, projected onto the exons encoding the domains of the protein. Exons (rectangles) are drawn to scale while introns (lines) are not to scale.

is its clinical heterogeneity, which ranges in severity from lethal to mild, or even asymptomatic forms. FVII is synthesized in the liver and is encoded by the FVII gene (*F7*) located on chromosome 13, 2.8 kb upstream of the FX gene. Plasma levels of FVII coagulant activity (FVII:C) and FVII antigen (FVII:Ag) are influenced by a number of genetic and environmental factors (sex, age, cholesterol and triglyceride levels) and it is also well known that FVII levels are modulated by *F7* polymorphisms. The majority of patients have concomitantly low levels of FVII:C and FVII:Ag, but several cases are characterized by normal or low borderline levels of FVII:Ag contrasting with lower levels of FVII:C. Most gene knockout mice made experimentally deficient in FVII develop normally, which suggests that complete lack of FVII is compatible with life (see Table 42.2).

Clinical manifestations and treatment

The severity of symptoms of FVII deficiency is variable and generally reported to be poorly correlated with plasma levels. Some patients do not bleed at all after major episodes of haemostasis. Life- or limb-endangering bleeding manifestations are relatively rare, the most frequent symptoms being epistaxis and menorrhagia. CNS bleeding was also reported to have high incidence (16%) in a series of 75 patients affected by FVII deficiency, the study concluding that the greatest risk factor for development of bleeding was trauma related to the birth process. However, these data were not confirmed by two subsequent large series of Italian and Iranian patients. Thrombotic episodes (particularly deep vein thrombosis) have also been reported in 3–4% of patients with FVII deficiency, particularly

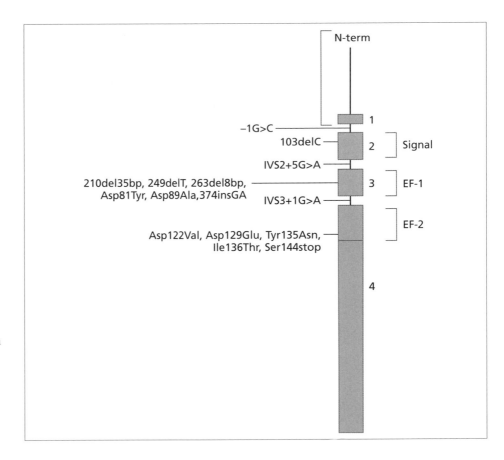

Figure 42.6 Schematic representation of the localization of the main mutations along the human *MCFD2* gene, projected onto the exons encoding the domains of the protein. Exons (rectangles) are drawn to scale while introns (lines) are not to scale.

in the presence of surgery and replacement treatment, but spontaneous thrombosis may also occur.

Lack of correlation between measured FVII:C *in vitro* and the clinical phenotype is well known and is probably due to the fact that only trace amounts of FVIIa are required to initiate coagulation *in vivo*. Empirical studies and mathematical modelling suggest that as little as 5 pmol/L (0.05% of normal FVII concentration) is sufficient to induce clot formation. None of the *in vitro* tests could differentiate between null and extremely low levels of FVII:C capable of initiating coagulation *in vivo*.

A number of therapeutic options can be offered to patients with FVII deficiency, including FFP, still used in developing countries, PCCs, plasma-derived FVII concentrates and recombinant FVIIa, which has to be considered the optimal replacement therapy because it can be used at very low dose (10–20 μg/kg). Prophylaxis has been a debated issue in FVII deficiency, especially because of the very short half-life of infused FVII in blood. *Ex vivo* studies have shown that infused recombinant FVIIa disappears quickly from the circulation but persists extravascularly bound to pericytes. These observations would support the feasibility of prophylaxis in FVII deficiency, but larger trials are needed to assess the optimal schedule.

The occurrence of frequent menorrhagic menses is almost invariably associated with iron deficiency and anaemia in women with the severe form of FVII deficiency. Pregnancy itself does not require special precautions and uncomplicated delivery is possible without prophylaxis. However, all cases of postpartum bleeding reported so far occurred in women with low FVII coagulant activity (< 15 units/dL) not receiving prophylaxis. Therefore, delivery should occur under the coverage of a short-term replacement.

Molecular defects

The molecular bases of FVII deficiency are more extensively characterized than those of other defects, perhaps due to the relatively high frequency of this defect and small size of the gene. Mutations are very heterogeneous: missense variants are the most frequent lesions (70–80%), splice-site changes are also well represented, while nonsense mutations and small deletions are rare, particularly in the homozygous condition. Mutations are located throughout the gene, suggesting that all domains are important in maintaining the overall structure and function of FVII. The previously available online database http://europium. csc.mrc.ac.uk/ allowed rapid access for researchers to the entire listing of *F7* mutations but is currently under revision; however, an updated overview of mutations is shown in Figure 42.7. The severe cases are all either homozygous or doubly heterozygous

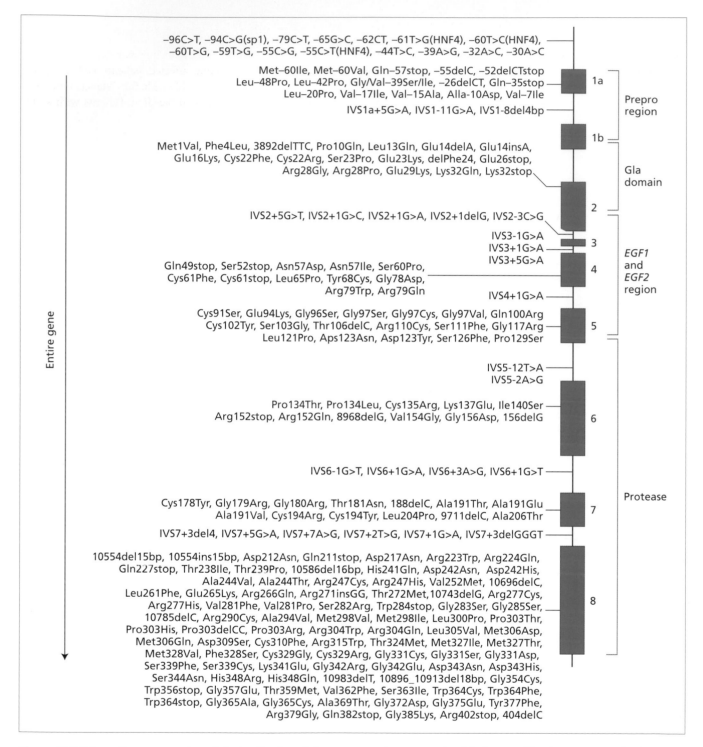

Figure 42.7 Schematic representation of the localization of the main mutations along the human FVII gene, projected onto the exons encoding the domains of the protein. Exons (rectangles) are drawn to scale while introns (lines) are not to scale. Gross deletion is indicated by the arrow.

for mutations that disrupt expression of the protein (e.g. deletions, insertions, splice junctions and promoter mutations), resulting in FVII:C levels typically less than 2% of normal. Individuals with a mild/moderate clinical phenotype are homozygous or doubly heterozygous for missense mutations; however, some missense mutations are also associated with a severe phenotype.

Frequent mutations (Ala294Val, 11125delC, Arg304Gln, Cys310Phe) identified among hundreds of patients with FVII deficiency by different groups are associated with a range of clinical severity and neither FVII:C nor gender provide an explanation for this heterogeneity, suggesting that other modifying factors may influence the different clinical manifestations in subjects carrying the same mutation. It is known that FVII levels are modulated by *F7* polymorphisms: different genotypes demonstrated up to fivefold differences in mean FVII levels. Tightly linked polymorphisms in the 5′ regulatory region regulate FVII levels and differential promoter activity *in vitro*; the p.Arg353Gln substitution in the catalytic domain, tightly associated with the decanucleotide insertion (g.−323 to −324insCCTATATCCT) and with the −401T allele in the promoter region, decreases FVII secretion, therefore reducing its plasma levels. The same effect is shown by the g.11293–11294insAA polymorphism in the 3′ untranslated region of *F7* that negatively affects the steady state of mRNA levels, leading to a reduction in FVII mRNA by 40%, which subsequently reduces FVII protein levels. An additional polymorphism, located in intron 7, is characterized by the presence of a variable number of 37-bp repeats. This polymorphism is reported to be associated with variable rates of FVII transcriptional activity according to the number of repeats present in the genotype. The peculiar presence of such repeated regions, and of polymorphic variation of repeats within *F7*, requires careful design of PCR primers to detect gene rearrangements when molecular diagnosis is performed.

Factor X deficiency

FX is a glycoprotein that plays a pivotal role in the coagulation cascade, being the first enzyme in the common pathway of thrombin formation. FX is mainly synthesized by the liver and is encoded by the *FX* gene, comprising 22 kb and located on chromosome 13, a few kilobases downstream of the *F7*. The clinical phenotypes of FX deficiency are characterized by concomitantly low levels of coagulant activity and antigen, or low coagulant activity contrasting with normal or low borderline antigen values. Mice rendered experimentally deficient in FX by targeted inactivation of the *FX* gene showed frequent embryonic lethality. Those who survived bled to death intra-abdominally at birth and in the CNS within the first 3–4 weeks of life (see Table 42.2).

Clinical manifestations and treatment

In FX deficiency the bleeding tendency may appear at any age, although the more severely affected patients (FX coagulant activity < 1%) present early in life with, for instance, umbilical-stump, CNS or gastrointestinal bleeding. Patients with severe deficiencies also commonly experience haemarthroses and haematomas. The most common bleeding symptoms reported at all levels of severity are epistaxis and menorrhagia. In FX deficiency there is reasonable correlation between the severity of clinical manifestations and residual FX activity, confirming animal study results.

Data from the United Kingdom Haemophilia Centre Doctors' Organisation (UKHCDO) registry shows that the proportion of patients with this deficiency who require treatment is much higher than that of other rare coagulation deficiencies. There is no specific FX product, plasma derived or recombinant, available as yet for treatment of patients with FX deficiency; hence current treatment is based on the administration of FFP and PCCs. However, these treatments could be associated with some complications stemming from the use of large amounts of plasma, particularly in children and elderly patients with cardiac disease, or because of the high concentrations of FII, FVII and FIX in PCCs that could be associated with a risk of thromboembolic events. To overcome this problem, a freeze-dried human coagulation FIX and FX concentrate with specified amounts of FX (and FIX) has been developed recently. Therapeutic options for the control of menorrhagia include both medical (e.g. antifibrinolytics, oral contraceptives, levonorgestrel intrauterine device and clotting factor replacement) and surgical (e.g. endometrial ablation and hysterectomy). Apart from menorrhagia, women with FX deficiency, as well as women with other RBDs, are likely to develop other gynaecological problems, such as corpus luteum haemorrhage or haemoperitoneum associated with ovulation, that may warrant the adoption of prophylactic treatment. Even if pregnancy is accompanied by increased concentrations of FX, women with severe FX deficiency and a history of adverse pregnancy outcomes, such as abortion, placental abruption or premature birth, may benefit from continuous replacement therapy. Finally, heterozygotes have also been reported to have bleeding after delivery that required treatment with FFP.

Molecular defects

The gene structure and organization is homologous to that of the other vitamin-K dependent proteins, with the exception of prothrombin, suggesting evolution from a common ancestor by a process of duplication and divergence. To date, 105 mutations comprising 85 missense, 14 insertions/deletions (three gross deletions plus 11 micro insertions/deletions), six splice site, two nonsense, and one in the 5′ flanking region have been reported

(Figure 42.8). Although most mutations are located in exon 8, the number of mutations located in each exon is proportional to the length of the exon itself, indicating the absence of a hotspot region on *FX* gene. Among the 105 mutations so far reported, only two were nonsense, and only one (C61X) was identified in the homozygous state in three unrelated patients.

Moreover, only a few of the entire group of missense mutations so far reported have been recurrent and found in more than one family from the same geographical area. In particular, Arg–1Thr, associated with a severe phenotype (FX coagulant activity < 1%), was identified in the homozygous state in four unrelated patients from Iran, while Gly380Arg, associated with intracranial haemorrhages, was identified in six homozygous patients from Costa Rica; Pro343Ser (FX Friuli), associated with reduced FX coagulant activity (4–9%), was identified in more than 10 patients from northern Italy. Other mutations, such as Gly–20Arg, Gly94Arg and Gly222Asp, all associated with a severe laboratory phenotype, have been reported from different groups worldwide.

To assess whether genotypic variations could have an influence on FX plasma level, four different polymorphisms located in the promoter region (a TTGTGA insertion between position −343A and −342G, a C/T polymorphism at position −222, a C/A polymorphism at position −220 and a C/T polymorphism at position −40) have been investigated but no association was found.

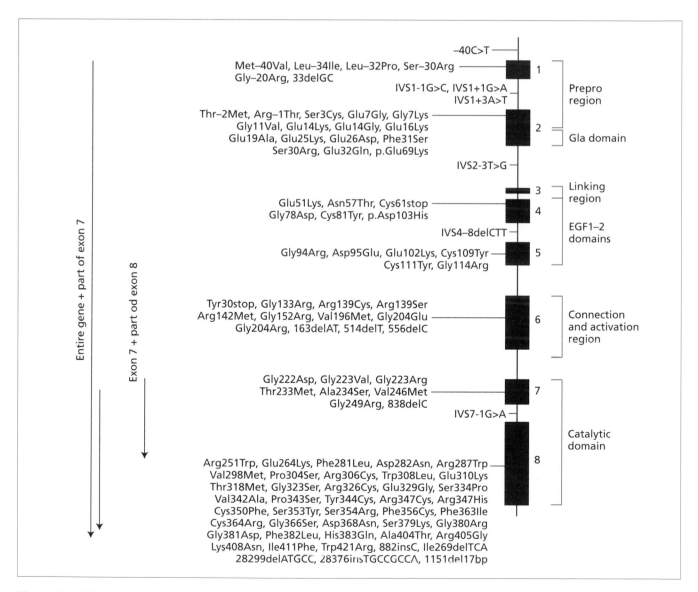

Figure 42.8 Schematic representation of the localization of the main mutations along the human FX gene, projected onto the exons encoding the domains of the protein. Exons (rectangles) are drawn to scale while introns (lines) are not to scale. Gross deletions are indicated by the arrows.

Factor XI deficiency

FXI deficiency is characterized by a decrease in the functional activity of this plasma protein, usually accompanied by correspondingly low FXI antigen levels. More rarely, normal or borderline levels of plasma FXI antigen are associated with a dysfunctional form of the protein. The estimated prevalence of the severe deficiency in most populations is about 1 in 1 million, but is reported to be much higher in Ashkenazi Jews, heterozygosity for FXI deficiency being as high as 8%.

FXI is mainly synthesized in the liver, although tiny amounts of transcript can also be detected in megakaryocytes and platelets. The protein is encoded by the *FXI* gene, comprising 23 kb and located on chromosome 4. The existence of a platelet FXI transcript, originating from the skipping of exon 5, was hypothesized for a long time but never confirmed by subsequent work. Nonetheless, recent data support the view that FXI transcripts undergo alternative splicing, leading to the synthesis of FXI isoforms whose physiological role and importance still need to be demonstrated. In knockout mice the loss of the gene coding for this factor is compatible with life, with no tendency for spontaneous bleeding (see Table 42.2).

Clinical manifestations and treatment

The relationship between FXI levels in plasma and the bleeding tendency is not as clear-cut as for other coagulation factor deficiencies. The phenotype of bleeding is not correlated with the genotype but with the site of injury. When a site of injury with local high fibrinolytic activity is involved (e.g. urogenital tract, oral cavity after dental extraction or tonsillectomy), the risk of bleeding is increased (49–67%) in comparison to sites with less local fibrinolytic activity (1.5–40%). Usually, patients with severe FXI deficiency (1% or less) are mildly affected and most bleeding manifestations are injury-related. Surprisingly, patients with low but detectable levels of FXI are also mild bleeders, so that clinical phenotypes are not strikingly different in these two groups. This observation, already made for Jewish patients, was recently confirmed in a series of Iranian non-Jewish patients with severe or moderate deficiency (FXI coagulant activity < 1 to 5%) and in patients with mild deficiency (6–30%). All patients were mild bleeders, but those symptoms that define the severity of the bleeding tendency, such as muscle haematomas and haemarthrosis, showed a similar frequency in the two groups of factor-deficient patients (about 25%). The most frequent symptoms were oral and postoperative bleeding, which occurred in more than 50% of patients. Women with FXI deficiency are prone to excessive bleeding during menstruation, but case series of women affected by severe FXI deficiency showed that 70% of pregnancies were uneventful, despite no prophylactic treatment. Also, patients with alloantibodies that inhibit FXI do not bleed spontaneously but only during surgery or trauma. Patients with inhibitors treated with FFP or FXI concentrates can suffer from prolonged bleeding if the presence of inhibitors is not diagnosed prior to surgery. After being exposed to plasma, 7 of 21 FXI-deficient Israeli patients homozygous for the Glu117stop mutation developed inhibitors to FXI. Recently, Zucker and colleagues showed that this also happened in an Italian woman homozygous for the same mutation after three injections of Rh immunoglobulin and without previous exposure to blood products.

Treatment is based on the use of antifibrinolytic agents, FFP, FXI concentrate and recombinant FVIIa, but care should be taken to reduce the risk of complications such as thrombotic events (especially when FXI concentrate or recombinant FVIIa is planned), volume overload, allergic reactions and development of inhibitors. Patients with partial deficiency of FXI who have no bleeding history do not require prophylactic treatment.

Molecular defects

To date, more than 180 mutations affecting *FXI* gene have been identified (Figure 42.9). These can be accessed on three different online databases:
• http://www.med.unc.edu/isth/mutations-databases/FactorXI_2007.html
• http://www.wienkav.at/kav/kar/texte_anzeigen.asp?ID=7137
• http:www.factorxi.com.
The high allelic heterogeneity of FXI deficiency is highlighted by the distribution of genetic defects throughout the whole gene. Missense mutations represent more than 60% of all variants, only seven of them being reported to lead to the dysfunctional form of the deficiency.

Two mutations are responsible for most cases of FXI deficiency in Ashkenazi Jews, while mutations are more varied in non-Jews. The so-called type II Jewish mutation is a stop codon in exon 5, compatible with the observation that patients homozygous for this defect usually have undetectable levels of FXI. The so-called type III Jewish mutation is a missense mutation in exon 9, leading to the Phe283Leu substitution. The mutation causes defective secretion of the protein from cells, but some FXI is ultimately produced so that these patients have measurable levels of FXI (about 10%). Type II/III compound heterozygosity is the commonest cause of severe to moderate FXI deficiency in Ashkenazi Jews.

Factor XIII deficiency

FXIII is a transglutaminase, is the last enzyme to be activated in the blood coagulation pathway and functions to cross-link the α and γ fibrin chains, resulting in a stronger clot with an increased resistance to fibrinolysis. The plasma factor consists of two catalytic A subunits (FXIII-A) and two carrier B subunits

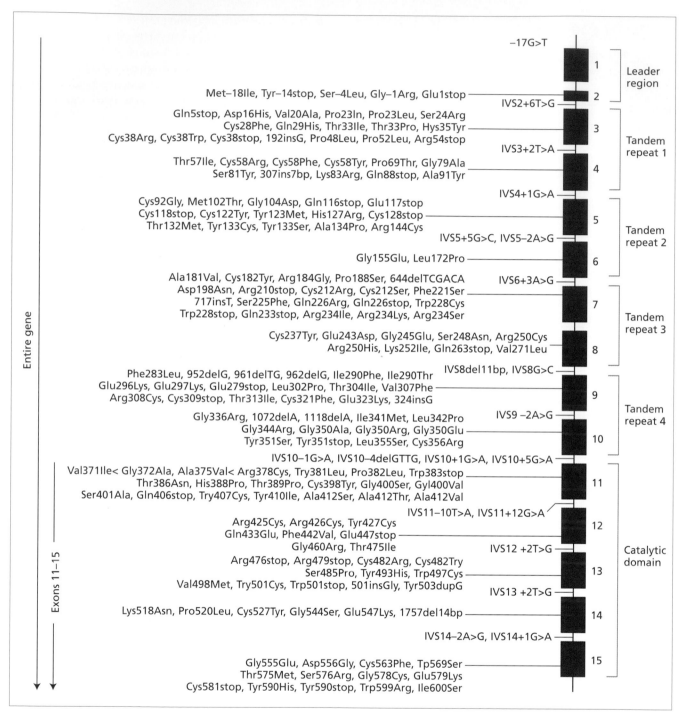

Figure 42.9 Schematic representation of the localization of the main mutations along the human FXI gene, projected onto the exons encoding the domains of the protein. Exons (rectangles) are drawn to scale while introns (lines) are not to scale. Gross deletions are indicated by arrows.

(FXIII-B). FXIII-A is synthesized in cells of bone marrow origin, while FXIII-B is produced in the liver. The corresponding genes are located on chromosomes 6 and 1. FXIII deficiency is probably, together with prothrombin deficiency, the rarest of the recessively transmitted coagulation factor deficiencies (1 in 2 million). In inherited FXIII deficiency, plasma levels of FXIII-A measured as functional activity or immunoreactive protein are usually extremely reduced, whereas the FXIII-B subunit is

Table 42.3 Classification of FXIII deficiency according to activity and antigen determinations of the FXIII subunits.

	FXIII-A deficiency		FXIII-B deficiency
	Quantitative defect	Qualitative defect	
Plasma activity	Reduced	Reduced	Moderately reduced
Plasma antigen A$_2$B$_2$	Reduced	Normal/near normal	Reduced
Plasma antigen A	Reduced	Normal/near normal	Moderately reduced
Platelet antigen A	Reduced	Normal/near normal	Normal
Platelet antigen B	> 30%	> 30%	Reduced

reduced but always at measurable levels. Table 42.3 shows the classification of FXIII deficiency according to activity and antigen determinations of the FXIII subunits.

Studies on homozygous null mice generated by deletion of exon 7 of the FXIII gene showed that these mice were fertile, although reproduction was impaired and bleeding episodes were associated with reduced survival (see Table 42.2). A new aspect of the relationship between FXIII and wound healing has recently been reported. Following an acute myocardial infarction in an experimental model, infarct expansion, heart failure and cardiac rupture were observed in FXIII-deficient mice, probably due to inadequate healing of the myocardial tissue. Spontaneous haemorrhagic events with subsequent inflammation and fibrosis were also reported in the heart tissue of FXIII-deficient mice, suggesting that low FXIII levels may impair cardiac healing and lead to complications in patients with acute myocardial infarction.

Clinical manifestations and treatment

Patients with FXIII-A deficiency have a bleeding tendency that is usually severe, particularly because of the early onset of life-threatening symptoms such as umbilical-cord and CNS bleeding. Bleeding from the umbilical stump in the first few days of life occurs in approximately 80% of patients, and CNS bleeding in up to 30%. Ecchymoses, haematomas and prolonged bleeding following trauma are also typical. Haemarthroses and intramuscular haematomas may appear unexpectedly, although less frequently. In a recent study made on the largest group of patients with severe FXIII deficiency (93 Iranians), the most frequent mucosal tract bleeding symptom was bleeding in the oral cavity (lips, tongue, gum) followed by menorrhagia and epistaxis. Gastrointestinal bleeding is not unusual. Soft-tissue bleeding such as spontaneous haematoma and haemarthrosis occur in a large proportion of patients. In women of reproductive age, 20% had intraperitoneal bleeding that occurred at the time of ovulation, in some cases leading to hysterectomy; 50% of women had at least one miscarriage during pregnancy. The same pattern of symptoms was also recently shown by Ivaskevicius and colleagues in an international registry formed mostly of European data, where joint bleeding is reported to be more commonly periarticular than intra-articular.

On the whole, the clinical impact of FXIII deficiency can shift from that of a very severe disease to that of a mild one, depending on the adoption of prophylactic treatment. All these symptoms usually lead to an early diagnosis, so that patients who survive are often treated prophylactically, starting early in life. Monthly prophylactic infusions of FXIII concentrate are also recommended in FXIII-A-deficient women who are pregnant in order to prevent bleeding and fetal loss. In fact, it was recently reported that among these women there were seven successful pregnancies and five had received FXIII replacement. Moreover, it was found that all women with deficiency of the FXIII-A subunit miscarried, with one exception, if replacement therapy was not given during pregnancy. These data suggest that implementation of replacement therapy is crucial for pregnancy and should commence as early as possible.

This approach to treatment is rendered simple and feasible by the fact that plasma levels of FXIII of 2–5% are sufficient to prevent bleeding, and that the long *in vivo* half-life of the factor (11–14 days) makes it possible to infuse cryoprecipitate or concentrates at intervals of 1 month or longer.

Because of the risk of blood-borne diseases, FFP and cryoprecipitate are less satisfactory for treatment or prophylaxis, and FXIII concentrate is recommended whenever available. A new recombinant FXIII-A$_2$ concentrate (rFXIII-A$_2$) has recently been manufactured in *Saccharomyces cerevesiae*. The rFXIII-A$_2$ homodimers associate in plasma with the endogenous FXIII-B to form the stable heterotetramer FXIII-A$_2$B$_2$. In a Phase I clinical trial, rFXIII-A$_2$, administered to 11 patients with FXIII deficiency, seemed to have a similar half-life and pharmacokinetics to those of the native protein and appeared to be safe. Only four cases of FXIII-B deficiency have been reported to date and the bleeding symptoms appear milder than in FXIII-A-deficient patients.

Molecular defects

More than 70 mutations within *F13A* have been published (Figure 42.10) and most of them are missense/nonsense point mutations. Multiple missense/nonsense mutations have also been reported for a number of codons (77, 260, 326, 413 and 541) with codon changes AAC/AAA and AAC/AAG. In the review by Ivaskevicius and colleagues, the two most frequent

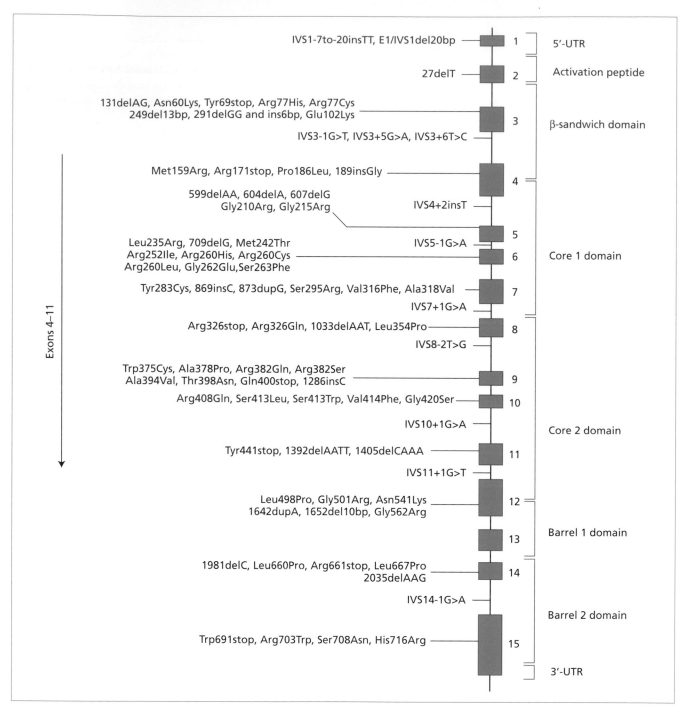

Figure 42.10 Schematic representation of the localization of the main mutations along the human FXIII-A gene, projected onto the exons encoding the domains of the protein. Exons (rectangles) are drawn to scale while introns (lines) are not to scale. Gross deletions are indicated by arrows.

mutations affecting *F13A* were found to be the IVS5–1G→A splice-site defect and the Arg661stop mutation. Haplotype analysis in four patients with the IVS5–1G→A mutation suggested a founder effect, while the concentration of Arg661stop mutation in Finland, Arg77Cys in Switzerland and Arg77His in Iran might also be due to founder effects, although the occurrence of these mutations at CpG dinucleotides raises the alternative possibility of independent origin.

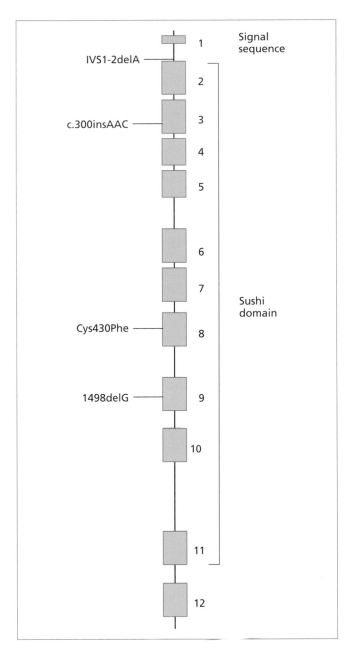

Figure 42.11 Schematic representation of the localization of the main mutations along the human FXIII-B gene, projected onto the exons encoding the domains of the protein. Exons (rectangles) are drawn to scale while introns (lines) are not to scale.

Mutations are scattered throughout the *F13A* gene and in a few studies the mutant proteins were expressed in cultured mammalian cell lines, showing that introduction of the mutation caused destabilization of protein structure and intracellular degradation.

Several polymorphisms in *F13A* have been identified. The most common are Val34Leu, Tyr204Phe, Pro564Leu, Val650Ile

and Glu651Gln. The Val34Leu variant is the most studied polymorphism, with the amino acid substitution occurring in the activation peptide sequence, three amino acids upstream from the thrombin-cleavage site. Studies have shown that the Leu34 allele variant promotes accelerated cleavage of the activation peptide once activated by thrombin and has been associated with a decreased risk of myocardial infarction. However, controversy has surrounded the role of Val34Leu in coronary artery disease, with the literature supporting both sides of the debate.

Only four mutations have been identified in *F13B* (Figure 42.11), a single-nucleotide deletion at the acceptor splice junction of intron A/exon 2 (IVS1(−2)delA), a Cys430Phe missense mutation, a G deletion in exon 9 and an AAC triplet insertion within codon Tyr80 in exon 3.

Vitamin K-dependent coagulation factors deficiency

The first case of vitamin K-dependent coagulation factors deficiency (VKCFD) was reported more than 40 years ago in a 3-month-old girl with multiple bruises and haemorrhages. The girl was studied further when she was 15 years old and was found to have immunologically measurable FII, FVII, FIX and FX that were lacking γ-carboxyglutamic acid residues. Vitamin K-dependent coagulation factors such as FII, FVII, FIX and FX require γ-carboxylation of glutamic acid residues at their Gla domains to enable binding of calcium and attachment to phospholipid membranes. The γ-carboxylation is catalysed by hepatic γ-glutamyl carboxylase (GGCX) and its cofactor reduced vitamin K (KH_2). During the reaction, KH_2 is converted to vitamin K epoxide (KO), which is recycled to KH_2 by the vitamin K epoxide reductase (VKOR) enzyme complex. Heritable dysfunction of GGCX or the VKOR complex results in the secretion of poorly carboxylated vitamin K-dependent coagulation factors, leading to combined deficiency of the vitamin K-dependent clotting factors. The γ-carboxylation of glutamic acid residues is also required for activity of the anticoagulant factors protein C, protein S and protein Z, and although protein S and protein C levels are low in VKCFD, there are no reports of venous or arterial thrombosis. Thus, the effect of VKCFD is clearly in the bleeding area. The GGCX and VKOR proteins are encoded by two corresponding genes: *GGCX* (13 kb, 15 exons) located on chromosome 2 and the unusually small *VKORC1* (5126 bp, three exons) located on chromosome 16; the latter gene was so named because of evidence suggesting that VKOR is a multisubunit complex. Studies on heterozygous mice carrying a null mutation for *GGCX* showed normal development and normal activity of the vitamin K-dependent coagulation factors, but only half of the γ-carboxylase-deficient mice developed to term and those delivered died due to massive intra-abdominal haemorrhages (see Table 42.2).

Clinical manifestations and treatment

VKCFD is a rare autosomal recessive bleeding disorder that often presents during infancy, although the routine administration of vitamin K may delay the diagnosis of VKCFD in neonates. Severe symptoms such as intracranial haemorrhage or umbilical stump bleeding are usually associated with factors levels below 5 units/dL. Severely affected children may also present with skeletal abnormalities such as nasal hypoplasia, distal digital hypoplasia, epiphyseal stippling and mild conductive hearing loss. Older patients can present with easy bruising and mucocutaneous or postsurgical bleeding.

Treatment with oral or parenteral vitamin K_1 should be started as soon as possible in all patients at diagnosis. However, some patients show insufficient response, and there are limited data on the effectiveness of prophylaxis with weekly administration of vitamin K_1 10 mg. In fact, massive parenteral doses of vitamin K do not always correct FII, FVII, FIX and FX activities, and there is clear biochemical evidence that the molecules are not fully carboxylated by such treatment. In this group of patients, factor replacement by virally inactivated FFP could also be used in cases of acute bleeding episodes or before surgery. PCC is the alternative choice when a rapid increase in clotting factor levels is necessary. However, PCCs have been associated with thrombosis and disseminated intravascular coagulation, and therefore should be used with caution in some patients.

Molecular defects

The rare VKCFD autosomal disorder arises from point mutations in either the *GGCX* (type I) or *VKOR* (type II) genes, the only exception being a kindred with a 14-bp deletion in intron 1 of *GGCX*. To date, few mutations have been described for the type I disorder: Asp31Asn, Trp157Arg, Leu394Arg, His404Pro, Arg485Pro, Trp501Ser, Thr591Lys and two recently identified splice-site mutations: a G→T transversion of the first nucleotide of intron 2 (c.1358+1G→T) and an A→G transversion of the third nucleotide of intron 11 (c.10363+3A→G). With regard to the Arg485Pro mutation, Rost and colleagues identified it in two patients originating from the same region in western Germany. Since VKCFD represents a rare entity, they hypothesized a founder effect that was strongly supported by further examination of three intragenic polymorphisms of *GGCX* (c.44–140_–127dup14 and c.44–32G→A in intron 1, and c.215–385G→C in intron 2) and five microsatellite markers surrounding the *GGCX* gene (D2S417, D2S2232, D2S388, D2S237 and D2S440). The only mutation identified so far leading to type II is the homozygous Arg98Trp mutation.

Concluding remarks

Molecular defects

In general, in these patients a defect in the DNA can be identified in the genes encoding the different coagulation factors. Combined FV and FVIII deficiency, explained by defects located in genes encoding transport proteins, is a typical exception. In each coagulation defect the mutations are multiple and the majority of them are private mutations, unique for any given patient. The unique nature of the mutations complicates the approach to the control of these diseases through prenatal diagnosis in families with affected members, because it renders necessary the actual identification of the underlying mutation in each kindred. Prevention of rare coagulation disorders through prenatal diagnosis of the underlying mutations is feasible in couples who have already had affected children. Primary prevention might be achieved by discouraging consanguineous marriages. Even though the cultural, religious and economic roots of this practice are deep in Muslim communities, consanguineous marriages are becoming much less frequent in large cities and among younger generations.

The relation between genotype and phenotype is not always clear-cut. Even though in general severe mutations predicting no protein production (stop codons, deletions, insertions, splicing abnormalities) are associated with severe factor deficiencies and severe clinical phenotypes, there are a number of cases with severe deficiencies and phenotypes associated with missense mutations. Usually, missense mutations are associated with milder phenotypes despite unmeasurable factor levels, probably because some protein is produced in these cases that cannot be detected with the currently available assays.

Expression of the mutations in cultured cell lines and characterization of the recombinant proteins has been useful for understanding how well-defined molecular lesions lead to structural abnormalities and to functional defects of the protein. In some cases expression studies have documented the mechanism whereby a mutant protein is synthesized normally but is not ultimately secreted in plasma from cells. In most cases impaired folding and/or conformational changes of the mutant protein leads to both intracellular and extracellular instability, which in turn causes factor deficiency in plasma. Expression work is still in its infancy and needs to be expanded, mainly in cases of missense mutations that appear of special functional interest when projected onto the crystal structure of the coagulation factors.

Treatment

Treatment of rare coagulation disorders is with the most purified blood product available that contains the missing factor. Because of the rarity of each factor deficiency, purified factor concentrates are not as freely available as they are for haemophilia A and B. Dosages and frequency of treatment depend on minimal haemostatic levels of the deficient factor, plasma half-life and type of bleeding episode. General recommendations for treatment on-demand, prophylaxis, pregnancy and delivery,

and for surgery of patients with rare coagulation disorders are summarized in Tables 42.4–42.6.

The avoidance of transmission of blood borne infectious agents is the primary requisite in the choice of replacement material. Solvent/detergent-treated plasma is an important

Table 42.4 Treatment of recessive coagulation disorders.

Deficient factor	Recommended trough levels	Plasma half-life	On demand
Fibrinogen	50–100 mg/dL	2–4 days	Cryoprecipitate (5–10 bags) SD-treated plasma (15–30 mL/kg) Fibrinogen concentrate (50–100 mg/kg)
Prothrombin	20–30%	3–4 days	SD-treated plasma (15–20 mL/kg) FIX concentrate and PCC (20–30 units/kg)
Factor V	10–20%	36 hours	SD-treated plasma (15–20 mL/kg)
Factor V and factor VIII	10–15%	FV 36 hours FVIII 10–14 hours	As for FV
Factor VII	10–15%	4–6 hours	FVII concentrate (30–40 mL/kg) PCC (20–30 units/kg) rFVIIa (15–30 μg/kg every 4–6 hours)
Factor X	10–20%	40–60 hours	SD-treated plasma (10–20 mL/kg) PCC (20–30 units/kg) FX/FIX concentrate (10–20 units/kg)
Factor XI	15–20%	50 hours	SD-treated plasma (15–20 mL/kg) FXI concentrate (15–20 units/kg)
Factor XIII	2–5%	9–12 days	Cryoprecipitate (2–3 bags) SD-treated plasma (3 mL/kg) FXIII concentrate (50 units/kg for high haemorrhagic events)
Vitamin K dependent			Vitamin K (10 mg i.v. or s.c. for minor bleeding)

PCC, prothrombin complex concentrate; rFVIIa, recombinant activated FVII; SD, solvent/detergent.

Table 42.5 General recommendations for long-term prophylaxis.

Deficient factor	Recommended trough levels	Plasma half-life	Reported dose schedule for successful long-term prophylaxis		
			Products	Dose	Frequency
Fibrinogen	50–100 mg/dL	2–4 days	Cryoprecipitate Fibrinogen concentrate	1 unit 3 units 30–100 mg/kg	Three times per week Every 7–10 days Every week
Prothrombin	20–30%	3–4 days	PCC	25–40 units/kg	Once per week
Factor V	10–20%	36 hours	SD-treated plasma	30 mL/kg	Twice per week
Factor V and factor VIII	10–15%	FV 36 hours FVIII 10–14 hours	No data	No data	No data

Table 42.5 *Continued*

Deficient factor	Recommended trough levels	Plasma half-life	Reported dose schedule for successful long-term prophylaxis		
			Products	Dose	Frequency
Factor VII	10–15%	4–6 hours	FFP	10–15 mL/kg	Twice per week
			pdFVII	10–50 units/kg	Three times per week
			rFVIIa	15–30 µg/kg	Two to three times per week
Factor X	10–20%	40–60 hours	PCC	30–40 units/kg	Two to three times per week
			FX/FIX concentrate	20–40 units/kg	One to two times per week in children
Factor XI	15–20%	50 hours	No data	No data	No data
Factor XIII	2–5%	9–12 days	Cryoprecipitate	2 units	Every 3 weeks
			SD-treated plasma	15–20 mL/kg	Every 4–6 weeks
			FXIII concentrate	10 units/kg	Every 4–6 weeks
Vitamin K			Vitamin K	10 mg	Once per week orally
dependent					

PCC, prothrombin complex concentrate; pdFVII, plasma-derived FVII; rFVIIa, recombinant activated FVII; SD, solvent/detergent.

Table 42.6 General recommendations for treatment during pregnancy and delivery and during surgery.

Deficient factor	Pregnancy/delivery		Surgery	
	Minimum level	Treatment	Minimum level	Treatment
Fibrinogen	> 150 mg/dL	Successful pregnancy in afibrinogenaemia is difficult without fibrinogen replacement therapy No strong data to support routine postpartum fibrinogen prophylaxis beyond the first 1–2 days	100 mg/dL	Fibrinogen concentrate (50–100 mg/kg) Antifibrinolytic agents (dental extraction)
Prothrombin	> 25%	No data	20–40%	SD-treated plasma (15–20 mL/kg) PCC (20–30 units/kg, higher doses for major surgery)
Factor V	15–25%	SD-treated plasma (15–20 mL/kg, until after delivery)	25%	SD-treated plasma (15–20 mL/kg)
Factor V and factor VIII		As for FV		As for FV
Factor VII	> 15–20%	Not required during pregancy, unless there is a bleeding history with previous pregnancies If FVII < 20%, peripartum prophylaxis should be considered	10–15%	FVII concentrate (30–40 mL/kg) PCC (20–30 units/kg) rFVIIa (15–30 µg/kg every 4–6 hours)
Factor X	10–20%	In severe FX deficiency and history of adverse outcome, replacement therapy to cover delivery (up to 3 days) is indicated	10–20%	SD-treated plasma (10–20 mL/kg) PCC (20–30 units/kg) FX(FIX) concentrate (10–20 units/kg)

Table 42.6 *Continued*

Deficient factor	Pregnancy/delivery		Surgery	
	Minimum level	Treatment	Minimum level	Treatment
Factor XI	15–20%	FXI levels 15–70 units/dL, with no bleeding history: give tranexamic acid for up to 3 days (first dose during labour) FXI levels < 15 units/dL: replacement therapy should be considered at the onset of labour	15–20%	Antifibrinolytic agents (250 mg/day)
Factor XIII	10%	FXIII concentrate: 250 units per 7 days in early period, 500 units per 7 days after 23 weeks Factor replacement should be given at delivery to maintain FXIII levels > 20%	5–10%	Cryoprecipitate (2–3 bags) SD-treated plasma (3 mL/kg) FXIII concentrate (10–20 units/kg)

PCC, prothrombin complex concentrate; rFVIIa, recombinant activated FVII; SD, solvent/detergent.

source of replacement that is recommended in the majority of these disorders; virus-inactivated concentrates, when commercially available, are also safe but expensive especially for developing countries. Non-virus-inactivated plasma and cryoprecipitate should be avoided if possible. Of course the treatment of choice may change depending on the facilities of the country where the patient is resident. Cost is the next most important determinant. Virally inactivated factor concentrates are available for several deficiencies and should be preferred when virally inactivated plasma is not available or repeated infusions causing fluid overload are needed, as may occur during surgery or in cases of bleeding in the CNS. An updated registry of the available clotting factor concentrates is published by the WFH (available at http://www.wfh.org/index.asp?lang=EN).

Acknowledgements

We would like to thank Professor P.M. Mannucci for his great supervision and all our colleagues who have helped us recently to develop a chapter on rare bleeding disorders in *Seminars of Thrombosis and Hemostasis*. Their revision of specific types of deficiency helped us to more accurately revise our present chapter. Thanks, therefore, to Philippe de Moerloose and Marguerite Neerman-Arbez, Stefano Lancellotti and Raimondo De Cristofaro, Rosanna Asselta and Marta Spreafico, Guglielmo Mariani and Francesco Bernardi, Stefano Duga and Ophira Salomon, Mehran Karimi, Zsuzsanna Bereczky, Nader Cohan and László Muszbek, and Benjamin Brenner, Amir A. Kuperman, Matthias Watzka and Johannes Oldenburg. We would also like to thank Isabella Garagiola and Roberta Palla for their help in writing the manuscript.

Selected bibliography

Acharya SS, Coughlin A, Dimichele DM (2004) Rare Bleeding Disorder Registry: deficiencies of factors II, V, VII, X, XIII, fibrinogen and dysfibrinogenemias. *Journal of Thrombosis and Haemostasis* **2**: 248–56.

Akhavan S, Luciani M, Lavoretano S *et al.* (2003) Phenotypic and genetic analysis of a compound heterozygote for dys- and hypoprothrombinemia. *British Journal of Haematology* **120**: 142–4.

Asakai R, Chung D, Davie E *et al.* (1991) Factor XI deficiency in Ashkenazi Jews in Israel. *New England Journal of Medicine* **325**: 153–8.

Asselta R, Tenchini ML, Duga S (2006) Inherited defects of coagulation factor V: the haemorrhagic side. *Journal of Thrombosis and Haemostasis* **4**: 26–34.

Auerswald G (2006) Prophylaxis in rare coagulation disorders: factor X deficiency. *Thrombosis Research* **118**: 29–31.

Bolton-Maggs P, Wan-Yin B, McGraw A *et al.* (1988) Inheritance and bleeding in factor XI deficiency. *British Journal of Haematology* **69**: 521–8.

Bolton-Maggs PH, Perry DJ, Chalmers EA *et al.* (2004) The rare coagulation disorders: review with guidelines for management from the United Kingdom Haemophilia Centre Doctors' Organization. *Haemophilia* **10**: 593–628.

Boneh A, Bar-Ziv J (1996) Hereditary deficiency of vitamin K-dependent coagulation factors with skeletal abnormalities. *American Journal of Medical Genetics* **65**: 241–3.

Brenner B, Sánchez-Vega B, Wu SM et al. (1998) A missense mutation in gamma-glutamyl carboxylase gene causes combined deficiency of all vitamin K-dependent blood coagulation factors. *Blood* **92**: 4554–9.

Chung KS, Bezeaud A, Goldsmith JC et al. (1979) Congenital deficiency of blood clotting factors II, VII, IX, and X. *Blood* **53**: 776–87.

De Cristofaro R, Carotti A, Akhavan S et al. (2006) The natural mutation by deletion of Lys9 in the thrombin A-chain affects the pKa value of catalytic residues, the overall enzyme's stability and conformational transitions linked to Na⁺ binding. *FEBS Journal* **273**: 159–69.

Degen SJ, Davie EW (1987) Nucleotide sequence of the gene for human prothrombin. *Biochemistry* **26**: 6165–77.

de Moerloose P, Neerman-Arbez M (2008) Treatment of congenital fibrinogen disorders. *Expert Opinion on Biological Therapy* **8**: 979–92.

de Visser MCH, Poort SR, Vos HL et al. (2001) Factor X Levels, polymorphisms in the promoter region of factor X, and the risk of venous thrombosis. *Thrombosis and Haemostasis* **85**: 1011–17.

Dewerchin M, Liang Z, Moons L et al. (2000) Blood coagulation factor X deficiency causes partial embryonic lethality and fatal neonatal bleeding in mice. *Thrombosis and Haemostasis* **83**: 185–90.

Duckers C, Simioni P, Spiezia L et al. (2008) Low plasma levels of tissue factor pathway inhibitor in patients with congenital factor V deficiency. *Blood* **112**: 3615–23.

Emsley J, McEwan PA, Gailani D (2010) Structure and function of factor XI. *Blood* **115**: 2569–77.

Furie B, Bochard BA, Furie BC (1999) Vitamin K-dependent biosynthesis of gamma-carboxyglutamic acid. *Blood* **93**: 1798–808.

Garagiola I, Palla R, Peyvandi F (2003) Pitfalls in molecular diagnosis in a family with severe factor VII (FVII) deficiency: misdiagnosis by direct sequence analysis using a PCR product. *Prenatal Diagnosis* **23**: 731–4.

Ghosh K, Shetty S, Mohanty D (1996) Inherited deficiency of multiple vitamin K-dependent coagulation factors and coagulation inhibitors presenting as haemorrhagic diathesis, mental retardation and growth retardation. *American Journal of Hematology* **52**: 67.

Giampaolo A, Vulcano F, Macioce G et al. (2005) Factor-V expression in platelets from human megakaryocytic culture. *British Journal of Haematology* **128**: 108–11.

Herrmann FH, Auerswald G, Ruiz-Saez A et al. (2006) Factor X deficiency: clinical manifestation of 102 subjects from Europe and Latin America with mutations in the factor X gene. *Haemophilia* **12**: 479–89.

Herrmann FH, Wulff K, Auerswald G et al. (2009) Factor VII deficiency: clinical manifestation of 717 subjects from Europe and Latin America with mutations in the factor 7 gene. *Haemophilia* **15**: 267–80.

Huntington JA (2005) Molecular recognition mechanisms of thrombin. *Journal of Thrombosis and Haemostasis* **3**: 1861–72.

Ichinose A (2001) Physiopathology and regulation of factor XIII. *Thrombosis and Haemostasis* **6**: 57–65.

Isetti G, Maurer MC (2007) Employing mutants to study thrombin residues responsible for factor XIII activation peptide recognition: a kinetic study. *Biochemistry* **46**: 2444–52.

Ivaskevicius V, Seitz R, Kohler HP et al. (2007) International registry on factor XIII deficiency: a basis formed mostly on European data. *Thrombosis and Haemostasis* **97**: 914–21.

Iwaki T, Sandoval-Cooper MJ, Paiva M et al. (2002) Fibrinogen stabilizes placental–maternal attachment during embryonic development in the mouse. *American Journal of Pathology* **160**: 1021–34.

Kadir R, Chi C, Bolton-Maggs P (2009) Pregnancy and rare bleeding disorders. *Haemophilia* **2**: 1–16.

Karimi M, Menegatti M, Afrasiabi A et al. (2008) Phenotype and genotype report on homozygous and heterozygous patients with congenital factor X deficiency. *Haematologica* **93**: 934–8.

Lak M, Sharifian R, Peyvandi F et al. (1998) Symptoms of inherited factor V deficiency in 25 Iranian patients. *British Journal of Haematology* **103**: 1067–9.

Lak M, Keihani M, Elahi F et al. (1999) Bleeding and thrombosis in 55 patients with inherited afibrinogenaemia. *British Journal of Haematology* **107**: 204–6.

Lak M, Peyvandi F, Ali Sharifian A et al. (2003) Pattern of symptoms in 93 Iranian patients with severe factor XIII deficiency. *Journal of Thrombosis and Haemostasis* **1**: 1852–3.

Lauer P, Metzener HJ, Zettlmeissl G et al. (2002) Targeted inactivation of the mouse locus encoding coagulation factor XIII-A: haemostatic abnormalities in mutant mice and characterization of the coagulation deficit. *Thrombosis and Haemostasis* **88**: 967–74.

Lee CA, Chi C, Pavord SR et al. (2006) The obstetric and gynaecological management of women with inherited bleeding disorders: review with guidelines produced by a taskforce of UK Haemophilia Centre Doctors Organization. *Haemophilia* **12**: 301–36.

Lee CJ, Lin P, Chandrasekaran V et al. (2008) Proposed structural models of human factor Va and prothrombinase. *Journal of Thrombosis and Haemostasis* **6**: 83–9.

Lovejoy AE, Reynolds TC, Visich JE et al. (2006) Safety and pharmacokinetics of recombinant factor XIII-A2 administration in patients with congenital factor XIII deficiency. *Blood* **108**: 57–62.

McVey JH, Boswell E, Mumford AD et al. (2001) Factor VII deficiency and the FVII mutation database. *Human Mutation* **7**: 3–17.

Mannucci PM, Levi M (2007) Prevention and treatment of major blood loss. *New England Journal of Medicine* **356**: 2301–11.

Mannucci PM, Duga S, Peyvandi F (2004) Recessively inherited coagulation disorders. *Blood* **104**: 1243–52.

Mariani G, Mazzucconi MG (1983) Factor VII congenital deficiency: clinical picture and classification of the variants. *Haemostasis* **13**: 169–74.

Mariani G, Herrmann FH, Dolce A et al. (2005) Clinical phenotypes and factor VII genotype in congenital factor VII deficiency. *Thrombosis and Haemostasis* **93**: 481–7.

Marty S, Barro C, Chatelain B et al. (2008) The paradoxical association between inherited factor VII deficiency and venous thrombosis. *Haemophilia* **14**: 564–70.

Miloszewski KJA (1999) Factor XIII deficiency. *British Journal of Haematology* **107**: 468–84.

Mitchell M, Mountford R, Butler R *et al.* (2006) Spectrum of factor XI (F11) mutations in the UK population: 116 index cases and 140 mutations. *Human Mutation* **27**: 829.

Monaldini L, Asselta R, Malcovati M *et al.* (2005) The DNA-pooling technique allowed for the identification of three novel mutations responsible for afibrinogenemia. *Journal of Thrombosis and Haemostasis* **3**: 2591–3.

Myers B, Pavord S, Kean L, Hill M, Dolan G (2007) Pregnancy outcome in factor XI deficiency: incidence of miscarriage, antenatal and postnatal haemorrhage in 33 women with factor XI deficiency. *BJOG: an International Journal of Obstetrics and Gynaecology* **114**: 643–6.

Nahrendorf M, Hu K, Frantz S *et al.* (2006) Factor XIII deficiency causes cardiac rupture, impairs wound healing, and aggravates cardiac remodelling in mice with myocardial infarction. *Circulation* **113**: 1196–202.

Nahrendorf M, Aikawa E, Figueiredo JL *et al.* (2008) Transglutaminase activity in acute infarcts predicts healing outcome and left ventricular remodelling: implications for FXIII therapy and antithrombin use in myocardial infarction. *European Heart Journal* **29**: 445–54.

Neerman-Arbez M, Antonarakis SE, Blouin JL *et al.* (1997) The locus for combined factor V–factor VIII deficiency (F5F8D) maps to 18q21, between D18S849 and D18S1103. *American Journal of Human Genetics* **61**: 143–50.

Neerman-Arbez M, Honsberger A, Antonarakis SE *et al.* (1999) Deletion of the fibrinogen alpha-chain gene (FGA) causes congenital afibrinogenemia. *Journal of Clinical Investigation* **103**: 215–18.

Négrier C, Rothschild C, Goudemand J *et al.* (2008) Pharmacokinetics and pharmacodynamics of a new highly-secured fibrinogen concentrate. *Journal of Thrombosis and Haemostasis* **6**: 1494–9.

Ni H, Denis CV, Subbarao S *et al.* (2000) Persistence of platelet thrombus formation in arterioles of mice lacking both von Willebrand factor and fibrinogen. *Journal of Clinical Investigation* **106**: 385–92.

Nichols WC, Valeri HT, Wheatley MA *et al.* (1999) ERGIC-53 gene structure and mutation analysis in 19 combined factors V and VIII deficiency families. *Blood* **93**: 2261–6.

Pechik I, Madrazo J, Mosesson MW *et al.* (2004) Crystal structure of the complex between thrombin and the central 'E' region of fibrin. *Proceedings of the National Academy of Sciences USA* **101**: 2718–23.

Perry DJ (1997) Factor X and its deficiency states. *Haemophilia* **3**: 159–72.

Peyvandi F, Mannucci PM (1999) Rare coagulation disorders. *Thrombosis and Haemostasis* **82**: 1380–1.

Peyvandi F, Mannucci PM, Asti D *et al.* (1997) Clinical manifestations in 28 Italian and Iranian patients with severe factor VII deficiency. *Haemophilia* **3**: 242–6.

Peyvandi F, Tuddenham EGD, Akhtari M *et al.* (1998) Bleeding symptoms in 27 Iranian patients with factor V and VIII combined deficiency. *British Journal of Haematology* **100**: 773–6.

Peyvandi F, Mannucci PM, Lak M *et al.* (1998) Congenital factor X deficiency: spectrum of bleeding symptoms in 32 Iranian patients. *British Journal of Haematology* **102**: 626–8.

Peyvandi F, Lak M, Mannucci PM (2002) Factor XI deficiency in Iranians: its clinical manifestations in comparison with those of classic hemophilia. *Haematologica* **87**: 512–14.

Peyvandi F, Garagiola I, Palla R, Marziliano N, Mannucci PM (2005) Role of the two adenine (g.11293–11294insAA) insertion polymorphism in the 3′ untranslated region of the factor VII (FVII) gene: molecular characterization of a patient with severe FVII deficiency. *Human Mutation* **26**: 455–61.

Pinotti M, Etro D, Bindini D *et al.* (2002) Residual factor VII activity and different haemorrhagic phenotypes in CRM(+) factor VII deficiencies (Gly331Ser and Gly283Ser). *Blood* **99**: 1495–7.

Platè M, Asselta R, Peyvandi F *et al.* (2007) Molecular characterization of the first missense mutation in the fibrinogen Aalpha-chain gene identified in a compound heterozygous afibrinogenemic patient. *Biochimica et Biophysica Acta* **1772**: 781–7.

Platè M, Asselta R, Spena S *et al.* (2008) Congenital hypofibrinogenemia: characterization of two missense mutations affecting fibrinogen assembly and secretion. *Blood Cells, Molecules and Diseases* **41**: 292–7.

Ragni MV, Lewis JH, Spero JA *et al.* (1981) Factor VII deficiency. *American Journal of Hematology* **10**: 79–88.

Rose T, Di Cera E (2002) Three-dimensional modelling of thrombin–fibrinogen interaction. *Journal of Biological Chemistry* **277**: 18875–80.

Rost S, Geisen C, Fregin A *et al.* (2006) Founder mutation Arg485Pro led to recurrent compound heterozygous GGCX genotypes in two German patients with VKCFD type. *Blood Coagulation and Fibrinolysis* **17**: 503–7.

Salomon O, Steinberg DM, Tamarin I *et al.* (2005) Plasma replacement therapy during labour is not mandatory for women with severe factor XI deficiency. *Blood Coagulation and Fibrinolysis* **16**: 37–41.

Salomon O, Steinberg DM, Seligshon U (2006) Variable bleeding manifestations characterize different types of surgery in patients with severe factor XI deficiency enabling parsimonious use of replacement therapy. *Haemophilia* **12**: 490–3.

Santagostino E, Mancuso ME, Morfini M *et al.* (2006) Solvent/detergent plasma for prevention of bleeding in recessively inherited coagulation disorders: dosing, pharmacokinetics and clinical efficacy. *Haematologica* **91**: 634–9.

Scanavini D, Girelli D, Lunghi B *et al.* (2004) Modulation of factor V levels in plasma by polymorphisms in the C2 domain. *Arteriosclerosis, Thrombosis and Vascular Biology* **24**: 200–6.

Soldà G, Asselta R, Ghiotto R *et al.* (2005) Type II mutation (Glu117stop) causes factor XI deficiency by inducing allele-specific mRNA degradation. *Haematologica* **90**: 1716–18.

Spohn G, Kleinridders A, Wunderlich FT *et al.* (2009) VKORC1 deficiency in mice causes early postnatal lethality due to severe bleeding. *Thrombosis and Haemostasis* **101**: 1044–50.

Sun H, Yang TL, Yang A *et al.* (2003) The murine platelet and plasma factor V pools are biosynthetically distinct and sufficient for minimal hemostasis. *Blood* **102**: 2856–61.

Sun MF, Ho D, Martincic D et al. (2007) Defective binding of factor XI-N248 to activated human platelets. *Blood* **110**: 4164.

Suori M, Koseki-Kuno S, Takeda N et al. (2008) Male-specific cardiac pathologies in mice lacking either the A or B subunit of factor XIII. *Thrombosis and Haemostasis* **99**: 401–8.

Thomas A, Stirling D (2003) Four factor deficiency. *Blood Coagulation and Fibrinolysis* **14** (Suppl. 1): S55–S57.

Titapiwatanakun R, Rodriguez V, Middha S, Dukek BA, Pruthi RK (2009) Novel splice site mutations in the gamma glutamyl carboxylase gene in a child with congenital combined deficiency of the vitamin K-dependent coagulation factors (VKCFD). *Pediatric Blood and Cancer* **53**: 92–5.

Tojo N, Miyagi I, Miura M et al. (2008) Recombinant human fibrinogen expressed in the yeast *Pichia pastoris* was assembled and biologically active. *Protein Expression and Purification* **59**: 289–96.

Triplett DA, Brandt JT, Batard MA et al. (1985) Hereditary factor VII deficiency heterogeneity defined by combined functional and immunochemical analysis. *Blood* **66**: 1284–7.

Tuddenham EGD, Cooper DN (1994) *The Molecular Genetics of Hemostasis and its Inherited Disorders*. Oxford University Press, Oxford.

Uprichard J, Perry DJ (2002) Factor X deficiency. *Blood Reviews* **16**: 97–110.

van't Hooft FM, Silveira A, Tornvall P et al. (1999) Two common functional polymorphisms in the promoter region of the coagulation factor VII gene determining plasma factor VII activity and mass concentration. *Blood* **93**: 3432–41.

Vollenweider F, Kappeler F, Itin C et al. (1998) Mistargeting of the lectin ERGIC-53 to the endoplasmic reticulum of HeLa cells impairs the secretion of a lysosomal enzyme. *Journal of Cell Biology* **142**: 377–89.

Vos HL (2006) Inherited defects of coagulation factor V: the thrombotic side. *Journal of Thrombosis and Haemostasis* **4**: 35–40.

Vos HL (2007) An online database of mutations and polymorphisms in and around the coagulation factor V gene. *Journal of Thrombosis and Haemostasis* **5**: 185–8.

Vu D, Neerman-Arbez M (2007) Molecular mechanisms accounting for fibrinogen deficiency: from large deletions to intracellular retention of misfolded proteins. *Journal of Thrombosis and Haemostasis* **5** (Suppl. 1): 125–31.

Weeterings C, de Groot PG, Adelmeijer J et al. (2008) The glycoprotein Ib–IX–V complex contributes to tissue factor-independent thrombin generation by recombinant factor VIIa on the activated platelet surface. *Blood* **112**: 3227–33.

Xue J, Wu Q, Westfield LA et al. (1998) Incomplete embryonic lethality and fatal neonatal haemorrhage caused by prothrombin deficiency in mice. *Proceedings of the National Academy of Sciences USA* **95**: 7603–7.

Zadra G, Asselta R, Tenchini ML et al. (2008) Simultaneous genotyping of coagulation factor XI type II and type III mutations by multiplex real-time polymerase chain reaction to determine their prevalence in healthy and factor XI-deficient Italians. *Haematologica* **93**: 715–21.

Zhang B, Kaufman RJ, Ginsburg D (2005) LMAN1 and MCFD2 form a cargo receptor complex and interact with coagulation factor VIII in the early secretory pathway. *Journal of Biological Chemistry* **280**: 25881–6.

Zhang B, McGee B, Yamaoka JS et al. (2006) Combined deficiency of factor V and factor VIII is due to mutations in either LMAN1 or MCFD2. *Blood* **107**: 1903–7.

Zhang B, Spreafico M, Zheng C et al. (2008) Genotype–phenotype correlation in combined deficiency of factor V and factor VIII. *Blood* **111**: 5592–600.

Zhu A, Raymond R, Zheng X et al. (1998) Abnormalities of development and hemostasis in γ-carboxylase deficient mice [Abstract]. *Blood* **92**: 152a.

Zucker M, Zivelin A, Teitel J et al. (2008) Induction of an inhibitor antibody to factor XI in a patient with severe inherited factor XI deficiency by Rh immune globulin. *Blood* **111**: 1306–8.

CHAPTER 43

Acquired coagulation disorders

43

Peter W Collins[1], Jecko Thachil[2] and Cheng-Hock Toh[2]

[1]Cardiff University School of Medicine, University Hospital of Wales, Cardiff, UK
[2]School of Clinical Sciences, University of Liverpool, Liverpool, UK

Introduction

Acquired disorders of haemostasis are a heterogeneous group of conditions with varied and often complex aetiologies. Patients may have multiple and overlapping causes for haemorrhagic symptoms and distinct conditions often have similar pathophysiologies. In order to manage acquired haemostatic failure it is important to understand the mechanisms by which haemostatic disturbance occurs and how these apply in different ways to a variety of conditions.

Systemic disease may present to haematologists with symptoms of bleeding or bruising or abnormalities of coagulation tests. Alternatively, patients with known disorders may need haematological input to manage symptoms or at the time of

Postgraduate Haematology: 6th edition. Edited by A. Victor Hoffbrand, Daniel Catovsky, Edward G.D. Tuddenham, Anthony R. Green
© 2011 Blackwell Publishing Ltd.

invasive procedures. Assessment of patients with symptoms of bleeding or bruising requires clinical review and laboratory investigation. Serial laboratory testing is often required because the haemostatic disturbance may evolve rapidly. The possibility of a congenital disorder should also be considered.

Haematologists are also often involved in the management of acutely bleeding patients who may have complex medical conditions and in whom bleeding is usually multifactorial. Critical to optimizing the management of these patients is a well-organized multidisciplinary team approach. Hospitals should have systems in place to respond rapidly to massive haemorrhage and hospital transfusion committees should establish protocols for these medical emergencies. Laboratories should be geared to producing accelerated full blood count (FBC) and coagulation results. The rapid supply of blood products and efficient transfer of these to the patient is vital to success. 'Fire drills' to test proficiency of response to emergencies are good practice in areas where massive haemorrhage often occurs, such as on labour wards and in casualty departments.

Tests of coagulation and point-of-care testing

Routine tests of haemostasis

To investigate a patient suspected of an acquired haemostatic defect, a platelet count will be required and examination of the blood film is often useful. Routine coagulation tests include the prothrombin time (PT), activated partial thromboplastin time (APTT), thrombin time (TT) and Clauss fibrinogen level. It is important that derived fibrinogen assays are not used because results are likely to be misleading in the context of acquired haemostatic defects.

If screening tests are abnormal, correction studies help to distinguish factor deficiencies from inhibitors. Comparison of TT with the reptilase time will establish whether abnormal results are due to heparin. Measurement of fibrin breakdown products, such as D-dimers, is required for investigation of possible disseminated intravascular coagulation (DIC). Further measurement of individual coagulation factor and von Willebrand factor (VWF) levels may be required. Assessment of platelet function may be useful in some circumstances through platelet aggregation studies, platelet nucleotides or a bleeding time, although these results may be difficult to interpret in the context of an acquired haemostatic defect. The role of global platelet function analysers remains to be defined but these are available in many hospitals.

Thromboelastography

This is a point-of-care test that assesses the viscoelastic properties of whole blood samples under low-shear conditions (Figure 43.1). Its main advantage is the global assessment of the different components of clot formation including platelets and coagulation factors. It has been used to guide blood product administration in patients undergoing liver transplantation and cardiopulmonary bypass. Other reported uses include the assessment of coagulation in liver disease, neonates, obstetrics and trauma as well as monitoring the effects of bypassing agents in haemophilia patients with inhibitors, although more studies are required to validate its role in these areas. The two main types of instruments are TEG and ROTEM, which measure the viscoelastic properties of an evolving clot in similar but distinct ways and then graphically display the changes to show all stages of the developing and dissolving clot. Different activators are available and heparinase cups can be used to investigate heparinized samples.

Thrombin generation assays

These tests measure the amount of thrombin generated over time following activation of a sample and may reflect an individual's coagulation potential. They are not available in routine practice. Assays are initiated by the addition of a trigger, usually tissue factor (TF), to recalcified plasma in the presence of phospholipids and thrombin is detected via cleavage of a chromogenic or fluorogenic substrate. When low concentrations of TF are used, contact activation must be inhibited by maize trypsin inhibitor. Several variations of these assays have been developed by varying the concentrations of TF, maize trypsin inhibitor, phospholipid and protein C-sensitizing reagents such as soluble thrombomodulin. Thrombin generation tests have been studied in the context of haemophilia, including monitoring of inhibitor bypass agent therapy. Other studies have examined thrombophilia and liver disease and monitoring of anticoagulant therapy and warfarin reversal. The clinical utility of many of these potential applications remains to be demonstrated.

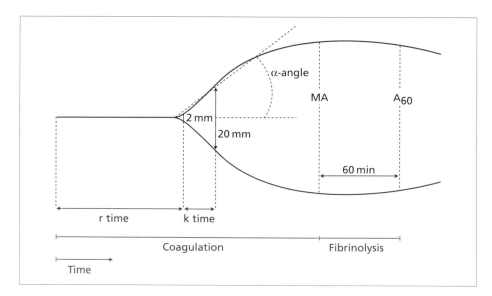

Figure 43.1 Representative thromboelastographic trace.

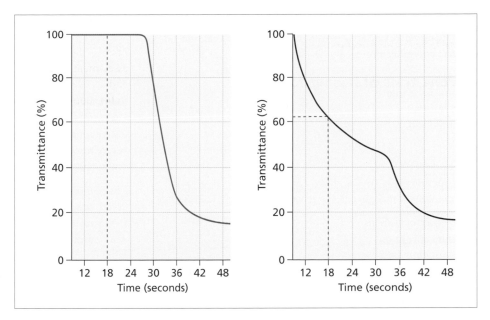

Figure 43.2 Representative normal and biphasic waveforms. Activated partial thromboplastin time waveform patterns: (a) normal; (b) biphasic. Dashed lines denote transmittance level at 18 s (TL18) as the quantitative index: (a) TL18 = 100; (b) TL18 = 63.

APTT biphasic waveform

The Multichannel Discrete Analyser is a coagulation analyser that generates an optical profile charting changes in light transmittance over time during the process of clot formation on the routine APTT. In contrast to the sigmoidal appearance of a normal APTT waveform, a 'biphasic' appearance correlates with acquired haemostatic dysfunction (Figure 43.2). The reliability of this method has been validated in several reports and correlates with the diagnosis of overt DIC according to the International Society for Thrombosis and Haemostasis (ISTH) criteria. This biphasic response is due to calcium-dependent complex formation between C-reactive protein and very low density lipoprotein, which has been shown to increase thrombin generation.

Activated clotting time

This test is predominantly used by anaesthetists to monitor anticoagulation with heparin during cardiopulmonary bypass (CPB) surgery. It uses whole rather than citrated blood and has a linear response at the high concentrations of heparin used during CPB. The APTT cannot be used because plasma is unclottable using this method at these heparin concentrations. Measured using a specialized analyser, the activated clotting time (ACT) reference range varies according to the method and usually falls within 70–180 s. During heparinization for CPB, the goal is to exceed 400–500 s. Off-pump cardiac surgery has been described using less anticoagulation and lower ACT reference ranges of 200–300 s.

Measurement of activated coagulation factors

Many publications have reported the measurement of activated coagulation factors and inhibitors during various clinical situations. Numerous assays and markers of coagulation are available, of which the commonest are thrombin–antithrombin complexes, prothrombin fragment 1+2 and plasmin–antiplasmin complexes. These assays are useful in a research context for understanding the pathogenesis of abnormal haemostasis but have not been shown to be useful in clinical practice.

Disseminated intravascular coagulation

DIC is characterized by the loss of localization or compensated control of intravascular activation of coagulation. Arising from diverse causes (Table 43.1), its pathology can manifest systemically and contribute to a worse prognosis for the patient. Uncoupling of the highly regulated balance between procoagulant, anticoagulant, profibrinolytic and antifibrinolytic processes can result in simultaneous bleeding and microvascular thrombosis at different vascular sites (Figure 43.3). Removal of the inciting cause is the best means of restoring haemostatic control but may not always be possible. Sepsis and malignancy account for more than half the cases of DIC.

Pathophysiology

There are several important themes in the pathophysiology of DIC (Figure 43.3): first is the central role played by the generation of thrombin; second, mechanisms that fuel and perpetuate thrombin generation become pathogenic in its dissemination; third is the parallel and concomitant activation of the inflammatory cascade; and fourth is the importance of the endothelial microvasculature in this process.

The excess bleeding in DIC is partly attributable to the depletion of coagulation factors and platelets. However, several other factors may contribute, including abnormal platelet function

Table 43.1 Clinical conditions associated with disseminated intravascular coagulation.

Sepsis/severe infection
Potentially any microorganism, including Gram-positive and
  Gram-negative bacteria, viruses, fungi and rickettsial infections
Malaria and other protozoal infections

Trauma
Serious tissue injury
Head injury
Fat embolism
Burns

Malignancy
Solid tumours
Haematological malignancies (e.g. acute promyelocytic leukaemia)

Obstetric complications
Placental abruption
Amniotic fluid embolism

Pre-eclampsia
Intrauterine fetal demise

Vascular abnormalities
Giant haemangiomas (Kasabach–Merritt syndrome)
Large vessel aneurysms (e.g. aortic)

Severe toxic or immunological reactions
Snake bites
Recreational drugs
Severe transfusion reactions
Transplant rejection

Miscellaneous
Severe pancreatitis
Heat stroke
ABO mismatch transfusion

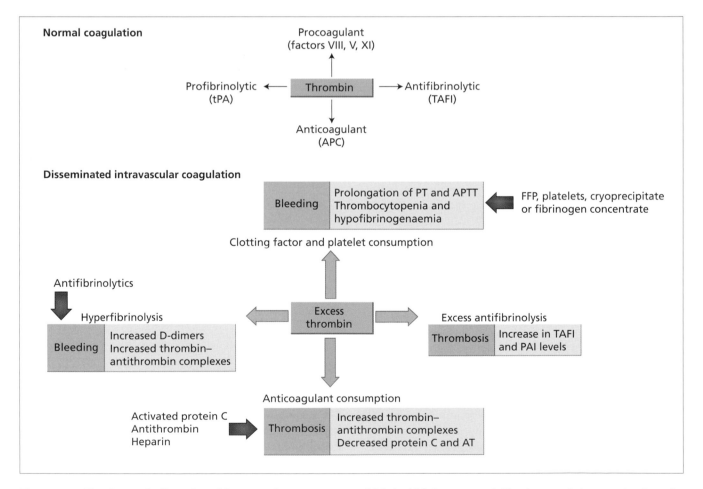

Figure 43.3 The changes in disseminated intravascular coagulation are compared with the normal coagulation. The excess thrombin generation in DIC leads to either bleeding or thrombosis (left) based on the predominant coagulation change (right) which has occurred. The therapeutic intervention in each setting is given by the arrow towards each double box. TAFI, thrombin activatable fibrinolysis inhibitor; PAI, plasminogen activator; AT, antithrombin.

due to renal dysfunction and decreased clotting factor synthesis due to liver impairment. Conversely, microvascular thrombosis can be precipitated by reduced levels of circulating anticoagulant proteins as well as loss of receptors, such as thrombomodulin, in the microvasculature. Endothelial dysfunction can also lead to the depletion of nitric oxide and result in uninhibited platelet activation.

Thrombin generation *in vivo*

The TF pathway plays a major role in initiating thrombin generation and different aetiologies promote this in different ways. In sepsis, the infecting microorganisms induce TF expression on monocytes and other inflammatory cells, while in trauma thromboplastin-like substances can be released from injured tissues like the brain. During obstetric complications, the placenta and amniotic fluid act as rich sources of TF and phospholipid while malignant cells release products with TF-like activity. Although the TF pathway is considered more important in thrombin generation, the contact pathway through factor (F)XII activation contributes to the pathological state by activation of the kallikrein–kinin system, causing vasodilatation and hypotension and activation of fibrinolysis.

Mechanisms for disseminating and sustaining thrombin generation

When the inciting insult is persistent or severe, the amount of thrombin generated becomes continuous and excessive. This can lead to consumption and depletion of both coagulation and anticoagulant factors. Increased exposure of negatively charged phospholipid surfaces facilitates the assembly and enhances the rate of coagulation reactions. Such surfaces, mainly rich in phosphatidylserine, are provided by externalization of the inner leaflet of cell membranes upon activation and apoptosis. Cell damage also leads to the generation of microparticles from platelets, monocytes and endothelial cells that increase the circulating surface area for coagulation reactions to occur. Phospholipid surfaces are also provided by very low density lipoprotein, which can increase several fold in severe sepsis to further enhance and sustain thrombin generation. Together, these mechanisms promote a spatially and temporally expanded response that is the hallmark of DIC.

Links between inflammation and coagulation

Once activated, the inflammatory and coagulation pathways interact to amplify the response. While cytokines and proinflammatory mediators such as tumour necrosis factor (TNF), interleukin (IL)-1 and high mobility group box protein (HMGB)-1 can induce activators of coagulation, thrombin and other serine proteases interact with protease-activated receptors (PARs) on cell surfaces to promote further activation and additional inflammation. When this process becomes generalized, it escapes the well-developed local checks and balances and results in a dysregulated undirected response that fuels a vicious cycle between inflammation and coagulation. Reactive oxygen species generated during sepsis and trauma can lead to further recruitment of neutrophils, cause lipid peroxidation and stimulate nuclear factor (NF)-κB to initiate the transcription of cytokine genes. An important role for the complement system has also been increasingly identified. Thrombin can convert C5 to C5a and the mannan-binding lectin pathway triggers coagulation by converting prothrombin to thrombin. C4b-binding protein of the complement pathway also binds and thus depletes free protein S, the cofactor for activated protein C.

Endothelial cell activation and dysfunction

Dysfunction and failure of the endothelium beyond the host adaptive response can lead to the development of DIC. The degree to which this occurs and the dominance of thrombotic or bleeding sequelae depend on genetic and other host-related factors. Damage to and activation of the endothelium downregulates and depletes its anticoagulant receptors, such as thrombomodulin and endothelial protein C receptor, exposes subendothelial collagen that binds activated platelets, and releases plasminogen activator inhibitor (PAI)-1 that inhibits fibrinolysis and ultra-large VWF multimers to increase platelet aggregation. *In vitro* studies show a downregulation of endothelial TF expression.

Clinical features

The perturbed coagulation associated with DIC can manifest clinically at any point in the spectrum from bleeding to thrombosis. Although bleeding, ranging from oozing at venepuncture sites to major gastrointestinal or intracranial haemorrhage, is the archetypal and most obvious manifestation of DIC, organ failure due to microvascular thrombosis is much more common and often unrecognized. For example, in meningococcal septicaemia and rarely pneumococcal infection, thrombosis of the adrenal vessels can lead to adrenal insufficiency and Waterhouse–Friderichsen syndrome.

Diagnosis

DIC is a clinicopathological syndrome and, as such, there is no single laboratory test that can confirm or refute the diagnosis. In clinical practice, the diagnosis is usually made by a combination of routinely available coagulation tests in a clinical situation where DIC is suspected. DIC must be differentiated from other acquired disorders of haemostasis (Table 43.2). The typical findings are a prolonged PT and APTT, elevated products of fibrin breakdown (e.g. D-dimer), thrombocytopenia and reduced fibrinogen. However, results within the normal range for these tests do not exclude a significant consumptive coagulopathy, especially because the acute-phase response results in shortening of the APTT and increased fibrinogen. A fall in platelet number within the normal range may also be significant.

Condition	Similarities	Differences
Liver disease	Bleeding common PT, APTT abnormal Platelet count low Fibrinogen low	D-dimer usually normal* FVIII levels not affected
Microangiopathic haemolytic anaemia (e.g. HELLP, TTP)	Microthrombi common Platelet count low	Bleeding uncommon Coagulation tests normal†
Hyperfibrinolysis	PT, APTT abnormal Fibrinogen low	Platelet count normal
Catastrophic antiphospholipid antibody syndrome	PT, APTT abnormal Platelet count low	Fibrinogen not low D-dimer normal‡
Massive transfusion	PT, APTT abnormal Fibrinogen low Platelet count low	D-dimer normal

Table 43.2 Differential diagnosis of disseminated intravascular coagulation (DIC).

*Unless additional disorders which increase the D-dimer coexist.
†Unless coexisting DIC.
‡Some antibodies can affect the D-dimer results.
HELLP, haemolysis, elevated liver enzymes, low platelet count (syndrome); TTP, thrombotic thrombocytopenic purpura.

It is also important to recognize that DIC is a dynamic process and thus interpreting a series of laboratory tests over time is more relevant than looking at a single set of results. The ISTH Sub-Committee of the Scientific and Standardization Committee on DIC has recommended the use of a scoring system for overt DIC (Table 43.3). This has been prospectively validated in various studies, indicating a very high sensitivity and specificity. A strong correlation between an increasing DIC score and mortality has been demonstrated. The optical light transmittance profile of the APTT, referred to as the biphasic waveform, has also been shown to correlate well with the overt DIC score. The biphasic waveform occurs independently of prolongation in the clotting times in patients with DIC.

Markers of increased thrombin generation (thrombin–antithrombin complexes) and increased fibrinolysis (plasmin–antiplasmin complexes) as well as endothelial markers have also been investigated as laboratory markers for DIC but single determinations are neither sensitive nor specific for DIC. More importantly, their general availability is limited due to practical considerations.

Treatment

The mainstay of treatment of DIC is to remove the underlying cause. However, DIC often continues even after appropriate treatment for the underlying condition. Supportive therapy with blood products may be necessary. Although the efficacy of blood product replacement has not been proven in randomized

Table 43.3 ISTH Sub-Committee of the Scientific and Standardization Committee on DIC recommended scoring system for overt disseminated intravascular coagulation (DIC).

1 Risk assessment: does the patient have an underlying disorder known to be associated with overt DIC?
 If yes, proceed
 If no, do not use this algorithm

2 Order global coagulation tests (platelet count, PT, fibrinogen, soluble fibrin monomers or FDPs)

3 Score global coagulation test results
 Platelet count ($\times 10^9$/L): > 100, score 0; < 100, score 1; < 50, score 2
 Elevated fibrin-related marker (e.g. soluble fibrin monomers or FDPs): no increase, score 0; moderate increase, score 2; strong increase, score 3
 Prolonged PT (s): < 3, score 0; > 3 but < 6, score 1; > 6, score 2
 Fibrinogen (g/L): > 1, score 0; < 1, score 1

4 Calculate score

5 Score ≥ 5 compatible with overt DIC. Repeat scoring daily

FDPs, fibrin degradation products; PT, prothrombin time.

controlled trials, it is a biologically rational option to replace both thrombin-promoting and thrombin-opposing proteins, particularly when there is significant depletion of these factors in a patient who is either bleeding or at risk of bleeding. In those patients not bleeding, transfusion of platelets or plasma in patients with DIC should not be undertaken based on laboratory results. There are no clinical or experimental data to suggest that platelet or plasma transfusions worsen the thrombotic process.

In patients with DIC and bleeding or at high risk of bleeding (e.g. after invasive procedures) and a platelet count less than 50×10^9/L, transfusion of platelets should be considered, especially because platelet function may be impaired. In bleeding patients with DIC and prolonged clotting times, fresh-frozen plasma (FFP) should be administered. If fluid overload is an issue, prothrombin complex concentrates (PCCs) could be considered but these will only correct vitamin K-dependent components. Activated PCCs should not be used because these can precipitate DIC. Severe hypofibrinogenaemia (< 1 g/L) requires the use of fibrinogen concentrate or cryoprecipitate to correct.

A recent large trial in patients with severe sepsis showed a non-significant benefit of low-dose heparin on mortality and suggested that this is continued in patients with DIC and abnormal coagulation parameters, in the absence of overt bleeding. Notably, these patients are at highest risk of venous thromboembolism due to immobility, recent surgery and a proinflammatory state. However, the role of heparin remains controversial and unproven.

Treatment with recombinant human activated protein C in adults with severe sepsis significantly reduced mortality at 28 days from 30.8% to 24.7% and should be considered in sepsis-related DIC. It is used as a 96-hour infusion and caution is required in patients with a platelet count less than 50×10^9/L due to the increased incidence of intracerebral haemorrhage. Although not licensed, (unactivated) protein C concentrate has been reported as useful in meningococcal septicaemia. No evidence exists to support the use of antithrombin or tissue factor pathway inhibitor concentrates.

The use of pro-haemostatic agents may be necessary in certain instances. There are some reports of the successful use of recombinant (r)FVIIa in patients with DIC and life-threatening bleeding. Antifibrinolytic agents, such as tranexamic acid and ε-aminocaproic acid, are not ideal treatments for DIC except if increased fibrinolysis with bleeding is observed (e.g. some cases of prostate cancer and giant haemangiomas).

Haemostatic dysfunction in acute promyelocytic leukaemia

Acute promyelocytic leukaemia (APL), in particular the microgranular variant (AML-M3v), is associated with major coagulation disturbance including DIC in at least 80% of cases. Although the introduction of all-*trans* retinoic acid (ATRA) and arsenic trioxide as differentiation agents has markedly reduced the rate of early haemorrhagic death and almost 90% of patients are cured, the 10% mortality from bleeding complications has not improved. Bleeding does not correlate with the clotting parameters but with a high white cell count.

The cause remains poorly understood and probably relates to enhanced proteolysis, including fibrinolysis and disruption of endothelial barrier integrity. APL blast cells express TF and can also stimulate the production of inflammatory cytokines, which can further amplify TF levels and promote thrombosis. Cancer procoagulant, a cysteine proteinase detected on APL blast cells, can activate FX independent of FVII. Both these procoagulants are noted to be progressively reduced once patients have been commenced on ATRA. ATRA has also been demonstrated to inhibit vascular endothelial growth factor (VEGF) production, which indirectly limits TF production. Annexin II expression is enhanced on the surface of the blast cells and can act as a cell surface receptor for plasminogen and its activator, tissue plasminogen activator (tPA). Elastase, cathepsin-G and proteinase-3 are present in the granules of the APL blasts and can directly degrade fibrinogen, α_1-antitrypsin, C1 esterase inhibitor and VWF, inducing the loss of high-molecular-weight multimers.

Management of the haemostatic abnormalities revolves around supportive care, including platelet transfusions to maintain a count of at least 30×10^9/L (or 50×10^9/L if the patient is bleeding) and the adequate replacement of fibrinogen to at least 1.5 g/L. The use of antifibrinolytic agents is supported by some evidence but remains controversial. Although markers of coagulation activation and fibrinolysis fall rapidly and completely following the start of ATRA therapy, there appears to be a slower resolution of procoagulant markers (up to 30 days). This may partly explain the clinical observation of thromboembolic events occurring in patients on ATRA, and thus prophylactic use of low molecular-weight heparin or other anticoagulants should be considered once bleeding manifestations have settled.

Vitamin K and related disorders

Vitamin K metabolism

Vitamin K ('K' denoting *Koagulation*) is a group of lipophilic and hydrophobic vitamins that are needed for the post-translational modification of proteins, mostly required for blood coagulation. All forms of vitamin K share a methyl-naphthoquinone ring but differ in the structures of the side-chain. Phylloquinone (vitamin K_1) is derived from plants and has a phytyl side-chain, while menaquinones (vitamin K_2), which differ in the constituent of the side-chain, are synthesized by bacteria in human and animal intestine. Menadione (vitamin K_3), a synthetic water-soluble derivative without a side-chain, has been withdrawn because its use often resulted in haemolytic anaemia and kernicterus, especially in patients with glucose 6-phosphate dehydrogenase deficiency.

Vitamin K is a cofactor for vitamin K-dependent carboxylase, an enzyme that catalyses the carboxylation of glutamic acid (Glu) residues in several proteins (Figure 43.4). A free cysteine residue in the carboxylase converts reduced vitamin K (KH_2) into a strong base that can extract hydrogen from the γ-carbon of glutamic acid. Subsequently, carbon dioxide is added to form γ-carboxyglutamic acid (or Gla). This reaction results in vitamin K 2,3-epoxide, which is recycled to reduced vitamin K by vitamin K epoxide reductase (VKOR), the enzyme inhibited by coumarin anticoagulants.

The Gla domains of the vitamin K-dependent coagulant and anticoagulant proteins (FII, FVII, FIX, FX and proteins C and S) allow calcium-dependent binding to negatively charged phospholipids of activated cell membranes. This enhances the rate of the enzymatic reactions. In the bones, carboxylation of the Gla protein osteocalcin is essential for incorporation of calcium into hydroxyapatite crystals. Retrospective studies suggest that long-term therapy with coumarin-based anticoagulants can affect vertebral bone density and fracture risk.

Vitamin K deficiency

Vitamin K deficiency can occur at any age but is more common in infants because vitamin K does not cross the pla-centa, breast milk has low levels and there is low colonic bacterial synthesis. The clinical presentation of vitamin K deficiency in infants is with bleeding. It was previously called 'haemor-rhagic disease of the newborn' but is now termed vitamin K deficiency bleeding (VKDB). Supplementation of vitamin K is necessary to reduce the risk of bleeding, especially in exclusively breast-fed babies. A single intramuscular injection of vitamin K 1 mg prevents VKDB; however, if oral replacement is used, prolonged administration is required, although the exact dose is still controversial.

In adults, vitamin K deficiency is uncommon due to recycling of the vitamin and an adequate gut flora. However, a poor dietary intake in combination with antibiotic therapy can cause deficiency. Other causes of vitamin K deficiency include malabsorption, cholestatic liver disease (poor enterohepatic circulation) and drugs such as anticonvulsants and warfarin.

Vitamin K-dependent coagulation factors in healthy full-term infants are about half of normal adult values. Adult values are reached by about 6 months except for protein C, which does not reach adult levels until adolescence. Coagulation tests should be compared with age-matched reference ranges to distinguish physiological and pathological deficiencies.

VKDB in young children has been classified into early, classical and late types. The clinical features are shown in Table 43.4. The diagnostic criteria for VKDB includes a PT more than four times control in the presence of at least one of (i) a normal platelet count, normal fibrinogen level and absent fibrinogen degradation products, (ii) normalization of coagulation tests after parenteral vitamin K administration or (iii) the presence of proteins induced by vitamin K absence or antagonism (PIVKA) in plasma. The presence of PIVKA without a coagulation deficit is a marker of subclinical vitamin K deficiency.

The treatment of a non-life-threatening bleed is with vitamin K_1 (phytomenadione) given slowly intravenously. A dose of 1–2 mg is enough to fully correct the deficiency in infants aged up to 6 months, higher doses offering no advantage in efficacy or speed of reversal. There have been reports of anaphylactic reactions with the parenteral form although these are rare. The

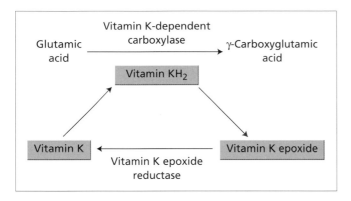

Figure 43.4 Vitamin K metabolism.

Table 43.4 Features of vitamin K-deficiency bleeding (VKDB).

	Early VKDB	Classical VKDB	Late VKDB
Presentation	First 24 hours of life	Days 2–7 of life	Day 8 to 6 months of life
Cause	Infants of mothers on vitamin K-inhibiting drugs	Inadequate feeding	Cholestasis or malabsorption syndromes
Clinical presentation	Severe, with intracranial and intrathoracic bleeds	Milder, with gastrointestinal or umbilical bleeds being common	Severe, with high incidence of intracranial bleeds with 'warning bleeds' in up to one-third
Incidence of intracranial haemorrhage	High	Rare	Very high

PT should improve within 48 hours and if this has not occurred after three doses, continuation of vitamin K in most cases is unlikely to help. Oral replacement may be used if there is no active bleeding and absorption is normal. Patients with severe bleeding should be treated with FFP or PCC.

Poisoning with warfarin follows the accidental ingestion of large doses of warfarin or compounds with similar properties. Diagnosis is suggested by poor correction of PT or International Normalized Ratio (INR) with normal doses of vitamin K. Serum assays of warfarin concentration can be undertaken for confirmation.

Haemostatic disturbance in liver disease (Figure 43.5)

Almost all procoagulant factors, natural anticoagulants and inhibitors of coagulation are synthesized in the liver. The liver is also involved in the clearance of activated clotting factors from the circulation. The effect of liver disease on haemostasis is therefore complex and a balance between procoagulant and antithrombotic changes (Figure 43.5; Table 43.5). Routine coagulation tests such as PT and APTT are commonly pro-

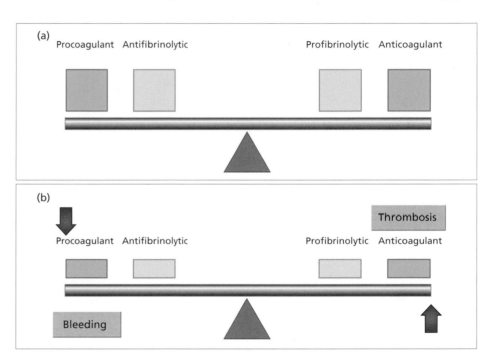

Figure 43.5 Haemostatic disturbance in liver disease. The haemostatic system in liver disease (bottom) compared with normal haemostasis (top). In normal healthy adults, the procoagulant and anticoagulant systems and the profibrinolytic and antifibrinolytic systems form a balance that is not easily disturbed. In patients with liver impairment, all four components are variably reduced and additional stimuli like infections or renal failure can upset the balance very easily, leading to either bleeding or thrombosis.

Table 43.5 Causes of increased bleeding tendency or coagulation abnormalities in liver disease.

Decreased coagulation factors	Hypofibrinogenaemia
Decreased synthesis	Impaired synthesis
Vitamin K deficiency	Loss into extravascular spaces (ascites)
Increased clearance	Increased catabolism
Abnormal coagulation factors due to hypocarboxylation	Loss due to massive haemorrhage
Decreased platelets	Dysfibrinogenaemia: abnormal sialic acid content
Sequestration in spleen or liver	Abnormal fibrinolysis
Thrombopoietin deficiency	Increased release and decreased clearance of tissue
Destruction due to toxins or antiplatelet antibodies or toxins	plasminogen activator
Toxic effect of alcohol on marrow	Decreased synthesis of α_2-antiplasmin, plasminogen and
Dysfunctional platelets	thrombin-activated fibrinolysis inhibitor
Altered platelet arachidonic acid metabolism	Infections
Defective signal transduction	Endogenous heparinoids: anti-FXa activity
Storage pool deficiency	Renal failure
Abnormalities of the platelet glycoprotein	Sinusoidal endothelial cell dysfunction
Increased platelet inhibitors nitric oxide and prostacyclin	Hypothermia

longed in liver disease but are only sensitive to decreases in procoagulant factors and hence are liable to overestimation of the haemostatic defect. Patients with liver disease have similar thrombin generation to healthy control individuals, when tests are performed in the presence of thrombomodulin to make them sensitive to protein C deficiency.

Acute hepatitis

Patients with acute hepatitis are often thrombocytopenic (platelets $100–150 \times 10^9$/L). The mechanism for this may be immune, due to concurrent hypersplenism or DIC. Platelet function may be impaired in acute hepatitis, although this is unlikely to be of clinical significance. In acute liver disease, hepatic biosynthesis of clotting factors is impaired and this may be reflected in a prolongation of coagulation tests. The PT and FV, FVII, antithrombin and protein C levels are the most sensitive to hepatic biosynthetic dysfunction. The PT and FVII level predict survival in acute liver disease. The plasma fibrinogen may be raised in acute hepatic disturbance as part of an acute-phase response. A low fibrinogen level is associated with a poor prognosis in this context. A pattern of reduced fibrinogen and increased fibrin degradation products seen in acute liver disease may be due to hyperfibrinolysis.

Chronic liver disease

Low platelet count and abnormal platelet function are also common in liver disease and have been thought to lead to bleeding. Mild to moderate thrombocytopenia is noted in up to 30% of patients with chronic liver disease and in up to 90% of patients with terminal liver disease. In patients with cirrhosis, this is frequently related to hypersplenism, secondary to portal hypertension. In addition, dietary problems, such as folate deficiency and the direct toxic effect of ethanol on megakaryocyte function, may contribute to thrombocytopenia. A more profound thrombocytopenia in patients with hepatitis C virus (HCV) infection may be autoimmune, although the response to steroids is poor; however, approximately half of adult such patients treated with interferon alfa responded with a rise in platelet count. Recently, a Phase II study using eltrombopag, an oral thrombopoietin receptor agonist, increased platelet counts in the majority of patients with cirrhosis associated with HCV infection to more than 100×10^9/L in a dose-dependent manner. Several platelet function abnormalities have also been demonstrated in liver disease. Despite this, recent evidence shows that VWF which binds to platelet glycoprotein is found to be increased tenfold and has been shown to support platelet adhesion despite reduced functional capacity. In addition, desmopressin did not show any efficacy in reducing blood loss in patients undergoing partial liver resection or liver transplantation.

Coagulation factor and natural anticoagulant synthesis is affected by chronic liver disease. FIX synthesis is usually reduced

less than that of FII, FVII, FX and protein C. The levels of these factors, especially FVII, have been demonstrated to fall proportionately with increasing severity of disease, with levels of FVII shown to be an independent predictor of survival (level below 34% associated with 93% mortality). Chronic liver impairment also leads to vitamin K deficiency, mainly by decreased absorption from the gut as a result of reduced bile salt secretion in cholestasis (parenteral vitamin K responsive) and decreased synthesis in parenchymal disease (parenteral vitamin K non-responsive). The PT, a test for the vitamin K-dependent factors, has been incorporated into prognostic indices of chronic liver disease, such as the Child–Pugh and Mayo End-Stage Liver Disease scores. Despite the prolongation of clotting tests such as PT and APTT, bleeding after liver biopsy or other potentially haemorrhagic procedure in patients with cirrhosis is rare, suggesting that these tests are not on their own indicative of the haemorrhagic tendency. Both these laboratory tests were developed to investigate coagulation factor deficiencies in patients with a bleeding history and as such they only measure the procoagulant factors. Overall, haemostasis is a complex interrelationship between endothelium, platelets, procoagulant proteins and inhibitors. The levels of such inhibitors (or anticoagulant proteins), antithrombin and proteins C and S are reduced in a similar manner to other clotting factors, thus potentially providing a net balance in haemostasis. Evidence for normal thrombin production in cirrhosis despite abnormal conventional coagulation tests has been recently demonstrated by thrombin generation tests, which include the other haemostatic parameters including platelets.

It is common practice to use the INR instead of the PT to access patients with liver disease. However, the INR is standardized for patients taking vitamin K antagonists and its use in patients who have liver disease requires determination of an international sensitivity index (ISI) relevant to liver disease. Recently, attempts have been made to use modifications of the INR called the INR$_{liver}$, which is free of the warfarin-based reference range.

Most patients with stable chronic liver disease have normal or increased fibrinogen, although in advanced disease fibrinogen falls. This may be due to impaired synthesis, loss into extravascular spaces (ascites), increased catabolism or massive haemorrhage. Some patients develop dysfibrinogenaemia due to increased activity of sialyltransferase expressed by immature hepatocytes generated during hepatic injury, which leads to low-molecular-weight fibrinogen with abnormal α-chains and higher sialic acid content. Dysfibrinogenaemia is reflected by a prolonged TT and/or reptilase time, with the fibrinogen antigen level reduced less than the Clauss fibrinogen. Cirrhosis can also be associated with accelerated fibrinolysis due to decreased clearance of tPA, and decreased synthesis of α_2-antiplasmin, plasminogen and thrombin-activatable fibrinolysis inhibitor (TAFI). However, the level of TAFI deficiency in cirrhosis is not associated with increased plasma fibrinolysis when a global test of fibrinolysis is employed. Also, the levels of plasminogen (a fibrinolytic) are reduced and those of PAI-1 (an antifibrinolytic) are high in liver disease, ultimately providing a balance for the fibrinolytic system. However, hyperfibrinolysis has been found to be a predictor of the first episode of upper gastrointestinal bleeding in cirrhotic patients with portal hypertension. This is due to delayed clotting activation because of the consumption of clotting factors and inhibition of fibrin polymerization and also secondary to reduced platelet adhesion and induction of platelet disaggregation.

Recent experiments have thrown light on non-haematological factors contributing to the bleeding diathesis in liver disease. These include bacterial infections, endogenous heparinoids, sinusoidal endothelial dysfunction and renal failure. Bacterial infections are a frequent coexisting problem in cirrhotic patients and are related to the degree of liver dysfunction. Infection is also an independent risk factor for variceal bleeding, with spontaneous bacterial peritonitis commonly preceding variceal bleeding and prophylactic antibiotic therapy shown to prevent early rebleeding. The endotoxins and inflammation due to infection can also release endogenous heparinoids from the endothelium and mast cells. These substances can have anti-FX activity that could in theory lead to bleeding. The dysfunction in sinusoidal endothelial cells makes them unable to respond to abrupt repeated increases in portal pressure (e.g. postprandial situations), which can lead to progressive dilatation of varices in cirrhosis. Life-threatening haemorrhage in patients with liver disease is often related more to portal hypertension (the localized coagulation problem is termed 'accelerated intravascular coagulation and fibrinolysis') than to net dysfunction of the clotting cascade, wherein the varices play a major part. Renal failure is also common in advanced liver disease (hepatorenal syndrome), which can impart a bleeding risk due to various reasons discussed separately. Hypothermia used as a therapeutic measure to prevent hepatic encephalopathy can reduce the enzymatic activity of plasma coagulation proteins and also has an effect on preventing the activation of platelets. Reduced hepatic clearance of activated clotting factors and lower synthesis of natural anticoagulants may predispose individuals with hepatic disease to DIC. This may occur following Gram-negative infection or in association with the insertion of a peritoneovenous shunt. Ascitic fluid should be discarded at the time of shunt insertion to prevent this complication.

The management of a bleeding patient with hepatic dysfunction depends on the site of bleeding and the haemostatic dysfunction. Clotting function should be assessed by means of the PT, APTT, TT, and fibrinogen and D-dimer levels, although the results should be interpreted in the clinical context before transfusions are undertaken. Vitamin K should be administered intravenously (10 mg daily for 3 days) to aid biosynthesis of vitamin K-dependent factors. The widespread practice of managing the coagulopathy of liver disease with transfusions of FFP, cryoprecipitate or platelets should only be considered in the presence of active bleeding. Large volumes of FFP may be required and this may present a management problem in patients with hepatic disease who are at risk of fluid overload. Platelet transfusion may be necessary, although platelet recovery may be reduced because of hypersplenism or immune-mediated destruction. There are no evidence-based guidelines to establish safe coagulation levels for liver biopsy and similar procedures and as such it is important to allow these only when the benefits outweighs the risks (transjugular route safer than percutaneous for liver biopsy). However, correction of the coagulopathy is particularly important before the placement of an intracranial pressure transducer in patients with hepatic encephalopathy. Spontaneous intracranial bleeding has been reported in such patients, though rarely, and this remains one of the principal concerns regarding abnormal coagulation in liver disease. In patients with evidence of increased fibrinolysis, antifibrinolytic drugs such as tranexamic acid should be considered.

Liver transplantation

The changes in the balance of haemostasis seen during liver transplantation are complex and multifactorial and can be due to surgical and non-surgical causes. Traditionally, the process of liver transplantation is split into three stages: stage I, the pre-anhepatic stage, which ends with the occlusion of the recipient's hepatic blood flow; stage II, the anhepatic phase, which ends with the reperfusion of the donor liver; and stage III, the reperfusion and neohepatic period. The risk of bleeding in the pre-anhepatic stage is related directly to the preoperative haemorrhagic risk related to the underlying liver disease. A reduction in procoagulant factors may also be seen, especially if large blood losses necessitate transfusion, leading to the dilution of clotting factors. During the second anhepatic stage, many studies have reported enhanced fibrinolytic activity. The lack of tPA clearance and the reduction in α_2-antiplasmin may be responsible for this enhanced primary fibrinolysis. The mechanism of the increase in tPA levels is most likely due to lack of hepatic clearance. Reperfusion of the liver during the post-anhepatic phase is the crucial point of the intervention where once again fibrinolysis seems to play a pivotal role. There is a dramatic increase after reperfusion in almost three-quarters of patients who undergo liver transplantation. Usually, hyperfibrinolysis subsides within an hour, but in damaged donor liver sustained increased fibrinolytic activity may be observed. The endothelium of the donor liver is an important source of tPA; the ischaemic damage to the graft during preservation may explain the dramatic increase in plasminogen activators. Trapping of platelets in the graft may also play a role in the bleeding tendency. After reperfusion, the release of heparin-like compounds has also been shown. In the postoperative period, a reduction in platelet count is related to platelet activation and blood loss in addition to low thrombopoietin levels. The levels of this hormone increase significantly on the first day after liver synthetic function is restored, with the platelet count normalizing in 2 weeks.

There is little evidence that one can predict the transfusion needs of a patient by examining the preoperative coagulation results. The profound coagulation abnormalities seen in fulminant hepatic failure should be corrected preoperatively. However, the correction of a mild coagulopathy in a patient with chronic liver disease prior to the operation is less likely to be of benefit. During surgery, the aim is to transfuse blood components to prevent the development of intractable coagulopathy. Whole-blood near-patient tests of haemostasis are often used in theatre to complement the tests performed in the coagulation laboratory. Many departments use algorithms based on coagulation and near-patient testing to guide FFP, red cell, cryoprecipitate and platelet transfusion during the procedure. Aprotinin can be administered to counteract the increase in fibrinolysis observed.

Hypercoagulability in liver disease

Tipping of the balance in the complex interplay between endogenous procoagulants and the anticoagulant system in liver disease can also lead to a hypercoagulable state that negates the generally believed notion of an 'autoanticoagulated state'. The hypercoagulable events may be clinically evident disease, as with portal vein thrombosis and venous thromboembolism, but in the microvasculature can be a major pathophysiological contributor to portopulmonary hypertension, liver fibrosis (termed 'parenchymal extinction' in this setting), thrombosis of extracorporeal circuits and progression of non-alcoholic steatohepatitis to cirrhosis. Hypercoagulation in liver disease may be related to poor flow, endothelial dysfunction and vasculopathy associated with a chronic inflammatory state, increased levels of FVIII and VWF, or decreased synthesis of the naturally occurring anticoagulant proteins. Hepatic fibrogenesis may be caused by tissue ischaemia and direct thrombin-mediated stellate cell activation by PAR-1 cleavage. FV Leiden mutation, protein C deficiency and increased expression of FVIII were associated with rapid progression to cirrhosis in chronic HCV. The association between hypercoagulation and increased fibrosis has led to experiments which have shown that interference with either the generation of thrombin or its downstream activity may reduce hepatic fibrosis.

Haemostatic disturbance in renal disease

Bleeding was a frequent cause of morbidity and mortality in patients with renal failure before the advent of dialysis. Common manifestations are gastrointestinal bleeding from angiodysplasia and peptic ulcers as well as prolonged bleeding from skin puncture sites. Subdural haematomas and haemorrhagic peri-

carditis are also seen but bleeding at the time of renal biopsy is rare. Bleeding is seen despite normal or elevated circulating levels of coagulation factors, suggesting that platelet abnormalities are the likely cause. This is supported by the finding of a prolonged bleeding time and reduced platelet aggregation to various agonists. Severe thrombocytopenia (platelets $< 50 \times 10^9$/L) secondary to renal failure is rare and its presence should suggest concomitant conditions such as HCV infection or vasculitis.

Platelet dysfunction with renal failure is multifactorial and can be divided into (i) intrinsic platelet defects, (ii) abnormal interaction of platelets with the endothelium, (iii) effects of uraemic toxins, (iv) effects of anaemia on platelets and (v) dialysis-related. Intrinsic platelet abnormalities reported in association with uraemia are shown in Table 43.6. The interaction between uraemic platelets and the endothelium can be markedly reduced, due partly to impaired VWF binding to platelets. As a result of excess urea, L-arginine is shunted to form guanidinosuccinic acid, which can upregulate endothelial production of nitric oxide, an inhibitor of platelet aggregation. Uraemic patients with prolonged bleeding times also have raised prostaglandin (PG)I_2 levels.

Anaemia-related haemostatic dysfunction is primarily a result of reduced displacement of platelets to the vessel wall by red cells. Decreased red cell number also results in reduced ADP release and decreased platelet interaction with collagen. Dialysis can improve bleeding symptoms and a likely explanation is the chronic low-level platelet activation associated with the procedure. Antifibrinolytic agents can help because fibrinogen fragments of fibrinolysis can interfere with platelet receptors. Antiplatelet drugs, antibiotics (especially those which can accumulate in renal failure) and heparin may contribute to the bleeding risk.

The bleeding time better correlates with clinical bleeding than tests of renal function, although measurement is rarely clinically useful. Adequate dialysis will improve symptoms and the bleeding time in most patients. Intravenous or intranasal

Table 43.6 Platelet abnormalities reported in uraemia.

Decreased GPIb complexes
Reduced serotonin and ADP in the granules
Increased levels of cyclic AMP
Defective ristocetin-induced platelet aggregation
Abnormal mobilization of free cytoplasmic calcium in response to agonists
Reduced release of arachidonic acid from membrane phospholipids
Decreased conversion of arachidonic acid to thromboxane A_2
Abnormal dense-granule and α-granule secretion
Abnormal cytoskeletal assembly
Deficient tyrosine phosphorylation

administration of desmopressin in conjunction with antifibrinolytics has also been used successfully to control uraemic bleeding. Although the response is brief (4–8 hours), the rapid onset of action is beneficial. Care is required to avoid hyponatraemia and fluid retention. Desmopressin is also thought to improve platelet function by the enhanced release of endothelial VWF multimers and also by increasing the levels of platelet glycoprotein (GP)Ib/IX.

Estrogen preparations have been used for a more prolonged effect, although the mechanism of action is not well understood. Correction of anaemia with recombinant human erythropoietin so that the haematocrit exceeds 30% improves platelet interaction with the vessel wall and has also been shown to increase the number of reticulated platelets. Other potentially beneficial effects of recombinant human erythropoietin include improved platelet intracellular calcium mobilization, increased expression of GPIb and improved platelet signal transduction. Cryoprecipitate transfusion for uraemic bleeding is going out of favour, although it may be tried if the patient is haemodynamically unstable.

Pregnancy-related haemostatic dysfunction

Normal pregnancy is associated with physiological changes in haemostasis, with increased levels of procoagulant proteins such as fibrinogen, VWF and FVIII and a fall in anticoagulants such as protein S. These changes partly contribute to the increased risk of venous thromboembolism during pregnancy.

Obstetric haemorrhage is the third most common cause of maternal death in the UK after venous thromboembolism and pre-eclampsia. The cause of bleeding is often multifactorial, with a combination of physical and acquired haemostatic defects. Consumption leads to depletion of platelets and coagulation factors, particularly fibrinogen. A particularly aggressive consumptive coagulopathy is seen with amniotic fluid embolus triggered by TF and phosphatidylserine, and is often fatal. Consumptive coagulopathy may also be triggered by placental abruption, intrauterine fetal death, pre-eclampsia and acute fatty liver of pregnancy. Once bleeding and resuscitation has started, a dilutional coagulopathy may exacerbate the haemostatic failure and contribute to the ongoing bleeding.

Treatment requires rapid recognition of bleeding and a coordinated response from obstetricians, midwives, anaesthetists and haematologists. Physical methods to control bleeding include the use of oxytocins to contract the uterus, B Lynch sutures, intrauterine balloon tamponade and uterine artery embolization. Assessment of haemostatic failure requires an urgent FBC and a coagulation screen that includes a Clauss fibrinogen because the PT and APTT may be normal despite a low fibrinogen. Blood product replacement is often required before the results of the blood test are available and empirical

replacement therapy may be necessary. In patients with severe haemostatic failure, a standard dose of FFP (15 mL/kg) is unlikely to be adequate to correct the haemostatic defect and the use of larger volumes should be anticipated. Fibrinogen should be maintained above at least 1.5 g/L and platelets above 50×10^9/L. Some centres now routinely use fibrinogen concentrate in obstetric haemorrhage to rapidly correct this clotting factor, although this product is not licensed in the UK. rFVIIa may be used if haemostasis cannot be secured by standard methods but will not be useful in the presence of low fibrinogen or thrombocytopenia.

As soon as bleeding has been controlled the patient is likely to be at high risk of venous thromboembolism; this should be assessed and appropriate prophylaxis started.

Haemostatic dysfunction associated with cardiopulmonary bypass surgery

Coronary artery bypass graft (CABG) surgery is associated with excessive bleeding in about 5% of cases. Reoperation for bleeding is required in 3–10% of cases, with a mortality of about 30%. Bleeding is more common with revision procedures. A surgically correctable source of bleeding is found in over half of cases. Bleeding due to haemostatic disturbances can be patient related or CPB related. Antiplatelet, anticoagulant or fibrinolytic drugs, particularly at the time of emergency CABG after stenting procedures, commonly contribute to perioperative bleeding. Despite its antiplatelet activity, aspirin has not been demonstrated to cause increased blood loss after CABG, and has been shown to reduce the risk of death by one-third.

Haemostatic abnormalities associated with CPB are related to the interaction of blood with the extensive non-endothelial bypass surfaces and retransfusion of pericardial blood. CPB decreases both the number and function of platelets. Platelet counts fall by 25–60% within 15 min of first passage of blood through the primed CPB circuit, in association with a prolonged bleeding time. This is due to the exposure of platelets to the high concentration of unfractionated heparin, the haemodilution caused by by the oxygenator primer and the non-biological extracorporeal surface. The platelet count rarely falls below 100×10^9/L and persistent or profound thrombocytopenia should prompt consideration of alternative causes including heparin-induced thrombocytopenia.

The observed changes in platelet function in patients undergoing CPB are due to modification of membrane components with loss of receptors, decrease in granule contents, aggregation to fibrinogen adsorbed onto the bypass circuit, mechanical trauma, exposure to hypothermia and heparin. CPB also results in increased numbers of platelet fragments and microparticles, denoting platelet activation. Following CPB, platelet function returns to normal within 1 hour, although the platelet count may take several days to normalize. Coagulation factors fall because of haemodilution, which can be exacerbated by use of cell-salvage systems. Fibrinolysis is also enhanced by returned blood from the pericardiotomy suction.

Blood component administration in patients with excessive bleeding related to CABG is generally empirical, with replacement of FPP and platelets. Near-patient whole-blood testing has been used to assess haemostasis and fibrinolysis in the context of cardiac surgery and has been shown to help rationalize blood product usage. The time delay in obtaining routine laboratory tests often limits their use in the acute management of bleeding patients. The off-licence use of PCCs and fibrinogen concentrates has also been reported. Case reports suggest that off-licence use of rFVIIa may be considered in patients who have failed standard treatment but randomized studies have not supported a role for its use as prophylactic treatment.

Aprotinin has been used to reduce bleeding during CPB by inhibition of fibrinolysis. Double-blind studies have consistently shown its effectiveness in reducing blood loss in comparison with tranexamic acid, α-aminocaproic acid and desmopressin. However, recent reports have shown a doubling of the risk of renal failure requiring dialysis in patients undergoing complex coronary artery surgery and a 55% increase in cardiovascular and cerebrovascular events. The current use of aprotinin is contentious and under intense debate.

Haemostatic dysfunction associated with trauma

Coagulopathy associated with trauma is multifactorial and the important initiators include tissue injury, loss of procoagulant factors and platelets, physiological and therapeutic haemodilution, inflammation, hypothermia and acidosis. The localization of coagulation to the sites of injury (in contrast to DIC of sepsis) has made some experts use the term 'acute coagulopathy of trauma-shock'. Tissue damage in trauma initiates coagulation via TF, with head injury causing release of brain-specific thromboplastins into the circulation. Increased fibrinolysis due to the direct release of tPA from the endothelium is also seen, together with abnormal fibrin polymerization that increases susceptibility to cleavage by plasmin.

Massive blood loss leads to deficiencies of haemostatic factors and up to half of the fibrinogen and one-third of platelets may be lost before treatment of the injury has begun. Tissue under-perfusion contributes to the coagulopathy by enhancing anticoagulation through activated protein C and fibrinolysis through reduced TAFI. Physiological filling of the vascular space with fluid from cellular and interstitial spaces, along with the administration of intravenous fluids and plasma-poor red cells, causes haemodilution to worsen the coagulopathy. Plasma expanders are also associated with anticoagulant effects such as reduced VWF levels and their use should be limited.

The presence of an abnormal coagulation test on arrival in the emergency department correlates with the severity of injury and the mortality rate. A raised PT is the most frequent abnormality (12.4% of patients) while a low platelet count is least frequent (5.6%). An abnormal PT and APTT increased the risk of mortality by 6.3-fold and 10.7-fold, respectively.

A guide to blood product support, with transfusion triggers, that may be used in conjunction with repeated laboratory tests is given in Table 43.7. Delay in obtaining coagulation and platelet count results dictates that empirical blood product replacement is often required. Recent observations, predominantly based on experience of battlefield trauma, have prompted recommendations for aggressive and early plasma and platelet replacement. This has been termed 'damage limitation resuscitation' (ratio of 1:1:1 for red cells, plasma and platelets). This strategy has been reported in non-randomized studies to improve outcome but definitive evidence is lacking for this approach. Issues such as hypothermia and acidosis need to be addressed by using prewarmed fluids and extracorporeal warming devices and appropriate resuscitation.

Table 43.7 Guide to blood product replacement in massive blood loss.

1 Control bleeding using surgical and/or radiological interventions
2 Restore an appropriate circulating blood volume
3 Control exacerbating factors: hypothermia and acidosis
4 Blood product support as detailed below

Red cells
Use O-negative red cells first
If no record of red cell antibodies, ABO- and Rh-compatible cross-matched blood should be available within 30 min (maximum 45 min)
Replace red cells as required to maintain circulating blood volume
Use blood warmer to avoid hypothermia

Fresh-frozen plasma
Transfuse FFP early to prevent coagulopathy to maintain PT and APTT < 1.5 times normal
If PT and APTT > 1.5 times normal FFP at doses > 15 mL/kg will be required

Platelet transfusion
One to two adult doses after 1.5–2 blood volume replacement (equivalent to 8–10 bags of red cells)
Aim for platelet count > 50×10^9/L

Fibrinogen
Cryoprecipitate (dose: two donation pools)
Fibrinogen concentrates (30–50 mg/kg)
Aim for fibrinogen level > 1.5 g/L

A randomized controlled trial of rFVIIa versus placebo in 301 patients with blunt and penetrating injuries showed a reduction in 2.6 RBC units transfused for the blunt trauma subgroup and a similar though non-significant trend in the penetrating injury subgroup. The incidence of adult respiratory distress syndrome was decreased in patients with blunt injury who received rFVIIa, although there were no differences in survival or in the incidence of thromboembolic events and multiorgan failure. In view of these data, use of rFVIIa in the management of trauma has to be considered on an individual basis.

Coagulopathy in massive blood loss

Massive blood loss is usually defined as 1 blood volume (about 5 L in an adult) in 24 hours or 50% blood volume in 3 hours or more than 150 mL/hour. The associated coagulopathy is complex and multifactorial. It is partly dilutional as blood is replaced with volume expanders and red cells but DIC, hypoxia, hypothermia and acidosis contribute in some clinical situations. Haemostatic management should be to maintain a platelet count of at least 75×10^9/L, a threshold that is likely to be reached after a 2-blood-volume transfusion. A higher platelet count of about 100×10^9/L will be needed in major trauma or central nervous system bleeding. Fibrinogen should be maintained above at least 1.5 g/L, a level that is likely to be reached after about a 1.5-blood-volume transfusion, assuming no significant additional consumptive coagulopathy.

Haemostatic therapy is to infuse platelets and FFP in volumes likely to maintain a safety margin above these critical levels. Hypofibrinogenaemia unresponsive to FFP may require cryoprecipitate or fibrinogen concentrate. It is important to predict ongoing dilution and consumption of coagulation factors and to replace these expectantly if bleeding continues. Regular measurement of FBC and coagulation screens (including Clauss fibrinogen) are important for monitoring replacement treatment, although often these are not available rapidly enough to guide initial management and empirical treatment may be required in the early phases (see Table 43.7).

Bruising

Purpura simplex (normal/easy bruising)

Distinguishing normal from pathological bruises may be difficult and individuals have variable thresholds for presenting for medical review. If bruising is not associated with other symptoms suggestive of a bleeding disorder and routine tests of coagulation (including VWF levels and platelet number) are normal, the patient can be reassured. Drugs such as non-steroidal anti-inflammatory agents or selective serotonin reuptake inhibitors are sometimes implicated.

Non-accidental bruising

Bruising is a common feature of non-accidental injury in both children and adults. Bruises that affect unusual sites, are in different stages of maturation or shaped like a hand or instrument should raise concern. In the case of children, appropriate liaison with child protection agencies should be undertaken, although the possibility of an underlying congenital or acquired bleeding disorder should also be thoroughly investigated. Self-harm may also present with bruising and should be suspected if the pattern of bruising is atypical. Deliberate ingestion of anticoagulants and long-acting vitamin K antagonists is also possible.

Senile purpura (atrophic or actinic purpura) and steroid-related purpura

Bruising is more common in elderly people due to atrophy of subcutaneous tissues and loss of collagen and elastin fibres in subcutaneous tissues. Blood vessels in the skin can be broken by minor trauma or shearing forces and typically purpura are seen on hands and forearms. If routine tests of platelet number and coagulation are normal, no further investigation is required. Long-term steroid use is also associated with bruising secondary to atrophy of collagen fibres supporting blood vessels.

Psychogenic purpura

Psychogenic purpura or Diamond–Gardner syndrome is a rare condition usually seen most commonly in women with psychological problems. It presents with painful ecchymotic lesions, mostly on the extremities and the face and rarely on less accessible parts of the body. The skin lesions can be preceded by paraesthesia or pain and are usually reported after surgery or minor trauma. The usual tests for haemostasis reveal no abnormalities. Diamond and Gardner suggested the possibility of a local reaction to the patient's own red cell stroma and gave it the name 'autoerythrocyte sensitization syndrome'.

Scurvy

Scurvy is caused by a lack of vitamin C (ascorbic acid), which is required for the hydroxylation of prolyl and lysyl residues in the formation of mature collagen. Vitamin C deficiency renders the collagen unable to self-assemble into rigid triple helices, resulting in blood vessel fragility and poor wound healing. The characteristic clinical finding is perifollicular haemorrhage but large ecchymoses can occur on the legs and trunk. Follicular hyperkeratosis and corkscrew hairs are other cutaneous features. Bleeding gums are also common. Scurvy is more common in people with poor nutrition, especially alcoholics. The diagnosis is made clinically although levels of plasma or leucocyte vitamin C can be measured. A prompt response to vitamin C treatment is also diagnostic.

Inherited disorders of collagen and elastic fibres

Ehlers–Danlos syndrome (EDS) is a group of dominantly inherited disorders of connective tissue characterized by lax hyperelastic skin, joint laxity and poor wound healing. There are six subtypes and subtype IV is associated with severe varicosities and spontaneous rupture of major blood vessels. Bruising is seen in 90% of patients with EDS and has also been reported in people with lax joints who do not fulfil the criteria of EDS. Although mild platelet and coagulation factor dysfunction has been reported in association with EDS, it is likely that these are coincidental. Some patients have a prolonged bleeding time and this can respond to DDAVP. Other disorders such as osteogenesis imperfecta and Marfan syndrome may also be associated with bruising. Recently, a pseudoxanthoma elasticum-like disorder has been described where deficiency of the vitamin K-dependent clotting factors was noted along with the typical excessive skin folding (or cutis laxa).

Haemostatic dysfunction associated with vasculitis

The vasculitides are a heterogeneous group of disorders characterized by inflammation within blood vessel walls of different organs. It is classified by the size of the blood vessel involved and can be associated with both thrombosis, for example Behçet's disease (see Chapter 46), and haemorrhage. The classic presentation of Henoch–Schönlein purpura is palpable purpura without thrombocytopenia or coagulopathy, arthritis/arthralgia, abdominal pain and renal disease. Henoch–Schönlein purpura is more commonly associated with bleeding than thrombosis.

Arteriovenous malformations

Hereditary haemorrhagic telangiectasia

Hereditary haemorrhagic telangiectasia (HHT) is a dominantly inherited, highly penetrant, familial disease in which telangiectasia develop on the skin and mucous membranes. Associated large arteriovenous malformations may occur in solid organs. International consensus diagnostic criteria have been developed based on epistaxis, mucocutaneous telangiectasia, visceral lesions and an affected first-degree relative. A patient is diagnosed as having 'definite HHT' when three crite-

ria are present, 'suspected HHT' when two criteria are present, or 'HHT unlikely' when only one criterion is present. All the offspring of an affected individual are at risk of having the disease since HHT may not manifest until late in life.

Mutations in the *ENG* gene (encoding endoglin) and *ALK1* gene (encoding activin receptor-like kinase 1) have been described. These genes encode proteins that are involved in signalling by the transforming growth factor (TGF)-β superfamily. In healthy endothelial cells, ALK-1 and endoglin cooperate in the TGF-β/Smad pathway. In HHT types 1 and 2, either endoglin or ALK-1 fail in cooperative signalling resulting in impaired TGF-β signalling. The latter can lead to a decreased capacity to form cord-like structures typical of the angiogenic process. This leads to dysregulation in the organization of the capillary network and arteriovenous malformation. Recently, it has also been shown that TGF-β1 has a biphasic effect on angiogenesis depending on its concentration. At high concentrations TGF-β1 inhibits VEGF-induced endothelial cell invasion and capillary lumen formation, whereas lower TGF-β1 concentrations potentiate VEGF activity. Increased levels of VEGF have been demonstrated in HHT (especially in patients who have frequent bleeds) and agents that inhibit VEGF, like thalidomide and bevacizumab, have been successful in treating severe HHT.

Cerebral, pulmonary and neurological involvement is described more commonly with *ENG* mutations, whereas liver involvement has been associated with *ALK1* mutations. Telangiectasia usually appears during the second and third decades of life but presentation at all ages has been described. Typical lesions are red 0.5–3 mm spots that blanch with pressure and are often noted on the skin of face and lips and mucosal surfaces of the tongue and mouth. Symptoms range from cosmetic and recurrent epistaxis and mouth bleeding to iron deficiency and intracranial haemorrhage. Epistaxis is seen in the majority of patients and is usually recurrent. Gastrointestinal bleeding from both upper and lower bowel and haematuria are also seen. Emboli, including septic emboli, may occur and antibiotic prophylaxis at the time of invasive procedures such as dental extraction is recommended. Occasionally bleeding can occur from internal organs without visible lesions.

Virtually all internal organs can be affected. The lungs develop pulmonary arteriovenous fistulae in about 30% of patients leading to haemoptysis, sometimes catastrophic, hypoxia, dyspnoea, high-output cardiac failure and clubbing. Transient ischaemic attacks, cerebral infarction and systemic emboli due to right-to-left shunting occur in about half of the patients with pulmonary arteriovenous fistulae. Pulmonary arteriovenous fistulae may worsen during pregnancy. Liver involvement is present in the majority of patients and, though often asymptomatic, can lead to cirrhosis, portal hypertension and high-output cardiac failure. Conjunctival telangiectasia may cause benign bleeds while more serious retinal bleeds can occur. Intracranial haemorrhage is associated with arteriovenous fistulae but embolization including septic emboli also commonly cause cerebral symptoms.

Screening tests in patients with mucocutaneous telangiectasia should include FBC, ferritin, liver function tests, chest radiography, liver ultrasound and contrast echocardiography (to identify pulmonary shunts). The role of gastrointestinal endoscopy and CT angiography or MRI of lung or brain in asymptomatic patients is unclear.

Treatment options for symptomatic lesions include local options such as laser therapy of skin and mucosal telangiectasia and embolization of arteriovenous malformations in lung or nervous system. Systemic treatment with estrogens and tranexamic acid may reduce bleeding symptoms.

Kasabach–Merritt syndrome

Kasabach–Merritt syndrome is a rare condition in which a vascular tumour (Kaposiform haemangioendothelioma) is associated with thrombocytopenia, hypofibrinogenaemia and bleeding, which can be life-threatening. The thrombocytopenia in Kasabach–Merritt syndrome is presumed to be due to platelet adhesion to the abnormally proliferating endothelium. This results in the activation of platelets with secondary consumption of clotting factors, including VWF, leading to systemic haemostatic failure. Excessive flow and shear rates secondary to arteriovenous shunting also contribute. The platelet count is often less than $20 \times 10^9/L$ and platelet half-life dramatically reduced. Intralesional bleeding can cause rapid enlargement of the haemangioma and can worsen the consumptive coagulopathy. Intralesional thrombosis may rarely occur, causing spontaneous resolution of some lesions. In addition to the thrombocytopenia and abnormal coagulation, some degree of microangiopathic haemolysis may be seen, suggesting intravascular coagulopathy. Management involves supportive care and, if possible, removal of the lesion. Steroids, interferon, chemotherapy with vincristine, radiotherapy and anti-angiogenic agents have been tried.

Microthromboembolic disease

Cholesterol embolism

Cholesterol embolism is a complication of widespread atherosclerotic disease. Rupture of an atherosclerotic plaque can occur spontaneously or, more commonly, at the time of vascular surgery or invasive procedures. Anticoagulant or fibrinolytic therapy can also weaken thrombi that usually prevent the release of cholesterol crystals. The characteristic presentation is with small limb-vessel occlusion with well-preserved peripheral pulses, which may occasionally lead to gangrene. Another common skin finding is livedo reticularis, where the cutaneous

venous plexus becomes visible because of increased amounts of desaturated venous blood. Organ involvement from cholesterol emboli is dependent on the vascular supply, with renal ischaemia being the commonest. The diagnosis of this condition is often missed unless the occurrence of the clinical features is related to the triggering procedure. Fundoscopy can reveal the presence of retinal cholesterol crystals (Hollenhorst plaques) in about 25% of cases. Biopsy of the cutaneous lesion or the affected organ is required for definitive diagnosis. The prostacyclin analogue iloprost has been used successfully in painful cutaneous necrotic lesions and renal insufficiency in a single report.

Fat embolism syndrome

Fat embolization is characterized by release of fat droplets into the systemic circulation after a traumatic or iatrogenic event. Its incidence depends on the bone involved (fractures of the femoral shaft > tibia or fibula > neck of femur), isolated or multiple fractures, age (10–40 years) and gender (occurs more in males). Although more common after lower limb fractures, fat embolism syndrome can also occur after liposuction, bone marrow harvesting, total parenteral nutrition, sickle cell crisis and pancreatitis. Classically, it presents with the triad of respiratory distress, mental status changes and petechial rash 24–48 hours after pelvic or long-bone fracture. The rash is pathognomonic and is seen usually on the conjunctiva, oral mucous membranes and upper body possibly due to embolization of fat droplets accumulating in the aortic arch. The diagnosis is made clinically because laboratory and radiographic diagnosis is nonspecific and inconsistent. Thrombocytopenia is common due to platelet activation and consumption into the thrombi. Management is mainly supportive with intensive care management to ensure haemodynamic stability. Aspirin and corticosteroids have also been shown to be helpful, although the use of heparin is controversial.

Warfarin-induced skin necrosis

Warfarin-induced skin necrosis is a rare condition that is due to microvascular thrombi provoked by a transient imbalance between procoagulant and anticoagulant factors. It most commonly affects the breasts, buttocks and thighs. It may occur on initiation of warfarin, especially in patients with heterozygous protein C or protein S deficiency because of the relatively shorter half-lives of the vitamin K-dependent proteins C and S compared with prothrombin. It is also seen in association with heparin-induced thrombocytopenia. It is prevented by bridging the initiation of warfarin with heparin and avoiding high loading doses. Treatment requires discontinuation of warfarin and starting therapeutic heparin. Intravenous infusions of protein C concentrate may also be used in the short term. Surgical débridement may be required in extensive cases.

Haemostatic dysfunction associated with paraproteinaemia and amyloidosis

Paraproteinaemia

Bleeding and thrombotic complications both occur in association with paraproteinaemias, although abnormalities in laboratory tests are found much more frequently than clinical effects. Bleeding is more common in Waldenström macroglobulinaemia and amyloidosis than multiple myeloma. Among myeloma patients, bleeding is most common in those with IgA paraproteinaemia. The circulating paraprotein in these conditions can (i) cause hyperviscosity and lead to arterial and retinal bleeds due to abnormal wall shear stress; (ii) inhibit or increase clearance of FVIII and VWF leading to von Willebrand disease or, less commonly, acquired haemophilia; (iii) impair platelet aggregation; (iv) inhibit fibrin polymerization; and (v) have heparin-like anticoagulant function that can be reversed by protamine. Management of these conditions is directed towards the underlying cause. Plasma exchange is of help as a temporary measure.

Amyloidosis

The pathophysiology of bleeding associated with systemic amyloidosis is multifactorial. The type of amyloidosis and the pattern of organ involvement are important determinants of the haemorrhagic tendency. AL amyloidosis, where liver and spleen involvement is frequent, is the commonest type associated with bleeding. Although FX deficiency is the most commonly found, decreased levels of all other factors, including VWF, have been reported. The coagulation factor deficiencies in these patients are thought to be due to adsorption onto amyloid fibrils. Abnormal fibrin polymerization and hyperfibrinolysis can also contribute to bleeding. Prolongation of the TT is the most common abnormality, seen in up to 90% of patients. A prolonged PT and APTT suggests FX deficiency.

Platelet dysfunction may also be seen, due to the binding of the amyloid light chains to the platelet membrane. Deposition of amyloid fibrils in the blood vessel wall and perivascular tissue may lead to impaired vasoconstriction and vessel fragility. This is exemplified by cerebral amyloid angiopathy, which can lead to intracerebral haemorrhage especially in elderly non-hypertensive individuals. The microvascular involvement also explains the 'raccoon eyes' (bilateral periorbital purpura from coughing or prolonged inverted positioning for lower gastrointestinal procedures) and the 'pinch purpura' (skin pinching leading to purpura). Several treatments have been described, including factor replacement with FFP or PCCs, platelet transfusion, DDAVP and rFVIIa. Severe FX deficiency can be difficult to manage and first-line therapy is with PCCs or FFP.

Acquired inhibitors of coagulation factors

Inhibitory autoantibodies to all coagulation factors have been described, although those against FVIII and VWF are most common.

Acquired haemophilia A

Acquired haemophilia A has an annual incidence of about 1.5 per million and usually affects older patients with a median age of about 75 years. It affects males and females equally, except in younger patients where there is a female preponderance associated with pregnancy. Acquired haemophilia A presents with a typical bleeding pattern that is distinct from that seen in congenital haemophilia. Widespread subcutaneous bleeding is common, as are muscle bleeds and gastrointestinal and genitourinary bleeding. Neurovascular compression may be limb-threatening. Haemarthroses are relatively uncommon. Fatal bleeding, such as intracranial, pulmonary, gastrointestinal and retroperitoneal, occurs in 8–22% of cases (Table 43.8). Patients remain at risk of severe bleeding until the inhibitor has been eradicated even if they present with mild bleeding. Acquired haemophilia A is associated with an underlying autoimmune (systemic lupus erythematosus or rheumatoid arthritis), malignant, lymphoproliferative or dermatological (pemphigoid) disease or pregnancy in about half of cases (Table 43.9). If acquired haemophilia A presents in association with pregnancy,

Table 43.8 Bleeding symptoms in patients with acquired haemophilia A.*

Site of bleeding	All bleeds at presentation (%)	Bleeds requiring treatment (%)
	N = 172	N = 65
Subcutaneous/skin	81	23
Muscle	45	32
Subcutaneous only	24	Not applicable
Gastrointestinal/ intra-abdominal	23	14
Genitourinary	9	18
Retroperitoneal/thoracic	9	5
Other	9	23
Postoperative	0	11
Joint	7	2
None	4	Not applicable
Intracranial haemorrhage	3	0
Fatal	9	No data

*Patients had often had multiple bleeds.
Source: data from Collins *et al.* (2007) and Morrison *et al.* (1993).

Table 43.9 Diseases associated with acquired haemophilia A.

	Green & Lechner (1981)	Morrison et al. (1993)	Collins et al. (2007)
Number of patients	215	65	150
Idiopathic (%)	46	55	63
Collagen, vascular and other autoimmune diseases (%)	18	17	17
Malignancy (%)	7	12	15
Skin diseases (%)	5	2	3
Possible drug reaction (%)	6	3	0
Pregnancy (%)	7	11	2

Source: data from Green & Lechner (1981), Morrison *et al.* (1993) and Collins *et al.* (2007).

it may recur in subsequent pregnancies and, if antenatal, the fetus may be affected.

Early diagnosis and urgent treatment of bleeding are key to successful management. The diagnosis is suggested by the clinical presentation and an isolated prolonged APTT. FVIII inhibitors are time and temperature dependent and in mixing studies normal plasma must be incubated for 1–2 hours otherwise the diagnosis may be missed. The diagnosis is confirmed by a low FVIII and positive Bethesda titre (Figure 43.6). In some cases diagnosis is complicated because all the intrinsic factors may be low due to inhibition of FVIII in the factor-deficient plasma used to assay other intrinsic factors. Dilution of the antibody will result in increased levels of the non-specifically reduced factors while FVIII remains low. It is important to exclude a lupus anticoagulant because this can also be associated with an apparently low FVIII and an APTT that does not correct with normal plasma. Acquired FVIII inhibitors have complex kinetics, so that not all FVIII is inhibited in a Bethesda assay. It is therefore often not possible to measure the inhibitor titre accu-

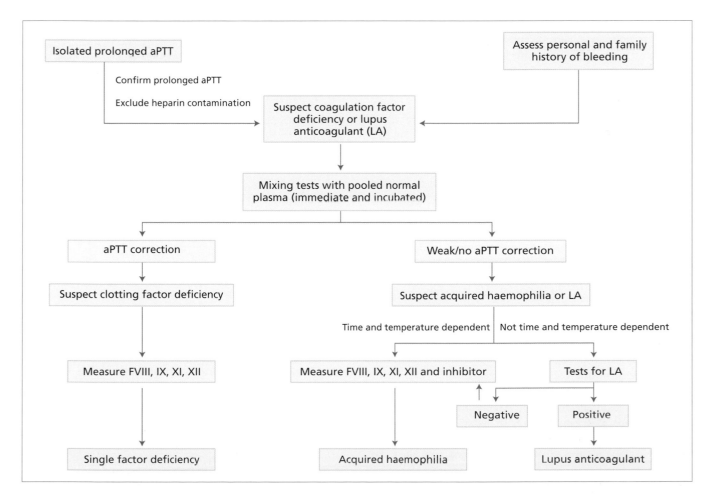

Figure 43.6 Diagnostic algorithm for an isolated prolonged APTT and possible acquired haemophilia A.

rately. The FVIII level and inhibitor titre are not predictive of the severity of the bleeding or response to treatment.

Treatment involves minimizing invasive procedures, protecting the patient from trauma, treatment of bleeds and eradication of the inhibitor. At present, the available therapies to treat bleeds are with bypassing agents, namely rFVIIa or the activated PCC FEIBA (factor eight inhibitor bypassing activity). Both agents appear to be equally efficacious. Multiple doses may be required to control bleeds and prevent recurrence. There is a risk of thrombosis associated with bypassing agents, particularly in elderly patients with risk factors for arterial thrombosis. FVIII is unlikely to be efficacious in acquired haemophilia A, although mild bleeds in patients with low-titre inhibitors and measurable FVIII may respond to desmopressin. Porcine FVIII has been used with good success in the past but is no longer available. The results of trials with a recombinant B domain-deleted porcine factor are awaited. If standard haemostatic treatment with bypassing agents fails, FVIII and immunoadsorption has been used with good effect, although this treatment modality is only available in a few specialized centres.

Immunosuppression should be started as soon as the diagnosis is made and is usually with either steroids alone or steroids plus a cytotoxic agent such as cyclophosphamide or azathioprine. A response is usually seen after 2–3 weeks but full remission takes a median of about 5 weeks. If first-line therapy fails, rituximab or combinations of cytotoxic agents may be used. Occasionally responses have been reported with ciclosporin. Intravenous immunoglobulin does not increase the response rate to other immunosuppressive agents.

Acquired von Willebrand disease

Acquired von Willebrand disease may be associated with an autoantibody, typically in the context of monoclonal gammopathy of undetermined significance, Waldenström macroglobulinaemia and other lymphoproliferative diseases, myeloproliferative disease and systemic lupus erythematosus. The antibody leads to either rapid clearance or functional inhibition of VWF. Low VWF:Ag, VWF:RCo and VWF:CB are found and measurement of the VWF propeptide may be useful in demonstrating rapid clearance. Mixing studies can be used to demonstrate the inhibitor.

Low VWF levels are also seen in hypothyroidism probably due to decreased synthesis, whereas increased VWF is associated with hyperthyroidism. Increased proteolysis of VWF in high-shear environments such as leaking cardiac values leads to a syndrome of acquired type 2A von Willebrand disease. VWF has also been reported in association with malignancy and it is suggested that it may be adsorbed onto malignant cells. Hydroxyethyl starches used as plasma expanders have been associated with bleeding secondary to VWF deficiency. Treatment options include DDAVP, VWF concentrates and, in patients with an inhibitory antibody, high-dose intravenous immunoglobulin.

Acquired factor V deficiency

Acquired inhibitors to FV may arise spontaneously but are usually associated with exposure to topical thrombin preparations that have trace amount of bovine FV. Laboratory findings are of prolonged PT and APTT that do not correct with normal plasma. Patients may respond to FFP and, in resistant cases, platelets may be useful because surface-bound FV appears to bypass the inhibitor.

Acquired protein S deficiency

Autoantibodies to protein S have been reported in association with infection, particularly chickenpox. Patients present with skin necrosis and DIC.

Prothrombin deficiency associated with lupus anticoagulant

Although lupus anticoagulants are typically associated with thrombosis, occasionally cross-reactivity with prothrombin can lead to a bleeding disorder. Acquired deficiencies of other procoagulant and antifibrinolytic proteins have occasionally been described. Bleeding manifestations are variable and some patients with markedly abnormal laboratory tests do not bleed.

Selected bibliography

Bevan DH (1999) Cardiac bypass haemostasis: putting blood through the mill. *British Journal of Haematology* **104**: 208–19.

Collins PW, Hirsch S, Baglin TP *et al.* (2007) Acquired hemophilia A in the United Kingdom: a 2-year national surveillance study by the United Kingdom Haemophilia Centre Doctors' Organisation. *Blood* **109**: 1870–7.

De Paepe A, Malfait F (2004) Bleeding and bruising in patients with Ehlers–Danlos syndrome and other collagen vascular disorders. *British Journal of Haematology* **127**: 491–500.

Eby C (2009) Pathogenesis and management of bleeding and thrombosis in plasma cell dyscrasias. *British Journal of Haematology* **145**: 151–63.

Falanga A, Rickles FR (2003) Pathogenesis and management of the bleeding diathesis in acute promyelocytic leukaemia. *Best Practice and Research. Clinical Haematology* **16**: 463–82.

Green D, Lechner K (1981) A survey of 215 non-hemophilic patients with inhibitors to Factor VIII. *Thrombosis and Haemostasis* **45**: 200–3.

Hess JR, Brohi K, Dutton RP (2008) The coagulopathy of trauma: a review of mechanisms. *Journal of Trauma* **65**: 748–54.

Hess JR, Lindell AL, Stansbury LG *et al.* (2009) The prevalence of abnormal results of conventional coagulation tests on admission to a trauma centre. *Transfusion* **49**: 34–9.

Huth-Kuhne A, Baudo F, Collins P *et al.* (2009) International recommendations on the diagnosis and treatment of patients with acquired haemophilia A. *Haematologica* **94**: 566–75.

Levi M, Toh CH, Thachil J, Watson HG (2009) Diagnosis and management of disseminated intravascular coagulation. *British Journal of Haematology* **145**: 24–33.

Levy JH, Dutton RP, Hemphill JC 3rd, Shander A *et al.* (2010) Multidisciplinary approach to the challenge of hemostasis. *Anesthesia and Analgesia* **110**: 354–64.

Lisman T, Leebeek FW, de Groot PG (2002) Haemostatic abnormalities in patients with liver disease. *Journal of Hepatology* **37**: 280–7.

Morrison AE, Ludlam CA, Kessler C (1993) Use of porcine factor VIII in the treatment of patients with acquired hemophilia. *Blood* **81**: 1513–20.

Noris M, Remuzzi G (1999) Uremic bleeding: closing the circle after 30 years of controversies? *Blood* **94**: 2569–74.

Stainsby D, Maclennan S, Thomas D, Isaac J, Hamilton PJ (2006) Guidelines on the management of massive blood loss. *British Journal of Haematology* **135**: 634–41.

Zangari M, Elice F, Fink L, Tricot G (2007) Hemostatic dysfunction in paraproteinemias and amyloidosis. *Seminars in Thrombosis and Hemostasis* **33**: 339–49.

CHAPTER 44

Thrombotic thrombocytopenic purpura and haemolytic–uraemic syndrome (congenital and acquired)

44

Pier M Mannucci, Flora Peyvandi and Roberta Palla

A. Bianchi Bonomi Hemophilia and Thrombosis Center, IRCCS Cà Granada, Ospedale Maggiore, Milan, Italy

Historical introduction

A brief historical sketch is useful for delineating the progress made in understanding these complex syndromes, which are difficult to diagnose. Thrombotic thrombocytopenic purpura (TTP) was first described in 1924 by Moschowitz in a previously healthy 16-year-old girl who died after an acute illness presenting with a pentad of signs and symptoms (anaemia, thrombocytopenia, fever, hemiparesis and haematuria). Post-mortem examination showed widespread thrombi in the terminal circulation of several organs, composed mainly of platelets. Over the next three decades, other cases were described, mainly, but not exclusively, in young or adult women. Some of these cases occurred in isolation (idiopathic), others in association with diseases or conditions (Table 44.1). It was understood that anaemia was due to massive intravascular haemolysis, in turn due to fragmentation (schistocytosis) of red cells that were forced by blood flow to pass through partially occluded vessels in the terminal circulation, and that thrombocytopenia was caused by consumption of platelets due to their widespread deposition in microvascular thrombi.

Thirty-one years after Moschowitz, the paediatric nephrologist Gasser described a syndrome that was called 'haemolytic–uraemic syndrome' (HUS) and which, in common with TTP, exhibited microangiopathic haemolytic anaemia, consumption thrombocytopenia and microvascular thrombosis, but which

differed because it occurred in very young children, with absent or minimal neurological symptoms but severe signs of renal damage. Subsequently, when larger series of patients with HUS and TTP were examined, it became apparent that a clear distinction between the two syndromes was often difficult. Although thrombocytopenia, microangiopathic haemolytic anaemia and ischaemic symptoms due to widespread formation of thrombi in the terminal circulation of several organs were consistent features, age and the prevalence of neurological over renal symptoms could not clearly differentiate TTP from HUS and vice versa. There were, for instance, recurrent forms which, in the same individual, presented sometimes with prevalent neurological symptoms (TTP) and on other occasions with renal symptoms (HUS). The term 'thrombotic microangiopathy' (TMA) was then proposed, intended to emphasize the common pathology of the two syndromes, with no implication on the prevalence of neurological or renal symptoms.

In the early 1980s, a major breakthrough in understanding the pathogenesis of TMAs strengthened the idea of the unitarian terminology. Even though it had been postulated for a long time that massive thrombus formation in the terminal circulation was due to the presence of 'toxic' substance(s) that aggregated platelets intravascularly, the putative aggregating agent had remained elusive. In 1982, Moake and others demonstrated, first in TTP and subsequently also in HUS, that the plasma of these patients contained highly thrombogenic forms of the multimeric glycoprotein von Willebrand factor (VWF), a major adhesive protein contained in endothelial cells, platelets and plasma. Abnormal VWF multimers of particularly high molecular weight (ultra-large) bind more avidly to platelet glycoprotein (GP)Ib and aggregate platelets in conditions of high shear

Postgraduate Haematology: 6th edition. Edited by A. Victor Hoffbrand, Daniel Catovsky, Edward G.D. Tuddenham, Anthony R. Green
© 2011 Blackwell Publishing Ltd.

stress in the terminal circulation. Accordingly, it was postulated that ultra-large VWF was the 'toxic' aggregating agent involved in the formation of occlusive thrombi in both TTP and HUS.

It remained to be explained why such ultra-large multimers, normally absent in the circulation, were present in patient plasma. The deficiency or dysfunction of one or more enzymes disposing of them physiologically was postulated but it was not until the late 1990s that Furlan and Tsai with their associates

Table 44.1 Conditions and diseases associated with TTP.

Pregnancy and post partum
Infections (particularly HIV)
Drugs (quinine and quinidine, ticlopidine, clopidogrel, ciclosporin, interferon alfa, statins)
Chemotherapy (mitomycin, cisplatin, gemcitabine)
Allogeneic bone marrow transplantation
Connective tissue disorders (lupus erythematosus and scleroderma)
Cardiac surgery

independently showed that the link between ultra-large VWF multimers and TTP was a metal ion-dependent plasma metalloproteinase of 190 kDa, identified in 2001 by Zheng and colleagues as a new (the 13th) member of the ADAMTS (*a* *d*isintegrin *a*nd *m*etalloprotease with *t*hrombospondin-1 repeats) family of metalloproteases and therefore called ADAMTS-13 (Figure 44.1). The only known physiological function of this protease, present in plasma and in platelets, is to regulate the size of VWF by cleaving ultra-large multimers as soon as they are secreted from endothelial cells into plasma (Figure 44.2), thereby preventing their circulation in plasma and role in platelet aggregation and thrombus formation. Most importantly, both the investigators made the intriguing observation that ADAMTS-13 was deficient in patients with TTP but measurable in normal amounts in those with HUS. This observation challenged the unitarian theory of TTP and HUS as different clinical manifestations of the same pathological process, and generated the paradigm that TTP is due to low levels of the VWF-cleaving protease, which however is not involved in the pathogenesis of HUS.

As often in clinical medicine, the paradigm was not sustained by the progress of knowledge. Not all cases of TMA diagnosed

Figure 44.1 Domain structure of ADAMTS-13. Pro, propeptide; TSP1, thrombospondin 1; CUB, complement components C1r/C1s, *u*rinary epidermal growth factor, *b*one morphogenetic protein-1.

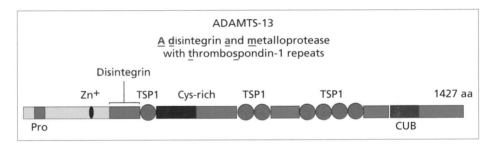

Figure 44.2 Interaction between VWF and ADAMTS-13 in plasma. VWF is secreted from endothelial cells as ultra-large multimers that anchor to endothelial cell surfaces and which are also released into the circulation. ADAMTS-13 cleaves a Tyr–Met bond in the A2 domain of VWF, severing the ultra-large multimers. Failure of cleavage leads to the persistence in plasma and on endothelial cells of ultra-large multimers, which tend to aggregate platelets, especially in conditions of high shear forces.

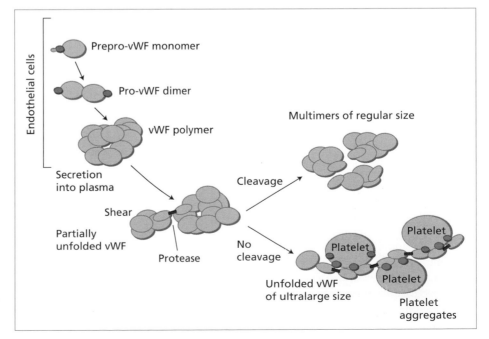

as TTP owing to the prevalence of neurological symptoms have low or undetectable levels of ADAMTS-13. On the other hand, even if most cases diagnosed as HUS due to the prevalence of renal symptoms have normal levels of ADAMTS-13 (particularly cases typically occurring in association with bloody diarrhoea), there are unequivocal cases of HUS, particularly the forms called atypical or diarrhoea-negative, characterized by low or undetectable protease levels. With this as historical background, we have decided to describe TTP separately from HUS in this chapter.

Thrombotic thrombocytopenic purpura

TTP is a rare disease, with an estimated incidence of 2–10 cases per million per year in all racial groups. Recently, greater awareness and perhaps improved diagnostic facilities give the impression that incidence is increasing. Even though both sexes may be affected, the syndrome is definitely more frequent in women (two-thirds of cases).

There are two different forms of TTP. Congenital TTP, caused by mutations in the ADAMTS-13 gene, is inherited as an autosomal recessive condition and is often, but not exclusively, clinically manifested at birth or during childhood. Acquired TTP can be differentiated into two types: autoimmune forms, due to autoantibodies against ADAMTS-13; and those probably secondary to massive endothelial activation with release of ultra-large VWF multimers in amounts exceeding the system's ability to degrade them, despite the presence of normal or only slightly reduced levels of ADAMTS-13 as measured with the currently available functional assay. Both these pathogenic situations are usually triggered by factors that cause massive endothelial activation. The most common physiological or pathological conditions present in the autoimmune forms are pregnancy, infections, autoimmune diseases and the use of drugs such as ticlopidine and clopidogrel. The most frequent conditions associated with the forms of TTP with normal or only slightly reduced levels of ADAMTS-13 (conventionally defined as levels above 10%) are metastatic tumours, organ transplantation (particularly allogeneic bone marrow transplantation and solid organ transplants) and the use of such drugs as ciclosporin, mitomycin and interferon alfa.

Mortality was very high (80–90%) until plasma exchange therapy was introduced, and is still unacceptably high (10–20%) despite the dramatic improvement due to the adoption of this therapeutic measure. Because of the variability of presenting symptoms and of the associated comorbid conditions (see Table 44.1), cases of TTP may be seen initially by a variety of physicians other than haematologists and pathologists, such as neurologists, nephrologists, oncologists and gynaecologists, and sometimes this hinders prompt recognition of the syndrome, an essential requisite for optimal management.

Pathology and pathogenesis

As mentioned above, the pathological basis of TTP is the widespread formation in the microcirculation of platelet thrombi, associated with relatively little endothelial cell injury and fibrin formation but with abundant intra-thrombus VWF. Microthrombi are found in several organs (mainly brain, kidney, myocardium, lung and pancreas), whereas grossly detectable thrombi, arterial or venous, are lacking. The present pathogenetic model implies that endothelial cells, activated by varied and often unidentified triggering agents, secrete large amounts of ultra-large uncleaved VWF, which aggregates platelets directly in conditions of high fluid shear stress and leads to massive intravascular platelet aggregation, ischaemic organ damage, consumptive thrombocytopenia and schistocytic anaemia. As mentioned above, two main mechanisms cause ADAMTS-13 deficiency in TTP: mutations in the gene that encodes the protease and the occurrence of autoantibodies against ADAMTS-13.

Congenital TTP

Congenital TTP is very rare (1 in 1 million) and represents 5% of all TTP cases. It usually occurs immediately after birth or during childhood, although some exceptions have been reported where the disease became manifest in adulthood or was still absent in the third decade of life. Congenital TTP is caused by homozygous or double heterozygous mutations in the *ADAMTS13* gene (located on chromosome 9q34) that affect protein secretion or function; it is inherited in autosomal recessive manner. To date, more than 80 mutations have been documented in patients with familial TTP. Analysis of the location of the mutations on the *ADAMTS13* gene reveals no evident hotspots. However, 75% of the missense mutations are found in the N-terminal part of the molecule, up to the spacer domain. Most (60%) of the identified mutations are missense; the remaining 40% (nonsense, frameshift and splicing mutations) generates truncated forms of the protein. Of those mutations analysed by *in vitro* expression studies (only 20–30% of the reported gene mutations), the majority cause severe ADAMTS-13 deficiency by decreasing its biosynthesis, intacellular trafficking and secretion and/or proteolytic activity. Also the spectrum of clinical presentation and course of congenital TTP is very wide. While some patients have neonatal disease onset and multiple recurrent episodes and develop progressive organ failure, others may only experience a single episode that develops in adulthood and which is very responsive to plasma infusion, leaving no residual organ damage. Moreover, there are cases from the same kindreds who present with very different clinical manifestations despite the same undetectable or barely detectable ADAMTS-13 activity and gene mutations: sibs with frequent and repeated episodes of TTP contrast with others who remain disease-free for prolonged periods or even lifelong.

Autoimmune TTP

Autoimmune TTP accounts for the majority of clinical cases and occurs in adults in the absence of any obvious triggering event. However, it can also arise secondary to other conditions, such as autoimmune diseases, infections, drug intake, pregnancy, sepsis, tumours and bone marrow transplantation. Autoimmune TTP is due to anti-ADAMTS-13 antibodies that inhibit the proteolytic activity of ADAMTS-13 and/or bind the protease to accelerate its clearance from plasma through opsonization and/or other yet unclear mechanisms. Anti-ADAMTS-13 antibodies are usually of IgG type, although in few cases autoantibodies of IgA and/or IgM isotype were also found. Epitope mapping of anti-ADAMTS-13 antibodies showed that autoantibodies found in the majority of patients (88%) are polyclonal (IgG4), with a primary epitope in the Cys-rich spacer. Indeed these domains have been shown to be essential for efficient VWF-cleaving activity of ADAMTS-13 and crucial in the interaction between VWF and the protease. However, subsequent studies have shown that cases of TTP are observed in patients with IgG molecules that also react with the TSP1 2–8 and CUB domains of ADAMTS-13, suggesting that autoantibodies with specificity towards more distal C-terminal domains of ADAMTS-13 may impair its function *in vivo*, probably taking part in the modulation of VWF binding. The higher incidence of autoimmune idiopathic TTP in specific ethnic groups such as Afro-Caribbeans, as well as the report of idiopathic TTP in two monozygotic twins both developing anti-ADAMTS-13 antibodies, strongly argue for a genetic predisposition even in the acquired form of the disease.

However, several observations fail to fit perfectly with this relatively straightforward mechanism of disease. Not all patients with bona fide TTP, as diagnosed by clinical criteria (thrombocytopenia and anaemia), have severe ADAMTS-13 deficiency and patients can present the characteristic features and clinical course of TTP without severe ADAMTS-13 deficiency or even with normal ADAMTS-13 activity levels. This may be explained by the inability of the functional assays available at present to reveal some types of ADAMTS-13 deficiency and/or by deficiency of VWF-cleaving proteases other than ADAMTS-13. Ultra-large VWF multimers, pivotal players in the presently accepted model of TTP, are not constantly detected in patient plasma. In some instances, there is an imbalance between their release into plasma from endothelial cells and excessive binding to platelets, so that even defective large multimers may be present in plasma. It is unclear why patients with sustained ADAMTS-13 deficiency, genetic or immunologically mediated, develop clinical symptoms and signs only sporadically. Still unknown factors that trigger excessive endothelial cell activation may be necessary for expression of the full clinical spectrum of the syndrome.

In summary, the prevailing paradigm holds that TTP is often the consequence of the defective processing of highly thrombogenic ultra-large multimers of VWF, which are secreted in excess by endothelial cells and which are not adequately disposed of because of congenital or immune-mediated dysfunction of ADAMTS-13 (see Figure 44.2). There are data suggesting that other possible mechanisms of disease, other than VWF and its cleaving processes, may be involved in the pathogenesis of TTP.

Clinical and laboratory findings

TTP occurs frequently, unheralded, in previously healthy individuals (acute idiopathic), but also in association with physiological or pathological conditions (see Table 44.1). The presence of thrombocytopenia and haemolytic anaemia, common to all TMAs, is essential for the diagnosis of TTP. Like HUS, TTP is a clinical diagnosis and biopsies are not necessary. Platelet count is often very low in the acute phase, with values of 20×10^9/L or less, and petechiae are frequently seen. Signs of microangiopathic haemolytic anaemia (haematocrit usually <20%) include the presence of schistocytes on peripheral blood smears, reticulocytosis, increased indirect bilirubin, low or unmeasurable haptoglobin and negative direct Coombs test. High serum lactate dehydrogenase (LDH), usually in excess of 1000 U/L, is a sensitive, albeit non-specific, sign of red cell destruction and necrosis of other tissues due to microthrombotic end-organ ischaemia and is an excellent diagnostic indicator and a parameter for monitoring evolution of the disease. Neurological symptoms (coma, stroke, seizures or focal signs such as motor deficits, diplopia and aphasia) typically fluctuate in presentation and severity as a result of the sustained formation and dissolution of thrombi in the cerebral microcirculation. Other symptoms or signs, such as headache, blurred vision, ataxia or mental status changes, are less typical. Even though only a minority of patients with TTP have elevated serum creatinine levels (>1.5 mg/dL), signs of renal involvement such as microscopic haematuria and proteinuria are frequent. High fever is not constant in TTP, despite the inclusion of this symptom in the original description. There is no or little alteration of coagulation and fibrinolysis, even though D-dimer levels are often moderately raised.

ADAMTS-13 assays

The possibility of using ADAMTS-13 data to manage TTP patients is based on the widespread availability of assays that are rapid, reliable and feasible for most clinical laboratories. Such tests includes assays of ADAMTS-13 activity, ADAMTS-13 antigen and neutralizing or non-neutralizing anti-ADAMTS-13 autoantibodies. Several assays of ADAMTS-13 activity have been developed. They are based on the degradation of purified, plasma-derived or recombinant VWF multimers or of synthetic VWF peptides by patient plasma and the direct or indirect detection of VWF cleavage products by ADAMTS-13 (Figure 44.3). A number of variables may interfere with assay results.

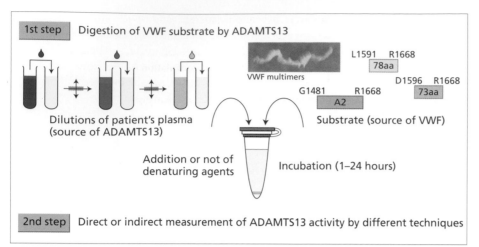

1st step   Digestion of VWF substrate by ADAMTS13

L1591   R1668
78aa

VWF multimers

D1596   R1668
73aa

G1481   R1668
A2

Dilutions of patient's plasma
(source of ADAMTS13)

Substrate (source of VWF)

Addition or not of
denaturing agents

Incubation (1–24 hours)

2nd step   Direct or indirect measurement of ADAMTS13 activity by different techniques

Figure 44.3 Principles of methods for the measurement of ADAMTS-13 activity. VWF multimers picture from Siedlecki CA, Lestini BJ, Kottke-Marchant K *et al.* (1996) Shear-dependent changes in the three-dimensional structure of human von Willebrand factor. *Blood* **88:** 2939–50.

1 All the assays measure ADAMTS-13 activity in static conditions and thus do not reflect the *in vivo* physiological blood flow conditions necessary for optimal ADAMTS-13 enzymatic activity.

2 Another important variable is that denaturating agents (i.e. guanidine HCl or 1.5 mol/L urea) are required to promote the susceptibility of VWF multimers to cleavage by ADAMTS-13.

3 The use of shorter peptides, instead of full-length VWF, in enzyme immunoassay-based methods has not solved the issue of intra- and inter-laboratory variability.

Immunoenzymatic assays employing different monoclonal and polyclonal antibodies to monitor plasma antigen levels of ADAMTS-13 are available.

With regard to the detection of anti-ADAMTS-13 autoantibodies, most of them are inhibitory and they can be titrated *in vitro* by classical mixing studies, using mixtures of heat-inactivated plasma from patients and normal plasma at 1:1 dilution or several dilutions. Less frequently, autoantibodies are non-neutralizing and promote the clearance of ADAMTS-13 from blood without inhibiting its activity. These non-neutralizing antibodies can be detected by Western blotting or ELISA assays.

Clinical utility of ADAMTS-13 testing

Analysis of a large cohort of patients with congenital TTP has revealed an age-dependent clustering of cases into two relatively distinct groups. As already mentioned before, about 50% of patients present within the first 5 years of life, but a second group remains without symptoms until 20–40 years of age (Figure 44.4). Examples of siblings with the same ADAMTS-13 mutations but markedly different clinical courses have also been reported. Whereas the first studies by Tsai and Lian and by Furlan and colleagues reported that all patients with acquired TTP had severe ADAMTS-13 deficiency, subsequent studies have shown that only a proportion of patients, ranging from 13 to 70%, develop TTP concomitant with severe ADAMTS-13

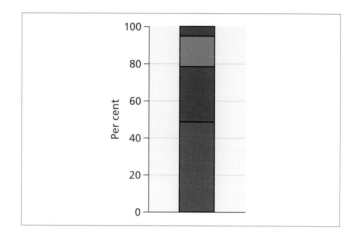

Figure 44.4 Age of disease onset in patients affected by congenital TTP showing percentages of patients (*N* = 78) with different age of TTP onset. Red indicates neonatal onset, orange intermediate onset (2 months to 18 years), green adult onset (>18 years) and light blue patients who reached adulthood without developing TTP episodes.

deficiency, thus challenging the previous observations that severely deficient activity of VWF-cleaving protease is a specific diagnostic marker for discriminating TTP from other microangiopathies. The current prevailing opinion is that while undetectable or very low plasma levels of enzymatic activity (<10%) unequivocally establish a diagnosis of inherited or acquired TTP, not all patients appropriately diagnosed with TTP on the basis of clinical and laboratory signs and symptoms have severe protease deficiency *in vitro*. The cases of TTP more frequently associated with normal or moderately reduced ADAMTS-13 levels (10–40% of normal) are those secondary to other diseases or conditions, such as allogeneic bone marrow transplantation, HIV infection, chemotherapy and metastatic cancer.

An important practical problem for the clinical haematologist is whether ADAMTS-13 testing during the acute phase of TTP helps to monitor plasma therapy and, more importantly, to predict such important short-term outcomes as clinical and laboratory remission or mortality. On the whole, the findings obtained to date fail to establish whether ADAMTS-13 and anti-ADAMTS-13 testing helps to identify patients with a higher likelihood of unfavourable outcomes. Other clinical and laboratory signs, more easily obtained than ADAMTS-13 and anti-ADAMTS-13, have been evaluated for their predictive value on the short-term outcomes of acute TTP. For instance, an index was developed based on age, haemoglobin and the presence of fever at presentation. Other authors have reported that platelet count and serum LDH are useful predictors of the response to plasma exchange during the acute episode.

After remission from an acute episode of TTP, approximately one-third of patients develop chronic recurrent disease. Hence it would be helpful to be able to predict the risk of relapse by using clinical and laboratory markers obtained at the time of the acute episode and/or during remission. Prospective and retrospective studies have shown that patients who present with undetectable ADAMTS-13 activity and detectable anti-ADAMTS-13 during the acute episode and/or during first remission are more likely to experience recurrences.

In summary, in order to diagnose TTP in the acute phase of the disease, it is not essential to assay ADAMTS-13 and to find very low or undetectable plasma levels. After having excluded other TMAs (see below), patients presenting with normal or moderately reduced ADAMTS-13 can still be appropriately diagnosed as TTP. The decision to implement plasma therapy (infusion in patients with inherited disease, exchange in acquired disease) does not warrant the availability of ADAMTS-13 values in real time. ADAMTS-13 testing appears to be more helpful as an index of relapse than as an index of diagnosis and short-term outcomes (remission and mortality rates), but larger prospective studies are warranted.

Differential diagnosis

Typical cases of HUS are distinguished from TTP by the occurrence of diarrhoeal prodromes and of more severe and persistent symptoms of renal impairment (see below). It is much more difficult to distinguish TTP from atypical HUS, except for the paradigmatic prevalence of neurological symptoms in the former and of renal failure in the latter. Other issues of differential diagnosis are concerned with conditions that present themselves as TMAs, all characterized by thrombocytopenia and microangiopathic haemolytic anaemia (Table 44.2). Therefore, accurate evaluation of the underlying conditions, symptoms and biological parameters is fundamental for determining the differential diagnosis and appropriate therapy.

Disseminated intravascular coagulation (DIC) can be distinguished by markedly increased levels of fibrin degradation products and D-dimer and, in decompensated cases, by the

Table 44.2 Clinical conditions other than TTP and HUS presenting as thrombotic microangiopathies.

Disseminated intravascular coagulation
Pre-eclampsia/HELLP syndrome
Scleroderma/systemic lupus erythematosus
Severe vasculitis
Catastrophic antiphospholipid antibody syndrome
Evans syndrome (autoimmune thrombocytopenia and haemolytic anaemia)
Heparin-induced thrombocytopenia
Disseminated malignancy

presence of hypofibrinogenaemia and prolonged prothrombin and activated partial thromboplastin times. The differential diagnosis also includes other TMAs such as pre-eclampsia and eclampsia, because pregnancy is one of the most frequent clinical associations of TTP. Malignant hypertension is less frequent, renal damage is not as severe and the degrees of anaemia and thrombocytopenia are more severe in TTP.

Tests of coagulation and fibrinolysis are usually abnormal in pre-eclampsia or eclampsia, albeit less markedly than in DIC. Abnormally high serum transaminases differentiate TTP from the so-called HELLP (haemolysis, elevated liver enzymes and low platelets) syndrome of pregnancy. Sometimes connective tissue disorders such as systemic lupus erythematosus and severe scleroderma present with widespread microvascular thrombosis, haemolytic anaemia, thrombocytopenia and fluctuating neurological symptoms. This situation may also occur in severe cases of the so-called catastrophic antiphospholipid antibody syndrome. These conditions may be distinguished from TTP because symptoms and signs are usually less severe, and laboratory tests such as antinuclear and anticardiolipin antibodies and lupus-like anticoagulant give positive results. Another element of differential diagnosis is the presence in these cases of venous and arterial thromboses in the major blood vessels.

Evans syndrome, due to the concomitant presence of anti-platelet and anti-erythrocyte antibodies, is distinguished by a positive Coombs test, lack of schistocytes and the usual absence of end-organ ischaemic symptoms. Severe ischaemic manifestations due to platelet thrombi are frequent features of heparin-induced thrombocytopenia, but TTP can be distinguished by not only lack of exposure to this drug but also the absence of haemolysis and schistocytosis. Disseminated malignancy is sometimes associated with thrombocytopenia and microangiopathic haemolytic anaemia. Until further investigations exclude or confirm the presence of metastatic cancer, it is not easy to distinguish TTP from this type of TMA.

What is the usefulness of ADAMTS-13 testing in the differential diagnosis of the aforementioned TMAs and TTP?

Table 44.3 Physiological and pathological states associated with mild to moderately severe deficiency of ADAMTS-13.

Age
Sex
Neonatal state
Pregnancy
Localized and metastatic cancer
HELLP syndrome
Liver cirrhosis
Inflammatory states
Postoperative period
Uraemia
Sepsis
Autoimmune diseases

Table 44.4 Variants of TTP.

Acute sporadic (or early relapsing)
   Idiopathic
   Antibody mediated
Chronic recurrent
   Inherited
   Antibody mediated

Complete deficiency of the protease clearly directs the diagnosis towards TTP, although severe deficiency of ADAMTS-13 has also been observed in 13% of typical HUS cases and 16% of DIC. Normal or reduced but detectable plasma levels of the protease do not help in the differential diagnosis because they may be found, albeit rarely, in TTP, typical HUS, other TMAs and several other unrelated conditions (Table 44.3).

Natural history (Table 44.4)

In approximately two-thirds of cases, TTP occurs only once (acute sporadic TTP). In more than one-third of patients, the disease tends to recur after periods of remission of the acute episode. Recurrence, defined as the re-emergence of clinical and laboratory signs and symptoms of TTP after remission of the initial acute episode, has a spectrum of presentations ranging from a single relapse to several episodes developing with variable frequency. Recurrences usually present with less severe clinical manifestations, perhaps because patients become alert to the first signs and symptoms of their disease, yet their quality of life is made gloomy by the perception of an impending risk.

The chronic recurrent forms may have a genetic basis or be associated with autoantibodies, whereas the forms associated with malignancy or transplantation usually present as acute

Table 44.5 Steps in the treatment of TTP.

Clinical diagnosis (based on severe thrombocytopenia, presence of schistocytes, high serum LDH)
Plasma infusion (30 mL/kg) until plasma exchange can be started
Daily plasma exchanges (3–6 L/day) until platelets are higher than 150×10^9/L for at least 2 days and LDH is normal
Adjuvant treatments: prednisone 1–2 mg/kg per day
Red cell transfusion as needed (avoid platelet transfusion, if possible)

episodes with a low propensity to recur (in part because of the high mortality rate).

In congenital TTP, ADAMTS-13 plasma levels are usually consistently below the limit of sensitivity of the assays available at present. It is not understood why in congenital but also in chronic recurrent TTP ADAMTS-13-deficient patients remain asymptomatic for prolonged periods of time (usually from 3 weeks to 3 months) and then thrombocytopenia and schistocytic anaemia herald the appearance of new symptoms of end-organ ischaemia.

Treatment

The modern management of TTP started with the serendipitous observations that plasma infusion improved the clinical course of TTP. Plasma exchange was subsequently found to be equally or more effective than plasma infusion. In 1991, the results of a prospective randomized clinical trial definitively confirmed the greater efficacy of plasma exchange over infusion, the clinical response rate being 78% in the former compared with 49% in the latter (mortality rates of 22% and 37%, respectively). Only recently, after the discovery of the role of VWF and its protease ADAMTS-13 in the pathogenesis of TTP, have these empirical treatments found a rationale. Plasma exchange may help by removing anti-ADAMTS-13 autoantibodies, the most frequent mechanism of acute sporadic TTP. Plasma exchange also helps to replace the deficient protease, infusion alone being probably sufficient in congenitally deficient cases with no associated autoantibody. Nevertheless, the efficacy of plasma therapies is still not fully explained, because exchange and/or infusion are definitely efficacious even in cases with normal plasma levels of ADAMTS-13 and no detectable autoantibody. A scheme summarizing the steps to be followed in the treatment of acute TTP is shown in Table 44.5.

Plasma therapy

Treatment with plasma should be initiated as soon as the clinical diagnosis is suspected (presence of schistocytic anaemia, severe thrombocytopenia and high serum LDH). There is as yet no evidence that ADAMTS-13 and autoantibody testing are necessary before starting therapy because, as mentioned above, there are unequivocal cases of TTP with normal levels of the protease. Moreover, the available assays are time-consuming, poorly standardized and results are not always specific for TTP.

Patients critically ill with TTP are often first admitted to hospitals without facilities for plasma exchange; in such circumstances, daily infusion of large amounts of fresh-frozen plasma (FFP) (30 mL/kg) should be started promptly, taking measures to avoid volume overload (see Table 44.5). Patients are best assisted in intensive care units, where renal failure, coma, seizures and such severe side-effects of plasma exchange as congestive heart failure and catheter-related bleeding, thrombosis and infections can be optimally managed. At least 1 plasma volume should be exchanged daily until platelets rise to 150×10^9/L or more, LDH is normal and schistocytes are no longer present on blood films. Daily treatment with plasma exchange must be continued for at least 3 days after remission has been obtained (see Table 44.5).

Treatment should be continued following this schedule for at least 10 days, whether or not early signs of clinical and laboratory improvement are observed. Daily exchanges for up to 1 month are sometimes necessary to achieve remission of TTP. It is not established whether discontinuation of plasma therapy should be abrupt or progressive. Cryoprecipitate-depleted plasma can be used instead of FFP if this fraction is available and convenient, but there is no evidence that this VWF-poor plasma is more effective than whole plasma. Plasma treated with virus-inactivation methods (e.g. solvent/detergent) should be preferred because it decreases the risk of infections associated with patient exposure to plasma from a large number of donors.

Patients with congenital TTP usually respond well to plasma infusion. A periodic plasma infusion every 2 weeks is sufficient to supply enough ADAMTS-13 to maintain low but measurable plasma levels of the protease and avoid platelet consumption, a consequence of the long plasma half-life of the enzyme. The intensity of plasma therapy cannot be tailored to each patient's case because of the lack of criteria for predicting short-term prognosis (risk of death and organ failure in the acute episode) based on the presenting features of the episode. In addition, congenital TTP often has a relapsing course, so that some patients are treated prophylactically with plasma infusions at regularly spaced intervals (every 5–7 days) in order to prevent further disease episodes. However, since relapse is not a constant finding and there are no well-established predictive factors, it is not clear which patients should undergo regular prophylaxis and what levels of ADAMTS-13 are necessary to attain remission of the acute episode and prevent recurrence. There is as yet no definite evidence that patients with congenital ADAMTS-13 deficiency develop alloantibodies, nor that an anamnestic response invariably occurs in patients with autoantibodies after they are treated with plasma.

Table 44.6 Suggested immunological treatments of refractory antibody-mediated TTP.

Prednisone: 1–2 mg/kg for at least 15 days, then tapering the drug over 45 days

Vincristine: 2 mg on day 1, then 1 mg on days 3, 6 and 9

Cyclophosphamide or azathioprine: 100–200 mg/day

Intravenous immunoglobulins

Immunoadsorption on staphylococcal protein A

Splenectomy

Anti-CD20 (rituximab)

Other therapies

Before the advent of plasma therapy, clinicians used many other treatment modalities to attempt to control the dramatic course of TTP. Their generally poor efficacy is apparent from the fact that only with the advent of plasma therapy has mortality dropped dramatically. Hence, these treatments should be generally attempted only when plasma therapy at full doses and for at least a fortnight provides no or minimal benefit (refractory TTP) (Table 44.6).

There is little or no theoretical or practical role for the use of antiplatelet agents, because these drugs (including aspirin) fail to inhibit shear/VWF-mediated platelet aggregation, the prevailing pathogenic mechanism of thrombus formation in TTP. Inhibitors of GPIb, by blocking binding of ultra-large VWF multimers to platelets, should perhaps be considered in the prevention or early management of chronic recurrent TTP, but in full-blown TTP they may increase the risk of thrombocytopenic bleeding. The immune pathogenesis of TTP may be tackled by using immunomodulating agents such as corticosteroids, cyclophosphamide, azathioprine, intravenous immunoglobulins and immunoadsorption on staphylococcal protein A (Table 44.6). Splenectomy has also been attempted.

In general, it is difficult to recommend a useful agent or procedure. Considering that autoantibodies are a frequent pathogenetic mechanism, large doses of prednisone (1–2 mg/kg) are often prescribed in addition to plasma exchange during the acute phase of TTP, tapering this treatment when remission is obtained (see Table 44.5). The same treatment may be considered in the chronic recurrent variant of TTP due to the persistence of autoantibodies. Efficacy of corticosteroids is not unequivocally demonstrated, and the adverse effects of prolonged intake of large doses are severe. Splenectomy is an alternative option in patients with chronic recurrent forms during remission, but carries a high risk of death in severely ill patients with acute TTP.

Another recent attempt to suppress the production of anti-ADAMTS-13 autoantibodies is based on a monoclonal antibody directed against CD20 antigen (rituximab). This therapy may be considered in the chronic recurrent forms, particularly those cases of TTP not responding to treatment with plasma exchange and refractory to other immunomodulating agents. The aim of treatment with rituximab is to block the production of anti-ADAMTS-13 antibodies by depleting B lymphocytes. Various studies have reported that this treatment plays an important role in producing prolonged remissions in chronic recurrent TTP. Published small series and case reports have described approximately 100 patients with refractory or relapsing idiopathic TTP treated with rituximab, usually at doses of $375\,mg/m^2$ every 7 days repeated for at least three or four cycles. Approximately 95% of reported patients have had a complete clinical and laboratory response within 1–3 weeks of starting treatment, including a normal ADAMTS-13 level and disappearance of anti-ADAMTS-13 antibodies. Mild acute reactions to ritixumab infusion were controlled by premedication with steroids, antihistamines and analgesics. More serious complications are relatively uncommon. One patient had transient cardiogenic shock and another had symptomatic gastrointestinal infection with *Strongyloides*. Relapses appear infrequent, occurring in approximately 10% of patients after intervals of 9 months to 4 years; all but one of these patients had a second prolonged complete remission on retreatment with rituximab. It remains to be demonstrated whether the complete B-lymphocyte depletion caused by this drug is without short- or long-term consequences for patients.

A forthcoming promising approach is replacement therapy with ADAMTS-13 concentrates. A recombinant preparation has been shown to improve the defective proteolysis of VWF *in vitro*, but clinical trials with this product have not yet started. Another pharmaceutical company is considering the clinical evaluation of a DNA aptamer meant to inhibit the binding between GPIb and ultra-large VWF multimers, thereby preventing intravascular platelet aggregation in the microcirculation.

Haemolytic–uraemic syndrome

The typical form of HUS called diarrhoea-related HUS, or D(+) HUS, is acquired and occurs acutely and sporadically after gastrointestinal infections with toxin-producing bacteria, particularly in infants and young children but sometimes also in adults. There are two forms of atypical HUS. One is familial, has a sporadic or chronic recurrent course and is due to the inherited deficiency of complement factor H or other complement components. It occurs mainly in infants or young children but at least one-third of cases also occur in adults. Another atypical form of HUS occurs at all ages in association with situations commonly seen also in association with TTP (Table 44.7).

Diarrhoea-related HUS

This acute syndrome almost always occurs as a single sporadic episode, heralded 2 days to 2 weeks before by bloody diarrhoea.

Table 44.7 Variants of HUS.

Typical
  Exotoxin-producing bacteria (*E. coli* 0157:H7, *Shigella dysenteriae*)
Atypical
  Inherited (complement factor deficiency)
  Acquired (post partum, drugs, bone marrow transplantation, chemotherapy) (see also Table 44.1)

The typical symptoms are severe renal failure with oligoanuria, jaundice and haemorrhagic signs such as petechiae, haemolytic anaemia and raised levels of serum LDH, but usually less marked than in TTP. Serum creatinine and urea are definitely more abnormal than in TTP, while the presence of ultra-large VWF is much less frequent than in TTP. Signs of compensated DIC, with higher plasma levels of D-dimer, are another distinctive feature. Neurological involvement is uncommon, although coma and seizures may occur in association with uraemia and severe hypertension.

Aetiology

The most common bacterial agent that causes the prodromal gastrointestinal infection is *Escherichia coli* type 0157:H7 or, less frequently, *Shigella dysenteriae* serotype I. These and other more rarely involved infectious agents produce similar forms of exotoxins called verotoxin, shiga toxin and shiga-like toxins. These toxins, after absorption from the gastrointestinal tract into the blood, have in common the property to bind to the glycosphingolipid membrane receptor globotriaosylceramide that is particularly dense in the glomerular capillary endothelial cells of infants, young children and elderly individuals. The toxin–receptor complex is endocytosed and thereby causes cytolysis and extensive endothelial swelling and desquamation, which in turn engenders massive thrombus formation in the renal microvasculature.

Pathology and pathogenesis

The pathology of diarrhoea-related HUS is characterized by more extensive endothelial injury and less VWF and more fibrin deposition in thrombi than in TTP. The behaviour of plasma VWF is also different, because ultra-large highly thrombogenic multimers are detectable less frequently during the acute phase of the disease. This phenomenon is thought to be due to the fact that VWF multimers leaking in excess into plasma from damaged endothelial cells bind avidly to GPIb on the platelet membrane and are thereby removed from plasma, particularly the multimers of larger size. There is quasi-unanimity of views that ADAMTS-13 is normal or only mildly reduced in the plasma of patients with this variant of HUS (Table 44.8).

Table 44.8 Clinical applications of ADAMTS-13 testing in TTP and HUS.

Stage	ADAMTS-13 deficiency (<10%)	Diagnostic implications
Acute phase	Yes	TTP/atypical HUS
	No	Typical HUS/TTP cannot be excluded
Remission	Yes	Risk of relapse

ADAMTS-13 levels are usually normal or only mildly reduced in the thrombotic microangiopathies listed in Table 44.2.

Natural history

In the great majority of cases, diarrhoea-related HUS is self-limiting, with much less tendency to early or late relapses than TTP. The acute episode is often accompanied by such severe renal failure that temporary haemodialysis is frequently required. Residual renal dysfunction is common after the acute episode and renal failure requiring maintenance dialysis or kidney transplantation occurs in approximately one-third of patients.

Treatment

During the diarrhoeal prodrome antimotility agents are contraindicated, because they favour the permanence of the bacterial toxins in the gastrointestinal lumen and their passage into blood. The role of antibiotics is controversial but in practice they are often used, with a strong indication for patients with evidence or suspicion of sepsis or *S. dysenteriae* infection. In cases of significant acute renal failure, early institution of dialysis is essential in order to reduce sequelae and death. Plasma exchange is usually not recommended in patients with typical HUS, whereas it is indicated in the atypical forms (see below), emphasizing again the similarities between this variant of HUS and TTP. A possible forthcoming approach to the prevention of toxin-induced HUS is vaccination against vero/shiga toxins of children who live in endemic areas.

Familial HUS

Autosomal recessive and dominant forms of familial HUS without diarrhoeal prodromes account for about 5–10% of all cases (Table 44.7). This variant is associated with a markedly severe impairment of renal function and with a high mortality rate (approximately one-third of the cases). Approximately half of the patients who survive acute disease require maintenance haemodialysis. Approximately 50% of patients with familial atypical HUS have mutations in one of the complement regulatory proteins factor H, factor I, MCP or factor B, resulting in excessive C3 activation, membrane deposition of this complement fraction and renal cell injury. A few patients have also

been described with autoantibodies against factor H. Patients with MCP mutations have a better prognosis than those with factor H mutations or no mutation. A recessively transmitted variant of familial HUS is very rare and is associated with very low levels of factor H in plasma and with the early onset of HUS in childhood. Dominantly transmitted variants are usually due to missense mutations in the gene encoding factor H, causing the production of normal amounts of a dysfunctional protein. Dominantly transmitted HUS is usually less severe than the recessive form, and occurs in late infancy or adulthood. Low serum C3 levels may be a simple and widely available method for diagnosing affected patients and detecting family members at risk.

Treatment of familial HUS is based on the replacement of factor H with FFP, combined with transient haemodialysis to attempt to control oligoanuria and uraemia. The outcome of kidney transplantation appears to correlate with the cause of complement dysregulation. Disease has not recurred in transplanted kidneys in patients with MCP mutations, presumably because the new kidney has protective levels of endogenous MCP. In contrast, kidney transplantation alone does not correct the deficiency of plasma factors made in the liver, and the outcome is poor in patients with factor H or factor I mutations owing to disease recurrence. However, combined liver and kidney transplantation may lead to a favourable long-term outcome for recurrent HUS associated with a factor H mutation. The severity of the disease warrants gene transfer as a therapeutic approach, but lack of animal models and of suitable vectors of the transgene have hindered this approach so far.

Atypical (non-diarrhoea-related) HUS

This form can only be distinguished from TTP by the absence of neurological symptoms and the predominance of renal symptoms. There are cases of atypical HUS associated with severe deficiency of ADAMTS-13, albeit less frequently than in TTP. Atypical HUS is often associated with the postpartum period or with the intake of several drugs (see Table 44.7). Individuals who have been treated for various illnesses by bone marrow transplantation make up a relatively large subgroup. Plasma therapy, using the same protocol recommended for TTP, is the treatment of choice.

Concluding remarks

In the last few years, TTP and HUS, known for several decades to clinicians and pathologists for their dire consequences, have witnessed spectacular improvements in knowledge of the pathogenesis and development of new diagnostic criteria and seen mortality and morbidity decrease. The pivotal role of VWF and of its major proteolytic enzyme in inducing microvascular platelet thrombi is evident, even though not all the variants of TTP, and particularly of HUS, fit this disease mechanism. Other proteins disposing of ultra-large highly thrombogenic forms of VWF may be involved. The development of laboratory methods to measure ADAMTS-13 in plasma has demonstrated that several types of TTP have very low levels of this protease. On the other hand, severe ADAMTS-13 deficiency is not found in all patients who have the appropriate clinical criteria for diagnosis of TTP (Table 44.8), questioning the significance of these criteria or the appropriateness of the currently available functional assays performed in non-physiological static conditions. The trigger(s) of full-blown TTP or HUS needs to be elucidated, because patients with constitutionally low levels of ADAMTS-13 or factor H may not manifest disease for long periods of time. It also remains to be understood which, and how many, cases respond to replacement therapy with protease concentrates, whether derived from plasma or made by recombinant DNA technologies. Meanwhile, the clinician confronted with the difficult treatment of these seriously ill patients should be cognizant that plasma therapy, mainly plasma exchange, remains the treatment of choice for all patients with clinically diagnosed TTP and the related syndrome called atypical HUS. Another important unresolved therapeutic problem is that of secondary prevention of the chronic recurrent forms. Various treatments have been tried, from chronic low-dose corticosteroids or other immunomodulatory agents (vincristine, immunoglobulins) to the more recent use of anti-CD20 monoclonal antibodies. There are anecdotal reports of the efficacy of all these agents, but their use is based on small series and reports are affected by publication bias. The prophylactic administration of plasma is plausible in the genetic forms, but much less so in the immune-mediated ones.

Diarrhoea-related HUS is now well characterized from an aetiological standpoint, so that it can be recognized and properly treated by paediatricians. A major problem remains the prevention of inherited HUS associated with factor H deficiency, because the long-term consequences of this scourge are dire. A suitable screening test is not yet available, even though there is the theoretical possibility of a DNA-based approach: most mutations are located in the exon encoding the most C-terminal short consensus repeat involved in binding factor H to complement C3b and to sialic acid molecules on host cells, thereby protecting host cells from excessive C3 activation.

There are numerous problems left to solve and, given the rarity of these conditions, clinical research on TTP and HUS must be necessarily multicentre.

Selected bibliography

Bell WR, Braine HG, Ness PM *et al.* (1991) Improved survival in thrombotic thrombocytopenic purpura–haemolytic uraemic syndrome. Clinical experience in 108 patients. *New England Journal of Medicine* 325: 398–403.

Bukowski RM, King JW, Hewlett JS (1977) Plasmapheresis in the treatment of thrombotic thrombocytopenic purpura. *Blood* 50: 413–17.

Furlan M, Robles R, Galbusera M *et al.* (1998) von Willebrand factor-cleaving protease in thrombotic thrombocytopenic purpura and the haemolytic–uraemic syndrome. *New England Journal of Medicine* 339: 1578–84.

George JN (2000) How I treat patients with thrombotic thrombocytopenic purpura–haemolytic uraemic syndrome. *Blood* 96: 1223–9.

Hovinga JA, Vesely SK, Terrell DR, Lämmle B, George JN (2010) Survival and relapse in patients with thrombotic thrombocytopenic purpura. *Blood* 115: 1500–11.

Levy GG, Nichols WC, Lian EC *et al.* (2001) Mutations in a member of the *ADAMTS* gene family cause thrombotic thrombocytopenic purpura. *Nature* 413: 488–94.

Mannucci PM, Lombardi R, Lattuada A *et al.* (1989) Enhanced proteolysis of plasma von Willebrand factor in thrombotic thrombocytopenic purpura and the haemolytic uraemic syndrome. *Blood* 74: 978–83.

Mannucci PM, Canciani MT, Forza I *et al.* (2001) Changes in health and disease of the metalloprotease that cleaves von Willebrand factor. *Blood* 98: 2730–5.

Manuelian T, Hellwage J, Meri S *et al.* (2003) Mutations in factor H reduce binding affinity to C3b and heparin and surface attachment to endothelial cells in hemolytic uremic syndrome. *Journal of Clinical Investigation* 111: 1181–90.

Moake J (1998) Moschcowitz, multimers, and metalloprotease. *New England Journal of Medicine* 339: 1629–31.

Moake JL (2002) Thrombotic microangiopathies. *New England Journal of Medicine* 347: 589–600.

Moake JL, Rudy CK, Troll JH *et al.* (1982) Unusually large plasma factor VIII: von Willebrand factor multimers in chronic relapsing thrombotic thrombocytopenic purpura. *New England Journal of Medicine* 307: 1432–5.

Moake JL, Turner NA, Stathopoulos NA, Nolasco LH, Hellums JD (1986) Involvement of large plasma von Willebrand factor (VWF) multimers and unusually large VWF forms derived from endothelial cells in shear stress-induced platelet aggregation. *Journal of Clinical Investigation* 78: 1456–61.

Moore JB, Hayward CPM, Warkentin TE *et al.* (2001) Decreased von Willebrand factor protease activity associated with thrombocytopenic disorders. *Blood* 98: 1842–6.

Remuzzi G, Ruggenenti P, Bertani T (1994) Thrombotic microangiopathy. In: *Renal Pathology* (CC Tisher, MM Brenner, eds), 2nd edn, p. 1154. Lippincott, Philadelphia.

Remuzzi G, Galbusera M, Noris M *et al.* (2002) Thrombotic thrombocytopenic purpura/haemolytic uraemic syndrome: von Willebrand factor cleaving protease (ADAMTS-13) is deficient in recurrent and familial thrombotic thrombocytopenic purpura and haemolytic uraemic syndrome. *Blood* 100: 778–85.

Rock GA, Shumak KH, Buskard NA *et al.* (1991) Comparison of plasma exchange with plasma infusion in the treatment of thrombotic thrombocytopenic purpura. Canadian Apheresis Study Group. *New England Journal of Medicine* 325: 393–7.

Ruggenenti P, Galbusera M, Cornejo RP *et al.* (1993) Thrombotic thrombocytopenic purpura: evidence that infusion rather than removal of plasma induces remission of the disease. *American Journal of Kidney Disease* **21**: 314–18.

Sadler JE (2008) Von Willebrand factor, ADAMTS-13, and thrombotic thrombocytopenic purpura. *Blood* **112**: 11–18.

Shelat SG, Ai J, Zheng XL (2005) Molecular biology of ADAMTS13 and diagnostic utility of ADAMTS13 proteolytic activity and inhibitor assays. *Seminars in Thrombosis and Hemostasis* **31**: 659–72.

Tripodi A, Peyvandi F, Chantarangkul V *et al.* (2008) Second international collaborative study evaluating performance characteristics of methods measuring the von Willebrand factor cleaving protease (ADAMTS-13). *Journal of Thrombosis and Haemostasis* **6**: 1534–41.

Tsai HM, Lian EC (1998) Antibodies to von Willebrand factor-cleaving protease in acute thrombotic thrombocytopenic purpura. *New England Journal of Medicine* **339**: 1585–94.

Upshwas JD (1978) Congenital deficiency of a factor in normal plasma that reverses microangiopathic hemolysis and thrombocytopenia. *New England Journal of Medicine* **298**: 1350–2.

Vesely SK, George JN, Lammle B *et al.* (2003) ADAMTS-13 activity in thrombotic thrombocytopenic purpura–haemolytic uraemic syndrome: relation to presenting features and clinical outcomes in a prospective cohort of 142 patients. *Blood* **102**: 60–8.

Zheng XL, Sadler JE (2008) Pathogenesis of thrombotic microangiopathies. *Annual Review of Pathology* **3**: 249–77.

Zheng X, Chung D, Takayama TK *et al.* (2001) Structure of von Willebrand factor-cleaving protease (ADAMTS-13), a metalloprotease involved in thrombotic thrombocytopenic purpura. *Journal of Biological Chemistry* **276**: 41059–63.

Heritable thrombophilia

45

Trevor Baglin

Cambridge University Hospitals NHS Trust, Addenbrookes Hospital, Cambridge, UK

Introduction

In most instances heritable thrombophilia is a late-onset genetic disease with low penetrance. There is no internationally accepted definition of thrombophilia. The term is sometimes used to describe disorders of haemostasis detected in the laboratory that appear to predispose to venous thrombosis. A clinical definition of heritable thrombophilia describes an inherited tendency for venous thrombosis, i.e. deep vein thrombosis (DVT) with or without associated pulmonary embolus. The incidence of a first episode of venous thrombosis is 1.5 per 1000 person-years, with a per-person lifetime incidence of 5%. Venous thrombosis is a multicausal disease. Understanding the genetic risk factors and gene–environment interactions is necessary to understand why an individual develops thrombosis at a specific point in time. Venous thrombosis is a disease in which genetic and acquired risk factors interact dynamically. Interaction occurs when two risk factors in combination produce an effect that exceeds the sum of their separate effects. Familial thrombophilia is a multiple gene disorder and family members may have more than one identifiable defect, probably in combination with additional candidate and totally unknown defects. It is likely that

this largely explains why a dichotomous testing strategy with a limited number of factors (e.g. presence or absence of FVR506Q) has limited predictive value, resulting in little if any clinical utility for most patients (clinical utility refers to the ability of a screening or diagnostic test to improve clinical outcome).

Deficiency of the natural anticoagulant antithrombin was the first reported inherited risk factor for venous thromboembolism. Since then deficiencies of the naturally occurring anticoagulants protein C and protein S have been linked with familial thrombosis. In recent years, several other potential thrombophilic risk factors have been investigated but only the F5G1691A (FVR506Q, factor V Leiden) and the F2G20210A gene mutations have been shown to be unequivocally associated with an increased risk of thrombosis, i.e. odds ratio (OR) of 2 or greater from case–control studies. In the 1980s and 1990s thrombophilia testing became common in unselected patients and their relatives despite the fact that there was no evidence that testing had clinical utility. It is now apparent that testing for heritable thrombophilia typically does not predict likelihood of recurrence in the majority of unselected patients with symptomatic venous thrombosis (Figure 45.1). Furthermore, testing for inherited thrombophilia did not reduce recurrence of venous thrombosis in a large cohort study. There is a low risk of thrombosis in affected asymptomatic relatives of patients with thrombophilic defects followed prospectively and the results of thrombophilia tests are frequently misinterpreted. Given these considerations the clinician must consider the

Postgraduate Haematology: 6th edition. Edited by A. Victor Hoffbrand, Daniel Catovsky, Edward G.D. Tuddenham, Anthony R. Green

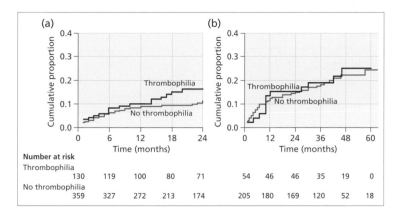

Figure 45.1 Cumulative recurrence of venous thrombosis in consecutive patients with and without heritable thrombophilia followed from the end of anticoagulation after a first episode of venous thrombosis in the first (a) and second (b) Cambridge cohort studies. The hazard ratio for recurrence in patients with thrombophilia compared with those without was 1.3 (95% CI 0.8–2.0) and 1.0 (95% CI 0.5–2.1), respectively. For ease of comparison, the point of 10% cumulative recurrence at 24

months is indicated on each chart. In the second cohort, patients with postoperative thrombosis were excluded, which may account for the apparent slightly higher recurrence rate. (For related publications on these cohorts, see Baglin *et al.* 2003 and Baglin T, Palmer CR, Luddington R, Baglin C (2008) Unprovoked recurrent venous thrombosis: prediction by D-dimer and clinical risk factors. *Journal of Thrombosis and Haemostasis* **6**: 577–82.)

potential clinical utility of testing for heritable thrombophilic defects in each individual patient or family affected by venous thrombosis.

Heritable thrombophilias associated with venous thrombosis

The heritable thrombophilias shown to be associated with at least a twofold increased risk of venous thrombosis are (i) deficiencies of the natural anticoagulants antithrombin, protein C and protein S, due to mutations in the corresponding genes *SERPINC1*, *PROC* and *PROS*, and (ii) two common mutations in genes encoding procoagulant factors, namely *F5G1691A* (FVR506Q, factor V Leiden) and *F2G20210A* (commonly referred to as the prothrombin gene mutation). The causal association between these heritable thrombophilias and venous thrombosis has been confirmed by comparing the prevalence of defects in patients with venous thrombosis and controls. In such studies measurement errors between cases and controls do not arise in relation to genotype and so the case–control study is the method of choice for measuring simple associations between genotype and disease. The prevalence of the heritable thrombophilias in cases and controls is shown in Table 45.1. The relative risk of venous thrombosis is estimated from the OR (the odds of the disease among those with the risk factor to the odds of the disease without the risk factor). The OR for each defect is indicated in Table 45.1. Deficiencies of antithrombin, protein C and protein S are rare and so the estimates of risks are uncertain but appear to be of the order of about a 10-fold increased risk of venous thrombosis. The FVR506Q and

Table 45.1 Prevalence of heritable thrombophilias shown to be associated with at least a twofold increased risk of venous thrombosis in patients and controls and relative risk of a first episode of venous thrombosis.

	General population	Consecutive patients with a first episode of venous thrombosis	Relative risk of venous thrombosis
Antithrombin	0.03%	1%	10–20
Protein C deficiency	0.3%	3%	10
Protein S deficiency	0.3%	3%	?–10
FVR506Q (FV Leiden)*	4%	15%	4
*F2G20210A**	2%	4%	2

*The prevalence of FVR506Q and *F2G20210A* is determined by ethnic origin as these mutations are only prevalent in whites.

F2G20210A occur much more frequently and so the estimates of risk are more certain.

Gene–environment interaction is present when the effect of genotype on disease risk depends on the level of exposure to an environmental factor. Heritable thrombophilia is subject to a strong gene–environment interaction. For example, there is a synergistic increase in risk of venous thrombosis due to an interaction between the factor V Leiden mutation and estrogen exposure. Another example is observed in patients with antithrombin deficiency where venous thrombosis frequently occurs when an affected patient is exposed to an environmental risk. This was evident in a study of families with type 1 antithrombin deficiency where the incidence of venous thrombosis was 20 times greater in affected family members but was strongly dependent on acquired risks. In this study the annual incidence of venous thrombosis in affected family members in any year in which they were exposed to surgery, trauma, plaster cast, hospitalization or immobilization was 20% (provoked venous thrombosis) but in any year in which there was no exposure the incidence was only 0.3% (i.e. unprovoked venous thrombosis rate). In this study the unprovoked venous thrombosis rate is only slightly, if at all, higher than the background incidence in the general population.

Antithrombin deficiency

The gene for antithrombin (*SERPINC1*) is located on the long arm of chromosome 1 and contains seven exons spanning 13.5 kb. Antithrombin (previously termed antithrombin III) is a glycoprotein (464 amino acids, 58 kDa, plasma concentration 2–3 μmol/L). Antithrombin is a serpin (*ser*ine *p*rotease *in*hibitor). Based on rates of inhibition, its primary targets are thrombin, factor (F)Xa and FIXa. Its concentration in the circulation is higher than that of prothrombin, and as only a fraction of prothrombin is converted to thrombin during coagulation, antithrombin is potentially present in vast excess over the protease, although the site will determine the local concentration of the enzyme and inhibitor. The plasma half-life of antithrombin is about 90 hours.

The serpin mechanism was confirmed by successful resolution of a crystal structure of the final serpin–protease complex by Jim Huntington in 2000. In contrast to the classical lock-and-key mechanism of protease inhibition, serpins form a stable covalent complex in which there is a dramatic conformational change in both the inhibitor and the inhibited protein that alters the properties of each, resulting in rapid clearance from the circulation. Antithrombin consists of three β-sheets and nine α-helices organized into an upper β-barrel domain and a lower helical domain. These two domains are bridged by the main structural feature of a serpin, the central A sheet (shown in red in Figure 45.2). The flexible reactive centre loop (RCL, shown in yellow) contains the scissile bond formed by the P1 arginine and P1′ serine. Amino acids in the RCL are designated P1, P2 and so forth moving towards the N-terminus of the peptide sequence and P1′, P2′ and so forth moving towards the C-terminus of the sequence. The length and flexibility of the loop renders it highly susceptible to proteolysis. Cleavage of the RCL by thrombin, FXa or FIXa produces a conformational change during which the RCL inserts as the central strand of the expanded central A sheet (Figure 45.2c). This results in translocation of the protease to the opposite pole

of the serpin. The incorporation of the RCL as the central strand produces a hyperstable molecule such that the protease is crushed by intermolecular clashes with the hyperstable serpin. Distortion of the active site architecture disrupts the catalytic triad and results in disorganization of almost 40% of the protease architecture. The poor inhibitory activity of the circulating native form of antithrombin is conferred by intramolecular contacts that restrain the RCL and orientate the P1 arginine away from attacking proteases (Figure 45.2a). Activation causing release of the RCL is dependent on binding of glycosaminoglycans to the 'heparin-binding site' located in the region of the D-helix (cyan in Figure 45.2). An initial low-affinity interaction induces high-affinity binding (referred to as the induced fit mechanism) and this produces a conformational change in the antithrombin that releases the RCL for protease attack (Figure 45.2b). Activation increases the rate of protease inactivation 1000-fold. Successful inhibition of the protease depends on a race between complete proteolysis of the RCL with release of the regenerated protease from the cleaved loop (the substrate pathway) and incorporation of the cleaved loop into the central A-sheet with resultant capture and crushing of the tethered protease (the inhibitory pathway). The rate of inhibition relative to the substrate reaction is defined as the stoichiometry of inhibition, where a value of 1 represents a perfect inhibitor and a value of 2 would indicate that half the reactions led to cleaved antithrombin and a regenerated protease. Some mutations in the *SERPINC1* gene produce a dysfunctional antithrombin molecule in which the insertion of the RCL into the central A-sheet is retarded, turning the molecule into a substrate rather than an inhibitor. This is an example of how this highly regulated mechanism of thrombin or FXa inhibition renders antithrombin susceptible to dysfunction through genetic mutation.

Two laboratory (intermediate) phenotypes of heritable antithrombin deficiency are recognized. Type 1 is characterized by a quantitative reduction of antithrombin, with a parallel reduction in function (measured as inhibitory activity) and level of protein in the plasma (measured immunologically as the antigenic level). Type 2 deficiency is due to the production of a qualitatively abnormal antithrombin protein with dysfunction due to disturbance of the complex inhibitory mechanism of protease inhibition by a mutation in *SERPINC1* gene. The functional activity is discrepantly low compared with the antigenic level. Type 2 deficiency is subclassified according to the nature of the functional deficit.

• Type 2 reactive site (RS): mutations alter the sequence of the RCL, reducing the ability to inhibit thrombin or FXa in the presence or absence of heparin in a laboratory assay.

• Type 2 heparin-binding site (HBS): mutations affect the ability of antithrombin to bind and be activated by glycosaminoglycans and therefore result in reduced ability to inhibit thrombin or FXa only in the presence of heparin in a laboratory assay. These mutations are typically located in the

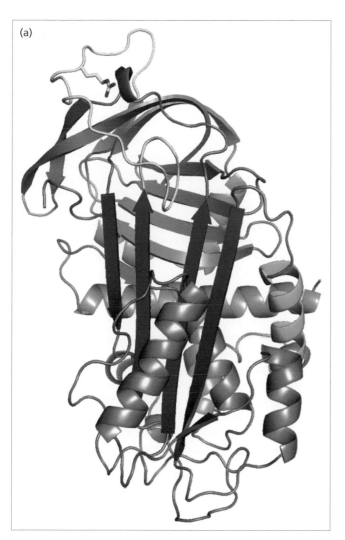

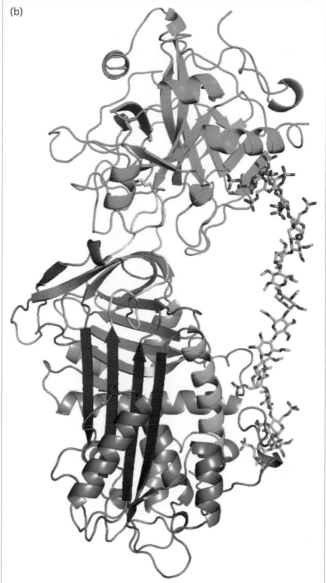

Figure 45.2 Model of thrombin destruction by antithrombin. Native antithrombin (a) circulates predominantly in an inert configuration with the reactive centre loop (RCL, shown in yellow) restrained on the C-sheet with the P1 arginine buried in a hydrophobic pocket and innaccesible to proteolytic attack. Binding of a glyscosaminoglycan such as heparin sulphate to helix D (shown in cyan) induces a conformational change in the molecule that results in closure of the central A-sheet (shown in red), release of the RCL and exposure of the P1 arginine for proteolytic attack by protease (shown in green) resulting in the formation of an encounter complex (b). A heparin chain is shown bridging antithrombin and thrombin. The heparin chain binds to the D-helix of antithrombin, inducing the conformational change and stabilizing the resultant encounter complex by binding to exosite II on thrombin. Cleavage of the RCL results in opening of the central A-sheet and incorporation of the cleaved loop as the central strand (c). This movement throws the protease to the opposite pole of the molecule where it is crushed by intermolecular clashes with antithrombin, which is now in a hyperstable conformation. Inhibition of the protease depends on incorporation of the cleaved loop into the central A-sheet with resultant capture and crushing of the tethered protease with distortion of the catalytic triad before completion of proteolysis of the RCL, which would release the protease. (Courtesy of Dr Jim Huntington, Department of Haematology, University of Cambridge.)

(c)

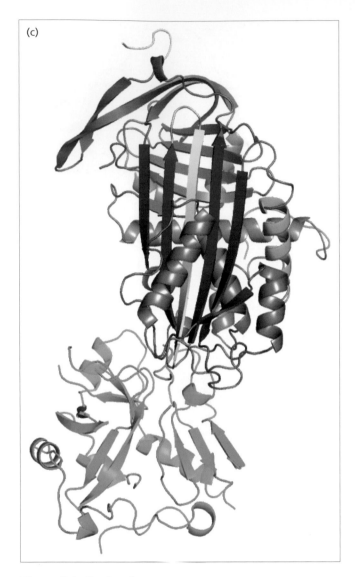

Figure 45.2 *Continued*

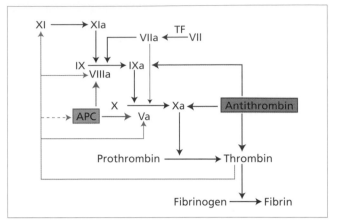

Figure 45.3 The thrombin explosion occurs in two phases: initiation and propagation. In the initiation phase, tissue factor (TF)–FVIIa generates small amounts of thrombin that enhances platelet activation (in conjunction with exposed subendothelial collagen at the site of vascular injury) and cleaves FV and FVIII to their active forms. The activation of FVa and FVIIIa amplifies thrombin generation and increasing concentrations of thrombin then lead to back-activation of FXI and the propagation phase. The activated forms of FV and FVIII are non-enzymatic cofactors that assemble and orientate the enzymes (FIXa and FXa) on the negatively charged surface of activated platelets. Antithrombin can neutralize the enzymatic coagulant factors FIXa, FXa and FIIa (thrombin). Thrombin bound to thrombomodulin cleaves protein C to its active form (APC), which proteolyses FVa and FVIIIa and dismantles the tenase (FVIIIa–FIXa) and prothrombinase (FVa–FIIa) complexes on phospholipid surfaces, which attenuates thrombin generation. Protein S is a cofactor for the APC-mediated inactivation of FVa and FVIIIa.

Protein C deficiency

The gene for protein C (*PROC*) is located on chromosome 2 and contains nine exons spanning 11 kb. Protein C is a vitamin K-dependent glycoprotein synthesized in the liver (419 amino acids, 62 kDa, plasma concentration 65 nmol/L). Its concentration in plasma is about 100 times less than that of antithrombin. The plasma half-life of protein C is about 6 hours.

Protein C is the zymogen precursor of activated protein C (APC). Protein C is activated by thrombin bound to thrombomodulin on the endothelial surface. This is facilitated by the endothelial protein C receptor (EPCR). APC acts as a physiological anticoagulant by cleaving the cofactors FVa and FVIIIa and so thrombin generation (which is dependent on FVa and FVIIIa cofactor activity) is attenuated (Figure 45.3). Protein S is a cofactor for APC-mediated inactivation of FVa and FVIIIa.

Protein C deficiency is classified into type 1 and 2 defects on the basis of functional and antigenic assays. The relative risk of thrombosis in relation to type 1 and the various type 2 defects has not been characterized. Most heritable protein C deficiency

designated 'heparin-binding site' in the region of the D helix of the molecule.

• Type 2 pleiotropic (PE): a single mutation produces multiple effects on the structure–function relationship of the molecule, often associated with low plasma levels due to either effects on secretion or instability.

Approximately 100 point mutations (missense, nonsense or insertions or deletions causing frameshifts) and several whole or partial gene deletions have been identified as causes of type 1 deficiency. Numerous point mutations causing qualitative type 2 deficiency have been identified. Homozygous type 1 deficiency and probably homozygous type 2 RS mutations are incompatible with life. Type 2 HBS and PE mutations are associated with a lower risk of thrombosis and are compatible with life.

is due to type 1 deficiency. The majority of type 1 defects are due to point mutations. Multiple type 2 defects have been reported involving the catalytic active site, the phospholipid-binding Gla domain, the propeptide cleavage activation site and sites of interaction with substrates or cofactors.

Protein S deficiency

The gene for protein S (*PROS*) is located on chromosome 3 and contains 15 exons spanning 80 kb. A pseudogene with approximately 95% homology is located adjacent to *PROS* and this can cause difficulty with identification of mutations within the *PROS* gene.

Protein S is a vitamin K-dependent glycoprotein produced in the liver, endothelial cells and megakaryocytes (676 amino acids, 69 kDa, plasma concentration of free protein 145 nmol/L). Protein S is a non-enzymatic cofactor for APC-mediated inactivation of FVa and FVIIIa. Approximately 60% circulates bound to C4b-binding protein and is inactive. The remaining 40%, designated free protein S, is uncomplexed and is the active form. Free protein S increases the affinity of APC for negatively charged phospholipid surfaces on platelets or the endothelium and increases complex formation of APC with the activated forms of FV (FVa) and FVIII (FVIIIa). However, the degree of C4b binding has not yet been shown to be a determinant of thrombosis risk. In addition to APC cofactor activity, protein S has an independent anticoagulant effect by acting as a cofactor for TFPI (tissue factor pathway inhibitor).

Protein S defects are divided into three types. In type I deficiency both total and free protein S levels are low (and functional activity is low if measured). In type III the total protein S level is normal but the free protein S level is low. Some type III deficiency is thought to be a phenotypic variation resulting from the same genetic mutations associated with classical type I deficiency. However, it is now apparent that many patients with an apparent type III phenotype do not have heritable protein S deficiency. This may be related to the increase in C4b levels with increasing age. Type II defects are characterized by reduced activity in the presence of normal total and free levels of protein S. Type II deficiency is difficult to diagnose because functional protein S assays are imprecise.

FVR506Q (factor V Leiden)

The gene for FV is located on chromosome 1, near the *SERPINC1* gene, and contains 25 exons spanning 80 kb. FV (2196 amino acids, 330 kDa, plasma concentration of free protein 30 nmol/L) is the cofactor for activation of prothrombin by FXa in the prothrombinase complex. The plasma half-life is 15 hours. It has no cofactor activity until cleaved by thrombin or FXa at Arg709, Arg1018 and Arg1545. In 1993, Bjorn Dahlbach and colleagues in Malmo described the phenomenon of resistance to APC in unrelated patients with venous thrombosis. Patient plasma was resistant to the anticoagulant effect of a fixed amount of added exogenous APC. The effect was measured by dividing the activated partial thromboplastin time (APTT) in the presence of added APC by the APTT in the absence of added APC. APC resistance was defined as a ratio less than 2.0. Further work confirmed that increased APC resistance cosegregated with thrombosis in families with familial venous thromboembolism. The following year it was reported by a team from Leiden that the majority of patients with familial APC resistance had the same point mutation in the gene for FV, a guanine to adenine transition at nucleotide 1691 in exon 10 of the *F5* gene. This is known as the FV Leiden mutation (FVR506Q). Mutant FV Leiden has normal procoagulant activity but substitution of glutamine for arginine at position 506 results in slower inactivation by APC. FVa is a cofactor for the assembly of the prothrombinase complex, the active component of which is the activated form of FX (FXa), which converts prothrombin to thrombin (Figure 45.3). FVa is generated from FV by cleavage by thrombin, thus providing a positive feedback loop for thrombin generation. Prothrombinase activity is dependent on FVa maintaining the integrity of the enzymatic complex unit on a phospholipid surface. Thus thrombin generation is rate limited by FVa, and inactivation of FVa by APC attenuates thrombin generation. Inactivation of FVa occurs through sequential cleavage of the protein at positions Arg306, Arg506 and Arg679 by APC. Initial cleavage at R506 is necessary for subsequent cleavage at R306 and R679. Mutation of these residues (*F5*G1691A, FVR506Q or FV Leiden; *F5*G1091C, FVA306T or FV Cambridge) results in resistance to inactivation by APC. APC resistance is observed in the laboratory as an impaired plasma anticoagulant response to APC added *in vitro*, usually with an APTT-based clotting test. However, nowadays the mutation is frequently detected by direct DNA analysis rather than by a clotting assay (see section on laboratory testing). The FVR506Q mutation is present in about 4% of the white population and about 15% of unselected consecutive patients with a first venous thrombosis. The prevalence is highest in northern Europeans. The mutation is infrequent in other populations. The high prevalence and founder effect suggests positive selection and this may relate to a favourable effect on embryo implantation and hence reproduction rather than a lower risk of fatal haemorrhage in females during childbirth, as originally thought.

APC also inactivates FVIIIa by cleavage at positions Arg336 and Arg562 but mutations affecting these sites in FVIII causing an increased risk of venous thrombosis have not been reported.

APC resistance in the absence of FVR506Q occurs in about 5% of patients with a history of venous thrombosis. This is often related to high FVIII levels or low FV levels, which may be found in association with the *F5*HR2 haplotype. There is evidence that APC resistance in the absence of FVR506Q is associated with venous thrombosis but defining the cause of resistance in individual patients has no clinical utility. Acquired APC resistance is explained by increased FVIII levels, pregnancy or estrogen exposure in some individuals.

*F2*G20210A

The gene for prothrombin is located on chromosome 2 and contains 14 exons spanning 21 kb. Prothrombin is a vitamin K-dependent protein synthesized in the liver (579 amino acids, 72 kDa, plasma concentration 2 μmol/L). Prothrombin is the zymogen precursor of thrombin.

A single nucleotide change, guanine to adenine at position 20210 in the 3′ untranslated region of the prothrombin gene (*F2*G20210A), is associated with elevated plasma prothrombin levels and an increased risk of venous thrombosis. This mutation was identified by the Leiden team when investigating candidate genes in the Leiden Thrombophilia Study cohort. The prevalence of the *F2*G20210A mutation is about 2% of whites, with a higher prevalence in southern compared with northern Europeans. The mutation increases the plasma level of prothrombin by about 30% but the mechanism has not been explained. No specific clotting test for the presence of the mutation has been described and diagnosis depends on detection of the genetic mutation by DNA analysis.

Candidate heritable thrombophilias

Peter Reitsma and Frits Rosendaal from Leiden have detailed the history of unravelling the genetic architecture of venous thrombosis risk. Initially, extended pedigrees of families with venous thrombosis were studied and plasma levels of natural anticoagulants were measured. With the advent of DNA technology, genes encoding the natural anticoagulant proteins were cloned and sequenced and hundreds of private mutations were reported, often with mutations found only in one family. Subsequently, the common public mutations (*F5*G1691A and *F2*G20210A) were found in case–control studies. Currently, common genetic markers in every gene encoding a protein involved in haemostasis are being studied in order to determine whether these markers are associated with thrombosis risk. Two types of genetic mutation cause venous thrombosis: those that reduce function (e.g. a mutation causing antithrombin deficiency) and those that increase function (e.g. FVR506Q, which renders the mutant protein resistant to inactivation, resulting in increased thrombin generation). The private mutations in *SERPINC1*, *PROC* and *PROS* and public mutations in *F5* and *F2* account for about 50% of the thrombosis risk attributable to genetic mutation. There are two approaches to identifying the remaining 50% of genetic mutations. A linkage study requires extended pedigree analysis and is limited by heterogeneity in the genetic cause of thrombosis in different families. This dilutes the apparent effect of a genetic mutation when data from different pedigrees are combined. The alternative approach is to use genetic markers of common risk alleles in association studies of unrelated individuals using genome-wide genotyping of a large set of single-nucleotide polymorphisms (SNPs). This approach relies on the principle that common diseases are explained by common risk alleles. The weakness of this approach is that there is little evidence that this principle is true. With this approach there is also a high risk of misidentifying a risk allele (type I error) due to multiple testing and in order to offset this it is necessary to raise the significance level of testing, which then leads to decreased sensitivity (type II error). Reitsma and Rosendaal suggest that a deep resequencing project may identify genetic factors and allow powerful genetic risk profiling. This hypothesis is supported by an initial proof of principle study showing that common SNPs which in isolation confer a very small risk of venous thrombosis (hazard ratio <1.5) interact synergistically to significantly increase the risk of venous thrombosis (hazard ratio >5.0 for four SNPs).

Other natural anticoagulants

Tissue factor pathway inhibitor (TFPI) is an inhibitor of FXa and tissue factor-bound FVIIa. TFPI knockout is embryonically lethal in mice. TFPI is predominantly extravascular and so measurement in plasma samples is not representative of total TFPI availability. In a few studies plasma TFPI levels were slightly lower in patients with venous thrombosis than in normal individuals and the low levels may be a mild risk factor for venous thrombosis. Protein Z is a vitamin K-dependent protein that circulates in complex with PZI (protein Z-dependent protease inhibitor) and catalyses the inhibition of FXa. A causal relationship between PZI and/or PZ deficiency and venous thrombosis has not been demonstrated. Heparin cofactor II, a serpin with a similar structure–function relationship to antithrombin, inhibits thrombin when activated by glycosaminoglycans. Heparin cofactor II knockout mice are healthy and do not develop spontaneous thrombosis but do have a shorter time to thrombosis in an arterial injury model. A relationship between heparin cofactor II deficiency and thrombosis in humans is uncertain. A relationship between thrombosis and mutations affecting thrombomodulin or EPCR has not been established.

Other procoagulant factors

Increased FVIII levels are associated with an increased risk of both venous and arterial thrombosis but a heritable basis for this, other than through ABO blood group effects on von Willebrand factor levels, has not been established. Elevated FIX and FXI levels are also associated with venous thrombosis risk but a heritable basis for high levels associated with venous thrombosis is not established. There is equivocal evidence for a causal relationship between fibrinogen levels and venous thrombosis. Approximately 300 examples of heritable dysfibrinogenaemia have been reported. The majority are asymptomatic or associated with increased bleeding and very few examples are considered to be genuinely associated with an increased tendency to thrombosis, which may be arterial or venous or a combination. Dysfibrinogenaemia has been found in less than 1% of patients with a history of venous thromboembolism. It is associated with postpartum thrombosis and an increased risk of pregnancy loss. The identification and characterization of rare dysfibrinogenaemias associated with thrombosis is beyond the capability of most coagulation laboratories. Polymorphisms in the prothrombin gene have been described that may further increase the risk of venous thrombosis associated with the *F2G20210A* mutation but the effect is mild. It was previously thought that deficiency of FXII was a risk factor for venous thromboembolism but subsequent investigation strongly indicates that this is unlikely. A polymorphism in the FXIII gene (FXIIIV341L) is significantly less common in patients with coronary heart disease than in control subjects and a protective effect for venous thromboembolism has been reported.

Fibrinolysis

A causal relationship between levels of individual specific proteins involved in regulating fibrinolysis has not been established. However, a global measure of fibrinolytic potential as measured by a plasma-clot lysis assay was associated with an approximately twofold increased risk of venous thrombosis in patients with clot lysis times above the 90th percentile of controls in the Leiden Thrombophilia Study. Analysis of the large MEGA (Multiple Environmental and Genetic Assessment) study confirmed this finding and demonstrated that hypofibrinolysis in combination with established acquired and genetic risk factors, such as FVR506Q, had a synergistic effect on venous thrombosis risk. A genetic basis for hypofibrinolysis in these patients was not investigated. Genetic mutation in the thrombin-activatable fibrinolytic inhibitor (TAFI) gene has not been linked to thrombosis risk, although plasma TAFI levels appeared to be weakly linked to thrombosis risk in some studies.

Homocysteine

Hyperhomocysteinaemia may be caused by genetic abnormalities but only the severe inherited abnormalities of homocysteine metabolism (homozygous cystathionine β-synthase deficiency and homozygous deficiency of methylenetetrahydrofolate reductase) result in congenital homocysteinuria associated with an increased risk of both arterial and venous thrombosis as well as premature atherosclerosis and mental retardation, epilepsy, and skeletal and eye problems. Half of patients present with venous or arterial thrombosis before the age of 30 years. The thermolabile variant of methylenetetrahydrofolate reductase

due to a common genetic mutation (C677T) is not a risk factor for venous thrombosis.

Treatment of patients with venous thrombosis and heritable thrombophilias

There is no evidence that heritable thrombophilia should influence the intensity of anticoagulation with heparin or warfarin. In patients with antithrombin deficiency, heparin resistance is infrequent and recurrence or extension of thrombosis while on treatment is no greater than that observed in individuals without antithrombin deficiency. Warfarin-induced skin necrosis is extremely rare, even in patients with protein C or S deficiency, such that most individuals with protein C or S deficiency do not develop skin necrosis. The intensity of maintenance therapy with warfarin should not be influenced by laboratory evidence of inherited thrombophilia. There is no evidence that recurrence on treatment is more likely in patients with heritable thrombophilia.

Long-term prospective cohort outcome studies have shown that finding a heritable thrombophilia does not predict recurrence in unselected patients after an episode of venous thrombosis. However, these studies were not powered to exclude an increased risk of recurrence specifically in relation to rare thrombophilias, such as antithrombin or protein C deficiency. Therefore, it remains uncertain if mutations in *SERPINC1*, *PROC* or *PROS* causing deficiency of the corresponding protein might predict a sufficiently high risk of thrombosis to justify long-term (lifelong) anticoagulation. Studies in thrombosis-prone families indicate a risk of recurrence that would justify long-term anticoagulation but these studies may not be representative of risk associated with the *SERPINC1*, *PROC* and *PROS* mutations per se but may be influenced by additional defects in the thrombosis-prone family members. Further studies are required to define the relative risk of recurrent events associated with the actual *SERPINC1*, *PROC* and *PROS* mutations.

Systematic reviews indicate a risk of 1.4 for recurrent venous thromboembolism in patients heterozygous for the FVR506Q mutation and 1.2–1.7 for the *F2G20210A* mutation. The authors concluded that the magnitude of the increase in risk was modest and by itself did not justify an extended duration of anticoagulation. An analysis of the MEGA study showed that testing for inherited thrombophilia did not reduce recurrence of venous thrombosis.

As a result of these observations, at present the following conclusions seem reasonable.
• Indiscriminate testing for heritable thrombophilias in unselected patients presenting with a first episode of venous thrombosis is not indicated.

• Decisions regarding duration of anticoagulation (lifelong or not) in unselected patients should be made with reference to whether a first episode of venous thrombosis was provoked, other risk factors, and risk of anticoagulant therapy-related bleeding, regardless of whether a heritable thrombophilia is known.
• Testing for heritable thrombophilias in selected patients, such as those with a strong family history of unprovoked recurrent thrombosis, may influence decisions regarding duration of anticoagulation. Unfortunately, in this regard identifying patients for testing is not straightforward as criteria for defining thrombosis-prone families have not been validated and the association between family history of thrombosis and detection of inherited thrombophilia is weak.

Treatment of venous thrombosis in unusual sites in patients with heritable thrombophilias

Upper limb DVT

More than 60% of episodes of upper limb DVT are associated with central venous catheters (CVC), with CVCs and cancer being the predominant risk factors. In patients without these factors heritable thrombophilias are found in one-third and there is an interaction between common thrombophilias and oral contraceptive exposure. The risk of recurrence is either not higher or marginally higher in patients with heritable thrombophilias but the absolute risk of recurrence in the presence of thrombophilia is less than 5% per year and 80% of patients are recurrence free 5 years after stopping anticoagulant therapy. Therefore thrombophilia testing is not recommended in patients with upper limb DVT.

Cerebral vein thrombosis

There is an association between thrombophilia and cerebral vein thrombosis, with an interaction between common thrombophilias, particularly *F2G20210A*, and oral contraceptive exposure. Overall the risk of recurrence of cerebral vein thrombosis is lower than previously thought, although it may be underestimated due to continuation of anticoagulant therapy in those patients thought to be at particular risk of recurrence. It has become common practice to test patients for heritable thrombophilia after cerebral vein thrombosis and some experts continue anticoagulation lifelong if there is a thrombophilic defect. In all patients acquired risks should be removed or minimized, for example combined oral contraceptive (COC) exposure and obesity. Therefore, testing for heritable thrombophilias after a first episode of cerebral vein thrombosis has unknown predictive value for recurrence and decisions regarding dura-

tion of anticoagulant therapy in relation to the results of testing are therefore not evidence based.

Retinal vein thrombosis

Vein occlusion is associated with hypertension, hypercholesterolaemia and diabetes. A relationship with heritable thrombophilia has not been established. Furthermore, it is uncertain if hypercoagulability is a contributory factor in this condition and there is no evidence that anticoagulant therapy is beneficial. Consequently, testing is not indicated in patients with retinal vein occlusion.

Intra-abdominal vein thrombosis

Myeloproliferative disorders, cirrhosis and surgery are strong risk factors for intra-abdominal venous thrombosis. The acquired JAK2 V617F mutation is a risk factor even in the absence of an overt myeloproliferative disorder, being found in about 15% of cases. No studies have investigated how the finding of a heritable thrombophilia should influence management. Therefore, testing for heritable thrombophilias after a first episode of intra-abdominal vein thrombosis has uncertain predictive value for recurrence and decisions regarding duration of anticoagulant therapy in relation to the results of testing are not evidence based. Many experts continue anticoagulation lifelong after intra-abdominal vein thrombosis as recurrence may be catastrophic.

Case finding

Testing for heritable thrombophilias in patients presenting with venous thrombosis allows case finding of affected asymptomatic family members. The rationale is that this permits avoidance of environmental risks (e.g. use of COCs by females) or provides an opportunity for targeted thrombophylaxis at times of unavoidable high risk (such as surgery). However, individual risk is affected by multiple genetic and environmental factors that will be different even among first-degree relatives. Prospective cohort studies have determined the annual risk of venous thrombosis in asymptomatic family members identified after testing unselected patients presenting with venous thrombosis. The studies included more than 3500 patient-years of observation. The annual risk of venous thrombosis in asymptomatic family relatives of index patients was 0.1% for those with *F2G20210A*, 0.6% for those with FVR506Q, about 2% for protein C and protein S deficiency, and 4% for antithrombin deficiency. High-risk periods contribute to approximately half of all events (provoked recurrence) in patients with FVR506Q and thrombophylaxis appears to reduce risk. In the EPCOT registry patients were referred to specialist centres for thrombophilia testing if they had a personal or family history of venous thrombosis. The incidence of thrombosis on study entry was determined retrospectively in asymptomatic relatives. The risk of venous thrombosis was 16 times higher in affected relatives, with the greatest risk in relatives of patients with deficiency of a natural anticoagulant or multiple defects. The highest risk was in individuals with antithrombin deficiency (1.7% per year) or combined defects (1.6% per year). Targeted case finding of relatives with 'severe' or 'high risk' thrombophilias, such as deficiency of antithrombin, protein C or protein S, has been suggested, although the clinical utility of such methods remains uncertain and contentious among experts.

Given uncertainty, some experts argue that it is reasonable to perform testing if it is anticipated that clinical management will be influenced, for example an intensified or extended period of prophylaxis during a high-risk period. If a family history suggests a high degree of genetic penetrance, then it might be reasonable to test a symptomatic patient and then their relatives with a view to enhanced prophylaxis at times of high risk in affected members, for example thrombophylaxis in pregnancy when there is a family history of pregnancy-associated thrombosis, or intensified or extended surgical thrombophylaxis when there is a history of thrombophylaxis failure in affected members. In all cases the risks, benefits and limitations of testing should be discussed in the context of explained inheritance and disease risk. The importance of this is demonstrated by reported anxiety after testing positive and an overestimated perception of risk. Simple methods for quantifying a positive family history do not discriminate patients with and without thrombophilia and therefore the decision to test for inherited thrombophilia cannot be accurately guided by the presence or absence of a family history.

Prevention of thrombosis associated with estrogen-containing hormone preparations

In some women heritable thrombophilia has already been established, while in others it is perceived that testing would enable informed decision-making regarding use of a COC or hormone-replacement therapy (HRT). However, the absolute risk of thrombosis is low and the fact that venous thrombosis has a multiple genetic basis with incomplete penetrance makes counselling in relation to genetic testing uncertain. In many instances an alternative effective contraceptive is acceptable. Similar principles apply to HRT, although the baseline risk is higher as the population is older. Rarely is there a therapeutic indication for HRT and in most instances there is only a weak indication. If HRT is considered essential, then a non-oral formulation is associated with a significantly lower risk of venous thrombosis.

A first-degree relative with a history of venous thrombosis is a relative contraindication to an estrogen-containing hormonal preparation. The risk is dependent on the circumstances of thrombosis in the relative. For example, a history of an elderly relative who developed venous thrombosis as a complication of cancer is not a contraindication. In contrast, a relative with unprovoked venous thrombosis, or specifically a sibling developing venous thrombosis while taking a COC, should be considered a strong contraindication. In families with known heritable thrombophilias the risk of venous thrombosis can be increased in unaffected members as well as affected and so a negative thrombophilia result does not exclude an increased risk of venous thrombosis. Therefore, decisions regarding use of COCs and whether thrombophilia testing is likely to be informative should be made with reference to individual clinical risk factors and the circumstances associated with venous thrombosis in the family.

Prevention of pregnancy-associated venous thrombosis

Pregnancy is associated with a fivefold to tenfold increased risk of venous thrombosis compared with non-pregnant women of comparable age, with an absolute risk of 1–2 per 1000 deliveries. The risk of thrombosis, compared with the general age-matched female population, is increased 100-fold in pregnancy in women with a previous thrombosis. Retrospective studies in women with previous venous thrombosis for whom detailed information on the type of thrombophilia was available indicate that the rate of recurrence is similar in women with and without thrombophilia, although studies excluded women with high-risk thrombophilias (anticoagulant deficiency, multiple defects). Thrombosis rarely occurs in women whose initial event is provoked. In general, the absolute risk of pregnancy-associated venous thrombosis in women with heritable thrombophilia with no previous history is small, but women with antithrombin deficiency or those homozygous for the FVR506Q or $F2$G20210A mutations or who are double heterozygotes should be regarded as being at higher risk. The number of women with these defects is very small.

In women with a previous history of venous thrombosis, the major factor in determining if prophylaxis should be given is whether prior venous thrombosis was provoked or not. If the episode was unprovoked, prophylaxis should be considered and thrombophilia testing is not required if prophylaxis is given. In women with a first provoked event, the decision to test should be influenced by the strength of the provocation, for example thrombosis associated with major trauma and subsequent immobility would not be an indication for prophylaxis or testing. In women with a first-degree relative with thrombosis, the decision to test should be influenced by whether the event in the relative was unprovoked or provoked and the strength of the provocation. If the event in the first-degree relative was associated with pregnancy or COC, then testing and finding thrombophilia should prompt consideration of prophylaxis, particularly if the symptomatic relative was known to have the same defect, especially deficiency of antithrombin or protein C. When testing in pregnancy is performed it is necessary to interpret the results with reference to the effect of pregnancy on the tests.

Pregnancy morbidity

There is evidence of an association between heritable thrombophilia and pregnancy morbidity, including early and late pregnancy loss, pre-eclampsia and intrauterine growth retardation. Randomized controlled trials with a no treatment or placebo arm in women with a history of pregnancy complications are in progress and results should be awaited before recommending that antithrombotic therapy is given to pregnant women based on testing for heritable thrombophilia.

Purpura fulminans

Purpura fulminans is a rare syndrome characterized by progressive haemorrhagic skin necrosis that occurs in neonates with congenital severe protein C deficiency at birth or in the first few days of life, and in association with infection in children and adults. The condition may occur in children without congenital anticoagulant deficiency following viral infections, with an onset within 10 days of infection. Acquired severe protein S deficiency has been reported in purpura fulminans following chickenpox infection. With bacterial infections disseminated intravascular coagulation (DIC) is often present, for example meningococcal infection. In patients with DIC or purpura fulminans due to sepsis, treatment with APC should be considered. In patients with very severe skin necrosis, testing for acquired protein C or S deficiency should be considered as plasma exchange may be beneficial. Neonates homozygous for protein C or S deficiency may be born with skin necrosis or DIC.

Oral vitamin K antagonist-induced skin necrosis

Oral vitamin K antagonist-induced skin necrosis, such as that seen with warfarin, is extremely rare, even in patients with protein C or S deficiency, such that most individuals with protein C or S deficiency do not develop skin necrosis. However, a high proportion of patients with vitamin K antagonist-induced necrosis have heritable protein C deficiency. The condition has been described in patients with other heritable thrombophilias. Vitamin K antagonist-induced necrosis associated with heritable thrombophilias tends to involve a central distribution.

Thrombophilia and arterial thrombosis

The genetic risk factors for venous thrombosis and arterial atherothrombosis overlap but the material contribution of each differs between the two diseases. Hypercoagulability resulting from variation in the genetic control of blood coagulation produces a greater material contribution to venous thrombosis. However, it is becoming increasingly recognized that both genetic and acquired risk factors are common denominators for venous and arterial thrombosis. In patients presenting with venous thrombosis before the age of 40 there appears to be an increased risk of acute myocardial infarction subsequently.

Evidence of an association between heritable thrombophilia and arterial thrombosis is limited to case reports and small studies. It is possible that heritable defects that result in increased coagulability increase the likelihood of atherothrombosis. However, the material contribution of heritable thrombophilia, as compared with established cardiovascular risk factors, is not sufficient to change therapy for primary and secondary prevention. Therefore, testing young patients for heritable thrombophilia after an arterial occlusive event is unhelpful. Because there is no established causal relationship and as treatment and secondary prevention should be in relation to established cardiovascular risk factors, thrombophilia testing is not recommended. In patients with arterial thrombosis at a young age that cannot be explained by conventional cardiovascular risk factors, various causes should be considered including antiphospholipid antibody syndrome, a cardiac or large-artery source of embolus, vasculitis, aneurysm, thoracic outlet syndrome or a collagen-vascular disorder causing arterial dissection.

Neonatal stroke

Heritable thrombophilic defects are associated with perinatal brain injury. The pathogenesis is thrombosis in either cerebral arteries or cerebral veins or sinuses. Secondary brain infarction results, with subsequent cystic change. Thrombophilia is not a significant risk factor for ischaemic stroke in adults, as it does not increase the risk of arterial thrombosis (but cerebral vein thrombosis can present as stroke). In the neonate the pathophysiology of stroke is quite different and thrombophilia may increase the risk of arterial thrombosis and stroke in the neonate or fetus. There are two potential explanations for this.
• The circulation in the neonate is different. In the adult venous blood is 'filtered' by the pulmonary circulation. In the fetus and

neonate the lungs are bypassed by the ductus arteriosus and so it is possible for clots arising in the venous system to bypass the lungs and occlude a cerebral artery.

• The blood coagulation system of the neonate is different to that of the adult. It is possible that the coagulability of blood in fetal and neonatal arteries is influenced by thrombophilic defects. However, this remains to be investigated.

Testing for defects may therefore identify a material contributory factor but does not typically inform management decisions. For example, anticoagulant therapy is not usually considered in children found to have a suffered a stroke in the neonatal period and there may be a significant time before a neurological deficit is recognized or the cause of stroke determined. In practice testing is sometimes performed in order to explain to parents why a stroke possibly occurred.

Laboratory methodology and testing strategy

The laboratory diagnosis of heritable thrombophilias is difficult as the tests are subject to considerable pre-analytical variables. Low levels of antithrombin, protein C and protein S occur in a variety of circumstances and test results and the clinical implications of both positive and negative results are frequently misinterpreted.

A full blood count and platelet count are useful indicators of general health and will identify myeloproliferative disorders that increase thrombotic risk. The APTT may detect some lupus anticoagulants but a sensitive assay should be used. The thrombin time will detect heparin contamination and the prothrombin time (PT) is useful for the interpretation of protein C and protein S levels. Testing is usually delayed until at least 1 month after completion of a course of anticoagulation with a vitamin K antagonist. Testing should be avoided during intercurrent illness and with use of COCs or HRT. Sometimes testing is performed during pregnancy and so interpretation of results must be made with reference to the effect of the pregnancy on results.

Functional assays should be used where accuracy and imprecision are acceptable. However, no single method will detect all defects. For example, a protein C chromogenic assay will not detect a dysfunctional protein C molecule with impaired phospholipid binding due to a mutation in the Gla domain. A clot-based protein C assay would be sensitive to this defect but imprecision of the assay would result in reduced sensitivity and specificity for other defects compared with a chromogenic assay. Similarly, the performance of antithrombin assays will be influenced by heparin, the pre-incubation time with heparin, use of FXa or thrombin as a substrate, the source of thrombin and the end-point detection method. For example, an assay utilizing a short heparin incubation time will detect heparin-

binding site defects, which may not be associated with an appreciably increased risk of venous thrombosis.

Even in families with characterized defects, a phenotypic assay may fail to accurately discriminate affected and non-affected individuals. True heritable deficiencies may not be detected and false-positive diagnoses are common.

Pre-analytical variables

Most assays are affected by clots in the sample. Antibody assays may be affected by atypical antibodies such as paraproteins, rheumatoid factor and heterophile antibodies. Chromogenic assays are subject to interference by lipaemia and haemolysis. Clot-based assays are subject to imprecision due to variation in the baseline clotting time and the levels of other factors.

Low levels of antithrombin, protein C or protein S may relate to age, sex, acquired illness or drug therapy and therefore interpretation requires knowledge of the patient's condition at the time of blood sampling. Interpretation of results in children must be with reference to the normal range for age.

Low levels of antithrombin, protein C or protein S suspected to be the result of heritable mutations should be confirmed on one or more separate samples. Demonstrating a low level in other family members supports a diagnosis of heritable deficiency and characterization of the genetic mutation can confirm the diagnosis and give some indication of thrombosis risk, particularly in the case of antithrombin deficiency.

General recommendations for laboratory tests and interpretation

• Testing at the time of acute venous thrombosis is not indicated as the utility and implications of testing need to be considered and the patient needs to be counselled before testing. As treatment of acute venous thrombosis is not influenced by test results, testing can be performed later.

• The PT should be measured to detect the effect of oral vitamin K antagonists, which will cause a reduction in protein C and S levels.

• Functional assays should be used to determine antithrombin and protein C levels.

• Chromogenic assays of protein C activity are less subject to interference than clotting assays and are preferable.

• Immunoreactive assays of free protein S antigen are preferable to functional assays. If a protein S activity assay is used in the initial screen, low results should be further investigated with an immunoreactive assay of free protein S.

• If an APC resistance assay is performed to detect FVR506Q, then the modified APC sensitivity test (predilution of the test sample in FV-deficient plasma), as opposed to the original APC sensitivity test, should be used as a phenotypic test for FV Leiden. If positive the mutation should be confirmed by a direct genetic test. An APC resistance assay is unnecessary if a direct genetic test for FV Leiden is used initially.

• Repeat testing for identification of deficiency of antithrombin, protein C and protein S is indicated and a low level should be confirmed on one or more separate samples. Deficiency should not be diagnosed on a single abnormal result.

• Rigorous internal quality assurance and participation in accredited external quality assessment schemes are mandatory.

• Thrombophilia testing must be supervised by experienced laboratory staff and the clinical significance of the results must be interpreted by an experienced clinician who is aware of all relevant factors that may influence individual test results in each individual case.

Antithrombin assays

The activity of antithrombin is measured as progressive activity towards thrombin in the absence of heparin (designated accordingly 'progressive activity') or in the presence of heparin against either thrombin or FXa (designated 'heparin cofactor activity'). Activity assays typically use a chromogenic substrate in which a small synthetic peptide is linked to *p*-nitroaniline. Cleavage of the peptide releases the *p*-nitroaniline, which turns yellow and can be measured quantitatively. Patient plasma is incubated with heparin and then an excess of thrombin or FXa is added. The heparin-activated antithrombin is complexed and neutralizes the excess thrombin or FXa. The remaining free protease quantified by cleavage of the chromogenic substrate is inversely proportional to the antithrombin level in patient plasma. Either thrombin or FXa with the appropriate chromogenic substrate can be used (Figure 45.4). The progressive assay is identical except that the patient plasma sample is not pre-incubated with heparin.

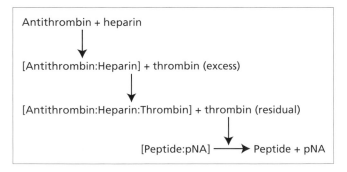

Figure 45.4 Chromogenic antithrombin heparin cofactor assay. Plasma (the source of antithrombin) is incubated with an excess of thrombin (human or bovine) in the presence of heparin. Thrombin is complexed and neutralized by heparin-activated antithrombin until all antithrombin is complexed. The residual thrombin is then detected by the chromogenic indicator. The concentration of antithrombin in the sample is inversely proportional to the residual thrombin concentration.

Interference by other proteases and inhibitors in the plasma sample is a potential problem. Interference by heparin cofactor II, another heparin-activated serpin, can be eliminated by using FXa or bovine thrombin as the target protease, as heparin cofactor II only inhibits human thrombin. The effect of other proteases in the patient plasma can be minimized by addition of a protease inhibitor such as aprotonin.

The total amount of antithrombin protein can be measured immunologically with antibodies, for example by ELISA. As antithrombin antigen levels may be normal or near normal in type II deficiency, immunological assays may fail to identify patients with these variants.

Antithrombin levels are slightly reduced in infants, during pregnancy, in women taking estrogen preparations and in some patients during heparin therapy. Levels also decrease with age and acquired low levels occur in liver disease, DIC, nephrotic syndrome, during L-asparaginase therapy, and in protein malnutrition and cachexia.

Protein C assays

Protein C defects are divided into type 1, with a reduced amount of functionally normal protein, and type 2, in which there is reduced activity due to a dysfunctional protein. In this case there is discordance between the functional and antigenic levels. The laboratory diagnosis of protein C deficiency is based on a functional assay. Most commercially available functional assays of protein C employ the specific activator Protac, a protein C activator derived from the venom of the southern copperhead snake (*Agkistrodon contortrix*). Chromogenic assays using a synthetic substrate for APC are simple to perform and can detect all type 1 defects and type 2 defects affecting the catalytic site. A chromogenic assay will not detect most other type 2 defects. Clotting assays utilizing the prolongation of either the PT or APTT after Protac activation have the capacity to detect other, but not all, type 2 defects but are subject to imprecision due to variation in the baseline clotting time and the levels of other factors, for example if there is a short APTT due to a high FVIII level, or the presence of the factor V Leiden mutation which results in a falsely low protein C activity due to APC resistance, or in the presence of a lupus anticoagulant. The diagnosis of protein C deficiency is problematic because of the wide overlap in protein C activity between heterozygous carriers and unaffected individuals. Protein C levels are not affected by pregnancy or estrogen exposure. Acquired low levels of protein C occur during anticoagulant therapy with oral vitamin K antagonists, vitamin K deficiency, DIC and liver disease.

Protein S assays

Protein S is usually quantified immunologically rather than measured functionally. Originally, free protein S was measured in plasma supernatant after precipitation of C4b-bound protein

S by polyethylene glycol (PEG). Nowadays PEG precipitation is not required as monoclonal antibodies that detect only free protein are used. Functional protein S assays are imprecise and are not used in the majority of coagulation laboratories.

Protein S levels are significantly lower in females, so much so that different normal reference ranges are required for males and females. There is a significant risk of a false-positive diagnosis of protein S deficiency in women. Protein S levels fall progressively during normal pregnancy and are reduced by estrogens. Acquired low levels of protein S occur during anticoagulant therapy with oral vitamin K antagonists, vitamin K deficiency, DIC and liver disease.

FVR506Q and APC resistance

Nowadays, the FVR506Q mutation is usually detected by direct mutation analysis. APC resistance assays typically utilize the APTT. Samples are tested with and without an added fixed concentration of APC. The clotting times are expressed as a sensitivity ratio, i.e. the APTT (seconds) of patient plasma plus APC divided by the APTT (seconds) of patient plasma without added APC; the lower the ratio, the greater the APC resistance. Platelet contamination and activation must be avoided as this will lead to APC resistance. The ratio can be normalized by dividing the patient's sensitivity ratio by the sensitivity ratio of a pooled normal plasma. If normalization is used, FVR506Q carriers should be excluded from the normal plasma pool. The APC resistance assay is abnormal not only in the presence of FVR506Q but with all other causes of heritable and acquired APC resistance and in individuals with a prolonged baseline APTT due to clotting factor deficiencies or anticoagulant therapy. It is therefore not specific for FVR506Q. Modification of the test by a 1 in 4 predilution of the test plasma in FV-deficient plasma increases the sensitivity and specificity of the assay for FVR506Q to almost 100% and this test is reliable if genetic analysis is not available.

*F2*G20210A

A laboratory clotting test with sensitivity and specificity for this mutation is not available and so detection is by direct mutation analysis.

Next-generation global thrombophilia tests

A test that predicts a high rate of recurrent venous thrombosis would be clinically useful. The clinical utility of such a test would be the identification of patients in whom the benefit of continued long-term anticoagulant therapy outweighed the risk. Patients with a first unprovoked venous thrombosis are at highest risk of recurrence but it is arguable if the level of risk estimated from clinical risk factors alone justifies long-term anticoagulation. A new generation of thrombophilia tests that

measure the degree of coagulability are now being investigated in clinical studies. These include biomarkers, such as D-dimer, which reflect the level of thrombin generation *in vivo*, and thrombin generation assays, which measure the capacity of a patient plasma sample to generate thrombin in response to a predefined coagulation trigger, for example low concentration tissue factor. It has now been demonstrated in several studies that the level of D-dimer or thrombin-generating potential correlates with risk of recurrent venous thrombosis. These tests appear to reflect different aspects of hypercoagulability and may be complementary in terms of clinical utility. However, it remains to be defined exactly how these tests should be used to stratify patient risk and influence clinical decisions regarding duration of anticoagulant therapy after an episode of venous thrombosis.

Counselling and genetic testing

Clinical utility refers to the ability of a screening or diagnostic test to prevent or reduce adverse health outcomes, including mortality, morbidity and disability. A test does not have inherent clinical utility; rather it is the adoption of a therapeutic or preventive intervention on the basis of the test result that influences health outcomes. Clinical utility can more broadly refer to any use of a test result to inform clinical decision-making, and this may include information considered important by individuals and families.

A large proportion of genetic counselling focuses on presenting risk information. Making sense of information can be difficult. Whenever a patient is offered an intervention there is a trade-off between benefit and risk. The benefit and risk information must be presented in ways that are relevant and understandable. In addition to the quantitative information, the qualitative aspect of risk is equally important. A relative risk does not indicate how likely it is than an outcome will occur, only how much relatively more or less likely it is. It is the absolute risk that indicates how likely an event will be. For example, the relative risk of venous thrombosis is increased twofold to sixfold in a female aged between 20 and 40 years who takes an estrogen-containing oral contraceptive (COC), depending on her age and the COC preparation. It is accepted that COC exposure increases the risk of venous thrombosis and some women presented with this information might choose not to use a COC as contraception, despite its proven efficacy and attractions. When informed that the risk would be 35-fold higher than the population baseline risk if the woman had the factor V Leiden mutation and used a COC, some women would again choose to avoid use of a COC. However, in order to make an informed decision it is necessary for the woman to know how likely it is she would suffer venous thrombosis if she did not use the COC and how much the absolute risk would change if she did use a COC. The population baseline risk of thrombosis is about 1 per 10 000 per year under the age of 40. If a woman used a COC it would increase about fourfold to about 4 per 10 000 per year. Clearly, the risk of venous thrombosis associated with COC use is very low. For a woman with the factor V Leiden mutation, her baseline risk of thrombosis would be about 1 per 2000 per year under the age of 40, a risk that is increased about fivefold compared with a woman without this mutation. If this woman were to take a COC, her absolute risk would increase from 1 per 2000 to 1 in 300, a risk that is increased about sevenfold for her but which is 35-fold greater than the population baseline risk. For many women an annual risk of 1 in 300 is acceptable given the proven efficacy, ease of use and other obvious advantages of a COC.

Selected bibliography

Allaart CF, Poort SR, Rosendaal FR, Reitsma PH, Bertina RM, Briet E (1993) Increased risk of venous thrombosis in carriers of hereditary protein C deficiency defect. *Lancet* **341**: 134–8.

Austin SK, Lambert JR (2008) The JAK2 V617F mutation and thrombosis. *British Journal of Haematology* **143**: 307–20.

Baglin T (2005) The measurement and application of thrombin generation. *British Journal of Haematology* **130**: 653–61.

Baglin T (2009) Communicating benefit and risk. *British Journal of Haematology* **146**: 31–3.

Baglin T, Luddington R, Brown K, Baglin C (2003) Incidence of recurrent venous thromboembolism in relation to clinical and thrombophilic risk factors: prospective cohort study. *Lancet* **362**: 523–6.

Baglin T (2010) Unravelling the thrombophilia paradox: from hypercoagulability to the prothrombotic state. *Journal of Thrombosis and Haemostasis* **8**: 228–33.

Bank I, Scavenius MP, Buller HR, Middeldorp S (2004) Social aspects of genetic testing for factor V Leiden mutation in healthy individuals and their importance for daily practice. *Thrombosis Research* **113**: 7–12.

Bauer KA (2001) Conventional fibrinolytic assays for the evaluation of patients with venous thrombosis: don't bother. *Thrombosis and Haemostasis* **85**: 377–8.

Bertina RM, Koeleman BP, Koster T et al. (1994) Mutation in blood coagulation factor V associated with resistance to activated protein C. *Nature* **369**: 64–7.

Besser M, Baglin C, Luddington R, van Hylckama Vlieg A, Baglin T (2008) High rate of unprovoked recurrent venous thrombosis is associated with high thrombin-generating potential in a prospective cohort study. *Journal of Thrombosis and Haemostasis* **6**: 1720–5.

Brill-Edwards P, Ginsberg JS, Gent M et al. (2000) Safety of withholding heparin in pregnant women with a history of venous thromboembolism. Recurrence of Clot in This Pregnancy Study Group. *New England Journal of Medicine* **343**: 1439–44.

Canonico M, Plu-Bureau G, Lowe GD, Scarabin PY (2008) Hormone replacement therapy and risk of venous thromboembolism in postmenopausal women: systematic review and meta-analysis. *British Medical Journal* **336**: 1227–31.

Chan WS, Dixon ME (2008) The 'ART' of thromboembolism: a review of assisted reproductive technology and thromboembolic complications. *Thrombosis Research* **121**: 713–26.

Christiansen SC, Cannegieter SC, Koster T, Vandenbroucke JP, Rosendaal FR (2005) Thrombophilia, clinical factors, and recurrent venous thrombotic events. *Journal of the American Medical Association* **293**: 2352–61.

Cohn DM, Vansenne F, Kaptein AA, De Borgie CA, Middeldorp S (2008) The psychological impact of testing for thrombophilia: a systematic review. *Journal of Thrombosis and Haemostasis* **6**: 1099–104.

Comp PC, Nixon RR, Cooper MR, Esmon CT (1984) Familial protein S deficiency is associated with recurrent thrombosis. *Journal of Clinical Investigation* **74**: 2082–8.

Coppens M, van Mourik JA, Eckmann CM, Buller HR, Middeldorp S (2007) Current practise of testing for inherited thrombophilia. *Journal of Thrombosis and Haemostasis* **5**: 1979–81.

Coppens M, Reijnders JH, Middeldorp S, Doggen CJ, Rosendaal FR (2008) Testing for inherited thrombophilia does not reduce recurrence of venous thrombosis. *Journal of Thrombosis and Haemostasis* **6**: 1474–7.

Dahlback B, Carlsson M, Svensson PJ (1993) Familial thrombophilia due to a previously unrecognized mechanism characterized by poor anticoagulant response to activated protein C: prediction of a cofactor to activated protein C. *Proceedings of the National Academy of Science USA* **90**: 1004–8.

Dentali F, Crowther M, Ageno W (2006) Thrombophilic abnormalities, oral contraceptives, and risk of cerebral vein thrombosis: a meta-analysis. *Blood* **107**: 2766–73.

De Stefano V (2004) Inherited thrombophilia and life-time risk of venous thromboembolism: is the burden reducible? *Journal of Thrombosis and Haemostasis* **2**: 1522–5.

De Stefano V, Martinelli I, Rossi E et al. (2006) The risk of recurrent venous thromboembolism in pregnancy and puerperium without antithrombotic prophylaxis. *British Journal of Haematology* **135**: 386–91.

Dudding TE, Attia J (2004) The association between adverse pregnancy outcomes and maternal factor V Leiden genotype: a meta-analysis. *Thrombosis and Haemostasis* **91**: 700–11.

Egeberg O (1965) Inherited antithrombin deficiency causing thrombophilia. *Thrombosis et Diathesis Haemorrhagica* **13**: 516–30.

Eriksson BI, Dahl OE, Rosencher N et al. (2007) Dabigatran etexilate versus enoxaparin for prevention of venous thromboembolism after total hip replacement: a randomized, double-blind, non-inferiority trial. *Lancet* **370**: 949–56.

Evans G, Luddington R, Baglin T (2001) Beriplex P/N reverses severe warfarin-induced overanticoagulation immediately and completely in patients presenting with major bleeding. *British Journal of Haematology* **115**: 998–1001.

Ferro JM, Canhao P, Stam J, Bousser MG, Barinagarrementeria F (2004) Prognosis of cerebral vein and dural sinus thrombosis: results of the International Study on Cerebral Vein and Dural Sinus Thrombosis (ISCVT). *Stroke* **35**. 664 70.

Flinterman LE, van Hylckama Vlieg A, Rosendaal FR, Doggen CJ (2008) Recurrent thrombosis and survival after a first venous thrombosis of the upper extremity. *Circulation* **118**: 1366–72.

Gopel W, Ludwig M, Junge AK, Kohlmann T, Diedrich K, Moller J (2001) Selection pressure for the factor-V-Leiden mutation and embryo implantation. *Lancet* **358**: 1238–9.

Greaves M, Baglin T (2000) Laboratory testing for heritable thrombophilia: impact on clinical management of thrombotic disease annotation. *British Journal of Haematology* **109**: 699–703.

Griffin JH, Evatt B, Zimmerman TS, Kleiss AJ, Wideman C (1981) Deficiency of protein C in congenital thrombotic disease. *Journal of Clinical Investigation* **68**: 1370–3.

Hellmann EA, Leslie ND, Moll S (2003) Knowledge and educational needs of individuals with the factor V Leiden mutation. *Journal of Thrombosis and Haemostasis* **1**: 2335–9.

Ho WK, Hankey GJ, Quinlan DJ, Eikelboom JW (2006) Risk of recurrent venous thromboembolism in patients with common thrombophilia: a systematic review. *Archives of Internal Medicine* **166**: 729–36.

Huntington JA (2003) Mechanisms of glycosaminoglycan activation of the serpins in hemostasis. *Journal of Thrombosis and Haemostasis* **1**: 1535–49.

James AH, Jamison MG, Brancazio LR, Myers ER (2006) Venous thromboembolism during pregnancy and the postpartum period: incidence, risk factors, and mortality. *American Journal of Obstetrics and Gynecology* **194**: 1311–15.

Janssen MC, den Heijer M, Cruysberg JR, Wollersheim H, Brdie SJ (2005) Retinal vein occlusion: a form of venous thrombosis or a complication of atherosclerosis? A meta-analysis of thrombophilic factors. *Thrombosis and Haemostasis* **93**: 1021–6.

Jennings I, Kitchen S, Woods TA, Preston FE (2005) Multilaboratory testing in thrombophilia through the United Kingdom National External Quality Assessment Scheme (Blood Coagulation) Quality Assurance Program. *Seminars in Thrombosis and Hemostasis* **31**: 66–72.

Kearon C, Julian JA, Kovacs MJ et al. (2008) Influence of thrombophilia on risk of recurrent venous thromboembolism while on warfarin: results from a randomized trial. *Blood* **112**: 4432–6.

Kenet G, Lütkhoff LK, Albisetti M et al. (2010) Impact of thrombophilia on risk of arterial ischemic stroke or cerebral sinovenous thrombosis in neonates and children: a systematic review and meta-analysis of observational studies. *Circulation* **121**: 1838–47.

Langlois NJ, Wells PS (2003) Risk of venous thromboembolism in relatives of symptomatic probands with thrombophilia: a systematic review. *Thrombosis and Haemostasis* **90**: 17–26.

Lisman T, de Groot PG, Meijers JC, Rosendaal FR (2005) Reduced plasma fibrinolytic potential is a risk factor for venous thrombosis. *Blood* **105**: 1102–5.

Marchiori A, Mosena L, Prins MH, Prandoni P (2007) The risk of recurrent venous thromboembolism among heterozygous carriers of factor V Leiden or prothrombin G20210A mutation. A systematic review of prospective studies. *Haematologica* **92**: 1107–14.

Martinelli I, Battaglioli T, Bucciarelli P, Passamonti SM, Mannucci PM (2004) Risk factors and recurrence rate of primary deep vein thrombosis of the upper extremities. *Circulation* **110**: 566–70.

Meltzer ME, Lisman T, Doggen CJ, de Groot PG, Rosendaal FR (2008) Synergistic effects of hypofibrinolysis and genetic and acquired risk factors on the risk of a first venous thrombosis. *PLoS Medicine* **5**: e97.

Middeldorp S, van Hylckama Vlieg A (2008) Does thrombophilia testing help in the clinical management of patients? *British Journal of Haematology* **143**: 321–35.

Munoz FJ, Mismetti P, Poggio R et al. (2008) Clinical outcome of patients with upper-extremity deep vein thrombosis: results from the RIETE Registry. *Chest* **133**: 143–8.

Poort SR, Rosendaal FR, Reitsma PH, Bertina RM (1996) A common genetic variation in the 3′-untranslated region of the prothrombin gene is associated with elevated plasma prothrombin levels and an increase in venous thrombosis. *Blood* **88**: 3698–703.

Prandoni P, Bilora F, Marchiori A et al. (2003) An association between atherosclerosis and venous thrombosis. *New England Journal of Medicine* **348**: 1435–41.

Reitsma PH, Rosendaal FR (2007) Past and future of genetic research in thrombosis. *Journal of Thrombosis and Haemostasis* **5** (Suppl. 1): 264–9.

Rey E, Kahn SR, David M, Shrier I (2003) Thrombophilic disorders and fetal loss: a meta-analysis. *Lancet* **361**: 901–8.

Robertson L, Wu O, Langhorne P et al. (2006) Thrombophilia in pregnancy: a systematic review. *British Journal of Haematology* **132**: 171–96.

Rosendaal FR (1999) Venous thrombosis: a multicausal disease. *Lancet* **353**: 1167–73.

Schulman S, Tengborn L (1992) Treatment of venous thromboembolism in patients with congenital deficiency of antithrombin III. *Thrombosis and Haemostasis* **68**: 634–6.

Spencer FA, Goldberg RJ (2005) Asymptomatic thrombophilia: a family affair. *Journal of Thrombosis and Haemostasis* **3**: 457–8.

Spencer FA, Emery C, Lessard D, Goldberg RJ (2007) Upper extremity deep vein thrombosis: a community-based perspective. *American Journal of Medicine* **120**: 678–84.

Spencer FA, Ginsberg JS, Chong A, Alter DA (2008) The relationship between unprovoked venous thromboembolism, age, and acute myocardial infarction. *Journal of Thrombosis and Haemostasis* **6**: 1507–13.

Tormene D, Simioni P, Pagnan A, Prandoni P (2004) The G20210A prothrombin gene mutation: is there room for screening families? *Journal of Thrombosis and Haemostasis* **2**: 1487–8.

van Boven HH, Vandenbroucke JP, Briet E, Rosendaal FR (1999) Gene–gene and gene–environment interactions determine risk of thrombosis in families with inherited antithrombin deficiency. *Blood* **94**: 2590–4.

van Sluis GL, Sohne M, El Kheir DY, Tanck MW, Gerdes VE, Buller HR (2006) Family history and inherited thrombophilia. *Journal of Thrombosis and Haemostasis* **4**: 2182–7.

Varga EA (2008) Genetic counseling for inherited thrombophilias. *Journal of Thrombosis and Thrombolysis* **25**: 6–9.

Verhovsek M, Douketis JD, Yi Q et al. (2008) Systematic review: D-dimer to predict recurrent disease after stopping anticoagulant therapy for unprovoked venous thromboembolism. *Annals of Internal Medicine* **149**: 481–90.

Vossen CY, Rosendaal FR (2006) Risk of arterial thrombosis in carriers of familial thrombophilia. *Journal of Thrombosis and Haemostasis* **4**: 916–18.

Vossen CY, Conard J, Fontcuberta J et al. (2004) Familial thrombophilia and lifetime risk of venous thrombosis. *Journal of Thrombosis and Haemostasis* **2**: 1526–32.

Acquired venous thrombosis

46

Beverley J Hunt[1] and Michael Greaves[2]

[1]Guy's and St Thomas' NHS Foundation Trust, London, UK
[2]School of Medicine and Dentistry, University of Aberdeen, Aberdeen, UK

Introduction

Deep vein thrombosis (DVT) is common, principally affecting the lower limbs. In many populations the annual incidence is around 1 per 1000 population. However, the disorder is highly age-dependent. For example, it is exceptional in childhood, has an incidence of the order of 1 per 10 000 population per year in young adults, and may reach 1% per annum in the very elderly. The incidence of pulmonary embolism is lower, possibly around 1 per 3000 population annually, although subclinical pulmonary embolism occurs frequently in subjects with lower limb proximal DVT. In patients who die in hospital there is evidence of pulmonary embolism in up to 20% of cases and in many it contributes to the cause of death. Clinically apparent pulmonary embolism occurs rarely when DVT is confined to calf veins, but if untreated calf vein thrombosis propagates to proximal veins in around 20% of cases, with an accompanying risk of significant pulmonary embolism. In some cases pulmonary embolism presents without identifiable DVT.

DVT is important because of the associated acute morbidity and risk of fatal pulmonary embolism, and also because of the potential long-term sequelae: a high risk of recurrent thrombosis, the development of chronic post-phlebitic symptoms, and pulmonary hypertension. The risk of recurrence after a first episode of apparently unprovoked proximal DVT of a lower limb is around 25% during the 5 years after discontinuation of oral anticoagulant therapy and is highest during the first few months. However, the risk is considerably lower when the first event was precipitated by a transient risk factor, such as a surgical procedure. When the first episode of thrombosis affects the deep veins, the symptoms of recurrence are most commonly those of DVT also. Similarly, recurrence after a first episode of pulmonary embolism is typically with further pulmonary embolism.

Chronic post-phlebitic symptoms in the leg range from minor itching and swelling to intractable ulceration. Some degree of post-phlebitic syndrome is present in around 30% of sufferers of previous lower limb DVT 10 years after the event. It is most frequent and severe after recurrent thrombosis and uncommon after DVT confined to the calf vessels. The risk of development of pulmonary hypertension after pulmonary embolism may have been underestimated previously. Symptomatic pulmonary hypertension may be present in around 4% of subjects and is more likely if there has been recurrent pulmonary embolism.

Vessels other than the deep veins of the limbs may be affected by thrombosis, including superficial limb veins, the intracranial venous sinuses and visceral veins. The pathogenesis of superficial thrombophlebitis may differ from that of DVT. Thrombosis of retinal veins also appears to have a different pathogenesis and natural history.

As described in the preceding chapter, venous thromboembolic episodes result from the interaction of multiple risk factors. These may be gene–environment interactions or multiple environmental or acquired risk factors. In this chapter, the acquired conditions that predispose to venous thromboembolism (VTE) are considered, although in most cases it is likely

Postgraduate Haematology: 6th edition. Edited by A. Victor Hoffbrand, Daniel Catovsky, Edward G.D. Tuddenham, Anthony R. Green
© 2011 Blackwell Publishing Ltd.

Table 46.1 Causal factors in acquired venous thromboembolism.

Inevitable/environmental
Increasing age
Pregnancy and post partum
Immobility, e.g. long-haul travel
Dehydration

Iatrogenic
Postoperative/immobilization
Indwelling venous devices
Pharmacological
    Estrogen related: combined oral contraceptive, hormone-
       replacement therapy, tamoxifen
    Chemotherapy
    Heparin
    Procoagulant treatment

Disease-related
Antiphospholipid syndrome
Cancer
    Myeloproliferative diseases
    Acute promyelocytic leukaemia
Inflammatory states
Haematological disease
    Paroxysmal nocturnal haemoglobinuria
    Thrombotic thrombocytopenic purpura
    Sickle cell disease
Intravenous drug abuse

that the individual genotype influences the likelihood of thrombosis in particular circumstances. In addition to the factors listed in Table 46.1, there has been recent interest in an association between VTE and artherosclerotic disease and the metabolic syndrome.

Pregnancy and venous thromboembolism

Around 1 in 1000 pregnancies is complicated by DVT or pulmonary embolism. Massive pulmonary embolism is the leading cause of pregnancy-related death in the UK. Although the postpartum phase has been considered to be the time of highest risk, overall at least as many episodes of VTE occur antepartum, including some in the first trimester. There are notable clinical features in pregnancy-related DVT: around 90% of thromboses affect the deep veins of the left lower limb and the vast majority of cases involve the iliofemoral vein from the time of presentation; thrombosis restricted to the deep veins of the calf is uncommon in pregnancy but is more common after birth. The left-sided predominance most likely relates to the anatomical relationship between the iliac artery and vein on that side. Many affected women develop post-phlebitic syndrome.

The pathogenesis of pregnancy-related VTE is multifactorial, as in other situations. For example, obesity may contribute. Unique factors include the raised intra-abdominal pressure and vascular compression caused by the gravid uterus, the suppressed systemic fibrinolytic capacity, the progressive increase in plasma concentrations of clotting factors from around 10 weeks' gestation, including factor (F)VIII and fibrinogen, and the fall in plasma concentration of the anticoagulant cofactor protein S. Tissue trauma from delivery contributes to the pathogenesis of post-partum VTE and operative delivery increases the risk further.

Although heritable thrombophilias contribute to the risk of pregnancy-related VTE, in around 70% of cases no hereditary thrombophilia can be identified and in 25% there is also no obvious risk factor other than otherwise normal pregnancy.

Immobility as a risk factor for venous thromboembolism

It is likely that venous stasis is a significant pathogenetic factor in VTE. For example, sitting still for 90 min reduces the flow through the popliteal vein by 50%. Immobility is a major contributor to hospital-acquired VTE, and is a factor in DVT in paralysed limbs and associated with splinting, for example in a plaster cast.

There has been considerable interest in the relationship between VTE and the physically cramped conditions encountered during travel, especially long-haul aircraft journeys. The term 'economy class syndrome' has been coined to encompass the occurrence of VTE during and after air travel. The level of risk of VTE has been exaggerated, partly due to media attention. Epidemiological data suggest a relative risk of around twofold, which persists for a few weeks after the journey. A similar level of risk applies to other modes of powered travel, including by road. Observational data indicate that the incidence of death from pulmonary embolism induced acutely by air travel is less than one in a million journeys. The duration of the flight is a factor, with some evidence that VTE risks begin to increase progressively with flight time of greater than 4 or 5 hours. As in other situations, the pathogenesis is multifactorial, for example the elderly and less mobile are more at risk. The contribution of the particular environmental conditions within a pressurized cabin, particularly hypobaric hypoxia, to hypercoagulability is disputed. At present it is reasonable to assume that any form of long-distance powered travel carries a low but increased risk of VTE and to recommend simple precautionary measures such as maintenance of hydration and calf exercises and ambulation in order to maintain venous flow in the lower limbs.

Iatrogenic venous thromboembolism

VTE is common in hospitalized subjects, despite the widespread adoption of physical and pharmacological methods of thrombophylaxis. As indicated above, immobility is probably a significant contributory factor. In postoperative patients and acutely ill medical patients, features of the acute-phase response, such as increased fibrinogen and FVIII concentrations in plasma, and reactive thrombocytosis also play a part. The highest prevalence of VTE occurs after major orthopaedic surgery to the lower limb. In hip replacement and knee replacement surgery subclinical DVT is frequently detectable by imaging, although there is evidence that clinically significant VTE may be becoming less common due to improvements in surgical techniques and materials, as well as wider use of thrombophylaxis.

Indwelling venous devices

Indwelling venous devices, such as Hickman catheters, are a significant cause of DVT, which may progress to complete occlusion of the superior vena cava. Up to 60% of patients with central venous catheters (CVCs) will develop a complication secondary to the device, thrombosis being one of the most common. Thrombosis associated with CVC may involve the catheter tip, the length of the catheter, the catheterized vessel in the upper limb, the central vasculature of the neck/mediastinum, or a combination of these. A higher incidence of thrombosis is seen in catheters with larger external diameters and those with a tip positioned distal to the superior vena cava. Other factors that predispose to a higher rate of catheter-related thrombosis include catheter infection, infusion of sclerosing chemotherapeutic agents, extrinsic vessel compression and a previous history of VTE.

Patients with CVC-related thrombosis may present with swelling and/or pain of the arm, neck or face. Some may present with symptoms suggestive of a pulmonary embolism or with catheter malfunction. Many of the symptoms are non-specific and for this reason imaging is required to confirm or exclude thrombosis. Contrast venography remains the reference standard for diagnosis of CVC-related thrombosis but this is invasive and may be painful. Ultrasonography is the most accurate non-invasive test, with a sensitivity and specificity of 93% and 95% respectively.

Treatment of CVC-related thrombosis remains poorly studied. There are several treatment options available: anticoagulation alone, systemic thrombolysis, low-dose local thrombolysis and catheter removal, or any combination of the above. Systemic thrombolysis may cause bleeding and should be avoided. Warfarin has been used to prevent catheter thrombosis in patients with cancer but appears to be ineffective and may result in increased bleeding. Almost all episodes of VTE in neonates are provoked by indwelling vascular devices.

Pharmaceuticals

Combined oral contraceptive

Iatrogenic VTE associated with use of the combined oral contraceptive is of particular importance because it affects healthy women in a young age group. The overall risk of VTE in a pill user is around fourfold to fivefold higher than in a non-pill user, although this is influenced greatly by the presence of some heritable thrombophilias, as described in the previous chapter. The risk is also increased by obesity and older age. Fortunately, the absolute risk remains acceptable because of the low background prevalence of thrombosis in women of childbearing age. Estrogen-containing preparations induce a state of reduced sensitivity to activated protein C, and this appears to be more marked with the third-generation contraceptives than second-generation preparations. (Most preparations in current use contain an equivalent dose of estrogen, usually 30–35 μg of ethinylestradiol. However, the progestagen content varies. In so-called second-generation oral contraceptives this is levonorgestrel, whereas in third-generation products it is desogestrel, gestodene or norgestimate.) There is convincing epidemiological evidence that the third-generation pills also carry a greater risk of clinical VTE. Progestagen-only oral contraceptives appear to carry a lower risk of VTE such that their use can be considered in women in whom the combined oral contraceptive is deemed to be contraindicated, for example due to previous VTE or presence of thrombophilia.

Hormone-replacement therapy

Hormone-replacement therapy (HRT) is also associated with VTE. In this case the absolute risk is higher due to the greater background prevalence of VTE in older women. Observational data indicate a very high rate of VTE in women with a previous history of venous thrombosis who embark upon HRT subsequently. Such is the level of risk that HRT is generally contraindicated in such women. If there are overwhelming indications for HRT (usually disabling menopausal symptoms) some clinicians consider warfarin thrombophylaxis alongside HRT in high-risk situations. Also, the procoagulant changes induced by transdermal preparations appear to be less marked, suggesting that they may be less likely to provoke VTE than oral formulations and may be considered in those thought to be at increased risk of VTE.

Chemotherapeutic agents

Use of chemotherapeutic agents and adjunctive therapies in malignancy has been linked to VTE. Notable examples are asparaginase in acute lymphoblastic leukaemia, thalidomide in myeloma and tamoxifen in breast cancer. Tamoxifen blocks estrogen receptors but has weak estrogenic activity and this may underly the association with VTE. Asparaginase inhibits protein synthesis, and markedly reduced plasma concentrations of antithrombin may be one mechanism of the prothrombotic state associated with its use. The pathogenesis of thrombosis associated with thalidomide has not been fully elucidated but it is noteworthy that some data suggest that aspirin may reduce the incidence of the complication. This potentially implicates platelets in the pathogenesis. It appears to be associated particularly with use of the agent in myeloma, rather than other indications.

Heparin-induced thrombocytopenia

Heparin-induced thrombocytopenia (HIT) is an important diagnosis because failure to recognize the syndrome carries a high risk of death from associated venous or arterial thrombosis. It is due to development of antibodies to a complex of heparin and platelet factor 4 that induces intravascular platelet activation and consumption. Typically, the platelet count begins to fall between 5 and 10 days after first exposure to heparin. In subjects with previous recent exposure it may occur earlier and very occasionally the thrombocytopenia develops after heparin has been discontinued. The condition may complicate heparin administered at any dose, including as perioperative thrombophylaxis and even when very low doses are used to maintain the patency of intravascular cannulae. Indeed, there are very occasional reports of a clinically identical syndrome developing in the absence of exposure to administered heparin. HIT is around 10-fold less common with low-molecular-weight preparations than with unfractionated heparin. The synthetic pentasaccharide fondaparinux appears unlikely to cross-react with HIT antibodies or to cause HIT. In contrast to other drug-related immune thrombocytopenias, the degree of thrombocytopenia is rarely severe and bleeding is not a feature. There may be systemic symptoms including fever and a local reaction at the heparin injection site, such as erythema or even skin necrosis after subcutaneous administration. Because of platelet activation there is often new thrombosis, and this may manifest before the platelet count reaches thrombocytopenic levels. When heparin has been administered to treat arterial disease the new thrombosis is most commonly arterial, and in treatment of DVT there is usually extension of the presenting thrombus, often with pulmonary embolism. Thrombotic stroke, myocardial infarction, visceral ischaemia and disseminated intravascular coagulation have all been reported.

Confirmatory laboratory tests are not entirely satisfactory. Immunoassays for heparin/platelet factor 4 are sensitive but lack specificity because a significant proportion of subjects treated with heparin have positive antibody tests but neither thrombocytopenia nor thrombosis. In contrast, bioassays which rely on activation of normal platelets in the presence of test plasma and a low concentration of heparin are specific but high sensitivity is difficult to achieve. Sensitivity is improved by use of platelet serotonin secretion as an end point and employment of donor platelets of proven sensitivity. Specificity

is achieved by the demonstration of a positive result with a low heparin concentration, which is absent in the presence of a high concentration. Because of the limitations of these confirmatory tests, monitoring of the platelet count and a high index of clinical suspicion are essential whenever heparin is administered.

The most practical approach to diagnosis outside the intensive care unit, where thrombocytopenia is common due to the other causes that may coexist with HIT, is the employment of a scoring algorithm based on the timing of onset of thrombocytopenia, presence or absence of new thrombosis, presence or absence of other potential cause of thrombocytopenia, and the degree of thrombocytopenia (the four T's algorithm). If the probability score is high, heparin should be stopped. When a high score is combined with an immunoassay, this results in improved sensitivity and specificity for HIT. Consideration of the antibody titre provides additional evidence, low-titre antibodies being less specific. A British Committee for Standards in Haematology guideline gives advice on the diagnosis and management of HIT using this approach.

When there is a noteworthy fall in the platelet count that cannot be accounted for in any other way, heparin, in all forms, must be discontinued. An alternative anticoagulant must be administered immediately as the risk of thrombosis persists for several days after heparin withdrawal. Warfarin given alone is contraindicated as massive thrombosis has been described in this situation, most likely due to the rapid fall in protein C caused by warfarin against a background severe prothrombotic state. Aspirin is insufficient. The antibody may cross-react with low-molecular-weight heparins and they should be avoided. Danaparoid is a mix of anticoagulant glycosaminoglycans, predominantly heparan sulphate and dextran sulphate, and has been used in HIT. There is a significant risk of cross-reactivity with the HIT antibody in vivo, which may not be predicted by in vitro testing. Lepirudin is used frequently in HIT. It carries no risk of cross-reactivity but there should be caution if used in the presence of renal impairment. Warfarin can be introduced once an adequate anticoagulant effect with the thrombin inhibitor has been established. Fondaparinux has been used, but experience is less than that with lepirudin and danaparoid.

The pathogenetic antibodies tend to become unmeasurable in the ensuing few months but further exposure to heparin should be avoided for at least 6 months.

Haemostatic treatments

Haemostatic treatments may induce thrombosis, most notably prothrombin complex concentrates. They should not be used to reverse the coagulopathy in severe liver impairment as major thrombosis has been reported, with disseminated intravascular coagulation and death in some cases. This is probably due to impaired clearance of activated clotting factors in liver failure.

Antiphospholipid syndrome

Antiphospholipid syndrome (APS) is an important thrombophilic condition because it is of high prevalence and is associated with considerable morbidity and mortality. The essential features are arterial or venous thrombosis or recurrent pregnancy loss or placental dysfunction occurring in a subject in whom laboratory tests for antiphospholipid antibody are positive. Diagnostic criteria have been established in order to standardize diagnosis for the purposes of clinical studies (Table 46.2).

Limb DVT, pulmonary embolism and ischaemic stroke are the principal thrombotic manifestations, but any vessel may be involved. A characteristic of APS in an individual patient is the tendency to cause recurrent problems in the same vascular bed. The full range of clinical features is not necessarily present. For example, women can have severe thrombotic events without pregnancy complications and those with pregnancy complications most commonly have no other manifestation. In addition to thrombosis and pregnancy failure, additional clinical and laboratory features are variably present in APS. These include mild thrombocytopenia and an unusual dermatological feature, livedo reticularis. Cardiac valvular abnormalities occur in up to 30% of patients, but are usually subclinical. Most commonly the mitral or aortic valve is affected, often with valve thickening or incompetence. However, haemodynamic changes as a consequence of valvular damage are rare. Exceptionally, the syndrome may manifest as widespread microvascular occlusion, with multiorgan failure, so-called catastrophic APS.

APS may occur with another chronic systemic autoimmune disease, usually systemic lupus erythematosus (SLE), when the term 'secondary antiphospholipid syndrome' is used. In primary APS there is no evidence for another relevant underlying condition.

Antiphospholipid antibodies

Antiphospholipid antibodies are a family of antibodies reactive with proteins that have the property of binding to negatively charged phospholipids. The most important is β_2-glycoprotein I (β_2-GPI), as pathogenic antibodies (i.e. those most strongly associated with clinical events) are most frequently reactive with this protein. β_2-GPI is a member of the complement control protein family. It has five domains. It is now known that antiphospholipid antibodies reactive with each of these five domains may occur but it is only those which recognize a specific epitope on domain I that are pathogenic. Antibodies to other proteins which have affinity for negatively charged phospholipid have been implicated in the syndrome, including protein C, protein S and annexin V.

The lupus anticoagulant (LA) is an *in vitro* phenomenon in which the antiphospholipid antibody slows clot formation, thereby lengthening the clotting time. This is probably due to impairment of the assembly of the components of prothrombinase on phospholipid due to interference by the antibody (Figure 46.1). LA is due to antibodies reactive to β_2-GPI/

Table 46.2 Diagnostic criteria in APS.

Clinical criteria*
Thrombosis: arterial, venous or microvascular thrombosis in any tissue or organ

Laboratory criteria*
Antiphospholipid antibody
IgG or IgM anticardiolipin antibodies at moderate or high concentration[†]; IgG or IgM anti-β_2-GPI >99th percentile *and/or*
Lupus anticoagulant

Pregnancy complications
Unexplained death of morphologically normal fetus at or beyond 10 weeks of gestation
Three or more unexplained consecutive miscarriages before 10 weeks
One or more premature births of a morphologically normal fetus before 34 weeks of gestation due to pre-eclampsia, eclampsia or severe placental insufficiency

*There must be at least one clinical and at least one laboratory criterion present. The laboratory test must be consistently positive on at least two occasions 12 weeks apart as transient antibodies may occur, for example in infection. Such antibodies are not usually associated with clinical events.
[†]Evidence on the definition of moderate/high concentration. In general, values of IgG anticardiolipin > 40 GPLU are considered to be moderate-titre antibodies; >99th percentile has been employed also. The significance of low-titre antibodies is less clear.

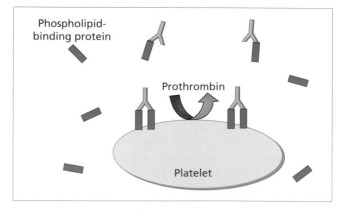

Figure 46.1 Antiphospholipid antibody binding: explanation for the lupus anticoagulant phenomenon.

phospholipid or to prothrombin/phospholipid. The β_2-GPI-dependent antibodies also bind in anticardiolipin assays, as the glycoprotein is present in test serum and often in assay reagents. LA due to prothrombin-reactive antibodies may be negative in anticardiolipin assays. Therefore some subjects with APS have LA and anticardiolipin and some LA only. Others have anticardiolipin without LA, due to the presence of non-β_2-GPI and non-prothrombin-dependent antibody or possibly to relative insensitivity of the coagulation assays for LA. Because antiphospholipid antibodies are so heterogeneous, a comprehensive laboratory approach is essential for their reliable detection. In most laboratories, ELISAs employing cardiolipin and coagulation-based assays for LA remain the principal diagnostic tools. ELISA for β_2-GPI may offer improved specificity. The pathogenicity of IgA anticardiolipin antibodies is disputed and their detection is not utilized routinely in diagnosis.

Pathogenic mechanisms in APS

The pathogenesis of pregnancy failure and thrombosis in APS is not fully understood. Animal experiments support a pathogenic role for antibodies to β_2-GPI. Important candidate mechanisms for thrombosis are antibody-induced concentration of prothrombin on phospholipid surfaces *in vivo* resulting in enhanced thrombin generation, interference with the activated protein C anticoagulant pathway, increased von Willebrand factor activity, and increased monocyte and endothelial tissue factor expression. Increased platelet activation and inhibition of fibrinolysis by antiphospholipid antibodies have also been proposed. In relation to pregnancy failure, again numerous pathogenic mechanisms have been proposed. It is noteworthy that early miscarriage is a common feature and occurs before full placentation. This raises doubts whether a thrombotic mechanism is causal. Therefore, it is of considerable interest that a body of evidence is accumulating for a role of complement activation in pregnancy loss in APS. Of particular note in this context, heparin is effective in preventing embryo loss in a murine model of APS and it does so through inhibition of complement rather than via an anticoagulant mechanism. This raises the possibility that similar mechanisms may be relevant to early pregnancy loss in women with APS. Placental dysfunction is the hallmark of second- and third-trimester complications of intrauterine fetal death, intrauterine growth restriction, pre-eclampsia and placental abruption. The aetiology of the placental dysfunction has been related to placental infarction and an acute atherosis in the maternal spiral arteries, although these are not universal features. One interesting hypothesis for the cause of placental insufficiency is displacement of annexin V from trophoblast by antiphospholipid antibodies, with resultant acceleration of thrombin generation on the exposed negatively charged phospholipid.

Laboratory diagnosis of antiphospholipid antibodies

In diagnosing APS it is essential to consider that antiphospholipid antibodies are not specific to the syndrome. In addition to transient antibodies, which may for example be triggered by intercurrent infection, some chronic infections are associated with antiphospholipid antibodies, such as syphilis and hepatitis C. Antiphospholipid antibodies may also be detected incidentally in healthy subjects and they occur in relation to use of some drugs, particularly chlorpromazine. These drug-induced and infection-related antibodies do not usually appear to be associated with the clinical thrombotic manifestations of APS. In some cases they appear to be neither β_2-GPI nor prothrombin dependent.

The diagnosis of APS relies on the demonstration of the persistent presence of either LA by coagulation tests or of antiphospholipid antibodies by solid-phase immunoassays for anticardiolipin and/or β_2-GPI. Reliance on just one type of assay may lead to false-negative assessment of antiphospholipid antibodies. Overall, among the commonly applied assays, it appears that those for LA associate most strongly with clinical events. In relation to solid-phase assays, high-titre antibodies and IgG antibodies associate more strongly with clinical manifestations than do IgM and lower-titre antibodies.

Coagulation assays (lupus anticoagulant tests)

The LA assay is a double misnomer for it is neither a test for SLE nor for an *in vivo* anticoagulant. LA tests are indirect assays that rely on slowing of the clotting time of plasma through interference by antiphospholipid antibodies. The tests most frequently employed are the activated partial thromboplastin time (APTT), the dilute Russell's viper venom time (DRVVT) and, less frequently now, the kaolin clotting time (KCT).

Platelet activation causes exposure of negatively charged phospholipid at the cell surface and therefore contamination of test plasma with platelets must be minimized, as these will limit the sensitivity of tests particularly when plasma must be stored frozen prior to testing. Platelet depletion may be achieved in various ways, most commonly by careful double centrifugation.

None of the above coagulation assays is specific for LA. Specificity and sensitivity are also reagent dependent. For example, some partial thromboplastin reagents are insensitive to LA. If the same reagent is employed for LA tests as in routine laboratory screening for coagulopathy, sensitivity to LA must be assured. Factors that lengthen or shorten clotting times (other than antiphospholipid antibodies) potentially intefere in LA tests. Examples are anticoagulant drugs and clotting factor deficiencies and inhibitors, which lengthen clotting times, and increased clotting factor levels, especially FVIII, which shortens the time to clotting in the APTT for example, potentially masking the presence of LA.

In order to reduce the risks of false interpretation, in addition to prolongation of clotting time in a phospholipid-dependent coagulation test, the criteria for LA positivity also include (i) evidence of an inhibitor demonstrated by mixing studies and (ii) confirmation of the phospholipid-dependent nature of the inhibitor. In principle, laboratory tests should employ a detection or screening stage (prolongation of the clotting time) and a confirmation stage showing (i) failure of correction of the prolongation when normal plasma is added in order to exclude factor deficiency as the cause of the prolongation and (ii) that the prolongation is phospholipid dependent, for example by showing that addition of excess phospholipid corrects the clotting time. To achieve this, and because no LA test consistently shows 100% specificity and sensitivity, more than one test system should be used for detection of LA. The prothrombin time and thrombin time should also be performed as they are not usually affected by the presence of LA and the results assist in the interpretation of LA tests, for example when there is undisclosed anticoagulant therapy.

The APTT is commonly employed as the initial screening test for LA. Its specificity for inhibitor detection is improved by inclusion of a mixing study with platelet-free normal pooled plasma. When prolongation of the APTT is due to coagulation factor deficiency, the clotting time corrects when the test is repeated on an equal mixture of patient and normal plasma, whereas the prolongation above normal may persist with LA, consistent with its inhibitory activity. However, correction in a mixing study does not exclude LA, as a weak antibody is obviously diluted out by addition of normal plasma and this may be sufficient to abolish its effect. Very occasionally LA causes enhancement of the prolongation of the APTT when normal plasma is added. This phenomenon has been called the lupus cofactor effect but is the exception rather than the rule. Inhibitors to clotting factors, usually FVIII, are associated with bleeding rather than thrombosis but also cause prolongation of the clotting times which may not be corrected by addition of normal plasma. Typically, FVIII inhibitors are time-dependent, unlike LA. Diagnostic confusion may arise due to LA that prolongs the APTT, causing erroneously low results in coagulation factor assays based on the APTT. A normal APTT is insufficient to exclude LA and additional tests must be performed.

The DRVVT does not involve the clotting factors of the extrinsic system, unlike the APTT, nor FVII, unlike the prothrombin time. Any inhibition of coagulant-active phospholipid in the test by LA results in a prolonged DRVVT. However, as is the case with all LA tests, it is not specific. Deficiencies of clotting factors, for example FII and FX due to warfarin therapy, will also prolong the DRVVT. The specificity of the test is improved by repeating it in the presence of a high concentration of phospholipid, which should result in partial or complete correction of the prolonged clotting time if it is due to LA. This phospholipid is conveniently provided as platelet membranes in which negatively charged phospholipid is exposed by freezing and thawing. In the presence of LA, the ratio of test to normal plasma clotting time is often in excess of 1.2, and corrects to less than 1.2, or at least partially, in the platelet neutralization procedure. As with all coagulation tests, because of variations in reagents and techniques it is essential that laboratories derive local normal ranges using a large number of plasma samples from healthy volunteers.

In the KCT no additional phospholipid is employed. The test therefore resembles the APTT in that it involves the extrinsic and common pathways of coagulation but the sensitivity to LA is enhanced because the small amount of phospholipid present is only that derived from residual platelets in the test sample and plasma lipids. The test is affected by clotting factor deficiencies and anticoagulants, but specificity can be improved by use of normal plasma mixing at more than one ratio to test plasma. LA is identified when the KCT fails to correct even after relatively large proportions of normal plasma are added, whereas in factor deficiency the KCT is corrected with small amounts of normal plasma.

Alternative tests for LA may be employed but are not in general use. They include the tissue thromboplastin inhibition test and clotting tests that use venoms other than Russell's viper venom. Examples are Taipan and Textarin venoms. Many laboratories rely on commercial assay kits for LA testing. It is essential that steps are taken to ensure internal and external quality assurance.

Solid-phase assays (for anticardiolipin and anti-β_2-GPI antibodies)

Solid-phase assays for antiphospholipid antibodies, such as the anticardiolipin ELISA, allow rapid processing of numerous serum samples and the results are not affected by factor deficiency or the use of anticoagulants. The introduction of international standards allows the calculation of anticardiolipin results in IgG or IgM antiphospholipid units (GPLU and MPLU, respectively) related to a given concentration of affinity-purified anticardiolipin immunoglobulin. Despite this, there remains a lack of precision, and comparability between laboratories using different assays is not ensured. Clinicians should be aware of the performance of the assay in use.

The detection of anticardiolipin allows the diagnosis of APS in a subject with an appropriate clinical history, even when LA is absent. However, the anticardiolipin assay is not a substitute for the LA test, nor does it confirm that LA is present due to the antibody heterogeneity referred to above. Furthermore, the clinical significance of low-titre anticardiolipin is doubtful. Thus, in cases where the anticardiolipin titre is less than 30 GPLU and tests for LA are negative, a diagnosis of APS may not be conclusive. Under these circumstances it is particularly important to consider other causes of thrombosis or miscarriage.

Specific assays for anti-β_2-GPI antibodies have been developed, and several commercial kits are available. Anti-β_2-GPI antibody assays may show higher precision and better correlation with the thromboembolic complications in APS and SLE than assays for anticardiolipin, and are less likely to show transient positive results in association with infection. Antiprothrombin antibodies generally exhibit poor specificity for venous thrombosis and recurrent fetal loss, and may be found in patients with infection, and are not included in the consensus criteria for diagnosis of APS.

The prevalence of antiphospholipid antibodies in subjects with thrombosis varies with selection criteria for testing. Because the risk of recurrent thrombosis appears to be great, antiphospholipid antibodies should be sought in subjects with arterial, venous or microvascular thrombosis where no other cause is apparent. Examples are younger subjects with ischaemic stroke in the absence of cardiovascular disease and subjects with unprovoked VTE.

The prevalence of persistent antiphospholipid antibodies among women with recurrent first-trimester miscarriage is around 15%, although a proportion of these are low-titre antibodies. In women with recurrent miscarriage due to APS the prospective fetal loss rate may be as high as 90%. In contrast, the prevalence of positive tests for antiphospholipid antibodies in unselected women of childbearing age is around 3% and they are not sensitive predictors of poor pregnancy outcome in women with no history of pregnancy complications. Because miscarriage is a common phenomenon, screening for antiphospholipid antibodies is not indicated after a single event. Maternal antiphospholipid antibodies may be downregulated during pregnancy, so tests are best performed preconceptually when possible. A small proportion of women with antiphospholipid antibodies also have anti-Ro antibodies. Their detection is important as anti-Ro is associated with a 2% risk of complete heart block in the fetus and a 10% chance of neonatal lupus.

Management of APS

Thrombosis

There is wide variability in severity of prothrombotic states between individuals with APS. The management of patients with antiphospholipid antibodies and previous thrombosis remains contentious. Retrospective observational studies suggested that these patients should remain on indefinite oral anticoagulation, maintaining an International Normalized Ratio (INR) of 3–4. However, subsequent prospective randomized studies indicate that a lower target INR of 2–3 is effective in preventing recurrent thrombosis in the majority of patients with previous venous thrombosis. There is less certainty in arterial thrombosis; for example, clinical observation suggests that there is a significant subpopulation of APS with small-vessel thrombosis, some evident as lacunar infarcts on magnetic resonance imaging, who appear to require a target INR of 3–4 to prevent recurrent cerebral thrombosis.

Immunosuppressive therapy is not generally indicated in primary APS other than in the very rare case where thrombosis recurs despite intensive anticoagulant therapy. Corticosteroids and other immunomodulatory therapies have been administered. An exception may be catastrophic APS when combination treatment with antithrombotics, corticosteroids and other immunomodulatory therapies such as rituximab are administered as potentially life-saving emergency measures.

Pregnancy

The management of recurrent fetal loss is based on the use of anticoagulation with empirical doses of heparin, usually low-molecular-weight heparin in the UK, often in combination with low-dose aspirin. Initial studies indicated that this approach increases the chance of a successful outcome of a healthy live birth from 30 to 70–80%, although the total number of cases in randomized studies is limited and trials have given conflicting results. Nevertheless, low-molecular-weight heparin prophylaxis has become standard, although some clinicians believe that combination antithrombotic therapy as a first line should be reserved for women with a previous history of fetal death while those with recurrent miscarriage should be given supporting care as first line, with aspirin or aspirin/heparin reserved for those with further pregnancy failure. Corticosteroids are ineffective and their use is associated with frequent maternal morbidity from hypertension, glucose intolerance and premature labour.

Thrombophylaxis for those with APS and a previous history of thrombosis is based again on use of low-molecular-weight heparin, although there is neither consensus on dosing nor the need to monitor therapy.

Venous thromboembolism and cancer

Cancer is a major risk factor for VTE. VTE is the major cause of morbidity and mortality after the cancer itself in patients with malignancy. It is estimated that almost 15% of cancer patients will have a thromboembolic event. Post-mortem studies have shown that thromboembolism is common in patients who die of cancer. Of all oncology patients, palliative-care inpatients have the highest risk of VTE with a DVT prevalence that may be as high as 50%, including bilateral deep vein thromboses. Chemotherapy may also increase that risk: thalidomide is a prominent example. The risk of thrombosis varies with type of cancer, ovarian, brain and pancreatic cancers having the highest rates. Lymphomas and leukaemias account for a significant proportion of thromboses as do colonic and lung cancers.

In Trousseau syndrome, the cancer-related phlebitis is recurrent and migratory and affects both the superficial and deep veins, in contrast to the more common association of lower limb DVT in cancer. Unusual sites such as arms and neck, as well as superficial veins of the thorax and abdomen may be involved. Typically, such a patient has an occult tumour, usually adenocarcinoma, although it is also a feature of acute leukaemia. In Trousseau syndrome, conventional anticoagulation often fails to prevent recurrent thromboses.

Prothrombotic changes associated with malignancies

In Table 46.3 the components of Virchow's triad are used to illustrate the features that lead to oncology patients having such a high risk of thrombosis. There are specific abnormalities unique to cancer patients, the so-called tumour procoagulants. Tumour procoagulants are surface molecules on cancer cells that activate coagulation. The two principal tumour cell procoagulants are tissue factor and cancer procoagulant. The latter directly activates FX without involvement of FVII. The increasing number of tumour procoagulants that have been described are listed on the International Society for Thrombosis and Haemostasis registry. APS has also been reported in malignancy, particularly in association with paraproteins.

Difficulties in management

Cancer patients with thrombosis are at particularly high risk of recurrent thrombotic events. Cohort and population-based studies have shown that the risk of recurrence after stopping anticoagulation in cancer patients is approximately double that in non-cancer patients. Treatment with anticoagulation in cancer patients is often unsuccessful, due to the high risk of recurrent VTE and major bleeding. Unfortunately, these risks are associated with oral anticoagulation intensities within the usual therapeutic range. The risks are greatest during the first

Table 46.3 Some pathogenic factors for thrombosis in cancer patients.

Stasis
Immobility
Extrinsic pressure, e.g. oedematous limbs

Vessel wall/endothelial perturbation
Cytokine release from tumours
Local tumour infiltration
Central venous catheter

Hypercoagulability
Dehydration
Cytokine-related prothrombotic changes
Tissue factor/cancer procoagulant expression on tumour cells
Disseminated intravascular coagulation
Increased platelet activation

few weeks of anticoagulation treatment and increase with cancer extent. Several studies have demonstrated significant increases in rates of bleeding, as high as 20% among cancer patients receiving oral anticoagulation. Within the palliative care setting, where patients have far more advanced disease, the bleeding incidence was higher, even with strict monitoring of anticoagulation. Oral anticoagulation in cancer patients is complicated further due to anorexia, vomiting, liver impairment and drug interactions. Moreover there may be frequent interruption to treatment due to thrombocytopenia and the need for invasive procedures, and venous access is often difficult in these patients especially if they have had previous chemotherapy through peripheral veins.

The decision to use oral anticoagulation in this group of patients should not be taken lightly and safe treatment requires intensive monitoring of INR and the burden of repeated blood tests. Disillusionment with the use of oral anticoagulation in cancer patients has led to trials assessing low-molecular-weight heparins in cancer. The CLOT trial randomized over 650 cancer patients with symptomatic proximal DVT and/or pulmonary embolism to treatment with dalteparin for 5–7 days and then randomization to either oral anticoagulation maintaining a target INR of 2.5 or dalteparin. In the dalteparin arm a full treatment dose was given for 1 month and then reduced to 75–80% of this dose. After 6 months there was a significantly reduced rate of recurrent VTE in the dalteparin group of 8.8% compared with 17.4% in the group with oral anticoagulation. Bleeding was also significantly reduced. A similar reduction in VTE was found in patients with cancer who entered the LITE study where treatment dose tinzaparin was compared with oral anticoagulation after VTE. These data support the use of low-molecular-weight heparin rather than warfarin in patients with cancer and VTE.

Thrombotic risk in polycythaemia rubra vera and essential (primary) thrombocythaemia

If left untreated, patients with polycythaemia vera (PV) have a median survival of 18 months, with the majority dying of vascular occlusion. The occlusive lesions may involve the larger vessels or the microvasculature. In PV, large-vessel events involve arteries and veins equally whereas in essential thrombocythaemia (ET) arteries are more commonly involved. A high proportion of thromboses occur in the cerebral circulation, although thrombosis widely distributed in the arterial and venous systems, including the splanchnic vessels, has been well documented. Hepatic vein and portal vein thromboses are more commonly associated with PV than ET. Indeed it has been reported that some patients with apparently idiopathic hepatic or portal vein thrombosis have subclinical myeloproliferative disease based on the finding of erythropoietin-independent erythroid colony growth in marrow culture or presence of JAK2 mutation. In PV there is good evidence that the incidence of vascular occlusion is positively related to the packed cell volume, with the lowest incidence in patients with good control of haematocrit. The role of thrombocytosis in risk of thrombosis in PV is disputed. The risk of thrombosis in PV also increases with advancing age and a past history of thrombosis.

ET is often diagnosed in the subclinical phase but a number of studies suggest that overall survival is determined principally by occurrence of thrombosis. In one study the rate of thrombosis ranged from around 2% per patient-year in those aged less than 40 to 15% in those aged greater than 60. In around 50% of cases of ET. the JAK2 V617F mutation is detectable. Whether subjects with the mutation are more likely to develop thrombosis is a subject of current investigation.

The pathogenesis of thrombosis in ET is poorly understood. Elevated platelet counts are implicated, with platelet counts greater than $600 \times 10^9/L$ being associated with increased incidence of vascular occlusion. Although treatment to reduce abnormal counts will reduce the frequency of events, a proportion of patients will still experience thrombosis. In addition, some patients with ET will remain thrombosis-free with no treatment to reduce their platelet count.

The microvascular events and vasomotor manifestations of both PV and ET almost certainly relate to quantitive and qualitative changes in platelets, for they are not seen in other forms of polycythaemia or thrombocytosis. It is possible that similar small-vessel occlusive and vasomotor changes seen in the feet and hands may also occur in other parts of the body. Erythromelalgia, a syndrome consisting of painful burning red extremities with normal peripheral pulses, is the characteristic vasomotor disturbance. Physical findings may be absent or there may be warmth, duskiness and mottled erythema of the involved areas. Livedo reticularis is occasionally found. In the digital vessels, usually of the toes but occasionally the fingers, the development of thrombosis can lead to digital ischaemia and gangrene. In relation to the cerebral circulation, a range of symptoms and signs including transient cerebral ischaemia, transient monocular blindness, migraine, headaches and seizures are seen. Both the cerebrovascular complications and erythromelalgia of myeloproliferative disease may respond promptly to low-dose aspirin and/or platelet cytoreduction.

Conventional risk factors for cardiovascular disease are implicated in the pathogenesis of thrombosis in ET, including hypertension, smoking, hypercholesterolaemia and diabetes, and should be considered in deciding whether cytoreductive therapy is indicated.

Acute promyelocytic leukaemia

In comparison with the severe haemorrhagic presentation in the majority of cases of acute promyelocytic leukaemia (APL), acute arterial thrombosis is a rare presenting feature. Thrombosis is associated with the microgranular variant of APL, which accounts for 25% of all cases, characterized by a paucity of myeloid granules and a lobulated monocytoid nucleus. The cells stain positive with Sudan black and myeloperoxidase and there is a high incidence of CD34 positivity. Vascular occlusion is more common when a high white cell count ($> 150 \times 10^9/L$) predisposes to leucostasis. It is thought that the leukaemic cells release procoagulants. It is important to recognize this variant of APL because the use of all-*trans* retinoic acid may increase the risk of thrombosis due to a further increase in peripheral white cell count exacerbating leucostasis.

Inflammation and thrombosis

Systemic inflammation is a potent prothrombotic stimulus (Table 46.4). Inflammation upregulates procoagulant factors, downregulates physiological anticoagulants, inhibits fibrinolytic activity and increases the platelet count. Inflammatory mediators promote coagulation by causing endothelial cell activation and increasing the expression of tissue factor. Endotoxin, tumour necrosis factor (TNF) and interferon-1α induce tissue factor expression primarily on monocytes/macrophages and probably in atherosclerotic plaques as well. Thrombin, a key enzyme in coagulation, also has cytokine-like activities for it augments leucocyte adhesion and can activate endothelium, leucocytes and platelets. Thrombin-mediated signalling through protease-activated receptor (PAR)-1 on vascular cells has recently been shown to mediate production of chemokines such as MCP-1, leading to recruitment of inflammatory cells including monocytes. Activation of these cells by thrombin increases the expression of negatively charged phospholipids such as phosphatidylserine on the surface of the cells, promoting surface procoagulant activity.

Interleukin (IL)-6 and its family of molecules mediate the acute-phase response. This increases liver synthesis of plasma proteins including fibrinogen and other coagulation proteins,

Table 46.4 Effects of inflammation on haemostasis.

Increased
Tissue factor expression
Surface procoagulant activity, negatively charged phospholipid
Platelet reactivity
Levels of fibrinogen and other coagulation proteins

Decreased
Thrombomodulin expression
Endothelial cell protein C receptor
Half-life of activated protein C
Protein Z
Fibrinolytic activity due to increased PAI-1
Endothelial gylcosaminoglycans

PAI, plasminogen activator inhibitor.

thus priming the blood coagulation system for action. IL-6 also increases platelet reactivity. Plasma levels of the recently discovered vitamin K-dependent anticoagulant protein Z, which acts by inhibiting FXa, fall during inflammation; thus protein Z appears to be a negative acute-phase protein.

Of all the physiological anticoagulant pathways, the protein C pathway appears to be the most influenced by inflammation. Thrombomodulin and endothelial cell protein C receptor are both downregulated by inflammatory cytokines such as TNF-α. There is inhibition of the promoter of the thrombomodulin gene as well as active pinocytosis to remove existing surface molecules, while neutrophil elastase readily cleaves thrombomodulin from the endothelial cell surface. Moreover, thrombomodulin is very sensitive to oxidation of an exposed methionine by oxidants produced by leucocytes. These observations have led to studies demonstrating apparent therapeutic value of activated protein C in subjects with multiorgan failure due to severe sepsis.

Endothelial cell activation occurs in inflammation. This causes downregulation of fibrinolytic activation by increased production of plasminogen activator inhibitor (PAI)-1. There may also be cleavage of glycosaminoglycans from the surface of the endothelium, so that there is loss of heparan sulphate and other molecules that activate antithrombin.

As a consequence of these changes, conditions that provoke an inflammatory response are associated with increased risk of venous thrombosis. These include inflammatory bowel disease, Behçet disease, systemic tuberculosis, SLE and diabetes. Atherosclerosis can be considered a chronic inflammatory state and has recently been associated with an increased incidence of venous thrombosis and, more recently, the metabolic syndrome has been implicated. Furthermore, epidemiological studies indicate an excess of minor illness, including infections, in the weeks preceding episodes of VTE. The association between inflammation and thrombosis emphasizes the need for thrombophylaxis in patients hospitalized on medical wards. Implementation of pharmacological thrombophylaxis has been inadequate in such patients.

Haematological prothrombotic states due to non-malignant diseases of the blood and bone marrow

Paroxysmal nocturnal haemoglobinuria (see Chapter 11)

Venous thrombosis occurs in up to 40% of patients with paroxysmal nocturnal haemoglobinuria (PNH) and represents a significant cause of morbidity and mortality. Frequently it is the presenting feature. Thrombosis most commonly occurs in the hepatic veins, portal veins and saggital sinus. Hepatic vein thrombosis leading to Budd–Chiari syndrome is the common-

est site and affects 15–25% of patients with PNH. Presentation is with pain in the right upper quadrant, jaundice and abdominal distension due to hepatomegaly and ascites. Thrombosis in splanchnic veins results in persistent abdominal pain, and symptoms and signs of intestinal obstruction may occur if infarction of the bowel ensues. Thrombosis of the splenic vein leads to splenomegaly and occasionally splenic rupture can occur. Portal vein thrombosis produces ascites and the later development of oesophageal varices. Saggital sinus thrombosis is the most frequent neurological complication. Symptoms include severe headache. There may be evidence of raised intracranial pressure, impaired conscious level and focal neurological signs. Occasionally, painful discoloured skin lesions occur when the dermal veins are affected. These lesions rarely ulcerate. Occasionally, skin lesions can resemble purpura fulminans; these can affect large areas of skin with necrosis and demarcation. Pregnancy in PNH is associated with an increased risk of fetal loss (40%) as a result of thrombosis and haemorrhage.

The pathogenesis of thrombosis in PNH remains uncertain. Platelets are capable of compensating for the decreased expression of decay accelerating factor (CD55) due to the presence of factor H, a similar protein, that is present within α-granules. In PNH there is also a deficiency of membrane inhibitor of reactive lysis (MIRL, CD59), a glycosylphosphatidylinositol (GPI) anchor-dependent protein. In the absence of CD59, platelet lysis is minimized by the release from the cell surface of excess membrane attack complex by exovesiculation. The externalized phosphatidyl serine on the microvesicles released into the circulation acts as the binding site for prothrombinase complex. It is likely that the release of procoagulant microvesicles contributes to the increased risk of venous thrombosis. Increased platelet activation and an increased sensitivity to aggregation by thrombin have also been described. Fibrinolysis is also affected in PNH. Urokinase-type plasminogen activator receptor is also a GPI-bound protein that is absent from PNH cells. It binds urokinase to the cell surface and converts plasminogen to plasmin.

Thrombotic thrombocytopenic purpura

See Chapter 44.

Sickle cell disease

In sickle cell disease the pathophysiology involves microvascular and macrovascular occlusion with sickled cells. There is also considerable clinical and post-mortem evidence of cerebral, pulmonary and placental thrombosis, suggesting a prothrombotic tendency in these patients. Additional evidence for a prothrombotic state is enhanced thrombin generation, as shown by increased levels of prothrombin fragment 1+2 and thrombin–antithrombin, in patients with sickle cell disease in their steady state when compared with age-matched controls. There is also evidence that sickled erythrocytes adhere more readily to vascular endothelium and strongly accelerate coagulation due to abnormal exteriorization of procoagulant anionic membrane phospholipids. Comparison of the coagulation and fibrinolytic pathways in sickle cell patients with ethnically matched controls has shown increased levels of von Willebrand factor during sickling, although it is not clear whether this is specific or part of the acute-phase reaction. Low levels of protein C, protein S and heparin cofactor II are well described. The aetiology of the reduction of these physiological anticoagulants is unclear. It may relate to impaired liver function from repeated hepatic sickling, whereas increased consumption has also been proposed as a cause. Low heparin cofactor II levels are also found in other chronic haemolytic anaemias such as thalassaemia intermedia, suggesting that chronic haemolysis may also lead to increased consumption of this protein. Nephrotic syndrome, sometimes associated with sickle nephropathy, leads to low antithrombin levels and a prothrombotic state.

Selected bibliography

Agnelli G, Becattini C (2010) Acute pulmonary embolism. *The New England Journal of Medicine* **363**: 266–74.

Arbuthnot C, Wilde JT (2006) Haemostatic problems in acute promyelocytic leukaemia. *Blood Reviews* **20**: 289–97.

Cannegieter SC, Doggen CJ, van Houwelingen HC, Rosendaal FR (2006) Travel-related venous thrombosis: results from a large population-based case control study. *PLoS Medicine* **3**: e307.

Cappellini MD (2007) Coagulation in the pathophysiology of haemolytic anaemias. *Hematology. American Society of Hematology Education Program* 74–8.

Carrier M, Lee AY (2009) Prophylactic and therapeutic anticoagulation for thrombosis: major issue in oncology. *Nature Clinical Practice. Oncology* **6**: 74–84.

Esmon CT (2003) Inflammation and thrombosis. *Journal of Thrombosis and Haemostasis* **1**: 1343–8.

Goldhaber SZ (2010) Risk factors for venous thromboembolism. *Journal of the American College of Cardiology* **56**: 1–7.

Greaves M, Machin SJ, Cohen H *et al.* (2000) Guidelines on the investigation and management of the antiphospholipid syndrome. *British Journal of Haematology* **109**: 704–15.

Harrison CN (2005) Platelets and thrombosis in myeloproliferative diseases. *Hematology. American Society of Hematology Education Program* 409–15.

Hillmen P (2008) The role of complement inhibition in PNH. *Hematology. American Society of Hematology Education Program* 116–23.

Keeling D, Davidson S, Watson HG (2006) The management of heparin-induced thrombocytopenia. *British Journal of Haematology* **133**: 259–69.

Pierangeli SS, Chen PP, Raschi E *et al.* (2008) Antiphospholipid antibodies and the antiphospholipid syndrome: pathogenic mechanisms. *Seminars in Thrombosis and Hemostasis* **34**: 236–50.

Prandoni P, Kahn SR (2009) Post-thrombotic syndrome: prevalence, prognostication and need for progress. *British Journal of Haematology* **145**: 286–95.

Robertson B, Greaves M (2006) Antiphospholipid syndrome: an evolving story. *Blood Reviews* **20**: 201–12.

CHAPTER 47

Management of venous thromboembolism

47

Beverley J Hunt

Thrombosis and Haemostasis King's College, London, UK
Guy's and St Thomas' NHS Foundation Trust, London, UK

Introduction and epidemiology

Venous thromboembolism (VTE), which comprises deep vein thrombosis (DVT) and pulmonary embolism (PE), is responsible for an estimated 60 000 deaths annually in the UK based on epidemiological modelling. The clinical incidence of VTE is about 1 per 1000 per annum in adults, with a slight preponderance in men. Two-thirds present as DVT and one-third as PE. The major outcomes are death, recurrent VTE, post-thrombotic syndrome, pulmonary hypertension and major bleeding due to anticoagulation. Within 1 month of diagnosis, about 6% of patients with DVT and 10% of those with PE die. The mortality rate for PE has been estimated to be as high as 30% in some patient groups due to the high failure rate of recognizing PE before death, with mortality rates being highest in those with cancer.

Despite the incidence of VTE increasing with age (1 per 10 000 per annum under 30 years of age and 5–6 per 1000 per annum by the age of 80), deaths also occur in the younger age group due to failure to consider the diagnosis. The increased numbers of VTE with ageing may relate to the increasing presence of other illnesses and also an inherent increased coagulability with ageing.

Postgraduate Haematology: 6th edition. Edited by A. Victor Hoffbrand, Daniel Catovsky, Edward G.D. Tuddenham, Anthony R. Green © 2011 Blackwell Publishing Ltd.

Approximately 60% of cases of fatal PE are hospital acquired, i.e. 32 000 per annum in the UK with 25 000 being preventable with appropriate thromboprophylaxis. Interestingly, more VTE is diagnosed in the 3 months following hospitalization than during admission. As a rule of thumb, in the natural history of post-orthopaedic surgery, the median time for DVT to present is 7 days after the event, with PE presenting 21 days postoperatively. Thus both cases and fatalities usually occur after hospital discharge, which is why 'hospital-acquired VTE' rather than 'hospital VTE' is considered appropriate. However, within hospital PE accounts for 10% of deaths.

Mechanisms

Virchow's triad described in 1859 remains the best model of venous thrombogenesis. Changes in blood flow, vessel wall or blood coagulability comprise the triad, and usually a combination of these are present. The multi-hit hypothesis of thrombosis recognizes that more than one factor is usually operating to cause VTE, although the number of factors required to cause thrombosis decreases with ageing. The major risk factors are given in Table 47.1. Immobility is the key factor in those who do not have major thrombophilias or vessel wall abnormalities, and increases the risk of VTE 10-fold. Just sitting still for 90 min reduces blood flow in the popliteal vein by 40%. The term 'seated immobility syndrome' (also known as SIT syndrome) has been coined to encompass VTE precipitated by prolonged

Table 47.1 Common risk factors for venous thromboembolism according to Virchow's triad.

Reduced or altered flow
Immobility
Seated immobility thrombosis (SIT) syndrome: travellers thrombosis, e-thrombosis
Previous venous thromboembolism
Surgery
Trauma

Prothrombotic changes
Increasing age
Pregnancy and the puerperium
COC, HRT and estrogen receptor-modulating drugs
Cancer
Genetic thrombophilia
Antiphospholipid syndrome
Myeloproliferative disease
Obesity
Surgery
Trauma

Damage to vein walls
Surgery
Trauma

COC, combined oral contraceptive; HRT, hormone-replacement therapy.

Table 47.2 Clinical scores used for predicting the probability of DVT prior to further testing.

Risk factors, symptoms or signs	Points
Active cancer (treatment ongoing or terminated within 6 months or palliative care)	1
Paralysis, paresis, recent plaster cast on the leg	1
Recent confinement to bed of more than 3 days or major surgery within 12 weeks	1
Localized tenderness along the deep venous system	1
Swelling of the entire leg	1
Calf circumference > 3 cm larger than the asymptomatic leg (measured 10 cm below the tibial tubercle)	1
Pitting oedema (more on the symptomatic side)	1
Collateral flow in superficial veins (not varicose veins)	1
Previous DVT	1
Alternative diagnosis as or more likely than DVT	−2

In the case of symptoms from both legs, the leg with the most pronounced symptoms is used.
Score > 2 points, high probability; score 1–2 points, medium probability; score < 1 point, low probability.
Source: Anderson *et al.* (2003) with permission

Diagnosis of venous thromboembolism

sitting, the term thus encompassing traveller's thrombosis and 'e-thrombosis' (caused by sitting at a computer workstation).

Diagnosis of venous thromboembolism

Diagnosis relies on the use of objective diagnostic methods. Over 80% of DVT episodes are clinically silent and often confined to the calf veins. The concern is that such asymptomatic DVT can become symptomatic and/or embolize. There is no way of predicting which patients will develop symptomatic VTE, and it is well recognized that significant numbers of massive fatal PE occur without warning and as a result of asymptomatic DVT. Thus the clinical approach to VTE is to maintain a high index of suspicion and to treat until the diagnosis is refuted or confirmed by objective testing.

Clinical presentation of PE depends on the size, location and number of emboli and the patient's underlying cardiorespiratory reserve. The classic triad of chest pain, haemoptysis and dyspnoea is present in less than 20% of patients, while 97% of patients with PE have at least one of the following: pleuritic chest pain, dyspnoea, respiratory rate above 20/min. Tachycardia and tachypnoea are the most frequent signs. A right-sided S3

sound, widely split second sound, the murmur of tricuspid regurgitation and an accentuated S2 closure sound may be found. Fever is present in 14%. Massive PE has a mortality of 18–33% and may present with shock, dyspnoea and confusion.

Chest radiography may show either nothing specific or the Westermark sign (dilatation of the pulmonary artery proximal to the emboli with sharp cut-off), while ECG may not show the classic signs of right ventricular strain such as P pulmonale and S1Q3T3. Arterial blood gases and transthoracic echocardiography have too low sensitivity The main role of these tests is to exclude other conditions, such as acute myocardial infarction. However, risk factors for VTE and clinical symptoms and signs with the highest predictive value can be assigned points that are added to obtain a clinical 'score' (Tables 47.2 and 47.3) that can be used as the first step in a diagnostic strategy to reduce costs and the requirement for invasive diagnostic procedures.

The next step is the measurement of fibrin D-dimers, which are split products of fibrin degraded by plasmin, where the D-fragments of two fibrin molecules still are covalently bound and often also in complex with the E-fragment. Several methods can be used, such as enzyme-linked immunosorbent assay (ELISA), whole-blood agglutination of erythrocytes, latex agglutination or immunofiltration. ELISA methods have the best sensitivity but are not practical for near-patient testing, whereas the others are semi-quantitative or qualitative methods. There are also quantitative automated latex methods. The

Table 47.3 Clinical scores used for predicting the probability of PE prior to further testing.

Risk factors, symptoms or signs	Points
Signs of DVT (swelling, tenderness)	3
Heart rate > 100	1.5
Immobilization > 2 days or recent surgery (< 4 weeks)	1.5
Previous objectively verified DVT	1.5
Haemoptysis	1
Cancer	1
Pulmonary embolism as or more likely than other diagnoses	3

Score > 6 points, high probability; score 2–6 points, medium probability; score < 2 points, low probability.
Source: Wells *et al.* (2001) with permission.

manual latex methods have lower sensitivity and negative predictive value for exclusion of DVT or PE. Each hospital should provide information on the sensitivity and specificity of the test chosen for D-dimers. In general, a D-dimer assay is used for its negative predictive value (i.e. to exclude VTE) when the clinical score indicates low clinical probability. A positive result cannot be used for confirmation of the diagnosis owing to low specificity. For this reason, D-dimer is not a useful test in pregnancy or after surgery or in acute illness or the elderly.

Whenever the clinical probability is high and/or the D-dimer test is positive, confirmation using diagnostic imaging techniques is necessary, aiming to use the most non-invasive method. In patients with massive PE and hemodynamic instability, rapid risk assessment is necessary and so bedside echocardiography has become the most popular tool. Spiral multislice chest computed tomography (CT) is also useful for identifying patients who may benefit from thrombolysis or embolectomy. Cardiac biomarkers, including troponin and the natriuretic peptides, are sensitive markers of right ventricular function. Low levels of troponin, B-type natriuretic peptide (BNP) and NT-terminal proBNP are highly sensitive for identifying patients with an uneventful clinical course. Multislice chest CT is useful not only for diagnosing or excluding PE but also for risk assessment. A right-to-left ventricular dimension ratio above 0.9 on the reconstructed CT four-chamber view identifies patients at increased risk of early death.

Objective diagnosis with imaging techniques

Venography was the gold standard for diagnosing DVT, but the diagnostic accuracy is dependent on a high-quality examination. The veins and possible thrombi have to be well visualized and interpreted by an experienced radiologist, as artefacts may be difficult to differentiate from thrombi. A non-ionic contrast medium with low osmolarity should be used to minimize side-effects and the risk of a post-venographic DVT. Caution is still needed with regard to renal failure.

Ultrasonography of the leg veins is non-invasive and has no contraindications and thus has largely replaced venography as the method of choice. Diagnostically, it depends on the skill of the operator and has lower sensitivity than venography, especially for the veins of the calf. The simplest variant is compression ultrasonography, where a cross-section of the vein is compressed with the transducer. A non-compressible vein is diagnostic for DVT. The pelvic veins are not accessible with this method and recurrent thrombosis is difficult to discern. The most sophisticated variant of the technique is colour Doppler, which can determinate flow in several venous segments simultaneously, although generally the sensitivity is higher for proximal than for distal DVT. Low clinical probability in combination with a negative ultrasonographic examination, including the common and superficial femoral veins, the popliteal vein and the trifurcation in the proximal part of the calf, is considered sufficient to exclude DVT. However, with medium clinical probability, a negative ultrasonographic examination should be repeated within 1 week and, if still negative at that point, DVT is satisfactorily excluded. Presentation with high clinical probability and negative ultrasonography requires further investigation with venography. Suspected recurrent DVT is better served by venography as a first-line investigation, for ultrasound has low sensitivity in this setting.

Objective verification of suspected PE has typically been obtained with ventilation–perfusion (V/Q) lung scanning, following a normal chest radiograph. Perfusion scanning with technetium-99m (^{99m}Tc) albumin macroaggregates is a sensitive but not very specific method. The specificity is improved by adding ventilation scanning, usually with xenon-133 (^{133}Xe) aerosol or ^{99m}Tc-labelled carbon particles (Technegas), considering a V/Q mismatch (negative ventilation and positive perfusion scan) indicative of PE. However, an embolus may cause bronchospasm and thereby a ventilation defect and, more importantly, a V/Q mismatch may occur with several other conditions, including tumours, pneumonia, atelectasis, chronic obstructive pulmonary disease and others, and it does not differ between old and new emboli. The interpretation of lung scans is difficult, especially with patients with low or intermediate probability for PE, and thus other methods should be preferred for concurrent cardiopulmonary disease. Treatment can safely be withheld if the perfusion scan is negative or with a low-probability scan in combination with low clinical probability. A high-probability lung scan, which should require perfusion defects corresponding to at least two segments, together with high clinical probability has a positive predictive value of more than 90%.

Spiral CT of the lungs has good interobserver agreement and the number of inconclusive examinations is definitely lower than with V/Q scanning. With multislice techniques and a slice thickness of 2 mm, adequate assessment of 93% of the segmental arteries and of 62% of the subsegmental arteries is achieved. Although the diagnostic accuracy for subsegmental PE is low with spiral CT, follow-up studies have shown that it was safe to withhold treatment on presentation of a negative examination.

If there is a high clinical probability for PE and a negative perfusion scan or negative spiral CT, one possibility is to investigate for thrombi in the legs with bilateral ultrasonography or otherwise to proceed with pulmonary angiography. With contrast medium of low osmolarity, pulmonary angiography was not associated with mortality and only 0.4% of serious complications in four studies with more than 3000 patients. Although pulmonary angiography is considered the gold standard for diagnosis of PE, there are both false-positive and false-negative results, and the interobserver variability is poor when the PE is located in subsegmental arteries. Nevertheless, the method appears to exclude with great certainty those PE that require therapy.

A novel possibility with high specificity and sensitivity for DVT and potential for PE is magnetic resonance imaging (MRI) direct thrombus imaging, which requires no contrast but relies on the formation of methaemoglobin in hypoxic trapped red cells within venous thrombi. This acts as an endogenous contrast agent when imaged using a T1-weighted magnetic resonance sequence – appearing as high signal.

Investigation for concomitant cancer

The prevalence of cancer is approximately 20% in many cohort studies of patients with VTE. In a minority the malignancy is occult at the time of VTE. However, there is no evidence that screening for malignancies in those with VTE decreases the mortality and morbidity in those who are detected to have cancer. Instead, directed examinations should be performed when suspicion is raised by clinical signs or symptoms. Underlying cancer should be considered in patients with bilateral DVT, concomitant deep and superficial vein thrombosis at separate locations or recurrent VTE despite anticoagulation.

Therapeutic agents

All agents discussed below have in common the obvious side-effect of bleeding.

Thrombolytic therapy

Streptokinase and recombinant tissue plasminogen activator are widely available fibrinolytic agents. Streptokinase, a glycoprotein purified from the supernatant of β-haemolytic streptococci, in complex with plasminogen, cleaves other plasminogen molecules to plasmin. This indirect action results in complex pharmacokinetic characteristics. Furthermore, streptokinase is immunogenic, which may cause allergic reactions as well as a reduced or absent response on repeated use or after a recent infection with streptococci. Recombinant tissue plasminogen activator is an autologous glycoprotein, produced commercially with recombinant DNA technology, and it has a direct enzymatic effect on plasminogen that is strongly enhanced by the presence of fibrin.

Anticoagulant therapy

For over 50 years, therapeutic anticoagulation was limited to the use of unfractionated heparin (UFH) and oral vitamin K antagonists. Although both are highly effective, both have major drawbacks, most notably their unpredictable pharmacokinetics, so that their use has become synonymous with monitoring. The arrival of new oral anticoagulants with predictable pharmacokinetics has led to great excitement.

Heparin

Heparin was first isolated between 1916 and 1922 by the medical students Jay McLean and Emmett Holt at Johns Hopkins University. As the source of the preparation was canine liver, it was named after the Greek word for liver, ηπαρ or *hepar*. In the 1930s it was used as an anticoagulant in human trials and its use became widespread after the Second World War.

UFH is a naturally occurring glycosaminoglycan produced by mast cells and basophils. The pharmaceutical product is derived from tissues rich in mast cells such as porcine intestine or bovine lung. UFH is a polymer of repeating disaccharide units, primarily comprising sulphated glucosamine and uronic acid with a heterogeneous mixture of differing chain lengths; most preparations have a mean molecular mass of 13–15 kDa.

A specific pentasaccharide sequence of the heparin molecule binds to antithrombin, inducing a conformational change and a 1000-fold increase in antithrombin activity. In turn, antithrombin inhibits thrombin and factor (F)Xa. Only the pentasaccharide sequence is required to generate anti-FXa activity, whereas a longer sequence of 18 saccharides, including the pentasaccharide, is necessary to bind thrombin to cause thrombin inhibition.

Heparins are only active when administered parenterally. UFH can be given intravenously or subcutaneously; intramuscular administration should be avoided as it can result in large haematomas. At typical therapeutic doses, the half-life of intravenous UFH is 45–60 min, demanding continuous intravenous infusion. Given subcutaneously UFH has a lower bioavailability than intravenous heparin; activity starts at 2 hours and lasts approximately 10 hours, necessitating twice-daily dosing.

A slight fall in platelet count (< 30% compared with baseline) occurs in up to one-third of patients within the first 4 days of starting heparin. This reversible dose-dependent phenomenon is not associated with bleeding or thrombotic complications and does not require cessation of heparin. More marked falls in platelet count (> 50% compared with baseline) should raise the possibility of heparin-induced thrombocytopenia (HIT). HIT is a life-threatening complication of heparin treatment and occurs in 0.3–6.5% of those receiving UFH. The onset is typically between 5 and 10 days after starting UFH unless heparin has previously been administered, in which case it may begin earlier. The cause is development of an IgG antibody to a complex of heparin and platelet factor 4, which is capable of activating and depleting platelets. Because the thrombocytopenia is due to platelet activation, patients with HIT are paradoxically at high risk of both venous and arterial thrombosis. Other features may include necrotizing skin changes at heparin injection sites or a history of anaphylactoid reactions to heparin injection. A clinical scoring system for suspected HIT is useful in determining the need for further investigation. The diagnosis of HIT may be confirmed by specific ELISA or by functional platelet studies. The treatment is immediate cessation of all types of heparins (including line flushes) and initiation of an alternative anticoagulant such as danaparoid, hirudin or fondaparinux at therapeutic doses. Platelet transfusion is contraindicated, and warfarin should not be started until the platelet count has recovered, as it may cause microvascular necrosis.

Prolonged use of UFH can lead to osteoporosis by increasing osteoclast activity and reducing osteoblast numbers; 2% of patients receiving treatment-dose UFH for more than 9 months developed vertebral fractures. The risk of osteoporosis is considerably lower for low-molecular-weight heparin than for UFH.

Low-molecular-weight heparin (LMWH) is produced by enzymatic or chemical depolymerization of UFH. Since its introduction in the late 1970s, LMWH has largely superseded UFH by virtue of its more predictable pharmacokinetic profiles, less frequent dosing and lower incidence of adverse effects. LMWH consists of a mixture of glycosaminoglycan chains of molecular mass 3000–5000 Da. LMWH has the same principal mode of action as UFH, but the inhibition of thrombin is reduced compared with the inhibition of FXa, as the former effect requires longer polysaccharide chains for binding to thrombin. The bioavailability after subcutaneous injection is better than for UFH and the effect is more predictable, due to less binding to plasma proteins. The half-life is also longer (3–5 hours), so that a once-daily subcutaneous injection is sufficient. Intravenous administration of LMWH is rarely used.

Treatment with UFH requires monitoring with the activated partial thromboplastin time (APTT), whereas with LMWH monitoring is rarely needed, with the main exception being renal failure when inhibition of activated FX (anti-FXa) is measured. Side-effects such as HIT and osteoporosis are less common with LMWH. Although there are differences in molecular range, sulphation, ratio of FXa to thrombin inhibition, and pharmacokinetic characteristics between different LMWH peparations, there is no evidence for clinically important differences between them.

Fondaparinux is a synthetic drug consisting of the antithrombin-binding pentasaccharide sequence found in the heparin molecule. The pentasaccharide binds the antithrombin molecule, causing a conformational change that enhances its activity against FXa. Because there are no additional saccharides to provide the necessary bridging function for thrombin binding, fondaparinux has no activity against thrombin. Fondaparinux is given as a subcutaneous injection and has a half-life of 17 hours, making it suitable for once-daily dosing. Clearance is exclusively renal, so dose adjustment in renal failure is required and it is not recommended in those with a creatinine clearance below 30 mL/min. Fondaparinux does not bind to platelet factor 4, so has no capacity to cause HIT.

Danaparoid is a heparinoid that consists of the glycosaminoglycans heparan sulphate, dermatan sulphate and chondroitin sulphate but without any heparin. Accordingly, it has low cross-reactivity with antibodies induced by heparin and it is therefore mainly used in patients with HIT. It is administered intravenously or subcutaneously and has an effect that is similar to UFH in the prevention and treatment of VTE.

Vitamin K antagonists

The vitamin K antagonists or coumarins were first isolated by Karl Paul Link at the University of Wisconsin in the 1930s. The observation that cows bled to death after eating mouldy clover had led Link's team to isolate the anticoagulant factor from the contaminated clover. Link later developed a synthetic coumarin derivative. This was patented by the Wisconsin Alumni Research Foundation who named it warfarin as a contraction of the organization's acronym, WARF, and the word coumarin. The use of coumarins became widespread in the 1940s.

There are two groups of vitamin K antagonists, the more commonly used coumarin derivatives and the indanediones, and their availability varies between countries. They exert their effect via inhibition of the enzymes vitamin K epoxide reductase and vitamin K reductase, which are required for the regeneration of KH_2 from vitamin K epoxide. The latter is generated when the vitamin K-dependent coagulation factors (FII, FVII, FIX and FX, as well as the physiological inhibitors protein C and protein S) undergo post-translational modification with γ-carboxylation of approximately 10 glutamic acid residues in the N-terminal Gla domain.

During treatment with vitamin K antagonists, typically three of these residues remain in the non-carboxylated state, which reduces the ability of these coagulation factors to bind calcium and to localize the coagulation process to phospholipid surfaces. The vitamin K antagonists are bound to plasma proteins, mainly albumin (98–99%), and are metabolized by the hepatic cytochrome P450 enzymatic system. Interactions with other drugs or food may occur at many levels (Table 47.4) and constitute a major disadvantage. There are a number of common genetic polymorphisms of the CYP2C9 enzyme primarily responsible for warfarin metabolism. The most common polymorphisms, CYP2C9*2 and CYP2C9*3, are each seen in around

Table 47.4 Mechanisms for drug interactions with vitamin K antagonists with typical examples of such drugs.

Enhancement of vitamin K pathway: vitamin K, lipid emulsions

Reduced endogenous synthesis of vitamin K: induced by antibiotics

Accelerated catabolism of coagulation factors: thyroid hormone, androgens

Decreased synthesis of coagulation factors: clofibrate

Decreased warfarin absorption due to binding: colestyramine

Increased absorption of warfarin: acarbose

Inhibition of cyclic interconversion of vitamin K: second-/ third-generation cephalosporins

Inhibition of cytochrome P450 (CYP3A4): clarithromycin

Inhibition of cytochrome P4502C9, S-enantiomer: sulfinpyrazone

Stereoselective inhibition of hydroxylation, R-enantiomer: cimetidine

Non-stereoselective clearance: amiodarone

Induction of hepatic enzymes: barbiturates, rifampicin

Displacement of protein binding: etoposide

Potentiation of the warfarin receptor effect: clofibrate

Antiplatelet effect: acetylsalicylic acid

10% of whites, and are associated with a reduced warfarin requirement.

A small proportion of individuals (< 1%) have a hereditary resistance to all coumarins mediated by reduced affinity of the coumarin receptor and require very large doses of coumarins (> 30 mg warfarin daily) to achieve an anticoagulant effect. Because of coumarin's unpredictable pharmacokinetics, treatment requires regular monitoring. This was initially with the prothrombin time (PT). With the widely adopted use of a standardized calibration system, the International Normalized Ratio (INR), the reliability of comparisons of treatment intensities at different laboratories has been improved. The INR from an individual sample is calculated using the formula $INR = (PT_{patient}/PT_{control})^{ISI}$.

Rare side-effects of vitamin K antagonists are skin necrosis, purple toe syndrome, rash and toxic hepatitis, whereas the adverse effect of warfarin on bone mineral density is debated. Skin necrosis can occur in approximately 1 in 5000 patients in early initiation of treatment, and is due to an imbalance between mildly depressed vitamin K-dependent coagulation factors and a more pronounced initial reduction of protein C and protein S, resulting in a hypercoagulable state with thrombus formation in small veins and venules in the dermis and subcutaneous fat. The purple toe syndrome is a very painful, burning, dark-blue discoloration of the toes and sides of the feet, probably due to cholesterol embolization from atherosclerotic plaques that have become friable owing to reduced fibrin deposition or haemorrhage into the plaques several weeks after initiation of anticoagulation. Skin rashes may be papular, vesicular or urticarial and often very itchy. Vitamin K antagonists also have a teratogenic effect, with skeletal malformations, optic atrophy and mental impairment, occurring in a small percentage of babies of exposed mothers.

Direct thrombin inhibitors

All are only active parenterally and are administered mainly by intravenous infusion. Hirudin is a 65-amino-acid polypeptide, originally discovered in the saliva of the medicinal leech *Hirudo medicinalis*. Two recombinant derivatives are available, lepirudin and desirudin. Hirudin is an irreversible direct thrombin inhibitor, binding to both the active and substrate-recognition sites of the thrombin molecule. As the clearance of hirudin is exclusively renal, the half-life is highly dependent on renal function. With normal renal function, hirudin has a half-life of 60 min after intravenous administration, but in those with end-stage renal failure the half-life can be as long as 300 hours. Hirudin is licensed for the treatment of thrombosis associated with HIT. Unfortunately, 40–70% of patients develop hirudin antibodies after a week of treatment; although they are rarely inhibitory, they may bind to hirudin and reduce renal clearance, resulting in a prolonged half-life.

Bivalirudin is a recombinant 20-amino-acid polypeptide analogue of hirudin. It binds to the substrate-binding site of thrombin, but unlike hirudin can be cleaved by thrombin itself, making bivalirudin a reversible thrombin inhibitor. Bivalirudin has a half-life of 25 min following intravenous injection. Because only a proportion of excretion is renal, clearance is less dependent on renal function than for hirudin. Argatroban is a small-molecule reversible thrombin inhibitor derived from the amino acid arginine with a half life of around 40 min; clearance is primarily hepatic. Because of their short half-lives, argatroban and bivalirudin have been used principally in the management of HIT and during percutaneous coronary procedures in patients at risk of HIT.

All these parenteral direct thrombin inhibitors require therapeutic monitoring, usually by APTT, with a typical target ratio of 2.0–2.5. The ecarin clotting time is a better alternative, but is less widely available. There is no specific reversal agent for these direct thrombin inhibitors. Options in bleeding patients include blood product support, activated prothrombin complex concentrates or recombinant activated FVII. Hirudin is not cleared by haemodialysis.

Oral direct thrombin inhibitors

Dabigatran

Dabigatran is a novel synthetic small-molecule direct thrombin inhibitor that binds reversibly to both fibrin-bound and free thrombin and has predictable pharmacokinetics and so does not require monitoring. It has a plasma half-life of 14–17 hours, permitting once-daily dosing. Clearance is predominantly renal, and dose adjustment in renal failure may be necessary.

Dabigatran causes prolongation of APTT, but not in a linear dose-dependent fashion; more accurate monitoring can be achieved using the ecarin clotting time. Dabigatran is licensed for thrombophylaxis after orthopaedic hip and knee replacement, and in clinical trials it has been shown to be non-inferior to warfarin in the management of VTE; patients randomized to dabigatran had fewer minor bleeds but more dyspepsia and more drug discontinuation. A Phase III study, RE-LY, evaluated the efficacy and safety of two different doses of dabigatran relative to warfarin in over 18 000 patients with atrial fibrilation. Dabigatran 110 mg was non-inferior to warfarin for the primary efficacy end point of stroke or systemic embolization, whereas dabigatran 150 mg was significantly more effective than warfarin or dabigatran 110 mg. Major bleeding occurred significantly less often with dabigatran 110 mg than warfarin; dabigatran 150 mg had similar bleeding to warfarin.

Oral direct factor Xa antagonists

Several oral direct FXa antagonists (i.e. they do not require antithrombin to exert their activity) are undergoing clinical trials; indeed rivaroxaban is now licensed for thrombophylaxis after orthopaedic joint replacement.

Rivaroxaban

Rivaroxaban has an oral bioavailability of 60–80% and has a rapid onset of action, reaching peak concentration at 3 hours and a half-life of 5–9 hours. Excretion is predominantly renal. In clinical trials where it was used as thrombophylaxis after orthopaedic hip and knee surgery, it was found to have superior efficacy to enoxaparin. Results from trials in other areas are awaited.

Novel anticoagulant drugs

There are a number of other novel oral anticoagulants in the pipeline, thus ensuring that the days of dependence on warfarin and heparin are numbered. Apixaban is an orally bioavailable small-molecule direct FXa inhibitor undergoing Phase III trials whose excretion is predominantly biliary and so it may be useful in renal failure. Others of interest include tecarfarin, a warfarin variant that is not metabolized by cytochrome P450 and thus has the potential to give more time in range.

Initial treatment of venous thromboembolism

Before treatment is started, blood samples for haemoglobin, platelet count, APTT and PT should be obtained for baseline assessment of the risk of bleeding. In addition, with anticipated treatment with LMWH, serum creatinine, and with thrombolytic therapy plasma fibrinogen and blood group and save, should also be performed. Thrombophilia screening is of no utility at this stage for the results do not usually affect immediate patient management. Moreover, false-positive results may

be obtained because levels of physiological anticoagulants are usually reduced at the time of an acute thrombus due to consumption.

Thrombolytic therapy

The most serious consequence of VTE is fatal PE. Many patients die before a diagnosis of PE has been made. Massive PE with unstable haemodynamics has a high mortality, but the prognosis improves dramatically with rapid lysis of the emboli. The benefit-to-risk ratio of thrombolysis in proximal DVT is as yet uncertain but it is recommended for unstable patients with PE, although these patients represent less than 5% of all patients hospitalized for PE. The streptokinase/urokinase PE thrombolysis trials showed that thrombolytic therapy successfully decreases pulmonary artery pressures acutely, with improvements in the lung scan and arteriogram at 12 and 24 hours, although there was no overall decrease in mortality in those receiving thrombolysis compared with those receiving heparin therapy. The use of thrombolytic treatment in patients with sub-massive PE is controversial.

Contraindications to thrombolysis include active internal bleeding, a stroke within 2 months, and an intracranial process such as neoplasm or abscess (Table 47.5). Relative contraindications include surgery within 10 days, uncontrolled hypertension

Table 47.5 Contraindications to thrombolytic therapy.

Absolute contraindications
Active internal bleeding
Known haemostatic disorder
Cerebrovascular accident, craniocerebral trauma or neurosurgery within 6 months
Active intracranial process

Relative contraindications
Major surgery, biopsy, puncture of non-compressible vessels, vaginal delivery, external heart massage or major trauma within 7 days
Vascular or eye surgery within 3 weeks
Gastrointestinal bleeding, acute pancreatitis or pericarditis within 3 months
Uncontrolled hypertension (diastolic ≥ 110 mmHg)
Age > 80 years
Diabetic retinopathy

In addition, caution should be observed during the first trimester of pregnancy, the first 20 hours of menstruation, bacterial endocarditis and where there are abnormal screening tests for haemostasis. Patients with previous treatment with streptokinase within 3–4 months are unlikely to respond to repeated treatment due to antibody formation. Adherence to these precautions and contraindications should be more strict for the treatment of DVT than of massive PE.

and pregnancy. Haemorrhagic complications are higher in patients with a recent invasive procedure such as pulmonary angiogram or placement of an inferior vena cava (IVC) filter. There is a reported incidence of intracranial haemorrhage of approximately 2%, with higher rates in the elderly and those with poorly controlled hypertension. The major haemorrhage rate ranges from 11 to 20%.

Heparin is discontinued 30 min before thrombolytic therapy and restarted 2–4 hours after its discontinuation. Regional or local infusion of fibrinolytic agents has not proved to be more effective, for bleeding complications are still prevalent. Antipyretics such as paracetamol may be given for febrile reactions and steroids for more pronounced allergic reactions, but prophylaxis with the latter does not provide any additional benefit.

With major haemorrhage, the infusion should be stopped and blood losses replaced. For patients undergoing streptokinase therapy, the situation is more complex. Because of the indirect pharmacokinetics, a paradoxical effect may occur if the infusion of streptokinase is slowed or stopped. More plasminogen will then become available for transformation to plasmin by already circulating streptokinase–plasminogen complexes. It is therefore vital to reduce the proteolytic potential, which can be done with aprotinin, an antiplasmin agent. Conventional inhibitors of fibrinolysis, such as tranexamic acid, are not effective as they only counteract plasminogen conversion to plasmin but do not inhibit already formed plasmin. With very low levels of fibrinogen and major haemorrhage, infusion of fibrinogen (concentrate or cryoprecipitate) is also indicated.

Plasma fibrinogen level should be monitored every 12–24 hours. If the level is not reduced whatsoever, it is unlikely that a thrombolytic effect is achieved. The target is approximately 0.2–1.0 g/L, but levels higher than 0.2 g/L do not exclude the risk of haemorrhage, and therapeutic levels do not provide a guarantee for removal of the thrombus.

Venous thrombectomy

There are insufficient data to evaluate the long-term benefit of surgical removal of the thrombus. The procedure is often combined with formation of an arteriovenous fistula to improve the flow, but there is not enough evidence to show that this increases the patency rate of the vein. Bleeding is common, often requiring transfusion, and a fatal outcome has been reported in up to 14%. The benefit of the treatment is that relief of symptoms is immediate, and it may be considered in the rare cases when loss of the limb is imminent.

Inferior vena cava filters

A temporary or permanent filter provides a tool to prevent further PE by reducing the risk during the first 12 days from 4.8% to 1.1%. However, PE can still occur in patients with IVC filters, and there is also a small risk of thrombosis at the site of

filter insertion. The primary indication for an IVC filter is the prevention of PE in patients with established VTE who have a contraindication to anticoagulation. Once the filter is in place, there is a tendency for clinicians to delay anticoagulation. However, anticoagulation should be considered in all patients with an IVC filter once a temporary contraindication to anticoagulation has passed. A large randomized trial showed no reduction in mortality or long-term risk of PE after 2 years of permanent indwelling catheters; indeed there was an increased risk of recurrent thrombosis.

Anticoagulant therapy

The objective of anticoagulant therapy in the acute phase is to prevent further progression of the thrombus as well as (further) PE. It is not sufficient to start treatment with vitamin K antagonists alone, because of the delay of about 5 days until they provide full anticoagulation. A once-daily treatment dose of subcutaneous LMWH can be given and will have immediate effect and so patients with DVT are usually managed as outpatients, unless they have renal failure where intravenous UFH is required. With UFH an initial intravenous bolus should be given and treatment is continued with intravenous infusion until anticoagulation with a coumarin, usually started simultaneously, has become effective. Treatment with UFH is targeted at an APTT of 2–2.5 times the upper limit of normal, which is measured 4 hours after starting the infusion and then at least once daily. With APTT below the target range, another bolus dose is given and the infusion rate is increased. Conversely, with APTT above the treatment range, the infusion may be halted for 30 min and should be restarted at a reduced rate.

Failure to reach the therapeutic APTT range is associated with a poor antithrombotic effect, whereas a possible association between long APTT results and bleeding complications is less evident. Occasionally, there may be difficulties in reaching a therapeutic APTT with inherited and acquired deficiencies of antithrombin. If the APTT is not prolonged despite increased doses of UFH, and especially if there is clinical deterioration, the antithrombin level should be measured and, if there is a deficiency, the addition of antithrombin, either by using fresh frozen plasma or antithrombin concentrates, should be considered. More often, a therapeutic APTT is not achieved despite normal antithrombin levels, but there is no evidence of clinical progression. This condition is believed to be caused by high levels of acute-phase proteins, such as FVIII or histidine-rich glycoprotein, which counteract the prolongation of APTT but apparently not the antithrombotic effect of heparin. Measurement of anti-FXa in these patients often demonstrates therapeutic levels and should be taken into account so that undue increment of the dose of heparin is avoided.

If the baseline APTT is prolonged, the reason may be presence of a lupus anticoagulant (mildly to moderately prolonged APTT) or congenital deficiency of FXII (severely prolonged

APTT for homozygous patients), and monitoring of treatment with UFH is often difficult. The alternatives are monitoring with anti-FXa or treatment with LMWH, which does not require monitoring.

Patients with suspected PE can be managed in the same way with LMWH subcutaneously and vitamin K antagonists orally. It is thus possible to give this treatment on an outpatient basis, but patient safety has so far not been demonstrated for outpatient management of PE in a randomized trial. Treatment for DVT with LMWH can be undertaken safely without hospitalization. Randomized trials have demonstrated equal effect and safety with LMWH injected once or twice daily. For hospitalized patients, LMWH is associated with a lower incidence of haemorrhage than treatment with UFH. In the case of very ill patients or with a high risk of bleeding, it still may be preferable to treat with UFH, infused intravenously, in view of the shorter half-life if the treatment has to be discontinued abruptly and protamine sulphate used to neutralize residual UFH. Interestingly, initial treatment with LMWH instead of UFH is associated with a reduced mortality during 3 months of follow-up due to an increased survival in the subgroup of patients with concomitant cancer.

Although the dose of LMWH is adjusted according to body weight, there are conflicting data regarding whether the dose should be increased linearly or 'capped' in obese patients. Patients with mild to moderate renal failure (serum creatinine 200–400 μmol/L) should have anti-FXa levels after 2–3 days at the time of peak concentration and, if above 1 unit/mL, the dose should be reduced. For patients with severe renal failure UFH is preferred.

Patients with VTE should be mobilized early, preferably within 1 day, unless thrombolytic therapy is given. Mobilization does not increase the risk of new PE, and pain and swelling of the leg diminish more rapidly than if the patients are immobilized for 1 week. Patients should wear compression stockings as soon as they are out of bed.

Primary prophylaxis (thrombophlyaxis)

A systematic review by the US Agency for Healthcare Quality and Research ranked PE as the most common preventable cause of hospital death, and thrombophylaxis as the number one strategy to improve patient safety in hospitals. Despite good clinical evidence of the efficacy and cost-effectiveness of thrombophylaxis, there has been failure of its implementation internationally.

Most inpatients have several risk factors for VTE. The baseline risk is estimated to be 5–15% for those adults who are acutely unwell in medical beds, with risks of about 50–60% in hip replacement surgery and severe stroke and nearly 100% in spinal cord injury/polytrauma cases. The arguments for using thrombophylaxis in all those at risk include the following.

- Despite the recognition of specific risk factors, it is impossible to predict exactly which individuals within a group at risk will have VTE.
- Screening with ultrasound has low sensitivity for DVT and is not cost-effective.
- Over 80% of DVT are clinically silent and often confined to the calf vein. The concern is that such asymptomatic DVT can become symptomatic and/or embolize. There is no way of predicting which patients will develop symptomatic VTE without warning and as a result of asymptomatic DVT.

Therefore in view of our inability to predict the exact individuals in a high-risk group who will develop VTE, the standard approach is to administer thrombophylaxis to all those at risk.

Efficacy and safety of thrombophylaxis

Many randomized clinical trials over the past 35 years have demonstrated the efficacy and safety of thrombophylaxis, summarized elegantly and regularly by the American College of Chest Physicians. The National Institute for Health and Clinical Excellence (NICE) have produced guidelines for the UK. Thrombophylaxis can be separated into mechanical and pharmacological methods.

Mechanical methods

Mechanical approaches include antiembolic stockings, intermittent pneumatic compression devices, mechanical foot pumps and IVC filters. All except IVC filters reduce the risk of DVT. IVC filters reduce the risk of embolism from an established DVT and can therefore be considered secondary prophylaxis. Antiembolic stockings apply graded circumferential pressure on the legs, greatest distally, which increase the velocity and volume of blood flow in the deep veins. They have a lower grade of compression compared with graduated compression stockings used in patients with post-thrombotic syndrome, and need to be fitted correctly to work effectively. Intermittent pneumatic compression causes sequential compression of the legs in a wave-like milking effect. Foot pumps squeeze the plexus of veins known as the venae comitantes of the lateral plantar artery and thus reduce venous stasis.

The poor quality, low number and poor end points of the studies of mechanical thrombophylaxis have been widely criticized. A recent well-conducted study showed that thigh-length stockings do not alter the risk of DVT after stroke but did have a 5% risk of skin breaks, ulcers, blisters and skin necrosis. Mechanical methods are contraindicated in patients with critical limb ischaemia, limb fractures and severe neuropathy, while ill-fitted stockings may cause oedema, arterial ischaemia and superficial thrombosis.

The key end point of the efficacy of thrombophylaxis is reduction in death rate due to PE, and to ascertain this requires thousands of patients in one or several trials, which would need to include post-mortem studies. Such studies have not been performed for mechanical thrombophylaxis. However, the main advantage of mechanical methods is that they do not produce an increased bleeding risk. Stockings and intermittent pneumatic compression act in a synergistic manner when combined with pharmacological agents in surgical patients. However, there is no evidence to suggest that there is any benefit when IVC filters are added to appropriate thrombophylaxis. Insertion is common in trauma patients who have a very high risk of VTE, but this has never been shown to be protective in a trial.

Pharmacological

UFH and LMWHs have been clearly shown to reduce the risk of death due to PE. The modern trials of pharmacological thrombophylaxis use a composite primary outcome measure of symptomatic and asymptomatic VTE. A meta-analysis of 46 trials of UFH thrombophylaxis in surgery showed that UFH, when compared with placebo, reduced the all-cause mortality from 4.2% to 3.2%. Fatal PE were reduced from 0.8% to 0.3%, symptomatic PE from 2.0% to 1.3% and DVT from 22% to 9%. However, bleeding events were significantly increased from 3.8 to 5.9%.

A problem with UFH is the need for frequent dosing. Thrice-daily dosing of UFH 5000 units was more effective in reducing the rate of VTE and especially PE, but the risk for major bleeding is significantly increased compared with twice-daily dosing. UFH has been largely superseded by LMWHs whose longer half-lives allow once-daily administration, although UFH remains the first choice in renal dysfunction, in which LMWH accumulates, causing increased bleeding, due to its long half-life and renal excretion. LMWH has been shown to reduce the risk of VTE by a similar amount as UFH (60–70%), with a similar bleeding risk compared with placebo.

Hospital-acquired VTE is more common in medical than surgical patients because medical patients are the commonest admissions. Indeed 70–80% of hospital-acquired fatal PE occurs in medical patients. Apart from being an older cohort, 40% of medical patients have more than one risk factor for VTE, including previous VTE, cancer, stroke, heart failure, chronic obstructive airways disease, sepsis and bed rest. Approximately 5000 acutely ill medical patients have been entered into randomized controlled trials comparing LMWH with placebo and studies comparing LMWH with UFH. For example, the MEDENOX study showed that enoxaparin 40 mg was superior to both enoxaparin 20 mg and placebo given for a median of 6 days to acutely ill medical patients. There was a significant reduction in DVT between 6 and 14 days in those patients who received enoxaparin 40 mg to 5.5%, compared with 15% who received placebo ($P < 0.001$). There were no significant differences in bleeding between the groups. Fondaparinux is also licensed for thrombophylaxis. Postoperative adjusted-dose oral vitamin K antagonists are unfashionable in Europe due to the unpredictable pharmacokinetics of warfarin leading to a significant risk of both over- and under-anticoagulation.

The evidence for using antiplatelet drugs in thrombophylaxis is based on methodologically flawed studies and has been shown to be inferior to LMWH. For example, in a trial of joint replacement randomized to aspirin or LMWH, the relative reduction in VTE risk of LMWH was 63% over aspirin. Moreover, aspirin is associated with an increased risk of bleeding, especially when combined with other methods. Its use in thrombophylaxis is not recommended in all the major guidelines.

For how long should thrombophylaxis be given?

The acute-phase response that produces a prothrombotic state persists for weeks after surgery. Although the risk of postoperative DVT is highest within the first few weeks after surgery, VTE complications may occur later. Extended prophylaxis for up to 35 days has been shown to reduce VTE in those with ongoing significant risk factors for VTE, and so LMWHs are licensed for extended use for 28–35 days in major hip, abdominal or cancer surgery, reducing the risk of VTE by a further 60% from 2.7% to 1.1%.

Secondary prophylaxis

After a VTE, if initial treatment with UFH or LMWH is not followed by a period of secondary prophylaxis, the risk of recurrence over 90 days is 29%. Secondary prophylaxis is usually given with vitamin K antagonists, commonly with warfarin. In some European countries, phenprocoumon or acenocoumarol is prescribed predominantly. Phenprocoumon has a half-life of 160 hours compared with 20–55 hours for warfarin, which may cause difficulties when the drug has to be eliminated quickly in case of overdose or haemorrhage. Acenocoumarol has a half-life of only 11 hours, and this does not result in a requirement for twice-daily dosing. Comparative studies with warfarin and acenocoumarol have demonstrated a similar effect and safety profile.

Treatment with a vitamin K antagonist should be started concomitantly with the initial anticoagulant therapy, or once the diagnosis of PE or DVT is established. The optimal intensity is an INR of 2.0–3.0, at least during the first 6 months after an episode of VTE. It may take 3–10 days to reach this target range and the maintenance dose varies from 1 to 20 mg daily. The time to reach the therapeutic range and to find the individual maintenance dose is shortened with higher initial dosing (warfarin 15 mg daily versus lower doses, or warfarin 10 mg vs. warfarin 5 mg) and by using a nomogram or computer software for the dose adjustments. The higher induction dose of 15 mg should be avoided in patients with a high risk of bleeding and is contraindicated in patients with deficiency of protein C or

S because of the increased risk of warfarin-induced skin necrosis.

The initial treatment with UFH or LMWH may be discontinued when the vitamin K antagonist has been given for at least 5 days and an INR of at least 2.0 has been achieved for two consecutive days. The secondary prophylaxis with vitamin K antagonists is then continued for a period that sometimes can be decided very shortly after the diagnosis of VTE, but which often requires reassessment due to the results of evaluation for thrombophilia or other investigations that may favour a longer treatment period. Conversely, bleeding complications or poor compliance may prompt a shortening of the planned treatment period. In order to improve the quality of anticoagulant therapy, it is crucial that the patient is followed properly as an outpatient.

Treatment is monitored by measuring the INR. Dose adjustments become more precise, with less INR results outside the therapeutic range, if decision support aids, such as nomograms, algorithms or computer software, are used. Staff in charge of dose adjustments should be trained and follow a large number of patients regularly. Well-motivated patients should be encouraged to perform self-testing with capillary blood sampling using a 'point-of-care' instrument and to be in charge of dose adjustments, with advantages in terms of less clinical complications. This requires some training and visits to an anticoagulant clinic a few times per year for comparison of the results with those obtained at the laboratory.

All patients who receive vitamin K antagonists should be informed about the following (printed information should also be provided).
- The risk of bleeding.
- Whom to contact whenever such symptoms occur.
- The risk of using acetylsalicylic acid and non-steroidal anti-inflammatory drugs, which impair platelet function, and about the alternatives that can be used. Although paracetamol interacts with warfarin, this is not clinically significant.
- Vast numbers of drugs interact with vitamin K antagonists so that the possibility of an interaction should be questioned for each new drug prescribed. Several herbal medicines, including St John's wort, ginseng and garlic, reduce the concentration of warfarin in blood.
- The effect of large amounts of dark green vegetables, which contain considerable amounts of vitamin K and may therefore neutralize the anticoagulant effect, but stressing that a regular intake of moderate amounts of vegetables is recommended.

Duration of secondary prophylaxis with oral vitamin K antagonists

The optimal duration of secondary prophylaxis is dependent on a risk–benefit analysis between avoidance of haemorrhagic complications and recurrent VTE. Meta-analyses have shown that a longer duration reduces the risk of recurrence, but treat-

Table 47.6 Factors associated with a higher risk of recurrence of venous thromboembolism.

Higher risk
Triggering risk factor not identified
Proximal DVT and/or PE
Presence of cancer

Thrombophilic defects
Deficiency of antithrombin, protein C or protein S
Homozygosity for FV Leiden or prothrombin G20210A
Antiphospholipid antibodies

Follow-up of the thrombotic disease
Persistently increased D-dimers
Remaining thrombus on ultrasound examination

Lower risk
Triggering risk factor removable or permanent
Distal DVT

Thrombophilic defects
Heterozygosity for FV Leiden
Heterozygosity for prothrombin G20210A

Follow-up of the thrombotic disease
Normalized level of D-dimers
Normalized ultrasound

ment for more than 6–12 months is associated with an increased risk of bleeding. Factors associated with a higher risk of recurrence are shown in Table 47.6. For the majority of patients, treatment of at least 6 months is recommended. Shorter treatment is indicated for a distal DVT and temporary risk factor, such as trauma, surgery or oral contraceptives (6 weeks), or for patients with a high risk of bleeding (3 months).

In randomized trials on the duration of secondary prophylaxis, there has typically been an annual incidence of 2–4% of major haemorrhage. One option to reduce this risk is to reduce the intensity of anticoagulant therapy, and studies on coumarins targeted at an INR of less than 2.0 have shown a favourable risk–benefit profile. Large randomized trials on low-intensity warfarin therapy in the extension of secondary prophylaxis after at least 3–6 months of treatment, targeted at the usual INR of 2.0–3.0, have shown that a prophylactic antithrombotic effect is obtained but perhaps less than with full intensity, although the annual incidence of major haemorrhage was only 0.9–1.0% and may be an option in some low-risk patients. However, secondary prophylaxis targeted at an INR of 1.5–2.0 was not tested in patients with active cancer, for whom even standard vitamin K antagonist therapy is often insufficient (see below).

A decision in favour of prolonged anticoagulation should be weighed against the cost and burden for the patient of monitor-

Table 47.7 Suggested duration of secondary prophylaxis in relation to presence of risk factors.

Condition	Duration
Thrombophilic defects not identified or unknown	
First event, distal DVT, provoked by temporary risk factor	6 weeks
First event, distal DVT with idiopathic or permanent risk factor, or any proximal DVT or PE	6 months or longer
As above with increased risk of bleeding	3 months
Single life-threatening event	12 months or longer
First event, active cancer	Until cancer resolved
Second event, contralateral DVT	As after the first event
Second event, ipsilateral or PE	12 months or longer
More than two events	Indefinitely
*Thrombophilic defects identified**	
Deficiency of antithrombin	Indefinitely
Deficiency of protein C or protein S	12 months or longer
Homozygous form of thrombophilic defect	Indefinitely[†]
Double heterozygous for thrombophilic defects	Indefinitely
Antiphospholipid syndrome	Indefinitely
Hyperhomocysteinaemia	As without[‡]
Elevated FVIII activity	6 months or longer
FV Leiden mutation, heterozygous	As without the defect
Prothrombin polymorphism, heterozygous	As without the defect
Life-threatening event and any defect	Indefinitely

*Independent of the event being provoked by a temporary or permanent risk factor, whenever the thrombophilic defect is permanent.
[†]Possibly excluding the homozygous form of prothrombin G20210A.
[‡]Consider the use of B vitamins thereafter.
Source: modified from Schulman (2003) with permission.

ing the treatment, effects on the quality of life in view of restrictions regarding diet and other concomitant medications and, finally, the fact that about 1% of patients annually will have a major haemorrhage. Suggestions for the duration of secondary prophylaxis are given in Table 47.7. However, a significant minority of patients may wish to stop coumarins and instead take thromboprophylaxis at times of haemostatic stress, for example prophylactic doses of LMWH at times of surgery or during long-haul air travel.

Although it is not clear that the risk of recurrence is higher after the second episode of VTE than after the first, recurrent DVT in the ipsilateral leg causes additional damage to the venous valves and increases the risk of post-thrombotic syndrome significantly. Patients with PE have a higher risk of recurrent symptomatic PE than do patients with initial DVT, and extension of secondary prophylaxis may thus be justified after recurrent PE. Patients with antiphospholipid syndrome have a high risk of recurrence without anticoagulation and therefore anticoagulation should be extended.

Cessation of vitamin K antagonists is often associated with an increment in prothrombin fragment 1+2 and D-dimers, independent of whether they were stopped abruptly or gradually, and so there seems to be no clinical benefit in stopping gradually.

Management in the case of bleeding or surgery

Excessive anticoagulation may be identified as an isolated prolonged INR above 4 or in combination with bleeding. Although elimination of one dose of the vitamin K antagonist, possibly followed by a reduction of the maintenance dose, may suffice in most cases, the addition of oral vitamin K_1 1 mg reduces the risk of bleeding. The reason for excessive anticoagulation should be investigated and may reveal an interaction with other drugs or irregular dosing.

In the case of major or life-threatening bleeding, reversal with vitamin K_1 is too slow, as only a weak effect is noticed after 2 hours and the full effect occurs after 6 hours. Replacement of the deficient vitamin K-dependent coagulation factors is necessary, but the volumes of fresh plasma required are so large (typically 2–3 L to reduce the INR from 4.0 to 1.5 in a patient with body weight of 80 kg) that there is a substantial risk of volume overload. Prothrombin complex concentrate is the agent of choice: it carries no risk of volume overload and has undergone viral inactivation to eliminate the risk of transmission of HIV or hepatitis B or C. A few cases with thromboembolic complications in association with the use of prothrombin complex concentrate have been reported, but the risk appears small as no complications were observed in prospective cohorts.

In patients with bleeding at INR levels within or below the therapeutic range, cancer should be suspected and investigations of the source are indicated.

For minor surgery, such as tooth extractions or dermatological surgery, anticoagulant therapy can be maintained within the therapeutic range. Randomized trials have shown an excellent prophylactic effect against bleeding complications after dental extractions if the patients were prescribed mouth rinses with the fibrinolytic inhibitor tranexamic acid every 6 hours.

For major surgery, the INR has to be reduced to below 1.5, either by complete interruption or by reduction in the vitamin K antagonist. Substitution with LMWH or UFH is given perioperatively until therapeutic INR has been regained.

Secondary prophylaxis with LMWH

Secondary prophylaxis with UFH twice daily subcutaneously, adjusted to prolong the APTT 1.5 times the normal value at 6 hours after injection, has been shown to be as effective as vitamin K antagonists. However, this never gained any popularity due to the requirement for two doses and adjustments. A meta-analysis of studies on secondary prophylaxis, comparing LMWHs with vitamin K antagonists, has shown that they are equally effective and safe. LMWH injected once daily subcutaneously may be the drug of choice for patients with a short treatment duration (6 weeks or less), with pronounced difficulties in achieving stable INR values, or when monitoring of the vitamin K antagonist is problematic. The dose of LMWH should be approximately 50% of the initial treatment dose and monitoring with anti-FXa is not required unless there is impairment of renal function or the patient is obese. The risk of osteoporosis with long-term LMWH is minimal and HIT is very rare.

Treatment of patients with cancer

In cohorts of unselected patients with VTE, the prevalence of cancer is about 20%. Even occult cancer increases the risk of thrombosis for several years until it becomes clinically manifest. The diagnosis and treatment of patients with VTE and known cancer differs somewhat from what has been described above. The diagnosis of DVT with ultrasonography or phlebography may become false positive due to obstruction of the iliac vein by a pelvic tumour mass or metastases, and CT may therefore be the diagnostic method of choice. Compression of a pulmonary artery by a tumour mass or tumour emboli may simulate perfusion defects by PE, both on lung scanning and on pulmonary angiography. Measurement of D-dimers may not be of any value in these patients, who typically have elevated levels even in the absence of VTE.

Initial treatment should preferably be given with LMWH in view of the survival benefit in patients with cancer over the following 3 months in comparison with those treated with UFH. Although patients with cancer have massive VTE more frequently than those without cancer, thrombolytic therapy is very hazardous, as the risk of bleeding is aggravated by necrosis in highly vascularized tumour tissue, erosion of normal tissues and thrombocytopenia due to bone marrow invasion by tumour or aplasia after chemotherapy. In some of these patients, the risk of bleeding is so pronounced that in the case of PE or massive DVT there is an indication for an IVC filter.

Long-term anticoagulation with coumarins in patients with cancer is unsatisfactory, because there is an increase in the annual risk of recurrence of 14–18% compared with patients without cancer and, paradoxically, an increase in major bleeding of 7–11%. For secondary prophylaxis, LMWH at a dose of 75% of the initial treatment dose may be a better alternative than vitamin K antagonists. Long-term LMWH may prolong survival in patients with cancer and VTE, and perhaps also in those without VTE. This does probably not apply to terminally ill patients but rather to those with an expected survival of at least 1 year. However, many questions remain to be answered: the mechanism for this effect, whether the effect is confined to certain types of cancer, the minimum treatment period required and the optimal dose of LMWH. Secondary prophylaxis should continue as long as active cancer is present, unless the severity of bleeding complications precludes treatment.

Venous thromboembolism in pregnancy

The incidence of VTE in association with pregnancy is 0.5–1.0 per 1000 with one to two fatal cases of PE in 100 000 pregnancies. DVT occurs commonly in the left iliofemoral vein. This may generate a clinical picture that is different from the one generally seen in DVT. The only symptoms may be abdominal cramps, sciatic back pain or fever. Objective diagnosis is even more important in the pregnant patient, as failure to treat an undiagnosed VTE as well as treatment of a false-positive diagnosis may cause harm.

Pressure from the uterus on the pelvic veins may simulate the effect of thrombosis on ultrasonography, particularly in the third trimester. These examinations are more accurate if the mother is resting on her side. The radiation dose from phlebography, ventilation–perfusion lung scanning, spiral CT or pulmonary angiography is so small that the possible risk for the child of future malignancy caused by radiation or hypothyroidism due to free iodine is substantially less than the risk of missing the diagnosis. These examinations should therefore be performed if they are considered to be important for the diagnosis, but obviously with all available precautions. MRI or direct thrombosis imaging is not known to cause any harm to the fetus and, if available, may be a useful diagnostic tool. D-dimers are not helpful in these patients, who often have increased levels, especially during twin pregnancies or pre-eclampsia.

Thrombolytic therapy may be considered for massive DVT or PE, but the risk of bleeding is particularly high if this is used shortly before or during the delivery or the puerperium. Thrombectomy for iliac or iliofemoral DVT can be performed safely, but there are no studies to show that this gives any better results than anticoagulant therapy.

Despite the lack of clinical trials of LMWHs during pregnancy, they are widely used because of their ease of administration and good safety profile. There is debate as to whether twice-daily administration is better than once daily, for the half-life of LMWH is shorter in pregnancy due to improved renal clearance. It is not clear whether anti-FXa levels need to be monitored in pregnancy; there have been no clinical trials to assess the level of anti-FXa activity required in pregnancy, so target levels are extrapolated from non-pregnant studies. After VTE some physicians continue with the treatment dose until the end of pregnancy, but usually secondary prophylaxis is carried on with a reduced dose of LMWH. Vitamin K antagonists should be avoided if possible because of an increased risk of fetal haemorrhage and because of teratogenic effects. Unlike coumarins, UFH and LMWH do not cross the placenta.

At the time of delivery, blood samples are taken on admission for platelet count, APTT and PT to evaluate the risk of bleeding, and LMWH administration ceased. According to current guidelines, based on expert opinion, regional anaesthesia cannot be commenced or terminated within 24 hours of a treatment dose of LMWH or 12 hours after the previous prophylactic dose of LMWH. After acute VTE in pregnancy, after birth the prophylaxis is continued for at least 6 weeks and with a total duration that is at least as long as would have been chosen for a non-pregnant patient with the same risk factors. Alternatively, coumarins can be given after delivery, and LMWH is then stopped when the INR is within 2.0–3.0 for at least 2 days and after a minimum of 5 days. Neither LMWH nor vitamin K antagonists are secreted in breast milk in any amounts that can have an effect on the baby, although it seems sensible to ensure that the neonate receives intramuscular vitamin K to prevent haemorrhagic disease of the newborn.

Women with inherited antithrombin deficiency require higher doses of heparin and regular anti-FXa activity monitoring. Administration of antithrombin concentrate should be considered in association with delivery to allow for safe cessation of LMWH.

The post-thrombotic syndrome

Thrombi that do not undergo thrombolysis or which are not removed rapidly will destroy venous valves in the healing process, where they are transformed into fibrous tissue. Venous return of blood becomes impaired, accompanied by increased venous pressure. Permeation of fluid to the extravascular space causes oedema and creates a perivascular barrier to plasma proteins, which reduces the transport of nutrients to the tissues and results in skin atrophy and, in the most severe cases, venous ulcers. This process takes between 1 and 5 years, sometimes even longer, and is seen in 30% of patients 2 years after an event. The tools available to reduce the risk of developing the post-thrombotic syndrome include the following.

• Thrombolytic therapy, which has limited use due to the risk of haemorrhage.

• Ensure that more than 50% of the time on coumarins is in the target range.

• Graduated compression stockings for 2 years after an episode of DVT reduce the incidence of post-thrombotic syndrome by half. It is not known if shorter or longer treatment would have

similar or more pronounced effects. Knee-high stockings are sufficient for the vast majority of patients; they should be of compression class II (20–30 mmHg), fitted individually and should be worn whenever the patient is not recumbent.

Chronic thromboembolic pulmonary hypertension

A prospective long-term follow-up study of patients after PE showed that 3.8% of patients at 2 years had evidence of chronic thromboembolic pulmonary hypertension, suggesting that it is a relatively common complication of PE. The diagnosis should be considered in those with dyspnoea after PE. Pulmonary endarterectomy is the first treatment of choice in patients with severe pulmonary hypertension, and it reduces pulmonary vascular resistance dramatically, although the perioperative mortality is 5–9%. Five-year survival of over 80% has been described.

Selected bibliography

Anderson DR, Kovacs MJ, Kovacs G *et al.* (2003) Combined use of clinical assessment and D-dimer to improve the management of patients presenting to the emergency department with suspected deep vein thrombosis (the EDITED Study). *Journal of Thrombosis and Hemostasis* 1: 645–51.

Baglin T (2010) Defining the population in need of thromboprophylaxis – making hospitals safer. *British Journal of Haematology* 149: 805–12.

British Committee for Standards in Haematology (2005) Guidelines on oral anticoagulation (warfarin): third edition, 2005 update. *British Journal of Haematology* 132: 277–85.

British Committee for Standards in Haematology (2006) Guidelines on the use of vena cava filters. *British Journal of Haematology* 134: 590–5.

British Committee for Standards in Haematology (2006) The management of heparin-induced thrombocytopenia. *British Journal of Haematology* 133: 259–69.

British Thoracic Society Standards of Care Committee Pulmonary Embolism Guideline Development Group (2003) British Thoracic Society guidelines for the management of suspected acute pulmonary embolism. *Thorax* 58: 470–84.

Caprini JA (2010) Risk assessment as a guide for the prevention of the many faces of venous thromboembolism. *American Journal of Surgery* 199 (1 Suppl.): S3–10. Review.

Cohen AT, Tapson VF, Bergmann JF *et al.* (2008) Venous thromboembolism risk and prophylaxis in the acute hospital care setting (ENDORSE study): a multinational cross-sectional study. *Lancet* 371: 387–94.

Connolly SJ, Ezekowitz MD, Yusuf S *et al.* (2009) Dabigatran versus warfarin in patients with atrial fibrillation. *New English Journal of Medicine* 361: 1139–51.

Geerts WH, Bergqvist D, Pineo GF *et al.* (2008) Prevention of venous thromboembolism: American College of Chest Physicians Evidence-Based Clinical Practice Guidelines (8th edition). *Chest* **133** (6 Suppl.): 381S–453S.

Hunt BJ (2009) The prevention of hospital-acquired venous thromboembolism in the United Kingdom. *British Journal of Haematology* **144**: 642–52.

Pengo V, Lensing AW, Prins MH *et al.* (2004) Incidence of chronic thromboembolic pulmonary hypertension after pulmonary embolism. *New England Journal of Medicine* **350**: 2257–64.

Prandoni P, Kahn SR (2009) Post-thrombotic syndrome: prevalence, prognostication and need for progress. *British Journal of Haematology* **145**: 286–95.

Schulman S (2003) Care of patients receiving long-term anticoagulant therapy. *New England Journal of Medicine* **349**: 675–83.

Thromboembolic Disease in Pregnancy and the Puerperium: Acute Management (Green-top 28). Available at http://www.rcog.org.uk/files/rcog-corp/uploaded-files/GT28ThromboembolicDisease2007.pdf

Thromboprophylaxis during Pregnancy, Labour and after Vaginal Delivery (Green-top 37). Available at http://www.rcog.org.uk/files/rcog-corp/uploaded-files/GT37Thromboprophylaxis2004.pdf

van der Heijden JF, Hutten BA, Büller HR, Prins MH (2002) Vitamin K antagonists or low-molecular-weight heparin for the long term treatment of symptomatic venous thromboembolism. *Cochrane Database of Systematic Reviews* (1): CD002001.

Wadelius M, Chen LY, Lindh JD *et al.* (2009) The largest prospective warfarin-treate dcohort supports genetic forecasting. *Blood* **113**: 784–92.

Wells PS, Anderson DR, Rodger M *et al.* (2001) Excluding pulmonary embolism at the bedside without diagnostic imaging: management of patients with suspected pulmonary embolism presenting to the emergency department by using a simple clinical model and D-dimer. *Annals of Internal Medicine* **135**: 98–107.

CHAPTER 48

Congenital platelet disorders

Maurizio Margaglione[1] and Paul RJ Ames[2]

[1]University of Foggia, Foggia, Italy
[2]Royal Preston Hospital, Preston UK

Introduction

In haemostasis, a sequence of local events culminates in spontaneous arrest of bleeding from a traumatized blood vessel. The normal haemostatic mechanisms are sufficient to seal any vascular discontinuity. Three closely linked biological systems are involved: platelets, blood vessels and coagulation proteins. Platelets, anucleate cells that are derived from the cytoplasm of bone marrow megakaryocytes, circulate in the bloodstream for about 7–10 days. In the resting state platelets do not normally interact with endothelial cells or other blood cells but do so when the vessel wall is disrupted. Adhesion to exposed subendothelial components allows platelet activation and release of active substances (e.g. ADP) from intracellular organelles that amplify and propagate activation and, finally, platelet aggregation that plugs the ruptured blood vessel. At this primary stage of haemostasis platelets stop bleeding from damaged blood vessels transiently and provide the surface which promotes blood coagulation that strengthens the platelet plug (the secondary phase of haemostasis). Clinically, abnormalities of platelet adhesion and aggregation exhibit a history of spontaneous and/or easy bruising and a prolonged skin bleeding time. The characteristic clinical features of abnormal bleeding due to platelet deficiencies are distinct from those seen in disorders of plasma coagulation factors (Table 48.1). The occurrence of superficial bleeding in patients with platelet disorders as opposed to the deeper bleeding in patients with clotting factor disorders is a useful clinical pointer, but it must be remembered that the activities of platelets and coagulation factors are closely related.

Bleeding associated with platelet abnormalities manifests as haemorrhages from small vessels. Petechiae usually develop on the skin and the visible mucous membranes, but they may be distributed throughout the body including internal organs. Characteristically, bleeding resulting from platelet diseases is immediate and transient, tends to stop promptly with local pressure and does not recur when the pressure is removed. When this pattern of bleeding occurs in the neonatal period, infancy and childhood, a congenital platelet disorder should be suspected. However, the disease may be clinically silent and the patient may enter adult life before bleeding occurs.

The family history may be of great importance, providing a characteristic pattern of inheritance, but it should be remembered that a negative family history does not exclude an inherited platelet abnormality, i.e. the family history is usually negative in autosomal recessive traits. A comprehensive medical history and a careful clinical examination of the patient presenting with a haemorrhagic disorder is crucial for the correct diagnosis. Subsequent laboratory tests chosen on the basis of the clinical information obtained will lead to a precise definition, where possible, of the platelet abnormality.

Congenital defects of platelets may give rise to bleeding syndromes of varying severity and are difficult to classify because of the rarity of many forms, the extreme heterogeneity, and also because of incomplete knowledge about a variety of diseases. Table 48.2 classifies congenital platelet disorders into two main groups: thrombocytopenias and thrombocytopathies. Each group is further divided according to specific criteria based on functional and biochemical defects. Such a classification, as others, should be viewed as tentative, because some disorders may be characterized by multiple pathogenetic factors whereas others are grouped together for convenience of classification rather than on their known pathophysiology.

Postgraduate Haematology: 6th edition. Edited by A. Victor Hoffbrand, Daniel Catovsky, Edward G.D. Tuddenham, Anthony R. Green
© 2011 Blackwell Publishing Ltd.

Table 48.1 Main specific clinical differences between diseases of coagulation factors and platelet disorders.

Findings	Disorders of coagulation	Platelets/vessels
Onset of bleeding	Delayed after trauma	Spontaneous or immediately after trauma
Mucosal bleeding	Rare	Common
Petechiae	Rare	Characteristic
Deep haematomas	Characteristic	Rare
Ecchymoses	Large and solitary	Small and multiple
Haemarthrosis	Characteristic	Rare
Bleeding from superficial cuts and scratches	Minimal	Persistent; often profuse
Sex of patient	80–90% male	Equal

Table 48.2 Classification of congenital platelet disorders.

Thrombocytopenia
Non-inherited thrombocytopenia
    Drugs and chemical agents
    Isoimmune thrombocytopenia
    Infiltration of bone marrow
    Infections
    Other causes
Inherited thrombocytopenias
    Thrombocytopenias with reduced platelet size
    Thrombocytopenias with normal platelet size
    Thrombocytopenias with increased platelet size

Thrombocytopathies
Disorders of platelet adhesion
Disorders of platelet signalling transduction
Disorders of platelet aggregation

Thrombocytopenias

Thrombocytopenia defines a subnormal number of platelets in the circulating blood, usually below 100×10^9/L. Acute thrombocytopenia is the most frequent cause of severe bleeding and the risk of haemorrhage is inversely proportional to the platelet count, with spontaneous bleeding occurring frequently at a platelet count below 20×10^9/L. When automated methods are used, 'artefactual thrombocytopenia' or pseudothrombocytopenia can be observed. Different mechanisms can cause a falsely low platelet reading. This may happen in patients with a wide variety of clinical disorders. Non-technical factors inducing pseudothrombocytopenia include paraproteinaemias, cold agglutinins, giant platelets, previous contact of platelets with foreign surfaces (i.e. dialysis membrane), lipaemia and EDTA-induced platelet clumping. The possibility of a pseudothrombocytopenia must be ruled out through manual counting and/or examination of an adequately stained blood film before concluding that a patient has true thrombocytopenia.

Congenital non-inherited thrombocytopenia

Congenital thrombocytopenia not ascribed to inherited causes may be the result of a series of pathogenetic mechanisms, most likely attributable to deficient marrow platelet production or enhanced platelet destruction.

Drugs and chemical agents
The maternal use of drugs and chemical agents may cause thrombocytopenia by suppressing platelet production, by damaging platelets directly or by inducing the formation of platelet antibodies. Maternal ingestion of ethanol, thiazides, chlorpropamide, tolbutamide, estrogens, steroids and other drugs may selectively suppress thrombopoiesis. Alkylating agents, antimetabolites or chemotherapeutic drugs capable of crossing the placenta may lead to severe thrombocytopenia in newborns as the result of a predictable suppression of the bone marrow. The maternal ingestion of quinine, quinidine, hydralazine or selected antibiotics known to induce immune-mediated thrombocytopenia may induce congenital immune-mediated thrombocytopenia. In these newborns, thrombocytopenia usually improves rapidly and very rarely gives rise to severe or fatal haemorrhages.

Alloimmune thrombocytopenia
Immune thrombocytopenia may also result from the placental transfer of platelet antibodies formed as the result of active immunization of the mother by fetal platelet isoantigens, if the fetus has inherited a paternal platelet-specific antigen that induces antibody formation. Transplacental passage of the maternal antibody, usually of the IgG isotype, may induce severe thrombocytopenia in the fetus. This usually occurs when the mother has PlA1-negative platelets and the fetus carries PlA1-positive platelets. Newborns may show petechiae and purpura, or more severe bleeding at the time of birth, or may appear normal at delivery and then manifest severe bleeding within the first week after birth. In this case, thrombocytopenia usually improves within 1 month but severe and fatal intracranial haemorrhages may occur.

Bone marrow infiltration
Congenital thrombocytopenia caused by bone marrow infiltration is extremely rare, being limited to cases of disseminated reticuloendotheliosis and congenital leukaemia. Thrombocytopenia with or without associated myeloid and

erythroid depression occurs in children with numerous infiltrative disorders, including solid tumours, myelofibrosis, Gaucher disease, Niemann–Pick disease and the mucopolysaccharidoses.

Infections

Thrombocytopenia, usually mild but sometimes very severe, is commonly seen in infected newborns and several mechanisms are probably responsible. In fact, impaired platelet production as a result of invasion of megakaryocytes, the destruction of circulating platelets and the formation of antigen–antibody complexes may explain many instances of thrombocytopenia associated with viral infections. Maternal infection with toxoplasma, cytomegalovirus, rubella, herpesviruses or hepatitis varicella, as well as recent maternal vaccinations (rubella), may induce congenital thrombocytopenia.

Other causes

Occasionally, children born to women with chronic idiopathic thrombocytopenic purpura manifest congenital thrombocytopenia. It is conceivable that autoantibodies causing the disease in the mother cross the placenta and bind fetal platelets. Other causes of congenital thrombocytopenia due to increased platelet consumption or destruction include common maternal disorders such as pre-eclampsia, systemic lupus erythematosus or other autoimmune diseases, especially if the woman has antiphospholipid antibodies. A moderate to severe thrombocytopenia has been observed in association with giant cavernous haemangioma, first described by Kasabath and Merritt, in which the consumption of platelets occurs primarily within the tumour. Thrombocytopenia is often found associated with coagulation abnormalities typical of disseminated intravascular coagulation and the severity tends to parallel the size of the vascular tumour.

Inherited thrombocytopenias

Several inherited diseases may present with thrombocytopenia as an accompanying feature of generalized bone marrow failure (e.g. Fanconi anaemia) or metabolic diseases causing marrow infiltration (e.g. Gaucher disease). These and other complex clinical syndromes (e.g. Noonan syndrome) are not discussed in this chapter. Inherited thrombocytopenias are very rare. In some of these diseases thrombocytopathy may coexist with thrombocytopenia (e.g. Bernard–Soulier syndrome, Wiskott–Aldrich syndrome). These diseases are discussed in the appropriate section according to the most prominent defect. As proposed by the Italian Working Group, both platelet size and the presence (syndromic) or absence (non-syndromic) of other clinical features, different from those deriving from platelet abnormalities, are helpful criteria for classifying inherited thrombocytopenias.

Inherited thrombocytopenias with reduced platelet size

Wiskott–Aldrich syndrome (WAS) is a rare (1 in 250 000) X-linked recessive disorder characterized by eczema, susceptibility to infections associated with defects in cellular and humoral immunity, and thrombocytopenia with reduced platelet size. The gene responsible for WAS maps to Xp11.4 and codes for a protein, WASp, expressed only in haemopoietic-derived cells and which is involved in the transduction of signals from the receptor to the actin cytoskeleton. Intermittent bleeding, recurrent bacterial and viral infections, and progressive eczema occur during the first months of life. Death at an early age commonly results from intracranial haemorrhage, infection or lymphoreticular malignancy. A number of kindreds have been reported in whom *X-linked thrombocytopenia* (XLT) occurred alone or in association with partial manifestations of WAS. XLT is caused by a mutation within the *WAS* gene. Patients with XLT mainly suffer from an isolated bleeding tendency.

Inherited thrombocytopenias with normal platelet size

Congenital deficiency of megakaryocytes is a rare form of thrombocytopenic purpura in the newborn and may occur with skeletal, renal or cardiac malformations. Isolated *congenital amegakaryocytic thrombocytopenia* is an autosomal recessive syndrome leading to bone marrow aplasia later in childhood. This disorder is associated with abnormalities in the expression or function of the thrombopoietin receptor c-Mpl, and a series of mutations in the c-Mpl gene (*THPO*) have been identified. Most commonly, associated skeletal anomalies are present. Bilateral agenesis of the radius is the most commonly associated abnormality, so called *thrombocytopenia with absent radius* (TAR) syndrome. The TAR syndrome is an autosomal recessive disease characterized by severe, even fatal, haemorrhagic manifestations. Although abnormalities in the thrombopoietin/c-Mpl signalling pathway have been suggested, no mutations have been found in genes coding for these proteins. In some infants, the ulna and humerus may also be absent and other skeletal abnormalities may occur. In addition, proximal radio-ulnar synostosis, syndactyly and other skeletal abnormalities are reported in association with an autosomal dominant congenital amegakaryocytic thrombocytopenia in patients carrying heterozygous mutations of the *HOXA11* gene. Less commonly, patients manifest cardiac and other minor defects. *Schulman–Upshaw syndrome*, which is caused by mutations in the *ADAMTS13* gene, is characterized by thrombotic thrombocytopenic purpura with neonatal onset (congenital microangiopathic haemolytic anaemia), thrombocytopenia and frequent relapses, and response to fresh plasma infusion.

Inherited thrombocytopenias with increased platelet size

Thrombocytopenias with increased platelet size are characterized by the presence of an increased platelet volume with a reduced number of platelets (megathrombocytopenia) and are the commonest inherited forms of thrombocytopenias. Among them, a series of diseases have been characterized at the molecular level, whereas other clinical entities still await clear identification of the molecular defect. Giant platelets and moderate thrombocytopenia are most frequently found in certain populations of Mediterranean extraction and may also be associated with other inherited or congenital syndromes, such as May–Hegglin anomaly, Bernard–Soulier syndrome and stomatocytosis. *May–Hegglin anomaly* is a rare autosomal dominant disease characterized by giant platelets and basophilic inclusions (Döhle bodies) within granulocytes. Large Döhle bodies are seen in peripheral blood and in bone marrow granulocytes, and most patients show mild neutropenia but no significant susceptibility to infection. About 50% of patients have significant thrombocytopenia deriving from ineffective thrombopoiesis, but the occurrence of life-threatening haemorrhage is rare. In patients suffering from May–Hegglin anomaly the platelets show not only a greatly increased (twice normal) volume but most of them also display bizarre morphology and hypergranularity. Closely related to the May–Hegglin anomaly is a group of other autosomal dominant diseases known as Sebastian, Fetchner and Epstein syndromes. Their main characteristic is the presence in almost all patients of giant platelets with thrombocytopenia. In addition, patients may develop sensorineural hearing loss, cataract and glomerulonephritis, and most of them display Döhle bodies. The exact classification of patients according to the presence or absence of the above-mentioned clinical signs is shown in Table 48.3. The molecular basis of these syndromes has been elucidated. All these clinical entities are caused by mutations that occur within a gene (*MYH9*) located on the long arm of chromosome 22 (22q13.1). This gene codes for the heavy chain of non-muscle myosin IIA (NMMHC-IIA), a protein involved in the contractile activity of the cytoskeleton.

Grey platelet syndrome (GPS) is a rare disorder inherited as an autosomal dominant trait, although recessive transmission has been shown. It is characterized by large platelets with a selective deficiency in the number and content of α-granules. As a result of this, platelets are either markedly hypogranular or agranular and display deficiency of α-granule proteins, such as fibrinogen, von Willebrand factor, thrombospondin, β-thromboglobulin and platelet factor 4. Recently, a missense mutation has been identified at position 759 in the *GATA1* gene that induces an amino acid change (Arg216Gln) which segregates in an X-linked fashion, suggesting that the *GATA1* gene is required for regulation of platelet α-granules. Thrombocytopenia is usually pronounced and severe bleeding may occur. *Mediterranean macrothrombocytopenia* is an asymptomatic disorder with moderate isolated thrombocytopenia and large platelets inherited as an autosomal dominant trait. The condition is characterized by mild or no clinical manifestations and normal bone marrow megakaryocytosis, platelet survival and *in vitro* platelet functions. Platelets from some patients suffering from Mediterranean macrothrombocytopenia show reduced expression of the GPIb/IX platelet receptor and heterozygous mutations within the GPIbα (*GP1BA*) or GPIbβ (*GP1BB*) genes have been described. Therefore, in these patients Mediterranean macrothrombocytopenia may be classified as a heterozygous form of Bernard–Soulier syndrome (see below). The remaining patients with Mediterranean macrothrombocytopenia do not show a reduction in the content of the GPIb/IX platelet receptor and the pathogenesis of this form remains to be clarified.

A thrombocytopenia resulting from enhanced platelet destruction may be present in *type 2B von Willebrand disease*. Patients suffering from this syndrome show a qualitative abnormality of plasma von Willebrand factor (VWF) such that VWF binds inappropriately to circulating platelets. The molecular bases are mutations within the VWF gene, usually in exon 28, that give rise to increased reactivity of VWF with the platelet receptor GPIb/IX. Clearance of the resulting VWF–platelet complexes leads to thrombocytopenia and the selective loss of the largest VWF multimers from plasma. In general, the degree of thrombocytopenia is moderate and bleeding is of variable severity. A mutation in the VWF gene has been identified in a kindred previously labelled *Montreal platelet syndrome*, a very rare platelet disorder characterized by giant platelets, reduced platelet count and spontaneous *in vitro* platelet aggregation; this

Table 48.3 Main clinical differences among syndromes due to mutations within the *MYH9* gene.

Disease	Macrothrombocytopenia	Renal desease	Hearing loss	Cataract	Leucocyte inclusion*
MHA	Present	Absent	Absent	Absent	Present
SBS	Present	Absent	Absent	Absent	Present
EPS	Present	Present	Present	Absent	Absent
FTS	Present	Present	Present	Present	Present

*Ultrastructural differences in leucocyte inclusions exist (see Balduini *et al.* 2003).

EPS, Epstein syndrome; FTS, Fetchner syndrome; MHA, May–Hegglin anomaly; SBS, Sebastian syndrome.

kindred has now been reclassified as having type 2B von Willebrand disease. Type 2B von Willebrand disease should be distinguished from the rare pseudo von Willebrand disease (or *platelet-type von Willebrand disease*). The defect in this autosomal dominant condition results from mutations in the gene encoding the GPIbα subunit of the platelet receptor GPIb/IX. The few mutations identified give rise to a gain of function of the platelet receptor and increase the affinity for VWF, resulting in spontaneous binding of platelets to VWF and leading to shortened platelet survival and thrombocytopenia. The reasons why most patients suffering from platelet-type von Willebrand disease show variable enlarged platelets remain unclear.

Other very uncommon causes of macrothrombocytopenia are *Jacobsen syndrome* and *Paris–Trousseau syndrome*. Both are syndromic diseases inherited as autosomal dominant traits and characterized by chromosomal deletion encompassing the same region of chromosome 11 (11q23.3–q24.2). A heterozygous deletion of the *FLI1* gene has been identified in unrelated children with deletions of 11q23 and Paris–Trousseau thrombocytopenia. Interestingly, in patients suffering from Jacobsen syndrome without thrombocytopenia, the chromosomal deletion did not include the *FLI1* gene, suggesting that deletion of this gene is responsible for the thrombocytopenia that occurs in most patients with Jacobsen and Paris–Trousseau syndromes.

Thrombocytopathies

Platelets have a complex ultrastructure comprising a multitude of molecules and the malfunctioning of any of these may give rise to a specific disease (Figure 48.1). Platelets participate in haemostasis by adhering to exposed elements of the subendothelial matrix. They then spread onto the subendothelial surface, become activated, release the contents of their storage organelles, and aggregate to each other. Abnormalities in any of these stages – adhesion, activation, secretion and aggregation – may give rise to congenital disorders of platelets. Patients suffering from any of these diseases usually show a bleeding diathesis with a prolonged bleeding time and a normal platelet count.

Disorders of platelet adhesion

The interaction of platelet receptors with elements of the subendothelium, collagen, fibronectin and blood components allows platelet adhesion to the subendothelium, but it also occurs through the bridging effect of VWF (Figure 48.2). A series of receptors have been identified on the platelet surface and they interact with one or more of these elements. The most important receptors are GPIb/IX and $\alpha_2\beta_1$ (previously known as GPIa/IIa). The $\alpha_2\beta_1$ receptor is one of the receptors on the platelet surface that binds collagen and is a member of the integrin β_1 subfamily. Other receptors for collagen are GPIV and GPVI. Binding of molecules to these receptors leads to the subsequent binding to other receptors, which serves to reinforce adhesion and to generate intracellular signals, such as calcium mobilization and protein phosphorylation.

Bernard–Soulier syndrome

Bernard–Soulier syndrome (BSS) is a bleeding disorder characterized by giant platelets on the blood smear, mild or moderate thrombocytopenia, and prolongation of the skin bleeding time disproportionate to the thrombocytopenia. BSS is a recessively inherited autosomal disorder and consanguinity is common in reported kindreds. Based on reported data, the frequency of BSS has been estimated to be approximately 1 in 1 million population. Bleeding may be severe and fatal haemorrhages may occur.

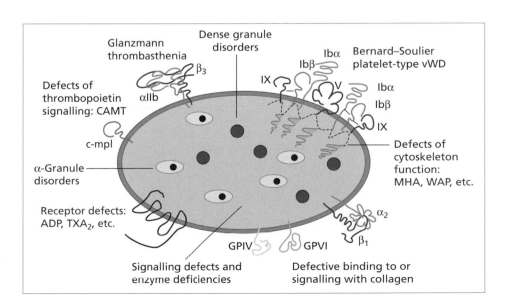

Figure 48.1 Schematic representation of the complex structure of platelets. Abnormalities of any platelet complex can lead to an alteration in a specific function.

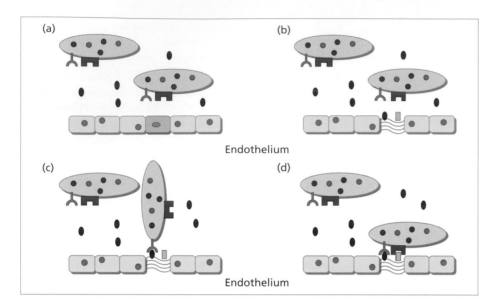

Endothelium

Endothelium

Figure 48.2 Platelets circulate in the bloodstream and do not interact with endothelial cells (a) unless the vessel wall is damaged (b). Adhesion of platelets to injured blood vessel wall (c) and spreading on it (d) are possible through the interaction of platelet receptors with their ligands and VWF–collagen.

Cutaneous haemorrhages and muscle and visceral bleeding are common. Epistaxis and menorrhagia may be difficult to control. Haemarthrosis has also been reported. Platelet counts range from as low as 20×10^9/L to near normal and, on the peripheral blood film, over 80% of platelets are usually larger than 2.5 μm, often up to 8.0 μm in diameter. The number of bone marrow megakaryocytes is usually normal.

Patients presenting with BSS show absent platelet agglutination in response to ristocetin (in the presence of human VWF) and normal aggregation, ATP secretion and thromboxane (Tx) B$_2$ formation in response to a variety of aggregating agents, and delayed response to thrombin. Biochemical and cellular factors contributing to these abnormalities have been clarified. Because of the defective binding with VWF, platelets in BSS do not agglutinate in response to ristocetin and have substantial reduction in their ability to adhere to sites of vascular injury where subendothelial VWF becomes exposed. As a consequence, plug formation, the primary haemostatic response, is impaired in BSS and increased and prolonged bleeding occurs. Variable levels of the GPIb–IX–V complex have been detected on the platelet surface of patients with BSS, some patients with BSS exhibiting nearly normal amounts (variant type of BSS). Despite the difference in glycoprotein content, the clinical bleeding problems and platelet functional and morphological abnormalities of these patients were indistinguishable from the classical BBS phenotype.

The GPIb–IX–V receptor complex provides the principal site mediating the interaction of platelets with the adhesive VWF. The entire cDNA sequences encoding the protein chains comprising this receptor have been deduced, allowing studies on the molecular basis of the syndrome. This complex consists of four proteins: the disulphide-linked α-chain (135 kDa) and β-chain

(25 kDa) of GPIb and the non-covalently associated subunits GPIX (22 kDa) and GPV (82 kDa). They all share structural and functional features suggesting a common evolutionary origin. Different transcripts encode the four polypeptide chains and, with the exception of that of GPIbβ, genes show continuous (intron-depleted) open reading frames. In addition, each element contains one or more homologous 24-amino-acid leucine-rich glycoprotein repeats. The genetic heterogeneity in the glycoprotein content of BSS patients shows that multiple molecular abnormalities may lead to a similar clinical disorder, and implies that BSS may be the result of defects within the subunits that hamper the coordinate expression of the complex on the platelet membrane. In this respect, BSS would resemble abnormalities of other multi-subunit complexes, in which a defect in a single subunit prevents the assembly and surface expression of the complex.

In addition to quantitative and qualitative abnormalities of the GPIbα gene, the recognized BSS phenotype has also been documented in patients with detrimental mutations within platelet GPIX and GPIbβ genes. Very few patients with a defect in one of the platelet receptors for collagen have been described. These patients show mild bleeding disorders and a selective impairment, at a variable extent, in collagen response, adhesion to subendothelial surfaces and collagen-induced platelet aggregation. Platelets have two major receptors for collagen, the α$_2$β$_1$ integrin, with a major role in adhesion of platelets to subendothelial surfaces, and GPVI, mainly involved in platelet activation. Thus, it is conceivable that collagen binding to platelets occurs through a multistep mechanism involving first the attachment of platelets to exposed collagen of the subendothelium in flowing blood by means of the α$_2$β$_1$ receptor and then platelet activation through a second receptor, GPVI.

Disorders of platelet signalling transduction

Platelets that adhere to the subendothelial surface become activated and begin the production or release of several intracellular messengers, which modulate a series of platelet responses such as calcium mobilization, protein phosphorylation and production of arachidonic acid. Activated platelets also release substances stored in their granules, some of which act in the recruitment of additional platelets and lead to the formation of the primary haemostatic plug (Figure 48.3). Several signalling mechanisms are involved in events that govern platelet responses, starting with platelet adhesion to injured blood vessel and leading to secretion and aggregation. Available evidence suggests that specific abnormalities in platelet signalling mechanisms may be the basis of platelet dysfunction, and the term 'platelet signalling disorders' defines a group of heterogeneous abnormalities in platelet secretion and signal transduction. Congenital defects of platelet signalling mechanisms are grouped together for convenience of classification rather than by the pathophysiology of specific diseases. Patients suffering from these defects represent the vast majority of subjects presenting with inherited thrombocytopathies.

Many platelet receptors are coupled to G proteins: $P2Y_1$ and TxA_2 receptors and thrombin act via $G_{\alpha q}$; prostaglandin recep-

tors activate whereas $P2Y_{12}$ receptors inhibit adenylate cyclase through G_s and G_{i2} respectively. Platelet activation by means of binding to receptors gives rise to hydrolysis of phosphoinositide by phospholipase (PL)C, leading to the formation of inositol trisphosphate, which in turn functions as a messenger to release calcium from intracellular stores. In addition, hydrolysis of phosphoinositide leads to the formation of diacylglycerol that activates protein kinase C. The activation of protein kinase C is thought to play a major role in platelet secretion and in the activation of the $\alpha_{IIb}\beta_3$ complex. Although defects in PLC activation, calcium mobilization and protein phosphorylation have been suggested in several patients, unique patients have been reported with deficiency in platelet $G_{\alpha q}$, G_s hyperfunction and reduced expression of $PLC\beta 2$.

Following stimulation, platelet PLA_2 mobilizes arachidonic acid from the phospholipid pool. The arachidonic acid is then metabolized by cyclooxygenase and thromboxane synthase to form TxA_2, a strong platelet-aggregating agent that is necessary for the secretion response. A defect in arachidonic acid mobilization and TxA_2 production has been identified in some patients. Few patients with impaired liberation of arachidonic acid have been described. Platelets in individuals with this defect show abnormal aggregation and secretion in response to a series of stimulating factors but normal production of TxA_2 in response to arachidonic acid. Several patients have been reported with deficiency of cyclooxygenase and show a slightly prolonged bleeding time and impaired platelet aggregation. In addition, a few patients show a defect in TxA_2 formation and present with a variable bleeding diathesis.

Disorders of platelet aggregation

Platelet aggregation may be defined as the interaction of activated platelets with one another and occurs after adhesion of platelets to the wall of the injured blood vessel. A series of factors are capable of inducing platelet aggregation and may be classified as primary and secondary platelet-aggregating agents. Primary aggregating agents are those factors, such as ADP, adrenaline and thrombin, able to directly induce platelet aggregation independently of their ability to release intraplatelet ADP or to induce the production of prostaglandins. Secondary aggregating agents are factors that induce aggregation of platelets through their ability to provoke the release reaction of ADP or the synthesis of prostaglandins. Accordingly, disorders due to impairment of platelet aggregation may be classified into defects of primary aggregation (Glanzmann thrombasthenia), selective impairment of platelet receptors (ADP, adrenaline) and defects of secondary aggregation (storage pool disease, selective impairment of platelet receptors such as thromboxane and collagen). *In vitro*, a series of substances are employed to challenge platelets and the manner in which they respond to these stimuli may be helpful for identifying specific thrombocytopathies (Table 48.4).

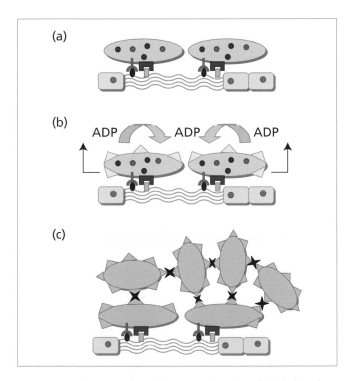

Figure 48.3 Platelets, after adhering to the subendothelial surface (a), become activated, release intracellular messengers (b) and aggregate each other leading to the formation of the primary haemostatic plug (c).

Table 48.4 Platelet response to aggregating agents in different thrombocytopathies.

Disorder	ADP	Adrenaline	Collagen	Arachidonic acid	Ristocetin
Bernard–Soulier	Normal	Normal	Normal	Normal	Absent
Pseudo von Willebrand disease	Normal	Normal	Normal	Normal	Increased at low doses
ADP receptor defect	Impaired	Impaired	Impaired	Impaired	Present
Adrenaline receptor defect	Normal	Impaired	Normal	Normal	Present
Collagen receptor defect	Normal	Normal	Impaired	Normal	Present
Defect of signal transduction	Variable impairment	Variable impairment	Variable impairment	Variable impairment	Present
Glanzmann thrombasthenia	Absent	Absent	Absent	Absent	Present
δ-Storage pool disorder	Impaired	Impaired	Impaired	Variable	Present
Thromboxane receptor defect	Impaired	Impaired	Impaired	Impaired	Present

Defects of primary aggregation: Glanzmann thrombasthenia

Glanzmann thrombasthenia (GT) is a bleeding diathesis marked by prolonged bleeding time, normal platelet count, and absence of platelet aggregation in response to platelet agonists such as ADP, collagen, arachidonic acid and thrombin. Platelet agglutination induced by ristocetin and VWF is normal. This congenital bleeding disorder is associated with impaired or absent clot retraction. GT is one of the less common of the congenital bleeding disorders (prevalence 1 in 1 million) and is transmitted as an autosomal recessive trait; consanguinity has been reported in affected kindreds. The clinical features are those expected with platelet dysfunction: easy and spontaneous bruising, mucosal membrane bleeding, subcutaneous haematomas, and petechiae. Rarely, patients suffer from intra-articular bleeding with resultant haemarthroses. Fatal haemorrhages have been reported.

Quantitative or qualitative (variant GT forms) abnormalities of the platelet $\alpha_{IIb}\beta_3$ integrin (also known as GPIIb/IIIa complex) have been shown to be responsible for this disorder. Mutations within the genes that code for $\alpha_{IIb}\beta_3$ subunits have been described in GT patients. As with other integrins, α_{IIb} and β_3 subunits are prominent integral components of the platelet membrane that form heterodimers containing specific sites for platelet–platelet cohesion. The $\alpha_{IIb}\beta_3$ integrin serves as a platelet receptor for fibrinogen, fibronectin, vitronectin and VWF. In addition, the $\alpha_{IIb}\beta_3$ integrin modulates, to some extent, calcium influx, cytoplasmic alkalinization, tyrosine kinase phosphorylation and clot retraction.

The clinical heterogeneity of GT has been stressed on the basis of platelet function testing or using crossed immunoelectrophoresis, Western blot, flow cytometry and fibrinogen binding. Type I GT is characterized by the lack of surface-detectable $\alpha_{IIb}\beta_3$ complex and a profound defect in platelet aggregation and clot retraction. At variance with type I, platelets of patients suffering from type II GT have detectable, but mark-

edly reduced, amounts of the $\alpha_{IIb}\beta_3$ receptor on their surface, usually 10–20% of normal values. Platelets manifest sufficient amounts of receptors to allow microaggregate formation, although there is still a profound defect in the ability to form large aggregates. Clot retraction is only moderately impaired. In addition, a series of patients with a variant form have been described who present near-normal levels of the $\alpha_{IIb}\beta_3$ complex, which is dysfunctional in that platelets, when activated, can neither aggregate nor bind fibrinogen. Extreme variability in the clinical symptoms is present, even among patients with similar degrees of platelet abnormality and prolongation of the bleeding time. In general, no aggregation abnormalities are detected in heterozygotes, but a decreased amount of the $\alpha_{IIb}\beta_3$ integrin has been reported, platelet content being approximately half of normal.

Selective impairment of platelet receptors

Defects of platelet ADP receptors have been characterized in a few patients and all suffered from a bleeding diathesis. On the platelet surface, different types of ADP receptors have been identified, including two G protein-coupled receptors, $P2Y_1$ and $P2Y_{12}$. The $P2Y_1$ receptor is responsible for the shape change of platelets and transient platelet aggregation, giving rise to centralization of platelet granules and formation of filopodia, while the $P2Y_{12}$ receptor is involved in amplification of the response and in the stabilization of platelet aggregates through full activation of the $\alpha_{IIb}\beta_3$ integrin. The $P2Y_{12}$ receptor defect is inherited as an autosomal recessive trait and most patients so far identified were born from consanguineous parents. In these patients, blunted platelet aggregation in response to ADP, with a retained shape change, has been reported. Only one patient has been briefly reported with a defect of the $P2Y_1$ receptor. This patient showed impaired platelet aggregation in response to ADP and other agonists.

The selective impairment of adrenaline (α_2-adrenergic) receptors has been associated with bleeding. A number of individuals with an impaired aggregation response to adrenaline and a congenital defect of platelet α_2-adrenergic receptors have been described and some of them presented a history of easy bruising.

Defects of secondary aggregation

Secondary aggregation disorders are more frequent than primary aggregation disorders and the most common in this category are the storage pool deficiency (SPD) syndromes. SPD syndromes may be classified in a system that takes into account the content of both dense and α granules (Figure 48.4). Thus δ-SPD identifies patients who show low platelet content of dense granules only. Patients with deficiency of both types of granules are designated $\alpha\delta$-SPD. Finally, patients presenting with reduced or absent platelet content of α-granules but normal levels of dense granules (α-SPD) are categorized as patients with GPS. The disorder is heterogeneous and the term SPD includes a group of disorders having as their common feature a diminution in secretable substances stored in platelet granules.

A storage pool disease is found as an associated defect in most of the patients carrying other rare syndromes, such as WAS and the TAR syndrome. However, the majority of patients presenting with an SPD have no associated diseases and are otherwise normal. The clinical features of this type of secondary aggregation disorder are those expected with a platelet function defect and consist of easy and spontaneous bruising, mucocutaneous haemorrhages, haematuria and epistaxis. Patients with δ-SPD or $\alpha\delta$-SPD usually have absent ADP- and adrenaline-induced secondary aggregation waves, although the primary waves are present. Patients with δ-SPD may present a severe or partial

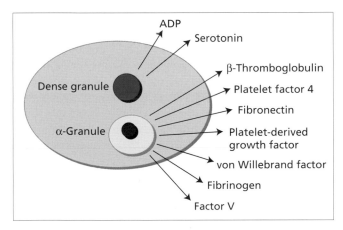

Figure 48.4 In platelets, granules are the storage site for substances that are important in the haemostatic process. The α-granules contain proteins involved in adhesion (fibronectin, VWF), cell–cell interaction (P-selectin) and in promoting coagulation (FV, platelet factor 4), whereas the content of dense granules is important in recruiting additional platelets (ADP, serotonin).

granule deficiency. Collagen-induced aggregation is absent or markedly reduced, whereas ristocetin-induced agglutination is normal. In several kindreds, the disorder appeared to be inherited as an autosomal dominant trait. However, in other families the type of inheritance could be not determined. In the absence of other congenital abnormalities or an associated α-granule deficiency, SPD is inherited as an autosomal dominant trait.

The other forms of δ-SPD coincident with other congenital abnormalities, such as TAR, are usually inherited as autosomal recessive traits, or as X-linked traits as in the case of WAS. An SPD is usually present in Hermansky–Pudlak syndrome and in Chédiak–Higashi syndrome. *Hermansky–Pudlak syndrome* (HPS) is a rare autosomal recessive inherited disorder characterized by the presence of oculocutaneous albinism, absence of platelet dense granules, and infiltration of ceroid-pigmented reticuloendothelial cells in the lung and the colon, leading to pulmonary fibrosis and inflammatory bowel disease. HPS results from the abnormal formation of intracellular vesicles. The impaired function of specific organelles indicates that the causative genes encode proteins operative in the formation of lysosomes and vesicles. HPS displays genetic heterogeneity and, so far, mutations in eight orthologous genes have been found in patients with this disease: *HPS1, HPS2 (AP3B1), HPS3, HPS4, HPS5, HPS6, HPS7 (DTNBP1)* and *HPS8 (BLOC1S3)*.

In *Chédiak–Higashi syndrome* (CHS) a variable degree of oculocutaneous albinism and a poor resistance to respiratory and cutaneous infections are usually found. The infections are generally fatal during infancy or in early childhood but patients may also die of a chronic lymphohistiocytic infiltration known as the accelerated phase during the second or third decades of life. CHS is extremely rare and is inherited as an autosomal recessive trait. Unlike HPS, CHS does not seem to display locus heterogeneity and the only gene proved to cause CHS, *LYST*, is located on chromosome 1q42.1–42.2. HPS and CHS both present findings typical of an SPD: bleeding of mucosae, epistaxis and spontaneous soft-tissue bruising. On the other hand, in *Quebec platelet disorder*, a rare autosomal dominant bleeding disease associated with abnormal proteolysis of α-granule proteins, platelets show increased stores of urokinase plasminogen activator and genetic studies implicate a major role for a mutation in an uncharacterized *cis* element near the urokinase plasminogen activator gene. Intraplatelet generation of plasmin is thought to trigger degradation of stored α-granule proteins, increasing risks for a number of bleeding symptoms, including delayed-onset bleeding after haemostatic challenges that responds only to fibrinolytic inhibitor therapy. Recently, Paterson *et al.* clarified the pathogenisis of the Quebec platelet disorder: a duplication of the PLAU gene.

Several patients have been described with selective impairment of the TxA$_2$ receptor, a mild lifelong disorder, exhibiting mucosal bleeding and easy bruising and defective platelet aggregation in respone to several agents but not thrombin. Autosomal dominant inheritance has been suggested in some cases.

Therapy

As a rule, there is no specific treatment for the vast majority of congenital platelet disorders. In congenital thrombocytopenias due to maternal use of drugs or chemical agents, thrombocytopenia recovers after a few days to a few weeks, as in the case of thiazide drugs. In surviving thrombocytopenic newborns infected with rubella or cytomegalovirus, platelets levels may return to normal after several months. In newborns with alloimmune congenital thrombocytopenia, platelets return to normal values in 14–21 days. Only severe cases need to be treated with washed platelets, corticosteroids or exchange transfusions. In general, the main treatments in patients with congenital platelet diseases are general measures aimed at avoiding bleeding and the use of supportive therapeutic approaches for controlling haemorrhage. However, since types and severity of bleeding vary in different patients, therapeutic approaches have to be individualized.

General measures

Education of patients is of great importance. Patients and their parents have to be instructed to avoid trauma. Regular dental care may be helpful in preventing gingival bleeding. Drugs that impair platelet functions, such as acetylsalicylic acid-containing medications, should be avoided. In women, oral contraceptives can be used to prevent menorrhagia. Local measures, such as the application of firm pressure in the case of epistaxis, will usually suffice in the event of mild bleeding.

Drugs

Antifibrinolytic agents are useful as an adjunctive measure to prevent and control mild or moderate bleeding and may stop menorrhagia and other mild bleeding manifestations from mucous membranes, such as epistaxis. In the case of more serious bleeding, antifibrinolytic drugs such as tranexamic acid may be used, either 15–25 mg/kg orally three times daily or 10 mg/kg i.v. three times daily.

Desmopressin (1-desamino-8-D-arginine vasopressin or DDAVP) is the mainstay of therapy of patients with congenital platelet defects. Depending on the platelet defect, administration of DDAVP may shorten the bleeding time. Intravenous, subcutaneous or intranasal administration of DDAVP increases factor VIII and VWF transiently by releasing them from storage sites and its use has been suggested to be of value in some patients presenting with congenital platelet defects, such as those with BSS, May–Hegglin anomaly, GPS, SPD and GT. The drug is usually administered at a dose of 0.3 μg/kg in 50 mL of saline by slow intravenous infusion (over 30 min) in order to avoid possible hypotensive effects. In general, since the response to DDAVP varies among patients but is constant in each patient, a test dose may be of value in identifying those patients who will benefit from this treatment in order to prevent or control future bleedings.

The use of recombinant activated factor VII (rFVIIa) has been proved to be helpful in the treatment of bleeding in haemophilic patients with inhibitors. Recently, administration of rFVIIa has been employed to stop bleeding in patients with congenital platelet disorders, such as BSS, SPD and GT. In addition, in thrombasthenics this drug has been employed to avoid bleeding during surgical procedures. However, adverse reactions have been described, such as venous thromboembolism and arterial ischaemia. Based on the evidence from the literature, rFVIIa is currently approved in Europe for prophylaxis and treatment of bleeding in patients with GT with antibodies to GPIIb/IIIa and/or HLA, and past or present refractoriness to platelet transfusion. The recommended dose is a bolus injection of 90 μg/kg at 2-hour intervals for a minimum of three doses.

A second generation of synthetic thrombopoietin agonists, including AMG 531 and eltrombopag, have shown great potential in the treatment of forms of thrombocytopenia, including immune thrombocytopenic purpura and chemotherapy-induced thrombocytopenia. It is conceivable that thrombopoietin agonists would be helpful in congenital thrombocytopenia with reduced plasma levels of endogenous thrombopoietin.

Platelet transfusions

Platelet transfusions, using platelets from HLA-matched donors when available, are employed to control severe haemorrhage in thrombocytopenic patients or in individuals with thrombocytopathies. Since the risk of post-traumatic as well as of spontaneous bleeding increases as the platelet count falls, spontaneous haemorrhage becomes common as platelet count drops below 20×10^9/L and is extremely likely at counts below 5×10^9/L. Extensive clinical experience has shown that control of bleeding is possible on achievement of an adequate elevation in the circulating platelet count. However, the coexistence of platelet dysfunction has to be taken into account in order to correctly calculate the dosage of platelets required. Platelet transfusions are effective in controlling bleeding but may be responsible for transmission of infectious diseases, febrile reactions or development of alloimmunization. In patients carrying thrombocytopathies, platelet transfusions should be employed only for the treatment of severe bleeding because of the risk of alloimmunization. The occurrence of platelet alloimmunization is more frequent in patients lacking a membrane glycoprotein, such as in BSS and GT. Alloantibodies develop because the deficient proteins are recognized as foreign and, in turn, induce refractoriness to platelet transfusion.

Other measures

Splenectomy has generally no effect in congenital thrombocytopathies and in thrombocytopenias but has proven effective in patients with WAS. Allogeneic bone marrow transplantation may provide, in theory, an effective cure for inherited disorders involving platelet count or function, restoring normal megakaryocytopoiesis. Transplants have been successfully performed with complete correction in patients with WAS and severe GT. However, the risks of such a drastic procedure still outweigh those related to bleeding tendency and it is therefore rarely required in patients suffering from congenital platelet disorders.

Conclusions

Over the last few years, a series of improvements to better understand the pathogenesis of congenital platelet disorders have been achieved. In several congenital platelet diseases, the gene responsible has been identified and several patients have been characterized at molecular level (Table 48.5). This information has allowed more accurate comprehension of congenital thrombocytopenias and thrombocytopathies. Careful collection of personal and family clinical data, physical examination and appropriate laboratory testing are of value for the evaluation of a patient presenting with bleeding due to congenital platelet disorders (Figure 48.5). Using this approach, in many instances it is possible to correctly identify the platelet defect. However, despite recent advances in knowledge, in most patients with a congenital bleeding disorder and impairment of platelet function, the underlying molecular mechanisms are still unknown. In the near future, one of the challenges will be to ameliorate our understanding of congenital platelet disorders in order to obtain powerful tools for prevention, diagnosis and therapy of bleeding. On the other hand, gene therapy may offer

Table 48.5 Genes involved in congenital platelet disorders.

Disorder	Gene	Locus
Wiskott–Aldrich syndrome	WAS	Xp11.4–p11.21
X-linked thrombocytopenia	WAS	Xp11.4–p11.21
Congenital amegakaryocytic thrombocytopenia	MPL	1p34
Congenital amegakaryocytic thrombocytopenia and radioulnar synostosis	HOXA11	7p15.2
Schulman–Upshaw syndrome	ADAMTS13	9q34
May–Hegglin anomaly and Sebastian, Epstein and Fetchner syndromes	MYH9	22q13.1
Mediterranean macrothrombocytopenia	GP1BA	17pter–p12
Jacobsen and Paris–Troussau syndromes	FLI1	11q24.1–q24.3
Bernard–Soulier syndrome	GP1BA	17pter–p12
	GP1BB	22q11.21–q11.23
	GP9	3q21.3
Pseudo von Willebrand disease	GP1BA	17pter–p12
ADP receptor defect	P2RY12	3q24–q25
	P2RY1	3q25.2
	P2RX1	17p13.3
Adrenaline receptor defect	ADRA2A	10q24–q26
Collagen receptor defect	ITGA2	5q11.2
Glanzmann thrombasthenia	ITGA2B	17q21.32
	ITGB3	17q21.32
Hermansky–Pudlak syndrome	HPS1	10q23.1–q23.3
	HPS2 (AP3B1)	5q14.1
	HPS3	3q24
	HPS4	22cen–q12.3
	HPS5	11p14
	HPS6	10q24.32
	HPS7 (DTNBP1)	6p22.3
	HPS8 (BLOC1S3)	19q13.32
Chédiak–Higashi syndrome	LYST	1q42.1–q42.2
Quebec platelet disorder	near PLAU locus	10q24
Thromboxane receptor defect	TBXA2R	19p13.3

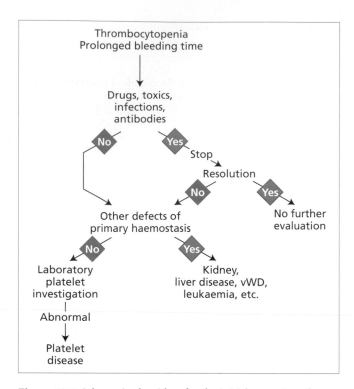

Figure 48.5 Schematic algorithm for the initial screening of patients with congenital platelet disorders.

a cure for congenital platelet disorders. Hopefully, improvements in such approaches will allow treatment of the majority of patients suffering from severe congenital platelet disorders.

Selected bibliography

Alamelu J, Liesner R (2010) Modern management of severe platelet function disorders. *British Journal of Haematology* **149**: 813–23.

Almeida A, Khair K, Hann I *et al.* (2003) The use of recombinant factor VIIa in children with inherited platelet function disorders. *British Journal of Haematology* **121**: 477–81.

American Society of Haematology ITP Practice Panel (1997) Diagnosis and treatment of idiopathic thrombocytopenic purpura: recommendations of the American Society of Haematology. *Annals of Internal Medicine* **126**: 319–26.

Arai M, Yamamoto N, Moroi M *et al.* (1995) Platelets with 10% of the normal amount of glycoprotein VI have an impaired response to collagen that results in a mild bleeding tendency. *British Journal of Haematology* **89**: 124–30.

Balduini CL, Noris P, Belletti S *et al.* (1999) *In vitro* and *in vivo* effects of desmopressin on platelet function. *Haematologica* **84**: 891–6.

Balduini CL, Iolascon A, Savoia A (2002) Inherited thrombocytopenias: from genes to therapy. *Haematologica* **87**: 860–80.

Balduini CL, Cattaneo M, Fabris F *et al.* (2003) Inherited thrombocytopenias: a proposed diagnostic algorithm from the Italian Gruppo di Studio delle Piastrine. *Haematologica* **88**: 582–92.

Bellucci S, Damaj G, Boval B *et al.* (2000) Bone marrow transplantation in severe Glanzmann's thrombasthenia with antiplatelet alloimmunization. *Bone Marrow Transplantation* **25**: 327–30.

Bernaciak J, Szczaluba K, Derwinska K *et al.* (2008) Clinical and molecular–cytogenetic evluation of a family with partial Jacobsen syndrome without thrombocytopenia caused by an ~5 Mb deletion del(11)(q24.3). *American Journal of Medical Genetics* **146A**: 2449–54.

Bizzaro N (2007) Pseudothrombocytopenia. In: *Platelets* (A Michelson, ed.), 2nd edn, pp. 999–1008. Elsevier Science, Boston.

Bolton-Maggs PHB, Chalmers EA, Collins PW *et al.* (2006) A review of inherited platelet disorders with guidelines for their management on behalf of the UKHCDO. *British Journal of Haematology* **135**: 603–33.

Cattaneo M (2002) Desmopressin in the treatment of patients with defects of platelet function. *Haematologica* **87**: 1122–4.

Cattaneo M (2005) The P2 receptors and congenital platelet function defects. *Seminars in Thrombosis and Hemostasis* **31**: 168–73.

Clark RH, Taylor LL, Wells RJ (1984) Congenital juvenile chronic myelogenous leukaemia: case report and review. *Pediatrics* **73**: 324–6.

D'Andrea G, Coalizzo D, Vecchione G *et al.* (2002) Glanzmann's thrombasthenia: identification of 19 new mutations in 30 patients. *Thombosis and Haemostasis* **87**: 1034–42.

Diamandis M, Paterson AD, Rommens JM *et al.* (2009) Quebec platelet disorder is linked to the urokinase plasminogen activator gene (PLAU) and increases expression of the linked allele in megakaryocytes. *Blood* **113**: 1543–6.

Favier R, Jondeau K, Boutard P *et al.* (2003) Paris–Trousseau syndrome: clinical, hematological, molecular data of ten new cases. *Thombosis and Haemostasis* **90**: 893–7.

Freson K, Jaeken J, Van Helvoirt M *et al.* (2003) Functional polymorphisms in the paternal expressed XLalphas and its cofactor ALEX decrease their mutual interaction and enhance receptor-mediated camp formation. *Human Molecular Genetics* **12**: 1121–30.

Gabbetta J, Vaidyula VR, Dhanasekaran DN *et al.* (2002) Human platelet Galphaq deficiency is associated with decreased Galphaq gene expression in platelets but not in neutrophils. *Thombosis and Haemostasis* **87**: 129–33.

Galbusera M, Noris M, Remuzzi G (2009) Inherited thrombotic thrombocytopenic purpura. *Haematologica* **94**: 166–70.

Geddis AE (2009) Congenital amegakaryocytic thrombocytopenia and thrombocytopenia with absent radii. *Hematology/Oncology Clinics of North America* **23**: 321–31.

George JN, Caen JP, Nurden AT (1990) Glanzmann's thromboasthenia: the spectrum of clinical disease. *Blood* **75**: 1383–95.

Hirata T, Kakizuka A, Ushikubi F *et al.* (1994) Arg60 to Leu mutation of the human thromboxane A2 receptor in a dominantly inherited bleeding disorder. *Journal of Clinical Investigation* **94**: 1662–7.

Introne W, Boissy RE, Gahl WA (1999) Clinical, molecular, and cell biological aspects of Chediak–Higashi syndrome. *Molecular Genetics and Metabolism* **68**: 283–303.

Jackson SC, Sinclair GD, Cloutier S *et al.* (2009) The Montreal platelet syndrome kindred has type 2B von Willebrand disease with the VWF V1316M mutation. *Blood* **113**: 3348–51.

Lillicrap D (2007) Von Willebrand disease – phenotype versus genotype: deficiency versus disease. *Thrombosis Research* **120** (Suppl. 1): S11–S16.

Lopez JA, Andrews RK, Afshar-Kharghan V *et al.* (1998) Bernard–Soulier syndrome. *Blood* **91**: 4397–418.

Mao GF, Vaiduyala VR, Kunapoli SP *et al.* (2002) Lineage-specific defect in gene expression in human platelet phospholipase C-beta2 deficiency. *Blood* **99**: 905–11.

Miller JL (1996) Platelet-type von Willebrand disease. *Thrombosis and Haemostasis* **75**: 865–9.

Molineux G, Newland A (2010) Development of romiplostim for the treatment of patients with chronic immune thrombocytopenia: from bench to bedside. *British Journal of Haematology* **150**: 9–20.

Nair S, Ghosh K, Kulkarni B *et al.* (2002) Glanzmann's thrombasthenia: updated. *Platelets* **13**: 387–93.

Nurden AT, Nurden P (2007) The grey platelet syndrome: clinical spectrum of the disease. *Blood Reviews* **21**: 21–36.

Ochs HD, Filipovich AH, Veys P *et al.* (2008) Wiskott–Aldrich syndrome: diagnosis, clinical and laboratory manifestations, and treatment. *Biology of Blood and Marrow Transplantation* **15** (1 Suppl.): 84–90.

Oury C, Lanaerts T, Peerlinck K (1999) Congenital deficiency of the phospholipase C coupled platelet P2Y1 receptor leads to mild bleeding disorder. *Thrombosis and Haemostasis* **82** (Suppl.): 20–1.

Paterson AD, Rommens JM, Bharaj B *et al.* (2010) Persons with Quebec platelet disorder have a tandem duplication of PLAU, the urokinase plasminogen activator gene. *Blood* **115**: 1264–6.

Pham A, Wang J (2007) Bernard–Soulier syndrome: an inherited platelet disorder. *Archives of Pathology and Laboratory Medicine* **131**: 1834–6.

Poon MC, d'Oiron R, Hann I *et al.* (2001) Use of recombinant factor VIIa (NovoSeven) in patients with Glanzmann thrombasthenia. *Seminars in Hematology* **38** (Suppl. 12): 21–5.

Rao AK, Willis J, Kowalska MA *et al.* (1988) Differential requirements for adrenaline induced platelet aggregation and inhibition of adenylate cyclase. Studies in familial α_2-adrenergic receptor defect. *Blood* **71**: 494–501.

Rao AK, Ghosh S, Sun L *et al.* (1995) Effect of mechanism of platelet dysfunction in response to DDAVP in patients with congenital platelet function defects. A double blind placebo-controlled trial. *Thombosis and Haemostasasis* **74**: 1071–8.

Rao AK, Jalagadugula G, Sun L (2004) Inherited defects in platelet signalling mechanisms. *Seminars in Thrombosis and Hemostasis* **30**: 525–35.

Rivera J, Lozano ML, Navarro-Núñez L, Vicente V (2009) Platelet receptors and signalling in the dynamics of thrombus formation. *Haematologica* **94**: 700–11.

Roberts I, Stanworth S, Murray NA (2008) Thrombocytopenia in the neonate. *Blood Reviews* **22**: 173–86.

Serrarens-Janssen V, Semmekrot B, Novotny V *et al.* (2008) Fetal/neonatal allo-immune thrombocytopenia (FNAIT): past, present, and future. *Obstetrical and Gynecological Survey* **63**: 239–52.

Shotelersuk V, Gahl WA (1998) Hermansky–Pudlak syndrome. Models for intracellular vesicle formation. *Molecular Genetics and Metabolism* **65**: 85–96.

Sola-Visner M, Sallmon H, Brown R (2009) New insights into the mechanisms of nonimmune thrombocytopenia in neonates. *Seminars in Perinatology* **33**: 43–51.

Stroncek DF, Rebulla P (2007) Platelet transfusions. *Lancet* **370**: 427–38.

Tubman VN, Levine JE, Campagna DR *et al.* (2007) X-linked grey platelet syndrome due to a GATA1 Arg216Gln mutation. *Blood* **109**: 3297–9.

van den Bemt PM, Meyboom RH, Egberts AC (2004) Drug-induced immune thrombocytopenia. *Drug Safety* **27**: 1243–52.

Wei ML (2006) Hermansky–Pudlak syndrome: a disease of protein trafficking and organelle function. *Pigment Cell Research* **19**: 19–42.

Weiss HJ, Lages B, Vicic W *et al.* (1993) Heterogeneous abnormalities of platelet dense granule ultrastructure in 20 patients with congenital storage pool deficiency. *British Journal of Haematology* **83**: 282–95.

Primary immune thrombocytopenia

49

Drew Provan and Adrian C Newland

Queen Mary University of London, London, UK

Introduction

Primary immune thrombocytopenia (ITP), previously called idiopathic thrombocytopenic purpura, is an autoimmune bleeding disorder that affects both children and adults. Until fairly recently, it was considered an autoantibody disorder in which platelets, opsonized with antiplatelet antibody, were removed prematurely by the reticuloendothelial system. More recently, studies have shown that in many patients there is a relative platelet underproduction that contributes to the thrombocytopenia seen in this disease.

Many patients have no clinical problems but bleeding may occur. ITP is unpredictable in its clinical course. To date, treatment has aimed at reducing the platelet destruction, mainly through immunosuppression. However, new thrombopoietin receptor agonists have been developed that enhance bone marrow platelet production. These newer targeted treatments are likely to be associated with less toxicity due to immunosuppression than traditional therapies.

Clinical features

The two principal forms of ITP, paediatric and adult, are quite distinct in their underlying cause and presentation. In children, ITP may follow a viral illness or immunization. The profound thrombocytopenia may be associated with extensive petechiae, purpura and bruises. There may also be bleeding from mucous membranes such as the nose or mouth. Despite the severity of the clinical features, most children need little treatment, and undergo spontaneous remission in the majority of cases. Around 15% will develop a more chronic form of the disease.

ITP in adults is much more insidious. There is generally no prodromal illness and the patient may be aware of petechiae or excessive bruising, and seek medical attention. ITP is often diagnosed by chance, for example during hospital admission for surgery or full blood count (FBC) is checked for other reasons. This is particularly true if the platelet count is not very low and there are no skin manifestations of thrombocytopenia.

ITP, particularly in adults, is heterogeneous. Many patients suffer few clinical problems related to their thrombocytopenia while others have major bleeding from the outset. The platelet count alone appears to be an unreliable predictor of outcome, and the clinical symptoms and signs of ITP are influenced by patient age, general health, comorbidities, medication and many other factors that have not been identified. In addition, there may be an acquired platelet dysfunction caused by antibody binding to an important region of the glycoprotein molecules on the platelet surface. Autoantibodies reacting with glycoprotein (GP)IIb/IIIa may affect platelet aggregation, and anti-GPIb/IX autoantibodies can impair platelet adhesion to the subendothelial matrix, causing unexpectedly severe bleeding for the level of platelet count. Other autoantibodies such as antiphospholipid antibodies occur in up to 30% of patients with

Postgraduate Haematology: 6th edition. Edited by A. Victor Hoffbrand,
Daniel Catovsky, Edward G.D. Tuddenham, Anthony R. Green
© 2011 Blackwell Publishing Ltd.

Table 49.1 New Consensus Terminology definitions.

Immune thrombocytopenia	Primary (old term 'idiopathic') Secondary (SLE, etc.)
Diagnosis	Requires platelet count $< 100 \times 10^9$/L
'Acute' and 'chronic' replaced by	'Newly diagnosed', 'persistent' and 'chronic' (see Figure 49.1)
Severe ITP	Where there is clinically relevant bleeding irrespective of platelet count
Refractory	Failed splenectomy or relapse *and* severe ITP or risk of bleeding

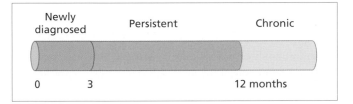

Figure 49.1 Stages of ITP using the new Consensus Terminology. After diagnosis until 3 months the patient is described as having newly diagnosed ITP. If the ITP persists beyond 3 months, it is termed persistent ITP and once the 12-month milestone has been reached the disease is described as chronic ITP.

ITP, and these may affect platelet and vascular function. However, in general, unlike the thrombocytopenia that accompanies bone marrow failure, serious bleeding is not common in patients with ITP. The reason for this is not completely understood, but is believed to be partly due to the large proportion of young (metabolically active) platelets present in ITP compared with other causes of thrombocytopenia. The other factor which is often overlooked is that the large platelets in ITP are not counted accurately by automated counters. The true platelet count in patients with ITP is therefore higher than the reading given when using an automated analyser.

Reaching a consensus on terminology

Until recently, comparing data from clinical studies in ITP has been made extremely difficult due to the inconsistent way in which terminology has been used. For example, the term 'refractory' has been interpreted in different ways. For some it implies the post-splenectomy patient who has failed to respond or who has relapsed. Others interpret the term to mean those who do not respond well to treatment irrespective of splenectomy status. Similarly, deciding what constitutes a 'complete response' to therapy differs from study to study, making comparisons of drug treatments fraught with problems.

In order to address this, a group of experts held a consensus meeting and agreed on the terminology that should be used in ITP. These have been published and will be used in all drug trials, and in the clinic, from now on. The key terminologies are listed in Table 49.1.

Chronic ITP implies disease that has been present for 12 months or more from diagnosis. Previously, the term 'chronic' applied to individuals who had ITP for 6 months or longer. However, because patients may remit between 6 and 12 months, the term 'chronic' has now been redefined to refer to those individuals whose ITP has been present for 12 months or greater (Figure 49.1).

Pathophysiology

ITP in adults is a typical organ-specific autoimmune disease and, in common with other autoimmune diseases, there is a skewing of the Th1/Th2 response towards Th1 (proinflammatory). These are disorders in which there are antibodies or cells (B cells, T cells, antigen-presenting cells, or others) that react against self antigens. These may cause disease if the target tissue is damaged. The binding of antibodies to target cells results in clearance of the antigen from the body. The normal adaptive response, such as that seen in microbial infection, results in complete removal of the non-self antigen. In autoimmune disease, however, there is continual production and incomplete clearance of the antigen, leading to perpetuation of the immune attack. In ITP the antigen is platelet glycoprotein, found on megakaryocytes and platelets.

Autoimmune disorders occur in around 5% of the population, although not all are symptomatic. In all, there are more than 80 distinct disorders, most of which are uncommon, apart from rheumatoid disease and autoimmune thyroiditis. Autoimmune diseases are clinical syndromes in which there is loss of tolerance to self, mediated by activation of T or B lymphocytes or other cells.

ITP is multifactorial

From studies of other autoimmune diseases, it is quite clear that ITP has a multifactorial basis, and that loss of tolerance to a self antigen alone is not sufficient to generate the autoimmune disorder. Patients probably require (i) a specific set of genetic determinants, such as polymorphisms within major histocompatibility complex (MHC), CTLA4, or other genes; (ii) dysregulation of the immune response (involving dendritic cells, T or B cells, or all three); and (iii) an environmental 'trigger'. The trigger may be infectious, for example a viral infection. Autoimmune disease arises only when all these determinants are present in an individual at the same time. This is further reinforced by the observation that self-reactive lymphocytes are commonly found in normal individuals. For example, siblings of patients who have autoimmune disorders are more likely to have autoantibodies themselves, with no overt evidence of autoimmune disease. This may be because they have not been exposed to the environmental trigger required to tip the balance towards autoimmune disease.

Antiplatelet antibodies and their targets

The autoantibodies involved in ITP are generally IgG, but IgA and IgM autoantibodies have been reported. Opsonized platelets are removed prematurely by the reticuloendothelial system via an Fc-dependent mechanism. In addition, the autoantibodies may impair megakaryocyte growth and development, platelet release and may also induce apoptosis of megakaryocytes. The overall result of this is failure of platelet production.

There are various assays for measuring antiplatelet antibodies. Looking for the presence of platelet-associated IgG is of no value since this is found in non-immune as well as immune thrombocytopenia. More sophisticated assays, such as the monoclonal antibody-specific immobilization of platelet antigens (MAIPA) assay, has greater specificity (90%) albeit with low sensitivity (50–65%). Using MAIPA, platelet-associated IgG and antigen capture assays, several platelet antigens have been characterized. These include GPIIb/IIIa ($\alpha_{IIb}\beta_3$, the fibrinogen receptor) and GPIb/IX (the von Willebrand receptor), which appear to be the most frequently involved. Less commonly, GPIa/IIa, GPIV and GPV are involved. Recent reports suggest that around 40% of autoantibodies are reactive to both GPIIb/IIIa and GPIb/IX. In terms of disease chronicity, GP-specific autoantibodies may be important in the pathogenesis of chronic ITP; from available data GPIIb/IIIa appears to play a major role in the development of chronic ITP in 30–40% of cases.

Which platelet epitopes are involved?

Research has shown that the 33-kDa chymotryptic core fragment of GPIIIa is a frequent target of the autoantibodies. Fujisawa and colleagues, using synthetic peptides corresponding to GPIIIa sequences, showed that in 5 of 13 sera from patients with chronic ITP, binding was to residues 721–744 or 742–762, corresponding to the carboxy-terminal of GPIIIa. Recently, Nieswandt and colleagues have examined the pathogenic effects of IgG monoclonal antibodies of different IgG subclasses against murine GPIIb/IIIa, GPIbα, GPIb/IX, GPV and CD31. Their findings suggest that, at least in mice, the antigenic specificity of the antiplatelet antibodies determines the pathogenic effects rather than the IgG subclass. They also demonstrated that antibodies against GPIb/IX caused thrombocytopenia through an Fc-independent mechanism, while that from autoantibodies against GPIIb/IIIa involved the Fc system.

So far we have focused our attention on the B cells in ITP. However, at the T-cell level, it has been demonstrated that T cells from patients with chronic ITP will proliferate in vitro to disulphide-reduced GPIIb/IIIa or the molecule's tryptic peptides. This suggested that autoreactive CD4$^+$ Th cells in chronic ITP need to recognize a modified GPIIb/IIIa molecule, implying that antigen-processing mechanisms within recipient antigen-presenting cells may be required to present GPIIb/IIIa autoantigens in the context of self HLA-DR molecules. Subsequently, mapping studies using six large (200 amino acids) recombinant fragments encoding different portions of the GPIIbα and GPIIIa chains showed that the T cells from patients with ITP recognized primarily the amino-terminal portion of the two GP chains (GPIIbα 18–259 and GPIIIa 22–262) and that these molecules also stimulated the production of antiplatelet autoantibodies. Ultimately, the GPIIIa molecule has been mapped for CD4$^+$ T-cell specificities by using 15-mer peptides of the GPIIIa chain and this has revealed several immunodominant peptides spanning the entire breadth of the molecule.

The role of *Helicobacter pylori* in the development of ITP

This Gram-negative microaerophilic bacterium is the main cause of gastritis and peptic ulcer disease. It has also been implicated in the development of gastric adenocarcinoma and mucosa-associated lymphoid tumours, and in some autoimmune disorders. A number of studies have shown improvement in platelet counts in ITP patients positive for *H. pylori* following eradication of the bacterium. However, the data from different studies are conflicting, with some centres showing a very high rate of response to eradication while others have a low rate. Further support for the involvement of *H. pylori* in ITP comes from studies which have shown that there is a reduction in the level of antiplatelet antibodies in plasma following eradication of the bacterium.

How *H. pylori* may initiate or perpetuate ITP is not known. Possibilities include molecular mimicry, where there is cross-reactivity between the antibody, bacterium and platelet antigens. The bacterial protein Cag-A may be the target antigen and research has shown that there is molecular mimicry between Cag-A and platelet-associated antibodies. Further evidence of involvement of bacterial antigens and ITP comes from the work of Semple and colleagues who showed that, in the presence of platelet autoantibodies, the lipopolysaccharide of Gram-negative bacteria can enhance platelet phagocytosis. Although the role of *H. pylori* is not fully elucidated, it is worth screening patients with ITP for the presence of the bacterium and eradicating with standard triple therapy to see whether the patient's platelet count responds.

In paediatric ITP, the underlying cause of thrombocytopenia is most likely molecular mimicry or immune complex deposition. In a typical case of molecular mimicry, the child generally suffers a trivial viral illness or receives an immunization. The antibody against the virus, by chance, recognizes an epitope on the platelet. This results in platelet opsonization followed by platelet destruction. An alternative mechanism involving immune complex formation occurs when immune complexes between antibody and viral antigen are adsorbed onto the platelet surface leading to the premature removal of the platelet. Immune complexes are transient phenomena and as far as we are aware do not cause ongoing platelet destruction.

T cells may also be involved

The role of T cells in the development of ITP is becoming clearer. That T cells are involved has been known for some time, since the autoantibodies in ITP are predominantly of the IgG subclass, and isotype switching from IgM to IgG requires T-cell help. However, some 40% of patients with chronic ITP have no detectible autoantibodies yet are thrombocytopenic and appear to have true ITP. CD8[+] T cells have been linked to the pathogenesis of many autoimmune diseases such as type 1 diabetes,

and recently it was shown that ITP patients have a direct CD8[+] T cell-mediated cytotoxicity that induces platelet destruction. At present, however, it is unknown whether cell-mediated platelet destruction contributes to the severity of disease or to the difficulty of treatment in some patients with ITP. However, recent studies by Wadenvik's group in Sweden suggests that in some patients with ITP, T cells may interact directly with platelets inducing platelet lysis (Figure 49.2).

Thrombopoietin levels in ITP

Since thrombopoietin (TPO) is the principal growth factor involved in platelet production, it might be expected that TPO levels would be raised in patients with ITP. Plasma TPO levels are undoubtedly elevated in patients with aplastic anaemia, chemotherapy-induced thrombocytopenia and other marrow failure syndromes. However, in ITP, levels of TPO are normal or only modestly elevated (Figure 49.3). The reason for this has been poorly understood until fairly recently.

The liver produces TPO at a constant rate and this binds to TPO receptors on platelets and megakaryocytes. The free (unbound) TPO is able to stimulate the bone marrow to generate sufficient platelets to counterbalance the natural daily platelet losses through platelet senescence. The key here appears to be the free TPO component. The greater this level, the more the bone marrow is driven to produce increased numbers of platelets. If the megakaryocyte mass and platelet numbers are increased, such as in ITP, TPO is bound to the receptors on these cells, leaving little free TPO to stimulate the bone marrow

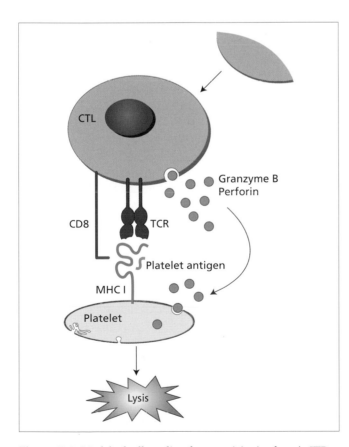

Figure 49.2 Model of cell-mediated cytotoxicity in chronic ITP. In the case of chronic ITP in the active phase, cytotoxic lymphocytes release toxic contents, such as granzyme B and perforin, and platelet lysis occurs.

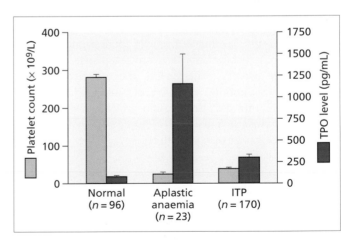

Figure 49.3 In normal individuals serum thrombopoietin (TPO) levels are low. In aplastic states, due to the absence of megakaryocytes and platelets (which bind TPO), TPO levels are high. In patients with ITP, the platelet count is low and TPO levels are normal or modestly elevated. This is believed to be due to absorption of free TPO by the increased megakaryocyte and platelet mass which is found in ITP. (From Nichol 1998 with permission.)

Table 49.2 Potential causes of thrombocytopenia in ITP.

Autoantibody opsonization of platelets leading to destruction by
  the reticuloendothelial system
Autoantibody opsonization of megakaryocytes, with inhibition of
  megakaryocyte growth, differentiation and platelet release
Autoantibody-induced megakaryocyte apoptosis
Relative thrombopoietin deficiency
Molecular mimicry and immune complex formation
T-cell direct lysis of platelets

Table 49.3 Investigation of suspected ITP.

Basic evaluation of ITP
Patient history
Family history
Physical examination
Full blood count
Peripheral blood film
Blood group (Rh) and reticulocyte count
Direct antiglobulin test
Quantitative immunoglobulin measurement
Bone marrow examination*

Helicobacter pylori
HIV
HCV

Tests that may be useful in selected cases
Antiphospholipid antibody (including anticardiolipin and lupus
  anticoagulant)
Antithyroid antibody and thyroid function
Pregnancy test
Antinuclear antibodies
Viral PCR for parvovirus and cytomegalovirus

Tests of unproven or uncertain benefit
Glycoprotein-specific antibody
Thrombopoietin assay
Reticulated platelet count
Indirect platelet-associated IgG
Bleeding time
Platelet survival study
Serum complement levels

*The need for bone marrow remains contentious and the
indications for performing this test are discussed in Table 49.4.

in patients with ITP. There is therefore a relative lack of TPO in patients with ITP, which compounds the platelet losses that occur through increased destruction of platelets by the reticuloendothelial system.

In summary, ITP is much more complex than originally believed, with several mechanisms leading to thrombocytopenia (Table 49.2).

Natural history of ITP

This has not been systematically studied. It is not clear which patients require treatment, whether treatment has any major beneficial effect on the patient, whether patients live longer, or whether treatment alters the natural history of the disease. For the majority of patients, ITP is a fairly minor disorder. Serious bleeding is not common and clinical sequelae of the disease are generally absent in patients with platelet counts above 30×10^9/L. There have been a few studies published looking at clinically relevant bleeding and platelet count. In normal individuals, there is a correlation between the platelet count and bleeding. The lower the platelet count, the more likely is bleeding. In ITP this is not the case, and most patients with ITP show little bleeding until the platelet count drops below 20×10^9/L. One study showed that no grade 4 bleeding occurred in patients with platelets greater than 10×10^9/L.

Diagnosis

Despite significant advances in our understanding of ITP, the diagnosis remains one of exclusion in both paediatric and adult ITP. A thorough history should be obtained, looking for diseases that might cause thrombocytopenia. The patient should be asked about bleeding during previous surgery or dentistry. The sites of bleeding should be determined. In children, the possibility of child abuse should be considered, although abused children will not generally have petechial haemorrhages or purpura, though they may have bruising.

A full physical examination should be normal apart from the expected clinical signs associated with thrombocytopenia. In addition to the 'dry purpura' of ITP, there should be an examination of the mucous membranes, including the mouth, and optic fundi looking for the presence of retinal haemorrhage. Enlargement of the liver, spleen or lymph nodes suggests an alternative diagnosis.

The laboratory investigation of ITP is straightforward. The FBC should confirm the isolated thrombocytopenia. There may be a degree of iron deficiency anaemia but this should be in proportion to the clinical history. There should be no abnormal white blood cells or red cell fragments in ITP. If the latter are found, the underlying diagnosis may be thrombotic thrombocytopenic purpura, a disorder that is far more serious than ITP and which requires urgent treatment. Table 49.3 outlines the most useful tests in the diagnosis of ITP, along with other tests that are either of limited value or no value.

Bone marrow examination

Previously, one of the mainstays of diagnosis was assessment of the bone marrow. The rationale behind this was the possibility of a patient having a marrow disorder such as leukaemia, lymphoma or infiltration. It was believed that detection of these by performing a bone marrow aspirate and trephine biopsy would aid diagnosis and management. However, studies to date have shown quite clearly that in patients with isolated thrombocytopenia, and with no atypical symptoms or signs, no cases of bone marrow pathology were detected. For this reason, recent guidelines do not recommend performing a bone marrow examination in such individuals. If patients fail to respond to, or relapse following, first-line treatment, then a bone marrow examination should be carried out. Similarly, if there is any hepatomegaly, splenomegaly, lymphadenopathy or any clinical or laboratory feature suggesting the presence of a disease other than ITP, a bone marrow examination should be performed. Bone marrow examination should also be performed if the patient is above the age of 60 years, since myelodysplasia becomes more likely, and myelodysplastic syndrome may resemble ITP. Finally, a bone marrow examination should possibly be carried out if splenectomy is being contemplated (Table 49.4), but in patients who have previously responded well to first-line therapies this test is probably unnecessary.

Cytologically, the bone marrow in ITP generally shows normal development and maturation of all cell lines. Megakaryocyte numbers are typically normal or increased. Increased numbers of small megakaryocytes may be a feature, suggesting increased proliferation of megakaryocytes required to compensate for the peripheral blood thrombocytopenia. What has not been appreciated until very recently is that the megakaryocytes may not be producing platelets at a sufficient rate, possibly through inhibition of platelet formation or release caused by the autoantibodies. In addition, MacMillan and others have shown that the binding of the glycoprotein autoantibodies may have other profound effects on thrombopoiesis, including the induction of apoptosis of megakaryocytes. The thrombocytopenia in ITP may therefore be due to peripheral destruction of platelets and a failure of production.

Table 49.4 Indications for bone marrow examination in ITP.

Failure to respond to, or relapse following, first-line therapy
Presence of atypical clinical or laboratory features
Age > 60 years
Before splenectomy (but see text)

Management

Major haemorrhage is the most feared event in patients with ITP. Over the years, attempting to prevent this by treating all patients with a platelet count below 30×10^9/L has led to over-treatment. However, catastrophic bleeding is not commonly seen and the main aim of treatment today has shifted away from trying to normalize the platelet count towards finding a strategy that will allow the patient to achieve a 'safe' platelet count. What constitutes a safe platelet count will vary from patient to patient, and also each patient with ITP will have differing requirements throughout their disease history. For example, a young patient with platelet count of 20×10^9/L should be safe to work and carry out normal day-to-day activities but would not be deemed safe if he or she wished to ski or undergo surgery. The safe platelet count would therefore be higher during these haemostatic challenges. So the one-size-fits-all approach has failed to work over the years and has caused increased morbidity and mortality in patients due to the adverse effects associated with many of the treatments in current use. When considering ITP treatments, we need to separate these into two major approaches: short-term and long-term treatments. These are discussed later.

There are many current treatments for ITP, although most have not been approved (licensed) for this indication. Those that do have a licence for ITP include corticosteroids, intravenous immunoglobulin (IVIg) and intravenous anti-D. All the others, of which there are many, have been used for many years but they have never undergone formal study and are not specifically approved for ITP. Even those that are licensed have variable licences, where the drugs are available in some European countries but not others. TPO receptor agonists are available in the USA and Australia but have not been fully approved in many other countries including the European Union.

All current treatments are of relatively low efficacy when used alone (around 30%), and all treatments address solely platelet destruction. They do this through a variety of different mechanisms but the net result is immunosuppression. The original rationale behind this was that in order to reduce the degree of autoantibody production, platelet opsonization and destruction by the reticuloendothelial system, the entire immune response should be suppressed. To some extent this works, although the treatments are purely palliative and once the treatment stops the platelet count drops to baseline levels once again. The disadvantage of immunosuppression is that, as well as reducing the level of antiplatelet antibody or diminishing the effectiveness of the reticuloendothelial system, normal immunity is suppressed. This can lead to infections and other complications. One study from 2001 showed quite clearly that, of the patients with ITP who died, at least half succumbed to infection caused by the immunosuppressive agents.

Traditionally, treatments have been grouped into first line, second line, third line, and so on depending on the disease stage in which they are used. These terms are not particularly useful clinically but do provide a guide as to which treatments to use initially and which should be used later.

First-line therapies comprise corticosteroids, IVIg and anti-D. These three treatments work fairly quickly (within 24–48 hours) and their efficacy rates are high at around 70–80%. The disadvantage of these and most of the other treatments is that the platelet count generally drops once the treatment is stopped. These treatments are seldom curative, and must be considered palliative therapies. In addition, IVIg and anti-D are pooled blood products.

If patients fail to respond to first-line treatment they may then be given a second-line drug, such as azathioprine or mycophenolate mofetil. These agents are much slower-acting and the efficacy rates are much lower than with first-line therapies (Table 49.5). As with first-line drugs, second- and third-line treatments are palliative.

Splenectomy is a surgical second-line option for patients who have relapsed after treatment with a first-line drug, although many clinicians prefer to defer splenectomy until later in the disease course. The rationale behind splenectomy is that the spleen is generally the main site of platelet destruction (and probably autoantibody production), so that removing the spleen prolongs the lifespan of the platelets and the platelet count rises. Although considered 'curative', splenectomy does not in fact cure ITP. Usually the autoantibodies remain and continue to opsonize the platelets. However, the main organ of platelet destruction has been removed and hence this is a form of phenotypic 'cure'.

Table 49.5 Treatment options after first-line therapy.

Non-approved second-line treatments
Azathioprine
Dexamethasone
Methylprednisolone
Ciclosporin
Mycophenolate mofetil
Cyclophosphamide
Danazol
Dapsone
Vincristine
Rituximab

Surgical second-line treatment
Splenectomy

Approved second-line treatments
Romiplostim
Eltrombopag

Short-term treatment

This refers to treatments lasting 2 weeks or more, which can be used when patients have a sudden drop in their platelet count leading to an unacceptably low platelet count, or when patients face haemostatic challenges such as planned surgery or dentistry or other high-risk activity, where the main risk is excessive bleeding. Patients are generally started on treatment 1 or 2 weeks prior to the event, with regular monitoring of platelet counts. Providing the counts reach a satisfactory level, the surgery or other procedure is carried out and the treatment is stopped shortly afterwards. By about 2 weeks the platelet count will have drifted back to baseline levels. Table 49.6 shows the target platelet counts for the most common procedures.

Long-term treatment

This is required when patients have an unsupported platelet count that is too low for normal day-to-day activities. Generally, these patients will have failed other therapies or, if they responded to corticosteroids, they require unacceptably high doses to maintain a safe count. In this setting the aim is not to achieve a specific count but rather to move the platelet count into a 'safe' zone. This will vary from patient to patient. In general, once platelets exceed $15-20 \times 10^9$/L the risk of bleeding is low. Older individuals, or those with comorbidities or previous bleeding, will generally require a higher platelet count.

As we have already seen, most of the existing treatments used for long-term platelet control have known toxicities. The aim with long-term treatment is to use a treatment that has acceptable levels of toxicity but which achieves the desired platelet count.

Role of splenectomy for long-term control of the platelet count

Splenectomy has been used as a treatment for ITP for many years. The procedure increases the lifespan of antibody-coated platelets and may reduce antibody production. Responses are seen in about two-thirds of patients who achieve a normal platelet count, and the response is often sustained with no additional therapy for at least 5 years. Even patients who do not have a complete response may still expect a partial or transient

Table 49.6 Target platelet counts for procedures.

Procedure	Target platelet count
Dentistry (non-invasive)	Splenectomy
Dentistry (fillings, local anaesthesia)	$\geq 30 \times 10^9$/L
Minor surgery	$\geq 50 \times 10^9$/L
Major surgery	$\geq 80 \times 10^9$/L

increase in platelet count. Around 14% of patients do not respond and approximately 20% of responders will relapse months or years later.

Postoperative complications of splenectomy

In a recent systematic analysis, the complication rates of splenectomy were 12.9% with laparotomy and 9.6% with laparoscopic splenectomy. The mortality rate is 1.0% with the open laparotomy procedure and 0.2% with laparoscopy.

Venous thromboembolism (VTE) may occur following splenectomy, particularly if the platelet count rises to 1000×10^9/L or more. ITP itself carries a small increased risk of VTE, although the exact level of risk is not known, but there may be an additive VTE effect in patients with ITP who undergo splenectomy. ITP patients should be evaluated for this risk and appropriate thrombophylaxis should be provided.

Predicting the response to splenectomy

Clinicians have long sought possible predictors of response to splenectomy. Potential predictors have included response to oral corticosteroids, IVIg and others. Indium-labelled autologous platelet scanning appears to be the most sensitive predictor of response to splenectomy. However, indium scanning is not available in every hospital but is limited to only a few centres worldwide.

Prevention of infection after splenectomy

Splenectomized patients are at long-term risk for opportunistic post-splenectomy infection (OPSI) with encapsulated bacteria. OPSI is often rapidly progressive and has a poor outcome. The main organisms responsible for sepsis in splenectomized patients are pneumococci (50%), meningococci and *Haemophilus influenzae*.

In order to prevent OPSI, patients should be given prophylactic polyvalent pneumococcal vaccine at least 4 weeks prior to, or 2 weeks after, splenectomy with revaccination according to local guidelines. *H. influenzae* b and meningococcal C conjugate vaccinations should also be administered prior to splenectomy. Revaccination in susceptible individuals for *H. influenzae* should be administered according to local guidelines. Vaccination status should be recorded in the case notes. In patients who have received rituximab in the past 6 months, vaccinations may not be effective due to B-cell depletion.

In the UK the Chief Medical Officer advises the long-term use of oral antibiotics in the form of phenoxymethylpenicillin 250–500 mg twice daily, or equivalent, or erythromycin 500 mg twice daily if the patient is allergic to penicillin. However, the need for lifelong antibiotic prophylaxis remains unproven.

Patients with refractory ITP

The term 'refractory' has caused confusion over the years due to a lack of agreement about whether the term should be used only for patients who have failed splenectomy. The new Terminology Consensus document published in 2009 defines refractory ITP as that where the patient has undergone splenectomy which has failed or relapsed, and who has 'severe' ITP (clinically relevant bleeding) or a risk of bleeding. Some 20% or more of adult patients fall into this category. Clinically, patients with refractory ITP pose a major challenge since, by definition, they are resistant to many of the treatments in current use. They often have low platelet counts, in addition to bleeding that is difficult to control since the disease is unresponsive to conventional therapies.

Is drug treatment needed?

Many adults with chronic refractory ITP are able to tolerate severe thrombocytopenia (platelet count as low as 10×10^9/L) relatively well, with near-normal quality of life. For patients who fail to respond to standard therapies and who require treatment, a limited number of options are available. The risks of continuing therapy should be discussed and evaluated with the patient and compared with the benefits that treatment may provide. Patients should be assessed for other possible causes of their thrombocytopenia, including drug-induced, infection, inherited thrombocytopenia and myelodysplastic syndromes. Instead of receiving further ineffective treatments, many patients choose to live with lower platelet counts and, providing they remain free of bleeding, a watching brief can be kept. If any bleeding does occur, the patient can be treated with rescue therapy such as IVIg in combination with intravenous corticosteroids or cyclophosphamide, aimed at raising the platelet count rapidly.

Rituximab

This chimeric monoclonal antibody targets the CD20 antigen on B cells and is licensed for B-cell non-Hodgkin lymphoma. There have been several studies of its use in ITP and other autoimmune haematological disorders. However, there are no randomized controlled studies and the drug has not been approved for use in ITP. Nonetheless, rituximab does appear to be effective in ITP, even when patients have failed multiple therapies. The largest review of rituximab in ITP was conducted by Arnold and colleagues, whose data suggest that around 60% of patients will respond to rituximab and approximately 40% of all patients will achieve a complete response. The responses are bimodal, with an early phase within 1–2 weeks and a second peak at about 6–8 weeks. Response duration varies from 2 months in partial responders to 5 years or more in about 15–20% of initially treated patients.

There are safety concerns with rituximab. For example, it should be used with caution in any patient who has positive hepatitis B core antibody status since hepatitis B may be reactivated. Adverse events associated with rituximab are usually mild or moderate, with a low incidence of infections. However, B- and T-cell repertoires do not return to normal even when B-cell numbers have normalized. Severe infectious complications, including *Mycoplasma pneumoniae* and *Aspergillus niger*, echovirus, papovavirus and cytomegalovirus, have been reported. There are also reports of over 50 cases of progressive multifocal leucoencephalopathy (PML) associated with rituximab treatment in patients with lymphoma and connective tissue disorders. The use of cyclophosphamide, a potent immunosuppressant, appears to increase the risk of PML.

In terms of dosing, instead of using standard lymphoma doses (375 mg/m^2 weekly for 4 weeks), lower doses of rituximab (100 mg i.v. weekly for 4 weeks) have been shown to be equally effective. Finally, rituximab in combination with high-dose dexamethasone has recently been explored as a first-line treatment option, and appears to be highly effective in treatment-naive patients.

Combination chemotherapy

This form of treatment may be effective for some patients with chronic refractory ITP. Recently, Tao and colleagues investigated a combination comprising intravenous cyclophosphamide on days 1–5 or 7 and prednisone on days 1–7, combined with vincristine on day 1, and one of the following: azathioprine on days 1 to 5 or 7 or etoposide on days 1–7. The overall response rate in the 31 patients treated was 67.9%, including a complete response in 41.9%; the therapy was well tolerated. Other combinations, such as CHOP and COP, have been used. However, the toxicities and side-effects of these therapies make them unpopular with both clinicians and patients.

Other treatments that have been used with variable success include alemtuzumab, stem cell transplantation and interferon alfa. These modalities of treatment have low efficacy and high toxicities and are best avoided, unless they are used within a trial setting.

New treatments: TPO receptor agonists

Because of the relative lack of TPO seen in ITP, as discussed earlier, there is the potential to use exogenous TPO in order to stimulate the bone marrow to generate more platelets. Early experience with recombinant human TPO (rhTPO) and recombinant human megakaryocyte growth and development factor (rhMGDF) yielded mixed results. The drugs appeared to be effective in raising the platelet count, but cross-reacting antibodies to the drugs neutralized endogenous TPO, making patients more thrombocytopenic than before the drug was given. For this reason development of rhTPO and rhMGDF ceased. More recently, rather than develop TPO receptor agonist drugs based on endogenous TPO, where there would be significant sequence homology and the potential for neutraliz-

ing antibodies to develop, pharmaceutical companies decided to create drugs with no sequence homology to the native TPO protein. Two TPO receptor agonists are now approved in the USA: one is a peptibody called romiplostim, and the other, eltrombopag, is a small non-peptide molecule. Both have been studied in patients with ITP both before and after splenectomy. The efficacy rates are encouraging in all patients, and since they do not involve immunosuppression and are not corticosteroid-based, they appear to offer many advantages over the drugs in current use. These drugs are likely to be used in place of the non-approved and relatively ineffective standard ITP therapies for non-pregnant adults, since the drugs have not been licensed for ITP in pregnancy or childhood. Studies in the latter have recently been approved in a number of countries in the European Union.

ITP in children

Children with ITP are treated based on clinical bleeding, quality of life and not just platelet count. Severe bleeding is uncommon in children with ITP, even when the platelet count is very low (< 10 × 10^9/L). The incidence of intracranial haemorrhage (ICH) in children with ITP is around 0.1–0.5%. As with adult ITP, there is no method to predict which children will develop ICH, and this complication has been reported even in children receiving treatment for ITP. In general, however, ICH is commoner in patients with refractory or resistant disease than at initial presentation. Investigation of childhood ITP is similar to that in adults, although the incidence of *H. pylori* infection is much lower and there is no need to screen for this.

'Watch and wait' policy

Around 70% of children with acute ITP do not have significant bleeding symptoms and can be managed without drug therapy. Admission to hospital should be reserved for children with clinically significant bleeding, such as severe epistaxis or gastrointestinal or other bleeding. Most children with minor, mild or moderate symptoms can be safely managed in the outpatient setting. The emphasis is towards treating symptoms rather than platelet counts, since the platelet count is a surrogate marker and does not accurately predict clinical outcome.

General measures for persistent and chronic ITP in children

The management of children with persistent/refractory ITP is much the same as for newly diagnosed ITP. Many children stabilize with an adequate platelet count (> 20–30 × 10^9/L) and have no symptoms unless injured. In children who are less than 10 years of age at diagnosis, spontaneous remission is likely to occur, and expectant management can continue depending on the risk of bleeding and the degree of activity restriction of the child. The onset of menstruation may be problematic and can be managed with antifibrinolytic agents and the combined contraceptive pill.

The optimal management of chronic ITP in childhood is not known. Treatment should be tailored to each individual child and situation, and therapy should be effective and it should not carry more risk than the untreated condition.

Treatment options in childhood ITP

Children with severe bleeding symptoms should be treated. Treatment should also be considered in children with moderate bleeding or those at increased risk of bleeding.

First-line treatment in children

The majority of children require no medical treatment, and can be managed using a 'watch-and-wait' policy. If treatment is deemed to be required, options include IVIg, anti-D and corticosteroids. The other drugs used in adult ITP are not suitable for childhood disease due to their toxicities and long-term sequelae.

IVIg raises the platelet count in more than 80% of children and does so more rapidly than steroids or no therapy. Transient side-effects are seen in 75% of children. Intravenous anti-D immunoglobulin can be given to Rh(D)-positive children as a short infusion and is useful in the outpatient setting. Mild extravascular haemolysis is common, with a mean drop in haemoglobin of 1 g/dL. Like IVIg, anti-D is a pooled blood product but it is derived from a smaller donor pool. The safety profile of anti-D is good with no reported transmission of infection to date. However, there have been reports of severe intravascular haemolysis leading to disseminated intravascular coagulation, most of which have been fatal. Prednisolone at a dose of 1–2 mg/kg daily for a maximum of 14 days is effective in around 75% of children (platelet count $> 50 \times 10^9$/L) within 72 hours. More prolonged high-dose corticosteroid regimens are associated with increased toxicity. There are data to suggest that higher doses of prednisolone (4 mg/kg) for shorter courses may be more effective and associated with fewer side-effects.

ITP in pregnancy

Thrombocytopenia occurs in 5% of pregnancies, but most of these cases are gestational rather than immune-mediated. The diagnosis of ITP involves the exclusion of other causes of thrombocytopenia during pregnancy. Patient history, physical examination, blood count and blood film examination are used as in non-pregnant patients. The work-up of a pregnant patient with ITP is essentially the same as that of a non-pregnant patient. There are some conditions specific to pregnancy and these should be considered when investigating a pregnant patient with thrombocytopenia (Table 49.7).

Table 49.7 Causes of maternal thrombocytopenia in pregnancy.

Gestational thrombocytopenia
Pre-eclampsia, HELLP syndrome, disseminated intravascular coagulation
Folate deficiency
Massive obstetric haemorrhage
Acute fatty liver

HELLP, haemolysis, elevated liver enzymes, low platelets.

Table 49.8 Investigation of suspected ITP in pregnancy.

Coagulation screening (prothrombin time, PT)
Activated partial thromboplastin time (APTT)
Fibrinogen assay
Liver function tests including bilirubin, albumin, total protein, transferases, γ-glutamyl transferase and alkaline phosphatase
Antiphospholipid antibodies, including anticardiolipin antibodies and lupus anticoagulant
SLE serology
Review of the peripheral blood film
Reticulocyte count
Bone marrow examination: not required to make the diagnosis of ITP in pregnancy

Laboratory investigation of ITP in pregnancy

ITP in pregnancy, as with other types of ITP, is a diagnosis of exclusion. All investigations carried out in pregnancy are aimed at excluding conditions that may result in thrombocytopenia. Some disorders such as thrombotic thrombocytopenic purpura and HELLP syndromes require urgent diagnosis and treatment since the mortality rates are high (Table 49.8).

Management of ITP in pregnancy

There should be close collaboration between the obstetrician, haematologist, obstetric anaesthetist and neonatologist. Treatment is largely based on the risk of maternal haemorrhage. Throughout the first two trimesters, treatment is initiated when the patient is symptomatic and/or when platelet counts fall below 20×10^9/L, or when it is necessary to produce an increase in platelet count to a level considered safe for procedures such as obstetric delivery or epidural anaesthesia. Patients with platelet counts of $20–30 \times 10^9$/L or more do not require routine treatment.

Delivery

A platelet count above 50×10^9/L is generally acceptable for standard vaginal or Caesarean delivery. For epidural anaesthesia a platelet count of 75×10^9/L is required, although this is not evidence-based.

Treatment options in pregnancy

The primary treatment options for maternal ITP are similar to those of other adult ITP patients, namely corticosteroids and IVIg. There is limited evidence for the use of intravenous anti-D, splenectomy and azathioprine. Other agents, such as vinca alkaloids, rituximab, danazol and most immunosuppressive drugs (apart from azathioprine), should not be used in pregnancy because of possible teratogenicity.

Corticosteroids

These are the most cost-effective option. Prednisolone is initially given at a dose of 10–20 mg/day and may then be adjusted to the minimum dose that produces a haemostatically effective platelet count. At least 90% of the administered dose of prednisone is metabolized in the placenta by 11β-hydroxlase, but high doses may have an effect on the fetus.

Intravenous immunoglobulin

If prolonged high-dose steroid therapy is required or significant side-effects occur, or a rapid platelet increase is required, IVIg should be considered. The conventional doses of IVIg and likely response rates are similar to those seen in non-pregnant patients.

Options for maternal ITP refractory to first-line treatment

As with non-pregnant adults, combining first-line treatments in the refractory patient may be appropriate in the weeks prior to delivery. High-dose methylprednisolone (1000 mg), possibly in combination with IVIg or azathioprine, has been suggested as a treatment for pregnant patients refractory to oral corticosteroids or IVIg. Azathioprine has been used for many years in the post-transplant setting and this drug appears to be safe in pregnancy though the response is generally slow. Splenectomy in pregnancy is rarely required but if essential is best carried out in the second trimester.

Management of the neonate (of mothers with ITP)

ITP in the neonate (from mothers with ITP) accounts for 3% of all cases of thrombocytopenia at delivery. The fetal or neonatal platelet count cannot be reliably predicted from the maternal platelet count. After delivery, a cord blood platelet count should be determined in all cases. Intramuscular injections (such as vitamin K) in the fetus should be avoided until the platelet count is known. Those infants with subnormal counts should be observed clinically and haematologically as the platelet count tends to fall further to a nadir between days 2 and 5 after birth.

Selected bibliography

Megakaryopoiesis
Broudy VC, Kaushansky K (1998) Biology of thrombopoietin. *Current Opinion in Pediatrics* **10**: 60–4.

Kaushansky K (1994) The mpl ligand: molecular and cellular biology of the critical regulator of megakaryocyte development. *Stem Cells* **12** (Suppl. 1): 91–6.

Kaushansky K (1995) Thrombopoietin: basic biology, clinical promise. *International Journal of Hematology* **62**: 7–15.

Kaushansky K (1998) Thrombopoietin. *New England Journal of Medicine* **339**: 746–54.

Kaushansky K (2005) The molecular mechanisms that control thrombopoiesis. *Journal of Clinical Investigation* **115**: 3339–47.

Kaushansky K (2008) Historical review: megakaryopoiesis and thrombopoiesis. *Blood* **111**: 981–6.

Autoimmune disease
Bao W, Bussel JB, Heck S *et al.* (2010) Improved regulatory T cell activity in patients with chronic immune thrombocytopenia treated with thrombopoietic agents. *Blood* [Epub ahead of print].

Davidson A, Diamond B (2001) Autoimmune diseases. *New England Journal of Medicine* **345**: 340–50.

Kamradt T, Mitchison NA (2001) Tolerance and autoimmunity. *New England Journal of Medicine* **344**: 655–64.

Mackay IR (2000) Science, medicine, and the future: tolerance and autoimmunity. *British Medical Journal* **321**: 93–6.

Maloy KJ, Powrie F (2001) Regulatory T cells in the control of immune pathology. *Nature Immunology* **2**: 816–22.

Sarzotti M (1997) Immunologic tolerance. *Current Opinion in Hematology* **4**: 48–52.

Sinha AA, Lopez MT, McDevitt HO (1990) Autoimmune diseases: the failure of self tolerance. *Science* **248**: 1380–8.

Taneja V, David CS (2001) Lessons from animal models for human autoimmune diseases. *Nature Immunology* **2**: 781–4.

ITP general
British Committee for Standards in Haematology (2003) Guidelines for the investigation and management of idiopathic thrombocytopenic purpura in adults, children and in pregnancy. *British Journal of Haematology* **120**: 574–96.

Fujisawa K, Tani P, O'Toole TE, Ginsberg MH, McMillan R (1992) Different specificities of platelet-associated and plasma autoantibodies to platelet GPIIb-IIIa in patients with chronic immune thrombocytopenic purpura. *Blood* **79**: 1441–6.

Gernsheimer T (2008) Epidemiology and pathophysiology of immune thrombocytopenic purpura. *European Journal of Haematology Supplementum* **69**: 3–8.

Kuhne T, Michaels LA (2008) *Helicobacter pylori* in children with chronic idiopathic thrombocytopenic purpura: are the obstacles in the way typical in paediatric haematology? *Journal of Pediatric Hematology/Oncology* **30**: 2–3.

Nichol JL (1998) Endogenous TPO (eTPO) levels in health and disease: possible clues for therapeutic intervention. *Stem Cells* **16** (Suppl. 2): 165–75.

Nieswandt B, Bergmeier W, Rackebrandt K, Gessner JE, Zirngibl H (2000) Identification of critical antigen-specific mechanisms in the development of immune thrombocytopenic purpura in mice. *Blood* **96**: 2520–7.

Provan D, Chapel HM, Sewell WA, O'Shaughnessy D (2008) Prescribing intravenous immunoglobulin: summary of Department of Health guidelines. *British Medical Journal* **337**: a1831.

Rodeghiero F, Ruggeri M (2008) Is splenectomy still the gold standard for the treatment of chronic ITP? *American Journal of Hematology* **83**: 91.

Rodeghiero F, Stasi R, Gernsheimer T *et al.* (2009) Standardization of terminology, definitions and outcome criteria in immune thrombocytopenic purpura of adults and children: report from an international working group. *Blood* **113**: 2386–93.

Stasi R, Provan D (2004) Management of immune thrombocytopenic purpura in adults. *Mayo Clinic Proceedings* **79**: 504–22.

Stasi R, Provan D (2008) *Helicobacter pylori* and chronic ITP. *Hematology. American Society of Hematology Education Program* 206–11.

Stasi R, Sarpatwari A, Segal JB *et al.* (2009) Effects of eradication of *Helicobacter pylori* infection in patients with immune thrombocytopenic purpura: a systematic review. *Blood* **113**: 1231–40.

Toxicities of current treatment

Portielje JE, Westendorp RG, Kluin-Nelemans HC, Brand A (2001) Morbidity and mortality in adults with idiopathic thrombocytopenic purpura. *Blood* **97**: 2549–54.

Development of novel TPO receptor agonists

Bussel JB, Cheng G, Saleh MN *et al.* (2007) Eltrombopag for the treatment of chronic idiopathic thrombocytopenic purpura. *New England Journal of Medicine* **357**: 2237–47.

Bussel JB, Provan D, Shamsi T *et al.* (2009) Effect of eltrombopag on platelet counts and bleeding during treatment of chronic idiopathic thrombocytopenic purpura: a randomized, double-blind, placebo-controlled trial. *Lancet* **373**: 641–8.

Bussel JB, Kuter DJ, Pullarkat V, Lyons RM, Guo M, Nichol JL (2009) Safety and efficacy of long-term treatment with romiplostim in thrombocytopenic patients with chronic ITP. *Blood* **113**: 2161–71.

Cines DB, Yasothan U, Kirkpatrick P (2008) Romiplostim. *Nature Reviews. Drug Discovery* **7**: 887–8.

George JN, Mathias SD, Go RS *et al.* (2009) Improved quality of life for romiplostim-treated patients with chronic immune thrombocytopenic purpura: results from two randomized, placebo-controlled trials. *British Journal of Haematology* **144**: 409–15.

Kuter DJ (2007) New thrombopoietic growth factors. *Blood* **109**: 4607–16.

Kuter DJ, Bussel JB, Lyons RM *et al.* (2008) Efficacy of romiplostim in patients with chronic immune thrombocytopenic purpura: a double-blind randomized controlled trial. *Lancet* **371**: 395–403.

Newland A (2008) Emerging strategies to treat chronic immune thrombocytopenic purpura. *European Journal of Haematology Supplementum* **69**: 27–33.

Newland A, Caulier MT, Kappers-Klunne M *et al.* (2006) An open-label, unit dose-finding study of AMG 531, a novel thrombopoiesis-stimulating peptibody, in patients with immune thrombocytopenic purpura. *British Journal of Haematology* **135**: 547–53.

Provan D, Newland A (2003) Idiopathic thrombocytopenic purpura in adults. *Journal of Pediatric Hematology/Oncology* **25** (Suppl. 1): S34–S38.

Provan D, Butler T, Evangelista ML, Amadori S, Newland AC, Stasi R (2007) Activity and safety profile of low-dose rituximab for the treatment of autoimmune cytopenias in adults. *Haematologica* **92**: 1695–8.

Haematological aspects of systemic disease

50

Atul B Mehta[1] and A Victor Hoffbrand[2]

[1]Royal Free Hospital, University College London School of Medicine London, UK
[2]Royal Free and University College Medical School, Royal Free Hospital, London, UK

Anaemia of chronic disease

The anaemia of chronic disease (ACD) is a common normochromic or mildly hypochromic anaemia that occurs in patients with a systemic disease (Table 50.1). It is characterized by a reduced serum iron and iron-binding capacity, and normal or raised serum ferritin with adequate iron stores (Table 50.2). It is not due to marrow replacement by tumour, bleeding, haemolysis or haematinic deficiency, although these often complicate it.

Pathogenesis

The key factor in the pathogenesis of chronic anaemia in the setting of inflammation, infection and malignancy is an increased level of hepcidin. Hepcidin binds to ferroportin and the complex serves to prevent transmembrane iron transport. The body utilizes this mechanism to reduce the supply of iron

to microorganisms, but it also results in the reduction of iron absorption from the intestine and the sequestration of iron within macrophages, reducing supply of iron to developing erythrocytes. Additional mechanisms result from increased levels of inflammatory cytokines, including interleukin (IL)-1, IL-6, tumour necrosis factor (TNF) and transforming growth factor (TGF)-β. These interact with accessory marrow stromal cells and with the erythroid progenitors themselves to reduce their sensitivity to erythropoietin. In this way, the marrow is attempting to aid the recruitment of pluripotent stem cells to produce white blood cells in order to combat infection/inflammation and possibly malignancy. These inflammatory cytokines have also been shown to reduce the circulating level of erythropoietin. However, the deficiency in erythropoietin is relative: although the plasma erythropoietin level in ACD remains inversely correlated with the haemoglobin, compared with patients with other types of anaemia and normal renal function it is inappropriately low. The plasma levels of TNF-α, IL-1 (IL-1α and IL-1β) and IL-6 are raised. TNF and IL-1 have been shown in experimental systems to reduce erythropoietin production by cultured hepatoma cells. In addition, IL-1α inhibits erythropoietin production by isolated serum-free perfused kidneys. A mild decrease in red cell lifespan occurs in

Postgraduate Haematology: 6th edition. Edited by A. Victor Hoffbrand, Daniel Catovsky, Edward G.D. Tuddenham, Anthony R. Green
© 2011 Blackwell Publishing Ltd.

Table 50.1 Conditions associated with anaemia of chronic disorders.

Chronic infections
Especially osteomyelitis, bacterial endocarditis, tuberculosis, abscesses, bronchiectasis, chronic urinary tract infections

Other chronic inflammatory disorders
Rheumatoid arthritis, juvenile rheumatoid arthritis, polymyalgia rheumatica, systemic lupus erythematosus, scleroderma, inflammatory bowel diseases, thrombophlebitis

Malignant diseases
Carcinoma (especially metastatic or associated with infection), lymphoma, myeloma

Others
Congestive heart failure, ischaemic heart disease, AIDS

Table 50.2 Haematological features of anaemia of chronic disease.

Haemoglobin	Not less than 9 g/dL
Mean corpuscular volume	Normal or mildly reduced (usually 77–82 fL)
Mean corpuscular haemoglobin	Usually normal; occasionally reduced
Serum iron	Reduced
Total iron-binding capacity (transferrin)	Reduced
Transferrin saturation	Mildly reduced
Serum ferritin	Normal or increased
Serum and urine hepcidin	Raised
C-reactive protein	Usually raised
Erythrocyte sedimentation rate	Usually raised

ACD but is at a level that could be compensated by a normal marrow. TNF has been shown to increase apoptosis in erythroid cells.

Inhibition of erythropoiesis

Both TNF and IL-1 inhibit erythropoiesis *in vitro* and it is likely that TNF increases apoptosis of bone marrow erythroid cells. Anaemia is observed in humans treated with TNF and in animals receiving either cytokine. The effect of IL-1 is probably mediated by interferon (IFN)-γ secreted by T lymphocytes, whereas TNF action is probably mediated by IFN-γ produced by marrow stromal cells. IL-6 and TGF-β may also have roles as mediators of ACD through inhibition of erythropoiesis.

Iron metabolism

A characteristic in ACD is the presence of a low serum iron with adequate reticuloendothelial iron stores, but with a reduction of iron granules in marrow erythroblasts. A fall in serum transferrin and a rise in serum ferritin occur as part of the acute-phase response. The fall in serum iron can occur as early as 24 hours after the onset of a systemic illness, and will persist during the course of a prolonged illness. The fall in serum iron results from an impaired flow of iron from cells (including intestinal mucosal cells, hepatocytes and macrophages) to plasma. This is due to increased secretion of hepcidin by hepatocytes in response to inflammation. Hepcidin inhibits release of iron from macrophages and iron absorption. Inflammation can cause a 100-fold increase in urinary hepcidin excretion. Microbial products may act on Kupffer cells to secrete IL-6, which then stimulates hepcidin secretion from hepatocytes. Low serum iron inhibits proliferation of microorganisms. Hepcidin secretion is also increased in iron overload. This seems unlikely to be due to a direct effect on hepatocytes. It is possible that iron in Kupffer cells or sinusoidal cells, like infection, stimulates production of cytokines, which act on hepatocytes.

In clinical specimens, there is a significant positive correlation between serum and urinary hepcidin and serum ferritin levels. The cytokines TNF, IL-1 and IFN-γ have all been shown to cause reduced serum iron and increased serum ferritin concentrations. The fall in serum iron is probably mainly, if not entirely, due to hepcidin. Anaemia usually reduces hepcidin secretion. In ACD, this effect is clearly abrogated by the effect of inflammation or malignancy increasing its secretion. Increased lactoferrin, occurring in response to inflammation and mediated by cytokines, competes with transferrin for iron and forms a complex that is taken up by macrophages in the liver and spleen. Increased intracellular apoferritin synthesis occurs in response to inflammation and malignancy and this too will bind iron. Both of these mechanisms reduce the amount of iron available for binding to serum transferrin.

Treatment

The severity of the anaemia correlates with the activity and severity of the underlying chronic disease. Successful therapy of this leads to a reduction in the levels of the mediator cytokines, increased erythropoietin production and reduced inhibition of erythropoiesis. Correction of the anaemia may take weeks or months. Pharmacological doses of recombinant erythropoietin have been used successfully to improve anaemia in patients with rheumatoid arthritis, cancer and myeloma. This observation suggests that inadequate erythropoietin production and its reduced action are more important than disturbed iron metabolism in the pathogenesis of ACD. It further suggests that the suppressive action of various cytokines can be overcome by use of pharmacological doses of erythropoietin. Iron therapy should be reserved for patients who have genuine iron deficiency.

Malignancy

Anaemia

Anaemia is the most frequent haematological abnormality in cancer patients and may be due to many causes (Table 50.3). ACD (see above) will affect almost all cancer patients at some stage of their illness. The degree of anaemia reflects the extent of the malignancy and may be worsened by the myelotoxic effects of chemotherapy. Plasma erythropoietin levels tend to be inappropriately low and therapy with recombinant erythropoietin can reduce transfusion requirements by improving the haemoglobin level in cancer patients undergoing chemotherapy.

Haemolysis

Warm antibody autoimmune haemolytic anaemia (AIHA) is most frequently found in association with the following malignant diseases: chronic lymphocytic leukaemia, Hodgkin disease and non-Hodgkin lymphoma. However, it has also been reported in association with solid tumours (e.g. carcinoma of the ovary). Cold-antibody AIHA is less common, but occurs in association with monoclonal cold agglutinins in chronic cold agglutinin disease, Waldenström macroglobulinaemia and myeloma.

Table 50.3 Causes of anaemia in cancer patients.

Type of anaemia	Associations
Anaemia of chronic disease	All neoplasms
Blood loss	Gastrointestinal neoplasms, gynaecological neoplasms
Haemolysis	
Immune	Ovarian carcinoma, lymphoma, others
Non-immune fragmentation syndrome	Mucin-secreting adenocarcinomas
Haemolysis: secondary to drugs	Mitomycin, ciclosporin, cisplatin
Pure red cell aplasia	Thymoma
Megaloblastic	Chemotherapy, folate deficiency, cobalamin deficiency (gastric carcinoma)
Leucoerythroblastic	Metastatic disease in bone marrow
Marrow hypoplasia	Chemotherapy/radiotherapy
Myelodysplasia	Chemotherapy/radiotherapy

Microangiopathic haemolytic anaemia (MAHA) with intravascular haemolysis may occur in association with disseminated carcinoma. An abrupt onset of anaemia and thrombocytopenia often occurs, with a leucoerythroblastic blood picture, reticulocytosis and red cell fragmentation. Renal failure may occur as a complication. Mucin-secreting adenocarcinomas (especially gastric), breast cancer and lung cancer are the most common underlying malignancies; in about one-third of patients with MAHA, it is the presenting feature of the tumour. Abnormal blood vessels may be within the tumour itself (or within metastatic tumour thrombi, especially in the lungs) or fibrin deposition may occur at other sites because of disseminated intravascular coagulation (DIC). Widely disseminated disease with bone marrow infiltration is almost always present and the outlook is poor. A syndrome resembling MAHA and idiopathic haemolytic–uraemic syndrome (HUS) has been reported with a number of chemotherapeutic agents and following allogeneic bone marrow transplantation. Principal among these is mitomycin, although cisplatin, carboplatin, bleomycin and ciclosporin have also been reported to be responsible. Immune complex deposition has been implicated in the pathogenesis.

Red cell aplasia

Acquired pure red cell aplasia is associated with a thymoma in approximately 50% of patients, although it complicates only approximately 5% of thymomas. Antibodies to erythroid precursors have been demonstrated in some patients, and removal of the thymoma (which is usually benign) leads to resolution of the anaemia in about half of those affected. Immunosuppressive therapy with cyclophosphamide, ciclosporin, steroids or plasma exchange may be helpful in patients who relapse. Red cell aplasia may also occur in a minority of patients with chronic lymphocytic leukaemia (CLL) or non-Hodgkin lymphoma and with large granular lymphocytic (LGL) leukaemia and as part of general marrow aplasia due to chemotherapy or radiotherapy.

Leucoerythroblastic anaemia

The blood film (Figure 50.1) shows the presence of erythroblasts and granulocyte precursors (e.g. myelocytes and myeloblasts). It is seen in primary myelofibrosis but is also frequent when there is marrow infiltration by tumour. This disturbs the marrow microvasculature and allows early release of the precursors. Marrow infiltration is most commonly observed in breast (Figure 50.2), prostate and haematological malignancies, but also in tumours of lung, thyroid, kidney and gastrointestinal tract and melanoma. It can also occur as a reflection of active bone marrow response to peripheral consumption (acute haemolysis, DIC, septicaemia, hypersplenism) or of extramedullary haemopoiesis (e.g. myelofibrosis or megaloblastic anaemia).

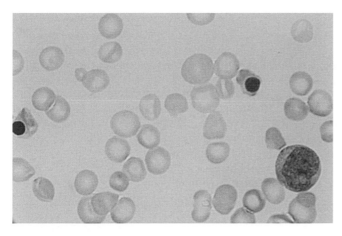

Figure 50.1 Nucleated red cells and an immature myeloid precursor in the peripheral blood film of a patient with a leucoerythroblastic anaemia.

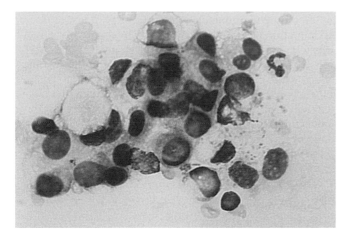

Figure 50.2 Bone marrow aspirate showing infiltration by metastatic breast carcinoma.

Other causes

Megaloblastic and dyserythropoietic anaemias are most commonly due to chemotherapy-induced disturbance of DNA synthesis within the bone marrow. Folate deficiency may also occur in patients with a poor diet and widespread disease. Cobalamin (vitamin B_{12}) deficiency due to underlying pernicious anaemia may complicate cancer of the stomach. Both chemotherapy and non-ionizing radiotherapy may lead to the development of myelodysplastic syndrome (MDS), which may progress to acute myeloid leukaemia (AML). Alkylating agents, especially melphalan and chlorambucil, nitrosoureas and epipodophyllotoxins in particular have been implicated, and there is evidence of a synergistic effect of these agents with small chronic doses of radiotherapy. The principal categories of patients affected are those who have received therapy for a haematological malignancy, but patients treated for non-haematological malignan-

cies (especially ovarian and gastrointestinal carcinoma) are also susceptible. The median latency prior to onset of MDS is 2–3 years and AML usually supervenes 6 months to 2 years later.

Treatment

Erythropoietin is effective in reversing anaemia in a proportion of patients with malignant disease, for example myeloma, lymphoproliferative disorders, MDS and carcinomas. It is recommended if the haemoglobin is less than 10 g/dL or in symptomatic patients with haemoglobin of 10–12 g/dL. Recombinant erythropoietin is not justified if the haemoglobin is above 12 g/dL as its use has been associated with an increased risk of thrombosis. The expression of both erythropoietin and its receptor is reported in a range of human tumours, including breast, prostate, colon, overy, uterine and head and neck squamous tumours. Caution is therefore advised in the use of recombinant erythropoietin to treat cancer-related and cancer treatment-related anaemia, and further studies are required. Dosage is 10 000 IU three times per week or 30 000 IU as a single weekly dose. The dose could be increased if there is no response (< 1 g/dL rise in 4 weeks).

Patients most likely to respond are those who have low pretreatment erythropoietin levels (< 100 mU/mL), well-preserved marrow function and normal/low levels of serum ferritin (< 400 ng/mL). A number of studies have demonstrated that erythropoietin therapy can lead to a reduced need for blood transfusion, better quality of life for patients and possibly improved overall outcome of anticancer therapy.

Polycythaemia

This is a rare complication of non-haematological malignancy. It usually arises through elaboration by tumour cells of erythropoietin and erythropoietin-like peptides. The tumours most commonly associated are renal cell carcinoma and hepatoma; others include uterine myoma, androgen-secreting ovarian tumours, phaeochromocytoma and cerebellar haemangioblastoma. Non-malignant conditions affecting these organs (e.g. renal cysts, viral hepatitis) may also rarely be associated.

White cells (Table 50.4)

Granulocytosis

Granulocytosis is a frequent manifestation of non-haematological malignancies. In part, the response is due to inflammation induced by the tumour. Interaction of tumour cells with host T lymphocytes and mononuclear phagocytic cells leads to the production of a range of cytokines, which induce white cell proliferation and differentiation. Tumour cells may also secrete specific agents that directly stimulate reactive proliferation. Cancer patients frequently have opportunistic infections, may bleed and are typically on a range of medications, all of which may influence the level of the white cell count.

943

Table 50.4 White cell changes in malignancy.

Neutrophils increased	Most, especially renal Hodgkin disease
Neutrophils decreased	Bone marrow infiltration Hypersplenism Treatment induced Chemotherapy/radiotherapy Large granular lymphocytic leukaemia
Basophils increased	Myeloproliferative disorders
Eosinophils increased	Hodgkin disease T-cell lymphomas Metastatic adenocarcinoma Other tumours (e.g. lung) Drug allergy Opportunistic infection
Monocytes increased	Carcinoma Hodgkin disease
Monocytes decreased	Treatment induced
Lymphocytes increased	Lymphoid malignancies Post splenectomy Opportunistic infection
Lymphocytes decreased	Treatment induced Radiotherapy/chemotherapy Lymphoma Opportunistic infection

Granulocytopenia

This is most frequently due to chemotherapy or radiotherapy but may also occur with widespread marrow infiltration, for example by lymphoma or due to LGL leukaemia.

Platelets

Thrombocytopenia (Table 50.5)

This may arise through decreased production or accelerated peripheral destruction and/or hypersplenism. The former may result from extensive marrow infiltration or be secondary to chemotherapy or radiotherapy. Hypersplenism is usually due to splenic infiltration by a haematological malignancy (e.g. lymphoma, CLL) but is rarely due to obstruction of the splenic or portal vein by hepatic and pancreatic malignancies. Increased destruction occurs with DIC. Immune thrombocytopenia may occur in association with haematological malignancy (CLL, lymphoma, MDS) and rarely may complicate solid tumours (e.g. breast, lung, ovary).

Table 50.5 Thrombocytopenia in patients with malignant disease.

Decreased production
Chemotherapy/radiotherapy
Marrow infiltration

Accelerated destruction
Hypersplenism
Disseminated intravascular coagulation
Drug-induced haemolytic–uraemic syndrome
Autoimmune thrombocytopenia

Thrombocytosis

A raised platelet count is frequently seen as a reactive phenomenon in patients with malignancy but is usually less than $1000 \times 10^9/L$ and is rarely of clinical significance.

Platelet function abnormalities

Impaired platelet function leading to excessive bleeding is primarily seen in myeloproliferative disorders (e.g. essential thrombocythaemia) and MDS. Paraproteins, especially IgM in Waldenström macroglobulinaemia and IgG in myeloma, are frequent causes of impaired platelet aggregation and adhesion. Increased platelet aggregation occurs in cancer patients when tumour cells release adenosine diphosphate (ADP), prostaglandins or thrombin. Increased platelet adhesiveness has also been reported, but is probably secondary to other coagulation changes.

Coagulation (Table 50.6)

A wide range of coagulation changes can occur in patients with malignant disease and can predispose to either haemorrhage or thrombosis. The distinction between activation of the coagulation part of the haemostatic pathway (i.e. DIC), which leads physiologically to activation of fibrinolysis (secondary fibrinolysis), and primary or direct activation of fibrinolysis may be difficult, and in some ways academic, in view of the intimate and dynamic relationship that exists between the coagulation and fibrinolytic pathways. These patients may also have other general medical problems, including infection; they may have undergone surgery, chemotherapy or radiotherapy and will typically be on a range of medications. All these factors may contribute to coagulation changes.

Disseminated intravascular coagulation

Chronic or compensated DIC is probably underdiagnosed in cancer patients. It occurs particularly in those with gastrointestinal, lung, pancreatic and breast neoplasms. Thrombosis, including migratory thrombophlebitis (Trousseau syndrome)

Table 50.6 Coagulation changes in malignancy.

Bleeding tendency
Disseminated intravascular coagulation, acute or chronic
Primary fibrinolysis
Acquired platelet function defect
Thrombocytopenia
Circulating anticoagulants/inhibitors

Treatment-related bleeding disorders
Thrombotic tendency
Venous stasis: bed rest, venous compression/invasion by tumours
Increased coagulation factors: FI, FV, FVII, FVIII, FIX, FXI
Decreased inhibitors of coagulation: low antithrombin, proteins
    C and S
Direct activation of coagulation by tumour cells: FVII, FX
Indirect activation: via trypsin release, mucin secretion,
    monocytes or endothelial damage
Increased platelet aggregability and adhesiveness
Thrombocytosis

Table 50.7 Circulating anticoagulants in malignancy.

Factor inhibitors
Factor V
Factor VII
Factor VIII

von Willebrand factor inhibitors
Paraproteinaemic disorders
Lymphoma
Myeloproliferative disorders
Chronic lymphocytic leukaemia

Others
Heparin-like anticoagulants: dysproteinaemias

and non-bacterial thrombotic endocarditis, is a more frequent manifestation of DIC than haemorrhage. In contrast, acute or uncompensated DIC is uncommon with solid tumours but occurs frequently with acute promyelocytic leukaemia (APL, FAB M3) and is associated with excessive bleeding. The triggering event in APL is likely to be release from the malignant promyelocytes of procoagulants and proteases, which may directly activate both coagulation and fibrinolysis. Tumour cells may activate coagulation by release of tissue factor (TF), which activates factor (F)VII. Direct activation of FX through the action of a cancer procoagulant has been reported in lung, kidney, colon and breast cancer. The sialic acid moiety of secreted mucin can directly activate FX, whereas the systemic release of trypsin in pancreatic tumours can also activate coagulation. Tumour cells may also activate the monocyte/macrophage system to produce procoagulant materials including TF and FX activators.

Primary fibrinolysis

This is less common as a cause of increased bleeding than DIC, but can occur, for example, in patients with prostatic cancer who undergo surgery. The release of proteases from leukaemic cells in both APL and monocytic leukaemia has been reported to induce fibrinolysis. Platelet counts tend to be higher than those seen in DIC, and fibrinogen levels are low, with raised fibrin degradation products (FDPs).

Acquired circulating anticoagulants (Table 50.7)

The most frequent is an acquired von Willebrand syndrome (both type 1 and type 2 disease) in patients with a paraprotein

or a B-lymphoid malignancy. A number of different mechanisms may operate. The paraprotein may be directed against an epitope within the FVIII–von Willebrand factor (VWF) molecule and inactivate it, or reduce its plasma half-life. Alternatively, immune complexes may form which bind non-specifically to FVIII–VWF and accelerate its clearance, or the malignant lymphoid cells may actually adsorb FVIII–VWF onto their surface. Paraproteins may also interfere with cross-linking of fibrin.

Treatment-induced bleeding disorders

Thrombocytopenia and MAHA may occur as a result of therapy (see below). Cancer patients with poor nutrition or who are on long-term antibiotics may develop vitamin K deficiency. L-Asparaginase induces defective hepatic protein synthesis and can lead not only to impaired production of coagulation factors but also to low levels of antithrombin, plasminogen and proteins S and C, and so give rise to thrombosis, most seriously of the cerebral veins. Mithramycin, which is used in the treatment of malignant hypercalcaemia, causes thrombocytopenia as well as platelet function defects, coagulation factor deficiencies and increased fibrinolytic activity.

Connective tissue disorders (Table 50.8)

Anaemia

ACD (see above) is the most common haematological abnormality seen in patients with rheumatoid arthritis (RA). Iron deficiency may coexist, particularly in patients taking non-steroidal anti-inflammatory agents. Folate deficiency may occur with severe disease and poor dietary intake. Warm-type AIHA with IgG and complement on the red cell surface is most frequently seen in systemic lupus erythematosus (SLE), although it can occur in the other connective tissue disorders, notably RA

Table 50.8 Haematological changes in connective tissue disorders.

Anaemia
Anaemia of chronic disease
Iron deficiency (drug-induced blood loss)
Folate deficiency
Sideroblastic anaemia
Pure red cell aplasia (PRCA), especially systemic lupus
   erythematosus (SLE)
Haemolytic anaemia: immune (especially SLE)/non-immune

White cells
Neutropenia (e.g. Felty syndrome)
Neutrophilia
Eosinophilia (e.g. Churg–Strauss syndrome, polyarteritis nodosa)

Platelets
Thrombocytopenia: immune/non-immune
Platelet dysfunction
Thrombotic thrombocytopenic purpura
Thrombocytosis

Pancytopenia
SLE

Coagulation
Lupus inhibitor
Specific factor deficiencies
Disseminated intravascular coagulation

Others
Myelofibrosis
Drug-related changes (e.g. aplastic anaemia due to gold,
   phenylbutazone; PRCA due to penicillamine)
Cryoglobulinaemia
Amyloidosis

and mixed connective tissue disorders. Sideroblastic anaemia has been reported in both SLE and RA, but MDS must be excluded. Pure red cell aplasia and dyserythropoietic anaemia with ineffective erythropoiesis are rare complications of SLE. Haemolysis can also occur as part of thrombotic thrombocytopenic purpura (TTP), complicating SLE.

White cells

The inflammatory process in connective tissue disorders can lead to a neutrophilia. Neutropenia is a feature of Felty syndrome, which is associated with splenomegaly in patients with RA. The pathogenesis is multifactorial and involves increased margination of neutrophils, sequestration of neutrophils within the enlarged spleen, and immune complex-mediated and humoral inhibition of granulopoiesis in the marrow. Antibodies

to mature neutrophils have also been reported in SLE. Lymphopenia occurs in both SLE and RA, and may be a measure of disease activity. Eosinophilia may be seen in SLE, RA, polyarteritis nodosa and Churg–Strauss syndrome. The pathogenesis is unknown, but presumably involves release of cytokines by T lymphocytes. Functional defects in polymorph and lymphocyte function have been reported in SLE and RA.

Platelets

Immune thrombocytopenia is a common manifestation of SLE and also occurs in mixed connective tissue disorders, scleroderma, RA and dermatomyositis. Autoantibodies to platelets may also impair platelet function. TTP is an association of SLE. Thrombocytosis is a non-specific reaction to inflammation and tissue damage in connective tissue disorders.

Coagulation

A wide diversity of coagulation changes may occur in patients with connective tissue disorders. In part, this may be due to liver and renal disease or to drug therapy. DIC has been reported in SLE patients who have high levels of circulating immune complexes and resulting angiopathy. The lupus anticoagulant (see Chapter 47) occurs as a complication in about 10% of patients with SLE and is associated with a thrombotic tendency, thrombocytopenia, recurrent miscarriages and pulmonary hypertension. Specific coagulation factor inhibitors encountered in patients with connective tissue disorders (especially SLE) include antibodies to VWF and to FVIII, FVII and fibrinogen.

Other changes

RA is one of the commonest causes of amyloidosis. An increased incidence of haematological malignancies (principally Hodgkin and non-Hodgkin lymphomas and B-lymphoproliferative disorders, including paraproteinaemias) has been noted in SLE, RA and, particularly, Sjögren syndrome. A wide range of haematological abnormalities also results from immunosuppressive therapy in these patients.

Renal disease (Table 50.9)

Anaemia

In acute renal failure, anaemia is commonly due to the drug or condition causing the renal failure, for example haemolysis due to sepsis or TTP. In chronic renal failure, anaemia is the most important haematological abnormality and its management has been revolutionized by the availability of recombinant human erythropoietin. Patients with acute or chronic renal failure

Table 50.9 Haematological changes in renal disease.

Anaemia
Failure of erythropoietin production
Haemolysis: haemolytic–uraemic syndrome (HUS), thrombotic
    thrombocytopenic purpura (TTP)
Iron deficiency
Folate deficiency
Hyperparathyroidism
Aluminium toxicity

Polycythaemia
Renal cell carcinoma
Other renal diseases (e.g. cysts, hydronephrosis, nephritic
    syndrome, renal transplantation)

Thrombocytopenia
HUS
TTP
Disseminated intravascular coagulation

Platelet function abnormalities
Abnormal aggregation to ADP, adrenaline, collagen
Decreased platelet adhesiveness
Reduced platelet factor 3 availability
Acquired storage pool defect
Abnormal prostaglandin metabolism
↑ Prostacylin
Defective platelet cyclooxygenase?

Coagulation
Hypocoagulability
↓ FXII, FXI, prothrombin
↓ FXII or inhibition
Hypercoagulopathy
↓ Protein C
↓ Antithrombin
↓ Fibrinolysis

develop a normochromic normocytic anaemia, with the presence of ecchinocytes (burr cells) in the blood film. The reticulocyte count is normal or slightly low, and the bone marrow shows normoblastic erythropoiesis without the erythroid hyperplasia expected at that level of anaemia. Patients who have undergone nephrectomy tend to be more severely anaemic than patients with polycystic disease. Reduced erythropoietin levels occur in renal failure and this is the dominant cause of anaemia.

An increase in serum creatinine above 133 μmol/L is associated with the loss of the normal inverse linear relation between plasma erythropoietin and haemoglobin concentration, but there is no direct correlation between reduction in glomerular filtration rate and impairment of renal erythropoietin production. Circulating inhibitors of erythropoiesis have also been

demonstrated. Chronic ambulatory peritoneal dialysis is more effective than haemodialysis in removing these inhibitors but, as recombinant erythropoietin can overcome these inhibitors, they are not of great clinical significance. Red cell survival is diminished in renal failure, but this is also a minor factor. Iron deficiency can arise through blood loss (exacerbated by haemodialysis). Folate deficiency arises in dialysed patients but is now prevented by prophylactic folic acid therapy. Renal failure is associated with elevated levels of 2,3-diphosphoglycerate and a right shift of the haemoglobin–oxygen dissociation curve.

Recombinant erythropoietin therapy can fully correct anaemia in renal failure. It can be administered intravenously, subcutaneously or intraperitoneally. The subcutaneous route is effective at lower doses, and it is usual to commence at 5–75 units/kg per week, given in two or three divided doses. Anaemia is corrected up to a level of 10–12 g/dL at a rate of 1 g/dL per month. Subclinical iron deficiency and impaired mobilization of storage iron are often present, so concomitant iron therapy is usually required. This can often be easily accomplished by the administration of intravenous iron, for example as iron dextran. An impaired response to recombinant erythropoietin should prompt a suspicion of iron, cobalamin or folate deficiency, haemolysis, infection, occult malignancy, aluminium toxicity or hyperparathyroidism. Hypertension occurs in about one-third of patients treated with recombinant erythropoietin and is dose dependent; the risk of thrombosis of an arteriovenous fistula is also increased.

The optimum dose of erythropoietin is one that restores the haemoglobin level to the normal or near-normal range and improves symptoms without increasing the risk of thrombosis; for most patients, this is approximately 12–12.5 g/dL and should not exceed 14 g/dL.

Polycythaemia

Secondary and inappropriate polycythaemia may result from either ectopic erythropoietin production by renal tumours or regional renal hypoxia (in benign disease and following renal transplantation), which disturbs physiological erythropoietin homeostasis. Up to 5% of patients with renal cell carcinoma have paraneoplastic polycythaemia.

Haemostatic abnormalities

Abnormal platelet function is probably due to the accumulation of toxic metabolites (e.g. guanidinosuccinic and phenolic acids). DDAVP (1-deamino-8-D-arginine vasopressin) therapy, which leads to the appearance of large multimers of VWF, can shorten the bleeding time in anaemic patients. Dysfibrinogenaemia has been reported rarely, whereas FDPs are often elevated and may prolong the thrombin time. Hypercoagulopathy with a predisposition to thrombosis can also occur, especially after recombinant erythropoietin therapy.

Haemodialysis with heparin anticoagulation can cause platelet activation. Fibrinolytic activity, antithrombin and protein C are all reduced in renal failure, and FV, FVII, FVIII:C and FX are increased. Thrombosis (particularly of the renal vein) is a particular feature of the nephrotic syndrome. Platelet hyperaggregability with increased plasma β-thromboglobulin is described and hypoalbuminaemia may enhance the synthesis of prostaglandins involved in platelet activation.

Endocrine disease (Table 50.10)

Both hyperthyroidism and hypothyroidism are associated with mild anaemia, which is usually normochromic and normocytic, but may be macrocytic in hypothyroidism. A raised mean corpuscular volume (MCV) can occur without anaemia in hypothyroidism, and low MCV has been described in thyro-

Table 50.10 Haematological changes in endocrine disease.

Red cells

Anaemia

Thyrotoxicosis (normochromic, normocytic or microcytic)

Hypothyroidism (normochromic, normocytic, occasionally macrocytic)

Diabetes mellitus (usually when complicated by infection, cardiac disease, renal failure, enteropathy)

Hyperparathyroidism (normochromic, normocytic)

Hypoadrenalism (normochromic, normocytic)

Hypogonadism (normochromic, normocytic)

Hypopituitarism (normochromic, normocytic)

Polycythaemia (pseudo)

Phaeochromocytoma

Cushing syndrome

White cells

Cushing syndrome: neutrophil leucocytosis

Phaeochromocytoma

Hyperthyroidism: lymphocytosis

Leucopenia: antithyroid drugs

Diabetes mellitus: impaired polymorph function

Platelets

Diabetes mellitus: abnormal platelet function

Hyperthyroidism

Coagulopathy

Diabetes mellitus: ↑ platelet aggregability, ↓ prostacyclin, ↑ FVIII, ↓ antithrombin

Estrogen therapy: ↑ FVIII, ↑ VWF

Cushing syndrome: ↑ FII, FIV, FIX, FXI, FXII

toxicosis. Thyroid hormones stimulate erythropoiesis, and tissue oxygen demands are increased in hyperthyroidism, whereas in hypothyroidism oxygen utilization is reduced. However, plasma volume is also increased and part of the anaemia in hypothyroidism is dilutional and/or due to defective iron utilization. Coexistent deficiencies of iron (due to menorrhagia or achlorhydria), folate and cobalamin must be excluded.

There is an increased incidence of pernicious anaemia in patients with hypothyroidism, hypoadrenalism and hypoparathyroidism. Antithyroid drugs (carbimazole, methimazole and propylthiouracil) can cause aplastic anaemia or agranulocytosis. Anaemia in patients with diabetes mellitus is usually due to complications of diabetes, although hyperglycaemia itself may lead to shortened red cell lifespan and decreased erythrocyte deformability. Polycythaemia (usually pseudo) can also occur with endocrine diseases. In anterior pituitary disease, androgen deficiency and adrenal insufficiency, a normochromic normocytic anaemia is common. Changes in leucocyte number and function are rarely of clinical significance, although many have been reported. Chemotaxis, phagocytosis and intracellular killing may all be disturbed in diabetes mellitus. Coagulation changes may contribute to a mild bleeding diathesis in hypothyroidism and to the thrombotic predisposition in diabetes mellitus.

Liver disease (Table 50.11)

Liver disease causes a greater range of haematological change than does disease in any other organ, with the exception of the bone marrow. The liver is an important source of erythropoietin in the fetus, and serves as a haemopoietic organ *in utero*; extramedullary haemopoiesis occurs within the adult liver only in pathological states (e.g. myelofibrosis, severe haemolysis or megaloblastic anaemia).

Anaemia

Anaemia occurs in up to 75% of patients with chronic liver disease. Portal hypertension often results in splenomegaly, which may cause haemodilution and pooling of red cells. Haemorrhage is a frequent complication, often due to oesophageal varices, and the red cell lifespan is shortened even in uncomplicated liver disease. Ferrokinetic studies suggest that the bone marrow response to anaemia is suboptimal, and many of the mechanisms that operate in ACD (see above) may be relevant. Macrocytosis occurs in approximately two-thirds of patients and erythropoiesis is macronormoblastic, indicating abnormal marrow function. Macrocytosis is particularly frequent in alcoholics, in whom reversible sideroblastic change may also occur. Target cells occur as the surface area of the cell increases, due to increased membrane lipid content without an increase in volume. Ecchinocytosis is fairly common because of

Table 50.11 Haematological changes in liver disease.

Red cells

Anaemia
Anaemia of chronic disease
Folate deficiency
Iron deficiency (blood loss)
Aplastic anaemia (viral hepatitis, rare)
Sideroblastic anaemia (alcohol)
Hypersplenism
Microangiopathy/disseminated intravascular coagulation (DIC) (rare)
Autoimmune (rare)
Zieve syndrome (rare)

Polycythaemia
Hepatocellular carcinoma (rare)
Infectious hepatitis (rare)

White cells

Neutrophilia
Infection
Haemorrhage
Malignancy
Haemolysis

Neutrophil function
Impaired chemotaxis (?due to lowered complement levels)

Neutropenia
Hypersplenism

Eosinophilia
Parasitic infestation
Chronic active hepatitis (rare)

Platelets

Thrombocytopenia
Hypersplenism, hepatic sequestration
DIC
Autoimmune (e.g. associated with viral hepatitis, primary biliary cirrhosis)
Post liver transplantation

Thrombocytosis
Hepatoma (rare)

Impaired platelet function
Inhibitory factors (including high-density lipoprotein and apolipoprotein E)

Other
Benign monoclonal gammopathy (biliary + other cirrhosis)
Cryoglobulinaemia (hepatitis B, hepatitis C, alcohol)

binding of the red cell membrane by abnormal high-density lipoproteins. In contrast, true acanthocytes are uncommon in uncomplicated liver disease, although they are a characteristic finding in 'spur-cell anaemia' (non-immune haemolytic anaemia in patients with alcoholic cirrhosis). Zieve syndrome, comprising haemolytic anaemia with hypertriglyceridaemia in patients with alcoholic liver disease, is also rare. Haemolysis due to the direct toxicity of copper ions on red cells is characteristically an early presentation of Wilson disease. Intracorpuscular changes are rare in liver disease. However, abnormal pyruvate kinase activity has been demonstrated in Zieve syndrome, and reduction of hepatocyte glucose-6-phosphate dehydrogenase (G6PD) levels in G6PD-deficient individuals, and in neonates, may exacerbate and prolong hyperbilirubinaemia with haemolysis. Viral hepatitis, including hepatitis A, B and C but most frequently hepatitis viruses yet to be fully characterized, may lead to a transient and mild pancytopenia or to severe aplastic anaemia.

Platelets and haemostasis

These are discussed in Chapter 39.

Liver transplantation

Orthotopic liver transplantation (OLT) is increasingly used for end-stage liver disease. Thrombocytopenia is frequently present prior to transplantation. The count tends to fall postoperatively despite platelet transfusions and this may be due to platelet sequestration in the transplanted liver. Immune thrombocytopenia has also been reported after OLT. Antibody-mediated haemolysis occurs in recipients of ABO-incompatible grafts, but the engrafted liver can also produce mild haemolysis due to anti-recipient ABO antibody. This is a form of humoral graft-versus-host disease (GVHD), but T cell-mediated GVHD has also been reported after OLT. Although aplastic anaemia is a rare complication of viral hepatitis, there are reports that it may occur in as many as 30% of patients transplanted for fulminant non-A, non-B viral hepatitis.

Infections (Tables 50.12 and 50.13)

Infection may produce a tremendous variety of haematological changes. Many of these are covered in other sections of this book.

Viruses

Anaemia
Haemolytic anaemia due to red cell autoantibody production, usually of the warm type, may occur, although cold-antibody syndromes have been reported in measles, influenza, infectious

Table 50.12 Haematological changes in viral infection.

Red cells

Anaemia

Autoimmune

  Measles

  Epstein–Barr virus (EBV)

  Hepatitis

  Cytomegalovirus (CMV)

  Human immunodeficiency virus (HIV)

  Others including herpesviruses, varicella, influenza

Non-immune

  Microangiopathic haemolytic anaemia

Reduced red cell production

  Marrow hypoplasia

  EBV (especially in X-linked lymphoproliferative syndrome)

  Hepatitis viruses

  HIV

  CMV (especially after renal or bone marrow transplantation)

  Others (rare) include togaviruses epidemic haemorrhagic fevers, dengue

Red cell aplasia

  Parvovirus B19, especially with haemolytic anaemia

White cells

Neutrophilia

  Especially HIV, influenza, hepatitis, rubella, adenoviruses, measles, mumps, CMV and EBV as part of nearly all viral infections

Neutropenia

  Aplasia (see above)

  Complicating myalgic encephalitis (?Enteroviruses, EBV)

Lymphocytosis

  Wide variety, especially early in course of infection

Malignant transformation

  HTLV-I, EBV, HIV

Platelets

Thrombocytosis (e.g. Kawasaki)

Thrombocytopenia

  Often history of viral prodrome in childhood immune thrombocytopenic purpura

  Autoimmune: EBV, hepatitis, rubella, CMV, HIV

  ↓ Production: aplasia (see above), measles, dengue, CMV, others

  ↑ Consumption: disseminated intravascular coagulation (DIC)/haemolytic–uraemic syndrome (see below)

Coagulation changes

DIC, especially varicella, vaccinia, rubella, arbovirus with/without microangiopathy, epidemic haemorrhagic fevers

Haemolytic–uraemic syndrome: coxsackievirus, mumps, echoviruses

Haemophagocytosis

Herpesviruses, adenoviruses, CMV

---

mononucleosis and mumps. Paroxysmal cold haemoglobinuria is rare and occurs in children due to Donath–Landsteiner IgG anti-P antibodies. Non-immune MAHA may be associated with TTP or DIC, which may be the result of viral infections.

Anaemia due to transient red cell aplasia is seen with parvovirus B19 infection in patients with haemolytic anaemias ('aplastic crisis'). This virus may also cause erythema infectiosum, or fifth disease, in children. It invades and destroys red cell progenitors and the aplasia is terminated when neutralizing IgM and IgG antibodies develop. If the virus attacks pregnant women, it may cross the placenta and cause spontaneous abortion or hydrops fetalis. Intravenous immunoglobulin therapy has been used for severe cases (e.g. in pregnancy, HIV infection and after bone marrow transplantation). Bone marrow aspirate shows characteristic giant erythroblasts.

Anaemia occurs with pancytopenia in virus-associated bone marrow aplasia, for example with hepatitis viruses. The presence of viruses, either within lymphocytes or on their cell surface, may lead to production of a range of cytokines (including TNF, IFN-α and IFN-γ), which inhibit haemopoietic cell proliferation *in vitro* and *in vivo*. This may cause a substantial reduction in erythropoiesis and is presumably the mechanism

underlying neutropenia and lymphopenia in viral infections. In infectious mononucleosis and other viral infections such as viral hepatitis, the virus infects B lymphocytes and the characteristic activated lymphocytes seen on the blood film are a reactive population of T cells.

Platelets

Thrombocytopenia may occur due to multiple mechanisms. Children with idiopathic thrombocytopenic purpura frequently give a history of a preceding viral illness, and autoantibody production is well described in infectious mononucleosis, rubella and cytomegalovirus infections. Reduction of bone marrow thrombopoiesis is frequently subclinical, but it is particularly important in virus-associated aplasia and dengue fever. Thrombocytosis can also occur in response to viral infections.

Bacterial, fungal and protozoal infections

Anaemia

ACD can occur in acute infections, overwhelming septicaemia and chronic or suppurative infection. Haemolytic anaemia is less common, but can occur through both immune (e.g. cold

Table 50.13 Haematological changes in bacterial, fungal and protozoal infections.

Anaemia

Anaemia of chronic disorders

Haemolytic

  Immune: *Mycoplasma*, malaria, syphilis (PCH), listeriosis

  Non-immune: *Clostridium perfringens* (toxin related),
    Bartonella bacilliformis (Oroya fever)

  Malaria/trypanosomiasis with microangiopathy/disseminated
    intravascular coagulation (DIC), septicaemia

  Haemolytic–uraemic syndrome: verotoxin-producing
    Escherichia coli and *Streptococcus pneumoniae*

Dilutional

  Splenomegaly (e.g. malaria, schistosomiasis)

Blood loss

  Helicobacter pylori, Ancylostoma

White cells

Neutrophilia

  Virtually any bacterial/fungal infection

Neutropenia

  Salmonella, Rickettsia, brucellosis, pertussis, disseminated
    tuberculosis (TB)

  Overwhelming septicaemia

Neutrophil function defects

  Rare (e.g. *Bacteroides*, endocarditis)

Lymphocytosis

  Whooping cough (*Bordetella pertussis*), *Rickettsia*

Lymphopenia

  TB, acute bacterial infections, brucellosis

Eosinophilia

  Aspergillosis, coccidioidomycosis, *Chlamydia*, streptococcal
    infections, *Ancylostoma*

Eosinopenia

  Common in acute *Bacteroides* infections

Monocytosis

  Subacute/chronic infections (e.g. disseminated TB, listeriosis)

Pancytopenia

  Bone marrow suppression (e.g. disseminated TB, listeriosis)

  Haemophagocytosis: septicaemia

  Peripheral destruction (e.g. DIC)

PCH, paroxysmal cold haemoglobinuria.

antibodies with anti-I specificity in *Mycoplasma* infection) and non-immune mechanisms. Direct red cell invasion frequently results in severe haemolysis in infections caused by *Bartonella baciliformis*, with elements of intravascular haemolysis (due to increased red cell fragility) and extravascular haemolysis. *Clostridium perfringens* produces an α-toxin (a lecithinase) and a θ-toxin, and *Staphylococcus aureus* an α-toxin, which act as

haemolysins to cause severe intravascular haemolysis. DIC and MAHA can occur in any severe bacterial, fungal or protozoal infection. HUS has been associated with a range of bacterial infections, including *Salmonella*, *Shigella* and *Campylobacter* spp., but most frequently with verotoxin-producing strains of *Escherichia coli*.

White cells

Neutrophilia is the most common manifestation. Circulating neutrophils constitute less than 5% of the total body pool, and the neutrophil response shows great individual variation, with no clear relationship to the severity of the infection. The term *leukaemoid reaction* is used to describe marked leucocytosis ($> 50 \times 10^9$/L), with circulating immature forms occurring in patients with non-leukaemic conditions, typically severe infection or haemolysis or with generalized malignancy. Such reactions are more common in children. Features that distinguish such a reactive leucocytosis from CML include the presence of toxic granulation, elevated leucocyte alkaline phosphatase, Döhle bodies, and the lack of twin peaks of neutrophils and myelocytes in the differential count. Neutropenia can also occur with virtually any bacterial infection, although it has been most frequently noted with *Salmonella*, *Rickettsia* and *Brucella*. Defects of neutrophil function may also occur.

Platelets

Thrombocytosis is frequent in patients with chronic infections, and during the convalescent phase of acute infections. Thrombocytopenia also occurs during severe bacterial or fungal infection, particularly where there is bloodstream invasion or in intensive care patients. Certain rickettsial infections (e.g. Rocky Mountain spotted fever) are almost always associated with thrombocytopenia. Accelerated platelet destruction is the most frequent mechanism and can arise through DIC or microangiopathy with platelet attachment to damaged endothelium. Immune destruction can also occur and circulating immune complexes may lead to thrombocytopenia. Decreased platelet production is a less common mechanism, but may occur (e.g. in disseminated tuberculosis). The inflammatory and procoagulant responses to infections are clearly related. TNF-α, IL-1α and IL-6 may activate coagulation and inhibit fibrinolysis, whereas thrombin may stimulate inflammatory pathways. In severe infection, the end result may be endovascular injury, DIC, multiorgan failure and death.

Haemostasis

DIC occurs frequently and may dominate the clinical picture in certain infections (e.g. bacterial meningitis). The acute-phase response that accompanies severe infection can lead to a rise in a range of coagulation factors, which may contribute to thrombotic manifestations. Suppurative thrombophlebitis, particularly in association with indwelling catheters, can occur in relation to both Gram-positive and Gram-negative infections.

In patients with systemic inflammation and organ failure due to acute infection, plasma protein C levels are reduced, and recombinant human activated protein C given as an intravenous infusion over 96 hours reduces the death rate but may be associated with increased risk of bleeding. Activated protein C promotes fibrinolysis and inhibits thrombosis and inflammation and reduces circulating levels of D-dimers and IL-6.

Malaria

Anaemia is the most prominent haematological manifestation of malarial infection. It is most marked with *Plasmodium falciparum*, which invades erythrocytes of all ages (*P. vivax* and *P. ovale* invade only reticulocytes, *P. malariae* only mature cells) and can give parasitaemia levels as high as 50%. Cellular disruption and haemoglobin digestion lead directly to haemolysis. Parasitized cells have an increased osmotic facility and lose deformability; they thereby become sequestered and destroyed within the spleen, which often becomes massively enlarged. Non-parasitized cells may then become sequestered within the spleen and a raised plasma volume contributes to the anaemia. In addition, malarial antigens may attach to non-parasitized red cells to give rise to a positive direct antiglobulin test and haemolysis via a complement-mediated immune response. Acute intravascular haemolysis with haemoglobinuria, often leading to renal failure ('blackwater fever'), occurs rarely in *P. falciparum* infection.

An inadequate bone marrow response to anaemia is seen with relative reticulocytopenia at times of active infection, with some recovery after effective therapy. TNF levels are typically elevated and ACD occurs. Leucocyte numbers may be slightly increased or normal, but leucopenia as a result of splenomegaly and impaired marrow function is characteristic. Eosinophilia is variable. Thrombocytopenia is seen in nearly 70% of *P. falciparum* infections and has multifactorial aetiology. Autoimmune mechanisms may operate as for red cells, splenic sequestration is a contributory factor, DIC (either acute as in blackwater fever, or low grade and chronic) is common, and ADP release from damaged red cells may lead to platelet activation and consumption.

Haemophagocytic lymphohistiocytosis (or haemophagocytic syndrome) (Table 50.14) (see also Chapters 10 and 17)

This may occur in association with a wide range of systemic illness including malignancies (e.g. lymphoma), infections (particularly viral, e.g. Epstein–Barr virus, HIV) and autoimmune diseases. It typically manifests as fever, splenomegaly and jaundice with cytopenias. It is particularly common in patients

Table 50.14 Conditions associated with reactive haemophagocytosis.

Infection
Viral (e.g. herpesviruses, adenoviruses, cytomegalovirus)
Bacterial, especially tuberculosis
Fungal

Tumours
Haematological
Others

Drugs
Phenytoin

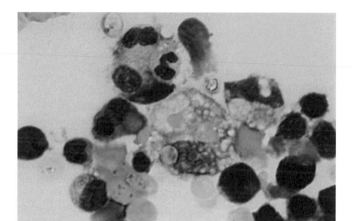

Figure 50.3 Bone marrow aspirate showing active haemophagocytosis, which in this patient antedated the development of high-grade non-Hodgkin lymphoma by 6 months.

who are immunosuppressed or who are acutely ill (e.g. septicaemic). A familial form is recognized (familial haemophagocytic lymphohistiocytosis; see Chapter 17) Macrophage activation syndrome is a variant form of haemophagocytic lymphohistiocytosis that occurs in children with juvenile RA. Pancytopenia is usual, although cytopenias affecting an individual cell lineage also occur, and coagulopathy due to associated DIC is frequently present. Abnormal liver function commonly coexists. The serum ferritin is usually markedly elevated. The bone marrow (Figure 50.3) shows the presence of increased numbers of histiocytes displaying haemophagocytosis. Myelofibrosis and/or marrow hypocellularity are present in a minority of cases. The underlying mechanisms are poorly understood. Excessive production of cytokines (e.g. IFN-γ and TNF-α) by dysregulated T cells has been demonstrated. In macrophage activation syndrome, increased levels of IL-6, IL-8, IL-12, IL-18 and macrophage inflammatory protein (MIP)-1α have also been reported. Treatment should be directed at the underlying disease process. Possible precipitating or complicating infection must be treated after appropriate cultures have been taken. Tuberculosis should be excluded. Immunosuppressive therapy (e.g. methylprednisolone) is appropriate if the condition occurs in the setting of an autoimmune condition. Anti-TNF antibody therapy has been successfully used in selected cases. Epstein–Barr virus-associated haemophagocytic lymphohistiocytosis may be indistinguishable from T-cell lymphoma and responds to chemotherapy, such as etoposide-containing regimens. The condition is usually of brief duration until recovery or, sometimes, death occurs.

Haematological aspects of pregnancy (Table 50.15)

Pregnancy poses a major physiological challenge to the human body and a number of haematological changes accompany it.

Table 50.15 Haematological changes during pregnancy.

Anaemia
Dilutional
Iron deficiency
Folic acid deficiency
Aplastic anaemia

White cells
Neutrophil leucocytosis

Platelets
Thrombocytopenia
Immune thrombocytopenic purpura
Eclampsia
Haemolytic–uraemic syndrome
Thrombotic thrombocytopenic purpura
HELLP syndrome (haemolysis, elevated liver enzymes, low platelet count)
Disseminated intravascular coagulation (DIC)
Drug induced

Coagulation
Coagulation factors: vitamin K-dependent factors FII, FVII, FIX, FXI, FX increased, FVIII increased, von Willebrand factor increased, fibrinogen increased
Coagulation inhibitors: protein C increased or no change, protein S decreased, antithrombin decreased or no change
Fibrinolytic activity decreased
DIC due to: abruptio placentae, intrauterine fetal death, amniotic fluid embolism, obstetric sepsis, eclampsia

Anaemia

Maternal plasma volume increases by approximately 50% during the first and second trimesters of pregnancy, whereas the corresponding increase in red cell mass is only 20–30%. A dilutional anaemia results, so that the lower limit of normal haemoglobin concentration is approximately 10.5 g/dL between 16 and 40 weeks of pregnancy. The increase in maternal red cell mass, transfer of iron to the fetus (which takes place largely in the third trimester) and blood loss during labour together impose a requirement of about 800 mg of iron, so that iron deficiency frequently arises in mothers with normal or reduced iron stores. Folic acid requirements are also raised during pregnancy (increased folate breakdown due to increased nucleic acid synthesis in mother and fetus) and routine supplementation is advised even during early pregnancy to prevent megaloblastic anaemia and neural tube defects in the fetus. A physiological rise in MCV of 5–10 fL occurs during normal pregnancy with pre-existing aplasia. AIHA occurring during pregnancy is typically severe and refractory to therapy.

White cells

A mild neutrophil leucocytosis with a left shift and occasional Döhle bodies occur during normal pregnancy.

Platelets

The normal range for the platelet count ($140–400 \times 10^9$/L) does not alter during pregnancy; thrombocytopenia occurring during pregnancy requires evaluation. Gestational thrombocytopenia complicates 8–10% of pregnancies and is characterized by mild thrombocytopenia occurring for the first time during pregnancy (platelets $80–150 \times 10^9$/L) and is usually not associated with neonatal thrombocytopenia or significant bleeding in the mother. Maternal immune thrombocytopenic purpura may antedate or present during pregnancy: it is often associated with increased levels of platelet-associated IgG, although this is a non-specific finding and the presence of serum platelet autoantibodies to platelet glycoproteins (GP)IIb/IIIa or GPIb/IX is more specific. The management of immune thrombocytopenic purpura is discussed in Chapter 49. Thrombocytopenia is regularly seen in pre-eclampsia. The mechanism is unknown, but increased aggregation is suggested, as low-dose aspirin therapy may reduce platelet consumption. TTP may occur at any time during pregnancy but typically it is before 24 weeks; the use of fresh-frozen plasma and plasma exchange has been shown to improve fetal outcome. HUS typically occurs within 48 hours of delivery in an otherwise normal pregnancy.

The potentially fatal syndrome of haemolysis, elevated liver enzymes and low platelets (HELLP) occurs in up to 10% of pregnancies complicated by eclampsia. The existence of coagulation abnormalities with red cell fragmentation suggests that microangiopathy, DIC and endothelial damage all have a role in its pathogenesis. Fetal and maternal outcomes are characteristically poor.

Basophilic stippling, crenated red cells and large platelets are characteristic peripheral blood findings in acute fatty liver of pregnancy.

Coagulation changes

Normal pregnancy is associated with a range of alterations to haemostatic components (see Table 50.15), which combine to give an increased risk of haemorrhage, thrombosis and DIC, occurring in up to 40% of patients with abruptio placentae, leading to haemorrhage and shock. Amniotic fluid embolism typically occurs during the course of a difficult delivery in a multiparous woman and rapidly leads to a picture of chronic low-grade DIC, with onset over a period of 1–2 weeks. Venous stasis resulting from the gravid uterus combines with the coagulation changes to make pregnancy a hypercoagulable state; operative delivery imposes an additional risk.

Haematological aspects of HIV infection (Table 50.16)

HIV infection and its treatment cause a range of haematological effects. The newer generation of treatments with highly active antiretroviral therapy (HAART) is changing the natural history of AIDS and increasingly turning it into a chronic disease. HAART is also less toxic, particularly to the marrow, than the treatments it has replaced in the developed world and the treatments that continue to be used to treat AIDS in the developing world.

Pathophysiology

The major mechanism by which HIV infection suppresses haemopoiesis is through the action of cytokines (e.g. IFN-γ, TNF-α). These are elaborated by activated lymphocytes in response to infection and have been shown to induce progenitor cell apoptosis and reduced growth of short-term marrow cultures. Direct infection of CD34 cells by HIV also occurs and cross-culture experiments have demonstrated that HIV infection impairs proliferation of CD34 cells from AIDS patients more than its effect on bone marrow stromal cells. Morphological evidence of ineffective myelopoiesis is seen in the marrow, with evidence of myelodysplasia in all three lineages. An increased number of plasma cells is also frequently observed.

Anaemia

This is the commonest abnormality, occurring in up to 80% of patients; it may be due to a range of factors (see Table 50.16).

Table 50.16 Haematological complications of HIV.

Pancytopenia, ineffective haemopoiesis, MDS
Anaemia
    Drugs: anti-HIV, supportive care (e.g. ganciclovir)
    Nutritional
    Bleeding/phlebotomy
    Anaemia of chronic disease
    Parvovirus
Thrombocytopenia
    Reduced platelet survival: antibodies, infection, splenomegaly, fever
    Reduced production: megakaryocyte differentiation reduced, CD34 reduction
Neutropenia: antibody mediated, drug induced
TTP/HUS/microangiopathy: usually treatment induced
Coagulation abnormalities
    Thrombosis
    Antiphospholipid antibodies plus anticardiolipin antibodies
    Protein S deficiency
Malignancy
    Lymphoma: non-Hodgkin/Burkitt-like, primary CNS, Hodgkin disease, others
    Myeloma
    Acute myeloid leukaemia

HUS, haemolytic–uraemic syndrome; MDS, myelodysplastic syndrome; TTP, thrombotic thrombocytopenic purpura.

HIV infection itself is a prominent cause of ACD. There is a reduction in erythropoiesis as a result of the mechanisms described above. Infiltration of the marrow by tumour, such as Hodgkin lymphoma, is much commoner among HIV-positive subjects than among the normal population. There is also a relative reduction in erythropoietin levels. Treatment of HIV infection by HAART will lead to an improvement in anaemia.

Other common causes include bleeding and infection. Certain infections, such as *Mycobacterium avium* and parvovirus B19, may directly involve the marrow and lead to decreased red cell production. Nutritional anaemia frequently arises from a defective diet and gastrointestinal disease (e.g. due to infection or drug toxicity) is common. Vitamin B_{12} defciency is seen in up to one-third of HIV-positive subjects and iron and folate deficiency are also common. Although treatment-induced anaemia is less common in the HAART era, treatment is a contributory factor in more than 50% of cases.

White cells

Leucopenia is frequently seen and predominantly due to lymphopenia. Neutropenia also occurs and is multifactorial. Granulocyte and monocyte production are reduced in HIV infection; drug-induced changes are common and autoimmune neutropenia also occurs. Granulocyte colony-stimulating factor has been successfully used to improve the neutrophil count in infected HIV-positive subjects. Defects in neutrophil and monocyte function have also been demonstrated.

Platelets

Thrombocytopenia is seen in up to 50% of HIV-infected patients. Reduced platelet production can occur for the reasons described above; however, it is usually due to increased platelet destruction. This is often antibody mediated (immune thrombocytopenia; see Chapter 49). HIV-specific antibodies have been shown to share a common epitope with antibodies against platelet GPIIb/IIIa. Non-specific absorption of immune complexes onto platelets also occurs and predisposes to immune thrombocytopenia. Reduced platelet production is common in HIV-positive subjects and direct infection of megakaryocytes by HIV has been described. Morphologically abnormal megakaryocytes are seen in the marrow. Other causes of thrombocytopenia include infection and microangiopathy. Both HUS and TTP are well described in the setting of HIV infection, particularly in the era before HAART. Treament of thrombocytopenia depends on the cause. Treatment of HIV infection using HAART frequently leads to improvement in the platelet count. Immune thrombocytopenia in HIV-infected subjects is treated in the same way as in the non-HIV population. However, immunosuppression carries particular risks and steroids should be used with extreme caution. Splenectomy is often effective, and anti-CD20 monoclonal antibody therapy may also be used.

Coagulation

Coagulation abnormalities can occur in the setting of infection and acute illness. Circulating coagulation inhibitors have also been described. Protein S deficiency is well described and predisposes to an increased risk of thrombosis. DIC is common in the setting of infection and HIV infection.

Other changes

Lymphoma is the commonest tumour in HIV-positive subjects (Chapter 35). Other haematological malignancies are also reported to occur with increased frequency, for example myeloma and AML. HIV-positive subjects who develop these malignancies often display a prolonged premalignant phase, with smouldering myeloma and myelodysplasia frequently reported.

Selected bibliography

Bernard GR, Vincent JL, Laterre P *et al.* (2001) Efficacy and safety of recombinant human activated protein C for severe sepsis. *New England Journal of Medicine* **344**: 699–709.

Bohlius J, Wilson J, Seidenfeld J *et al.* (2006) Recombinant human erythropoietins and cancer patients: updated meta-analysis of 57 studies including 9353 patients. *Journal of the National Cancer Institute* **98**: 708–14.

Dallalio G, Fleury T, Neans RT (2003) Serum hepicidin in clinical specimens. *British Journal of Haematology* **122**: 996–1000.

Ganz T (2003) Hepicidin, a key regulator of iron metabolism and mediation of anaemia of inflammation. *Blood* **102**: 783–8.

Guan X, Chen L (2008) Role of erythropoietin in cancer related anaemia: a double-edged sword? *Journal of International Medical Research* **36**: 1–8.

Ludwig H, Rai KR, Blade J *et al.* (2002) Management of disease related anaemia in patients with multiple myeloma or chronic lymphocytic leukaemia: epoietin treatment recommendations. *Haematology Journal* **3**: 121–30.

McRae KR, Samuels P, Schreiber AD (1992) Pregnancy associated thrombocytopenia: pathogenesis and management. *Blood* **80**: 2697–714.

Malaria Working Party of the General Haematology Task Force of British Committee for Standards in Haematology (1997) The laboratory diagnosis of malaria. *Clinical and Laboratory Haematology* **19**: 165–70.

Nemeth E, Valore EV, Territo M *et al.* (2003) Hepicidin, a putative mediator of anaemia of inflammation, is a type II acute phase protein. *Blood* **101**: 2461–3.

Papadaki HA, Kritkos HD, Valatas V *et al.* (2002) Anemia of chronic disease in rheumatoid arthritis is associated with increased apoptosis of bone marrow erythroid cells: improvement following anti-tumour necrosis factor-α therapy. *Blood* **100**: 474–82.

Sloand E (2005) Hematologic complications of HIV infection. *AIDS Reviews* **7**: 187–96.

Weiss G, Goodnough LT (2005) Anemia of chronic disease. *New England Journal of Medicine* **352**: 1011–23.

Haematological aspects of tropical diseases

51

Imelda Bates[1] and Ivy Ekem[2]

[1]Liverpool School of Tropical Medicine, Liverpool, UK
[2]University of Ghana Medical School, Accra, Ghana

Introduction

For the purposes of this chapter, 'tropical diseases' refers to infectious diseases occurring predominantly in tropical areas. The chapter has been divided into two sections, covering tropical diseases in which organisms can be visualized in the blood or bone marrow and those that cause secondary haematological abnormalities.

Around the world, 1 in 35 people (i.e. 2.9% of the population) are migrants, moving mostly from poorer to richer countries. In the UK, net international migration contributed to 68% of the population growth in 2005 and travelling migrants are responsible for a major component of imported tropical infections. Rapid increases in worldwide travel mean that haematologists need to know about the tropical diseases that can cause haematological abnormalities and be able to take relevant travel histories from patients. They also need to be aware of ethnic variations in reference ranges to avoid wasting resources on unnecessary investigations and to avoid causing undue anxiety for the patient.

Ethnic variations in reference ranges

The white blood cell count and relative and absolute neutrophil counts are lower in black people, Yemenite Jews, Palestinians

Postgraduate Haematology: 6th edition. Edited by A. Victor Hoffbrand, Daniel Catovsky, Edward G.D. Tuddenham, Anthony R. Green
© 2011 Blackwell Publishing Ltd.

and Saudi Arabians than in white people. After the age of 1 year, Africans have lower counts than West Indians or black Americans (Table 51.1). This is due to the non-white populations having a greater number of neutrophils in the storage pool. Stimulation of a neutrophil response in these ethnic groups leads to rises in the neutrophil count to the same level as white populations irrespective of the baseline level. Indian, Chinese and Southeast Asian populations have the same white blood cell and neutrophil counts as white northern Europeans. The platelet counts in healthy West Indians and Africans may be 10–20% lower than in Europeans living in the same environment. It is not clear whether there are true ethnic variations in eosinophil counts but counts of up to 2×10^9/L have been described in healthy blood donors in Africa. Interpretation of variations in blood counts should therefore take account of the individual's ethnic background.

Tropical diseases with organisms in peripheral blood or bone marrow

Malaria

Epidemiology and biology

Four species of plasmodia cause malaria in humans: *Plasmodium falciparum*, *P. vivax*, *P. ovale* and *P. malariae*. *Plasmodium falciparum* is by far the most dangerous and causes the greatest mortality and morbidity. Over 80% of *P. falciparum* infections in the UK are acquired in sub-Saharan Africa, while 85% of *P. vivax* infections are acquired in South Asia, especially India and Pakistan. In 2007, 1548 cases of malaria were reported in the

Table 51.1 Automated white cell (WBC) and neutrophil counts in adults of different ethnic origins (95% ranges).

	Male		Female	
	WBC ($\times 10^9$/L)	Neutrophil count ($\times 10^9$/L)	WBC ($\times 10^9$/L)	Neutrophil count ($\times 10^9$/L)
White	3.7–9.5	1.7–6.1	3.9–11.1	1.7–7.5
Afro-Caribbean	3.1–9.4	1.2–5.6	3.2–10.6	1.3–7.1
African	2.8–7.2	0.9–4.2	3.0–7.4	1.3–3.7

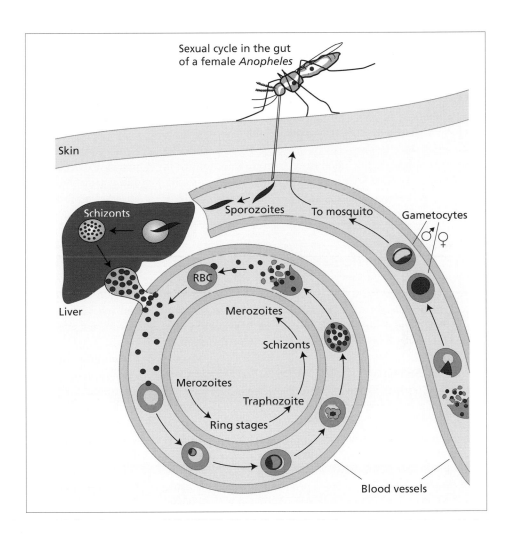

Figure 51.1 Life cycle of the malarial parasite.

UK, of which 1139 (73%) were due to *P. falciparum* and 256 (16%) to *P. vivax*; there were five deaths. Malaria rates were highest in immigrants returning from visits to their countries of origin and accounted for one-third of all reports. The majority of travellers (81%) had not taken malaria prevention tablets.

Malaria is transmitted by the bite of an infected female *Anopheles* mosquito. The infecting agent is the sporozoite and thousands of these spindle-shaped cells may be injected by a single bite. Infrequently, transmission may also occur through blood transfusion, bone marrow transplantation and transplacentally (0.5% of all UK cases). There have also been reports of

malaria transmission in aircraft or near airports in temperate zones due to infected mosquitoes being brought to non-malarious areas.

Within a few hours of an infected bite, the sporozoites enter the hepatocytes, where they divide (Figure 51.1). Rupture of the hepatocyte releases the parasites into the blood where they attach to red cell membranes using specific receptors. The parasites feed on the red cell stroma, and the digestion products form the characteristic brown pigment (haemozoin) that accumulates in phagocytic cells. In the red cells asexual replication of the trophozoites (ring forms) occurs, giving rise to erythrocyte schizonts. The schizonts mature into merozoites and are released into the circulation to reinfect other red cells. The periodicity of this release varies with the species and is responsible for the classical cyclical nature of malaria fevers. Relapses, which can occur months or years after the primary illness, are characteristic of infection with *P. vivax* and *P. ovale*, and are due to maturation of persistent hypnozoites in the liver.

A few of the trophozoites develop into male and female banana-shaped gametocytes and are taken up by the mosquito at a blood meal. Inside the midgut of the mosquito, they undergo sexual reproduction and sporozoites migrate to the salivary glands, ready to infect another host when the mosquito bites.

Unlike the schizonts of *P. vivax*, *P. ovale* and *P. malariae*, those of *P. falciparum* are not commonly seen in the peripheral blood of the human host. This is because *P. falciparum*-infected cells have surface cytoadherence molecules that enable them to be sequestered in the deep tissues. Therefore *P. falciparum* schizonts only appear in the blood in very severe infections or in splenectomized patients. Sequestration is responsible for some of the severe clinical consequences of *P. falciparum* malaria, such as cerebral malaria.

Clinical features

The time between the infected bite and the appearance of clinical symptoms and parasites in the peripheral blood varies between species. It is 7–30 days (mean 10 days) in *P. falciparum* but can be months, or even years, with other species, particularly *P. vivax* and *P. ovale*, because of their hypnozoite stage. The dormancy time of hypnozoites varies with the different strains.

Maximal immunity to malaria takes around 10 years to develop and is lost over the course of 1–5 years if the individual leaves a malarious area and is no longer exposed to infections. This is often not appreciated by students or immigrants from malaria-endemic countries, who are more prone to severe attacks of malaria when they return home after a prolonged period in a non-malarious area.

All four *Plasmodium* species produce factors that cause release of tissue cytokines, especially from leucocytes. These cytokines produce fever and contribute to anaemia through marrow suppression. Splenomegaly is a common feature of acute malaria and mild jaundice may also occur secondary to haemolysis. Other clinical features vary with different species.

Plasmodium falciparum

Plasmodium falciparum is the only species associated with complicated and severe disease. Death may occur after a single exposure to malaria, particularly in those with no immunity such as non-immune travellers or young children in endemic countries. Despite this, the majority of infections cause a self-limiting febrile illness. Recurrent fevers and other symptoms of malaria may be due to either recrudescence of blood forms that persist between attacks or to reinfection with a new strain or species. Recurrent attacks with different strains lead to the development of clinical immunity but not necessarily to complete clearance of parasites. Parasites may therefore be detected in a high proportion of adults in endemic areas who are clinically asymptomatic.

In addition to fever with rigors, nausea and hot and cold phases, *P. falciparum* infection can also present with diarrhoea and cough (Table 51.2). Serious complications include severe anaemia, cerebral involvement and failure of major organs such as kidneys and liver.

During pregnancy, immunity to malaria is reduced and parasite density increases. Even if parasites cannot be visualized in the peripheral blood, they may be sequestered in the placenta and compromise fetal development. *Plasmodium falciparum* is therefore an important cause of low birth weight in neonates and anaemia in pregnant women. Both of these factors have a detrimental effect on the later development of the infant.

Plasmodium malariae

The incubation period of *P. malariae* may be several weeks. It is associated with recurrent fever, anaemia and enlargement of the liver and spleen. Without treatment, recrudescences may occur with decreasing severity over many years. Clinical symptoms of malaria have been reported up to 30 years after the initial infection.

Plasmodium vivax *and* Plasmodium ovale

These species cause a similar clinical picture with bouts of fever occurring periodically up to 5 years after the initial infection. These are relapses, due to reinvasion of red cells by hypnozoites,

Target organ	Clinical features	Potential common misdiagnosis
Gastrointestinal	Diarrhoea, vomiting	Traveller's diarrhoea
Respiratory	Cough, pulmonary oedema	Pneumonia, cardiac failure
Neurological	Delirium, coma, convulsions, focal neurological signs	Encephalitis, meningoencephalitis
Renal	Oliguria, haemoglobinuria	Nephritis
Hepatic	Jaundice, hypoglycaemia	Hepatitis
Haematological	Anaemia, splenomegaly	Viral infection, lymphoma

Table 51.2 Clinical features of *P. falciparum* malaria infection.

rather than recrudescences, which are due to incomplete treatment of the primary infection. The trigger for hypnozoites to reactivate after dormancy is unknown.

Haematological abnormalities

Normochromic normocytic anaemia is common, particularly in children, but the degree and rapidity of onset are very variable. The haemoglobin may fall by up to 2 g/dL each day. In malaria-endemic regions, chronic anaemia due to nutritional deficiencies, intestinal helminths, HIV and haemoglobinopathies may be compounded by the effects of malaria. In chronically anaemic patients, the oxygen dissociation curve is shifted to the right so they are better able to tolerate further falls in haemoglobin. The clinical effects of anaemia in malaria are therefore due to a combination of the degree and rate of fall of haemoglobin.

The anaemia associated with malaria has multiple aetiologies. Red cells containing parasites are removed from the circulation by the reticuloendothelial system. There is also accelerated destruction of non-parasitized cells and dyserythropoiesis in the bone marrow. Both parasitized and non-parasitized red cells lose deformability and the high shear rates in the spleen enhance their removal by that organ. In acute malaria reticulocyte response is suppressed. Erythropoietin levels are usually elevated, although occasionally they are less than anticipated for the degree of anaemia.

Uncommon complications of malaria that can exacerbate the anaemia are hyperreactive malarial splenomegaly and 'blackwater fever'. Hyperreactive malarial splenomegaly is characterized by massive splenomegaly with hypersplenism (see later) and occurs as a result of a disordered immune response to malaria. Blackwater fever is associated with severe intravascular haemolysis with haemoglobinuria, and can lead to acute renal failure. It has been associated with antimalarial drugs, particularly quinine, and may be more common in individuals with glucose-6-phosphate dehydrogenase (G6PD) deficiency.

The high prevalence of severe anaemia in areas with intense malaria transmission has generally been ascribed to malaria, but recent studies in Malawian children have suggested that the anaemia is multifactorial, with bacteraemia, malaria, hookworm, HIV and deficiencies of G6PD, vitamin A and vitamin B_{12}, but not iron and folate deficiency, being important.

Case fatality rates of children with severe anaemia in Africa are 9–18% and mortality rises steeply at haemoglobin concentrations of less than 4 g/dL. Severe decompensated malarial anaemia can be accompanied by hypovolaemia and acidosis and therefore requires urgent intravenous rehydration and blood transfusion. The high risk of transfusion-transmissible infections in poorer countries makes it especially important to prevent and adequately treat the milder forms of anaemia so that transfusions can be avoided. Antimalarial prophylaxis, presumptive malarial treatment and insecticide-treated bednets are valuable in reducing malaria infections and anaemia in specific groups, such as pregnant women and young children, in endemic countries.

The white cell count in malaria is usually normal but may be raised in severe disease. Other white cell changes that have been described in malaria include a leucoerythroblastic response, monocytosis, eosinopenia and a reactive eosinophilia during the recovery phase. Neutrophil activation, indicated by raised leucocyte elastase levels, may be apparent in severe malaria. Mild thrombocytopenia with counts around 100×10^9/L is common. It is due to increased splenic clearance and is associated with increased platelet turnover and raised thrombopoietin levels. Pancytopenia without massive splenomegaly has also been described.

The bone marrow of patients with acute malaria due to any of the four species shows prominent dyserythropoiesis. This may persist for weeks after the acute infection and is caused by intramedullary cytokines produced by the infection. Erythrophagocytosis and macrophages containing malaria pigment are frequently seen in marrow samples from malaria patients.

Although malaria is associated with thrombocytopenia and activation of the coagulation cascade and fibrinolytic system, bleeding and haemorrhage are uncommon even though the prothrombin and partial thromboplastin times may be prolonged. The trigger for this activation is unknown but there is evidence that it may be a combination of procoagulant cytokines and parasitized erythrocytes, which can directly activate coagulation pathways. Disseminated intravascular coagulation (DIC) is not important in the pathogenesis of severe malaria. Fibrinogen levels are often increased and there is rapid fibrinogen turnover with consumption of antithrombin and factor (F)XIII, and increased fibrin degradation products (FDPs). Microparticle formation from platelets, red cells and macrophages also causes widespread activation of blood coagulation. Malaria has recently been found to result in increased levels of circulating active von Willebrand factor (VWF).

Haematological indicators of a poor prognosis in severe malaria include:
- leucocytosis $> 12 \times 10^9$/L;
- severe anaemia (packed cell volume < 15%);
- thrombocytopenia $< 50 \times 10^9$/L;
- prolonged prothrombin time (> 16 s);
- prolonged partial thromboplastin time (> 40 s);
- reduced fibrinogen (< 2 g/L);
- hyperparasitaemia > 100 000/μL (high mortality > 500 000/μL);
- > 20% of parasites are pigment-containing trophozoites and schizonts;
- > 5% of neutrophils contain visible malaria pigment.

Genetic haematological protection mechanisms

Plasmdium vivax needs Duffy blood group antigen as a receptor to enter red cells. This antigen is absent in at least two-thirds of black races who consequently have a natural resistance to infection with *P. vivax*. The protective effect of HbAS against the life-threatening complications of malaria is well recognized. Similar but less marked protection is associated with other red cell genetic abnormalities such as G6PD deficiency, α thalassaemia trait and HbC trait.

Diagnosis
Microscopy

Direct visualization of parasites by light microscopy using a combination of thick and thin blood films is the gold-standard diagnostic technique for malaria (Table 51.3 and Figure 51.2). A Romanowsky stain (e.g. Field, Giemsa, Leishman) pH 7.2 is used so that the parasite cytoplasm stains blue and the nuclear chromatin red. A thick blood film should be used as the first screening tool as it allows larger volumes of blood to be examined than the thin film. However, the parasites appear distorted due to the process of lysing the red cells so this method cannot be used for parasite morphology and speciation. A thin blood film allows visualization of undistorted parasites and of the size and shape of the red cells but has low sensitivity because of the small amount of blood that can be examined.

The disadvantages of basing a diagnosis of malaria on blood film examination include the following.

• A negative film does not exclude malaria: at least three films taken during episodes of fever should be examined and even if these are negative it does not entirely exclude the diagnosis especially in the presence of antimalarial drugs.

• A positive film does not prove that symptoms are due to malaria: asymptomatic parasitaemia is common in adults from endemic areas.

• Parasites, particularly *P. falciparum* gametocytes, may be washed off the slide during staining; bulk staining of slides may result in transfer of parasites between slides.

• Parasite density does not necessarily correlate with disease severity, although heavy parasitaemia (> 5% of red cells infected) indicates a poor prognosis.

Malaria pigment may persist in phagocytic cells for several weeks after an acute attack and may be helpful in retrospective diagnosis of malaria. Automated haematology analysers may produce an abnormal pattern on the white cell differential count histogram. Debris below the white cell threshold may be due to malaria parasites and manual examination of blood films is indicated if this pattern is flagged up by the analyser.

Antigen detection

Rapid diagnostic tests for malaria are based on detection of the malaria antigen histidine-rich protein (HRP)2 or parasite lactate dehydrogenase (pLDH). They have been incorporated into immunochromatographic antigen-capture kits for rapid diagnosis. The sensitivity of these dipstick strip tests approaches that of thick film microscopy (i.e. 0.002% parasitaemia equivalent to 100–200 parasites/μL of blood). HRP2 protein may remain positive for 14 days after successful treatment and false positives due to rheumatoid factor have been reported. pLDH

Table 51.3 Differentiating features of human *Plasmodium*/*Babesia* species in stained thin blood films.

	P. falciparum	P. malariae	P. vivax	P. ovale	Babesia *sp.*
Appearance of infected red blood cells (size and shape)	Both normal	Normal shape; size normal or smaller	1.5–2 times larger than normal; shape normal or oval	As for *P. vivax*, but some have irregular edges	Both normal
Red cells with multiple parasites/cell	Common	Rare	Occasional	As for *P. vivax*	Common
Stages present in peripheral blood	Rings and gametocytes; occasionally schizonts	All stages	All stages	As for *P. vivax*	Only rings and rare pear-shaped forms ('Maltese cross'); no gametocytes
Ring form (young trophozoite)	Delicate small ring; scanty cytoplasm; sometimes at the edge of red cell ('accolé form')	Ring one-third of the diameter of cell; heavy chromatin dot; vacuole sometimes 'filled in'	Ring one-third to half of the diameter of cell; heavy chromatin dot	As for *P. vivax*	Resembles ring of *P. falciparum*; look for pear-shaped structure
Gametocyte	'Crescent' or 'sausage' shape is characteristic	Round or oval; dark coarse pigment	Round or oval	Round or oval (smaller than *P. vivax*)	No gametocyte

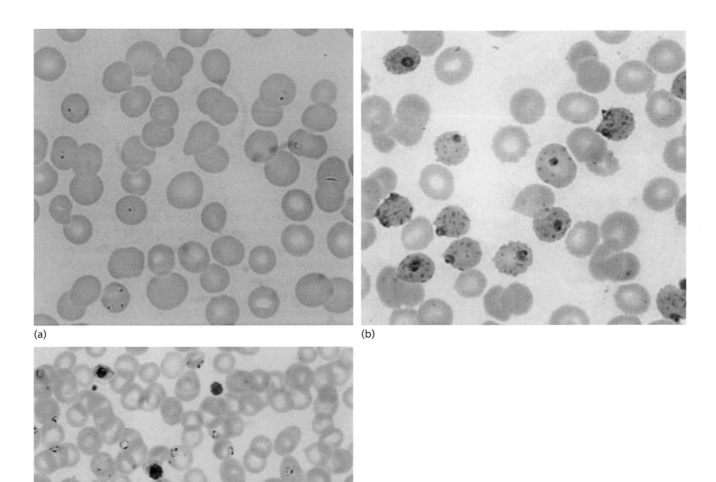

(a)

(b)

(c)

Figure 51.2 Stages in the life cycle of *Plasmodium falciparum* in Giemsa-stained thin films; the cells are not enlarged or decolorized: (a) delicate early ring forms; (b) ring forms with prominent Maurer's clefts; and (c) ring forms and early and late schizonts (schizonts are not commonly seen in the peripheral blood).

is only produced by viable parasites so it becomes negative 2–3 days after successful treatment. None of these kits are able to provide quantitative information about parasitaemia but some are able to distinguish between *P. falciparum* and other species.

Potential uses of malaria antigen detection tests include:
- confirmation of malaria diagnosis on a blood film;
- detection of *P. falciparum* when the microscopist is inexperienced (e.g. on-call or emergency situations);
- determination of species when there is a possibility of mixed infection;
- monitoring response to treatment (not HRP2 based tests).

Antibody detection

Malarial antibodies can remain in the blood after the eradication of parasites, so their detection is not useful for diagnosis in the acute attack. The main uses of malarial antibody detection are for excluding malaria as a cause of recurrent fever, for population surveys and as a screening test for blood transfusion purposes.

DNA-based methods

DNA probes have been developed for malaria diagnosis but their use is generally restricted to research and epidemiological surveys.

Haematological implications of treatment for falciparum malaria

Chloroquine was the first-line treatment for malaria in many countries for decades and was generally well tolerated. However, widespread parasite resistance has now seriously restricted its use and it is therefore being superseded by newer drugs, often in combination, to reduce the development of resistance. Some antimalarial drugs have significant haematological side-effects, as described below.

Pyrimethamine is used in combination with a long-acting sulphonamide, such as sulfadoxine (as in Fansidar). It is a dihydrofolate reductase inhibitor and may therefore induce megaloblastic anaemia and other cytopenias. The sulphur component of these combinations may rarely cause cytopenias and methaemoglobinaemia.

Dapsone acts by inhibiting the synthesis of dihydrofolic acid and is used as part of a fixed combination with proguanil or chlorproguanil. It may be associated with haemolytic anaemia, methaemoglobinaemia and eosinophilia.

Primaquine, an inhibitor of protein synthesis, is active against the hypnozoites of *P. vivax* and the gametocytes of *P. falciparum*. It causes oxidant haemolysis in patients with G6PD deficiency and, rarely, methaemoglobinaemia.

Quinine is usually reserved for life-threatening infections especially in endemic countries. It acts by disrupting the food vacuole of the parasite. Rarely, it is associated with immune thrombocytopenia and severe intravascular haemolysis.

Mefloquine, halofantrine and artemisinin-related compounds do not commonly cause significant haematological side-effects. A combination of artemether and lumefantrine (Coartem or Riamet) is commonly used as first-line treatment in endemic areas. It has no major haematological side-effects.

Some antibacterial drugs, such as doxycycline, clindamycin, trimethoprim and sulphonamides, have also been used for their antimalarial effect and may be associated with haematological side-effects.

For malaria due to *P. vivax*, *P. ovale* and *P. malariae*, chloroquine is still widely used for treatment as resistance is generally low; primaquine is added to prevent relapses in vivax and ovale malaria.

Babesiosis

Epidemiology and biology

Babesiosis is not a tropical disease but is briefly described here as it can be confused with malaria. Babesiosis is endemic in the northeastern and upper midwestern regions of the USA and is found sporadically in other parts of the USA, Europe, Asia, Africa and South America. It is primarily a disease of animals and rarely infects humans. It is due to a protozoan parasite transmitted by the bite of the ixodid tick. Following the bite, the organisms penetrate red cells, where they take on an oval, round or pear shape and multiply by budding. The erythrocytic ring forms of *Babesia microti* and *B. divergens* may be confused with malaria *P. falciparum* rings, but they do not produce pigment or cause alterations in red cell morphology. A minority of organisms take on a folded shape and are thought to be gametocytes.

Babesia bovis, *B. microti* and *B. divergens* are responsible for the majority of human infections, which range from asymptomatic to severe and occasionally are fatal. Most of the cases reported from Europe have been due to *B. divergens* and

occurred in patients without a functioning spleen. In North America almost all the cases have been due to *B. microti*, which usually produces a subclinical infection. Specific laboratory diagnosis of babesial infection is made by morphological examination of Giemsa-stained blood smears, serology and amplification of babesial DNA using polymerase chain reaction (PCR).

Clinical features

The incubation period varies from 1 to 4 weeks, and the severity and progression of the clinical features vary with the infecting species. Most patients have no recollection of a tick bite. The disease presents with fever, prostration, mild hepatosplenomegaly and haemolytic anaemia with jaundice and haemoglobinuria. Severe complications, including acute tubular necrosis, respiratory distress and DIC, and a fulminant fatal course has been described in patients who are splenectomized, immunosuppressed, infected with HIV or elderly.

Haematological abnormalities

The anaemia may be mild to moderately severe and is due to parasite-induced abnormalities in the red cell membrane. Haemolytic anaemia, which may last for several weeks, is a prominent feature of babesiosis, particularly in splenectomized individuals. Although the haemolysis is due to complement or antibody coating of the red cells, the direct antiglobulin test (DAT) is usually negative. Haptoglobin levels are reduced and the reticulocyte count is increased. The presence of parasitaemia needs to be interpreted with caution as parasites may persist for months after the resolution of symptoms and the level of parasitaemia does not parallel the severity of disease (see Table 51.3). Babesia parasites may be confused with Pappenheimer bodies in splenectomized patients with active haemolysis. Thrombocytopenia may occur in severe cases. Total white cell counts are usually normal or low.

Haematological implications of treatment for babesiosis

The combination of atovaquone and azithromycin is the treatment of choice for mild or moderate babesiosis, whereas clindamycin and quinine and exchange transfusion are indicated for severe disease. Atovaquone has been associated with anaemia and neutropenia; azithromycin and clindamycin have been associated with neutropenia and thrombocytopenia.

Filariasis

Epidemiology and biology

There are two groups of human filariasis: those that occur in the blood (lymphatic filariasis) and those that occur in the skin (onchocerciasis). Only lymphatic filariasis is considered in this chapter, as it is associated with detectable organisms in the peripheral blood.

Two species of filarial worms cause lymphatic filariasis in humans and are relevant for haematologists, *Wuchereria ban-*

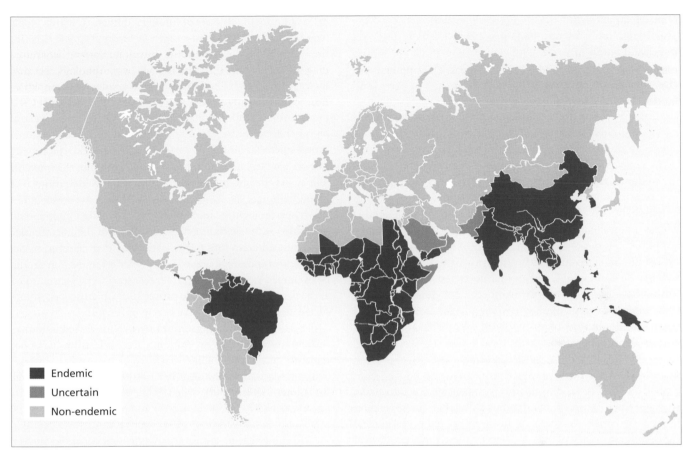

Figure 51.3 Global distribution of lymphatic filariasis.

crofti and *Brugia malayi*. They have different geographical distributions, with *W. bancrofti* being the most widespread. More than 90% of infections due to *W. bancrofti* are found in Asia, although it also occurs in Africa, America and the Pacific Islands. Filariasis due to *B. malayi* occurs in China, Indo-China, Thailand, Malaysia, Indonesia, the Philippines and south-west India (Figure 51.3).

The worms are 4 cm (male) to 10 cm (female) in length and can live for over 10 years in the lymphatics. Microfilariae, which are 250–300 μm long, are produced by the female worm and released into the blood after 3–8 months, where they may live for up to 1 year. Microfilariae densities can reach 10 000/mL but are usually much lower. They exhibit daily periodicity in the blood and this timing is designed to match the biting habits of their mosquito vectors, culicine and anopheline mosquitoes. The microfilariae develop in the mosquito and pass into the proboscis, ready to be injected into another human.

Clinical presentation

There is wide variation in the presenting features of lymphatic filariasis, which may occur 6 months or more after the infective bite. The symptoms and signs are due to lymphangitis. There are recurrent bouts of fever with heat, redness and pain over lymphatic vessels. In fair-skinned people, the lymphangitis can be seen to spread distally (i.e. the opposite direction to septic lymphangitis). In *W. bancrofti* infection, these repeated episodes of inflammation eventually result in the typical chronic picture of filariasis, including hydrocele, lymphoedema and elephantiasis, chyluria and tropical pulmonary eosinophilia. The clinical picture in *B. malayi* infection is similar but it does not cause hydrocele or chylous urine.

Other filariae with blood-inhabiting larvae
Loa loa

This occurs in the rain-forest belt of Africa, especially West Africa. The adult worms migrate through the subcutaneous tissues, including the conjunctiva, and occasionally can be seen passing across the eye.

Mansonella perstans

This is a non-pathogenic and common infection of people in Africa. These organisms may therefore coexist in the blood with *W. bancrofti* but can be distinguished by their smaller size and absence of a sheath.

Mansonella ozzardi

This is also probably non-pathogenic and occurs in the West Indies and South America.

Haematological abnormalities

Eosinophilia is the major and most frequent haematological abnormality produced by lymphatic filariasis. Tropical pulmonary eosinophilia is an unusual complication of filariasis and is due to an immunological hyperresponsiveness to microfilariae in the lungs. It is more common in men than women. Although microfilariae are absent from the blood in this syndrome, they may be seen in lung biopsies and adult worms can be visualized in lymphatics on ultrasound. There is an extreme eosinophilia, with eosinophil counts of greater than 10×10^9/L; the level of eosinophilia is not related to the severity of symptoms. In tropical pulmonary eosinophilia, diethylcarbamazine treatment reduces the eosinophil count and produces resolution of symptoms. This rapid response to treatment distinguishes filariasis from other causes of marked eosinophilia, such as helminths that affect the lungs (*Ascaris, Strongyloides, Schistosoma* subsp. *trichinosis* and *Toxocara*).

Diagnosis of filariasis

The adult worms residing in the lymphatics are inaccessible, so diagnosis is based on finding microfilariae in the peripheral blood. The level of filaraemia is inversely related to the clinical signs because much of the damage is due to immunological responses to the microfilariae rather than to the organisms themselves. Furthermore, the presence of microfilariae does not necessarily mean that they are causing clinical problems and, conversely, a lack of microfilariae in the blood does not exclude a diagnosis of filariasis. The peripheral blood findings must therefore be assessed in the context of the clinical picture.

To optimize the chances of finding scanty microfilariae in the blood, the sample should be taken at the appropriate time for the expected peak concentration of microfilariae (i.e. around midnight or midday for nocturnally and diurnally periodic forms respectively). There are many techniques for demonstrating microfilariae in the laboratory. The simplest method is a wet preparation of fresh blood. Microfilariae will survive in venous blood collected into EDTA for 2 days at room temperature. Motile microfilariae can be seen on a slide under low power and can be counted in a counting chamber. Numbers of microfilariae may be low, requiring concentration techniques such as blood filtering.

For species identification, thick and thin blood films should be stained with Giemsa or haematoxylin and the microfilariae differentiated according to the pattern of their sheaths, nuclei distribution and size (Figure 51.4). The edges of the film should be examined carefully as microfilariae tend to be concentrated at the periphery and are easily missed if the microscopist immediately uses high power in the centre of the film.

Detection of circulating antigen by enzyme-linked immunosorbent assay (ELISA) or immunochromatography (ICT) has replaced microscopy for the diagnosis of bancroftian, but not brugian, filariasis. An antigen ICT card test is available for the detection of *W. bancrofti*, which does not react with other filariae and is highly sensitive (100%) and specific (92%). Filarial DNA can be detected by PCR, and ultrasound scans can help identify adult worms within the lymphatic system. Serological tests are not very helpful as most individuals from endemic areas have antibodies to crude filarial antigens and there is cross-reactivity with other filariae and nematodes.

Haematological implications of treatment for filariasis

Oral diethylcarbamazine is the drug of choice in all forms of lymphatic filariasis, including subclinical infection. Alternative

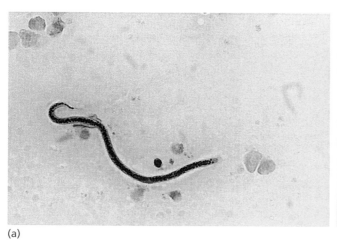

(a)

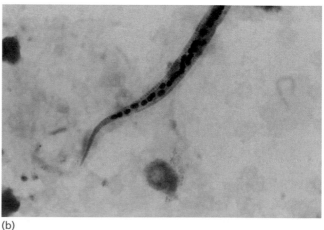

(b)

Figure 51.4 Microfilariae of *W. bancrofti* in thick film: (a) microfilaria showing the negative impression of the sheath (× 365); (b) tail of the microfilaria showing that the nuclei do not extend into the tail (× 912).

964

treatments include combinations of albendazole and ivermectin. None of these drugs has common, serious haematological side-effects. It has recently been discovered that depletion of *Wolbachia* endobacteria, a symbiont of *Onchocerca*, by tetracycline antibiotics leads to long-lasting sterility of adult female worms.

African trypanosomiasis (sleeping sickness)

Epidemiology and biology

African sleeping sickness is caused by the haemoflagellate protozoa *Trypanosoma brucei gambiense* in West and Central Africa, and *T. brucei rhodesiense* in eastern Africa (Figure 51.5). These parasites are fusiform in shape, 12–35 µm long and morphologically indistinguishable from each other. The disease is transmitted by the bite of the tsetse fly, which is only found in Africa. The trypanosomes multiply by fission in the vicinity of the infected bite and are then disseminated by the bloodstream. Congenital transmission has also been described.

The distribution of African sleeping sickness is determined by the ecological limits of the tsetse fly vector and lies in the region between Senegal and Somalia in the north and the Kalahari and Namibian deserts in the south. Sleeping sickness is an important public health problem in Central African

Republic, Chad, Democratic Republic of Congo, Côte d'Ivoire, Guinea, Malawi, Uganda and United Republic of Tanzania. During recent epidemic periods the prevalence reached 50% in several villages in the Democratic Republic of Congo, Angola and southern Sudan. Improved surveillance has reduced the number of new cases over the last decade.

Clinical features

The bite of a tsetse fly is very painful and causes a small indurated lesion that may persist for some days. The local multiplication of the trypanosomes may cause a marked inflammatory reaction (a chancre) that regresses after 2–3 weeks. Entry of the trypanosomes into the bloodstream is associated with fever, which tends to be less marked in West African trypanosomiasis than in the East African variety. East African trypanosomiasis is primarily a disease of cattle and only enters human hosts by accident. It is therefore less well tolerated than West African sleeping sickness, having a more aggressive course and intense symptoms.

The early stages of sleeping sickness can be associated with prominent lymphadenopathy, particularly of the posterior cervical nodes, and mild splenomegaly. These features may be suggestive of infectious mononucleosis, tuberculous lymphadenitis or a lymphoproliferative disorder. Severe anaemia, haemorrhages and petechiae may occur at this stage.

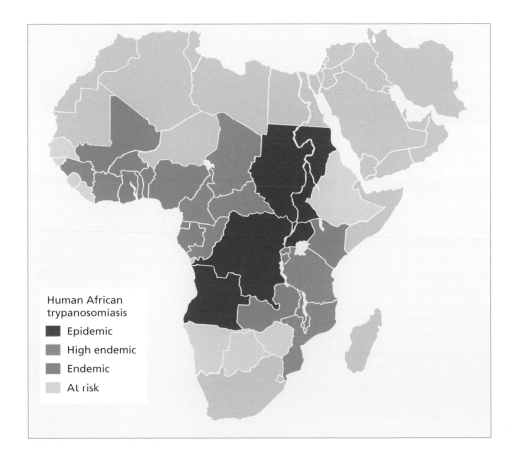

Figure 51.5 Global distribution of African trypanosomiasis.

Both types of African sleeping sickness cause a protracted febrile illness which, despite the name, is not always associated with drowsiness. Death is inevitable if the disease is left untreated. As the disease progresses parasitaemia decreases, trypanosomes invade the central nervous system (CNS) and neurological disturbances due to inflammatory chronic meningoencephalitis supervene. In West African trypanosomiasis, the disease runs its course over several years but in East African trypanosomiasis infection CNS involvement may occur within weeks.

Haematological abnormalities

The aetiology of the anaemia in sleeping sickness is multifactorial but primarily due to phagocytic removal of immune complex-coated red cells from the circulation. Trypanosomes liberate haemolytic factors that contribute to this process, and increases in plasma volume cause a dilutional anaemia. There is a failure to incorporate iron into red cell precursors and the resulting dyserythropoiesis means that the bone marrow is unable to compensate for the fall in haemoglobin. There may be a moderate leucocytosis with increased monocytes, lymphocytes and plasma cells. Mott morular cells have also been described in sleeping sickness. The bone marrow is hypercellular, with areas of gelatinous degeneration.

As the disease advances, a bleeding tendency may develop due to thrombocytopenia, vascular injury and coagulopathy. Platelet dysfunction has also been described and is manifest as clumping and abnormal aggregation responses. DIC with raised FDPs may occur in the later stages. Although some of these haematological changes can be linked to the non-specific polyclonal activation of B cells, overall the mechanisms underlying these are not well understood.

Diagnosis of sleeping sickness

Trypanosomes can be seen on stained thin blood films but the number of trypanosomes in the circulation can vary considerably and is often low, so concentration techniques are usually required. Quantitative buffy coat method is the technique of choice for diagnosis of African sleeping sickness. This involves concentrating the trypanosomes at the plasma–platelet interface in a special microhaematocrit tube using differential centrifugation. Parasites are identified by labelling with the fluorescent marker acridine orange.

Wet preparations of fluid aspirated from the lymph nodes, bone marrow or cerebrospinal fluid (CSF) may also reveal live motile organisms. This technique is more likely to be productive in the case of infection with *T. brucei rhodesiense* than *T. brucei gambiense*. The organisms are fragile so care must be taken not to damage them when making the smears.

The highly specific and sensitive serological card agglutination test for trypanosomiasis (CATT) may be used in conjunction with a direct visualization method. If these tests are positive,

then CSF examination is mandatory to determine the stage of the illness.

Haematological implications of treatment for African sleeping sickness

Pentamidine and suramin are the drugs of choice for the early stages of West and East African trypanosomiasis respectively. They have a cure rate of around 90% but are only able to achieve modest CSF concentrations so they cannot be used for later stages of the disease. The most common haematological side-effects of pentamidine are leucopenia, thrombocytopenia and anaemia. Suramin has serious side-effects, including haemolytic anaemia and bone marrow toxicity.

Melarsoprol, an arsenic-based compound, has been the drug of choice for late-stage sleeping sickness but is highly toxic, with a mortality of 4–12%. Its main adverse effect is a fatal encephalopathic syndrome; haematological toxicity is not a particular problem.

Eflornithine is expensive but is of benefit in late-stage sleeping sickness, particularly West African disease; 25–50% of patients treated with this drug exhibit bone marrow toxicity with pancytopenia.

American trypanosomiasis (Chagas disease)

Epidemiology and biology

Chagas disease is caused by a haemoflagellate protozoa, *T. cruzi*, which is transmitted by triatomine bugs that infest poor-quality housing. It can also be transmitted through blood transfusions and congenitally. It is restricted to a region in the Americas between Argentina and the southern states of the USA.

Clinical features

The incubation period is usually a couple of weeks but may be up to several months if transmission was through blood transfusion. In the acute phase, swelling at the site of entry of the organism, a chagoma, may be accompanied by fever, mild hepatosplenomegaly and local or generalized lymphadenopathy. The trypanosomes multiply intracellularly in muscle tissue, particularly the heart, colon and oesophagus. Once infection has occurred, the organisms will be present for life unless treatment is given. The chronic phase of the disease is associated with heart disease in 30% of infected individuals, which is manifest as arrhythmias and cardiomegaly. A small proportion of individuals also have clinical involvement of the gastrointestinal tract and other hollow organs resulting in loss of peristalsis, organomegaly and organ failure. Asymptomatic infection is common and poses a problem for blood transfusion services in endemic areas, so some countries routinely screen blood for American trypanosomiasis.

Diagnosis of Chagas disease

Although similar methods to those used for African trypanosomiasis can be helpful for diagnosis, serological tests are more commonly used as the primary diagnostic tool. They are based on enzyme immunoassay or immunofluorescent antibody test and have good sensitivity. PCR may also be useful but is not in routine use.

Haematological implications of treatment for American trypanosomiasis

There are only two effective drugs for the treatment of *T. cruzi* infection, nifurtimox and benznidazole. Major haematological side-effects are not common with either drug, although agranulocytosis has been reported with benznidazole.

Leishmaniasis

Epidemiology and biology

Visceral and cutaneous leishmaniases are caused by protozoan flagellates that are transmitted through the infective bite of a phlebotomine sandfly. Following an infected bite, parasites spread from the inoculation site to the mononuclear phagocytic system. Only the visceral form (kala-azar) is associated with organisms in haemopoietic tissues and thus is considered here. Visceral leishmaniasis is due to the species *Leishmania donovani* and *L. infantum* and is found in 47 countries throughout the world, with extension limits from 45° N to 32° S; 90% of cases are in Bangladesh, India, Nepal, Sudan and Brazil (Figure 51.6). The number of cases of visceral leishmaniasis, particularly around the Mediterranean basin in southern Europe, has increased in association with HIV-related immunosuppression.

Clinical features

The clinical expression of leishmaniasis depends on both the genotypic potential of the parasite and the immunological response of the patient. Incubation period varies from days to years but is generally 2–6 months. Onset can be sudden with high fever, or gradual with intermittent fever. Diarrhoea, joint pains, weight loss and bleeding gums occur in the acute phase. This is followed by progressive muscle wasting, protuberant abdomen, fever, weight loss, anaemia and hepatosplenomegaly. The splenomegaly appears early and the spleen increases in size in relation to the duration of the disease, so that eventually it may reach into the left hyopchondrium. In immunocompromised patients, such as transplant recipients and those with advanced HIV disease, kala-azar behaves like an opportunistic infection.

Haematological abnormalities

Normochromic normocytic anaemia is a frequent and clinically significant feature of visceral leishmaniasis and haemoglobin levels of 7–10 g/dL are common. The massive splenic enlargement results in hypersplenism with consequent pancytopenia. Liver dysfunction with jaundice, ascites and deranged coagulation may occur in the late stages and has a poor prognosis. The bleeding tendency may be exacerbated by thrombocytopenia. In all patients with unexplained splenomegaly, pancytopenia or fever, a high index of suspicion of leishmaniasis needs to be maintained to prevent fatalities.

Diagnosis of leishmaniasis

Definitive diagnosis is based on detection of the parasites, or their DNA, in smears of bone marrow, splenic aspirate or fluid aspirated from enlarged lymph nodes.

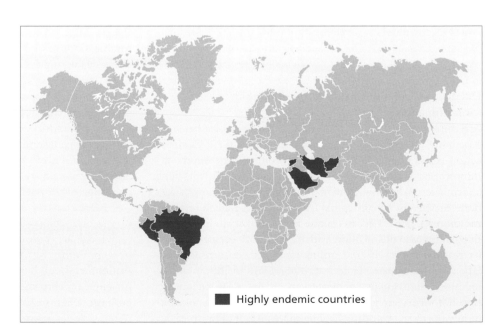

Figure 51.6 Global distribution of visceral leishmaniasis.

■ Highly endemic countries

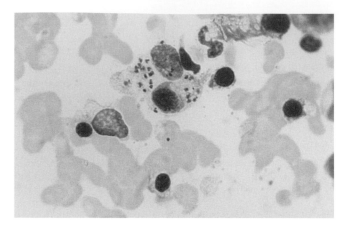

Figure 51.7 Bone marrow aspirate of leishmaniasis infection showing a macrophage containing numerous organisms. The presence of both a nucleus and a small paranuclear kinetoplast gives the organisms their characteristic 'double-dot' appearance (MCG ×940).

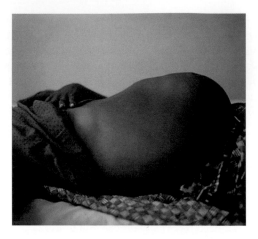

Figure 51.8 Patient with massive splenomegaly due to hyperreactive malarial splenomegaly.

On microscopy *Leishmania* are usually seen as intracellular amastigotes in mononuclear cells but can also be seen extracellularly (Figure 51.7). They are 2–6 μm in diameter and contain a nucleus lying close to the rod-shaped kinetoplast, and an internal flagellum. Using a Romanowsky stain, the nucleus and kinetoplast stain purple and can be clearly distinguished. Amastigotes can be seen in both bone marrow aspirates and in trephine-impression smears. They are rarely seen in peripheral blood and then only in buffy coat preparations.

Direct microscopic visualization is less sensitive than molecular diagnosis, particularly when there is co-infection with HIV. PCR can be performed on lesion aspirate, marrow, blood and biopsy material. The indirect fluorescent antibody tests ELISA and DAT are useful for detecting antibodies to visceral leishmaniasis, but results may be inconclusive in immunosuppressed patients.

Haematological implications of treatment for leishmaniasis

For the last 80 years, the treatment of leishmaniasis has been based on pentavalent antimonials, although their mode of action is still unclear. Sodium stibogluconate is the most commonly used antimonial. It can be associated with worsening anaemia and thrombocytopenia, although its most serious detrimental effects are on cardiac function. Resistance levels to antimonials are high in some countries including India, Bangladesh, Brazil and Sudan, so other options such as amphotericin, paromomycin and miltefosine need to be considered. HIV co-infected patients do not respond well to antimonials so for these individuals amphotericin is the drug of choice. Amphotericin can produce haematological side-effects, commonly normocytic normochromic anaemia, but its most serious

toxicity is related to renal, cardiac, neurological and hepatic dysfunction. Side-effects can be reduced by using the liposomal preparation. Immunocompromised patients may require prophylaxis to prevent relapses.

Non-specific haematological abnormalities associated with tropical diseases

Hypersplenism

Hypersplenism is a syndrome characterized by splenomegaly and cytopenias. Tropical infections associated with massive splenomegaly include hyperreactive malarial splenomegaly, visceral leishmaniasis, schistosomiasis and trypanosomiasis (Figure 51.8). The cytopenias in hypersplenism are due to a combination of sequestration and haemodilution. The degree of expansion of plasma volume is proportional to the size of the spleen, and can be improved by splenectomy. The thrombocytopenia and neutropenia are rarely severe enough to cause clinical problems. Most of the thrombocytopenia is due to pooling in the spleen which, when massively enlarged, can hold up to 90% of the platelet mass. Neutropenia is the result of increased marginalization of granulocytes. Treatment of the underlying disorder generally leads to regression of the splenomegaly with resolution of the haematological abnormalities.

Tropical diseases associated with changes in the full blood count

Anaemia

Anaemia of chronic disease is a common and non-specific finding in many types of tropical infections. Some infections are responsible for specific types of anaemia. For example, hookworm infection contributes to iron deficiency anaemia, and megaloblastic anaemia secondary to parasite consumption of vitamin B_{12} is a feature of infection with the tapeworm *Diphyllobothrium latum*. Intraerythrocytic parasites, such as those that cause malaria and babesiosis, may be associated with significant intravascular haemolysis.

White cell abnormalities

Severe infections particularly due to bacteria may cause a neutrophilia and a leukaemoid reaction with circulating myeloid precursors and neutrophils with toxic granulation, vacuolation and Döhle body formation. Lymphocytosis with neutropenia, splenomegaly, nose bleeds, rash and neurological complications is a feature of rickettsial diseases (e.g. typhus, Q fever, trench fever). Some, such as trench fever, may persist for many years and are transmissible in blood transfusions. The absence of neutrophilia in the presence of marked fever is a particular feature of typhoid. Lymphocytosis or monocytosis may also be present in typhoid; other clinical features include hepatosplenomegaly and, in severe disease, haemorrhage from ileal ulcers exacerbated by DIC. Helminths and other predominantly tropical organisms that invade tissues may be associated with a significant eosinophilia ($> 0.5 \times 10^9$/L). Such diseases include loiasis, lymphatic filariasis, schistosomiasis, trichinosis, toxocariasis, strongyloidiasis, hydatid disease, oriental liver flukes and guinea worm.

Tropical infections with fever and haemorrhage

Relapsing fever

Relapsing fevers are borne by either lice or ticks. Louse-borne relapsing fever is endemic in the horn of Africa and Rwanda. Tick-borne relapsing fever has a wider distribution through Africa, the Mediterranean basin and the Middle East. They have a relapsing course and severe disease is characterized by fever with jaundice, neutrophilia, thrombocytopenia and DIC. There is a marked bleeding tendency, with petechial haemorrhage and epistaxis. Spiral organisms (*Borrelia* spp.) can be seen in the blood. Relapsing fevers respond well to tetracycline but this must be given with care as it can generate a severe life-threatening Jarisch–Herxheimer reaction.

Viral haemorrhagic fevers

These are caused by arenaviruses, filoviruses, bunyaviruses and flaviviruses and are classified according to their reservoir hosts and their primary means of transmission. They are divided into:
• rodent-associated viruses (e.g. Lassa fever, hantaviruses);
• arthropod-borne viruses (e.g. dengue, yellow fever and Chikungunya viruses);
• unknown vectors or hosts (e.g. Marburg, Ebola).
They often occur in epidemics, have human-to-human transmission and may only be suspected if a relevant travel history is elicited from the patient. Dengue and yellow fever are becoming increasingly important imported infections.

Dengue

The four types of dengue virus belong to a group of flaviviruses and are transmitted by *Aedes* mosquitoes. Dengue is endemic in tropical areas of Asia, Africa, South America and the Caribbean and is particularly virulent in Southeast Asia, including Thailand and Vietnam. There has been a resurgence of the disease as a result of urbanization, poverty, the demise of *Aedes* eradication programmes and increasing travel.

Primary infection occurs in young children and is usually asymptomatic. Older children and adults develop acute fever, headache and myalgia ('breakbone fever'). Leucopenia may accompany this stage of the illness. Severe complications may arise in those who have had previous dengue infection. These include hypotensive shock, marked thrombocytopenia with spontaneous bleeding, neutropenia, bone marrow hypoplasia and abnormal megakaryocytopoiesis.

Lassa fever, Ebola virus and Marburg virus

These are endemic in equatorial Africa and are important because they cause potentially fatal infections and have the ability to spread from person to person. Only about 10% of infected individuals become ill. Of these 1–2% develop fatal disease. The clinical features of these three haemorrhagic fevers are similar and are characterized by headache, fever and oesophagitis. Spontaneous bleeding occurs in 25% of hospitalized patients and is thought to be due to abnormal platelet function. Case reports suggest that treatment with ribavirin may be helpful.

Yellow fever

Yellow fever virus is transmitted by *Aedes* mosquitoes and exists throughout equatorial Africa, and northern and central southen America. It invades hepatocytes, causing hepatocellular dysfunction and jaundice. Fever, myalgia and back pain may be followed by jaundice, bleeding and, in the most severe cases, renal failure.

Selected bibliography

Malaria

Francischetti IM, Seydel KB, Monteiro RQ (2008) Blood coagulation, inflammation and malaria. *Microcirculation* 15: 81–107.

Ghosh K, Shetty S (2008) Blood coagulation in falciparum malaria: a review. *Parasitology Research* 102: 571–6.

Groot E, de Groot PG, Fijnheer R, Lenting PJ (2007) The presence of active von Willebrand factor under various pathological conditions. *Current Opinion in Hematology* 14: 284–9.

Health Protection Agency Advisory Committee on Malaria Prevention guidelines. Available at http://www.nathnac.org/pro/clinical_updates/importedmalaria_250408.htm

WHO malaria treatment guidelines. Available at http://www.who. int/malaria/docs/TreatmentGuidelines2006.pdf

Babesiosis

Vannier E, Gewurz BE, Krause PJ (2008) Human babesiosis. *Infectious Disease Clinics of North America* **22**: 469–88, viii–ix.

Filariasis

Hoerauf A (2006) New strategies to combat filariasis. *Expert Review of Antiinfective Therapy* **4**: 211–22.

African trypanosomiasis (sleeping sickness)

World Health Organization. Information on African trypanosomiasis (sleeping sickness). Available at http://www.who.int/mediacentre/factsheets/fs259/en/ (accessed 4 March 2009).

Viral haemorrhagic fevers

Centers for Disease Control Special Pathogens Branch. Information on viral hemorrhagic fevers. Available at http://www.cdc.gov/ncidod/dvrd/Spb/mnpages/dispages/vhf.htm (accessed 4 March 2009).

World Health Organization. Information on viral hemorrhagic fevers. Available at http://www.who.int/topics/haemorrhagic_fevers_viral/en/ (accessed 4 March 2009).

General

Bain BJ (2006) *Blood Cells: A Practical Guide*, 4th edn. Wiley-Blackwell, Oxford.

Calis JC, Phiri KS, Faragher EB *et al.* (2008) Severe anaemia in Malawian children. *New England Journal of Medicine* **358**: 888–99.

Cheesbrough M (2005) *District Laboratory Practice in Tropical Countries. Parts 1 and 2. Tropical Health Technology*, 2nd edn. Cambridge University Press, Cambridge.

Cook GC, Zumla A (eds) (2009) *Manson's Tropical Diseases*, 22nd edn. Saunders/Elsevier, Edinburgh.

Lewis SM, Bain BJ, Bates I (eds) (2006) *Dacie and Lewis Practical Haematology*, 10th edn. Churchill Livingstone, London.

Neonatal haematology

52

Irene AG Roberts

Centre for Haematology, Imperial College London, London, UK

Developmental haemopoiesis

Haemopoiesis begins in the yolk sac in the third week of gestation and moves sequentially to the aorta–gonad–mesonephros (AGM) by 5 weeks' gestation, the liver by 6–8 weeks and the bone marrow around the 11th week of gestation. The AGM involutes early in the first trimester and the liver is the principal site of haemopoiesis until the end of the third trimester. The predominant lineage during fetal life is erythropoiesis but platelets and all types of leucocyte found in adult blood are also seen from as early as 4–5 weeks' gestation.

There are a number of differences between erythropoiesis in neonates and adults: red cell morphology is distinctive with large numbers of crenated red cells, particularly in preterm neonates (Figure 52.1); red cell lifespan is reduced (35–50 days in preterm infants, 60–70 days in term infants); susceptibility to oxidant-induced injury is increased because of differences in the glycolytic and pentose phosphate pathways; the erythropoietin response to anaemia is blunted; and specific embryonic and fetal globin chains are synthesized (Table 52.1). The first globin chain produced is ε-globin, followed by α- and γ-globin chains. Haemoglobin F (HbF, $\alpha_2\gamma_2$) is produced from 4–5 weeks' gestation and is the predominant haemoglobin until after birth. Adult haemoglobin (HbA, $\alpha_2\beta_2$) is produced from 6–8 weeks' gestation, but remains at low levels until after birth. In term babies, the average HbF at birth is 70–80%, the HbA is 25–30%,

Postgraduate Haematology: 6th edition. Edited by A. Victor Hoffbrand, Daniel Catovsky, Edward G.D. Tuddenham, Anthony R. Green
© 2011 Blackwell Publishing Ltd.

there are small amounts of HbA_2 and sometimes a trace of Hb Barts (γ_4).

Immediately after birth, rates of haemoglobin synthesis and red cell production fall in response to the sudden increase in tissue oxygenation at birth. In term babies, the haemoglobin reaches a mean of 13–14 g/dL at 4 weeks and 9.5–11 g/dL at 7–9 weeks of age. Studies of well preterm infants show a steeper fall in haemoglobin, reaching a mean of 6.5–9 g/dL at 4–8 weeks of age. The reticulocyte count falls after birth as erythropoiesis is suppressed and increases to normal values at 6–8 weeks of age. The blood volume at birth varies with gestational age and the timing of clamping of the cord. In term infants, the average blood volume is 80 mL/kg and in preterm infants 106 mL/kg (range 85–143 mL/kg). Term and preterm babies have adequate stores of iron, folic acid and vitamin B_{12} at birth. However, stores of both iron and folic acid are lower in preterm infants and are depleted more quickly, leading to deficiency after 2–4 months if the recommended daily intakes are not maintained.

Neonatal anaemia

Definition and pathophysiology

Any neonate with a haemoglobin of less than 13 g/dL at birth should be considered anaemic and may require investigation (Figure 52.2). However, it is important to be aware that the haemoglobin concentration is affected by the site of sampling (it is up to 4 g/dL lower in venous than in heel-prick samples in

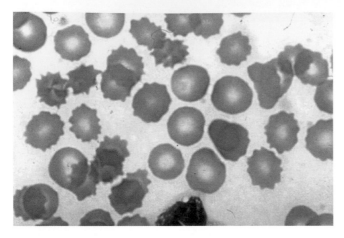

Figure 52.1 Typical erythrocyte morphology in a preterm neonate. Crenated red cells are a normal feature of the blood film of preterm neonates during the first few weeks of life. This film is from a neonate born at 26 weeks' gestation and shows the number of crenated cells present in neonates under 28 weeks' gestation. The numbers of these cells is inversely proportional to gestational age at birth.

Table 52.1 Composition of haemoglobins in the human embryo, fetus and neonate.

Haemoglobin	Globin chains		Gestation
	α-Globin gene cluster*	β-Globin gene cluster*	
Embryonic			
Hb Gower 1	ξ_2	ε_2	From 3–4 weeks
Hb Gower 2	α_2	ε_2	
Hb Portland	ξ_2	γ_2	From 4 weeks
Fetal			
HbF	α_2	γ_2	From 4 weeks
Adult			
HbA	α_2	β_2	From 6–8 weeks
HbA$_2$	α_2	δ_2	From 30 weeks

*The α-globin gene cluster is situated on chromosome 16 and the β-globin gene cluster on chromosome 11. Note that fetuses and neonates with α-thalassaemia major, who are unable to synthesize α-globin chains, will have Hb Portland as well as Hb Barts (β_4), detectable by haemoglobin electrophoresis or HPLC.

the first few days of life) and the timing of the clamping of the cord (around 3 g/dL higher after late clamping). The clinical significance of neonatal anaemia depends on whether the baby is able to maintain adequate tissue oxygenation. This in turn depends on the position of the haemoglobin–oxygen dissocia-

Table 52.2 Common causes of neonatal anaemia.

Reduced red cell production
Diamond–Blackfan anaemia
Congenital viral infections, e.g. parvovirus, cytomegalovirus
Congenital dyserythropoietic anaemia
Pearson syndrome

Increased red cell destruction (haemolysis)
Alloimmune: haemolytic disease of the newborn (Rh, ABO, Kell, other)
Red cell membrane disorders, e.g. hereditary spherocytosis
Red cell enzyme deficiencies, e.g. pyruvate kinase deficiency
Some haemoglobinopathies, e.g. α-thalassaemia major, HbH disease

Blood loss
Occult haemorrhage before or around birth, e.g. twin–twin, fetomaternal
Internal haemorrhage, e.g. intracranial, cephalhaematoma
Iatrogenic, due to frequent blood sampling

Anaemia of prematurity
Impaired red cell production plus reduced red cell lifespan

tion curve, which is principally determined by the concentrations of HbF and 2,3-diphosphoglycerate (2,3-DPG); a high HbF and low 2,3-DPG both shift the curve to the left, i.e. the affinity of haemoglobin for oxygen is increased and less oxygen is released to the tissues. This is the situation just after birth and may be more of a problem for very preterm babies as their HbF levels are greater than 90%. Over the first few months of life, 2,3-DPG levels rise and HbF levels fall so that the haemoglobin–oxygen dissociation curve gradually shifts to the right, the oxygen affinity of haemoglobin falls and oxygen delivery to the tissues increases, ameliorating the effects of the falling haemoglobin.

Causes of neonatal anaemia

Anaemia may be caused by reduced red cell production, increased red cell destruction (haemolysis) or blood loss (Table 52.2).

Neonatal anaemia due to reduced red cell production
The main diagnostic clues to reduced red cell production are the combination of a low reticulocyte count ($< 20 \times 10^9$/L) with a negative direct antiglobulin test (Coombs test). The most common causes are congenital parvovirus infection and genetic red cell aplasias, particularly Diamond–Blackfan anaemia (DBA).

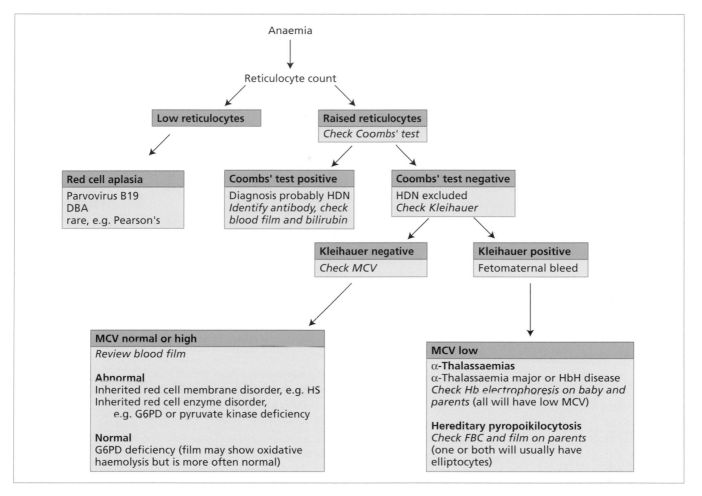

Figure 52.2 A diagnostic algorithm for neonatal anaemia. The most useful screening tests for investigating unexplained neonatal anaemia are the reticulocyte count, the Coombs test and the mean corpuscular volume (MCV) of the red cells. DBA, Diamond–Blackfan anaemia; G6PD, glucose-6-phosphate dehydrogenase; HDN, haemolytic disease of the newborn; HS, hereditary spherocytosis.

Parvovirus B19 and fetal/neonatal anaemia

Maternal infection with parvovirus B19 can cause severe fetal anaemia and in 9% of cases leads to intrauterine death. The baby has marked reticulocytopenia (often $< 10 \times 10^9$/L) and thrombocytopenia may also occur. The diagnosis is made by maternal serology and demonstration of B19 DNA in the fetus or neonate by dot-blot hybridization or polymerase chain reaction (PCR) of peripheral blood (bone marrow aspiration for morphology and parvovirus B19 PCR may be necessary in difficult cases). Severe cases require intrauterine transfusion but have a good long-term outcome if they survive to delivery.

Genetic red cell aplasia

Apart from DBA, the genetic causes of congenital red cell aplasia are extremely rare. They include congenital dyserythropoietic anaemia (CDA) and Pearson syndrome; the other inherited bone marrow failure syndromes, such as Fanconi anaemia, are almost never present at birth. DBA, which occurs in five to seven babies per million live births, has a clear family history in 20% of cases (autosomal dominant or recessive) and appears to be sporadic in the remaining 80%. It usually presents as increasing anaemia over the first few weeks or months of life but more severe cases manifest as second-trimester anaemia or hydrops fetalis. Around 40% of infants have associated congenital anomalies, particularly craniofacial dysmorphism, neck anomalies and thumb malformations similar to those seen in Fanconi anaemia. The blood film shows normochromic red cells with an absence of polychromasia and nucleated red cells despite severe anaemia (Figure 52.3). Reticulocytopenia is usually severe but automated reticulocyte counts of $20–30 \times 10^9$/L are sometimes seen. Erythroid precursors are absent in the bone marrow aspirate. These features are diagnostic of DBA if parvovirus infection is excluded. Raised red cell levels of adenosine deaminase (ADA) in the patient and/or parents may be useful

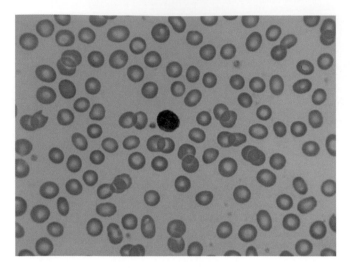

Figure 52.3 Blood film from a neonate with Diamond–Blackfan anaemia. This baby presented with fetal anaemia at 20 weeks' gestation and received intrauterine transfusion. At birth, the baby had normochromic anaemia and the blood film showed a complete absence of polychromasia and nucleated red cells, despite a haemoglobin of 7 g/dL.

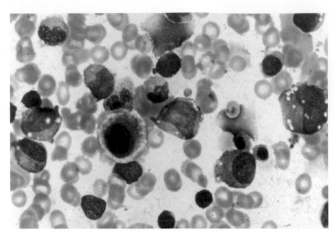

Figure 52.4 Pearson syndrome. Bone marrow aspirate from a neonate with Pearson syndrome showing typical vacuolation of erythroblasts and a dysplastic megakaryocyte.

for confirming the diagnosis, although normal red cell ADA levels do not exclude DBA. Recent studies indicate that DBA is due to defects in structural ribosomal proteins (RP). At present mutations in six genes (*RPS19*, *RPS24*, *RPS17*, *RPL5*, *RPL11* and *RPL35a*) have been identified and account for about 50% of DBA cases, *RPS19* mutations being the commonest (25% of all DBA). In the neonatal period, the only treatment of DBA is red cell transfusion, although steroids are used in older infants and children.

The other genetic causes of congenital red cell aplasia, CDA and Pearson syndrome, can be distinguished from DBA by marrow morphology. In Pearson syndrome, which is caused by mutations in mitochondrial DNA and presents with normochromic anaemia, neutropenia, thrombocytopenia and failure to thrive in the first few weeks of life, there is highly characteristic vacuolation of early erythroid cells on the marrow aspirate (Figure 52.4). Unfortunately, the prognosis for children with Pearson syndrome is very poor, with few surviving beyond the second year of life. Mutations in codanin-1 and SEC23B have recently been shown to be responsible for many, but not all, cases of type I and II CDA respectively.

Neonatal anaemia due to increased red cell destruction (haemolysis)

The main diagnostic clues suggesting a haemolytic anaemia are increased numbers of reticulocytes and/or circulating nucleated red cells (Figure 52.5), unconjugated hyperbilirubinaemia, a positive Coombs test (if immune) and characteristic changes in the morphology of the red cells on a blood film (e.g. hereditary spherocytosis; Figure 52.5). The main cause of immune haemolytic anaemia is haemolytic disease of the newborn. The main causes of non-immune neonatal haemolysis are red cell membrane disorders, red cell enzymopathies and, occasionally, haemoglobinopathies (Table 52.2).

Immune haemolysis, including haemolytic disease of the newborn

The principal alloantibodies causing haemolytic disease of the newborn are those against rhesus antigens (anti-D, anti-c and anti-E), anti-Kell, anti-Kidd (J^k), anti-Duffy (F^y) and antibodies of the MNS blood group system, including anti-U. Anti-D is the most frequent alloantibody causing significant haemolytic anaemia, affecting 1 in 1200 pregnancies. Anti-Kell antibodies are less common but can cause severe fetal and neonatal anaemia as they inhibit erythropoiesis as well as causing haemolysis. Most babies with haemolytic disease of the newborn present with jaundice and/or anaemia; in severe cases there is hepatosplenomegaly and/or skin deposits due to extramedullary haemopoiesis. ABO haemolytic disease occurs only in offspring of women of blood group O and is confined to the 1% of such women who have high-titre IgG antibodies. Haemolysis due to anti-A is more common (1 in 150 births) than that due to anti-B. In contrast with anti-rhesus antibodies, both anti-A and anti-B usually cause hyperbilirubinaemia without significant anaemia; however, hydrops has occasionally been described. The blood film in ABO haemolytic disease characteristically shows very large numbers of spherocytes with little or no increase in nucleated red cells (see Figure 52.5a); this contrasts with rhesus haemolytic disease of the newborn, in which there are few spherocytes and large numbers of circulating nucleated red cells (see Figure 52.5b).

Figure 52.5 Haemolytic disease of the newborn. (a) Blood film from a baby with rhesus haemolytic disease of the newborn due to anti-D showing polychromasia and large numbers of nucleated red cells but relatively few spherocytes. (b) Blood film from a neonate with ABO haemolytic disease of the newborn due to anti-A showing very large numbers of spherocytes, polychromasia and no nucleated red cells.

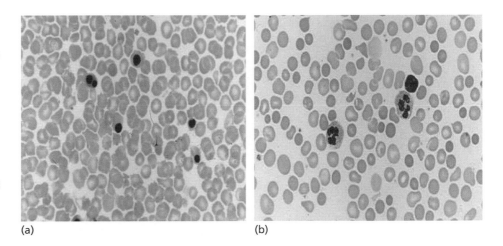

(a)   (b)

Management of haemolytic disease of the newborn

All neonates at risk should have cord blood taken for measurement of haemoglobin, bilirubin and a Coombs test and should remain in hospital until hyperbilirubinaemia and/or anaemia have been properly managed. Rhesus-alloimmunized infants with haemolysis should receive phototherapy from birth, as the bilirubin can rise steeply; this prevents the need for exchange transfusion in some infants. In haemolytic disease due to anti-Kell, anaemia is usually more prominent than jaundice and minimal phototherapy may be necessary despite severe anaemia. ABO haemolytic disease of the newborn usually just requires phototherapy as anaemia is uncommon. The indications for exchange transfusion in haemolytic disease of the newborn are:

• severe anaemia (haemoglobin < 10 g/dL at birth); and/or
• severe or rapidly increasing hyperbilirubinaemia.

The British Committee for Standards in Haematology (BCSH) have published useful guidelines for neonatal exchange transfusion. Intravenous immunoglobulin has been used to reduce the need for exchange transfusion but the value of this approach remains to be proven in clinical trials. Neonates with haemolytic disease due to anti-rhesus antibodies may develop 'late' anaemia at a few weeks of age, requiring 'top-up' transfusion; irradiated blood must be used for infants previously receiving intrauterine transfusion to prevent the risk of transfusion-associated graft-versus-host disease. Recombinant erythropoietin sometimes prevents the need for top-up transfusion for late anaemia but is not effective when haemolysis is brisk. Folic acid (500 μg/kg daily) should be given to all babies with haemolysis until they reach 3 months of age.

Neonatal haemolytic anaemia due to red cell membrane disorders

In neonates, these disorders present with jaundice and moderate anaemia (usually due to hereditary spherocytosis), as an incidental finding on routine blood films in the absence of jaundice or anaemia (usually hereditary elliptocytosis) or, occasionally, as severe transfusion-dependent haemolytic anaemia with a characteristic low mean corpuscular volume (MCV) of 50–60 fL (usually due to hereditary pyropoikilocytosis). The main clues are a family history and an abnormal blood film, as red cell membrane disorders can nearly always be recognized by the characteristic shape of the red cells (Figure 52.6a). Identification of the exact type of membrane abnormality may require specialized investigations. The osmotic fragility test is of limited value in neonates and recent data indicate that the dye binding test is more useful. If the clinical phenotype is severe and family history or family studies are unhelpful, red cell membrane electrophoresis is indicated to clarify the diagnosis (on pretransfusion blood samples to minimize diagnostic confusion due to transfused cells).

Hereditary spherocytosis occurs in 1 in 5000 live births to parents of northern European extraction. It is caused by mutations in the genes for spectrin, ankyrin, protein 4.1 or protein 3 and is usually inherited in an autosomal dominant fashion. The blood film shows spherocytes and is identical to that of ABO haemolytic disease (Figure 52.6b). Neonatal anaemia due to hereditary spherocytosis is usually moderate (haemoglobin 7–10 g/dL); it is not uncommon for affected neonates to require one or two transfusions during the neonatal period before a transfusion-free plateau haemoglobin of 8–10 g/dL is achieved after a few months. *Hereditary elliptocytosis*, which is caused by different mutations in the genes for spectrin, ankyrin or protein 4.1, usually has no clinical manifestations in the neonate apart from elliptocytes on the blood film. However, neonates who are homozygous or compound heterozygous for hereditary elliptocytosis mutations have severe haemolytic anaemia. The most common form is *hereditary pyropoikilocytosis*, which causes severe transfusion-dependent haemolytic anaemia. The diagnosis is easily made from the low MCV and blood films of the baby (which show bizarre fragmented red cells and microspherocytes; see Figure 52.6a), and both parents (one or both of whom

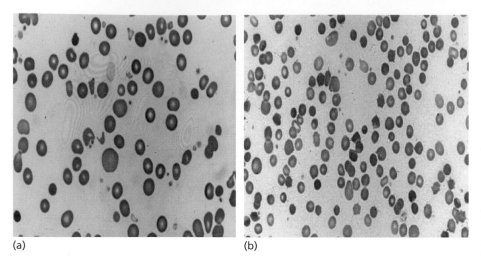

Figure 52.6 Red cell membrane disorders. (a) Blood film from a baby with hereditary pyropoikilocytosis showing microspherocytes, red cell fragments and polychromasia. (b) Blood film from a neonate with hereditary spherocytosis showing large numbers of spherocytes and polychromasia.

usually has elliptocytosis). Red cell transfusion is necessary until the child is old enough to undergo splenectomy, to which there is an excellent response.

Neonatal haemolysis due to red cell enzymopathies

The commonest inherited red cell enzymopathies presenting in the neonatal period are glucose-6-phosphate dehydrogenase (G6PD) deficiency and pyruvate kinase deficiency. *G6PD deficiency* has a high prevalence in individuals from Central Africa (20%) and the Mediterranean (10%). In neonates, G6PD deficiency nearly always presents with jaundice within the first few days of life; the vast majority of affected neonates are boys, as the *G6PD* gene is on the X chromosome. The jaundice is often severe, whereas anaemia is uncommon. The blood film is usually completely normal but in the small number of neonates with anaemia due to G6PD deficiency the blood film shows typical changes of oxidative haemolysis. The diagnosis is made by assaying G6PD on a peripheral blood sample. The pathogenesis of the jaundice is unclear as most babies with G6PD deficiency have no evidence of haemolysis. Management of neonatal G6PD deficiency requires close monitoring of the bilirubin to prevent kernicterus, particularly when interactions with other risk factors for neonatal hyperbilirubinaemia are present, such as Gilbert syndrome or hereditary spherocytosis, and also the counselling of the babies' parents regarding which medicines, chemicals and foods may precipitate haemolysis. For the vast majority of patients there is no chronic haemolysis and no anaemia and therefore folic acid supplements are not indicated.

Pyruvate kinase deficiency is the second most common inherited red cell enzymopathy in neonates and is transmitted in an autosomal recessive fashion. It is clinically heterogeneous, varying from anaemia severe enough to cause hydrops fetalis to a mild unconjugated hyperbilirubinaemia. In severe cases, the jaundice has a rapid onset within 24 hours of birth and exchange transfusion may be required. The diagnosis is made by measur-

ing pretransfusion red cell pyruvate kinase activity; in mild cases enzyme activity may be relatively modestly reduced making the diagnosis difficult and it is often useful to assay levels in the parents for confirmation. The blood film is sometimes distinctive but more often shows non-specific changes of non-spherocytic haemolysis. Management in the neonatal period depends on the severity of the jaundice and anaemia; some, but not all, children are transfusion dependent and folic acid supplements should be given to prevent deficiency due to chronic haemolysis.

The other red cell enzymopathies are rare. The most important in the neonatal period is *triosephosphate isomerase deficiency*, as one-third of patients present with neonatal haemolytic anaemia, often many months before the devastating neurological features of this disorder become apparent. Another cause of acute haemolysis confined to the neonatal period is *infantile pyknocytosis*. This poorly understood condition, which is probably due to transient glutathione peroxidase deficiency, usually presents at 1–6 weeks of age, produces moderately severe anaemia requiring one to two red cell transfusions, shows changes of oxidative haemolysis on the blood film (Figure 52.7) and resolves by 6–12 weeks of age. Measurement of glutathione peroxidase levels in affected neonates may be useful (parental levels are normal) but the diagnosis is usually easily made from the blood film.

Neonatal haemolysis due to haemoglobinopathies

The only haemoglobinopathy that presents typically in the neonatal period is α-thalassaemia major, as all four α-globin genes are deleted. Occasional non-thalassaemic structural α- and γ-globin gene mutations, which are clinically completely silent in adults and children, cause transient neonatal haemolytic anaemia in the neonate because they are unstable (e.g. Hb Hasharon, Hb Poole), whereas the major β-globin haemoglobinopathies (sickle cell disease and β-thalassaemia major) rarely manifest clinically in neonates.

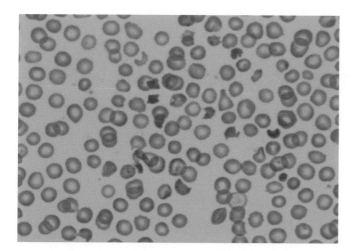

Figure 52.7 Infantile pyknocytosis. Blood film from a neonate with infantile pyknocytosis and a low level of erythrocyte glutathione peroxidase showing pyknocytes, fragmented red cells, polychromasia and occasional spherocytes.

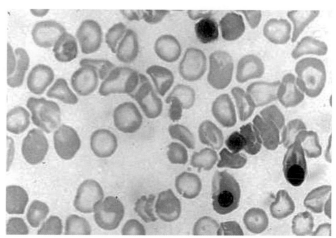

Figure 52.8 α-Thalassaemia major. Blood film from a neonate with α-thalassaemia major, born at 28 weeks' gestation, showing severe hypochromia, microcytosis, target cells, polychromasia and nucleated red cells.

α-Thalassaemia major predominantly affects families of Southeast Asian, Mediterranean or Middle Eastern origin, and presents with second-trimester fetal anaemia or hydrops fetalis, which is fatal within hours of delivery. The only long-term survivors of α-thalassaemia major are those who have received intrauterine transfusions followed by regular postnatal transfusions and/or a bone marrow transplant. There is also a high incidence of hypospadias and limb defects in survivors and others have severe neurological problems. If intrauterine transfusions are delayed until anaemia is severe, neonatal pulmonary hypoplasia is a cause of early mortality. The diagnosis of α-thalassaemia major should be suspected in any case of severe fetal anaemia that presents in the second trimester, and any case of hydrops fetalis with severe anaemia in which the parents come from high-prevalence areas, particularly Southeast Asia. Checking the blood counts of the parents will immediately identify whether they are at risk of having a child with α-thalassaemia major: both parents will have hypochromic microcytic red cell indices, with MCV usually below 74 fL and mean corpuscular haemoglobin (MCH) usually less than 24 pg. The diagnosis of α-thalassaemia major is confirmed by haemoglobin electrophoresis or HPLC (which shows Hb Barts, Hb Portland and sometimes HbH; HbF and HbA are absent); the blood film shows hypochromic microcytic red cells with vast numbers of circulating nucleated red cells (Figure 52.8).

Neonatal anaemia due to blood loss

Blood loss as a cause of neonatal anaemia may be very obvious (e.g. a cephalhaematoma or rupture of the cord) or be concealed and easy to miss unless specifically sought (e.g. fetomaternal bleeds). Usually, the most serious blood loss occurs prior to delivery and important causes of this are twin–twin transfusion and fetomaternal blood loss. *Twin–twin transfusion* occurs

in monochorionic twins with monochorial placentas. If the bleeding is chronic, there may be a marked difference in birth weight between twins: the donor twin is smaller, pale, lethargic and may have overt cardiac failure; the recipient twin may be plethoric, with hyperviscosity and hyperbilirubinaemia and polycythaemia.

Fetomaternal haemorrhage occurs spontaneously or secondary to trauma usually in the third trimester. Most episodes involve very small quantities of blood (0.5 mL or less) but acute loss of more than 20% of the blood volume may cause intrauterine death, circulatory shock or hydrops. Diagnostic clues are anaemia at birth in an otherwise well baby with no or minimal jaundice. The most useful diagnostic tests are a Coombs test to exclude immune haemolysis, a reticulocyte count to exclude red cell aplasia, a Kleihauer test on maternal blood to quantify the number of HbF-containing fetal red cells in the maternal circulation and a blood film (Figure 52.9). Blood loss around the time of delivery is usually due to obstetric complications (e.g. placenta praevia, placental abruption); in these circumstances, the babies are often extremely ill, with circulatory shock, anaemia worsening rapidly after birth, large numbers of circulating nucleated red cells and disseminated intravascular coagulation (DIC).

Anaemia of prematurity

The normal fall in haemoglobin in preterm neonates has been termed 'physiological anaemia of prematurity', as it does not appear to be associated with any abnormalities in the baby. The pathogenesis is not fully elucidated but contributory factors include the reduced lifespan of fetal erythrocytes, the relatively low erythropoietin concentration, the rapid growth rate and iatrogenic blood loss. Routine supplementation of preterm

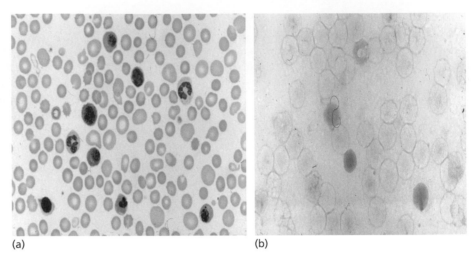

Figure 52.9 Fetomaternal haemorrhage. (a) Blood film from a neonate with a haemoglobin of 5 g/dL at birth due to a large fetomaternal haemorrhage; the main features are the marked polychromasia, large numbers of nucleated red cells and normal red cell morphology. (b) Kleihauer test showing HbA-containing maternal 'ghost' cells and pink-staining HbF-containing fetal cells.

(a)

(b)

neonates with folic acid and iron means that nutritional deficiency rarely plays a role. The diagnosis is usually straightforward: a well preterm baby with a slowly falling haemoglobin, unremarkable blood film showing normochromic/normocytic red cells, slightly low reticulocytes (20×10^9/L) and no nucleated red cells.

Management of anaemia of prematurity and the role of erythropoietin

The severity of anaemia of prematurity and thereby the need for red cell transfusion can be reduced by (i) limiting iatrogenic blood loss by appropriate use of blood tests; (ii) administering iron and folate supplements to all preterm infants (iron 3 mg/kg daily from 4–6 weeks of age or iron-fortified formula with 0.5–0.9 mg/dL of iron and folic acid 50 μg daily or 500 μg once weekly); and (iii) judicious use of erythropoietin. The many controlled trials of recombinant erythropoietin for prevention of neonatal anaemia have been reviewed extensively. Erythropoietin reduces the number of transfusions in relatively well infants with low transfusion requirements, but not in sick preterm infants who have a need for frequent phlebotomy and multiple transfusions. The main roles for recombinant erythropoietin in neonates are in ameliorating the anaemia in infants who have received intrauterine transfusions for alloantibody-mediated anaemia and in preterm babies of Jehovah's Witnesses. The usual dose is 300 μg/kg of epoetin beta by subcutaneous injection three times per week, starting in the first week of life, together with oral iron supplements.

Indications for red cell transfusion in neonatal anaemia

The BCSH recently revised their guidelines for transfusion of fetuses, neonates and older children; the guidelines contain recommendations about the products and indications for red cell transfusion in neonates. These are consensus guidelines and need to be adapted for use in each individual neonatal intensive

Table 52.3 Causes of neonatal polycythaemia.

Intrauterine growth restriction
Maternal hypertension
Maternal diabetes
Chromosomal disorders: trisomy 21, 18 or 13
Twin–twin transfusion
Delayed clamping of the cord
Endocrine disorders: thyrotoxicosis, congenital adrenal
    hyperplasia

care unit, depending on the case mix of babies, as adherence to strict neonatal transfusion guidelines reduces both the number of transfusions and donor exposure.

A simple diagnostic approach to neonatal anaemia

Red cell disorders associated with neonatal or fetal anaemia present in three main ways: with a low haemoglobin, with jaundice due to haemolysis or with hydrops. A diagnostic algorithm to help identify which of these causes is most likely, which can be excluded and what further investigations are most appropriate is shown in Figure 52.2.

Neonatal polycythaemia

For both term and preterm infants, polycythaemia can be defined as a central venous haematocrit of greater than 0.65, as there is an exponential rise in blood viscosity above this level. However, even at haematocrits greater than 0.70, only a minority of neonates have clinical signs of hyperviscosity, such as lethargy, hypotonia, hyperbilirubinaemia and hypoglycaemia. Causes of polycythaemia are shown in Table 52.3. Treatment is controversial and is not necessary in infants with very minor symptoms (e.g. borderline hypoglycaemia or poor peripheral perfusion). Infants with neurological signs and a haematocrit greater than 0.65 should have a partial exchange transfusion (using a crystalloid solution such as normal saline) to reduce the haematocrit to 0.55.

White cell disorders

Normal values

In the neonate, normal values for leucocytes, particularly neutrophils, are affected by a number of factors including gestational age, postnatal age, antenatal history, perinatal history and ethnic origin. Neutrophil counts in healthy babies increase for the first 12 hours then fall to a nadir at 4 days of age. The neutrophil count is higher in capillary samples and after vigorous crying; it is lower in neonates of African origin. Healthy preterm babies often have circulating myeloblasts and lymphoblasts, although these usually form less than 5% of the white cell differential count.

Neutropenia

A pragmatic approach is to consider a neutrophil count at birth of less than 2×10^9/L as abnormal and worth monitoring, and a neutrophil count during the first month of life of less than 0.7×10^9/L as significant enough to merit further investigation.

Causes of neutropenia

The commonest cause of neutropenia at birth in preterm neonates is reduced neutrophil production, secondary to intra-uterine growth restriction or maternal hypertension. Most affected neonates also have thrombocytopenia and increased erythropoiesis (polycythaemia and/or increased circulating nucleated red cells), secondary to fetal tissue hypoxia. The neutropenia resolves spontaneously usually within a few days of birth. The commonest cause of neutropenia in term infants is bacterial or viral infection. Other important causes of neutropenia are alloimmune neutropenia and severe congenital neutropenia (SCN) due to failure of neutrophil production (e.g. Kostmann syndrome), both of which predispose to severe neonatal infection.

Alloimmune neutropenia is the neutrophil equivalent of haemolytic disease of the newborn and alloimmune thrombocytopenia, and may affect 3% of all deliveries. It occurs when fetal neutrophils express paternally derived neutrophil-specific antigens absent on maternal neutrophils and against which the mother produces IgG neutrophil alloantibodies. The causative antibodies are usually anti-NA1 or -NA2. It presents in the first few days of life with fever and infections of the respiratory tract, urinary tract and skin, particularly due to *Staphylococcus aureus*, and the mainstay of treatment is antibiotics. The diagnosis is made by demonstrating antineutrophil antibodies in the mother and baby, which react against paternal, but not maternal, neutrophil antigens. The neutropenia is self-limiting, usually resolving within 1–2 months.

Congenital and inherited neonatal neutropenias should be sought when the neutropenia is prolonged, if there is a relevant family history or consanguinity or if the baby has typical dysmorphic features (e.g. thumb/radial abnormalities in Fanconi anaemia). SCN is the most likely cause in the neonatal period. Infants usually present with severe infections and a marked neutropenia ($< 0.2 \times 10^9$/L), often with a compensatory monocytosis. The diagnosis is made by the severity of the neutropenia, the bone marrow appearance (arrest of differentiation at the myelocyte/promyelocyte stage) and the absence of antineutrophil antibodies. The inheritance of SCN can be autosomal recessive or dominant or X-linked. Mutations in *ELA2* (neutrophil elastase) are the most common cause of SCN, but other causes include mutations in *GFI1* (growth factor-independent protein 1) and *WAS* (Wiskott–Aldrich syndrome protein, WASp). Recently, homozygous mutations in the *HAX1* gene were found to explain the SCN in the original Kostmann family but this appears to be a rare cause of the disease.

Congenital leukaemias

The most common forms of congenital leukaemia are acute monoblastic leukaemia and acute megakaryoblastic leukaemia; acute megakaryoblastic leukaemia is particularly common in babies with Down syndrome. The babies present with signs of anaemia, thrombocytopenia and/or skin lesions caused by leukaemic infiltration. The blood film and bone marrow aspirate show large numbers of primitive blast cells. The prognosis is extremely poor; few are cured by chemotherapy and bone marrow transplantation may be the best option. Around 5–10% of neonates with Down syndrome have a transient megakaryoblastic leukaemia also known as transient abnormal myelopoiesis or transient myeloproliferative disorder (TMD), characterized by leucocytosis and circulating blast cells (Figure 52.10). TMD develops in fetal life and nearly always presents in the first week of life. Most cases spontaneously resolve within 2–3 months and no treatment is indicated, but 20–30% subsequently develop acute megakaryoblastic leukaemia within the first 5 years of life. Mutations in the *GATA1* gene are found in virtually all cases of TMD and acute megakaryoblastic leukaemia associated with Down syndrome.

Haemostasis and thrombosis in the newborn

Bleeding and thrombotic problems are relatively common in neonates, particularly in those who are preterm and/or sick, and

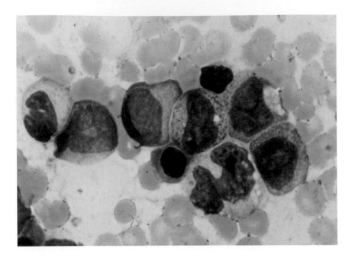

Figure 52.10 Transient leukaemia in a neonate with Down syndrome. Leucoerythoblastic blood film showing increased numbers of blast cells, which spontaneously returned to normal by 2 months of age.

the number of genetic and acquired causes of thrombophilia that can be identified in neonates and their families is rising.

Developmental haemostasis

Coagulation proteins are present at measurable levels from the 10th week of gestation and gradually rise during fetal life. They do not cross the placenta, or do so in very small amounts, and therefore need to be independently synthesized by the fetus. 'Normal values' in the neonate vary not only with gestational but also with postnatal age. Data for babies at less than 30 weeks' gestation derive from fetoscopy samples: levels of the vitamin K-dependent factors (FII, FVII, FIX and FX) and of FXI and FXII are all low (< 40% of adult values) and remain so during the first month of life. In contrast, even in preterm babies (> 30 weeks), levels of FV, FXIII and fibrinogen are normal at birth and levels of F VIII and von Willebrand factor (VWF) are normal or increased. Platelet counts at birth in term and preterm neonates are within the normal adult range. Many studies have found impaired function of neonatal platelets *in vitro* in term and preterm infants; the most consistent abnormalities are reduced aggregation in response to adrenaline, ADP and thrombin. Their significance in clinical practice is unclear as the bleeding time is normal in term and preterm infants (≤ 135 s).

Screening tests for bleeding disorders

Nearly all significant bleeding disorders in neonates can be identified using simple screening tests; exceptions are FXIII deficiency and platelet function disorders. It is often helpful to test both parents for coagulation abnormalities to help identify inherited disorders as there is considerable overlap between the deficiency states and the lower limit of normal. The most useful screening tests in neonates are the prothrombin time (PT), activated partial thromboplastin time (APTT), thrombin time (TT), fibrinogen and platelet count. Bleeding times are generally unhelpful in neonates and investigation of platelet function abnormalities is often deferred until a few months of age when platelet aggregometry and PFA-100 become practical.

Inherited coagulation disorders

The commonest inherited disorders presenting in the neonatal period are FVIII deficiency (haemophilia A), which has a frequency of 1 in 5000 male births, and FIX deficiency (haemophilia B), which occurs in 1 in 30 000 male births.

Factor VIII deficiency

Almost 40% of patients with inherited FVIII deficiency present in the neonatal period. The clinical signs include intracranial haemorrhage, cephalohaematomas and bleeding after circumcision or from venous or arterial puncture sites. As in adults, the diagnosis is made by finding an isolated prolonged APTT and reduced FVIII clotting activity. Acute management of the bleeding neonate with haemophilia requires intravenous administration of recombinant FVIII (50–100 units/kg twice daily) to achieve FVIII levels of 1.0 unit/mL. As the half-life of FVIII is shorter than in adults, more frequent dosing or a continuous FVIII infusion may be required. For neonates with intracranial bleeding treatment with FVIII should continue for at least 2 weeks. Fibrin glue may be useful in circumcision-associated bleeds. For patients diagnosed prenatally, vaginal delivery is safe provided that no difficulties are anticipated and vacuum extraction is avoided. The role of prophylactic FVIII administration to haemophiliac newborns following difficult delivery to reduce the risk of intracranial bleeding (1–4%) is controversial but is increasingly used. Prophylactic FVIII should also be used for a newborn haemophiliac when a previous sibling has had a major intracranial bleed.

Factor IX deficiency

Deficiency of FIX is clinically indistinguishable from FVIII deficiency. As FIX levels are also low in liver disease and vitamin K deficiency, it is important to recheck FIX levels at 6 weeks and 6 months of age if the diagnosis is in doubt. Neonates with bleeding are treated with recombinant FIX concentrate (100 units/kg i.v. once daily, monitored to achieve a FIX level of 1.0 IU/mL).

von Willebrand disease in neonates

The two forms of von Willebrand disease (vWD) that can present in neonates are type 2B vWD, which presents with thrombocytopenia and bleeding is uncommon, and type 3 vWD, which has a clinical phenotype similar to haemophilia as levels of both VWF and FVIII are low. The inheritance in type 3 vWD is autosomal recessive. The diagnosis is made by measuring VWF, FVIII and the pattern of VWF multimers. At present, type 3 vWD is treated with intermediate purity FVIII (Haemate-P is the most commonly used product).

Factor XIII deficiency

This rare autosomal recessive disorder usually presents with delayed bleeding from the umbilical cord during the first 3 weeks of life. The diagnosis is made by measuring clot solubility in 5 mol/L urea solution as a screening test followed by a specific FXIII assay; molecular tests for the common mutations are also available. The routine diagnostic coagulation screen is normal. Bleeding is treated with FXIII concentrate; cryoprecipitate (10 mL/kg) can also be used.

Acquired disorders of coagulation

Causes of acquired coagulopathy in neonates include vitamin K deficiency, DIC, liver disease, metabolic disorders, extracorporeal membrane oxygenation and giant haemangioendotheliomas (Kasabach–Merritt syndrome).

Vitamin K deficiency

Levels of vitamin K-dependent procoagulant factors (FII, FVII, FIX and FX), protein C and protein S are low at birth because of poor placental transfer of vitamin K, low vitamin K stores at birth, low vitamin K in breast milk and the lack of bacterial vitamin K synthesis in the sterile neonatal gut. Vitamin K deficiency can lead to haemorrhagic disease of the newborn, also known as vitamin K deficiency bleeding (VKDB). Early VKDB presents in the first 24 hours of life with severe gastrointestinal and intracranial haemorrhage. It is usually due to maternal medication that interferes with vitamin K, for example anticonvulsants (phenobarbital, phenytoin), antituberculous therapy and oral anticoagulants. Classical VKDB presents at 2–7 days in 0.25–1.7% of babies who have not received prophylactic vitamin K at birth, especially if breast-fed or with poor oral intake. Late VKDB occurs between 2 and 8 weeks after birth and presents with sudden intracranial haemorrhage in an otherwise well breast-fed term baby or in babies with liver disease.

The diagnosis of VKDB is usually made by an isolated prolonged PT, which corrects following vitamin K administration. If doubt remains, assays of the inactive form of FII (decarboxyprothrombin; PIVKA II) can be used to confirm the diagnosis. Treatment of VKDB is vitamin K 1 mg intravenously or subcutaneously with fresh-frozen plasma only in severe haemorrhage. Classic and late VKDB can be prevented by a single intramuscular dose of vitamin K or, slightly less effectively, by weekly 1-mg oral doses of vitamin K over the first 12 weeks of life (in exclusively breast-fed infants neither single oral dose vitamin K nor daily very low dose vitamin K 25 μg are effective in preventing classic VKDB). Some studies, but not others, suggest a link

between intramuscular vitamin K at birth and later childhood malignancies. In healthy babies, the choice of which route of administration is increasingly being left to parents. However, infants of mothers taking drugs that inhibit vitamin K (e.g. warfarin) are at risk of early VKDB and these babies should receive intramuscular vitamin K 1 mg as soon as possible after birth.

Disseminated intravascular coagulation

The main triggers of DIC in neonates are severe hypoxia and/or acidosis and sepsis. It occurs in sick neonates and presents with generalized bleeding, including pulmonary haemorrhage and oozing from venepuncture sites. The usual pattern of coagulation abnormalities in neonatal DIC is prolongation of the PT, APTT and TT, together with low platelets and fibrinogen. D-dimers are increased but are not specific and can be found in healthy neonates with no evidence of coagulopathy. The most important aspect of management of DIC is treatment of the underlying cause. Blood product replacement is indicated for clinical bleeding, aiming to maintain the platelet count above 30×10^9/L and fibrinogen greater than 1 g/L.

Neonatal thrombocytopenia

Thrombocytopenia occurs in 1–5% of all neonates and up to 50% of neonates who are preterm and sick. It usually presents in one of two clinical patterns: early thrombocytopenia (within 72 hours of birth) and late thrombocytopenia (after 72 hours of life) (Table 52.4). The most frequent causes of early thrombocytopenia in preterm infants are intrauterine growth restriction and maternal hypertension or diabetes; the most frequent causes in term infants are neonatal alloimmune thrombocytopenia (NAITP) and thrombocytopenia secondary to maternal immune thrombocytopenic purpura (ITP). The most common causes of late thrombocytopenia are sepsis and necrotizing enterocolitis.

Neonatal alloimmune thrombocytopenia

This is the platelet equivalent of haemolytic disease of the newborn and affects around 1 in 1000 pregnancies. It is frequently severe (platelet count < 30×10^9/L) and occurs in the first pregnancy in almost 50% of cases. Thrombocytopenia results from transplacental passage of maternal platelet-specific antibodies to human platelet antigens (HPA), which the mother lacks but which the fetus inherits from the father. In 80% of cases, these are anti-HPA-1a antibodies and in 10–15% anti-HPA-5b; occasional cases are due to anti-HPA-3a. HLA-DRB3*0101-positive women are 140 times more likely to make anti-HPA-1a than HLA-DRB3*0101-negative women. Intracranial haemorrhage occurs in 10% of cases, with long-term neurodevelopmental sequelae in 20% of survivors.

The diagnosis is made by demonstrating platelet antigen incompatibility between mother and baby and anti-HPA anti-

Table 52.4 Causes of neonatal thrombocytopenia.

Early (< 72 hours)
Placental insufficiency (PET, IUGR, diabetes)
Neonatal alloimmune thrombocytopenia
Birth asphyxia
Perinatal infection (group B *Streptococcus*, *Escherichia coli*, *Listeria*)
Congenital infection (CMV, toxoplasmosis, rubella)
Maternal autoimmune (ITP, SLE)
Severe rhesus HDN
Thrombosis (renal vein, aortic)
Aneuploidy (trisomy 21, 18, 13)
Congenital/inherited (TAR, Wiskott–Aldrich)

Late (> 72 hours)
Late-onset sepsis and necrotizing enterocolitis
Congenital infection (CMV, toxoplasmosis, rubella)
Maternal autoimmune (ITP, SLE)
Congenital/inherited (TAR, Wiskott–Aldrich)

CMV, cytomegalovirus; HDN, haemolytic disease of the newborn; ITP, idiopathic thrombocytopenic purpura; IUGR, intrauterine growth restriction; PET, pre-eclampsia; SLE, systemic lupus erythematosus; TAR, thrombocytopenia with absent radii.

bodies in the mother. Transfusion with HPA-compatible platelets is recommended for neonates with platelet counts below 30×10^9/L and/or those with bleeding. Intravenous IgG (total dose 2 g/kg, over 2–5 days) may be useful if thrombocytopenia is prolonged. Prenatal management of NAITP is controversial. Most centres have abandoned the invasive approach, except in very high risk cases, as this relies on fetal blood sampling plus fetal transfusion with HPA-compatible platelets, which carries a risk of preterm delivery and fetal death. Instead, most centres now use a non-invasive approach relying on maternal intravenous IgG therapy during the second half of pregnancy.

Neonatal autoimmune thrombocytopenia

This is secondary to transplacental passage of maternal platelet autoantibodies in maternal ITP and systemic lupus erythematosus (SLE), which affects 1–5 in 10 000 pregnancies. Around 10% of infants develop thrombocytopenia, which is severe in less than 1%. In babies with severe thrombocytopenia, intravenous IgG is usually effective. In some cases neonatal thrombocytopenia is prolonged and may last 6–8 weeks before spontaneously resolving.

Indications for platelet transfusion

A number of countries have published consensus guidelines to help decide the indications for platelet transfusion in term and preterm neonates. In general, platelet transfusion is not considered necessary in well babies if the platelet count is above 20–30×10^9/L. Most groups agree that the threshold for transfusing sick babies, particularly preterm babies in the first few weeks of life, should be higher ($30–50 \times 10^9$/L).

Neonatal thrombosis: physiology and developmental aspects

Neonates have an increased risk of thrombosis (2.4 per 1000 hospital admissions) compared with older infants and children. This is largely due to the physiologically low levels of many of the inhibitors of coagulation and the frequent use of indwelling vascular catheters. Concentrations of antithrombin, heparin cofactor II and protein C are decreased at birth; protein S levels are also low but overall protein S activity is normal as it exists mainly in its free active form due to the virtual absence of its binding protein (C4b-BP) in neonates. Levels of plasminogen at birth are only 50% of adult values so neonates have a reduced ability to generate plasmin in response to fibrinolytic agents.

Screening tests for thrombophilia in neonates

The only inherited deficiencies for which there is a proven role in neonatal thrombosis are deficiencies in proteins C and S, which cause purpura fulminans. FV Leiden and the prothrombin 20210A promoter mutation (prothrombin[20210A]) have not yet been reported to cause neonatal thrombotic problems in isolation. Recent guidelines from the Haemostasis and Thrombosis Task Force of the BCSH state that congenital thrombophilia should be considered and screened for in any child with:
• clinically significant thrombosis, including spontaneous thrombotic events, unanticipated or extensive venous thrombosis, ischaemic skin lesions or purpura fulminans; and
• a positive family history of neonatal purpura fulminans.

The screening tests that should be performed in all suspected cases of thrombophilia include protein C activity, protein S, antithrombin, FV Leiden and prothrombin[20210A]. In addition, babies with thrombosis born to mothers with SLE and/or antiphospholipid syndrome should be tested for lupus anticoagulant, as antiphospholipid antibodies may cross the placenta and are a rare cause of neonatal thrombosis in such babies. The relevance of serum liporotein a and the MTHFR genotype to neonatal management is unclear at present.

Inherited thrombotic disorders in neonates

Proteins C and S deficiency

Protein C deficiency occurs in 1 in 160 000–360 000 births. Affected babies usually present within hours or days of birth with purpura fulminans, in which there is DIC and rapidly progressive life-threatening haemorrhagic necrosis due to dermal vessel thrombosis or cerebral, renal vein or ophthalmic thrombosis. The diagnosis of protein C deficiency is made by the clinical picture and undetectable levels of protein C (< 0.01 units/mL) in the patient, together with heterozygote levels in the parents. Protein C-deficient heterozygotes rarely present as neonates and have low protein C levels, which may overlap with the lower limit of normal in the first few months of life, delaying diagnosis until 6 months or later. Treatment is with protein C concentrate (40 units/kg, aiming to maintain a plasma level > 0.25 units/mL). Protein S deficiency presents with identical features; levels of protein S are undetectable (< 0.01 units/mL) and treatment is with fresh-frozen plasma (10–20 mL/kg) to maintain a plasma protein S in excess of 0.25 units/mL.

Antithrombin deficiency

Homozygous antithrombin deficiency usually presents later in childhood but neonatal deep venous thrombosis and inferior vena cava thrombosis have been reported. Heterozygous antithrombin deficiency is more common (1 in 2000–5000 births); it usually presents in the second decade of life but neonatal presentation with aortic thrombosis, myocardial infarction and cerebral dural sinus thrombosis may occur.

Acquired thrombotic problems in neonates

The most common risk factors for neonatal thrombosis are an intravascular catheter and shock, secondary to sepsis, hypoxaemia or hypovolaemia. Thrombosis particularly affects the renal veins, the aorta, aortic arch or cerebral vessels. Catheter-related thrombosis causes more than 80% of venous thromboses and more than 90% of arterial thromboses. The diagnosis is made by Doppler ultrasound or contrast angiography. Treatment of catheter-related thrombosis depends on the severity and extent of thrombosis. The first step is prompt removal where possible. If signs progress despite catheter removal, unfractionated heparin or low-molecular-weight heparin should be started using a dosing regimen adapted for neonates. Thrombolytic therapy with urokinase or tissue plasminogen activator has been used successfully for catheter-related thrombosis in neonates, but experience in preterm neonates is very limited. It is important to maintain fibrinogen at levels less than 1 g/L and the platelet count greater than 50×10^9/L in neonates receiving thrombolytic therapy, and heparin (starting dose 28 units/kg per hour) is often given to maintain vessel patency after thrombolytic therapy, although there is no evidence that this is beneficial. Excellent guidelines for antithrombotic therapy in neonates are regularly updated by the American College of Chest Physicians.

Selected bibliography

Andrew M (1997) The relevance of developmental haemostasis to haemorrhagic disorders of newborns. *Seminars in Perinatology* **21**: 70–85.

Anwar R, Minford A, Gallivan L *et al.* (2002) Delayed umbilical bleeding. A presenting feature for factor XIII deficiency: clinical features, genetics, and management. *Pediatrics* **109**: E32143.

Bishara N, Ohls RK (2009) Current controversies in the management of anaemia of prematurity. *Seminars in Perinatology* **33**: 29–34.

British Committee for Standards in Haematology Haemostasis and Thrombosis Task Force (2002) The investigation and management of neonatal haemostasis and thrombosis. *British Journal of Haematology* **119**: 295–309.

British Committee for Standards in Haematology Transfusion Task Force. Transfusion guidelines for neonates and older children. Available at www.bcshguidelines.com/

Brown K (2000) Haematological consequences of parvovirus B19 infection. *Baillière's Best Practice and Research. Clinical Haematology* **13**: 245–59.

Bussel JB, Sola-Visner M (2001) Current approaches to the evaluation and management of the fetus and neonate with imune thrombocytopenia. *Seminars in Perinatology* **33**: 35–42.

Chalmers EA, Williams MD, Richards M *et al.* (2005) Management of neonates with inherited bleeding disorders: a survey of current UK practice. *Haemophilia* **11**: 186–7.

Dzierzak E, Speck NA (2009) Of lineage and legacy: the development of mammalian haematopoietic stem cells. *Nature Immunology* **9**: 129–36.

Israels SJ, Cheang T, McMillan-Ward EM *et al.* (2001) Evaluation of primary hemostasis in neonates with a new *in vitro* platelet function analyzer. *Journal of Pediatrics* **138**: 116–19.

Kulkarni R, Ponder KP, James AH *et al.* (2006) Unresolved issues in diagnosis and management of inherited bleeding disorders in the perinatal period: a White Paper of the Perinatal Task Force of the Medical and Scientific Advisory Council of the National Hemophilia Foundation, USA. *Haemophilia* **12**: 205–11.

Lallemand AV, Doco-Fenzy M, Gaillard DA (1999) Investigation of nonimmune hydrops fetalis: multidisciplinary studies are necessary for diagnosis. Review of 94 cases. *Pediatric and Developmental Pathology* **2**: 432–9.

Monagle P, Chalmers E, Chan A *et al.* (2009) Antithrombotic therapy in neonates and children. American College of Chest Physicians Evidence-Based Clinical Practice Guidelines, 8th edition. *Chest* **133** (6 Suppl.): 887S–968S.

New H, Stanworth SJ, Engelfriet CP *et al.* (2009) Neonatal transfusions. *Vox Sanguis* **96**: 62–85.

Puckett RM, Offringa M (2000) Prophylactic vitamin K for vitamin K deficiency bleeding in neonates. *Cochrane Database of Systematic Reviews* **4**: CD002776.

Roberts IAG (2008) The changing face of haemolytic disease of the newborn. *Early Human Development* **84**: 515–23.

Roberts I, Stanworth S, Murray NA (2008) Thrombocytopenia in the neonate. *Blood Reviews* **22**: 173–86.

Shearer MJ (2009) Vitamin K deficiency bleeding (VKDB) in early infancy. *Blood Reviews* **23**: 49–59.

Sohan K, Billington M, Pamphilon D, Goulden N, Kyle P (2002) Normal growth and development following *in utero* diagnosis and treatment of homozygous alpha-thalassaemia. *BJOG: an International Journal of Obstetrics and Gynaecology* **109**: 1308–10.

Watts TL, Roberts IAG (1999) Haematological abnormalities in the growth-restricted infant. *Seminars in Neonatology* **4**: 41–54.

Webb D, Roberts I, Vyas P (2007) Haematology of Down syndrome. *Archives of Disease in Childhood* **92**: F503–F507.

Wee LY, Fisk NM (2002) The twin–twin transfusion syndrome. *Seminars in Neonatology* **7**: 187–202.

Normal values

	Males	Females	Males and females
Haemoglobin	13.5–17.5 g/dL	11.5–15.5 g/dL	
Red cells (erythrocytes)	4.5–6.5×10^{12}/L	3.9–5.6×10^{12}/L	
PCV (haematocrit)	40–52%	36–48%	
MCV			80–95 fL
MCH			27–34 pg
MCHC			20–35 g/dL
White cells (leucocytes)			
Total			4.0–11.0×10^9/L
Neutrophils			2.5–7.5×10^9/L
Lymphocytes			1.5–3.5×10^9/L
Monocytes			0.2–0.8×10^9/L
Eosinophils			0.04–0.44×10^9/L
Basophils			0.01–0.1×10^9/L
Platelets			150–400×10^9/L
Red cell mass	30 ± 5 mL/kg	27 ± 5 mL/kg	
Plasma volume	45 ± 5 mL/kg	45 ± 5 mL/kg	
Serum iron			10–30 μmol/L
Total iron-binding capacity			40–75 μmol/L (2.0–4.0 g/L as transferrin)
Serum ferritin*	40–340 μg/L	14–150 μg/L	
Serum vitamin B_{12}*			160–925 ng/L
Serum folate*			3.0–15.0 μg/L
Red cell folate*			160–640 μg/L

*Normal ranges differ with different commercial kits.
MCH, mean corpuscular haemoglobin; MCHC, mean corpuscular haemoglobin concentration; MCV, mean corpuscular volume; PCV, packed cell volume.

Postgraduate Haematology: 6th edition. Edited by A. Victor Hoffbrand, Daniel Catovsky, Edward G.D. Tuddenham, Anthony R. Green
© 2011 Blackwell Publishing.

World Health Organization classification of tumours of the haematopoietic and lymphoid tissues

Myeloproliferative neoplasms

Chronic myelogenous leukaemia, *BCR–ABL1* positive
Chronic neutrophilic leukaemia
Polycythemia vera
Primary myelofibrosis
Essential thrombocythaemia
Chronic eosinophilic leukaemia, not otherwise specified
Mastocytosis
    Cutaneous mastocytosis
    Systemic mastocytosis
    Mast cell leukaemia
    Mast cell sarcoma
    Extracutaneous mastocytoma
Myeloproliferative neoplasms, unclassifiable
Myeloid and lymphoid neoplasms associated with eosinophilia and abnormalities of *PDGFRA*, *PDGFRB* or *FGFR1*
    Myeloid and lymphoid neoplasms associated with *PDGFRA* rearrangement
    Myeloid neoplasms associated with *PDGFRB* rearrangement
    Myeloid and lymphoid neoplasms with *FGFR1* abnormalities

Myelodysplastic/myeloproliferative neoplasms

Chronic myelomonocytic leukaemia
Atypical chronic myeloid leukaemia, *BCR–ABL1* negative
Juvenile myelomonocytic leukaemia
Myelodysplastic/myeloproliferative neoplasms, unclassifiable
    Refractory anaemia with ringed sideroblasts (RARS) associated with marked thrombocytosis*

Postgraduate Haematology: 6th edition. Edited by A. Victor Hoffbrand, Daniel Catovsky, Edward G.D. Tuddenham, Anthony R. Green
© 2011 Blackwell Publishing.

Myelodysplastic syndromes

Refractory cytopenia with unilineage dysplasia
    Refractory anaemia
    Refractory neutropenia
    Refractory thrombocytopenia
Refractory anaemia with ring sideroblasts
Refractory cytopenia with multilineage dysplasia
Refractory anaemia with excess blasts
Myelodysplastic syndromes associated with isolated del(5q)
Myelodysplastic syndromes, unclassifiable
Myelodysplastic syndromes in children

Acute myeloid leukaemia

Acute myeloid leukaemia (AML) with recurrent genetic abnormalities
    AML with t(8;21)(q22;q22), *RUNX1–RUNX1T1*
    AML with inv(16)(p13.1q22) or t(16;16)(p13.1;q22), *CBFB–MYH11*
    Acute promyelocytic leukaemia with t(15;17)(q22;q11–12), *PML–RARA*
    AML with t(9;11)(p22;q23), *MLLT3–MLL*
    AML with t(6;9)(p23;q34), *DEK–NUP214*
    AML with inv(3)(q21q26.2) or t(3;3)(q21;q26.2), *RPN1–EVI1*
    AML (megakaryoblastic) with t(1;22)(p13;q13), *RBM15–MKL1*
    AML with mutated *NPM1**
    AML with mutated *CEBPA**
Acute myeloid leukaemia with myelodysplasia-related changes
Therapy-related myeloid neoplasms
Acute myeloid leukaemia, not otherwise categorized
    AML with minimal differentiation
    AML without maturation
    AML with maturation
Acute myelomonocytic leukaemia
Acute monoblastic and monocytic leukaemia

Acute erythroid leukaemia
   Acute erythroid leukaemia, erythroid/myeloid
   Acute pure erythroid leukaemia
Acute megakaryoblastic leukaemia
Acute basophilic leukaemia
Acute panmyelosis with myelofibrosis
Myeloid sarcoma
Myeloid proliferations related to Down syndrome
   Transient abnormal myelopoiesis
   Acute myeloid leukaemia associated with Down syndrome
Blastic plasmacytoid dendritic cell neoplasm
Acute leukaemias of ambiguous lineage
   Acute undifferentiated leukaemia
   Acute biphenotypic leukaemia

Precursor lymphoid neoplasms

B lymphoblastic leukaemia/lymphoma
B lymphoblastic leukaemia/lymphoma, not otherwise specified
B lymphoblastic leukaemia/lymphoma with recurrent cytogenetic/molecular genetic abnormalities
   B lymphoblastic leukaemia/lymphoma with t(9;22) (q34;q11.2), BCR–ABL1
   B lymphoblastic leukaemia/lymphoma with t(11q23), MLL rearranged
   B lymphoblastic leukaemia/lymphoma with t(12;21) (p13;q22), TEL–AML1 (ETV6–RUNX1)
   B lymphoblastic leukaemia/lymphoma with hyperdiploidy
   B lymphoblastic leukaemia/lymphoma with hypodiploidy (hypodiploid ALL)
   B lymphoblastic leukaemia/lymphoma with t(5;14)(q31;q32), IL3–IGH
   B lymphoblastic leukaemia/lymphoma with t(1;19) (q23;p13.3), E2A–PBX1 (TCF3–PBX1)
T-lymphoblastic leukaemia/lymphoma

Mature B-cell neoplasms

Chronic lymphocytic leukaemia/small lymphocytic lymphoma
B-cell prolymphocytic leukaemia
Splenic marginal zone lymphoma
Hairy cell leukaemia
Splenic lymphoma/leukaemia, unclassifiable
   Splenic diffuse red pulp small B-cell lymphoma*
   Hairy cell leukaemia variant*
Lymphoplasmacytic lymphoma
   Waldenström macroglobulinaemia
Heavy chain diseases
   Alpha heavy chain disease
   Gamma heavy chain disease
   Mu heavy chain disease
Plasma cell myeloma

Solitary plasmacytoma of bone
Extraosseous plasmacytoma
Extranodal marginal zone B-cell lymphoma of mucosa-associated lymphoid tissue (MALT lymphoma)
Nodal marginal zone B-cell lymphoma
   Paediatric type nodal marginal zone lymphoma
Follicular lymphoma
   Paediatric type follicular lymphoma
Primary cutaneous follicle centre lymphoma
Mantle cell lymphoma
Diffuse large B-cell lymphoma (DLBCL), not otherwise specified
   T-cell/histiocyte-rich large B-cell lymphoma
   DLBCL associated with chronic inflammation
   EBV-positive DLBCL of the elderly
Lymphomatoid granulomatosis
Primary mediastinal (thymic) large B-cell lymphoma
Intravascular large B-cell lymphoma
Primary cutaneous DLBCL, leg type
ALK-positive large B-cell lymphoma
Plasmablastic lymphoma
Primary effusion lymphoma
Large B-cell lymphoma arising in HHV8-associated multicentric Castleman disease
Burkitt lymphoma
B-cell lymphoma, unclassifiable, with features intermediate between DLBCL and Burkitt lymphoma
B-cell lymphoma, unclassifiable, with features intermediate between DLBCL and classical Hodgkin lymphoma

Mature T-cell and NK-cell neoplasms

T-cell prolymphocytic leukaemia
T-cell large granular lymphocytic leukaemia
Aggressive NK-cell leukaemia
Systemic EBV-positive T-cell lymphoproliferative disease of childhood (associated with chronic active EBV infection)
Hydroa vaccineforme-like lymphoma
Adult T-cell leukaemia/lymphoma
Extranodal NK/T-cell lymphoma, nasal type
Enteropathy-associated T-cell lymphoma
Hepatosplenic T-cell lymphoma
Subcutaneous panniculitis-like T-cell lymphoma
Mycosis fungoides
Sézary syndrome
Primary cutaneous anaplastic large-cell lymphoma
Primary cutaneous aggressive epidermotropic CD8-positive cytotoxic T-cell lymphoma*
Primary cutaneous γδ T-cell lymphoma
Primary cutaneous small/medium CD4-positive T-cell lymphoma*
Peripheral T-cell lymphoma, not otherwise specified
Angioimmunoblastic T-cell lymphoma

Anaplastic large-cell lymphoma, ALK positive
Anaplastic large-cell lymphoma, ALK negative*

Hodgkin lymphoma

Nodular lymphocyte-predominant Hodgkin lymphoma
Classical Hodgkin lymphoma
    Nodular sclerosis classical Hodgkin lymphoma
    Lymphocyte-rich classical Hodgkin lymphoma
    Mixed cellularity classical Hodgkin lymphoma
    Lymphocyte depleted classical Hodgkin lymphoma

Histiocytic and dendritic cell neoplasms

Histiocytic sarcoma
Langerhans cell histiocytosis
Langerhans cell sarcoma
Interdigitating dendritic cell sarcoma
Follicular dendritic cell sarcoma
Dendritic cell tumour, not otherwise specified
Indeterminate dendritic cell tumour
Fibroblastic reticular cell tumour

Post-transplant lymphoproliferative disorders

Early lesions
    Reactive plasmacytic hyperplasia
    Infectious mononucleosis-like
Polymorphic post-transplant lymphoproliferative disorder
Monomorphic post-transplant lymphoproliferative disorder (B- and T/NK-cell types)*
Classical Hodgkin lymphoma-type post-transplant lymphoproliferative disorder

*These represent provisional entities or provisional subtypes of other neoplasms. They are provisional because there are insufficient data to support their being a definite entity, significant controversies about their defining features and/or uncertainty about whether they are unique or closely related to other definite entities. Further classify according to the lymphoma they resemble.

Index

Postgraduate Haematology: 6th edition. Edited by A. Victor Hoffbrand, Daniel Catovsky, Edward G.D. Tuddenham, Anthony R. Green
© 2011 Blackwell Publishing Ltd.